Practical **Thoracic Pathology**

Diseases of the Lung, Heart & Thymus

Practical Thoracic Pathology

Diseases of the Lung, Heart & Thymus

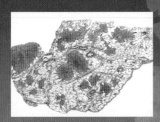 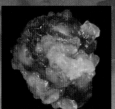 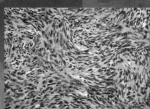 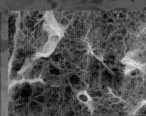 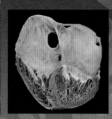

Allen P. Burke, MD

Professor
Department of Pathology
University of Maryland School of Medicine
Baltimore, Maryland
The Joint Pathology Center
National Capital Region Medical Directorate
Silver Spring, Maryland

Marie-Christine Aubry, MD

Professor of Laboratory Medicine & Pathology
Consultant, Division of Anatomic Pathology
Mayo Clinic
Rochester, Minnesota

Joseph J. Maleszewski, MD

Associate Professor of Laboratory Medicine & Pathology
Associate Professor of Medicine
Consultant, Divisions of Anatomic Pathology,
    Cardiovascular Diseases, and Medical Genetics
Mayo Clinic
Rochester, Minnesota

Borislav A. Alexiev, MD

Associate Professor
Department of Pathology
Northwestern University Feinberg School of Medicine
Chicago, Illinois

Fabio R. Tavora, MD, PhD

Associate Medical Director
Argos Laboratory
Head of Anatomic Pathology
Messejana Heart and Lung Hospital
Fortaleza, Brazil

. Wolters Kluwer

Philadelphia • Baltimore • New York • London
Buenos Aires • Hong Kong • Sydney • Tokyo

Acquisitions Editor: Ryan Shaw
Product Development Editor: Kate Heaney
Production Project Manager: David Orzechowski
Manufacturing Coordinator: Beth Welsh
Marketing Manager: Dan Dressler
Design Coordinator: Stephen Druding
Production Service: SPi Global

Library of Congress Cataloging-in-Publication Data
Names: Burke, Allen, editor. | Alexiev, Borislav, editor. | Aubry, Marie-Christine, 1966- editor. | Maleszewski, Joseph J., editor. | Tavora, Fabio, editor.
Title: Practical thoracic pathology : diseases of the lung, heart, and thymus / [edited by] Allen P. Burke, Borislav Alexiev, Marie-Christine Aubry, Joseph Maleszewski, Fabio Tavora.
Description: Philadelphia : Wolters Kluwer, [2017] | Includes bibliographical references and index.
Identifiers: LCCN 2016015387 | ISBN 9781451193510
Subjects: | MESH: Thoracic Diseases—pathology | Lung Diseases—pathology | Heart Diseases—pathology | Lymphatic Diseases—pathology
Classification: LCC RC756 | NLM WF 970 | DDC 616.2/407—dc23 LC record available at https://lccn.loc.gov/2016015387

RRS1606

To my family, to the clinicians and radiologists who help me make reasonable diagnoses, to my pathology colleagues, and to the many patients whose illnesses are described and depicted in this book.
Allen P. Burke

To all who have guided me along this journey, my teachers and mentors, my friends and colleagues, my residents and fellows, my family and parents, and above all my husband.
Marie-Christine Aubry

To Bill Edwards for his constant mentorship, support, and encouragement. To my wife, Brooke – a wellspring of patience and optimism. And our children, Emma and Joseph – sources of endless joy.
Joseph J. Maleszewski

To my wife Anna – it's a privilege to share my life and love with you. And to my children Alexander and Julia – your growth provides a constant source of joy and pride.
Borislav A. Alexiev

To Iusta, a woman of love and letters. To Andre and Igor: may they always have strong lungs and warm hearts.
Fabio R. Tavora

Contributors

Borislav A. Alexiev, MD
Associate Professor
Department of PathologyNorthwestern University
    Feinberg School of Medicine
Chicago, Illinois

Marie-Christine Aubry, MD
Professor of Laboratory Medicine & Pathology
Consultant, Division of Anatomic Pathology
Mayo Clinic
Rochester, Minnesota

Jennifer M. Boland, MD
Assistant Professor of Laboratory Medicine and Pathology
Consultant, Division of Anatomic Pathology
Mayo Clinic
Rochester, Minnesota

Allen P. Burke, MD
Professor
Department of Pathology
University of Maryland School of Medicine
Baltimore, Maryland
The Joint Pathology Center
National Capital Region Medical Directorate
Silver Spring, Maryland

Marisa Dolhnikoff, MD, PhD
Professor
Department of Pathology
Sao Paulo University Medical School
Sao Paulo, Brazil

Amy Duffield, MD, PhD
Assistant Professor of Pathology
Johns Hopkins Medical Institutions
Baltimore, Maryland

Seth Kligerman, MD
Associate Professor
Department of Radiology and Nuclear Medicine
University of Maryland School of Medicine
Medical Director of Magnetic Resonance Imaging
University of Maryland Medical Center
Baltimore, Maryland

Rima Koka, MD, PhD
Assistant Professor
Department of Pathology
University of Maryland School of Medicine
University of Maryland Medical Center
Baltimore, Maryland

Brandon T. Larsen, MD, PhD
Assistant Professor
Department of Pathology
University of Arizona College of Medicine
Banner – University Medical Center Tucson
Tucson, Arizona

Teklu Legesse, MD
Department of Pathology
University of Maryland Medical Center
Baltimore, Maryland

Michael Lewin-Smith, MB, BS
The Joint Pathology Center
National Capital Region Medical Directorate
Silver Spring, Maryland

Juliana Magalhães Cavalcante, MD
Staff Pathologist
Argos Laboratory
Fortaleza, Brazil

Joseph J. Maleszewski, MD
Associate Professor of Laboratory Medicine & Pathology
Associate Professor of Medicine
Consultant, Divisions of Anatomic Pathology, Cardiovascular
    Diseases, and Medical Genetics
Mayo Clinic
Rochester, Minnesota

Haresh Mani, MD
Pathologist
Department of Pathology
Inova Fairfax Hospital
Falls Church, Virginia

Thais Mauad, MD, PhD
Associate Professor
Department of Pathology
Sao Paulo University Medical School
Sao Paulo, Brazil

Andre L. Moreira, MD, PhD
Professor
Department of Pathology
New York University Langone Medical Center
New York, New York

Cleto D. Nogueira, MD
Associated Medical Director
Argos Laboratory
Fortaleza, Brazil

Adina Paulk, MD
Resident
Department of Anatomic and Clinical Pathology
University of Maryland Medical Center
Baltimore, Maryland

Bobbi S. Pritt, MD, MSc
Medical Director, Clinical Parasitology
Department of Laboratory Medicine and Pathology
Mayo Clinic
Rochester, Minnesota

Anja C. Roden, MD
Associate Professor of Laboratory Medicine and Pathology
Consultant, Division of Anatomic Pathology
Mayo Clinic
Rochester, Minnesota

Fabio R. Tavora, MD, PhD
Associate Medical Director
Argos Laboratory
Head of Anatomic Pathology
Messejana Heart and Lung Hospital
Fortaleza, Brazil

Andre C. Teixeira, MD
Staff Pathologist, Argos Laboratory
Assistant Professor, Unichristus School of Medicine
Fortaleza, Brazil

Eunhee S. Yi, MD
Professor of Laboratory Medicine and Pathology
Consultant, Division of Anatomic Pathology
Mayo Clinic
Rochester, Minnesota

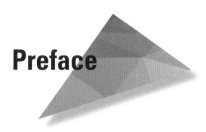

Major changes mark the second edition of "Practical Cardiovascular Pathology." Since the publication of the first book, we decided to expand the volume to include the lung and thymus. Much of this desire derived from our involvement in teaching residents and fellows in lung and mediastinal pathology as well as cardiac pathology. Our efforts in maintaining up-to-date lectures on new classifications in neoplastic and nonneoplastic lung disease led to the development of many of the chapters in the first section. Of course this book is a much larger undertaking than the last, requiring additional editors. We are indebted to MC Aubry and Joe Maleszewski for their huge contributions. Without their help, and the help of Bob Alexiev, this new volume would not have been thinkable. We also expanded the individual author list to include dozens of experts, tapping on expertise from Mayo Clinic, Baltimore, New York, and Brazil from a variety of institutions. In this area also we are grateful to our Mayo coeditors for seeking out the necessary breadth of expertise.

Our goal in this second edition is to fill a niche in the market for a pathology text that has reasonable depth, fits in one volume, and includes all structures in the thorax except the esophagus and bony structures. A semantic issue involving the title is the use of the word "thymus" instead of "mediastinum." Although all areas of the mediastinum were covered except the esophagus, "thymus" was chosen as tumors and conditions of the thymus were emphasized in the second section.

Areas of recent developments in pulmonary pathology is an in-depth assessment of updated classifications of interstitial lung disease and carcinomas of the lung, with an intent to remain unbiased in discussing pros and cons of divergent approaches. Similarly for the thymus, we wanted to objectively present different points of view for the classification of epithelial tumors. In the case of carcinomas of the lung and thymus, and mesotheliomas of the pleura, the TNM classification (as of the time this book is in press) is in transition, but the upcoming staging, which should be published later this year or next, is presented in the chapters devoted to these entities with comparison to the current staging system.

The subject of the genetics of lung cancer is a moving target, and any review will be somewhat out-of-date as soon as the ink dries and the book is in press. Nevertheless, this important area is presented in some depth with the practicing pathologist in mind, focusing on current guidelines for genetic testing and what likely lies ahead.

The interpretation of nonneoplastic lung disease in general is facilitated by correlation with imaging studies and is greatly improved with interaction and mutual learning from our radiology colleagues, whom we frequently consult before committing to a diagnosis. How often are we led astray by incomplete clinical information, and only pointed to the correct diagnosis by obtaining imaging and clinical data? We are indebted in this book to Seth Kligerman, for his contributions to imaging in interstitial lung disease, as well as a separate chapter on the subject. Many of the chapters in the lung section include sections of radiologic findings and explain radiologic findings that correlate with pathologic diagnosis.

One objective in formulating this book was ease of use as a reference text. In the lung volume, there is a first section that introduces a "pattern" diagnosis approach, which provides differential diagnoses that are addressed in individual chapters in following sections. The result is a certain degree of redundancy, with numerous cross-references, which we believe will facilitate location of diagnostic entities in the differential diagnosis of a particular histologic finding.

The cardiac section (which formed the entire first edition) has been significantly changed with extensive reorganization of the material. The classification system of cardiomyopathy, for example, is complex and largely dependent on clinical and genetic material and has changed significantly over the past 10 years. For this reason, this sections was completely rewritten. Furthermore, the understanding of genetics of cardiomyopathy and sudden death has evolved tremendously. Because cardiovascular pathology requires knowledge of clinical cardiology, the cardiac volume discusses clinical correlation even more than the pulmonary and mediastinal sections. Our goal in the heart section was to maintain the "practical" nature of the first edition, while updating the material and making it even more relevant to day-to-day pathologic practice as a reference text.

We hope that residents, community pathologists, forensic pathologists, and academic pathologists who occasionally review thoracic pathologic materials find this volume to be a practical reference source for difficult and not-so-difficult diagnostic problems. Because of the depth of many of the chapters, we would also hope that some subspecialty pathologists may also find the book of use. We hope this book helps practicing pathologists and those in training in the difficult areas of thoracic pathology, by providing a reference that answers in a more efficient or usable way than what is currently available.

Allen P. Burke
Marie-Christine Aubry
Joseph J. Maleszewski
Borislav A. Alexiev
Fabio R. Tavora

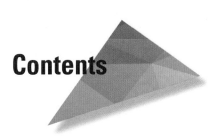

Contents

PART 2
Mediastinum

PART 3
Heart

Practical **Thoracic Pathology**

Diseases of the Lung, Heart & Thymus

SECTION ONE
APPROACH TO DIAGNOSIS

1 Normal Anatomy and Histology, Specimen Processing, Pathologic Reporting, and Artifacts

Allen P. Burke, M.D., and Joseph J. Maleszewski, M.D.

Pulmonary Anatomy and Histology

General Features and Development

The respiratory system broadly includes the acini, which are primarily responsible for gas exchange, and the airways and blood vessels that deliver the gases and blood, respectively, to such.

The lungs begin development as bilateral and symmetric structures; they acquire asymmetry through development and therefore ultimately exhibit sidedness (situs). Pulmonary sidedness is determined by the position of the morphologic right and left lungs, which is largely driven by the relative position of the pulmonary arteries and bronchi. In normal sidedness (situs solitus), the right mainstem bronchus is short and eparterial, meaning that the right pulmonary artery travels anterior to the right upper and intermediate bronchi. The left upper lobe bronchus is longer and hyparterial, passing inferior to the left pulmonary artery (Fig. 1.1).

Airways

Airways can be categorized by structure/size (large cartilaginous and small noncartilaginous) and by function. The latter categorization divides airways into those that are responsible for transmitting gas to and from the units of gas exchange (conducting airways) and those that actually contain gas exchange units (respiratory airways). Regardless of classification, the airways begin at the trachea and end at the respiratory bronchiole.

The trachea enters the thoracic inlet, just distal to the larynx, along with vascular structures, esophagus, muscles, vagus and phrenic nerves, and thoracic duct. The trachea divides into the right and left bronchi, with a more acute angle to midline on the right (20 degrees) than on the left (35 degrees), leading to a propensity for aspirated material to enter the right bronchus. In addition to transmitting air to and from the acini, they also provide an important protective role, both immunologic and physical, with their lymphoid, epithelial, and mucociliary structures.

The airways are lined by respiratory epithelium, under which is the muscular layer. The bronchi have a cartilaginous and fibrous layer under the muscularis and mucus glands between the muscularis and cartilage (submucosa). The respiratory epithelium consists of mucus-secreting goblet cells, ciliated cells, scattered neuroendocrine cells, and a basal layer. Additionally, there is a population of pulmonary brush cells, which differ ultrastructurally from ciliated cells, thought to be involved in fluid absorption.[1] The ciliated cells are important in mucous transit and the clearance of particulate matter from the airways back to the environment. Ultrastructurally, the cilia consist of nine doublets that surround a central pair (Fig. 1.2). Dynein arms (inner and outer) join the peripheral doublets, and radial spokes connect the peripheral doublets to the central pair. Identification of these normal structures is critical in the evaluation for primary ciliary dyskinesia.

All epithelial cells express cytokeratins, including cytokeratin 7; in addition, the basal cells express p40 and p63. TTF-1 expression is limited to respiratory bronchioles, which contain Clara cells (surfactant-producing cells), and to alveolar lining cells (pneumocytes). In general, the number of goblet and ciliated cells decreases in the distal airways, and the respiratory bronchioles are composed primarily of basal and Clara cells.

Lobation and Lung Segments

The left and right lung lobes are separated by interlobar fissures, usually one on the left and two on the right (Fig. 1.1). Oblique fissures, on each right and left lung, divide the upper and lower lobes and travel from the upper lateral to lower medial lungs. A horizontal fissure on the right separates the upper and middle lobes. Incomplete development or absence of the horizontal fissure is a common variant, resulting in a two-lobed right lung.[2] This is why lung laterality is best assigned by the relationship of the bronchus and pulmonary artery, rather than lobation.

There are 19 bronchopulmonary segments: 10 on the right and 9 on the left, owing to fusion of the apical and posterior segments of the left upper lobe (Table 1.1). Secondary pulmonary lobules (Fig. 1.3), the smallest unit recognized by high-resolution computed tomography (CT), are 1.0- to 2.5-cm polyhedral collections of acini (see below) served by terminal bronchioles. They are bounded by the pleura and the interlobular septa.

Alveoli

Each secondary lobule contains between 10 and 15 acini (the functional units), which include all the alveoli containing structures distal to the terminal bronchiole. The alveoli are the sac-like structures involved in gas exchange and receive air from the upstream airways. The alveoli themselves measure ~200 μm across. Some alveolar sacs arise directly from respiratory bronchioles without connections through primary lobules.

The histologic features in two dimensions do not readily allow for distinction between the various alveolar compartments. Respiratory bronchioles may be seen adjacent to alveoli, whereas bronchioles are generally seen on cross section.

The lining cells of the terminal bronchioles and alveoli are composed of TTF-1–positive Clara cells in the former and pneumocytes in the latter. Mature type I pneumocytes are flattened, attenuated squamous cells with abundant cytoplasm, and small nuclei are generally not visible in normal sections and cover over 95% of the alveolar surface. They are attached to one another by desmosomes and occluding junctions. Pneumocytes with the ability to regenerate are type II pneumocytes, which have surfactant production capability. They are cuboidal and cover a much smaller surface area (<5%), despite the fact that they are actually more numerous than type I pneumocytes.

Approach to Histologic Evaluation of Peripheral Lung Tissue

When evaluating lung tissue, starting at low magnification helps to characterize the overall architecture and pattern of any pathology. Identification of bronchovascular bundles, small airways, interlobular septa, alveolar septa, and pleural surfaces should also be done at this

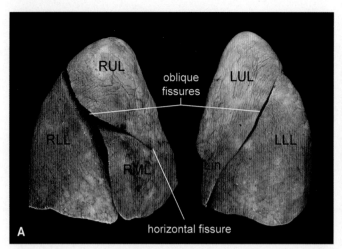
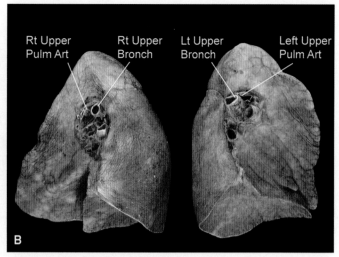

FIGURE 1.1 ▲ Gross pulmonary anatomy. **A.** Normal lobation pattern. **B.** Normal relationship of the pulmonary artery and bronchus. A morphologic right lung shows the pulmonary artery anterior to the upper lobe bronchus, while a morphologic left lung shows the pulmonary artery superior to the upper lobe bronchus.

time (Figs. 1.4 to 1.7). Patterns of pathology can help to establish a differential diagnosis.

Bronchiolocentric processes occur around the bronchioles, while angiocentric lesions occur around the adjacent muscular pulmonary arteries. Septal and paraseptal patterns of disease/injury follow the interlobular septa that bound the pulmonary lobules. Lymphatics are present along the pleura, bronchovascular bundles, and interlobular septa, which will all tend to be involved in diseases with a lymphatic distribution. Consolidative processes will fill the airspaces and make the lung look more "solid." Finally, diffuse interstitial diseases can involve virtually all of the nonairspace regions of the pulmonary microanatomy. Although the limits of the secondary lobules cannot usually be clearly seen in normal lung, the parenchyma around the bronchovascular bundles is generally centrilobular or centriacinar and that alveoli near pleural surfaces or lobular septa are peripheral.

Pulmonary Arteries

The pulmonary trunk branches into the right and left pulmonary arteries. The right pulmonary artery, longer than the left, travels beneath the aortic arch before entering the lung hilum. The arteries divide into lobar and segmental branches, with names similar to the bronchopulmonary segments that they feed. The bronchial arteries arise from the thoracic aorta just distal to the arch, directly either from the aorta or from the intercostal arteries, and usually with one on the right and two on the left.

Histologically, pulmonary arteries are identified adjacent to the bronchi and in bronchovascular bundles toward the periphery. Normally, there is little intima, and the media is thin (10% or less of the diameter of the artery) (Fig. 1.8). There may be concentric intimal thickening (or hyalinosis) as a result of aging or increased arterial pressures. Typically, the artery is similar in diameter to the accompanying airway. The proximal arteries accompanying the bronchi (main pulmonary arteries and lobar arteries) are elastic, with concentric elastic lamellae, seen best on elastic stains. There is a gradual transition to muscular arteries accompanying segmental bronchi and bronchioles.

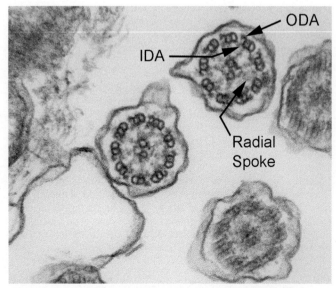

FIGURE 1.2 ▲ Ciliary ultrastructure. Nine outer doublets radiate around a central pair and are connected to such via radial spokes. Inner dynein arms (IDA) and outer dynein arms (ODA) are visible extending from the outer doublets. Absences or abnormalities of these dynein arms are the most common morphologic finding in cases of primary ciliary dyskinesia.

TABLE 1.1   Lung Segments

Lobe	Segments
Right upper	Apical
	Posterior
	Anterior
Right middle	Lateral
	Medial
Right lower	Superior
	Medial basal
	Anterior basal
	Lateral basal
	Posterior basal
Left upper	Apicoposterior
	Anterior
	Superior lingular
	Inferior lingular
Left lower	Superior
	Medial basal
	Anterior basal
	Lateral basal
	Posterior basal

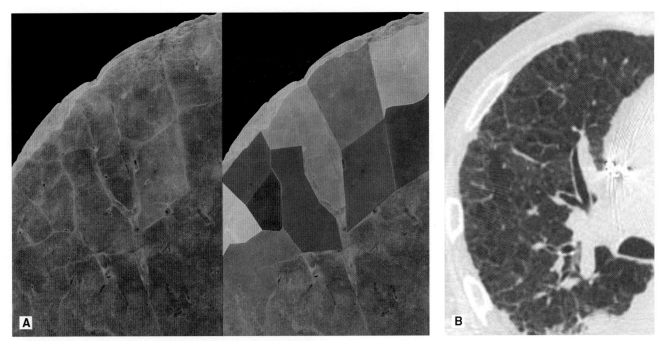

FIGURE 1.3 ▲ Secondary pulmonary lobules. **A.** These polygonal lobules are bounded by the interlobular septa and pleura. **B.** The secondary lobules (sometimes called "pulmonary lobule") are the smallest recognizable organizational unit identified by high-resolution CT scan (seen here in this case of pulmonary venoocclusive disease).

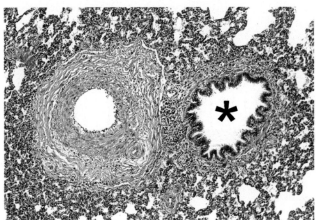

FIGURE 1.4 ▲ Bronchovascular bundle. The airways (*asterisk*) travel with muscular pulmonary arteries and are of similar caliber.

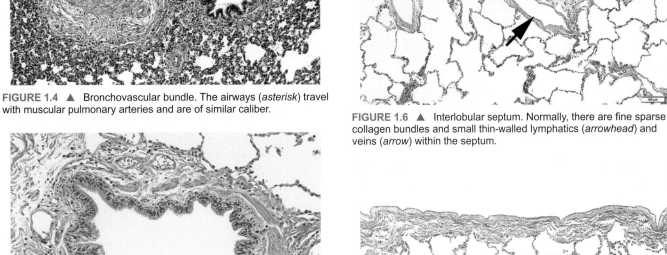

FIGURE 1.6 ▲ Interlobular septum. Normally, there are fine sparse collagen bundles and small thin-walled lymphatics (*arrowhead*) and veins (*arrow*) within the septum.

FIGURE 1.5 ▲ Cross section of bronchiole. In this transbronchial biopsy, there was a complete cross section of a bronchiole. Often, only tangential or partial sections are present. Note the normal serrated border in the collapsed state. There is little inflammation and collagen between the respiratory epithelium and muscle wall (lamina propria).

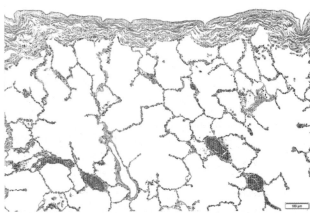

FIGURE 1.7 ▲ Pleura. The pleural surface is relatively thin, composed of collagen, elastin, and a mesothelial lining.

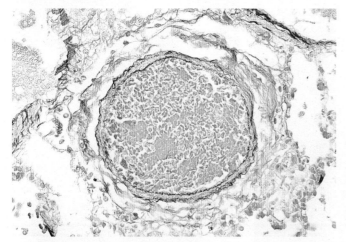

FIGURE 1.8 ▲ Muscular pulmonary artery. The media is <10% of the total vessel diameter and is bounded by defined internal and external elastic membranes.

Muscular pulmonary arteries have a distinct internal and external elastic lamina, unlike bronchial arteries, which tend to have only a distinct internal elastic membrane with a more fragmented external elastic membrane (like all other systemic muscular arteries).

Pulmonary Veins

The pulmonary veins travel in the interlobular septa. The media of the veins is less organized than the discrete media of the arteries and frequently contains smooth muscle bundles rather than layers. There is more elastic tissue in the adventitia in veins, compared to arteries. There is no discrete internal and external elastic lamina. With increased pulmonary venous pressure, there may be accentuation of the elastic tissue, with a thicker inner elastic layer mimicking an internal elastic lamina (so-called arterialization of veins). Like in arteries, aging and interstitial lung disease may cause hyalinization or intimal thickening of the wall in distal veins.

Types of Specimens, Processing, and Reporting

Transbronchial Forceps Biopsy

The most frequent tissue sampling of lung parenchyma is performed by transbronchial biopsy, which was first introduced in the early 1960s with a rigid bronchoscope, and later in the 1970s with flexible bronchoscopy. Risks include bleeding and pneumothorax, with thrombocytopenia and mechanical ventilation considered to be relative contraindications. The tissue is obtained via forceps biopsy, and is blind, as the catheter is advanced as far as possible. For this reason, biopsies for focal lesions are generally performed under fluoroscopy, and CT guidance is also possible.[3] Optimally, 4 to 10 fragments are obtained, with higher numbers recommended for focal lesions (Fig. 1.9).[4] Fragments are usually about 3 mm, unless jumbo forceps with rigid bronchoscopy are used, which may increase the diagnostic yield in interstitial lung disease. Concomitant suction catheter aspiration can result in higher diagnostic yields.[5] Histologic samples are generally from peripheral lung, as opposed to endobronchial biopsies. A sample of histologic findings in pathologic reporting is presented in Table 1.2. There are no specific processing requirements; shaking the container to minimize specimen atelectasis has anecdotally been recommended, similar to larger specimens (Fig. 1.10A).[6]

Transbronchial Cryobiopsy

This relatively new technique relies on utilization of a bronchoscopically delivered cryoprobe that transbronchial freezes the subjacent

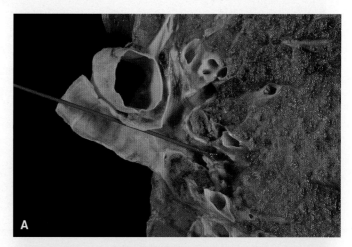

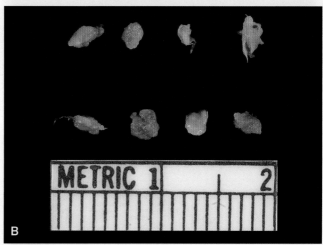

FIGURE 1.9 ▲ Transbronchial biopsy (forcep method). **(A)** The bioptome is placed into the airway and is lodged peripherally before **(B)** 6 to 8 samples are taken.

parenchyma. The stuck on tissue is then retracted with the cryoprobe. It has the advantages, over forcep biopsy, of less crush artifact, better architectural preservation, and larger samples (Fig. 1.10B). Some studies have reported more hemorrhage with this modality than traditional forcep methods.[7] Preliminary studies suggest that this technique can have additional utility in the diagnosis of interstitial lung diseases, which typically necessitated surgical (wedge) lung biopsy (see below).[8]

Endobronchial Biopsy

Endobronchial biopsies are generally performed with the same bronchoscope as transbronchial biopsies, but are used for proximal lesions, which are directly visualized through the bronchoscope. In such samples, alveolated parenchyma may be absent/scant with the specimen largely limited to bronchial mucosa and submucosa. The presence of the various layers present (respiratory epithelium, lamina propria, muscularis mucosa, submucosa with mucus glands, cartilage) should be mentioned in the pathology report, along with pathologic alterations.

Transthoracic Core Biopsies

These are usually performed under CT guidance for tumors or masses. Tissue sampling is critical in obtaining tumor for potential molecular markers; therefore, procedures to minimize sectioning of paraffin blocks are paramount. Typically, a 17- or an 18-gauge needle is used

TABLE 1.2   Pathologic Reporting of Nonneoplastic Transbronchial Biopsies in Native Lung Biopsies

Number of Tissue Fragments	Number with Lung Parenchyma, Number with Airway
Alveolar spaces	Intra-alveolar fibrin (not procedure related), indicative of acute lung injury
	Acute inflammation (airway, intra-alveolar)
	Histiocytes (intra-alveolar vs. interstitial); type (foamy, anthracotic pigment, iron pigment, fine dusty pigment, vacuolated)
	Eosinophils
	Organizing pneumonia
	Proteinaceous material (pulmonary alveolar proteinosis)
	Mucus (exclude adjacent neoplasm vs. mucus plugging with extravasation)
	Edema fluid
Alveolar septa	Mononuclear inflammation (note distribution relative to bronchovascular bundles and venules)
	Acute inflammation (note relation with hemorrhage and possible capillaritis)
	Organizing pneumonia
	Pneumocytes (normal, reactive, viral inclusions)
	Smooth muscle cell hyperplasia or fibrosis
	Hyaline membranes
	Vacuolated pneumocytes (suggestive of amiodarone exposure)
Bronchovascular bundles	Granulomas (well or poorly formed and location)
	Squamous metaplasia (especially endobronchial biopsies)
	Vascular changes (intimal thickening, thrombi)
Interlobular septa	Edema
	Fibrosis
	Thickened veins
	Venous recanalization

to produce multiple tissue cores (Fig. 1.10C).[9] Common complications include pneumothorax (most of which resolve spontaneously) and hemoptysis.

Cytologic Specimens

In many cases of transbronchial biopsy, concomitant cytologic specimens are obtained, especially in the evaluation of masses or nodules. These include bronchial washes, brushes, and needle aspirates of either central tumors or mediastinal lymph nodes, which can be sampled via bronchial and esophageal endoscopy (Fig. 1.10D). It is a matter of choice whether to combine samples into one case accession or separate biopsies from cytologic specimens obtained in one bronchoscopic session.

Bronchoalveolar lavage (BAL) is often performed as an adjunct to diagnosis of inflammatory lung disease as well as malignancies.

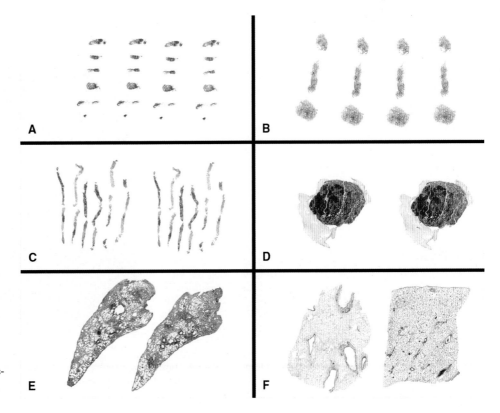

FIGURE 1.10 ▲ Relative sizes of lung specimens sampled for histology. **A.** Transbronchial forcep biopsy. **B.** Transbronchial cryobiopsy. **C.** Needle core biopsy. **D.** Bronchoalveolar lavage (BAL) cell block. **E.** Surgical wedge resection. **F.** Pneumonectomy, lobectomy, or autopsy.

Typically, about 100 mL is infused, either in an affected area or right middle lobe or lingula in diffuse disease, which is most easily accessed in a supine patient. Total numbers of leukocytes are expressed per unit volume with a differential count, and organisms are identified by routine special stains. BAL is useful for the diagnosis of cytomegalovirus, herpes, pneumocystis, and fungal infections and may be useful in the diagnosis of sarcoidosis, hypersensitivity pneumonitis, and idiopathic pulmonary fibrosis, although the findings are nonspecific. Pneumoconioses may be diagnosed by the identification of silicates or asbestos bodies.

Wedge Biopsies

Open lung biopsy is commonly used for the diagnosis of most forms of interstitial lung disease and is generally performed by minimally invasive techniques, such as video-assisted thoracoscopic surgery (VATS) (Fig. 1.10E). In order to minimize the artifact of specimen atelectasis, injection of the parenchyma with formalin using a needle is often recommended. Inking the pleura is generally not necessary, unless there is a possibility of extension through the pleura in cases of peripheral lung cancer resection.[10] The histologic assessment of margins for tumor may be difficult in cases of stapled parenchymal resection margins.[10,11] Careful removal of staples with assessment of the margin is recommended. Cytologic assessment of margins has also been espoused before removing the staples.[12]

In the case of wedge biopsies for interstitial lung disease, it is recommended that multiple regions (upper and lower lobes) be sampled, such that the distribution of the process can be ascertained. Reporting of biopsies for interstitial lung disease involves enumeration of histologic patterns of injury (to be discussed in the following chapters), with the formulation of a clinicopathologic diagnosis following the acquisition and integration of radiographic and clinical data (see Chapter 16).

Lobectomy

In lobectomy specimens, the pathologist or assistant should attempt to distend the tissue from a vascular or airway at the surgical margin, which should be assessed in cases of tumor for staging purposes. The size and nature of nodules and relationship and distance to pleural and resection margins should be recorded. Any peribronchial lymph nodes should be evaluated. The total number of lymph nodes obtained for cancer resections is critical for staging, and peribronchial nodes in lobectomies need to be carefully dissected and counted.

Pneumonectomy

Complete lung resections are performed for proximal lung cancers, certain infections, and during allotransplantation in patients who are surgical candidates with adequate respiratory reserve in the contralateral lung (Fig. 1.10F). Optimally, the lung should be distended with formalin to prevent specimen atelectasis, and all lymph nodes must be submitted for histologic assessment. Vascular and bronchial margins are necessary for tumor staging in the case of resection for malignancy.

Pleural Surfaces

The state of the pleura is important to describe, including the presence of adhesions, fibrosis, puckering, exudates, anthracosis, and "cobblestoning" (retraction caused by interstitial fibrosis). It is especially important in cancer resections to note any puckering, which could represent visceral pleural invasion, and the presence of shaggy tissue or obvious portions of chest wall (skeletal muscle or bone). It is useful to refer to the operative summary to determine if a part of endothoracic fascia was resected near a tumor, because an additional margin is thus created. Pleural surfaces need not be inked if there is underlying tumor, as the intact pleura is not a margin. However, if there is attached chest wall, then determination of margins with inking is essential in determining the proper tumor stage.

Autopsy

In order to assess histologic changes at autopsy, perfusion fixation is especially important, because of the added effect of autolysis on postmortem atelectasis. In general, it is not difficult to directly deliver formalin into the trachea or individually in the mainstem bronchi to distend the distal parenchyma. With adequate distention of the lungs, fixation is generally sufficient within a few minutes following clamping of the trachea or bronchi. Optimal visual inspection of the lungs occurs by placing the lungs with the hilum up and performing serial parasagittal sections with a sharp knife at ~1 cm intervals.

Histologic Artifacts

Specimen Atelectasis

Specimen atelectasis refers to collapse of the alveolar spaces after biopsy or resection, or postmortem. This effect can be minimized by gentle agitation of small specimens or formalin injection/distension of larger specimens. With practice, it is possible to distinguish alveolar collapse from areas of consolidation (Fig. 1.11). Cytokeratin staining can occasionally be useful in this regard. Specimen atelectasis also makes especially difficult the distinction between in situ and invasive low-grade adenocarcinoma (Chapter 74).

Procedural Fibrin Versus Acute Lung Injury

It may be difficult to distinguish procedural hemorrhage with fibrin coagulation from acute lung injury and pathologic deposition. In general, procedural hemorrhage will demonstrate intact red blood cells and fine fibrillar fibrin strands indicative of recent formation (Fig. 1.12). Organization will also be absent in procedure-related changes.

Vascular Tunneling

A common artifact in lung biopsies is procedural intussusception of vessels, especially arteries, mimicking intimal thickening (Fig. 1.13).

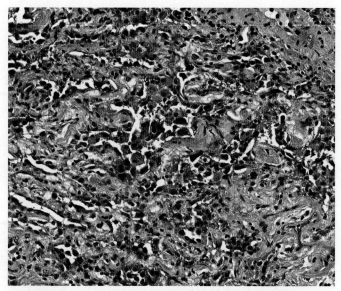

FIGURE 1.11 ▲ Specimen atelectasis. If the airspaces are not expanded, the alveolar structures collapse, making interpretation difficult. In this case, alveolar septal inflammation and reactive pneumocytes are discernable, allowing a diagnosis of subacute lung injury.

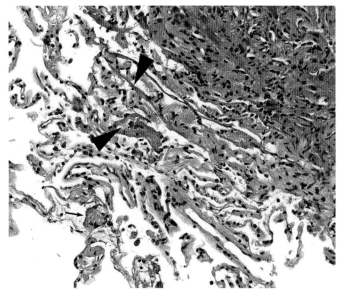

FIGURE 1.12 ▲ Procedural fibrin. There are intact fibrin strands (*arrowheads*) and scattered erythrocytes. In the absence of pneumocyte hyperplasia or other findings, the fibrin is likely due to the forceps trauma.

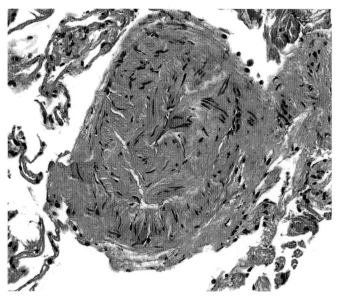

FIGURE 1.13 ▲ Arterial telescoping. Artifactual intussusception of normal arteries may result in an appearance mimicking intimal thickening.

REFERENCES

1. Reid L, Meyrick B, Antony VB, et al. The mysterious pulmonary brush cell: a cell in search of a function. *Am J Respir Crit Care Med.* 2005;172(1):136–139.
2. Meenakshi S, Manjunath KY, Balasubramanyam V. Morphological variations of the lung fissures and lobes. *Indian J Chest Dis Allied Sci.* 2004;46(3):179–182.
3. Hautmann H, Henke MO, Bitterling H. High diagnostic yield from transbronchial biopsy of solitary pulmonary nodules using low-dose CT-guidance. *Respirology.* 2010;15(4):677–682.
4. Gilman MJ, Wang KP. Transbronchial lung biopsy in sarcoidosis. An approach to determine the optimal number of biopsies. *Am Rev Respir Dis.* 1980;122(5):721–724.
5. Peschke A, Wiedemann B, Höffken G, et al. Forceps biopsy and suction catheter for sampling in pulmonary nodules and infiltrates. *Eur Respir J.* 2012;39(6):1432–1436.
6. Travis WD, Colby TV, Koss MN, et al. Handling and analysis of bronchoalveolar lavage and lung biopsy specimens with approach to patterns of lung injury. *ARP Atlases.* 2007;1:17–47.
7. Rubio ER, le SR, Whatley RE, et al. Cryobiopsy: should this be used in place of endobronchial forceps biopsies? *Biomed Res Int.* 2013;2013:730574.
8. Hagmeyer L, Theegarten D, Wohlschläger J, et al. The role of transbronchial cryobiopsy and surgical lung biopsy in the diagnostic algorithm of interstitial lung disease. *Clin Respir J.* 2015.
9. Tsai IC, Tsai WL, Chen MC, et al. CT-guided core biopsy of lung lesions: a primer. *AJR Am J Roentgenol.* 2009;193(5):1228–1235.
10. Marchevsky AM. Problems in pathologic staging of lung cancer. *Arch Pathol Lab Med.* 2006;130(3):292–302.
11. Goldstein NS, Ferkowicz M, Kestin L, et al. Wedge resection margin distances and residual adenocarcinoma in lobectomy specimens. *Am J Clin Pathol.* 2003;120(5):720–724.
12. Sawabata N, Karube Y, Umezu H, et al. Cytologically malignant margin without continuous pulmonary tumor lesion: cases of wedge resection, segmentectomy and lobectomy. *Interact Cardiovasc Thorac Surg.* 2008;7(6):1044–1048.

2 Pathologic Changes Involving Alveolar Septa and Interstitium

Allen P. Burke, M.D., and Fabio R. Tavora, M.D., Ph.D.

Inflammation

The most common type of inflammation in the alveolar septa is a mixture of mononuclear cells, including lymphocytes (usually predominantly T cells), macrophages, and plasma cells. If a pattern is recognizable, it is important to mention if it appears bronchiolocentric (Figs. 2.1 and 2.2) or perivascular (Fig. 2.3). There is often reactive pneumocyte hyperplasia, which indicates organizing lung injury of various causes and stages. The organizing lung injury may show discrete areas of organizing pneumonia.

The differential diagnosis of chronic interstitial pneumonitis (a nonspecific pattern of diagnosis) is outlined in Table 2.1.

Neutrophilic inflammation is less common and may be seen in infection (Fig. 2.4) and in areas close to an infarction. It is a hallmark of autoimmune injury (capillaritis, Fig. 2.5) and may be seen in alloimmune injury as well (antibody-mediated rejection).

Other components of interstitial inflammation may include eosinophils, seen in allergic or in eosinophilic pneumonia and to a lesser degree in hypersensitivity pneumonitis.

Fibroblasts and Collagen

Chronic inflammation may progress to interstitial fibrosis in a variety of settings, including interstitial pneumonias, organizing lung injury, and hypersensitivity pneumonitis. Initially, there are fine strands of collagen in a cellular matrix (Fig. 2.6), which may become more collagenized or form localized areas with organizing pneumonia (Fig. 2.7). Type II pneumocyte hyperplasia is typical when there is early collagen

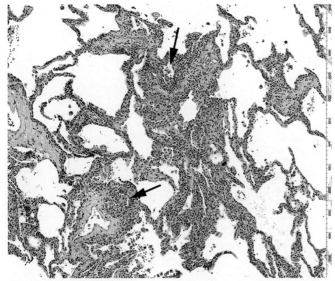

FIGURE 2.1 ▲ Chronic interstitial inflammation, peribronchiolar. The bronchioles are difficult to discern in the inflammation and are identified by their perivascular location (*arrows*). The patient's ultimate clinico-pathologic diagnosis was nonspecific interstitial pneumonia with areas of organizing pneumonia.

deposition. Denser collagen may occur with organizing diffuse alveolar damage (Fig. 2.8) or smoking-related fibrosis. Dense acellular collagen, often with "naked" granulomas, is typical of sarcoidosis, although the scarring is not typically within alveolar capillaries.

Elastosis

Elastosis is an extremely common finding especially in localized reactions to tumors and pneumothorax. Caps of elastosis in the apices ("apical caps") are present in most lungs of older people. When diffuse, the term "pleuroparenchymal fibroelastosis" is used. Elastosis does not typically demonstrate an alveolar septal distribution but is associated with alveolar collapse and loss of normal architecture.

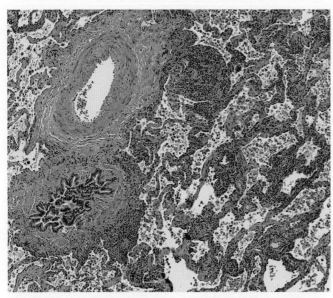

FIGURE 2.2 ▲ Chronic interstitial inflammation, peribronchiolar. There is a large bronchovascular bundle on the left. The ultimate diagnosis was probable hypersensitivity pneumonitis.

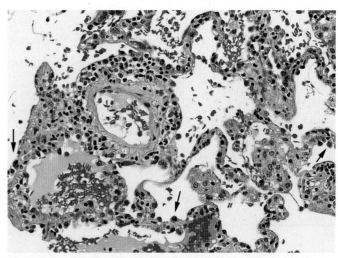

FIGURE 2.3 ▲ Chronic interstitial inflammation interstitial and perivascular. There is mild reactivity to alveolar lining cells (*arrows*). The patient had an undifferentiated connective tissue syndrome and interstitial cellular infiltrates that responded to steroids. The clinicopathologic diagnosis was interstitial pneumonia associated with rheumatoid arthritis.

Smooth Muscle Cells

In addition to forming collagen and elastic fibers, regenerative fibroblasts may transform into smooth muscle cells, forming diffuse interstitial thickening or small nodules (Fig. 2.9). Smooth

TABLE 2.1

Pattern, High Magnification	Pattern, Lower Magnification/ Accompanying Features	Possible Clinicopathologic Diagnoses
Chronic interstitial inflammation[a]	Predominantly peribronchiolar	Hypersensitivity pneumonitis (poorly formed granulomas, OP) Chronic bronchiolitis, including infectious NSIP COP
Chronic interstitial inflammation[a]	Indeterminate pattern, perivascular	Infection Organizing diffuse alveolar damage (often with loose fibrosis) NSIP COP Drug reaction Autoimmune lung injury in CTD (i.e., lupus pneumonitis) Alloimmune lung injury
Capillaritis		Autoimmune (MPA, lupus and other CTD, Goodpasture) Early infarction Infection
Interstitial inflammation with fibrosis	With or without OP	NSIP Autoimmune CTD Drug reaction Organizing lung DAD (may have areas of loose fibrosis mimicking OP)

[a]Reactive pneumocytes are common and are a result of alveolar injury of various causes. OP, organizing pneumonia; COP, cryptogenic organizing pneumonia; CTD, connective tissue disease; MPA, microscopic polyangiitis; NSIP, nonspecific interstitial pneumonia.

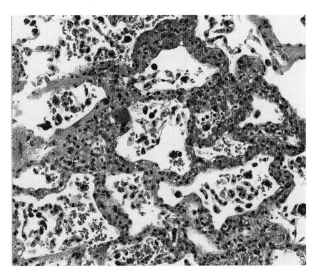

FIGURE 2.4 ▲ Acute interstitial inflammation. There is acute and chronic alveolar septal inflammation with early necrosis and alveolar hemosiderin macrophages. The patient had fungal sepsis and areas of hematogenous spread of *Aspergillus* in the lung. The findings could represent early infarct from angioinvasive aspergillosis with resulting capillary congestion.

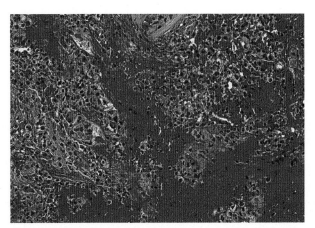

FIGURE 2.5 ▲ Acute interstitial inflammation, capillaritis. The patient had acute lung injury secondary to microscopic polyangiitis, ANCA-positive.

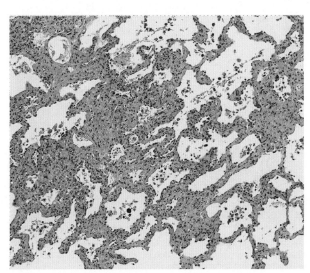

FIGURE 2.6 ▲ Chronic interstitial inflammation with type II pneumocyte hyperplasia and early fibrosis. The clinicopathologic diagnosis was hypersensitivity pneumonitis in a patient with birds as pets.

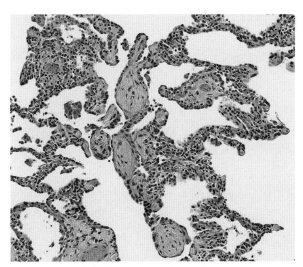

FIGURE 2.7 ▲ Chronic interstitial inflammation with patchy organizing pneumonia. The clinicopathologic diagnosis was cryptogenic organizing pneumonia.

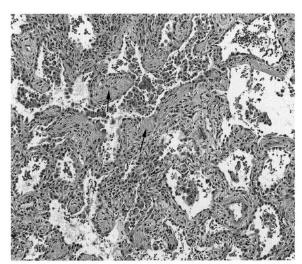

FIGURE 2.8 ▲ Diffuse interstitial inflammation with focal fibrosis (*arrows*) and diffuse type II pneumocyte hyperplasia. The clinicopathologic diagnosis was organizing diffuse alveolar damage.

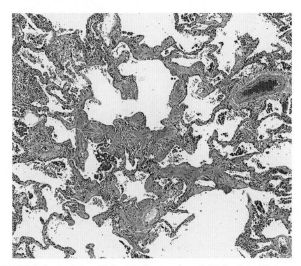

FIGURE 2.9 ▲ Interstitial smooth muscle cell thickening. There are bundles of smooth muscle cells in the interstitium, with early remodeling of the alveolar architecture. The clinicopathologic diagnosis was idiopathic pulmonary fibrosis, with diagnostic changes of usual interstitial pneumonia in subpleural locations.

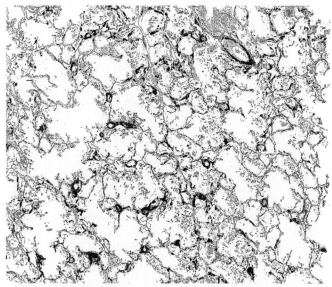

FIGURE 2.10 ▲ Diffuse alveolar calcification. The patient developed sepsis with acute and chronic renal failure, resulting in early diffuse alveolar damage with calcification of damaged alveolar septa.

muscle cell proliferation is especially common in idiopathic interstitial pneumonias and bronchiolocentric conditions. Occasionally, smooth muscle cell nodules are incidental findings of unclear cause.

Calcification and Ossification

Alveolar wall calcification is uncommon and associated with the combination of chronic renal failure, alveolar injury, and secondary hyperparathyroidism (Fig. 2.10). Nodules of ossification are very common in patients with idiopathic interstitial pneumonias in areas of fibrosis (Fig. 2.11).

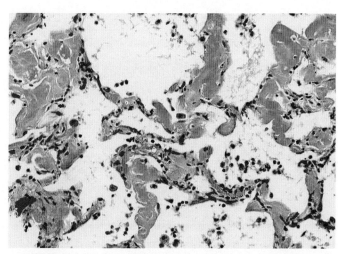

FIGURE 2.12 ▲ Interstitial amyloidosis. The patient died with cardiac amyloidosis, ATTR type, with areas of interstitial amyloid deposits in the lung.

Amyloid

Amyloidosis takes several forms in the lungs, including a diffuse interstitial type (Fig. 2.12), and is usually associated with systemic amyloidosis (see Chapter 27).

Congestion and Infarct

Capillaries may be filled with blood (chronic congestion, Fig. 2.4) in cases of venous hypertension and infarction or may contain round clear spaces consistent with fat embolism (Fig. 2.13). In later stages of infarcts, the alveolar septa may be infarcted, with loss of nuclear detail (Fig. 2.14).

Megakaryocytes

Megakaryocytes are commonly trapped in the alveolar capillaries in sepsis and other conditions resulting in thrombocytosis and are particularly common in autopsies (Fig. 2.15).

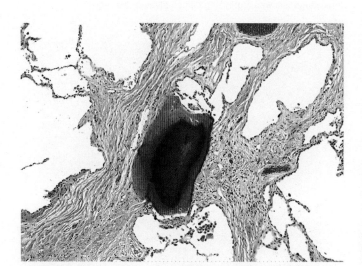

FIGURE 2.11 ▲ Pulmonary ossification. Areas of bony metaplasia in fibrotic lung are common, especially in the idiopathic interstitial pneumonias.

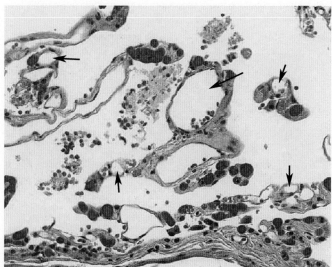

FIGURE 2.13 ▲ Diffuse fat embolism. The alveolar capillaries are widened by empty spaces. Fat stain on frozen sections is necessary prior to processing for a definitive diagnosis.

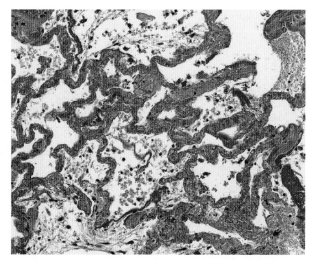

FIGURE 2.14 ▲ Pulmonary infarct. In later stages of infarction, the alveolar septa are necrotic. There is pulmonary congestion with increased red cells in the interstitium.

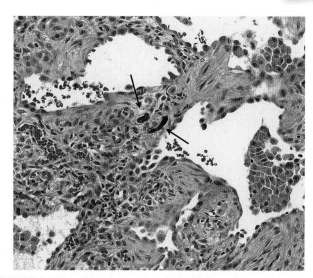

FIGURE 2.15 ▲ Megakaryocytes. Interstitial megakaryocytes (*arrows*) are common in sepsis and other systemic conditions that stress the bone marrow.

3 Pathologic Processes Involving the Alveolar Spaces

Allen P. Burke, M.D., and Haresh Mani, M.D.

General

Alveolar pathology involves filling of alveolar spaces with acellular material (fluid, blood, protein, or matrix) or cells.

Edema

Transudates occur in the alveolar spaces generally in the absence of alveolar injury, but in the presence of venous hypertension (e.g., heart failure) and osmotic changes. The alveolar spaces are filled with light-staining homogenous pink material, sometimes with tiny vacuoles, in the absence of fibrillar or granular structures (Fig. 3.1). Often, however, the edema fluid dissolves during tissue processing leaving empty-appearing alveolar spaces. Presence of dilated lymphatics and veins in interlobular septa and subpleural locations may then offer a clue to diagnosis, in the correct clinical setting.

Hemorrhage

As with fibrin, procedural hemorrhage is a common artifact. In order to suspect true hemorrhage, evidence of hemosiderin-laden macrophages (occurring in a few days, Fig. 3.2) or early phases of organization should be found. Pulmonary hemorrhage may be acute or chronic.

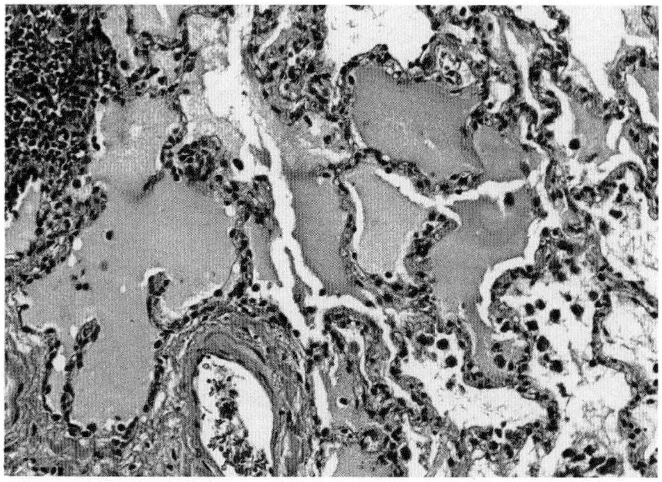

FIGURE 3.1 ▲ Pulmonary edema. There is a finely flocculent homogenous pink transudate filling the alveolar septa, with artifactual separation from the walls. There is no granularity or crystals to suggest proteinosis. Alveolar lining cells are nonreactive, and a fibrillary or ropy appearance to suggest fibrin is absent.

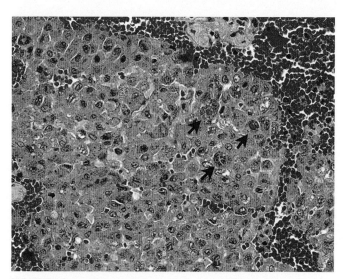

FIGURE 3.2 ▲ Pulmonary hemorrhage. In addition to intra-alveolar blood, there are scattered hemosiderin macrophages (*arrows*). Pulmonary alveolar lining cells are enlarged, and there are nonpigmented macrophages as well.

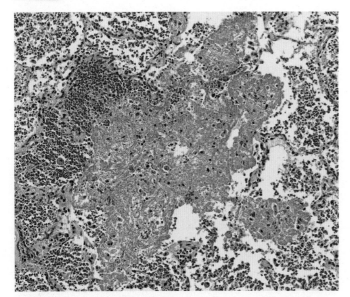

FIGURE 3.3 ▲ Intra-alveolar fibrin secondary to pneumonia. There is little acute inflammation, and the fibrin is fibrillar, with few red cells and dispersed inflammatory cells.

Surgical biopsies are rarely, if ever, performed to evaluate acute hemorrhage; more often, the pathologist may be asked to evaluate bronchoalveolar lavage (BAL) specimens in this setting. One must be cautious in interpreting iron stains on BAL specimens since so-called smoker's macrophages also contain fine iron. Siderophages, on the other hand, contain coarse iron granules of varying sizes.

The differential diagnosis of pulmonary hemorrhage is discussed in Chapter 32.

Fibrin

Fibrin is a common intra-alveolar process that should never be overlooked. Again, intact fibrin strands and red cells usually represent a procedural artifact. Early pathologic fibrin may maintain a fibrillar structure, but inflammatory cells are interspersed through it without layering or intact red cells (Figs. 3.3 and 3.4). Later, fibrin will show organization with endothelial cells at the periphery. A special form of fibrin mixed with

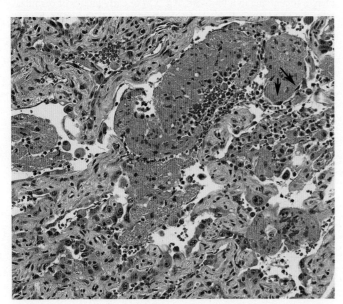

FIGURE 3.4 ▲ Intra-alveolar fibrin, early organization. There are scattered endothelial cells around the fibrin (arrows). There was focal acute lung injury in a lung resection for carcinoma, the injury being of uncertain etiology, but likely infectious.

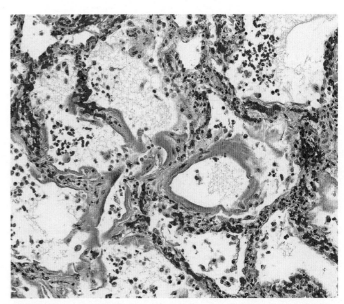

FIGURE 3.5 ▲ Hyaline membranes. These are a form of fibrin deposition that results from diffuse lung injury, desquamation of the alveolar lining, and pneumocyte necrosis.

necrotic alveolar lining cells results in hyaline membranes (Fig. 3.5; see Chapter 4). Fibrin may be focal and inconspicuous, usually accompanied by neutrophils, in areas of acute lung injury. The fibrin seen around pneumocystis pneumonia typically shows minute floccular clear spaces corresponding to the fungal organisms (Fig. 3.6). In general, any biopsy with acute lung injury should be stained for organisms (acid fast bacilli, gomori methenamine silver, tissue gram) and, if indicated, immunohistochemical stains for viruses. In practice, presence of prominent alveolar fibrin should raise a differential diagnosis of diffuse alveolar damage, acute fibrinous and organizing pneumonia, and pulmonary hemorrhage syndromes.

Alveolar Proteinosis

The intra-alveolar proteinaceous material is easily overlooked on small biopsy and is finely granular with larger eosinophilic crystals in the background that are either inconspicuous (Fig. 3.7) or obvious. The presence of relatively acellular alveolar proteinaceous material should

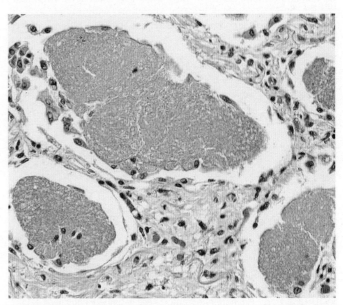

FIGURE 3.6 ▲ Pneumocystis pneumonia. The alveoli are filled with pneumocystis organisms that mimic the appearance of fibrin. There is a finely flocculent appearance corresponding to the organisms, which must be stained for visualization.

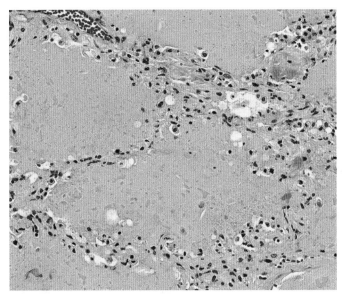

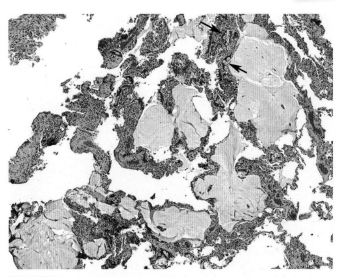

FIGURE 3.9 ▲ Intra-alveolar mucin (mucinous metaplasia). In some cases of small airway disease, hyperplastic reactive lining cells may undergo goblet cell hyperplasia (*arrows*) and secrete mucus into the airspaces.

FIGURE 3.7 ▲ Alveolar proteinosis. There is a granular eosinophilic material filling the alveolar spaces, within which are scattered larger eosinophilic granules.

prompt a GMS stain to exclude *Pneumocystis jiroveci* pneumonia. True pulmonary alveolar proteinosis (PAP) is caused by accumulation of surfactant components in the alveoli and terminal airways due to insufficient surfactant clearance by macrophages (Chapter 31).

Blue Bodies and Corpora Amylacea

Blue bodies are intra-alveolar lightly calcified hematoxylinophilic concretions that are found in a variety of conditions. In addition to calcium carbonate, they contain mucopolysaccharides and iron.[1] Much more common than blue bodies are corpora amylacea, which are similar in appearance to those seen in the prostate and brain and which are likewise of unknown significance (Fig. 3.8). These may rarely accumulate in large numbers resulting in mass-like lesions.[2]

Intra-alveolar Mucin

Collections of mucin may travel into relatively normal lung from mucinous tumors and obstructed airways. These appear similar to

"mucocele-like lesions" in other organs such as the breast (Fig. 3.9). If there are small airway changes in a nearby focus, the lesion is not significant, but intramucinous tumor cells and mucinous adenocarcinoma in situ should be carefully excluded.

Neutrophils

Intra-alveolar neutrophils generally indicate lung injury resulting in intermixed fibrin, which can be fine in early stages and denser in later stages. Suppurative pneumonia is highly suggestive of bacterial pneumonia. In cases of neutropenia, only intra-alveolar fibrin with reactive pneumocytes may be present.

Macrophages

Intra-alveolar macrophages are extremely common in cases of lung disease that result in any airway obstruction or remodeling due to fibrosis. Hemorrhage may result in hemosiderin macrophages, either by small occult hemorrhages in venous hypertension caused by heart failure or mitral stenosis or by other forms of localized hemorrhage. Finely pigmented macrophages that are often relatively cohesive are typical of smoking (Fig. 3.10) and are seen in excessive numbers in respiratory bronchiolitis

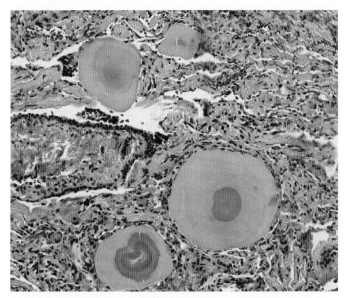

FIGURE 3.8 ▲ Corpora amylacea. Concentric intra-alveolar nodules that resemble blue bodies but are larger, not calcified, and more eosinophilic, are nonspecific findings.

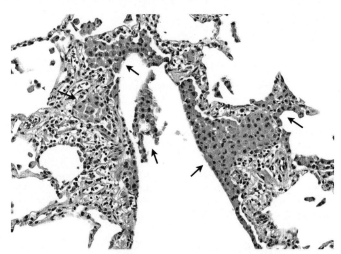

FIGURE 3.10 ▲ Smokers' macrophages. The terminal bronchiole contains clusters of macrophages that form cohesive aggregates that contain very fine barely visible pigment (*arrows*). The finding was incidental in a trauma victim with emergent thoracotomy.

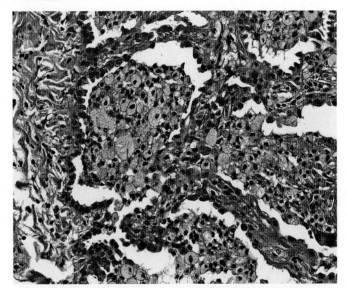

FIGURE 3.11 ▲ Foam cell macrophages. The alveolar septa are mildly thickening, and there is reactivity of the pneumocytes. The foam cell macrophages are indicative of ingested lipid by the scavenger cells, usually the result of obstruction.

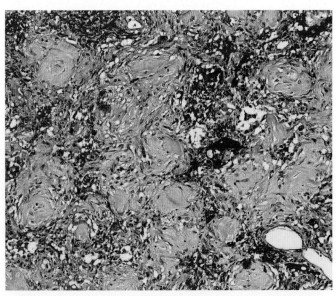

FIGURE 3.12 ▲ Organizing alveolar lung injury. Diffuse alveolar damage, at around 2 weeks, shows predominantly loose fibrosis, which can have a rounded appearance due to filling of alveolar spaces, when the alveolar architecture has not been destroyed.

and desquamative interstitial pneumonia. Foamy macrophages filled with lipid are typical of obstruction (Fig. 3.11). Nonpigmented macrophages accumulate in a variety of conditions, including acute lung injury (when they can mimic granulomas), congenital surfactant deficiency (when they mimic desquamative interstitial pneumonia), and noninfectious pneumonia. Dust-laden macrophages are typical of pneumoconioses and are present in a centrilobular (peribronchiolar) location (see Chapter 61).

Histiocyte accumulations in the lung are discussed in Chapter 98.

Eosinophils

Intra-alveolar eosinophils, when numerous, raise the possibility of eosinophilic pneumonia, which in early stages resembles bacterial pneumonia with eosinophils and later stages organizing pneumonia. Typically, patients present acutely with rapidly progressive respiratory failure that responds to steroid treatment. However, steroid treatment can reduce or eliminate the eosinophil population, leaving behind sheets of pale to pink histiocytes on biopsy material.

Loose Fibrosis

Although generally considered an interstitial or airway-related process, loose fibrosis can fill alveolar airspaces in the organizing phase of diffuse alveolar damage (Fig. 3.12). Alveolar and bronchiolar filling by fibromyxoid plugs typifies an organizing pneumonia pattern and is much more common than loose fibrosis. An organizing pneumonia pattern of injury is nonspecific and may be seen following lung injury of any etiology (e.g., infection, hemorrhage, connective tissue disease related, aspiration, drug toxicity, and idiopathic).

REFERENCES

1. Koss MN, Johnson FB, Hochholzer L. Pulmonary blue bodies. *Hum Pathol.* 1981;12(3):258–266.
2. Dobashi M, et al. Histopathological study of corpora amylacea pulmonum. *Histol Histopathol.* 1989;4(2):153–165.

4 Diffuse Alveolar Damage

Marie-Christine Aubry, M.D., and Allen P. Burke, M.D.

Terminology

Diffuse alveolar damage (DAD) is an acute lung injury involving predominantly the interstitium and characterized by two overlapping histologic phases, acute or exudative, and organizing or proliferative (Table 4.1). It is the common histologic finding in patients with adult respiratory distress syndrome (ARDS) (Chapter 21) and acute interstitial pneumonia (AIP) (Chapter 19).

Radiologic Findings

Imaging in patients with DAD corresponds to the underlying disease and is generally similar across different etiologies. Radiographic findings include diffuse bilateral infiltrates, often with "whiteout" of the lungs, with diffuse ground-glass opacities by computed tomography. These findings often obscure underlying processes that may predispose to diffuse alveolar damage, such as idiopathic interstitial fibrosis and areas of consolidation caused by infectious processes.

Tissue Sampling

Patients with DAD are usually assessed by bronchoalveolar lavage and culture. Transbronchial biopsies may be helpful in excluding granulomatous disease, malignancy, and infections but are limited due to sampling. Open lung biopsy is generally done only in cases refractory to therapy without clear cause, in order to exclude infections, capillaritis,

TABLE 4.1 Histologic Phases of Diffuse Alveolar Damage

Phase	Other Designations	Time Frame After Injury	Histologic Features
Early	Acute, exudative	12 h–3 d	Capillary congestion Interstitial edema Intra-alveolar edema Intra-alveolar fibrin
		3–7 d	Hyaline membranes Interstitial myofibroblasts Sparse interstitial inflammation Reactive pneumocytes with atypia
Late	Proliferative, organizing	1–2 wk	Cuboidal (hobnail) pneumocyte hyperplasia Squamous metaplasia, often with atypia Interstitial fibro- and myofibroblasts with loose collagen and inflammation (granulation tissue), and interstitium
Fibrotic	—	>3–4 wk	Remodeling with cystic change Interstitial fibrosis Intimal thickening, arteries and veins

other causes of diffuse alveolar hemorrhage, and, rarely, amniotic or fat embolism. Occasionally, frozen sections are requested in order to establish that representative tissue is present,[1] as autopsy studies have shown that DAD may be regional.[2]

Microscopic Findings

The two phases of DAD are the exudative (acute) phase and the proliferative (organizing) phase.[3] In addition, some patients survive without significant sequelae or may develop fibrotic lung disease. The histologic findings of the two phases and the fibrotic sequelae are present in Table 4.1.

Early findings in the exudative phase are edema, both interstitial and alveolar with capillary congestion, indistinguishable from other causes of pulmonary edema and congestion. The histologic hallmark of acute DAD is **hyaline membranes**, which develop 24 hours after the beginning of symptoms (Fig. 4.1). They are densely eosinophilic, thick linear structures that line denuded alveolar walls. They are composed of plasma proteins such as fibrinogen, immunoglobulin and complement, and surfactant components. The proliferative phase becomes prominent after 1 to 2 weeks. It is characterized by **interstitial** thickening, resulting from the **proliferation of fibroblasts** and **myofibroblasts** admixed with varying numbers of inflammatory cells, including neutrophils. The cells are embedded in a myxoid stroma rich in acid mucopolysaccharides. Hyperplastic type II pneumocytes characterized by a cuboidal morphology often line the alveolar septa and may show marked nuclear atypia (Fig. 4.2A). Remnants of hyaline membranes can also be seen lining alveolar spaces; however, at this stage, they are often very focal. Squamous metaplasia of terminal bronchiolar epithelium may be prominent, and the cells may show considerable cytologic atypia with enlarged, vesicular nuclei and prominent nucleoli (Fig. 4.2B). The cytologic atypia of the hyperplastic pneumocytes and the squamous cells can be interpreted as malignant on preparations from sputa, bronchoalveolar lavage, or, more rarely, transbronchial biopsy specimens.[4] Myofibroblastic proliferation progresses with intra-alveolar and interstitial loose fibrosis.

DAD is a pattern of acute lung injury that is **nonspecific** since it can result from numerous causes and a specific etiology usually determined clinically (Table 4.2).[5-8] Exceptions are infections that can be diagnosed histologically such as pneumocystis, cytomegalovirus (CMV), and adenovirus (Chapters 39 and 42).

The diagnosis of DAD is commonly posed at autopsy and readily recognizable on surgical lung biopsies. But DAD can also be diagnosed on transbronchial biopsies as hyaline membranes are distinctive and unique to DAD.[9] The reported sensitivity is, however, relatively low (~50%).[10]

TABLE 4.2 Causes of Diffuse Alveolar Damage

Sepsis
Pulmonary infections
   Pneumocystis
   Viruses (influenza, adenovirus, CMV, SARS)
   Legionella, mycoplasma
Shock
Connective tissue disease
Inhalants (smoke, oxygen, paint remover)
Drugs
   Chemotherapeutic agents (bleomycin, methotrexate, etc.)
   Others (amiodarone, gold, etc.)
   Illicit (heroin, other opiates)
Radiation
Stem cell or solid organ transplantation
Acute exacerbation of UIP/idiopathic pulmonary fibrosis
Others
Idiopathic (acute interstitial pneumonia)

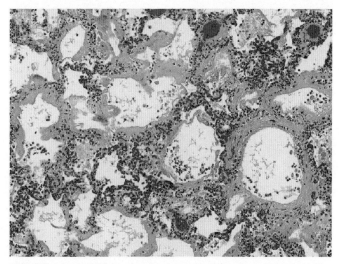

FIGURE 4.1 ▲ Diffuse alveolar damage, acute stage. There are diffuse hyaline membranes with loss of alveolar lining cells.

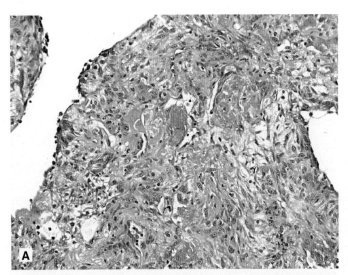
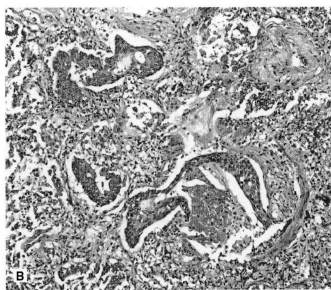

FIGURE 4.2 ▲ Diffuse alveolar damage, organizing (proliferative) phase. **A.** There is thickening of the alveolar septa, which are lined by reactive pneumocytes. There is minimal residual fibrin. **B.** Diffuse alveolar damage, with squamous metaplasia. Squamous metaplasia is common and, in this instance, associated with intra-alveolar fibrin deposition.

In addition to the two recognized phases of diffuse alveolar damage, a subset of patients survive and develop chronic fibrotic lung disease, which is relatively little studied. It is characterized by cystic remodeling and interstitial and intra-alveolar fibrosis, that is typically heterogeneous[1] (Figs. 4.3 and 4.4). In the final stage of organization, the parenchyma can be markedly altered by fibrosis and result in irregularly shaped airspaces, which are variably sized, but often small and slit-like. If the process continues for a sufficient period of time, honeycomb changes can be seen. However, a follow-up computer tomography study of survivors of acute respiratory syndrome showed most frequently a reticular pattern, with a striking anterior distribution, without significant cystic change.[11]

An autopsy study has shown that in 10% of cases of "diffuse" alveolar damage, the distribution is not diffuse but regional, most frequently in the upper lobes. The patients with regional alveolar damage did not differ significantly from those with diffuse alveolar injury, including the need for mechanical ventilation, and had the development of organizing localized lesions, arguing against an early phase of diffuse alveolar damage.[2]

Other histologic features of may be seen, including vascular thrombi, intimal thickening of vessels (in later stages), areas of superimposed bronchopneumonia, and calcification, especially if there is renal failure. Thrombi in small arteries are an almost constant associated finding. They are usually formed in situ, secondary to endothelial injury.

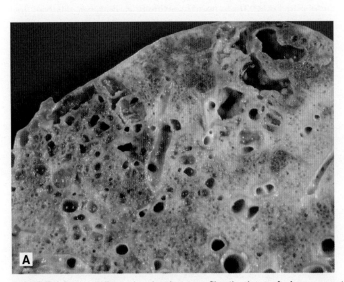
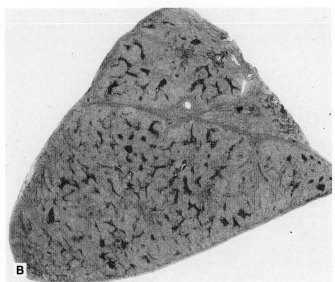

FIGURE 4.3 ▲ Diffuse alveolar damage, fibrotic phase. **A.** A gross section at autopsy demonstrates irregular scarring and small cysts. **B.** There is diffuse fibrosis at lowest magnification. There is, an addition, diffuse hemorrhage, which was secondary to extracorporeal membrane oxygenation therapy.

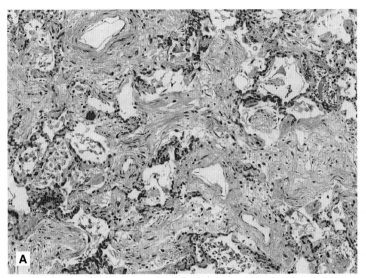
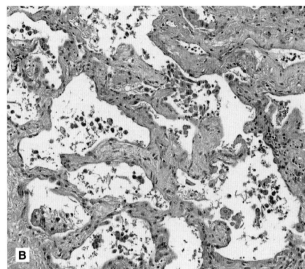

FIGURE 4.4 ▲ Diffuse alveolar damage, fibrotic phase. **A.** There is diffuse interstitial and intra-alveolar fibrosis. The patient had bleomycin-induced diffuse alveolar damage, which began 1.5 months prior to death. **B.** A different patient with diffuse fibrosis that is primarily interstitial, with early cystic remodeling.

Differential Diagnosis

The **differential diagnosis** of DAD includes other acute lung injuries such as organizing pneumonia (OP), acute and fibrinous organizing pneumonia (AFOP), and so-called acute eosinophilic pneumonia (AEP) (Table 4.3) as well as other predominantly interstitial lung diseases such as usual interstitial pneumonia (UIP) and nonspecific interstitial pneumonia (NSIP).

OP (Chapter 5) tends to be patchier and bronchiolocentric, and the proliferating fibroblasts are predominantly intraluminal rather than interstitial. Hyaline membranes and vascular thrombi are not seen. Prominent pneumocyte hyperplasia and squamous metaplasia are uncommon.

AFOP describes a histologic pattern with overlapping features between DAD and OP.[12] Histologically, airspace fibrin with varying amounts of OP and pneumocyte hyperplasia dominate. Patients with AFOP have similar clinical presentation and outcome as patients with DAD.

UIP (Chapter 17) is characterized by its temporal variegation and is mostly fibrotic with collagen fibrosis causing architectural distortion and honeycomb change. The proliferating fibroblasts form small foci at the interface between the fibrosis and normal-appearing lung.

NSIP (Chapter 17) and DAD can be occasionally difficult to distinguish. In NSIP, the interstitial fibrosis tends to be more collagen than fibroblasts and associated with more chronic inflammation. Prominent pneumocyte hyperplasia is also uncommon. However, in the initial description of NSIP, a couple of cases were thought to be advanced stage of DAD.[13]

AEP (Chapter 26), as defined by Tazelaar et al., is **acute and organizing DAD** with increased (although quantity not specified) numbers of interstitial and alveolar **eosinophils.**[14] This distinction is important since patients with AEP respond to steroids in contrast to patients with DAD.

Pathogenesis

Electron microscopic studies of lungs with DAD have shown the presence of both epithelial and endothelial injuries.[15] In the exudative phase, type 1 pneumocytes become necrotic and slough from the septa, leaving a denuded basement membrane. Endothelial cells show swelling with widened intercellular junctions. Occasionally, they undergo necrosis with denudation of the capillary basement membrane. These injuries lead to an increase in vascular permeability resulting in widening of the septa by edema, fibrin, and red cells and the formation of hyaline membranes; eventually, interstitial fluid escapes into the alveolar spaces. In the proliferative phase, the widening of the septa results, in part, from the proliferation of mesenchymal and epithelial cells. Fibroblasts and myofibroblasts proliferate within the interstitium and are admixed with inflammatory cells such as lymphocytes, plasma cells, and macrophages. Usually, only small amounts of collagen and elastic fibers are laid down in the interstitium. In all cases, there is a marked proliferation of type 2 pneumocytes.

TABLE 4.3 Contrasting Histologic Features of DAD, UIP, NSIP, OP, and AEP

Pathologic Features	DAD	UIP	NSIP	OP	AEP	AFOP
Pattern	Interstitial	Interstitial	Interstitial	Airspace	Interstitial	Airspace
Temporal appearance	Uniform	Heterogeneous	Uniform	Uniform	Uniform	Uniform
Interstitial inflammation	Scant	Scant	Usually prominent	Variable	Prominent eosinophils	Variable
Collagen fibrosis	Occasionally late stage	Patchy	Variable, diffuse	No	No	No
Fibroblast proliferation	Diffuse interstitial	Patchy fibroblast foci	Occasional	Patchy airspace	Diffuse interstitial	Patchy airspace
Honeycomb changes	Rare	Yes	Rare	No	Rare	No
Hyaline membranes	Yes	No	No	No	Yes	No
Fibrinous exudate	No	No	No	No	No	Yes airspace
Increased eosinophils	No	No	No	No	Yes	No

Two other mechanisms play an important role in the interstitial thickening. The first involves an incorporation of intra-alveolar exudates into the alveolar walls. The cytoplasmic processes of type 2 pneumocytes extend along the surface of the basement membrane and cover cells and debris overlying the basement membrane, incorporating this material into the septum. The second consists of partial to complete collapse of alveoli with permanent apposition of alveolar septa. The collapse occurs when the epithelial basement membrane is denuded. The proliferating type 2 pneumocytes, therefore, cover a collapsed portion of alveoli rather than relining intact and expanded alveoli. These mechanisms contribute to the thickening of septa and help explain the restructuring of the lung as part of the repair process and the formation of honeycomb areas.

The contribution of epithelial and endothelial injury to the pathogenesis of DAD has been well established. However, the mechanisms underlying the cellular injury still remain unclear.[5] Studies have concentrated on the role of inflammatory cells with emphasis on neutrophils and macrophages. These cells accumulate in the interstitium and alveolar spaces and, through the secretion of cytokines, are thought to contribute not only in direct cell injury but also to the initiation of repair mechanisms. The clinical and histologic picture most likely results from the complex interplay of these various cytokines. Some cytokines have a proinflammatory role, such as interleukin-1, interleukin-6, and interleukin-8, tumor necrosis factor-alpha, and monocyte chemoattractant protein, and others a reparative/fibrotic role, such as transforming growth factor, platelet-derived growth factor, basic fibroblast growth factor and, interleukin-4, interleukin-10, and interleukin-13. However, DAD can be induced in the absence of neutrophils and seen in patients with profound neutropenia. This suggests that other mechanisms are involved.

Other studies have concentrated on the process of apoptosis as a major contributor to the development of DAD. Apoptosis, directly observed by nick end-labeling method, or by the expression of p53 and WAF1, has been predominantly localized to type 2 pneumocytes.[16] It is most prominent in the acute stage of DAD. The expression of BAX protein, which promotes apoptosis, is increased and widespread in type 2 pneumocytes and interstitial myofibroblasts.[17] Apoptosis is induced by DNA damage. Several known causes of DAD, such as radiation and infection, can induce apoptosis by causing DNA damage. However, possible causes of DNA damage in idiopathic cases remain unknown.

Genetic factors likely contribute to the susceptibility of patients developing DAD with several genetic polymorphisms or variants discovered in genes involved in apoptosis, regulation of inflammation, epithelial cell injury, or effects of infection by certain pathogens.[18]

Practical Points

▶ DAD is a pattern of acute lung injury that involves the interstitium of the lung.

▶ DAD varies morphologically according to duration of disease and can be classified as acute/exudative and organizing/proliferative.

▶ DAD can be diagnosed on transbronchial biopsy as hyaline membranes are diagnostic of the disease.

▶ DAD is nonspecific and etiologies need to be correlated clinically with the exception of infectious etiologies identified morphologically.

REFERENCES

1. Castro CY. ARDS and diffuse alveolar damage: a pathologist's perspective. *Semin Thorac Cardiovasc Surg.* 2006;18:13–19.
2. Yazdy AM, Tomashefski JF Jr, Yagan R, et al. Regional alveolar damage (RAD). A localized counterpart of diffuse alveolar damage. *Am J Clin Pathol.* 1989;92:10–15.
3. Thille AW, Esteban A, Fernandez-Segoviano P, et al. Chronology of histological lesions in acute respiratory distress syndrome with diffuse alveolar damage: a prospective cohort study of clinical autopsies. *Lancet Respir Med.* 2013;1:395–401.
4. Ogino S, Franks TJ, Yong M, et al. Extensive squamous metaplasia with cytologic atypia in diffuse alveolar damage mimicking squamous cell carcinoma: a report of 2 cases. *Hum Pathol.* 2002;33:1052–1054.
5. Ware LB, Matthay MA. The acute respiratory distress syndrome. *N Engl J Med.* 2000;342:1334–1349.
6. Parambil JG, Myers JL, Aubry MC, et al. Causes and prognosis of diffuse alveolar damage diagnosed on surgical lung biopsy. *Chest.* 2007;132:50–57.
7. Parambil JG, Myers JL, Ryu JH. Diffuse alveolar damage: uncommon manifestation of pulmonary involvement in patients with connective tissue diseases. *Chest.* 2006;130:553–558.
8. Katzenstein AL, Myers JL, Mazur MT. Acute interstitial pneumonia. A clinicopathologic, ultrastructural, and cell kinetic study. *Am J Surg Pathol.* 1986;10:256–267.
9. Leslie KO, Gruden JF, Parish JM, et al. Transbronchial biopsy interpretation in the patient with diffuse parenchymal lung disease. *Arch Pathol Lab Med.* 2007;131:407–423.
10. Rao VK, Ritter J, Kollef MH. Utility of transbronchial biopsy in patients with acute respiratory failure: a postmortem study. *Chest.* 1998;114:549–555.
11. Desai SR, Wells AU, Rubens MB, et al. Acute respiratory distress syndrome: CT abnormalities at long-term follow-up. *Radiology.* 1999;210:29–35.
12. Beasley MB, Franks TJ, Galvin JR, et al. Acute fibrinous and organizing pneumonia: a histological pattern of lung injury and possible variant of diffuse alveolar damage. *Arch Pathol Lab Med.* 2002;126:1064–1070.
13. Katzenstein AL, Fiorelli RF. Nonspecific interstitial pneumonia/fibrosis. Histologic features and clinical significance. *Am J Surg Pathol.* 1994;18:136–147.
14. Tazelaar HD, Linz LJ, Colby TV, et al. Acute eosinophilic pneumonia: histopathologic findings in nine patients. *Am J Respir Crit Care Med.* 1997;155:296–302.
15. Katzenstein AL. Pathogenesis of "fibrosis" in interstitial pneumonia: an electron microscopic study. *Hum Pathol.* 1985;16:1015–1024.
16. Guinee D Jr, Fleming M, Hayashi T, et al. Association of p53 and WAF1 expression with apoptosis in diffuse alveolar damage. *Am J Pathol.* 1996;149:531–538.
17. Guinee D Jr, Brambilla E, Fleming M, et al. The potential role of BAX and BCL-2 expression in diffuse alveolar damage. *Am J Pathol.* 1997;151:999–1007.
18. Matthay MA, Ware LB, Zimmerman GA. The acute respiratory distress syndrome. *J Clin Invest.* 2012;122:2731–2740.

5 Organizing Pneumonia

Allen P. Burke, M.D., and Teklu Legesse, M.D.

Terminology

Organizing pneumonia (OP) is a histologic "pattern" that denotes a subacute phase of lung injury characterized by loose fibrosis that is reasonably discrete and circumscribed.[1] The term "BOOP" (bronchiolitis obliterans organizing pneumonia) is used by some[2] and discouraged by others.[3] The true frequency of bronchiole-related OP may be underestimated due to sampling or sectioning artifact, but it seems fairly certain that a large proportion of OP occurs in the interstitium remote from the airways, favoring the term "OP" over "BOOP." Idiopathic OP is termed "cryptogenic organizing pneumonia" or "idiopathic BOOP" and is discussed in Chapter 19. OP or BOOP should not be confused with obliterative bronchiolitis, bronchiolitis obliterans syndrome, or constrictive bronchiolitis (see Chapter 37), all of which are immune-related airway destructive processes and histologically distinct from OP.

Microscopic Findings

OP is characterized by nodules of myofibroblasts within a background of extracellular matrix and collagen (Fig. 5.1). These nodules are sometimes called "Masson bodies," a term ascribed to Masson years after he published histologic findings of the lungs of patients with acute rheumatic fever.[4] OP is either within the bronchioles ("polypoid bronchiolitis obliterans") (Fig. 5.2), adjacent to the bronchioles (Fig. 5.3), or within the interstitium. If there is coalescence into a nodule, or if airways are not readily identified, relationship to airway is indeterminate (Fig. 5.4). There may be associated granulomas adjacent to or within the organizing pneumonia

(Fig. 5.5). Fibrin is occasionally present, in which case, the term "acute and organizing pneumonia" may be used. Granulation tissue may occur, but usually, the lesion is often composed almost completely of fibroblasts, ground substance, and chronic inflammation, with little neovascularity. There may be focal reactive pneumocyte hyperplasia, but widespread pneumocyte changes with diffuse interstitial loose fibrosis are more typical of diffuse alveolar damage than OP (Fig. 5.6). There may be adjacent interstitial inflammation, especially in hypersensitivity pneumonitis, as well as adjacent fibrosis, with an NSIP-like pattern, especially in COP.

Differential Diagnosis

The OP "pattern" is invariable in cryptogenic organizing pneumonia and organizing infectious or aspiration pneumonia (Figs. 5.7 and 5.8). It is typically seen as a component of hypersensitivity pneumonitis, drug-induced lung injury, autoimmune lung injury such as rheumatoid lung disease, alloimmune lung injury, and allergic lung injury (eosinophilic pneumonia) (Table 5.1). OP may be present to a lesser degree in virtually any condition with lung injury, including Wegener granulomatosis, pneumoconiosis, ECMO-related lung injury, and NSIP. OP is a characteristic of "acute fibrinous and organizing pneumonia," a recently described interstitial lung disease that is a variant of acute interstitial pneumonia (see Chapter 19). OP may be present in areas of lung not grossly involved by honeycombing in idiopathic pulmonary fibrosis (UIP). Areas of OP are frequently seen in patients with emphysema (Fig. 5.9), and adjacent to tumors, presumably

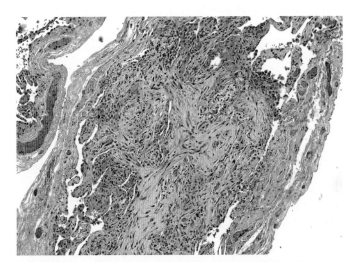

FIGURE 5.1 ▲ Organizing pneumonia, high magnification. The nodule (occasionally termed "Masson body") is composed of myofibroblasts in a loosely collagenized matrix.

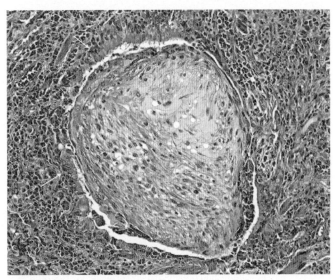

FIGURE 5.2 ▲ Organizing pneumonia, polypoid bronchiolitis obliterans. In this case, the Masson body fills a bronchiole.

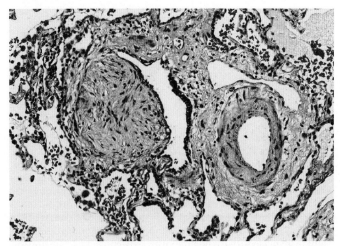

FIGURE 5.3 ▲ Organizing pneumonia, adjacent to bronchiole. The area of OP extrudes in the bronchiolar lumen. The associated artery is at the right.

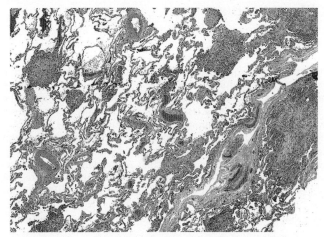

FIGURE 5.4 ▲ Organizing pneumonia, multifocal. There are numerous interstitial areas of OP, which are indeterminate for airway location, which are not clearly evident.

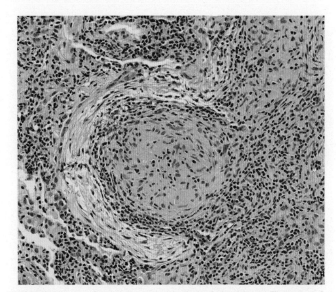

FIGURE 5.5 ▲ Organizing pneumonia and granuloma. The area of OP wraps around the granuloma in the center. OP and poorly formed granulomas are characteristic of hypersensitivity pneumonitis. In this patient, there were multiple well- and poorly formed granulomas forming a mass, but cultures and special stains were negative.

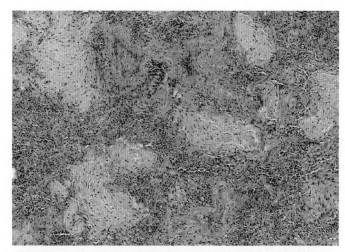

FIGURE 5.6 ▲ Organizing pneumonia pattern in diffuse alveolar damage. In healing DAD, the high magnification mimics organizing pneumonia. However, clinically and radiologically, the overall picture was that of ARDS.

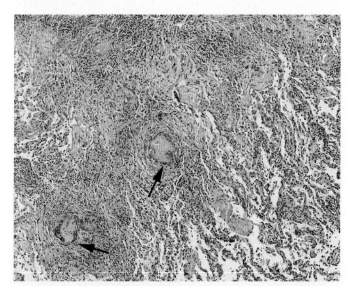

FIGURE 5.7 ▲ Organizing aspiration pneumonia. There are foreign body macrophage giant cells around aspirated starch grains (*arrows*).

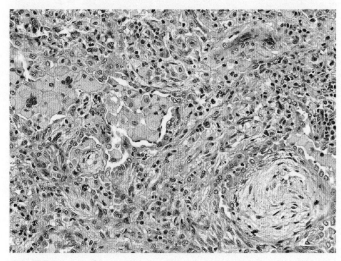

FIGURE 5.8 ▲ Organizing pneumonia, postobstructive. In addition to OP, there are intra-alveolar collections of foamy macrophages.

TABLE 5.1   Conditions in Which the OP Pattern is Frequently Present

Condition	Associated Findings
Cryptogenic OP	May have areas of NSIP
Hypersensitivity pneumonitis	Bronchiolocentric chronic inflammation, poorly formed granulomas
Organizing infectious pneumonia	Areas of acute pneumonia (fibrin, neutrophils)
Organizing aspiration pneumonia	Aspirated material, areas of acute pneumonia
Organizing postobstructive pneumonia	Foamy macrophages
Eosinophilic pneumonia	Eosinophils, acute pneumonitis (fibrin)
OP forming solitary nodules clinically mimicking tumors	None; are presumably postinfectious
Autoimmune connective tissue diseases, especially rheumatoid arthritis	None; acute lung injury, capillaritis, NSIP (variable)
Drug-induced lung injury, subacute phase	None; may show acute lung injury as well
Graft-versus-host disease, subacute phase	Interstitial inflammation with lymphocytes and neutrophils, bronchiolar inflammation; may show acute lung injury as well
NSIP, cellular type especially	Interstitial fibrosis, temporally uniform
Diffuse alveolar damage, organizing phase	Hyaline membranes if overlap with acute phase and fibrosis mimicking NSIP if overlap with fibrotic phase
Neoplasia, especially epithelial tumors	OP variably seen in the periphery of tumors, presumably by organizing injury due to obstruction

NSIP, nonspecific interstitial pneumonia.

TABLE 5.2   Histologic Differential Diagnosis of OP

Pattern of Injury	Distinguishing Features
Granuloma	Lack of fibroblasts, loose collagen, and extracellular matrix; presence of macrophages with lymphocytes; granulomas may be intermixed with OP, however
DAD, organizing	May be difficult or impossible to distinguish on small biopsies; diffuse vs. localized process
Fibroblast focus	Present adjacent to cystic honeycombing; may be difficult to distinguish in nonfibrotic areas of UIP, however
Constrictive bronchiolitis[a]	Dense fibrosis that surrounds bronchiole eventually destroying the airway, with mucosal granulation tissue in subacute phase

[a]Termed bronchiolitis obliterans syndrome in the context of graft-versus-host disease, obliterative bronchiolitis in lung transplant patients, and constrictive bronchiolitis in autoimmune conditions.

by a variety of mechanisms including obstruction and infection. OP may be the only finding in masses resected from patients with suspected neoplasms, especially in those with known cancers who are being investigated for possible metastatic disease. In these cases, OP is likely the consequence of an infectious or obstructive process.

Thus, the histologic differential diagnosis of OP is very broad and includes granulomatous inflammation, diffuse alveolar damage, fibroblastic foci, and constrictive bronchiolitis (Table 5.2). The distinction among these entities may be difficult on small biopsies and rests on the identification of loose fibrosis in the absence of inflammation and widespread acute or resolving lung injury.

REFERENCES

1. Cordier JF. Organising pneumonia. *Thorax*. 2000;55(4):318–328.
2. Katzenstein AL, Mukhopadhyay S, Myers JL. Diagnosis of usual interstitial pneumonia and distinction from other fibrosing interstitial lung diseases. *Hum Pathol*. 2008;39(9):1275–1294.
3. American Thoracic Society/European Respiratory Society International Multidisciplinary Consensus Classification of the Idiopathic Interstitial Pneumonias. This joint statement of the American Thoracic Society (ATS), and the European Respiratory Society (ERS) was adopted by the ATS board of directors, June 2001 and by the ERS Executive Committee, June 2001. *Am J Respir Crit Care Med*. 2002;165(2):277–304.
4. Herbut PA, Manges WE. The "Masson body" in rheumatic pneumonia. *Am J Pathol*. 1945;21(4):741–751.

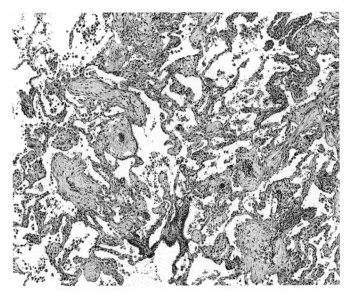

FIGURE 5.9 ▲ Organizing pneumonia in emphysema. This explanted lung showed emphysema patchy organizing pneumonia and respiratory bronchiolitis.

6 Alveolar Pneumocytes, Reactive and Metaplastic Changes

Allen P. Burke, M.D.

Acute Reactive Changes

Alveolar lining cells are denuded and regenerative in acute alveolar injury. Histologic features of regeneration include nuclear enlargement, cytoplasmic enlargement, and cytoplasmic vacuolization. Extensive vacuolization that involves macrophages as well is typical of amiodarone toxicity and Hermansky-Pudlak syndrome. Reactive pneumocytes persist from acute to organizing stage of alveolar injury (Figs. 6.1 to 6.3). In some cases, the changes suggest viral cytopathic effects.

Chronic Reactive Changes

With loss of fibrin and transformation of the interstitium to a more restive, fibrotic state, type II pneumocytes are less atypical but maintain a crowded configuration with cuboidal shape. In this phase, they are most difficult to distinguish from preneoplastic changes, such as atypical adenomatous hyperplasia (AAH). AAH tends to be relatively circumscribed and uniform, whereas reactive changes are more diffuse and show areas typical of reactive fibrosis (Figs. 6.4 to 6.7).

Mucinous and Squamous Metaplasia

Squamous metaplasia is a reactive feature in both acute lung injury, such as diffuse alveolar damage and acute respiratory distress syndrome, as well as chronic lung injury (Fig. 6.8). In the latter, it is typically seen in the variegated lining of remodeled cystic cavities in usual interstitial pneumonia.

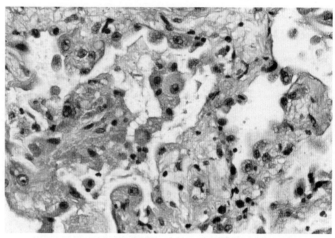

FIGURE 6.2 ▲ Acute pneumocyte hyperplasia, alloimmune lung injury. The patient had a bone marrow transplant, cutaneous graft-versus-host disease, and lung infiltrates. Biopsy showed interstitial inflammation and edema and markedly reactive pneumocytes.

Mucinous metaplasia is a feature of chronic airway disease and bronchiectasis and may spread into surrounding airways in cases of peribronchiolar metaplasia (Fig. 6.9). Because goblet cells are a normal component of proximal airways, the term hyperplasia is more appropriate in larger airways. The extravasated mucus may raise concern for mucinous adenocarcinoma, but the clearly reactive nature of mucus gland hyperplasia in the reactive airways suggests that the process is benign.

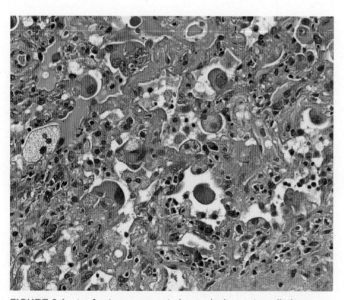

FIGURE 6.1 ▲ Acute pneumocyte hyperplasia, acute radiation pneumonitis. A variety of acute lung injury can result in reactive atypia in regenerating pneumocytes. The lining cells are markedly enlarged with vacuolated cytoplasm and prominent nucleoli. In addition, there is inflammation in the thickened alveolar septa.

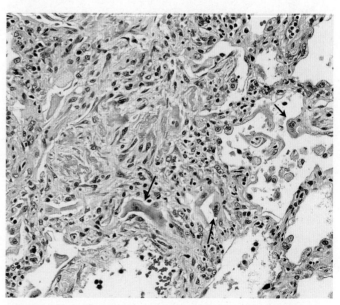

FIGURE 6.3 ▲ Organizing acute alveolar injury, acute interstitial pneumonia. At this phase, there is loose interstitial fibrosis admixed with fibrin. Some markedly atypical pneumocytes remain (arrows).

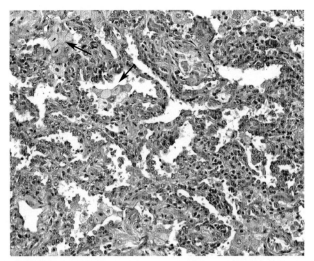

FIGURE 6.4 ▲ Organizing lung injury, localized, with diffuse pneumocyte hyperplasia. The area was adjacent to organizing pneumonia and empyema. In addition to diffuse interstitial thickening with regenerating pneumocytes, there are focal foam cell macrophages indicative of a degree of obstruction (*arrows*).

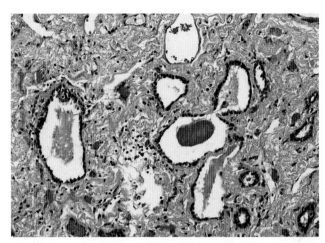

FIGURE 6.7 ▲ Reactive pneumocyte hyperplasia, in area of radiation fibrosis. In this example, the pneumocytes form acinar structures in a background of dense scar. An absence of atypia excludes acinar adenocarcinoma, and evaluation in the context with the entire specimen is helpful, as the remaining tissue demonstrated diffuse interstitial fibrosis.

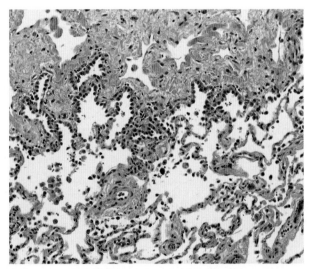

FIGURE 6.5 ▲ Paraseptal pneumocyte hyperplasia. Reactive pneumocytes are common adjacent to areas of fibrosis in the pleura or, in this case, the interlobular septum.

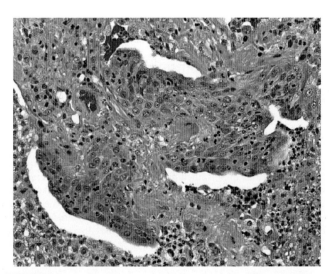

FIGURE 6.8 ▲ Squamous metaplasia, organizing diffuse alveolar damage. There are multiple foci of squamous metaplasia within organizing fibrin exudate.

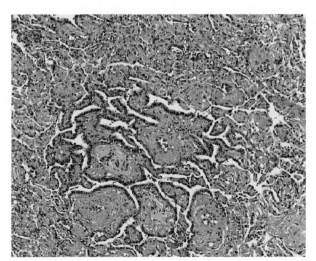

FIGURE 6.6 ▲ Peribronchiolar metaplasia with diffuse pneumocyte hyperplasia. In areas of scarring around destroyed airways, the regenerating pneumocytes may extend into the surrounding lung. In contrast to atypical adenomatous hyperplasia, the alveolar architecture is lost.

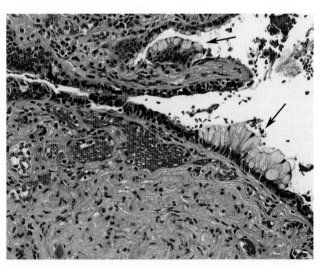

FIGURE 6.9 ▲ Mucinous metaplasia. Another area demonstrates hyperplastic and stratified mucus cells (*arrows*), which produce an abundance of mucus, which may spill into surrounding airspaces.

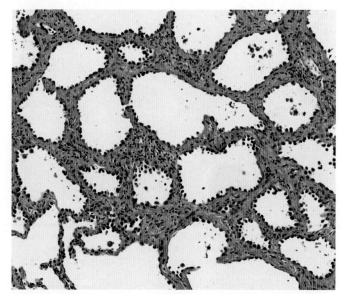

FIGURE 6.10 ▲ Atypical adenomatous hyperplasia. There is uniform thickening of alveolar septa and uniformly crowded cuboidal pneumocytes with minimal atypia.

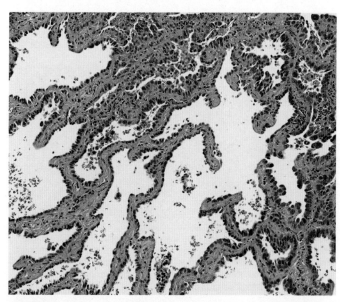

FIGURE 6.11 ▲ Adenocarcinoma in situ. The degree of crowding and atypia exceeds that seen in the previous slide. The changes can be similar to reactive hyperplasia. It is helpful to evaluate the adjacent findings; in this case, the AIS merged with areas of invasive acinar adenocarcinoma.

Cystic Honeycombing

A hallmark feature of a honeycomb cyst is the variable lining, alternating from reactive pneumocytes to respiratory or squamous lining to denuded airways with fibroblast foci.

Pulmonary Interstitial Emphysema

Increased air pressure results in subcutaneous emphysema or pneumatosis in various organs, including the lung parenchyma. Tracking of air within the parenchyma is termed pulmonary interstitial emphysema, a term usually used in the context of infants on mechanical ventilation, or paraseptal emphysema. Macrophage giant cells often line air within the interstitium. In adults, interstitial or paraseptal emphysema may be seen in interstitial lung disease and patients on mechanical ventilation.

Neoplastic Nonmucinous Pneumocyte Proliferations

Atypical adenomatous hyperplasia and adenocarcinoma in situ may be difficult to separate from reactive conditions on purely histologic grounds (Figs. 6.10 and 6.11). In general, the alveolar septa are uniform and mildly thickened with AAH, and the lesion is relatively circumscribed, corresponding to a ground-glass nodule on CT imaging.

7 Patterns of Airway Injury

Allen P. Burke, M.D., and Haresh Mani, M.D.

Bronchiolocentric Inflammation

On low magnification, bronchiolocentric inflammation is identified by inflammation around small airways with or without reactive lymphoid hyperplasia, granulomas, or fibrosis (Figs. 7.1 and 7.2). A variety of insults involve the airways, including infections (especially bacterial and viral pneumonias), drug reactions, allo- and autoimmune lung injury, hypersensitivity pneumonitis, and inhalational injury. Inflammation can be primarily neutrophilic in bacterial infections (Fig. 7.3) or eosinophilic in drug reaction (Fig. 7.4). Various types of bronchiolitis are discussed in Chapter 39.

Constrictive Bronchiolitis

Inflammation of the bronchiole that progresses to mucosal denudation, fibrosis, and obliteration of the airway is termed constrictive bronchiolitis. Constrictive bronchiolitis surrounds, rather than fills, the lumen, resulting in extrinsic compression of the airway. It is most frequently related to inhalational injury, autoimmune connective tissue diseases, and alloimmune disease (termed "obliterative bronchiolitis" in allografts and "bronchiolitis obliterans syndrome" in bone marrow transplant patients). Histologically, the process progresses in phases from destructive bronchiolar inflammation, predominantly T-cell mediated, to peribronchiolar fibrosis with or without peribronchiolar metaplasia, followed by obliteration and scarring of bronchioles (Figs. 7.5 to 7.7). In the final phase, airways may be difficult to discern, having been replaced by nodules of scar and smooth muscle adjacent to the pulmonary artery branch.

Bronchiectasis

Dilatation of the major airways, or bronchiectasis, is more common than distal dilatation (bronchiolectasis). There are two major pathways to bronchiectasis - inflammatory and noninflammatory. Chronic infections may damage the airway wall, usually at the level of the bronchus, resulting in a massively dilated structure (Fig. 7.8). Recurrent pneumonias in patients with cystic fibrosis make

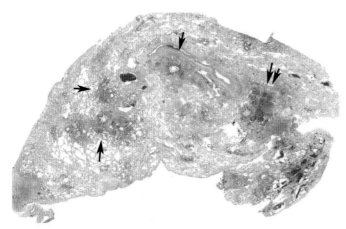

FIGURE 7.1 ▲ Bronchiolocentric inflammation. In this example, there is more extensive fibrosis and inflammation around airways (*arrows*), with focal lymphoid nodules (*double arrows*).

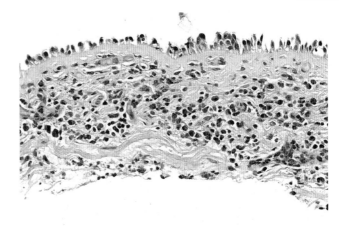

FIGURE 7.4 ▲ Eosinophilic bronchiolitis. The biopsy shows intense eosinophilic inflammation in the mucosa under the lamina propria. The patient had a reaction to an antibiotic, which resolved after cessation.

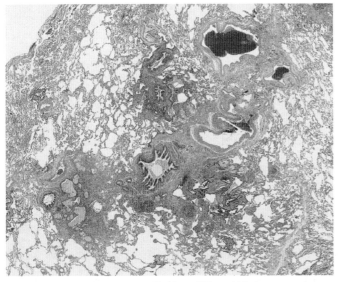

FIGURE 7.2 ▲ A higher magnification of Figure 7.1 shows scarring, inflammation around airways with peribronchiolar metaplasia, and mucus in surrounding alveoli. The patient had a long history of war-related inhalational exposure.

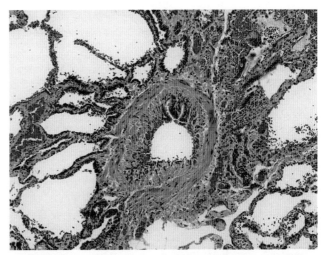

FIGURE 7.5 ▲ Constrictive bronchiolitis with peribronchiolar metaplasia. There is focal denuding of the bronchiole, peribronchiolar fibrosis, and peribronchiolar metaplasia in the surrounding alveoli. The patient had Sjögren syndrome and obstructive lung disease. Other connective tissue disease associated with constrictive bronchiolitis include rheumatoid arthritis, scleroderma, lupus erythematosus, inflammatory myositis syndrome, and mixed connective tissue disease.

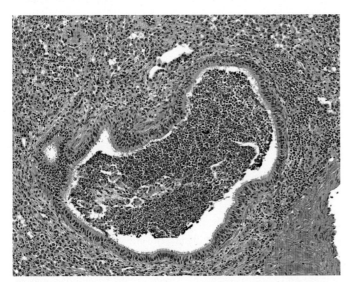

FIGURE 7.3 ▲ Acute bronchiolitis. The patient sustained thoracic trauma in a motor vehicle accident and had recurrent pneumonias and empyema.

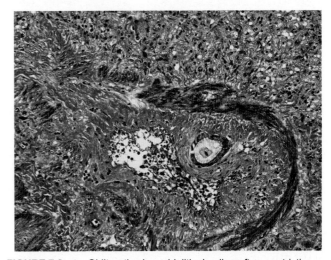

FIGURE 7.6 ▲ Obliterative bronchiolitis. In allografts, constrictive bronchiolitis is termed "obliterative bronchiolitis" and has similar histologic features as in autoimmune, alloimmune, or drug-induced disease. Masson trichrome stain shows marked fibrosis within the muscularis, obliterating the lumen.

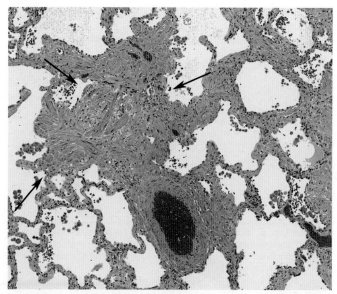

FIGURE 7.7 ▲ Constrictive bronchiolitis with airway destruction. The specimen was a lung explanted for scleroderma-related lung disease, which included restrictive lung disease as well as obstructive changes with mosaic attenuation on CT scan. Many airways were obliterated and replaced by smooth muscle cell nodules (*arrows*). The artery is seen at the bottom.

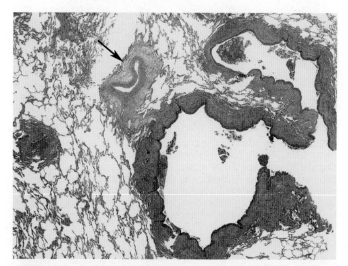

FIGURE 7.8 ▲ Bronchiectasis. There is a markedly dilated, inflamed airway. Note the difference in size compared to the artery in the same bronchovascular bundle (*arrow*).

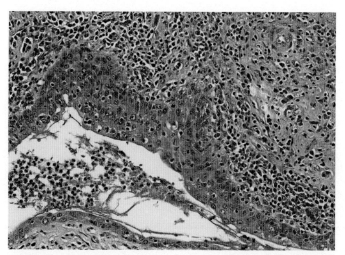

FIGURE 7.9 ▲ Chronic bronchitis with squamous metaplasia. Squamous metaplasia is common in the airways of smokers as well as patients with recurrent bronchitis.

them especially prone to the development of bronchiectasis (see Chapter 34).

Chronic irritation to the mucosa may result in squamous metaplasia (Fig. 7.9), whether from recurrent pneumonias or smoking-related irritation. Noninflammatory bronchiectasis is called "traction bronchiectasis" by radiologists, and is caused by the extrinsic pressure on the airways by surrounding fibrosis. It is common in fibrosing interstitial pneumonias, especially usual and nonspecific interstitial pneumonias, but may be seen in sarcoidosis, radiation fibrosis, as well as other fibrosing lung diseases. Histologically, the airway is intact but is much larger than normal and may extend to the pleural surface.

Peribronchiolar Metaplasia

Peribronchiolar metaplasia refers to extension of respiratory mucosa in alveolar airspaces around a bronchiole. Typically, there is some inflammatory destruction of the bronchiole. It is not specific for primary airway-related diseases and has been described in interstitial fibrosis and chronic obstructive lung disease as well. Occasionally it is the dominant finding in small airway disease, and is associated with autoimmune connective tissue disease and smoking.[1] In small biopsies and on frozen sections, extensive peribronchiolar metaplasia should not be mistaken for a well-differentiated adenocarcinoma. Unlike in adenocarcinomas, the lining cells in peribronchiolar metaplasia are ciliated.

REFERENCE

1. Fukuoka J, et al. Peribronchiolar metaplasia: a common histologic lesion in diffuse lung disease and a rare cause of interstitial lung disease: clinicopathologic features of 15 cases. *Am J Surg Pathol*. 2005;29(7):948–954.

8 Pathologic Changes in Pulmonary Vessels

Allen P. Burke, M.D., and Joseph J. Maleszewski, M.D.

Arterial Changes, Elastic Pulmonary Arteries

Thromboembolism

Thrombus within the central pulmonary arteries is typically related to embolic phenomena and is most frequently seen at autopsy.

Recurrent pulmonary embolism (chronic thromboembolic pulmonary disease) may cause "narrowing" of the pulmonary trunk and main pulmonary arteries and sometimes requires endarterectomy and surgical excision. Rarely, in situ thrombosis may be present due to atherosclerosis, vasculitis, or a pulmonary artery malignancy.

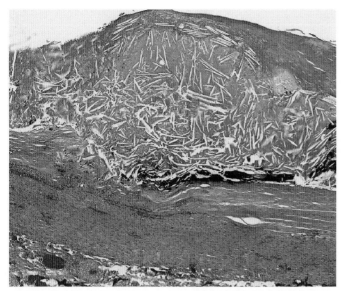

FIGURE 8.1 ▲ Chronic thromboembolic disease with superimposed atherosclerosis, pulmonary artery. Atheroma formation occurs only in long-standing pulmonary hypertension in the proximal pulmonary arterial circulation.

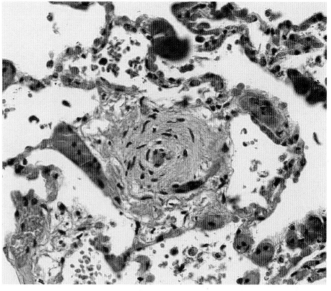

FIGURE 8.3 ▲ Muscularization of pulmonary arteriole. This is a hallmark of persistent pulmonary hypertension of the newborn but may also occur in severe pulmonary hypertension in adults.

Atherosclerosis

The pulmonary circulation is resistant to the development of atherosclerosis, probably secondary to the different pressures and hemodynamics when compared to the systemic circuit. The exception to this rule occurs in patients with pulmonary arterial hypertension (PAH), who may develop typical features of atherosclerosis, including lipid-rich atheromas (Fig. 8.1). Typically, there is associated dilatation of the pulmonary artery in addition to atheroma in the setting of pulmonary arterial hypertension. There will invariably be other long-standing changes of pulmonary hypertension, including right ventricular hypertrophy and other findings of cor pulmonale. Pulmonary arterial atherosclerosis is essentially a diagnosis made at autopsy.

Arteritis

Vasculitis of the main pulmonary arteries is rare. Takayasu disease may involve the proximal pulmonary circulation, although much less frequently than the aorta. The histologic findings are similar to that seen in the aorta and its branches. Typically, this includes a granulomatous

medial infiltrate, with intimal and adventitial fibrosis. Necrotizing arteritis may rarely occur in patients with Behçet disease (Fig. 8.2).

Pulmonary Arterial Dissection

Spontaneous dissection of the proximal pulmonary arteries is a rare complication of severe, chronic arterial pulmonary hypertension of any cause. The main pulmonary artery is usually the site of involvement, and extension to the branch arteries is uncommon. Rare reports of dissection occurring as a complication of aneurysm formation (caused by infection, trauma, or connective tissue diseases) have been reported. Rupture of the dissection may occur, leading to hemopericardium and/or tamponade.

Arterial Changes, Muscular Pulmonary Arteries

Muscularization of Arterioles

Muscularization of arterioles, proximal to the alveolar capillary bed, is a feature of persistent pulmonary hypertension of the newborn (Fig. 8.3) (see Chapter 13).

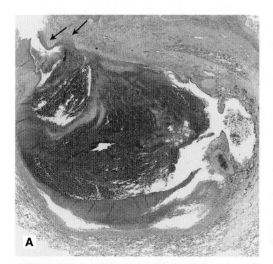

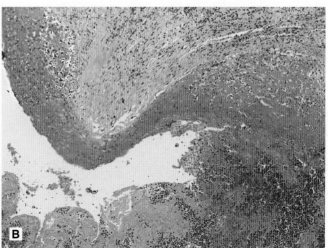

FIGURE 8.2 ▲ Behçet disease and necrotizing pulmonary arteries. **A.** The pulmonary artery demonstrated fibrinoid necrosis (*arrows*), which resulted in a pseudoaneurysm that ruptured into the mainstem bronchus (*right*) causing massive hemoptysis. **B.** A higher magnification of the artery with fibrinoid necrosis.

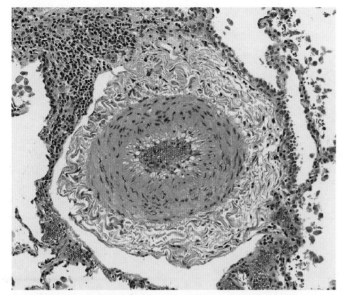

FIGURE 8.4 ▲ Medial hypertrophy. The smooth muscle of the media is markedly thickened, without significant intimal changes.

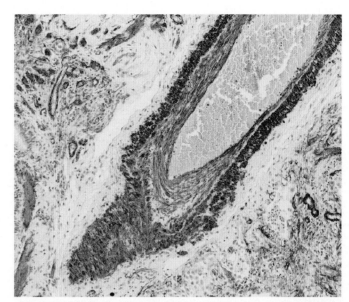

FIGURE 8.6 ▲ Intimal thickening, actin immunohistochemical stain. The intima is rich in smooth muscle cells.

Medial Hypertrophy

Medial hypertrophy of pulmonary arteries is defined as a medial thickness >10% of the diameter (or 20% if both sides are measured) (Fig. 8.4). Medial hypertrophy is nonspecific and may be present in pre- and postcapillary causes of pulmonary hypertension. Thickened small muscular arterial branches may occur in the periphery, especially as a reaction to interstitial lung process, and are not necessarily reflective of increased arterial pressures.

Intimal Thickening

The normal arterial intima is composed of endothelial cells overlying a basement membrane above the internal elastic membrane, with a few myofibroblasts. Therefore, it is normally barely discernable histologically. Intimal thickening occurs in pulmonary hypertension, as part of thrombosis or as a reaction to surrounding lung injury (Figs. 8.5 and 8.6).

Intimal thickening with scattered myofibroblasts is generally reactive or secondary to thrombosis. The presence of intimal thickening has been noted frequently in patients with interstitial lung disease. Eccentric intimal thickening is in this category and is generally ascribed to thrombosis. (Eccentric thickening is often defined as significant thickening of one part of the vessel wall, with an arc of artery without intimal change or with thickening less than the medial thickness.)

Concentric elastotic intimal thickening, akin to onion skinning as seen in renal vessels, is indicative of irreversible pulmonary hypertension and is invariably associated with plexiform lesions.

Thromboembolism

In contrast to more proximal vessels, thrombosis in small muscular arteries may be due to in situ thrombosis as often as embolism. Hypercoagulable states, especially antiphospholipid syndrome, may predispose to diffuse thrombosis of the pulmonary vessels. The histologic findings may show acute platelet-rich thrombi (Fig. 8.7), healing fibrin-rich thrombi (Fig. 8.8), or predominantly healed, recanalized thrombi (Fig. 8.9).

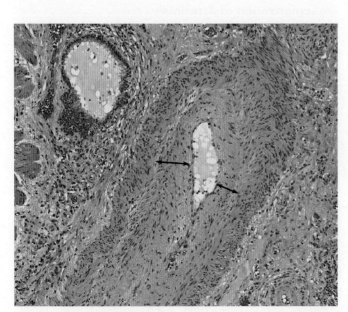

FIGURE 8.5 ▲ Intimal thickening. In this case, the intima (*arrows*) was thickened by smooth muscle cells. The patient had mitral stenosis and secondary venous hypertension, which may also cause changes in the arterial circulation.

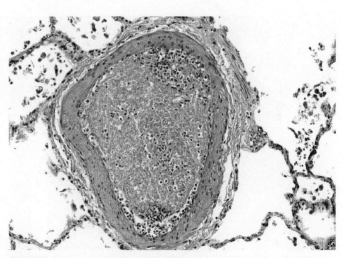

FIGURE 8.7 ▲ Acute thrombus. The artery is filled primarily with platelets. The patient had antiphospholipid syndrome and died with multiple arterial thrombi in various organs.

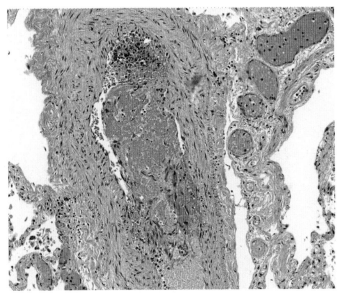

FIGURE 8.8 ▲ Acute and organizing thrombus. The thrombus is primarily made of fibrin, with organization indicated by endothelial cells in and around the thrombus.

Plexiform Arteriopathy

Plexiform arteriopathy denotes the presence of peculiar "glomeruloid" lesions in small muscular branch arteries (Fig. 8.10). These lesions are present in primary pulmonary arterial hypertension as well as some secondary forms of pulmonary arterial hypertension, such as long-standing left-to-right shunts, portal hypertension, connective tissue diseases, human immunodeficiency virus, and certain drugs and toxins. In many cases of primary pulmonary arterial hypertension, the proximal pulmonary arteries show secondary findings of intimal thickening and muscular hypertrophy or may be relatively normal.

Arteritis

Arteritis of muscular pulmonary arteries occurs in two settings. In primary pulmonary hypertension, arteritis can be found in ~25% of cases and is thought to be a precursor lesion of plexiform arteriopathy. Muscular arteritis may also be present in granulomatosis with

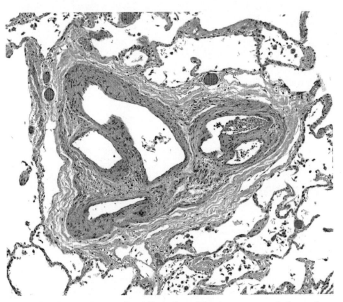

FIGURE 8.9 ▲ Recanalized thrombus. There are several channels, each with a smooth muscle media, within the larger artery.

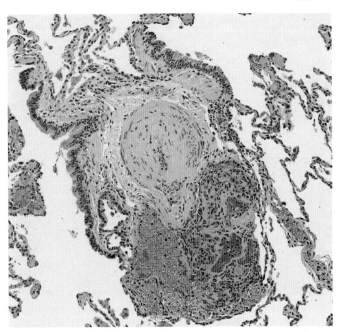

FIGURE 8.10 ▲ Plexiform lesion. This lesion occurs primarily in severe primary pulmonary hypertension, or long-standing intracardiac shunts. The plexiform lesion branches from small muscular arteries 50 to 100 μm in diameter, which are accompanied by bronchioles. The artery above the plexiform lesion shows marked intimal thickening. The airway is also evident. There are dilated capillaries around the lesion, which is a frequent finding "dilatation lesion."

polyangiitis (Wegener granulomatosis), although the necrotizing granulomatous inflammation is the dominant clinical finding, along with small vessel vasculitis (capillaritis). Necrotizing arteritis with fibrinoid necrosis typical of polyarteritis nodosa rarely occurs in the lung.

Capillary Changes

Capillaritis

Neutrophilic inflammation of the pulmonary capillaries is caused by either immune-mediated mechanisms marked by complement and immunoglobulin deposition or pauci-immune inflammation mediated by antineutrophil cytoplasmic autoantibodies (ANCA). Capillaritis-like changes may also be seen early in pulmonary infarcts and in patients with alloimmune vascular injury (antibody-mediated rejection). Histologically, there is intra-alveolar hemorrhage, marked by red blood cells and hemosiderin-laden macrophages, and interstitial neutrophils. If no alveolar hemorrhage is noted, other causes of capillaritis should be considered. Occasionally, neutrophils can be present in the alveolar spaces as well, with a paucity of fibrin, in contrast to bacterial pneumonia.

Capillary Hemangiomatosis

Capillary hemangiomatosis is an exceptionally rare condition marked by proliferation of capillaries in the alveolar septa. It is a relatively uncommon form of pulmonary hypertension. Elastic stains may show layers of capillaries on both sides of the alveolar wall. On low magnification, there is patchy hemorrhage.

Miscellaneous

Fat embolism may result in diffuse dilatation of capillaries in the alveolar septa. Fat embolism should be distinguished from bone marrow embolism that occurs in larger vessels (typically small muscular arteries), the latter demonstrating trilineage hematopoiesis. Megakaryocytes are a frequent finding in autopsies and wedge biopsies of the lung, especially in patients who are septic.

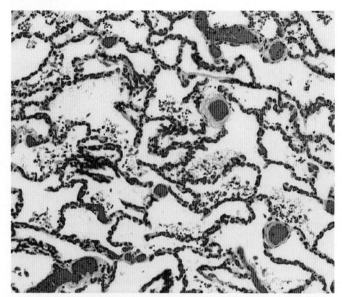

FIGURE 8.11 ▲ Passive congestion. At autopsy, the dependent portions of the lung show capillaries and small vessels distended with red cells. The finding is not pathologic.

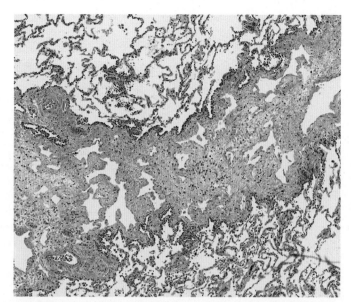

FIGURE 8.12 ▲ Lymphatic dilatation, secondary to obstruction. The lobular septum is thickened with prominent dilated lymphatic dilatation. The underlying process was arteriovenous malformation.

Venous Changes

Pulmonary Venous Hypertensive Changes

Dependent congestion in autopsy lungs results in capillaries distended with erythrocytes (Fig. 8.11). The most common venous changes encountered in wedge biopsies and autopsies are those of chronic outflow obstruction, which is most often caused by left-sided heart disease (e.g., mitral valve stenosis). The changes of chronic pulmonary congestion include edema, fibrosis, and thickening of the interlobular septa (where the pulmonary veins reside) (Fig. 8.12). The veins will show increased elastic tissue and variable intimal thickening (Fig. 8.13). In addition, there are frequently scattered intra-alveolar hemosiderin-laden macrophages consistent with occult microhemorrhages as a result of increased capillary pressures.

Pulmonary Venoocclusive Disease

Pulmonary venoocclusive disease is a rare cause of pulmonary hypertension, manifest by primary obstruction of pulmonary outflow within the pulmonary veins. The intimal damage to the veins results in thrombosis and recanalization, with secondary septal fibrosis. Recanalized thrombi within pulmonary veins are considered pathognomonic (see Chapter 66).

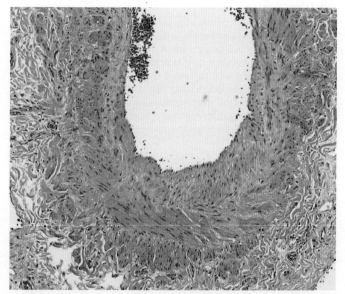

FIGURE 8.13 ▲ Venous hypertrophy. The wall of the vein is thickened, with mild fibrosis near the luminal surface.

9 Approach to the Diagnosis of Nonneoplastic Parenchymal Lung Nodules

Allen P. Burke, M.D., Marie-Christine Aubry, M.D., and Haresh Mani, M.D.

Poorly Formed Granulomas

Granulomas in the lung parenchyma are generally classified as poorly or well formed. Poorly formed granulomas are a hallmark of hypersensitivity to inhaled allergens. They are indistinct collections of lymphocytes with macrophages, typically giant cells. Poorly formed granulomas are generally near the bronchovascular bundles and are often associated with interstitial inflammation (Fig. 9.1).

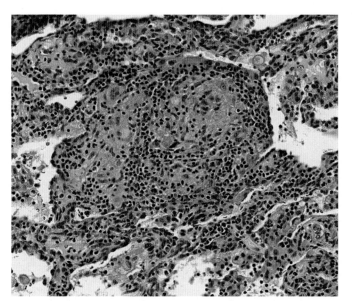

FIGURE 9.1 ▲ Poorly formed granuloma. The interstitium contains chronic inflammation with granulomatous inflammation in the center (epithelioid macrophages with a few giant cells).

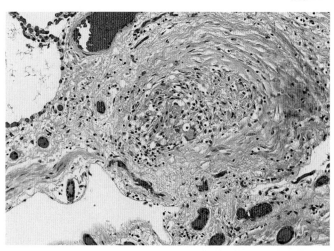

FIGURE 9.2 ▲ Well-formed granuloma, sarcoid. There is a discrete collection of macrophages and lymphocytes. The surrounding fibrosis favors sarcoid over infection but is nonspecific.

Well-Formed Granulomas

Well-formed granulomas are found in sarcoid or infections, usually fungal or mycobacterial. sarcoid and infections (Table 9.1). There is a compact collection of epithelioid histiocytes with a discrete border

(Fig. 9.2) and a subpopulation of T lymphocytes. Sarcoid granulomas are found in a lymphatic distribution in the bronchovascular bundles, interlobular septa, and subpleural space. Fibrosis is a characteristic of sarcoid granulomas (Fig. 9.3). Infectious granulomas are, in contrast, asymmetric and occur randomly in the parenchyma. Further, presence of significant lymphoplasmacytic inflammation favors an infectious etiology. Well-formed granulomas of any cause, but especially sarcoid, may contain mineral deposits (Schaumann bodies), which should not

TABLE 9.1   Histologic Features of Pulmonary Granulomas

Diagnosis	Necrosis	Multiplicity	Contour	Lymphatic Distribution	Neutrophils	Multinucleated Macrophages	Necrotizing Vasculitis	Distinguishing Features
Sarcoidosis	10%–20%[a]	100%	Regular (100%)	70%–100%	Absent	100%	Absent	Diffuse, symmetric
Mycobacterial infection[b]	75%	90%	Regular (2/3)	20%	80%	100%	Absent	Positive AFB stain (about 50%)
Histoplasmosis	>90%	75%	Regular (80%)	<5%	50%	80%–90%	Absent	Positive GMS stain (>90%, but requires careful review)
Coccidioidomycosis	>90%	80%	Regular (90%)	<5%	90% also, frequent eosinophils	90%	Absent	Positive GMS stain (>90%)
Blastomycosis	>90%	80%	Irregular (75%)	<5%	100%	50%–80%	Absent	Positive GMS stain (>90%)
Talc granulomas	Absent	100%	Regular	Absent	Infrequent	100%	Absent	Birefringent crystals
Granulomatosis with polyangiitis	100%	>90%	Irregular (100%)	0	100% (usually with apoptosis)	60%	20%–50%	Apoptotic neutrophils causing basophilic necrosis
Idiopathic (unexplained)	>95%; abundant in 75%[c]	80%	Regular (60%)	<20%	50%	80%	Absent	Are presumed infections; some will demonstrate NTM DNA by PCR
Rheumatoid nodule	100%	60%	Irregular (60%)	0	80%	100%	Absent	History and serology
Hyalinizing granuloma	Absent	50%	Regular	Absent	Absent	Absent	Absent	IgG4-related histologic features

Percentages are approximate. For further histologic features distinguishing fungal infections, see Chapter 41 and 44.
[a]Necrosis in sarcoid is usually inconspicuous and central in the granuloma.
[b]Nontuberculous (atypical) mycobacterial granulomas are more frequently encountered as lung nodules than tuberculosis. Histologic features are different in infections in immunocompromised patients, and discrete nodules are not as common (see Chapter 40).
[c]Idiopathic nonnecrotizing granulomatous disease is synonymous with sarcoidosis and is typically bilateral and symmetric. Solitary idiopathic necrotizing granulomas are common. Well-formed granulomas that do not have necrosis and that form solitary lung nodules are rare.
NTM, nontuberculous mycobacteria; PCR, polymerase chain reaction.
Adapted in part from Mukhopadhyay S, Wilcox BE, Myers JL, et al. Pulmonary necrotizing granulomas of unknown cause: clinical and pathologic analysis of 131 patients with completely resected nodules. *Chest.* 2013;144:813–824.

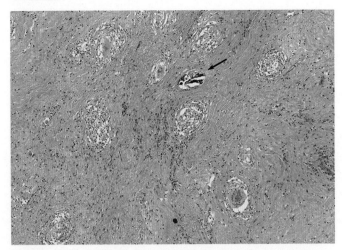

FIGURE 9.3 ▲ Granulomas with scarring, sarcoid. In the fibrotic phase of sarcoid, the granulomas are embedded in fibrosis, a finding very atypical for infection. There may be mineralization in sarcoid or other types of granulomas (Schaumann body, *arrow*).

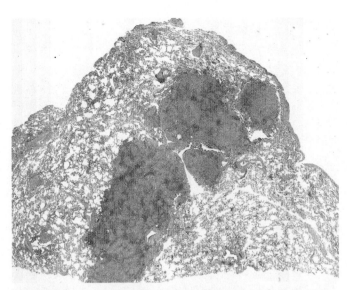

FIGURE 9.5 ▲ Necrotizing granuloma. Necrotizing infectious granulomas are random, without a lymphatic or peribronchiolar distribution. This case represented histoplasmosis.

be mistaken for pneumoconiosis (Fig. 9.3). Asteroid bodies are also nonspecific features of well-formed granulomas (Fig. 9.4).

Necrotizing Granulomas

Necrosis is a common feature of well-formed granulomas and is suggestive of an infectious process (Figs. 9.5 and 9.6). Special stains for mycobacteria and fungi should be performed on all well-formed granulomas, regardless of the presence of necrosis. Conversely, sarcoid granulomas may occasionally undergo central necrosis.

There are variants of granulomatous nodules with central necrosis that typically occur in rheumatologic conditions. Rheumatoid nodules are areas of necrosis with a macrophage infiltrate, often with peripheral palisading. The necrosis in rheumatoid nodules is typically amphophilic (Fig. 9.7). Necrotizing granulomatous nodules of Wegener granulomatosis (granulomatosis with polyangiitis) have basophilic zones of necrosis (due to the presence of karyorrhectic debris) often surrounded by neutrophils and neutrophilic microabscesses (Fig. 9.8).[1,2]

Hyalinizing Granuloma

Hyalinizing granulomas are rare discrete parenchymal nodules with a similar histologic appearance as sclerosing mediastinitis (Fig. 9.9). The name is a misnomer, since granulomas are not a feature. They may be single or multiple and may measure up to 10 cm in size. The histologic features of hyalinizing granulomas are those of IgG4-related sclerosing conditions. There are collagenous bands in a storiform or lamellar pattern, in an inflammatory background that surrounds lymph nodes, nerves, and vessels, with inflammatory destruction of veins. Inflammation may be sparse and manifest only at the periphery of the nodules. There may be an association between hyalinizing granuloma and elevated serum levels of autoantibodies against antinuclear antigens, and serum IgG4.[3,4]

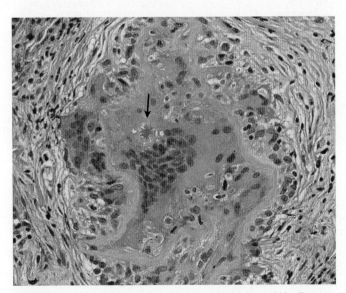

FIGURE 9.4 ▲ Well-formed granuloma, sarcoid. Asteroid bodies are nonspecific, but a not uncommon finding in sarcoid.

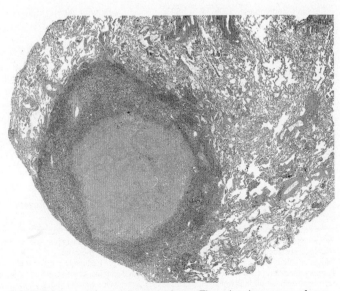

FIGURE 9.6 ▲ Necrotizing granuloma. There is a large area of central necrosis. Although suggestive of an infectious etiology, all cultures were negative.

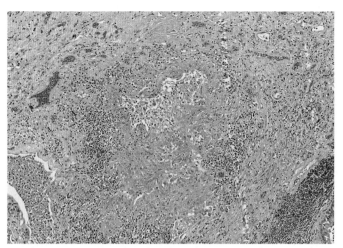

FIGURE 9.7 ▲ Rheumatoid nodule. Necrobiotic nodules may occur in the lung parenchyma in patients with autoimmune connective tissue diseases, especially rheumatoid arthritis. The histologic features are nondescript; in this case, there was no peripheral palisading as is frequently seen.

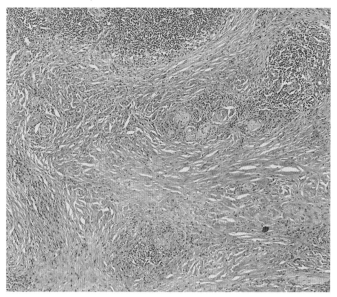

FIGURE 9.9 ▲ Hyalinizing granuloma. There is storiform dense fibrosis surrounding vessels typical of sclerosing IgG4-related disease.

Focal Scars and Smooth Muscle Cell Nodules

Patchy interstitial scars may occur in the setting of interstitial lung disease, normal lungs, and emphysema. In smoking-related lung disease, the diagnosis of pulmonary Langerhans cell histiocytosis (PLCH) should be considered, especially if there is adjacent cystic change (Fig. 9.10A) and the shape of the scar is *stellate* or cicatricial. Sometimes, the nodule is composed primarily of smooth muscle cells. In such cases, an obliterated bronchiole secondary to small airway disease should be considered (Fig. 9.10B). However, it is important to note that focal fibrosis can occur in normal lungs and may have no identifiable etiology.

Organizing Pneumonia

Organizing pneumonia is often mistaken for a neoplasm on imaging. In contrast to dense scars, loose intraalveolar fibromyxoid plugs is

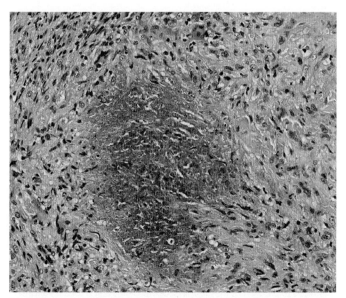

FIGURE 9.8 ▲ Necrotizing nodule of Wegener granulomatosis. Basophilic necrosis is typical Wegener granulomatosis (granulomatosis with polyangiitis), due to apoptotic death of collections of neutrophils.

characteristic in a subacute phase of lung injury, which, when discrete, is termed "organizing pneumonia." There are numerous causes, including infections, auto- and alloimmunity, hypersensitivity, and drugs. Occasionally, the main finding in an excision for a solitary lung nodule is organizing pneumonia. The histologic hallmark is that of discrete nodules of fibroblasts (Masson bodies) in a proteoglycan matrix. If the lesion is polypoid and extending into a bronchiolar lumen, the appearance may be more that of granulation tissue. An organizing pneumonia reaction can be seen in other conditions, such as Wegener granulomatosis, pneumoconiosis, and inflammatory pseudotumors. Presence of organizing pneumonia in a small biopsy does not exclude a neoplasm, since the organization may be a secondary reaction to adjacent tumor.

Inflammatory Pseudotumor

There are several related terms for lung nodules that are composed of variable amounts of mixed chronic inflammation and fibroblasts. Plasma cell granuloma denotes a lesion that is predominantly inflammatory, and inflammatory myofibroblastic tumor denotes one that is composed more of spindled cells. These tumors are most frequent in children and young adults and may be bronchiolocentric. There is an association with systemic inflammation[5] and IgG4-related disease.[6] Low-grade lymphomas also need exclusion.

Histologically, inflammatory myofibroblastic tumors (pseudotumors) are inflammatory masses, often with entrapped TTF-1–positive pneumocyte rests. In contrast to organizing pneumonia, the fibroblastic reaction is cellular, without background matrix, and does not form small discrete nodules. However, areas of organizing pneumonia are not uncommon at the periphery of inflammatory pseudotumors.

Nodular Lymphoid Hyperplasia

Diffuse hyperplasia of bronchial-associated lymphoid tissue (BALT) is a feature of immunodeficiency syndromes and is part of the spectrum of lymphocytic bronchiolitis. Occasionally, reactive lymphoid hyperplasia can cause a discrete lesion in the lung, mimicking a neoplasm clinically. Histologically, there may be multiple areas of lymphoid hyperplasia with germinal centers (Figs. 9.11 and 9.12). Unlike in marginal zone lymphoma, nodular lymphoid hyperplasia lacks Dutcher bodies and lymphoepithelial lesions. However, the distinction between localized marginal zone lymphoma and reactive hyperplasia is difficult and may require clonality and cytogenetic studies for differentiation.

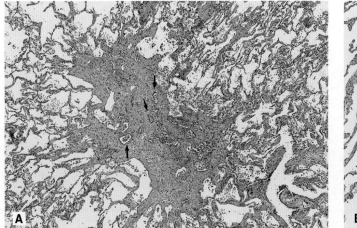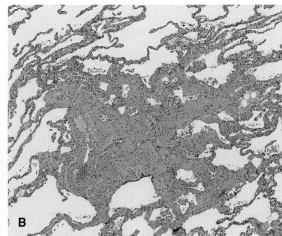

FIGURE 9.10 ▲ Focal scar. **A.** In a variety of background processes, there may be occasional areas of fibrosis with a spiculated, scarring mimicking malignancy. "Stellate" scars are typical of pulmonary Langerhans cell histiocytosis, although in this case, immunohistochemical stains were negative for CD1a and S100 protein. There are scattered entrapped tubular pneumocyte inclusions (*arrows*), which are common in inflammatory and mesenchymal proliferations of the lung. **B.** Focal scar, smooth muscle cell rich. Nodules of smooth muscle cells may be found in interstitial lung diseases or otherwise normal lungs. In some cases, the causes are not known. End stages of constrictive bronchiolitis may occasionally appear as smooth muscle cell scars.

Intrapulmonary lymph nodes are usually subpleural in location and are usually seen in middle-aged or older patients with a history of cigarette smoking or organic dust exposure. They typically border on the pleura or interlobular septa and lack a capsule. There are often only primary follicles without germinal centers, although the latter may be seen. Histiocytes containing dust pigment and birefringent silica particles are often prominent, and many lesions contain hyalinized silicotic nodules and ectatic lymphatics, suggesting that these "lymph nodes" develop secondary to lymphatic obstruction by organic dust.

Rounded Atelectasis

Rounded (or round) atelectasis represents prominent folding of the pleura with invagination into the underlying lung. Most cases are incidental findings on chest x-ray or CT scans, which show pleural-based masses, most frequently the posterior surface of the lower lobe, often with a "comet tail" sign. The cause is unknown but may be related to organizing pleural effusion or inflammatory process. The pleural fibrosis is superficial to the elastic layer of the pleura, which shows wrinkling and infolding (Fig. 9.13). Following excision, the mass may "disappear" due to release of the entrapped lobule, and careful sampling of thickened pleura and interlobular septa is required to establish a diagnosis.

Apical Cap

Apical caps are nearly ubiquitous, especially in advanced age, and result from pleural fibroelastosis with minimal extension in to the parenchyma. Extensive elastosis with parenchymal involvement is sometimes called pleuroparenchymal fibroelastosis.

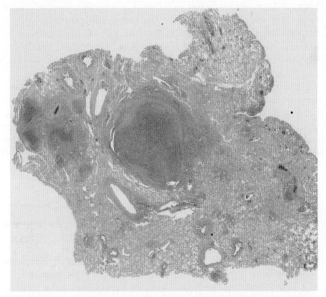

FIGURE 9.11 ▲ Nodular lymphoid hyperplasia. Tumor-like masses may result from marked bronchial-associated lymphoid hyperplasia. In this case, there were several nodules, with one dominant mass.

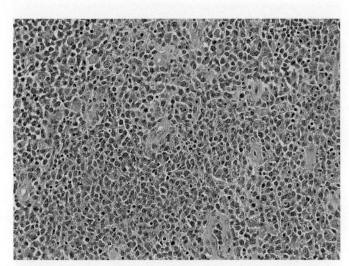

FIGURE 9.12 ▲ A higher magnification of the previous figure demonstrates expansion of the germinal center. Although a localized form of marginal zone lymphoma was suspected, it could not be confirmed. In any event, localized marginal zone lymphomas of the lung have an excellent prognosis.

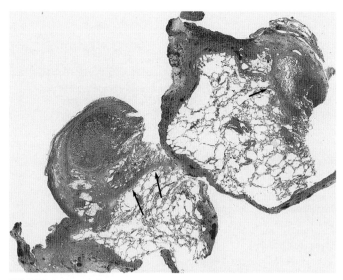

FIGURE 9.13 ▲ Rounded atelectasis. There is pleural fibrosis with septal fibrous bands extending into the parenchyma (*arrows*) giving a rounded appearance.

Amyloidosis

Pulmonary amyloidosis may be either localized to the lung or may be secondary to systemic amyloidosis. Nodular amyloidosis is a rare cause of pulmonary nodule (see Chapter 30).

REFERENCES

1. Mukhopadhyay S, Wilcox BE, Myers JL, et al. Pulmonary necrotizing granulomas of unknown cause: clinical and pathologic analysis of 131 patients with completely resected nodules. *Chest.* 2013;144:813–824.
2. Aubry MC. Necrotizing granulomatous inflammation: what does it mean if your special stains are negative? *Mod Pathol.* 2012;25(suppl 1):S31–S38.
3. Chapman EM, Gown A, Mazziotta R, et al. Pulmonary hyalinizing granuloma with associated elevation in serum and tissue IgG4 occurring in a patient with a history of sarcoidosis. *Am J Surg Pathol.* 2012;36:774–778.
4. Schlosnagle DC, Check IJ, Sewell CW, et al. Immunologic abnormalities in two patients with pulmonary hyalinizing granuloma. *Am J Clin Pathol.* 1982;78:231–235.
5. Yi E, Aubry MC. Pulmonary pseudoneoplasms. *Arch Pathol Lab Med.* 2010;134:417–426.
6. Zen Y, Kitagawa S, Minato H, et al. IgG4-positive plasma cells in inflammatory pseudotumor (plasma cell granuloma) of the lung. *Hum Pathol.* 2005;36:710–717.

10 Pulmonary Computed Tomography

Seth Kligerman, M.D., and Allen P. Burke, M.D.

Chest CT: General Aspects

Technical Considerations

Advances in CT technology over the past few decades have let to improvements in both spatial and temporal resolution. Most modern multidetector CT (MDCT) scanners can provide isotropic voxel sizes of <1 cm, and even newer scanners can image patients with isotropic voxels of 0.5 mm. In addition, the temporal resolution of most modern MDCT scanners is <300 ms, and newer technologies allow for effective temporal resolutions as low as 66 ms.[1] This rapid temporal resolution can be paired with dual-source (two x-ray tubes) or long z-axis (256 to 320 slices) technology to allow for acquisition of the entire chest in <3 seconds and in some instances in <1 second. These advances in both spatial and temporal resolution allow for accurate assessment of both the lung parenchyma and distal airways at radiation doses <1 mSv.[2]

As the CT scanner emits photons, these particles are attenuated as they travel through the patient before reaching the detectors on the other side of the scanner. Various types of material will attenuate the beam in different ways, and these differences are manifest as grayscale images. For instance, photons easily travel through air and appear black, while metal blocks nearly all photons and will appear white. This attenuation has a scale called Hounsfield units (HU), which, although relatively standardized, can demonstrate some degree of variability depending on the scanner type, kilovoltage used, and scan image parameters such as slice thickness and kernel of reconstruction. According to the scale, water is set at 0 HU and air is set at −1,000 HU. There are no upper limits of attenuation. Fat, which attenuates fewer photons than water but more than air, has an HU around −100 HU, and soft tissue (muscle, solid organs, etc.), which attenuates more photons than water but less than bone, has an attenuation value that can range from 40 to 100 HU. Bone metal attenuates the most photons and appears relatively white.

Glossary of Selected Radiologic Terms

Nodules and Masses

The only difference between a nodule and a mass is size. A nodule is a focal opacity measuring up to 3 cm in diameter, and a mass is a lesion measuring >3 cm in diameter.[3] Nodules and masses can be rounded, lobulated, speculated, or poorly defined. Current terminology suggests the division of nodules into two main categories, solid and subsolid. Subsolid nodules can be composed of only ground-glass attenuation (Table 10.1) or be composed of both solid and ground-glass component. A nodule is a nonspecific finding and can be seen in numerous disease states ranging from inflammation to malignancy (Table 10.2). Although most nodules found on CT are benign, follow-up imaging is often necessary to assess for changes over time.

TABLE 10.1 Causes of Diffuse Ground-Glass Opacity

Acute	Subacute to Chronic
Pulmonary edema	Organizing pneumonia
Pulmonary hemorrhage	Hypersensitivity pneumonitis
Infections	Infections
Pneumocystis pneumonia	Pneumocystis pneumonia
Cytomegalovirus pneumonia	
Herpes simplex pneumonia	
Diffuse alveolar damage, exudative phase	Diffuse alveolar damage, organizing and fibrotic phases
Acute respiratory distress syndrome	
Acute interstitial pneumonia	
Acute eosinophilic pneumonia	Nonspecific interstitial pneumonia

TABLE 10.2   Differential Diagnosis of Pulmonary Nodules

Neoplasm Malignant	Neoplasm Benign	Infection	Inflammatory	Congenital
Non–small cell lung cancer Adenocarcinoma Squamous cell carcinoma Large cell carcinoma	Hamartoma Papilloma	Fungal[a] Coccidioidomycosis Cryptococcus Blastomycosis Histoplasmosis Nocardia	Intraparenchymal lymph node Mucus plugging[a] Organizing pneumonia	Intrapulmonary bronchogenic cyst Congenital pulmonary airway malformation
Small cell lung cancer	Chondroma	Bacteria Tuberculosis[a]	Focal fibrosis/scarring	Arteriovenous malformation
Carcinoid tumor Metastasis[a] Lymphoma[a] Lymphomatoid granulomatosis	Solitary fibrous tumor Lipoma Benign metastasizing leiomyoma[a]	Granuloma Round pneumonia Lung abscess	Amyloidoma Pulmonary infarct Granulomatosis with polyangiitis[a]	Sequestration Bronchial atresia with mucoid impaction
Carcinomas of salivary gland origin	Inflammatory myofibroblastic tumor	Parasitic Hydatid cyst	Rheumatoid nodule[a]	

[a]Often multiple.

Pinpointing the exact etiology of nodules or masses can be very difficult and relies on size, number, tissue composition and morphology, and distribution. Although size is not a reliable indicator of benignity, in general, the larger a nodule is, the greater the chance of malignancy.[4] Nodules measuring <4 mm in diameter have less than a 1% chance of being malignant, while nodules around 8 mm in diameter have a 10% to 20% change of being malignant.[5] In terms of likelihood ratio (LR), solitary nodules <1 cm in diameter, nodules between 1.1 and 2 cm, nodules between 2.1 and 3 cm, and masses >3 cm have an LR of malignancy of 0.52, 0.74, 3.67, and 5.23, respectively. Nonetheless, over 90% of nodules measuring <2 mm in diameter are benign.[6]

The presence of macroscopic fat in a nodule is almost always indicative of a benign tumor, most notably a hamartoma, although ~50% of hamartomas contain no visible fat on CT. In very rare instances, fat can be seen within malignant lesions, namely primary pulmonary or metastatic liposarcomas.

Most calcified nodules are benign, and there are six patterns of calcification of a pulmonary nodule, including diffuse, central, laminated, "popcorn like," amorphous, and punctate. Except for amorphous and punctate calcifications, the other patterns of calcification within a nodule or mass suggest that it is benign. Most calcified nodules seen on CT are due to prior granulomatous infection, and one usually sees numerous, small, well-defined calcified nodules. Popcorn-like calcifications can be seen in both hamartomas and amyloidomas. Amorphous or punctate calcifications have no real pattern or distribution with the nodule and appear as single or multiple flecks of calcification with a lesion. This pattern should raise the possibility of malignancy.[7]

In the case of a solid solitary pulmonary nodule with soft tissue attenuation, a smooth contour and ovoid shape are suggestive of a benign process, while a spiculated or ragged margin and a more complex, nonrounded shape suggests a malignant process (Figs. 10.1 and 10.2). However, there is significant overlap between these findings, and the presence of a smooth, ovoid nodule does not exclude the diagnosis of malignancy. Other findings suggestive of malignancy include vascular convergence, surrounding pleural retraction, and air bronchograms within a nodule. Cavitation can be seen with certain malignancies such as squamous cell carcinoma but can be seen with certain infections, vasculitis, and inflammatory conditions.[5] In general, nodules or masses with a thicker cavity wall are more likely to be malignant than those with a thinner cavitary wall.

Subsolid nodules, either pure ground-glass opacity (pGGO) nodules or mixed-solid and ground-glass opacity (mGGO) nodules, are less common than solid nodules but have a higher likelihood of being malignant. However, in non–lung cancer screening situations, short-term follow-up is important as in one study nearly 40% of pGGO and 50% of mGGO nodules resolved or significantly decreased in size on repeat CT performed 3 months later.[8] Nodules that persist on follow-up imaging have a high incidence of malignancy with one study demonstrating that 75% of persistent subsolid nodules were in the adenocarcinoma spectrum ranging from adenocarcinoma in situ (AIS) to invasive adenocarcinoma, while another 6% were atypical adenomatous hyperplasia (AAH).[9] However, persistent subsolid nodules can also represent focal areas of fibrosis or organizing pneumonia in about 20% of cases.[5]

In general, it can be difficult to differentiate between these benign and malignant etiologies. With pGGO nodules, growth over time can often be difficult to assess because of the long doubling time of AIS,

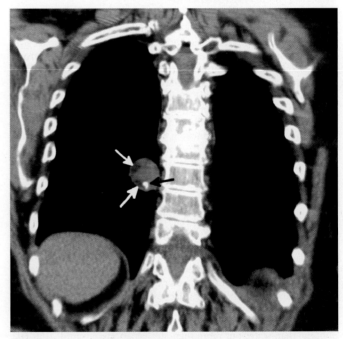

FIGURE 10.1 ▲ Imaging characteristics of a benign lung nodule. Image from a coronal CT obtained in a 69-year-old woman shows a solitary, well-rounded nodule with areas of macroscopic fat (*white arrows*) and a chunky calcification (*black arrow*). The findings are diagnostic of a pulmonary hamartoma, which is a benign nodule.

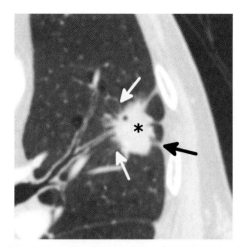

FIGURE 10.2 ▲ Imaging characteristics of a malignant nodule. Axial CT image through the lingual in a 72-year-old man with a long history of smoking shows a 2.4-cm nodule (*asterisk*). The nodule has a spiculated margin (*white arrows*) and causes mild retraction of the adjacent pleural surface (*black arrow*). Close interval follow-up CT showed no change in the lesion, which was subsequently shown to represent a squamous cell carcinoma on biopsy.

although lung cancers can occur in any lobe, they are still more common in the upper lobes, on the right greater than the left.[4,10] On the other hand, metastatic lesions, which are often multiple, are more common in the lower lobes due to increased blood flow to this area. In addition, metastases tend to be well rounded and located peripherally rather than centrally.

Ground-Glass Opacities

On CT, ground-glass opacity (GGO) occurs when there is increased lung attenuation through which the underlying airway and vessels remain visible (Fig. 10.2).[3] Ground-glass opacity itself is a nonspecific finding with numerous etiologies, and differentiation between these causes on imaging can be difficult. However, answering questions about its distribution can help to provide a differential diagnosis on imaging.

Focal or multifocal patchy areas of GGO are often due to areas of acute infection or inflammation in the lung, which usually resolve without issue. Persistent focal areas of pure GGO should raise the possibility of neoplastic disease, usually representing adenocarcinoma in situ or minimally invasive adenocarcinoma and are discussed below.

Diffuse GGO has a wide differential and differs based on whether the finding is acute or chronic. If the patient is acutely ill, diffuse GGO is often due to pulmonary edema and is characterized by more central GGO with areas of septal thickening. Diffuse pulmonary hemorrhage can have a similar appearance but is much less common and tends not to be as centrally located as edema. Acute lung injury (including acute interstitial pneumonia, acute respiratory distress syndrome, and acute exacerbations of usual interstitial pneumonia) often demonstrates diffuse GGO and consolidation that is lower lobe predominant and often spares the anterior portion of the lung.[13] Opportunistic infections manifest by diffuse GGO include CMV, PCP, HSV, and RSV pneumonia and can have an appearance similar to etiologies of DAD.

If the diffuse GGO is subacute or chronic, examination of the distribution of the ground-glass opacity is important as certain diseases tend to occur in lower lung zones such as nonspecific interstitial pneumonia (NSIP), while others are usually more pronounced in the upper lung zones such as hypersensitivity pneumonitis (HP).[14] Others may have no appreciable zonal distribution such as certain cases of organizing pneumonia (OP) or chronic eosinophilic pneumonia.[13,15] It is also important to evaluation the axial distribution of the GGO. NSIP and OP tend to be more pronounced peripherally and along the bronchovascular bundles, while fibrotic HP is more pronounced centrally.[14] Bilateral disease is common in most diffuse lung disease that leads to GGO. However, unilateral disease can be seen with OP.[13] Other clues to

which can exceed 2 years. Therefore, indicators other than growth, such as the presence of internal air bronchograms, pleural retraction, increasing density, and/or vascular convergence within a ground-glass nodule, assume greater importance in suggesting the diagnosis of a lesion along the adenocarcinoma spectrum.[10] Interestingly enough, unlike solid nodules, a rounded shape is more associated with malignancy in subsolid nodules, probably because well-differentiated adenocarcinomas with lepidic growth show relatively little scarring. In some instances, a small solid component may be present if areas of alveolar collapse or fibroblastic proliferation are present. However, any solid component should raise concern for a more invasive lesion. Changes in size and morphology may occur very slowly and require comparison with CT images performed over many years (Fig. 10.3).

Location or nodules can help with determining their underlying cause. For instance, perifissural nodules are most likely benign lymphatic tissue and have an extremely low incidence of malignancy. In three large lung cancer screening studies, of 1,098 perifissural nodules, not a single one was malignant.[4,11,12] In terms of lobar location,

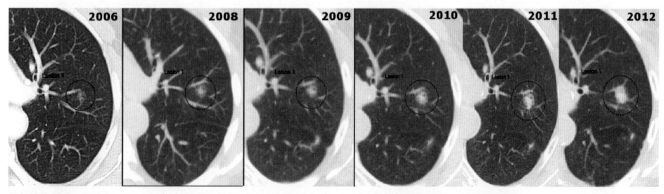

FIGURE 10.3 ▲ Slow growth of a lung adenocarcinoma over 6 years. Axial CT images through the left upper lobe in a 51-year-old woman with a history of smoking show a slow but progressive increase in size and density of the left upper lobe nodule (*circles*). In 2006, the 1.2-cm nodule is purely ground glass in attenuation (**left-most image**). In 2009, the 1.2-cm nodule demonstrates both ground-glass and solid components (**middle image**). In 2012, the 2.1-cm nodule is completely soft tissue in attenuation. Notice that the size of the nodule does significantly change over the first 3 years and the only detectable change is the increase in attenuation. Once the solid component forms, which reflects more invasive tumor, the growth of the nodule accelerates.

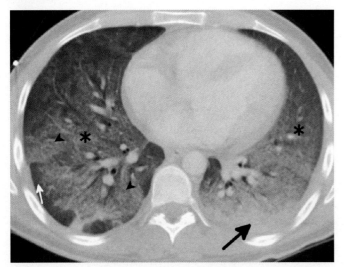

FIGURE 10.4 ▲ Axial CT image in a 24-year-old man with diffuse alveolar hemorrhage from Goodpasture syndrome shows diffuse ground-glass opacity (GGO, *asterisks*), which leads to increased areas of lung attenuation. However, the GGO does not obscure the underlying lung architecture. In addition to the GGO, there is an area of more dense consolidation at the left base (*arrow*). This consolidation obscures the underlying lung architecture. In addition, there are areas of interlobular (*white arrow*) and intralobular (*black arrowheads*) septal thickening due to resorption of blood product.

the underlying etiology depend on the presence or absence of findings of fibrosis, which include reticulation, traction bronchiectasis, and/or honeycombing, which are discussed below. Although some degree of GGO may be present in UIP/IPF, it should not be a predominant finding.

Consolidation

Consolidation is an area of homogeneous increase in attenuation that obscures the underlying architecture of the lung[3] (Fig. 10.4). The differential diagnosis is very broad, including neoplastic, infectious, and inflammatory conditions. In cases of diffuse lung disease, consolidation is often present in organizing pneumonia and in causes of DAD,

although this finding is often intermixed with areas of GGO. Although uncommon, decreased attenuation within an area of consolidation can occur and is suggestive of lipoid pneumonia.[3] Areas of high attenuation consolidation can be seen in amiodarone toxicity.

Septal Thickening

On thin-section CT scans, interlobular septal thickening may be smooth or nodular. Smooth interlobular septal thickening occurs when the lymphatics or veins in the secondary pulmonary lobule become dilated and the septum itself becomes edematous. Although it may occur in isolation, smooth septal thickening is commonly associated with GGO in cases of diffuse lung disease, and its presence can help narrow the differential diagnosis. Pulmonary edema, *Pneumocystis jiroveci* pneumonia (PCP), and diffuse alveolar hemorrhage are all causes of smooth septal thickening. Interlobular septal thickening with GGO can also occur in both DAD and organizing pneumonia (OP).[13]

Nodular septal thickening should raise the possibility of lymphatic invasion or infiltration (Fig. 10.5A). This is most commonly associated with lymphangitic carcinomatosis, although this can also lead to smooth septal thickening. Sarcoidosis and silicosis also lead to nodular septal thickening, although the nodularity often predominates. Rare causes of nodular septal thickening include Kaposi sarcoma, lymphoid interstitial pneumonia, and amyloidosis.

Human lymphatic vessels extend deep inside the pulmonary lobule in association with bronchioles, intralobular arterioles, or small pulmonary veins, and these intralobular lymphatics are usually contiguous with the lymphatics in the interlobular septa.[16] In certain instances, both the interlobular and intralobular septa become thickened. A "crazy paving" pattern is a descriptive designation for thickening of these septa superimposed on a ground glass. It was originally reported in patients with alveolar proteinosis (Fig. 10.5B) but has a broad differential diagnosis (Fig. 10.5B).

Reticulation

"Reticulation" denotes thin, peripheral linear opacities that produce an appearance resembling a net (Fig. 10.6). Reticular densities typical imply interstitial fibrosis of variable cause and are prominent in the interstitial pneumonias that lead to fibrosis. Pathologically, they are thought to represent interlobular septal thickening, intralobular lines, intralobular areas of fine fibrosis, and the cyst walls of honeycombing.[3]

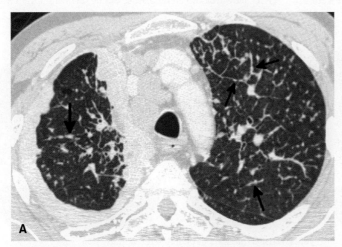

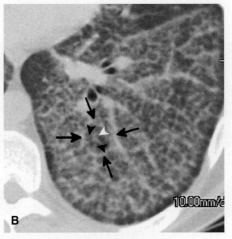

FIGURE 10.5 ▲ **A.** Nodular septal thickening. Axial CT image in a patient with metastatic renal cell carcinoma shows bilateral nodular septal thickening (*black arrows*) consistent with lymphangitic carcinomatosis. **B.** Crazy paving pattern. Axial CT image in a 42-year-old man with pulmonary alveolar proteinosis shows interlobular (*black arrows*) and intralobular (*black arrowheads*) septal thickening superimposed on diffuse ground-glass opacity creating a "crazy paving" pattern. The intralobular septa radiate outward from the center of the secondary pulmonary lobule (*white arrowhead*) and usually communicate with the more peripheral interlobular septa.

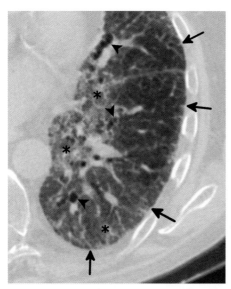

FIGURE 10.6 ▲ Reticulation in a 63-year-old man with idiopathic pulmonary fibrosis. Axial CT image demonstrates thin, peripheral linear densities consistent with reticulation (*arrows*) and dilation of the peripheral airways due to traction bronchiectasis (*arrowheads*). Honeycombing is absent, and there is patchy ground-glass opacity (*asterisks*). This was determined to be a possible UIP pattern on CT, and subsequent open lung biopsy demonstrated UIP on pathology.

Traction Bronchiectasis

There are numerous causes of bronchiectasis and bronchiolectasis, which can be due to prior injury, chronic infection, or chronic inflammation or can be congenital in etiology.[17] However, when the large and small airways are pulled open by surrounding fibrosis, traction bronchiectasis and bronchiolectasis are diagnosed, respectively. Traction bronchiectasis is a finding suggestive of fibrotic lung disease and is common in UIP, NSIP, and the fibrotic phases of sarcoid and hypersensitivity pneumonitis[14] (Fig. 10.7). Traction bronchiectasis can also be seen in the fibrotic phase of DAD and in certain cases of organizing pneumonia, which progress to fibrosis.[13]

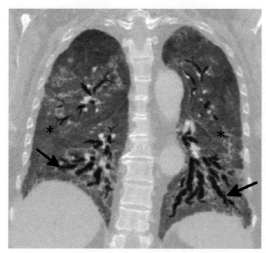

FIGURE 10.7 ▲ Traction bronchiectasis in a 47-year-old woman with scleroderma. Coronal 5-mm thick minimum intensity projection image shows marked dilation of the bronchi due to surrounding fibrosis (*arrows*). The bronchiectasis and ground-glass opacity (*asterisks*) are more severe in the lower lobe. Open lung biopsy demonstrated both nonspecific interstitial pneumonia and organizing pneumonia.

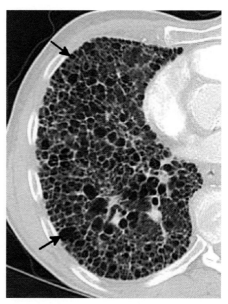

FIGURE 10.8 ▲ Honeycombing in a 67-year-old man with idiopathic pulmonary fibrosis. Axial image through the right lower lobe shows extensive subpleural predominant cystic change (*arrows*). The finding was most severe at the lung bases, and the cystic structures are stacked on top of one another. Although the interobserver agreement between radiologists for the presence of honeycombing on CT is only moderate, the findings in this case are classic and should obviate the need for open lung biopsy.

Honeycombing

Honeycombing is both a radiologic and pathologic term. By CT imaging, it denotes subpleural clustered cystic air spaces, typically of 3 to 10 mm in diameter, with well-defined walls (Fig. 10.8). The finding of multiple layers or stacked, subpleural cysts with definable walls is more definitive than a single layer.[3] Honeycombing on CT does not necessarily correlate with pathologic honeycombing, and pathologic findings in areas of honeycombing on CT also include traction bronchiectasis and paraseptal emphysema.[18] This heterogeneity of etiologies on imaging can lead to discrepancies in the diagnosis of honeycombing as interobserver agreement between expert thoracic radiologists on what meets the radiologic criteria for honeycombing is only moderate. However, the presence of lower-lobe predominant honeycombing is an important finding on imaging as its presence is highly correlated with a UIP pattern on histology and often obviates the need for open lung biopsy.[19]

Micronodules

Micronodules describe the presence of numerous small nodules measuring 3 mm or less[3] (Fig. 10.9). These nodules occur in three distinct patterns: centrilobular, perilymphatic, and random. Although direct visualization of the small airways is not possible on CT in normal individuals, they can become visible in certain disease states. In the vast majority of cases, centrilobular nodules on CT are secondary to increased soft tissue and/or inflammation in or around the respiratory bronchioles in the center of the secondary pulmonary lobule. In most instances, centrilobular nodules are a focal or patchy finding due to an infectious bronchiolitis. However, in certain inhalational diseases, such as hypersensitivity pneumonitis and respiratory bronchiolitis, upper-lobe predominant centrilobular nodularity is often present, which can help make the diagnosis.

Perilymphatic nodules occur along the bronchovascular bundles, septa, or periphery of the lung as this corresponds to the location of the pulmonary veins and lymphatics. Perilymphatic nodules are most commonly seen in sarcoidosis and silicosis. Lymphangitic carcinomatosis can lead to perilymphatic nodules, but septal thickening is often present, a finding that is often mild or absent in sarcoidosis and silicosis.

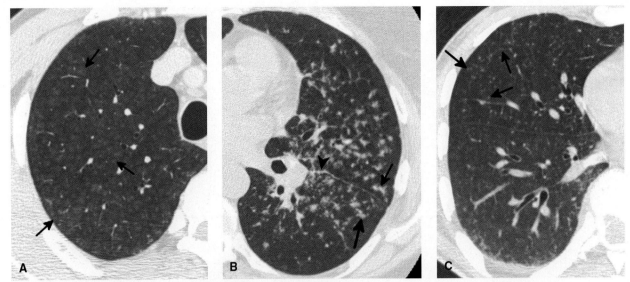

FIGURE 10.9 ▲ Different patterns of micronodules. **A.** Axial image through the right upper lobe in a patient with hypersensitivity pneumonitis demonstrates ill-defined ground-glass nodules in the center of the secondary pulmonary lobule consistent with centrilobular nodules (*arrows*). These nodules spare the lung periphery and bronchovascular bundles. **B.** Axial CT image through the left lung shows perihilar predominant micronodules, which stud the broncho-vascular bundles (*arrows*) and fissures (*arrowhead*) consistent with a perilymphatic distribution in this patient with sarcoidosis. **C.** Axial CT image though the right lung shows diffuse micronodules without appreciable pattern (*arrows*) consistent with a random distribution due to hematogenous dissemination in a patient with miliary tuberculosis.

Random micronodules are diffusely distributed throughout the secondary pulmonary lobule. They are indicative of a hematogenous spread of disease and usually occur with metastatic disease or miliary tuberculosis.

Reticulonodular Pattern

A reticulonodular pattern is a finding on chest radiograph used to describe the interposition of both reticulation and micronodularity.[3] With thin-section CT, the reticulation and micronodularity can be easily separated, and the differential diagnosis can be broken down based on the distribution of the nodules (centrilobular, perilymphatic, or random) and type of septal thickening (smooth or nodular) as described above.

Mosaic Attenuation Pattern and Air Trapping

Mosaic attenuation is a common finding on CT and is defined as heterogeneous areas of differing lung attenuation (Fig. 10.10). A mosaic attenuation has a broad differential diagnosis including diseases that affect

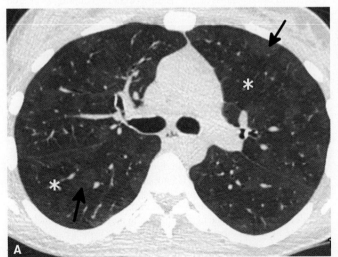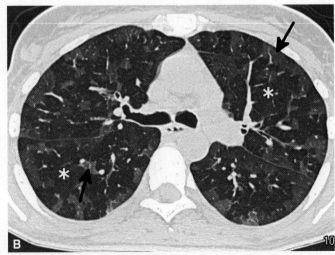

FIGURE 10.10 ▲ Mosaic attenuation and air trapping in a 40-year-old woman with constrictive bronchiolitis due to rheumatoid arthritis. **A.** Axial image through the carina shows a pronounced mosaic attenuation with areas of relative decreased attenuation (*asterisks*) adjacent to areas of relative increased attenuation (*arrows*). The paucity of vessels in the more lucent lung suggests that it is abnormal. **B.** Expiratory image performed at the same level shows a further increase in attenuation in the denser areas of the lung (*arrows*) seen in **(A)**, which is the expected finding on expiration imaging due to the presence of less air. However, the more lucent lung does not change in attenuation (*asterisks*) due to obstruction of the small airways. This increased conspicuity between the relatively normal (*arrows*) and abnormal (*asterisks*) lung on expiration confirms the findings of air trapping on expiratory CT.

the small airways, the pulmonary vasculature, the alveoli, and the interstitium, alone or in combination. Causes of small airways disease that lead to mosaic attenuation on CT are numerous and include constrictive bronchiolitis, respiratory bronchiolitis, hypersensitivity pneumonitis, asthma, and infectious bronchiolitis.[20] Chronic thromboembolic pulmonary hypertension (CTEPH) and pulmonary arterial hypertension (primary pulmonary hypertension) are the most common vascular etiologies to lead to a mosaic attenuation on CT. Diffuse ground-glass opacities interspersed with areas of normal lung attenuation can lead to a mosaic pattern. This can be seen in acute (e.g., infection, pulmonary edema), subacute (e.g., organizing pneumonia), or chronic settings (e.g., fibrotic diseases). There are numerous imaging findings that can help one differentiate between these different etiologies, although this is not always an easy task. In general, paucity of small vessels in the hyperlucent lung suggests either a small airways etiology due to hypoxic vasoconstriction or CTEPH due to arteriolar obstruction. Differentiation between these two can be made by assessing the large airways, which are often abnormal in the setting of small airways disease. In cardiovascular etiologies, there are often signs of right ventricular hypertrophy or pulmonary artery enlargement. In causes due to GGO, septal thickening or signs of fibrosis can help make narrow the differential diagnosis.

However, one of the best ways to differentiate small airways disease from other forms of mosaic attenuation is through the demonstration of air trapping on expiratory imaging. On expiratory CT in normal patients, the lungs should show a diffuse increase in attenuation (be more grey) since less air is present. However, in patients with small airways disease, air cannot readily escape in the regions where the small airways are obstructed. Because of this, the attenuation of the involved segments remains relatively unchanged when compared to the inspiratory scan. The difference in attenuation between the normal and abnormal areas becomes much more pronounced, and air trapping can be diagnosed (Fig. 10.10B). In patients with a mosaic attenuation not related to abnormalities of the small airways, expiration imaging will usually lead to a diffuse increase in attenuation throughout the entire lung.

Halo Sign (and Reverse)

The halo sign is used to describe ground-glass opacity, classically due to pulmonary hemorrhage, surrounding a nodule or mass (Fig. 10.11).[21] It is most commonly associated with angioinvasive infections such as aspergillosis in a severely immunocompromised patient. However, hemorrhage metastasis (melanoma, renal cell carcinoma, angiosarcoma, etc.),

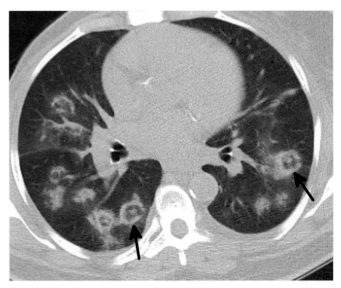

FIGURE 10.12 ▲ Reverse halo sign in a 31-year-old woman with cryptogenic organizing pneumonia. Axial image through the midlung zones shows circular areas of consolidation with central ground-glass opacity (arrows). The reverse halo sign was first described with organizing pneumonia but, like the halo sign, has a broad differential diagnosis.

granulomatosis with polyangiitis, and pulmonary infarction can all lead to a halo sign. In some instances, a halo sign has been described with adenocarcinoma of the lung where more solid, invasive areas of adenocarcinoma are surrounded by areas of adenocarcinoma in situ.

The reversed halo sign is the converse, namely an area of ground-glass opacity surrounded by consolidation (Fig. 10.12). It was initially reported to be specific for organizing pneumonia but has been reported in other conditions, including infections and pulmonary infarcts.[22] Similar to the halo sign, this sign represents a finding and not a diagnosis.

Pathologic Situations Where CT Findings Are Especially Important

General

When evaluating lung biopsies for diffuse lung disease, whether transbronchial or wedge biopsies, it is exceedingly helpful for the pathologist to interact with the clinician and radiologist, in order to have a differential diagnosis with which to assess the histologic findings. That being said, it is also critical for the pathologist to avoid overreliance on clinical and imaging features, which are nonspecific. With practice, a descriptive diagnosis that is reasonable and helpful for directing patient care, and that outlines the salient histologic patterns, gives a differential diagnosis, and comments about imaging features (when relevant), is routinely achievable, especially on wedge biopsy material.

One of the most important concerns is to identify areas of potential infection or acute lung injury, especially when there is extensive GGO on CT. Any areas of fibrin should be distinguished from procedural hemorrhage, by identifying other features of acute lung injury. These should be stained for microorganisms, and a differential diagnosis explaining their presence should be mentioned. Similarly, in areas of hemorrhage with hemosiderin macrophages, capillary inflammation with neutrophils should be carefully excluded, to rule out or confirm a diagnosis of capillaritis, which also can manifest at GGO on CT.

Cryptogenic Organizing Pneumonia Versus Organizing Diffuse Alveolar Damage

Histologically, the dominant features of cryptogenic organizing pneumonia (COP) are nodules of organizing pneumonia, with variable interstitial inflammation and fibrosis. In contrast to DAD, fibrin and

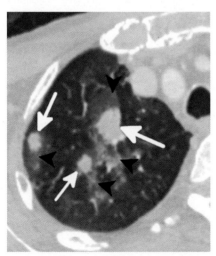

FIGURE 10.11 ▲ Halo sign in a 41-year-old man with metastatic angiosarcoma. Axial CT image through the right upper lobe shows well-defined nodules (white arrows) surrounded by areas of ground-glass opacity (arrowheads) due to hemorrhage. Although classically described with angioinvasive Aspergillus infection, there halo sign has a differential diagnosis.

acute lung injury are absent. In some cases, however, there may be large areas of organizing pneumonia with minimal fibrin, and the differential diagnosis is organizing DAD, versus acute and organizing pneumonia. In such cases, the CT imaging findings of dominant ground glass, especially in the upper lobes, is helpful to favor organizing DAD. In some cases where the distinction seems arbitrary, the term "acute fibrinous and organizing pneumonia" has been used.[23]

COP Versus NSIP

In wedge biopsies of patients with diffuse parenchymal lung disease, there is often a mixture of organizing pneumonia and NSIP patterns. In such cases, a descriptive diagnosis with a differential of clinicopathologic entities is appropriate in the pathologic diagnostic report. If imaging findings favor areas of consolidation and nodular densities, then a diagnosis of COP is more likely than that of NSIP, which shows a predominantly reticular and ground-glass pattern without subpleural sparing.

COP Versus UIP

There is some evidence that a subset of patients (probably less than one-third) with COP do not respond to steroids and progress to interstitial fibrosis, either NSIP or UIP pattern. In some wedge biopsies, there may be a predominance of organizing pneumonia with patchy fibrosis in a nonspecific pattern in the upper lobes and a pattern in the lower lobe with peripheral honeycombing and some features of UIP. In such cases, again, a descriptive diagnosis is best, and correlation with imaging findings helpful in a differential diagnosis.

UIP Versus NSIP

The classic differential diagnosis in chronic interstitial pneumonia is that of UIP versus NSIP. The CT algorithm for the diagnosis of UIP is presented in Table 10.2, and the histologic features to distinguish these two entities are further described in Chapter 17.

HP Versus NSIP or UIP

The CT imaging characteristics distinguishing these three entities are discussed above; the radiologic distinction of these three entities, regardless of knowledge of autoimmune or inhalational risk factors of the patient, has been recently reviewed. Histologically, HP is dominated by interstitial inflammation that is bronchiolocentric, with relatively minor components of organizing pneumonia and small if any, poorly formed granulomas. In later stages, there is variable interstitial fibrosis with remodeling that may be confused with NSIP or UIP.

REFERENCES

1. Meyer M, Haubenreisser H, Raupach R, et al. Initial results of a new generation dual source CT system using only an in-plane comb filter for ultra-high resolution temporal bone imaging. *Eur Radiol.* 2015;25:178–185.
2. Khawaja RD, Singh S, Gilman M, et al. Computed tomography (CT) of the chest at less than 1 mSv: an ongoing prospective clinical trial of chest CT at submillisievert radiation doses with iterative model image reconstruction and iDose4 technique. *J Comput Assist Tomogr.* 2014;38:613–619.
3. Hansell DM, Bankier AA, MacMahon H, et al. Fleischner Society: glossary of terms for thoracic imaging. *Radiology.* 2008;246:697–722.
4. McWilliams A, Tammemagi MC, Mayo JR, et al. Probability of cancer in pulmonary nodules detected on first screening CT. *N Engl J Med.* 2013;369:910–919.
5. Truong MT, Ko JP, Rossi SE, et al. Update in the evaluation of the solitary pulmonary nodule. *Radiographics.* 2014;34:1658–1679.
6. Winer-Muram HT. The solitary pulmonary nodule. *Radiology.* 2006;239:34–49.
7. Erasmus JJ, Connolly JE, McAdams HP, et al. Solitary pulmonary nodules: Part I. Morphologic evaluation for differentiation of benign and malignant lesions. *Radiographics.* 2000;20:43–58.
8. Oh JY, Kwon SY, Yoon HI, et al. Clinical significance of a solitary ground-glass opacity (GGO) lesion of the lung detected by chest CT. *Lung Cancer.* 2007;55:67–73.
9. Kim HY, Shim YM, Lee KS, et al. Persistent pulmonary nodular ground-glass opacity at thin-section CT: histopathologic comparisons. *Radiology.* 2007;245:267–275.
10. Kligerman S, White C. Imaging characteristics of lung cancer. *Semin Roentgenol.* 2011;46:194–207.
11. Ahn MI, Gleeson TG, Chan IH, et al. Perifissural nodules seen at CT screening for lung cancer. *Radiology.* 2010;254:949–956.
12. de Hoop B, van Ginneken B, Gietema H, et al. Pulmonary perifissural nodules on CT scans: rapid growth is not a predictor of malignancy. *Radiology.* 2012;265:611–616.
13. Kligerman SJ, Franks TJ, Galvin JR. From the radiologic pathology archives: organization and fibrosis as a response to lung injury in diffuse alveolar damage, organizing pneumonia, and acute fibrinous and organizing pneumonia. *Radiographics.* 2013;33:1951–1975.
14. Kligerman SJ, Groshong S, Brown KK, et al. Nonspecific interstitial pneumonia: radiologic, clinical, and pathologic considerations. *Radiographics.* 2009;29:73–87.
15. Jeong YJ, Kim KI, Seo IJ, et al. Eosinophilic lung diseases: a clinical, radiologic, and pathologic overview. *Radiographics.* 2007;27:617–637; discussion 637–9.
16. Sozio F, Rossi A, Weber E, et al. Morphometric analysis of intralobular, interlobular and pleural lymphatics in normal human lung. *J Anat.* 2012;220:396–404.
17. Cantin L, Bankier AA, Eisenberg RL. Bronchiectasis. *AJR Am J Roentgenol.* 2009;193:W158–W171.
18. Staats P, Kligerman S, Todd N, et al. A comparative study of honeycombing on high resolution computed tomography with histologic lung remodeling in explants with usual interstitial pneumonia. *Pathol Res Pract.* 2015;211:55–61.
19. Wells AU. The revised ATS/ERS/JRS/ALAT diagnostic criteria for idiopathic pulmonary fibrosis (IPF)—practical implications. *Respir Res.* 2013;14(suppl 1):S2.
20. Ryu JH, Myers JL, Swensen SJ. Bronchiolar disorders. *Am J Respir Crit Care Med.* 2003;168:1277–1292.
21. Lee HL, Ryu JH, Wittmer MH, et al. Familial idiopathic pulmonary fibrosis: clinical features and outcome. *Chest.* 2005;127:2034–2041.
22. Godoy MC, Viswanathan C, Marchiori E, et al. The reversed halo sign: update and differential diagnosis. *Br J Radiol.* 2012;85:1226–1235.
23. Beasley MB, Franks TJ, Galvin JR, et al. Acute fibrinous and organizing pneumonia: a histological pattern of lung injury and possible variant of diffuse alveolar damage. *Arch Pathol Lab Med.* 2002;126:1064–1070.

11 Congenital Cysts and Malformations

Haresh Mani, M.D., and Jennifer M. Boland, M.D.

Overview

Most surgical lung specimens from children are resections of cystic lesions and malformations, which are usually treated by excision of the abnormal lobe. The different cystic lesions and malformations often have overlapping radiographic features and clinical presentation, so the pathologist plays a key role in diagnosis and classification (Table 11.1).

The most commonly excised lung lesions from children are congenital pulmonary airway malformations (CPAMs). Other encountered malformations include bronchial atresia, intralobar and extralobar sequestrations, infantile lobar emphysema (congenital lobar overinflation), and bronchopulmonary foregut malformations. Bronchial atresia or some form of airway obstruction in utero may play a role in the pathogenesis of many of these malformations. The pathologic pattern may be determined by the timing of the obstructive event during lung development, as well as the level and completeness of obstruction.[1-3]

Clinical and Radiologic Findings

Children with congenital cysts and malformations of the lung are most often born at term. If the lesion is large, it may cause respiratory distress at birth due to compression or hypoplasia of the surrounding normal lung with subsequent respiratory compromise. Alternatively, if the surrounding lung is functioning normally, the child may be asymptomatic at birth and may present later in infancy or childhood with respiratory symptoms. Some lesions are asymptomatic and discovered incidentally, whereas others may present with symptoms and signs of pneumonia.

Radiographically, CPAMs, sequestrations, and lobar overinflation are usually limited to one lobe. They may appear as lucencies, densities, or cystic lesions on imaging. Sequestrations have a characteristic systemic vascular supply that is often apparent on imaging.

Congenital Pulmonary Airway Malformation

Terminology

CPAMs were formerly known as congenital cystic adenomatoid malformations (CCAM), but CPAM is now considered the preferred term for these lesions, since these lesions are "cystic" in only three of the five types and "adenomatoid" in only one type (type 3).

Incidence

As a group, they are the most common developmental lung malformation, with an incidence of about 1 in 5,000 live births.[4]

Localization

Over 90% of CPAMs are restricted to a single lobe; involvement of multiple lobes should alert the pathologist to other possibilities such as pleuropulmonary blastoma (PPB).

Clinical Findings

In a single-institution analysis of 172 cases of CPAM, the most common presenting symptoms were respiratory distress in infants under 6 months of age (40%) and recurrent pneumonia in older children (75%). Associated anomalies were seen in 47% of children, the most frequent being sequestration (71%) in association with type 2 CPAM. Mortality was 5%; risk factors for mortality were respiratory failure, sepsis, respiratory assistance requirements, and severe associated comorbidities.[5]

Classification

CPAMs have been classified into five major clinicopathologic types[4,6] conceptually based on the putative anatomic level of the abnormality, that is, tracheobronchial to peripheral acinar. In a large series of CPAM, all histologic types were found; type 1 was the most frequent (70%), followed by type 2 (24%).[5]

Type 0 CPAM

The lesion historically described as type 0 CPAM is essentially synonymous with acinar dysplasia.[7] These are extremely rare catastrophic developmental abnormalities that lead to profound pulmonary hypoplasia and are incompatible with life (see Chapter 12). This abnormality may be seen in term and premature infants and is associated with cardiovascular abnormalities and dermal hypoplasia. Grossly, the lungs are small and firm with a diffusely granular surface. Microscopically, there are no acini, and the lesion consists of bronchus-like structures with muscle, glands, and numerous cartilage plates.

Type 1 CPAM

Type 1 CPAM, the large or predominant cyst type, is the most common type of CPAM in most series. It presents primarily in the neonatal period but can be seen in older children and even adults. It is amenable to surgery and has a good prognosis. Grossly, type 1 CPAM is characterized by single or multiple large cysts (3 to 10 cm in diameter) surrounded by smaller cysts and compressed normal parenchyma.

Microscopically, the cysts recapitulate proximal bronchi, being lined by ciliated, pseudostratified columnar epithelium with underlying fibromuscular tissue and focal cartilage plates. The epithelium usually shows a characteristic "sawtooth" architecture (Fig. 11.1). Almost half the cases show foci of mucous cells in the epithelial lining, which resemble benign gastric foveolar cells in most cases (Fig. 11.2). Identification of this mucigenic epithelium is strong evidence that the cystic lesion is a type 1 CPAM and thus can be useful in classification. The presence of mucigenic epithelium should always be reported if identified, since these mucous cells are recognized to be precursors for the rare examples of adenocarcinoma that have been described in association with type 1 CPAM.[8]

Type 2 CPAM

Type 2 CPAM conceptually recapitulates smaller bronchi and bronchioles, being composed therefore of medium-sized cysts. While historically

TABLE 11.1   Features of CPAM and Sequestration

	Synonyms	Incidence, Associations	Clinical/Prognosis	Characteristic Features
Type 0 CPAM	Acinar dysplasia	Rare	Neonates, incompatible with life	Small, firm, retracted lungs
Type 1 CPAM	Large cyst type	Most common	Neonatal, older children, good prognosis	Sawtooth cysts, mucinous metaplasia
Type 2 CPAM	Medium cyst type	Associated with bronchial atresia, sequestration; 20% with extrapulmonary anomalies	Follows associated conditions, if present	Evenly distributed cysts that blend with surrounding lung; rhabdomyomatous dysplasia (occasional)
Type 3 CPAM	Small cyst/solid type	Rare	Neonatal, male predominance	Resembles immature lung
Type 4 CPAM	Peripheral acinar type	Rare; may be a form of regressed PPB	Newborns, young children	Thin-walled alveolar septa-like cyst walls; may appear similar to PPB, but without immature blastemal elements
Extralobar sequestration	—	Hydrops, polyhydramnios CPAM type 2, pulmonary hypoplasia, diaphragmatic hernia Uncommon	Prenatal, <3 mo; uncommon	Left hemithorax most common, then right hemithorax, mediastinum, and subdiaphragmatic; systemic feeder artery and venous drainage; outside normal pleural envelopment
Intralobar sequestration	—	Common	Childhood to adult	Systemic feeder artery; venous drainage pulmonary; lower lobes predominate, fibrosis; within normal pleural envelopment

PPB, pleuropulmonary blastoma.

thought to represent only 10% to 15% of cases of CPAM, it has likely been largely under recognized. Type 2 CPAM is a pattern observed in various other entities including bronchial atresia, intralobar sequestration, and extralobar sequestration. Therefore, recognition of the type 2 CPAM pattern should lead to careful consideration of these other entities, since some authors believe that essentially all cases of type 2 CPAM pattern are a result of intrauterine bronchial atresia or sequestration.

About 20% of cases of type 2 CPAM pattern may have other associated congenital anomalies involving renal, cardiovascular, pulmonary, skeletal, and/or nervous systems,[4,9] resulting in poor outcomes.

The type 2 lesion is composed of evenly distributed cysts measuring 0.5 to 2.0 cm in diameter that blend with the adjacent normal parenchyma (Fig. 11.3). Typically, there are bronchiole-like structures lined by cuboidal to columnar epithelial cells with a thin, underlying, fibromuscular layer (Fig. 11.4). These structures can be distinguished from normal bronchioles in that they lack a smooth muscle wall and lack an accompanying pulmonary artery branch. These bronchiole-like cystic structures may be back to back or may be more widely scattered with intervening alveolated parenchyma. Mucous cells and cartilage plates are absent except as components of "entrapped" normal bronchi.

A subgroup of cases showing type 2 CPAM pattern will have so-called rhabdomyomatous dysplasia, characterized by ribbons of striated muscle fibers throughout the lesion, in association with the cysts, between alveolar ducts and around blood vessels (Fig. 11.5). Reported cases of associated rhabdomyosarcoma probably represent primary pleuropulmonary blastoma (PPB) rather than arising secondarily within type 2 CPAM.

Type 3 CPAM

Type 3 CPAM, the small cyst or solid type, is the originally described congenital cystic adenomatoid malformation.[10] It is very rare (<5% of cases), usually presents in the first days to weeks of life, and has a male predominance. It tends to be large, is associated with maternal polyhydramnios and fetal anasarca, and has a high mortality rate. Grossly, it consists of a large, bulky, parenchymal mass involving an entire lobe or even an entire lung, with significant mass effect that may result in hypoplasia of the uninvolved lung. Cysts are typically uniform and <0.2 cm in diameter.

Microscopically, the lesion resembles an immature lung devoid of bronchi. There are irregular bronchiole-like structures lined with cuboidal epithelial cells surrounded by alveolar ducts and saccules that are also lined by cuboidal cells, imparting an "adenomatoid" appearance

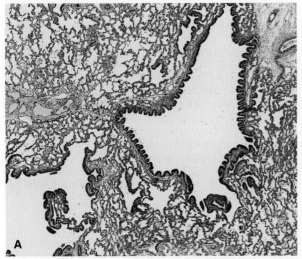
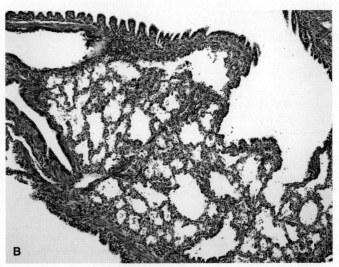

FIGURE 11.1 ▲ Type 1 CPAM. **A.** There are cysts of various sizes, lined by a sawtooth pattern of bronchial epithelial cells. **B.** Higher magnification demonstrating cyst lining and adjacent alveolar spaces.

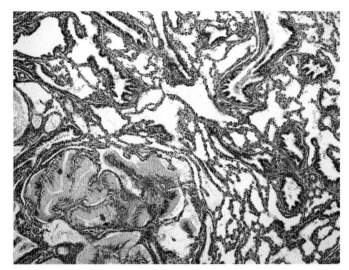

FIGURE 11.2 ▲ Type 1 CPAM. Foci of mucigenic epithelium (**lower left**) that gastric foveolar cells may arise in type 1 CPAM, and are thought to be the precursor to rare examples of mucinous adenocarcinoma that arise from CPAM.

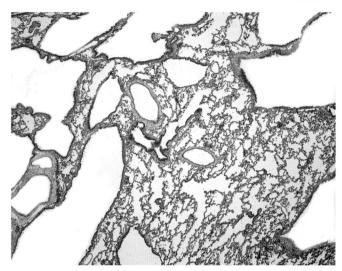

FIGURE 11.4 ▲ Type 2 CPAM. The larger cysts are lined by columnar and cuboidal epithelium and have a thin fibromuscular layer but no true bronchial wall.

(Fig. 11.6). There is a paucity of blood vessels; mucous cells, cartilage, and rhabdomyomatous dysplasia are usually not present.

Type 4 CPAM

Type 4 CPAM, the peripheral acinar cyst type, resembles the distal acinus. This variant may present in newborns or in young children (usually <5 years of age) with respiratory distress or pneumothorax, with some cases being detected incidentally.[4,11] Imaging may show large air-filled cysts with mediastinal shift and pneumothorax. Grossly, large thin-walled collapsible cysts are present at the periphery of the lobe and appear to be lined by a smooth membrane (Fig. 11.7). Microscopically, the cysts are lined predominantly by flattened to cuboidal alveolar-type epithelial cells (Fig. 11.7), the underlying wall being composed of loose to fibrous mesenchyme with prominent arteries and arterioles.

Recently, it has been recognized that type 4 CPAM bears a striking resemblance to cystic (type 1) PPB (see Chapter 93). Before rendering a diagnosis of type 4 CPAM, resection specimens should be entirely submitted to look for immature mesenchymal cells and blastemal elements in the fibrovascular septa to exclude a type 1 PPB. Some authorities believe that all type 4 CPAMs represent type 1 PPBs[12] and propose that lesions that do not show immature mesenchymal cells in the fibrovascular cyst walls are actually regressed type 1 PPBs rather than type 4 CPAM.[13] Thus, follow-up for type 4 CPAMs should be similar to that for type 1 PPBs. This recognition is important, since some patients with PPBs will have *DICER1* germline mutations that may be familial.[14]

Bronchogenic Cyst

A bronchogenic cyst is a developmental cyst that occurs most frequently in the hilar or middle mediastinal area, although it may be present in a midline location from the subcutaneous region of the suprasternal area to the retroperitoneum.[15–18] It is usually detected incidentally and is often asymptomatic. Symptoms, when present, may relate to mechanical obstruction of the tracheobronchial tree or esophagus, secondary infection, hemorrhage, or perforation.

A bronchogenic cyst is a discrete, extrapulmonary mass that may be attached to, but does not communicate with, the tracheobronchial tree. Grossly, it is of variable size, usually 1.0 to 5.0 cm in infants but may be much larger in adults. It is filled with serous fluid that may be

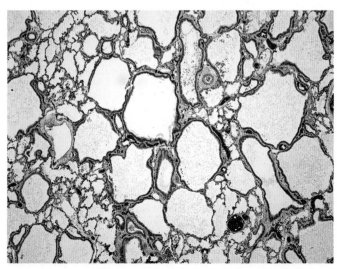

FIGURE 11.3 ▲ Type 2 CPAM. The cysts are uniform and blend into surrounding lung.

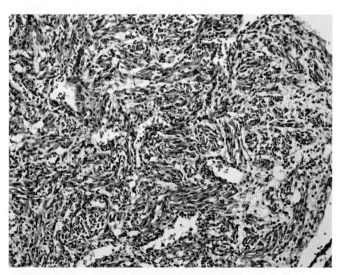

FIGURE 11.5 ▲ Type 2 CPAM, rhabdomyomatous dysplasia. Striated muscle fibers may be seen throughout the lesion, between alveolar ducts and around blood vessels.

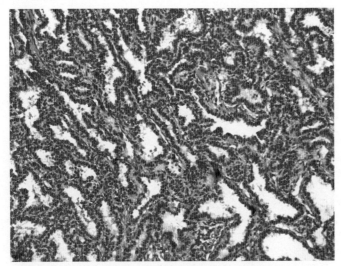

FIGURE 11.6 ▲ Type 3 CPAM. The lesion resembles relatively normal immature lung. The uniform cysts give an "adenomatoid" appearance.

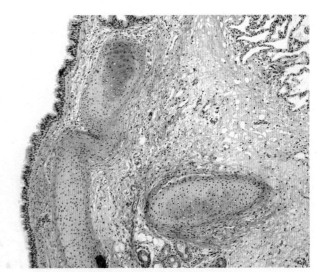

FIGURE 11.8 ▲ Bronchogenic cyst. The wall of the cyst contains cartilage and is lined by respiratory epithelium.

turbid (if infected) or hemorrhagic. It is lined respiratory epithelium that overlies a wall composed of fibromuscular connective tissue with seromucinous glands and cartilage plates recapitulating the wall of a bronchus (Fig. 11.8).

The majority of thoracic bronchogenic cysts arise in the mediastinum, while intrapulmonary bronchogenic cysts are relatively rare.

Sequestration

Definition

Pulmonary sequestration is a mass of nonfunctioning pulmonary tissue that has no identifiable bronchial communication and that receives its blood supply from one or more anomalous systemic arteries.

Extralobar Pulmonary Sequestration

Extralobar sequestrations are discrete masses of lung parenchyma outside the normal pleural investment and, similar to bronchogenic cysts, are not connected to the tracheobronchial tree. They are thought to originate from an outpouching of the foregut, separate from the

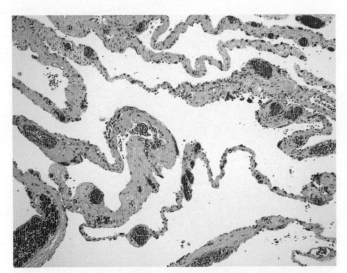

FIGURE 11.7 ▲ Type 4 CPAM. Peripheral thin-walled cysts may mimic cystic pleuropulmonary blastoma but lack blastemal and immature elements; some consider type 4 CPAM to represent "regressed PPB."

normally developing lung that then loses its connection with the foregut, isolating the parenchyma from the tracheobronchial tree.

Extralobar sequestrations are diagnosed prenatally in about 25% of cases, and about 60% of these patients present by 3 months of age with dyspnea and cyanosis due to mass effect, although older children may be asymptomatic.[9] They may be associated with fetal nonimmune hydrops, anasarca, and maternal polyhydramnios. More than 65% of cases of extralobar sequestration have other associated anomalies including type 2 CPAM pattern, bronchogenic cyst, cardiovascular malformations, bronchopulmonary–foregut connection, pectus excavatum, absence of pericardium, and diaphragmatic hernia with concomitant pulmonary hypoplasia.[19,20] In the absence of severe associated anomalies, prognosis and survival is usually good.

Typically, an extralobar sequestration is a single ovoid to triangular lesion ranging from 0.5 to 15 cm in diameter. In Conran's analysis of 50 cases, 48% were located in the left hemithorax, 20% in the right hemithorax, 8% in the anterior mediastinum, 6% in the posterior mediastinum, and 18% beneath the diaphragm.[9] Grossly, these lesions are invested by their own pleura, and subpleural lymphatics may be prominent; cut surface resembles normal pulmonary parenchyma but may appear cystic in the presence of associated type 2 CPAM pattern. The blood supply to the extralobar sequestration is through a direct branch of the thoracic or abdominal aorta in over 75% of cases, with the remaining cases being supplied by either smaller systemic arteries or the pulmonary artery.[21] Venous drainage is also usually through the systemic circulation.

Microscopically, extralobar sequestrations consist of uniformly dilated and tortuous bronchioles, alveolar ducts, and alveoli in a normal acinar pattern. About 50% of cases will show a type 2 CPAM pattern, consisting partially or entirely of back-to-back, dilated, bronchiole-like structures, and may also show rhabdomyomatous dysplasia. Lymphatics are unremarkable in the majority of cases but may be dilated and increased in number beneath the pleura and around bronchovascular bundles, occasionally resembling congenital pulmonary lymphangiectasia (see Chapter 13). Rarely, secondary inflammation or infarction may be present.

Intralobar Sequestration

Intralobar sequestration is more common than extralobar sequestration and may be seen in both children and adults.[22] As the name suggests, intralobar sequestration consists of a portion of lung within the normal pleural investment that is isolated (sequestered) from the tracheobronchial tree and is supplied by a systemic artery[23] (Fig. 11.9). It has historically been hypothesized that most intralobar sequestrations form following repeated episodes of pneumonia involving a particular lung

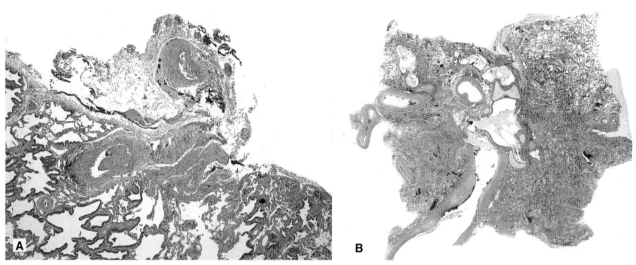

FIGURE 11.9 ▲ Intralobar sequestration, feeder arteries. **A.** The feeder artery enters through the pleura. **B.** In this case, it arose from the aorta.

segment. During these episodes, systemic artery branches increase their blood supply to the inflamed segment, gradually become hypertrophic and replace the pulmonary artery supply to the affected portion.[21] This would explain the fact that these lesions typically show systemic arterial supply and also that almost all intralobar sequestrations occur in the lower lobes, since pulmonary ligament arteries course between the mediastinum and the lower lobes of the lung.[24] Venous drainage occurs through the pulmonary veins in 95% of cases. While the number of intralobar sequestrations that are truly congenital is quite controversial, it seems that at least a subset are clearly congenital in origin, which can be conceptualized as bronchial atresia with a systemic vascular supply.[25,26]

Grossly, the sequestered segment of lung displays findings that may be expected in a setting of recurrent inflammation. There is variable pleural thickening with adhesions between mediastinal structures, the diaphragm, and the parietal pleura. The cut surface shows dense fibrous parenchyma, which may contain variably sized (1 mm to 5.0 cm) cysts filled with thin to viscid fluid. Microscopically, the pulmonary parenchyma is distorted by chronic inflammation and fibrosis, with the cysts likely representing bronchiolectasis or dilated alveoli. A type 2 CPAM pattern is present in a subset of cases. Arteries may show medial hypertrophy, thrombosis, and arteritis, likely due to exposure to high systemic pressures.

Bronchial Atresia

Bronchial atresia is an entity seen almost exclusively in infants, although cases have been reported in children up to 13 years of age (median, 4 years) with symptoms of chronic cough and fever, often related to the recurrent pneumonia noted in more than 90% of cases.[27] The atretic bronchus is connected to the right lower lobe, left upper lobe, and right upper lobe in decreasing order of frequency. Histologically, the affected bronchus may be obstructed by circumferential or eccentric luminal fibrosis with or without abnormalities of the cartilage plates and filled with mucin to create a "mucocele." The fibrosis may be the result of in utero inflammation in the neonate or possibly postpartum inflammation in the case of children and adults. In bronchial stenosis, the lumen may be intrinsically narrowed or extrinsically compressed. Intrinsic causes include postinflammatory fibrosis or intraluminal masses such as aspirated meconium or other foreign material, bronchial adenoma, ectopic thyroid tissue, or bronchial mucosal web. Extrinsic causes of bronchial stenosis include peribronchial masses such as teratoma and bronchogenic cyst, enlarged or abnormally located pulmonary arteries, and cardiac or left atrial enlargement. It is often difficult to demonstrate bronchial atresia/stenosis unless a dissecting microscope is used and the lesion looked for carefully. The presence of an intrabronchial mucocele is helpful. Given that bronchial atresia can be quite

subtle, especially if it involves a sublobar bronchus, the presence of a type 2 CPAM pattern without systemic vascular supply (sequestration) should alert the pathologist to possible occult bronchial atresia.

Infantile (Congenital) Lobar Emphysema/ Congenital Lobar Overinflation

Infantile (congenital) lobar emphysema (ILE) may more correctly be referred to as congenital lobar overinflation since a true loss of parenchyma, as is typical of emphysema, is not seen. ILE occurs due to overdistension of a pulmonary lobe, thought to be the result of a partial postnatal obstruction of the associated bronchus with resultant air trapping behind the point of obstruction. The condition may also be restricted to a segment rather than involving the whole lobe, and these patients can be cured by segmentectomy.

The condition presents with respiratory distress in the first 6 months of life in over 80% of cases, with about 50% presenting in the first week.[28] Imaging studies reveal a hyperlucent lobe or a lobe of normal lucency that occupies a disproportionate part of the hemithorax, with mediastinal shift and compression of the uninvolved lobes. Associated anomalies are present in 5% to 40% of patients, and 70% of these anomalies are cardiovascular.[29,30] The upper lobes are involved in over 95% of cases, with multiple lobe involvement occurring in about 15% of cases.[28] Lower lobe involvement is rare and may be secondary to bronchial obstruction by granulation tissue following mucosal trauma in premature infants receiving mechanical ventilation.[31]

Grossly, the lobe is hyperexpanded in vivo but may collapse and appear grossly normal after resection. Thus, correlation with preoperative imaging findings is often necessary to correctly classify this abnormality. The supplying bronchus may reveal stenosis, atresia, or intrinsic obstruction, although many cases may be caused by extrinsic bronchial obstruction, so the bronchus may appear grossly normal. Microscopically (Fig. 11.10), the lung displays a uniform overdistension of apparently normally developed acini with alveolar saccules and alveoli 3 to 10 times the normal size but with radial alveolar counts (RAC) similar to those of age-matched controls. A polyalveolar form has also been described characterized by normal alveolar size but increased alveolar numbers as documented by RACs that are two standard deviations beyond the mean of age-matched controls.[28] This polyalveolar form may be considered a localized form of pulmonary hyperplasia.[3]

Interstitial Pulmonary Emphysema

As the name suggests, interstitial pulmonary emphysema (IPE) is the dissection of interstitial septa by air. Air tracks around bronchovascular

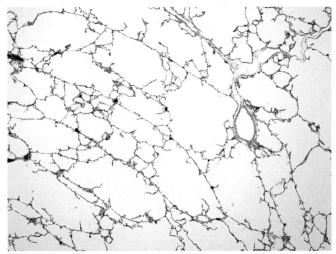

FIGURE 11.10 ▲ Infantile lobar emphysema. There is uniform over-distension of acini.

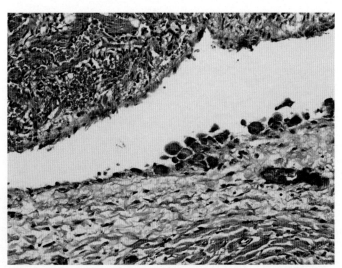

FIGURE 11.12 ▲ Persistent interstitial pulmonary emphysema. When IPE persists, there is a giant cell reaction to the dissecting air.

bundles and along interlobular septa as the result of rupture of alveoli, usually in association with mechanical ventilation. Peripheral dissection of air may lead to pneumothorax, whereas medial dissection could cause pneumomediastinum and pneumopericardium. Early administration of surfactant and the limited use of high-pressure ventilation have significantly reduced the incidence of IPE. Risk factors include infants with lower APGAR scores, increased surfactant utilization, and higher inspired oxygen concentration.[32] IPE has also been reported in 20% of patients dying of acute asthma, following cardiopulmonary resuscitation, and in association with a variety of infectious diseases.[33]

IPE is classified as acute (typically <7 days' duration) or persistent IPE (PIPE) and may be localized to a single lobe or diffusely distributed.[34] Grossly, there are subpleural air blebs and round to oval air spaces along interlobular septa and around bronchovascular bundles. Unlike congenital pulmonary lymphangiectasia (see Chapter 13), air cysts typically do not spread laterally subpleurally and do not involve lymphatics. Microscopically, the cysts of acute IPE are unlined and compress the adjacent blood vessels and acini (Fig. 11.11). Subpleural lymphatics are rarely involved and appear unremarkable.

PIPE occurs when acute IPE lasts more than a few days. The cysts of PIPE may be localized to a single lobe or, when seen in association with bronchopulmonary dysplasia, may diffusely radiate through most

or all of the lobes.[34] PIPE is grossly characterized by multiple 0.1- to 0.3-cm cysts localized to the interlobular septa and extending radially from the hilum to the pleura. Cysts in the localized form of PIPE tend to be larger than those in lungs that are diffusely involved, occasionally as large as 5 cm. Microscopically, the cysts are composed of a thin to thick fibrous connective tissue wall intermittently "lined" with multinucleated foreign body giant cells, the pathognomonic feature of PIPE (Fig. 11.12). The adjacent parenchyma is usually compressed. The diffuse form of PIPE may show parenchymal organization of associated bronchopulmonary dysplasia. The lack of subpleural extension, absence of an endothelial lining, and the presence of giant cell reaction to air help differentiate PIPE from CPL.

Peripheral Cysts of the Lung

Peripheral, air-containing cysts of the lung are exceedingly rare. They have been described in neonates, infants, and young children, usually in association with Down syndrome as a result of pulmonary infarction or in association with idiopathic spontaneous pneumothorax.[35] Occlusion of the pulmonary artery in infants can result in peripheral infarction of the lung, which, with necrosis and organization, can produce subpleural cysts of varying size. Gonzalez et al.[36] reported peripheral cysts in 18 of 98 patients with Down syndrome and suggested that the cysts are an intrinsic feature of the disease that may result from reduced postnatal production of peripheral small air passages and alveoli. The 0.2- to 1.0-cm air-filled cysts are located beneath the pleura and are formed of vascular fibrous connective tissue walls lined by alveolar lining cells. The cysts communicate with more centrally located bronchioles and alveolar ducts. The cysts resemble those seen in the upper lobes of adult males with idiopathic spontaneous pneumothorax and have also been noted in a case of ILE.[28]

REFERENCES

1. Kunisaki SM, Fauza DO, Nemes LP, et al. Bronchial atresia: the hidden pathology within a spectrum of prenatally diagnosed lung masses. *J Pediatr Surg.* 2006;41:61–65; discussion 61–5.
2. Riedlinger WF, Vargas SO, Jennings RW, et al. Bronchial atresia is common to extralobar sequestration, intralobar sequestration, congenital cystic adenomatoid malformation, and lobar emphysema. *Pediatr Dev Pathol.* 2006;9:361–373.
3. Langston C. New concepts in the pathology of congenital lung malformations. *Semin Pediatr Surg.* 2003;12:17–37.
4. Stocker JT. Congenital pulmonary airway malformation—a new name for and an expanded classification of congenital cystic adenomatoid malformation of the lung. *Histopathology.* 2002;41:424–430.

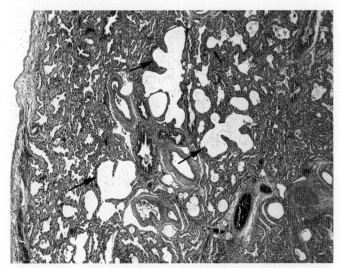

FIGURE 11.11 ▲ Interstitial pulmonary emphysema. Cysts of acute IPE (*arrows*) are unlined and compress the adjacent blood vessels and acini.

5. Giubergia V, Barrenechea M, Siminovich M, et al. Congenital cystic adenomatoid malformation: clinical features, pathological concepts and management in 172 cases. *J Pediatr (Rio J)*. 2012;88:143–148.
6. Stocker JT, Madewell JE, Drake RM. Congenital cystic adenomatoid malformation of the lung. Classification and morphologic spectrum. *Hum Pathol*. 1977;8:155–171.
7. Rutledge JC, Jensen P. Acinar dysplasia: a new form of pulmonary maldevelopment. *Hum Pathol*. 1986;17:1290–1293.
8. Mani H, Shilo K, Galvin JR, et al. Spectrum of precursor and invasive neoplastic lesions in type 1 congenital pulmonary airway malformation: case report and review of the literature. *Histopathology*. 2007;51:561–565.
9. Conran RM, Stocker JT. Extralobar sequestration with frequently associated congenital cystic adenomatoid malformation, type 2: report of 50 cases. *Pediatr Dev Pathol*. 1999;2:454–463.
10. Ch'In KY, Tang MY. Congenital adenomatoid malformation of one lobe of a lung with general anasarca. *Arch Pathol (Chic)*. 1949;48:221–229.
11. Mani HS, Shilo K, Galvin JR, et al. Clinicopathologic study of type 4 congenital pulmonary airway malformation: evidence for distal acinar origin. *Mod Pathol*. 2007;20:326A.
12. Hill DA, Jarzembowski JA, Priest JR, et al. Type I pleuropulmonary blastoma: pathology and biology study of 51 cases from the international pleuropulmonary blastoma registry. *Am J Surg Pathol*. 2008;32:282–295.
13. Messinger YH, Stewart DR, Priest JR, et al. Pleuropulmonary blastoma: a report on 350 central pathology-confirmed pleuropulmonary blastoma cases by the International Pleuropulmonary Blastoma Registry. *Cancer*. 2015;121:276–285.
14. Hill DA, Ivanovich J, Priest JR, et al. DICER1 mutations in familial pleuropulmonary blastoma. *Science*. 2009;325:965.
15. Sauvat F, Fusaro F, Jaubert F, et al. Paraesophageal bronchogenic cyst: first case reports in pediatric. *Pediatr Surg Int*. 2006;22:849–851.
16. Mehta RP, Faquin WC, Cunningham MJ. Cervical bronchogenic cysts: a consideration in the differential diagnosis of pediatric cervical cystic masses. *Int J Pediatr Otorhinolaryngol*. 2004;68:563–568.
17. Zvulunov A, Amichai B, Grunwald MH, et al. Cutaneous bronchogenic cyst: delineation of a poorly recognized lesion. *Pediatr Dermatol*. 1998;15:277–281.
18. Cao DH, Zheng S, Lv X, et al. Multilocular bronchogenic cyst of the bilateral adrenal: report of a rare case and review of literature. *Int J Clin Exp Pathol*. 2014;7:3418–3422.
19. Datta G, Tambiah J, Rankin S, et al. Atypical presentation of extralobar sequestration with absence of pericardium in an adult. *J Thorac Cardiovasc Surg*. 2006;132:1239–1240.
20. Lucaya J, Garel L, Martin C. Clinical quiz. Extralobar sequestration, esophageal bronchus (bronchopulmonary foregut malformation). *Pediatr Radiol*. 2003;33:665–666.
21. Stocker JT. Sequestrations of the lung. *Semin Diagn Pathol*. 1986;3:106–121.
22. Wei Y, Li F. Pulmonary sequestration: a retrospective analysis of 2625 cases in China. *Eur J Cardiothorac Surg*. 2011;40:e39–e42.
23. Frazier AA, Rosado de Christenson ML, Stocker JT, et al. Intralobar sequestration: radiologic-pathologic correlation. *Radiographics*. 1997;17:725–745.
24. Stocker JT, Malczak HT. A study of pulmonary ligament arteries. Relationship to intralobar pulmonary sequestration. *Chest*. 1984;86:611–615.
25. Yamanaka A, Hirai T, Fujimoto T, et al. Anomalous systemic arterial supply to normal basal segments of the left lower lobe. *Ann Thorac Surg*. 1999;68:332–338.
26. Walford N, Htun K, Chen J, et al. Intralobar sequestration of the lung is a congenital anomaly: anatomopathological analysis of four cases diagnosed in fetal life. *Pediatr Dev Pathol*. 2003;6:314–321.
27. Landing BH, Wells TR. Tracheobronchial anomalies in children. *Perspect Pediatr Pathol*. 1973;1:1–32.
28. Mani H, Suarez E, Stocker JT. The morphologic spectrum of infantile lobar emphysema: a study of 33 cases. *Paediatr Respir Rev*. 2004;5(suppl A):S313–S320.
29. Moideen I, Nair SG, Cherian A, et al. Congenital lobar emphysema associated with congenital heart disease. *J Cardiothorac Vasc Anesth*. 2006;20:239–241.
30. Ozcelik U, Gocmen A, Kiper N, et al. Congenital lobar emphysema: evaluation and long-term follow-up of thirty cases at a single center. *Pediatr Pulmonol*. 2003;35:384–391.
31. Miller KE, Edwards DK, Hilton S, et al. Acquired lobar emphysema in premature infants with bronchopulmonary dysplasia: an iatrogenic disease? *Radiology*. 1981;138:589–592.
32. McAdams RM. Risk factors and clinical outcomes of pulmonary interstitial emphysema in extremely low birth weight infants. *J Perinatol*. 2006;26:521–522; author reply 522–523.
33. O'Donovan D, Wearden M, Adams J. Unilateral pulmonary interstitial emphysema following pneumonia in a preterm infant successfully treated with prolonged selective bronchial intubation. *Am J Perinatol*. 1999;16:327–331.
34. Stocker JT, Madewell JE. Persistent interstitial pulmonary emphysema: another complication of the respiratory distress syndrome. *Pediatrics*. 1977;59:847–857.
35. Stocker JT. Postinfarction peripheral cysts of the lung. *Pediatr Pathol*. 1987;7:111–117.
36. Gonzalez OR, Gomez IG, Recalde AL, et al. Postnatal development of the cystic lung lesion of Down syndrome: suggestion that the cause is reduced formation of peripheral air spaces. *Pediatr Pathol*. 1991;11:623–633.

12 Pulmonary Hypoplasia

Jennifer M. Boland, M.D., and Marie-Christine Aubry, M.D.

Definition

Pulmonary hypoplasia (PH) is an incomplete development of the lung, primarily due to a decreased amount of alveolated parenchyma, although the number of airways is also decreased.[1] This leads to abnormally low lung weight and small size, and usually a decreased alveolar radial count, which is a measure used to estimate number of alveoli per unit area.[1,2] The reported incidence of PH in the general population ranges between 9 and 14/10,000 births.[3,4] The estimated prevalence of some degree of PH from neonatal autopsy series ranges between 7% and 26%,[3,5] and involvement may vary from an isolated lobe to complete involvement of bilateral lungs.[5]

Etiology and Pathogenesis

PH can be primary or secondary.[1,6] Primary PH is characterized by isolated PH in the absence of other congenital anatomic abnormalities. It is thought to be extremely rare at 0.8 to 1.6 per 10,000 births[3,4] and can be caused by a catastrophic congenital developmental abnormality such as acinar dysplasia.[7] Other embryologic defects of the lung or vascular tissue may cause PH, or it may be secondary to an in utero vascular accident. Some examples of primary PH may show no obvious histopathologic abnormalities but have an abnormally low lung weight to body weight ratio and/or radial alveolar count (see below).[6] Most cases of primary PH are sporadic, although familial cases have been reported.[8,9] Primary PH may involve a unilateral lung.[5]

TABLE 12.1 Causes of Pulmonary Hypoplasia

Thoracic etiologies	• Diaphragmatic hernia
	• Hydrops fetalis with pleural effusions
	• Intrathoracic tumor or cystic lesion (Chapter 11)
	• Chronic elevation of the diaphragm with cavity compression
	  • Abdominal mass
	  • Ascites
	• Obstruction of the upper respiratory tract

Extrathoracic etiologies	• Oligohydramnios
	  • Premature rupture of membranes
	  • Anuric genitourinary anomalies
	    • Renal agenesis
	    • Polycystic disease
	    • Outflow obstruction
	• Neuromuscular and central nervous disorders
	  • Anencephaly
	• Skeletal disorders
	  • Chondrodystrophies/skeletal dysplasia
	  • Osteogenesis imperfecta
	• Chromosomal abnormalities

The vast majority of PH is secondary to another fetal abnormality (Table 12.1). Normal fetal lung growth is dependent on a number of physical factors including adequate intrathoracic space, sufficient volume of amniotic fluid, normal fetal breathing movements, and balance of fluid volume/pressure. Thus, any fetal, maternal, or placental abnormalities that interfere with these factors may potentially lead to PH. These abnormalities classically cause either intrathoracic or extrathoracic compression of the lungs with subsequent impairment of lung development (congenital diaphragmatic hernia, thoracic cysts and masses, etc.) or decreased amount of amniotic fluid reaching the alveolated parenchyma in utero (urogenital abnormalities, upper airway abnormalities, anencephaly, premature rupture of membranes, etc.).[1,10,11]

Clinical Presentation, Radiology, and Outcome

The clinical presentation and outcome of PH vary with its severity. Most cases are rapidly lethal,[2,6] with a mortality rate of 50% to 80%.[4] However, there are some sublethal forms,[6] and the clinical manifestations of PH depend on the severity of the respiratory underdevelopment, which in turn depends on the underlying etiology and the gestational age of occurrence. For example, as would be expected, survival of infants with PH due to premature rupture of membranes depends on the gestational age at which rupture occurred.[12] One study of fetuses and infants experiencing sudden unexplained death found a high incidence of PH and brainstem hypodevelopment, suggesting that subclinical cases of PH occur, possibly due to developmental issues involving the brainstem, and this may put infants at risk for sudden unexplained death.[13]

The clinical presentation of PH may vary from the classic lethal form with severe respiratory failure and hypoxemia leading to early neonatal death[6] to less severe forms characterized by respiratory insufficiency with hemorrhage, bronchopulmonary dysplasia, or even mild respiratory symptoms in some cases. In most secondary cases of PH, the etiology is clear and the diagnosis of PH is easily made. However, some cases of primary PH may present with hypoxia and clear small lung fields, and it may be unclear that PH is the underlying cause, with other entities such as congenital heart disease and persistent fetal circulation entering the differential diagnosis.[6] At birth, PH due to a space-occupying lesion is suspected in infants with respiratory distress who have decreased breath sounds on one side and contralateral shift of the heart sounds. Primary treatment is surgical excision/repair of the mass lesion (if present) with subsequent supportive care to provide oxygenation while pulmonary growth occurs.[6,14] Outcome will depend on the severity of the hypoplasia and ability for the lung to maintain

adequate gas exchange.[6] If PH is the result of decreased amniotic fluid or other etiologies, the infant will have small clear lung fields on chest radiograph.[6] Treatment is supportive with mechanical ventilation as needed, which is commonly complicated by air leaks with pneumothorax and pulmonary interstitial emphysema.[6] Extracorporeal membrane oxygenation (ECMO) may be successfully used for patients with PH, with survival observed in infants having lung volumes at least 45% predicted for age-matched controls.[15]

Predicting PH on prenatal imaging is challenging. 2-D ultrasound has many limitations, but in the setting of a congenital diaphragmatic hernia, the lung-to-head ratio (LHR) is a valid predictor of PH survival rates, with 0% survival if LHR is <0.6 and 100% survival if if >1.4 (intermediate values associated with a wide survival range of 38% to 61%).[4,16,17] The effects of gestational age can be controlled by comparing the observed LHR to the predicted LHR for gestational age (observed to expected LHR).[18] 3-D ultrasound is better for evaluating PH, with a sensitivity of 92% to 94% and specificity of 82% to 84%.[4,19,20] The prenatal diagnosis of a treatable underlying disorder is important, as this may lead to the consideration of in utero prenatal treatment to potentially reverse or decrease the severity of PH.

Pathologic Findings

The morphologic appearance of PH varies, and some of this variation may be explained by the gestational age at which the underlying cause occurred. Thus, it is important to have some understanding of normal lung development (Table 12.2; Fig. 12.1).[21]

TABLE 12.2 Stages of Normal Lung Development

Stage	Specific Development
Embryonic stage: 22 d to 6–8 wk, development of proximal airways	Day 22: Pulmonary primordium develops from ventral aspect of the foregut. Day 26: Division of right and left "lung buds" Day 33: Pulmonary lobe development—main bronchi with division into 3 right branches and 2 left branches Day 41: Formation of the bronchopulmonary segments by asymmetric dichotomy Day 48: Completion of the first generation of bronchi—as the airways develop, the adjacent mesenchyme develops into blood vessels, smooth muscle, and connective tissue
Pseudoglandular stage: 6–8 to 16 wk, development of conducting airways	Continuation of the bronchial development until completion Respiratory channels are smooth walled with blind ending, lined by cuboidal epithelium, separated by sparsely cellular thick interstitial septa. Capillaries are found in the epithelial tissue
Canalicular stage: 17th to 28th wk, acinar development	Development of the acinus with further subdivision of the airways between the terminal bronchioles and the periphery with increase in the radial alveolar count Thinning of the airway epithelium and development of the distal pulmonary circulation, which allows for gas exchange. Capillaries develop in a subepithelial orientation. Type II pneumocytes differentiate.
Saccular stage: 28th to 36th wk, development of sites for gas exchange	Subdivision of saccules and production of surfactant starting 32–36 wk Completion of the vascularization and thinning of the interstitium with rapid increase in the gas exchange surface
Alveolar stage: 36th wk to term (and up to 4–8 y of age), increase in surface area for gas exchange	Development of alveoli. Majority of alveoli formed after birth, mostly in the first 2 y. The epithelial lining becomes thinner, type I pneumocytes develop, and adjacent capillaries bulge into the alveolar lumen. Preacinar arteries and veins develop along with the major airways and the intra-acinar arteries and veins develop within the alveoli.

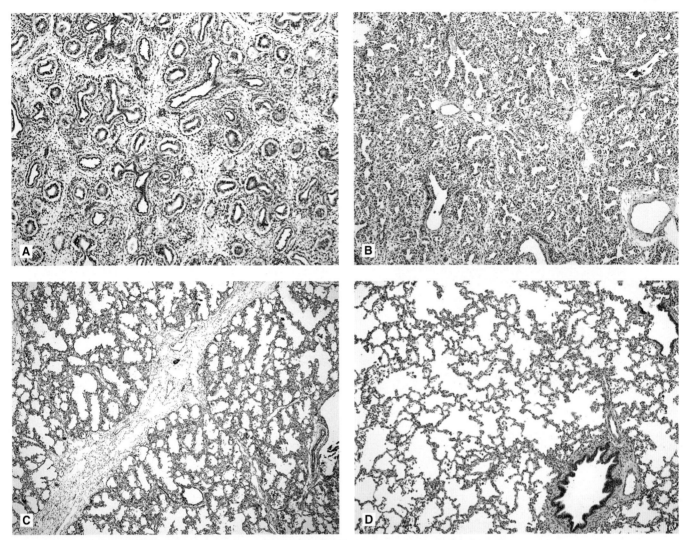

FIGURE 12.1 ▲ Representative photomicrographs of fetal lungs at different stages of development.
A. Pseudoglandular stage: The conducting airways are forming, represented by tubules lined by cuboidal epithelium and separated by abundant hypovascular mesenchymal tissue. **B.** Canalicular stage: Acinar structures
appear, with associated increased vascularity of the stroma. **C.** Saccular stage: The airspace walls thin and
become more compact, with closer approximation of the interstitial capillaries to the acinar epithelium. **D.** Alveolar
stage: Terminal airspaces have thin walls containing a single capillary directly opposed to the pneumocytes, and
there is secondary branching of the alveolar walls.

Grossly, at autopsy, lungs in PH appear to have normal anatomy
with normal lobation but are often conspicuously small compared
to the other organs (Fig. 12.2). When assessing for PH, the most
important diagnostic criteria is the lung weight to body weight ratio
(LBWR). The normal mean LBWR is 0.018 ± 0.003, with a range
of 0.012 to 0.025. For gestational age <28 weeks, PH is diagnosed
if the LBWR is 0.015 or less.[4] For gestations of 28 weeks or greater,
LBWR <0.012 is used to diagnose PH.[2,4] When a borderline LBWR is
observed (0.013 to 0.017), evaluation using another method such as
radial alveolar count may be helpful to further support or refute the
diagnosis of PH.

Some authors have suggested that LBWR may not be accurate in
secondary disease states, which may artificially increase lung weight,
including conditions that cause pulmonary edema, hemorrhage, or
infection.[22] Therefore, these authors have recommended assessing
lung volume instead of lung weight, especially in cases that have a
risk factor for PH (rupture of membranes, chromosomal abnormalities, etc.) but a normal LBWR.[4,22] This can be performed by inflating
the lungs at standardized pressure, with volumes determined by a
water immersion method.[22] More studies are needed to confirm these
findings.

Radial alveolar count (RAC) is considered another objective measurement of lung development, as it assesses the number of alveoli,
which is unaffected by any state of expansion. The mean RAC is
dependent on gestational age; therefore, values should be compared
to a chart of average/standard deviation for a given age.[23] The measurement of RAC is performed by dropping a perpendicular line
from the center of a terminal bronchiole to the edge of the acinus
(pleura or interlobular septum) and counting the number of alveoli
traversed by the line.[23] Since the most dramatic increase in RAC
takes place after 32 weeks, this measure of PH is more useful at later
stage of development (i.e., late secular and alveolar). The RAC should
be compared to mean for gestational age, and a value <75% of the
mean could be suggestive of PH.[2] However, it should be noted that
alveolar simplification with decreased RAC can be observed secondary to many other causes, including chronic neonatal lung disease
of prematurity and other developmental/chromosomal abnormalities (Down syndrome, etc.), and thus, a decreased RAC alone is not
diagnostic of PH.

Histologically, hypoplastic lungs often appear immature for gestational age but may otherwise show no diagnostic abnormalities (Fig.
12.3). This immaturity is usually easy to recognize when severe, and the

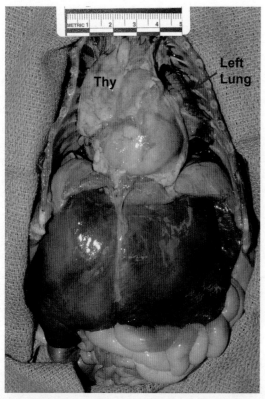

FIGURE 12.2 ▲ Gross photographs of an infant born at 36 weeks, with pulmonary hypoplasia secondary to bilateral multicystic dysplastic kidneys and resultant anhydramnios. The hypoplastic lungs are very small for gestational age (lung weight to body weight ratio = 0.0065) and barely visible behind the heart and thymus. (Thy, thymus)

but often have alveolar simplification (decreased number of alveoli per unit area/volume), which can be detected by performing a radial alveolar count.[1] Careful examination of the interstitium should also be performed, since alveolar stage lungs have very thin septa with a single capillary directly under the pneumocytes, whereas saccular stage lungs have a thicker interstitium with more interstitial mesenchymal tissue. After 16 weeks (postpseudoglandular stage), acinar complexity and maturation may be impaired, but airway branching remains unaffected. Since growth of vessels parallels airway development, PH also results in abnormalities of the vascular bed, including a decrease in the number of vessels, an increase in the smooth muscle of the arterial wall with increased wall thickness, and peripheral extension of smooth muscle into the smaller arteries.[15]

It should be noted that there may be secondary superimposed histologic patterns in patients with PH, especially those who survive for some period after birth. These secondary changes could include hyaline membrane disease,[10] pulmonary interstitial emphysema, infection, and chronic neonatal lung disease of prematurity. Presence of these secondary changes depends on the gestational age at birth, need for mechanical ventilation, and other complications of the child's clinical course. These conditions may partially obscure changes in the background lung, alter lung weight and RAC, and make diagnosis of PH much more challenging.

Practical Points

▶ PH is an incomplete development of the lung, which is diagnosed by a decreased lung weight to body weight ratio. Decreased radial alveolar count is another measurement that may be useful in the diagnosis of PH.

▶ PH is most often secondary to an underlying etiology resulting in decreased thoracic space with lung compression, or decrease in amniotic fluid. Rarely, PH may be primary.

▶ Grossly, hypoplastic lungs usually appear anatomically normal although much smaller in comparison to other intrathoracic organ. Histologically, the lung often appears more immature than expected for the gestational age or shows alveolar simplification.

most severe forms may have total agenesis of acinar structures, resembling the pseudoglandular phase of fetal development.[7] If PH develops before 16 weeks gestational age, bronchiolar branching, cartilage development, acinar complexity, and maturation are all reduced, and vascularization and thinning of the air–blood barrier retarded. However, the histologic immaturity may be much more difficult to recognize in less severe cases, when lungs may appear quite histologically normal

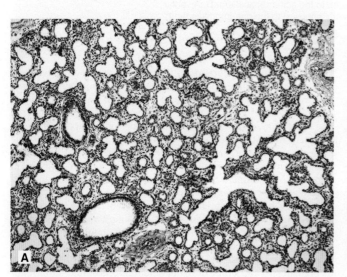

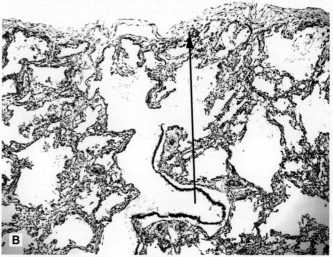

FIGURE 12.3 ▲ The microscopic appearance of hypoplastic lungs is variable. Lungs often show obvious immaturity for gestational age (**A**, 32 weeks fetus, but lungs resemble canalicular phase of development). Other cases are more subtle, with alveolar simplification (**B**), best detected by performing a radial alveolar count (indicated by the *arrow*, only three alveoli traversed when crossing from terminal bronchiole to pleural surface).

REFERENCES

1. Reale FR, Esterly JR. Pulmonary hypoplasia: a morphometric study of the lungs of infants with diaphragmatic hernia, anencephaly, and renal malformations. *Pediatrics.* 1973;51(1):91–96.
2. Askenazi SS, Perlman M. Pulmonary hypoplasia: lung weight and radial alveolar count as criteria of diagnosis. *Arch Dis Child.* 1979;54(8):614–618.
3. Lauria MR, Gonik B, Romero R. Pulmonary hypoplasia: pathogenesis, diagnosis, and antenatal prediction. *Obstet Gynecol.* 1995;86(3):466–475.
4. Vergani P. Prenatal diagnosis of pulmonary hypoplasia. *Curr Opin Obstet Gynecol.* 2012;24(2):89–94.
5. Abrams ME, Ackerman VL, Engle WA. Primary unilateral pulmonary hypoplasia: neonate through early childhood—case report, radiographic diagnosis and review of the literature. *J Perinatol.* 2004;24(10):667–670.
6. Swischuk LE, Richardson CJ, Nichols MM, et al. Primary pulmonary hypoplasia in the neonate. *J Pediatr.* 1979;95(4):573–577.
7. Davidson LA, Batman P, Fagan DG. Congenital acinar dysplasia: a rare cause of pulmonary hypoplasia. *Histopathology.* 1998;32(1):57–59.
8. Frey B, Fleischhauer A, Gersbach M. Familial isolated pulmonary hypoplasia: a case report, suggesting autosomal recessive inheritance. *Eur J Pediatr.* 1994;153(6):460–463.
9. Green RA, Shaw DG, Haworth SG. Familial pulmonary hypoplasia: plain film appearances with histopathological correlation. *Pediatr Radiol.* 1999;29(6):455–458.
10. Nakamura Y, Funatsu Y, Yamamoto I, et al. Potter's syndrome associated with renal agenesis or dysplasia. Morphological and biochemical study of the lung. *Arch Pathol Lab Med.* 1985;109(5):441–444.
11. Nakamura Y, Harada K, Yamamoto I, et al. Human pulmonary hypoplasia. Statistical, morphological, morphometric, and biochemical study. *Arch Pathol Lab Med.* 1992;116(6):635–642.
12. van Teeffelen AS, van der Ham DP, Oei SG, et al. The accuracy of clinical parameters in the prediction of perinatal pulmonary hypoplasia secondary to midtrimester prelabour rupture of fetal membranes: a meta-analysis. *Eur J Obstet Gynecol Reprod Biol.* 2010;148(1):3–12.
13. Ottaviani G, Mingrone R, Lavezzi AM, et al. Infant and perinatal pulmonary hypoplasia frequently associated with brainstem hypodevelopment. *Virchows Arch.* 2009;454(4):451–456.
14. Porter HJ. Pulmonary hypoplasia—size is not everything. *Virchows Arch.* 1998;432(1):3–6.
15. Thibeault DW, Haney B. Lung volume, pulmonary vasculature, and factors affecting survival in congenital diaphragmatic hernia. *Pediatrics.* 1998;101(2):289–295.
16. Metkus AP, Filly RA, Stringer MD, et al. Sonographic predictors of survival in fetal diaphragmatic hernia. *J Pediatr Surg.* 1996;31(1):148–151; discussion 151–152.
17. Lipshutz GS, Albanese CT, Feldstein VA, et al. Prospective analysis of lung-to-head ratio predicts survival for patients with prenatally diagnosed congenital diaphragmatic hernia. *J Pediatr Surg.* 1997;32(11):1634–1636.
18. Jani J, Nicolaides KH, Keller RL, et al. Observed to expected lung area to head circumference ratio in the prediction of survival in fetuses with isolated diaphragmatic hernia. *Ultrasound Obstet Gynecol.* 2007;30(1):67–71.
19. Gerards FA, Twisk JW, Fetter WP, et al. Two- or three-dimensional ultrasonography to predict pulmonary hypoplasia in pregnancies complicated by preterm premature rupture of the membranes. *Prenat Diagn.* 2007;27(3):216–221.
20. Vergani P, Andreani M, Greco M, et al. Two- or three-dimensional ultrasonography: which is the best predictor of pulmonary hypoplasia? *Prenat Diagn.* 2010;30(9):834–838.
21. Sherer DM, Davis JM, Woods JR Jr. Pulmonary hypoplasia: a review. *Obstet Gynecol Surv.* 1990;45(11):792–803.
22. De Paepe ME, Shapiro S, Hansen K, et al. Postmortem lung volume/body weight standards for term and preterm infants. *Pediatr Pulmonol.* 2014;49(1):60–66.
23. Emery JL, Mithal A. The number of alveoli in the terminal respiratory unit of man during late intrauterine life and childhood. *Arch Dis Child.* 1960;35:544–547.

13 Congenital Pulmonary Vascular Disease

Allen P. Burke, M.D., and Jennifer M. Boland, M.D.

Persistent Pulmonary Hypertension of the Newborn

Etiology and Clinical Findings

Persistent pulmonary hypertension of the newborn (PPHN) is characterized by markedly increased pulmonary vascular resistance without clear etiology. It is likely a heterogeneous group of disorders with various causes. Its estimated incidence is 1.9 per 1,000 live births.[1]

In utero, pulmonary vascular resistance is fairly high and falls rapidly with expansion of the lungs at birth, an 8- to 10-fold increase in pulmonary blood flow, and closure of the ductus arteriosus and fossa ovalis. The failure of arteriolar relaxation and hypoxemia constitutes PPHN. It is associated with impaired function of endothelial nitric oxide synthase and an increase in oxidative stress.[2]

Risk factors for PPHN include Black and Asian race, male gender, and maternal obesity, asthma, and diabetes.[3]

Clinically, infants are cyanotic and hypoxemic with markedly elevated pulmonary arterial pressures. There is poor cardiac output, which may lead to cardiogenic shock. By definition, there is a lack of cardiac shunting due to congenital defects, and persistent elevations of pulmonary vascular resistance cause right-to-left shunting across the ductus arteriosus or foramen ovale. Pulmonary hypertension caused by diseases of prematurity is considered a separate entity; therefore, PPHN is general not diagnosed in infants born <34 weeks gestation.

Conditions that predispose to PPHN include intrapartum asphyxia, infection, pulmonary hypoplasia, and congenital heart disease (excluding intracardiac shunts). There is an association with material use of nonsteroidal anti-inflammatory drugs, which is also implicated in premature ductal closure.[4,5]

Recently, PPHN has been grouped into three etiologic categories[6] (Table 13.1). Although meconium aspiration syndrome is frequently mentioned in conjunction with PPHN, the frequency of PPHN in series of patients with meconium aspiration is low. Deaths are not related to PPHN, but rather intrauterine asphyxia with neurologic deficits, or associated congenital anomalies.[7]

Radiologic Findings

Chest x-ray is helpful in excluding associated conditions, including consolidation typical of meconium aspiration syndrome, congenital diaphragmatic hernia, and congenital pulmonary airway malformations (CPAMs). Pulmonary arterial hypertension is manifest by decreased vascular markings. Typically, the cardiac silhouette is normal.

Tissue Sampling

The diagnosis of PPHN is generally made clinically, based on pulmonary hypertension in a term infant, without structural heart disease. The diagnosis is confirmed at autopsy, by demonstration of extension of smooth muscle into distal arterioles.[8]

TABLE 13.1   Persistent Pulmonary Hypertension of the Newborn, Classification by Etiology

Pathophysiologic Grouping	Associated Conditions and Findings
Pulmonary vasoconstriction	Meconium aspiration syndrome Pneumonia Neurologic disease Hypothermia Hypoglycemia
Anatomic decrease in vascular bed	Pulmonary hypoplasia Diaphragmatic hernia
Idiopathic	Arterial remodeling (muscular hypertrophy and muscular extension) Maternal NSAID use (intrauterine NSAID exposure)

Microscopic Findings

The hallmark of PPHN, especially the idiopathic type, is diffuse extension of medial smooth muscle to the precapillary pulmonary arteries[9,10] (Fig. 13.1). Fully muscularized vessels extend as far as the intra-acinar arteries, which are normally nonmuscular at birth. In addition, there is medial hypertrophy of more proximal muscular arteries and arterioles. Morphometric analysis may be helpful in demonstrating medial hypertrophy.[11] There are often superimposed changes related to infectious complications, including pneumonia and alveolar injury (diffuse alveolar damage). Significant meconium aspiration should lead to a diagnosis of meconium aspiration syndrome.

It is not entirely clear if the pulmonary vasculature in cases of PPHN associated with vasospasm or pulmonary hypoplasia shows similar features to the idiopathic form, including muscularization and medial hypertrophy. In a baboon model, neither meconium aspiration nor intrauterine asphyxia resulted in physiologic or histologic changes of PPHN.[12]

Immunohistochemical Stains

Immunohistochemical staining for smooth muscle actin highlights extension of muscular vessels into the alveolar septa (Fig. 13.2).

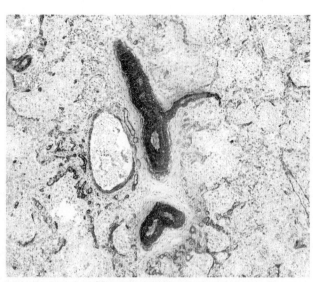

FIGURE 13.2 ▲ Pulmonary hypertension of the newborn. Immunohistochemical staining for smooth muscle actin demonstrates marked medial hypertrophy.

Differential Diagnosis

At autopsy, the main concern is to exclude associated conditions, such as congenital heart defects, pulmonary malformations, and alveolar capillary dysplasia (see below). From a clinical standpoint, the differential diagnosis includes congenital heart disease with left to right shunts, bronchopulmonary dysplasia and respiratory distress syndrome (seen in earlier gestational age), sepsis, and surfactant deficiency. Therefore, it is important for the autopsy pathologist to document an absence of evidence for these alternative conditions, in order to support a diagnosis of PPHN.

Prognosis and Treatment

Therapy includes treatment of any detected underlying causes, sedation, ventilation, and pharmacologic measures aimed at dilating the pulmonary vessels.[1,2] Efforts to maintain cardiac output and oxygenation may include extracorporeal membrane oxygenation (ECMO). The mortality is ~10%.[1]

Alveolar Capillary Dysplasia
Background and Clinical Findings

Alveolar capillary dysplasia is a rare lethal condition that was originally described in 1981 as a congenital absence of normal capillary ingrowth in the alveolar septa.[13] Forty cases had been reported by 2000.[14] Since then, there have been more than a dozen additional cases, some with emphasis on misaligned pulmonary veins as a component of the disease.[15] The term "alveolar capillary dysplasia with misalignment of pulmonary veins" has been used to reinforce both components of the malformation.

Related conditions include severe developmental abnormalities such as acinar dysplasia and congenital alveolar dysplasia, both of which lead to severe and generally lethal pulmonary hypoplasia.[16]

A family history of similar disease has been reported in a little over 10% of cases, with several reports in siblings.[14] There is no gender predominance, although one review found a 2:1 female bias.[17] Most infants are full term, with presentations similar to PPHN, including respiratory distress and cyanosis. One-half of patients present within 24 hours, although symptoms may occur as late as 6 weeks. There is a high rate of extrapulmonary anomalies, most commonly involving the gastrointestinal tract (40% of patients) or genitourinary tract (one-third).[17]

The genetic basis for familial disease has been linked to mutations in the *FOXF1* gene[18] located on chromosome 16q24.1. The mechanism involves microdeletion resulting in haploinsufficiency.[19,20]

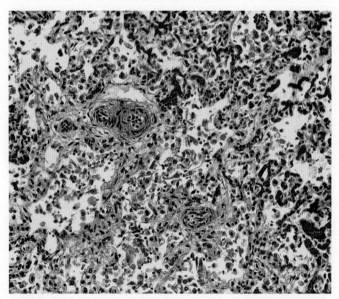

FIGURE 13.1 ▲ Pulmonary hypertension of the newborn. Vessels within the capillary walls (alveolar septa) are focally thickened and muscularized.

Radiologic Findings

Chest radiograph may show normal findings, pneumothoraces, reticular markings, and granular, patchy, or diffuse opacities. Decreased pulmonary vascular markings are rarely seen. Echocardiography demonstrates a right-to-left shunt.[17]

Tissue Sampling

Fewer than one in three cases are diagnosed by open lung biopsy, the remainder diagnosed at autopsy, often in patients with suspected PPHN.[17,18]

Microscopic Findings

The two histopathologic hallmarks of this disease are decreased capillaries in the alveolar septa and misplaced veins in the bronchovascular bundles (Fig. 13.3). Rare capillaries that are present in the alveolar septa are often centrally located, without the proper apposition to the type 1 pneumocytes required to facilitate gas exchange. The histologic appearance is that of alveolar septa with sparse capillaries (Fig. 13.4). Secondary changes of alveolar capillary dysplasia may include muscularization of distal arterioles and medial hypertrophy of small arteries. Bronchovascular bundles should normally only contain an airway, artery, and lymphatics; veins are normally localized to the interlobular septa, so presence of veins in the bronchovascular bundles is distinctly abnormal. The misplaced veins may be patchy, leading to a diagnosis of PPHN on biopsy and alveolar capillary dysplasia at autopsy. The misplaced veins are usually present between the arteries and airways.

Immunohistochemical Studies

Two cases of alveolar capillary dysplasia were evaluated immunohistochemically for CD117, showing decreased CD117-positive spindle cells in the alveolar septa, in contrast to controls. This finding was interpreted as a lack of interstitial cells forming the pulmonary capillaries.[21] The diagnostic utility of this finding has not been reproduced at this time.

Differential Diagnosis

Clinically, alveolar capillary dysplasia is not distinguishable from PPHN. Pathologically, there is an overlap with PPHN, the diagnosis depending on the finding of misaligned veins within the bronchovascular bundles and abnormal paucity of alveolar capillaries.

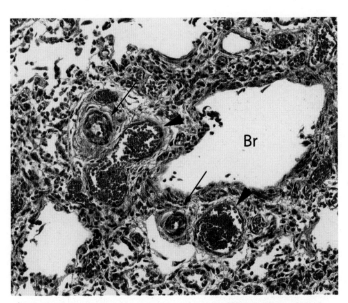

FIGURE 13.3 ▲ Alveolar capillary dysplasia with misalignment of pulmonary veins. The bronchiole (Br) is denuded secondary to autolysis in this autopsy specimen. The small arteries (*arrows*) are present with the thin-walled veins (*arrowheads*) in the bronchovascular bundle.

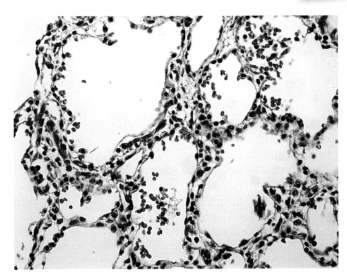

FIGURE 13.4 ▲ Alveolar capillary dysplasia. Note the paucity of identifiable capillaries in the alveolar septa.

Prognosis and Treatment

Alveolar capillary dysplasia is a uniformly lethal disease, with lung transplantation the only theoretical definitive treatment. There are rare reports of prolonged life, up to 7 months.[22] Treatment includes high-frequency oscillatory ventilation, infusion of magnesium sulfate, dopamine, dobutamine, nitric oxide inhalation therapy, and ECMO, similar to PPHN.[14,23]

Pulmonary Lymphangiomatosis

Terminology and Clinical Findings

Lymphangiomatosis is a progressive disease of an abnormal and extensive proliferation of lymph channels that typically involves multiple sites, most frequently the skeleton, abdomen (especially spleen), and thorax. When the predominant symptoms occur from involvement of the lungs, the term pulmonary lymphangiomatosis is used. "Lymphangiomatosis" is distinguished from localized or isolated lymphangiomas, which, in the thorax, are typically limited to the pericardium or pleura and do not involve lung parenchyma. The designation "thoracic lymphangiomatosis" denotes lesions of the lung, pleura, heart, or thymus.[24] Rarely, lymphangiomatosis is confined to the lung without imaging evidence of lesions outside the lungs and pleura.[25]

Patients typically become symptomatic as children, often with bone fractures, ascites, chylous pleural effusions, and gastrointestinal complaints. With isolated pulmonary involvement, the mean age at presentation is 10 years, with bilateral lower lobe infiltrates, with mixed obstructive and restrictive lung parameters.[25] Occasionally, the dominant presenting symptom is disseminated intravascular coagulation[24,26] (Table 13.2).

TABLE 13.2 **Presenting and Associated Features of Thoracic Lymphangiomatosis**

Feature	Rate
Chylothorax	49%
Pulmonary infiltrates	45%
Bone lesions	39%
Splenic lesions	15%
Disseminated intravascular coagulation	9%
Skin lesions	7%

Data from Alvarez OA, Kjellin I, Zuppan CW. Thoracic lymphangiomatosis in a child. *J Pediatr Hematol Oncol.* 2004;26:136–141.

Radiologic Findings

Chest radiographs typically demonstrate lower lung opacities and reticular densities. If there is concomitant bone involvement, lytic lesions may be present in the ribs and vertebrae.[27] There is frequently a mediastinal mass that may involve surrounding structures. The lesions are typically described as sharply defined, nonenhanced cystic lesions on MR and CT scans.[28]

Tissue Sampling

Open lung biopsy is the most definitive means of diagnosis.[25] The diagnosis has been reportedly established by transbronchial biopsy.[29]

Microscopic Findings

Histologically, there is a proliferation of lymphangioma-like vessels, present in lymphatic distribution, especially along the pleura and interlobular septa. The lymphatic vessels are lined by endothelial cells that express factor VIII-related antigen, CD31, *Ulex europaeus* lectin, and D2-40 (Fig. 13.5).[25,27] D2-40 expression has been described in a case of mediastinal lymphangiomatosis.[30] There is prominent smooth muscle in the interstitium of the lymphatic proliferation that expresses actin, desmin, and progesterone receptor. In contrast to lymphangioleiomyomatosis, the intervening cells are negative for HMB-45.

Differential Diagnosis

Despite the similar name, there are few histologic and clinical features that pulmonary lymphangiomatosis shares with lymphangioleiomyomatosis. The latter is a disease of childbearing women and is a PEComa characterized by multiple lung cysts and a proliferation of HMB-45-positive smooth muscle cells (see Chapter 71). An even more rare condition, primary pulmonary lymphangiectasia,[31] may cause diagnostic difficulties.

Prognosis and Treatment

Treatment of localized or isolated lymphangiomas includes surgery, pleurectomy, pleurodesis, thoracic duct ligation, radiation therapy, and percutaneous doxycycline.[27] For diffuse disease, intravenous interferon has been attempted, but patients must continue infusions indefinitely. Steroids, tamoxifen, and propranolol are other systemic therapies that have variable success.[26,32] Lung transplantation may be necessary in progressive diffuse disease.[33] There is evidence that presentation in adulthood imparts a better outcome.[34] The overall mortality in children is 39%, compared to 0% in adults.[24]

Primary Pulmonary Lymphangiectasia

Primary pulmonary lymphangiectasia is a rare disease of children associated with chronic bronchial infections, obstructive lung symptoms, hyperinflated lungs, and dilated lymphatics within the bronchovascular bundles on biopsy or wedge resection. Similar to lymphangiectasis in other organ sites, secondary causes of lymphatic dilatation are excluded before a diagnosis of idiopathic process is applied.

A series of over 2,000 infant autopsies showed that just under 0.5% demonstrated pulmonary features of lymphangiectasia. A majority of these patients had obstruction at the left of the heart, usually in the form of total anomalous pulmonary venous connections, indicating that in most cases pulmonary lymphangiectasia is secondary.[35]

The findings of primary pulmonary lymphangiectasia (PPL) include septal edema and prominent lymphatics, which are nonspecific and may be seen in pulmonary outflow obstruction of a variety of causes. In contrast to lymphangiomatosis, the dilated vessels do not form anastomosing channels with intervening smooth muscle bundles or significant fibrosis.

Pulmonary Arteriovenous Malformations

Background

Pulmonary arteriovenous malformations (PAVMs) are congenital connections between arteries and veins, often with an aneurysmal component. In most patients, PAVMs are a manifestation of Osler-Weber-Rendu syndrome (hereditary hemorrhagic telangiectasia, or HHT). The incidence of PAVM reflects that of HHT, whose incidence is estimated to be about one in 5,000, or 0.02% of the population. About 30% of patients with HHT have pulmonary involvement.[36] In one study, 25 of 31 patients with PAVM had other clinical findings of HHT.[37]

Clinical and Imaging Findings

General clinical findings of HHT include telangiectasias, especially involving the face, fingers, and oral cavity; epistaxis; family history; and AVMs, which most commonly involve the gastrointestinal tract, followed by the lung, liver, brain, and spine.[36] There is no gender predominance. Most patients with symptomatic pulmonary involvement are diagnosed prior to the age of 20 years. The patients may be followed for many years prior to treatment, which may occur in the fourth and fifth decades.[37]

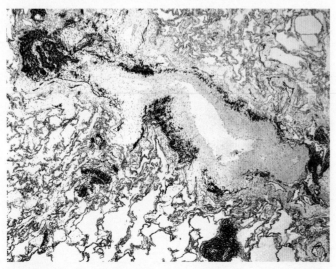

FIGURE 13.5 ▲ Lymphangiomatosis. A D2-40 immunohistochemical stain shows a proliferation of lymphatics.

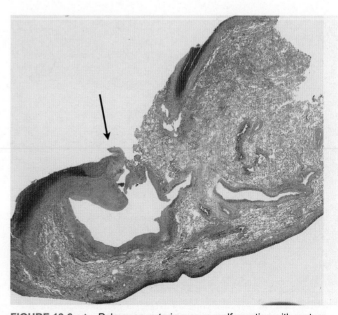

FIGURE 13.6 ▲ Pulmonary arteriovenous malformation with rupture into the pleural cavity. There are dilated vessels, with one aneurysm, that ruptured into the pleural cavity (*arrow*), resulting in hemorrhagic pleuritis.

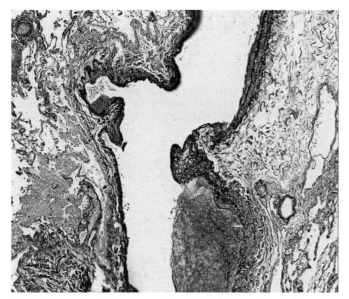

FIGURE 13.7 ▲ Pulmonary arteriovenous malformation. A junction of artery and vein shows the artery at the top, with distinct media, entering a venous channel below with marked intimal thickening.

Pulmonary AVMs are often clinically silent. Pulmonary symptoms occur in about one-half of patients and include dyspnea, hemoptysis, clubbing, and cyanosis. Embolic phenomena related to paradoxical embolism are frequent and include stroke and cerebral abscess. Rupture of PAVM with hemothorax is rare but a potentially lethal complication, which may be the presenting symptom (Fig. 13.6). Massive intraparenchymal hemorrhage is another rare complication.[38]

Imaging Findings

Pulmonary AVMs are frequently multiple, and most frequently involve the periphery of the lower lobes. The modality of choice for direct embolization treatment is helical CT angiography, which identifies the feeder arteries amenable to embolization, and established right-to-left shunting.[37] Over one-third of patients have enlarged bronchial, phrenic, or internal mammary arteries.[37] On imaging, the mean size is 20 mm, with a range of 8 to 40 mm. For most lesions, there is a single feeding artery, although there may be two and, rarely, three separate vessels entering the lesion. Other imaging techniques, such as endobronchial ultrasound, have been used to detect PAVM.[39]

Pathologic Findings

Histologically, PAVMs consist of dilated, tortuous vessels, both arteries and veins (Fig. 13.6). The venous channels typically are thickened, with increased elastic tissue (Fig. 13.7). In most sections, the communications between the arteries and veins are not apparent. The diagnosis is generally established prior to surgical excision, and many cases are treated with embolization alone, without pathologic sampling.

Treatment

Treatment consists of embolization treatment or surgical excision or a combination of both modalities.[36,37,40,41]

REFERENCES

1. Walsh-Sukys MC, Tyson JE, Wright LL, et al. Persistent pulmonary hypertension of the newborn in the era before nitric oxide: practice variation and outcomes. *Pediatrics.* 2000;105:14–20.
2. Ng C, Franklin O, Vaidya M, et al. Adenosine infusion for the management of persistent pulmonary hypertension of the newborn. *Pediatr Crit Care Med.* 2004;5:10–13.
3. Hernandez-Diaz S, Van Marter LJ, Werler MM, et al. Risk factors for persistent pulmonary hypertension of the newborn. *Pediatrics.* 2007;120:e272–282.
4. Talati AJ, Salim MA, Korones SB. Persistent pulmonary hypertension after maternal naproxen ingestion in a term newborn: a case report. *Am J Perinatol.* 2000;17:69–71.
5. Tarcan A, Gurakan B, Yildirim S, et al. Persistent pulmonary hypertension in a premature newborn after 16 hours of antenatal indomethicin exposure. *J Perinat Med.* 2004;32:98–99.
6. Teng RJ, Wu TJ. Persistent pulmonary hypertension of the newborn. *J Formos Med Assoc.* 2013;112:177–184.
7. Dargaville PA, Copnell B; Australian and New Zealand Neonatal Network. The epidemiology of meconium aspiration syndrome: incidence, risk factors, therapies, and outcome. *Pediatrics.* 2006;117:1712–1721.
8. Codispoti M, Burns JE, Haworth SG, et al. Persistent pulmonary hypertension of the newborn associated with pulmonary atresia and intact interventricular septum. *Heart.* 1999;82:531–533.
9. Tsai CE, Chou YH, Tsou KI, et al. Persistent pulmonary hypertension of the newborn associated with excessive pulmonary arterial muscularization: report of an autopsy case. *J Formos Med Assoc.* 1993;92:842–844.
10. Patterson K, Kapur SP, Chandra RS. Persistent pulmonary hypertension of the newborn: pulmonary pathologic aspects. *Perspect Pediatr Pathol.* 1988;12:139–154.
11. Ohara T, Ogata H, Tezuka F. Histological study of pulmonary vasculature in fatal cases of persistent pulmonary hypertension of the newborn. *Tohoku J Exp Med.* 1991;164:59–66.
12. Cornish JD, Dreyer GL, Snyder GE, et al. Failure of acute perinatal asphyxia or meconium aspiration to produce persistent pulmonary hypertension in a neonatal baboon model. *Am J Obstet Gynecol.* 1994;171:43–49.
13. Janney CG, Askin FB, Kuhn C, III. Congenital alveolar capillary dysplasia—an unusual cause of respiratory distress in the newborn. *Am J Clin Pathol.* 1981;76:722–727.
14. Al-Hathlol K, Phillips S, Seshia MK, et al. Alveolar capillary dysplasia. Report of a case of prolonged life without extracorporeal membrane oxygenation (ECMO) and review of the literature. *Early Hum Dev.* 2000;57:85–94.
15. Galambos C, Sims-Lucas S, Abman SH. Three-dimensional reconstruction identifies misaligned pulmonary veins as intrapulmonary shunt vessels in alveolar capillary dysplasia. *J Pediatr.* 2013.
16. Cazzato S, di Palmo E, Ragazzo V, et al. Interstitial lung disease in children. *Early Hum Dev.* 2013;89(suppl 3):S39–S43.
17. Li N, Zhou XH, Chen HW, et al. [Alveolar capillary dysplasia: a case report and review of literature]. *Zhonghua Er Ke Za Zhi.* 2010;48:674–679.
18. Castilla-Fernandez Y, Copons-Fernandez C, Jordan-Lucas R, et al. Alveolar capillary dysplasia with misalignment of pulmonary veins: concordance between pathological and molecular diagnosis. *J Perinatol.* 2013;33:401–403.
19. Zufferey F, Martinet D, Osterheld MC, et al. 16q24.1 microdeletion in a premature newborn: usefulness of array-based comparative genomic hybridization in persistent pulmonary hypertension of the newborn. *Pediatr Crit Care Med.* 2011;12:e427–e432.
20. Nogee LM. Genetic basis of children's interstitial lung disease. *Pediatr Allergy Immunol Pulmonol.* 2010;23:15–24.
21. Chang KT, Rajadurai VS, Walford NQ, et al. Alveolar capillary dysplasia: absence of CD117 immunoreactivity of putative hemangioblast precursor cells. *Fetal Pediatr Pathol.* 2008;27:127–140.
22. Ahmed S, Ackerman V, Faught P, et al. Profound hypoxemia and pulmonary hypertension in a 7-month-old infant: late presentation of alveolar capillary dysplasia. *Pediatr Crit Care Med.* 2008;9:e43–e46.
23. Hung SP, Huang SH, Wu CH, et al. Misalignment of lung vessels and alveolar capillary dysplasia: a case report with autopsy. *Pediatr Neonatol.* 2011;52:232–236.
24. Alvarez OA, Kjellin I, Zuppan CW. Thoracic lymphangiomatosis in a child. *J Pediatr Hematol Oncol.* 2004;26:136–141.
25. Tazelaar HD, Kerr D, Yousem SA, et al. Diffuse pulmonary lymphangiomatosis. *Hum Pathol.* 1993;24:1313–1322.
26. Tamay Z, Saribeyoglu E, Ones U, et al. Diffuse thoracic lymphangiomatosis with disseminated intravascular coagulation in a child. *J Pediatr Hematol Oncol.* 2005;27:685–687.
27. Ramani P, Shah A. Lymphangiomatosis. Histologic and immunohistochemical analysis of four cases. *Am J Surg Pathol.* 1993;17:329–335.
28. Oztunc F, Koca B, Adaletli I. Generalised lymphangiomatosis in an 8-year-old girl who presented with cardiomegaly. *Cardiol Young.* 2011;21:465–467.
29. Ostertag H. Transbronchial biopsy in pulmonary lymphangiomatosis. *Am J Surg Pathol.* 1995;19:241–242.
30. Ikeda J, Morii E, Tomita Y, et al. Mediastinal lymphangiomatosis coexisting with occult thymic carcinoma. *Virchows Arch.* 2007;450:211–214.

31. Barker PM, Esther CR, Jr, Fordham LA, et al. Primary pulmonary lymphangiectasia in infancy and childhood. *Eur Respir J.* 2004;24:413–419.

32. Ozeki M, Fukao T, Kondo N. Propranolol for intractable diffuse lymphangiomatosis. *N Engl J Med.* 2011;364:1380–1382.

33. Kinnier CV, Eu JP, Davis RD, et al. Successful bilateral lung transplantation for lymphangiomatosis. *Am J Transplant.* 2008;8:1946–1950.

34. Espinosa V, Martin-Achard A, Guinand O. Diffuse pulmonary lymphangiomatosis: case report and literature review. *Rev Med Suisse.* 2012;8:1125–1129.

35. France NE, Brown RJ. Congenital pulmonary lymphangiectasis. Report of 11 examples with special reference to cardiovascular findings. *Arch Dis Child.* 1971;46:528–532.

36. Begbie ME, Wallace GM, Shovlin CL. Hereditary haemorrhagic telangiectasia (Osler-Weber-Rendu syndrome): a view from the 21st century. *Postgrad Med J.* 2003;79:18–24.

37. Brillet PY, Dumont P, Bouaziz N, et al. Pulmonary arteriovenous malformation treated with embolotherapy: systemic collateral supply at multidetector CT angiography after 2–20-year follow-up. *Radiology.* 2007;242:267–276.

38. Supakul N, Fan R, Karmazyn B. A case report: pulmonary venous malformation complicated with pulmonary hemorrhage. *J Pediatr Surg.* 2012;47:e35–e38.

39. Kuo CH, Wang CH, Kuo HP. Pulmonary arteriovenous malformation of Osler-Weber-Rendu syndrome diagnosed by endobronchial ultrasound. *Respirology.* 2007;12:295–298.

40. Georghiou GP, Berman M, Vidne BA, et al. Pulmonary arteriovenous malformation treated by lobectomy. *Eur J Cardiothorac Surg.* 2003;24:328–330.

41. Wechsler J, Jedlicka V, Kerwitzer J, et al. A case of a pulmonary arteriovenous malformation treated by lobectomy. *Acta Chir Hung.* 1999;38:53–55.

14 Lung Disease in Premature Infants

Thais Mauad, M.D., Ph.D., and Jennifer M. Boland, M.D.

Background

One out of every nine live births in the United States and Europe occurs at <37 weeks of gestation, and rates of preterm births are increasing. In countries like the United States, 90% of preterm infants survive, resulting in a high rate of lung disease related to prematurity.

Pulmonary complications of preterm births are seen most frequently in extremely preterm infants (<28 weeks of gestation) and very preterm infants (28 to 31 weeks of gestation). In general, infants born during the canalicular or early saccular stage of lung development have the greatest risk of developing early pulmonary disease and later pulmonary morbidity.

Bronchopulmonary dysplasia (BPD) is the most common chronic lung disease observed as a complication of prematurity. Further, preterm birth predisposes the development of adult respiratory disease, such as asthma and chronic obstructive pulmonary disease.[1]

Stages of Lung Development and Prematurity

The embryonic lung buds appear as early as 3 to 4 weeks of embryonic life. This bud is an outgrowth of the ventral wall of the primitive foregut, the laryngotracheal groove. The stages of lung development are outlined in Chapter 12.

In the *canalicular* stage (16 to 28 weeks gestation), respiratory bronchioles, alveolar ducts, and primitive alveoli are formed. There is differentiation of type I and type II pneumocytes and the formation of the alveolar capillary barrier. At 24 weeks of intrauterine life, surfactant protein is detected, an important milestone in lung growth and maturation. The canalicular stage is characterized by enlargement of the peripheral airways and the formation of saccules (dilatation of the acinar tubules) and thinning of the alveolar walls. There is also incremental increase in surfactant production.[2,3]

The majority of the gas exchange surface is formed during the *saccular–alveolar stage*, occurring at 27 to 28 weeks of gestation and later. The formation of double capillary walled secondary septa and multiplication of alveoli continue rapidly up to 2 to 3 years after birth.[4] A series of hormones, growth factors, and transcriptional factors are involved in each stage of maturation, and deciphering the molecular biology of the developing lung is very important to advance the process of lung regeneration.[5]

It is estimated that there are 20 to 50 million of alveoli at birth, increasing to 300 to 800 million in adulthood. Alveolar size and surface area increase until after adolescence. Postnatal microvascular maturation occurs up to 2 to 3 years of age, involving fusion of double-walled capillaries into mature single layer alveolar walls, allowing for optimal gas exchange. From age 2 years to young adulthood, lung compartments grow in proportion to lung volume and also linearly with body weight.[6]

When preterm delivery occurs at 24 weeks, surfactant deficiency leading to respiratory distress inevitably occurs.[4,6]

Respiratory Distress Syndrome

Definition

Respiratory distress syndrome (RDS) is immature lung disease in a preterm infant resulting from insufficient surfactant.

Incidence and Risk Factors

The overall incidence of RDS is increasing, in part related to the steep rise in the number of multiple births over the past decades. Advances in medical technology and management (antenatal corticosteroids, artificial surfactant, and protective or noninvasive ventilator strategies) have led to increase in the survival of extremely preterm babies born during the late canalicular stage of lung development, when the thinning of the epithelium in terminal bronchioles permits gas exchange and sustains life, but before the terminal airspaces have formed. Survival before this stage of maturation is only possible when extracorporeal oxygenation is provided (margin of viability).[7]

The incidence of RDS decreases with gestational age at birth and is about 70% in infants <32 weeks' gestation.[7]

Males tend to have higher incidence and severity of RDS because of increased circulating androgens, which delays lung maturation. Black infants develop RDS less frequently, and with less severity, compared to other races. Maternal diabetes, caesarean section, and perinatal asphyxia are associated with increased rates of RDS, whereas prolonged rupture of membranes and chronic fetal stress tend to decrease the incidence of RDS. Antenatal administration of corticosteroids decreases the incidence of RDS, but it is believed also to impair microvascular maturation and cause lung growth arrest.[8]

Surfactant Physiology and RDS Pathogenesis

Similar to a soap bubble, the alveolus is characterized by high surface tension generated by molecular forces at an air–liquid interface. The physical integrity of the alveolus is maintained by surfactant, composed mostly of phospholipid, especially phosphatidylcholine, which has surface tension–lowering properties. The surfactant proteins

A, B, and C constitute 10% of the pulmonary surfactant and facilitate the formation of phospholipid films at the air–liquid interface. They also function as host defense proteins.[8]

Surfactant is secreted by type II pneumocytes and stored in lamellar bodies. Secretion of surfactant is promoted by physical stretch of the lungs. The extruded phospholipid combines with four surface active proteins (surfactant proteins A, B, C, and D) to form an ordered complex lattice, known as tubular myelin, which is pivotal to lower alveolar surface tension and prevent acinar collapse.

Surfactant appears in the fetal lung by 23 to 24 weeks of gestation, but adequate physiologic amounts of surfactant are not secreted until 35 weeks of gestation, when the incidence of RDS decreases significantly. In the very immature infant, an excessively compliant chest wall and weakness of the respiratory muscles also contribute to alveolar collapse.

Alveolar collapse causes alteration in the relationship between ventilation and perfusion, producing a pulmonary shunt with hypoxemia and metabolic acidosis and pulmonary vasoconstriction. Pulmonary hypertension may produce left-to-right shunt through a patent foramen ovale and ductus arteriosus, worsening the hypoxemia. Pulmonary blood flow eventually increases due to the persistence of the ductus arteriosus and reduction in pulmonary vascular resistance, culminating in the accumulation of fluid and proteins in the alveolar spaces.[9]

Clinical Findings

Neonates with RDS typically present with nonspecific tachypnea, expiratory grunting, nasal flaring, cyanosis, and intercostal retractions. Radiologically, the lungs show decreased lung expansion, symmetric generalized consolidation, effacement of normal pulmonary vessels, and air bronchograms.[9]

Pathologic Findings

Macroscopically, the lungs appear solid and congested, with diffuse atelectasis, sometimes being referred as lung hepatization. There may be grossly discernable areas of collapsed alveoli intermingled with distended ones, especially when artificial ventilation has taken place.

Microscopically, hyaline membranes are the characteristic lesions of RDS (Fig. 14.1). Hyaline membranes appear as early as 3 to 4 hours after birth, but are usually well established by 12 to 24 hours. They are smooth, homogeneous, eosinophilic membranes that line the terminal bronchioles and alveolar ducts. They are composed of fibrin, debris from dead epithelial cells, and plasma exudate.

The clearance of hyaline membranes occurs by alveolar macrophages, when hyaline membranes detach from the alveolar or bronchiolar walls

and organize into the acinar lumen or are organized into the alveolar septa.[8] During the organizing phase, there is associated alveolar septal thickening by type 2 pneumocyte hyperplasia, often accompanied by interstitial fibroblastic proliferation and edema. Coexisting infection may lead to increased numbers of neutrophils, but marked inflammatory infiltrates are generally not observed in isolated RDS.

Treatment

Progress in medical management, particularly the use of surfactant replacement therapy and efficient mechanical ventilation, has improved survival of very low birth neonates (23 to 24 weeks of gestation). Optimal treatment includes acceleration of prenatal lung maturation with steroid therapy, early treatment with continuous positive airway pressure, and minimally invasive modes of surfactant administration, including aerosolized delivery that does not require tracheal intubation.[10,11]

Chronic Lung Disease of Prematurity and Bronchopulmonary Dysplasia

Incidence and Risk Factors

Chronic lung disease of prematurity (CLDP, also known as bronchopulmonary dysplasia—BPD) occurs most frequently in infants with birth weights <1,000 to 1,500 g who were treated for RDS. CLDP develops in 10% to 40% of very low-weight and extremely low-weight infants.

Clinical Definition

The National Institute for Child Health and Human Development Network defined diagnostic criteria for CLDP/BPD in children with gestational age less or greater than 32 weeks. Patients are categorized according to the severity of their disease, that is, the necessity and extent of oxygen supplementation received for at least 28 postnatal days.[12]

Incidence

With the increase in survival of preterm infants, the incidence of CLDP has also increased. Nearly 70% of the extremely immature infants develop CLDP/BPD.[13]

Etiology

The etiology of CLDP/BPD is multifactorial. Preterm lungs have poorly developed airway-supporting structures, surfactant deficiency, decreased compliance, poorly developed antioxidant mechanisms,

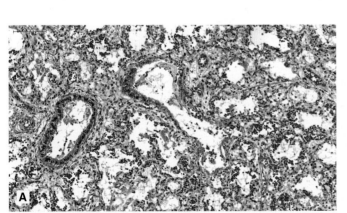
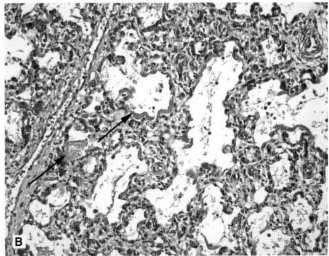

FIGURE 14.1 ▲ Respiratory distress syndrome. **A.** Lung of a premature infant with hyaline membranes; homogenous deposition of fibrin along the alveolar duct and alveolar walls. **B.** Observe the immature aspect of the alveolar septa, with double-layered capillary walls. *Arrows* point to hyaline membranes.

and inadequate fluid clearance. Inflammation caused by mechanical ventilation, oxygen toxicity, and infection may also play an important role in its development.

Clinical Findings

Most infants that go on to develop CLDP are ventilator-dependent, preterm babies with severe RDS requiring surfactant therapy. The evolution to CLDP/BPD is recognized at 2 weeks of age, as pulmonary function deteriorates rather than improves. Infants are usually tachypneic, with audible crackles, and may have mild to severe retractions, remaining ventilator dependent.

Most infants gradually improve during the next 3 to 4 months, and oxygen requirements tend to decrease, although infants with severe CLDP/BPD may remain ventilator dependent. Infants with the severe form of the disease may also develop hypertension and cor pulmonale. Increased pulmonary resistance may affect lymphatic drainage and exacerbate interstitial edema. Anastomoses between pulmonary and systemic vessels may worsen pulmonary hypertension.

Imaging

In the early phase, chest radiograph becomes diffusely hazy with ground-glass shadows, indicating inflammation and edema, with normal or low volumes. The chest radiograph of patients with later stages of BPD shows hyperinflation, streaky densities, or cystic areas, an appearance that has come to be called "bubbly lungs."[14]

Pathologic Findings

The pathologic changes observed in CLDP have changed over time, with the advent of exogenous surfactant supplementation and more advantageous mechanical ventilation strategies. The main characteristic of "modern BPD" in the era of advanced therapies is disruption or arrested acinar development, leading to alveolar simplification (Fig. 14.2). Lungs show an oversimplified acinar morphology due to decreased alveolar septation and hypoplasia, which can be confirmed using radial alveolar count (see Chapter 12).[8] Protective management

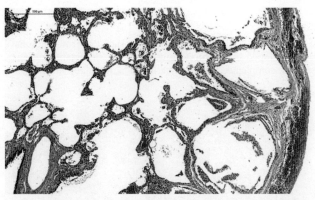

FIGURE 14.2 ▲ Bronchopulmonary dysplasia (chronic lung disease of prematurity). The alveolar spaces are simplified and enlarged, with mild septal thickening near the pleural surface.

and surfactant therapy have reduced the incidence of necrotizing bronchiolitis and septal fibrosis as initially described in BPD, such that "classic BPD" is uncommonly observed today.

Microvascular development is altered in patients with CLDP. Affected lungs show a dysmorphic pattern of vascular organization with prominent "corner" vessels, adjacent dilated vessels, sparse capillaries in some alveolar walls, and dilated and abundant capillaries in others.[15] These structural changes suggest that altered distal vascular growth or abnormal physiologic regulation of intrapulmonary arteriovenous anastomotic vessels may contribute to the pathobiology of severe BPD, which appears similar to that observed in alveolar capillary dysplasia/misalignment of pulmonary veins. The persistence of intrapulmonary arteriovenous anastomotic vessels contributes to intrapulmonary shunt with resultant hypoxemia, pulmonary edema, and possibly pulmonary hypertension in severe BPD.[16]

Whether infants with CLDP have been treated with prenatal steroids and/or surfactant, they still show impaired alveolar development, an abnormal capillary morphology, and an interstitium with variable cellularity caused by a proliferation of fibroblasts.[15]

REFERENCES

1. Islam JY, Keller RL, Aschner JL, et al. Understanding the short and long-term respiratory outcomes of prematurity and bronchopulmonary dysplasia. *Am J Respir Crit Care Med.* 2015;192:134–156.
2. Inselman LS, Mellins RB. Growth and development of the lung. *J Pediatr.* 1981;98:1–15.
3. Kimura J, Deutsch GH. Key mechanisms of early lung development. *Pediatr Dev Pathol.* 2007;10:335–347.
4. Joshi S, Kotecha S. Lung growth and development. *Early Hum Dev.* 2007;83:789–794.
5. Kho AT, Bhattacharya S, Tantisira KG, et al. Transcriptomic analysis of human lung development. *Am J Respir Crit Care Med.* 2010;181:54–63.
6. Burri PH. Structural aspects of postnatal lung development—alveolar formation and growth. *Biol Neonate.* 2006;89:313–322.
7. Anderson MR. Update on pediatric acute respiratory distress syndrome. *Respir Care.* 2003;48:261–276; discussion 276–278.
8. Agrons GA, Courtney SE, Stocker JT, et al. From the archives of the AFIP: lung disease in premature neonates: radiologic–pathologic correlation. *Radiographics.* 2005;25:1047–1073.
9. Cornfield DN. Acute respiratory distress syndrome in children: physiology and management. *Curr Opin Pediatr.* 2013;25:338–343.
10. Lopez E, Gascoin G, Flamant C, et al. Exogenous surfactant therapy in 2013: what is next? Who, when and how should we treat newborn infants in the future? *BMC Pediatr.* 2013;13:165.
11. Sweet DG, Halliday HL, Speer CP. Surfactant therapy for neonatal respiratory distress syndrome in 2013. *J Matern Fetal Neonatal Med.* 2013;26(suppl 2):27–29.
12. Jobe AH, Bancalari E. Bronchopulmonary dysplasia. *Am J Respir Crit Care Med.* 2001;163:1723–1729.
13. Baker CD, Abman SH. Impaired pulmonary vascular development in bronchopulmonary dysplasia. *Neonatology.* 2015;107:344–351.
14. Turcios NL, Fink RJ, eds. *Pulmonary Manifestations of Pediatric Diseases.* 1st ed. Philadelphia, PA: Saunders Elsevier; 2009:348.
15. Coalson JJ. Pathology of bronchopulmonary dysplasia. *Semin Perinatol.* 2006;30:179–184.
16. Galambos C, Sims-Lucas S, Abman SH. Histologic evidence of intrapulmonary anastomoses by three-dimensional reconstruction in severe bronchopulmonary dysplasia. *Ann Am Thorac Soc.* 2013;10:474–481.

15 Pediatric Interstitial Lung Disease and Hermansky-Pudlak Syndrome

Allen P. Burke, M.D., and Jennifer M. Boland, M.D.

Pediatric Interstitial Lung Disease

Terminology and Classification

Children's interstitial lung disease (ChILD) can generally be divided into disorders more prevalent in infancy and those that can that can occur anytime during childhood but are more commonly seen in older children (>2 years).[1-3] Diffuse lung diseases of infancy include disorders of surfactant metabolism, alveolar growth abnormalities (deficient alveolarization), diffuse developmental disorders (conditions that catastrophically affect alveolar development or vascular development), and several specific conditions of unknown etiology (neuroendocrine cell hyperplasia of infancy [NEHI] and pulmonary interstitial glycogenosis [PIG]).[1-3]

There are a variety of primary and secondary disorders that may occur throughout childhood, which can be classified based on the presence of an underlying systemic disease and the host immune status.[1,3] There are also disorders that may masquerade as interstitial lung disease in children, including various causes of pulmonary hypertension, lymphatic disorders, vasculitis, and congestive heart disease.[1,3] ChILD with a known genetic basis includes alveolar capillary dysplasia (see Chapter 13), surfactant disorders, disorders of macrophages resulting in alveolar proteinosis, and usual interstitial pneumonia (UIP).[4,5] The last entity rarely occurs in children; familial IPF and its genetic basis are discussed in Chapter 17.

Interstitial lung diseases that primarily involve infants are generally classified separately from those occurring in children and adolescents (Table 15.1).[1-3,6,7] For older children and young adults, a classification similar to that used in adults has been proposed.[6] However, idiopathic interstitial pneumonias (acute interstitial pneumonia, UIP, nonspecific interstitial pneumonia [NSIP], and respiratory bronchiolitis-interstitial lung disease) rarely if ever occur in young children. A particularly confusing factor is the historical use of "desquamative interstitial pneumonia," or DIP, for one of the typical histologic appearances of congenital surfactant disorders. The use of terms such as "cryptogenic alveolitis," DIP, and early interstitial pneumonia in the context of pediatric lung disease is now obsolete.[8] The term DIP should be reserved for the typical smoking-related interstitial lung disease seen in adults (Chapter 18).

Incidence

The incidence of pediatric interstitial lung disease has been estimated at 3 to 4 per million.[7,8] Prior to routine genetic testing, the frequency of familial pediatric interstitial lung disease (ILD) was less than 25%.[8]

Disorders of Surfactant Metabolism

Clinical Features

Infants with congenital disorders of surfactant metabolism classically present with a syndrome similar to neonatal respiratory distress syndrome (NRDS)/hyaline membrane disease, occurring in a term infant (rather than the typical premature infant where NRDS would be expected due to functional surfactant deficiency).[9] Symptoms include respiratory distress with cough and tachypnea.[9] There is generally hypoxemia with diffuse bilateral infiltrates on chest radiographs and CT scans,[7] which may include ground-glass opacities, "crazy paving" pattern, or complete whiteout of the bilateral lung fields. However, as more is learned about surfactant-related disorders and genetic testing for causative mutations is more readily available, it is becoming apparent that the clinical course is variable, and some children may present after infancy or even into teenage years and young adulthood with chronic pulmonary disease.[9]

TABLE 15.1 Classification of Pediatric Interstitial Lung Disease[a]

Condition (Diseases of Infancy in Bold)	Comment
Diffuse developmental disorders (i.e., dysplasias) **Acinar dysplasia** **Congenital alveolar dysplasia** **Alveolar capillary dysplasia with misalignment of pulmonary veins**	Acinar and alveolar dysplasias are rare, associated with pulmonary hypoplasia (see Chapter 12). Acinar dysplasia resembles arrest at pseudoglandular phase of development; alveolar dysplasia resembles arrest at saccular phase. Alveolar capillary dysplasia (see Chapter 13)
Surfactant disorders	See Table 15.2
Alveolar growth abnormalities (AGA)	Alveolar simplification often with cystic change, most commonly observed in context of chronic lung disease of prematurity (see Chapter 14); similar changes may occur in trisomy 21 and congenital heart disease.
Pulmonary interstitial glycogenosis	Glycogen-rich mesenchymal cells in the interstitium; usually occurs as a secondary change (nonspecific change), but may be idiopathic
Neuroendocrine cell hyperplasia of infancy	Normal histologic findings; increased bombesin-secreting neuroendocrine cells in >75% of airways, >10% of airway epithelium
Cryptogenic organizing pneumonia	Overlaps with adult disease (see Chapter 19)
Hypersensitivity pneumonitis	Overlaps with adult disease (see Chapter 23)
Eosinophilic lung disease	Loeffler syndrome (transient infiltrates, often precipitated by parasitic infection) Eosinophilic pneumonitis (acute and chronic); dramatic response to corticosteroids
Diffuse alveolar hemorrhage syndromes	See Chapter 29
Systemic disorders	Collagen vascular disease Storage diseases Sarcoidosis Langerhans cell histiocytosis

[a]A similar classification for interstitial lung disease as used in adults has also been applied to children, although the idiopathic interstitial pneumonias occur rarely if at all in infants and young children. The table presents those that occur with any frequency in children[6].
Modified from Cazzato S, et al. Interstitial lung disease in children. *Early Hum Dev.* 2013;89(suppl. 3):S39–S43.

TABLE 15.2   Genetic Basis for Children's Interstitial Lung Disease

Genetic Syndrome	OMIM	Gene, Chromosomal Location, Mechanism	Inheritance	Pathology	Age at Onset and Clinical Course
SP-B deficiency	#265120 SMDP1	SFTPB 2p12-p11.2 Loss of function	Autosomal recessive	Surfactant dysfunction	Neonatal onset, severe, fatal
ABCA3 deficiency	#610921 SMDP3	ABCA3 16p13.3 Loss of function	Autosomal recessive	Surfactant dysfunction	Neonatal to childhood onset, variable
SP-C dysfunction	#610913 SMDP2	SFTPC 8p21 Toxic gain in function	Autosomal dominant	Surfactant dysfunction	Neonatal to young adult, variable
Brain–thyroid–lung syndrome	#610978	TTF1 (NKX2.1) 14q13.3 Haploinsufficiency	Autosomal dominant, sporadic	Surfactant dysfunction	Newborn, hypothyroid, variable
GM-CSF receptor deficiency, α chain	#300770 SMDP4	CSF2RA Xp22.32, Yp11.3 Loss of function	Autosomal recessive	Alveolar proteinosis	Childhood, variable
Lysinuric protein intolerance	#222700	SLC7A7 14q11.2 Loss of function	Autosomal recessive	Alveolar proteinosis	Infancy to childhood, hyperammonemia, progressive course
Alveolar capillary dysplasia (see Chapter 13)	#265380	FOXF1 16q24.1 Haploinsufficiency	Autosomal dominant, sporadic	Misalignment of pulmonary veins, alveolar capillary dysplasia	Neonatal, severe, and fatal

Adapted from Nogee LM. Genetic basis of children's interstitial lung disease. *Pediatr Allergy Immunol Pulmonol.* 2010;23(1):15–24

Etiology and Genetics of Surfactant-Related Disorders

Most genetic interstitial lung diseases of infancy are attributed to genes that encode proteins involved in surfactant metabolism (Table 15.2). These include ABCA3 (ATP-binding cassette transporter protein A3), SP-B, SP-C, and TTF-1 (thyroid transcription factor 1), also known as NKX2.1, which is involved in transcription of surfactant proteins.[5,7]

Surfactant is a mixture of lipids and proteins whose function is to reduce alveolar surface tension. It is produced by type II pneumocytes within lamellar bodies and secreted by exocytosis. The lipid portion, largely disaturated phosphatidylcholine, requires hydrophobic proteins SP-B and SP-C in addition to more hydrophilic proteins SP-A and SP-D. Because surfactant is catabolized by alveolar macrophages by a mechanism dependent on GM-CSF (granulocyte–monocyte colony-stimulating factor) signaling, macrophage defects may also result in lung disease, usually resembling pulmonary alveolar proteinosis (PAP). In adults, PAP occurs from antibodies to GM-CSF (see Chapter 28), whereas in infants and children, the defect is usually genetic.[5,7]

The first described mutation resulting in NRDS involves the gene encoding SP-B (*SFTPB*), which is a very rare cause of surfactant deficiency inherited in an autosomal recessive fashion. *SFTPB* mutation results in loss of function of the protein and severe loss of surfactant activity. Infants are usually full term, with symptoms of respiratory distress occurring within hours. Most children die within 3 months. Two-thirds of patients harbor a frameshift mutation in *SFTPB*.[4,5]

The next mutation that was discovered involved the gene encoding SP-C (*SFTPC*), which is inherited in an autosomal dominant pattern. The clinical course is much more variable, and thus, this mutation can present in older children or even adults, at which time the lung can show significant fibrosis and remodeling. In contrast to SP-B mutations, the altered amino acid sequence of SP-C protein results in misfolding and an increase in the protein and accumulation of hydrophobic epitopes in the endoplasmic reticulum, causing pneumocyte apoptosis and interstitial inflammation.

More recently, mutations in *ABCA3* have been described, which have actually been found to be the most common cause of inherited surfactant deficiency currently known. The mutation is inherited in an autosomal recessive fashion. The ABC transporters hydrolyze ATP to move proteins across membranes and are most highly expressed in lung, where they are localized to lamellar bodies of surfactant within the alveolar type II cells. Initial reports documented a highly lethal disease resembling SP-B deficiency.[4,5] More recently, less lethal mutations

have been discovered resulting in a milder clinical course,[10] and thus the clinical presentation and severity are thought to be quite variable.

TTF-1/NKX2.1 is necessary for the transcription of SP-A, SP-B, SP-C, as well as ABCA3. As it is also expressed in the thyroid gland and basal ganglia, it is not surprising that mutations in *TTF-1/NKX21* also cause extrapulmonary disease, including hypothyroidism and neurologic manifestations, resulting in the "brain–thyroid–lung" syndrome.[4,5] Mutations typically result in haploinsufficiency, with deletions of one allelic gene copy.[5]

The failure of macrophages to catabolize surfactant may also result in pediatric lung disease, usually with an onset in childhood (Table 15.2). Mutations in the genes coding GM-CSF receptor α (*CSF2RA*), in addition to lysinuric protein, result in a histologic pattern of alveolar proteinosis that is often indistinguishable from the more common antibody-mediated form seen in adults (Fig. 15.1).[5,10]

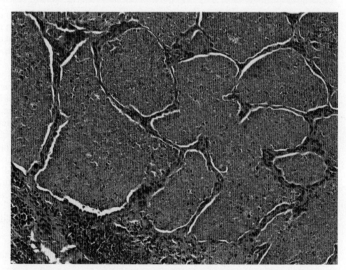

FIGURE 15.1 ▲ Pulmonary alveolar proteinosis, 6-year-old child. The appearance is similar to that seen in adults, with alveoli filled with granular, largely acellular proteinaceous material. The molecular basis for the patient's lung disease was not elucidated.

Mutations in the gene encoding surfactant protein A2 (*SFTPA2*) have been reported to result in familial IPF in young adults.[7] More commonly, familial IPF is caused by genes in telomerase proteins (*TERT, TERC*) (see Chapter 17).

Microscopic Findings

The histologic features of congenital surfactant deficiency are variable, and many observed patterns have been reported. The most commonly observed patterns have features resembling DIP, PAP, NSIP, endogenous lipid pneumonia, and "chronic pneumonitis of infancy."[2,9–11] Other terms such as "fibrosing alveolitis" and "early interstitial pneumonia" have been applied to pediatric ILD without clear definitions.[8] Teenagers and young adults with fibrotic interstitial lung disease have also been found to have mutations in the surfactant deficiency–related genes, with a pattern that resembles UIP.[12] Therefore, it seems prudent to not use these diagnoses (DIP, PAP, NSIP) in infants and young children to avoid confusion with their adult counterparts. Instead, a description of the observed findings may be more helpful with a comment that these patterns have been observed in congenital disorders of surfactant metabolism, and genetic testing may be helpful in this regard.

Most classic cases of surfactant deficiency disorders occurring in infancy/during the neonatal period show type 2 pneumocyte hyperplasia with accumulation of granular proteinaceous debris in the alveolar spaces, associated with cholesterol clefts and increased alveolar foamy macrophages (Fig. 15.2). Depending on the proportion of proteinaceous debris and intra-alveolar macrophages, the appearance may closely resemble PAP (simulating the adult antibody-mediated form) or DIP (simulating the disease seen in adult smokers, but lacking the cytoplasmic brown-black pigment). This pattern resembling DIP or PAP is most often associated with abnormalities in SP-B or ABCA3.[9] In cases that may be less symptomatically severe and thus present later in life, the histologic pattern is different. Older infants/young children often show more interstitial fibrosis and mild interstitial chronic inflammation, while the type 2 pneumocyte hyperplasia and the amount of intra-alveolar lipoproteinaceous material may diminish. The lipoproteinaceous debris is PAS positive, which can be helpful to identify it in cases where it is not particularly prominent, or to differentiate it from edema fluid and hyaline membranes, which are PAS negative. This more chronic phase likely correlates to what has been described as "chronic pneumonitis of infancy"[2] and may resemble NSIP, and these patterns are more commonly associated with mutations affecting SP-C.[9]

Electron microscopy (EM) may be used as an adjunctive test in the evaluation of possible genetic disorders of surfactant metabolism. While a normal EM evaluation does not exclude a surfactant deficiency disorder, abnormal lamellar bodies are sometimes observed, especially in patients with *ABCA3* or *SPB* mutations. This may include lack of normal mature lamellar bodies and abnormal cytoplasmic electron-dense bodies (which may be within the lamellar bodies), or lamellar bodies may show abnormal packaging (multiple grouped together) or abnormally rigid lamellation.[13]

Neuroendocrine Cell Hyperplasia of Infancy
Clinical Features

NEHI is one of the rare interstitial lung diseases of unknown etiology that is only seen in infants and young children.[9] It was described as the histologic correlate of the clinical disorder "persistent tachypnea of infancy."[1] This is characterized by persistent tachypnea, hypoxia usually requiring supplemental oxygen, chest retractions, and crackles on chest auscultation.[1] Cough and wheezing are not often observed, and children do not typically have respiratory failure requiring intubation.[1,9] Chest imaging abnormalities are also commonly seen, including ground-glass opacities accentuated in the right middle lobe and lingua, and areas of hyperlucency/air trapping.[1,3,14] Prognosis is generally good with no mortality observed, but there is a poor response to steroids and bronchodilators, so treatment is generally supportive with supplemental oxygen.[1,9,14] Most children have symptomatic improvement as they age, although some may have persistent symptoms.[1,9,14]

Microscopic Findings

The most characteristic feature of NEHI is that the pulmonary symptoms and chest imaging findings seem out of proportion to the histopathologic findings.[9,14] In fact, initial review of H&E slides from infants with NEHI appears histologically normal in most cases (Fig. 15.3), or shows at most minimal chronic inflammatory infiltrates around the bronchioles.[1] The diagnosis is made by performing a stain for neuroendocrine cells (NECs), which must show increased numbers in the airways to be diagnostic of NEHI (generally, patients with NEHI have NECs in >70% of airway cross-sections, and NECs constitute >10% of cells in airway as highlighted by the neuroendocrine stain).[14] Bombesin is the recommended stain to evaluate for NEHI, as it is considered the most sensitive for airway NECs in infancy.[1] Alternative neuroendocrine markers (chromogranin, synaptophysin) may be used to support the diagnosis of NEHI if the diagnostic criteria are met. However, they are not considered sufficiently sensitive to exclude the diagnosis, which requires bombesin staining.[1]

It should be noted that secondary airway NEC hyperplasia can occur due to a number of factors (infection, bronchopulmonary

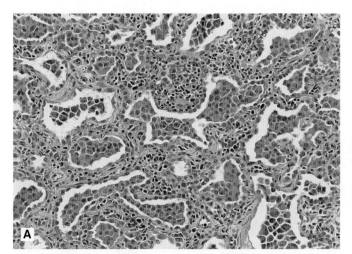
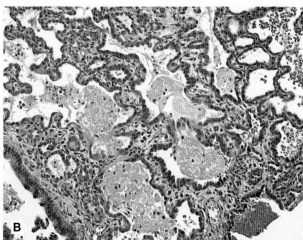

FIGURE 15.2 ▲ Interstitial lung disease in congenital surfactant deficiency. **A.** The interstitial expansion is caused by fibroblasts, scattered lymphocytes and mononuclear cells, and the alveolar spaces are filled with nonpigmented macrophages ("DIP-like"). **B.** This example of ABCA3 deficiency shows pronounced type 2 pneumocyte hyperplasia, interstitial fibrosis, and alveolar lipoproteinaceous debris ("PAP-like").

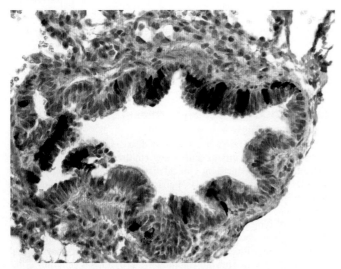

FIGURE 15.3 ▲ Neuroendocrine cell hyperplasia of infancy. Bombesin immunostain highlights the increased number of neuroendocrine cells within the airways.

dysplasia, acute lung injury, cystic fibrosis, cigarette smoke exposure, living at increased altitude, sudden infant death syndrome, etc.).[1,9,14] Therefore, the diagnosis of NEHI requires correlation with the typical clinical and radiographic findings, which includes clinical exclusion of secondary causes of NEC hyperplasia. NEHI should also only be diagnosed in an otherwise essentially normal biopsy, since other histologic findings would point to an alternative diagnosis.[9]

Pulmonary Interstitial Glycogenosis

Clinical Findings

PIG was described initially as an idiopathic form of neonatal interstitial lung disease, characterized by tachypnea, hypoxia, and diffuse bilateral pulmonary infiltrates with hyperinflation.[15] In its idiopathic form, PIG seems to have an excellent clinical outcome with resolution in most cases and often responds favorably to steroid therapy.[15] Since that time, PIG has been described as a presumably secondary finding in lung parenchyma with a multitude of other primary abnormalities, including alveolar capillary dysplasia, congenital alveolar dysplasia, infection, alveolar growth abnormalities, bronchopulmonary dysplasia,

congenital lobar overinflation, or in the lung parenchyma adjacent to a mass lesion.[11] Therefore, it seems that PIG may occur as a nonspecific reactive phenomenon only observed in infancy.

Microscopic Findings

Histologically, PIG is characterized by interstitial expansion by an increased number of immature mesenchymal cells, which contain abundant cytoplasmic glycogen (Fig. 15.4).[15] These cells are usually short spindled to ovoid-shaped cells with bland nuclei and moderate pale cytoplasm. The cytoplasmic glycogen can be highlighted by PAS stain and can also be seen by EM.[15] It is thought that PIG causes respiratory symptoms by diffusion impairment; therefore, it should be mentioned in the pathology report even if it is not the primary abnormality, as it can exacerbate underlying diseases and is steroid responsive.

Hermansky-Pudlak Syndrome

Terminology

The term "Hermansky-Pudlak syndrome" (HPS) was initially applied for an autosomal recessive disorder characterized by tyrosinase-positive oculocutaneous albinism, bleeding diathesis, and systemic manifestations. Pulmonary fibrosis associated with HPS is called Hermansky-Pudlak syndrome–associated interstitial pneumonia (HPSIP), as the histologic and pathologic features differ from UIP.[16]

Etiology

Systemic manifestations result from the liposomal accumulation of ceroid lipofuscin in macrophages of the lungs, heart, kidneys, and intestines. Nine genes have been associated with HPS, mutations of which show differing clinical manifestations.[16] The interstitial fibrosis in HPS results from alveolar injury related to the accumulation of ceroid lipofuscin, both within alveolar macrophages and pneumocytes, and activation of macrophages with increased concentrations of cytokines in alveolar fluid.[17] The exact mechanism of lung injury is unclear.

Clinical

HPSIP has a similar clinical course as idiopathic pulmonary fibrosis (IPF) and is the major cause of morbidity and mortality. Onset of pulmonary fibrosis is typically in the fourth decade of life, with death within one decade.[18–23] HPSIP is a restrictive lung disease with a decrease in forced vital capacity (FVC), forced expiratory volume in one second (FEV1), total lung capacity (TLC), and diffusing capacity for carbon monoxide (DLCO).

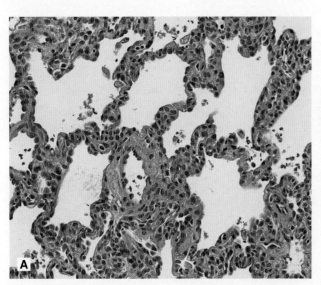
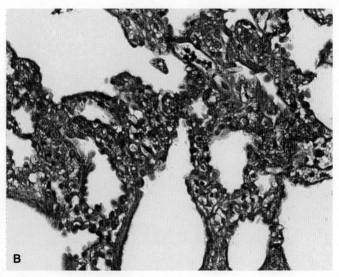

FIGURE 15.4 ▲ Pulmonary interstitial glycogenosis. **A.** There is a population of bland immature ovoid mesenchymal cells in the interstitium. **B.** PAS stain without diastase shows abundant cytoplasmic glycogen.

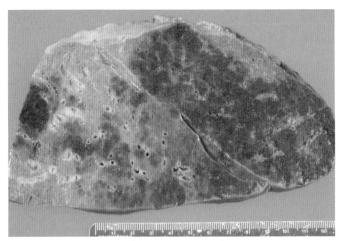

FIGURE 15.5 ▲ Hermansky-Pudlak syndrome, gross findings at explant. There is patchy dense fibrosis with intervening relatively normal areas. Cysts or honeycomb change is not obvious. The uninvolved areas appear dark and hemorrhagic, secondary to extracorporeal membrane oxygenation (ECMO) therapy prior to transplant.

Radiologic Findings

High-density CT scans show diffuse ground-glass opacity with findings of superimposed fibrosis including peripheral reticulation and bronchiectasis. In addition, scattered parenchymal and subpleural cystic lesions may cause a bizarre pattern of pulmonary fibrosis, which is atypical for both IPF and NSIP.[16]

Pathology

The gross findings of explants from patients with HPSIP show "bosselation" or "cobblestoning" of the pleural surfaces (similar to UIP), firm or rubbery consistency of lung tissue due to diffuse interstitial fibrosis (Fig. 15.5), and diffuse fibrosis in all lung fields, with occasional cyst or bullous formation, particularly in the upper lung fields.[24–27]

The histopathologic appearance of HPSIP was first described in 1976 by Davies and Tuddenham as "cryptogenic fibrosing alveolitis,"[28] or IPF. In 1979, Garay et al.[29] described ceroid-like material within alveolar macrophages under both light microscopy and EM.

Although HPS has been included as a condition that can result in the histologic features of UIP,[30] there are key histologic differences between the two entities. In HPSIP (Fig. 15.6), there is a zonal, homogenous distribution without the typical patchwork random distribution of UIP, and fibroblast foci are typically absent. Unlike UIP, HPSIP is characterized histologically by giant lamellar body formation and swelling in type II pneumocytes, which can be seen by light microscopy as well as ultrastructurally.[25]

Prognosis

There is currently no effective treatment for HPSIP.[20,31] The first case of lung transplant for HPSIP was reported in 2005,[24] and this is currently the treatment of choice for eligible patients.

REFERENCES

1. Deterding RR, et al. Persistent tachypnea of infancy is associated with neuroendocrine cell hyperplasia. *Pediatr Pulmonol.* 2005;40(2):157–165.
2. Katzenstein AL, et al. Chronic pneumonitis of infancy. A unique form of interstitial lung disease occurring in early childhood. *Am J Surg Pathol.* 1995;19(4):439–447.
3. Kurland G, et al. An official American Thoracic Society clinical practice guideline: classification, evaluation, and management of childhood interstitial lung disease in infancy. *Am J Respir Crit Care Med.* 2013;188(3):376–394.
4. Nogee LM. Genetics of pediatric interstitial lung disease. *Curr Opin Pediatr.* 2006;18(3):287–292.
5. Nogee LM. Genetic basis of children's interstitial lung disease. *Pediatr Allergy Immunol Pulmonol.* 2010;23(1):15–24.
6. Dishop MK. Paediatric interstitial lung disease: classification and definitions. *Paediatr Respir Rev.* 2011;12(4):230–237.
7. Cazzato S, et al. Interstitial lung disease in children. *Early Hum Dev.* 2013;89(suppl. 3):S39–S43.
8. Dinwiddie R, Sharief N, Crawford O. Idiopathic interstitial pneumonitis in children: a national survey in the United Kingdom and Ireland. *Pediatr Pulmonol.* 2002;34(1):23–29.
9. Deutsch GH, et al. Diffuse lung disease in young children: application of a novel classification scheme. *Am J Respir Crit Care Med.* 2007;176(11):1120–1128.
10. Wert SE, Whitsett JA, Nogee LM. Genetic disorders of surfactant dysfunction. *Pediatr Dev Pathol.* 2009;12(4):253–274.
11. Rice A, et al. Diffuse lung disease in infancy and childhood: expanding the chILD classification. *Histopathology.* 2013;63(6):743–755.

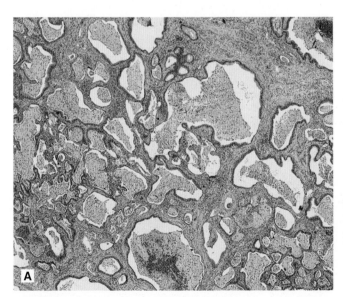
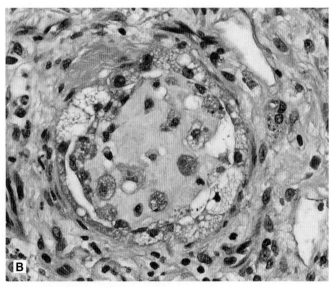

FIGURE 15.6 ▲ Hermansky-Pudlak syndrome, microscopic findings. **A.** At low magnification, there is cystic remodeling, with interstitial fibrosis, mucus and inflammation within the spaces. **B.** At higher magnification, the pneumocytes are reactive and contain vacuoles, as a result of ceroid lipofuscin accumulation. The macrophages show similar cytoplasmic vacuoles.

12. Young LR, et al. Usual interstitial pneumonia in an adolescent with ABCA3 mutations. *Chest.* 2008;134(1):192–195.

13. Edwards V, et al. Ultrastructure of lamellar bodies in congenital surfactant deficiency. *Ultrastruct Pathol.* 2005;29(6):503–509.

14. Young LR, et al. Neuroendocrine cell distribution and frequency distinguish neuroendocrine cell hyperplasia of infancy from other pulmonary disorders. *Chest.* 2011;139(5):1060–1071.

15. Canakis AM, et al. Pulmonary interstitial glycogenosis: a new variant of neonatal interstitial lung disease. *Am J Respir Crit Care Med.* 2002;165(11):1557–1565.

16. Choi J, et al. Hermansky-Pudlak syndrome-associated interstitial pneumonia: pathologic and imaging findings. *Pathol Case Rev.* 2013;18(3):111–114.

17. Rouhani FN, et al. Alveolar macrophage dysregulation in Hermansky-Pudlak syndrome type 1. *Am J Respir Crit Care Med.* 2009;180(11):1114–1121.

18. Avila NA, et al. Hermansky-Pudlak syndrome: radiography and CT of the chest compared with pulmonary function tests and genetic studies. *AJR Am J Roentgenol.* 2002;179(4):887–892.

19. Brantly M, et al. Pulmonary function and high-resolution CT findings in patients with an inherited form of pulmonary fibrosis, Hermansky-Pudlak syndrome, due to mutations in HPS-1. *Chest.* 2000;117(1):129–136.

20. Gahl WA, et al. Genetic defects and clinical characteristics of patients with a form of oculocutaneous albinism (Hermansky-Pudlak syndrome). *N Engl J Med.* 1998;338(18):1258–1264.

21. Anderson PD, et al. Hermansky-Pudlak syndrome type 4 (HPS-4): clinical and molecular characteristics. *Hum Genet.* 2003;113(1):10–17.

22. Bachli EB, et al. Hermansky-Pudlak syndrome type 4 in a patient from Sri Lanka with pulmonary fibrosis. *Am J Med Genet A.* 2004;127A(2):201–207.

23. Gochuico BR, et al. Interstitial lung disease and pulmonary fibrosis in Hermansky-Pudlak syndrome type 2, an adaptor protein-3 complex disease. *Mol Med.* 2012;18:56–64.

24. Lederer DJ, et al. Successful bilateral lung transplantation for pulmonary fibrosis associated with the Hermansky-Pudlak syndrome. *J Heart Lung Transplant.* 2005;24(10):1697–1699.

25. Nakatani Y, et al. Interstitial pneumonia in Hermansky-Pudlak syndrome: significance of florid foamy swelling/degeneration (giant lamellar body degeneration) of type-2 pneumocytes. *Virchows Arch.* 2000;437(3):304–313.

26. Pierson DM, et al. Pulmonary fibrosis in Hermansky-Pudlak syndrome. A case report and review. *Respiration.* 2006;73(3):382–395.

27. Reynolds SP, Davies BH, Gibbs AR. Diffuse pulmonary fibrosis and the Hermansky-Pudlak syndrome: clinical course and postmortem findings. *Thorax.* 1994;49(6):617–618.

28. Davies BH, Tuddenham EG. Familial pulmonary fibrosis associated with oculocutaneous albinism and platelet function defect. A new syndrome. *Q J Med.* 1976;45(178):219–232.

29. Garay SM, et al. Hermansky-Pudlak syndrome. Pulmonary manifestations of a ceroid storage disorder. *Am J Med.* 1979;66(5):737–747.

30. American Thoracic Society/European Respiratory Society International Multidisciplinary Consensus Classification of the Idiopathic Interstitial Pneumonias. This joint statement of the American Thoracic Society (ATS), and the European Respiratory Society (ERS) was adopted by the ATS board of directors, June 2001 and by the ERS Executive Committee, June 2001. *Am J Respir Crit Care Med.* 2002;165(2):277–304.

31. O'Brien K, et al. Pirfenidone for the treatment of Hermansky-Pudlak syndrome pulmonary fibrosis. *Mol Genet Metab.* 2011;103(2):128–134.

SECTION THREE
DIFFUSE PARENCHYMAL LUNG DISEASES

16 Diffuse Parenchymal Lung Disease: Classification and Concepts

Marie-Christine Aubry, M.D., and Allen P. Burke, M.D.

Terminology

Diffuse parenchymal lung disease (DPLD), also known as interstitial lung disease, encompasses a broad heterogeneous group of nonneoplastic disorders that affect the lung parenchyma, predominantly the interstitium but also to some extent the airspaces, peripheral airways, and vessels. This includes not only diseases with known etiologies and/or well-defined clinical pathologic features such as pneumoconiosis, sarcoidosis, pulmonary Langerhans cell histiocytosis (PLCH), or lymphangioleiomyomatosis (LAM) (Table 16.1) but also a group of diseases referred to as "idiopathic interstitial pneumonia" (IIP).[1,2]

IIP is used for a subset of DPLD of unknown cause (Table 16.2).[3] Historically, the concept of IIP began with the description of rapidly progressive, idiopathic interstitial fibrosis with mononuclear inflammation ("Hamman-Rich syndrome").[4,5] The recognition that the alveolar spaces were affected in organization of interstitial lung disease led to the term "diffuse fibrosing alveolitis,"[6] which was categorized as secondary to inhalational agents or drugs and idiopathic.[7] Subsequently, the term "cryptogenic fibrosing alveolitis" was used by clinicians usually for chronic interstitial pneumonias, but they occasionally included more acute processes. Idiopathic pulmonary fibrosis (IPF) was introduced as a synonym for cryptogenic fibrosing alveolitis, and soon both terms came to encompass several pathologic entities including usual interstitial pneumonia (UIP), desquamative interstitial pneumonia (DIP), nonspecific interstitial pneumonia (NSIP), diffuse alveolar damage (DAD), and organizing pneumonia (OP), leading to much confusion in the classification of IIP. In 2002, IPF was officially restricted to cases of UIP. In the United States, cryptogenic fibrosing alveolitis is not used, leaving IPF as the sole clinical term for patients with a histologic diagnosis of UIP.

The other major contributing factor to the confusion of the IIP classification has been the use of different terms by clinicians and pathologists. The 2002 ATS/ERS multidisciplinary consensus classification established a new classification that correlates both the clinical and pathologic diagnoses.[1] This classification was recently updated (Table 16.2).[8]

The consensus classification provides the basis for a multidisciplinary clinical–radiologic–pathologic diagnosis with the purpose of improving the accuracy of the diagnosis. Indeed, there is not a high level of reproducibility among pathologists in assessing interstitial lung disease.[9,10] The increased interactions between pathologists, radiologists, and clinicians have shown to improve the overall diagnosis compared to each group individually.[11] Nevertheless, there remains a subset of unclassifiable IIP, for various reasons such as inadequate pathology; major discordance between the pathologic, radiologic, or clinical findings; or prior treatment effect.

Incidence

The prevalence of all DPLD is ~81 per 100,000 people.[12] The most common diagnosis is pulmonary fibrosis (not otherwise specified), with a prevalence of 30 per 100,000, without sex predilection. Occupational lung disease is by far more common in men than women, with a prevalence of 21 per 100,000 in men. DPLD associated with connective tissue disease is seen at a prevalence of ~10 per 100,000 and is somewhat higher in women. Pulmonary sarcoidosis' prevalence is 9 per 100,000 without gender predilection.[12]

Pulmonary Function Tests

Typically, DPLD results in restrictive lung defects, which are manifested by decreased forced vital capacity (FVC) and impaired gas change. In contrast to obstructive lung disease, the ratio of the FEV1 (forced expiratory

TABLE 16.1 Diffuse Parenchymal Lung Disease, Classification

Etiology	Examples
Hereditary	Familial interstitial pneumonia
	Hermansky-Pudlak syndrome
Inhalational, inorganic (pneumoconiosis)	Silicosis
	Asbestosis
	Berylliosis
Inhalational, organic	Hypersensitivity pneumonitis
Connective tissue diseases (autoimmune)	Systemic sclerosis
	Polymyositis—dermatomyositis
	Systemic lupus erythematosus
	Rheumatoid arthritis
Drug induced	Chemotherapeutic drugs (e.g., bleomycin)
	Antiarrhythmic drugs (e.g., amiodarone)
	Statins
	Antibiotics
Granulomatous	Sarcoidosis
Others	Pulmonary Langerhans cell histiocytosis
	Lymphangioleiomyomatosis
Idiopathic interstitial pneumonias	See Table 16.2.

TABLE 16.2 Classification of Idiopathic Interstitial Pneumonias

Histologic Diagnosis	Clinical Diagnosis
Major idiopathic interstitial pneumonias	
Usual interstitial pneumonia[a]	Idiopathic interstitial fibrosis
Nonspecific interstitial pneumonia[a]	(Idiopathic) nonspecific interstitial pneumonia
Organizing pneumonia[b]	Cryptogenic organizing pneumonia
Diffuse alveolar damage[b]	Acute interstitial pneumonia
Respiratory bronchiolitis[c]	Respiratory bronchiolitis interstitial lung disease
Desquamative interstitial pneumonia[c]	Desquamative interstitial pneumonia
Rare idiopathic interstitial pneumonias	Lymphoid interstitial pneumonia
	Pleuroparenchymal fibroelastosis
Unclassifiable IIP	

[a]Categorized as chronic fibrosing interstitial pneumonia.
[b]Categorized as acute/subacute interstitial pneumonia.
[c]Categorized as smoking-related interstitial pneumonia.

volume in 1 second) to the FVC is relatively spared, as there is a concomitant decrease in FVC. The mechanism of decreased FVC, total lung volume, and FEV1 is directly related to the mechanical effects of scarring of the lung parenchyma. There are several types of DPLD with an obstructive component, characterized by decreases in FEV, especially at one second or in midexhalation, as a fraction of FVC, and bronchiolar hyperreactivity. These include sarcoidosis, hypersensitivity pneumonia, PLCH, and LAM.

Tissue Sampling

If imaging and clinical features are not diagnostic of a given DPLD, open lung biopsy is performed, usually by video assistance (VATS, or video-assisted thoracoscopic surgery). It has been estimated that, in over 50% of patients, a diagnosis of IPF can be made on the basis of clinical and imaging findings, obviating the need for lung biopsy.[13] However, in the more general group of patients with DPLD, tissue biopsy confirmation is necessary in a far higher proportion of patients due to variability in interpretation of CT scans.[14] Recommendations by the American Thoracic Society[1] include biopsies obtained at the edge of grossly abnormal areas to include normal areas, avoidance of the tips of the lingula or right middle lobe, sampling of more than one lobe (preferably upper and lower), and deep biopsies, of 3 to 5 cm in greatest dimension. Avoidance of the lingula is important, as honeycomb remodeling may occur here is a relatively nonspecific finding and does not necessarily suggest a diagnosis of UIP.

Bronchoalveolar lavage (BAL) may be helpful in the diagnosis of ILD.[15] In cases of sarcoidosis, there is a predominance of T lymphocytes with a high CD4/CD8 ratio. Hypersensitivity pneumonia shows a lymphocytosis with predominant CD8 cells. Idiopathic pulmonary fibrosis (UIP) shows more neutrophils and eosinophils. The clinical utility of these distinctions is, however, of limited value.[15]

Transbronchial biopsies can be useful in the diagnosis of DPLD.[15–18] Indeed, some of these diseases have unique features that may be recognizable on small biopsies, although these tend to be rare diseases, such as pulmonary alveolar proteinosis, amyloidosis, and LAM, or with a low yield, such as PLCH. Of all the IIP, DAD can be diagnosed with confidence on a small biopsy if hyaline membranes are recognized. Some authors have argued that UIP can also be diagnosed on transbronchial biopsies, but this remains controversial.[19]

Idiopathic Interstitial Pneumonias

Terminology

The classification of idiopathic interstitial pneumonias (IIP) has evolved since the 1940s. Initially, Liebow and Carrington described 5 subgroups: UIP, bronchiolitis obliterans with interstitial pneumonia (BIP, an obsolete term), DIP, lymphoid interstitial pneumonia (LIP), and giant cell interstitial pneumonia (GIP).[20,21] GIP has been abandoned from the classification of IIP as all cases usually have an identifiable etiology, most commonly exposure to hard metals. LIP is regarded by most as a variant of lymphoid hyperplasia, along with follicular bronchiolitis and nodular lymphoid hyperplasia. As such, it is almost never idiopathic, occurring in patients with autoimmune disorders or HIV infection. LIP was described before NSIP was introduced in 1994,[22] and now, most cases of what has been called LIP would be classified as NSIP. Many therefore have argued for removing LIP from the classification of IIP; however, since it is an interstitial process that enters the differential diagnosis of other IIP, it has remained in the updated classification of IIP. With the introduction of NSIP, the new classification in 1998 included four major groups: acute interstitial pneumonia (AIP), DIP—respiratory bronchiolitis–interstitial lung disease (RB-ILD), UIP, and NSIP.[2] The American Thoracic Society/European Respiratory Society (ATS/ERS) categorization of ILD in 2002 emphasized the need to combine clinical, imaging, and pathologic data to form six specific clinicopathologic diagnoses. In addition to previous entities, cryptogenic organizing pneumonia (COP) was added, and the entities of DIP and LIP were preserved (Table 16.2).[1,8] The most recent ATS/ERS classification[8] divided the IIP into major, rare, and unclassifiable, adding a new rare IIP, idiopathic pleuroparenchymal fibroelastosis. The major IIPs were further categorized into chronic fibrosing (IPF/UIP and NSIP), acute/subacute (AIP/DAD, OP/COP), and smoking related (RB/RB-ILD and DIP). Although RB/RB-ILD and DIP have an identifiable etiology, that is, smoking, these disorders remain in this latest consensus classification. Two new rare histologic diseases were introduced; however, these were not included as new IIPs as the question remains whether these histologic patterns are simply variants of existing IIPs. These new histologic diseases are acute fibrinous and organizing pneumonia (AFOP) and bronchiolocentric interstitial pneumonia.

Acute and Subacute IIPs

These IIPs have an acute (AIP/DAD) or subacute (OP/COP) presentation or may represent an acute exacerbation of an existing chronic IIP. Histologically, all these have in common the proliferation of fibroblasts. Fibroblasts, in the lung, are a marker of acute lung injury. In DAD/AIP, the fibroblasts typically cause septal thickening. In contrast, in OP/COP, the fibroblasts form intraluminal plugs filling small airways and alveolar spaces. In acute exacerbation, most often DAD, but also OP, will be superimposed on a chronic IIP.

AFOP is not included as a separate IIP, but morphologically, it represents an acute lung injury with overlapping features between DAD and OP. Indeed, there is an airspace proliferation of fibroblasts like OP but admixed with a fibrinous exudate that may mimic the hyaline membranes of DAD. Clinically, AFOP shares features similar to AIP.[23]

Chronic Fibrosing IIPs

Chronic fibrosing IIPs, namely, UIP/IPF and NSIP, are characterized by varying proportions of interstitial fibrosis and chronic inflammation. UIP is typically distinguished from NSIP based on its geographic and temporal variegation. The temporal variegation lies in the recognition of fibrosis of different transitioning age, with early (or acute) fibrosis in the form of fibroblast foci and old collagen fibrosis ultimately resulting into honeycomb lung. Fibroblast foci being comprised of fibroblasts need to be distinguished from the fibroblastic proliferation of DAD and OP. This distinction can be nearly impossible in cases of acute exacerbation of UIP/IPF. However, in general, fibroblastic foci form small dome-shaped proliferation arising in the interstitium. By definition, fibroblastic foci are few and scattered, compared to the more diffuse proliferation of fibroblasts in DAD. Fibroblast foci protrude into the airspace and are lined by cuboidal epithelial cells. They are not located entirely within the airspaces as seen in OP. Furthermore, the fibroblastic plugs in OP are usually not lined by prominent reactive pneumocytes. Katzenstein et al. best defined fibroblast foci as follows:

> Fibroblast foci are composed of small dome-shaped collections of spindle-shaped fibroblasts and myofibroblasts within myxoid stroma. They are present in the interstitium, and their surface is covered by hyperplastic alveolar lining cells. Because of their myxoid stroma, they are easily recognizable at low magnification.[24]

Histologically, honeycomb lung is characterized by enlarged restructured airspaces with thick fibrotic walls, containing inspissated mucous, often rich in acute and chronic inflammatory cells. Honeycombing by itself is nonspecific and can potentially be the result of a number of diseases, not only UIP.[24]

REFERENCES

1. American Thoracic Society/European Respiratory Society International Multidisciplinary Consensus Classification of the Idiopathic Interstitial Pneumonias. This joint statement of the American Thoracic Society (ATS), and the European Respiratory Society (ERS) was adopted by the ATS board of directors, June 2001 and by the ERS Executive Committee, June 2001. *Am J Respir Crit Care Med.* 2002;165(2):277–304.
2. Katzenstein AL, Myers JL. Idiopathic pulmonary fibrosis: clinical relevance of pathologic classification. *Am J Respir Crit Care Med.* 1998;157(4 pt 1):1301–1315.
3. Kim DS, Collard HR, King TE Jr. Classification and natural history of the idiopathic interstitial pneumonias. *Proc Am Thorac Soc.* 2006;3(4):285–292.
4. Hamman L, Rich AR. Acute diffuse interstitial fibrosis of the lungs. *Bull Johns Hopkins Hosp.* 1944;74:177–212.

5. Hamman L, Rich AR. Fulminating diffuse interstitial fibrosis of the lungs. *Trans Am Clin Climatol Assoc.* 1935;51:154–163.
6. Scadding JG. Fibrosing alveolitis. *Br Med J.* 1964;2(5410):686.
7. Scadding JG. Diffuse pulmonary alveolar fibrosis. *Thorax.* 1974;29(3):271–281.
8. Travis WD, Costabel U, Hansell DM, et al. An official American Thoracic Society/European Respiratory Society statement: update of the international multidisciplinary classification of the idiopathic interstitial pneumonias. *Am J Respir Crit Care Med.* 2013;188(6):733–748.
9. Lettieri CJ, Veerappan GR, Parker JM, et al. Discordance between general and pulmonary pathologists in the diagnosis of interstitial lung disease. *Respir Med.* 2005;99(11):1425–1430.
10. Flaherty KR, Andrei AC, King TE Jr, et al. Idiopathic interstitial pneumonia: do community and academic physicians agree on diagnosis? *Am J Respir Crit Care Med.* 2007;175(10):1054–1060.
11. Flaherty KR, King JE Jr, Raghu G, et al. Idiopathic interstitial pneumonia: what is the effect of a multidisciplinary approach to diagnosis? *Am J Respir Crit Care Med.* 2004;170(8):904–910.
12. Coultas DB, Hubbar R. Epidemiology of idiopathic pulmonary fibrosis. In: Lynch JPI, ed. *Idiopathic Pulmonary Fibrosis, Lung Biology in Health and Disease.* New York, NY: Marcel Dekker; 2004:772.
13. Hunninghake GW, Zimmerman MB, Schwartz DA, et al. Utility of a lung biopsy for the diagnosis of idiopathic pulmonary fibrosis. *Am J Respir Crit Care Med.* 2001;164(2):193–196.
14. Aziz ZA, Wells AU, Hansell DM, et al. HRCT diagnosis of diffuse parenchymal lung disease: inter-observer variation. *Thorax.* 2004;59(6):506–511.
15. Reynolds HY. Use of bronchoalveolar lavage in humans—past necessity and future imperative. *Lung.* 2000;178(5):271–293.
16. Katzenstein AL, Askin FB. Interpretation and significance of pathologic findings in transbronchial lung biopsy. *Am J Surg Pathol.* 1980;4(3):223–234.
17. Poletti V, Patelli M, Poggi S, et al. Transbronchial lung biopsy and bronchoalveolar lavage in diagnosis of diffuse infiltrative lung diseases. *Respiration.* 1988;54(suppl 1):66–72.
18. Leslie KO, Gruden JF, Parish JM, et al. Transbronchial biopsy interpretation in the patient with diffuse parenchymal lung disease. *Arch Pathol Lab Med.* 2007;131(3):407–423.
19. Berbescu EA, Katzenstein AL, Snow JL, et al. Transbronchial biopsy in usual interstitial pneumonia. *Chest.* 2006;129(5):1126–1131.
20. Liebow AA, Carrington DB. The interstitial pneumonias. In: Simon M, Potchen EJ, LeMay M, eds. *Frontiers of Pulmonary Radiology.* New York, NY: Grune & Stratteon; 1969:102–141.
21. Liebow AA. Definition and classification of interstitial pneumonias in human pathology. *Progr Respir Res.* 1975;8:1–33.
22. Katzenstein AL, Fiorelli RF. Nonspecific interstitial pneumonia/fibrosis. Histologic features and clinical significance. *Am J Surg Pathol.* 1994;18(2):136–147.
23. Beasley MB, Franks TJ, Galvin JR, et al. Acute fibrinous and organizing pneumonia: a histological pattern of lung injury and possible variant of diffuse alveolar damage. *Arch Pathol Lab Med.* 2002;126(9):1064–1070.
24. Katzenstein AL, Mukhopadhyay S, Myers JL. Diagnosis of usual interstitial pneumonia and distinction from other fibrosing interstitial lung diseases. *Hum Pathol.* 2008;39(9):1275–1294.

17 Chronic Fibrosing Idiopathic Interstitial Pneumonias

Marie-Christine Aubry, M.D., Allen P. Burke, M.D., and Seth Kligerman, M.D.

Usual Interstitial Pneumonia/Idiopathic Pulmonary Fibrosis

Terminology

Usual interstitial pneumonia (UIP) is a form of diffuse parenchymal lung disease characterized by patchy subpleural and basal remodeling of lung tissue with honeycomb change. UIP is a pathologic process, also referred to as pattern, that can be seen in a variety of clinical settings such as connective tissue disease (CTD) and drug toxicity.

Familial pulmonary fibrosis and Hermansky-Pudlak syndrome also cause pulmonary fibrosis similar to UIP.

UIP is most commonly seen as the pathologic correlate of idiopathic pulmonary fibrosis (IPF). By definition, IPF requires the exclusion of other known causes of diffuse parenchymal lung disease and the presence of UIP by high-resolution computed tomography (HRCT) or by surgical lung biopsy.

General Clinical Features

The prevalence and incidence of IPF are difficult to ascertain due to lack of large-scale studies and the variations in the definition of IPF over the years. Therefore, the estimates of incidence and prevalence are quite broad with reported incidence ranging between 4.6 and 16.3 per 100,000 and prevalence between 2 and 42.7 per 100,000.

Although by definition IPF is idiopathic, there are several potential risk factors described, including cigarette smoking, chronic aspiration, advanced age, male gender, family history of chronic lung disease, and exposures. Environmental exposures linked to the development of IPF include metal dust, wood dust, livestock, textile dust, stone and sand, and wood fires.[1] Genetic factors also play a role as a familial history of IPF can be elicited in about 5% of patients. Criteria for considering familial pulmonary fibrosis are varied, but in general, there must be features of UIP by HRCT with or without histologic confirmation in at least two first-degree family members, or a confirmed case of UIP with a history of two other affected relatives. Autosomal dominance is suspected in most cases. Age of onset is younger than that of nonfamilial IPF, and disease progression is more rapid. There are no consistent imaging or histologic differences between familial and nonfamilial forms of the disease.[2] Heterozygous mutations in *TERT, TERC, SFTPC,* and *FTPA2* account for about 20% of familial interstitial pneumonias.[3]

These cases are still classified as idiopathic interstitial pneumonias.

In IPF, men are more commonly affected than are women, and the mean age at onset is around 60 years, with a history of prior respiratory symptoms typically measured in months to years. The symptoms are not specific and comprise exertional dyspnea and nonproductive cough. Physical exam typically reveals bibasilar inspiratory crackles qualified as Velcro-like. Digital clubbing is common. In young adults, the diagnosis of UIP should raise the possibility of familial disease, occult collagen vascular disease, or occult inhalational exposure. Pulmonary function tests reveal restriction with decreased lung volumes and total lung capacity, normal or increased FEV1/FVC (unless the patient has combined chronic obstructive pulmonary disease), and/or decreased diffusing capacity.

Radiologic Findings

HRCT may be used to diagnose IPF in the absence of pathology if all features of UIP are identified. These features include (1) subpleural, basal predominance, (2) reticular abnormalities, (3) honeycombing with or without traction bronchiectasis, and (4) the absence of atypical features (Fig. 17.1).[4,5] The atypical features that are described as inconsistent with UIP include an upper lobe predominance, peribronchovascular predominance, micronodules, discrete cysts

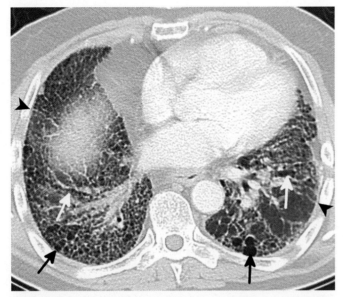

FIGURE 17.1 ▲ Usual interstitial pneumonia. UIP pattern. Axial CT image through the lower lobes in a 59-year-old man shows extensive lower lobe predominant honeycombing (*black arrows*) with reticulation (*arrowheads*) and traction bronchiectasis (*white arrows*). The CT findings are consistent with a UIP pattern, which obviates the need for open lung biopsy.

distinct from honeycombing, mosaic attenuation representing air trapping, or consolidation. Although extensive ground-glass opacity is also considered an atypical feature, it can be seen in cases of accelerated IPF. Honeycombing is a hallmark of UIP and appears as stacked subpleural cysts.[6] Surgical biopsies are typically performed in cases of HRCT

atypical features, often the lack of honeycombing. Histology-proven UIP is demonstrated in up to 25% of these cases.[5]

Prognosis and Treatment

Patients with IPF have a progressive illness that is eventually fatal, and the only treatment is lung transplant. There is currently no proven pharmacologic treatment for IPF. Therefore, IPF needs to be distinguished from all other IIPs, in particular from NSIP since NSIP has a better prognosis. The 5-year survival for IPF is 30% to 50%, with slight improvement among patients with "discordant" UIP (present in only 1 or 2 lobes on biopsy).[7] In another study, IPF had a median survival of 40 months after diagnosis, with a 1- and 3-year mortality rate of 17% and 43%, respectively. This is in contrast to patients with UIP related to a specific etiology such as autoimmune CTD; survival was far better, with a median survival of 143.8 months, 1-year mortality rate of 7.9%, and 3-year mortality of 13.9%.[8] Other factors that may affect survival negatively in patients with IPF include male gender, combined emphysema, pulmonary hypertension, carbon monoxide diffusing capacity of < 60%, and decline in the FVC over 6 to 12 months.

Most patients with IPF experience a slowly progressive decline. Some patients may experience rapid progression, remain stable for many years, or experience sudden acute worsening of their symptoms known as accelerated or acute exacerbation of IPF. Lung cancer is a known complication of patients with IPF but does not seem to impact the overall survival of these patients.

Gross Findings

External examination demonstrates typical features of "cobblestone" pleura, caused by interstitial fibrosis (Fig. 17.2A). Cut section demonstrates patchy scarring, usually with cysts, in a predominantly subpleural distribution (Fig. 17.2B). Findings are more prominent in the lower lobes. When the upper lobes are involved, the abnormalities will be more prominent in the lower zones.

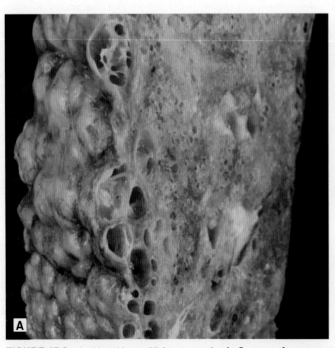

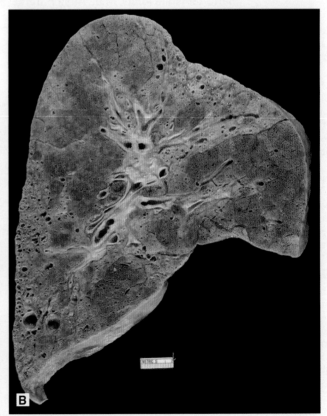

FIGURE 17.2 ▲ Usual interstitial pneumonia. **A.** Gross surface appearance of UIP. A bosselated "cobblestone" appearance is typical of UIP. **B.** On cut section, there is fibrosis with cystic change, most prominent under the pleural surfaces.

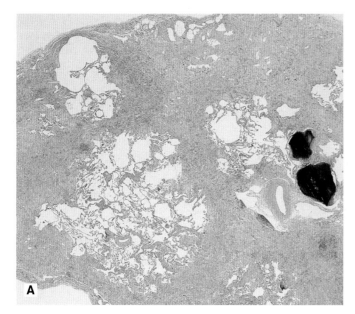

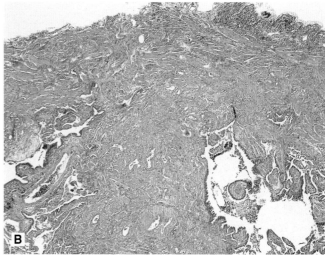

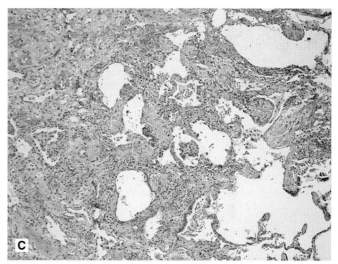

FIGURE 17.3 ▲ Usual interstitial pneumonia. **A.** The low power photomicrograph emphasizes the heterogeneity of UIP with subpleural and paraseptal distribution of the infiltrates and juxtaposition of honeycombing with normal lung. Bone metaplasia is a common finding in the areas of fibrosis. Prominent smooth muscle hyperplasia in lieu of fibrosis can also be seen **(B)**. **C.** Away from the fibrosis and honeycombing, the interstitial thickening is less pronounced, blending with normal lung. Fibroblastic foci are typically found in these less involved areas of the lung.

Microscopic Findings

The diagnosis of UIP stems on the presence of three major histologic features: (1) fibrosis with architectural distortion (with or without honeycombing) in a subpleural and/or paraseptal distribution, (2) patchy involvement, and (3) fibroblast foci (Fig. 17.3). These features should be present, for a definitive pathologic diagnosis, in the absence of several negative histologic features: granulomas, predominant airway-centered disease, and prominent interstitial inflammation away from honeycombed areas. The overall appearance of UIP is strikingly heterogeneous due to the juxtaposition of scarred lung next to normal lung, of marked fibrosis and architectural distortion next to mild interstitial fibrosis, and of old collagen fibrosis next to young cellular fibrosis in the form of fibroblast foci. This heterogeneity is extremely helpful for the differential diagnosis with other fibrosing parenchymal lung diseases, in particular nonspecific interstitial pneumonia (NSIP). This heterogeneity is appreciable with the naked eye and at very low power. Honeycomb lung is characterized by enlarged airspaces with thick fibrotic wall, lined by reactive bronchiolar epithelium or occasionally squamous metaplastic epithelium. In the areas of fibrosis, it is common to see other features such as ossification and smooth muscle cell hyperplasia.

The interface between the collagen fibrosis and the normal or less involved lung is where the fibroblast foci are typically found. They are composed of fibroblasts forming small dome-shaped lesions. The fibroblasts are arranged in a linear arrangement and present in a pale myxoid stroma. The foci are lined by cuboidal epithelial cells (Fig. 17.4). Increased numbers of fibroblast foci have been associated with worse outcome in some studies.

Although fibroblast foci need to be distinguished from other acute lung injuries such as diffuse alveolar damage (DAD) and organizing pneumonia (OP), in patients with accelerated IPF, DAD or OP is present, superimposed on the underlying UIP.

Chronic inflammation is present but normally overshadowed by the fibrosis. Peribronchiolar lymphoid aggregates may be seen; however, any significant peribronchiolar airway-centered fibrosis and inflammation should raise the consideration of alternative diagnosis such as chronic hypersensitivity pneumonia (HP). The dilated airspaces of honeycombing are often filled with mucus and acute inflammation and do not constitute acute bronchopneumonia (Fig. 17.5).

Occasionally, prominent airspace accumulation of eosinophils resembling eosinophilic pneumonia can be present. The significance of this finding is unclear but can be seen in cases of UIP related to drug toxicity.

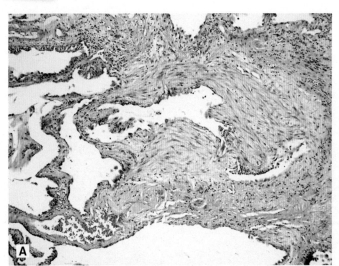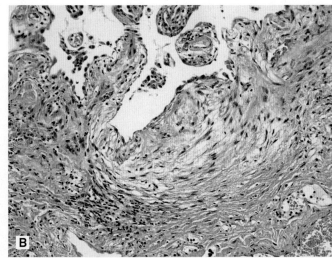

FIGURE 17.4 ▲ Usual interstitial pneumonia. Several examples of fibroblast foci. They are composed of bland spindle cells in a linear arrangement within a mucoid stroma. They are lined by cuboidal cells (**A**). These foci can be inconspicuous (**B**).

In a smoker, airspace accumulation of smokers' macrophages is common and may resemble desquamative interstitial pneumonia (DIP-like). Vascular remodeling secondary to the fibrosis is typical in UIP. Common vascular changes include intimal fibrosis and medial hypertrophy of arteries with variable intimal thickening. Veins and venules may also be affected resulting in increased alveolar septal capillaries and hemosiderin deposition resulting in pulmonary veno-occlusive disease (PVOD)-like changes. These findings lead to pulmonary hypertension, which, however, needs clinical confirmation with echocardiogram.[9]

Occasionally, in cases of multiple lung biopsies, histologic features of UIP may be seen in one site while features of NSIP may be seen in another. This has been referred to as "discordant" UIP, but for practical purpose, the final diagnosis may simply be UIP.

UIP is a common histologic finding in patients with autoimmune CTD, including rheumatoid arthritis, followed by systemic sclerosis, Sjogren syndrome, dermatomyositis–polymyositis, and undifferentiated CTD.[8] Often, UIP in CTD is identical to UIP in IPF. In one series, the histologic findings of UIP in 9 patients with rheumatoid arthritis

(4), polymyositis–dermatomyositis (2), mixed CTD (1), systemic lupus erythematosus (1), and systemic sclerosis (1) were compared to those of 99 patients with IPF.[10] In this study, the number of fibroblastic foci was significantly greater in the IPF group.[10] However, by itself, this feature cannot be used to distinguish CTD-associated UIP from UIP in IPF. Additional findings of follicular bronchiolitis and pleural lymphoid inflammation are seen at higher rates and raise the possibility of CTD.

Tissue Sampling

Open or video-assisted stereoscopic lung biopsy is most important in those patients with an uncertain diagnosis and those thought unlikely to have IPF by HRCT.[11] Lungs should be sampled at the edge of grossly abnormal areas avoiding of the tips of the lingula or right middle lobe and sampling of more than one lobe of 3 to 5 cm in greatest dimension is recommended.[12] Overall, it has been estimated that fewer than 15% of patients with IPF have tissue diagnosis by open biopsy.[13] Although most authorities stress the need for wedge biopsies, there is some utility to transbronchial biopsy in the diagnosis of interstitial lung disease.[14] However, findings must be interpreted with caution, as most of the features that are typical of UIP depend on overall distribution and subpleural findings, which are not commonly found in transbronchial specimens.

Occasionally, explanted lungs from patients with UIP who have undergone transplantation will be the first specimen available for pathology examination. There have been two studies comparing open biopsies with explant pathology in patients with UIP, and these have shown some differences between both. Indeed, honeycombing is universal in explants and present to a lesser degree in biopsies.[15,16] NSIP-like areas also appear to be more common in explants. Another finding described in explants is interstitial emphysema. Interstitial emphysema is well described as a complication in neonates, with or without mechanical ventilation. It is not as recognized in adults, especially in the context of interstitial lung disease.[17] Interstitial emphysema (Chapter 46) results from air dissecting into the lung's soft tissue and, histologically, appears as cysts lined by fibrous tissue and histiocytic reaction with foreign body–type giant cells.

Malignancy in UIP

Lung carcinomas occur with increased frequency in patients with IPF (9% to 38%) and are typically peripherally located in areas of scarring.[18,19] The location of the tumors in the areas of scarring suggests that the fibrotic process itself may play a role in tumor genesis. Earlier studies

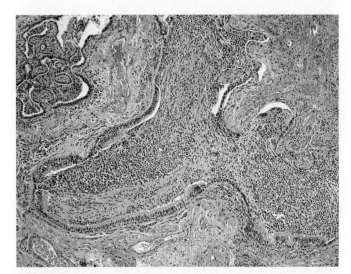

FIGURE 17.5 ▲ Usual interstitial pneumonia. In honeycombing, airspaces are enlarged and will fill with mucin and neutrophils, which may mimic a bronchopneumonia.

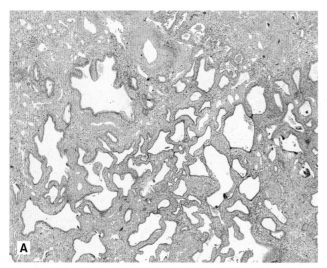 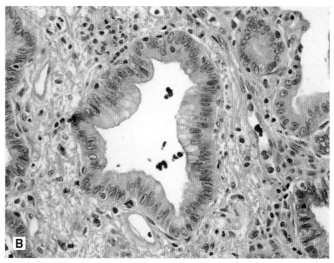

FIGURE 17.6 ▲ Usual interstitial pneumonia with adenocarcinoma. **A.** Increased glandular proliferation with architectural complexity in the area of honeycomb change raises the concern for adenocarcinoma. **B.** At higher magnification, the glands are lined by cylindrical, mostly mucinous, nonciliated cells. The nuclei are enlarged with pseudostratification and nuclear overlapping.

suggested a predominance of adenocarcinoma. However, in later studies, about two-thirds are squamous carcinomas, seen mostly in older men. As squamous cell carcinomas are typically not located peripherally, the atypical location of these tumors further supports the role of fibrosis in the pathogenesis of these cancers. The tumors are also more likely multiple than in patients without IPF.[18–20] The challenge for pathologists lies in two distinct clinical scenarios. The first is that the diagnosis of lung cancer is suspected and an underlying UIP not recognized before surgery. It will therefore fall on the pathologist to not only diagnose the cancer but also recognize the presence of UIP. Finding a squamous cell carcinoma in an area of peripheral fibrosis should raise the diagnosis of UIP. The second and most challenging scenario is the incidental finding of lung cancer in a biopsy taken for a diagnosis of interstitial lung disease. It may be extremely difficult to distinguish reactive epithelial atypia, glandular or squamous, from an incipient lung cancer. Recognizing the architectural complexity of the cell proliferation and cell atypia is key (Fig. 17.6).

Nonspecific Interstitial Pneumonia

Terminology

NSIP was first defined as an interstitial lung disease that differed from UIP clinically, histologically, and prognostically and that had a multiplicity of background etiologies.[21] In contrast to UIP, NSIP patients have a relatively short onset of symptoms, often have a recent systemic inflammatory illness, and have a good prognosis. There is no evidence that NSIP represents an early phase of UIP as suggested in earlier studies.[15,22,23] Originally, NSIP was seen as a common pathway from a variety of insults, including acute lung injury, inhalational exposures, and especially inflammatory CTD.[21]

More recently, it was recognized that NSIP is, similar to IPF, a distinct clinicopathologic entity in addition to a pathologic diagnosis. A consensus panel established that there are patients with idiopathic interstitial lung disease, in whom clinical, radiologic, and pathologic findings have excluded other diffuse parenchymal lung disease.[3,23] These include the other idiopathic interstitial pneumonias, specifically UIP/IPF, OP/cryptogenic OP (COP), respiratory bronchiolitis (RB)/respiratory bronchiolitis–interstitial lung disease (RBILD), DIP and DAD/acute interstitial pneumonia (AIP), as well as HP.

Clinical Findings

There is no known gender predominance, as the percentage of males ranges from 30% to 69% across series.[4,21,23–32] The mean age at presentation in these series was from 43 to 57 years, generally somewhat younger than the mean age for UIP. In one study, patients with the cellular type of NSIP were younger than those with the fibrotic type.[33] NSIP can also occur in children, in contrast to UIP.

About 25% of patients have constitutional symptoms, including weight loss, fever, and arthralgias.[23] The mean duration of symptoms is 6 to 18 months, with some series showing much longer durations, especially those with fibrotic NSIP.[25,28] The most common symptom is dyspnea, followed by cough. Similar to UIP, there is restrictive lung impairment and reduced diffusing capacity for carbon monoxide.[22]

Idiopathic NSIP denotes the absence of a specific etiology, which may be present in over 40% of patients. These etiologies include most commonly connective tissue, other autoimmune diseases, exposure to environmental antigens, and drug toxicity. Occasionally, the discovery of the etiology may become apparent after the histologic diagnosis of NSIP is made.[33–35]

Imaging Findings

Similar to UIP, NSIP is associated with symmetric, lower lobe predominant fibrosis with reticulation, traction bronchiectasis, and lower lobe volume loss (Fig. 17.7). Unlike UIP, GGO is a predominant feature of NSIP and is seen in 76% to 100% of cases. The etiology of this GGO is thought to represent either areas of fine interstitial fibrosis or areas of OP. Classically, the ground-glass opacity spares the periphery of the lung. This subpleural sparing is uncommon in UIP, but its absence does not exclude NSIP as a diagnosis. Consolidation may be present and often represents areas of OP or DAD. Radiologic honeycombing should be absent or minimal. Nodules, cysts, and areas of low attenuation are uncommon and should point one toward other diagnoses. Because many cases of NSIP are associated with CTD, it is important to look for associated findings that may suggest an underlying CTD such as esophageal dilation, pleural/pericardial effusions, and musculoskeletal abnormalities.

Tissue Sampling

Wedge biopsy of multiple lobes of the lung is recommended for the diagnosis of NSIP. NSIP should not be diagnosed on transbronchial biopsies as the histologic findings are not specific enough to allow it. Bronchoalveolar lavage cytology may show an increase in lymphocytes in over 50% of cases.

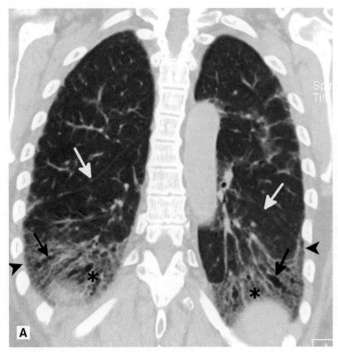

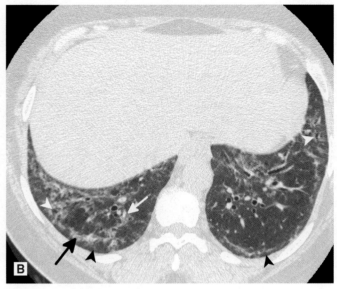

FIGURE 17.7 ▲ Nonspecific interstitial pneumonia, CT findings. **A.** Coronal CT shows lower lobe predominant ground-glass opacity (*asterisks*), reticulation (*arrowheads*), and traction bronchiectasis (*arrows*) and inferior displacement of the major fissures (*white arrow*), findings all consistent with lower lobe fibrosis. Patchy areas of GGO are also seen in the upper lobes. Honeycombing is absent. **B.** Axial CT shows lower lobe predominant peripheral (*black arrows*) and peribronchovascular (*white arrow*) ground-glass opacity with associated traction bronchiectasis (*white arrowheads*). In addition, there is sparing of the very subpleural portion of the lung (*black arrowheads*), a finding that is commonly associated with NSIP.

Gross Findings

In contrast to UIP, the cut surfaces of lungs with NSIP show a relative scarcity of cysts, sometimes a more central location of scarring, and diffuse uniform fibrosis (Fig. 17.8). The pleural surface may be bosselated, but the "cobblestone" pattern typical of UIP is less pronounced.

Microscopic Findings

Broadly, NSIP is characterized by the presence of diffuse inflammation and fibrosis, of variable degree, thickening the alveolar septa and lacking features of other idiopathic interstitial pneumonias or fibrotic lung diseases due to specific etiologies. Specifically, there is spatial uniformity of the inflammation and fibrosis, reflecting a uniform temporal onset, in contrast to UIP. At the cellular end of NSIP, there is more inflammation than fibrosis (Fig. 17.9). There is usually a mild diffuse hyperplasia of alveolar pneumocytes, but marked atypia as seen in acute lung injury is absent. The composition of the inflammatory infiltrate is varied, predominantly lymphocytes, but plasma cells occasionally may be more prominent. In contrast, in NSIP, predominantly fibrotic, the interstitial thickening is mostly composed of collagen fibrosis with mild chronic inflammation (Fig. 17.10). The fibrosis may cause architectural distortion and even some focal microscopic honeycombing, but overall, the features remain uniform, field to field, without the variegation typical of UIP. Because there is frequently a mixture of cellular areas and fibrosis in NSIP,[33] the simple diagnosis of NSIP is made.[36] However, in cases where the fibrosis is prominent, adding the qualifier of "with fibrosis" provides additional information as to potential response to treatment and prognosis. If OP appears to be superimposed on a background of NSIP, then a second diagnosis of OP should be rendered. Furthermore, fibroblast foci as seen in UIP can be observed, but they should be rare and the overall appearance of the infiltrates remains uniform.

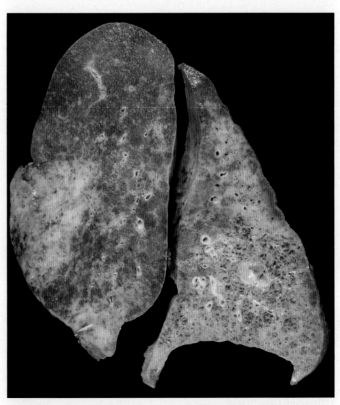

FIGURE 17.8 ▲ Nonspecific interstitial pneumonia, explant. There is patchy predominantly lower lung zone fibrosis with no significant subpleural honeycombing.

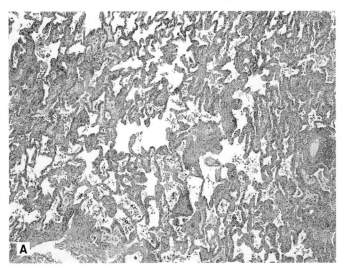 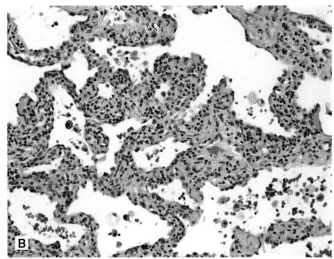

FIGURE 17.9 ▲ Nonspecific interstitial pneumonia, cellular type. **A.** Low-power magnification shows diffuse septal thickening mostly by a chronic inflammatory infiltrate. **B.** The chronic inflammatory infiltrate is composed of a mixture of lymphocytes and plasma cells.

Prognosis and Treatment

The treatment of NSIP includes steroids and other immunosuppressive medications, to which it responds better than UIP. In general, NSIP has a far better prognosis than UIP. Most patients will experience stable disease with response to treatment. Some will experience complete recovery, while a minority may progress and die of their disease. The reported survival has been varied, with reported five-year survival of 70%,[24] 82%,[23] and 88%.[27] Ten-year survival ranges from 65%[24] to 73%.[23] Fifteen-year survival is around 50%.[24] Series with the worse outcomes most likely included patients with UIP based on the description of honeycombing on imaging. The extent of fibrosis on histology appears to be a predictor of survival. Indeed, several studies have shown a vast superiority in survival, especially long term, of cellular NSIP as compared to fibrotic NSIP, with a spread of 28 percentage points at 80 months,[28] 55 percentage points at 10 years,[33] and 65 percentage points at 7 years.[27,28,32,37]

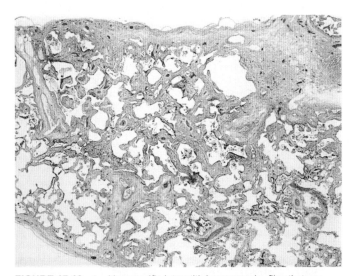

FIGURE 17.10 ▲ Nonspecific interstitial pneumonia, fibrotic type. There is marked interstitial fibrosis, but overall, the changes remain homogenous across the lobules.

Differential Diagnosis

The main differential diagnosis of UIP is with NSIP. Other diagnostic considerations include idiopathic pleuroparenchymal fibroelastosis (IPPFE) (Chapter 20), HP with fibrosis (Chapter 23), and asbestosis (Chapter 56). The distinguishing histologic feature of NSIP is a uniform temporal appearance, and if fibroblast foci or OP-like areas are seen, they are always very focal and inconspicuous. Similarly, honeycomb changes are only seen infrequently and blend with the adjacent collagen fibrosis of the fibrotic type of NSIP, in contrast to UIP.

"Fibrosing" HP is said to resemble UIP because it can have a heterogeneous aspect with honeycomb changes. However, this disease not only involves mainly the superior lobes but also is more bronchiolocentric in distribution. The airways will be chronically inflamed and scarred by fibrosis with bronchiolar metaplasia. The identification of giant cells and/or poorly formed nonnecrotizing granulomas in the wall of the airways is a clue to the diagnosis.

The fibrosis in asbestosis is different from UIP. It is an important distinction since UIP/IPF may occur in patients with exposure to asbestos.[38] Indeed, the fibrosis of asbestosis tends to be more airway centered, extending toward the periphery of the lobules. It can result in architectural distortion and honeycombing but not with the degree of heterogeneity of UIP. Furthermore, fibroblast foci are rare. But most importantly, in order to make the diagnosis of asbestosis, asbestos bodies need to be identified within the fibrotic lung.

IPPFE has only recently been introduced in the classification of IIPs. Like UIP, the fibrosis involves the pleura and subpleural space. In contrast to UIP, the fibrosis is elastotic and does cause as much architectural distortion. Fibroblast foci are inconspicuous.

If other specific parenchymal diseases have been ruled out, yet the chronic fibrosing interstitial pneumonia does not meet the diagnostic criteria of UIP or shows several atypical features, a diagnosis of chronic fibrosing interstitial pneumonia, not otherwise specified, is made with a comment regarding the histologic findings and potential differential diagnosis.

The diagnosis of NSIP may be challenging. Based on one study assessing interobserver variability in diagnosing interstitial lung disease, NSIP had one of lower kappa ratings and was confused with a host of other "patterns," including DAD (Chapter 4), OP (Chapter 5), and HP (Chapter 23), even among experts.[39] Other important differential diagnosis includes DIP (Chapter 18) and lymphoid interstitial pneumonia (LIP) (Chapter 20). Furthermore, NSIP may show several histologic features that are not specific to NSIP and shared with other interstitial lung diseases.[3,40] As such, the diagnosis of NSIP is often considered a diagnosis of exclusion.

The distinction with late phase of DAD can be challenging. In fact, in the original description of NSIP,[21] two cases were thought to be late phase of DAD based on retrospective review of the clinical histories. Morphologically, the fibrosis in DAD is more cellular being composed of fibroblasts and less collagen. But in a late phase of DAD, collagen increases along with a chronic inflammatory infiltrate. So the history may be the main clue in this distinction as patients with DAD typically have an acute onset of their symptoms and not uncommonly require mechanical ventilation.

Since OP can be a minor morphologic component of NSIP or be superimposed on NSIP, the distinction between OP and NSIP may be difficult. In OP, there may be septal thickening by a chronic inflammatory component but usually limited to the areas of the intraluminal fibroblastic plugs. In the areas away from the airspace plugs, the alveolar septa appear normal.

The distinction between NSIP in a smoker with DIP-like changes and DIP is controversial. However, it is overall thought that the interstitial fibrosis of DIP, when present, is quite distinctive, hyaline in nature, and paucicellular with no inflammation.

REFERENCES

1. King TE Jr. Clinical advances in the diagnosis and therapy of the interstitial lung diseases. *Am J Respir Crit Care Med.* 2005;172(3):268–279.
2. Lee HL, Ryu JH, Wittmer MH, et al. Familial idiopathic pulmonary fibrosis: clinical features and outcome. *Chest.* 2005;127(6):2034–2041.
3. Travis WD, Costabel U, Hansell DM, et al. An official American Thoracic Society/European Respiratory Society statement: update of the international multidisciplinary classification of the idiopathic interstitial pneumonias. *Am J Respir Crit Care Med.* 2013;188(6):733–748.
4. Elliot TL, Lynch DA, Newell JD Jr, et al. High-resolution computed tomography features of nonspecific interstitial pneumonia and usual interstitial pneumonia. *J Comput Assist Tomogr.* 2005;29(3):339–345.
5. Lee HY, Lee KS, Jeong YJ, et al. High-resolution CT findings in fibrotic idiopathic interstitial pneumonias with little honeycombing: serial changes and prognostic implications. *AJR Am J Roentgenol.* 2012;199(5):982–989.
6. Raghu G, Collard HR, Egan JJ, et al. An official ATS/ERS/JRS/ALAT statement: idiopathic pulmonary fibrosis: evidence-based guidelines for diagnosis and management. *Am J Respir Crit Care Med.* 2011;183(6):788–824.
7. Flaherty KR, Toews GB, Travis WD, et al. Clinical significance of histological classification of idiopathic interstitial pneumonia. *Eur Respir J.* 2002;19(2):275–283.
8. Song JW, Do KH, Kim MY, et al. Pathologic and radiologic differences between idiopathic and collagen vascular disease-related usual interstitial pneumonia. *Chest.* 2009;136(1):23–30.
9. Kim EJ, Elicker BM, Maldonado F, et al. Usual interstitial pneumonia in rheumatoid arthritis-associated interstitial lung disease. *Eur Respir J.* 2010;35(6):1322–1328.
10. Flaherty KR, Colby TV, Travis WD, et al. Fibroblastic foci in usual interstitial pneumonia: idiopathic versus collagen vascular disease. *Am J Respir Crit Care Med.* 2003;167(10):1410–1415.
11. Hunninghake GW, Zimmerman MB, Schwartz DA, et al. Utility of a lung biopsy for the diagnosis of idiopathic pulmonary fibrosis. *Am J Respir Crit Care Med.* 2001;164(2):193–196.
12. American Thoracic Society/European Respiratory Society International Multidisciplinary Consensus Classification of the Idiopathic Interstitial Pneumonias. This joint statement of the American Thoracic Society (ATS), and the European Respiratory Society (ERS) was adopted by the ATS board of directors, June 2001 and by the ERS Executive Committee, June 2001. *Am J Respir Crit Care Med.* 2002;165(2):277–304.
13. The diagnosis, assessment and treatment of diffuse parenchymal lung disease in adults. Introduction. *Thorax.* 1999;54(suppl 1):S1–S14.
14. Berbescu EA, Katzenstein AL, Snow JL, et al. Transbronchial biopsy in usual interstitial pneumonia. *Chest.* 2006;129(5):1126–1131.
15. Katzenstein AL, Zisman DA, Litzky LA, et al. Usual interstitial pneumonia: histologic study of biopsy and explant specimens. *Am J Surg Pathol.* 2002;26(12):1567–1577.
16. Todd NW, Scheraga RG, Galvin JR, et al. Lymphocyte aggregates persist and accumulate in the lungs of patients with idiopathic pulmonary fibrosis. *J Inflamm Res.* 2013;6:63–70.
17. Staats P, Kligerman S, Todd N, et al. A comparative study of honeycombing on high resolution computed tomography with histologic lung remodeling in explants with usual interstitial pneumonia. *Pathol Res Pract.* 2015;211(1):55–61.
18. Aubry MC, Myers JL, Douglas WW, et al. Primary pulmonary carcinoma in patients with idiopathic pulmonary fibrosis. *Mayo Clin Proc.* 2002;77(8):763–770.
19. Kawasaki H, Nagai K, Yokose T, et al. Clinicopathological characteristics of surgically resected lung cancer associated with idiopathic pulmonary fibrosis. *J Surg Oncol.* 2001;76(1):53–57.
20. Goto T, Maeshima A, Oyamada Y, et al. Idiopathic pulmonary fibrosis as a prognostic factor in non-small cell lung cancer. *Int J Clin Oncol.* 2014;19(2):266–273.
21. Katzenstein AL, Fiorelli RF. Nonspecific interstitial pneumonia/fibrosis. Histologic features and clinical significance. *Am J Surg Pathol.* 1994;18(2):136–147.
22. Kim MY, Song JW, Do KH, et al. Idiopathic nonspecific interstitial pneumonia: changes in high-resolution computed tomography on long-term follow-up. *J Comput Assist Tomogr.* 2012;36(2):170–174.
23. Travis WD, Hunninghake G, King TE Jr, et al. Idiopathic nonspecific interstitial pneumonia: report of an American Thoracic Society project. *Am J Respir Crit Care Med.* 2008;177(12):1338–1347.
24. Bjoraker JA, Ryu JH, Edwin MK, et al. Prognostic significance of histopathologic subsets in idiopathic pulmonary fibrosis. *Am J Respir Crit Care Med.* 1998;157(1):199–203.
25. Cottin V, Donsbeck AV, Revel D, et al. Nonspecific interstitial pneumonia. Individualization of a clinicopathologic entity in a series of 12 patients. *Am J Respir Crit Care Med.* 1998;158(4):1286–1293.
26. Daniil ZD, Gilchrist FC, Nicholson AG, et al. A histologic pattern of nonspecific interstitial pneumonia is associated with a better prognosis than usual interstitial pneumonia in patients with cryptogenic fibrosing alveolitis. *Am J Respir Crit Care Med.* 1999;160(3):899–905.
27. Flaherty KR, Travis WD, Colby TV, et al. Histopathologic variability in usual and nonspecific interstitial pneumonias. *Am J Respir Crit Care Med.* 2001;164(9):1722–1727.
28. Jegal Y, Kim DS, Shim TS, et al. Physiology is a stronger predictor of survival than pathology in fibrotic interstitial pneumonia. *Am J Respir Crit Care Med.* 2005;171(6):639–644.
29. Johkoh T, Müller NL, Colby TV, et al. Nonspecific interstitial pneumonia: correlation between thin-section CT findings and pathologic subgroups in 55 patients. *Radiology.* 2002;225(1):199–204.
30. Monaghan H, Wells AU, Colby TV, et al. Prognostic implications of histologic patterns in multiple surgical lung biopsies from patients with idiopathic interstitial pneumonias. *Chest.* 2004;125(2):522–526.
31. Nagai S, Handa T, Tabuena R, et al. Nonspecific interstitial pneumonia: a real clinical entity? *Clin Chest Med.* 2004;25(4):705–715, vi.
32. Nicholson AG, Colby TV, du Bois RM, et al. The prognostic significance of the histologic pattern of interstitial pneumonia in patients presenting with the clinical entity of cryptogenic fibrosing alveolitis. *Am J Respir Crit Care Med.* 2000;162(6):2213–2217.
33. Travis WD, Matsui K, Moss J, et al. Idiopathic nonspecific interstitial pneumonia: prognostic significance of cellular and fibrosing patterns: survival comparison with usual interstitial pneumonia and desquamative interstitial pneumonia. *Am J Surg Pathol.* 2000;24(1):19–33.
34. Kinder BW, Collard HR, Koth L, et al. Idiopathic nonspecific interstitial pneumonia: lung manifestation of undifferentiated connective tissue disease? *Am J Respir Crit Care Med.* 2007;176(7):691–697.
35. Suffredini AF, Ognibene FP, Lack EE, et al. Nonspecific interstitial pneumonitis: a common cause of pulmonary disease in the acquired immunodeficiency syndrome. *Ann Intern Med.* 1987;107(1):7–13.
36. Todd NW, Marciniak ET, Sachdeva A, et al. Organizing pneumonia/nonspecific interstitial pneumonia overlap is associated with unfavorable lung disease progression. *Respir Med.* 2015;109(11):1460–1468.
37. Nagai S, Kitaichi M, Itoh H, et al. Idiopathic nonspecific interstitial pneumonia/fibrosis: comparison with idiopathic pulmonary fibrosis and BOOP. *Eur Respir J.* 1998;12(5):1010–1019.
38. Churg A. Asbestos-related disease in the workplace and the environment: controversial issues. *Monogr Pathol.* 1993;36:54–77.
39. Nicholson AG, Addis BJ, Bharucha H, et al. Inter-observer variation between pathologists in diffuse parenchymal lung disease. *Thorax.* 2004;59(6):500–505.
40. Flaherty KR, King TE Jr, Raghu G, et al. Idiopathic interstitial pneumonia: what is the effect of a multidisciplinary approach to diagnosis? *Am J Respir Crit Care Med.* 2004;170(8):904–910.

18 Smoking-Related Idiopathic Interstitial Pneumonias

Allen P. Burke, M.D., Fabio R. Tavora, M.D., Ph.D., Seth Kligerman, M.D., and Marie-Christine Aubry, M.D.

Respiratory Bronchiolitis—Interstitial Lung Disease

Terminology

Respiratory bronchiolitis (RB) and desquamative interstitial pneumonia (DIP) form a spectrum of smoking-related lung disease that is characterized by inflammation of the small airways, aggregates of cohesive finely pigmented macrophages within alveolar spaces, and variable degrees of interstitial fibrosis (Table 18.1). The term "respiratory bronchiolitis" is considered a pathologic pattern by the ATS/ERS and "respiratory bronchiolitis-associated interstitial lung disease" a clinicopathologic designation.

It was first appreciated in 1974 that "clusters of pigmented alveolar macrophages [are] present in the lungs of all smokers …"[1] The term RBILD was introduced by Myers and Katzenstein[2] and subsequently used by Yousem et al.[3] The initial report involved 6 heavy cigarette smokers with lung infiltrates, cough, dyspnea, and histologic features on open lung biopsy of inflammation with macrophage infiltrates of the terminal airways and airspaces.[2] Another entity related to smoking is pulmonary Langerhans cell histiocytosis (PLCH), which is discussed separately in Chapter 24.

Whether or not RBILD and DIP are considered a single entity or two different ones is debated. In some classifications, they are considered the same entity[4,5]; in the latest ATS-ERS (American Thoracic Society–European Respiratory Society) nomenclature, they are separated into two entities under "smoking-related interstitial pneumonia" since the clinical and radiologic presentations differ.[6] A DIP pattern may be present in pediatric interstitial lung disease related to surfactant deficiency, but this entity is unrelated to smoking-related DIP. Rarely, other agents have been reported as causing a DIP-like reaction, which include dust inhalation, drug reactions, and other inborn error of metabolism other than surfactant deficiency.[7–10] An even small number of patients have no identifiable cause and are never smokers.[11]

Clinical Findings

Pathologists most commonly see respiratory bronchiolitis in resection specimens for lung cancers as an incidental finding. In rare cases, the condition presents as a form of interstitial lung disease with pulmonary symptoms, abnormal pulmonary function tests, and imaging abnormalities, especially reticular densities and ground-glass opacities. It is then described as respiratory bronchiolitis-associated interstitial lung disease (RBILD). RBILD presents with nonspecific complaints such as dyspnea and new or changed cough. It usually affects current smokers in the fourth and fifth decades of life with average exposures of more than 30 pack-years of cigarette smoking. Men are more often affected than women; in contrast to DIP, finger clubbing is usually absent.[2,6,12] In Fraig et al.'s study, RB was found in some patients many years after cessation of smoking, including 42% after 3 years and 33% after 5 years.[13]

Radiologic Findings

The HRCT findings of RBILD include centrilobular nodules, patchy ground-glass attenuation, and airway thickening. Upper lobe centrilobular emphysema is common.[12] Upper lobe predominant centrilobular nodules can have an appearance similar to nonfibrotic hypersensitivity pneumonia (Fig. 18.1).

TABLE 18.1   Fibrosing Lung Diseases Associated with Smoking, Various Terms Used by Radiologists, Clinicians, and Pathologists

Designation	Explanation
RB; RB-ILD	No requirement of fibrosis, although chronic interstitial inflammation typical; emphasis on intra-alveolar and distal bronchiolar accumulation of finely pigmented macrophages; RB used by pathologists for the pathologic findings; RBILD used by clinicians for the clinical and radiologic findings
RB-ILD with fibrosis	Pathologic term introduced by Yousem in 2006, bland acellular interstitial fibrosis in otherwise typical RB-ILD. Not used clinically
Airspace enlargement with fibrosis (AEF)	Pathologic term introduced by Kawabata et al. in 2008 to emphasize interstitial fibrosis in areas of smoking-related emphysema. Mentioned in the differential diagnosis of RBILD and DIP in the ATS/ERS consensus classification (Travis et al.[6])
Smoking-related interstitial fibrosis (SRIF)	Term introduced by Katzenstein. Similar morphology to AEF
PLCH	Reactive fibrosis forming cysts and stellate scars in areas of Langerhans cell infiltrates (see Chapter 24)
Combined pulmonary fibrosis and emphysema (syndrome)	Term used by radiologists to designated smokers with emphysema in upper lobes and usually UIP/IPF in lower lobes
Smoking-related ILD	Radiologic term for variety of changes that can be seen by CT (emphysema, RB-ILD, DIP, and PLCH)
Smoking-related lung changes (injury)	Pathologist terminology to encompass mixture of nonspecific background changes related to smoking on biopsies or autopsy samples

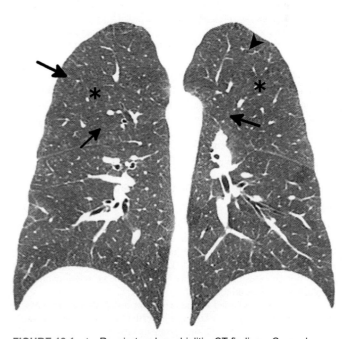

FIGURE 18.1 ▲ Respiratory bronchiolitis, CT findings. Coronal 50-mm-thick minimum intensity projection image shows upper lobe predominant ground-glass opacity (*asterisks*), centrilobular nodules (*arrows*), and emphysema (*arrowhead*). The lung attenuation is diffusely heterogeneous. Although similar imaging findings can be seen in nonfibrotic hypersensitivity pneumonia, the smoking history confirms the diagnosis of respiratory bronchiolitis. There are large collections of cohesive brown macrophages adjacent to airways.

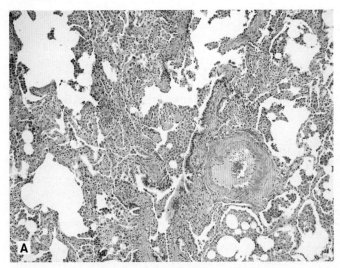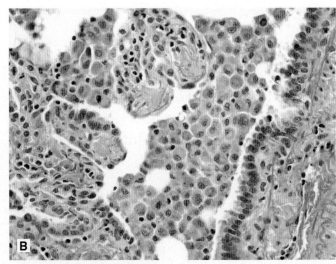

FIGURE 18.2 ▲ Respiratory bronchiolitis. **A.** At low power, RB is characterized by airspace accumulation of pigmented macrophages, which are more prominent within the lumen of the small airway and decrease in density in the alveolar spaces away from the airway. **B.** The pigment of smoking is brown-black and finely granular.

Tissue Sampling

Smoking-related lung disease is often diagnosed by computed tomography and only occasionally will be the major finding at wedge biopsy. Bronchoalveolar lavage fluid contains alveolar macrophages with golden-, brown-, or black-pigmented inclusions typical of those seen in smokers. A modest increase in neutrophils may also be present.[12]

Microscopic Findings

The pathologic lesion of RBILD is RB. At low power, RB displays a patchy bronchiolocentric distribution characterized by airspace accumulation of pigmented (smoker's) macrophages within distal bronchioles and adjacent alveolar spaces (Fig. 18.2). The macrophages contain a finely granular brown pigment. Peribronchiolar chronic inflammation and fibrosis may be present in the areas of RB and extend into adjacent alveolar septa with bronchiolar metaplasia of the pneumocytes.[3]

Prognosis and Treatment

The reported 5-year mortality is <5% and presumably related to other conditions.[14] A follow-up study of biopsied patients with RBILD showed that although mortality is low, improvement (either symptomatic or on pulmonary function testing) occurs in a minority of patients. Furthermore, some patients who stopped smoking or received immunosuppressive treatment had progressive disease.[15]

Desquamative Interstitial Pneumonia

Terminology

DIP is usually considered to be a more extensive form of RBILD in which the pigmented macrophages fill alveolar spaces diffusely throughout larger areas of the lung. Although it is considered a smoking-related disease, along with RBILD,[6] there are a slightly higher proportion of cases in which there appears to be no relationship with smoking, as compared to RBILD.

DIP was first included in the classification of idiopathic interstitial pneumonias in 1969.[16] DIP was described as an interstitial pneumonia morphologically distinct from usual interstitial pneumonia (UIP) and later shown to have significantly better survival than UIP.[17] Initially, the intra-alveolar cells were thought to be desquamated reactive pneumocytes; thus the terminology of "desquamative" in the diagnosis of DIP.

Clinical Findings

Although considered one of the rarest of interstitial pneumonias,[18] the true incidence depends on its distinction from the much more common smoking-related lung disease, RBILD. DIP affects cigarette smokers at a mean age of about 40 to 50 years.[3,19] Sex predilection reflects smoking trends, and most studies show a male predominance.[3,17,20-22] Although in most series about 90% of patients are smokers,[3,22] one study reported a rate of only 60%.[20] Similar to RBILD, there is an insidious onset of dry cough and dyspnea that may progress to respiratory failure. Digital clubbing develops in about 50% of patients.[17] Lung physiology confirms normal lung volumes or a mild restrictive abnormality, and the carbon monoxide diffusing capacity is moderately decreased.[12]

Radiologic Findings

Ground-glass opacification is present on CT in all cases of DIP, reflects the presence of partial alveolar filling by macrophages, and is present to a greater degree than in RBILD (Fig. 18.3). The ground-glass distribution is most frequent in the lower zones (73%) followed by peripheral (59%) and patchy (23%) distributions; this distribution differs from RBILD, which is more upper lobe predominant.[23] In addition, there are frequent irregular linear opacities with a reticular pattern, usually limited and confined to the lung bases. Limited honeycombing is seen in less than one-third of cases and is usually peripheral.[12]

Microscopic Findings

The distinctive features of DIP are its uniform appearance at low power, in contrast to UIP, and accumulation of numerous pigmented alveolar macrophages within the distal airspaces (Fig. 18.4). The macrophages, similar to those seen in RBILD, have abundant cytoplasm containing finely brown granular pigment. The macrophages are often confluent and may be multinucleated. Eosinophils are often admixed with the macrophages (Fig. 18.4). The alveolar septa are thickened by mild, bland fibrosis, sparse inflammatory infiltrate, mostly plasma cells, and reactive cuboidal pneumocytes.[12] Prominent diffuse fibrosis and focal honeycombing as originally described by Carrington[17] is not a recognized feature of DIP in the ATS/ERS consensus statement. However, some authors accept that more prominent fibrosis may be seen in DIP (Fig. 18.5).[18] Lymphoid follicles with germinal centers are commonly seen (Fig. 18.4), centered on the bronchioles as well as in the distal interstitium and pleura, and are a useful diagnostic feature.

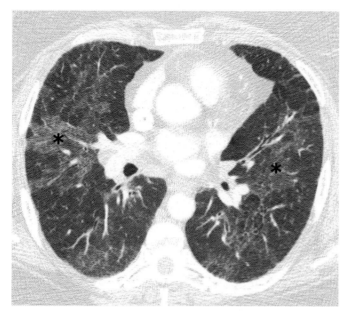

FIGURE 18.3 ▲ Desquamative interstitial pneumonia, CT findings. Axial CT image through the midlung zones shows patchy areas of ground-glass opacity (*asterisks*), which persisted over many months. Open lung biopsy demonstrated DIP.

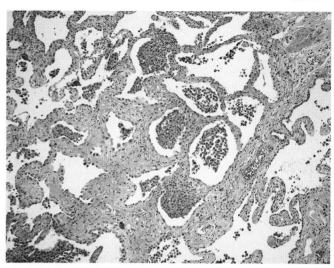

FIGURE 18.5 ▲ Desquamative interstitial pneumonia. DIP with more prominent interstitial fibrosis. The fibrosis has a hyaline appearance and contains scarce inflammation.

Prognosis and Treatment

In a seminal study from more than 25 years ago, mortality among patients with DIP was 27.5%, with a mean survival of 12.2 years. A review of more recent studies shows an overall mortality of 6% to 30%.[18] In one study of 31 patients, only 1 patient died due to progression of disease.[24] In Ryu et al.'s[22] series of 23 patients, 3 patients died of disease progression and 2 of cancer. In contrast to RBILD, there is more severe interstitial disease on pulmonary function tests, and progressive respiratory disease is frequent.[3] Treatment is corticosteroids, which is generally initially effective.[18] In a follow-up radiologic study of 31 patients, not histologically documented, 5 developed honeycombing by CT imaging, and 4 patients developed lung cancers. The progression of DIP into a fibrosing interstitial disease, either by imaging

or histologic findings at explant, may be difficult to discern from the development of smoking-related fibrosis.[18]

Fibrosis Related to Smoking

Terminology

The concept of smoking-induced fibrosis is not new, and was first documented in 1974 in a histomorphometric study of over a thousand autopsied lungs. This study showed a 40-fold increase in interstitial fibrosis in smokers as compared to nonsmokers, with a dose-dependent relationship with pack-year history.[25] Since these patients are smokers, it is not surprising that this localized fibrosis is typically accompanied by RB. In his series of RBILD, Yousem et al.[26] reported fibrosis as a key feature to distinguish incidental RB from RBILD, hence their suggested terminology of RBILD with fibrosis. However, they also identified a small subgroup of patients in their series that were asymptomatic, without features of an interstitial lung disease. This combination of findings has now been described by several different

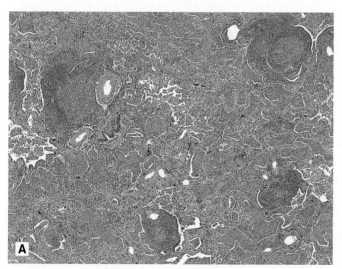

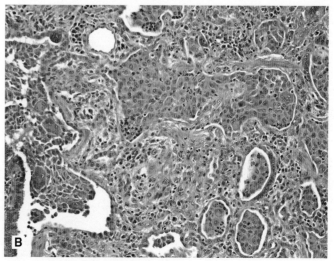

FIGURE 18.4 ▲ Desquamative interstitial pneumonia. **A.** At low power, DIP is a diffuse interstitial and airspace process. Scattered lymphoid follicles with germinal centers are seen. **B.** At higher power, the pigmented macrophages appear cohesive and many eosinophils are admixed. The reactive pneumocytes are uniform and cuboidal. The alveolar septa are mildly thickened by inflammatory cells, mostly plasma cells.

terminologies including *airspace enlargement with fibrosis* (AEF),[27] *smoking-related interstitial fibrosis* (SRIF),[28] and more recently RB with fibrosis (RBF).[29]

Basically, all three describe findings of interstitial fibrosis and RB in heavy smokers, often in association with dilated or emphysematous airspaces, which should be distinguished from RBILD and DIP. The term "SRIF" is useful in emphasizing the fact that fibrosis with a characteristic histologic appearance is a component of smoking-related lung injury. The most recent consensus classification on IIPs prefers the terminology of AEF.[6]

Furthermore, this incidental smoking-related fibrosis needs to be distinguished from combined pulmonary fibrosis and emphysema (CPFE). CPFE represents usually the combination of IPF/UIP [Chapter 17] with centrilobular emphysema [Chapter 44].[23,30] In 2005, Cottin et al. coined the term "combined pulmonary fibrosis and emphysema," sometimes called "combined pulmonary fibrosis and emphysema syndrome."[31,32] That same year, Grubstein et al.[33] described 8 smokers with bullous emphysema in the upper lobes, and interstitial fibrosis resembling UIP in the lower lobes, and suggested that smoking can result in pulmonary fibrosis as well as emphysema.

The pathologic implications are that some smokers with IPF/UIP may have emphysema or SRIF in addition to typical findings of UIP. Similarly, smokers may have SRIF but not IPF/UIP or RBILD/DIP. Therefore, it is critical as a pathologist, when presented with histologic findings of interstitial fibrosis and RB, to know the exact clinical and radiologic context of the findings before making a definitive diagnosis.

In this chapter, we use SRIF for this concept of smoking-induced fibrosis and to encompass all studies on the topic using alternate terminology of AEF and RBF. Table 18.1 outlines some of the terms used by clinicians, radiologists, and pathologists for conditions that are caused by smoking and that cause interstitial fibrosis.

Incidence and Clinical Findings

The exact incidence is not known, but studies suggest that SRIF likely occurs in the majority of cigarette smokers. The reported mean age varies between 44 and 65 years, likely based on the study's methodology. Although found in mild smokers, SRIF is more prevalent in moderate to heavy smokers (>30 pack-years). Typically, these findings are incidental, and patients do not have symptoms attributable to SRIF, and no restriction is identified on pulmonary function test.

Radiologic Findings

High-resolution CT descriptions of SRIF are sparse. The most comprehensive study is by Reddy et al. who describe patchy mild reticular opacities in the upper and midlung zones, in association with emphysema. Ground-glass opacities are often present. In contrast to RB/RBILD, no centrilobular ground-glass nodules were identified.[29]

Tissue Sampling

Smoking-related fibrotic changes are most frequently encountered as incidental findings adjacent to tumors excised in patients who are smokers. Occasionally, wedge biopsies of smokers with diffuse parenchymal lung disease may show these changes as incidental and unrelated to primary reason for the lung biopsy. Therefore, it is very important to correlate the pathologic findings with the clinical and radiologic context of the biopsy.

Gross Findings

There are few studies of gross findings of SRIF. Kawabata et al. describe these as variously sized, thin-walled cysts, different than honeycombing, which has thicker walls. These were often associated with areas of centrilobular emphysema.[27]

Microscopic Findings

On low magnification, there are varying degrees of interstitial fibrosis, in a background of centrilobular emphysema and RB (Fig. 18.6). The distribution is variable, often subpleural but also seen deeper in the lung, centered on small bronchioles. The interstitial fibrosis is characteristic, being paucicellular, bland, and hyaline, amyloid-like with scarce interstitial inflammation (Fig. 18.6). Peribronchiolar metaplasia or honeycombing is extremely rare and reported in cases

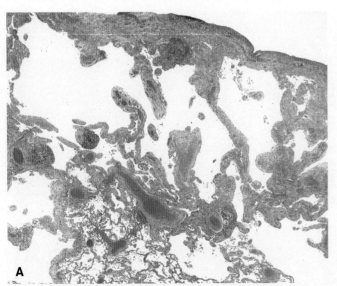
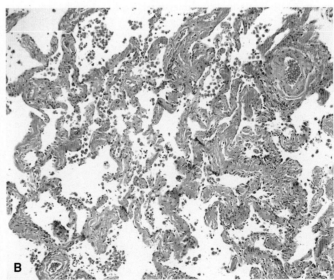

FIGURE 18.6 ▲ Smoking-related interstitial fibrosis. **A.** At low magnification, SIRF within the apex of the upper lobe is a localized process, associated with centrilobular emphysema. **B.** The interstitium shows varying degrees of interstitial thickening, usually mild to moderate, without significant architectural distortion or honeycombing. The fibrosis appears hyaline and inflammation is sparse. RB is present.

of prominent fibrosis. Fibroblast foci are rare, if present. The findings are typically localized.

Prognosis and Treatment

Follow-up on patients with SRIF is scant and short term. However, all studies have reported similar findings. No patients experienced progressive disease.[26,28,34]

Differential Diagnosis

The differential diagnosis of the RB includes nonspecific accumulations of intra-alveolar macrophages without pigment, which may occur in all forms of interstitial lung disease, especially NSIP and UIP.[13,35]

Furthermore, the smoker's pigment of macrophages in RB and DIP needs to be distinguished from hemosiderin-laden macrophages seen in patients with prior hemorrhage or with heart failure. Hemosiderin forms refractile intracellular blocky pigment that differs from the fine dust characteristic of the brown pigment of RB.[18]

RB and DIP-like changes are nonspecific histologic findings, seen in smokers with various lung diseases such as lung cancer, UIP, and PLCH. The histologic diagnosis of RB/RBILD and DIP thus requires ruling out clinically, radiologically, or histologically any other lung disease that may be responsible for the patient's clinical presentation.

Differentiating RB/RBILD from DIP may be challenging. Although it is convenient to consider RB as macrophages within the airways, and DIP extending into "distal alveoli,"[13] it is in practice difficult to distinguish the two, and occasionally a diagnosis of RB/DIP may be rendered. DIP should have more diffuse septal thickening than RB/RBILD. Also, lymphoid follicles are more common in DIP than RB/RBILD.[20]

The presence of significant fibrosis in DIP and its distinction from nonspecific interstitial pneumonia with DIP-like changes remain controversial. However, some authors suggest that fibrosis may be prominent in DIP. Furthermore, the fibrosis in DIP is distinct from that of NSIP, being bland and hyaline, with scarce inflammation, similar to the fibrosis of SRIF.[18] Furthermore, the lymphoid follicles and intra-alveolar eosinophils are more typical of DIP than NSIP. In the context of fibrosis in DIP, a mild amount of honeycomb may be acceptable, but DIP should lack the temporal variegation typical of UIP.

The main distinction between SRIF and RBILD and DIP lies in the clinical presentation. Indeed, SRIF is an incidental finding usually seen in lung specimens resected for cancers.

Typically, in RBILD and DIP, emphysema is not a prominent histologic finding, in contrast to SRIF.

PLCH [Chapter 24] enters the differential diagnosis of RB/ILD, DIP, and SIRF. The main distinctive feature of PLCH is the presence of centrilobular stellate-shaped fibrotic nodules, containing a mixed inflammatory infiltrate.

The presence of eosinophils may so be prominent in some cases of DIP as to raise a diagnosis of eosinophilic pneumonia (EP) [Chapter 26]. The clinical and radiologic findings are quite different between EP and DIP. Furthermore, histologically, the eosinophils in EP form microabscesses and are admixed in a fibrinous exudate, or occasionally with organizing pneumonia.

REFERENCES

1. Niewoehner DE, Kleinerman J, Rice DB. Pathologic changes in the peripheral airways of young cigarette smokers. *N Engl J Med.* 1974;291(15):755–758.
2. Myers JL, et al. Respiratory bronchiolitis causing interstitial lung disease. A clinicopathologic study of six cases. *Am Rev Respir Dis.* 1987;135(4):880–884.
3. Yousem SA, Colby TV, Gaensler EA. Respiratory bronchiolitis-associated interstitial lung disease and its relationship to desquamative interstitial pneumonia. *Mayo Clin Proc.* 1989;64(11):1373–1380.
4. King TE Jr. Clinical advances in the diagnosis and therapy of the interstitial lung diseases. *Am J Respir Crit Care Med.* 2005;172(3):268–279.
5. Myers JL, Katzenstein AL. Beyond a consensus classification for idiopathic interstitial pneumonias: progress and controversies. *Histopathology.* 2009;54(1):90–103.
6. Travis WD, et al. An official American Thoracic Society/European Respiratory Society statement: update of the international multidisciplinary classification of the idiopathic interstitial pneumonias. *Am J Respir Crit Care Med.* 2013;188(6):733–748.
7. Herbert A, et al. Desquamative interstitial pneumonia in an aluminum welder. *Hum Pathol.* 1982;13(8):694–699.
8. Corrin B, Price AB. Electron microscopic studies in desquamative interstitial pneumonia associated with asbestos. *Thorax.* 1972;27(3):324–331.
9. Freed JA, et al. Desquamative interstitial pneumonia associated with chrysotile asbestos fibres. *Br J Ind Med.* 1991;48(5):332–337.
10. Aoki Y, et al. Desquamative interstitial pneumonitis accompanied by a variety of autoimmune abnormalities in an individual with a history of asbestos exposure. *Nihon Kokyuki Gakkai Zasshi.* 1998;36(8):717–721.
11. Bressieux-Degueldre S, et al. Idiopathic desquamative interstitial pneumonia in a child: a case report. *BMC Res Notes.* 2014;7:383.
12. American Thoracic Society/European Respiratory Society International Multidisciplinary Consensus Classification of the Idiopathic Interstitial Pneumonias. This joint statement of the American Thoracic Society (ATS), and the European Respiratory Society (ERS) was adopted by the ATS board of directors, June 2001 and by the ERS Executive Committee, June 2001. *Am J Respir Crit Care Med.* 2002;165(2):277–304.
13. Fraig M, et al. Respiratory bronchiolitis: a clinicopathologic study in current smokers, ex-smokers, and never-smokers. *Am J Surg Pathol.* 2002;26(5):647–653.
14. Kim DS, Collard HR, King TE Jr. Classification and natural history of the idiopathic interstitial pneumonias. *Proc Am Thorac Soc.* 2006;3(4):285–292.
15. Portnoy J, et al. Respiratory bronchiolitis-interstitial lung disease: long-term outcome. *Chest.* 2007;131(3):664–671.
16. Liebow AA, Carrington DB. The interstitial pneumonias. In: Simon M, Potchen EJ, LeMay M, eds. *Frontiers of Pulmonary Radiology.* New York, NY: Grune & Stratteon; 1969:102–141.
17. Carrington CB, et al. Natural history and treated course of usual and desquamative interstitial pneumonia. *N Engl J Med.* 1978;298(15):801–809.
18. Tazelaar HD, Wright JL, Churg A. Desquamative interstitial pneumonia. *Histopathology.* 2011;58(4):509–516.
19. Godbert B, Wissler MP, Vignaud JM. Desquamative interstitial pneumonia: an analytic review with an emphasis on aetiology. *Eur Respir Rev.* 2013;22(128):117–123.
20. Craig PJ, et al. Desquamative interstitial pneumonia, respiratory bronchiolitis and their relationship to smoking. *Histopathology.* 2004;45(3):275–282.
21. Tubbs RR, et al. Desquamative interstitial pneumonitis. Cellular phase of fibrosing alveolitis. *Chest.* 1977;72(2):159–165.
22. Ryu JH, et al. Desquamative interstitial pneumonia and respiratory bronchiolitis-associated interstitial lung disease. *Chest.* 2005;127(1):178–184.
23. Attili AK, et al. Smoking-related interstitial lung disease: radiologic-clinical-pathologic correlation. *Radiographics.* 2008;28(5):1383–1396; discussion 1396–1398.
24. Kawabata Y, et al. Desquamative interstitial pneumonia may progress to lung fibrosis as characterized radiologically. *Respirology.* 2012;17(8):1214–1221.
25. Auerbach O, Garfinkel L, Hammond EC. Relation of smoking and age to findings in lung parenchyma: a microscopic study. *Chest.* 1974;65(1):29–35.
26. Yousem SA. Respiratory bronchiolitis-associated interstitial lung disease with fibrosis is a lesion distinct from fibrotic nonspecific interstitial pneumonia: a proposal. *Mod Pathol.* 2006;19(11):1474–1479.
27. Kawabata Y, et al. Smoking-related changes in the background lung of specimens resected for lung cancer: a semiquantitative study with correlation to postoperative course. *Histopathology.* 2008;53(6):707–714.
28. Katzenstein AL, et al. Clinically occult interstitial fibrosis in smokers: classification and significance of a surprisingly common finding in lobectomy specimens. *Hum Pathol.* 2010;41(3):316–325.
29. Reddy TL, Mayo J, Churg A. Respiratory bronchiolitis with fibrosis. High-resolution computed tomography findings and correlation with pathology. *Ann Am Thorac Soc.* 2013;10(6):590–601.
30. Wiggins J, Strickland B, Turner-Warwick M. Combined cryptogenic fibrosing alveolitis and emphysema: the value of high resolution computed tomography in assessment. *Respir Med.* 1990;84(5):365–369.
31. Cottin V, et al. Combined pulmonary fibrosis and emphysema: a distinct underrecognised entity. *Eur Respir J.* 2005;26(4):586–593.

32. Portillo K, Morera J. Combined pulmonary fibrosis and emphysema syndrome: a new phenotype within the spectrum of smoking-related interstitial lung disease. *Pulm Med.* 2012;2012:867870.
33. Grubstein A, et al. Concomitant upper-lobe bullous emphysema, lower-lobe interstitial fibrosis and pulmonary hypertension in heavy smokers: report of eight cases and review of the literature. *Respir Med.* 2005;99(8): 948–954.
34. Churg A, Muller NL, Wright JL. Respiratory bronchiolitis/interstitial lung disease: fibrosis, pulmonary function, and evolving concepts. *Arch Pathol Lab Med.* 2010;134(1):27–32.
35. Travis WD, et al. Idiopathic nonspecific interstitial pneumonia: prognostic significance of cellular and fibrosing patterns: survival comparison with usual interstitial pneumonia and desquamative interstitial pneumonia. *Am J Surg Pathol.* 2000;24(1):19–33.

19 Acute and Subacute Idiopathic Interstitial Pneumonias

Marie-Christine Aubry, M.D., Allen P. Burke, M.D., and Seth Kligerman, M.D.

Cryptogenic Organizing Pneumonia

Terminology

One of the first uses of a term related to "organizing pneumonia (OP)" in the context of interstitial lung disease was by Liebow and Carrington, who designated "bronchiolitis obliterans with clinical interstitial pneumonia" as one of the five idiopathic interstitial pneumonias (IIPs).[1] The concept of cryptogenic organizing pneumonia (COP) originated in 1983, when Davison et al. described a clinicopathologic entity afflicting eight patients with malaise, weight loss, elevated sedimentation rate, and diffuse lung infiltrates.[2] COP defined a noninfectious, steroid-responsive condition histologically mimicking postinfectious organizing pneumonia; airway or bronchiolar involvement was not stressed. Interestingly, in the same year (1983), Davison and Epstein described "relapsing organizing pneumonitis" in a patient with CREST syndrome.[3] Soon thereafter, Epler et al. described a larger series of 50 patients with histologic documented "bronchiolitis obliterans with patchy organizing pneumonia," which was likewise idiopathic and noninfectious and steroid responsive. This series marked the first use of the term "bronchiolitis obliterans organizing pneumonia," or BOOP.[4] The authors emphasized the intraluminal morphology of BOOP nicely describing the histologic finding of "polypoid masses of granulation tissue in lumens of small airways, alveolar ducts, and some alveoli" while recognizing the restrictive physiology on lung function, as seen in interstitial lung disease.

The predominant airspace nature of BOOP led many authors to question its validity as an interstitial lung disease. Furthermore, the bronchiolitis obliterans of BOOP was unfortunately confused with a completely different and purely obstructive airway disease called constrictive bronchiolitis, also known as bronchiolitis obliterans.

The American Thoracic Society and European Respiratory Society maintained BOOP as an IIP since BOOP can clinically present as and enters the differential diagnosis of IIPs. Due to the confusion generated by the terminology, they also suggested dropping the BO part of BOOP and use the terminology of COP to designate a disease that is idiopathic and histologically characterized by "organization within alveolar ducts and alveoli *with or without* organization within bronchioles."[5]

Clinical Findings

COP is generally a disease of subacute onset, usually <3-month duration. Overall, it represents between 4% and 12% of IIPs.[6] There is an equal sex distribution, and more patients are nonsmokers than smokers.[5] The mean age at onset is 55 years.[5] Patients present with shortness of breath and cough, which may be productive with clear sputum. Systemic symptoms are common. Finger clubbing is rare, and there is often increased C-reactive protein and sedimentation rate.[5] Lung parameters show usually a restrictive defect with moderately reduced carbon monoxide transfer factor, mild airflow obstruction, and mild hypoxemia.[5]

The diagnosis of *cryptogenic* OP requires a lack of association with other diseases such as hypersensitivity pneumonitis, infection, tumors, drugs, connective tissue diseases, rejection, aspiration, and eosinophilic pneumonia (EP) (Chapter 26).[6]

Radiologic Findings

There are numerous CT patterns described with OP ranging from a focal nodule to diffuse fibrotic lung disease. Although focal disease can occur, most patients with COP and secondary OP present with a diffuse parenchymal abnormality.

Series have shown that high-resolution computed tomography (HRCT) shows ground-glass opacities (GGO) (60% to 85%) and consolidation (70% to 90%) that may be peribronchovascular or peripheral (Fig. 19.1).[4,5,7] These are often patchy with lower zone predominance.[6] In 90% of cases, there are air bronchograms in the areas of consolidation.[5] The distribution may be subpleural or peribronchial, with small nodules involving bronchovascular bundles. In 15%, the radiologic presentation is that of multiple large nodules.[5] Rarely, COP may mimic lung cancer, presenting as a single nodule with irregular borders with positive emission tomography (PET) positivity.[8] The reverse halo sign is typical but not pathognomonic. Pleural effusion is uncommon. In contrast to nonspecific interstitial pneumonia (NSIP) or usual interstitial pneumonia (UIP), there is no volume loss or honeycombing.[9]

Tissue Sampling

In the appropriate clinical and radiologic confirm, a transbronchial biopsy may be sufficient to confirm the diagnosis of OP.[10] However, an open lung or video-assisted thoracoscopic surgery is the preferred method of tissue sampling if a broader differential diagnosis is considered clinically. Bronchoalveolar lavage (BAL) shows increased lymphocyte proportion of total cells, up to 40%, and decreased CD4/CD8 ratio, similar to NSIP.[9]

Microscopic Findings

The histologic findings are those of OP (Chapter 5). The dominant feature is the proliferation of fibroblast/myofibroblast in a loose myxoid stroma forming intraluminal plugs (Fig. 19.2). There may be an associated chronic interstitial inflammation, with reactive pneumocytes, and increased alveolar macrophages, some of which may be foamy. However, these findings are limited to the areas of lung with the intraluminal fibroblast plugs. Away from these airspace changes, the lung parenchyma appears normal. Occasionally, there is increased collagen deposition within the intraluminal plugs and replacement of the fibroblasts (Fig. 19.3). Over time, this collagen fibrosis may get incorporated into the alveolar septa. These features may pertain to a worse prognosis.[11] Fibrin may be focally present but not conspicuous.

Prognosis and Treatment

The treatment of COP is steroids, which result in clearing of symptoms in the majority of patients. Although the radiologic abnormalities are

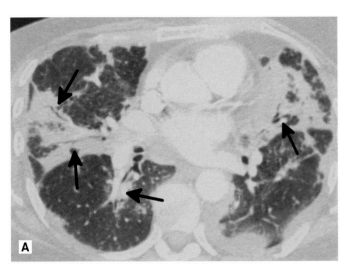
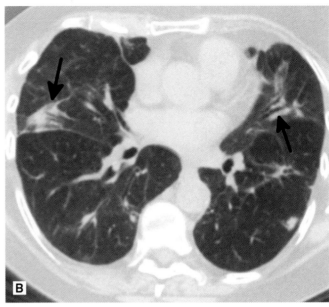

FIGURE 19.1 ▲ Organizing pneumonia. **A.** Axial CT image 2 weeks after initiation of therapy shows bilateral peribronchovascular consolidation (*black arrows*), one of many imaging patterns that can be seen with OP. **B.** CT scan 2 months later after initiation of corticosteroids shows marked improvement in peribronchovascular consolidation (*arrows*). On imaging, OP can have numerous imaging findings ranging from an isolated nodule to diffuse parenchymal fibrosis.

thought to typically resolve, a study suggests that some residual findings may persist in the majority of patients.[7] There may be recurrence after cessation of steroid therapy, or if reduced below 14 mg/day. Deaths due to COP are considered rare.[6] The concept of progression of COP to fibrotic lung disease is controversial and not well documented. One study comparing progressive COP with steroid-responsive COP found that progressive disease histologically had scarring and remodeling of the background lung parenchyma, without honeycombing.[11] From this study, it is not possible to ascertain if some patients had preexisting fibrotic lung disease. Indeed, patients with UIP diagnosed on explant may have a prior wedge biopsy with prominent areas of "BOOP."[12] Therefore, in general, most cases of COP described as progressing to

UIP may have an initial wrong diagnosis.[5] However, in the series from Yousem et al., there were a few cases that had a premortem biopsy and autopsy, confirming the absence of a chronic fibrosing lung disease such as NSIP or UIP, therefore supporting the concept of fibrosing OP.

Acute Interstitial Pneumonia

Terminology

Acute interstitial pneumonia (AIP) was initially described by Katzenstein et al. to designate a disease that differed from chronic interstitial pneumonia by an acute onset and rapid course.[13] AIP was likely "Hamman-Rich syndrome" based on this initial description of

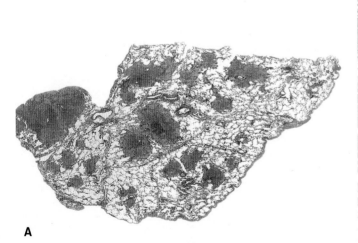
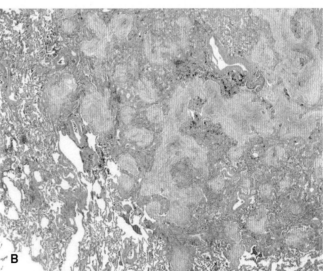

FIGURE 19.2 ▲ Cryptogenic organizing pneumonia. **A.** Whole mounted section shows the patchy, predominantly airspace distribution of OP. **B.** At low magnification, the airspaces are filled with proliferating fibroblasts in a myxoid background. The adjacent alveolar septa are mildly thickened by inflammation. However, away from the intraluminal plugs, the lung parenchyma appears normal.

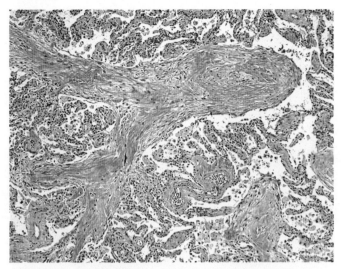

FIGURE 19.3 ▲ Cryptogenic organizing pneumonia with fibrosis. The photomicrograph illustrates the deposition of collagen within the intraluminal plugs of OP, replacing the more typical loose fibrosis of proliferating fibroblasts in myxoid stroma.

four patients with rapidly fatal interstitial fibrotic lung disease.[14] The underlying pathology is diffuse alveolar damage (DAD), morphologically indistinct from DAD due to an identifiable underlying cause (Chapters 4 and 21).[5,15–17]

Clinical Findings

The initially reported eight cases of AIP were characterized by sudden onset of respiratory symptoms, leading to respiratory failure and death, usually within 2 months of onset.[13] Subsequent series have shown that the median time from first symptom to severe dyspnea is <3 weeks.[5,17] Patients may have a prior systemic illness suggestive of inflammatory etiology. AIP occurs over a wide age range, with a mean age of ~50 years, without gender predilection. Pulmonary function tests show a restrictive pattern with reduced diffusing capacity, and hypoxemia develops early and progresses rapidly to respiratory failure.[5]

Radiologic Findings

The acute phase of DAD manifests as relatively diffuse but patchy GGO with areas of consolidation and septal thickening, which is most severe in the dependent portions of the lungs (Fig. 19.4). Focal areas of spared, normal-attenuation, secondary lobules adjacent to the involved lung are a common finding and create a geographic appearance. Bronchiectasis is absent or very mild in this phase and usually coincides with a transition to the organizing phase of the disease. As the lung injury progresses, findings of fibrosis may rapidly develop including reticulation and traction bronchiectasis.[5]

If a patient survives, consolidation and GGO slowly improve and may completely resolve. However, up to 85% of patients have some degree of residual fibrosis, and although the fibrosis usually involves <25% of the lung, it can occasionally be extensive and debilitating.

Gross Findings

The lungs of patients dying with AIP resemble those of patients dying of DAD due to an underlying etiology. They are heavy and diffusely lacking in aeration. Additional findings as a result of treatments and complications before death, including pneumonia and extracorporeal membrane oxygenation (ECMO), may include areas of consolidation and hemorrhage.

Microscopic Findings

The histologic features of AIP are those of DAD due to any cause (Chapter 4). In the acute or early phase, hyaline membranes and denudation and regeneration of pneumocytes dominate (Fig. 19.5). In the organizing or late phase of DAD, fibroblast/myofibroblast proliferation dominates, and hyaline membranes are rare (Fig. 19.5). The myofibroblast proliferation will cause thickening and distortion of the alveolar septa. In the organizing phase, there may be some areas of organizing pneumonia, characterized by focal airspace proliferation of the fibroblasts.[18] Reactive pneumocytes show marked nuclear atypia and cytoplasmic enlargement and may mimic viral cytopathic effects. Fibrin thrombi in small muscular arteries and squamous metaplasia of bronchiolar epithelium are common.[18] Special stains for fungi and *Pneumocystis jiroveci* are indicated, as well as correlation with cultures.[18]

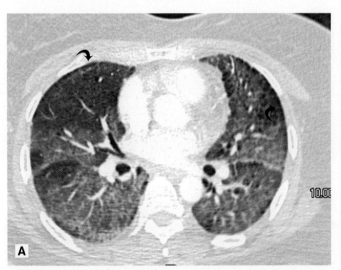
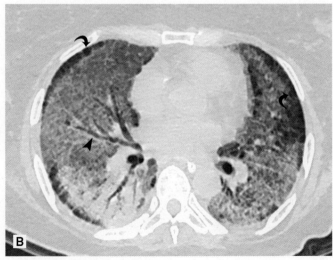

FIGURE 19.4 ▲ Acute interstitial pneumonia. **A.** Axial CT image through the midlung zone shows basilar predominant ground-glass opacity (GGO) with relative sparing of the anterior lungs. Underlying paraseptal emphysema is present (*curved arrows*). **B.** CT image 4 days later shows worsening GGO with right basilar consolidation. Bronchiectasis (*arrowheads*) and paraseptal emphysema (*curved arrows*) have increased in size, likely due to surrounding alveolar collapse and developing fibrosis.

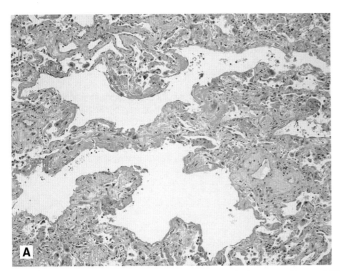
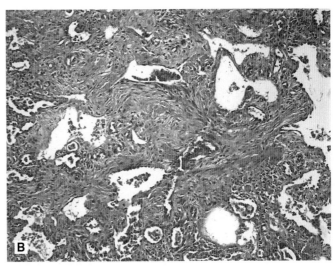

FIGURE 19.5 ▲ Acute interstitial pneumonia. **A.** In acute phase of DAD, hyaline membranes and prominent reactive pneumocytes predominate. The hyaline membranes line the alveolar septa, which are mildly thickened by reactive pneumocytes. **B.** High power of organizing phase of DAD. The alveolar septa are thickened by a fibroblast proliferation with narrowing of the alveolar spaces. The hyaline membranes are no longer visible.

Tissue Sampling

DAD is one of the diffuse parenchymal diseases that can be diagnosed on a transbronchial biopsy since hyaline membranes are pathognomonic to the diagnosis (Fig. 19.6). However, when hyaline membranes are no longer present, distinguishing the different acute lung injuries on a small biopsies may be challenging and require a wedge biopsy. BAL fluid contains increased total cells, hemorrhage in the form of red blood cells, and/or hemosiderin, neutrophils, and occasionally increased lymphocytes. Atypical reactive pneumocytes and fragments of hyaline membranes may be seen.[5]

Prognosis and Treatment

AIP is a highly aggressive disease with an acute fatality rate of up to 70%.[18] Most deaths occur between 1 and 2 months of illness onset. The natural history in survivors is variable, including patients who fully recover, patients who suffer multiple relapses, and a small number who develop chronic interstitial lung disease.[19] Some survivors with persistent fibrotic lung disease likely had previously unrecognized fibrotic lung disease, which presented with accelerated disease.[20]

Acute Fibrinous and Organizing Pneumonia (AFOP)

In 2002, Beasley et al. described a new histologic pattern of acute lung injury as a possible variant of DAD.[21] Acute fibrinous and organizing pneumonia (AFOP) was felt to be distinct from DAD, OP, and acute eosinophilic pneumonia (AEP) and, as with DAD and OP, could occur in an idiopathic clinical setting. In the initial description, there were 17 cases defined as a "dominant histologic pattern of intra-alveolar fibrin with organization" (Fig. 19.7). Three patients had autoimmune connective tissue disease, one amiodarone exposure, and three possible inhalant exposure. The overall outcome was similar to AIP, with 10 of 17 patients dying within the follow-up period. AFOP is currently recognized as a rare histologic pattern in the most recent consensus classification.[17]

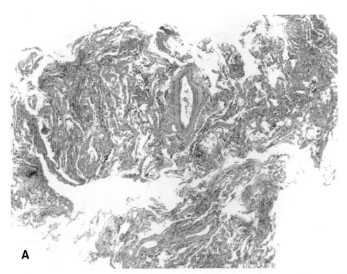
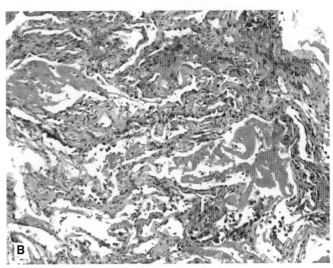

FIGURE 19.6 ▲ Acute interstitial pneumonia. Transbronchial biopsy of DAD. **A.** At low power, the fragments of alveolated parenchyma show mild septal thickening and airspace hyaline material. **B.** At higher power, hyaline membranes are easily identifiable. The alveolar septa are mildly thickened due to prominent reactive pneumocytes.

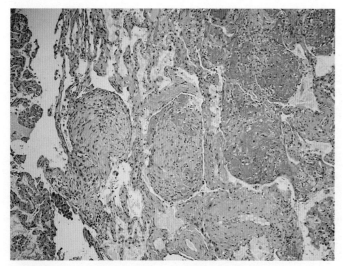

FIGURE 19.7 ▲ Acute fibrinous organizing pneumonia. Histologically, both airspace proliferating fibroblasts and fibrinous exudate are seen, admixed together. The fibrinous exudate fills the airspace and does not form membranes lining the septa like in DAD.

It has not been included as a specific IIP as it remains unclear if AFOP is simply a morphologic variant of existing IIPs, specifically AIP and COP.

Acute Exacerbation of Chronic Fibrosing Interstitial Pneumonias

Definition and Causes

Patients with fibrosing interstitial pneumonia, idiopathic and not, are prone to the development of acute lung injury. Acute exacerbation may occur at any time point in the course of the patient's chronic lung disease, or may be the initial manifestation, in which case both acute and chronic phases are diagnosed simultaneously. The criteria for clinical diagnosis are outlined in Table 19.1.[22] Although typically associated with UIP/idiopathic pulmonary fibrosis (IPF), acute exacerbation of NSIP also occurs,

TABLE 19.1 Diagnosis of Acute Exacerbation of Idiopathic Fibrotic Lung Disease[a]

Previous or concurrent diagnosis of idiopathic pulmonary fibrosis (or idiopathic NSIP)
Unexplained worsening or development of dyspnea within 30 days
High-resolution computed tomography with new bilateral ground-glass opacities and/or consolidation, superimposed on honeycomb pattern consistent with usual interstitial pneumonia pattern, or pattern consistent with NSIP
No evidence of pulmonary infection by endotracheal aspirate or bronchoalveolar lavage
Clinical exclusion of
    Left heart failure
    Pulmonary embolism
    Conditions associated with ARDS

[a]Adapted from and initially applied to idiopathic pulmonary fibrosis,[22] also applies to NSIP, idiopathic or associated with collagen vascular disease.[23,24]

both in the idiopathic form and NSIP associated with rheumatologic autoimmune diseases, and with chronic hypersensitivity pneumonia (HP).[20,23–25] The rate of acute exacerbation in UIP/IPF varies widely with estimates between 10% and 21%.[22,26] In Park et al.'s series, 8% of patients with idiopathic NSIP and 4% of patients with collagen vascular disease–associated NSIP developed acute exacerbation.[23] Predisposing factors for acute exacerbation of UIP/IPF include surgery and lung biopsy, never smoking, and low forced vital capacity.[26–28] Hypothetical causes of acute exacerbation of IPF (and presumably NSIP) include viral infections, subclinical or microaspiration of gastric contents, and unknown lung stresses.[22] In some cases, patients may present with AIP, and underlying fibrotic lung disease is subsequently diagnosed by biopsy or autopsy.[20]

Radiologic Findings

The main CT features of acute exacerbations of fibrosing interstitial pneumonias include bilateral ground-glass opacities (a constant feature) and consolidation (seen in three-fourths of patients) superimposed on a reticular pattern and traction bronchiectasis with or without honeycombing representing underlying fibrotic lung disease (Fig. 19.8).

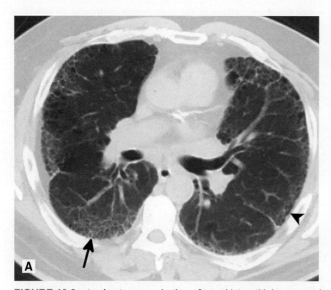
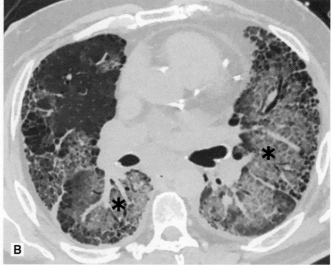

FIGURE 19.8 ▲ Acute exacerbation of usual interstitial pneumonia. **A.** Axial CT image below the carina 2 months prior to admission shows honeycombing lower lobe and peripheral predominant reticulation (*arrow*) and honeycombing (*arrowhead*). **B.** Axial CT image at the same level 6 days after admission for worsening dyspnea demonstrates development of diffuse ground-glass opacity (*asterisks*). Diffuse alveolar damage was shown on bronchoscopic biopsy. The patient died 6 days later.

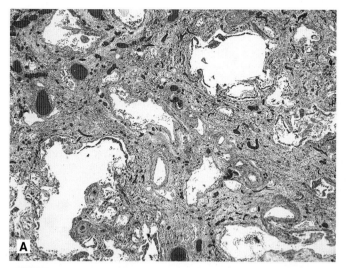
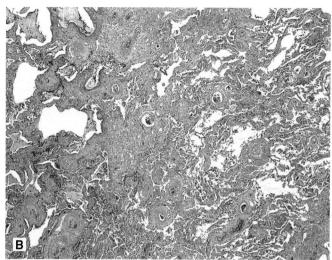

FIGURE 19.9 ▲ Acute exacerbation of usual interstitial pneumonia. **A.** Low-power photomicrograph of the peripheral honeycombing of UIP. **B.** Away from the honeycombing, the alveolar septa remain abnormal due to thickening by proliferating fibroblasts and hyaline membranes (*arrows*) due to superimposed DAD.

The ground-glass opacities and consolidation that indicate the acute injury are diffuse in 54% of the cases, multifocal in 21%, and peripheral in 25%.[29]

Pathologic Findings

There are few studies of the histologic findings of acute exacerbation of UIP. The largest series of open lung biopsies used broad clinical criteria, relied heavily on the presence of GGO by CT imaging, and most patients had a relatively short duration of illness.[30] In this series, many of the patients had OP histologically, and some had "large areas of fibroblast foci." However, most series show DAD to be the most common pattern.

Gross and histologic features of acute exacerbation of UIP are thus those of UIP including subpleural honeycombing in basal lung areas, with the superimposed acute lung injury (Fig. 19.9). Often, the findings of the superimposed acute lung injury are best seen in upper lung zones, away from the zones most involved by UIP. Similar findings are seen in acute exacerbation of NSIP, although the gross and microscopic features of the underlying chronic fibrotic lung disease differ and are those of NSIP (see Chapter 17).

There are many challenges in recognizing an acute exacerbation of UIP or NSIP. Depending on the site biopsy, the chronic or the acute disease may predominate. Therefore, when making a diagnosis of UIP or NSIP, one should always look for features of a superimposed DAD or OP. Similarly, when making a diagnosis of DAD or OP, one should rule out an underlying fibrotic interstitial lung disease. Distinguishing DAD and OP from fibroblast foci in UIP can also be challenging.[30,31] The identification of hyaline membranes is extremely helpful in confirming DAD superimposed on UIP. However, recognizing the diffuse septal thickening by the fibroblasts in the center of the lobules, away from the peripheral honeycombing, also assists with the diagnosis of DAD. OP, in contrast to the fibroblast foci of UIP, appears entirely intraluminal and typically not lined by epithelial cells.

Prognosis

Acute exacerbation has a negative impact on patients with UIP/IPF. In a survival comparison of patients with UIP without and with acute exacerbation, mean survival time was 35 versus 22 months.[6] The mortality in some series is as high as 78%.[22] The lack of follow-up studies has impaired our knowledge of the natural course of the disease.[30] In series in which acute lung injury with hyaline membranes is documented, prognosis is dismal.[30]

Acute exacerbation of fibrotic lung disease in patients with collagen vascular disease may have a worse prognosis than acute exacerbations

of idiopathic NSIP and is typically associated with rheumatoid lung disease.[23]

Differential Diagnosis

DAD, OP, and AFOP are characterized histologically by proliferating myofibroblasts/fibroblasts and need to be distinguished from each other. Hyaline membranes are pathognomonic of DAD and are extremely useful in the differential diagnosis. In OP, in contrast to DAD, the proliferation of fibroblasts is typically patchy and predominantly within the airspaces. The presence of fibrinous thrombi and prominent reactive pneumocyte hyperplasia are also features that favor DAD. In AFOP, the proliferation of fibroblasts is similar to OP but differs from OP by the presence of a prominent fibrinous exudate admixed with the fibroblasts.

OP may be confused with NSIP (Chapter 17) and hypersensitivity pneumonia (Chapter 23).[32] Indeed, NSIP may frequently show areas of organizing pneumonia. Features favoring the latter include lack of significant interstitial inflammation away from the areas of intraluminal fibroblast proliferation. Small foci of OP are often present in HP. However, in HP, other histologic findings are clues to the correct diagnosis including cellular interstitial pneumonia, typically bronchiolocentric, and poorly formed granulomas. In granulomatous inflammation due to infection, it is very common to see granulomas admixed with OP; however, the granulomas are more important to the diagnosis and etiology than the OP.

Eosinophilic pneumonia (Chapter 26) also enters the differential diagnosis with OP and DAD since both OP and DAD may be patterns found in EP. The distinguishing feature is the presence of numerous eosinophils in EP.

In IgG4-related disease (Chapter 51), OP may be one of the underlying morphologic features. The main histologic clue is the presence of a marked lymphoplasmacytic infiltrate within the OP and presence of increased IgG4 plasma cells.

With DAD/AIP, the important differential diagnosis includes infections that may cause DAD.[5] Indeed, several viruses, including herpes simplex, measles, adenovirus, respiratory syncytial virus, and cytomegalovirus, can result in DAD and have distinctive nuclear and/or cytoplasmic inclusions identifiable on H&E stain (Chapter 39). DAD is also a pattern of injury seen in *P. jiroveci* pneumonia (Chapter 42); therefore, performing a special stain in any potentially immunocompromised host is indicated to rule out this infection. Other causes of DAD need to be ruled out clinically, mainly connective tissue disease, drug toxicity, and other types of infections not identifiable histologically.[33,34]

DAD may complicate other injuries such as capillaritis (Chapter 47), especially in patients with rheumatologic disorders. It is important to recognize the features of capillaritis and make the diagnosis as the prognosis and treatment will differ from that of DAD alone. Capillaritis is defined by intra-alveolar hemorrhage with hemosiderin macrophages and alveolar septal neutrophils with necrosis.

REFERENCES

1. Liebow AA, Carrington DB. The interstitial pneumonias. In: Simon M, Potchen EJ, LeMay M, eds. *Frontiers of Pulmonary Radiology.* New York, NY: Grune & Stratteon;1969:102–141.
2. Davison AG, Heard BE, McAllister WAC, et al. Cryptogenic organizing pneumonitis. *Q J Med.* 1983;52(207):382–394.
3. Davison AG, Epstein O. Relapsing organising pneumonitis in a man with primary biliary cirrhosis, CREST syndrome, and chronic pancreatitis. *Thorax.* 1983;38(4):316–317.
4. Epler GR, Colby TV, McLoud TC, et al. Bronchiolitis obliterans organizing pneumonia. *N Engl J Med.* 1985;312(3):152–158.
5. American Thoracic Society/European Respiratory Society International Multidisciplinary Consensus Classification of the Idiopathic Interstitial Pneumonias. This joint statement of the American Thoracic Society (ATS), and the European Respiratory Society (ERS) was adopted by the ATS board of directors, June 2001 and by the ERS Executive Committee, June 2001. *Am J Respir Crit Care Med.* 2002;165(2):277–304.
6. King TE Jr, Clinical advances in the diagnosis and therapy of the interstitial lung diseases. *Am J Respir Crit Care Med.* 2005;172(3):268–279.
7. Lee JW, Lee KS, Lee HY, et al. Cryptogenic organizing pneumonia: serial high-resolution CT findings in 22 patients. *AJR Am J Roentgenol.* 2010;195(4):916–922.
8. Maldonado F, Daniels CE, Hoffman EA, et al. Focal organizing pneumonia on surgical lung biopsy: causes, clinicoradiologic features, and outcomes. *Chest.* 2007;132(5):1579–1583.
9. Nagai S, Kitaichi M, Itoh H, et al. Idiopathic nonspecific interstitial pneumonia/fibrosis: comparison with idiopathic pulmonary fibrosis and BOOP. *Eur Respir J.* 1998;12(5):1010–1019.
10. Dina R, Sheppard MN. The histological diagnosis of clinically documented cases of cryptogenic organizing pneumonia: diagnostic features in transbronchial biopsies. *Histopathology.* 1993;23(6):541–545.
11. Yousem SA, Lohr RH, Colby TV. Idiopathic bronchiolitis obliterans organizing pneumonia/cryptogenic organizing pneumonia with unfavorable outcome: pathologic predictors. *Mod Pathol.* 1997;10(9):864–871.
12. Katzenstein AL, Zisman DA, Litzky LA, et al. Usual interstitial pneumonia: histologic study of biopsy and explant specimens. *Am J Surg Pathol.* 2002;26(12):1567–1577.
13. Katzenstein AL, Myers JL, Mazur MT. Acute interstitial pneumonia. A clinicopathologic, ultrastructural, and cell kinetic study. *Am J Surg Pathol.* 1986;10(4):256–267.
14. Hamman L, Rich AR. Acute diffuse interstitial fibrosis of the lungs. *Bull Johns Hopkins Hosp.* 1944;74:177–212.
15. Katzenstein AL, Mukhopadhyay S, Myers JL. Diagnosis of usual interstitial pneumonia and distinction from other fibrosing interstitial lung diseases. *Hum Pathol.* 2008;39(9):1275–1294.
16. Katzenstein AL, Myers JL. Idiopathic pulmonary fibrosis: clinical relevance of pathologic classification. *Am J Respir Crit Care Med.* 1998;157(4 pt 1):1301–1315.
17. Travis WD, Costabel U, Hansell DM, et al. An official American Thoracic Society/European Respiratory Society statement: update of the international multidisciplinary classification of the idiopathic interstitial pneumonias. *Am J Respir Crit Care Med.* 2013;188(6):733–748.
18. Myers JL, Katzenstein AL. Beyond a consensus classification for idiopathic interstitial pneumonias: progress and controversies. *Histopathology.* 2009;54(1):90–103.
19. Vourlekis JS, Brown KK, Cool CD, et al. Acute interstitial pneumonitis. Case series and review of the literature. *Medicine (Baltimore).* 2000;79(6):369–378.
20. Marais CE, Frazier AA, Burke A. Idiopathic acute lung injury: acute interstitial pneumonia and exacerbation of nonspecific interstitial fibrosis. *Pathol Case Rev.* 2013;18(3):115–119.
21. Beasley MB, Franks TJ, Galvin JR, et al. Acute fibrinous and organizing pneumonia: a histological pattern of lung injury and possible variant of diffuse alveolar damage. *Arch Pathol Lab Med.* 2002;126(9):1064–1070.
22. Collard HR, Moore BB, Flaherty KR, et al. Acute exacerbations of idiopathic pulmonary fibrosis. *Am J Respir Crit Care Med.* 2007;176(7):636–643.
23. Park IN, Kim DS, Shim TS, et al. Acute exacerbation of interstitial pneumonia other than idiopathic pulmonary fibrosis. *Chest.* 2007;132(1):214–220.
24. Suda T, Kaida Y, Nakamura Y, et al. Acute exacerbation of interstitial pneumonia associated with collagen vascular diseases. *Respir Med.* 2009;103(6):846–853.
25. Olson AL, Huie TJ, Groshong SD, et al. Acute exacerbations of fibrotic hypersensitivity pneumonitis: a case series. *Chest.* 2008;134(4):844–850.
26. Song JW, Hong SB, Lim CM, et al. Acute exacerbation of idiopathic pulmonary fibrosis: incidence, risk factors and outcome. *Eur Respir J.* 2011;37(2):356–363.
27. Kondoh Y, Taniguchi H, Kitaichi M, et al. Acute exacerbation of interstitial pneumonia following surgical lung biopsy. *Respir Med.* 2006;100(10):1753–1759.
28. Chida M, Kobayashi S, Karube Y, et al. Incidence of acute exacerbation of interstitial pneumonia in operated lung cancer: institutional report and review. *Ann Thorac Cardiovasc Surg.* 2012.
29. Silva CI, Müller NL, Fujimoto K, et al. Acute exacerbation of chronic interstitial pneumonia: high-resolution computed tomography and pathologic findings. *J Thorac Imaging.* 2007;22(3):221–229.
30. Churg A, Müller NL, Silva CIS, et al. Acute exacerbation (acute lung injury of unknown cause) in UIP and other forms of fibrotic interstitial pneumonias. *Am J Surg Pathol.* 2007;31(2):277–284.
31. Churg A, Wright JL, Tazelaar HD. Acute exacerbations of fibrotic interstitial lung disease. *Histopathology.* 2011;58(4):525–530.
32. Nicholson AG, Addis B, Bharucha H, et al. Inter-observer variation between pathologists in diffuse parenchymal lung disease. *Thorax.* 2004;59(6):500–505.
33. Hozumi H, Nakamura Y, Johkoh T, et al. Acute exacerbation in rheumatoid arthritis-associated interstitial lung disease: a retrospective case control study. *BMJ Open.* 2013;3(9):e003132.
34. Torre O, Harari S. Pleural and pulmonary involvement in systemic lupus erythematosus. *Presse Med.* 2011;40(1 pt 2):e19–e29.

20 Rare Idiopathic Interstitial Pneumonias

Allen P. Burke, M.D., Marie-Christine Aubry, M.D., and Seth Kligerman, M.D.

Idiopathic Pleuroparenchymal Fibroelastosis

Background

Idiopathic pleuroparenchymal fibroelastosis (PPFE) was initially described in 2004 as a form of idiopathic interstitial pneumonia characterized by predominantly upper lobe subpleural scarring with elastosis.[1] Recently, it was recognized as a rare form of idiopathic interstitial pneumonia by the American Thoracic Society/European Society of Respiratory Diseases.[2,3] It has also been described as "idiopathic pulmonary upper lobe fibrosis."[4] A related, if not identical, disease was previously described as idiopathic progressive pulmonary fibrosis[5] or "Amitani disease" in the Japanese literature. Although initially described in native lungs in patients with normal immune function, PPFE has also been reported in bone marrow transplant recipients[6,7] and in lung allografts as a manifestation of restrictive allograft syndrome.[8,9]

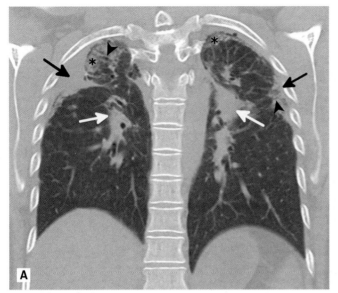
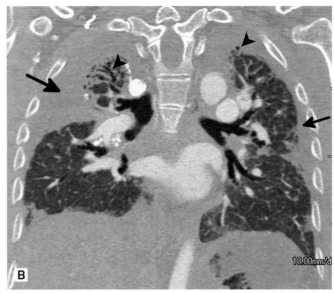

FIGURE 20.1 ▲ Progression of idiopathic pleuroparenchymal fibroelastosis (PPFE) in a 26-year-old woman. **A.** Coronal CT shows upper lobe predominant pleuroparenchymal thickening (*black arrows*) and ground-glass opacity (*asterisks*) with findings of upper lobe fibrosis including superior displacement of the hila (*white arrows*) and traction bronchiectasis (*arrowheads*). **B.** Coronal CT image 4 years later shows worsening upper lobe fibrosis with increasing traction bronchiectasis (*arrowheads*) and worsening upper lobe pleuroparenchymal thickening (*arrows*). IPPFE was confirmed after lung transplant.

Clinical Findings

PPFE has no gender predilection. It has been described in several patients with prior chemotherapy, including cyclophosphamide,[1,10] and has been reported in twins.[1] There is no clear association with smoking.[4,11] Symptoms include dyspnea, shortness of breath, and nonproductive cough.[11] A history of recurrent infections is common. Pneumothorax and pneumomediastinum occur spontaneously or as a complication of treatment and appear more common in PPFE in the setting of bone marrow transplantation.[4,7,11] Some patients have incidental pleural thickening noted on chest radiograph years prior to disease manifestation.[10] Pulmonary function tests show restrictive ventilatory impairment and decrease diffusion capacity.

Radiologic Findings

Imaging by computed tomography demonstrates apical pleural fibrotic changes.[7,9] The parenchyma typically shows reticular opacities with thickened subpleural parenchyma and interlobular septal thickening[4] (Fig. 20.1). Upper lobe volume loss, architectural distortion with traction bronchiectasis, and honeycombing, involving the upper lobe, have also been described.

Tissue Sampling

Because of pleural distribution, transbronchial biopsy is not useful in the diagnosis of PPFE. Diagnosis is made primarily by wedge lung biopsy, typically video-assisted, or at explant, in patients with restrictive allograft syndrome.[9] The diagnosis is frequently made first at autopsy.[9,11]

Histologic Findings

The process involves the upper lobes and superior segments of the lower and middle lobes or lingula. The pleura may show remarkable thickening by dense collagen fibrosis (Fig. 20.2). Invariably, there is prominent subpleural fibroelastosis that may form acellular masses and infiltrate around intact alveolar spaces (Fig. 20.2). The elastosis appears as slate gray fibrillar deposits, which are highlighted by lowering the microscope condenser. Elastic stains demonstrate the elastic fibers by

silver impregnation. The junction between the elastotic areas and more central lung tissue is usually abrupt, and the lung parenchyma away from the fibroelastosis appears normal.[4] Rare fibroblast foci at the leading edge of the fibroelastosis have been reported. Histologic findings of prior pneumothorax are common. Reactive pneumocytes forming small entrapped glands are common and should not be overdiagnosed as adenocarcinoma (Fig. 20.2).

The histologic findings of PPFE associated with restrictive allograft syndrome include other manifestations of chronic rejection with obliterative bronchiolitis, acute and organizing diffuse alveolar damage, organizing pneumonia, nonspecific interstitial pneumonia-like fibrosis, and acute bronchopneumonia.[9]

Differential Diagnosis

The differential diagnosis includes apical cap and usual interstitial pneumonia (UIP) (Chapter 17). Apical cap is histologically composed of fibroelastosis similar to PPFE. However, apical cap is a localized process involving the apex of a lobe, usually the upper lobe. PPFE shares with UIP a peripheral subpleural distribution with traction bronchiectasis and honeycombing. However, in contrast to UIP, PPFE is an upper lobe–predominant disease. Furthermore, elastotic changes are not a feature of UIP, fibroblast foci are rare in PPFE, and histologic findings in PPFE are temporally homogeneous.

Prognosis and Treatment

Most patients develop progressive disease.[4] Approximately 50% of patient die of disease or require transplant within 5 years, with death occurring between 5 months and 12 years after diagnosis.[1,7,10,11]

Lymphocytic Interstitial Pneumonia

Lymphocytic interstitial pneumonia (LIP) is also considered a rare IIP. LIP was described as an interstitial lung disease before nonspecific interstitial pneumonia. Since the introduction of NSIP, the diagnosis of LIP has become rare and usually limited to patients with known autoimmune disease or with immunodeficiency (Chapter 36).

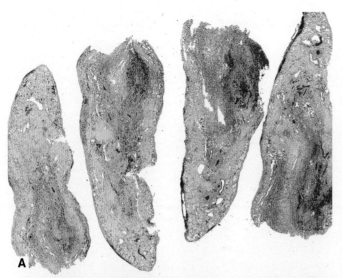

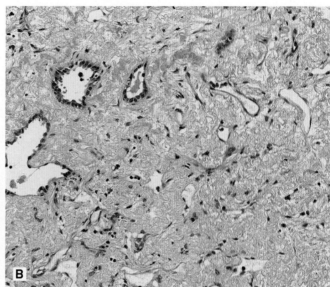

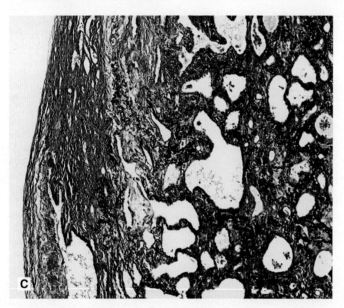

FIGURE 20.2 ▲ Pleuroparenchymal fibroelastosis, low magnification. **A.** There is a subpleural fibroelastotic process that appears pale pink and nearly involves the entire sections, sparing the central portion. **B.** Reactive pneumocytes forming small glands and tubules are entrapped in the elastosis. **C.** The elastic stain highlights the elastosis in the lung distinct from the pleural fibrosis.

REFERENCES

1. Frankel SK, et al. Idiopathic pleuroparenchymal fibroelastosis: description of a novel clinicopathologic entity. *Chest.* 2004;126(6):2007–2013.
2. Travis WD, et al. An official American Thoracic Society/European Respiratory Society statement: update of the international multidisciplinary classification of the idiopathic interstitial pneumonias. *Am J Respir Crit Care Med.* 2013;188(6):733–748.
3. Ryerson CJ, Collard HR. Update on the diagnosis and classification of ILD. *Curr Opin Pulm Med.* 2013;19(5):453–459.
4. Watanabe K, et al. Rapid decrease in forced vital capacity in patients with idiopathic pulmonary upper lobe fibrosis. *Respir Investig.* 2012;50(3):88–97.
5. Fraisse P, et al. Idiopathic progressive pleuropulmonary fibrosis. Apropos of 2 cases. *Rev Pneumol Clin.* 1984;40(2):139–143.
6. Fujikura Y, et al. Pleuroparenchymal fibroelastosis as a series of airway complications associated with chronic graft-versus-host disease following allogeneic bone marrow transplantation. *Intern Med.* 2014;53(1):43–46.
7. von der Thusen JH, et al. Pleuroparenchymal fibroelastosis in patients with pulmonary disease secondary to bone marrow transplantation. *Mod Pathol.* 2011;24(12):1633–1639.
8. Hirota T, et al. Pleuroparenchymal fibroelastosis as a manifestation of chronic lung rejection? *Eur Respir J.* 2013;41(1):243–245.
9. Ofek E, et al. Restrictive allograft syndrome post lung transplantation is characterized by pleuroparenchymal fibroelastosis. *Mod Pathol.* 2013;26(3):350–356.
10. Becker CD, Gil J, Padilla ML. Idiopathic pleuroparenchymal fibroelastosis: an unrecognized or misdiagnosed entity? *Mod Pathol.* 2008;21(6):784–787.
11. Reddy TL, et al. Pleuroparenchymal fibroelastosis: a spectrum of histopathological and imaging phenotypes. *Eur Respir J.* 2012;40(2):377–385.

21 Acute Respiratory Distress Syndrome

Marie-Christine Aubry, M.D., and Allen P. Burke, M.D.

Definition

Acute respiratory distress syndrome (ARDS) is defined clinically and is, as such, not a pathologic term. Until recently, the clinical diagnostic criteria of the American-European Consensus Conference (AECC) were used, namely, bilateral pulmonary infiltrates on chest radiograph, a ratio of the partial pressure of arterial oxygen to the fraction of inspired oxygen (PaO_2/FiO_2) of <200, and absence of clinical evidence of left atrial hypertension (if measured, the pulmonary capillary wedge pressure is ≤18 mm Hg). The term "acute lung injury" was a synonym, with a higher cutoff of PaO_2/FiO_2 set at 300.[1] The criteria have been modified by the "Berlin Definition," an initiative of the European Society of Intensive Care Medicine with endorsement by the American Thoracic Society and the Society of Critical Care Medicine[2] (Table 21.1). The new criteria grade the degree of ARDS largely based on the PaO_2/FiO_2 into three groups, and remove the term "acute lung injury." These changes resulted in a better predictive validity for mortality than the prior AECC criteria.

Clinical Findings

The estimated incidence of ARDS in the United States is 17 to 64 per 100,000 population per year.[3] Patients with ARDS typically present with rapid (within 1 week) onset of respiratory failure, with profound dyspnea and tachypnea, usually requiring mechanical ventilation. Arterial hypoxemia refractory to treatment with supplemental oxygen is a characteristic feature.

A risk factor is usually present (Table 21.2). The presence of multiple predisposing factors increases the risk, as does the presence of underlying chronic lung disease. Sepsis represents the highest risk for progression to ARDS. Nearly 50% of patients with severe sepsis and septic shock will require endotracheal intubation and mechanical ventilation because of ARDS.[4]

Severe burns, such as those experienced by US servicemen suffering casualties in Iraq and Afghanistan, result in ARDS in about one in three patients.[5]

The risk for developing ARDS after general surgery has been estimated at 0.2%. Preoperative risk factors for ARDS development included American Society of Anesthesiologist status 3 to 5 (odds ratio [OR] 19), emergent surgery (OR 9), renal failure (OR 2), chronic obstructive pulmonary disease (OR 2), and intraoperative erythrocyte transfusion (OR 5).[6]

After thoracotomy for lung cancer, the risk is <2% of overall for the development of ARDS, but increases dramatically if there is preoperative computed tomographic evidence of interstitial pulmonary fibrosis.[5]

Among viral pneumonias, A/H1N1 influenza infection results in severe ARDS with poor response to routine treatment.[7]

Pathogenesis

ARDS is thought to be the result of dysregulated inflammation, which causes the accumulation and increased activity of leucocytes and platelets. This leads to abnormal permeability of the endothelial–epithelial alveolar wall and activation of the coagulation pathways. Different pathways are disrupted such as the VE–cadherin bonds and may be potential therapeutic targets. Resolution of the process is dependent on macrophages and monocytes, and lymphocytes, to remove debris and resolve inflammation through activation of anti-inflammatory pathways.[8]

Radiologic Findings

Chest radiographs are characterized by bilateral air–space opacifications. They are most often diffuse, but can predominantly involve upper or lower lung zones. Chest computed tomographic scans show bilateral, symmetric areas of ground-glass attenuation, usually diffuse, but occasionally patchy. The majority of patients will also have bilateral areas of air–space consolidation, mostly diffuse or with a basal predominance.

Microscopic Findings

The pathologic correlate of ARDS is typically thought of as diffuse alveolar damage,[9,10] which is the most common finding on open lung biopsy[11,12] (see Chapter 4) (Table 21.3). Because lung biopsies may be associated with increased risk complications in patients with ARDS, they are not routinely performed, unless there is persistent ARDS of unknown etiology.

TABLE 21.1 The Berlin Definition of ARDS

Timing	Within 1 week of known clinical insult or new or worse worsening respiratory symptoms
Chest imaging	Bilateral opacities—not explained by effusions, lung collapse, or nodules
Origin of edema	Respiratory failure—not cardiac failure or fluid overload
	Need objective assessment to exclude hydrostatic edema
Oxygenation	
Mild ARDS	PaO_2/FIO_2 >200 and ≤ 300 mm Hg with PEEP or CPAP ≥5 cm H_2O
Moderate ARDS	PaO_2/FIO_2 >100 and ≤ 200 mm Hg with PEEP ≥ 5 cm H_2O
Severe ARDS	PaO_2/FIO_2 ≤ 100 mm Hg with PEEP ≥ 5 cm H_2O

Imaging: Chest X-ray or CT scan.
CPAP, continuous positive airway pressure; FIO₂, fraction of inspired oxygen; PaO₂, partial pressure of arterial oxygen; PEEP, positive end-expiratory pressure.

TABLE 21.2 Causes of ARDS

- Sepsis
- Severe trauma (with shock)
- Multiple transfusions
- Acute pancreatitis
- Drug overdose
- Cardiopulmonary bypass
- Infection
  - Virus—Influenza
  - Bacterial
  - Fungal and parasites—Pneumocystis
- Aspiration of stomach content
- Pulmonary contusion
- Fat emboli
- Inhalational injury
- Reperfusion injury
- Near drowning

TABLE 21.3 Histologic Findings in ARDS

- Diffuse alveolar damage (most common), acute and organizing
- Capillaritis, with or without superimposed diffuse alveolar damage
- Other pulmonary hemorrhage syndromes
- Acute fibrinous and organizing pneumonia
- Fungal infection, for example, pneumocystis
- Viral pneumonia
- Bacterial pneumonia
- Fat or amniotic fluid embolism with or without superimposed diffuse alveolar damage

For a detailed description of histologic features of diffuse alveolar damage, see Chapter 4.

Other reported morphologic findings, other than diffuse alveolar damage, include viral, fungal, or bacterial pneumonia, diffuse alveolar hemorrhage with or without capillaritis, and eosinophilic pneumonia.[11,12] For these reasons, routine use of special stains for organisms and careful evaluation for capillaritis are important in the assessment of open lung biopsies in patients with ARDS. Despite the fact that a significant proportion of biopsies showed findings other than typical diffuse alveolar damage, alterations in treatment did not affect overall survival.[12] Other reported histologic findings include pulmonary embolism, organizing pneumonia and acute fibrinous and organizing pneumonia.[13] Since many histologic processes have been associated with ARDS, a pathological diagnosis has not been included in the new Berlin definition of ARDS.

Prognosis and Treatment

Therapy for ARDS relies on the identification and treatment of a specific underlying etiology, if present, and support of the lungs with appropriate ventilation measures. Mortality rates have declined over time with improved therapy and vary with the severity of the clinical syndrome (20% to 40%).[3,6] Usually, mortality results from multiorgan failure, but it can also be related to the primary lung disease. In a prospective study, most early deaths were caused by the underlying illness, most late deaths were related to sepsis, and only 16% of deaths were thought to be caused by primary respiratory failure.[14] In patients who survive, many will experience a return of their pulmonary function to near normal with only mild residual impairments resulting in restriction obstruction or impaired diffusion capacity.

REFERENCES

1. Bernard GR, Artigas A, Brigham KL, et al. The American-European Consensus Conference on ARDS. Definitions, mechanisms, relevant outcomes, and clinical trial coordination. *Am J Respir Crit Care Med.* 1994;149:818–824.
2. Ranieri VM, Rubenfeld GD, Thompson BT, et al. Acute respiratory distress syndrome: the Berlin definition. *JAMA.* 2012;307:2526–2533.
3. Sharma S. Acute respiratory distress syndrome. *BMJ Clin Evid.* 2007;2007.
4. Sevransky JE, Levy MM, Marini JJ. Mechanical ventilation in sepsis-induced acute lung injury/acute respiratory distress syndrome: an evidence-based review. *Crit Care Med.* 2004;32:S548–S553.
5. Saito H, Minamiya Y, Nanjo H, et al. Pathological finding of subclinical interstitial pneumonia as a predictor of postoperative acute respiratory distress syndrome after pulmonary resection. *Eur J Cardiothorac Surg.* 2011;39:190–194.
6. Blum JM, Stentz MJ, Dechert R, et al. Preoperative and intraoperative predictors of postoperative acute respiratory distress syndrome in a general surgical population. *Anesthesiology.* 2013;118:19–29.
7. Witczak A, Prystupa A, Kurys-Denis E, et al. Acute respiratory distress syndrome (ARDS) complicating influenza A/H1N1v infection—a clinical approach. *Ann Agric Environ Med.* 2013;20:820–822.
8. Matthay MA, Ware LB, Zimmerman GA. The acute respiratory distress syndrome. *J Clin Invest.* 2012;122:2731–2740.
9. Capelozzi VL. What have anatomic and pathologic studies taught us about acute lung injury and acute respiratory distress syndrome? *Curr Opin Crit Care.* 2008;14:56–63.
10. Hoelz C, Negri EM, Lichtenfels AJ, et al. Morphometric differences in pulmonary lesions in primary and secondary ARDS. A preliminary study in autopsies. *Pathol Res Pract.* 2001;197:521–530.
11. Barbas CS, Capelozzi VL, Hoelz C, et al. Impact of open lung biopsy on refractory acute respiratory failure. *J Bras Pneumol.* 2006;32:418–423.
12. Patel SR, Karmpaliotis D, Ayas NT, et al. The role of open-lung biopsy in ARDS. *Chest.* 2004;125:197–202.
13. Beasley MB, Franks TJ, Galvin JR, et al. Acute fibrinous and organizing pneumonia: a histological pattern of lung injury and possible variant of diffuse alveolar damage. *Arch Pathol Lab Med.* 2002;126:1064–1070.
14. Montgomery AB, Stager MA, Carrico CJ, et al. Causes of mortality in patients with the adult respiratory distress syndrome. *Am Rev Respir Dis.* 1985;132:485–489.

22 Pulmonary Sarcoidosis

Allen P. Burke, M.D., Marie-Christine Aubry, M.D., and Seth Kligerman, M.D.

Definition

Sarcoidosis is a systemic disease characterized histologically by the presence of nonnecrotizing granulomas, with lung involvement occurring in up to 90% of patients. The etiology of sarcoidosis is thought to be multifactorial but ultimately remains unknown.[1]

Pathophysiology

The stimulus for granuloma formation involves antigen-presenting cells, human leukocyte antigen (HLA) class II molecules, and T-cell receptors.[1] Several HLA-DR, DQ, and DP alleles have been shown to increase the risk of sarcoidosis in a race-dependent way.[1] Mutations in non–HLA-related proteins have been shown to be associated with sarcoidosis, including butyrophilin-like 2 (BTNL2) in Caucasians.

The granuloma in sarcoidosis is composed of epithelioid histiocytes and giant cells derived from monocytes and CD4⁺ T lymphocytes. Experimental studies have shown important roles for interleukin-γ, interferon-α, and tumor necrosis factor (TNF) in the development of these granulomas. Bioinformatic studies have shown an involvement of the STAT1 pathway (signal transducer and activator of transcription 1). The identification of the inciting antigen has remained elusive, but recurrence in transplant patients indicates that host immunity and an exogenous factor are both necessary for the development of sarcoidosis. Candidates for the trigger of sarcoidosis include a variety of proteins, especially those related to *Mycobacterium tuberculosis*, and other antigens based on ethnicity and geography.

Clinical Findings

Sarcoidosis is more prevalent in African American than in Caucasians and Asians. There is no sex predilection, and patients are usually young, between 20 and 50 years old. The clinical presentation of sarcoidosis varies according to the organ(s) of involvement. Most patients are asymptomatic at diagnosis. Symptoms are nonspecific. Systemic symptoms are common and include low-grade fever, night sweats, and fatigue. Pulmonary symptoms, when present, include dyspnea and cough. Occasionally, spontaneous pneumothorax may be the initial presentation.[2,3] Pulmonary function tests may show restriction due to parenchymal lung involvement and/or obstruction. Obstruction may be caused by endobronchial disease, bronchial stenosis, distortion of airways, or increased airway reactivity.

Pulmonary hypertension occurs in 5% to 15% of asymptomatic patients, 50% of patients with symptomatic pulmonary sarcoidosis, and at higher frequencies in patients requiring transplant. The etiology of pulmonary hypertension in pulmonary sarcoidosis is multifactorial and includes vascular involvement and interstitial fibrosis.[4–7]

Radiologic Findings

Pulmonary sarcoid is staged by radiographic findings of mediastinal lymph nodes and lung fields (Table 22.1; Figs. 22.1 and 22.2). Reticulonodular densities correspond to granulomatous infiltrates. Stage 4 disease is characterized by cystic change, and traction bronchiectasis, corresponding to fibrosis. Lymph nodes are thought to regress in size with more advanced disease, secondary to scarring.

Gross Findings

At explant or autopsy, pulmonary sarcoidosis is typically bilateral and symmetric. Areas of granulomatous inflammation in the parenchyma resemble consolidation, typically centrally predominating over peripheral lesions. Scarring occurs in a lymphatic distribution (bronchovascular bundles, interlobular septa, and pleura), also with a central predominance. Scarring can cause secondary bronchiectasis and cystic change, but in contrast to idiopathic pulmonary fibrosis, subpleural cysts are uncommon (Fig. 22.3).

Tissue Sampling

The diagnosis is made either by finding of nonnecrotizing granulomas on bronchial biopsy or by biopsy of mediastinal lymph nodes. The latter can be accomplished by mediastinoscopy or by transbronchial needle aspiration (TBNA). The yield of TBNA is increased if there is endobronchial ultrasound (EBUS) guidance and as high as 90% in enlarged lymph nodes.[1] The rate of positive bronchial biopsy is 40% (Fig. 22.4).[8] The yield of finding granulomas in bronchial biopsies is high due to the common airway involvement by the granulomas in sarcoidosis.

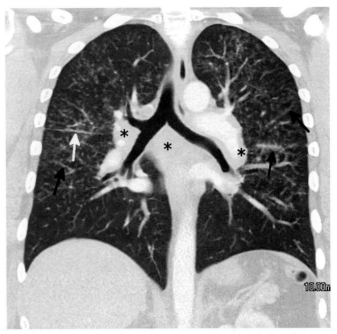

FIGURE 22.1 ▲ Sarcoidosis in a 34-year-old man with shortness of breath. Coronal CT image demonstrates mild and upper lung predominant perilymphatic micronodules with studding of the peribronchovascular interstitium (*black arrows*) and fissures (*white arrow*). In addition, there is bulky, symmetric mediastinal and hilar lymphadenopathy (*asterisks*), which confirm the diagnosis.

Microscopic Findings

Sarcoidosis is characterized by the presence of well-formed nonnecrotizing granulomas. There are two phases of pulmonary involvement, which usually overlap: an active, granulomatous phase and a fibrotic phase.[9] In a wedge biopsy, the characteristic lymphatic distribution of the nonnecrotizing granulomas, with exquisite

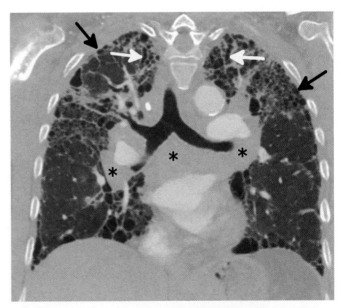

FIGURE 22.2 ▲ Sarcoidosis leading to fibrosis in a 58-year-old woman. Coronal CT image shows mild and upper lung predominant fibrosis with traction bronchiectasis (*white arrows*), reticulation, and subpleural honeycombing-like cystic spaces (*black arrows*). Bulky mediastinal and hilar lymphadenopathy (*asterisks*) is also present.

TABLE 22.1   Clinical Stages of Pulmonary Sarcoidosis, by Chest Radiograph

Stage 0	No mediastinal lymphadenopathy or lung infiltrates
Stage 1	Bilateral hilar lymphadenopathy
Stage 2	Bilateral hilar lymphadenopathy and reticulonodular infiltrates
Stage 3	Bilateral pulmonary infiltrates alone (without lymphadenopathy)[a]
Stage 4	Fibrocystic sarcoidosis typically with upward hilar retraction, cystic and bullous changes

[a]In the fibrotic phase of pulmonary sarcoid, there is often fibrosis of lymph nodes histologically, with few granulomas, without enlargement.

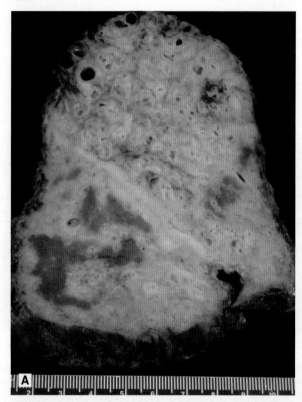

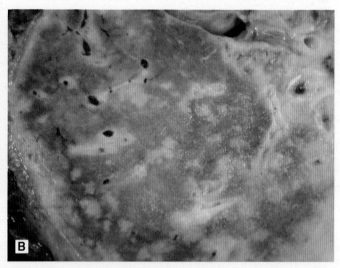

FIGURE 22.3 ▲ Sarcoidosis, explant lung. **A.** There is massive fibrosis, with accentuation in the septal, pleural, and bronchocentric regions (lymphatic distribution). Bronchi are diffusely dilated. **B.** A higher magnification demonstrates fibrosis along the lymphatic pathways.

involvement of the bronchovascular bundles, pleural surface, and interlobular septa, is easily appreciated (Fig. 22.5). This is a diagnostic hallmark of sarcoidosis. The remainder of the lung parenchyma is spared. An inflammatory process with prominent inflammation of the interstitium or organizing pneumonia is typically absent. The granulomas are comprised of epithelioid histiocytes with occasional

multinucleated giant cells (Fig. 22.6). Lymphocytes are sparse, usually forming a thin rim. The multinucleated giant cells often contain various inclusions and calcifications that are not specific to sarcoidosis (Fig. 22.5). Rarely, the granulomas may contain central punctate necrosis (Fig. 22.6). In a subset of cases, the granulomas may coalesce to form large nodules in so-called nodular sarcoidosis. In fibrotic sarcoidosis, the fibrosis is hyalinized and lacks inflammation. It gradually surrounds the granulomas inflammation and typically remains limited to the lymphatic pathways. Eventually, the granulomas may be entirely replaced by fibrosis except for scattered residual multinucleated giant cells (Fig. 22.7). Vascular involvement by granulomas may be prominent (Fig. 22.8). When veins are involved, pulmonary venoocclusive disease like changes may occur. These include fibrous occlusion of venules, best appreciated with an elastic stain (Fig. 22.8), and capillary proliferation with hemosiderosis.

Necrotizing Sarcoid Granulomatosis

Necrotizing sarcoid granulomatosis has a similar clinical presentation to classic sarcoidosis. However, it appears to be almost entirely restricted to the lung. In the original description of this entity, there was emphasis that it may represent a form of nodular sarcoid with severe vascular involvement.[10] The lack of data from large series limits our understanding of this entity; however, the evidence suggests necrotizing sarcoid granulomatosis is a variant of sarcoidosis.[11,12] On imaging, there are single or multiple large nodules,[13] frequently with pleural involvement.[14] Histologically, necrotizing sarcoid granulomatosis is characterized by large areas of necrosis in a background of nonnecrotizing granulomas, usually confluent forming large nodules. The necrosis is usually eosinophilic and devoid of abundant nuclear debris; however, it may be more basophilic raising the diagnosis of granulomatosis with polyangiitis (GPA). The remainder of the lung parenchyma will typically display the usual features of classic sarcoidosis, that is,

FIGURE 22.4 ▲ Transbronchial biopsy showing nonnecrotizing granulomas surrounded by hyaline fibrosis.

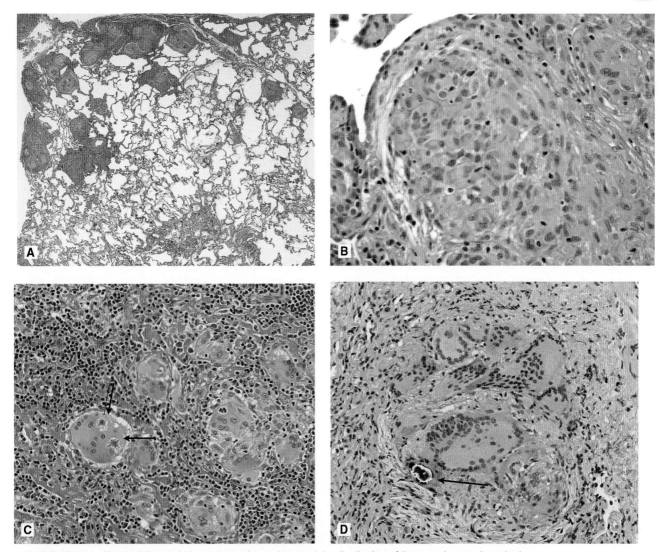

FIGURE 22.5 ▲ Wedge biopsy. **A.** Low power shows the exquisite distribution of the granulomas along the lymphatic pathways. The granulomas are thus located along the pleural surface, interlobular septa, and in the bronchovascular bundle. The remainder of the lung parenchyma is normal. **B.** At high power, the granuloma is composed of epithelioid histiocytes. **C.** Asteroid bodies (*arrows*) may be present in sarcoid granulomas but are nonspecific. **D.** Mineralized inclusions (*arrow*) in sarcoid granulomas are common and should not be confused with exogenous particles.

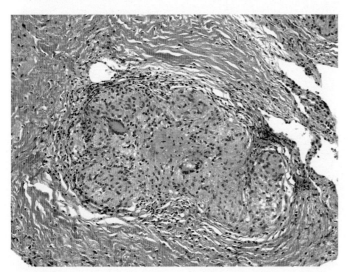

FIGURE 22.6 ▲ Granuloma with central punctate necrosis. This granuloma was otherwise present in a histologic background typical for sarcoidosis.

nonnecrotizing granulomas along lymphatic pathways. Vascular involvement by granulomas leading to vascular occlusion is a typical finding.[4,6]

Special Studies

Biopsy samples of lung showing granulomas, either necrotic or not, should be stained for fungi and acid-fast bacilli. Correlation with microbiologic studies (serologies, smear, and cultures) may be necessary to rule out infection.

Differential Diagnosis

The differential diagnoses of sarcoidosis include other diseases characterized by granulomas such as infection mainly mycobacterial and fungal (Chapters 40 and 41), hypersensitivity pneumonia (Chapter 23), occupational diseases such as berylliosis (Chapter 58), talc granulomatosis, and, in the case of necrotizing sarcoid granulomatosis, GPA (Chapter 48). As noted above, infection is ruled out with appropriate stains and microbiologic studies. Usually, in infection, the granulomas are not exquisitely lymphangitic in distribution and are often associated with other inflammatory responses such as bronchiolitis, interstitial inflammation, or organizing pneumonia. Fibrosis as seen in sarcoidosis

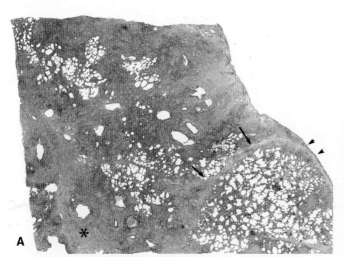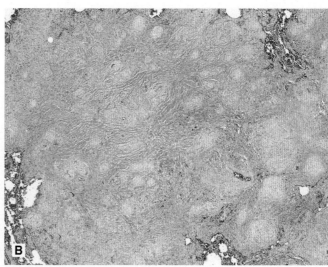

FIGURE 22.7 ▲ Sarcoidosis with fibrosis. **A.** At low magnification, the dense fibrosis follows the lymphatic pathways in the pleura (*arrowheads*), interlobular septum (*arrows*), and centrally around airways (*asterisk*). **B.** The fibrosis is hyalinized, gradually replacing the histiocytes within the granuloma.

is unusual with infection. Although granulomas are present in hypersensitivity pneumonia, they are usually poorly formed, limited to the airways and associated with chronic bronchiolitis and interstitial pneumonia. Berylliosis is indistinguishable from sarcoidosis. The diagnosis relies on establishing exposure to beryllium by the clinical history or tissue analysis, evidence of lung disease clinically and radiologically, and evidence of hypersensitivity to beryllium with lymphocyte proliferation tests. Talc granulomatosis is characterized histologically by foreign body giant cell proliferation within the interstitium and vessels, in contrast to the well-formed granulomas along the lymphatic pathways of sarcoidosis. Talc differs from the usual inclusion bodies seen in sarcoidosis by its characteristic sheet-like crystalline shape that is polarizable. In GPA, the necrosis differs from necrotizing sarcoid granulomatosis by being geographic and "dirty" due to the abundant nuclear debris of the neutrophils. Although granulomatous inflammation of the vessels is present

in GPA, true necrotizing vasculitis with fibrinoid necrosis is typically absent in necrotizing sarcoid granulomatosis.

Treatment and Prognosis

Treatment of sarcoid includes observation, steroids, methotrexate, azathioprine, leflunomide, mycophenolate, and, in intractable cases, infliximab.[1] However, patients may be refractory to treatment and require lung transplant. Up to 20% of patients with pulmonary sarcoid may develop progressive fibrotic disease. Patients with pulmonary hypertension have an especially poor prognosis.[7] Sarcoid frequently recurs in allografts. Pulmonary function does not appear to be compromised in the short term, and recurrence does not significantly shorten graft survival.[15–17] The inflammatory cells in the granulomas have been demonstrated to originate from the recipient.[16]

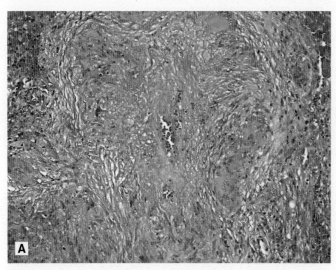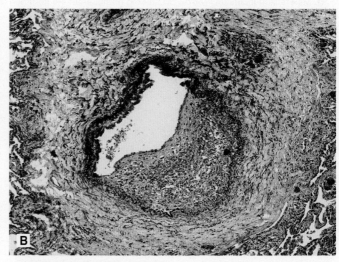

FIGURE 22.8 ▲ Involvement of vessels in sarcoidosis, both by granulomas and fibrosis. **A.** Vessel entirely replaced by granulomas with near-complete occlusion. **B.** Fibrous occlusion of vein (elastic stain).

REFERENCES

1. Baughman RP, Culver DA, Judson MA. A concise review of pulmonary sarcoidosis. *Am J Respir Crit Care Med.* 2011;183:573–581.
2. Akelsson IG, Eklund A, Skold CM, et al. Bilateral spontaneous pneumothorax and sarcoidosis. *Sarcoidosis.* 1990;7:136–138.
3. Sharma SK, Pande JN, Mukhopadhay AK, et al. Bilateral recurrent spontaneous pneumothoraces in sarcoidosis. *Jpn J Med.* 1987;26:69–71.
4. Hoffstein V, Ranganathan N, Mullen JB. Sarcoidosis simulating pulmonary veno-occlusive disease. *Am Rev Respir Dis.* 1986;134:809–811.
5. Jones RM, Dawson A, Jenkins GH, et al. Sarcoidosis-related pulmonary veno-occlusive disease presenting with recurrent haemoptysis. *Eur Respir J.* 2009;34:517–520.
6. Nunes H, Uzunhan Y, Freynet O, et al. Pulmonary hypertension complicating sarcoidosis. *Presse Med.* 2012;41:e303–e316.
7. Nunes H, Humbert M, Capron F, et al. Pulmonary hypertension associated with sarcoidosis: mechanisms, haemodynamics and prognosis. *Thorax.* 2006;61:68–74.
8. Kieszko R, Krawczyk P, Michnar M, et al. The yield of endobronchial biopsy in pulmonary sarcoidosis: connection between spirometric impairment and lymphocyte subpopulations in bronchoalveolar lavage fluid. *Respiration.* 2004;71:72–76.
9. Gal AA, Koss MN. The pathology of sarcoidosis. *Curr Opin Pulm Med.* 2002;8:445–451.
10. Churg A, Carrington CB, Gupta R. Necrotizing sarcoid granulomatosis. *Chest.* 1979;76:406–413.
11. Le Gall F, Loeuillet L, Delaval P, et al. Necrotizing sarcoid granulomatosis with and without extrapulmonary involvement. *Pathol Res Pract.* 1996;192:306–313; discussion 314.
12. Popper HH, Klemen H, Colby TV, et al. Necrotizing sarcoid granulomatosis—is it different from nodular sarcoidosis? *Pneumologie.* 2003;57:268–271.
13. Niimi H, Hartman TE, Muller NL. Necrotizing sarcoid granulomatosis: computed tomography and pathologic findings. *J Comput Assist Tomogr.* 1995;19:920–923.
14. Arfi J, Kerrou K, Traore S, et al. F-18 FDG PET/CT findings in pulmonary necrotizing sarcoid granulomatosis. *Clin Nucl Med.* 2010;35:697–700.
15. Milman N, Burton C, Andersen CB, et al. Lung transplantation for end-stage pulmonary sarcoidosis: outcome in a series of seven consecutive patients. *Sarcoidosis Vasc Diffuse Lung Dis.* 2005;22:222–228.
16. Ionescu DN, Hunt JL, Lomago D, et al. Recurrent sarcoidosis in lung transplant allografts: granulomas are of recipient origin. *Diagn Mol Pathol.* 2005;14:140–145.
17. Muller C, Briegel J, Haller M, et al. Sarcoidosis recurrence following lung transplantation. *Transplantation.* 1996;61:1117–1119.

23 Hypersensitivity Pneumonia

Marie-Christine Aubry, M.D., Allen P. Burke, M.D., and Seth Kligerman, M.D.

Hypersensitivity Pneumonia
Terminology and Definition

Hypersensitivity pneumonia, also known as hypersensitivity pneumonia[1,2] and extrinsic allergic alveolitis,[3] is an interstitial lung disease that results from an immunologic reaction to various inhaled antigens (Table 23.1). The exposure may not be readily recognized clinically, and therefore, pathology becomes essential to the diagnosis. Although a specific combination of histologic features may lead to a histologic diagnosis of hypersensitivity pneumonia, in many instances, the pathology is not entirely specific[4] and other morphologic features may be present, including the so-called bronchiolocentric interstitial pneumonias, such as airway-centered interstitial fibrosis, idiopathic bronchiolocentric interstitial pneumonia.[5–7]

Pathogenesis

The pathogenesis of hypersensitivity pneumonia is obscure. Only a small proportion of patients exposed to offending agents develop the disease. A Th1-predominant immune response has been shown in the acute phase of hypersensitivity pneumonia, whereas a Th2-predominant immune response may factor in the development of the fibrotic form of the disease, similar to other fibrosing lung diseases.[8] Other pathogenetic features in common with idiopathic pulmonary fibrosis include the up-regulation of proteins involved in apoptosis in bronchiolar epithelial cells.[9]

Epidemiology

In the United Kingdom, the incidence of hypersensitivity pneumonia has been estimated nearly 1 per 100,000 person-years, with a threefold increased risk for death over the general population.[3]

In a series of interstitial lung disease from Mexico in the 1980s, after excluding patients with autoimmune collagen vascular disease and inorganic exposures, over two-thirds of patients with interstitial lung disease were diagnosed with hypersensitivity pneumonia (pigeon breeder's lung). The high incidence was attributed to the custom of having pigeons fly freely in the home as pets.[10]

Clinical

Between two-thirds and 90% of patients are women, with a mean age at presentation of about 50 years for the acute form and 60 years for the fibrotic form.[11] There is no association with cigarette smoking.[3] Most patients have symptoms for a year or longer. In approximately two-thirds of patients, an inciting antigen is found and may be derived from a wide variety of fungal, bacterial, animal, or chemical sources including birds, household mold, thermophilic bacteria linked to contaminated humidifiers, and hay.

The clinical presentation of hypersensitivity pneumonia can be acute, subacute, or chronic. Acute hypersensitivity pneumonia occurs following exposure to a large amount of antigen. Patients develop severe dyspnea, cough, fever, and chills usually within 4 to 8 hours of exposure.[2] The symptoms resolve rapidly after removal of exposure and recur with re-exposure to the antigen. Typically, a biopsy is not performed as it is not necessary for the diagnosis.

The subacute and chronic presentations result from prolonged exposure to small amounts of antigen, which may not be evident to the patient, and therefore the diagnosis becomes more problematic, commonly leading to a biopsy. These patients have a more insidious onset of shortness of breath, with nonproductive cough. They may also develop fever, fatigue, and malaise. Chronic hypersensitivity pneumonia may progress into pulmonary fibrosis.[2,11–14]

Upon examination of the chest, tachypnea and inspiratory crackles are found in all clinical presentations of hypersensitivity pneumonia. Wheezing may occur and lead to a misdiagnosis of asthma. In chronic hypersensitivity pneumonia progressing to fibrosis, digital clubbing and manifestations of pulmonary hypertension with cor pulmonale may occur.

Pulmonary function tests are characterized by a predominantly restrictive physiology, increase residual volume due to air trapping, decrease diffusion capacity, and hypoxemia.[4]

TABLE 23.1 Etiologic Agents of Hypersensitivity Pneumonia and Their Associated Clinical Diseases

Antigens	Source	Disease
Bacteria		
Saccharopolyspora rectivirgula	Moldy hay	Farmer's lung
Thermoactinomyces vulgaris	Moldy hay and compost, water reservoirs, humidifiers	Farmer's lung, mushroom-worker's disease, humidifier lung
Thermoactinomyces sacchari	Moldy sugar cane, moldy compost	Bagassosis, mushroom-worker's disease
Thermoactinomyces candidus	Humidifier, house dust, air conditioner	Ventilation pneumonitis, humidifier lung
Mycobacterium immunogenum	Water-based cutting fluids	Metal working–associated HP
Mycobacterium avium complex	Hot tub mist, mold	Hot tub lung
Fungi		
Absidia corymbifera	Silage	Farmer's lung
Aspergillus clavatus	Moldy barley	Malt worker's lung
Aspergillus fumigatus	Moldy barley, Esparto grass, Cork dust	Malt worker's lung, stipatosis, suberosis
Penicillium glabrum	Cork dust	Suberosis
Cryptostroma corticale	Moldy maple bark	Maple bark stripper's lung
Pullularia	Humidifiers, moldy sawdust, sauna water	Humidifier lung, sequiosis, sauna taker's lung
Alternia	Wood dust	Woodworker's lung
Penicillium casei	Moldy cheese	Cheese washer's lung
Penicillium citreonigrum	Peat moss	Peat moss worker's lung
Trichosporon cutaneum	Contaminated old houses	Summer-type HP
Amoebae		
Acanthamoeba castellanii + polyphaga	Water mist	Humidifier lung
Bacterial product		
Bacillus subtilis enzymes	Detergent	Detergent worker's lung
Insect product		
Sitophilus granarius (wheat weevil)	Grain	Wheat weevil's lung, Miller's lung
Animal proteins		
Avian proteins	Feathers, bird droppings	Pigeon breeder's lung, bird fancier's lung, poultry worker's lung
Urine protein	Rats and gerbils	Laboratory worker's lung
Animal fur dust	Animal pelts	Furrier's lung
Chemicals		
Isocyanates[a]	Paint, resins and glues, polyurethane foams, rubber and plastic manufacturing	Chemical worker's lung
Pyrethrum	Insecticides	Pyrethrum pneumonitis
Acid anhydrides[b]	Epoxy resins	Epoxy resin lung

[a]TDI, toluene diisocyanate; HDI, hexamethylene diisocyanate; MDI, methylene bisphenyl isocyanate.
[b]PHA, phthalic anhydride; PMDA, pyromellitic anhydride.

Laboratory Detection of Antibodies

Specific IgG-precipitating serum antibodies are detected in 30% to 75% of patients[4,10,11,15] and may be used to identify the causal antigen. They are especially useful in the acute form of hypersensitivity pneumonia. Because precipitins are markers of exposure, however, they do not indicate disease and are frequently present in asymptomatic persons. False negatives are also common due to variation in standardization of reagents and in serum antibody levels.[2] In one study, the sensitivity of precipitin testing among groups of patients with known exposure was 75% for microbial antigens and 52% for avian antigen.[4]

In vitro testing of patient lymphocyte proliferation in response to the presumptive antigen is an adjunct diagnostic test that is largely a research tool.[16] Challenge studies may be a useful adjunct in diagnosis but are rarely performed in the clinical setting and may be limited by lack of standardized reagents.[2]

Clinical Diagnostic Criteria

There are no unequivocal diagnostic clinical criteria for hypersensitivity pneumonia short of inhalational challenge, which is not widely used in the clinic.[17] Clinical criteria include reproduction of the symptoms by environmental provocation or laboratory-controlled inhalation of the causative antigen (inhalational challenge), CT findings typical of hypersensitivity pneumonia, progression of restrictive lung disease with symptoms over 6 months, and positive antibodies.[16] A predominance of lymphocytes on bronchoalveolar lavage (BAL) is a supporting evidence of the diagnosis but nonspecific.[18]

Imaging

In the acute phase, confluent opacities may mimic infection or edema. Nodules with areas of ground-glass opacities predominate in the subacute phase, with mosaic perfusion pattern and air trapping on expiratory imaging (Fig. 23.1).[19]

Small poorly defined centrilobular nodules and thin-walled cysts may also be present. Reticular or linear opacities, traction bronchiectasis, and honeycomb change resembling usual interstitial pneumonia (UIP) are seen in about half of patients and occur in the chronic phase of disease when fibrosis develops[2,4] (Fig. 23.2).

Bronchoalveolar Lavage

BAL will typically show >25% of lymphocytosis, a CD4/CD8 ratio of <1.0, and >1% of mast cells in the acute phase.[20]

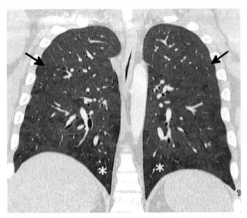

FIGURE 23.1 ▲ Coronal CT scan image in a 28-year-old man with multiple birds shows upper lobe-predominant centrilobular nodules (*arrows*) with diffuse ground-glass opacity areas of relative hypoattenuation in the lower lobes (*asterisks*) creating a mosaic attenuation. This constellation of findings can be seen with either respiratory bronchiolitis or subacute hypersensitivity pneumonia (HSP). The history, lack of smoking history, and subsequent biopsy all confirmed the diagnosis of hypersensitivity pneumonitis.

Gross Pathology

The gross pathology of hypersensitivity pneumonia is usually assessed in explant lungs from patients at a fibrotic stage of hypersensitivity pneumonia. The gross features include fibrosis, which may be central or peripheral, and honeycombing with pleural cobblestoning. Findings are usually more prominent in the upper lung zones (Fig. 23.2).

Microscopic Pathology

A classical triad of bronchiolocentric cellular chronic interstitial inflammation, chronic bronchiolitis, and poorly formed nonnecrotizing granulomatous in the peribronchiolar interstitium characterizes hypersensitivity pneumonia.[2] Others emphasize a similar "triad" of peribronchiolar inflammation, poorly formed granulomas, and organizing intraluminal fibrosis (organizing pneumonia).[21]

Not all these features are always present. The most prevalent finding is the cellular chronic interstitial pneumonia, which is similar to nonspecific interstitial pneumonia (NSIP) (Fig. 23.3).[2,18] The interstitial thickening is mostly the result of lymphocytes and plasma cells. Eosinophils and neutrophils, if present, are sparse.

Organizing pneumonia is seen in about half of the patients (Fig. 23.3).[4] There is frequently peribronchiolar lymphoid hyperplasia (Fig. 23.3), although follicular bronchiolitis with germinal centers is uncommon.[4] Peribronchiolar metaplasia is present in about half of biopsies.[4]

The granulomas of hypersensitivity pneumonia are typically loose clusters of epithelioid macrophages or isolated multinucleated giant cells in the walls of the bronchioles but may also be seen in the alveolar spaces (Fig. 23.4). Well-formed granulomas are inconspicuous and should raise consideration for other diagnosis.[4] There may also be interstitial giant cells or granulomas and Schaumann bodies. There should be an absence of changes suggestive of infection or other forms of interstitial lung disease.[10]

In the fibrosing phase of hypersensitivity pneumonia, the histologic features may resemble UIP with interstitial fibrosis and honeycombing in the peripheral lung (Fig. 23.5). However, there is also more peribronchiolar fibrosis and upper lobe involvement than in typical UIP.[4,15,16,22,23] In some instances, only peribronchiolar fibrosis is present or the fibrosis has the pattern of fibrotic NSIP. The identification of poorly formed granulomas in the areas of fibrosis aids in the diagnosis

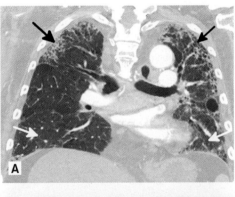

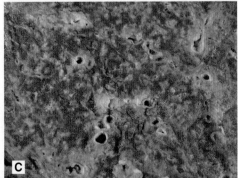

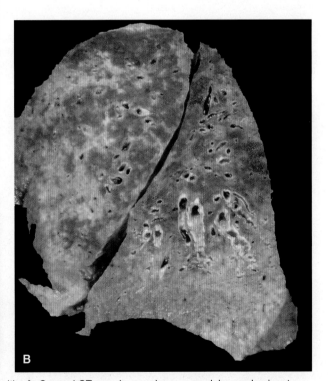

FIGURE 23.2 ▲ Fibrotic hypersensitivity pneumonitis. **A.** Coronal CT scan image shows upper lobe-predominant reticular opacities with honeycombing (*black arrows*). The lower lobes are relatively spared (*white arrows*). **B.** The explant shows fibrosis both central and peripheral with some traction bronchiectasis. **C.** A higher magnification shows centrilobular nodules. The patient had a long-standing history of exposure to birds and clinical findings of hypersensitivity pneumonitis years before transplant.

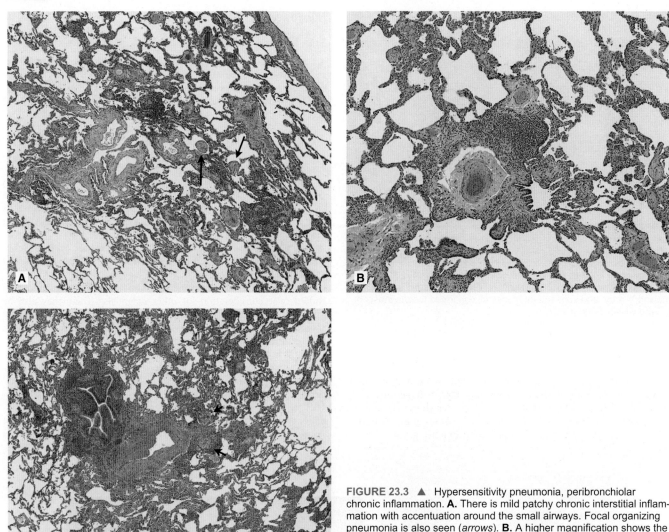

FIGURE 23.3 ▲ Hypersensitivity pneumonia, peribronchiolar chronic inflammation. **A.** There is mild patchy chronic interstitial inflammation with accentuation around the small airways. Focal organizing pneumonia is also seen (*arrows*). **B.** A higher magnification shows the peribronchiolar inflammation, that is, chronic bronchiolitis. **C.** There is peribronchiolar inflammation with poorly formed granulomas (*arrows*).

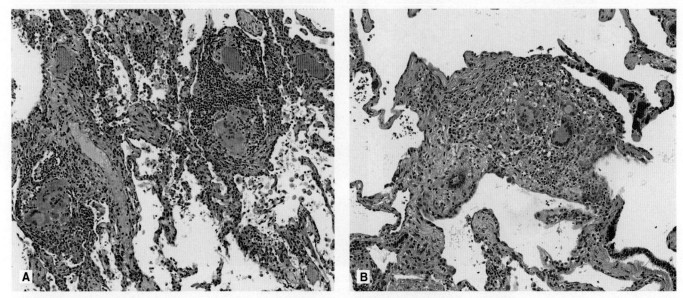

FIGURE 23.4 ▲ Hypersensitivity pneumonitis, granulomas. **A.** The granulomas are loose and poorly formed and, in this case, predominantly composed of multinucleated giant cells. **B.** Another example of poorly formed granuloma of hypersensitivity pneumonitis.

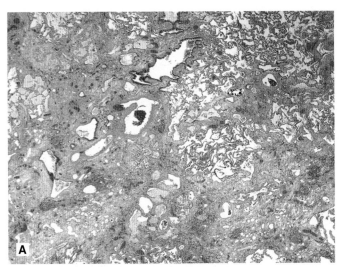 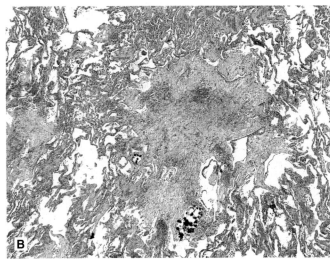

FIGURE 23.5 ▲ Fibrotic hypersensitivity pneumonia. **A.** Low-power photomicrograph shows a fibrosing interstitial pneumonia with peripheral distribution and early honeycombing, resembling usual interstitial pneumonia (UIP). **B.** In contrast to UIP, in fibrotic hypersensitivity pneumonitis, the airways are also involved by fibrosis.

of fibrotic hypersensitivity penumonia. As fibrosis influences patient outcome (see "Treatment and Prognosis" section), it is important to report the finding and pattern in the pathology report.

In hot tub lung disease, the main distinction with other causes of hypersensitivity pneumonia is the larger and better formed nonnecrotizing granulomas.[11,24] Mycobacteria are usually not identified with histochemical stains.

As described in Chapter 19, acute exacerbation may complicate hypersensitivity pneumonia usually in its fibrotic stage. Histologically, diffuse alveolar damage is superimposed on the chronic changes of fibrosis with chronic inflammation and poorly formed granulomas.[25,26]

Differential Diagnosis

Lung biopsies from patients with well-established clinical diagnoses of hypersensitivity pneumonia occasionally show histological features that overlap with NSIP (Chapter 17). The distinction with NSIP is based on the accentuation of the chronic inflammation around the small airways with a chronic bronchiolitis and the presence of poorly formed granulomas. However, even when a diagnosis of NSIP is rendered, a history of exposure should be ruled out clinically.

Fibrotic hypersensitivity pneumonia may resemble UIP (Chapter 17) histologically. Occasional poorly formed granulomas may be found incidentally in lung resections including in cases of typical UIP. In order to consider a diagnosis of fibrotic hypersensitivity pneumonia in a biopsy with features of UIP, histologic findings more typical of hypersensitivity pneumonia need to be identified.[17] These included airway-centered fibrosis and upper lobe predominance.

Patients, particularly older women, may develop bronchiectasis with infection by atypical mycobacteria. Histologically, the small airways show prominent chronic inflammation with nonnecrotizing granulomas. However, usually, the small airways are also dilated (bronchiolectasis) and the granulomas better formed. Also, there is no significant cellular interstitial pneumonia as with hypersensitivity pneumonia.

Several studies have been published emphasizing a pattern of inflammation and fibrosis centered on the airways, so-called bronchiolocentric interstitial pneumonias. *Idiopathic bronchiolocentric interstitial pneumonia* describes a centrilobular chronic inflammation with small airway fibrosis, in the absence of granulomas, a history of autoimmune

disease, or metal exposure. The exact nature of idiopathic bronchiolocentric interstitial pneumonia without clinical or histologic features of hypersensitivity is unknown, but there is a suggestion of a relatively poor prognosis.[5] *Airway-centered interstitial fibrosis* describes an interstitial process characterized by prominent airway-centered fibrosis with extensive bronchiolar metaplasia.[5] Many of the patients in that series had a possible history of exposure and therefore likely represented a form of fibrosing hypersensitivity pneumonia without the airway-centered granulomas.

Treatment and Prognosis

The clinical course associated with hypersensitivity pneumonia is variable. With early diagnosis and avoidance of the offending antigen, the prognosis tends to be favorable and permanent respiratory impairment can be avoided. Rapid recovery of pulmonary function is typical of acute hypersensitivity pneumonia.[11]

Antigen avoidance is the cornerstone of therapy and is often curative in patients for whom a specific antigen source is identified. Corticosteroids are useful in accelerating the rate of recovery. Lung function improves over a period of months and years, but abnormalities may persist in nearly half of patients. Repeated symptomatic attacks, older age, cigarette smoking, and the presence of established fibrosis and honeycomb change at the time of diagnosis are associated with a more aggressive course.[2] In fibrotic hypersensitivity pneumonia, lung transplantation may be the only therapeutic alternative.

The survival rate of hypersensitivity pneumonia is variable, depending on the population studied and rate of biopsy diagnosis. In hospitalized patients, a 25% 15-year survival rate for fibrotic hypersensitivity pneumonia was reported, compared to over 80% 15-year survival rate for the nonfibrotic form of disease.[15] A similar study of shorter follow-up showed, at 108 months, a 52% versus 97% survival rate for the two groups, respectively.[11] In the classic study of Perez-Padilla et al.[10], there was 71% four-year survival rate for patients with pigeon breeder's lung disease.

In a series of biopsy that documented hypersensitivity pneumonia, 7 of 9 patients with a UIP pattern on biopsy died of the disease, 5 of the 7 patients with a fibrotic form of NSIP died of the disease, and all of 5 patients with a cellular NSIP-like pattern improved.[27] In a more recent series documented by open lung biopsy, 0/24 patients with purely cellular hypersensitivity pneumonia died of their disease, 16 of the 18 patients with a UIP-like pattern died of the disease, 4 of 4 patients with a fibrotic NSIP-like pattern died of the disease, and 2 of 3 patients with only peribronchiolar fibrosis at the time of biopsy died of the disease.[22] The studies emphasize the importance of fibrosis on biopsy in predicting outcome.

REFERENCES

1. Herbst JB, Myers JL. Hypersensitivity pneumonia: role of surgical lung biopsy. *Arch Pathol Lab Med.* 2012;136:889–895.
2. Myers JL. Hypersensitivity pneumonia: the role of lung biopsy in diagnosis and management. *Mod Pathol.* 2012;25(suppl 1):S58–S67.
3. Solaymani-Dodaran M, West J, Smith C, et al. Extrinsic allergic alveolitis: incidence and mortality in the general population. *QJM.* 2007;100:233–237.
4. Trahan S, Hanak V, Ryu JH, et al. Role of surgical lung biopsy in separating chronic hypersensitivity pneumonia from usual interstitial pneumonia/idiopathic pulmonary fibrosis: analysis of 31 biopsies from 15 patients. *Chest.* 2008;134:126–132.
5. Yousem SA, Dacic S. Idiopathic bronchiolocentric interstitial pneumonia. *Mod Pathol.* 2002;15:1148–1153.
6. de Carvalho ME, Kairalla RA, Capelozzi VL, et al. Centrilobular fibrosis: a novel histological pattern of idiopathic interstitial pneumonia. *Pathol Res Pract.* 2002;198:577–583.
7. de Souza RB, Borges CT, Capelozzi VL, et al. Centrilobular fibrosis: an underrecognized pattern in systemic sclerosis. *Respiration.* 2009;77:389–397.
8. Kishi M, Miyazaki Y, Jinta T, et al. Pathogenesis of cBFL in common with IPF? Correlation of IP-10/TARC ratio with histological patterns. *Thorax.* 2008;63:810–816.
9. Jinta T, Miyazaki Y, Kishi M, et al. The pathogenesis of chronic hypersensitivity pneumonitis in common with idiopathic pulmonary fibrosis: expression of apoptotic markers. *Am J Clin Pathol.* 2010;134:613–620.
10. Perez-Padilla R, Salas J, Chapela R, et al. Mortality in Mexican patients with chronic pigeon breeder's lung compared with those with usual interstitial pneumonia. *Am Rev Respir Dis.* 1993;148:49–53.
11. Hanak V, Golbin JM, Ryu JH. Causes and presenting features in 85 consecutive patients with hypersensitivity pneumonitis. *Mayo Clin Proc.* 2007;82:812–816.
12. Glazer CS, Rose CS, Lynch DA. Clinical and radiologic manifestations of hypersensitivity pneumonitis. *J Thorac Imaging.* 2002;17:261–272.
13. Morell F, Roger A, Reyes L, et al. Bird fancier's lung: a series of 86 patients. *Medicine (Baltimore).* 2008;87:110–130.
14. Yoshizawa Y, Ohtani Y, Hayakawa H, et al. Chronic hypersensitivity pneumonitis in Japan: a nationwide epidemiologic survey. *J Allergy Clin Immunol.* 1999;103:315–320.
15. Vourlekis JS, Schwarz MI, Cherniack RM, et al. The effect of pulmonary fibrosis on survival in patients with hypersensitivity pneumonitis. *Am J Med.* 2004;116:662–668.
16. Hayakawa H, Shirai M, Sato A, et al. Clinicopathological features of chronic hypersensitivity pneumonitis. *Respirology.* 2002;7:359–364.
17. Katzenstein AL, Mukhopadhyay S, Myers JL. Diagnosis of usual interstitial pneumonia and distinction from other fibrosing interstitial lung diseases. *Hum Pathol.* 2008;39:1275–1294.
18. Vourlekis JS, Schwarz MI, Cool CD, et al. Nonspecific interstitial pneumonitis as the sole histologic expression of hypersensitivity pneumonitis. *Am J Med.* 2002;112:490–493.
19. Hartman TE. The HRCT features of etrinsic allergic alveolitis. *Semin Respir Crit Care Med.* 2003;24:419–426.
20. Chan AL, Juarez MM, Leslie KO, et al. Bird fancier's lung: a state-of-the-art review. *Clin Rev Allergy Immunol.* 2012;43:69–83.
21. American Thoracic Society/European Respiratory Society International Multidisciplinary Consensus Classification of the Idiopathic Interstitial Pneumonias. This joint statement of the American Thoracic Society (ATS), and the European Respiratory Society (ERS) was adopted by the ATS board of directors, June 2001 and by the ERS Executive Committee, June 2001. *Am J Respir Crit Care Med.* 2002;165:277–304.
22. Churg A, Sin DD, Everett D, et al. Pathologic patterns and survival in chronic hypersensitivity pneumonitis. *Am J Surg Pathol.* 2009;33:1765–1770.
23. Akashi T, Takemura T, Ando N, et al. Histopathologic analysis of sixteen autopsy cases of chronic hypersensitivity pneumonitis and comparison with idiopathic pulmonary fibrosis/usual interstitial pneumonia. *Am J Clin Pathol.* 2009;131:405–415.
24. Khoor A, Leslie KO, Tazelaar HD, et al. Diffuse pulmonary disease caused by nontuberculous mycobacteria in immunocompetent people (hot tub lung). *Am J Clin Pathol.* 2001;115:755–762.
25. Churg A, Wright JL, Tazelaar HD. Acute exacerbations of fibrotic interstitial lung disease. *Histopathology.* 2011;58:525–530.
26. Olson AL, Huie TJ, Groshong SD, et al. Acute exacerbations of fibrotic hypersensitivity pneumonitis: a case series. *Chest.* 2008;134:844–850.
27. Ohtani Y, Saiki S, Kitaichi M, et al. Chronic bird fancier's lung: histopathological and clinical correlation. An application of the 2002 ATS/ERS consensus classification of the idiopathic interstitial pneumonias. *Thorax.* 2005;60:665–671.

24 Pulmonary Langerhans Cell Histiocytosis

Marie-Christine Aubry, M.D., Anja C. Roden, M.D., and Allen P. Burke, M.D.

Terminology

Pulmonary Langerhans cell histiocytosis (PLCH) is an interstitial lung disease characterized by an abnormal proliferation of Langerhans cells. While Langerhans cell histiocytosis (see Chapter 92) may involve the lung as part of a systemic hematopoietic neoplasm, PLCH is distinct in that it occurs mainly in smoking adults in whom pulmonary involvement is the sole or predominant manifestation of the disease.[1,2]

PLCH is a rare disease; precise data regarding prevalence are not available, partly because it is not always biopsied or histologically documented. A large series of hundreds of patients undergoing surgical lung biopsies for diffuse lung disease reported PLCH in 4% to 5% of biopsies for interstitial lung disease.[3] In a series of PLCH diagnosed on clinical and radiologic findings, the incidence was nearly 7%.[4]

Pathogenesis

PLCH, in contrast to systemic LCH, has been considered a nonneoplastic process.[5] PLCH is thought to be a manifestation of an immune response to an unknown exogenous antigen related to cigarette smoke.[6,7] Since only a small percentage of cigarette smokers develop PLCH, underlying host factors must be a factor.[8] Cigarette smoking is associated with an increase in dendritic cells and Langerhans cells in the alveolar epithelium[9,10] and induces the secretion of bombesin-like peptides by pulmonary neuroendocrine cells.[11] Oligoclonal expansion would contribute to the maintenance of Langerhans cells at the sites of disease.[5] Recently, *BRAF V600E* mutation and BRAF expression have been reported in a subset (up to 28%) of PLCH suggesting that some cases do represent a true clonal process and might be true neoplasms.[12]

Although classified as an interstitial lung disease, PLCH affects small airways, explaining the exquisite bronchiolocentric distribution of the nodules. The cystic lesions are thought to arise from the destruction of the bronchioles.[13,14]

Clinical

PLCH affects young adults between the ages of 20 and 70 years, with a median age of 33 years.[7] There is no gender predilection, but there may be a predominance in Caucasians.[8] As nearly all patients are current or former smokers, PLCH is considered a form of smoking-related interstitial lung disease. Most patients with PLCH are symptomatic. Spontaneous pneumothorax occurs in nearly 25% of patients. Extrapulmonary involvement is rare in PLCH.[7] Pulmonary function tests are variable. The most common abnormality is reduced diffusion capacity. Restriction, obstruction, or mixed ventilatory defects are also seen.

Radiologic Findings

The coexistence of upper lung nodules and cysts in a smoker is highly suggestive of PLCH (Fig. 24.1).[15] Cystic lesions are the most common high-resolution CT feature and measure from <10 mm in diameter to 20 mm. Cysts are often seen in association with nodules, although reticulonodular densities are relatively uncommon. The cysts occur predominantly in upper lung zones.[8] Rarely, PLCH can present as a solitary macronodule or an obstructing endobronchial tumor.[16,17]

Tissue Sampling

PLCH is generally diagnosed by wedge lung biopsy, although the diagnosis may be made on transbronchial or transthoracic needle biopsy with the support of immunohistochemical studies.[7] Bronchoalveolar lavage may show increased Langerhans cells, stained with Giemsa stain or by immunohistochemistry.[18]

Pathologic Findings

Grossly, PLCH is characterized by multiple grayish-white irregular nodules, usually < 1 cm, with surrounding cystic areas (Fig. 24.2).[8] The findings involve predominantly the upper lobes.

Histologically, at low magnification, the defining feature of PLCH is the presence of bronchiolocentric nodules with a stellate configuration (Fig. 24.3). The morphology of the nodules varies. Early lesions are cellular with peribronchiolar interstitium and adjacent alveolar

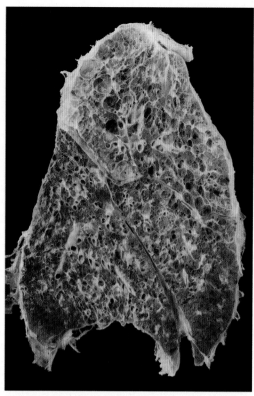

FIGURE 24.2 ▲ PLCH at autopsy. All lobes are involved although changes are most severe in the upper lobe. White fibrotic stellate shape nodules are seen associated mostly with variable-sized cysts.

septa thickened by clusters of Langerhans cell admixed with variable numbers of eosinophils, neutrophils, lymphocytes, macrophages, and fibroblasts (Figs. 24.4 and 24.5). Eosinophils are often numerous and can form eosinophilic abscesses, but may also be completely absent. In some cases, neutrophils are a conspicuous component of the inflammation. Macrophages usually containing smokers' pigment are found within the interstitium and surrounding airspaces, imparting a "desquamative interstitial pneumonia (DIP)-like" appearance to

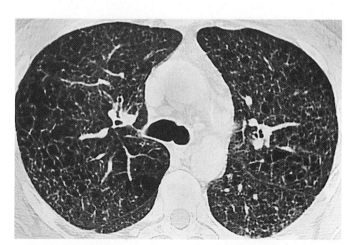

FIGURE 24.1 ▲ CT scan of PLCH showing small irregular shaped nodules and multiple thin-walled cysts.

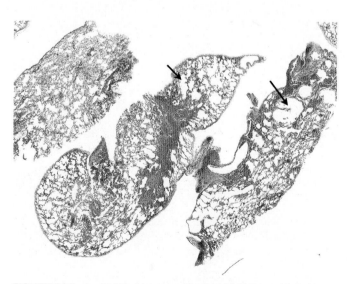

FIGURE 24.3 ▲ PLCH at low magnification. Multiple centrilobular stellate-shaped nodules associated with cystic changes (*arrows*).

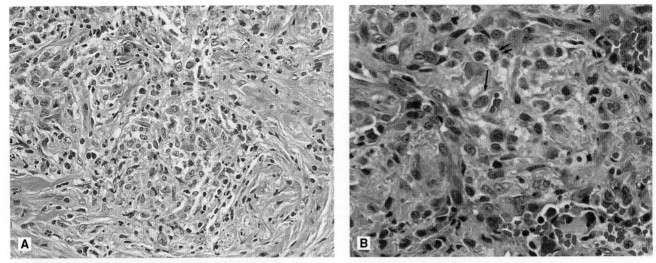

FIGURE 24.4 ▲ PLCH, Langerhans cells. **A.** There are scattered eosinophils. **B.** Langerhans cells are characterized by indistinct cytoplasmic borders (*arrows*) with irregular shaped, grooved nuclei (*double arrow*).

the process. As the lesions progress, they become more fibrotic and less cellular. Typically, fibrosis develops in the center of the nodules with the most cellular areas extending in the periphery (Fig. 24.6). The fibrosis may be cellular resembling organizing pneumonia. Ultimately, the nodules become completely fibrotic with scant inflammatory cells and no diagnostic Langerhans cell (Fig. 24.7). In this scenario, a presumptive diagnosis of PLCH can be made, with a note that correlation with imaging is recommended for definitive diagnosis.

Paracicatricial airspace enlargement (irregular or scar emphysema) affecting surrounding airspaces is a characteristic finding in fibrotic lesions and accounts for most of the "cysts" seen on imaging (Figs. 24.2 and 24.3).[13,14] At this stage, PLCH may be confused with chronic fibrosing interstitial pneumonias, in particular usual interstitial pneumonia (UIP).

Langerhans cells are 12 to 15 μm with pale pink cytoplasm, grooved nuclei, and poorly defined cell borders (Fig. 24.3). Electron microscopy

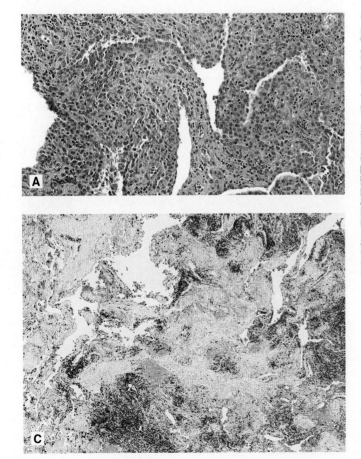

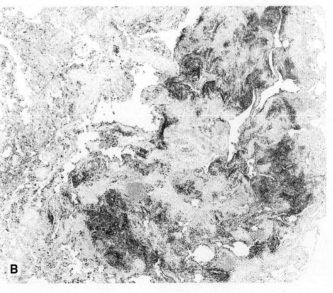

FIGURE 24.5 ▲ **A.** In this example, there is expansion of the alveolar walls by PLCH with reactive pneumocytes lining the intervening spaces. **B.** A low magnification showing patchy S100 positivity. **C.** Slightly higher magnification showing patchy CD1a positivity.

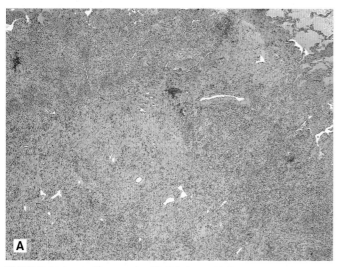 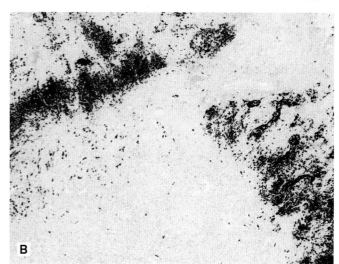

FIGURE 24.6 ▲ Progressing PLCH. **A.** As PLCH nodules progress, the center becomes more fibrotic. **B.** Langerhans cells are present at the periphery (anti-CD1a).

demonstrates Langerhans or Birbeck granules, which are 100- to 400- by 35- to 45-nm rods with a pentalaminar appearance.[8] Langerhans cells are demonstrated immunohistochemically by their expression of S100 protein, CD1a, and langerin (Figs. 24.5 and 24.6). The number of Langerhans cells varies widely with the progression of the disease. Conversely, the presence of Langerhans cells is nonspecific, as they are increased in COPD, lung cancer, and interstitial lung diseases; therefore, the diagnosis of PLCH hinges on the recognition of these cells in the appropriate background.[19]

Differential Diagnosis

The differential diagnosis for PLCH is broad. In an advanced and fibrotic stage, UIP enters the differential diagnosis (Chapter 17). In contrast to PLCH, UIP is a predominantly lower lobe disease and with peripheral subpleural distribution.

The DIP-like reaction associated with PLCH may be so prominent as to render the diagnostic lesions of PLCH almost inconspicuous.

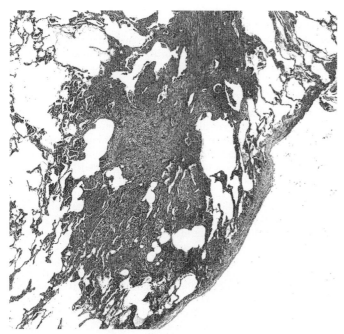

FIGURE 24.7 ▲ Old PLCH. The nodule is entirely composed of fibrosis with scattered lymphocytes. No Langerhans cells are present.

In DIP (Chapter 18), HRCT is characterized by ground-glass opacities without the characteristic cysts and nodules of PLCH. As DIP is a diagnosis of exclusion, other diseases such as PLCH need to be ruled out histologically. Searching for bronchiolocentric stellate shape nodules is key to diagnosing PLCH.

Eosinophilic pneumonia (EP) (Chapter 26) enters the differential diagnosis because of the numerous eosinophils that may be seen in PLCH. EP is characterized by intra-alveolar accumulation of macrophages and eosinophils admixed with a fibrinous exudate and lacks the bronchiolocentric nodules and clusters of Langerhans cells seen in PLCH.

Prognosis and Treatment

The natural history of PLCH ranges from spontaneous regression to progressive respiratory insufficiency and death. Disease-specific mortality is between 10% and 20% with median survivals around 13 years.[20] The prognosis is often hard to predict, but older age, marked airflow limitation with air trapping and reduced diffusion capacity, and pulmonary hypertension are associated with worse prognosis. There is also an association between PLCH and other malignancies such as lung cancer, smoking being the shared risk factor. Treatment of PLCH is smoking cessation.[21] Steroids are often used with limited anecdotal evidence of efficacy. Transplantation is an option but PLCH may recur in allografts. Reports of remission after chemotherapy, such as 2-chlorodeoxyadenosine, likely refer to systemic Langerhans cell histiocytosis (see Chapter 92).[22] With the presence of *BRAF V600E* mutation in a subset of PLCH, perhaps targeted therapy may play a role in the treatment of these patients.

REFERENCES

1. Goicochea L, Frazier AA, Todd N, et al. Pulmonary Langerhans cell histiocytosis and smoking-related lung disease. *Pathol Case Rev.* 2013;18:132–137.
2. Suri HS, Yi ES, Nowakowski GS, et al. Pulmonary Langerhans cell histiocytosis. *Orphanet J Rare Dis.* 2012;7:16.
3. Gaensler EA, Carrington CB. Open biopsy for chronic diffuse infiltrative lung disease: clinical, roentgenographic, and physiological correlations in 502 patients. *Ann Thorac Surg.* 1980;30:411–426.
4. Vassallo R, Ryu JH. Pulmonary Langerhans' cell histiocytosis. *Clin Chest Med.* 2004;25:561–571, vii.
5. Yousem SA, Colby TV, Chen YY, et al. Pulmonary Langerhans' cell histiocytosis: molecular analysis of clonality. *Am J Surg Pathol.* 2001;25:630–636.
6. Tazi A, Bonay M, Grandsaigne M, et al. Surface phenotype of Langerhans cells and lymphocytes in granulomatous lesions from patients with pulmonary histiocytosis X. *Am Rev Respir Dis.* 1993;147:1531–1536.

7. Travis WD, Borok Z, Roum JH, et al. Pulmonary Langerhans cell granulo-matosis (histiocytosis X). A clinicopathologic study of 48 cases. *Am J Surg Pathol.* 1993;17:971–986.

8. Abbott GF, Rosado-de-Christenson ML, Franks TJ, et al. From the archives of the AFIP: pulmonary Langerhans cell histiocytosis. *Radiographics.* 2004;24: 821–841.

9. Soler P, Tazi A, Hance AJ. Pulmonary Langerhans cell granulomatosis. *Curr Opin Pulm Med.* 1995;1:406–416.

10. Casolaro MA, Bernaudin JF, Saltini C, et al. Accumulation of Langerhans' cells on the epithelial surface of the lower respiratory tract in normal subjects in association with cigarette smoking. *Am Rev Respir Dis.* 1988;137:406–411.

11. Vassallo R, Ryu JH, Colby TV, et al. Pulmonary Langerhans'-cell histiocytosis. *N Engl J Med.* 2000;342:1969–1978.

12. Roden AC, Hu X, Kip S, et al. BRAF V600E expression in Langerhans cell histiocytosis: clinical and immunohistochemical study on 25 pulmonary and 54 extrapulmonary cases. *Am J Surg Pathol.* 2014;38:548–551.

13. Kambouchner M, Basset F, Marchal J, et al. Three-dimensional characteriza-tion of pathologic lesions in pulmonary Langerhans cell histiocytosis. *Am J Respir Crit Care Med.* 2002;166:1483–1490.

14. Myers JL, Aubry MC. Pulmonary Langerhans cell histiocytosis: what was the question? *Am J Respir Crit Care Med.* 2002;166:1419–1421.

15. Attili AK, Kazerooni EA, Gross BH, et al. Smoking-related interstitial lung disease: radiologic-clinical-pathologic correlation. *Radiographics.* 2008;28:1383–1396; discussion 1396–1398.

16. Khoor A, Myers JL, Tazelaar HD, et al. Pulmonary Langerhans cell histio-cytosis presenting as a solitary nodule. *Mayo Clin Proc.* 2001;76:209–211.

17. O'Donnell AE, Tsou E, Awh C, et al. Endobronchial eosinophilic granuloma: a rare cause of total lung atelectasis. *Am Rev Respir Dis.* 1987;136:1478–1480.

18. Takizawa Y, Taniuchi N, Ghazizadeh M, et al. Bronchoalveolar lavage fluid analysis provides diagnostic information on pulmonary Langerhans cell his-tiocytosis. *J Nippon Med Sch.* 2009;76:84–92.

19. Marchal-Somme J, Uzunhan Y, Marchand-Adam S, et al. Dendritic cells accumulate in human fibrotic interstitial lung disease. *Am J Respir Crit Care Med.* 2007;176:1007–1014.

20. Vassallo R, Ryu JH, Schroeder DR, et al. Clinical outcomes of pulmonary Langerhans'-cell histiocytosis in adults. *N Engl J Med.* 2002;346:484–490.

21. Mogulkoc N, Veral A, Bishop PW, et al. Pulmonary Langerhans' cell histio-cytosis: radiologic resolution following smoking cessation. *Chest.* 1999;115: 1452–1455.

22. Aerni MR, Aubry MC, Myers JL, et al. Complete remission of nodular pul-monary Langerhans cell histiocytosis lesions induced by 2-chlorodeoxy-adenosine in a non-smoker. *Respir Med.* 2008;102:316–319.

25 Aspiration Pneumonia

Allen P. Burke, M.D., Fabio R. Tavora, M.D., Ph.D., and Marie-Christine Aubry, M.D.

Aspiration and Aspiration Pneumonia

Clinical and Radiologic Findings

Recurrent aspiration of gastric contents, or chronic occult aspiration, is a common, often silent, process that especially affects infants with feeding problems, adults with neurologic deficits, and patients with decreased gastroesophageal motility and acid reflux. Recurrent aspi-ration is known to cause lung disease and recurrent pneumonia and may also be a contributing factor in exacerbating chronic lung dis-eases, such as idiopathic pulmonary fibrosis (IPF), chronic obstruc-tive lung disease, chronic rejection in lung transplant patients, and cystic fibrosis.

In a series of patients with lung infiltrates and pulmonary symptoms that could not be explained by routine evaluation, almost half showed pulmonary aspiration by overnight scintigraphy, which correlated pos-itively with obstructive sleep apnea and recurrent pneumonias.[1]

Gastroesophageal reflux disease (GERD) is a proven risk factor for recurrent microaspiration, which may cause lung injury. Unfortunately, there are no reliable widely used diagnostic tests for microaspira-tion. Proximal esophageal acid detection by pH monitoring is widely available but lacks sensitivity. Impedance monitoring measures both acid and nonacid reflux episodes and is therefore more sensitive.[2] In fact, experimental studies have shown that microaspiration is a fairly common phenomenon and can be seen in up to 40% of normal indi-viduals and in up to 70% of people with neurologic alterations or obstructive sleep apnea. However, normal people tend to clear such aspirations without sequelae.[3,4] Aspiration pneumonia generally results from a single large event and is a common autopsy finding in debili-tated patients with neurologic defects or other predisposing factors.

Common presenting symptoms of aspiration-induced lung disease include dyspnea, fever, and cough. There is a history of recurrent pneu-monia in about 25% of patients. In addition to reflux and neurologic disease, drug use is an additional predisposing factor.[5] The most com-mon clinical settings for aspiration are presented in Table 25.1.

Chest radiograph shows bilateral infiltrates or nodules in about half, with unilateral findings in the other half. Areas most prone to aspiration are the right middle and lower lobes, due to the anatomic configuration of the bronchi. However, these vary depending on the patient's position at the time of aspiration (e.g., sleep patterns). In some cases, nodules may be solitary and raise a clinical concern for malig-nancy. Computed tomography (CT) in patients with prominent small airway involvement typically shows centrilobular nodules in depen-dent portions of the lung. In aspiration pneumonia, imaging often demonstrates airspace disease (ground glass or consolidation), reticu-lar densities, and nodules.

Cytologic Findings

The presence of lipid-laden macrophages in bronchoalveolar lavage, especially when quantitatively high, is suggestive of a diagnosis of recurrent aspiration, both in children[6,7] and in adults.[8]

Gross and Histologic Findings

Aspiration pneumonia is characterized by patchy areas of consolida-tion (Fig. 25.1). Abscess formation is not uncommon.

The histologic findings of aspiration depend on the type and amount of aspirated material. Aspiration of a large bolus of acid gas-tric content causes diffuse alveolar damage (Chapter 4). Aspiration of recurrent small amount of food or pills usually causes acute and orga-nizing pneumonia with multinucleated foreign body giant cell reaction and suppurative granulomas. Chronic bronchiolitis may be the pre-dominant histologic finding secondary to chronic occult aspiration.[9] A definitive diagnosis rests on the identification of foreign material within the giant cells or suppurative granulomas (Figs. 25.2 to 25.4).[5] The most common vegetable matter seen in chronic aspiration is the starch grain or granule, found in legumes, including peas, beans, and lentils. The starch granule is about 100 μ in length (Fig. 25.3), is eosinophilic and well demarcated and oval, and eventually degenerates as macro-phages engulf the material (Fig. 25.4). Other foreign materials that may be seen in aspiration include cellulose (Fig. 25.5), crospovidone (Fig. 25.6), Kayexalate (Fig. 25.7),[10] and talc (Fig. 25.8), each with characteristic histologic features. If foreign material is not present,

TABLE 25.1 Most Common Aspiration Material and ClinicoPathologic Findings

Material	ClinicoPathologic Findings
Gastric acid aspiration	Major cause of diffuse alveolar damage in patients with neurologic impairment
	Atelectasis
	May lead to lung abscess
Recurrent "microaspiration"	Chronic airway disease
	Bronchiectasis
	Interstitial fibrosis associated with foci of organizing pneumonia
Hydrocarbons	Especially common in children, it produces rapid symptoms: congestion, hemorrhage, edema, and hyaline membrane formation
Food aspiration	Most commonly vegetable matter (seeds), skeletal muscle, fat tissue, or fragments of bone
	Acute exudative response in <24 h
	Chronic changes include foreign body giant cell reaction and organizing pneumonia.
	Fibrosis and calcification can occur at later stages.
	Recurrent aspiration can lead to diffuse bronchiolitis in a miliary form.
Drugs	Tablet components (cellulose, crospovidone, talc, etc.) may be found alone or in association with food material.
	Some of the components may be birefringent on polarization.
	Kayexalate has a distinctive histologic appearance—large dark PAS-positive basophilic glassy particles.
Oil (exogenous lipid)	Mineral, vegetable, and animal oil can all be aspirated into the lung.
	Mineral oil used in drugs is the most common agent in exogenous lipid pneumonia.
	Microscopically, the droplets are usually dissolved by tissue processing, and one can see as circular negative images within the tissue and commonly associated with giant cells.

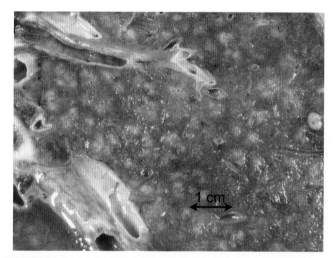

FIGURE 25.1 ▲ Aspiration pneumonia, autopsy. Gross findings are patchy areas of consolidation, especially in dependent portions of the lung.

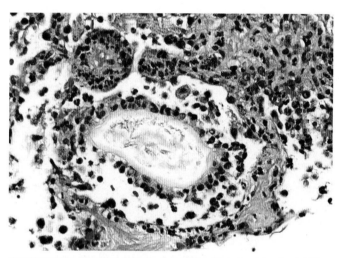

FIGURE 25.3 ▲ Aspirated starch granule. The starch is about 100 μ in length and has elicited an acute inflammatory reaction.

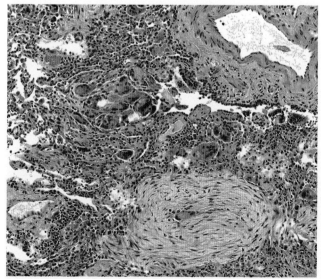

FIGURE 25.2 ▲ Aspiration pneumonia. There is organizing pneumonia with scattered multinucleated giant cells. Even if no foreign material is found, the finding is suggestive of aspiration.

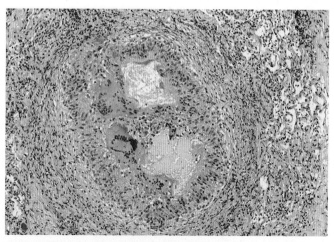

FIGURE 25.4 ▲ Aspirated foreign material. There is a multinucleated giant cell reaction to acellular debris, which by size and shape may represent degenerated starch grains.

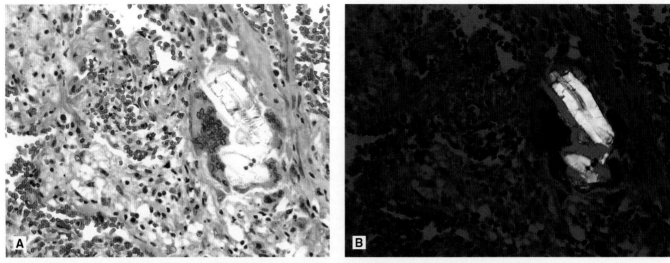

FIGURE 25.5 ▲ Aspirated cellulose. **A.** Microcrystalline cellulose aspiration of ground pills forming gray rod-like sheet material. **B.** Typical longitudinal central groove of microcrystalline cellulose under polarized light.

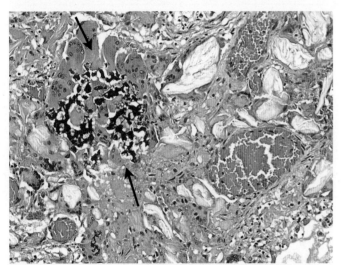

FIGURE 25.6 ▲ Polyvinylpyrrolidone (PVP). PVP and related compounds are found in adhesives and toothpaste and is the most widely used excipient in pharmaceuticals. The material forms hematoxylinophilic irregular deposits in this case surrounded by macrophage giant cells (*arrows*).

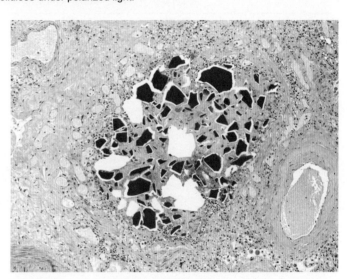

FIGURE 25.7 ▲ Kayexalate aspiration. There are crystals within an airway. There is autolysis of the mucosa secondary to autopsy artifact.

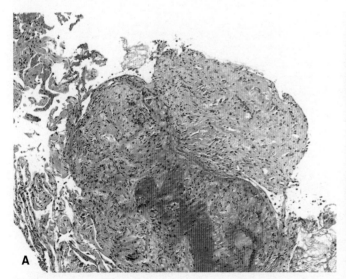

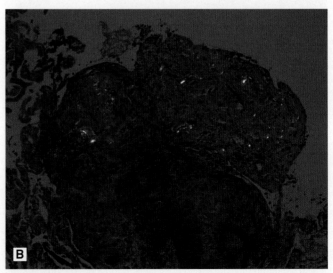

FIGURE 25.8 ▲ Talc granulomas, transbronchial biopsy. **A.** High magnification photomicrograph demonstrates nonnecrotizing granulomas. **B.** Viewed under polarized light, talc crystals are readily identified.

a histologic diagnosis of aspiration pneumonia cannot be made, although can be surmised with clinical documentation of aspiration and exclusion of other causes of lung disease.[11]

Aspiration pneumonia may result in an infectious process due to superinfection by bacteria from the oropharynx or bacteria found in aspirated matter. Histologically, the features are those of an acute bronchopneumonia, often necrotizing, and foreign material may or may not be present.[11]

Recurrent Aspiration and Idiopathic Pulmonary Fibrosis

Gastroesophageal reflux may play a role in advancing the course of disease as well as causing symptoms in patients with IPF. A high prevalence of reflux has been found among patients with IPF.[12,13] The clinical impact of reflux on IPF disease progression is unclear, and the benefits of antireflux surgery have not been entirely substantiated. However, it is believed that a subset of patients with IPF benefit from antireflux therapy.[2]

Recurrent Aspiration in Lung Transplantation

Because the median survival of lung transplant patients is only around 5 years, there is active interest in the role of microaspiration in the development of chronic rejection (obliterative bronchiolitis), which is the main complication limiting allograft survival.[2] There is some evidence that acid reflux increases after transplant and contributes to lung dysfunction and that reflux surgery may improve lung symptoms and slow the progression of, or even reverse obliterative bronchiolitis.[14–16]

Recurrent Aspiration in Children

Oropharyngeal aspiration and silent aspiration occurs in about one-third of children with feeding difficulties and is associated with neurologic impairment, developmental delay, and enteral feeding. A significant proportion of these children develop aspiration lung disease.[17] Many children are still not adequately diagnosed or treated for aspiration until permanent lung damage has occurred.[18] The histologic features of aspiration lung disease in children have not been characterized.

Endogenous Versus Exogenous Lipid Pneumonia

Lipid (or lipoid) pneumonia refers to the accumulation of lipid within inflammatory cells (typically macrophages) within airspaces of the lung. Lipid pneumonia is generally categorized as endogenous or exogenous. Endogenous lipid pneumonia refers to lipid formed by the breakdown of cells and is a general indication of obstruction. Extracellular lipid in endogenous lipid pneumonia typically accumulates as cholesterol crystals. In contrast, exogenous lipid pneumonia is caused by the inhalation of fats and oils, especially mineral oils. Exogenous lipid pneumonia is characterized by accumulations of extracellular lipid in the form of large vacuoles lined by macrophage giant cells. So-called idiopathic lipid pneumonia has been reported in patients with either endogenous or exogenous lipid pneumonia having no predisposing etiologies.[19,20]

Endogenous Lipid Pneumonia

Clinical Findings

The clinical features of endogenous lipid pneumonia are dominated by the inciting process, usually obstruction of a large airway. The most common cause of obstruction is by a relatively slow-growing neoplasm. Postobstructive pneumonia may be the initial presentation of tumor or an incidental finding at imaging or pathologic examination of resection lung cancers. Subsequent high-resolution imaging or bronchoscopy uncovers the endoscopic obstructive lesion. Central carcinomas are frequently accompanied by distal infiltrates seen on CT scans that may include postobstructive atelectasis or pneumonia, or collapse of the entire lung. Bronchogenic carcinomas arising in the middle and lower lobes are more likely to be obstructed than those of the upper lobes.[21] Patients with lung cancers and significant postobstructive pneumonias have an overall worse postoperative prognosis than uncomplicated tumors.[22]

Recurrent infections, such as fungal pneumonias, can occasionally have a prominent component of foam cells and cholesterol crystals especially in the background of myelomonocytic leukemia.[23]

Radiologic Findings

Endogenous lipoid pneumonia typically manifests as areas of consolidation distal to a centrally occluded airway. Unlike exogenous lipid pneumonia, opacities with low attenuation characteristic of lipid are not frequently present.[24] Radiographically, it may be difficult to distinguish postobstructive changes from malignancy, especially in recurrent and treated carcinomas. Magnetic resonance imaging is able to differentiate tumor from pneumonia, using heavily weighted T2 imaging.[25]

Gross Findings

Lipid pneumonia is also called "cholesterol pneumonia" or "golden pneumonia." Grossly, the consolidated parenchymal has a yellowish coloration due to the accumulation of lipid in the alveolar spaces.[18]

Microscopic Findings

Histologically, there are intra-alveolar lipid-filled macrophages and occasionally eosinophilic proteinaceous material derived from degenerating cells (Fig. 25.9). The macrophages contain a foamy, finely vacuolated cytoplasm. Cholesterol clefts indicating the presence of free cholesterol crystals are frequently present. Organizing pneumonia and bronchiolectasis, other features of obstruction, are commonly seen (Fig. 25.9).

Endogenous lipoid pneumonia is typical of obstructive pneumonia. However, there are other histologic findings often seen in tumor resections distal to the obstruction. These include organizing pneumonia, bronchiectasis, bronchiolectasis, mucous plugging with mucus extravasation, lymphatic dilatation, abscess formation, and atelectasis.

Differential Diagnosis

The differential diagnosis of endogenous lipoid pneumonia includes exogenous lipid pneumonia. Exposure to certain medications can lead to the airspace accumulation of foamy macrophages such as with amiodarone. In contrast to endogenous lipid pneumonia, with exposure to amiodarone, the pneumocytes lining the alveolar septa will also contain foamy cytoplasm (Fig. 25.10). Histologically, genetic disorders of surfactant metabolism will often display foamy histiocytes; however, other findings such as proteinaceous exudate, interstitial inflammation, and fibrosis may also be seen. Some systemic metabolic and storage diseases may involve the lung, particularly Niemann-Pick disease (Fig. 25.11), glycogen storage disease, and mucopolysaccharidoses. In these diseases, the presence of foamy alveolar macrophages is common. However, in contrast to endogenous lipoid pneumonia, the foamy macrophages will also be found within the alveolar and interlobular septa and pleura.[26]

Exogenous Lipid Pneumonia

General

Exogenous lipid pneumonia is the result of the inhalation of animal fats or mineral or vegetable oils. It was initially described almost a century ago in four patients with a prolonged history of laxative ingestion.[27] Historically, the prevalence of exogenous pneumonia was due to the practice of self-treatment of mineral oil over a long period by adults and the dropping of oil into the nose of sick, recumbent children. Aspiration of fats or oils may occur with chronic use of petroleum-based lubricants and decongestants, lip gloss, and occupational inhalational exposure

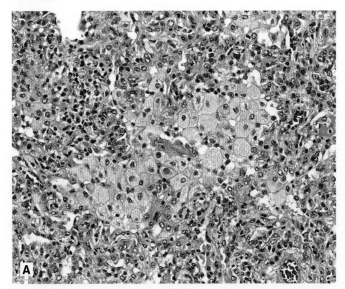

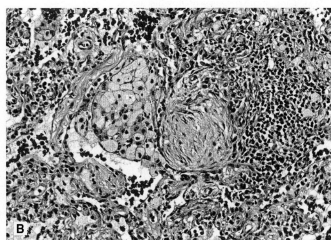

FIGURE 25.9 ▲ Endogenous lipid pneumonia. **A.** There are foam cells mixed with chronic inflammation, an incidental finding in a resection specimen for endoluminal tumor. **B.** Other features of obstruction such as organizing pneumonia were also seen.

vegetable oils, paints, and pesticides.[28,29] In parts of the Middle East and Africa, force-feeding of infants with dairy products high in lipid results in exogenous lipid pneumonia.[30,31] There is a clinical overlap with recurrent aspiration, as patients with neurologic deficits, children and adults with chronic reflux, and children with cleft palate are at risk for exogenous lipoid pneumonia, similar to aspiration and aspiration pneumonia[28,29,32]

Clinical

Aspiration of lipids may result in acute lung injury, if large amounts are inhaled, but more commonly causes subacute lung injury and chronic lung changes. Acute exogenous lipid pneumonia manifests clinically as cough, dyspnea, and low-grade fever that usually resolve with supportive therapy.[28] In contrast, patients with chronic exogenous lipid pneumonia are afebrile, and asymptomatic in half of cases, and are identified because of an incidentally detected abnormality on radiologic imaging. The other half of patients with chronic lipid pneumonia have low-grade pulmonary symptoms with a duration of months to years.[28]

Most patients with exogenous lipid pneumonia are in the sixth to seventh decade of life; have an anatomic or neurologic deficits predisposing to aspiration, such as alcohol abuse, cerebral infarction, recent surgery, esophageal cancer, tracheotomy, drug use, or encephalopathy[28]; and have a history of topical application or ingestion of lipids. Fewer than half of patients have an elevated white blood cell count. The history of aspiration is often elicited after initial evaluation and lung biopsy.

Radiologic Findings

Computed tomographic findings of exogenous lipid pneumonia include ground glass and consolidative opacities in one or more lung segments, typically in a peribronchovascular distribution in the lower lobes. There is often thickening of interlobular septa.[24,28] The combination of septal thickening and ground glass has been referred to as "crazy-paving" pattern.[24] The most characteristic CT finding is the presence of negative (fat) attenuation values within areas of consolidation.[33]

Tissue Sampling

The diagnosis can be suggested on transbronchial biopsies (Fig. 25.12). Most often, open or thoracoscopic wedge biopsy is required for

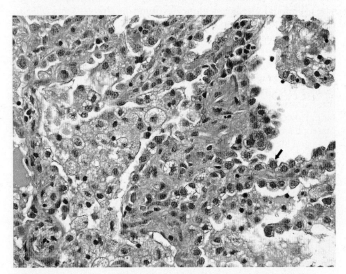

FIGURE 25.10 ▲ Lung biopsy from patient on amiodarone. The alveolar spaces contain vacuolated macrophages. Note that many of the pneumocytes lining the alveolar septa also have a vacuolated cytoplasm.

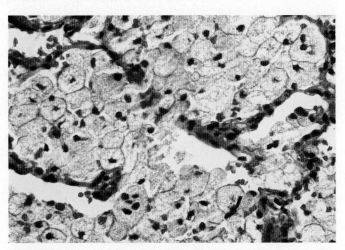

FIGURE 25.11 ▲ Patient diagnosed with Niemann-Pick disease. The alveolar spaces were filled with foamy macrophages. These macrophages could also be found in the interstitium.

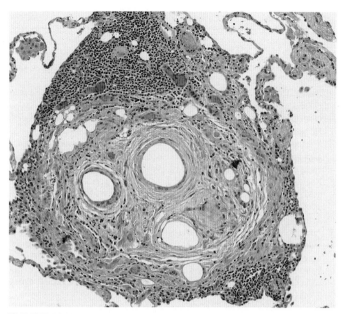

FIGURE 25.12 ▲ Transbronchial biopsy showing the histologic features of exogenous lipid pneumonia.

definitive diagnosis.[28] The predominance of foamy macrophages in bronchoalveolar lavage specimens is supportive of the diagnosis.

Microscopic Findings

In the subacute phase, there is a predominance of foamy macrophages filling the alveolar spaces, which are often destroyed (Fig. 25.13). The vacuoles of these foamy macrophages are typically larger than those of endogenous lipid pneumonia. In the chronic phase, there is the formation of lipogranulomas, peribronchiolar fibrosis, progressive destruction of alveolar architecture, and septal scarring. The lipogranulomas are characterized by large vacuoles surrounded by foreign body giant cells (Fig. 25.13). There may be other changes of aspiration, such as organizing pneumonia and bronchiectasis.[34] The differential diagnosis includes artifactual vacuoles and spaces caused by biopsy artifact (Fig. 25.14).

Prognosis and Treatment

When diagnosed in the acute phase, most patients improve after control of aspiration. However, patients with long-term symptoms rarely get better.[28] There is little consensus on treatment other than avoiding the offending agent. In cases of diffuse pulmonary damage, whole-lung lavage, systemic corticosteroids, and thoracoscopy with surgical debridement have been attempted with various successes.[24]

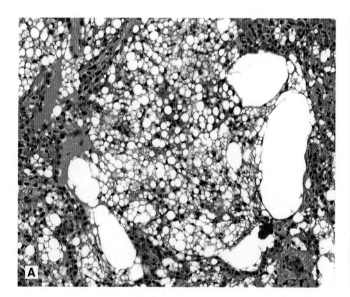

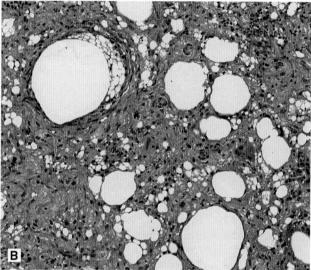

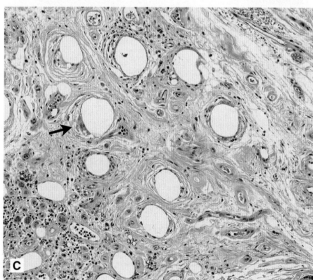

FIGURE 25.13 ▲ Exogenous lipid pneumonia. **A.** The airspace is distended by numerous alveolar macrophages filled with lipid vacuoles. Although some of the vacuoles are smaller as seen in endogenous lipid pneumonia, most are larger and typical of exogenous lipid pneumonia. **B.** With chronic aspiration, the background becomes more chronically inflamed and fibrosis. **C.** The lipid vacuoles are surrounded by foreign body multinucleated giant cells (*arrow*).

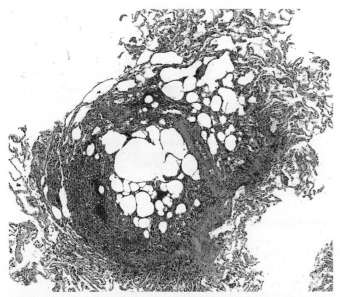

FIGURE 25.14 ▲ Biopsy artifact. Artifact may result in holes resembling lipid vacuoles. There are no macrophage giant cells lining the holes, which are not discrete and round like lipid droplets.

Practical Points

▶ Sometimes incorrectly termed "lentil granulomas," one of the more common histologic signs of aspiration of food is a foreign body reaction to microscopic starch grains, which occur in lentils and other legumes.

▶ Kayexalate is recognizable as rhomboid-shaped dark blue or purpose crystals with internal stripes akin to Venetian blinds.

▶ Talc is a hydrated magnesium silicate that is used in industry, is found in baby powder and detergent, and occurs as an adulterant in illegal drugs, especially heroin. It may occur in the lungs both in airways and in vessels and cause a granulomatous reaction.

▶ Common pitfalls in aspirated material include endogenous inclusions in granulomas, including crystals that polarize (calcium oxalate and carbonate) and those that do not (Schaumann bodies).

REFERENCES

1. Ravelli AM, Panarotto MB, Verdoni L, et al. Pulmonary aspiration shown by scintigraphy in gastroesophageal reflux-related respiratory disease. *Chest.* 2006;130(5):1520–1526.
2. Sweet MP, Patti MG, Hoopes C, et al. Gastro-oesophageal reflux and aspiration in patients with advanced lung disease. *Thorax.* 2009;64(2):167–173.
3. Beal M, Chesson A, Garcia T, et al. A pilot study of quantitative aspiration in patients with symptoms of obstructive sleep apnea: comparison to a historic control group. *Laryngoscope.* 2004;114(6):965–968.
4. Huxley EJ, Viroslav J, Gray WR, et al. Pharyngeal aspiration in normal adults and patients with depressed consciousness. *Am J Med.* 1978;64(4):564–568.
5. Mukhopadhyay S, Katzenstein AL. Pulmonary disease due to aspiration of food and other particulate matter: a clinicopathologic study of 59 cases diagnosed on biopsy or resection specimens. *Am J Surg Pathol.* 2007;31(5):752–759.
6. Ahrens P, Noll C, Kitz R, et al. Lipid-laden alveolar macrophages (LLAM): a useful marker of silent aspiration in children. *Pediatr Pulmonol.* 1999;28(2):83–88.
7. Knauer-Fischer S, Ratjen F. Lipid-laden macrophages in bronchoalveolar lavage fluid as a marker for pulmonary aspiration. *Pediatr Pulmonol.* 1999;27(6):419–422.
8. Adams R, Ruffin R, Campbell D. The value of the lipid-laden macrophage index in the assessment of aspiration pneumonia. *Aust N Z J Med.* 1997;27(5):550–553.
9. Barnes TW, Vassallo R, Tazelaar HD, et al. Diffuse bronchiolar disease due to chronic occult aspiration. *Mayo Clin Proc.* 2006;81(2):172–176.
10. Gonzalez-Cuyar LF, Cresswell NB, Burke AP. Sodium polystyrene sulfonate (Kayexalate) aspiration. *Diagn Pathol.* 2008;3:27.
11. Yousem SA, Faber C. Histopathology of aspiration pneumonia not associated with food or other particulate matter: a clinicopathologic study of 10 cases diagnosed on biopsy. *Am J Surg Pathol.* 2011;35(3):426–431.
12. Raghu G, Freudenberger TD, Yang S, et al. High prevalence of abnormal acid gastro-oesophageal reflux in idiopathic pulmonary fibrosis. *Eur Respir J.* 2006;27(1):136–142.
13. Salvioli B, Belmonte G, Stanghellini, V, et al. Gastro-oesophageal reflux and interstitial lung disease. *Dig Liver Dis.* 2006;38(12):879–884.
14. Hadjiliadis D, Duane Davis R, Steele MP, et al. Gastroesophageal reflux disease in lung transplant recipients. *Clin Transplant.* 2003;17(4):363–368.
15. Palmer SM, Miralles AP, Howell DN, et al. Gastroesophageal reflux as a reversible cause of allograft dysfunction after lung transplantation. *Chest.* 2000;118(4):1214–1217.
16. Abbassi-Ghadi N, Kumar S, Cheung B, et al. Anti-reflux surgery for lung transplant recipients in the presence of impedance-detected duodenogastroesophageal reflux and bronchiolitis obliterans syndrome: a study of efficacy and safety. *J Heart Lung Transplant.* 2013;32(6):588–595.
17. Weir KA, McMahon S, Taylor S, et al. Oropharyngeal aspiration and silent aspiration in children. *Chest.* 2011;140(3):589–597.
18. de Benedictis, FM, Carnielli VP, de Benedictis D. Aspiration lung disease. *Pediatr Clin North Am.* 2009;56(1):173–190, xi.
19. Sharma A, Ohri S, Bambery P, et al. Idiopathic endogenous lipoid pneumonia. *Indian J Chest Dis Allied Sci.* 2006;48(2):143–145.
20. Lococo F, Cesario A, Porziella V, et al. Idiopathic lipoid pneumonia successfully treated with prednisolone. *Heart Lung.* 2012;41(2):184–187.
21. Fishman JE, Schwartz DS, Sais GJ, et al. Bronchogenic carcinoma in HIV-positive patients: findings on chest radiographs and CT scans. *AJR Am J Roentgenol.* 1995;164(1):57–61.
22. Haraguchi S, Koizumi K, Tanimura S, et al. Surgical results of lung cancer associated with postobstructive pneumonia. *Ann Thorac Cardiovasc Surg.* 2009;15(5):297–303.
23. Itoh Y, Segawa H, Kito K, et al. Lipoid pneumonia with chronic myelomonocytic leukemia. *Pathol Res Pract.* 2009;205(2):143–147.
24. Betancourt SL, Martinez-Jimenez S, Rossi SE, et al. Lipoid pneumonia: spectrum of clinical and radiologic manifestations. *AJR Am J Roentgenol.* 2010;194(1):103–109.
25. Bourgouin PM, McLoud TC, Fitzgibbon JF, et al. Differentiation of bronchogenic carcinoma from postobstructive pneumonitis by magnetic resonance imaging: histopathologic correlation. *J Thorac Imaging.* 1991;6(2):22–27.
26. Dishop MK. Diagnostic pathology of diffuse lung disease in children. *Pediatr Allergy Immunol Pulmonol.* 2010;23(1):69–85.
27. Laughlen GF. Studies on pneumonia following naso-pharyngeal injections of oil. *Am J Pathol.* 1925;1(4):407–414, 1.
28. Baron SE, Haramati LB, Rivera VT. Radiological and clinical findings in acute and chronic exogenous lipoid pneumonia. *J Thorac Imaging.* 2003;18(4):217–224.
29. Baron HC, Shafiroff BG. Acute lipoid pneumonitis due to aspiration of pressurized paint droplets. *Dis Chest.* 1959;36:434–437.
30. Dossing M, Khan JH. Nasal or oral oil application on infants: a possible risk factor for adult bronchiectasis. *Eur J Epidemiol.* 1995;11(2):141–144.
31. Al-Malki TA. Lung resections in bronchiectasis due to lipoid pneumonia: a custom-design approach. *East Afr Med J.* 2000;77(4):203–205.
32. Kurlandsky LE, Vaandrager V, Davy CL, et al. Lipoid pneumonia in association with gastroesophageal reflux. *Pediatr Pulmonol.* 1992;13(3):184–188.
33. Marchiori E, Zanetti G, Mano CM, et al. Exogenous lipoid pneumonia. Clinical and radiological manifestations. *Respir Med.* 2011;105(5):659–666.
34. Papla B, Urbańczyk K, Gil T, et al. Exogenous lipoid pneumonia (oil granulomas of the lung). *Pol J Pathol.* 2011;62(4):269–273.

26 Eosinophilic Pneumonia and Related Conditions

Allen P. Burke, M.D.

Eosinophilic Lung Disease

Terminology

Eosinophilic lung disease forms a rare spectrum of idiopathic and secondary conditions that may be acute or chronic processes. Eosinophilic pneumonia is the most common form. Clinically, eosinophilic lung diseases are classified by etiology, the largest group being idiopathic. Idiopathic eosinophilic lung diseases are divided into simple pulmonary eosinophilia (which has no real pathologic counterpart), acute eosinophilic pneumonia, chronic eosinophilic pneumonia, and idiopathic hypereosinophilic syndrome. Eosinophilic lung diseases of known cause include drug-related eosinophilic pneumonias (with no histologic differences from the idiopathic group), a group of infectious processes (allergic bronchopulmonary aspergillosis/fungal disease, bronchocentric granulomatosis, parasitic infections), and vasculitis (allergic angiitis and granulomatosis, or Churg-Strauss syndrome). The latter group of diseases is discussed in other chapters in this book. Table 26.1 outlines the clinical classification of eosinophilic lung disease.

In cases of pathologically documented eosinophilic lung disease, the most common is idiopathic chronic eosinophilic pneumonia, followed by drug-induced eosinophilic pneumonia and acute eosinophilic pneumonia. The largest relatively recent series of histologically documented eosinophilic pneumonia described five acute and six chronic cases, and a distinction between idiopathic and drug-induced disease was not made.[1]

Eosinophilic infiltrates in the bronchioles and bronchi may also result in respiratory symptoms and are generally considered separately from eosinophilic pneumonia as eosinophilic bronchitis or bronchiolitis. It has recently been demonstrated that eosinophilic pneumonia and bronchitis may coexist, however.[2]

Simple Pulmonary Eosinophilia

Simple pulmonary eosinophilia is sometimes called "Löffler syndrome," although in the initial reports Löffler himself included parasitic infection.[3] Because simple pulmonary eosinophilia is rarely biopsied, the pathologic features are not well characterized, but are typically described as interstitial eosinophils and pulmonary edema.[4] Patients are by definition asymptomatic and are found incidentally to have migrating lung opacities that are nonsegmental, peripheral, and with ill-defined margins and that spontaneously clear within 1 month. The diagnosis rests on the finding of peripheral eosinophilia in conjunction with lack of symptoms, imaging findings, and absence of other conditions, including infections and parasitic disease. Some patients eventually developed symptoms leading to a specific diagnosis, such as parasitic lung disease, drug-induced lung disease, or allergic bronchopulmonary lung disease.[5]

Etiology

As noted above, eosinophils may accumulate in the lung due to infectious, allergic reactions, or toxic insults or be a response to unknown stimuli. The list of exposures and conditions associated with pulmonary eosinophilia is long (Table 26.2).[6]

The mechanism by which eosinophils cause tissue damage involves the Charcot-Leyden crystal protein, an eosinophil lysophospholipase encoded by the CLC gene, in addition to eosinophil cationic protein, a ribonuclease that possesses neurotoxic, helminthotoxic, and ribonucleolytic properties.[4,9]

Acute Eosinophilic Pneumonia

Clinical Features

The incidence of eosinophilic pneumonia is unknown, because the diagnosis is not often pathologically documented. It is considered rare, as most series contain only a few cases.[1,10] The original description of Allen et al. entailed a total of four patients.[11] Series of over six patients

TABLE 26.1 Classification of Eosinophilic Lung Diseases

Eosinophilic lung diseases of unknown cause
Simple pulmonary eosinophilia (Löffler syndrome)
Acute eosinophilic pneumonia (idiopathic)
Chronic eosinophilic pneumonia (idiopathic)
Idiopathic hypereosinophilic syndrome

Eosinophilic lung diseases of known cause
Drug reactions (usually eosinophilic pneumonia, acute or chronic)
Allergic bronchopulmonary fungal disease
Bronchocentric granulomatosis
Parasitic infections

Eosinophilic vasculitis (Churg-Strauss syndrome)

TABLE 26.2 Causes of Eosinophilic Pneumonia

Inhalational	Other exposures
Scotchgard	Cigarettes smoke
Methylchloroform	Red spider allergens
Stainless steel dust containing 0.1% nickel	Radiographic contrast
Dust	L-tryptophan (eosinophilia–myalgia syndrome)
Fireworks	

Drugs	Infectious
acetaminophen	*Parasitic infections*
aspirin	*Toxocara canis*
bleomycin	*Filariasis*
carbamazepine	*Ascaris lumbricoides*
chlorpromazine	*Paragonimus westermani*
chlorpropamide	*Fungal infections*
cromolyn sodium	*Aspergillus species*
dantrolene	*Trichosporon terrestre*
daptomycin	*Trichosporon cutaneum*
gold	*Trichoderma viride*
hydralazine	*Viral/chlamydial infections*
loxoprofen	HIV
methotrexate	Coxsackie A2 virus
minocycline	Chlamydia ("pertussoid" eosinophilic pneumonia)
naproxen	
nitrofurantoin	*Bacterial infections*
penicillin	*Mycobacterium tuberculosis*
pentamidine	*Pseudomonas maltophilia*
quinidine	
salazopyrin	**Immunologic diseases**
sulfadoxine	Rheumatoid diseases
sulfasalazine	Sarcoidosis
tamoxifen	
tolfenamic acid	

From references 4, 6, 7, 8.

TABLE 26.3 Criteria for the Clinical Diagnosis of Eosinophilic Pneumonia

Major criteria
Symptoms (cough, fever, dyspnea)
Peripheral infiltrates (patchy, nodular, nonsegmental, shifting, recurrent)
Transbronchial or wedge biopsy showing interstitial or alveolar eosinophils[a]

Minor criteria
Peripheral eosinophilia (>0.4 × 10^9/L)
Eosinophilia in BAL (usually > 25%)[a]
Steroid responsiveness

Nonexcluding criteria
Presence of allergic symptoms, atopy, or asthma
Drug or medication history

Excluding criteria
ABPA, bronchocentric granulomatosis, sarcoidosis, Hodgkin lymphoma, hypereosinophilic syndrome, parasitic infections, bacterial infections, fungal infections

The criteria for chronic eosinophilic pneumonia is duration more than 1–2 months, or recurrence. Otherwise the disease is considered acute. ABPA, allergic bronchopulmonary aspergillosis.
[a]Many or most publications currently accept BAL eosinophilia in the absence of biopsy findings.
Adapted from Matsuda Y, Tachibana K, Sasaki Y, et al. Tracheobronchial lesions in eosinophilic pneumonia. *Respir Investig.* 2014;52(1):21–27.

are based on clinical, imaging, and bronchoalveolar lavage (BAL) findings alone with histologic documentation.[2,12]

Most patients are adults, with a wide range from the third to the eighth decades, with a mean age about 30 years.[1,12] There is no apparent gender predilection.[12] Over one-half of patients are current or recent smokers.[12] A series of three children with acute eosinophilic pneumonia has been reported.[10]

Acute eosinophilic pneumonia is a febrile illness characterized by diffuse pulmonary infiltrates and eosinophilia in BAL fluid (usually > 25% eosinophils).[6] The clinical diagnostic criteria are outlined in Table 26.3. The duration of illness is generally <1 month (classically < 1 week), with severe hypoxemia (usually < 60 mm Hg on room air). Infectious processes exclude the diagnosis of eosinophilic pneumonia.[11,12] The mean white count is 22 × 10^9/L with a mean eosinophil count of 5%.[12] Respiratory failure may progress to ventilatory dependence.[6] There is typically spontaneous improvement especially to treatment with steroids, without relapses. By definition, if relapses occur, a diagnosis of chronic eosinophilic pneumonia is made.

In contrast to other forms of eosinophilic lung disease, peripheral eosinophil counts are normal in about 50% of patients.[1,4,10] A peripheral eosinophil count over 10 × 10^9/L (10,000/μL) has been reported in a patient with fulminant eosinophilic pneumonia.[6]

A history of medication use is common; four of five patients in the series of Umeki et al. were on antibiotics.[1] A causative association between medication use and eosinophilic lung injury can only be presumed if there is a positive in vitro drug-stimulated lymphocyte transformation test,[13] or if there is a positive drug challenge after resolution of symptoms.[1] The term "idiopathic" is generally not applied to cases of eosinophilic pneumonia if there is a suspicion of drug reaction.[12]

A few patients with acute eosinophilic pneumonia have inhalational exposures, such as tear gas, marijuana, and dust.[1,10] Four of 22 patients in one series[12] had recent inhalational exposures, to home renovation, tear gas, and gasoline fumes. There may be a slight increase in incidence in the summer and fall.[12]

In contrast to chronic eosinophilic pneumonia, a history of asthma is generally absent, indicating chronic eosinophilic lung disease by definition.[5] In 2 of 22 patients with acute eosinophilic pneumonia fulfilling diagnostic criteria, there was a history of atopy without asthma.[12]

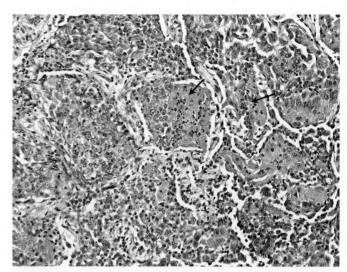

FIGURE 26.1 ▲ Acute eosinophilic pneumonia. There is acute pneumonitis with numerous interstitial and intra-alveolar eosinophils (*arrows*).

Radiologic Findings

Radiologically, acute eosinophilic pneumonia mimics hydrostatic pulmonary edema. On chest radiograph, there are bilateral reticular densities, with or without patchy consolidation, and pleural effusions. On CT scans, there are bilateral patchy areas of ground-glass opacity, sometimes accompanied by interlobular septal thickening, consolidation, and poorly defined nodules.[4]

Microscopic Findings

As with simple pulmonary eosinophilia, a pathologic diagnosis is often not made, because of the short course of duration and response to steroids. The diagnosis typically rests on clinical and BAL findings.[6] It has been suggested recently that biopsy is unnecessary for the diagnosis.[12] In cases of biopsy-proven acute eosinophilic pneumonia, the histologic findings are those of acute pneumonitis with intra-alveolar fibrin and acute lung injury (Figs. 26.1 to 26.3); eosinophils are found in the interstitium and alveolar spaces.[1] There may be associated acute alveolar injury with hyaline membranes, in cases of severe lung injury.

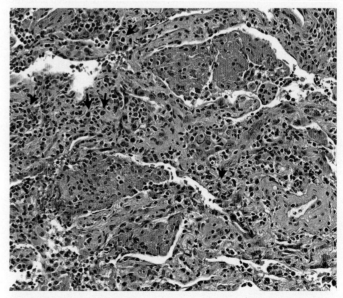

FIGURE 26.2 ▲ Acute eosinophilic pneumonia. There are marked reactive changes to alveolar pneumocytes. There are scattered intra-alveolar eosinophils (*arrows*).

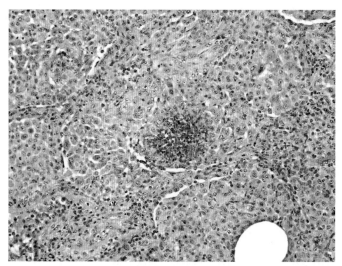

FIGURE 26.3 ▲ Acute eosinophilic pneumonia, with abundant macrophages. There may be marked accumulation of macrophages in the alveolar spaces, which are generally nonpigmented. There are numerous eosinophils with an abscess-like aggregate in the center.

The findings on BAL include increased eosinophils (mean 42 to 51).[11,12] The other cellular components include macrophages, neutrophils, and lymphocytes, in descending order.[12]

Differential Diagnosis

Clinically, the differential diagnosis includes acute lung injury due to diffuse alveolar damage in the absence of eosinophilic damage (e.g., acute respiratory distress syndrome or acute interstitial pneumonia).[12] Some patients may demonstrate an acute eosinophilic pneumonia in response to *Paragonimus westermani* infection[7] or to amiodarone toxicity.[14] In cases of transbronchial biopsies, any numbers of eosinophils in the alveolar walls or alveolar space, without or without associated fibrin and acute lung injury, is supportive of the diagnosis. An acute infection, either bacterial or especially parasitic, may be accompanied by an eosinophilic reaction and should be in the differential diagnosis. There is often a prominent macrophages response in the alveoli, but pigment characteristic of desquamative interstitial pneumonia or respiratory bronchiolitis is absent.

The differential diagnosis of eosinophilia in BAL fluid includes interstitial pneumonias and HIV-associated pneumonia, in addition to eosinophilic lung diseases. Normal bronchoalveolar fluid contains around 90% alveolar macrophages, 10% lymphocytes, and only occasional neutrophils or eosinophils. Any eosinophil count over 5% to 10% is considered abnormal.[6] In cases of eosinophilic pneumonia, the eosinophil count is invariably over < 15% with a mean of 55%.[1,12] Eosinophilic in lavage fluid is uncommon in adult respiratory distress syndrome (a common clinical differential diagnosis), lung cancer, or community-acquired pneumonia or in immunocompromised persons without AIDS.[6]

Treatment and Prognosis

The prognosis of acute eosinophilic pneumonia is excellent, with 25% of patients recovering spontaneously and the remainder responding to steroids.[12] Supportive care including intubation with mechanical ventilation may be necessary in some patients.[6] Antibiotics are frequently given empirically initially prior to a definitive diagnosis.

Chronic Eosinophilic Pneumonia

Clinical Features

Chronic eosinophilic pneumonia is a slowly progressing disease characterized by pulmonary symptoms of several months duration.[15] The subacute presentation is frequently marked by constitutional symptoms and treatment for presumed bronchopneumonia. Most patients are adults, with a slight female predominance in some, but not all, series.[15–17] Almost 50% of patients have a history of atopy, especially asthma.[15] Pulmonary function tests usually show restrictive defects. Peripheral blood eosinophilia is usually elevated and is variable. Acute phase reactants are typically elevated in the serum and blood, and there may be an increase in serum IgE levels.[4] The most characteristic diagnostic finding is the presence of markedly elevated eosinophils in the BAL, typically over 25%, with a range of 14% to 75%.[1,10,18]

Approximately 50% of patients are smokers, and pulmonary symptoms include shortness of breath and cough in all. There may be a history of drug exposure, including antibiotics.[1] There has been a single series of chronic eosinophilic pneumonia in five children, aged 5 to 14 years.[10] All had markedly elevated peripheral eosinophil counts, and three had a history of asthma.

About one in 20 patients with chronic eosinophilic pneumonia have tracheobronchial nodules, which histologically demonstrate eosinophilic infiltrates.[2]

Radiologic Findings

The classic CT finding of chronic eosinophilic pneumonia is nonsegmental peripheral airspace consolidation that was initially termed "photographic negative shadow of pulmonary edema."[19] This finding was subsequently found in fewer than one-third of patients, however, if defined as opacification limited to the outer third of the lung fields.[15] More frequently, there are areas of central consolidation in addition to peripheral airspace consolidation. Mediastinal adenopathy occurs in about one-half of patients.[16]

Histologic Findings

Histologically, chronic eosinophilic pneumonia shows organizing lung injury with eosinophils and forms a spectrum with acute eosinophilic pneumonia (Figs. 26.4 and 26.5). Although the spectrum of acute lung injury with hyaline membranes, interstitial eosinophilic inflammation with reactive pneumocytes, and organizing pneumonia with intra-alveolar and interstitial eosinophils outlines the evolution of eosinophilic lung injury, progression to fibrosis has not been documented, mirroring the clinical findings of resolution in most patients.

Similar with acute eosinophilic pneumonia, the diagnosis may be made entirely by clinical and cytologic findings. Open lung biopsy is more diagnostic than transbronchial biopsy, which may show only

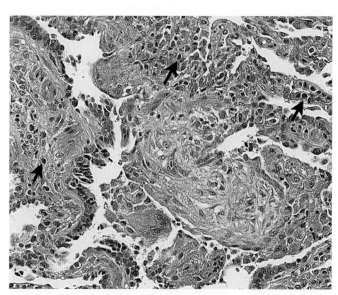

FIGURE 26.4 ▲ Organizing pneumonia, secondary to chronic eosinophilic pneumonia. There is organizing pneumonia near an airway (so-called bronchiolitis obliterans organizing pneumonia) in addition to intra-alveolar eosinophils (*arrows*).

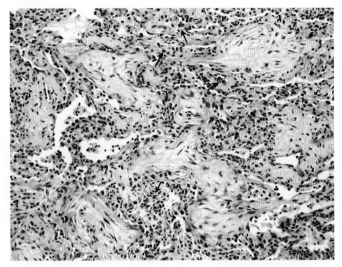

FIGURE 26.5 ▲ Eosinophilic pneumonia, transbronchial biopsy, related to daptomycin therapy. There is organizing pneumonia with scattered eosinophils (*arrows*).

scattered intra-alveolar eosinophils.[15] A biopsy is more likely to be performed if there is relatively minor peripheral eosinophilia or a borderline increase on lavage specimens.

Histologic examination typically shows accumulation of eosinophils and lymphocytes in the alveoli and interstitium, with an organizing pneumonia pattern. Eosinophilic abscesses and bronchiolitis obliterans occur less frequently.[15] The differential diagnosis includes amiodarone toxicity, which can result in both and acute and chronic form of eosinophilic pneumonia, as well as infections, especially parasitic.[14]

Treatment and Follow-up

With steroid treatment, most patients have an excellent long-term prognosis.[17] There are few follow-up radiologic studies, but clearing of consolidation is the rule without progression to fibrotic lung disease.[16,17] Relapses occur in up to 50% of patients but are equally as responsive to steroids as the initial illness.[17] In children, most patients develop chronic asthma, and half have abnormal CT scans, with interstitial opacities, cysts, or mild bronchiectasis.[10]

Hypereosinophilic Syndrome

Definition

Hypereosinophilic syndrome, in contrast to other eosinophilic lung diseases, denotes that presence of symptomatic eosinophilic infiltrates in multiple organs, resulting from eosinophilic-related tissue damage. The skin is most frequently involved, followed by the lung, gastrointestinal tract, and heart (see Chapter 164).[20] There is an overlap with Churg-Strauss syndrome (allergic granulomatosis with eosinophilia), which is defined by the presence of either large-vessel or small-vessel vasculitis, often with ANCA positivity. Churg-Strauss angiitis of the lung is discussed separately in Chapter 49.

Hypereosinophilic syndrome is classified as the myeloproliferative variant, lymphocytic variant, and idiopathic variant.[21] Pulmonary involvement has been described in all variations of the syndrome.[22,23]

Clinical Features

Idiopathic hypereosinophilic syndrome is rare, the incidence estimated at 0.036 per 100,000 persons per year.[20] It is characterized by prolonged peripheral idiopathic eosinophilia and organ dysfunction-related eosinophil-associated tissue damage. Classic diagnostic criteria include persistent eosinophilia of 1,500 cells per mm³ for more than 6 months, the absence of known causes of eosinophilia, and multiorgan system dysfunction.[24] Onset usually occurs in the third or fourth decade of life,

with a male female ratio of 7:1.[25] Pulmonary involvement occurs in up to 40% of patients, mostly from pulmonary edema or thromboembolic disease. The BAL fluid eosinophilia can be as high as 73%.[26]

At CT, idiopathic hypereosinophilic syndrome is characterized by single or multiple nodules with a surrounding ground-glass opacity halo.[4]

Histologic Findings

There are few histologic descriptions of pulmonary involvement in idiopathic hypereosinophilic syndrome. Pulmonary involvement is typically diagnosed by hypereosinophilia in BAL specimens.[26,27] Few available descriptions suggest that there are no differences from eosinophilic pneumonia, other than the presence of extrapulmonary involvement.[4,20,24]

REFERENCES

1. Umeki S. Reevaluation of eosinophilic pneumonia and its diagnostic criteria. *Arch Intern Med.* 1992;152(9):1913–1919.
2. Matsuda Y, Tachibana K, Sasaki Y, et al. Tracheobronchial lesions in eosinophilic pneumonia. *Respir Investig.* 2014;52(1):21–27.
3. Löffler W. Flüchtige Lungeninfiltrate mit Eosinophilie. *Klin Wochenschr.* 1935;14(9):297–299.
4. Jeong YJ, Kim KI, Seo IJ, et al. Eosinophilic lung diseases: a clinical, radiologic, and pathologic overview. *Radiographics.* 2007;27(3):617–637; discussion 637–639.
5. Allen JN, Davis WB. Eosinophilic lung diseases. *Am J Respir Crit Care Med.* 1994;150(5 pt 1):1423–1438.
6. Hogan TF, Riley RS, Thomas JG. Rapid diagnosis of acute eosinophilic pneumonia (AEP) in a patient with respiratory failure using bronchoalveolar lavage (BAL) with calcofluor white (CW) staining. *J Clin Lab Anal.* 1997;11(4):202–207.
7. Boland JM, Vaszar LT, Jones JL, et al. Pleuropulmonary infection by *Paragonimus westermani* in the United States: a rare cause of Eosinophilic pneumonia after ingestion of live crabs. *Am J Surg Pathol.* 2011;35(5):707–713.
8. Schaad UB, Rossi E. Infantile chlamydial pneumonia—a review based on 115 cases. *Eur J Pediatr.* 1982;138(2):105–109.
9. Akuthota P, Weller PF. Eosinophils and disease pathogenesis. *Semin Hematol.* 2012;49(2):113–119.
10. Giovannini-Chami L, Hadchouel A, Nathan N, et al. Idiopathic eosinophilic pneumonia in children: the French experience. *Orphanet J Rare Dis.* 2014;9(1):28.
11. Allen JN, Pacht ER, Gadek JE, et al. Acute eosinophilic pneumonia as a reversible cause of noninfectious respiratory failure. *N Engl J Med.* 1989;321(9):569–574.
12. Philit F, Etienne-Mastroïanni B, Parrot A, et al. Idiopathic acute eosinophilic pneumonia: a study of 22 patients. *Am J Respir Crit Care Med.* 2002;166(9):1235–1239.
13. Oishi Y, Sando Y, Tajima S, et al. Indomethacin induced bulky lymphadenopathy and eosinophilic pneumonia. *Respirology.* 2001;6(1):57–60.
14. Larsen BT, Vaszar LT, Colby TV, et al. Lymphoid hyperplasia and eosinophilic pneumonia as histologic manifestations of amiodarone-induced lung toxicity. *Am J Surg Pathol.* 2012;36(4):509–516.
15. Jederlinic PJ, Sicilian L, Gaensler EA. Chronic eosinophilic pneumonia. A report of 19 cases and a review of the literature. *Medicine (Baltimore).* 1988;67(3):154–162.
16. Mayo JR, Müller NL, Road J, et al. Chronic eosinophilic pneumonia: CT findings in six cases. *AJR Am J Roentgenol.* 1989;153(4):727–730.
17. Mochizuki Y, Kobashi Y, Nakahara Y, et al. Chronic eosinophilic pneumonia—a follow-up study of 12 cases. *Nihon Kokyuki Gakkai Zasshi.* 2002;40(11):851–855.
18. Carrington CB, Addington WW, Goff AM, et al. Chronic eosinophilic pneumonia. *N Engl J Med.* 1969;280(15):787–798.
19. Gaensler EA, Carrington CB. Peripheral opacities in chronic eosinophilic pneumonia: the photographic negative of pulmonary edema. *AJR Am J Roentgenol.* 1977;128(1):1–13.
20. Gotlib J. World Health Organization-defined eosinophilic disorders: 2012 update on diagnosis, risk stratification, and management. *Am J Hematol.* 2012;87(9):903–914.
21. d'Elbee JM, Parrens M, Mercié P, et al. Hypereosinophilic syndrome—lymphocytic variant transforming into peripheral T-cell lymphoma with severe oral manifestations. *Oral Surg Oral Med Oral Pathol Oral Radiol.* 2013;116(3):e185–e190.

22. Valent P, Horny HP, Bochner BS, et al. Controversies and open questions in the definitions and classification of the hypereosinophilic syndromes and eosinophilic leukemias. *Semin Hematol.* 2012;49(2):171–181.

23. Valent P, Klion AD, Horny HP, et al. Contemporary consensus proposal on criteria and classification of eosinophilic disorders and related syndromes. *J Allergy Clin Immunol.* 2012;130(3):607–612 e9.

24. Chusid MJ, Dale DC, West BC, et al. The hypereosinophilic syndrome: analysis of fourteen cases with review of the literature. *Medicine (Baltimore).* 1975;54(1):1–27.

25. Spry CJ, Davies J, Tai PC, et al. Clinical features of fifteen patients with the hypereosinophilic syndrome. *Q J Med.* 1983;52(205):1–22.

26. Slabbynck H, Impens N, Naegels S, et al. Idiopathic hypereosinophilic syndrome-related pulmonary involvement diagnosed by bronchoalveolar lavage. *Chest.* 1992;101(4):1178–1180.

27. Lim KS, Ko J, Lee SS, et al. A case of idiopathic hypereosinophilic syndrome presenting with acute respiratory distress syndrome. *Allergy Asthma Immunol Res.* 2014;6(1):98–101.

27 Pulmonary Amyloidosis

Marie-Christine Aubry, M.D., and Allen P. Burke, M.D.

Definition

Amyloidosis is a heterogeneous group of disorders that share one feature in common: deposition of amyloid, a protein in an abnormal beta-pleated form, within the interstitium of various organs.[1] Histologically, amyloid is an amorphous eosinophilic material by routine H&E stain and characteristically apple green when stained with Congo red (the current gold standard) under cross-polarized light. By ultrastructural studies, the fibrils are nonbranching, indefinite in length, and with a diameter varying between 7.5 and 10 nm. Although amyloid is histologically quite uniform, chemically it is heterogeneous with over 30 distinct proteins described and the basis of amyloid classification (Table 27.1). The most common proteins are AL, AA, and ATTR (transthyretin). They account for 90% of all amyloidosis.

AL represents complete immunoglobulin light chains, the terminal fragments or both, and most are λ light chains. This type of amyloid is found in primary systemic amyloidosis and complicates clonal B-cell dyscrasias, including up to 15% of multiple myeloma. It is also present in some forms of localized amyloidosis.

AA, amyloid-associated protein, is derived from a larger precursor protein, serum amyloid A, synthesized by the liver in inflammatory condition such as rheumatoid arthritis, IBD, tuberculosis, and osteomyelitis. AA amyloid can also be deposited in cases of malignant neoplasms such as renal cell carcinoma and Hodgkin lymphoma. Finally, it is also seen in some forms of hereditary amyloidosis.

ATTR, the amyloid form of transthyretin (or prealbumin), is a normal serum protein that can accumulate with age (wild-type amyloidosis) or owing to an underlying structural alteration in the protein that makes it more amylogenic than usual. Typing the amyloid is central to the treatment and prognosis of amyloidosis.[2]

Clinical Features

Pulmonary involvement by amyloid is rare, and with few exceptions, the amyloid is AL type.[3,4] The histologic manifestations of pulmonary amyloidosis include (1) diffuse alveolar septal amyloidosis, (2) nodular pulmonary amyloidosis, and (3) tracheobronchial amyloidosis.

Diffuse alveolar septal amyloidosis is usually systemic and present in patients with primary amyloidosis with or without associated plasma cell disorder and rarely with senile, secondary, or hereditary amyloidosis or in patients with renal failure on long-term hemodialysis.[3,5] Typically, lung involvement is an incidental finding as these patients rarely manifest

TABLE 27.1 Classification of Amyloidosis

Major Fibril Protein	Clinical Syndrome	Associated Diseases/Organ Involvement
AL (Ig light chains)	Primary systemic amyloidosis	Immunocyte dyscrasia (multiple myeloma, monoclonal gammopathy, occult dyscrasia)
AL (Ig light chains)	Local nodular amyloidosis	Lung, larynx, skin, bladder, tongue
AH (Ig heavy chain)	Primary systemic amyloidosis	Immunocyte dyscrasia (multiple myeloma, monoclonal gammopathy, occult dyscrasia)
AA	Reactive systemic amyloidosis	Chronic inflammatory diseases (rheumatoid arthritis, ankylosing spondylitis, IBD)
AA	Hereditary amyloidosis such as familial Mediterranean fever	Amyloid nephropathy
ATTR (normal)	Senile systemic amyloidosis	Predominantly cardiac involvement
ATTR (mutated)	Hereditary amyloidosis such as familial amyloid neuropathies, familial amyloidotic cardiomyopathy	Predominantly polyneuropathy and cardiac involvement
AFib (fibrinogen Aα)	Hereditary amyloidosis	Predominantly renal involvement
ALys (lysozyme)	Hereditary amyloidosis	Predominantly renal and GI involvement
AApoAI or II	Hereditary amyloidosis	Predominantly renal, liver, and cardiac involvement
Aβ$_2$m (β$_2$ microglobulin)	Hemodialysis-associated amyloidosis	Chronic renal failure with long-term dialysis
Aβ	Focal senile amyloidosis of the prostate Focal senile amyloidosis of the brain Nonfamilial Alzheimer disease Sporadic cerebral amyloid angiopathy	Brain only
AANF (atrial natriuretic factor)	Focal senile amyloidosis of the heart	Heart only
A Cal (calcitonin)	Localized to the thyroid	Medullary carcinoma
AIAPP (islet amyloid peptide)	Localized to the islet of Langerhans	Type II diabetes

pulmonary symptoms. However, in a small subset of patients, diffuse alveolar septal amyloidosis presents with no extrapulmonary involvement, thus representing a form of localized amyloidosis.[6] In this clinical context, patients present mainly with a clinical picture of interstitial lung disease. Therefore, these patients primarily complain of progressive shortness of breath and show restriction on pulmonary function tests. In rare cases, the amyloid deposition is predominantly vascular, and patients have clinical findings of pulmonary hypertension or diffuse alveolar hemorrhage.[7] If the amyloid extends to the pleural surface, the clinical picture is dominated by recurrent chronic pleural effusions.

Nodular pulmonary amyloidosis is the most common form of pulmonary amyloidosis, a localized process to the lung, historically referred to as benign amyloidoma.[3] Nodular pulmonary amyloidosis has been described in association with low-grade lymphomas, mainly marginal zone lymphomas of mucosa-associated lymphoid tissue (MALT).[8] A recent study suggests that nodular pulmonary amyloidosis is part of a spectrum of lymphoproliferative disorders.[9] Patients with nodular amyloidosis present in their sixth decade (range 48 to 80) and have no sex predilection. Some patients present with a history of autoimmune disease such as Sjögren syndrome or prior MALT lymphoma. The nodules are usually discovered incidentally and the clinical differential diagnosis of granulomatous or metastatic disease considered. In most patients, the process remains localized without evidence of a systemic process.[10]

Tracheobronchial amyloidosis is rare.[3] As the name implies, amyloid is confined to the tracheobronchial tree and may extend to the larynx. Patients are usually in their fifth to sixth decade (reported age range 35 to 85 years). The association of tracheobronchial amyloidosis with Sjögren syndrome has been reported.[11] Patients, when symptomatic, usually present with stridor, wheezing, hemoptysis, or recurrent pulmonary infections.

Radiologic Findings

In **diffuse alveolar septal amyloidosis**, radiologic exams show bilateral reticulonodular interstitial opacities, commonly predominant in the lower lung zones.[12] The presumptive clinical diagnosis is interstitial lung disease, and a lung biopsy is necessary for the diagnosis. Bilateral pleural effusions may dominate the radiologic picture. In patients with systemic disease such as Sjögren syndrome, the lung disease is often cystic[13] (Fig. 27.1).

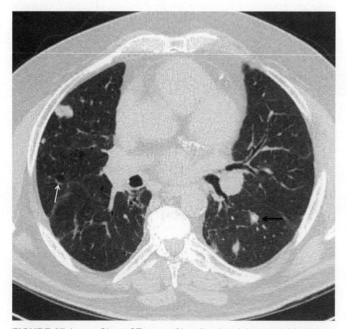

FIGURE 27.1 ▲ Chest CT scan of localized nodular amyloidosis in a patient with connective tissue disease. Multiple lung nodules, some partially calcified (*black arrow*), are identified along with a few thin-walled cysts (*white arrow*).

Nodular pulmonary amyloidosis is characterized by one or more well-circumscribed lobulated nodules, ranging in size from < 0.5 to 5 cm. These nodules may become calcified[12] (Fig. 27.1).

Tracheobronchial amyloidosis leads to airway thickening with luminal narrowing and associated postobstructive changes of atelectasis, pneumonia, or long-term bronchiectasis.[12]

Serum amyloid P (SAP) scintigraphy may be used to determine extent of amyloid involvement to differentiate between localized and systemic disease and monitor treatment response. As SAP is a protein component of all types of amyloid, it can be radiolabeled with iodine-123, injected, and will equilibrate with the existing deposits of amyloid in the body.[12]

FDG-PET scanning may show significant uptake in patients with pulmonary amyloidosis with or without associated hematologic malignancies.[14]

Tissue Sampling

The type of biopsy will depend on the clinical presentation. In patients with diffuse alveolar septal amyloidosis, the diagnosis of amyloidosis may be achieved by transbronchial biopsy.[15] If the clinical picture is predominated by pleural effusions, a pleural biopsy may be performed. Patients with nodular amyloidosis may undergo a transbronchial or transthoracic needle biopsy depending on the location and accessibility of the nodule. In some circumstances, a surgical biopsy may be the biopsy of choice. Lesions in tracheobronchial amyloidosis are directly visualized and biopsied by bronchoscopy.

Pathologic Findings

In **diffuse alveolar septal amyloidosis**, amyloid deposits thicken the alveolar septa and the wall of the vessels (Figs. 27.2 and 27.3). The deposits are usually diffuse but may be focal and mild and often easiest to appreciate within the vessel walls. Rarely, reactive lymphoid hyperplasia, such as follicular bronchiolitis or lymphocytic interstitial pneumonia, is present, often in association with an autoimmune disease such as Sjögren syndrome. Pleural involvement with associated pleural effusion may occur. The differential diagnosis on lung biopsy is with a fibrotic interstitial lung disease such as fibrotic nonspecific interstitial pneumonia (NSIP). Usually, fibrosis appears more fibrillary and not amorphous, and with NSIP, interstitial chronic inflammation is more prominent. The distinction between fibrosis and amyloid is made with histochemical stains such as Congo red (Fig. 27.2) or sulfated Alcian blue. In patients presenting with pulmonary hypertension, the amyloid extensively and predominantly involves vessels with severe luminal narrowing of the pulmonary vasculature.

The nodules of **nodular pulmonary amyloidosis** are composed of the typical amorphous eosinophilic material of amyloid (Fig. 27.4). Foreign body giant cells are frequently seen engulfing the amyloid. Amyloid may undergo calcification or bone metaplasia.

There are a variety of lymphoid proliferations that may accompany nodular amyloidosis. Small aggregates of plasma cells and lymphocytes are often present within the amyloid. There is frequently an infiltrate of plasma cells at the periphery that shows light chain restriction.[9] If the lymphoplasmacytic infiltrate is dense with lymphangitic spread and lymphocytes appear atypical, the diagnosis of a low-grade lymphoma needs to be considered (Fig. 27.5), or there may be adjacent nodular lymphoid hyperplasia.

The differential diagnosis of pulmonary nodular amyloidosis includes mainly light chain deposition disease and pulmonary hyalinizing granuloma. In light chain deposition disease, the morphologic findings are identical to those of nodular amyloidosis with the exception of a negative Congo red stain.[16] This should still prompt for additional ancillary study such as mass spectrometry to confirm the diagnosis. Pulmonary hyalinizing granuloma is characterized by thick ropy collagen bundles arranged in a lamellar configuration (Fig. 27.6). Ossification, calcification, or foreign body giant cells are absent.

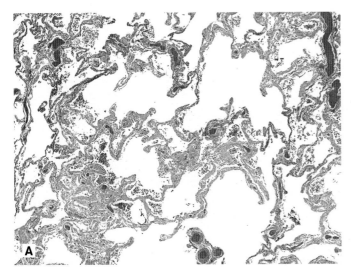

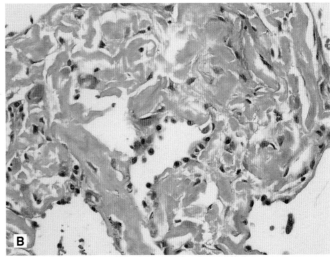

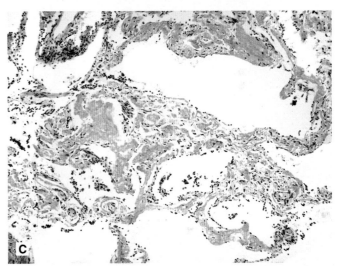

FIGURE 27.2 ▲ Septal amyloidosis. **A.** Diffuse alveolar septal amyloidosis causing mild septal thickening, mimicking a fibrosing interstitial pneumonia. **B.** A higher magnification shows the septa are thickening by an amorphous eosinophilic material without significant inflammatory cells. A giant cell reaction is absent and is uncommon in contrast to nodular amyloidosis. **C.** Amyloid is congophilic by regular light.

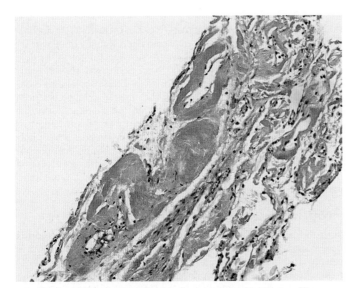

FIGURE 27.3 ▲ Septal amyloidosis, transbronchial biopsy. The diagnosis should be suspected if there are masses of interstitial acellular eosinophilic material, especially around vessels as in this case.

Although other fibrotic processes may ossify and calcify, foreign body giant cells will not be seen and prove to be a very useful diagnostic feature of amyloidosis.

In **tracheobronchial amyloidosis**, the amyloid deposition usually forms flat plaques or nodules within the large airways (Fig. 27.7). The plaques or nodules may be single or multiple, localized, or diffuse. In case of a single nodule, it may mimic carcinoma with airway obstruction. The amyloid is localized in and expands the submucosa of the bronchus (Fig. 27.8). It typically surrounds glands and cartilage. Foreign body giant cells as well as calcification and bone metaplasia are common findings.

Ancillary Studies

The gold standard for the diagnosis of amyloid is the Congo red stain, which stains the amyloid with a pink-red color and more specifically results in a green birefringence when viewed in cross-polarized light (Fig. 27.2).[1] The execution of this stain may be challenging and known to result in false-positive or false-negative results. The best outcome results from performing the stain on a 10-μm section. Other histochemical stains may be used such as sulfated Alcian blue, crystal or methyl violet, and thioflavin T, which stain either the amyloid itself or the amyloid matrix. Sulfated Alcian blue has the advantage of staining fibrosis in a rust color distinct from the green color of amyloid and useful in

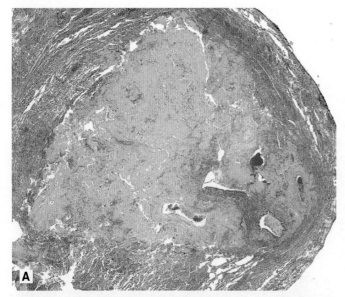

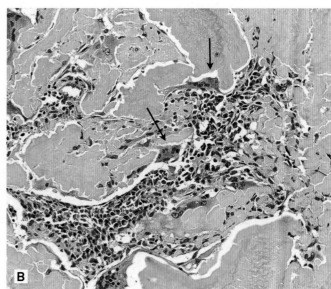

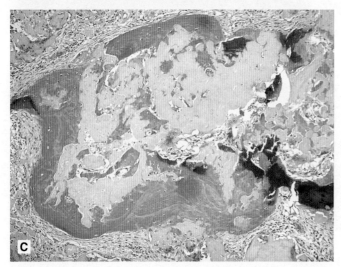

FIGURE 27.4 ▲ Nodular amyloidosis. **A.** There is an ill-defined nodule predominantly composed of amyloid. **B.** Multinucleated giant cells (*arrows*), many engulfing the amyloid, are commonly seen and a clue to the nature of the eosinophilic material. Indeed, this type of reaction is not seen with fibrosis. **C.** In nodular amyloidosis, the amyloid often displays osseous metaplasia and calcification.

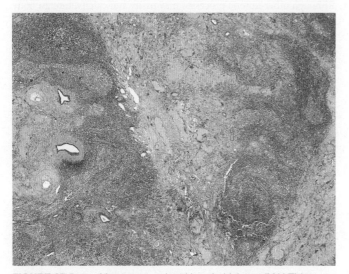

FIGURE 27.5 ▲ Mucosa-associated lymphoid tissue (MALT) lymphoma with amyloid deposition. Lymphoma needs to be considered in the diagnosis of nodular amyloidosis when the lymphoid or lymphoplasmacytic infiltrate is dense and prominent with a lymphangitic growth pattern.

the differential diagnosis with fibrosis (Fig. 27.5). Amyloid is metachromatic with the crystal or methyl violet and fluorescent by thioflavin T.

Currently, in the lung, a study using mass spectrometry (the gold standard for subtyping amyloid) has been performed systematically only in pulmonary nodular amyloidosis.[9] In diffuse septal amyloidosis and tracheobronchial amyloidosis, the amyloid subtype has been determined using other methods. Based on the combination of the findings in these studies, the amyloid in diffuse septal amyloidosis is most commonly AL and the light chain typically lambda. It has rarely been reported as ATTR, AA, or β2-microglobulin.[1] In nodular pulmonary amyloidosis, the amyloid is almost always AL, with rare exception of ATTR,[17] and in contrast to diffuse septal amyloidosis, it is predominantly kappa often with codeposition of heavy chains.[9]

Prognosis and Treatment

Since the majority of patients with **diffuse alveolar septal amyloidosis** have systemic disease in the setting of primary amyloidosis, death is usually attributed to cardiac amyloidosis and only rarely (about 10%) to lung involvement. Primary amyloidosis has a poor prognosis with median survival of ~16 months. In the rare cases of lung involvement by senile, hereditary, or secondary amyloidosis, the prognosis is significantly better, with median survival of 4 to 5 years. Amyloidosis leading to pulmonary hypertension has uniformly been fatal, usually as a result of right heart failure. Treatment is dependent on the

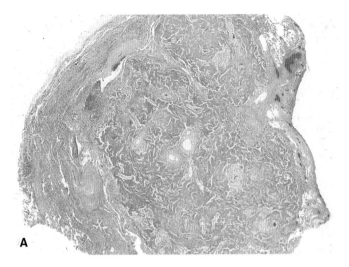

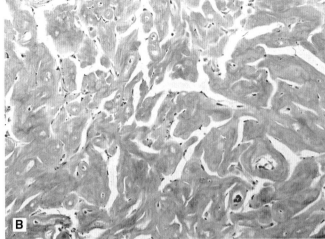

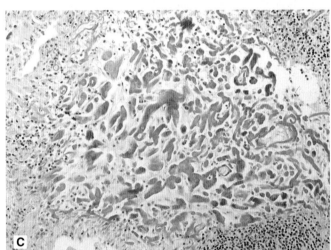

FIGURE 27.6 ▲ Hyalinizing granuloma. **A.** There is a well-defined nodule composed of thick, hyalinized, collagen bundles in a lamellar arrangement with an appearance similar to sclerosing mediastinitis. **B.** Note the absence of multinucleated giant cells. **C.** The sulfated Alcian blue stain is very helpful in the differential diagnosis with nodular amyloidosis as fibrosis appears rusty red in contrast to amyloid, which appears "sea foam" blue.

amyloid subtype and disease. Thus, patients with primary amyloidosis will be treated with chemotherapy and considered for stem cell transplantation, while patients with hereditary amyloidosis require liver transplantation.[1,2]

In **nodular pulmonary amyloidosis**, patients may experience recurrence of amyloid pulmonary nodules or MALT lymphoma in other sites. None developed systemic amyloidosis in the largest series to date.[9]

The course of **tracheobronchial amyloidosis** is not always benign, as deaths due to respiratory failure or pneumonia have been reported. Treatment is usually local management with bronchoscopic or surgical resection, or laser therapy if the patient is symptomatic.[11]

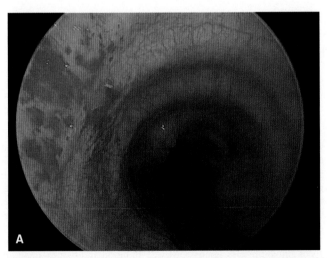

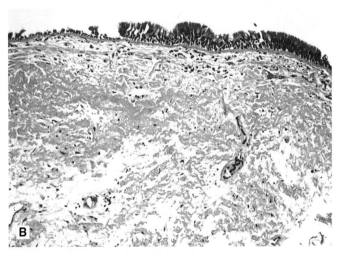

FIGURE 27.7 ▲ Tracheobronchial amyloidosis. **A.** Tracheobronchial amyloidosis forming submucosal nodules, apparent on bronchoscopy (photograph courtesy of Dr. F. Maldonado). **B.** By light microscopy, the submucosa is expanded by the amyloid.

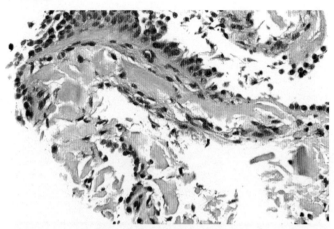

FIGURE 27.8 ▲ Tracheobronchial amyloidosis, endobronchial biopsy. There is amorphous pink material under the basement membrane. The diagnosis is often suggested by clinical findings and needs to be confirmed by Congo red staining (not shown).

Practical Points

▶ Pulmonary amyloidosis has several histologic presentations, diffuse septal, nodular, and tracheobronchial amyloidosis, associated with variable clinical syndromes with variable outcome and treatment.

▶ Morphologically, amyloid is an amorphous eosinophilic material that needs to be distinguished from fibrosis. The presence of giant cells and Congo red stain positivity support a diagnosis of amyloidosis.

▶ Amyloidosis may be associated with pulmonary lymphoid hyperplasia, such as nodular lymphoid hyperplasia and lymphocytic interstitial pneumonia, or lymphoma.

▶ Subtyping of amyloid is critical to the management of the patient. Mass spectrometry-based proteomic analysis is currently the optimal method.

REFERENCES

1. Buxbaum JN. The systemic amyloidoses. *Curr Opin Rheumatol.* 2004;16: 67–75.
2. Picken MM. Modern approaches to the treatment of amyloidosis: the critical importance of early detection in surgical pathology. *Adv Anat Pathol.* 2013;20:424–439.
3. Utz JP, Swensen SJ, Gertz MA. Pulmonary amyloidosis. The Mayo Clinic experience from 1980 to 1993. *Ann Intern Med.* 1996;124:407–413.
4. Gillmore JD, Hawkins PN. Amyloidosis and the respiratory tract. *Thorax.* 1999;54:444–451.
5. Ogoshi T, Kawanami T, Yatera K, et al. Dialysis-related amyloidosis with diffuse parenchymal lung involvement. *Intern Med.* 2012;51:3303–3304.
6. BoydKing A, Sharma O, Stevenson K. Localized interstitial pulmonary amyloid: a case report and review of the literature. *Curr Opin Pulm Med.* 2009;15:517–520.
7. Dingli D, Utz JP, Gertz MA. Pulmonary hypertension in patients with amyloidosis. *Chest.* 2001;120:1735–1738.
8. Lim JK, Lacy MQ, Kurtin PJ, et al. Pulmonary marginal zone lymphoma of MALT type as a cause of localised pulmonary amyloidosis. *J Clin Pathol.* 2001;54:642–646.
9. Grogg KL, Aubry MC, Vrana JA, et al. Nodular pulmonary amyloidosis is characterized by localized immunoglobulin deposition and is frequently associated with an indolent B-cell lymphoproliferative disorder. *Am J Surg Pathol.* 2013;37:406–412.
10. Xu L, Frazier A, Burke A. Isolated pulmonary amyloidomas: report of 3 cases with histologic and imaging findings. *Pathol Res Pract.* 2013;209: 62–66.
11. Inaty H, Folch E, Stephen C, et al. Tracheobronchial amyloidosis in a patient with Sjogren syndrome. *J Bronchol Interv Pulmonol.* 2013;20:261–265.
12. Aylwin AC, Gishen P, Copley SJ. Imaging appearance of thoracic amyloidosis. *J Thorac Imaging.* 2005;20:41–46.
13. Baqir M, Kluka EM, Aubry MC, et al. Amyloid-associated cystic lung disease in primary Sjogren's syndrome. *Respir Med.* 2013;107:616–621.
14. Baqir M, Lowe V, Yi ES, et al. 18F-FDG PET scanning in pulmonary amyloidosis. *J Nucl Med.* 2014;55:565–568.
15. Kline LR, Dise CA, Ferro TJ, et al. Diagnosis of pulmonary amyloidosis by transbronchial biopsy. *Am Rev Respir Dis.* 1985;132:191–194.
16. Khoor A, Myers JL, Tazelaar HD, et al. Amyloid-like pulmonary nodules, including localized light-chain deposition: clinicopathologic analysis of three cases. *Am J Clin Pathol.* 2004;121:200–204.
17. Roden AC, Aubry MC, Zhang K, et al. Nodular senile pulmonary amyloidosis: a unique case confirmed by immunohistochemistry, mass spectrometry, and genetic study. *Hum Pathol.* 2010;41:1040–1045.

28 Pulmonary Alveolar Proteinosis

Allen P. Burke, M.D., and Fabio R. Tavora, M.D., Ph.D.

Classification and Terminology

Rosen, Castleman, and Liebow described pulmonary alveolar proteinosis (PAP) more than 50 years ago.[1] Currently, there are three main forms of PAP: hereditary, secondary, and autoimmune, the last type by far the most frequent (Table 28.1).[2,3] Autoimmune PAP has previously been termed "idiopathic," "acquired," or the "adult type" of PAP.

Etiology

All three types of PAP have in common impaired clearance of surfactant by alveolar macrophages, which normally catabolize surfactant via the granulocyte–monocyte colony–stimulating factor (GM-CSF) receptor.[2]

Various mutations have been associated with congenital PAP, the rarest form, including mutations in the CSF2RA and CSF2RB genes, encoding alpha and beta chains of the GM-CSF receptor, respectively,

mutations in the SFTPB (surfactant protein B) gene, and the gene encoding for ABC transporter A3.[2,3] The majority of congenital pulmonary alveolar proteinoses are transmitted by autosomal recessive inheritance.[2]

Secondary PAP (5% to 10% of cases) is caused by, or associated with, a variety of neoplastic, inhalational, and infectious processes (Table 28.2). The etiology of PAP in these conditions is unclear, but presumed related to toxic effects on macrophages and usually not related to autoantibodies to GM-CSF receptor.[2] In the case of hematologic conditions, defective expression of GM-CSF receptor has been described.[4] In the case of indium exposure and PAP, there may be an autoimmune mechanism involving autoantibodies to GM-CSF.[5–7]

Patients with idiopathic PAP (up to 90% of cases) have high levels of autoantibodies against GM-CSF in blood and tissues, including the pulmonary alveolar fluid.[8] These antibodies bind to epitopes on the GM-CSF molecule, blocking the interaction of GM-CSF with its receptor and critically impairing the process of surfactant clearance

TABLE 28.1   Classification of PAP

	Congenital	Autoimmune	Secondary
Etiology	Genetic mutations in pathway related to surfactant expression	Autoantibodies to GM-CSF	Infections or inhaled particles CSF-GM defects (hematologic malignancies) Autoantibodies to GM-CSF (indium exposure)
Age at presentation	Newborn	Adult	Adult; children with leukemias
Treatment	None (transplant)	Total lung lavage, exogenous GM-CSF	Treatment of underlying condition

in the lung.[8] This impairment involves decreased ability of macrophages for adhesion, chemotaxis, microbicidal activity, phagocytosis, and phagolysosome fusion.[3] These mechanisms have been studied in knockout mice defective in the GM-CSF or GM-CSF receptor genes. These genetically altered animals develop a disease similar to PAP, and surprisingly few infectious complications.[9]

Incidence

The prevalence of autoimmune PAP is between 3.7 and 6.2 cases per million.[2,3,10] The corresponding incidence has been estimated at 0.36 new cases per 1 million persons each year.[10]

Clinical Findings

Infants with congenital PAP characteristically present with an acute onset of rapidly progressive respiratory distress immediately after birth.[3]

Adults with PAP typically complain of progressive dyspnea (mean duration, 7 to 10 months) and dry or minimally productive cough.[8] Less common signs and symptoms include fatigue, weight loss, low-grade fever, chest pain, and hemoptysis.[8] Up to a third of patients are asymptomatic, with diagnosis made incidental on imaging.[2] Pulmonary function studies show mild restrictive parameters, and there is diffused diffusion capacity resulting in hypoxemia.[2] There may be associated infections, although it may be unclear if these are secondary to the PAP or the inciting cause. Typical opportunistic infections occurring in patients with PAP include *Nocardia*, Candida spp., cryptococcosis, aspergillosis, cytomegalovirus, mycobacteria, histoplasmosis, pneumocystis, and *Streptococcus pneumoniae*.

TABLE 28.2   Secondary PAP, Associated Conditions

Hematopoietic Disorders
Myelodysplastic syndrome
Acute myeloid leukemia
Chronic myelogenous leukemia
Chronic lymphocytic leukemia
Fanconi anemia

Autoimmune Disorders
Psoriasis
Amyloidosis
Immunoglobulin G monoclonal gammopathy

Immunodeficiency
Human immunodeficiency virus
Thymic alymphoplasia
Immunoglobulin A deficiency
Immunosuppression for organ transplant
Severe combined immunodeficiency disorder

Inhalation
Silica
Cotton
Cement
Fiberglass
Titanium
Aluminum
Indium tin oxide
Cellulose
Nitrogen dioxide

Infections
Nocardia
Cytomegalovirus
Pneumocystis jirovecii
Histoplasma capsulatum
Cryptococcus neoformans
Mycobacterium tuberculosis
Mycobacterium avium—intracellulare

In adults, there is a male predominance of about 1.7:1.[2,3,8] The mean age at presentation is between 40 and 50 years. The smoking rate was initially described as 70%, but this figure has decreased to 57%.[3]

Serologic Findings

Serum chemistry shows elevated lactate dehydrogenase in 82% of cases, a nonspecific finding. The autoantibodies to GM-CSF that are present in autoimmune PAP are polyclonal and consist of neutralizing IgG1, IgG2, and small amounts of IgG3 and IgG4.[3] They are found in the blood as well as in bronchoalveolar lavage (BAL) fluid. Healthy individuals can have low levels of GM-CSF autoantibodies, but the risk of PAP is increased if the GM-CSF antibody level is more than 5 μg/mL.[3] The latex agglutination test is the most widely used, with a sensitivity and specificity of 100% and 98%, respectively.[3] Anti-IgG anti-GM-CSF autoantibodies have been described in PAP secondary to exposure to indium.[5–7]

Radiologic Findings

There is often clinicoradiologic disparity between the moderate clinical symptomatology of PAP and the more impressive radiographic.[8] The CT appearance of "crazy paving," defined as a network of smoothly thickened septal lines superimposed on areas of ground-glass opacity, is considered classic for PAP.[8] These features are typically widespread and bilateral. The "crazy-paving" pattern has also been described in lipoid pneumonia (see Chapter 25).

Bronchoalveolar Lavage

Grossly, the BAL fluid may be milky and opaque and settles into a sediment layer with a clear overlying supernatant. Biochemical analysis shows the presence of phospholipids; surfactant proteins A, B, and D; and phosphatidylcholine and phosphatidylglycerol. Microscopically, there are enlarged foamy macrophages with intracytoplasmic diastase–resistant, periodic acid–Schiff-positive inclusions.

Ultrastructurally, insoluble material in BAL sediment includes tubular multilamellated structures, resembling myelin, fused-membrane multilamellated structures, and occasional crystals.[11]

Histologic Findings

PAP is characterized by the intra-alveolar accumulation of lipoproteinaceous PAS-positive material. The PAP material varies suggestive stages of organization. Initially, there is diffuse amorphous finely granular eosinophilic material without internal structure (Figs. 28.1 and 28.2).

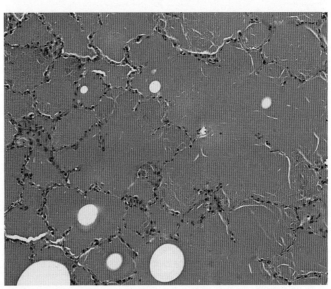

FIGURE 28.1 ▲ Pulmonary alveolar proteinosis. The alveolar spaces are completely filled with homogenous eosinophilic material. The white spaces are artifact.

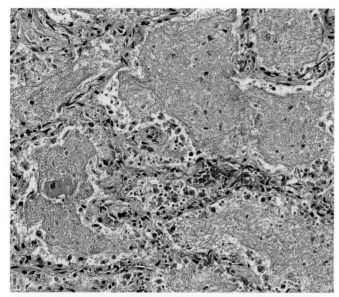

FIGURE 28.2 ▲ Pulmonary alveolar proteinosis. The material in this example is more granular, with scattered mononuclear inflammatory cells. The interstitium is mildly thickened.

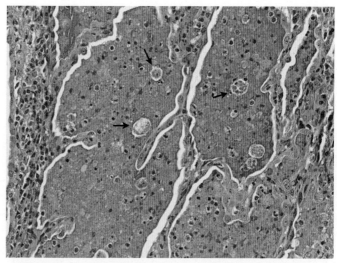

FIGURE 28.4 ▲ Pulmonary alveolar proteinosis. In this example, there is focal interstitial inflammation, as well as typical findings of PAP. This open biopsy was performed in a child with viral pneumonia and secondary PAP that resolved spontaneously with eradication of the infection.

Eventually, some of the material coalesces into darker, homogeneous eosinophilic globules, resulting in a biphasic appearance (Fig. 28.3). There are occasional mononuclear inflammatory cells in the material. There is at later stages the accumulation of cholesterol crystals and scattered macrophages that often appear swollen (Fig. 28.4). PAS shows weak positivity that is diastase resistant (Fig. 28.5). The alveolar walls may be normal or slightly thickened by type 2 pneumocyte hyperplasia and variable combinations of chronic inflammatory cells. Interstitial inflammation is more marked if there is PAP secondary to viral pneumonitis (Fig. 28.4). The proteinaceous material may be inconspicuous and easily missed on transbronchial biopsy (Fig. 28.6).

Differential Diagnosis

The differential diagnosis of intra-alveolar eosinophilic material includes primarily fibrin and edema fluid. Fibrin may appear somewhat granular and typically is not present diffusely throughout the alveolar spaces, unless associated with pneumocystis pneumonia in immunocompromised patients. Therefore, GMS staining for fungi may be indicated to distinguish PAP from pneumocystis pneumonia. The presence of cholesterol crystals and aggregated protein globules are distinctive features of PAP. Neutrophils are typically absent in the PAP, which are typically found admixed with fibrin secondary to bacterial pneumonias. Amyloid appears homogeneous, without granularity or inflammation, and is present in the interstitium. Edema fluid is pale and translucent and lacks the granularity of PAP.

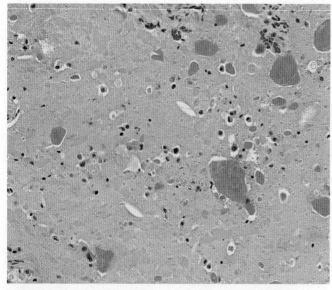

FIGURE 28.3 ▲ Pulmonary alveolar proteinosis. In addition to granular material, there are aggregated globules of denser, eosinophilic inclusions.

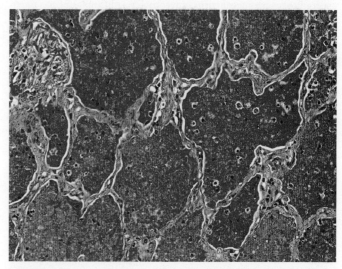

FIGURE 28.5 ▲ Pulmonary alveolar proteinosis. A PAS stain after diastase demonstrates change of color to a darker red.

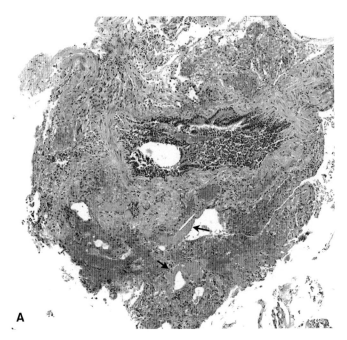

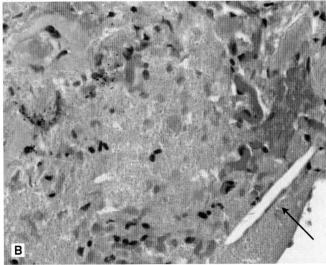

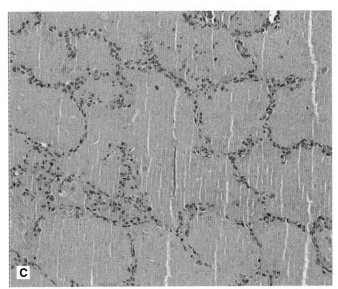

FIGURE 28.6 ▲ **A.** Pulmonary alveolar proteinosis, transbronchial biopsy. A transbronchial diagnosis performed in a patient with unexplained ground-glass opacities demonstrates a small area of proteinaceous material (*arrow*). **B.** Pulmonary alveolar proteinosis, transbronchial biopsy. A higher magnification shows an area of granular material and a cholesterol crystal (*arrow*). **C.** Pulmonary alveolar proteinosis. A wedge biopsy performed to confirm the diagnosis shows typical features of PAP.

Prognosis and Treatment

Clinical remission or spontaneous resolution occurs in the minority of patients, the remainder requiring treatment. There is no effective treatment for congenital PAP other than supportive measures or lung transplantation. Secondary PAP is treated by removal of the inciting agent from the patient's environment or treatment of the hematologic or infectious cause. Patients with idiopathic PAP are treated with sequential therapeutic whole-lung lavage; administering exogenous GM-CSF or suppressing the neutralizing antibody may be used concurrently or as an alternate to whole-lung lavage. Exogenous GM-CSF can be given systemically or by aerosol.[3]

Approximately 63% of patients with idiopathic PAP require whole lung lavage (WLL) within 5 years of diagnosis.[8] Although it is generally considered a benign condition, it is believed that overall survival is less than that of the general population.[2] The 5- and 10-year survival rates have been estimated at 75% and 68%, respectively.[12]

REFERENCES

1. Rosen SH, Castleman B, Liebow AA. Pulmonary alveolar proteinosis. *N Engl J Med.* 1958;258(23):1123–1142.
2. Ben-Dov I, Segel MJ. Autoimmune pulmonary alveolar proteinosis: clinical course and diagnostic criteria. *Autoimmun Rev.* 2014;13(4–5):513–517.
3. Khan A, Agarwal R. Pulmonary alveolar proteinosis. *Respir Care.* 2011;56(7): 1016–1028.
4. Dirksen U, Hattenhorst U, Schneider P, et al. Defective expression of granulocyte–macrophage colony-stimulating factor/interleukin-3/interleukin-5 receptor common beta chain in children with acute myeloid leukemia associated with respiratory failure. *Blood.* 1998;92(4):1097–1103.
5. Costabel U, Nakata K. Pulmonary alveolar proteinosis associated with dust inhalation: not secondary but autoimmune? *Am J Respir Crit Care Med.* 2010;181(5):427–428.
6. Cummings KJ, Donat WE, Ettensohn DB, et al. Pulmonary alveolar proteinosis in workers at an indium processing facility. *Am J Respir Crit Care Med.* 2010;181(5):458–464.

7. Lison D, Delos M. Pulmonary alveolar proteinosis in workers at an indium processing facility. *Am J Respir Crit Care Med.* 2010;182(4):578; author reply 578–579.

8. Frazier AA, Franks TJ, Cooke EO, et al. From the archives of the AFIP: pulmonary alveolar proteinosis. *Radiographics.* 2008;28(3):883–899; quiz 915.

9. Seymour JF, Begley CG, Dirksen U, et al. Attenuated hematopoietic response to granulocyte–macrophage colony-stimulating factor in patients with acquired pulmonary alveolar proteinosis. *Blood.* 1998;92(8):2657–2667.

10. Presneill JJ, Nakata K, Inoue Y, et al. Pulmonary alveolar proteinosis. *Clin Chest Med.* 2004;25(3):593–613, viii.

11. Gilmore LB, Talley FA, Hook GE. Classification and morphometric quantitation of insoluble materials from the lungs of patients with alveolar proteinosis. *Am J Pathol.* 1988;133(2):252–264.

12. Seymour JF, Presneill JJ. Pulmonary alveolar proteinosis: progress in the first 44 years. *Am J Respir Crit Care Med.* 2002;166(2):215–235.

29 Diffuse Alveolar Hemorrhage

Allen P. Burke, M.D., and Marie-Christine Aubry, M.D.

Terminology and General Concepts

Diffuse alveolar hemorrhage (DAH) is caused by a group of disorders that result in hemorrhage originating in the alveoli and involving the lungs diffusely. DAH needs to be distinguished from localized pulmonary hemorrhage and hemorrhage secondary to other diseases (Table 29.1). This distinction is determined in part based on the clinical and radiologic findings. It is an important distinction in assessing for a potential etiology.

TABLE 29.1 Alveolar Hemorrhage: Classification and Etiologies

I. Localized alveolar hemorrhage
  Neoplasm (lung cancer)
  Fungus ball
  Pulmonary infarct
  Bronchiectasis/bronchitis
  Arteriovenous malformation
II. Diffuse alveolar hemorrhage, secondary
  Venous hypertension due to cardiovascular diseases with left heart
    failure or pulmonary venous occlusive disease
  Renal failure with volume overload
  Coagulopathies/anticoagulant therapy
  Diffuse alveolar damage
  Vascular neoplasm (angiosarcoma, Kaposi sarcoma)
III. Diffuse alveolar hemorrhage, primary
  ANCA-related vasculitis
    Granulomatosis with polyangiitis
    Microscopic polyangiitis
    Eosinophilic granulomatosis with polyangiitis
  Connective tissue disease
    Systemic lupus erythematosus
    Rheumatoid arthritis
    Polymyositis
    Systemic sclerosis
    Mixed connective tissue disease
  Other immune complex–mediated vasculitis
    Mixed cryoglobulinemia
    Henoch-Schönlein purpura (IgA nephropathy)
    Behçet disease
    Goodpasture syndrome
    Drugs
      Retinoic acid
      Diphenylhydantoin
      Propylthiouracil
      Crack cocaine
      Penicillamine
  Bone marrow transplantation
  Idiopathic/isolated capillaritis
  Idiopathic pulmonary hemosiderosis

Most cases of primary DAH are due to an immune capillary injury, often resulting in capillaritis.[1,2] Capillaritis is commonly associated with glomerular disease and is discussed in detail in Chapter 47. The term "pulmonary–renal syndrome" refers to the acute onset of renal failure (generally in patients with autoimmune connective tissue diseases) and DAH of any cause.[3]

DAH in Autoimmune Disorders

DAH has been described in most autoimmune disorders that involve the lung (see Chapter 47). Capillaritis is the most frequent cause of alveolar hemorrhage in these patients, followed by acute alveolar injury and thrombotic microangiopathy (TMA). In some cases, there is no histologic finding other than hemorrhage. Drugs used in the treatment of autoimmune diseases may precipitate DAH by immune-mediated mechanisms or direct lung toxicity. DAH usually occurs when there is active symptomatic disease. The mean duration of underlying autoimmune disease before onset of DAH varies and has been reported 15.7 months in systemic lupus erythematosus (SLE)[4] and 6.4 years in systemic sclerosis.[5]

DAH is an uncommon complication of anti-neutrophil cytoplasmic antibody (ANCA)-related vasculitis, namely, granulomatosis with polyangiitis (Wegener granulomatosis),[6,7] microscopic polyangiitis,[8] and eosinophilic granulomatosis with polyangiitis (Churg-Strauss syndrome).[9] These conditions are discussed in Chapters 48 and 49.

DAH in patients with SLE is usually caused by capillaritis[10] and less frequently TMA.[11] The true incidence of various types of underlying pathology in DAH associated with lupus and other autoimmune diseases is probably unknown, however, since lung biopsies are often not performed. An autopsy-proven case of DAH in a patient with mixed connective tissue disease demonstrated hemorrhage without vasculitis or acute lung injury.[12] D-penicillamine, an immunosuppressive drug frequently prescribed in patients with Sjögren syndrome, rheumatoid arthritis, and systemic sclerosis may rarely result in DAH (see below). Like other autoimmune disease, DAH in systemic sclerosis has three most frequent causes, capillaritis, TMA (typically with scleroderma renal crisis), and penicillamine-related hemorrhage,[13] and occurs more frequently when there is pulmonary fibrosis[5] or after steroid treatment.[3] The histologic changes of TMA are generally seen in the kidney and rarely documented in lung biopsies. DAH has been described in patients with Sjögren syndrome,[14] cryoglobulinemia,[15,16] and rheumatoid arthritis,[1] the latter isolated to the lung.

Anti-glomerular basement membrane (GBM) disease (Goodpasture syndrome) is characterized by alveolar hemorrhage. Most patients are young, and there is an association with cigarette smoking. Chronic lung disease is rare in anti-GBM disease, although chronic renal failure is common. Renal outcome is relatively favorable, however, in the subgroup of patients with predominant pulmonary involvement.[17]

DAH in Antiphospholipid Syndrome

DAH is a rare complication of antiphospholipid syndrome (APS). As of 2014, fewer than 30 cases had been reported.[18,19] Previously, it was thought that microthrombi were the cause of the bleeding into the alveolar spaces. More recent data show that capillaritis is the predominant pathology.[20–22] The exact mechanism of neutrophil activation and recruitment, which are increased in bronchoalveolar lavage (BAL) fluid, is unknown.[19,23] APS-associated DAH is defined, in a patient with established APS and no other cause of DAH, as bilateral pulmonary infiltrates and BAL fluid containing gross blood or >20% hemosiderin-laden macrophages.[18] The predominant inflammatory cell in the BAL fluid is the neutrophil. DAH carries a very poor prognosis in the setting of APS.[18]

In cases of DAH associated with APS, hematologic features of disseminated intravascular coagulation, such as thrombocytopenia, elevated fibrin split products, and schistocytes on peripheral blood smear, are not necessarily present.[18] "Catastrophic antiphospholipid syndrome" (CAPS) is characterized by disseminated intravascular thrombosis resulting in multiorgan failure and ischemic injury and often DAH. Patients with CAPS develop hemoptysis, respiratory failure, microangiopathic hemolytic anemia, thrombocytopenia, elevated fibrin degradation products, and renal failure.[24] Histologic features of TMA are present in the renal biopsies in patients with CAPS.[23]

Drug-Related DAH

A number of medications have been associated with DAH, with a variety of mechanisms. Up to one-third of patients with Graves disease treated with propylthiouracil develop positive serum ANCA, usually against myeloperoxidase. Fewer than 5% of ANCA-positive patients develop small-vessel vasculitis of the skin or lungs, the latter resulting in DAH.[25–27]

Another drug associated with immune-related vasculitis is D-penicillamine, which can result in the formation of an anti-GBM autoantibody and a Goodpasture-like syndrome[5] as well as ANCA-mediated vasculitis.[3,28] Because patients receiving penicillamine often have conditions predisposing to vasculitis, it is difficult to ascribe the DAH to the drug, although vasculitis has been reported in patients on penicillamine for Wilson disease,[29] and DAH is more common in scleroderma patients taking penicillamine than those not on the drug.[5] Coumadin treatment may predispose to DAH, especially when given with other drugs that may inhibit its metabolism[30,31] or in cases of overdose.[32] Transplant patients receiving sirolimus and everolimus may experience DAH that appears related to administration of the drug.[33,34] Other drugs associated with DAH include leflunomide, often with methotrexate,[35] which is also associated with pauci-immune glomerulonephritis (leflunomide–pulmonary–renal syndrome); etanercept[36]; nitrofurantoin,[37] which also causes a microangiopathic reaction[38]; etanercept[36]; and the tyrosine kinase inhibitor nilotinib.[39]

Various inhaled agents have been associated with DAH, including cocaine,[40] trimellitic anhydride,[41] and aluminum hydroxide generally unnatural deaths.[42]

Isolated Capillaritis Causing DAH

In rare cases, seronegative biopsy-proven capillaritis has been reported in the absence of autoimmune diseases or renal involvement. In this rare group of patients, prognosis appears favorable.[2]

Thrombotic Microangiopathy and DAH

The primary thrombotic microangiopathic syndromes (thrombotic thrombocytopenic purpura and hemolytic uremic syndrome) rarely result in DAH, despite the presence of diffuse microvascular thrombi. Disseminated intravascular coagulation is also not associated with DAH, other than in context with CAPS.

Secondary TMA is relatively common in autoimmune collagen vascular syndromes and may also occur after solid organ, bone marrow, or stem cell transplant.[43] "Scleroderma renal crisis" is characterized by TMA and the abrupt onset of renal failure, usually with hypertension, and may be complicated by DAH.[13,44] Patients with SLE may develop TMA with overlapping clinical features, which may be precipitated by nitrofurantoin therapy.[38]

TMA is characterized by renal failure and microangiopathic hemolytic anemia in addition to DAH.[3,43,45–48] Pathologically, TMA is diagnosed in kidney biopsies in the presence of acute endothelial swelling and fibrin–platelet-rich microthrombi in glomerular capillaries and interstitial arterioles, progressing to onion skinning.[11] The histopathologic characteristics of TMA in lung biopsies have not been fully described, however.

Secondary TMA, in contrast to thrombotic thrombocytopenic purpura, is not usually caused by decreases in von Willebrand factor–cleaving metalloprotease (ADAMTS13).[47]

Secondary DAH in Immunocompromised Patients

Immunocompromised patients with lung diseases (especially pneumonias) frequently undergo BAL for diagnostic purposes, usually to exclude opportunistic infections. Over one-third of these patients will show BAL findings consistent with DAH.[49] A variety of infectious and neoplastic processes have been associated with DAH in this setting, none significantly more than another, including bacterial pneumonias, CMV pneumonia, *Pneumocystis jiroveci* pneumonia, aspergillosis, mycobacterial infection, lung cancer, and Kaposi sarcoma.[49] Interestingly, over 50% of patients have no predisposing cause, other than immunosuppression, for the presence of DAH.[49]

Secondary DAH in Transplant Patients

DAH is relatively common after transplantation, occurring in 2.5% of bone marrow transplant patients, especially allogeneic.[50–52] DAH is also a known complication of solid organ transplants, including heart, kidney, and liver. The cause overlaps with other immunocompromised patients and includes infection and unknown causes.[49] Transplantation is also associated with the development of TMA, induced by endothelial cell injury caused by the toxic effects of high-dose chemoradiotherapy.[43] There may also be a direct alloimmune-related endothelial injury predisposing to DAH.[53]

Clinical

Hemoptysis is the major sign of DAH. It may develop suddenly or over a period of days to weeks. Hemoptysis may be absent in the initial phase of disease in up to one-third of patients,[10] in which case diagnostic suspicion is established after sequential BAL reveals worsening RBC counts.[54]

The clinical findings in DAH are varied and often depend on the underlying conditions. Because of frequent comorbidities, the diagnosis may be missed, resulting in delayed treatment. In addition to hemoptysis, there may be anemia and signs of hypoxemia.[55,56]

Radiologic Findings in DAH

Chest radiography shows bilateral interstitial opacities, and computed tomography scans reveal bilateral and diffuse ground-glass pulmonary parenchymal opacities with interlobular septal thickening.[33,35]

Bronchoalveolar Lavage

BAL has been called the "gold standard" for diagnosis of DAH[56] and is often the basis for diagnosis.[35] Hemosiderin-filled macrophages and plentiful erythrocytes are found in lavage fluid. Grossly, the fluid is pink or red, and over 90% of patients have >30% hemosiderin macrophages, determined by staining with Prussian blue or Perls iron.[17] Often, blood is encountered during bronchoscopic examination, in the absence of endobronchial lesion explaining the hemorrhage.[33] There are two methods of determining hemorrhage, one incorporating strength of staining (Golde score) and a simplified method using percent of staining macrophages; in the latter, a <20% is considered negative for DAH, and >60% indicative of severe DAH.[49] Over three-fourths of fluids will have elevated neutrophils in the case of DAH caused by anti-GBM disease.[17]

In many patients with the diagnosis of DAH, the finding of increasing red blood cells in lavage fluid is the only diagnostic criterion in addition to clinical and radiologic findings.[57,58]

Gross Findings, DAH

At autopsy, lungs are heavy and hemorrhagic, with zonal areas of blood, which appears red in fresh specimens (Fig. 29.1) and brown after fixation. Hemorrhagic areas may extend to interlobar and segmental septa.

Microscopic Findings

The microscopic features of DAH are nonspecific. There are three general patterns: alveolar hemorrhage without other abnormalities (so-called bland DAH) (Fig. 29.2); DAH with capillaritis (Fig. 29.3); and diffuse alveolar damage (DAD) with hyaline membranes and superimposed hemorrhage. Often, there is a combination of the latter two features (capillaritis and DAD, Fig. 29.4),[10] in which case both diagnoses should be rendered. The unifying feature is the presence of hemorrhage, which can be recent with red cells admixed with fibrin and/or older and organized with hemosiderin macrophages within alveolar spaces, and occasionally in the interstitium, admixed with proliferating fibroblasts like seen in organizing pneumonia. Capillaritis may be quite

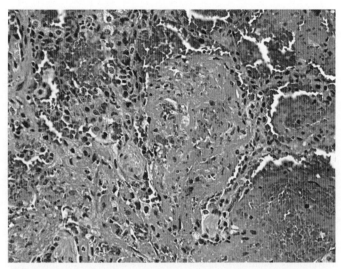

FIGURE 29.2 ▲ Diffuse alveolar hemorrhage. The airspace is filled with fibrin admixed with red cells. Scattered fibroblasts are seen in the fibrin suggesting early organization. A few hemosiderin-laden macrophages are also present in the fibrin (H&E, 200×).

subtle. It is patchy and characterized by slight expansion of the alveolar septa by neutrophils, many of which are undergoing apoptosis. Rarely, small arterioles or venules may show fibrinoid necrosis of their wall with a necrotic neutrophilic infiltrate.

Identifying an underlying injury such as capillaritis and acute lung injury, or assists with identification of a potential etiology, which ultimately requires correlation with clinical and serologic findings. Most etiologies of primary DAH will be associated with capillaritis. Goodpasture syndrome is more typically characterized by bland type of DAH. Bland type of DAH has been associated with mixed connective tissue disease[12] and SLE.[10] DAD with or without capillaritis has been described mostly in patients with SLE or in cases of drug toxicity[30,59] often with reactive pneumocytes.[41]

In many cases of DAH, the diagnosis is made by clinical, bronchoscopic, radiologic, and BAL findings. The use of wedge lung biopsy has been discouraged in patients with DAH due to bleeding complications in ill patients.[60] However, bronchoscopic biopsies have a low yield for the diagnosis of capillaritis due to sampling.

Immunofluorescence (IF) plays little role in the etiologic diagnosis of primary DAH. Its main value is in the diagnosis of Goodpasture syndrome. As in the kidney, the IF in the lung will display linear deposits of IgG in the capillary membrane (Fig. 29.5). Otherwise, the IF is not sensitive or specific with various deposits of immunoglobulin or complement reported in different connective tissue disease, ANCA-related vasculitis as well as nonimmune diseases such as idiopathic pulmonary fibrosis.[61]

Differential Diagnosis

The first differential diagnosis is to separate procedural related blood from true alveolar hemorrhage. In a wedge biopsy, true alveolar hemorrhage is composed of red cells admixed with fibrin.[62] The fibrin can show early organization with fibroblasts seen at the periphery of the fibrin plug. The adjacent alveolar septa are often mildly thickened and the pneumocytes reactive. This is in contrast to procedural related blood where the airspaces are flooded with red cells only, without fibrin. The presence of hemosiderin-laden macrophages further clenches the diagnosis of DAH. However, this raises another differential diagnosis. Indeed, hemosiderin needs to be distinguished from the more common pigment, smoker's pigment seen in respiratory bronchiolitis and desquamative interstitial pneumonia. Hemosiderin is coarse, more golden, and refractile compared to smoker's pigment, which is brown-black and finely granular (Fig. 29.6).

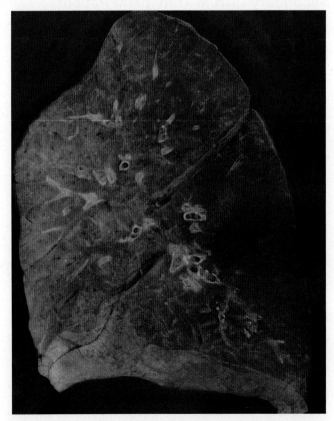

FIGURE 29.1 ▲ DAH at autopsy. Diffuse implies bilateral and all lobes. Grossly, the hemorrhagic areas are patchy in that not the entire lobe or lung is involved. Fresh, the hemorrhage appears *dark red*.

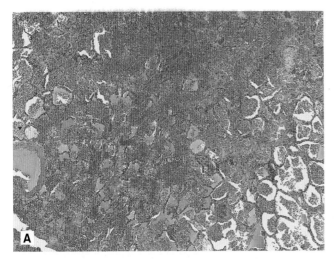

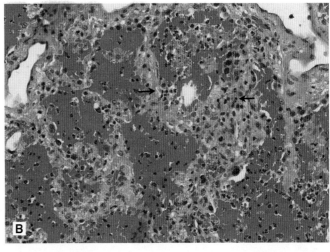

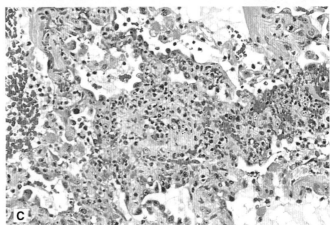

FIGURE 29.3 ▲ DAH with capillaritis in a patient with antiphospholipid syndrome. Capillaritis can be quite subtle. **A.** Low-power magnification shows DAH, mostly red cells with focal fibrin and some septal thickening. **B.** Focally, pockets of neutrophils centered on alveolar septa are seen (*arrows*). At a minimum, the neutrophils should show necrosis for a diagnosis of capillaritis. **C.** Alveolar septal disruption can be seen (H&E, 200×).

Both hemosiderin and smoker's pigment contain iron and thus will be positive with the iron stain.[63]

Some malignancies may present as DAH, specifically angiosarcoma (Fig. 29.7).[64] Therefore, before assuming that the DAH represents a nonneoplastic process, it is important to assess for the presence of malignancy.

The differential diagnosis with capillaritis is acute pneumonia/bronchopneumonia. Typically, with infection, the epicenter of the neutrophilic infiltrate is the airspace and the infiltrate tends to be diffuse. In contrast, in capillaritis, the epicenter of the infiltrate is the alveolar septa with some spilling in the alveolar space and the infiltrate is patchier, often subtle.

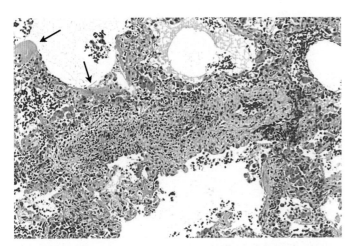

FIGURE 29.4 ▲ DAH with capillaritis and diffuse alveolar damage in a patient with systemic lupus erythematosus. Hyaline membranes (*arrows*) are present along with a neutrophilic infiltrate, which in this case involves the wall of the arteriole (H&E, 100×).

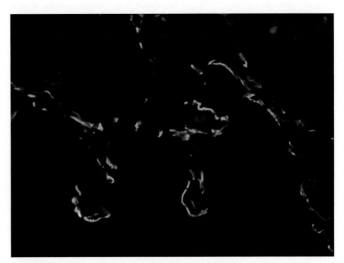

FIGURE 29.5 ▲ Immunofluorescence in Goodpasture syndrome. The IgG shows linear staining of the alveolar septa.

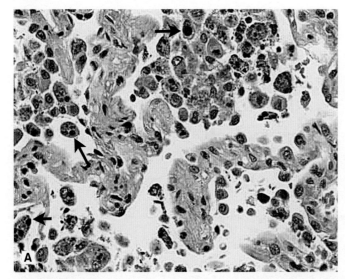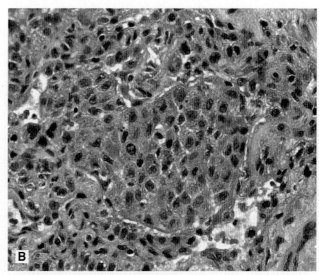

FIGURE 29.6 ▲ **A.** Hemosiderin, localized alveolar hemorrhage. The iron pigment is coarse, golden, and refractile (*arrows*). **B.** In contrast, the smoker's pigment in smoking-related lung disease (respiratory bronchiolitis, desquamative interstitial pneumonia) is fine and granular and may show fine blue granules on iron stain (not shown).

Prognosis and Treatment

The prognosis of DAH depends on the underlying cause. In patients with lupus, factors associated with an increased mortality include the need for mechanical ventilation, concomitant infection, and requirement of cyclophosphamide therapy.[10] DAH resulting in pulmonary–renal syndrome in systemic sclerosis imparts a dismal prognosis.[5] Prognosis in DAH related to APS is guarded, but remission is possible in a substantial proportion of patients with aggressive, multimodality therapy.[18] Drug-related DAH may be successfully treated with cessation of the offending agent and intravenous steroids.[40]

In general, the treatment of DAH is treatment of the underlying condition. In autoimmune DAH, steroids are indicated[12] with the addition of cyclophosphamide, rituximab, plasmapheresis, mycophenolate mofetil, and intravenous gamma globulin as needed.[4,18,65–67] Topical instillation of recombinant factor VII may be used for intractable bleeding,[68] as well as extracorporeal membrane oxygenation, in case of respiratory failure.[69]

Idiopathic Pulmonary Hemosiderosis

Idiopathic pulmonary hemosiderosis is a rare condition characterized by pulmonary hemorrhage of unknown cause. It is, by definition, a diagnosis of exclusion, after histologic features of capillaritis and acute lung injury have been excluded, clinical evaluation has ruled out toxin and drug etiologies, and rheumatologic evaluation is negative for autoimmune disorders. In some patients with the diagnosis of idiopathic pulmonary hemosiderosis, autoimmune disorders develop after initial symptoms, especially rheumatoid arthritis.[70]

Most patients with a diagnosis of idiopathic pulmonary hemosiderosis are children. Grossly, the lungs are pigmented due to hemosiderosis, and microscopically, there is overwhelming iron deposition, in the absence of vasculitis. Clinically, there may be cyclical symptoms, with remissions and acute exacerbations. There may be episodes of neutropenia followed by increased blood eosinophilia.[71] Recurrence after transplant has been reported.[72]

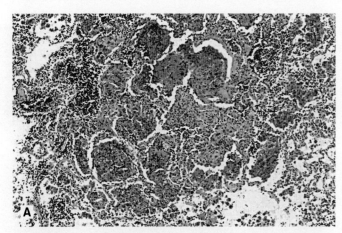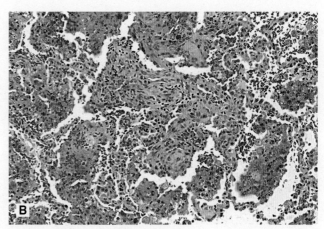

FIGURE 29.7 ▲ Metastatic angiosarcoma. **A.** Focal perivascular interstitial thickening in background of diffuse alveolar hemorrhage. **B.** At high power, the thickening is the result of atypical cells forming vascular channels. The patient was found to have a cardiac angiosarcoma.

REFERENCES

1. Schwarz MI, Zamora MR, Hodges TN, et al. Isolated pulmonary capillaritis and diffuse alveolar hemorrhage in rheumatoid arthritis and mixed connective tissue disease. *Chest.* 1998;113:1609–1615.
2. Jennings CA, King TE Jr, Tuder R, et al. Diffuse alveolar hemorrhage with underlying isolated, pauciimmune pulmonary capillaritis. *Am J Respir Crit Care Med.* 1997;155:1101–1109.
3. Naniwa T, Banno S, Sugiura Y, et al. Pulmonary-renal syndrome in systemic sclerosis: a report of three cases and review of the literature. *Mod Rheumatol.* 2007;17:37–44.
4. Canas C, Tobon GJ, Granados M, et al. Diffuse alveolar hemorrhage in Colombian patients with systemic lupus erythematosus. *Clin Rheumatol.* 2007;26:1947–1949.
5. Bar J, Ehrenfeld M, Rozenman J, et al. Pulmonary-renal syndrome in systemic sclerosis. *Semin Arthritis Rheum.* 2001;30:403–410.
6. Gomez-Gomez A, Martinez-Martinez MU, Cuevas-Orta E, et al. Pulmonary manifestations of granulomatosis with polyangiitis. *Rheumatol Clin.* 2014;10(5):288–293.
7. Toma C, Belaconi I, Dumitrache-Rujinski S, et al. Rapidly progressive pattern of granulomatosis with polyangiitis (Wegener's)—clinical case. *Chest.* 2014;145:223A.
8. Mackay J. Rapidly progressive pulmonary haemorrhage in a case of microscopic polyangiitis. *BMJ Case Rep.* 2011;2011:pii:bcr0620114336.
9. Jagadeesh LY, Sangle SR, Verma H, et al. Alveolar haemorrhage in eosinophilic granulomatosis and polyangiitis (Churg-Strauss). *Clin Rheumatol.* 2014;33(8):1177–1179.
10. Zamora MR, Warner ML, Tuder R, et al. Diffuse alveolar hemorrhage and systemic lupus erythematosus. Clinical presentation, histology, survival, and outcome. *Medicine (Baltimore).* 1997;76:192–202.
11. Song D, Wu LH, Wang FM, et al. The spectrum of renal thrombotic microangiopathy in lupus nephritis. *Arthritis Res Ther.* 2013;15:R12.
12. Horiki T, Fuyuno G, Ishii M, et al. Fatal alveolar hemorrhage in a patient with mixed connective tissue disease presenting polymyositis features. *Intern Med.* 1998;37:554–560.
13. Nanke Y, Akama H, Yamanaka H, et al. Progressive appearance of overlap syndrome together with autoantibodies in a patient with fatal thrombotic microangiopathy. *Am J Med Sci.* 2000;320:348–351.
14. Tomita Y, Mori S, Arima N, et al. Rapidly progressive pulmonary fibrosis following the onset of diffuse alveolar hemorrhage in Sjogren's syndrome: an autopsy case report. *Intern Med.* 2012;51:295–299.
15. Amital H, Rubinow A, Naparstek Y. Alveolar hemorrhage in cryoglobulinemia—an indicator of poor prognosis. *Clin Exp Rheumatol.* 2005;23:616–620.
16. Gomez-Tello V, Onoro-Canaveral JJ, de la Casa Monje RM, et al. Diffuse recidivant alveolar hemorrhage in a patient with hepatitis C virus-related mixed cryoglobulinemia. *Intensive Care Med.* 1999;25:319–322.
17. Lazor R, Bigay-Game L, Cottin V, et al. Alveolar hemorrhage in anti-basement membrane antibody disease: a series of 28 cases. *Medicine (Baltimore).* 2007;86:181–193.
18. Cartin-Ceba R, Peikert T, Ashrani A, et al. Primary antiphospholipid syndrome-associated diffuse alveolar hemorrhage. *Arthritis Care Res (Hoboken).* 2014;66:301–310.
19. Koolaee RM, Moran AM, Shahane A. Diffuse alveolar hemorrhage and Libman-Sacks endocarditis as a manifestation of possible primary antiphospholipid syndrome. *J Clin Rheumatol.* 2013;19:79–83.
20. Erkan D, Espinosa G, Cervera R. Catastrophic antiphospholipid syndrome: updated diagnostic algorithms. *Autoimmun Rev.* 2010;10:74–79.
21. Deane KD, West SG. Antiphospholipid antibodies as a cause of pulmonary capillaritis and diffuse alveolar hemorrhage: a case series and literature review. *Semin Arthritis Rheum.* 2005;35:154–165.
22. Asherson RA, Cervera R, Wells AU. Diffuse alveolar hemorrhage: a non-thrombotic antiphospholipid lung syndrome? *Semin Arthritis Rheum.* 2005;35:138–142.
23. Rangel ML, Alghamdi I, Contreras G, et al. Catastrophic antiphospholipid syndrome with concurrent thrombotic and hemorrhagic manifestations. *Lupus.* 2013;22:855–864.
24. Vieregge GB, Harrington TJ, Andrews DM, et al. Catastrophic antiphospholipid syndrome with severe acute thrombotic microangiopathy and hemorrhagic complications. *Case Rep Med.* 2013;2013:915309.
25. Sghiri R, Ouertani M, Ben Hsine H, et al. Prevalence of antineutrophil cytoplasmic antibodies during treatment with benzylthiouracil. *Pathol Biol (Paris).* 2009;57:410–414.
26. El-Fakih R, Chehab BM, Shaver T. Thionamide-induced vasculitis: a case of alveolar haemorrhage secondary to propylthiouracil. *J Intern Med.* 2008;264:610–612.
27. Irani F, Elkambergy H, Naraharisetty K, et al. Propylthiouracil-induced leucocytoclastic vasculitis with pulmonary hemorrhage treated with plasmapheresis. *Am J Med Sci.* 2009;337:470–472.
28. Sharma R, Jain S, Kher V. ANCA-associated Goodpasture's syndrome in a patient with rheumatoid arthritis on penicillamine. *Indian J Nephrol.* 2012;22:45–47.
29. Bienaime F, Clerbaux G, Plaisier E, et al. D-Penicillamine-induced ANCA-associated crescentic glomerulonephritis in Wilson disease. *Am J Kidney Dis.* 2007;50:821–825.
30. Hashemi-Sadraei N, Sadrpour S, Baram D, et al. Sirolimus-associated diffuse alveolar hemorrhage in a renal transplant recipient on long-term anticoagulation. *Clin Nephrol.* 2007;68:238–244.
31. Itoh M, Oh-Ishi S, Nemoto K, et al. A case of diffuse alveolar hemorrhage associated with tegafur plus uracil and warfarin therapy. *Clin Med Insights Case Rep.* 2011;4:73–77.
32. Klenner AF, Friesecke S, Schaper C, et al. Diffuse alveolar hemorrhage with acute respiratory distress syndrome associated with phenprocoumon therapy. *Blood Coagul Fibrinolysis.* 2008;19:813–815.
33. Khalife WI, Kogoj P, Kar B. Sirolimus-induced alveolar hemorrhage. *J Heart Lung Transplant.* 2007;26:652–657.
34. Junpaparp P, Sharma B, Samiappan A, et al. Everolimus-induced severe pulmonary toxicity with diffuse alveolar hemorrhage. *Ann Am Thorac Soc.* 2013;10:727–729.
35. Carloni A, Piciucchi S, Giannakakis K, et al. Diffuse alveolar hemorrhage after leflunomide therapy in a patient with rheumatoid arthritis. *J Thorac Imaging.* 2008;23:57–59.
36. Khaja M, Menon L, Niazi M, et al. Diffuse alveolar hemorrhage and acute respiratory distress syndrome during treatment of rheumatoid arthritis with etanercept. *J Bronchology Interv Pulmonol.* 2012;19:228–231.
37. Boggess KA, Benedetti TJ, Raghu G. Nitrofurantoin-induced pulmonary toxicity during pregnancy: a report of a case and review of the literature. *Obstet Gynecol Surv.* 1996;51:367–370.
38. Lopez-Lopez L, Rivera-Rodriguez N, Vila LM. Nitrofurantoin-induced microangiopathic haemolytic anaemia and thrombocytopaenia in a patient with systemic lupus erythematosus. *BMJ Case Rep.* 2012;2012:pii: bcr-2012-006507.
39. Donatelli C, Chongnarungsin D, Ashton R. Acute respiratory failure from nilotinib-associated diffuse alveolar hemorrhage. *Leuk Lymphoma.* 2014;55(10):2408–2409.
40. Bouchi J, el Asmar B, Couetil JP, et al. [Alveolar hemorrhage after cocaine inhalation]. *Presse Med.* 1992;21:1025–1026.
41. Rivera M, Nicotra MB, Byron GE, et al. Trimellitic anhydride toxicity. A cause of acute multisystem failure. *Arch Intern Med.* 1981;141:1071–1074.
42. Sinha US, Kapoor AK, Singh AK, et al. Histopathological changes in cases of aluminium phosphide poisoning. *Indian J Pathol Microbiol.* 2005;48:177–180.
43. Shimoni A, Yeshurun M, Hardan I, et al. Thrombotic microangiopathy after allogeneic stem cell transplantation in the era of reduced-intensity conditioning: the incidence is not reduced. *Biol Blood Marrow Transplant.* 2004;10:484–493.
44. Guillevin L, Berezne A, Seror R, et al. Scleroderma renal crisis: a retrospective multicentre study on 91 patients and 427 controls. *Rheumatology (Oxford).* 2012;51:460–467.
45. Abudiab M, Krause ML, Fidler ME, et al. Differentiating scleroderma renal crisis from other causes of thrombotic microangiopathy in a postpartum patient. *Clin Nephrol.* 2013;80:293–297.
46. Badwal S, Kotwal J, Varma PP. Unusual case of pulmonary renal syndrome with autopsy findings. *Indian J Pathol Microbiol.* 2013;56:294–296.
47. Mal H, Veyradier A, Brugiere O, et al. Thrombotic microangiopathy with acquired deficiency in ADAMTS 13 activity in lung transplant recipients. *Transplantation.* 2006;81:1628–1632.
48. Takatsuka H, Takemoto Y, Okamoto T, et al. Thrombotic microangiopathy following allogeneic bone marrow transplantation. *Bone Marrow Transplant.* 1999;24:303–306.
49. De Lassence A, Fleury-Feith J, Escudier E, et al. Alveolar hemorrhage. Diagnostic criteria and results in 194 immunocompromised hosts. *Am J Respir Crit Care Med.* 1995;151:157–163.
50. Lewis ID, DeFor T, Weisdorf DJ. Increasing incidence of diffuse alveolar hemorrhage following allogeneic bone marrow transplantation: cryptic etiology and uncertain therapy. *Bone Marrow Transplant.* 2000;26:539–543.

51. Carreras E, Diaz-Ricart M. The role of the endothelium in the short-term complications of hematopoietic SCT. *Bone Marrow Transplant.* 2011;46:1495–1502.

52. Nadir Y, Brenner B. Thrombotic complications associated with stem cell transplantation. *Blood Rev.* 2012;26:183–187.

53. Tichelli A, Gratwohl A. Vascular endothelium as 'novel' target of graft-versus-host disease. *Best Pract Res Clin Haematol.* 2008;21:139–148.

54. von Ranke FM, Zanetti G, Hochhegger B, et al. Infectious diseases causing diffuse alveolar hemorrhage in immunocompetent patients: a state-of-the-art review. *Lung.* 2013;191:9–18.

55. De Los Santos R, Cedeno de Jesus S, Jimenez Rodriguez B, et al. Diffuse hemorrhage alveolar metastases: a rare cause of lung pancreatic carcinoma. *Chest.* 2014;145:298A.

56. Erdogan D, Kocaman O, Oflaz H, et al. Alveolar hemorrhage associated with warfarin therapy: a case report and literature review. *Int J Cardiovasc Imaging.* 2004;20:155–159.

57. Tanawuttiwat T, Harindhanavudhi T, Hanif S, et al. Amiodarone-induced alveolar haemorrhage: a rare complication of a common medication. *Heart Lung Circ.* 2010;19:435–437.

58. Vandewiele B, Vandecasteele SJ, Vanwalleghem L, et al. Diffuse alveolar hemorrhage induced by everolimus. *Chest.* 2010;137:456–459.

59. Borders CW III, Bennett S, Mount C, et al. A rare case of acute diffuse alveolar hemorrhage following initiation of amiodarone: a case report. *Mil Med.* 2012;177:118–120.

60. Cordier JF, Cottin V. Alveolar hemorrhage in vasculitis: primary and secondary. *Semin Respir Crit Care Med.* 2011;32:310–321.

61. Magro CM, Morrison C, Pope-Harman A, et al. Direct and indirect immunofluorescence as a diagnostic adjunct in the interpretation of nonneoplastic medical lung disease. *Am J Clin Pathol.* 2003;119:279–289.

62. Colby TV, Fukuoka J, Ewaskow SP, et al. Pathologic approach to pulmonary hemorrhage. *Ann Diagn Pathol.* 2001;5:309–319.

63. Tazelaar HD, Wright JL, Churg A. Desquamative interstitial pneumonia. *Histopathology.* 2011;58:509–516.

64. Adem C, Aubry MC, Tazelaar HD, et al. Metastatic angiosarcoma masquerading as diffuse pulmonary hemorrhage: clinicopathologic analysis of 7 new patients. *Arch Pathol Lab Med.* 2001;125:1562–1565.

65. Haupt ME, Pires-Ervoes J, Brannen ML, et al. Successful use of plasmapheresis for granulomatosis with polyangiitis presenting as diffuse alveolar hemorrhage. *Pediatr Pulmonol.* 2013;48:614–616.

66. Nguyen T, Martin MK, Indrikovs AJ. Plasmapheresis for diffuse alveolar hemorrhage in a patient with Wegener's granulomatosis: case report and review of the literature. *J Clin Apher.* 2005;20:230–234.

67. Krause ML, Cartin-Ceba R, Specks U, et al. Update on diffuse alveolar hemorrhage and pulmonary vasculitis. *Immunol Allergy Clin North Am.* 2012;32:587–600.

68. Heslet L, Nielsen JD, Nepper-Christensen S. Local pulmonary administration of factor VIIa (rFVIIa) in diffuse alveolar hemorrhage (DAH)—a review of a new treatment paradigm. *Biologics.* 2012;6:37–46.

69. Lee JH, Kim SW. Successful management of warfarin-exacerbated diffuse alveolar hemorrhage using an extracorporeal membrane oxygenation. *Multidiscip Respir Med.* 2013;8:16.

70. Lemley DE, Katz P. Rheumatoid-like arthritis presenting as idiopathic pulmonary hemosiderosis: a report and review of the literature. *J Rheumatol.* 1986;13:954–957.

71. Cohen S. Idiopathic pulmonary hemosiderosis. *Am J Med Sci.* 1999;317:67–74.

72. Calabrese F, Giacometti C, Rea F, et al. Recurrence of idiopathic pulmonary hemosiderosis in a young adult patient after bilateral single-lung transplantation. *Transplantation.* 2002;74:1643–1645.

30 Chronic Bronchitis

Allen P. Burke, M.D.

General Terminology

Chronic bronchitis is a descriptive term, when used pathologically, that indicates chronic inflammation of large airways of any cause (Fig. 30.1). In clinical practice, it refers to a constellation of symptoms related to inflammation and hypersecretion in large and small airways, often sharing causes that result in emphysema and/or asthma (Table 30.1). Interestingly, although the inflammatory component of chronic obstructive lung disease (COPD) involves small airways as prominently as bronchi, the term "chronic bronchiolitis" is generally used for processes restricted to small airways (such as obliterative, constrictive, and follicular bronchiolitis) and not in the context of COPD. The pathologic findings that are specific for asthma or emphysema are described in subsequent chapters.

Etiology and Pathogenesis

Chronic bronchitis is characterized pathologically by chronic inflammation and mucous gland hyperplasia resulting in narrowing of the airway and hypersecretion and involves bronchioles as well as bronchi.[1] Chronic bronchitis is a complication of exposures to particulate matter, especially tobacco smoke, but may also result from allergic hyperreactive airway disease (chronic asthma). Regardless of the cause, recurrent infections frequently exacerbate the condition and contribute to gradual decline in lung function. Airflow obstruction results from physical narrowing of the airway, epithelial remodeling, and airway collapse secondary to alteration of airway surface tension. Chronic bronchitis is at one end of the classic COPD spectrum, with emphysema on the other, and most patients lie somewhere in between.[2] Studies in animal models suggest that chronic bronchitis resembles the natural defense against viral infection and therefore is in a way an exaggerated normal immune response.[3]

Clinical Features

The diagnosis of chronic bronchitis is entirely clinical and is based on symptoms of bronchial hypersecretion, chronic productive cough, expectoration, and phlegm production. A generally held definition for chronic bronchitis is chronic cough and sputum production for at least 3 months per year for at least two consecutive years, in the absence of other known causes.[2] It is often separated into patients with or without airway obstruction on pulmonary function tests and presence of asthma or emphysema. Population estimates of the prevalence of chronic bronchitis vary by population and definition, and range from 3.4% to 22% of the population, with current and former smokers at the higher end.[2]

Acute exacerbations of chronic bronchitis affect a significant proportion of patients with chronic bronchitis and are usually related to bacterial infection.[4] Patients with chronic bronchitis are more susceptible to this than those at the emphysema or asthma ends of the spectrum.[5]

Radiologic Findings

Neither chest radiograph nor high-resolution computed tomography is particularly useful in the diagnosis of patients with chronic bronchitis, other than excluding other diseases. A variety of computed tomography findings can be observed, but they are considered nonspecific, subjective, and poorly reproducible. The finding of bronchial wall thickening, for example, is neither particularly sensitive nor specific for chronic bronchitis.[6]

Microscopic Findings

Because chronic bronchitis is clinically diagnosed, tissue sampling is not performed for establishing the diagnosis. However, transbronchial biopsies may be performed to rule out specific infections, eosinophilic bronchitis or bronchiolitis, or other causes of airway inflammation, such as sarcoidosis. The general features of chronic bronchitis and bronchiolitis are chronic inflammation in the respiratory epithelium, extending into the submucosa and smooth muscle, with increase in submucosal glands and goblet cells, especially in the distal bronchioles (Figs. 30.2 and 30.3). There may be superimposed acute inflammation corresponding typically to bacterial superinfection (Fig. 30.4). Although there are frequently coexisting features of asthma, including mucous plugging and thickened basement membrane, eosinophilic inflammation of the lamina propria is only mild. Increased mucous production may result in extravasation into the surrounding airspaces, in which case a mucinous adenocarcinoma should be excluded by careful histologic inspection (Fig. 30.5). Airway mucus attracts neutrophils, and presence of neutrophils within luminal mucus does not imply acute bronchitis/bronchiolitis.

There have been several studies investigating the histologic findings in chronic bronchitis, generally in the patients with COPD. Tissue samples in these studies are not procured for diagnostic purposes, but for a variety of indications, such as volume reduction, or removal of masses. Patients with chronic bronchitis have greater mucosal inflammation in airways >2 mm luminal diameter and greater submucosal inflammation around mucous glands in bronchi larger than 4 mm diameter.[1] In studies of smaller airways (bronchioles), smokers without chronic bronchitis had more neutrophils, CD8-positive T lymphocytes, and macrophages compared to nonsmokers with and smokers with chronic bronchitis.[7] Bronchiolar lymphocytic inflammation is related to mucous metaplasia (increase in goblet cells).[8] In the small airways, the degree of inflammation (including neutrophils, macrophages, T lymphocytes, B lymphocytes, and lymphoid follicles) and amount of luminal mucus show a stepwise increase with the progression of COPD.[9] A link between epithelial mucin dysregulation and airflow obstruction has been established.[10]

The *Reid Index* is a mathematical formula that estimates the degree of mucous metaplasia and is defined as ratio between the thickness of the submucosal glands and the thickness between the epithelium and cartilage that covers the bronchi. The Reid Index is not of diagnostic use, but it has value in research.[11,12]

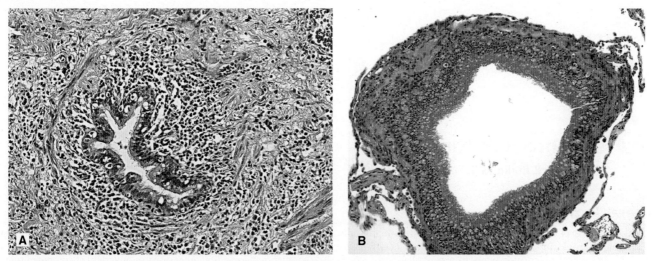

FIGURE 30.1 ▲ Chronic bronchiolitis. **A.** Inflammation involves epithelium, lamina propria, and smooth muscle layer. There is no increase in goblet cells in this example. **B.** In this example, there is diffuse hyperplasia of goblet cells.

TABLE 30.1 Syndromes of Chronic Bronchitis, Asthma, and Emphysema

	Chronic Bronchitis	Asthma	Emphysema
Etiology	Irritation to airway (smoking, infections, etc.)	Allergens (most common) Drugs, infections (triggers)	Cigarette smoking, other exposures, alpha-1 antitrypsin deficiency
Pathophysiology	Inflammation, hypersecretion with mucous gland hyperplasia, relatively fixed obstruction	Reversible obstruction by hyperreactive airways, smooth muscle hyperplasia	Destruction of alveolar walls
Symptoms	Productive cough	Wheezing, dyspnea	Dyspnea
Overlaps	Emphysema (large); asthma (small)	Small overlap with chronic bronchitis and emphysema	Chronic bronchitis (large); asthma (small)
Lung volume	Mildly increased	Increased (reversible)	Increased (irreversible)
Pulmonary arterial hypertension	Infrequent	Absent	Common
Small airway disease, irreversible	Common	Infrequent	Common

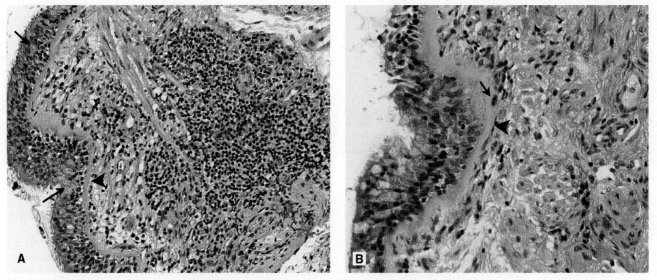

FIGURE 30.2 ▲ **A.** Chronic bronchiolitis. There is some increase in goblet cells (*arrows*) and a thickened basement membrane (*arrowhead*). The inflammation extends into the smooth muscle wall. Eosinophils are not prominent. **B.** Chronic bronchiolitis. A higher magnification demonstrates rare eosinophils (*arrow*) and thick basement membrane (*arrowhead*).

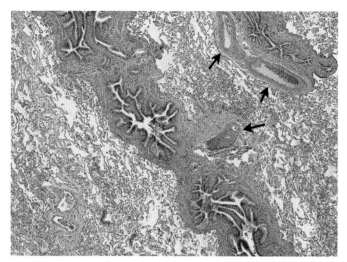

FIGURE 30.3 ▲ Chronic bronchiolitis. There is a thickened wall caused by inflammation, mild fibrosis, and epithelial proliferation. The arrows point to the accompanying arteries of the bronchovascular bundles (*arrows*), which had resulted in thickened small airways visible on CT scan in this patient.

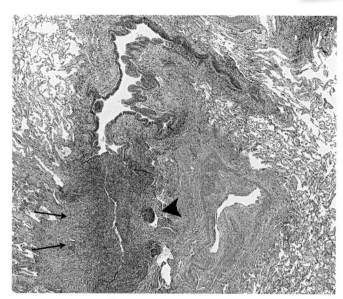

FIGURE 30.4 ▲ Chronic bronchiolitis with acute inflammation. There is an area of destruction of respiratory mucosa (*arrows*), with focal lymphoid aggregates (*arrowhead*).

Ultrastructural Findings

The axonemes of the bronchial cilia may possess ultrastructural abnormalities in patients with chronic bronchitis, especially smokers.[13] Mucous metaplasia has been documented ultrastructurally as an increase in goblet cells and a decrease in Clara cells in the distal airways.[14]

Prognosis and Treatment

Chronic bronchitis results in a decreased quality of life, because of acute infectious exacerbations and symptomatic decline in lung function. There may also be a decrease in overall mortality.[2] Treatment includes smoking cessation, chest physical therapy, and inhaled beta-adrenergic agents and glucocorticosteroids. Oral medications used to treat chronic bronchitis include mucolytics, expectorants, methylxanthines, anticholinergics, phosphodiesterase inhibitors, and antioxidants. Except for macrolide antibiotics, which have a variety of effects in addition to antimicrobial properties, administration of antibiotics is not indicated for the treatment of chronic bronchitis, unless there is an acute exacerbation in the form of bacterial infection.[4]

Eosinophilic Bronchitis and Bronchiolitis

Airway eosinophilic infiltration may be seen in asthma, nonasthmatic eosinophilic bronchitis, allergic bronchopulmonary aspergillosis, drug reactions, and chronic obstruction lung disease, in addition to primary eosinophilic lung disease (eosinophilic pneumonia and eosinophilic granulomatosis with polyangiitis). However,

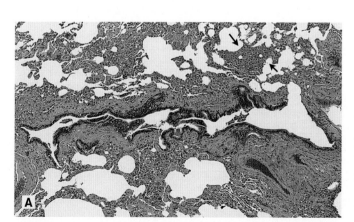

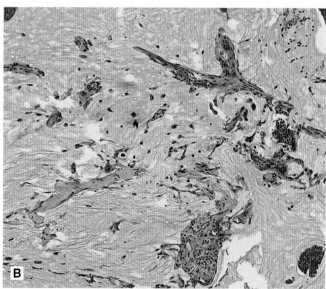

FIGURE 30.5 ▲ **A.** Chronic bronchiolitis. There is bronchiolar epithelial proliferation and inflammation. **B.** Chronic bronchiolitis with mucus extravasation. A different area showed mucus extravasation, which had formed a mass visible on CT scan; the mass was excised for suspicion of tumor.

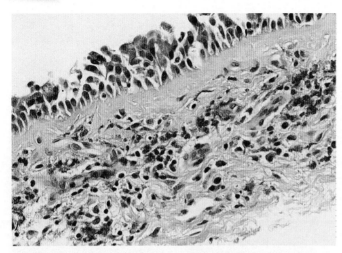

FIGURE 30.6 ▲ Eosinophilic bronchiolitis. There are prominent eosinophils in the lamina propria, under the thickened basement membrane.

the degree of airway eosinophil infiltration may not correlate with symptoms and disordered airway function in these conditions. In contrast to asthma, nonasthmatic eosinophilic bronchitis is not associated with variable airflow limitation or airway hyperresponsiveness, and there is more pronounced tissue eosinophilia within respiratory epithelium. The condition can be transient, episodic, or persistent. The reason for the absence of asthmatic symptoms in eosinophilic bronchitis is unclear but may due to the location of mast cells within the airway epithelium in eosinophilic bronchitis, and within airway smooth muscle in asthma. The diagnosis is made by pathologic confirmation of eosinophilic airway inflammation, after other causes for chronic cough are ruled out on clinical and radiologic grounds. Unlike asthma, in which there are luminal mucous plugs with eosinophils and little tissue eosinophilia, eosinophilic bronchitis is characterized by a dense infiltrate of eosinophils under the basement membrane (Fig. 30.6) without mucous plugging. The cough usually responds well to treatment with inhaled corticosteroids, with long-term prednisone treatment occasionally necessary.[15,16] Eosinophilic bronchitis may also be a rare manifestation of graft versus host disease.[17]

More recently, eosinophilic inflammation in the bronchioles has been reported (so-called eosinophilic bronchiolitis or hypereosinophilic obliterative bronchiolitis).[18,19] The definition of eosinophilic bronchiolitis includes peripheral eosinophilia, increased eosinophils in bronchial lavage fluid, and obstructive symptoms, the latter resulting in a good deal of overlap with chronic asthma.[20] Similar to eosinophilic bronchitis, there is a predominance of tissue eosinophilia in the bronchiolar wall, as opposed to eosinophil-rich mucus plugs characteristic of asthma. In contrast to eosinophilic pneumonia, the infiltrates are limited to the airways, although airway involvement may occur in the former.[21] Both eosinophilic bronchiolitis and asthma share numerous other histologic features, including increased goblet cells (mucous metaplasia), thickened basement membranes, and chronic inflammation. However, bronchiolar eosinophilia is more likely to be secondary to other eosinophilic lung diseases than primary eosinophilic bronchiolitis.

Plastic Bronchitis

Plastic bronchitis is a rare disease in which there is the formation of large gelatinous, rubbery, or rigid branching airway casts.[22] The casts may be composed mainly of fibrin and inflammation with eosinophils, typically seen in asthma or cystic fibrosis, of primarily of mucus, often seen in patients with palliated congenital heart disease. In addition to cystic fibrosis, asthma, and congenital heart disease, plastic bronchitis has been reported in patients with pneumonia, lymphangiomatosis, allergic bronchopulmonary aspergillosis, bronchiectasis, sickle cell disease, and smoke inhalation. Involvement of major airways can be life threatening. The casts have been classified as inflammatory (type I) or acellular (type II); the former are often associated with bronchial disease and acute presentations, whereas the latter are characteristic of congenital heart disease and are more often chronic and recurrent.

REFERENCES

1. Mullen JB, Wright JL, Wiggs BR, et al. Reassessment of inflammation of airways in chronic bronchitis. *Br Med J.* 1985;291:1235–1239.
2. Kim V, Criner GJ. Chronic bronchitis and chronic obstructive pulmonary disease. *Am J Respir Crit Care Med.* 2013;187:228–237.
3. Holtzman MJ, Tyner JW, Kim EY, et al. Acute and chronic airway responses to viral infection: implications for asthma and chronic obstructive pulmonary disease. *Proc Am Thorac Soc.* 2005;2:132–140.
4. Blasi F, Ewig S, Torres A, et al. A review of guidelines for antibacterial use in acute exacerbations of chronic bronchitis. *Pulm Pharmacol Ther.* 2006;19:361–369.
5. Wilson R. Evidence of bacterial infection in acute exacerbations of chronic bronchitis. *Semin Respir Infect.* 2000;15:208–215.
6. Zompatori M, Sverzellati N, Gentile T, et al. Imaging of the patient with chronic bronchitis: an overview of old and new signs. *Radiol Med.* 2006;111:634–639.
7. Saetta M, Turato G, Baraldo S, et al. Goblet cell hyperplasia and epithelial inflammation in peripheral airways of smokers with both symptoms of chronic bronchitis and chronic airflow limitation. *Am J Respir Crit Care Med.* 2000;161:1016–1021.
8. Kim V, Kelemen SE, Abuel-Haija M, et al. Small airway mucous metaplasia and inflammation in chronic obstructive pulmonary disease. *COPD.* 2008;5:329–338.
9. Hogg JC, Chu F, Utokaparch S, et al. The nature of small-airway obstruction in chronic obstructive pulmonary disease. *N Engl J Med.* 2004;350:2645–2653.
10. Innes AL, Woodruff PG, Ferrando RE, et al. Epithelial mucin stores are increased in the large airways of smokers with airflow obstruction. *Chest.* 2006;130:1102–1108.
11. Reid L. Chronic bronchitis and emphysema. *Adv Intern Med.* 1964;12:256–294.
12. Reid L. Measurement of the bronchial mucous gland layer: a diagnostic yardstick in chronic bronchitis. *Thorax.* 1960;15:132–141.
13. Verra F, Escudier E, Lebargy F, et al. Ciliary abnormalities in bronchial epithelium of smokers, ex-smokers, and nonsmokers. *Am J Respir Crit Care Med.* 1995;151:630–634.
14. Ebert RV, Terracio MJ. The bronchiolar epithelium in cigarette smokers. Observations with the scanning electron microscope. *Am Rev Respir Dis.* 1975;111:4–11.
15. Brightling CE. Chronic cough due to nonasthmatic eosinophilic bronchitis: ACCP evidence-based clinical practice guidelines. *Chest.* 2006;129:116S–121S.
16. Brightling CE. Cough due to asthma and nonasthmatic eosinophilic bronchitis. *Lung.* 2010;188(suppl 1):S13–S17.
17. Akhtari M, Langston AA, Waller EK, et al. Eosinophilic pulmonary syndrome as a manifestation of GVHD following hematopoietic stem cell transplantation in three patients. *Bone Marrow Transplant.* 2009;43:155–158.
18. Takayanagi N, Kanazawa M, Kawabata Y, et al. Chronic bronchiolitis with associated eosinophilic lung disease (eosinophilic bronchiolitis). *Respiration.* 2001;68:319–322.
19. Cordier JF, Cottin V, Khouatra C, et al. Hypereosinophilic obliterative bronchiolitis: a distinct, unrecognised syndrome. *Eur Respir J.* 2013;41:1126–1134.
20. Poletti V. Eosinophilic bronchiolitis: is it a new syndrome? *Eur Respir J.* 2013;41:1012–1013.
21. Matsuda Y, Tachibana K, Sasaki Y, et al. Tracheobronchial lesions in eosinophilic pneumonia. *Respir Investig.* 2014;52:21–27.
22. Madsen P, Shah SA, Rubin BK. Plastic bronchitis: new insights and a classification scheme. *Paediatr Respir Rev.* 2005;6:292–300.

31 Bronchiectasis

Allen P. Burke, M.D.

Definition

Bronchiectasis is a descriptive term for irreversibly dilated, thickened, and inflamed bronchi. Diffuse bronchiectasis is a hallmark of cystic fibrosis. Non–cystic fibrosis bronchiectasis is caused by recurrent infections of diverse causes, resulting in bacterial colonization of the lower respiratory tract, inflammation, and frequent exacerbations.[1] Bronchiectasis syndromes are occasionally divided into three groups: cystic fibrosis, primary ciliary dyskinesia (PCD), and non–cystic fibrosis bronchiectasis.[2]

The term "traction bronchiectasis" or "bronchiolectasis" is primarily used by radiologists and indicates peripheral bronchiolectasis caused by diffuse interstitial lung disease with fibrosis and is not a primary inflammatory process. The term "bronchiolectasis" is infrequently used by pathologists and may be a histologic feature of honeycomb lung.

Incidence

The incidence of bronchiectasis has declined in developed countries with the decrease in prevalence of pertussis and other illnesses prevented by vaccination, and bacterial and tuberculous pneumonia. The true incidence is difficult to ascertain and depends on location and diagnostic assessment. Based on diagnostic reporting, the annual incidence in Finland was estimated at 3.9 per 100,000, with a range of 0.5 at age 0 to 14 years to 10.4 at 65 years.[3] Estimates for the United States are far higher, at 4 per 100,000 at ages 18 to 34 to over 100 per 100,000 over age 65.[4] In South Korea, a full 9% of patients were diagnosed with bronchiectasis by screening CT scans of volunteers.[5]

Etiology

Bronchiectasis is the result of recurrent respiratory infections, with a variety of underlying conditions, including genetic diseases, socioeconomic factors, and subtle alterations in immune function. A list of the more common entities is shown in Table 31.1. Central bronchiectasis

TABLE 31.1 **Bronchiectasis, Causes, and Associations**

Congenital systemic diseases	Cystic fibrosis
	Ciliary dyskinesia
Immunodeficiency syndromes	HIV
	Chronic granulomatous disease
	Combined variable immunodeficiency
Lung diseases	Tuberculosis
	Asthma, including allergic bronchopulmonary aspergillosis
	Chronic aspiration
	Lipoid pneumonia
	Recurrent pneumonias
	Emphysema with alpha-1 antitrypsin disease[6]
	Congenital cystic malformation
	Tracheobronchomegaly
	Williams-Campbell syndrome
Rheumatologic disease	Systemic sclerosis
	Rheumatoid arthritis
	Sjögren syndrome
GI disorders	Inflammatory bowel disease
	Gastroesophageal reflux

is typical, if not pathognomonic, of allergic bronchopulmonary aspergillosis.[7] Chronic aspiration, asthma, primary immune deficiency syndromes (e.g., chronic granulomatous disease, common variable immunodeficiency), and ciliary dyskinesia are potential causes for recurrent infections resulting in bronchiectasis. The largest single group is idiopathic. In a retrospective study throughout the country of Ireland, causes of non–cystic fibrosis–related bronchiectasis were idiopathic (32%), postpneumonia (17%), immune deficiency (16%), recurrent aspiration (16%), primary ciliary dyskinesia (9%), chronic aspiration with immune deficiency (5%), post foreign body inhalation (2%), tracheomalacia (1%), and obliterative bronchiolitis (1%).[8] Bronchiectasis is prevalent in adults with chronic obstructive lung disease and recurrent pneumonia and is associated with poorer lung function, more frequent exacerbations, and a higher rate of *Pseudomonas* infections.[9]

An underlying disorder is identified in the majority of children with bronchiectasis, including infections (17%), primary immunodeficiency (16%), aspiration (10%), ciliary dyskinesia (9%), congenital malformation (3%), and secondary immunodeficiency (3%).[10]

In developed countries, a history of tuberculosis and advanced age are associated with bronchiectasis.[5] In developing countries, children with bronchiectasis are more likely to have underlying lung disease (especially asthma), chronic sinusitis, immunodeficiency, central nervous system disorders predisposing to aspiration, and cardiac conditions compared to the normal population.[11] Lipoid pneumonia following aspiration of oils is a common predisposing factor in some parts of Africa and the Middle East[12].

Patients with autoimmune disorders, including rheumatoid arthritis, Sjögren syndrome, relapsing polychondritis, and inflammatory bowel disease are more likely to develop bronchiectasis.[13] The mechanisms are diverse and include immunosuppression, lung involvement, and esophageal hypomotility. Patients with systemic sclerosis and bronchiectasis are characterized by an older age, a high frequency of hiatus hernia, increased respiratory infections, a low incidence of anti-Ro/SS-A, and high frequency of anti-smooth muscle antibodies.[14] Bronchiectasis in rheumatoid arthritis often occurs in patients with severe, long-standing nodular disease and causes recurrent pulmonary infections that may result in fatal respiratory failure.[15]

Primary Ciliary Dyskinesia

PCD is a rare autosomal recessive disease manifest by structural and functional abnormalities of the motile cilia. Disease-causing mutations in at least 16 genes have already been identified, including biallelic mutations in multiple genes.[16] Pathologic diagnosis rests on ultrastructural absence of dynein arms of the ciliary microtubules. However, up to 30% of patients may have normal ultrastructure, in whom genetic tests, ciliary motility, and nasal nitric oxide production studies may establish a diagnosis.

The estimated incidence of PCD is conservatively estimated at 1 per 15,000 births. Chronic infections of the ears, sinuses, and lungs are associated with organ laterality defects, typically situs inversus, in ~50% of cases. There are typically recurrent episodes of respiratory tract infections. Pulmonary function tests show generally obstructive impairment. Lung biopsy shows nonspecific inflammation. Bronchiectasis (usually with situs inversus) is typical on chest imaging. Male infertility due to immotile spermatozoa is often present.

Given the heterogeneity and the rarity of the disorder, therapy is not evidence based and analogous with the treatment for cystic fibrosis.[17,18]

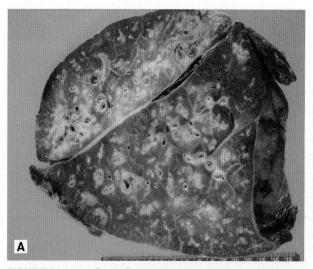
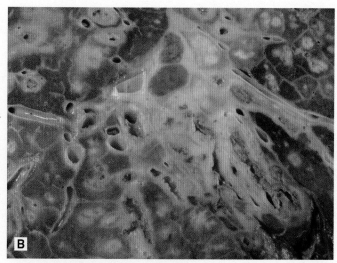

FIGURE 31.1 ▲ Cystic fibrosis. **A.** An explanted lung shows prominent airways with extensive peribronchial consolidation. **B.** A higher magnification shows irregular dilated airways with patchy surrounding consolidation.

Cystic Fibrosis

Cystic fibrosis is an autosomal recessive disease caused by dysfunction of the cystic fibrosis transmembrane conductance receptor (CFTR) protein, resulting in an imbalance of chloride secretion and sodium absorption and airway surface dehydration.[19]

The prevalence of cystic fibrosis is ~1 in 25,000 in Caucasians, and between one-fourth and one-fifth that in African Americans and Asians.[19] The diagnosis is made by the finding of two *CFTR* pathogenic allelic variants, two abnormal quantitative pilocarpine iontophoresis sweat chloride values (>60 mEq/L), or transepithelial nasal potential difference measurements characteristic of CF.[20] Of the thousands known, the most common mutation is ΔF508, which results in classic cystic fibrosis if homozygous. There is a spectrum of severity of disease phenotype depending on allele pairing. Certain mutations in the *CFTR* gene cause *congenital absence of the vas deferens* and infertility in males, without cystic fibrosis, and no disease in females.

Pulmonary disease is the most important cause of morbidity and mortality in cystic fibrosis. Pulmonary remodeling in cystic fibrosis includes bronchiectasis, mucoid impaction, atelectasis, fibrosis, and hypervascularity. Biopsies in children with cystic fibrosis show thickened basement membranes, inflammation with neutrophils, increase in smooth muscle, and an increase in submucosal glands, changes that predate structural changes.[21] Eventually, there is the development of diffuse bronchiectasis, with recurrent infections, and pus-filled cysts (Figs. 31.1 and 31.2). Colonization of dilated bronchi by bacteria, especially *Pseudomonas aeruginosa* and *Burkholderia cepacia* negatively affects clinical outcome.[22,23] Neutrophil-dominated inflammation persists in the majority of patients. Sputum neutrophil elastase levels are higher in patients with severe lung disease and contribute to decreased lung function and bronchiectasis.[24]

Pathogenesis of Bronchiectasis

Infections in bronchiectasis cause erosion and weakening of the airway and breakdown of the resistance to infection, including ciliary function, active transport of sodium and chloride, and production of antibacterial peptides. A vicious cycle ensues, with bacterial overgrowth, chronic inflammation, and formation of cytokines and proteases that further dilated the airway.[1] Adults with bronchiectasis may have low levels of IgG3, circulating B lymphocytes, helper T cells, and neutrophil oxidative function.[25]

Clinical and Radiologic Findings

Patients with bronchiectasis develop productive cough, often with dyspnea and wheezing. Patients with congenital disease such as cystic fibrosis and common variable immunodeficiency present in childhood. Symptoms may begin months after an initial infection, and recurrent pneumonia is typical. The radiologic gold standard for the diagnosis of bronchiectasis is computed tomography. Depending on the etiology, there may be unilobar involvement or multilobular involvement, typically of the lower lobes.[11] The most common lobes are the left lower lobe (also frequently involved in aspiration), right middle lobe, and right lower lobes.[26] Imaging of bronchiectasis is often classified by shape of the dilated airway (Table 31.2). In children with

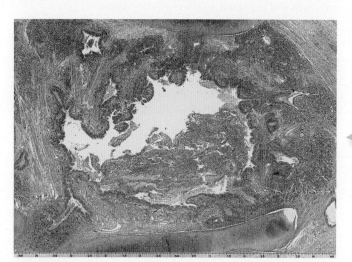

FIGURE 31.2 ▲ Cystic fibrosis. A histologic section demonstrates a dilated airway with intense peribronchial inflammation.

TABLE 31.2 Pathologic and Imaging Features of Bronchiectasis

Pathologic Description[a]	Radiologic Terms
Cylindrical (regular)	Cylindrical bronchiectasis
	Enlarge, nontapering airways >1.5× diameter of accompanying artery
Fusiform	Varicose bronchiectasis
	Dilated airways with irregular outlines
Globular (sacculated)	Cystic bronchiectasis, with grape-like clusters

[a]Historical use primarily.

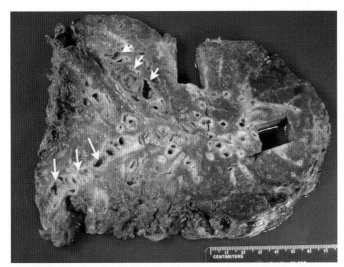

FIGURE 31.3 ▲ Bronchiectasis, explanted lung. There is diffuse airway dilatation, without significant consolidation. The bronchi are tortuous and focally extend to near the pleural surface (*arrows*). The patient suffered diffuse airway injury following inhalation of smoke in a house fire.

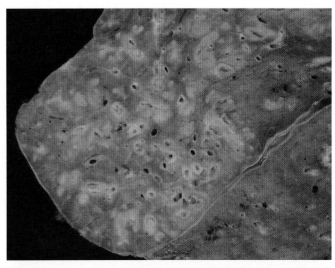

FIGURE 31.4 ▲ Bronchiectasis, explanted lung. The lung had been transplanted as a donor lung 1.5 years prior, and the patient's course was complicated by bronchial stenosis, stenting, and recurrent infections leading to bronchiectasis.

common variable immunodeficiency, the most common abnormality was mosaic attenuation, indicative of air trapping.[27]

Bronchoalveolar Lavage

Whether caused by cystic fibrosis, PCD, or other causes, BAL fluid in bronchiectasis is characterized by increased cell counts, with a predominance of neutrophils.[28] Most patients have positive bacterial and fungal cultures for pathogens, including *Haemophilus influenza*, *Mycoplasma pneumoniae*, *S. pneumoniae*, *Aspergillus fumigatus*, and *P. aeruginosa*. Nonpathogenic bacteria, such as nontuberculous mycobacteria, may contribute to the local inflammatory process.

Gross Findings

There are three classic types of bronchiectasis (Table 31.2): cylindrical, fusiform (varicose with constrictions), and sacculated bronchiectasis.[29] Surgical treatment is currently uncommon, although the pathologist will encounter bronchiectasis at autopsy (Fig. 31.2) and explant

(Figs. 31.3 and 31.4). There may be enlarged mediastinal lymph nodes, as well as areas of hemorrhage.

Microscopic Findings

Histologically, dilated bronchi are thickened by chronic inflammation, with variable erosion and destruction of underlying smooth muscle and cartilage (Figs. 31.5 and 31.6). The inflammation extends to bronchioles and may result in bronchiolectasis, acute bronchiolitis, and acute bronchopneumonia. There is often filling of airways by inflammatory debris and mucus, which may extend into adjacent alveoli. Squamous metaplasia may line the cystically dilated bronchus (Fig. 31.7). Follicular bronchiectasis has excessive formation of lymphoid tissue, and there is formation of follicles and nodes within walls of diseased bronchi. Ectatic airways may be colonized by Aspergillus organisms, with or without a surrounding granulomatous response (bronchocentric granulomatosis, see Chapter 33) (Fig. 31.8). Peribronchial fibrosis is common, especially distally. As with any chronic fibrotic process, there may be neuroendocrine hyperplasia and the formation of reactive carcinoid tumorlets.[30]

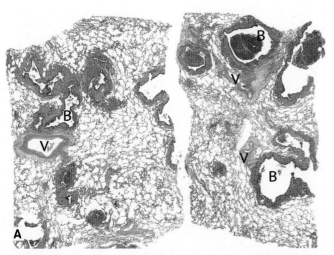
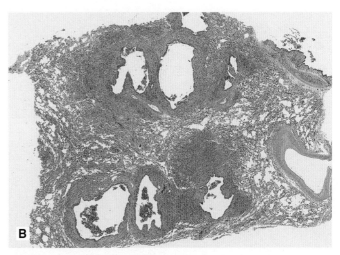

FIGURE 31.5 ▲ Bronchiectasis, explanted lung. **A.** Most bronchi (B) are ectatic compared to arterial vessels (V). The patient was immunosuppressed secondary to treatment of myasthenia gravis and suffered from recurrent pseudomonas pneumonias that progressed to bronchiectasis, which recurred in the transplanted lung (see Fig. 31.4). **B.** A higher magnification demonstrates pneumonia surrounding the ectatic airways.

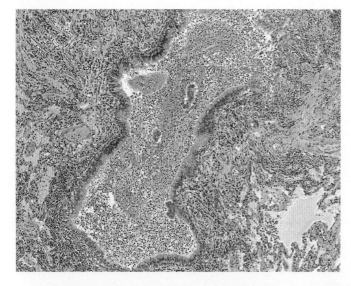

FIGURE 31.6 ▲ Bronchiectasis. There is superimposed acute bronchopneumonia with focal destruction of the bronchial wall.

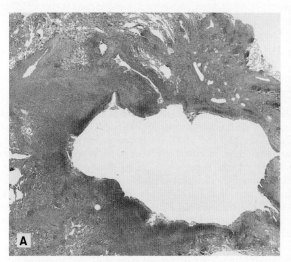
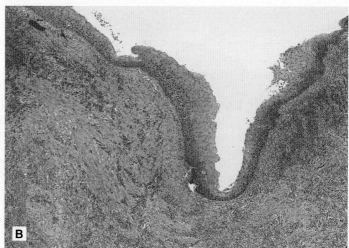

FIGURE 31.7 ▲ Bronchiectasis, allergic bronchopulmonary aspergillosis. **A.** Low magnification shows a cystic space, not recognizable as bronchus, with surrounding fibrosis and lymphoid aggregates. **B.** On higher magnification, the wall is lined by squamous epithelium.

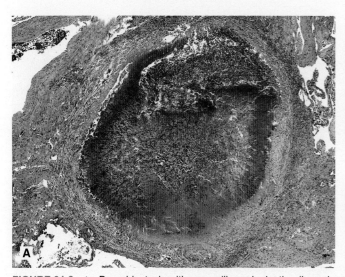
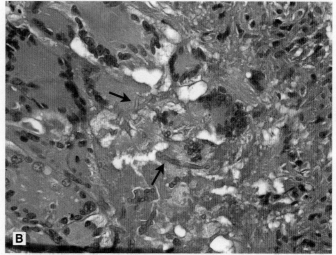

FIGURE 31.8 ▲ Bronchiectasis with aspergillus colonization (bronchocentric granulomatosis). **A.** Low magnification demonstrates bronchus filled with necrotic material and inflammation. **B.** A high magnification shows hyphae (*arrows*) with a giant cell reaction.

Prognosis and Treatment

Treatment is supportive and includes antibiotics for underlying infections, mucoactive therapy, and anti-inflammatory agents. Surgery is used as a last resort in cases of intractable infection and abscess formation or in cases of lipoid pneumonia.[12,31]

REFERENCES

1. Whitters D, Stockley R. Immunity and bacterial colonisation in bronchiectasis. *Thorax.* 2012;67:1006–1013.
2. Flight WG, Jones AM. Cystic fibrosis, primary ciliary dyskinesia and non-cystic fibrosis bronchiectasis: update 2008–11. *Thorax.* 2012;67:645–649.
3. Saynajakangas O, Keistinen T, Tuuponen T, et al. Evaluation of the incidence and age distribution of bronchiectasis from the Finnish hospital discharge register. *Cent Eur J Public Health.* 1998;6:235–237.
4. Weycker D, Edelsberg J, Oster G, et al. Prevalence and economic burden of bronchiectasis. *Clin Pulm Med.* 2005;12:205–209.
5. Kwak HJ, Moon JY, Choi YW, et al. High prevalence of bronchiectasis in adults: analysis of CT findings in a health screening program. *Tohoku J Exp Med.* 2010;222:237–242.
6. Fahim A, Wilmot R, Hart SP. Emphysema and bronchiectasis secondary to alpha-1 antitrypsin deficiency. *J Coll Physicians Surg Pak.* 2013;23:224–225.
7. Kang EY. Large airway diseases. *J Thorac Imaging.* 2011;26:249–262.
8. Zaid AA, Elnazir B, Greally P. A decade of non-cystic fibrosis bronchiectasis 1996–2006. *Ir Med J.* 2010;103:77–79.
9. Ni Y, Shi G, Yu Y, et al. Clinical characteristics of patients with chronic obstructive pulmonary disease with comorbid bronchiectasis: a systemic review and meta-analysis. *Int J Chron Obstruct Pulmon Dis.* 2015;10:1465–1475.
10. Brower KS, Del Vecchio MT, Aronoff SC. The etiologies of non-CF bronchiectasis in childhood: a systematic review of 989 subjects. *BMC Pediatr.* 2014;14:4.
11. Banjar HH. Clinical profile of Saudi children with bronchiectasis. *Indian J Pediatr.* 2007;74:149–152.
12. Al-Malki TA. Lung resections in bronchiectasis due to lipoid pneumonia: a custom-design approach. *East Afr Med J.* 2000;77:203–205.
13. Boyton RJ. Regulation of immunity in bronchiectasis. *Med Mycol.* 2009;47(suppl 1):S175–S182.
14. Soto-Cardenas MJ, Perez-De-Lis M, Bove A, et al. Bronchiectasis in primary Sjogren's syndrome: prevalence and clinical significance. *Clin Exp Rheumatol.* 2010;28:647–653.
15. Shadick NA, Fanta CH, Weinblatt ME, et al. Bronchiectasis. A late feature of severe rheumatoid arthritis. *Medicine (Baltimore).* 1994;73:161–170.
16. Zariwala MA, Omran H, Ferkol TW. The emerging genetics of primary ciliary dyskinesia. *Proc Am Thorac Soc.* 2011;8:430–433.
17. Boon M, Jorissen M, Proesmans M, et al. Primary ciliary dyskinesia, an orphan disease. *Eur J Pediatr.* 2013;172:151–162.
18. Boon M, Smits A, Cuppens H, et al. Primary ciliary dyskinesia: critical evaluation of clinical symptoms and diagnosis in patients with normal and abnormal ultrastructure. *Orphanet J Rare Dis.* 2014;9:11.
19. Accurso FJ. Update in cystic fibrosis 2005. *Am J Respir Crit Care Med.* 2006;173:944–947.
20. Moskowitz SM, Chmiel JF, Stemen DL, et al. CFTR-related disorders. *GeneReviews.* 2008. Available from http://www.ncbi.nlm.nih.gov/books/NBK1250/
21. Regamey N, Jeffery PK, Alton EW, et al. Airway remodelling and its relationship to inflammation in cystic fibrosis. *Thorax.* 2011;66:624–629.
22. Sagel SD, Gibson RL, Emerson J, et al. Impact of *Pseudomonas* and *Staphylococcus* infection on inflammation and clinical status in young children with cystic fibrosis. *J Pediatr.* 2009;154:183–188.
23. Madeira A, dos Santos SC, Santos PM, et al. Proteomic profiling of Burkholderia cenocepacia clonal isolates with different virulence potential retrieved from a cystic fibrosis patient during chronic lung infection. *PLoS One.* 2013;8:e83065.
24. Sagel SD, Sontag MK, Accurso FJ. Relationship between antimicrobial proteins and airway inflammation and infection in cystic fibrosis. *Pediatr Pulmonol.* 2009;44:402–409.
25. King PT, Hutchinson P, Holmes PW, et al. Assessing immune function in adult bronchiectasis. *Clin Exp Immunol.* 2006;144:440–446.
26. Karakoc GB, Yilmaz M, Altintas DU, et al. Bronchiectasis: still a problem. *Pediatr Pulmonol.* 2001;32:175–178.
27. van de Ven AA, van Montfrans JM, Terheggen-Lagro SW, et al. A CT scan score for the assessment of lung disease in children with common variable immunodeficiency disorders. *Chest.* 2010;138:371–379.
28. Kapur N, Grimwood K, Masters IB, et al. Lower airway microbiology and cellularity in children with newly diagnosed non-CF bronchiectasis. *Pediatr Pulmonol.* 2012;47:300–307.
29. Moulton BC, Barker AF. Pathogenesis of bronchiectasis. *Clin Chest Med.* 2012;33:211–217.
30. Canessa PA, Santini D, Zanelli M, et al. Pulmonary tumourlets and microcarcinoids in bronchiectasis. *Monaldi Arch Chest Dis.* 1997;52:138–139.
31. Amorim A, Gamboa F, Azevedo P. New advances in the therapy of non-cystic fibrosis bronchiectasis. *Rev Port Pneumol.* 2013;19:266–275.

32 Asthma

Marie-Christine Aubry, M.D., and Allen P. Burke, M.D.

Incidence

Asthma has a high prevalence, affecting 6% to 10% of the US population. Although present in all age groups, the prevalence of asthma is higher in children. Women and blacks are also more likely to develop asthma over the course of their life.[1] Allergic diseases, such as asthma, have markedly increased in the past half century and are associated with urbanization.[2]

Clinical

Asthma almost always starts in childhood, upon sensitization to common inhaled allergens, such as house dust mites, cockroaches, animal dander, fungi, and pollens. In addition to atopy, other potential risk factors include secondhand exposure to smoking, respiratory infections, obesity, and some occupations. Clinically, asthma may present as sudden onset of bronchoconstriction and wheezing that may be life-threatening "asthma attacks," or have a more indolent course. Patients may complain of cough, tightness of chest, and breathlessness, and these symptoms characteristically are variable and triggered by factors such as exercise, infection, allergens, and drugs. Other clinical conditions are seen in patients with asthma and may cause exacerbation of their asthma. These include eosinophilic pneumonia (Chapter 26), eosinophilic granulomatosis with polyangiitis (aka Churg-Strauss syndrome) (Chapter 49), rhinosinusitis, and allergic bronchopulmonary aspergillosis (Chapter 33). Although there may be some overlap in airway obstruction and reversibility with chronic obstructive pulmonary diseases, these two conditions are considered separate clinically. The diagnosis of asthma is based on a compatible clinical history, spirometry confirming response to bronchodilators, response to trial of steroids, and positive exercise test.

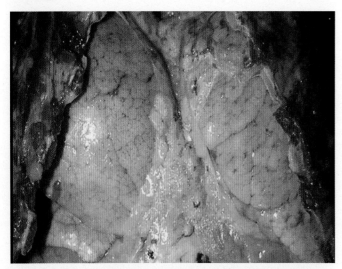

FIGURE 32.1 ▲ Autopsy lungs, patient dying from acute asthma attack "status asthmaticus." The lungs are hyperinflated, such that they nearly approach at midline after removal of the chest wall.

Pathophysiology

The hallmarks of asthma are reversible airflow obstruction, nonspecific bronchial hyperreactivity, and chronic airway inflammation. Dendritic cells take up allergens, process antigens, and present them to naive helper T cells, resulting in the activation of allergen-specific Th2 cells. Also involved are Th17 and Th9 T lymphocytes, which produce IL-17A, IL-17F, and IL-22, inducing airway inflammation and smooth muscle contraction.

Radiologic Findings

During an attack, chest x-rays may show hyperinflation, bronchial thickening, and focal atelectasis, or be completely normal. Complications such as consolidation and pneumomediastinum can also been seen on chest x-ray.[3]

High-resolution computed tomography is useful in patients with chronic or recurring symptoms to exclude possible associated disease such as allergic bronchopulmonary aspergillosis (see Chapter 33) and bronchiectasis (see Chapter 31). Expiratory scans are useful in demonstrating a mosaic pattern of lung attenuation with lucent areas representing air trapping.

Gross Findings

At autopsy, lungs are usually hyperinflated when death was caused by an acute attack (Fig. 32.1). There may be secondary changes of bronchiectasis and pneumomediastinum.

Microscopic Findings

The cytologic and histologic features seen in asthma are not specific to asthma and may be present in other conditions such as chronic bronchitis and bronchiectasis (Chapters 30 and 31). Furthermore, there are two pathologic variants of asthma with differing histologic findings, eosinophilic and noneosinophilic asthma.[4]

Cytologic specimens from patient with asthma contain various bodies related to goblet cell hyperplasia and increased mucous production such as creola bodies and Curschmann spirals.[5-7] Creola bodies are composed of ciliated columnar cells sloughed from the bronchial mucosa that may mimic adenocarcinoma in adult sputa.[8] Curschmann spirals are coiled strands of mucus that have extruded from hyperplastic mucus glands (Fig. 32.2). In the eosinophilic variant of asthma, eosinophils are numerous and associated with Charcot-Leyden crystals (Fig. 32.2). These crystals appear as eosinophilic rhomboid structures, the result of aggregated eosinophilic granules. In noneosinophilic variant, eosinophils are not present. Increased mast cells are present in both types.

Histologically, the segmental and subsegmental bronchi are typically affected. The bronchial epithelium is often denuded. When intact, goblet cell hyperplasia is seen. Basal membrane thickening is variable and absent in the noneosinophilic variant. The smooth muscle is hypertrophic and, in cases of fatal asthma, hyperplastic (Fig. 32.3). The layer of submucosal glands is thicker, and submucosal glands contain more mucous cells (Fig. 32.4). Inflammation is prominent, a mixture of lymphocytes and mast cells, and eosinophils, in cases of eosinophilic asthma. In wedge biopsies of a subset of patients with severe refractory asthma, interstitial granulomas are present in addition to the airway histologic findings. This constellation of findings has been coined "asthmatic granulomatosis".[9] Patients with fatal asthma have more prominent mucous plugging and goblet cell hyperplasia than that of nonfatal asthma (Fig. 32.5).[10] A prominent neutrophilic infiltrate has also been reported to be characteristic in sudden-onset fatal asthma.

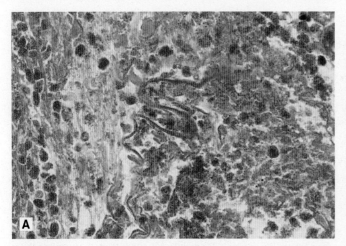

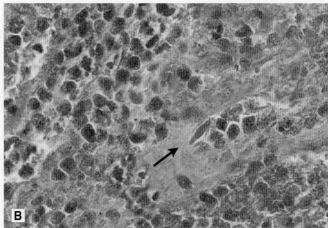

FIGURE 32.2 ▲ **A.** Curschmann spiral. The spiral is an elongated, serpiginous mucus strand. **B.** Charcot-Leyden crystal (*arrow*). Rhomboid-shaped crystal in a background of necrotic eosinophils.

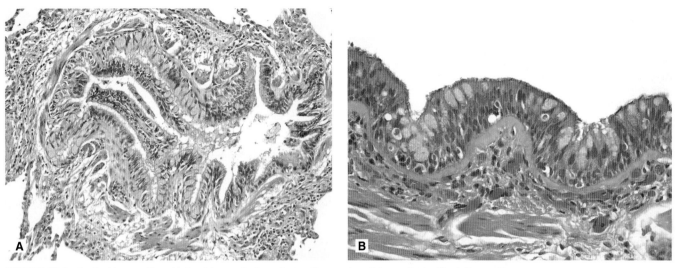

FIGURE 32.3 ▲ **A.** Airway with goblet cell hyperplasia and smooth muscle cell hyperplasia. The inflammation is mixed with predominance of eosinophils. **B.** High power of the airway mucosa demonstrating thickened basal membrane.

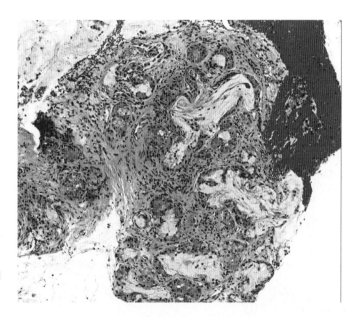

FIGURE 32.4 ▲ Mucus gland hyperplasia. There is typically increased number of mucus glands in the submucosal gland layer in patients with asthma.

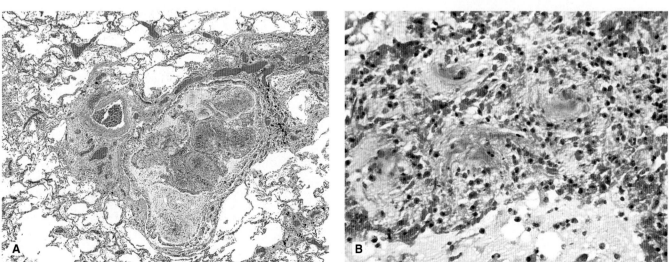

FIGURE 32.5 ▲ **A.** In fatal asthma, the airways are distended by mucus plugs. **B.** The plugs contain numerous eosinophils, most of which are degranulated or necrotic.

Treatment and Prognosis

The cornerstone of the treatment is to control the asthma. The goals are to decrease the severity of the symptoms and decrease the risk and number of attacks, with minimal side effects from treatment (https://www.nhlbi.nih.gov/files/docs/guidelines/asthma_qrg.pdf). The outcome of patients with asthma depends on its severity and early and successful management.[11]

REFERENCES

1. *Asthma: Data, Statistics, and Surveillance.* National Center for Environmental Health; 2013. Available from http://www.cdc.gov/asthma/asthmadata.htm.
2. Alfven T, Braun-Fahrlander C, Brunekreef B, et al. Allergic diseases and atopic sensitization in children related to farming and anthroposophic lifestyle—the PARSIFAL study. *Allergy.* 2006;61:414–421.
3. Gillies JD, Reed MH, Simons FE. Radiologic findings in acute childhood asthma. *J Can Assoc Radiol.* 1978;29:28–33.
4. Berry M, Morgan A, Shaw DE, et al. Pathological features and inhaled corticosteroid response of eosinophilic and non-eosinophilic asthma. *Thorax.* 2007;62:1043–1049.
5. Gleich GJ. The pathology of asthma: with emphasis on the role of the eosinophil. *N Engl Reg Allergy Proc.* 1986;7:421–424.
6. Molinari M, Ruiu A, Biondi M, et al. Hyperdense mucoid impaction in allergic bronchopulmonary aspergillosis: CT appearance. *Monaldi Arch Chest Dis.* 2004;61:62–64.
7. Sakula A. Charcot-Leyden crystals and Curschmann spirals in asthmatic sputum. *Thorax.* 1986;41:503–507.
8. Yamada Y, Yoshihara S. Creola bodies in infancy with respiratory syncytial virus bronchiolitis predict the development of asthma. *Allergol Int.* 2010;59:375–380.
9. Wenzel SE, Vitari CA, Shende M, et al. Asthmatic granulomatosis: a novel disease with asthmatic and granulomatous features. *Am J Respir Crit Care Med.* 2012;186:501–507.
10. Aikawa T, Shimura S, Sasaki H, et al. Marked goblet cell hyperplasia with mucus accumulation in the airways of patients who died of severe acute asthma attack. *Chest.* 1992;101:916–921.
11. Koh MS, Irving LB. Evidence-based pharmacologic treatment for mild asthma. *Int J Clin Pract.* 2007;61:1375–1379.

33 Allergic Bronchopulmonary Aspergillosis

Joseph J. Maleszewski, M.D., Marie-Christine Aubry, M.D., and Allen P. Burke, M.D.

Definition

Allergic bronchopulmonary aspergillosis (ABPA) is a term used to describe exacerbation of underlying airway injury, usually in the setting of asthma or cystic fibrosis, by exposure and subsequent hypersensitivity to *Aspergillus*-associated antigens.

While *Aspergillus* is far and away the most common offending agent, other fungi (e.g., *Candida albicans*, *Curvularia* sp., *Helminthosporium* sp., *Torulopsis glabrata*, *Saccharomyces cerevisiae*, and *Trichosporon beigelii*) are known to produce antigens that have been associated with similar clinical and pathologic features. Hence, ABPA can be considered more broadly under the term "allergic bronchopulmonary fungal disease."

Epidemiology

Most patients with ABPA have an underlying chronic airway condition, with asthma being the most common and cystic fibrosis being the second. Hypersensitivity to *Aspergillus* is a relatively common phenomenon, occurring in ~25% of those with asthma. ABPA is less common, affecting anywhere between 1% and 13% of asthmatics and ~10% of those with cystic fibrosis.[1,2] Steroid-dependent asthmatics appear to be at higher risk for ABPA than do nonsteroid-dependent asthmatics.

Rarely, ABPA can affect individuals without clinical evident airway disease.[3] Those patients with congenital immunodeficiencies or chronic granulomatous disease are also at increased risk for developing ABPA.[4]

Clinical, Laboratory, and Radiologic Features

Symptoms

Most patients with ABPA present with worsening of their underlying lung disease. Exacerbation of symptoms of asthma, such as increased cough, wheezing, and expectoration of sputum plugs often occurs. Episodic fever and/or hemoptysis may also occur. These symptoms often occur despite aggressive antiasthmatic medications. Over the years, a list of major and minor criteria that combine these symptoms has been created to aide in rendering a diagnosis in those patients with asthma (Table 33.1). Modifications have been made to evaluate other patients (such as those with cystic fibrosis) as well. A subset of patients with ABPA may also have symptoms of chronic sinusitis, which may indicate concurrent allergic fungal sinusitis.

The clinical presentation is divided into five stages (Table 33.2). Stage I is considered the acute phase, characterized by fever, cough, chest pain, hemoptysis, and/or sputum production. Stage II is remission in which the patient is usually asymptomatic or has had stabilization of their asthma. Stage III is exacerbation, where symptoms of the acute phase may return or laboratory/radiologic evidence of the disease is again apparent. In stage IV, there is persistent severe asthma that is corticosteroid dependent. Patients with stage V disease will usually exhibit cyanosis and extreme dyspnea. These end-stage patients will usually also have radiologically or pathologically evident fibrosis.

Serologic and Hypersensitivity Testing

Patients with ABPA will almost invariably have elevated total serum IgE concentration, as well as antibodies (IgE or IgG) directed against fungal organisms (most commonly *Aspergillus fumigates*). Cutaneous hypersensitivity to fungal antigens is also a common finding, with ABPA patients demonstrating an almost immediate wheal-and-flare reaction.

Microbiology

The most common offending organism in ABPA is *Aspergillus fumigates*. While it is sometimes possible to culture such from sputum, the finding is neither sensitive nor specific for the diagnosis on its own.

Imaging

Chest radiography can range from normal in the early stages of the disease to central and upper lung zone infiltrates in later phases. Mucoid impaction of the proximal airways may result in band-like opacities

TABLE 33.1   Diagnostic Criteria for ABPA

Major Criteria
Asthma
Cutaneous reactivity to *Aspergillus* or fungal antigens
Total serum IgE > 1,000 ng/mL
Elevated serum anti-*Aspergillus* (IgE and/or IgG)
Central bronchiectasis[a]

Minor Criteria
Radiologic pulmonary infiltrates
Peripheral eosinophilia (>500/mm³)
Precipitating antibodies to *Aspergillus*

[a]If not present, a diagnosis of seropositive allergic bronchopulmonary aspergillosis can be made.

extending from the hilum. Inflamed and thickened bronchi may also result in "ring signs/shadows," in a similar distribution. High-resolution computed tomography (HRCT) scans offer better assessment of the pattern and distribution. The central distribution of the bronchiectasis is perhaps the most characteristic sign of ABPA, radiologically.[6] Additional findings include mosaic attenuation, centrilobular nodules, and tree-in-bud opacities.

Treatment and Prognosis

The prognosis and treatment of patients with ABPA are largely driven by the clinical stage (Table 33.2), with the poorest prognosis seen in stages IV and V. Patients with stage I disease are typically managed with oral steroids, with imaging and sequential serum IgE levels to monitor for response. Most patients with uncomplicated disease will respond to the steroid and enter into remission (stage II). Some patients develop recurrence after initial response (Stage III). Those patients who progress to more advanced disease (stage IV) become steroid dependent and ultimately may develop end-stage (stage V) disease with hypercapnic respiratory failure and possibly heart failure (cor pulmonale).

Pathologic Features

Pathologic features of ABPA can be evaluated at the time of autopsy, explantation, lobectomy, or biopsy. Lung biopsy is usually not requisite for the diagnosis, but it can be helpful in cases of atypical presentation. Bronchoalveolar lavage is also sometimes done, usually

if respiratory status is stable, and there is some evidence for its therapeutic role.[7]

Gross Pathology

The gross pathology largely mirrors what is seen on high-resolution CT, namely, cylindrical bronchiectasis of the proximal airways involving the middle and upper lungs. Mucoid impaction is commonly identified, with the airways occluded by mucus. When significant occlusion is present, downstream atelectasis can result.

Histopathology

Transbronchial biopsies typically show nonspecific findings reflective of bronchiectasis (see Chapter 31), with changes of chronic reactive airway disease. At low power, the lung tissue in a wedge biopsy will usually exhibit an airway-centered process. At higher power, there will be obvious airway inflammation, increased eosinophils in the lamina propria, and airway wall smooth muscle hyperplasia. The airway lumina will often contain so-called allergic-type mucin (Fig. 33.1). This mucin is characteristically laminated with eosinophils (both whole cells and inflammatory cell debris) and mucoid material. Hyphal forms, commonly fragmented, can be identified within the mucus using a histochemical stain such as Grocott-methamine silver (GMS). There may be areas of either organizing or eosinophilic pneumonia present as well. The airway walls will often exhibit squamous metaplasia, owing to the chronic injury.

Sputum in cases of ABPA will demonstrate allergic-type mucus with Curschmann spirals and Charcot-Leyden crystals (see Chapter 32). The presence of fungi is variable and tends to consist of occasional fragmented hyphae.

Bronchocentric Granulomatosis

An uncommon reaction termed *bronchocentric granulomatosis* can develop in the context of ABPA. This tissue reaction is characterized by necrotizing granulomatous inflammation with partial destruction of the airway wall (Figs. 33.2 and 33.3). The accompanying inflammatory infiltrate is usually dense with a prominent eosinophilic component. Often, there is relatively abrupt transition from normal bronchial mucosa to the lesional area. Fungal hyphae may be identified within the airway necrosis. Histochemical stain such as GMS stain is usually required as the organisms are often rare and fragmented (Fig. 33.4).

TABLE 33.2   Clinical Stages of ABPA

Stage	Findings		
	Clinical	**Serologic**	**Radiologic**
I	Fever, cough, chest pain, hemoptysis, and sputum production	Elevated serum IgE	Normal or upper/middle lobe infiltrates
II	Asymptomatic/stable asthma	Normal or elevated serum IgE	No infiltrates
III	Similar to stage I	Elevated serum IgE	Upper/middle lobe infiltrates
IV	Persistent severe asthma	Normal or elevated serum IgE	With or without infiltrates
V	Cyanosis and severe dyspnea	Normal or elevated serum IgE	Cavitary lesions, extensive bronchiectasis, and fibrosis

Adapted from Patterson R, Greenberger PA, Halwig JM, et al. Allergic bronchopulmonary aspergillosis. Natural history and classification of early disease by serologic and roentgenographic studies. *Arch Intern Med.* 1986;146:916–918, Ref. 5.

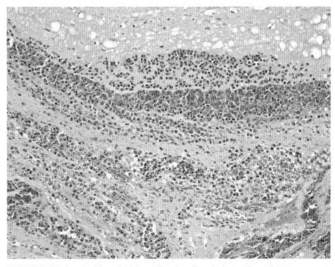

FIGURE 33.1 ▲ Mucoid impaction in allergic bronchopulmonary aspergillosis. The biopsy is mainly composed of so-called allergic mucin. The mucin contains layers of acellular mucin alternating with cellular mucin. The cells within the mucin are eosinophils, many of which are necrotic and degranulated.

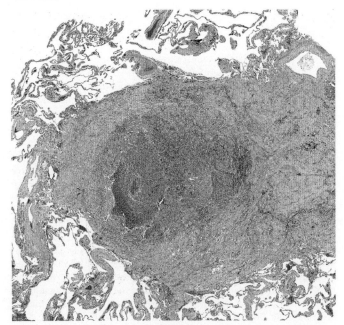

FIGURE 33.2 ▲ A medium-power photomicrograph exhibiting airway destruction by dense inflammation with vague granulomatous features (so-called bronchocentric granulomatosis).

Bronchocentric granulomatous inflammation may also occur in the setting of entities such as bronchogenic carcinoma, nonfungal infections, rheumatologic disease, and other granulomatous diseases (e.g., granulomatosis with polyangiitis, chronic granulomatous disease). This manifestation of lung injury differs from bronchocentric granulomatosis seen in patients with ABPA as it is often associated with necrotizing granulomatous inflammation involving the lung parenchyma, eosinophils are variable, and there may be other specific histologic features such as a necrotizing vasculitis or nonfungal infections.

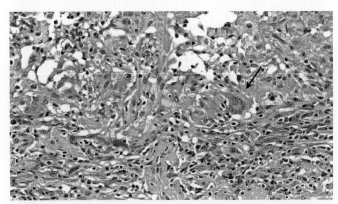

FIGURE 33.3 ▲ High-power photomicrograph of dense airway wall inflammation with increased eosinophils and rare giant cells (*arrow*).

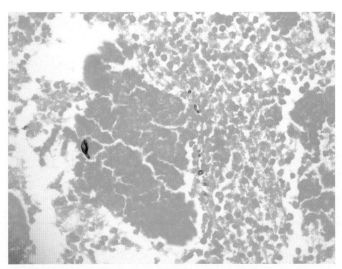

FIGURE 33.4 ▲ In the lumen, among the necrotic eosinophils, fragments of hyphae are identified (GMS stain).

Differential Diagnosis

Virtually all causes of inflammation with increased eosinophils and granulomatous disease can be included in the differential diagnosis for ABPA. These include, but are not limited to, eosinophilic pneumonia, drug reactions, infections, eosinophilic granulomatosis with polyangiitis (Churg-Strauss), and granulomatosis with polyangiitis (Wegener granulomatosis).

It is important to emphasize that ABPA is not considered a manifestation of invasive fungal disease (i.e., angioinvasive aspergillosis), because it represents a hypersensitivity reaction to the antigens of the fungus.

REFERENCES

1. Greenberger PA. Clinical aspects of allergic bronchopulmonary aspergillosis. *Front Biosci.* 2003;8:S119–S127.
2. Zander DS. Allergic bronchopulmonary aspergillosis: an overview. *Arch Pathol Lab Med.* 2005;129:924–928.
3. Glancy JJ, Elder JL, McAleer R. Allergic bronchopulmonary fungal disease without clinical asthma. *Thorax.* 1981;36:345–349.
4. Eppinger TM, Greenberger PA, White DA, et al. Sensitization to *Aspergillus* species in the congenital neutrophil disorders chronic granulomatous disease and hyper-IgE syndrome. *J Allergy Clin Immunol.* 1999;104:1265–1272.
5. Patterson R, Greenberger PA, Halwig JM, et al. Allergic bronchopulmonary aspergillosis. Natural history and classification of early disease by serologic and roentgenographic studies. *Arch Intern Med.* 1986;146:916–918.
6. Agarwal R, Khan A, Garg M, et al. Pictorial essay: allergic bronchopulmonary aspergillosis. *Indian J Radiol Imaging.* 2011;21:242–252.
7. Khalil KF. Therapeutic bronchoalveolar lavage with conventional treatment in allergic bronchopulmonary aspergillosis. *J Coll Physicians Surg Pak.* 2015;25:359–362.

34 Diseases of the Trachea and Bronchi

Joseph J. Maleszewski, M.D., and Allen P. Burke, M.D.

Introduction

Diseases of the trachea can result in stenosis, malacia (softening of the trachea), and tracheomegaly and involve congenital, infectious, and neoplastic processes (Table 34.1). Neoplastic entities will be discussed later in the book.

Conditions that Result in Stenosis

Congenital Stenosis

Tracheal stenosis in infants is rare. There may be generalized hypoplasia, funnel-shaped narrowing tapering to stenosis just proximal to the carina, or segmental stenosis. Severe tracheal stenosis resulting in atresia occurs in two in 100,000 newborns and requires a tracheoesophageal fistula for spontaneous breathing.[1]

More than half of the infants who manifest clinical symptoms show a long-segment stenosis, most commonly caused by complete tracheal rings producing a "napkin-ring" stenosis.[2] Vascular rings caused by congenital aortic arch anomalies and bronchogenic cysts may result in extrinsic compression of the trachea. Tracheal stenosis is more prevalent in infants with Down syndrome and may be associated with bronchial abnormalities and pulmonary agenesis.[3]

When limited in length, tracheal stenosis is amenable to resection with anastomosis. A variety of surgical options have been recommended.[4]

Relapsing Polychondritis

Relapsing polychondritis is an autoimmune disorder characterized by recurrent progressive inflammatory episodes involving cartilage of the ear, nose, larynx, peripheral joints, and tracheobronchial tree. In addition to stenosis, tracheomalacia can also occur. The disease generally presents in young adulthood. Respiratory tract involvement occurs in up to 50% of patients, is uncommon at presentation, and carries a poor prognosis. The larynx and subglottic trachea are most involved initially, with progression to the distal trachea and bronchi, often with patchy involvement.

Histopathologically, the disease is characterized by mixed acute and chronic inflammation in and around the cartilage. Tracheal stenosis occurs when there is fibrosis and contraction of the airway and may be severe. Loss of structural cartilaginous support may result in tracheobronchomalacia. The process is centered on the cartilage and therefore spares the posterior membranous wall of the trachea, unless there is constrictive fibrosis.[5,6]

Severe stenosis may necessitate tracheostomy in addition to steroid therapy. Stenting to the level of the tracheal bifurcation may also be required.[7]

Amyloidosis

Pulmonary amyloidosis occurs in three forms (see Chapter 27): diffuse interstitial amyloidosis, nodular amyloidosis, and tracheobronchial deposits of submucosal amyloid. Tracheobronchial amyloidosis occurs in only 1.1% of patients with amyloid.[8] Computed tomography demonstrates nodular and irregular narrowing of the tracheal lumen. Pulmonary manifestations include lobar or segmental collapse, recurrent pneumonia, bronchiectasis, and obstructive hyperinflation.[8] There may be secondary mural calcification or ossification of the lesions, leading to confusion with tracheobronchopathia osteochondroplastica, although there is no sparing of the posterior membrane.

Sarcoidosis

Although distal bronchial involvement is common in sarcoidosis, the larynx and upper trachea are affected in only in 1% to 3% of patients, with a slightly higher rate of involvement of the distal trachea and mainstem bronchi. Narrowing of the airway is caused by extrinsic compression by paratracheal lymph nodes or may be the result of thickening of the mucosa and submucosa by sarcoid granulomas. The classic endobronchial finding is the raised "cobblestone" appearance of the mucosa.[5] Positive biopsies show granulomas, typically non-necrotizing, in the lamina propria or submucosa (see Chapter 22).

Granulomatosis with Polyangiitis

Airway involvement is found in 15% to 55% of patients with granulomatosis with polyangiitis (GPA, Wegener granulomatosis) (see Chapter 48) and is more frequent in women younger than 30 years.[9]

TABLE 34.1   Diseases Affecting the Trachea and Proximal Bronchi

Conditions that result in tracheobronchial narrowing
Congenital stenosis
Relapsing polychondritis
Amyloidosis
Sarcoidosis
Systemic autoimmune diseases
- Wegener granulomatosis
- Ulcerative colitis
Tracheopathia osteoplastica
IgG4-related disease
Postintubation

Tracheobronchomalacia
Congenital
COPD
Trauma
Cystic fibrosis
Polychondritis

Tracheobronchomegaly (Mounier-Kuhn disease)
Miscellaneous congenital conditions
Tracheal bronchus
Accessory cardiac bronchus
Congenital bronchial atresia

Infections
Viral
Fungal
Bacterial

Benign tumors
Solitary papillomas
Recurrent respiratory papillomatosis
Hamartomas
Granular cell tumor

Malignant tumors
Squamous cell carcinoma
Adenoid cystic carcinoma
Metastatic tumors
- Local extension: thyroid, esophagus, larynx, lung
- Hematogenous: melanoma, renal cell, breast

More distal thickening in the segmental and subsegmental bronchi is present in almost 75% of patients.[10] Subglottic stenosis is the most frequent airway manifestation in GPA, seen in 9 of 10 patients in one series.[10]

Histopathologically, endobronchial biopsies of tracheobronchial GPA show necrosis, giant cells, vasculitis, capillaritis, and microabscesses. Slightly more than one-third of biopsies show features supportive of the diagnosis, whereas the remainder show nonspecific inflammation or are normal.[9]

Inflammatory Bowel Disease

Tracheobronchial involvement of Crohn disease is rare and can manifest as airway obstruction, including luminal narrowing from the subglottic trachea to the proximal main bronchus.[11] Large airway involvement may also complicate ulcerative colitis, as diffuse sclerosing tracheobronchitis.[12] Histologic features are nonspecific and show acute and chronic tracheitis with mucosal ulceration, diffuse and chronic submucosal inflammation, and fibrosis.

Tracheopathia Osteoplastica (Tracheobronchopathia Osteochondroplastica)

Tracheobronchopathia osteochondroplastica is an idiopathic disease of the trachea and large bronchi characterized by submucosal fibro-osseous nodules projecting into the lumens of the airways. Only 0.1% of all endobronchial biopsies show features consistent with the disease.[13] Patients are usually elderly and generally asymptomatic but may complain of nonproductive cough and dyspnea. By computed tomography, small submucosal osteocartilaginous nodules of high density consistent with calcium are present in the cartilaginous portion of the airways sparing the posterior portion (Fig. 34.1).

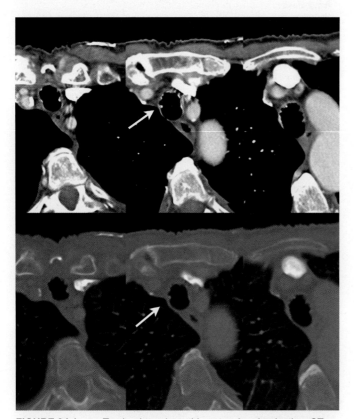

FIGURE 34.1 ▲ Tracheobronchopathia osteochondroplastica. CT scan shows projections into the tracheal lumen (*arrows*) some of which are of bone density. The anterior distribution and sparing of the posterior membranous trachea are evident.

Endobronchial or endotracheal biopsy is diagnostic in 70% of patients with the disease but frequently requires multiple biopsies, because the bony lesions are difficult to grasp with the bioptome.[14] Autopsy studies have shown osseous and cartilaginous nodules in the tracheal submucosa and lamina propria. Serial sections of the nodules have demonstrated continuity between the submucosal lesions and the tracheal cartilaginous rings only a minority of cases. Squamous metaplasia is common in the overlying mucosa.[14]

The differential diagnosis includes relapsing polychondritis and tracheobronchial amyloidosis. If dystrophic ossification or chondroid metaplasia involving the submucosa or lamina propria is found, the diagnosis of tracheobronchopathia osteochondroplastica can be assumed. Calcification of airway cartilage may be normal in old age, particularly in women, but are not associated with soft tissue ossification. Similarly, relapsing polychondritis results in degeneration and secondary calcification of the cartilage, but block-like calcification and nodular calcifications of the lamina propria and submucosa are absent. Amyloidosis has been reported in a subset of patients with tracheobronchopathia osteochondroplastica; therefore, Congo red staining can be a useful adjunct.

Tracheobronchial Tuberculosis

Tuberculosis is in the differential diagnosis of diffuse tracheobronchial thickening. Tracheobronchial tuberculosis has been reported in 10% to 40% of patients with pulmonary parenchymal tuberculosis through bronchoscopic examination[15] (see Chapter 40). In over half of patients, there are parenchymal lesions with paratracheal or peribronchial lymphadenopathy. In the remainder of the patients, a lack of parenchymal lesions suggests direct submucosal spread of mycobacterium along the peribronchial lymphatic channels. Sputum cytology has a relatively low yield, but high-resolution computed tomography is more sensitive in demonstrating tubercular involvement of tracheobronchial tree.

Endobronchial tuberculosis is more prevalent in young female patients. There is typically involvement of the long segment of the distal trachea and proximal bronchi. The endoscopic gross appearance has been classified as actively caseating, edematous–hyperemic, fibrostenotic, tumorous, granular, ulcerative, and bronchitic, with the granular and caseating types more likely to yield positive culture.[16] The fibrostenotic type accounts for < 10% of cases. Fibrosis with luminal narrowing or obstruction is more frequent in the left main bronchus.[5] Some degree of stenosis may develop in up to 90% of patients with endobronchial tuberculosis despite antimicrobial treatment. Imaging findings may occasionally mimic bronchogenic carcinoma, necessitating biopsy to for definitive diagnosis.[5]

Bronchoscopic biopsy is considered the most reliable method for confirmation of the diagnosis of endobronchial tuberculosis, with 30% to 84% sensitivity.[15] Granulomatous inflammation (with or without necrosis) as well as necrosis without overt granulomatous inflammation are considered diagnostic. Other nonspecific findings include edema of the lamina propria, nodular fibrosis, and chronic bronchial inflammation with linear fibrosis.[16]

IgG4-Related Disease

Tracheobronchial stenosis is a rare manifestation of pulmonary IgG4-related disease.[17] More commonly, bronchovascular bundles in the lung parenchyma are involved[18,19] (Chapter 51). IgG4 disease may result in a mediastinal mass (sclerosing mediastinitis) that infiltrates the trachea[20] and, occasionally, diffuse bronchial wall thickening.[21] Airway involvement is typically but not invariably accompanied by bilateral hilar lymphadenopathy.[22] Endobronchial or endotracheal biopsy may disclose features typical of IgG4-related disease, namely, storiform fibrosis, entrapment of veins and lymphoid tissue, and lymphocytic infiltrate with abundant IgG4-positive plasma cells (Fig. 34.2).

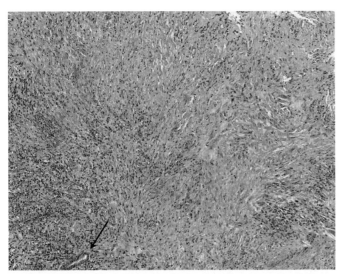

FIGURE 34.2 ▲ IgG4-related disease. There is a dense fibroinflammatory process composed of thick collagen bands in a vaguely storiform pattern, with a background of chronic inflammation. An entrapped mucous gland of the trachea is seen at the bottom left (*arrow*).

Postintubation Tracheal Stenosis

Tracheal stenosis is a serious complication of prolonged intubation that frequently requires surgery if long or multisegmental.[23] With the implementation of low-pressure cuffs, the incidence has been reduced to <1%.[23]

Histopathologically, there is squamous metaplasia, chronic inflammation and fibrosis in the lamina propria (Fig. 34.3), osseous metaplasia of cartilage (which can be a normal finding in the elderly), and dense scarring around the cartilaginous rings.[24] The mechanism of injury is initial necrosis of the mucosa, followed by granulation tissue formation, fibrosis, and cicatrization.

Tracheal wall thickening can also be caused by granulation tissue and scar formation around stents placed for various causes of stenosis, including tuberculosis.[25]

Broncholithiasis

Although not a cause of diffuse tracheobronchial thickening, broncholithiasis may distort the lumen of a proximal bronchus and cause stenosis. The underlying abnormality is usually calcified granulomatous lymphadenopathy caused by tuberculous or fungal infection. Calcified material perforates and obstructs the airway, which leads to postobstructive changes of atelectasis, pneumonitis, mucous impaction, and bronchiectasis. Broncholithiasis is more common in the right lung, especially the right middle lobe.[5]

Tracheo- and Bronchomalacia

Congenital Tracheomalacia

Tracheomalacia is caused by increased compliance and excessive collapsibility of the central airway caused by weakness of the supporting cartilage and occurs in ~1 in 2,100 children.[26] Severe tracheomalacia in children has been termed "major airway collapse" and can be classified into three groups. The first, congenital tracheomalacia without airway compression includes cases caused by severe prematurity, esophageal atresia, tracheoesophageal fistula, mucopolysaccharidoses, and Larsen syndrome. The second group is caused by extrinsic compression, such as that from vascular anomalies, cysts, tumors, and thymus or thyroid enlargement. The third type is associated with major airway collapse and refers to acquired malacia arising from prolonged ventilatory support, tracheotomy, or severe tracheobronchitis.[27]

Congenital tracheomalacia is exceedingly rare. Most clinical cases of tracheomalacia in which the trachea has been studied have cartilage plate deficiency rather than cartilage that is abnormally pliant. There is an increased risk in trisomy 21 of laryngomalacia (50%), tracheomalacia (33%), tracheal bronchus (17%), and bronchomalacia (17%). Other associations in infants include polychondritis, compressive cardiovascular anomalies, Larsen syndrome, and various chondrodystrophies.[4,28]

Clinically, the diagnosis of tracheomalacia is made by collapse of the trachea during expiration. Sudden exacerbation of symptoms may occur during induction of anesthesia.[29] Treatment includes surgical aortopexy to suspend the anterior wall of the trachea, stenting, long-term positive pressure ventilation, and tracheostomy.[30]

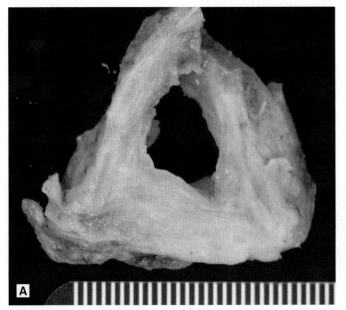
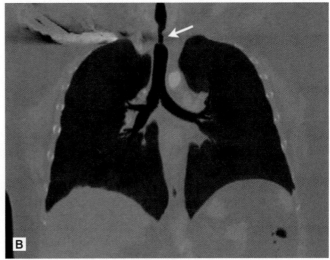

FIGURE 34.3 ▲ Postintubation tracheal stenosis. **A.** The gross specimen of the resected trachea shows marked scarring. The posterior membrane is at the bottom. **B.** CT scan showing narrowing (*arrow*).

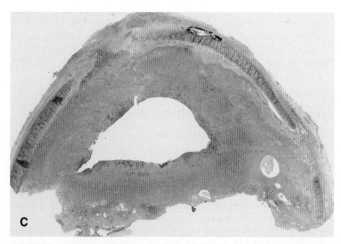

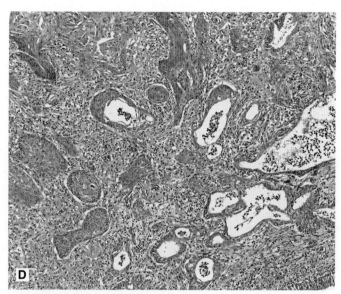

FIGURE 34.3 (*Continued*) ▲ **C.** Microscopic section demonstrating fibrosis. The cartilaginous segment is at the bottom. **D.** There is marked inflammation and squamous metaplasia of submucosal glands.

Chronic Obstructive Lung Disease

Using criteria of >50% reduction in the cross-sectional area of the tracheal lumen at end-expiration, tracheobronchomalacia occurs in 7% to 53% of patients with chronic obstructive lung disease and often correlates with the degree of emphysema.[31-33]

Histopathologic studies have shown atrophy of the bronchial cartilage in emphysema, with mild chronic inflammation presumably caused by irritation of cigarette smoke.[34]

Trauma and Iatrogenic

Analogous to tracheal stenosis, prolonged intubation may result in central airway disease manifested as tracheomalacia, especially in premature infants with respiratory distress syndrome.[35] Tracheotomy also increases the risk of tracheomalacia[35] as does any trauma causing loss of cartilage, such as external trauma and surgery, including transplantation.

Recurrent infection

Chronic infections of the airway generally result in ectasia of the bronchi (bronchiectasis), more so than the trachea (see Chapter 36). Of the causes of bronchiectasis, cystic fibrosis shows manifestations of tracheomalacia in 15% of children and up to 70% of adults (Fig. 34.4) and is associated with pseudomonal infection.[26,36]

Tracheobronchomegaly (Mounier-Kuhn Disease)

Tracheobronchomegaly is characterized by marked dilatation of the trachea and main bronchi and is usually congenital (Mounier-Kuhn syndrome). The cause is believed to be atrophy of the longitudinal elastic fibers and thinning of the muscularis mucosa resulting in diverticula and tracheomalacia, possibly mediated by inflammation. The trachea is greater than 21 × 23 mm in women and greater than 25 × 27 mm in men.

On imaging, there is tracheobronchial luminal dilatation, often associated with a corrugated appearance of the tracheal wall and tracheal diverticulosis. Bronchiectasis and tracheobronchomalacia are also common.[5]

Histologically, there are decreased elastic fibers in the submucosal connective tissue; diffuse chronic inflammation, primarily comprised of CD4+ cells; and increased metalloproteases, which may play an etiologic role.[37]

Miscellaneous Congenital Conditions

Tracheal Bronchus

Tracheal bronchus refers to a congenitally abnormal bronchus originating from the trachea and is present in 3.7% of patients with congenital heart disease and 0.3% of patients without. The anomalous origin is usually located in the right lateral wall of the trachea within 2 cm of the carina and may predispose to recurrent infections.[5]

Accessory Cardiac Bronchus

An accessory cardiac bronchus is a supernumerary bronchus from the inner wall of the right main bronchus or an intermediate bronchus that advances toward the pericardium. It is more uncommon than tracheal bronchus (0.08%). Recurrent infection or hemoptysis can develop in a small percentage of patients.[5]

Bronchial Atresia

Bronchial atresia is a rare anomaly that characteristically presents with a pulmonary nodule and hyperinflation of the lung distal to the nodule.[38] Computed tomography scans demonstrated mucoceles, bronchial occlusions, parenchymal hyperinflation, and cysts.[39] Patients are usually young men without symptoms with incidental involvement of the apical–posterior segment of the left upper lobe. Occasionally, patients complain of fever, cough, or shortness of breath, resulting from postobstructive infections. Surgical excision is reserved for symptomatic cases.[40] Histopathologic findings are nonspecific in resected specimens and including extravasation mucus and peribronchial fibrosis (Fig. 34.5).

Miscellaneous Infections

Viral

The most common viral infection of the trachea is herpetic tracheitis, which generally occurs in immunosuppressed patients.[41,42] Biopsy may demonstrate intracytoplasmic inclusions seen on routine stains and in situ hybridization. Cytomegalovirus tracheitis has been described in an AIDS patient.[43] In children, influenza A is frequently found in cultures taken from patients with bacterial tracheitis, indicating coinfection.[44]

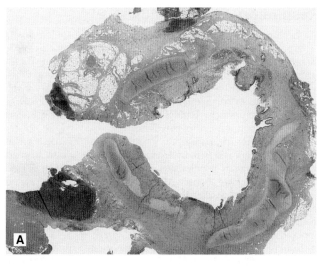

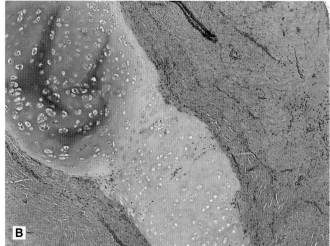

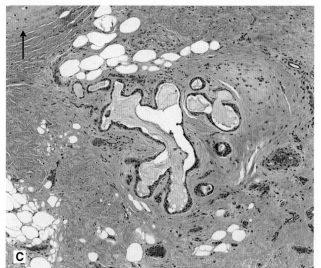

FIGURE 34.4 ▲ Tracheobronchomalacia, cystic fibrosis. **A.** A low magnification shows the mainstem bronchus. **B.** A higher magnification demonstrates necrosis of the cartilage and surrounding fibrosis. **C.** Submucosal glands show scarring, fibrosis, and squamous metaplasia. A portion of the cartilage is seen at the *arrow*.

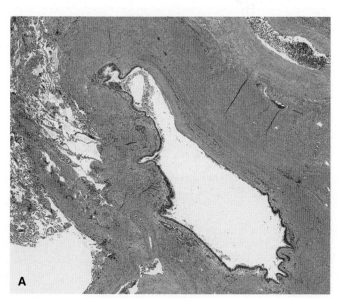

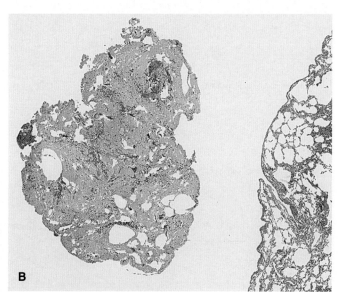

FIGURE 34.5 ▲ Bronchial atresia. This condition, although congenital, is often manifested in adulthood. The diagnosis rests on CT findings, and histologic features are nonspecific. **A.** Portion of bronchus with surrounding fibrosis. **B.** Fragments of the lung (**right**) and mucocele (**left**) that were removed in the surgical procedure.

Fungal

Large airway involvement by aspergillosis includes intrabronchial aspergilloma in nonimmunocompromised patients, allergic bronchopulmonary aspergillosis (see Chapter 33) in asthma patients, semi-invasive chronic necrotizing bronchial aspergillosis, and acute invasive tracheobronchitis. Acute fungal tracheobronchitis caused by aspergillosis results in ulcers and pseudomembranes. Nonspecific tracheobronchial wall thickening with smooth or nodular luminal narrowing is occasionally seen on CT scan.[45] Biopsies show ulceration of the surface respiratory epithelium, intense submucosal inflammation, and hyphae that are mostly superficial within the fibrin exudate. Other fungi can result in tracheitis, including Mucor, especially in immunocompromised patients (Fig. 34.6).

Bacterial

Bacterial tracheitis in the pediatric population results in acute upper airway obstruction and croup-like symptoms, with fever and severe cough. The diagnosis is generally made by direct visualization of the trachea via bronchoscopy.[46] The mean age is approximately 7 years of age, with more than 50% of patients requiring intubation. *Moraxella catarrhalis*, *Staphylococcus aureus*, *Streptococcus pneumoniae*, and *Haemophilus influenzae* are the most common isolates. Influenza A viral infection is a predisposing factor in three-fourths of patients.[44] Biopsy is generally not performed in the evaluation and treatment of bacterial tracheitis.

Respiratory Papillomatosis

Tracheobronchial papillomatosis (laryngotracheal papillomatosis) is believed to be acquired by vaginal transmission during childbirth in infants and via oral routes in adults. The disease generally involves the larynx, with extension to the trachea and lungs occurring in a minority of patients, indicating relatively poor prognosis. Pulmonary involvement by respiratory papillomatosis is discussed in Chapter 66. Because the course is typified by multiple recurrences, the current preferred term is "recurrent respiratory papillomatosis."

Childhood recurrent respiratory papillomatosis manifests on average at age 4 years and is more likely to involve the glottis than adult recurrent respiratory papillomatosis. Tracheal involvement is associated with younger age at onset. Almost two-thirds of children are boys. The course is more accelerated than in adults, with an average of 2.3 surgical procedures per year in the initial course, compared to only one in adults. Involvement of trachea or lungs occurs in 10% of children, as opposed to 3% of adults.

In adult recurrent respiratory papillomatosis, the average age is 34.0 years, also with a male predominance.[47] Occasionally, the disease is diagnosed in advanced age.[48]

The most common HPV types are 6 and 11, with coinfection not uncommon. In adults, HPV11 is associated with a more aggressive course.[47]

Histologically, the lesions resemble condylomas from other sites (Fig. 34.7).

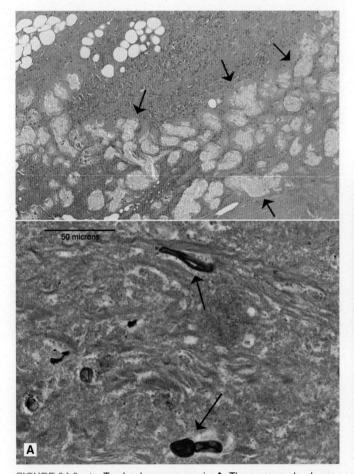

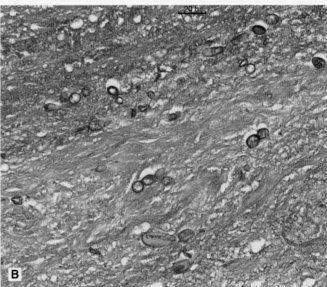

FIGURE 34.6 ▲ Tracheal mucormycosis. **A.** The mucous glands are necrotic (*arrows*, above). Hyphae are seen by Gomori methenamine–silver staining (*arrows*, below). **B.** The hyphae may often be seen with routine staining.

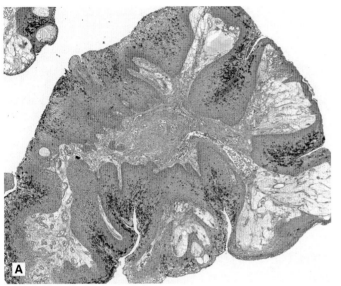
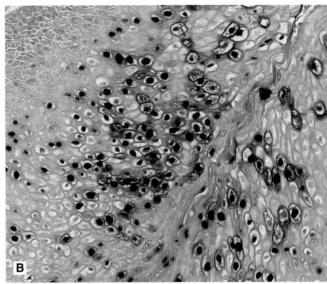

FIGURE 34.7 ▲ Respiratory papillomatosis, trachea. **A.** The lesions resemble a condyloma on low magnification (in situ hybridization for low-risk HPV). **B.** Higher magnification demonstrates hybridization signal in basally located nuclei.

REFERENCES

1. Krause U, Rodel RM, Paul T. Isolated congenital tracheal stenosis in a pre-term newborn. *Eur J Pediatr.* 2011;170(9):1217–1221.
2. Rimell FL, Stool SE. Diagnosis and management of pediatric tracheal steno-sis. *Otolaryngol Clin North Am.* 1995;28(4):809–827.
3. Yokoo N, et al. A case of Toriello-Carey syndrome with severe congenital tracheal stenosis. *Am J Med Genet A.* 2013;161(9):2291–2293.
4. Jaquiss RD. Management of pediatric tracheal stenosis and tracheomalacia. *Semin Thorac Cardiovasc Surg.* 2004;16(3):220–224.
5. Kang EY. Large airway diseases. *J Thorac Imaging.* 2011;26(4):249–262.
6. Kwong JS, Muller NL, Miller RR. Diseases of the trachea and main-stem bronchi: correlation of CT with pathologic findings. *Radiographics.* 1992;12(4):645–657.
7. Nakayama T, et al. Tracheal stenosis due to relapsing polychondritis man-aged for 16 years with a silicon T-tube covering the entire trachea. *Ann Thorac Surg.* 2011;92(3):1126–1128.
8. O'Regan A, et al. Tracheobronchial amyloidosis. The Boston University experience from 1984 to 1999. *Medicine (Baltimore).* 2000;79(2):69–79.
9. Daum TE, et al. Tracheobronchial involvement in Wegener's granulomato-sis. *Am J Respir Crit Care Med.* 1995;151(2 Pt 1):522–526.
10. Lee KS, et al. Thoracic manifestation of Wegener's granulomatosis: CT find-ings in 30 patients. *Eur Radiol.* 2003;13(1):43–51.
11. Henry MT, Davidson LA, Cooke NJ. Tracheobronchial involvement with Crohn's disease. *Eur J Gastroenterol Hepatol.* 2001;13(12):1495–1497.
12. Wilcox P, et al. Airway involvement in ulcerative colitis. *Chest.* 1987;92(1):18–22.
13. Jabbardarjani HR, et al. Tracheobronchopathia osteochondroplastica: pre-sentation of ten cases and review of the literature. *Lung.* 2008;186(5):293–297.
14. Leske V, et al. Tracheobronchopathia osteochondroplastica: a study of 41 patients. *Medicine (Baltimore).* 2001;80(6):378–390.
15. Lee JH, et al. Endobronchial tuberculosis. Clinical and bronchoscopic fea-tures in 121 cases. *Chest.* 1992;102(4):990–994.
16. Ozkaya S, et al. Endobronchial tuberculosis: histopathological subsets and microbiological results. *Multidiscip Respir Med.* 2012;7(1):34.
17. Ryu JH, et al. Spectrum of disorders associated with elevated serum IgG4 levels encountered in clinical practice. *Int J Rheumatol.* 2012;2012:232960.
18. Zen Y, et al. IgG4-related lung and pleural disease: a clinicopathologic study of 21 cases. *Am J Surg Pathol.* 2009;33(12):1886–1893.
19. Matsui S, et al. Respiratory involvement in IgG4-related Mikulicz's disease. *Mod Rheumatol.* 2012;22(1):31–39.
20. Noh D, Park CK, Kwon SY. Immunoglobulin G4-related sclerosing dis-ease invading the trachea and superior vena cava in mediastinum. *Eur J Cardiothorac Surg.* 2014;45(3):573–575.
21. Umeda M, et al. A case of IgG4-related pulmonary disease with rapid improvement. *Mod Rheumatol.* 2012;22(6):919–923.
22. Yamamoto H, et al. IgG4-related airway involvement which developed in a patient receiving corticosteroid therapy for autoimmune pancreatitis. *Intern Med.* 2011;50(24):3023–3026.
23. Bagheri R, et al. Outcome of surgical treatment for proximal long segment post intubation tracheal stenosis. *J Cardiothorac Surg.* 2013;8:35.
24. Welkoborsky HJ, et al. Microscopic examination of iatrogenic subglottic tracheal stenosis: observations that may elucidate its histopathologic origin. *Ann Otol Rhinol Laryngol.* 2014;123(1):25–31.
25. Eom JS, et al. Tracheal wall thickening is associated with the granulation tissue formation around silicone stents in patients with post-tuberculosis tracheal stenosis. *Yonsei Med J.* 2013;54(4):949–956.
26. Fischer AJ, et al. Tracheomalacia is associated with lower FEV1 and Pseudomonas acquisition in children with CF. *Pediatr Pulmonol.* 2014;49(10):960–970.
27. Mair EA, Parsons DS. Pediatric tracheobronchomalacia and major airway collapse. *Ann Otol Rhinol Laryngol.* 1992;101(4):300–309.
28. Kugler C, Stanzel F. Tracheomalacia. *Thorac Surg Clin.* 2014;24(1):51–58.
29. Okuda Y, et al. Airway obstruction during general anaesthesia in a child with congenital tracheomalacia. *Eur J Anaesthesiol.* 2000;17(10):642–644.
30. McNamara VM, Crabbe DC. Tracheomalacia. *Paediatr Respir Rev.* 2004;5(2):147–154.
31. Inoue M, et al. Incidence of tracheobronchomalacia associated with pul-monary emphysema: detection with paired inspiratory-expiratory multi-detector computed tomography using a low-dose technique. *Jpn J Radiol.* 2009;27(8):303–308.
32. Ochs RA, et al. Prevalence of tracheal collapse in an emphysema cohort as measured with end-expiration CT. *Acad Radiol.* 2009;16(1):46–53.
33. Sverzellati N, et al. Airway malacia in chronic obstructive pulmonary dis-ease: prevalence, morphology and relationship with emphysema, bronchiec-tasis and bronchial wall thickening. *Eur Radiol.* 2009;19(7):1669–1678.
34. Thurlbeck WM, et al. Bronchial cartilage in chronic obstructive lung disease. *Am Rev Respir Dis.* 1974;109(1):73–80.
35. Carden KA, et al. Tracheomalacia and tracheobronchomalacia in children and adults: an in-depth review. *Chest.* 2005;127(3):984–1005.
36. McDermott S, et al. Tracheomalacia in adults with cystic fibrosis: deter-mination of prevalence and severity with dynamic cine CT. *Radiology.* 2009;252(2):577–586.
37. Mitterbauer A, et al. Clinical-radiological, histological and genetic analyses in a lung transplant recipient with Mounier-Kuhn syndrome and end-stage chronic obstructive pulmonary disease. *Clin Respir J.* 2015;9(3):375–379.
38. Finck S, Milne EN. A case report of segmental bronchial atresia: radiologic evaluation including computed tomography and magnetic resonance imag-ing. *J Thorac Imaging.* 1988;3(1):53–57.

39. Wang Y, et al. Congenital bronchial atresia: diagnosis and treatment. *Int J Med Sci.* 2012;9(3):207–212.
40. Nordstrom CR, et al. Bronchial atresia with relapsing pulmonary infection in a middle-aged man. *Respir Care.* 2001;46(6):601–603.
41. Alvarez-Uria, G., et al. Herpetic tracheitis and polybacterial pneumonia in an immunocompetent young man is herpes tracheitis involved in the pathogenesis of bacterial pneumonia? *J Clin Virol.* 2008;41(2):164–165.
42. McCarthy DW, et al. Herpetic tracheitis and brachial plexus neuropathy in a child with burns. *J Burn Care Rehabil.* 1999;20(5):377–381.
43. Imoto EM, et al. Central airway obstruction due to cytomegalovirus-induced necrotizing tracheitis in a patient with AIDS. *Am Rev Respir Dis.* 1990;142(4):884–886.
44. Bernstein T, Brilli R, Jacobs B. Is bacterial tracheitis changing? A 14-month experience in a pediatric intensive care unit. *Clin Infect Dis.* 1998;27(3):458–462.
45. Franquet T, et al. Aspergillus infection of the airways: computed tomography and pathologic findings. *J Comput Assist Tomogr.* 2004;28(1):10–16.
46. Al-Mutairi B, Kirk V. Bacterial tracheitis in children: approach to diagnosis and treatment. *Paediatr Child Health.* 2004;9(1):25–30.
47. Omland T, et al. Risk factors for aggressive recurrent respiratory papillomatosis in adults and juveniles. *PLoS One.* 2014;9(11):e113584.
48. Shibuya H, et al. An adult case of multiple squamous papillomas of the trachea associated with human papilloma virus type 6. *Intern Med.* 2008;47(17):1535–1538.

35 Small Airways Disease, General Aspects

Fabio R. Tavora, M.D., Ph.D., and Allen P. Burke, M.D.

Bronchiolitis, General Concepts

Small airway disease refers to a number of lesions that mainly involve the bronchioles, described as segments of <2 mm in diameter (Fig. 35.1), a definition mainly derived from the radiology literature. The term "bronchiolitis" may sometimes be confusing to clinicians because it may be applied both as a descriptive term indicating inflammation of distal bronchioles and as a final pathologic diagnosis. Rarely, a surgical pathologist will encounter a biopsy or surgical specimen with no histologic alteration of small airways, in patients with clinically documented small airway disease. Therefore, a pathologic diagnosis of bronchiolitis only has a meaning when linked to the clinical and radiologic context.[1]

Bronchiolitis was first described more than 100 years ago with the term "bronchiolitis obliterans," which has evolved to a varied terminology that sometimes differs in the clinical, radiology, and pathology literature.[2,3] Bronchiolitis may be an isolated pathologic finding but often is secondary to diseases affecting other parts of the airways or lung parenchyma. Inflammation of bronchioles is a finding present in a large variety of lung lesions, and this may add to the confusion of the terminology. The term "small airway disease" is a generic descriptive term (often used by radiologists) that encompasses several

histologic appearances. A classification based on main histologic appearance, inflammatory cell type, and extent of disease is summarized in Table 35.1.

The histologic findings of the main types of bronchiolitis overlap and the causes and clinical manifestations are extremely varied. In children younger than 2 years of age, bronchiolitis is usually acute, is associated with several viruses (respiratory syncytial virus, enterovirus, and rhinovirus), and is rarely biopsied.[3–7]

Chronic "cellular" bronchiolitis in adults is usually diagnosed on high-resolution computed tomography and is associated mainly with collagen vascular disease, infection, and allograft rejection. Follicular bronchiolitis, or chronic peribronchial inflammation with lymphoid follicles, is especially frequent in adults with collagen vascular disease (classically Sjögren syndrome), and immunocompromised states, and less often hypersensitivity pneumonia and as a reaction to neoplasia. Respiratory bronchiolitis is directly related to tobacco exposure. Constrictive bronchiolitis is a late phase of diffuse bronchiolitis and is associated with collagen vascular disease, fume exposure, or drug reaction or is idiopathic.[8] Table 35.2 shows the main causes of histologic types of chronic bronchiolitis. Small airway disease in hypersensitivity pneumonitis and asthma is discussed in Chapters 23 and 32. Follicular bronchiolitis is discussed more comprehensively in Chapter 36.

Radiologic Findings

Most patients with small airway disease are diagnosed clinically with high-resolution computed tomography imaging. While the findings are nonspecific regarding either etiology or the histologic appearance of bronchiolitis, it provides clues to the presence of an underlying bronchiolar disorder.[3] Bronchioles are not seen on imaging in healthy state, but air trapping, distal insufflation, or thickening of the bronchiolar wall on HRCT yields indirect evidence of small airway disease.[9]

Direct signs of bronchiolitis include centrilobular thickening, peripheral nodules, so-called tree-in-bud opacities, and bronchiolectasis. Some authors argue that the presence of *tree-in-bud* opacities favors an infectious etiology to the bronchiolitis.[10] Tree-in-bud opacities may be caused by vascular thickening as well, for example, by microembolization and peribronchiolar fibrosis. Indirect signs of small airway disease are caused by obstruction of the bronchioles and subsequent underperfused lung from compensatory vasoconstriction, the appearance known as *mosaic attenuation* pattern on HRCT (see Chapter 10).[10,11] The second indirect sign is air trapping that can be accentuated on expiratory CT.

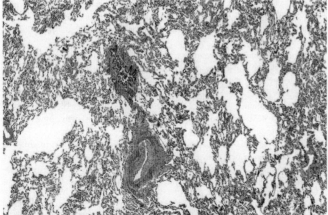

FIGURE 35.1 ▲ Normal lung. The distal bronchovascular bundle shows similar diameter of the bronchiole and arteriole, with minimal fibrous tissue surrounding the mucosa, and no inflammatory infiltrates. There is mild nonspecific intimal thickening of the artery.

TABLE 35.1   Histologic Classification of Small Airway Disease

Classification	Main Histologic Findings
Cellular bronchiolitis (acute, chronic, and eosinophilic)	Chronic bronchiolitis shows mainly lymphocytic infiltrates with mild fibrosis with reactive hyperplasia of respiratory epithelium. Long-term disease may lead to constrictive bronchiolitis and sometimes squamous metaplasia. Acute reveals neutrophils, necrotic debris and purulent material. In children, bronchiolitis is usually acute and seldom biopsied. A predominance of eosinophils may lead to the consideration of eosinophilic bronchiolitis (see Chapters 26 and 30).
Respiratory bronchiolitis	Cellular lymphocytic predominant infiltrates within the bronchiolar walls and surrounding tissue associated with collections of pigment-rich macrophages in the lumen and adjacent alveoli. Minimal to mild fibrosis is usually seen surrounding bronchioles.
Follicular bronchiolitis	Peribronchiolar lymphoid hyperplasia that extends into surrounding lung parenchyma with prominent germinal centers
Diffuse panbronchiolitis	Inflammation of all layers of the wall or respiratory bronchioles. There is transmural infiltration of the bronchiole and surrounding lung interstitium along with macrophages, plasma cells, and lymphocytes.
Constrictive bronchiolitis	Narrowing of bronchioles by submucosal and peribronchiolar fibrosis associated with lymphocytic infiltrates
Granulomatous bronchiolitis	Depending on the etiology, granulomas can be well or poorly formed, with or without necrosis, and generally are also present in the surrounding parenchyma, especially along the septa and pleura.
Cryptogenic organizing pneumonia	Plugs of granulation tissue and fibroblasts within a myxoid or edematous stroma, located within bronchiolar lumens, in association with surrounding lymphocytic inflammation.

Clinical Findings

Multiple syndromes can lead to manifestations of diffuse pulmonary disease affecting the distal bronchiolar tree. Some well-defined entities are discussed in separate chapters (asthma, follicular bronchiolitis, hypersensitivity pneumonitis, organizing pneumonia, transplant-associated constrictive bronchiolitis).

In general terms, clinical characteristics cannot be predicted by histologic findings, which can be very subtle in small airway disease. Pathologic changes in the distal bronchioles may cause both restrictive and obstructive symptoms, depending on the stage of the disease, on etiology, and on compartments involved.

TABLE 35.2   Etiologic Considerations of Small Airway Disease

Diagnosis	Possible Etiologies
Acute bronchiolitis	Viral infections (RSV, enterovirus, rhinovirus) Changes adjacent to bronchopneumonia Bronchocentric fungal infections Exposure to fumes Granulomatosis with polyangiitis—Wegener (rare)
Chronic bronchiolitis	Posttransplant Infection Collagen vascular disease Asthma GVHD Aspiration pneumonia
Follicular bronchiolitis	Collagen vascular disease (Sjögren, RA, lupus, IBD)
Diffuse panbronchiolitis	Idiopathic Familial with association with HLA Bw54
Granulomatous bronchiolitis	Sarcoidosis Hypersensitivity pneumonitis Middle lobe syndrome Infection Aspiration pneumonia Vasculitides (Wegener granulomatosis, IBD, etc.)
Constrictive bronchiolitis	Inhalation injury (gases, fumes, dust, organic substances) Bone marrow transplantation Lung transplantation (chronic rejection) Healed infection Drug reactions Collagen vascular disease IBD Idiopathic
Eosinophilic bronchiolitis	Various etiologies, including asthma, allergies, drug and idiopathic (see Chapter 30)

Cellular bronchiolitis is usually associated with infection, with a clinical presentation characterized by acute onset of cough, dyspnea, wheezing, sneezing, chest wall retractions, and cyanosis in some cases.[12-14] Acute infectious bronchiolitis has a short period of symptoms. Chronic diseases may also be associated with cellular bronchiolitis, such as in collagen vascular diseases. Constrictive bronchiolitis is associated with dyspnea, fatigue, low oxygenation, and nonproductive cough with associated obstructive pulmonary function pattern.[15] Chronic bronchiolitis can evolve to peribronchiolar scarring and peribronchiolar metaplasia and is associated with a restrictive pulmonary test pattern, dyspnea, and cough.[16]

Microscopic Findings

Acute bronchiolitis is characterized by mixed inflammation rich in neutrophils and rare to occasional eosinophils in association with sloughed epithelium and necrotic cellular debris within the alveolar spaces. There is a continuum between acute and chronic bronchiolitis, which has a predominance of lymphocytes with variable peribronchiolar fibrosis and bronchiolar metaplasia of surrounding alveoli (Figs. 35.2 to 35.4). In both acute and chronic bronchiolitis, the inflammation extends into the surrounding tissue. Other chronic changes are smooth muscle cell hypertrophy, increased goblet cells, and basement membrane thickening.

In cases of either acute or chronic bronchiolitis, if the disease is primary to the bronchioles (i.e., not secondary to parenchymal injury), the term cellular bronchiolitis can be helpful as a morphologic descriptor. The process may be associated with intraluminal polyps or constrictive (fibrotic) changes. The two most common types of cellular bronchiolitis are follicular bronchiolitis and respiratory bronchiolitis.

Follicular bronchiolitis as a special type of chronic airway disease shows the presence of lymphoid follicles with germinal centers around bronchiolar walls that are often thickened and also infiltrated by lymphocytes (Figs. 35.5 and 35.6) (see Chapter 36). The third form of chronic bronchiolitis is the granulomatous type. As in other types of bronchiolitis, there are several etiologies associated with this form, including hypersensitivity pneumonitis and bronchiolitis associated with immunodeficiency syndromes. In cases of aspiration, extraneous material sometimes is appreciated in association with necrotic debris and abscess formation.

Respiratory bronchiolitis (smoker's type) is common as incidental finding. There is accumulation of pigmented macrophages within the bronchiolar walls and surrounding alveolar lumina and parenchyma (Fig. 35.7). The overall architecture is usually mildly distorted by fibrosis, and the bronchiolar walls are mildly thickened and tortuous.

Constrictive bronchiolitis may be the end stage of chronic bronchiolitis or be a de novo phenomenon associated with various immune-related injuries. The diagnosis is based on severe bronchiolar wall

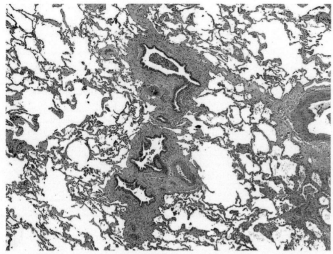

FIGURE 35.2 ▲ Bronchiolar fibrosis, incidental finding in a case of primary lung adenocarcinoma (not shown). Note increase in fibrous tissue with remodeling of the airway. There is no significant inflammation.

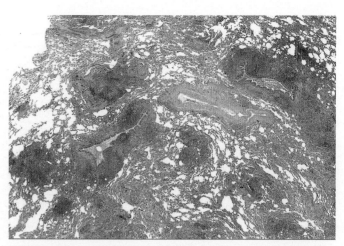

FIGURE 35.5 ▲ Follicular bronchiolitis, low power. Case of inflammatory bowel disease–associated follicular bronchiolitis. Observe lymphoid follicles in a bronchiolocentric distribution with occasional germinal centers.

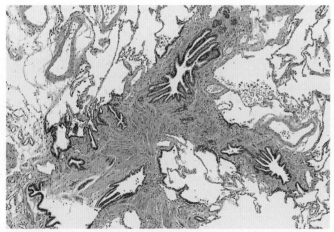

FIGURE 35.3 ▲ Small airway disease characterized by fibrosis of the bronchiolar wall, disordered architecture of the airway, and peribronchiolar metaplasia. There is minimal lymphocytic inflammation.

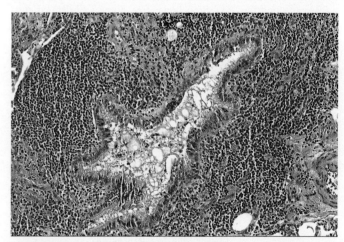

FIGURE 35.6 ▲ Follicular bronchiolitis, high power. Lymphoid hyperplasia and expanding bronchiolar wall.

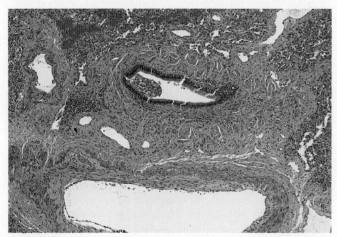

FIGURE 35.4 ▲ High-power view of bronchovascular bundle showing mild bronchiolar fibrosis. Note fibrous tissue separating epithelium from muscular layer of bronchiolar wall associated with mild chronic inflammation.

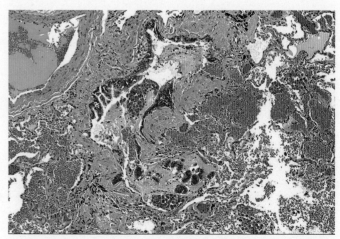

FIGURE 35.7 ▲ Respiratory bronchiolitis. There is airway disease characterized by bronchiolar fibrosis. Note also accumulation of pigmented macrophages within bronchiolar lumen and adjacent alveoli.

fibrosis, smooth muscle hyperplasia, and obliteration of the lumen that can be diffuse or patchy, making the diagnosis often difficult. There is variable amount of inflammation that decreases with the severity of the process.

Bronchiolitis Associated with Inhalational Injury

Significant airway injury can be seen in patients exposed to gases, fumes, and dusts. In an acute phase, severe and life-threatening symptoms may occur, including severe hypoxia, laryngospasm, and asphyxia.[3,17] Nitrogen dioxide is the prototype inhalant that leads to acute disease that later develops into constrictive bronchiolitis. In the acute phase, it causes diffuse alveolar damage that in weeks to months develops into severe obstruction and later fibrosis of the airways. Several other gases and volatile compounds have been reported in association with the development of constrictive bronchiolitis, including sulfur, diacetyl, chlorine, and phosgene.[3,12,15]

Recently, there have been reports of constrictive bronchiolitis in soldiers with inhalational exposure in Iraq, especially to sulfur mine fires.[18]

Drug-Induced Bronchiolitis

Lung toxicity due to drug therapy is characterized by several morphologic patterns that are usually nonspecific and rarely limited to the bronchioles (see Chapter 59). Historically, the use of penicillamine or gold in the treatment of rheumatoid arthritis (RA) has been implicated in small airway toxicity.[19] Since RA can also be associated with bronchiolitis itself, it is hard to determine if the therapy or the disease process is responsible for the changes.[1,15] More recently, the use of the anti-CD20 drug rituximab has been associated with a constrictive form of bronchiolitis.[20-22]

Diffuse Panbronchiolitis

The term "diffuse panbronchiolitis" refers to a unique form of chronic injury to the bronchioles almost exclusively seen in Japanese men, usually in their fourth or fifth decade.[23,24] Many descriptions of the disease show association with chronic sinusitis and/or bronchiectasis, suggesting a disorder of the ciliary system.[25] Clinical associations with rheumatologic and autoimmune diseases such as ulcerative colitis, allergic angiitis, myasthenia gravis, IgA nephropathy, and common variable immunodeficiency have been described.[26-28] Patients usually present with progressive obstructive symptoms and episodes of infection.

The lungs are usually hyperinflated and also show bronchiectasis. Occasional foci of bronchopneumonia can be seen in surgical specimens. The main histologic findings are of the triad of severe bronchiolocentric inflammation, lymphoid hyperplasia, and interstitial macrophage foam cells. However, these findings are also seen in other airway disorders and are not specific of diffuse panbronchiolitis. The differential diagnoses include other airway processes such as chronic bronchitis, hypersensitivity pneumonia, follicular bronchiolitis, and constrictive bronchiolitis.

REFERENCES

1. Visscher DW, Myers JL. Bronchiolitis: the pathologist's perspective. *Proc Am Thorac Soc.* 2006;3:41–47.
2. Poletti V, Costabel U. Bronchiolar disorders: classification and diagnostic approach. *Semin Respir Crit Care Med.* 2003;24:457–464.
3. Garibaldi BT, Illei P, Danoff SK. Bronchiolitis. *Immunol Allergy Clin North Am.* 2012;32:601–619.
4. Harasawa M. [Infectious bronchitis—acute bronchiolitis in patients with chronic respiratory tract diseases and in infants]. *Kokyu To Junkan.* 1974;22:508.
5. Rutishauser M, Hollander G. [Changes in the small airways as a long-term sequela of acute bronchiolitis and a pre-stage of chronic obstructive airway disease in adults]. *Schweiz Med Wochenschr.* 1983;113:1540–1544.
6. Pagtakhan RD, Reed MH, Chernick V. Is bronchiolitis in infancy an antecedent of chronic lung disease in adolescence and adulthood? *J Thorac Imaging.* 1986;1:34–40.
7. Flaherman VJ, Ragins AI, Li SX, et al. Frequency, duration and predictors of bronchiolitis episodes of care among infants ≥32 weeks gestation in a large integrated healthcare system: a retrospective cohort study. *BMC Health Serv Res.* 2012;12:144.
8. de Carvalho ME, Kairalla RA, Capelozzi VL, et al. Centrilobular fibrosis: a novel histological pattern of idiopathic interstitial pneumonia. *Pathol Res Pract.* 2002;198:577–583.
9. Hansell DM. HRCT of obliterative bronchiolitis and other small airways diseases. *Semin Roentgenol.* 2001;36:51–65.
10. Devakonda A, Raoof S, Sung A, et al. Bronchiolar disorders: a clinical-radiological diagnostic algorithm. *Chest.* 2010;137:938–951.
11. Kang EY, Woo OH, Shin BK, et al. Bronchiolitis: classification, computed tomographic and histopathologic features, and radiologic approach. *J Comput Assist Tomogr.* 2009;33:32–41.
12. Poletti V, Zompatori M, Cancellieri A. Clinical spectrum of adult chronic bronchiolitis. *Sarcoidosis Vasc Diffuse Lung Dis.* 1999;16:183–196.
13. Wu XY, Luo ZX, Fu Z, et al. [Clinical analysis of 28 cases of bronchiolitis obliterans]. *Zhongguo Dang Dai Er Ke Za Zhi.* 2013;15:845–849.
14. Pardo J, Panizo A, Sola I, et al. Prognostic value of clinical, morphologic, and immunohistochemical factors in patients with bronchiolitis obliterans-organizing pneumonia. *Hum Pathol.* 2013;44:718–724.
15. Lynch JP 3rd, Weigt SS, DerHovanessian A, et al. Obliterative (constrictive) bronchiolitis. *Semin Respir Crit Care Med.* 2012;33:509–532.
16. Colby TV. Bronchiolitis. Pathologic considerations. *Am J Clin Pathol.* 1998;109:101–109.
17. Matsuse T, Oka T, Kida K, et al. Importance of diffuse aspiration bronchiolitis caused by chronic occult aspiration in the elderly. *Chest.* 1996;110:1289–1293.
18. King MS, Eisenberg R, Newman JH, et al. Constrictive bronchiolitis in soldiers returning from Iraq and Afghanistan. *N Engl J Med.* 2011;365:222–230.
19. Turner-Warwick M. Adverse reactions affecting the lung: possible association with D-penicillamine. *J Rheumatol Suppl.* 1981;7:166–168.
20. Ergin AB, Fong N, Daw HA. Rituximab-induced bronchiolitis obliterans organizing pneumonia. *Case Rep Med.* 2012;2012:680431.
21. Lorillon G, Robin M, Meignin V, et al. Rituximab in bronchiolitis obliterans after haematopoietic stem cell transplantation. *Eur Respir J.* 2011;38:470–472.
22. Urun Y, Dincol D, Kumbasar OO. Rituximab-related cryptogenic organizing pneumonia and late onset neutropenia in a patient with non-Hodgkin lymphoma: report of two rare complications and review of the literature. *J BUON.* 2012;17:602–603.
23. Randhawa P, Hoagland MH, Yousem SA. Diffuse panbronchiolitis in North America. Report of three cases and review of the literature. *Am J Surg Pathol.* 1991;15:43–47.
24. Fisher MS Jr, Rush WL, Rosado-de-Christenson ML, et al. Diffuse panbronchiolitis: histologic diagnosis in unsuspected cases involving North American residents of Asian descent. *Arch Pathol Lab Med.* 1998;122:156–160.
25. Chen W, Shao C, Song Y, et al. Primary ciliary dyskinesia complicated with diffuse panbronchiolitis: a case report and literature review. *Clin Respir J.* 2014;8:425–430.
26. Maekawa R, Shibuya H, Hideyama T, et al. [A case of myasthenia gravis with invasive thymoma associated with diffuse panbronchiolitis, alopecia, dysgeusia, cholangitis and myositis]. *Rinsho Shinkeigaku.* 2014;54:703–708.
27. Ginori A, Barone A, Bennett D, et al. Diffuse panbronchiolitis in a patient with common variable immunodeficiency: a casual association or a pathogenetic correlation? *Diagn Pathol.* 2014;9:12.
28. Tossier C, Pilette C, Guilleminault L, et al. Diffuse panbronchiolitis and IgA nephropathy. *Am J Respir Crit Care Med.* 2014;189:106–109.

36 Follicular Bronchiolitis and Lymphoid Interstitial Pneumonia

Allen P. Burke, M.D., Fabio R. Tavora, M.D., Ph.D., and Seth Kligerman, M.D.

Overview and Terminology

Follicular bronchiolitis and lymphoid interstitial pneumonia (LIP) are part of a spectrum of related inflammatory lung conditions, the former emphasizing airway and the latter, interstitial localization. Nodular lymphoid hyperplasia, inflammatory pseudotumor, Castleman disease, and IgG4-related disease in the lung are considered related entities.[1]

The term "lymphoid interstitial pneumonia" originates in the 1960s, with Liebow's classification of interstitial pneumonias (see Chapter 16), whereas "follicular bronchiolitis" is somewhat more recent, with the first series published in the 1980s.[2] Histologic features of both entities overlap, with the predominant pattern (bronchiolar vs. interstitial) dictating the proper designation.[3] In fact, "LIP" is now considered rare[4] and is even considered by some to be an obsolete term.[5] The predisposing conditions to both entities are presented in Tables 36.1 and 36.2.

Follicular bronchiolitis is a reactive B-cell proliferation centered on small airways, and "LIP" is a diffuse interstitial process with a typical cystic appearance on chest CT scans.[6] Both conditions are associated with immunodeficiency and autoimmune disorders and often overlap. However, peribronchiolar inflammation with germinal centers (the histologic definition of follicular bronchiolitis) may have a variety of causes and is seen as a minor histologic component in diverse diseases, whereas LIP is a more homogeneous clinicopathologic entity closely associated with autoimmune disorders (especially Sjögren disease) and HIV/AIDS.

Follicular Bronchiolitis

Clinical Features

From the time of Yousem et al.'s initial series in the 1980s, it was apparent that follicular bronchiolitis, as seen on lung biopsies, formed three clinicopathologic entities.[2] The largest group was that associated with autoimmune collagen vascular disease, especially rheumatoid arthritis and Sjögren syndrome. A second important group comprised patients with inherited immunodeficiency syndromes. The third group is heterogeneous and includes hypersensitivity and infectious conditions causing reactive lymphoid hyperplasia in the small airways.[2] In the largest recent series of biopsy-documented follicular bronchiolitis, 2 of 12 patients had connective tissue disorders (Sjögren syndrome and undifferentiated connective-tissue disease (CTD), respectively), two had common variable immunodeficiency (CVID) syndrome, and the remaining two-thirds had no apparent underlying condition.[3] The latter finding highlights the nonspecificity of reactive follicles surrounding airways in biopsies of patients with clinically heterogeneous processes. Follicular bronchiolitis has also been described in patients with HIV,[7] although the interstitial inflammatory component is typically emphasized in association with HIV (LIP).

Clinically, patients typically have frequent pulmonary infections. Most patients have some degree of dyspnea and cough, and abnormal chest radiographs are common. Bronchoscopic findings are usually nondiagnostic. Respiratory function tests show variable results, but a restrictive pattern may be present. By CT scan, nodular or micronodular lung densities with prominent, thickened distal airways, often with areas of ground-glass opacities or consolidation, are present.[3]

Microscopic Findings

Follicular bronchiolitis is largely a descriptive diagnosis. By definition, only distal cartilaginous bronchi and bronchioles are involved; reactive hyperplasia around more proximal bronchiectatic airways or follicular lymphoid hyperplasia in the context of prominent acute or necrotizing inflammation is not considered follicular bronchiolitis.

Histologically, follicular bronchiolitis is characterized by lymphoid follicular hyperplasia of small airways, often with reactive germinal centers that may coalesce (Figs. 36.1 to 36.3).[2] Other findings and diagnoses may be present, depending on the clinical setting, including emphysema, respiratory bronchiolitis, carcinoid tumors, and granulomas.[3] In general, acute inflammation is minimal, unless there is superimposed infection.

Differential Diagnosis

Lymphoid follicles, typically without germinal centers, are not uncommon in diffuse interstitial lung diseases, such as usual or nonspecific interstitial pneumonia, as well as localized inflammatory processes. Lymphoid follicles may occur in proximal airways and occasionally result in masses (Figs. 36.4 and 36.5).

The major clinicopathologic entity in the differential diagnosis is LIP, which is often considered part of the same disease (see below). The most important entity in the histologic differential diagnosis is marginal zone B-cell lymphoma and nodular lymphoid hyperplasia. Although lymphoepithelial lesions are characteristic of lymphoma, they may also be seen in reactive processes (Fig. 36.6). Immunohistochemical studies and flow cytometry are required to exclude low-grade lymphoma.[8] In general, lymphomas demonstrate a single or few dominant masses, in

TABLE 36.1 Conditions Associated with Lymphoid Interstitial Pneumonia

Autoimmune collagen vascular diseases
Sjögren syndrome
Rheumatoid arthritis
Systemic lupus erythematosus

Other immunologic disorders
Autoimmune hemolytic anemia
Pernicious anemia
Myasthenia gravis
Hashimoto thyroiditis
Primary biliary cirrhosis
Celiac disease

Immunodeficiency
HIV/AIDS (pediatric)
Common variable immunodeficiency

Drug-induced/toxic exposure
Dilantin

Reprinted from Travis WD, Galvin JR. Non-neoplastic pulmonary lymphoid lesions. *Thorax.* 2001;56:964–971, with permission.

TABLE 36.2 Conditions Associated with Follicular Bronchiolitis

Autoimmune collagen vascular diseases, especially rheumatoid arthritis
Immunodeficiency syndromes
Lymphoproliferative disorders
Middle lobe syndrome
Bronchiectasis

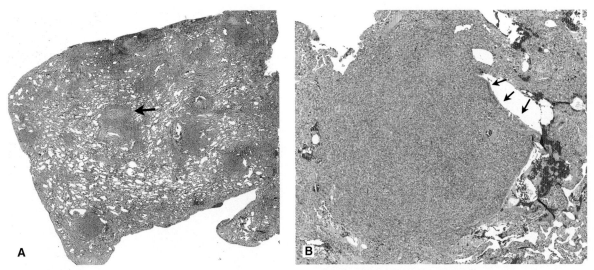

FIGURE 36.1 ▲ Follicular bronchiolitis child with HIV. **A.** Low magnification demonstrates patchy inflammation with scattered germinal centers (*arrow*). **B.** A higher magnification of a reactive lymphoid follicle distorting the airway (*arrows*).

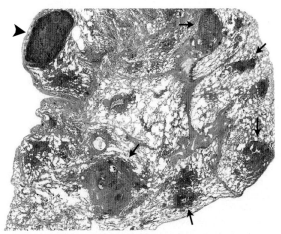

FIGURE 36.2 ▲ Follicular bronchiolitis. A low magnification demonstrates peribronchiolar lymphoid hyperplasia (*arrows*) and a subpleural intraparenchymal lymph node with reactive changes (*arrowhead*). The patient had recurrent *Moraxella* infection and some clinical features of immunodeficiency.

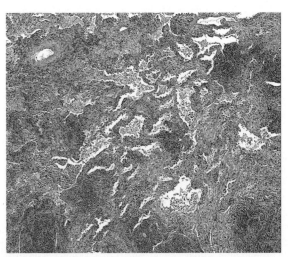

FIGURE 36.4 ▲ Follicular hyperplasia in postobstructive pneumonia. The finding was incidental to an obstructing squamous carcinoma. There is diffuse lymphoid hyperplasia with lymphoid aggregates, although reactive germinal centers are absent.

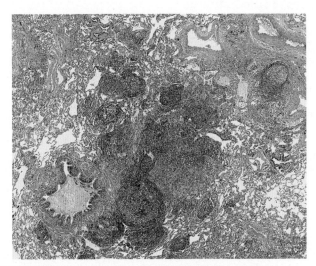

FIGURE 36.3 ▲ Follicular bronchiolitis. Woman with diffuse lymphoid infiltrates underwent open lung biopsy revealing airway-centered lymphoid follicle with reactive germinal centers. Subsequently, she developed autoimmune syndrome with some features of Sjögren syndrome.

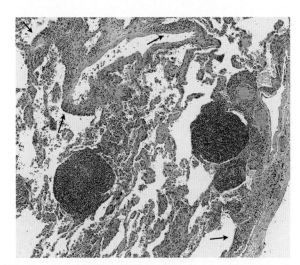

FIGURE 36.5 ▲ Localized follicular hyperplasia with lymphocytic interstitial inflammation. The patient underwent surgical resection of a lung mass, possible carcinoma. Histologically, there were lymphoid follicles with inflammation extending into the interstitium (*arrows*). The features resemble nodular lymphoid hyperplasia, but the interstitial inflammation is unusual.

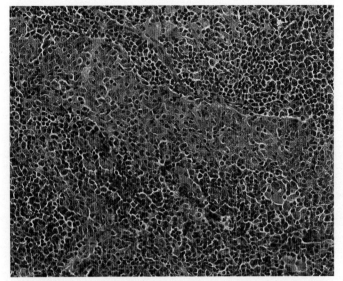

FIGURE 36.6 ▲ Lymphoepithelial lesion, without evidence of lymphoma. The finding was an incidental lesion within a pseudotumor adjacent to a resected carcinoma.

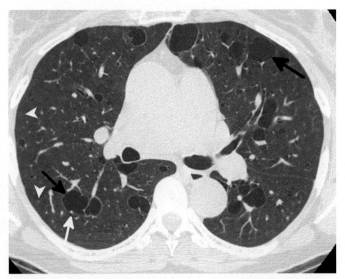

FIGURE 36.7 ▲ Lymphocytic interstitial pneumonia, high-resolution computed tomography. Lymphoid interstitial pneumonia (LIP) in a 45-year-old woman with Sjögren syndrome. Axial CT through the midlung zones shows numerous parenchymal cysts (*black arrows*). Vessels can be seen coursing along the sides of many of the cysts (*white arrow*). A few centrilobular nodules are present (*arrowheads*), likely representing areas of follicular bronchiolitis.

contrast to follicular bronchiolitis, in which there is diffuse small airway involvement with a dominant lesion. Follicular bronchiolitis may occur as the pulmonary manifestation of Castleman disease.[9]

Prognosis and Treatment

The treatment of follicular bronchiolitis includes steroids and azathioprine if patients with underlying connective tissue disease. Most patients improve.[3] A man with histologically confirmed progression to LIP has been reported.[10]

Pulmonary Nodular Lymphoid Hyperplasia

Nodular lymphoid hyperplasia of the lung was initially introduced as a term for localized airway-centered reactive follicular hyperplasia by Kradin and Mark.[11] Like follicular bronchiolitis, it is a reactive lymphoid proliferation with germinal centers that is centered on small airways. However, it differs from follicular bronchiolitis in that there are only one or few masses. It is unclear whether nodular lymphoid hyperplasia of the lung is a discrete entity. In the largest series with molecular analysis, the authors postulated that nodular lymphoid hyperplasia is part of the spectrum of LIP.[12] Of 14 cases, only 1 was diffuse (therefore difficult to distinguish from follicular bronchiolitis) and more than half only one mass. In this series, no patient developed or had molecular evidence for marginal zone lymphoma.[12]

The mean size of nodules of nodular lymphoid hyperplasia is 2.1 cm. Histologically, there are reactive germinal centers with mantle zones and plasma cells (Fig. 36.7). Reactive lymphadenopathy may be present in the mediastinum.[13]

Lymphoid Interstitial Pneumonia

Overview

LIP as a diagnostic entity has undergone a gradual transformation from a relatively common type of interstitial pneumonia to a rare condition that is seen most frequently in patients with Sjögren syndrome, other autoimmune disorders, and immunodeficiency states. Because chronic interstitial inflammation is nonspecific, in many patients the most diagnostic feature is diffuse cystic change with interstitial markings on computed tomography scans, and histologically the presence of interstitial inflammation with or without follicular bronchiolitis. Although "lymphoid interstitial pneumonia" is probably the most prevalent term, synonyms include "lymphocytic interstitial pneumonia"[13,14] and "lymphoid interstitial pneumonitis".[15] Because there may be granulomas in the infiltrate of LIP in patients with immunodeficiency syndromes, the term "granulomatous lymphocytic lung disease" is sometimes used in this setting.[16]

Clinical Findings

Lymphocytic interstitial pneumonia is currently diagnosed almost exclusively in patients with autoimmune collagen vascular diseases and immunodeficiency syndromes.[6] There is a female predominance and no association with smoking.[6] It is rare in HIV-infected adults, but in children under the age of 13, it is one of the defining criteria for AIDS.[13] Patients are symptomatic from a few months to years, with cough, dyspnea, weight loss, fever, chest pain, and arthralgias. Pulmonary function tests usually demonstrate a restrictive ventilatory defect.[13]

High-resolution computed tomography findings consist of diffuse ground-glass opacities, ill-defined centrilobular nodules, bronchovascular thickening, interlobular septal thickening, and scattered thin-walled cysts (Fig. 36.7). The cysts may be seen in up to 80% of the patients and are typically few in number and measure <3 cm in diameter.[17]

Microscopic Findings

Bronchoalveolar lavage (BAL) specimens demonstrate lymphocytosis.[6] Histologically, lymphocytic interstitial pneumonia is characterized by a marked infiltrate of T lymphocytes and plasma cells in the alveolar septa with reactive pneumocyte hyperplasia (Figs. 36.8 to 36.10). Follicular bronchiolitis is generally present, composed of B-lymphocyte–rich follicles usually with scattered germinal centers.[18] There may be a considerable population of B cells in the interstitium as well.[19] Poorly formed nonnecrotizing granulomas may be seen, especially when associated with immunodeficiency syndromes (see below). The frequency of Epstein-Barr virus (EBV) is high in HIV-infected children with LIP.[20] In other older series, EBV was detected in adults with LIP as well.[18,19] However, in a recent series of LIP occurring in patients with Sjögren syndrome and other autoimmune diseases, EBV as an association was not even mentioned.[6]

Differential Diagnosis

Lymphocytic interstitial pneumonia must be differentiated histologically from malignant lymphoma, follicular bronchiolitis, nodular lymphoid hyperplasia, and infection. It must also be distinguished from other interstitial lung disorders such as nonspecific interstitial pneumonia, organizing pneumonia, and usual interstitial pneumonia.[4] Currently, from a practical standpoint, radiologic correlation is essential, as the diagnosis is typically rendered in the setting of typical cystic

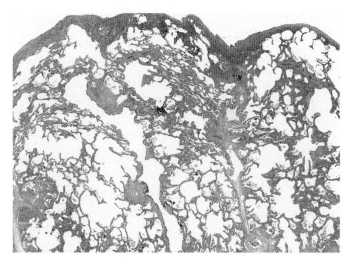

FIGURE 36.8 ▲ Interstitial pneumonia in Sjögren syndrome. A low magnification shows patchy interstitial inflammation and vague cystic change, which is better appreciated on computed tomography scans.

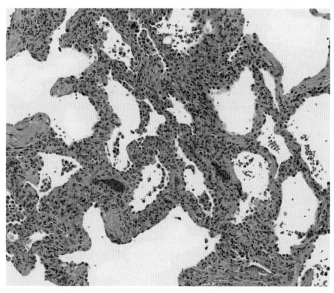

FIGURE 36.9 ▲ Interstitial pneumonia in Sjögren syndrome. A higher magnification shows dense interstitial inflammation; in this case, peribronchiolar inflammation was not prominent, and there is overlap with cellular nonspecific interstitial pneumonia.

changes on CT scans. The most useful histologic finding is the presence of diffuse follicular bronchiolitis, which is relatively rare in other conditions, given the lack of specificity of interstitial infiltrates.

Prognosis and Treatment

The treatment of LIP is corticosteroids, and in the case of lack of response to steroids, other cytotoxic drugs, including cyclophosphamide, azathioprine, colchicine, and cyclosporine A.[6] The overall survival is difficult to estimate, due to the low incidence of the disease and varied underlying conditions. In one series, the median survival was only 12 years, but the cause of death was related to pulmonary involvement in fewer than one-half of cases.[6] Two patients without underlying autoimmune diseases progressed to "end-stage lung disease" without histologic documentation; it is unclear if these biopsies may have better been classified as nonspecific interstitial pneumonia.[6]

One patient with Sjögren syndrome and LIP developed low-grade marginal zone lymphoma of the parotid gland that was successfully treated surgically.[6]

Granulomatous Lymphocytic Interstitial Lung Disease

LIP is part of the spectrum of interstitial lung disease in patients with CVID. In contrast to LIP associated with childhood HIV or autoimmune disorders, granulomas are characteristic, leading to the sometimes-used designation "granulomatous lymphocytic interstitial lung disease." Epstein-Barr virus is not believed to be involved in the pathogenesis of lymphomas or interstitial pneumonia in CVID.[16]

Clinically, respiratory symptoms are common in CVID and may be the initial manifestation. In addition to LIP, infections of the lung and low-grade marginal zone lymphomas are increased in incidence in patients with CVID. To further complicate the clinical and histologic differential diagnosis, autoimmune disorders, such as Sjögren syndrome, and granulomatous infections may complicate CVID.

Imaging is key in distinguishing LIP from other pulmonary processes in patients with CVID. The computed tomographic findings are similar to that seen in LIP from other causes, with the important

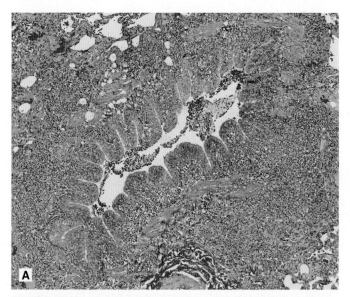

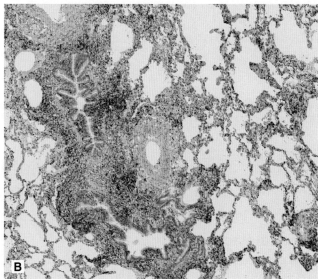

FIGURE 36.10 ▲ Follicular bronchiolitis with lymphoid interstitial pneumonia, child with HIV. **A.** A low magnification shows marked bronchiolar inflammation. **B.** A CD3 stain demonstrates peribronchiolar and interstitial T lymphocytes.

difference that cystic change characteristic of Sjögren syndrome is usually not present. The dominant findings are related to small airway disease, with diffuse bilateral centrilobular micronodules and air trapping. In addition, interstitial disease is manifest on chest CT by areas of ground-glass opacification and later by reticular densities and, uncommonly, honeycombing indicative of advanced interstitial fibrosis.

A lymphocyte-predominant BAL is typical of LIP in CVID patients, but nonspecific, as it is also seen in hypersensitivity pneumonitis, drug-induced lung disease, and sarcoidosis. Flow cytometry and gene rearrangement studies may be useful in excluding lymphoma on BAL fluid.

The histologic appearance of LIP in granulomatous lymphocytic interstitial lung disease (GLILD) is no different from LIP of other causes. Transbronchial biopsies are limited by sampling error but may show follicular bronchiolitis, interstitial inflammation, and granulomas that point to the diagnosis of LIP. If only one or two components are present, a descriptive diagnosis is rendered, with a differential diagnosis including LIP or granulomatous interstitial lung disease (ILD). The granulomas are sarcoid-like, nonnecrotizing, and relatively well circumscribed. Similar granulomatous inflammation may occur in the liver, kidneys, and gastrointestinal tract.

The histologic differential diagnosis of GLILD includes granulomatous infection, and special stains for mycobacteria and fungi should complement microbiologic studies. Hypersensitivity pneumonitis has many overlapping histologic features, except that reactive follicles are typically absent. Sarcoid may also mimic GLILD but is generally a distinct clinical syndrome and not related to CVID. Lymphoma (marginal zone, bronchial-associated lymphoid tissue type) is suspected if there is destruction of lung architecture or extension into the parietal pleura and confirmed by immunohistochemical and flow cytometric studies.

In patients with CVID, GLILD is associated with shortened survival, and when present, respiratory failure is the most common cause of death.[21]

Practical Points

▶ Follicular bronchiolitis, lymphoid interstitial pneumonia, and granulomatous LIP are part of a spectrum of inflammatory lung conditions, generally associated with autoimmune diseases, immunodeficiency syndromes, and collagen vascular diseases.

▶ Follicular bronchiolitis is particularly associated with Sjögren syndrome. Imaging shows micronodular densities, ground-glass opacities, and consolidations.

▶ In contrast to follicular bronchiolitis, LIP usually shows cystic changes on CT scans and also peripheral interstitial involvement.

▶ Lymphoproliferative disorders should be excluded in cases of LIP.

REFERENCES

1. Tian X, Yi ES, Ryu JH. Lymphocytic interstitial pneumonia and other benign lymphoid disorders. *Semin Respir Crit Care Med.* 2012;33:450–461.
2. Yousem SA, Colby TV, Carrington CB. Follicular bronchitis/bronchiolitis. *Hum Pathol.* 1985;16:700–706.
3. Aerni MR, Vassallo R, Myers JL, et al. Follicular bronchiolitis in surgical lung biopsies: clinical implications in 12 patients. *Respir Med.* 2008;102:307–312.
4. Travis WD, Costabel U, Hansell DM, et al. An official American Thoracic Society/European Respiratory Society statement: update of the international multidisciplinary classification of the idiopathic interstitial pneumonias. *Am J Respir Crit Care Med.* 2013;188:733–748.
5. Myers JL, Katzenstein AL. Beyond a consensus classification for idiopathic interstitial pneumonias: progress and controversies. *Histopathology.* 2009;54:90–103.
6. Cha SI, Fessler MB, Cool CD, et al. Lymphoid interstitial pneumonia: clinical features, associations and prognosis. *Eur Respir J.* 2006;28:364–369.
7. Shipe R, Lawrence J, Green J, et al. HIV-associated follicular bronchiolitis. *Am J Respir Crit Care Med.* 2013;188:510–511.
8. Herbert A, Walters MT, Cawley MI, et al. Lymphocytic interstitial pneumonia identified as lymphoma of mucosa associated lymphoid tissue. *J Pathol.* 1985;146:129–138.
9. Hwangbo Y, Cha SI, Lee YH, et al. A case of multicentric Castleman's disease presenting with follicular bronchiolitis. *Tuberc Respir Dis (Seoul).* 2013;74:23–27.
10. Terada T. Follicular bronchiolitis and lymphocytic interstitial pneumonia in a Japanese man. *Diagn Pathol.* 2011;6:85.
11. Kradin RL, Mark EJ. Benign lymphoid disorders of the lung, with a theory regarding their development. *Hum Pathol.* 1983;14:857–867.
12. Abbondanzo SL, Rush W, Bijwaard KE, et al. Nodular lymphoid hyperplasia of the lung: a clinicopathologic study of 14 cases. *Am J Surg Pathol.* 2000;24:587–597.
13. Travis WD, Galvin JR. Non-neoplastic pulmonary lymphoid lesions. *Thorax.* 2001;56:964–971.
14. King TE Jr. Clinical advances in the diagnosis and therapy of the interstitial lung diseases. *Am J Respir Crit Care Med.* 2005;172:268–279.
15. Harley W, Horton JM, Corbin RP. Recurrent pneumococcal pneumonia in an HIV-positive patient with lymphoid interstitial pneumonitis. *South Med J.* 1992;85:1015–1016.
16. Fernandez Perez ER. Granulomatous lymphocytic interstitial lung disease. *Immunol Allergy Clin North Am.* 2012;32:621–632.
17. Silva CI, Flint JD, Levy RD, et al. Diffuse lung cysts in lymphoid interstitial pneumonia: high-resolution CT and pathologic findings. *J Thorac Imaging.* 2006;21:241–244.
18. Swigris JJ, Berry GJ, Raffin TA, et al. Lymphoid interstitial pneumonia: a narrative review. *Chest.* 2002;122:2150–2164.
19. Barbera JA, Hayashi S, Hegele RG, et al. Detection of Epstein-Barr virus in lymphocytic interstitial pneumonia by in situ hybridization. *Am Rev Respir Dis.* 1992;145:940–946.
20. Andiman WA, Eastman R, Martin K, et al. Opportunistic lymphoproliferations associated with Epstein-Barr viral DNA in infants and children with AIDS. *Lancet.* 1985;2:1390–1393.
21. Bates CA, Ellison MC, Lynch DA, et al. Granulomatous-lymphocytic lung disease shortens survival in common variable immunodeficiency. *J Allergy Clin Immunol.* 2004;114:415–421.

37 Constrictive Bronchiolitis

Fabio R. Tavora, M.D., Ph.D., and Allen P. Burke, M.D.

Historical Background

Constrictive (obliterative) bronchiolitis is a clinicopathologic entity of diverse causes denoting inflammation and fibrosis of bronchioles, usually concentric, resulting in obliterative changes. It is a subset of small airway disease characterized by progressive fibrosis limited to small airways. Both "constrictive" and "obliterative" bronchiolitis are used as clinical as well as pathologic designations. The first series with pathologic documentation appeared in 1977, at which time Geddes et al. reported six patients, five with rheumatoid arthritis, with progressive small airway disease leading to respiratory failure. In four autopsied patients from this series, the term "obliterative bronchiolitis" was used to describe fibrotic small airways in the absence of features of asthma or chronic bronchitis.[1] Soon thereafter, Turton et al. reported 10 patients with "obliterative bronchiolitis" defined clinically (without pathologic confirmation) as obstructive small airway disease in nonsmokers that did not respond to steroid treatment.[2] In 1985, Epler et al. reported a pathologic series of bronchiolitis obliterans and contrasted the favorable prognosis of the group with organizing pneumonia to the unfavorable one of obliterative bronchiolitis.[3] For this reason, constrictive bronchiolitis is not to be confused with "bronchiolitis obliterans organizing pneumonia" (cryptogenic organizing pneumonia; Chapter 19), which has dramatically different clinical, imaging, and pathologic findings.[4] Unfortunately, the term "bronchiolitis obliterans" has been used interchangeably with constrictive bronchiolitis, necessitating careful evaluation of the older publications to distinguish concentric bronchiolitis from organizing pneumonia.[5] Because of the potential confusion with organizing pneumonia, the term "constrictive" may be a preferred term over "obliterative," although the latter term is entrenched, especially in the transplant literature (Table 37.1).

There are three major clinical settings of constrictive bronchiolitis: first is the disease that occurs in native lungs and is often associated with autoimmune diseases or inhalational exposure (see Table 37.1); the second form occurs in patients with stem cell transplants and is a chronic form of graft versus host disease (see Chapter 54); and the third is the hallmark of chronic allograft dysfunction in lung transplant patients (see Chapter 53).[6,7] The current chapter is devoted to primary constrictive bronchiolitis (the first of the three groups).

Pathogenesis

The initial insult in constrictive bronchiolitis is inflammation of the epithelium and subepithelial structures with aberrant tissue repair mechanism that leads to progression over time to marked narrowing of the lumen, or even obliteration. The remodeling of the airways is considered generally a consequence of immune responses that chronically lead to fibrosis.[8] Because 50% or more of patients had evidence of rheumatologic disorders, autoimmunity is likely a role in many patients.[1] Studies of patients with bronchiolar constriction and ataxia–telangiectasia suggest that IgA deficiency and T-cell dysfunction may also lead to chronic inflammation and fibrosis in the bronchioles,

perhaps triggered by bacterial or viral infections.[5] Acquired and inherited hypogammaglobulinemias predispose to bronchiolar inflammation in the form of follicular bronchiolitis or diffuse panbronchiolitis but typically without significant fibrosis. Because a similar, if not identical, syndrome to constrictive bronchiolitis occurs after inhalation of smoke and particulate matter, direct injury to the airway epithelium may trigger an immunologically mediated fibrosing bronchiolitis. Although the pathogenesis of transplant-related obliterative bronchiolitis has been extensively studied (see Chapter 53), the pathogenesis of idiopathic constrictive bronchiolitis or the diseases unrelated to lung transplant or bone marrow transplantation is less understood.[9]

Incidence

Constrictive bronchiolitis is rare; in one series of 2,500 native open lung biopsies, the diagnosis was rendered in 0.4% (10 cases).[3]

Clinical Findings

The most important symptoms of constrictive bronchiolitis are nonproductive cough, dyspnea, and signs of airflow obstruction, including wheezing, with slow progression over months to years.[1,2,10] Recurrent infections are common. Pulmonary function test findings include obstructive pattern with forced expiratory volume in 1 second (FEV1) of <60% predicted, air trapping, and clinical exclusion of other causes of obstruction. Rarely, there are predominantly restrictive parameters.[11] Typically (or even by definition), there is no improvement following inhaled bronchodilators or steroids.[12,13] In contrast, cryptogenic organizing pneumonia usually responds to steroid therapy.[3]

Evidence of rheumatologic or autoimmune disease, especially rheumatoid arthritis, is found in variable proportion of patients with constrictive bronchiolitis, ranging from 50% to 83%[1,2] to 20% to 27%.[11,14] In addition to rheumatoid arthritis, there is an association between inflammatory bowel disease, systemic lupus erythematosus, Sjögren syndrome, systemic sclerosis, dermatomyositis, and IgA nephropathy with constrictive bronchiolitis[4,14] (Table 37.2). Paraneoplastic pemphigus, an autoimmune disease that may complicate lymphomas

TABLE 37.1 Terminology of Primary Fibrotic Small Airway Disease

Term	Usage
Constrictive bronchiolitis	Pathologic term (especially not transplant related); also used clinically (especially occupational and autoimmune)
Obliterative bronchiolitis (OB)	Pathologic term, especially transplant related
	Used synonymously for constrictive bronchiolitis, but somewhat more general, including nonfibrotic phase
Obliterative bronchiolitis syndrome or Bronchiolitis obliterans syndrome (BOS) (more common)	Clinical designation, usually transplant-related or chronic graft versus host disease
Bronchiolitis obliterans	Obsolete clinical term for non–transplant-related constrictive bronchiolitis and term for clinical transplant-related constrictive bronchiolitis
	Term to be avoided pathologically, as suggests bronchiolitis obliterans organizing pneumonia (a different clinicopathologic entity)

TABLE 37.2 Constrictive Bronchiolitis, Clinical Associations[a]

Type of Association	Specific Association
Autoimmune	Rheumatoid arthritis (most common)
	Systemic lupus erythematosus
	Inflammatory bowel disease
	Sjögren syndrome
	Dermatomyositis
	IgA nephropathy
	Paraneoplastic pemphigus
Immunodeficiency syndromes	Ataxia–telangiectasia
	Acquired and hereditary hypogammaglobulinemia
	HIV
Toxic exposure	Ammonia gas
	Sulfur mine fire smoke
	Dust storms
	Smoke (combat, incinerators)
	Carbon monoxide
	Nitrogen dioxide/silo gas
	Polymethylene polyphenol isocyanate
	Fiberglass
	Diacetyl
	Coffee-flavoring chemicals
Chronic infections	Viral
	Atypical mycobacteria
	Other bacterial infections
Ingested toxins	*Sauropus androgynus* leaves (used for weight reduction)

[a]Excluding transplant related.

and other malignancies, usually affects large airways, but a constrictive bronchiolitis related to autoantibodies directed against plakin proteins occasionally occurs and may cause respiratory failure.[15] Up to one-third of patients with constrictive bronchiolitis have autoantibodies without overt collagen vascular disease.[11] A further discussion of airway disease in patients with autoimmune disorders is presented in Chapter 50.

Chronic mycobacterial and mycoplasma infection may also predispose to constrictive bronchiolitis,[14] as well as viral and bacterial infections in immunodeficiency syndromes, especially ataxia–telangiectasia.[5] In contrast to ataxia–telangiectasia, which is associated with constrictive bronchiolitis, other inherited immunodeficiency syndromes, especially those associated with hypogammaglobulinemia, are more likely to result in follicular bronchiolitis (as seen in some patients with HIV disease) or diffuse panbronchiolitis. Constrictive bronchiolitis has rarely been reported in HIV infection, however.[4]

The rate of inhalational exposure in reported series of constrictive bronchiolitis is variable. There were no cases of inhalation in early series[2] and the largest clinicopathologic study reported just fewer than one-third with inhalational exposure, including two patients with histologic features of hypersensitivity pneumonitis.[11] More recently, it is believed that occult exposure may underlie a relatively larger proportion of obliterative bronchiolitis.[16] A recent report of Middle East war veterans described a series of pathologically documented constrictive bronchiolitis related to inhalation of particulate matter from a combination of sulfur mine fires, incinerated waste, dust storms, and combat smoke.[17] This series differed from previous reports of obliterative bronchiolitis in that the presenting symptom was dyspnea without significant cough, most patients did not have obstructive parameters, and the illustrated histologic findings were relatively subtle with minimal fibrosis, concomitant arterial intimal changes, and interstitial silicoanthracotic deposits.[17] There have also been series of obliterative or constrictive bronchiolitis in fiberglass workers and those working in coffee-processing facilities.[18–20]

The chemical diacetyl is used in artificial butter flavoring and posed aerosolized occupational risk in popcorn plant workers in the early 2000s. Fixed airway obstruction was reported in clusters of plant workers, with histologic confirmation of constrictive bronchiolitis in only a handful of cases,[21] with only one illustrated example.[22]

Smoking is not considered a risk factor for constrictive bronchiolitis and is associated with reactive airway disease and respiratory bronchiolitis instead. Most series of constrictive bronchiolitis either exclude smokers or have no smokers[2,13] or consist of fewer than 50% of patients with a significant smoking history.[11,17]

Ingested drugs are rarely associated with constrictive bronchiolitis and include penicillamine (see Chapter 59) and Sauropus androgynus, a Malaysian bush, which is eaten raw as an anorexigen.[4,23]

The major clinical differential diagnoses include cryptogenic organizing pneumonia, sarcoidosis, and respiratory bronchiolitis interstitial lung disease. Less commonly, pulmonary lymphangitic carcinomatosis, primary marginal cell lymphoma, lymphomatoid granulomatosis, and diffuse idiopathic pulmonary neuroendocrine cell hyperplasia can mimic constrictive bronchiolitis.

Imaging Findings

Chest x-ray may show hyperinflation. High-resolution CT scans show areas of decreased density reflecting air trapping and mosaic attenuation on expiratory films, often with marked bronchial wall thickening.[22] There is usually a paucity of ground-glass opacities, which would be more suggestive of organizing pneumonia.[9] High-resolution computerized tomography studies can be normal, especially in occupational exposure,[16] but show small centrilobular nodules in 64% of patients with idiopathic obliterative bronchiolitis or that associated with immune dysfunction.[14]

Histologic Features

There is no consensus on the histologic definition of constrictive bronchiolitis. The lack of a need for histologic confirmation for diagnosis[2] hampers the development of reproducible histologic criteria,

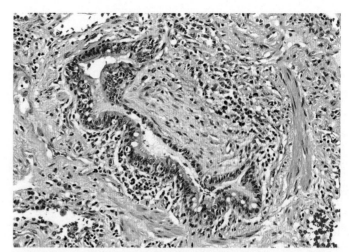

FIGURE 37.1 ▲ Early constrictive bronchiolitis. There is one segmental cellular fibrosis on one aspect of a bronchiole. There is focal flattening of the respiratory mucosa, but it is still intact.

and biopsy may not demonstrate diagnostic findings, even on wedge biopsies.

The earliest change is nondiagnostic and consists of eccentric or partial fibrosis around the bronchiolar lumen that progresses from loose to dense scarring (Figs. 37.1 and 37.2). In later phases, a standard definition is "concentric narrowing of the bronchiolar lumen, mural scarring, smooth muscle hyperplasia, and mucus stasis"[13] (Figs. 37.3 to 37.5). From a practical standpoint, the fibrosis is most marked between the muscle layer and the respiratory epithelium, and smooth muscle cell hyperplasia is difficult to assess and therefore use as a diagnostic criterion (Fig. 37.4). A "cellular" phase progressing to a "constrictive" phase has been described.[4,14] Cellular infiltrates associated with epithelial sloughing maybe seen in an acute phase and be associated with intraluminal buds resembling organizing pneumonia that later can progress to constrictive fibrosis. Markopoulou et al. define obliterative bronchiolitis as inflammatory narrowing with variable fibrosis, classified as adventitial (outside the muscle layer), subepithelial (within the muscle layer), and minimal mural fibrosis (visible with special stains).[11] A reliable criterion for constrictive bronchiolitis is the finding of fibrosis with or without granulation tissue, partly destroying the respiratory

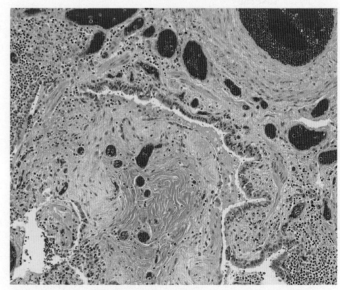

FIGURE 37.2 ▲ Constrictive bronchiolitis, later stage. There is eccentric fibrosis with loss of respiratory epithelium along the fibrotic segment.

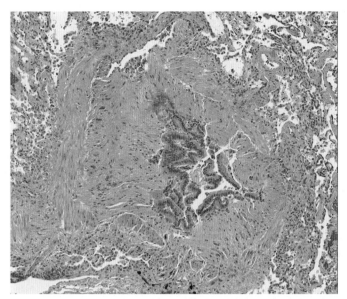

FIGURE 37.3 ▲ Constrictive bronchiolitis, concentric. There is loose fibrosis surrounding the bronchiole, with intact respiratory epithelium. The fibrosis is typically between the epithelium and the smooth muscle bundles of the bronchiolar wall. The epithelium is intact, but the lumen is irregular.

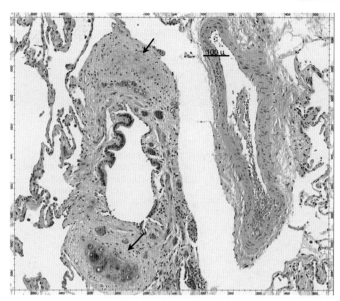

FIGURE 37.5 ▲ Constrictive bronchiolitis with cartilaginous metaplasia. There is eccentric fibrosis with partly denuded respiratory epithelium and focal cartilage in the bronchiolar wall (*arrow*).

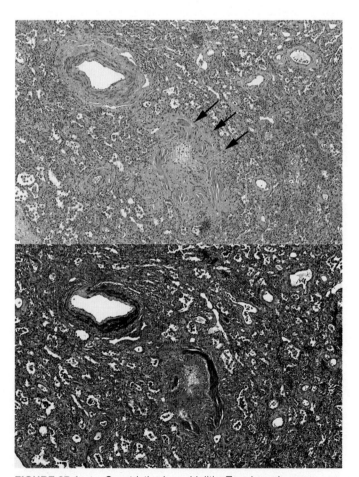

FIGURE 37.4 ▲ Constrictive bronchiolitis. **Top**, bronchovascular bundle showing area of bronchiole with complete obliteration. The muscular layer can still be seen (*arrows*). In some cases, a Masson trichrome stain can help identify the former bronchiolar wall **(bottom)**.

mucosa, with or without obliteration of the lumen. Importantly, loose fibrotic plugs typical of organizing pneumonia are not features of constrictive (obliterative) bronchiolitis.

In a series of environmental exposure predominantly from toxic fumes, the histologic findings have been described as relatively mild, with fibrosis between the epithelium and the muscle layer seen best with Masson trichrome staining.[17] The scarcity of findings in patients with clinical constrictive bronchiolitis following diacetyl exposure was underscored in a series of three thorascopic wedge biopsies, which showed diagnostic lesions in only two, one of which involved a single airway. Diagnostic findings in this small series included submucosal fibrosis with narrowing of the bronchiolar lumina with only mild inflammation; mucostasis and rare granulomas were also sometimes present.[22]

Because of the patchy nature of the disease,[24] transbronchial biopsies can often be noncontributory, similar to diagnosing obliterative bronchiolitis in transplant biopsies.[25] Concentric luminal narrowing with mild subepithelial collagen deposition may be the only finding in a surgical biopsy early in the disease. In contrast, late in the disease, the scar maybe so prominent that one cannot identify the outline of the former bronchiolar wall, sometimes making the diagnosis difficult. Immunohistochemical stains for smooth muscle actin and Masson trichrome stains can facilitate localization of the destroyed airways in advanced cases. Additionally, the use of elastic stains such as the van Gieson may help highlight the bronchiolar architecture, especially in cases lacking inflammation.[26] Surgical (thorascopic) lung biopsy has a higher yield than does transbronchial biopsy but is infrequently performed for diagnosis of small airway disease.[12]

Histologic Differential Diagnosis

The histologic diagnosis, as mentioned above, is limited by sampling. Reliance on imaging and pulmonary function studies for the clinical diagnosis has led to a paucity of histologic data. The major differential diagnoses include other idiopathic bronchiolocentric lung diseases (see below) (Table 37.3), sarcoidosis, and rare examples of lymphangitic carcinoma and neuroendocrine cell hyperplasia that result in small airway narrowing. In the latter condition, endocrine cells are difficult to identify without immunohistochemical staining for endocrine granules, such as synaptophysin[4]; there is little fibrosis or inflammation, as the bronchiolar occlusion is more the result of muscular reaction. Uncommon disorders that overlap somewhat clinically and pathologically with

TABLE 37.3 Histopathology Differential Diagnosis of Constrictive Bronchiolitis

Pathologic Diagnosis	Histologic Features and Differentiation from Constrictive Bronchiolitis
Organizing pneumonia	Bronchiolar or alveolar plugs of loose fibrosis
	Lack of concentric bronchiolar fibrosis
Airway-centered interstitial fibrosis	Often involves entire secondary lobule
	Absence of isolated obliterated bronchioles
Peribronchiolar metaplasia	Usually a secondary finding in small airway or interstitial lung disease
	Does not show obliterated bronchioles or bronchiolar constriction
Hypersensitivity pneumonitis or	Absence of obliterated bronchioles
	Loose fibrosis plugging adjacent or away from bronchioles
Idiopathic bronchiolocentric interstitial pneumonia	No circumferential fibrosis
	Poorly formed granulomas (hypersensitivity pneumonitis)

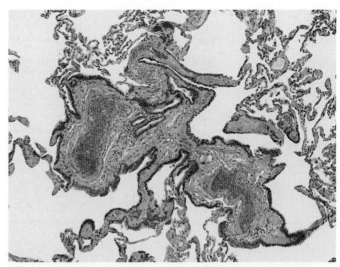

FIGURE 37.6 ▲ Peribronchiolar metaplasia. There are areas where the native bronchiole is absent, possibly indicating constrictive bronchiolitis, and the peribronchiolar extension is evident.

constrictive bronchiolitis include follicular bronchiolitis (see Chapter 36), which is seen in HIV infection, Sjögren syndrome and other rheumatologic lung disease, X-linked agammaglobulinemia, and common variable immunodeficiency.[27] Granulomatous–lymphocytic interstitial lung disease is a related process that also affects patients with common variable immunodeficiency, marked by interstitial inflammation with granulomas, as well as follicular bronchiolitis.[28]

Airway-Centered Interstitial Fibrosis and Centrilobular Fibrosis

Usual interstitial pneumonia and nonspecific interstitial pneumonia are generally distinct both clinically and pathologically from constrictive bronchiolitis, because they primarily involve the lung parenchyma, not the small airways. Although it was appreciated decades ago that small airway disease may be a component of idiopathic pulmonary fibrosis,[29] bronchiolar disease is secondary and pulmonary function tests generally show restrictive, not obstructive parameters. Occasional idiopathic forms of fibrotic lung disease may be primarily bronchiolocentric and have been termed "airway-centered interstitial fibrosis"[30] and "centrilobular fibrosis."[31] Although bronchioles are often narrowed and distorted in these conditions, they are not overtly obstructed by dense fibrosis, and instead of subepithelial fibrosis, there is more adventitial scarring. Illustrations of these entities actually more likely show bronchiolectasis and peribronchiolar metaplasia, as opposed to true constrictive bronchiolitis, and the whole secondary lobule is often scarred. Furthermore, imaging in idiopathic centrilobular or airway-centered fibrosis is not typical of constrictive bronchiolitis, in that there is little or no hyperinflation, air trapping, or increased bronchovascular markings.[30]

Peribronchiolar Metaplasia

Peribronchiolar metaplasia denotes extension of respiratory epithelium along alveolar septa around bronchioles (Fig. 37.6) and is a common secondary finding in interstitial lung disease. About one-half of biopsies of usual interstitial pneumonia, nonspecific interstitial pneumonia, desquamative interstitial pneumonia, and hypersensitivity pneumonitis show peribronchiolar metaplasia; it is less frequent in respiratory bronchiolitis.[32] It has been described as the sole finding in open lung biopsies and therefore as a novel form of small airway disease in a series of fifteen patients.[32] In these patients, there was an association with collagen vascular disease and inhalational exposure, similar to constrictive bronchiolitis. Histologic features that overlapped with constrictive bronchiolitis included peribronchiolar fibrosis in 11 cases, although

"constrictive change" was considered to be only minor, with narrowing of the lumen in only two cases. Although it is tempting to consider idiopathic peribronchiolar metaplasia as a variant of constrictive bronchiolitis, the computed tomography findings in this series of patients were not typical of constrictive bronchiolitis, and most patients had primarily restrictive or mixed pulmonary function tests.[32]

Hypersensitivity Pneumonitis

Hypersensitivity pneumonitis (Chapter 23) is in a certain sense the prototypic small airway disease, being probably second most common in frequency after reactive airway disease in chronic bronchitis and emphysema. Therefore, it is in the differential diagnosis of any type of small airway disease. Some series of constrictive bronchiolitis patients have a few cases that seem to overlap with hypersensitivity pneumonitis, in that there are poorly formed granulomas.[11] However, hypersensitivity pneumonitis by definition has a prominent interstitial component. Furthermore, the airway changes in hypersensitivity pneumonitis are more frequently chronic inflammation and peribronchiolar metaplasia, without concentric fibrosis. The fibrosis seen in hypersensitivity pneumonitis is more that of loose fibrosis (organizing pneumonia) that is adjacent to airways or within the alveolar spaces. Radiologic features of hypersensitivity pneumonitis not typical of constrictive bronchiolitis include areas of ground-glass opacities (corresponding to organizing pneumonia histologically) and poorly defined centrilobular nodules; air trapping and mosaic attenuation are seen in both entities.

Idiopathic Bronchiolocentric Interstitial Pneumonia

Yousem and Dacic described a form of small airway disease as "idiopathic bronchiolocentric interstitial pneumonia."[33] This series of patients had primarily restrictive lung disease with histologic features that overlapped with hypersensitivity pneumonitis, but (by definition) without granulomas. Although small airway fibrosis was described as "peribronchiolar fibrosis with coexistent bronchiolar and goblet cell metaplasia" or "microscopic honeycomb change," the histologic illustration was similar to that of extensive peribronchiolar metaplasia. The 10 patients in this series had an unusually aggressive course, with many progressive to fibrotic lung disease.[33]

Prognosis and Treatment

The prognosis is generally poor for cases of established fibrous obliteration of lumina. Irrespective of etiology, most patients worsen and die within months to few years,[4,10,34] although patients may remain stable for long periods with persistent disease.[13] The most common treatment is long-term steroid and other immunosuppressive agents.[35] Lung transplantation has been attempted with variable success rates.[36–38] In constrictive bronchiolitis caused by occupational inhalation, symptoms of cough may improve after cessation of exposure, but dyspnea often does not, and many patients require lung transplant.[22]

REFERENCES

1. Geddes DM, Corrin B, Brewerton DA, et al. Progressive airway obliteration in adults and its association with rheumatoid disease. *Q J Med.* 1977;46:427–444.
2. Turton CW, Williams G, Green M. Cryptogenic obliterative bronchiolitis in adults. *Thorax.* 1981;36:805–810.
3. Epler GR, Colby TV, McLoud TC, et al. Bronchiolitis obliterans organizing pneumonia. *N Engl J Med.* 1985;312:152–158.
4. Lynch JP III, Weigt SS, DerHovanessian A, et al. Obliterative (constrictive) bronchiolitis. *Semin Respir Crit Care Med.* 2012;33:509–532.
5. Ito M, Nakagawa A, Hirabayashi N, et al. Bronchiolitis obliterans in ataxia-telangiectasia. *Virchows Arch.* 1997;430:131–137.
6. Jonigk D, Merk M, Hussein K, et al. Obliterative airway remodeling: molecular evidence for shared pathways in transplanted and native lungs. *Am J Pathol.* 2011;178:599–608.
7. Belperio JA, Weigt SS, Fishbein MC, et al. Chronic lung allograft rejection: mechanisms and therapy. *Proc Am Thorac Soc.* 2009;6:108–121.
8. Jonigk D, Theophile K, Hussein K, et al. Obliterative airway remodelling in transplanted and non-transplanted lungs. *Virchows Arch.* 2010;457:369–380.
9. Barker AF, Bergeron A, Rom WN, et al. Obliterative bronchiolitis. *N Engl J Med.* 2014;370:1820–1828.
10. Kelly K, Hertz MI. Obliterative bronchiolitis. *Clin Chest Med.* 1997;18:319–338.
11. Markopoulou KD, Cool CD, Elliot TL, et al. Obliterative bronchiolitis: varying presentations and clinicopathological correlation. *Eur Respir J.* 2002;19:20–30.
12. Ryu JH, Myers JL, Swensen SJ. Bronchiolar disorders. *Am J Respir Crit Care Med.* 2003;168:1277–1292.
13. Kraft M, Mortenson RL, Colby TV, et al. Cryptogenic constrictive bronchiolitis. A clinicopathologic study. *Am Rev Respir Dis.* 1993;148:1093–1101.
14. Homma S, Sakamoto S, Kawabata M, et al. Comparative clinicopathology of obliterative bronchiolitis and diffuse panbronchiolitis. *Respiration.* 2006;73:481–487.
15. Hasegawa Y, Shimokata K, Ichiyama S, et al. Constrictive bronchiolitis obliterans and paraneoplastic pemphigus. *Eur Respir J.* 1999;13:934–937.
16. Kreiss K. Occupational causes of constrictive bronchiolitis. *Curr Opin Allergy Clin Immunol.* 2013;13:167–172.
17. King MS, Eisenberg R, Newman JH, et al. Constrictive bronchiolitis in soldiers returning from Iraq and Afghanistan. *N Engl J Med.* 2011;365:222–230.
18. Cullinan P, McGavin CR, Kreiss K, et al. Obliterative bronchiolitis in fibreglass workers: a new occupational disease? *Occup Environ Med.* 2013;70:357–359.
19. Chen CH, Tsai PJ, Wang WC, et al. Obliterative bronchiolitis in workers laying up fiberglass-reinforced plastics with polyester resin and methylethyl ketone peroxide catalyst. *Occup Environ Med.* 2013;70:675–676.
20. Centers for Disease C and Prevention. Obliterative bronchiolitis in workers in a coffee-processing facility – Texas, 2008–2012. *MMWR Morb Mortal Wkly Rep.* 2013;62:305–307.
21. Kanwal R, Kullman G, Piacitelli C, et al. Evaluation of flavorings-related lung disease risk at six microwave popcorn plants. *J Occup Environ Med.* 2006;48:149–157.
22. Akpinar-Elci M, Travis WD, Lynch DA, et al. Bronchiolitis obliterans syndrome in popcorn production plant workers. *Eur Respir J.* 2004;24:298–302.
23. Chang H, Wang JS, Tseng HH, et al. Histopathological study of Sauropus androgynus-associated constrictive bronchiolitis obliterans: a new cause of constrictive bronchiolitis obliterans. *Am J Surg Pathol.* 1997;21:35–42.
24. Couture C, Colby TV. Histopathology of bronchiolar disorders. *Semin Respir Crit Care Med.* 2003;24:489–498.
25. Hopkins PM, Aboyoun CL, Chhajed PN, et al. Prospective analysis of 1,235 transbronchial lung biopsies in lung transplant recipients. *J Heart Lung Transplant.* 2002;21:1062–1067.
26. Rice A, Nicholson AG. The pathologist's approach to small airways disease. *Histopathology.* 2009;54:117–133.
27. Costa-Carvalho BT, Wandalsen GF, Pulici G, et al. Pulmonary complications in patients with antibody deficiency. *Allergol Immunopathol (Madr).* 2011;39:128–132.
28. Park JH, Levinson AI. Granulomatous-lymphocytic interstitial lung disease (GLILD) in common variable immunodeficiency (CVID). *Clin Immunol.* 2010;134:97–103.
29. Fulmer JD, Roberts WC, von Gal ER, et al. Small airways in idiopathic pulmonary fibrosis. Comparison of morphologic and physiologic observations. *J Clin Invest.* 1977;60:595–610.
30. Churg A, Myers J, Suarez T, et al. Airway-centered interstitial fibrosis: a distinct form of aggressive diffuse lung disease. *Am J Surg Pathol.* 2004;28:62–68.
31. de Carvalho ME, Kairalla RA, Capelozzi VL, et al. Centrilobular fibrosis: a novel histological pattern of idiopathic interstitial pneumonia. *Pathol Res Pract.* 2002;198:577–583.
32. Fukuoka J, Franks TJ, Colby TV, et al. Peribronchiolar metaplasia: a common histologic lesion in diffuse lung disease and a rare cause of interstitial lung disease: clinicopathologic features of 15 cases. *Am J Surg Pathol.* 2005;29:948–954.
33. Yousem SA, Dacic S. Idiopathic bronchiolocentric interstitial pneumonia. *Mod Pathol.* 2002;15:1148–1153.
34. Perez T, Remy-Jardin M, Cortet B. Airways involvement in rheumatoid arthritis: clinical, functional, and HRCT findings. *Am J Respir Crit Care Med.* 1998;157:1658–1665.
35. Weigt SS, Wallace WD, Derhovanessian A, et al. Chronic allograft rejection: epidemiology, diagnosis, pathogenesis, and treatment. *Semin Respir Crit Care Med.* 2010;31:189–207.
36. Pigula FA, Griffith BP, Zenati MA, et al. Lung transplantation for respiratory failure resulting from systemic disease. *Ann Thorac Surg.* 1997;64:1630–1634.
37. Redel-Montero J, Bujalance-Cabrera C, Vaquero-Barrios JM, et al. Lung transplantation for bronchiolitis obliterans after allogenic bone marrow transplantation. *Transplant Proc.* 2010;42:3023–3025.
38. Lai RS, Wang JS, Wu MT, et al. Lung transplantation in bronchiolitis obliterans associated with vegetable consumption. *Lancet.* 1998;352:117–118.

38 Bacterial Pneumonias

Allen P. Burke, M.D., and Marie-Christine Aubry, M.D.

Community-Acquired Pneumonia

Clinical Findings

Pneumonia is the most common cause of death from infectious diseases worldwide. Community-acquired pneumonia is believed to result, in most cases, from endogenous infection originating from oropharyngeal colonization. Bacteria such as *Streptococcus pneumoniae*, *Staphylococcus aureus*, *Haemophilus influenzae*, *Moraxella catarrhalis*, and *Streptococcus pyogenes* are found in the upper respiratory tracts of asymptomatic individuals.[1] In cases of *S. aureus* pneumonia, skin lesions are frequently present and are believed to be an additional source of endogenous pneumonia.

Inhalation of aerosolized respiratory or gastrointestinal secretions from infected persons is an uncommon route of infection for bacterial pneumonias. It is the most frequent method of spread for mycobacterial pneumonia (Chapter 40), mycoplasma pneumonia, and chlamydial (chlamydophila) pneumonia. Rarely, bacteria such as *Yersinia pestis*, *Francisella tularensis*, and *Bacillus anthracis* are causes of exogenous pneumonia. *Legionella pneumophila* is acquired by inhalation of infected water droplets from commercial sources such as cooling towers or air conditioning systems.

The most common symptom is cough, followed by sputum production, dyspnea, and chest pain. Chest x-ray typically shows an area of consolidation, with multilobar involvement in one-third of patients. An interstitial pattern is uncommon and associated with atypical pneumonia.

Complications occur in <25% of patients and include respiratory failure requiring mechanical ventilation, septic shock, and empyema.

The mortality of community-acquired pneumonia that requires hospitalization is 10%, and is higher in elderly patients and patients with comorbidities, bacteremia, and multidrug-resistant pathogens.[2]

Etiology

The most common causes of community-acquired pneumonia requiring hospitalization are the "typical" bacteria: *S. pneumoniae* (the most common in all series), *H. influenzae* (usually the second most common), *Serratia marcescens*, *S. aureus*, *Klebsiella pneumoniae*, *M. catarrhalis*, enterobacteriaceae, and enterococci. In nonhospitalized patients, atypical bacteria (*Mycoplasma pneumoniae* and *Chlamydophila pneumoniae*) are the most common. *Legionella pneumophila* is a common cause in some series and usually occurs in outbreaks.[3] The age at presentation is not associated with the infectious agent.[2]

Laboratory Diagnosis

The standard method of diagnosis is that of sputum culture. Blood cultures are frequently positive in cases of staphylococcal and streptococcal infection. Single or paired serology is typically the diagnostic test for atypical pneumonias. The diagnosis of *L. pneumophila* is based on urine antigen testing, as culture is difficult.[4]

Rapid molecular testing is available in respiratory pathogen panels for *M. pneumoniae*, *C. pneumoniae*, and *Bordetella pertussis*.

Open lung biopsy is rarely performed in cases of community-acquired pneumonia. However, in some cases, a noninfectious etiology can be established and appropriate treatment instituted.[5]

Nosocomial (Hospital-Acquired) Bacterial Pneumonias

Clinical Findings

Nosocomial pneumonia is defined as a pneumonia that is acquired by patients at least 2 to 3 days after being hospitalized. Most hospital-acquired pneumonias occur in patients on assisted ventilation (aka as ventilator-associated pneumonia) who have been on prior antibiotics. The risk is proportional to the duration of mechanical ventilation with an overall risk of about 50%. There is a high mortality of between 40% and 50%.[6,7]

The diagnosis is generally made clinically and based on new and persistent pulmonary opacities, purulent respiratory secretions, systemic signs of inflammatory response, and fever.[8] Most occur within the first week after tracheotomy, with a median onset of 20 days after admission to the intensive care unit.[8]

The treatment is broad-spectrum antibiotics, which may be ineffectual due to the increase in multidrug-resistant organisms, especially *Acinetobacter* and *Staphylococcus*. Surgical intervention with pleural decortication may be required, if there is the development of abscesses with empyema.[7]

Etiology

When patients are admitted to the hospital, there is a shift in the bacteria colonizing the upper respiratory tract, from predominantly Gram-positive bacteria to Gram-negative bacteria.[9] Tracheostomy performed for assisted breathing is associated with an increased risk for pneumonia, especially Gram-negative bacteria. Although tracheal aspirates show colonization with Gram-negative bacilli in the majority of hospitalized patients, preintubation tracheal cultures do not reliably predict the development of pneumonia.[8]

The specific agent is often not identified. The most frequent isolates in ventilator-associated pneumonia are *Acinetobacter baumannii*, *Pseudomonas aeruginosa*, *Escherichia coli*, *S. aureus*, *Proteus mirabilis*, *K. pneumoniae*, and *H. influenzae*.[6,8,10,11]

Laboratory Diagnosis

The diagnosis is confirmed by quantitative culture of bronchoalveolar lavage fluid.[12] Thresholds for identification of etiologic pathogens are typically 1,000 cfu/mL for protected specimen brush and 1,000,000 cfu/mL for tracheal aspirates.[8]

Tissue Gram stains of lower airway endotracheal aspirates show a good correlation with culture, with a negative Gram stain yielding a high negative predictive value, especially for Gram-positive cocci.[13] The detection of intracellular organisms in bronchoalveolar lavage fluids is also diagnostically useful.[14]

Transbronchial or open lung biopsy is rarely performed for the diagnosis of nosocomial pneumonia.

Bacterial Pneumonia in Immunosuppressed Patients

Transplant-Related Pneumonias

Bacterial infections are the most frequent cause of pneumonia in transplant patients. Viral infections and pneumocystis pneumonia are also common and are usually treated prophylactically, especially early after transplantation (Chapters 39 and 42).

Pneumonia in transplant patients, similar to immunocompetent patients, may be community acquired or nosocomial. In solid organ transplants, the rate is ~10 episodes of pneumonia per 1,000 recipients/year. A specific diagnosis is made in about two-thirds of patients. Bacterial causes are by far the most frequent and show a high rate of multidrug resistance when hospital acquired. Graft rejection or dysfunction occurs in about 20% of patients.[15]

Bacteria that result in transplant-related pneumonia include *S. pneumoniae*, *H. influenzae*, *M. catarrhalis*, *S. aureus*, *Nocardia*, *Mycobacterium tuberculosis*, *C. pneumoniae*, and *Veillonella* species. In hospital-acquired multidrug-resistant cases, the most frequent organisms are *P. aeruginosa*, Enterobacteriaceae, *S. aureus*, *A. baumannii*, *Stenotrophomonas maltophilia*, and *Burkholderia cepacia*.[15,16]

Chemotherapy and Neutropenia-Related Pneumonias

Neutropenia is the most important risk factor for pneumonia in patients with hematologic and solid malignancies. Neutrophils are sensitive to alkylating agents and nucleoside analogues and neutropenia is defined as severe when blood counts are below 500/mL.[17]

Infections are the leading cause for nonrelapse mortality in cancer patients. Despite early empirical antibiotic therapy, infection-related mortality in neutropenic cancer patients is 4% to 7%.[18]

The bacterial causes of pneumonias in cancer patients include common respiratory pathogens such as *S. pneumoniae*, *S. aureus*, and *H. influenza* as well as Gram-negative enteric organisms, including *Pseudomonas* spp., *K. pneumoniae*, *E. coli*, *Enterobacter cloacae*, *S. maltophilia*, *Citrobacter* spp., *S. marcescens*, *A. baumannii*-complex, and *Proteus* spp.[18-20]

Pneumonia Caused by Gram-Positive Cocci

Streptococcus pneumoniae

Typical pneumococcal pneumonia presents as a lobar consolidation, although focal consolidation also occurs. The inflammatory infiltrate consists of a mixture of polymorphonuclear neutrophils and macrophages. In the early stages of the infection, organisms are present in the infiltrate, and fibrin strands and leukocytes are intact. Most treated pneumococcal pneumonia resolve without sequelae, but cavitary disease may occur.

Historically, a specific diagnosis of *S. pneumoniae* can be made by applying polyvalent antiserum to capsular polysaccharide on sputum smears or tissue implants (the *Quellung reaction*). This procedure also works for other encapsulated bacteria such as *K. pneumoniae*.

Group A Streptococcal Pneumonia (S. pyogenes)

S. pyogenes is a rare cause of community-acquired pneumonia.[4] Abscess formation and empyema, sometimes with bronchopleural fistula formation, are more commonly seen than in pneumonias caused by *S. pneumoniae*.

Viridans Streptococci

Classified variously (sometimes as *Streptococcus milleri*), α-hemolytic streptococci may occasionally result in pneumonias and lung abscesses. They are frequently isolated from patients with empyema.[21] The in-hospital mortality rate for patients with empyema is 4% to 15%.[21] Approximately 40% of patients require surgical intervention, in the form of pleural decortication.

Neisseria meningitides

Pneumonia can rarely occur in patients with sepsis secondary to *N. meningitides*, resulting in abscesses and empyema.[22,23]

Staphylococcus aureus

Historically, *S. aureus* pneumonia was recognized as a complication of influenza outbreaks. Currently, it is an uncommon cause of community-acquired pneumonia.[4,24] *Staphylococcus aureus* is emerging as a relatively common cause of nosocomial pneumonia, being the most common Gram-positive nosocomial pathogen, but less frequent than Gram-negative pneumonia.[25]

Occasional necrotizing community-acquired pneumonias have been reported with methicillin-resistant *S. aureus*, often associated with skin lesions.[26] High virulence is associated with the formation of toxins such as Panton-Valentine leukocidin that cause extensive tissue necrosis. Strains forming this toxin are becoming more frequently resistant to methicillin and are associated with a high mortality.[27,28]

Botryomycosis

Infections with *S. aureus* can result in a chronic granulomatous inflammatory response around clusters of organisms resembling sulfur granules of actinomycosis, which typically involve the skin. Rarely, viscera including the lung are involved.[29] Other bacteria can cause botryomycosis, primarily Gram-negative rods.

Gram-Negative Bacterial Pneumonias

Pseudomonas aeruginosa

Pseudomonas pneumonia is typically a nosocomial infection and often spreads from aspirated stomach contents or hematogenously from other sources of infection.

Chronic pseudomonas infection occurs in the majority of cystic fibrosis patients and may result in cavitary lesions and empyema.[30]

Haemophilus influenzae

Haemophilus influenzae pneumonia typically results in focal or lobar consolidations and is rarely fatal. It is the second most common typical bacterial cause of community-acquired pneumonia, after *S. pneumoniae*.[4]

Haemophilus influenzae type b was previously the most common serotype isolated from respiratory infections. With the use of vaccines against this type, there has been an emergence of invasive infection with nontypable *H. influenzae* causing severe and even fatal pneumonia in children and elderly immunocompetent patients.[31-33]

Klebsiella pneumoniae and Other Enterobacteriaceae

Enterobacteriaceae (enteric Gram-negative bacilli) are opportunistic infections in immunosuppressed patients and patients with alcoholism, diabetes mellitus, chronic obstructive lung disease or on ventilators. The mode of transmission is secondary to colonization of the oropharynx and aspiration of secretions. Necrosis, abscess formation, and empyema occur more frequently than in pneumococcal pneumonia. Bacteremia is associated with a poor prognosis.

Legionella pneumonia

Legionella pneumophila and *L. micdadei* cause a community-acquired pneumonia after exposure to the pathogen in water droplets from ventilation systems or water towers and are the causes of nearly 10% of community-acquired pneumonia.[3]

Nonpneumophila species including *L. micdadei* and *L. bozemanii* are relatively common opportunistic infections in immunosuppressed patients, including stem cell and solid organ transplants.[34] The urine antigen test developed for *L. pneumophila*[35] may not be positive in some species, and the appearance on acid fast bacilla (AFB) stain may occasionally be mistaken for mycobacteria.[36-38]

Acinetobacter baumannii

Acinetobacter baumannii has become a leading cause of nosocomial infections and, in some series, the most common form of bacterial pneumonia.[25] There are few pathologic studies of *Acinetobacter* pneumonia, but there may be abscesses, and organisms, which are very short and confused with cocci, may be present. There may be prominent suppuration and focal hyaline membranes.[39]

Community-acquired *Acinetobacter* pneumonia is rare, although may be relatively common in indigenous populations in tropical and subtropical regions.[40]

Other Bacterial Pneumonias

Gram-Positive Bacilli

Rhodococcus (Corynebacterium) equi is an equine pathogen that commonly causes pneumonia in foals. In humans, *R. equi* may rarely result in pneumonia in both immunocompetent and immunosuppressed patients.[41–45] Chest radiographs usually show a unilobar opacity that may spread to other lobes or cavitate, and mimic tuberculosis. Abscesses and empyema may occur.[46]

Anthrax is a highly transmissible respiratory disease caused by *B. anthracis* resulting from exposure to spores. It manifests as cutaneous pustules, gastrointestinal disease, septicemia, and pneumonia, the last via inhalation of spores that germinate and multiply in the mediastinal lymph nodes. Pulmonary involvement is secondary and is characterized by hemorrhage and edema. The most prominent autopsy finding is that of enlarged, hemorrhagic lymph nodes in the tracheobronchial regions. Pneumonia can occasionally be secondary to gastrointestinal involvement.[47]

Pneumonia has also been reported secondary to *Bacillus cereus*, an organism related to *B. anthracis*, in both immunocompetent and immunocompromised patients, especially if the anthrax toxin is elaborated.[48,49]

Mycoplasma

Pneumonia caused by *M. pneumoniae* and *C. pneumoniae* (see below) constitutes most of the so-called atypical pneumonias, characterized by lesser degrees of fever, a relatively benign course, and difficulty culturing on routine media. It is a frequent cause of community-acquired pneumonia, especially those that do not require hospitalization. The diagnosis has traditionally been made by serology, although both organisms are now represented in respiratory pathogen panels using molecular techniques.

Mycoplasma may rarely cause severe and fulminant pneumonia, occasionally resulting in death. Pathologic findings show lymphoplasmacytic bronchiolitis and organizing pneumonia.[50–52]

Chlamydia

The most common chlamydial pneumonia is that caused by *C. pneumoniae*. *Chlamydia trachomatis* and *Chlamydia psittaci* primarily cause pneumonia in infants and owners of pet birds, respectively. Pathologic features are nonspecific, and not well studied, due to the generally good prognosis.

Coxiella Pneumonia

Q fever is caused by infection due to *Coxiella burnetii*, an organism that was generally classified as a rickettsia and more currently a Gram-negative rod related to *Legionella* spp. Approximately 5% of patients with the disease develop lower respiratory infection.

Pathologic Findings

Bacterial infection results in intra-alveolar collections of fluid, fibrin, and leukocytes, which cause areas of consolidation (Table 38.1). Grossly, consolidation may be lobar (Fig. 38.1) as typically seen in

TABLE 38.1 Characteristics of Selected Bacterial Pneumonias

Organism	Species Notes	Relative Occurrence in Immunocompetent Patients	Abscesses/ Cavitation	Empyema	Notes
Streptococcus pneumoniae	Can be identified by capsule (Quellung)	Frequent	Occasional, especially with bacteremia	Infrequent	Empyema common with viridans infection
Staphylococcus aureus	Coagulase positive	Infrequent, may be increasing	Frequent (especially PVL)	Frequent	Toxin producing (e.g., PVL) causes extensive necrosis.
Bacillus anthracis	Some overlap with toxin-forming *B. cereus*	Frequent	Infrequent	Infrequent	Hemorrhage and edema, especially of paratracheal and peribronchial lymph nodes
Rhodococcus equi	Previously corynebacterium	Frequent	Frequent	Occasional	Malakoplakia
Enterobacteriaceae	*Klebsiella, E. coli, Serratia* Quellung reaction with encapsulated *K. pneumoniae*	Rare	Frequent	Frequent	Vasculitis, especially with *Serratia*
Pseudomonas aeruginosa		Rare	Frequent	Common, especially in CF patients	Vasculitis, with organisms in vessel wall, thrombi, and infarcts
Burkholderia cepacia	Prev. pseudomonas	Rare	Necrotizing nodules	Common	Associated with cystic fibrosis
Burkholderia pseudomallei	Prev. pseudomonas	Frequent in endemic areas (Southeast Asia)	Necrotizing nodules	Occasional	Causes melioidosis
Moraxella catarrhalis	Gram—coccobacilli Prev. *Neisseria* and *Branhamella*	Frequent	Rare	Rare	Mild disease
Acinetobacter baumannii	Many previous names	Occasional, especially in tropics	Frequent	Frequent	Common opportunistic pathogen
Legionella spp.	*L. pneumophila*; nonpneumophila spp.	Common (typically pneumophila and longbeachae spp.)	Infrequent	Uncommon, except nonpneumophila spp., in immunocompromised patients	Extensive apoptosis/karyorrhexis of inflammatory exudate Vasculitis

PVL, Panton-Valentine leukocidin.

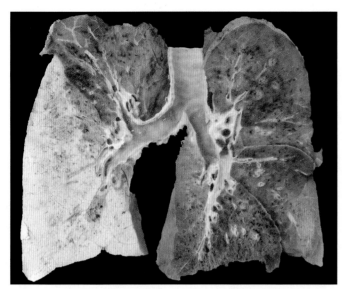

FIGURE 38.1 ▲ Lobar pneumonia. The entire left lower lobe is involved by a consolidative process, sharply demarcated from the left upper lobe at the fissure.

pneumococcal lobar pneumonia or patchy as in bronchopneumonia (Fig. 38.2). Smaller areas of consolidation may be difficult to distinguish from surrounding lung parenchyma, especially in early stages. Areas of consolidation may result in necrotic cavities and abscess formation (Fig. 38.3) and empyema (Fig. 38.4).

The gross term "red hepatization" has been used to designate the early phase of consolidation, corresponding histologically to intact intra-alveolar erythrocytes, fibrin, and neutrophils, with desquamated pneumocytes (Fig. 38.5). Colonies of bacteria may be visible. "Gray hepatization" follows several days later, when the lungs are darker and firmer, and there is degeneration of intra-alveolar leukocytes and red cells with appearance of macrophages. Ultimately, resolution of the exudate occurs. In some patient, the histologic process evolves into organizing pneumonia (Chapters 5). The development of diffuse interstitial fibrosis in the healed phase of bacterial pneumonia is exceptional.[53]

Some organisms may exhibit particular histologic findings. In *Legionella* pneumonia, the inflammatory infiltrate is generally composed of neutrophils, but an intense apoptotic degeneration often makes distinction of the cell type difficult (Fig. 38.6). Macrophages may

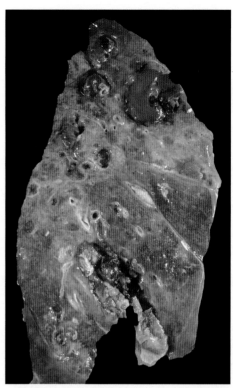

FIGURE 38.3 ▲ Necrotizing pneumonia with multiple hemorrhagic cavities and abscesses.

also be numerous. Small pulmonary vessels may show inflammation without additional vascular abnormality.[54] *R. equi* may cause an unusual histiocytic inflammatory process resulting in malakoplakia, with histiocytes containing the typical intracytoplasmic Michaelis-Gutmann

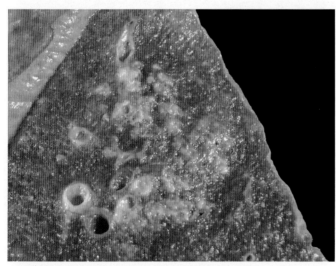

FIGURE 38.2 ▲ Bronchopneumonia. In contrast to a lobar pneumonia, bronchopneumonia is characterized by multifocal areas of consolidation centered on the airways.

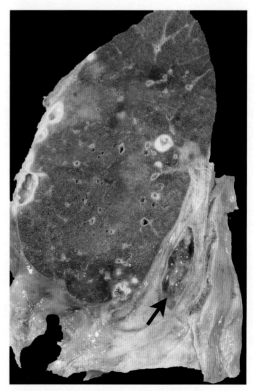

FIGURE 38.4 ▲ Pneumonia with abscesses and empyema. There are scattered subpleural abscesses and an empyema cavity (*arrow*).

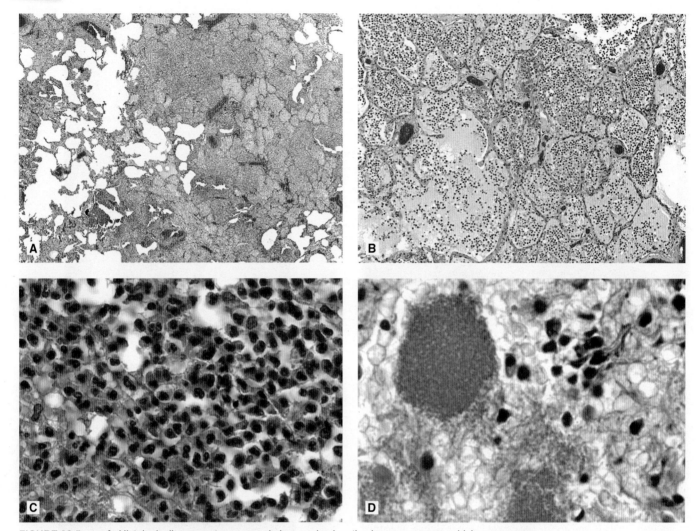

FIGURE 38.5 ▲ **A.** Histologically, an acute pneumonia is a predominantly airspace process, which may appear patchy. **B.** The airspaces are filled by fibrin admixed with numerous inflammatory cells. **C.** The inflammatory cells are mostly neutrophils. **D.** Colonies of bacteria can often be seen on H&E.

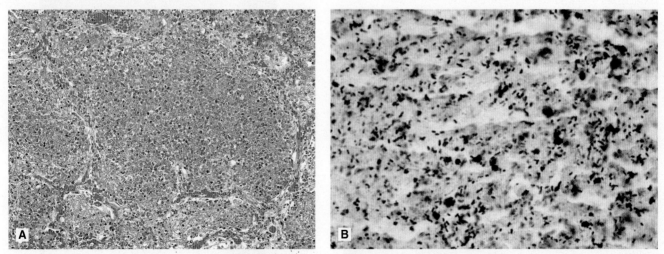

FIGURE 38.6 ▲ **A.** In *Legionella* pneumonia, neutrophils typically undergo significant apoptosis. **B.** A Warthin-Starry stain assists with the identification of the organisms.

bodies.[55] Q fever pneumonia is characterized histologically by numerous alveolar macrophages containing *C. burnetii* that can be demonstrated immunohistochemically within large cytoplasmic vacuoles.[56,57]

Pneumonia may be complicated by **abscess formation**. This is the result of necrosis with tissue destruction by the acute inflammation. Abscess formation is commonly seen in *Pseudomonas*, *Klebsiella*, and *Serratia* pneumonia. Furthermore, prominent vascular inflammation, with or without necrosis of the vessels, with thrombosis and pulmonary infarct may be seen with these organisms. Commonly, bacteria may be present within the vessels.[58-61] This may lead to another complication of pneumonia, which is **bacteremic dissemination** to other organs, including the brain, heart valves, and joints, resulting in meningitis, endocarditis, and septic arthritis. Another complication of pneumonia is **empyema**. Empyema occurs in ~1% of community-acquired cases. Clinically, empyema is defined by the presence of microorganisms in pleural fluid, Gram stain, or culture; pleural pH < 7.2 associated with radiographic features of empyema; or frank pus in the pleural space at the time of thoracoscopy. The pathologic definition is that of purulent inflammation within the pleural cavity with presence of microorganisms histologically or clinically proven. The most common pathogen is *Streptococcus*, especially *S. milleri* (viridans) (50%).

The histologic appearance of pneumonia differs in neutropenic patients. Indeed, there is abundant hemorrhage with fibrin, but acute inflammation is absent. Bacteria may be seen without cellular reaction and are usually present within macrophages.[58]

Special Stains for Organisms

Special stains are helpful in identifying intracellular organisms in autopsy and biopsy samples of immunocompromised patients. Brown-Hopps stains are best for general bacteria, whereas Brown-Brenn staining is superior for Gram-positive bacteria. Bacteria are also well stained by Gomori methenamine staining normally used for fungi. Steiner or Warthin-Starry stains are helpful for small organisms such as *Legionella* (Fig. 38.6), *Yersinia*, *Francisella*, and *Brucella*, and poorly staining acid-fast bacilli. Some nonmycobacterial species can stain for AFB, such as *Legionella* spp., mimicking mycobacterial infection.

REFERENCES

1. Winther FO, Horthe K, Lystad A, et al. Pathogenic bacterial flora in the upper respiratory tract of healthy students. Prevalence and relationship to nasopharyngeal inflammatory symptoms. *J Laryngol Otol.* 1974;88: 407–412.
2. Cilloniz C, Polverino E, Ewig S, et al. Impact of age and comorbidity on cause and outcome in community-acquired pneumonia. *Chest.* 2013;144:999–1007.
3. Arancibia F, Cortes CP, Valdes M, et al. Importance of *Legionella pneumophila* in the etiology of severe community-acquired pneumonia in Santiago, Chile. *Chest.* 2014;145:290–296.
4. Diaz A, Barria P, Niederman M, et al. Etiology of community-acquired pneumonia in hospitalized patients in Chile: the increasing prevalence of respiratory viruses among classic pathogens. *Chest.* 2007;131:779–787.
5. Dunn IJ, Marrie TJ, MacKeen AD, et al. The value of open lung biopsy in immunocompetent patients with community-acquired pneumonia requiring hospitalization. *Chest.* 1994;106:23–27.
6. Ranjan N, Chaudhary U, Chaudhry D, et al. Ventilator-associated pneumonia in a tertiary care intensive care unit: analysis of incidence, risk factors and mortality. *Indian J Crit Care Med.* 2014;18:200–204.
7. Behnia M, Logan SC, Fallen L, et al. Nosocomial and ventilator-associated pneumonia in a community hospital intensive care unit: a retrospective review and analysis. *BMC Res Notes.* 2014;7:232.
8. Rello J, Lorente C, Diaz E, et al. Incidence, etiology, and outcome of nosocomial pneumonia in ICU patients requiring percutaneous tracheotomy for mechanical ventilation. *Chest.* 2003;124:2239–2243.
9. Johanson WG, Pierce AK, Sanford JP. Changing pharyngeal bacterial flora of hospitalized patients. Emergence of gram-negative bacilli. *N Engl J Med.* 1969;281:1137–1140.
10. Inchai J, Pothirat C, Liwsrisakun C, et al. Ventilator-associated pneumonia: epidemiology and prognostic indicators of 30-day mortality. *Jpn J Infect Dis.* 2015;68:181–186.
11. Ali S, Waheed K, Iqbal ZH. Microbiological pattern of ventilator associated pneumonia. *J Ayub Med Coll Abbottabad.* 2015;27:117–119.
12. Kirtland SH, Corley DE, Winterbauer RH, et al. The diagnosis of ventilator-associated pneumonia: a comparison of histologic, microbiologic, and clinical criteria. *Chest.* 1997;112:445–457.
13. Gottesman T, Yossepowitch O, Lerner E, et al. The accuracy of Gram stain of respiratory specimens in excluding *Staphylococcus aureus* in ventilator-associated pneumonia. *J Crit Care.* 2014;29:739–742.
14. Torres A, El-Ebiary M, Fabregas N, et al. Value of intracellular bacteria detection in the diagnosis of ventilator associated pneumonia. *Thorax.* 1996;51:378–384.
15. Giannella M, Munoz P, Alarcon JM, et al. Pneumonia in solid organ transplant recipients: a prospective multicenter study. *Transpl Infect Dis.* 2014;16:232–241.
16. Dizdar OS, Ersoy A, Akalin H. Pneumonia after kidney transplant: incidence, risk factors, and mortality. *Exp Clin Transplant.* 2014;12:205–211.
17. Evans SE, Ost DE. Pneumonia in the neutropenic cancer patient. *Curr Opin Pulm Med.* 2015;21:260–271.
18. Neumann S, Krause SW, Maschmeyer G, et al. Primary prophylaxis of bacterial infections and *Pneumocystis jiroveci* pneumonia in patients with hematological malignancies and solid tumors: guidelines of the Infectious Diseases Working Party (AGIHO) of the German Society of Hematology and Oncology (DGHO). *Ann Hematol.* 2013;92:433–442.
19. Cordani S, Manna A, Vignali M, et al. Bronchoalveolar lavage as a diagnostic tool in patients with hematological malignancies and pneumonia. *Infez Med.* 2008;16:209–213.
20. Inai K, Iwasaki H, Noriki S, et al. Frequent detection of multidrug-resistant pneumonia-causing bacteria in the pneumonia lung tissues of patients with hematological malignancies. *Int J Hematol.* 2007;86:225–232.
21. Ahmed RA, Marrie TJ, Huang JQ. Thoracic empyema in patients with community-acquired pneumonia. *Am J Med.* 2006;119:877–883.
22. Romero-Gomez MP, Rentero Z, Pano JR, et al. Bacteraemic pneumonia caused by Neisseria meningitidis serogroup Y. *Respir Med Case Rep.* 2012;5:23–24.
23. Glikman D, Matushek SM, Kahana MD, et al. Pneumonia and empyema caused by penicillin-resistant Neisseria meningitidis: a case report and literature review. *Pediatrics.* 2006;117:e1061–e1066.
24. Centers for Disease Control and Prevention (CDC). Severe methicillin-resistant *Staphylococcus aureus* community-acquired pneumonia associated with influenza—Louisiana and Georgia, December 2006–January 2007. *MMWR Morb Mortal Wkly Rep.* 2007;56:325–329.
25. Tan L, Sun X, Zhu X, et al. Epidemiology of nosocomial pneumonia in infants after cardiac surgery. *Chest.* 2004;125:410–417.
26. Napolitano LM, Brunsvold ME, Reddy RC, et al. Community-acquired methicillin-resistant *Staphylococcus aureus* pneumonia and ARDS: 1-year follow-up. *Chest.* 2009;136:1407–1412.
27. Morgan MS. Diagnosis and treatment of Panton-Valentine leukocidin (PVL)-associated staphylococcal pneumonia. *Int J Antimicrob Agents.* 2007;30:289–296.
28. Rojo P, Barrios M, Palacios A, et al. Community-associated *Staphylococcus aureus* infections in children. *Expert Rev Anti Infect Ther.* 2010;8:541–554.
29. Ariza-Prota MA, Pando-Sandoval A, Garcia-Clemente M, et al. Primary pulmonary botryomycosis: a bacterial lung infection mimicking lung cancer. *Int J Tuberc Lung Dis.* 2013;17:992–994.
30. Mohan K, Lakshman V, Fothergill JL, et al. Empyema due to a highly transmissible *Pseudomonas aeruginosa* strain in an adult cystic fibrosis patient. *J Med Microbiol.* 2010;59:614–616.
31. Hu H, He L, Dmitriev A, et al. The role of *Haemophilus influenzae* type b in fatal community-acquired pneumonia in Chinese children. *Pediatr Infect Dis J.* 2008;27:942–944.
32. Zacharisen MC, Watters SK, Edwards J. Rapidly fatal *Haemophilus influenzae* serotype f sepsis in a healthy child. *J Infect.* 2003;46:194–196.
33. Fukushima K, Doi H, Hamaguchi S, et al. Fulminant pneumonia caused by nontypable *Haemophilus influenzae*. *Intern Med.* 2013;52:1755.
34. Wright AJ, Humar A, Gourishankar S, et al. Severe Legionnaire's disease caused by Legionella longbeachae in a long-term renal transplant patient: the importance of safe living strategies after transplantation. *Transpl Infect Dis.* 2012;14:E30–E33.

35. Yu VL, Stout JE. Rapid diagnostic testing for community-acquired pneumonia: can innovative technology for clinical microbiology be exploited? *Chest.* 2009;136:1618–1621.

36. Waldron PR, Martin BA, Ho DY. Mistaken identity: *Legionella micdadei* appearing as acid-fast bacilli on lung biopsy of a hematopoietic stem cell transplant patient. *Transpl Infect Dis.* 2015;17:89–93.

37. Miller ML, Hayden R, Gaur A. *Legionella bozemanii* pulmonary abscess in a pediatric allogeneic stem cell transplant recipient. *Pediatr Infect Dis J.* 2007;26:760–762.

38. Chow JW, Yu VL. *Legionella*: a major opportunistic pathogen in transplant recipients. *Semin Respir Infect.* 1998;13:132–139.

39. Koshimizu N, Sato M, Gemma H, et al. [An autopsy case of fulminant community-acquired pneumonia due to *Acinetobacter baumannii*]. *Kansenshogaku Zasshi.* 2009;83:392–397.

40. Davis JS, McMillan M, Swaminathan A, et al. A 16-year prospective study of community-onset bacteremic Acinetobacter pneumonia: low mortality with appropriate initial empirical antibiotic protocols. *Chest.* 2014;146:1038–1045.

41. Enriquez Rodriguez AI, Garcia Clemente M, Buchelli Ramirez HL. Severe pneumonia caused by *Rhodococcus equi* with hematogenous spread to the central nervous system in an immunocompromised patient. *Arch Bronconeumol.* 2015;51:203–204.

42. Gelfand MS, Cleveland KO, Brewer SC. *Rhodococcus equi* pneumonia in a patient with fludarabine-treated chronic lymphocytic leukemia and CD4-lymphopenia. *Am J Med Sci.* 2010;340:80–81.

43. Khan MY, Ali S, Baqi S. *Rhodococcus equi* pneumonia in a live related renal transplant recipient. *J Pak Med Assoc.* 2013;63:635–638.

44. Ng S, King CS, Hang J, et al. Severe cavitary pneumonia caused by a non-equi *Rhodococcus* species in an immunocompetent patient. *Respir Care.* 2013;58:e47–e50.

45. Shahani L. *Rhodococcus equi* pneumonia and sepsis in an allogeneic haematopoietic stem cell transplant recipient. *BMJ Case Rep.* 2014;2014.

46. Rose R, Nord J, Lanspa M. Rhodococcus empyema in a heart transplant patient. *Respirol Case Rep.* 2014;2:42–44.

47. Meric M, Willke A, Muezzinoglu B, et al. A case of pneumonia caused by *Bacillus anthracis* secondary to gastrointestinal anthrax. *Int J Infect Dis.* 2009;13:e456–e458.

48. Avashia SB, Riggins WS, Lindley C, et al. Fatal pneumonia among metalworkers due to inhalation exposure to *Bacillus cereus* Containing *Bacillus anthracis* toxin genes. *Clin Infect Dis.* 2007;44:414–416.

49. Hoffmaster AR, Hill KK, Gee JE, et al. Characterization of *Bacillus cereus* isolates associated with fatal pneumonias: strains are closely related to *Bacillus anthracis* and harbor B. anthracis virulence genes. *J Clin Microbiol.* 2006;44:3352–3360.

50. Nishikawa A, Mimura K, Kanagawa T, et al. Thrombocytopenia associated with Mycoplasma pneumonia during pregnancy: case presentation and approach for differential diagnosis. *J Obstet Gynaecol Res.* 2015;41:1273–1277.

51. Izumikawa K, Izumikawa K, Takazono T, et al. Clinical features, risk factors and treatment of fulminant *Mycoplasma pneumoniae* pneumonia: a review of the Japanese literature. *J Infect Chemother.* 2014;20:181–185.

52. Kannan TR, Hardy RD, Coalson JJ, et al. Fatal outcomes in family transmission of *Mycoplasma pneumoniae. Clin Infect Dis.* 2012;54:225–231.

53. Carlon GC, Dickinson PC, Goldiner PL, et al. *Serratia marcescens* pneumonia. *Arch Surg.* 1977;112:1220–1224.

54. Winn WC Jr, Myerowitz RL. The pathology of the Legionella pneumonias. A review of 74 cases and the literature. *Hum Pathol.* 1981;12:401–422.

55. Mule A, Petrone G, Santoro A, et al. Pulmonary malakoplakia at early stage: use of polymerase chain reaction for detection of *Rhodococcus equi. Int J Immunopathol Pharmacol.* 2012;25:703–712.

56. Botelho-Nevers E, Singh S, Chiche L, et al. Effect of omeprazole on vacuole size in *Coxiella burnetii*-infected cells. *J Infect.* 2013;66:288–289.

57. Sauer JD, Shannon JG, Howe D, et al. Specificity of *Legionella pneumophila* and *Coxiella burnetii* vacuoles and versatility of *Legionella pneumophila* revealed by coinfection. *Infect Immun.* 2005;73:4494–4504.

58. Goldstein JD, Godleski JJ, Balikian JP, et al. Pathologic patterns of *Serratia marcescens* pneumonia. *Hum Pathol.* 1982;13:479–484.

59. Tillotson JR, Lerner AM. Characteristics of nonbacteremic Pseudomonas pneumonia. *Ann Intern Med.* 1968;68:295–307.

60. Rose HD, Heckman MG, Unger JD. *Pseudomonas aeruginosa* pneumonia in adults. *Am Rev Respir Dis.* 1973;107:416–422.

61. Fetzer AE, Werner AS, Hagstrom JW. Pathologic features of pseudomonal pneumonia. *Am Rev Respir Dis.* 1967;96:1121–1130.

39 Viral Pneumonias

Allen P. Burke, M.D., and Marie-Christine Aubry, M.D.

Overview

Viral Pneumonias in Immunocompetent Patients

Viral infections account for 5% to 34% of community-acquired pneumonias.[1] Because many cases of community-acquired pneumonias are pathogenically undetermined, the rate of viral cause may be higher. With the onset of molecular testing, the frequency of viral detection in community-acquired pneumonia is almost one-third.[2] In addition, viral infections often precede bacterial pneumonias, and viruses and bacteria are both identified in patients with pneumonia in about 5% of cases.[3,4]

Clinically, viral pneumonias are less likely to cause expectoration and cough than bacterial pneumonias, although there is no difference in the degree of fever.[1] Patients tend to be older and frailer and have a higher likelihood of cardiac disease.[4,5] There is no significant difference in the radiographic appearance of bacterial and viral pneumonias.[1]

The most common organisms are influenza A and B, human parainfluenza virus, respiratory syncytial virus (RSV), and adenovirus.[1,6] With the use of expanded molecular panels, other viruses, such as metapneumovirus, coronavirus, and rhinovirus, have been implicated.[2–4]

The pathologic findings of viral pneumonias in immunocompetent patients, which are usually self-limited, are not well studied, as pathologic sampling is not performed for diagnosis.

Viral Pneumonias in the Immunosuppressed and Hospitalized Patient

Nosocomial pneumonias in immunocompetent patients are usually bacterial,[7] with the exception of cytomegalovirus (CMV) pneumonia. Nosocomial viral infections are however common in immunocompromised patients, especially in organ transplant patients, patients with chemotherapy-induced immunosuppression, and neutropenic patients with HIV/AIDS.

The most common viral pneumonia in immunocompromised patients is CMV pneumonia. Because of the high likelihood of reactivation of CMV, solid organ transplant patients are routinely given prophylaxis in the initial stages after transplant, either with ganciclovir or valganciclovir.[8–11] In open lung biopsies performed for unexplained lung opacities in immunocompromised patients, CMV is detected by light microscopy and immunohistochemistry in 3% to 6% of biopsies.[12–14]

RSV also causes pneumonia in immunosuppressed patients, with a mortality rate between 10% and 20%.[15,16] A number of other viral pneumonias occur in the immunocompromised, including varicella, HSV, and metapneumoviruses.[17-19]

Laboratory Diagnosis of Viral Pneumonias

The diagnosis of pneumonia is generally made in the microbiology laboratory, except in instances of open lung biopsy in immunocompromised patients, in which viral inclusions are identified by H&E, immunohistochemistry, or in situ hybridization. In addition to histology, cell culture techniques, serology, polymerase chain reaction (PCR), and electron microscopy are all important in diagnosing viral pneumonias.

Viruses require live cells for cultivation and are more difficult than bacteria to isolate from clinical samples. The traditional viral culture uses shell vials that take up to 5 days, are labor intensive, and suffer from a lack of sensitivity.

The least expensive method of diagnosing a viral cause of a patient with pneumonia is the detection of seroconversion for a specific viral antigen, with a fourfold rise in IgG titers.[1] This method requires a delay of weeks, however, and serial testing of the patient's serum.

A more rapid test is the direct immunofluorescence assay performed on nasopharyngeal swabs for influenza virus types A and B, parainfluenza virus types 1 to 3, adenovirus, and RSV.[4,6]

Nasopharyngeal samples can also be subjected to PCR and nucleotide amplification for pathogens such as influenza A and B, human metapneumovirus (HMPV), RSV, rhinovirus, parainfluenza 1 to 4, coronaviruses (OC43, 229E, and NL63), and adenoviruses.[2,4] Expanded molecular respiratory pathogen panels detect up to 20 pathogens, including 3 bacteria, with a turnaround time of hours.[20]

Although not used routinely in the clinical setting, electron microscopy may be critical in outbreaks of unknown etiology, as it was in the Hendra virus, Nipah virus, and coronavirus outbreaks in 1994, 1999, and 2003, respectively.

Influenza Pneumonia

Clinical

Influenza accounts for 14% to 64% of viruses detected in patients hospitalized for pneumonia.[1,2,4,6] There are no particular clinical features that distinguish influenza from other viral pneumonias.[4]

Influenza virus belongs to the Orthomyxoviridae family of RNA viruses. Types A and B are associated with significant human disease. Influenza A viruses are further classified based on the antigenicity of their hemagglutinin and neuraminidase surface glycoproteins, of which there are 16 and 9 subtypes, respectively. Only subtypes HI, H2, and H3 and subtypes Nl and N2 have established stable lineages in the human population since 1918. There have been few human outbreaks of avian flu H5N1 (Ng), and an epidemic of a swine virus of the H1N1 subtype occurred in 2009.[21]

Gross Findings

Reported pathologic findings are based largely on autopsies that are skewed toward fatal cases, which represent a small fraction of infections. For example, in the H1N1 outbreak, only 5% of cases were fatal in the southern Indian region of Hyderabad.[21]

Autopsied lungs are heavy, with subpleural hemorrhages. The mucosa of the trachea and bronchi are hemorrhagic and swollen, and the cut surfaces of the lungs show diffuse hemorrhagic consolidations.[21] Bloody pleural effusions are common.[22]

Microscopic Findings

Inflammatory changes occur in both the airways and lung parenchyma. There is chronic inflammation in the walls of the bronchi and bronchioles, with acute bronchiolitis and necrosis of bronchiolar mucosa. The parenchyma shows diffuse alveolar damage with hyaline membranes, expansion of the alveolar septa by edema and chronic inflammation, and intra-alveolar edema and hemorrhage.[21] No viral inclusions are identified (Table 39.1).

As is typical of alveolar injury of any cause, the diffuse alveolar damage associated with influenza pneumonia evolves through an acute exudative phase in the first 2 weeks and an organizing phase in patients dying in the 3rd week or later.[22]

Respiratory Syncytial Virus

Clinical

RSV is a member of the RNA virus family Paramyxoviridae. Of the two groups (A and B), the subgroup A strains are associated with more severe infections. RSV is the most common cause of bronchiolitis and pneumonia among infants and children under 1 year of age[23] and accounts for 7% to 10% of viral infections of the lower respiratory tract in immunocompetent adults.[1,2,4] In immunocompetent children, RSV pneumonia is rarely lethal (Table 39.2).[24,25]

Approximately 60% of adults with severe RSV pneumonia are immunocompromised. Symptoms are nonspecific and include cough, dyspnea, fever, expectoration, and flu symptoms.[26]

Pathologic Findings

The major histopathologic changes described in fatal RSV infections include necrotizing bronchiolitis, interstitial pneumonia, and diffuse alveolar damage. Giant cells are occasionally present and contain irregular, intracytoplasmic, eosinophilic inclusions surrounded by a clear halo. Immunohistochemical stains are helpful in identifying the inclusions, which are present in alveolar pneumocytes[27,28] (Table 39.2).

Human Parainfluenza Virus

Clinical

Human parainfluenza viruses are common viral causes of community-acquired pneumonia, particularly in children, usually under 5 years of age. The most frequent symptoms are cough and rhinorrhea.[29]

In adults with viral pneumonia, parainfluenza virus accounts for 10% to 50% of viruses detected.[1,4,6]

Pathologic Findings

Parainfluenza viral infection is rarely fatal, unless patients are immunocompromised. Autopsy studies show interstitial inflammation with organizing diffuse alveolar damage. In the majority, there are multinucleated giant cells with intracytoplasmic viral inclusions. These are

TABLE 39.1 Common Lower Respiratory Viruses Not Forming Inclusions

Family	Virus	Histologic Tissue Reaction	Ultrastructural Appearance
Orthomyxoviridae (RNA)	Influenza	Necrotizing bronchitis and bronchiolitis Diffuse alveolar damage	Pleomorphic enveloped filamentous nucleocapsids, 80–100 nm, budding at the plasma membrane
Coronaviridae (RNA)	SRAS corona virus	Interstitial pneumonia, diffuse alveolar damage	Spherical, enveloped virions, 75–160 nm in cytoplasmic vesicles
Bunyaviridae (RNA)	Hantavirus	Pulmonary edema, diffuse alveolar damage	Rarely detected in tissue granulofilamentous nucleocapsids in endothelial cells

TABLE 39.2   Common Lower Respiratory Viruses Forming Inclusions

Family	Virus	Histologic Appearance of Inclusion	Histologic Tissue Reaction	Ultrastructural Appearance
Adenoviridae (DNA)	Adenovirus	Smudgy, nuclear	Necrotizing bronchiolitis, diffuse alveolar damage	70–90 nm nucleocapsids with a dense core in cell nuclei, sometimes in paracrystalline arrays
Herpesviridae (DNA)	Cytomegalovirus Herpes simplex Varicella zoster	Nuclear and cytoplasmic, prominent halo Glassy, amphophilic, intranuclear inclusions, present in multiple cell types, occasionally with giant cells	Necrotizing bronchopneumonia, diffuse alveolar damage	100 nm viral nucleocapsids Tegument surrounds the nucleocapsids (cytoplasmic inclusion).
Paramyxoviridae (RNA) *Paramyxovirinae*	Measles Parainfluenza Human metapneumovirus	Ill-defined cytoplasmic inclusions, in multinucleated cells (fused bronchiolar cells and pneumocytes)[a]	Interstitial pneumonia, diffuse alveolar damage, necrotizing bronchiolitis	Enveloped filamentous nucleocapsids, 125–250 nm, in plasmalemma, with 18 nm buds into extracellular space
Pneumovirinae	Human metapneumovirus Respiratory syncytial virus			Spherical, enveloped 90–130 nm particles with 14 nm nucleocapsids

[a]Warthin-Finkeldey giant cells typical of measles are formed of macrophages, do not have inclusions, and are present in lymphoid tissues and spleen, and not the lung.

indistinguishable from measles and RSV inclusions, and a diagnosis generally rests on molecular testing. In autopsy samples, the inclusions may also be difficult to distinguish from herpetic inclusions, but immunohistochemical staining should readily detect inclusions of HSV or varicella zoster virus.[30] Ultrastructure will demonstrate intracytoplasmic inclusions contained fuzzy-form nucleocapsids.

Adenovirus

Clinical

Adenovirus infections are a common cause of respiratory and enteric illnesses of late infancy and childhood. In neonates, adenovirus infections are rare, carrying a high morbidity and mortality rate (Table 39.2).[31]

The mean age of children hospitalized for adenoviral pneumonia is 3 years. The most common respiratory symptoms are cough, rhinorrhea, and dyspnea. Approximately one-fifth of patients require intensive care, but most children recover without sequelae.[32]

In adolescents and adults, adenovirus accounts for 5% of community-acquired pneumonia.[3] The diagnosis is made by molecular analysis of nasopharyngeal swabs, similar to other respiratory viruses, or by identification of characteristic adenovirus-like cytopathic effects on cultured Hep-2 cells directly inoculated with the specimen sample.[3]

The most frequent symptom in adults with adenoviral pneumonia is cough and dizziness, with relatively less frequent rhinorrhea, as compared to adenoviral infections limited to the upper respiratory tract. Differential leukocyte count often reveals monocytosis.[33]

In immunocompromised patients, adenovirus can result in pulmonary consolidation. The diagnosis is made by identification of the virus from the respiratory tract or by the finding of adenoviral viremia ($>1 \times 10^5$ copies/mL). Open lung biopsy is rarely performed. The mortality is high.[34]

Pathologic Findings

Fatal cases of adenoviral pneumonia in immunocompromised patients show diffuse alveolar damage with abundant neutrophils.[35] There is also necrotizing bronchitis, bronchiolitis, and interstitial pneumonia. Characteristic smudgy intranuclear inclusions are identified in pneumocytes, which can be characterized as adenoviral inclusions by immunohistochemistry for viral protein or in situ hybridization for viral genome (Fig. 39.1).[36]

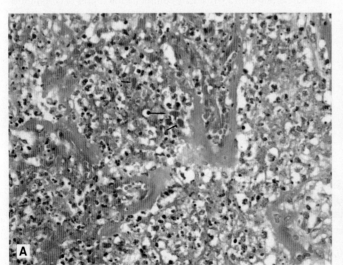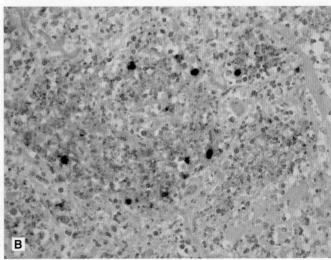

FIGURE 39.1 ▲ Adenovirus pneumonia. **A.** Viral inclusions are typically found in the areas of necrosis. The nuclear inclusions result in a smudgy appearance of the infected cells (*arrows*). **B.** In situ hybridization confirms the nature of the inclusions.

Cytomegalovirus

Clinical

CMV infection is highly prevalent and generally ranges from asymptomatic disease to mononucleosis-like syndrome. Severe life-threatening CMV disease is well documented in immunocompromised patients. Rarely, CMV causes symptomatic pneumonia in otherwise healthy persons (Table 39.2).[37]

Pneumonia secondary to CMV is common in transplants, usually after routine antiviral prophylaxis with ganciclovir has been discontinued.

Nosocomial ventilator-associated pneumonia is caused by CMV in almost one-third of patients and may be diagnosed by open lung biopsy.[38]

Pathologic Findings

CMV pneumonia is typically associated with organizing diffuse alveolar damage. Immunohistochemical staining for the viral antigen is positive in both the nuclear and cytoplasmic inclusions, facilitating the diagnosis (Fig. 39.2). Immunohistochemical staining may also show scattered cells in lungs from patients with CMV viremia without pneumonia.[39]

Herpes Simplex Virus

Clinical

Herpes simplex pneumonia is not infrequent in immunocompromised patients and may be underrecognized in immunocompetent patients as well. Symptoms include fever, dyspnea, and productive cough, and severe leukocytosis is typical. Survival is poor in both immunocompetent and immunosuppressed patients, despite ganciclovir therapy (Table 39.2).[17]

Pathologic Findings

In cases of herpetic pneumonia, concomitant herpetic tracheitis and esophagitis are common, as well as visceral dissemination.[40] The diagnosis may be facilitated by immunohistochemical stains (Fig. 39.3).[39] Airway-centered necrosis with diffuse alveolar damage is common in open lung biopsy specimens.[17]

Varicella Zoster Virus

Clinical

Varicella zoster, unlike herpes virus, can be transmitted by direct aerosol contact, as virions are present in the sputum of infected

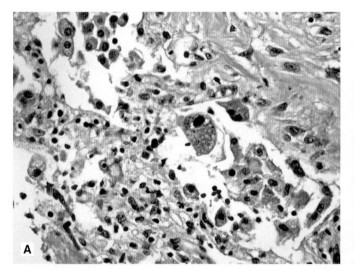

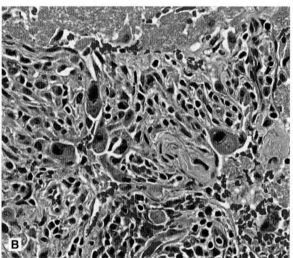

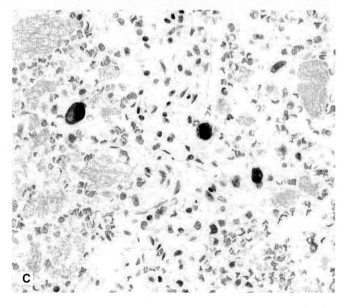

FIGURE 39.2 ▲ Cytomegalovirus pneumonia. **A.** Detached enlarged cells, probably pneumocyte, with nuclear inclusion with surrounding halo ("owl's eye"). Small granular inclusions are present in the cytoplasm as well. **B.** The infected cells have nuclear and cytoplasmic inclusions and are present in organizing alveolar damage. **C.** Immunohistochemical staining is positive.

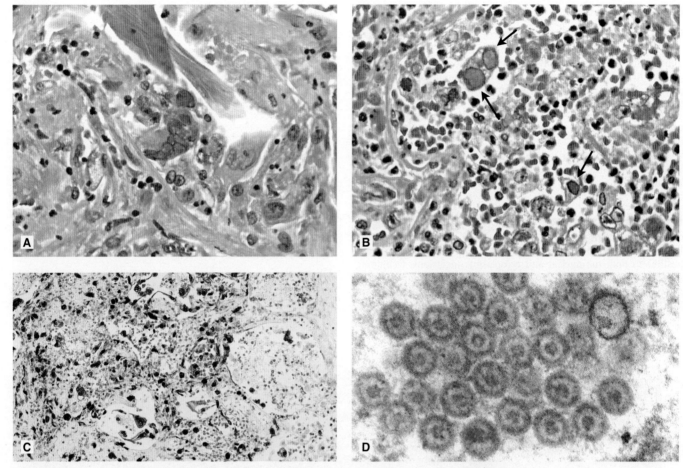

FIGURE 39.3 ▲ Herpes simplex pneumonia. **A.** The glassy inclusions are present in a giant cell. **B.** Detached cells show typical diffuse glassy nuclear inclusions (*arrows*). The infected cells are typically in areas of acute inflammation. **C.** Immunohistochemical stains show abundant positivity, including cells that do not appear on routine stains to harbor inclusions. **D.** By ultrastructure, the capsids contain a dark core.

patients. Adults are ~25 times more likely to develop pneumonia than children during an episode of cutaneous infection (chickenpox). The incidence of varicella pneumonia has declined significantly since universal childhood vaccination for varicella was implemented in 1995. In immunocompromised patients and pregnant women, however, varicella pneumonia is a serious complication of varicella zoster virus, with mortality rates of 30% to 50% (Table 39.2).[18]

Patients present with a zoster rash, followed by respiratory symptoms that may result in respiratory failure. Prognosis appears to be worse in patients with deep tracheal and bronchial ulcerations.[18]

Pathologic Findings

Grossly, there are often necrotic, hemorrhagic lesions on the visceral pleura that resemble cutaneous pox. In fatal cases, there are extensive mucosal airway ulcerations from the pharynx to the main bronchi.[18] Microscopically, there are multiple findings, including interstitial pneumonia, necrotic microabscesses, necrotizing bronchiolitis with hemorrhage, and diffuse alveolar damage. Immunohistochemical staining will demonstrate intranuclear inclusions that are difficult to ascertain on routine microscopy, within giant cells, typically in necrotic foci. Infected cells include respiratory epithelial cells, pneumocytes, fibroblasts, and capillary endothelial cells.

Other Viral Pneumonias

Coronavirus SARS

Severe acute respiratory syndrome is caused by coronavirus (SARS-CoV) that initially spread through southern China and other parts of Asia and North America in 2002–2003.[22] Pathologically, fatal cases show diffuse alveolar damage in the exudative or organizing phase, depending on the duration of illness (Table 39.1).[41]

Rhinovirus

In children with pneumonia or bronchiolitis, rhinovirus, together with RSV and parainfluenza virus, is the most common viral isolate.[42] The diagnosis is generally made by nucleic acid testing of nasopharyngeal aspirates, which frequently demonstrates mixed viral infections, especially with RSV.[43] In adults, rhinovirus is detected in about 14% of patients with community-acquired pneumonia.[4]

The histology of rhinoviral pneumonia is not known, as severe disease or fatal cases in immunocompromised patients have not yet been reported.

Metapneumovirus

HMPV is the cause of about 7% of childhood respiratory infections and generally affects infants at a mean age of 1.6 years. The most common

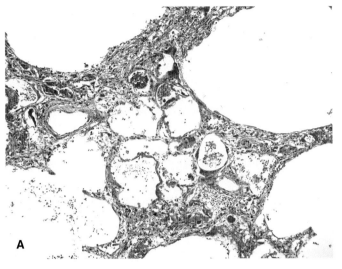

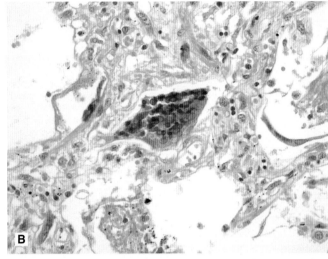

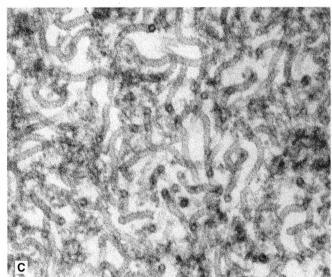

FIGURE 39.4 ▲ Measles pneumonia. **A.** In a background of diffuse alveolar damage, several large multinucleated giant cells are identified. **B.** The nuclei of the giant cells contain eosinophilic inclusions. **C.** Ultrastructurally, the viral particles form filamentous nucleocapsids.

symptoms are cough, fever, rhinitis, vomiting, and diarrhea.[44] In adults, HMPV is detected in up to 25% of viral community-acquired pneumonias (Table 39.2).[4]

In children and adults with underlying hematologic malignancies, HMPV pneumonia can be severe, causing areas of consolidation, although fatal disease is rare.[19,45,46]

The bronchoalveolar lavage specimens show degenerative changes and ill-defined eosinophilic cytoplasmic inclusions within epithelial cells and multinucleated giant cells. There are few reports of histologic features of HMPV pneumonia.

Measles (Rubeola) Pneumonia

Historically, measles pneumonia was nearly as important as influenza, because of high rate of aerosol transmission. A large outbreak of measles pneumonia predated the 1918 influenza epidemic.[47] With the current vaccine, measles pneumonia is rarely encountered. In infants who are not yet vaccinated, measles exposure and infection can result in adult respiratory distress syndrome.[48] Fatal measles pneumonia in immunosuppressed patients with HIV/AIDS has been reported (Table 39.2).[49]

There are two types of multinucleated giant cells that characterize measles infection. Warthin-Finkeldey giant cells are not seen in the

lung and are macrophage derived. Epithelial giant cells in the lung are formed by fusion of bronchiolar epithelial cells or pneumocytes and contain eosinophilic inclusion that can be identified by immunofluorescence or immunohistochemistry (Fig. 39.4).

REFERENCES

1. de Roux A, Marcos MA, Garcia E, et al. Viral community-acquired pneumonia in nonimmunocompromised adults. *Chest.* 2004;125:1343–1351.
2. Lieberman D, Shimoni A, Shemer-Avni Y, et al. Respiratory viruses in adults with community-acquired pneumonia. *Chest.* 2010;138:811–816.
3. Cao B, Huang GH, Pu ZH, et al. Emergence of community-acquired adenovirus type 55 as a cause of community-onset pneumonia. *Chest.* 2014;145: 79–86.
4. Johnstone J, Majumdar SR, Fox JD, et al. Viral infection in adults hospitalized with community-acquired pneumonia: prevalence, pathogens, and presentation. *Chest.* 2008;134:1141–1148.
5. Cilloniz C, Polverino E, Ewig S, et al. Impact of age and comorbidity on cause and outcome in community-acquired pneumonia. *Chest.* 2013;144: 999–1007.
6. Diaz A, Barria P, Niederman M, et al. Etiology of community-acquired pneumonia in hospitalized patients in chile: the increasing prevalence of respiratory viruses among classic pathogens. *Chest.* 2007;131:779–787.

7. Rello J, Lorente C, Diaz E, et al. Incidence, etiology, and outcome of nosocomial pneumonia in ICU patients requiring percutaneous tracheotomy for mechanical ventilation. *Chest.* 2003;124:2239–2243.

8. Kalil AC, Mindru C, Botha JF, et al. Risk of cytomegalovirus disease in high-risk liver transplant recipients on valganciclovir prophylaxis: a systematic review and meta-analysis. *Liver Transpl.* 2012;18:1440–1447.

9. Mitsani D, Nguyen MH, Kwak EJ, et al. Cytomegalovirus disease among donor-positive/recipient-negative lung transplant recipients in the era of valganciclovir prophylaxis. *J Heart Lung Transplant.* 2010;29:1014–1020.

10. Osorio JC, Medina RD, Patino N, et al. Significance of cytomegalovirus prophylaxis strategies and development of cancer in kidney transplant recipients. *Transplant Proc.* 2011;43:3380–3382.

11. Sullivan T, Brodginski A, Patel G, et al. The role of secondary cytomegalovirus prophylaxis for kidney and liver transplant recipients. *Transplantation.* 2015;99:855–859.

12. Haverkos HW, Dowling JN, Pasculle AW, et al. Diagnosis of pneumonitis in immunocompromised patients by open lung biopsy. *Cancer.* 1983;52:1093–1097.

13. Cheson BD, Samlowski WE, Tang TT, et al. Value of open-lung biopsy in 87 immunocompromised patients with pulmonary infiltrates. *Cancer.* 1985;55:453–459.

14. Browne MJ, Potter D, Gress J, et al. A randomized trial of open lung biopsy versus empiric antimicrobial therapy in cancer patients with diffuse pulmonary infiltrates. *J Clin Oncol.* 1990;8:222–229.

15. Abdallah A, Rowland KE, Schepetiuk SK, et al. An outbreak of respiratory syncytial virus infection in a bone marrow transplant unit: effect on engraftment and outcome of pneumonia without specific antiviral treatment. *Bone Marrow Transplant.* 2003;32:195–203.

16. Team RSVOI. Contributing and terminating factors of a large RSV outbreak in an adult hematology and transplant unit. *PLos Curr.* 2014;6.

17. Chong S, Kim TS, Cho EY. Herpes simplex virus pneumonia: high-resolution CT findings. *Br J Radiol.* 2010;83:585–589.

18. Inokuchi R, Nakamura K, Sato H, et al. Bronchial ulceration as a prognostic indicator for varicella pneumonia: case report and systematic literature review. *J Clin Virol.* 2013;56:360–364.

19. Godet C, Le Goff J, Beby-Defaux A, et al. Human metapneumovirus pneumonia in patients with hematological malignancies. *J Clin Virol.* 2014;61:593–596.

20. Salez N, Vabret A, Leruez-Ville M, et al. Evaluation of four commercial multiplex molecular tests for the diagnosis of acute respiratory infections. *PLoS One.* 2015;10:e0130378.

21. Bal A, Suri V, Mishra B, et al. Pathology and virology findings in cases of fatal influenza A H1N1 virus infection in 2009–2010. *Histopathology.* 2012;60:326–335.

22. Ng WF, To KF, Lam WW, et al. The comparative pathology of severe acute respiratory syndrome and avian influenza A subtype H5N1—a review. *Hum Pathol.* 2006;37:381–390.

23. Tabatabai J, Prifert C, Pfeil J, et al. Novel respiratory syncytial virus (RSV) genotype ON1 predominates in Germany during winter season 2012–13. *PLoS One.* 2014;9:e109191.

24. Shachor-Meyouhas Y, Zaidman I, Kra-Oz Z, et al. Detection, control, and management of a respiratory syncytial virus outbreak in a pediatric hematology–oncology department. *J Pediatr Hematol Oncol.* 2013;35:124–128.

25. Lukic-Grlic A, Bace A, Lokar-Kolbas R, et al. Clinical and epidemiological aspects of respiratory syncytial virus lower respiratory tract infections. *Eur J Epidemiol.* 1999;15:361–365.

26. Reina J, Lopez C. Respiratory infections caused by respiratory syncytial virus in the adult population: description of 16 cases. *Med Clin (Barc).* 2013;141:163–166.

27. Johnson JE, Gonzales RA, Olson SJ, et al. The histopathology of fatal untreated human respiratory syncytial virus infection. *Mod Pathol.* 2007;20:108–119.

28. Welliver TP, Garofalo RP, Hosakote Y, et al. Severe human lower respiratory tract illness caused by respiratory syncytial virus and influenza virus is characterized by the absence of pulmonary cytotoxic lymphocyte responses. *J Infect Dis.* 2007;195:1126–1136.

29. Villaran MV, Garcia J, Gomez J, et al. Human parainfluenza virus in patients with influenza-like illness from Central and South America during 2006–2010. *Influenza Other Respir Viruses.* 2014;8:217–227.

30. Lewis VA, Champlin R, Englund J, et al. Respiratory disease due to parainfluenza virus in adult bone marrow transplant recipients. *Clin Infect Dis.* 1996;23:1033–1037.

31. Soileau SL, Schneider E, Erdman DD, et al. Case report: severe disseminated adenovirus infection in a neonate following water birth delivery. *J Med Virol.* 2013;85:667–669.

32. Chen SP, Huang YC, Chiu CH, et al. Clinical features of radiologically confirmed pneumonia due to adenovirus in children. *J Clin Virol.* 2013;56:7–12.

33. Hwang SM, Park DE, Yang YI, et al. Outbreak of febrile respiratory illness caused by adenovirus at a South Korean military training facility: clinical and radiological characteristics of adenovirus pneumonia. *Jpn J Infect Dis.* 2013;66:359–365.

34. Lee YJ, Palomino-Guilen P, Babady NE, et al. Disseminated adenovirus infection in cancer patients presenting with focal pulmonary consolidation. *J Clin Microbiol.* 2014;52:350–353.

35. Mayeur N, Srairi M, Tetu L, et al. Lethal hemorrhagic alveolitis after adenovirus pneumonia in a lung transplant recipient. *Heart Lung.* 2012;41:401–403.

36. Simsir A, Greenebaum E, Nuovo G, et al. Late fatal adenovirus pneumonitis in a lung transplant recipient. *Transplantation.* 1998;65:592–594.

37. Grilli E, Galati V, Bordi L, et al. Cytomegalovirus pneumonia in immunocompetent host: case report and literature review. *J Clin Virol.* 2012;55:356–359.

38. Papazian L, Fraisse A, Garbe L, et al. Cytomegalovirus. An unexpected cause of ventilator-associated pneumonia. *Anesthesiology.* 1996;84:280–287.

39. Oda Y, Okada Y, Katsuda S, et al. Immunohistochemical study on the infection of herpes simplex virus, human cytomegalovirus, and Epstein–Barr virus in secondary diffuse interstitial pneumonia. *Hum Pathol.* 1994;25:1057–1062.

40. Ramsey PG, Fife KH, Hackman RC, et al. Herpes simplex virus pneumonia: clinical, virologic, and pathologic features in 20 patients. *Ann Intern Med.* 1982;97:813–820.

41. Franks TJ, Chong PY, Chui P, et al. Lung pathology of severe acute respiratory syndrome (SARS): a study of 8 autopsy cases from Singapore. *Hum Pathol.* 2003;34:743–748.

42. Tran DN, Trinh QD, Pham NT, et al. Human rhinovirus infections in hospitalized children: clinical, epidemiological and virological features. *Epidemiol Infect.* 2015:1–9.

43. Xiang Z, Gonzalez R, Xie Z, et al. Human rhinovirus C infections mirror those of human rhinovirus A in children with community-acquired pneumonia. *J Clin Virol.* 2010;49:94–99.

44. Nor'e SS, Sam IC, Mohamad Fakri EF, et al. Phylogenetic analysis of human metapneumovirus among children with acute respiratory infections in Kuala Lumpur, Malaysia. *Trop Biomed.* 2014;31:562–566.

45. Chu HY, Renaud C, Ficken E, et al. Respiratory tract infections due to human metapneumovirus in immunocompromised children. *J Pediatric Infect Dis Soc.* 2014;3:286–293.

46. Wang Y, Ji W, Chen Z, et al. Comparison of severe pneumonia caused by human metapneumovirus and respiratory syncytial virus in hospitalized children. *Indian J Pathol Microbiol.* 2014;57:413–417.

47. Morens DM, Taubenberger JK. A forgotten epidemic that changed medicine: measles in the US Army, 1917–18. *Lancet Infect Dis.* 2015;15:852–861.

48. Piastra M, Onesimo R, De Luca D, et al. Measles-induced respiratory distress, air-leak and ARDS. *Eur J Clin Microbiol Infect Dis.* 2010;29:181–185.

49. Okamura A, Itakura O, Yoshioka M, et al. Unusual presentation of measles giant cell pneumonia in a patient with acquired immunodeficiency syndrome. *Clin Infect Dis.* 2001;32:E57–E58.

40 Pulmonary Tuberculosis and Atypical Mycobacterial Infection

Fabio R. Tavora, M.D., Ph.D., and Allen P. Burke, M.D.

Mycobacterium Tuberculosis

Microbiology

Tuberculosis has been known as a human disease for several millennia. It is a pulmonary and systemic disease caused by *Mycobacterium tuberculosis* complex species. The *M. tuberculosis* complex consists of seven organisms: *M. tuberculosis, M. bovis, M. africanum, M. microti, M. canetti, M. caprae,* and *M. pinnipedii.* In humans, tuberculosis is overwhelmingly caused by *M. tuberculosis,* with a small fraction of disease cause by *M. bovis* and *M. africanum.*[1]

Epidemiology

In 2013, there were about 9 million new cases of active tuberculosis, and about 20% of those involve coinfection with HIV.[2] In 2001, a total of 15,989 cases of TB were reported to the Centers for Disease Control and Prevention (CDC) from the 50 states and the District of Columbia, a number which decreased to 9,582 cases in 2013, a rate of 3.0 cases per 100,000 persons (http://www.cdc.gov/tb/statistics). Despite the overall decline in the number of cases of tuberculosis, the percentage of extrapulmonary disease and drug-resistant forms has remained constant or increased.[3] Furthermore, despite advances in antimicrobial therapy, tuberculosis still accounts for millions of deaths worldwide, with an estimated annual death toll of 1.58 million.[4,5]

Clinical Features

In general terms, pulmonary infection by *M. tuberculosis* can be divided in latent and active infection (Table 40.1). Because of differences in treatment and prognosis, drug-resistant tuberculosis is often considered separately.

The clinical features of pulmonary tuberculosis include productive chronic cough, weight loss, intermittent fever, night sweats, and hemoptysis.[6] About 5% of active cases may become resistant to regular regimens.

In 4% of cases, diagnosis is not made until death. These patients were more likely older, Caucasian, and drug addicts.[7]

Latent Tuberculosis

Latent infection is manifest only by a positive tuberculin skin test,[8] which relies on measurement of host immune response.[9]

Newer tests relying on interferon-γ release assays have no cross-reactivity with prior vaccine exposure and have a higher positive predictive value for the subsequent development of active disease.[9] Overall, ~2% of the population in the United States have a positive skin test, a rate that is higher in foreign born (from high-risk countries), intravenous drug addicts, homeless persons, and those with known contact with an infected individual.[9] It has also been estimated (of particular interest to practicing pathologists) that the staff of laboratories and necropsy rooms are estimated to be between 100 and 200 times more likely than the general public to develop latent or active tuberculosis.[10]

Latent infection suggests an absence of prior active disease and therefore a normal chest radiograph. However, patients in the "latent" category often include those with abnormal chest x-rays indicative of healed, untreated tuberculosis placing them in a high-risk category for postprimary or reactivation tuberculosis.[9] Any evidence of acute infection by clinical, radiologic, or microbiologic means indicates active disease in a patient with a positive skin test done for screening purposes.

Although it is often stated that *M. tuberculosis* organisms persist in an inactive state in granulomas in the latent phase, this fact has never been directly demonstrated.[5] An autopsy study utilizing multiple molecular techniques (including in situ polymerase chain reaction [PCR]) showed nucleotide sequences specific for *M. tuberculosis* in the lungs, spleens, kidneys, and livers, all at about the same rate, of patients with presumed latent tuberculosis. Cells infected included endothelium, pneumocytes, macrophages, Bowman parietal cells, and proximal tubular cells. Interestingly, none was found in granulomas, inflammatory infiltrates, or fibrosis.[11]

Active Tuberculosis

Active disease has traditionally been classified into two groups: disease progressing from the initial infection (primary tuberculosis) and disease occurring years after initial infection, with reactivation. Since many patients do not neatly fall into either category, current clinical classifications separate patients into latent, active, and drug-resistant tuberculosis.[12] Because, however, some pathologic differences have been espoused between primary tuberculosis and postprimary tuberculosis, they will be considered separately.

TABLE 40.1 Classifications of Clinical Tuberculosis

Latent vs. active	"Latent" denotes disease detected only by evidence of immune response (skin test, interferon-γ release assays). "Active" indicates presence of organisms detected by culture, smear, histology and AFB stain, or molecular testing, regardless of skin testing.
Primary vs. reactivation (active disease)	*Primary* indicates symptomatic disease occurring at the initial time of exposure, often in children. *Reactivation,* or *postprimary,* indicates an asymptomatic interval, as determined by history. "Reactivation" tuberculosis can also be used if there is radiologic evidence of "old" disease in a patient with new onset symptoms. Most patients with reactivation tuberculosis have apparently normal immune status, but there are a number of predisposing conditions. Patients are highly infectious and often have cavitary disease. The distinction between primary and reactivation tuberculoses is currently often not made.
Primary vs. accelerated	"Accelerated" tuberculosis is generally used in patients with immunosuppression and, unlike reactivation TB, frequently involves nonpulmonary sites.
Miliary tuberculosis	"Miliary" denotes hematogenous (and sometimes lymphatic) dissemination of tuberculosis resulting in miliary pattern on chest radiograph or CT scan and typically involves the liver, spleen, and bone marrow; diagnosis is often missed during life. Skin tests are negative because of altered T-cell immunity to the mycobacterial antigens.
Drug-resistant active infection	Drug resistance is determined by automated liquid culture system, or molecular probes for rifampicin resistance, a surrogate for multidrug resistance.

Primary Tuberculosis

The initial infection (primary tuberculosis) begins when bacilli are inhaled into the lungs where they induce a granulomatous inflammatory response. The organisms rapidly spread from the lung to lymph nodes and hematogenously. The infection is typically self-limited with the development of effective cell-mediated immunity and resolves in 6 to 8 weeks, either leaving no trace or resulting in healed lesions on chest radiograph. In a small percentage of individuals, the initial infection progresses to pleuritis, if the granuloma ruptures into the pleura; extensive consolidative pneumonia; enlargement of mediastinal lymph nodes, causing bronchial obstruction and postobstructive pneumonia; rupture of a tuberculous focus into a bronchus, leading to extensive endobronchial spread; or rupture of a tuberculous focus into a pulmonary blood vessel with hematogenous spread.[1,13] Primary tuberculosis is usually seen in children.[13]

Postprimary (Reactivation)

Reactivation tuberculosis occurs in patients previously sensitized to *M. tuberculosis*. Genetic studies suggest that susceptibility to primary and postprimary tuberculosis may be governed by different genes.[14]

It is believed that 80% of cases of tuberculosis in the United States are the result of reactivated latent infection.[9] The diagnosis of reactivation depends on history of prior skin test, history or remote exposure, or findings on chest radiograph more typical of previous disease. In otherwise healthy patients with latent disease, there is a 5% to 10% chance over a lifetime of developing active disease,[9] a number that is reduced to 1% with antimicrobial prophylaxis.[15] In patients with HIV infection prior to effective therapy, there was a 7% yearly risk of developing tuberculosis.[8]

The fact that the risk of "reactivation" tuberculosis increases dramatically with acquired immune deficiency is at odds with the concept that reactivation requires a strong cellular immune response.[13] For this reason, and because tuberculosis that results from reactivation of a latent infection is not always clinically distinguishable from tuberculosis that results from recent exposure,[9] the distinction between reactivation and primary tuberculosis is not always made. The term "accelerated" tuberculosis has been substituted for "reactivation" in referring to disease developing in immunocompromised patients, in essence placing immunosuppression-related tuberculosis in a category of primary disease.[13]

In addition to immunosuppression, reactivation rates are increased if there is malnutrition, debilitation, alcoholism, poorly controlled diabetes mellitus, smoking, low body weight, silicosis, immunosuppression, the postpartum period, gastrectomy, chronic hemodialysis, and jejunoileal bypass surgery, although in most patients no predisposing factor can be identified.[1,9,16] Evidence of untreated tuberculosis on chest x-ray and recent contact with an infected person imparts the greatest risk for reactivation.[1]

Postprimary tuberculosis in patients with normal immunity is generally confined to the lung, does not spread to lymph nodes or distant sites, and does not spontaneously regress. It is characterized by cavities in the lung that produce massive numbers of organisms resulting in high infectivity.[17] It occurs more commonly in adults and usually involves the apical and posterior segments of the upper lung lobes and the superior segments of the lower lobes.[16]

Miliary Tuberculosis

Miliary tuberculosis occurs in 2% of tuberculosis. It is variably considered a form of primary (accelerated) or reactivation tuberculosis, depending on the patient's exposure history and immune status.[3] Risk factors overlap with reactivation disease and include prior infection with tuberculosis, coinfection with HIV, treatment with immunosuppressive agents, diabetes mellitus, and alcoholism. Unlike other types, miliary tuberculosis relatively frequently is misdiagnosed during life, and the diagnosis is first made at autopsy in 33% of patients.[3] Once considered a disease of children, it is increasingly seen in adults. There is a bimodal distribution, with one peak in children and adolescents and the other in the elderly. The mortality is estimated at 18% to 30%.[18]

The tuberculin skin test has been reported to be almost always negative miliary tuberculosis.[3] There is believed to be an inadequacy of effector T-cell response to the organism. The clinical manifestations are extremely variable and range from subtle, systemic symptoms to a fulminant process with adult respiratory distress syndrome (see Chapter 21).[3] In a series from India, 5% of patients treated in intensive care for acute respiratory distress syndrome had tuberculosis as the underlying cause.[19]

Miliary tuberculosis represents a relatively large proportion of extrapulmonary disease (over 20%) and involves the liver, spleen, bone marrow, and meninges most frequently, in addition to the lungs.[18]

Immunocompromised Patients

The risk of developing tuberculosis is as high as 20% in patients with AIDS.[7] In HIV disease, there are radiologic and pathologic differences compared to reactivation tuberculosis in immunocompromised patients. Imaging of the lung may show subtle or even absent findings. Small and diffuse opacities on lung imaging, pleural effusions, and hilar lymphadenopathy may be the only findings. Pulmonary cavities are uncommon, resulting in a lower likelihood for transmission of infection by aerosolization.[13]

In general, tuberculosis in HIV disease has a higher frequency of negative tuberculin skin tests than non–HIV-related tuberculosis (61% vs. 10%). Other clinical differences include a higher rate of extrapulmonary involvement (60% vs. 28%), a higher rate of diffuse or miliary infiltrates (60% vs. 32%), a higher rate of hilar lymphadenopathy (20% vs. <5%), a higher rate of normal chest radiographs despite pulmonary involvement (15% vs. <1%), a lower rate of focal infiltrates (35% vs. 68%), and a lower rate of cavities (18% vs. 67%).[1] These differences corroborate the concept that reactivation tuberculosis is different from the accelerates disease seen in immunocompromised patients.[17]

Pathologically, compared to tuberculosis in immunocompetent individuals, there is more likely to be necrosis, organisms are more numerous, and giant cells, well-formed granulomas, and lymphocytes are less common.[17,20]

In transplanted lungs, tuberculosis can be the result of primary infection, reactivation of latent infection, or transmission from the donor. The overall rate of tuberculosis in transplant patients is 6%, one-half are diagnosed in the explanted lung, and the remainder occur after transplant, often with a favorable course.[21] In contrast, the course can be rapid, with atypical findings of abscesses and necrosis, numerous bacilli in the necrotic tissue, and an absence of granulomas.[22]

Radiologic Findings

The computed tomographic findings of active tuberculosis include centrilobular nodules and branching linear structures of bronchiolar thickening, giving the classic a tree-in-bud appearance, lobular consolidation, cavitation, and bronchial wall thickening.[23] The findings of inactive or regressed tuberculosis include calcified nodules and irregular linear opacities. Tuberculomas present with solid nodules with an occasional ground-glass periphery that may mimic neoplasia. Atypical CT findings include basilar infiltrates, military patterns, pleural-based consolidations, and scattered small parenchymal nodules.[23] Healed primary tuberculosis appears as calcified parenchymal nodules and may be associated with calcified hilar lymph nodes.[16] Miliary tuberculosis is manifest by a mixture of both sharply and poorly defined nodules of 1 to 2 mm, disseminated throughout the lobes associated with diffuse reticulation.[16]

Pathologic Findings
General

Since tissue diagnosis is not often used (and not required) to the diagnosis of pulmonary tuberculosis, the surgical pathologist rarely encounters a case of a "de novo" diagnosis. The identification of positive patients relies mainly on the tuberculin test and interferon-γ release assay and for latent infection and sputum microscopy and culture in liquid medium with subsequent drug susceptibility testing in active cases. PCR tests and histopathology are considered only supplementary tests.[5,9]

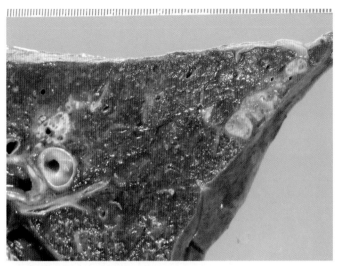

FIGURE 40.1 ▲ Primary tuberculosis. The Ghon complex is a pleural-based granuloma with granulomatous hilar node in the same lobe.

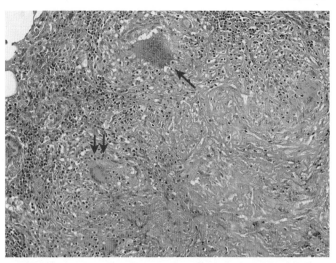

FIGURE 40.3 ▲ Tuberculous granuloma. Macrophage giant cells are common and are of the "Langhans" (*double arrow*) and foreign body type (*arrow*).

Primary Tuberculosis

The characteristic finding of primary pulmonary tuberculosis is a granuloma, surrounded by macrophage giant cells and lymphocytes, with central necrotic cavity. The lesion is typically peripheral, and the accompanying granulomas in the hilar lymph nodes produce the classic *Ghon complex* on imaging (Fig. 40.1). The primary nodule is usually solitary, but there may be multiple and bilateral lesions.

The granulomas typically cluster, with normal surrounding lung (Fig. 40.2).[13] Later lesions may show fibrosis surrounding the granuloma, but the persistence of macrophages indicates active disease.[17] The type of macrophage giant cell is classically described as the Langhans type (nuclei distributed peripherally in a horseshoe pattern), although the feature is nonspecific (Fig. 40.3). When found, bacilli are typically centrally located and, if there is necrosis, usually in the necrotic area. Eosinophils and plasma cells may be intermixed within the peripheral lymphoid infiltrate. The central necrotic core is where bacilli are present, although culture is more sensitive than special stains.[24]

Postprimary (Reactivation) Tuberculosis in Immunocompetent Individuals

Classically, reactivation tuberculosis is characterized by cavities partly filled with soft, partly liquid material surrounded by irregular fibrosis. Indeed, the initial use of the term "caseation" was applied to these gross lesions, specifically the material within them, and was not related to the microscopic necrosis within the granulomas. Cavitary lesions are commonly peripheral and range from 2 to 10 cm, typically in the most aerated areas of the lung, in the upper lobes. Calcification, pleural fibrosis and adhesions, and erosion into the bronchi are common, but hilar lymphadenopathy is not conspicuous. In general, postprimary tuberculosis begins as areas of consolidation, rather than discrete granulomas.[17]

Histologically, granulomas are not prominent, but there is necrotizing lipid pneumonia, cystic degeneration, macrophage giant cells (classically of the Langhans type), and infarction. Acid-fast bacilli are found in areas of necrosis and within foamy alveolar macrophages. Referring to reactivation tuberculosis, Rich is said to have written, in 1951: "It has been found by all who have studied early human pulmonary lesions that they represent areas of gaseous pneumonia rather than nodular tubercles."[13]

Miliary Tuberculosis

In patients with miliary tuberculosis, the diagnosis is usually made by culture and radiographic findings. Biopsies of the lymph nodes and bone marrow, and less commonly the lung and liver, may show diagnostic necrotizing granulomas in those patients without typical radiographs.[25]

In the lung, there are typical necrotizing granulomas, 1 to 5 mm in diameter, with macrophage giant cells at the periphery, with inflammation in the surrounding interstitium (Fig. 40.4A). At autopsy, the granulomas are disseminated, and also involve the liver, kidneys, spleen, and other organs. Acid-fast bacilli (AFB) are readily demonstrated.[3]

AFB Staining and Detection of Bacilli

The organisms are often few, especially in immunocompetent patients, and require review of the entire slide at 40× or oil immersion magnification. At least two blocks should be stained,[26] or all blocks with granulomas or necrosis. Bacilli are not visualized by routine staining. The property of acid fastness is related to the carbon chain length of the mycolic acid found in all species of mycobacteria. Acid-fast staining demonstrates tiny, curved, wine-red organisms (about 2 to 2.5 μM) (Fig. 40.4B). Fluorescent staining as is routinely performed on cytologic smear preparations, such as the auramine-O test, may increase

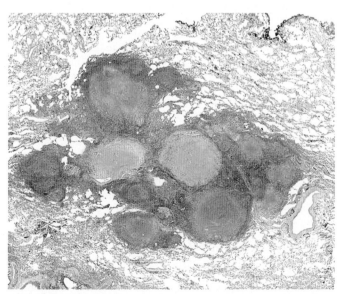

FIGURE 40.2 ▲ Primary tuberculosis. The granulomas are necrotizing and often clustered.

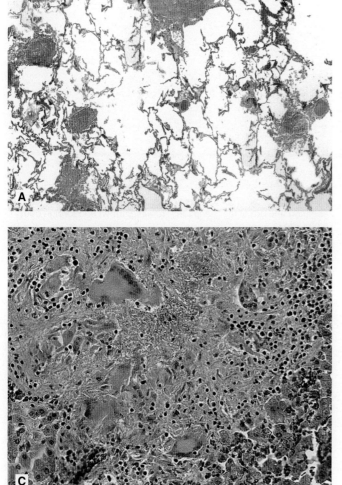

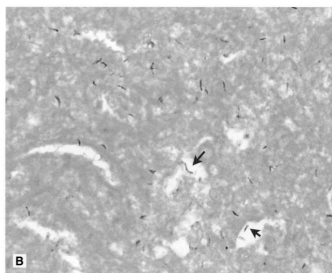

FIGURE 40.4 ▲ Miliary tuberculosis, autopsy. **A.** The lung showed numerous granulomas in the interstitium. The diagnosis was not suspected during life. **B.** Oil immersion, acid-fast bacillus stain (100×). There are numerous acid-fast bacilli. The *red* color of the organisms can be seen where there is no background necrosis (*arrows*). **C.** There was liver involvement (shown) as well as granulomas in the mediastinal lymph nodes, spleen, and bone marrow (not shown).

sensitivity.[27] It has been demonstrated by comparative quantitative PCR testing that many bacilli are missed by acid-fast stains,[28] underscoring the need for culture of all samples of suspected tuberculosis, even when organisms or even granulomas are absent.

In some cases, the pathologist will be asked to perform molecular studies for *M. tuberculosis* in paraffin sections showing necrotizing granulomas, when culture was inadvertently not performed, or in cases where the diagnosis was not suspected and no fresh tissue saved. PCR sequencing assay is sensitive down to as few as 100 AFB in paraffin samples,[29] although validated clinical tests on tissue samples are difficult to come by and the test generally has to be done on a research basis or by contacting the Centers for Disease Control and Prevention.

There is an inverse correlation between the extent of granuloma formation and the number of acid-fast bacilli identified by special staining. In a study of transbronchial biopsies positive for tuberculosis, 71% of well-formed granulomas with few AFB occurred in patients who were immunocompetent, 63% of granulomas with poorly formed granulomas and numerous AFB occurred in immunosuppressed patients, and there were few if any with a strong positive correlation between the extent of granulomas and organisms.[20] In lesions without well-formed granulomas, necrosis is generally extensive. It is imperative, therefore, that the suspicion of tuberculosis should remain high in the presence of necrotic tissue without obvious granulomas and that staining for AFB be performed in all such biopsies.

Biopsy Diagnosis of Tuberculosis

The first line of diagnosis for tuberculosis is acid-fast staining and culture of sputum or gastric aspirates. The AFB stain test requires 5,000 to 10,000 bacteria/mL for detection, is unable to distinguish between tuberculosis and atypical mycobacteria, and has a limited sensitivity (22% to 78% depending on clinical situation).[4] When necessary, bronchoscopy is performed to obtain bronchoalveolar lavage specimen, usually with transbronchial biopsy, to increase the yield of diagnosis. Bronchoscopy is necessary in up to one-third of patients, more often in limited and noncavitary disease.[30,31] In some patients, transcutaneous biopsy may be helpful in establishing a tissue diagnosis if bronchoscopy is negative.[4]

Transbronchial biopsy yields diagnostic tissue in ~30% to 60% of patients with negative sputum culture.[31] Ultrasound guidance may increase the yield of positive AFB smears by fine needle aspiration, bronchoalveolar lavage fluid, and biopsies, with a positive rate of over 80% for all three procedures combined.[30,32]

Histologically, in positive biopsies of non-HIV patients, there are necrotizing granulomas in about two-thirds of cases and nonnecrotizing granulomas in about one-third, with fewer than 5% showing necrosis only[4] (Fig. 40.5).

In negative transbronchial biopsies, findings are typically nonspecific chronic inflammation or organizing pneumonia. In up to 15% of biopsies, diagnoses other than tuberculosis are made, including

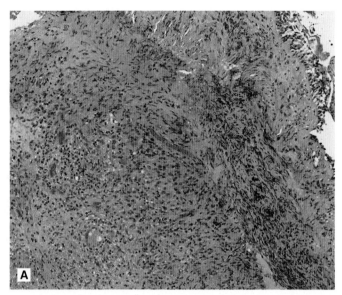 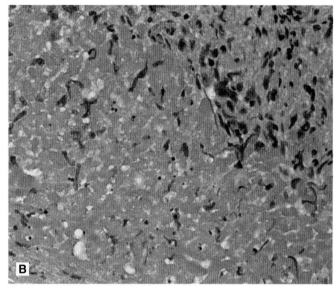

FIGURE 40.5 ▲ Tuberculosis, transbronchial biopsy. **A.** Low magnification with necrotizing granuloma and portion of the airway (**upper right**). **B.** Interface between necrosis and granulomatous inflammation.

pneumocystis pneumonia, fungal infections, nocardia, atypical mycobacterial infection, and neoplasms.[33]

Mediastinal involvement by tuberculosis can be diagnosed by mediastinoscopic biopsy in the majority of cases. Right paratracheal involvement is especially common.[34]

In cases of tuberculous pleuritis, the number of bacilli in the pleural fluid is low, with positive cultures found in <25% of cases. Pleural biopsy shows granulomatous inflammation in ~60% of patients, with diagnostic yield increasing to 90% if multiple biopsies with tissue culture are performed.[35]

Surgical Resection Specimens

The pathologist may receive an open or thoracoscopic wedge biopsy for the evaluation of a localized lung nodule, which may occasionally demonstrate necrotizing granulomas due to unsuspected tuberculosis.[36] Acid-fast staining will usually demonstrate organisms, although occasionally there is a positive culture after tissue staining is negative.[24] Necrotizing granulomas with negative stains are not usually caused by tuberculosis, but are more often caused by atypical mycobacterial infection, fungal infections, and noninfectious processes.[24]

Surgical procedures done for therapeutic, as opposed to diagnostic indications, include debridement of necrotic lung tissue, debridement of bronchopleural fistulas, pleural decortications (Fig. 40.6), excision of mycetomas, and the excision of infected tissue in the case of multidrug-resistant tuberculosis.[37,38] Other than the last example, in which the histologic features are those of granulomatous infection, findings are typically nonspecific and include fibrosis, chronic inflammation, postobstructive changes, granulation tissue, and chronic pleuritis.

Differential Diagnosis

The differential diagnoses of necrotizing granulomas include atypical mycobacterial infection, fungal infection, sarcoidosis, autoimmune diseases such as rheumatoid nodule, granulomatosis with polyangiitis, and idiopathic granuloma.[39] The diagnosis is established by special stains, culture, and clinical and serologic findings.[24]

In cases of necrosis without well-formed granulomas, typically occurring in immunocompromised patients, the major differential diagnosis is another type of infection, necessitating special stains and culture. Tuberculous pneumonitis may also mimic diffuse alveolar damage, raising the differential diagnosis of acute respiratory distress syndrome (see Chapter 21).

Atypical Mycobacterial Infection

Classification

Nontuberculous mycobacteria (atypical or environmental mycobacteria) are of universal distribution and found mainly in soil, water sources, and decomposed plants. There are more than 150 species of mycobacteria and likely more will be discovered. Atypical mycobacteria have been classically classified into two categories: slow growing or rapid growing. The former group has the *M. avium* complex (*M. avium* and *M. intracellulare*) as the most important group, whereas the rapid-growing mycobacteria include *M. abscessus* and *M. fortuitum*.

Epidemiology

Atypical mycobacterial infection is rare, but the true incidence and prevalence of nontuberculous mycobacterial pulmonary infections is unknown, since isolation by culture does not necessarily indicate clinical infection. One study demonstrated that only one-fifth of pulmonary isolates likely represented significant pulmonary disease.[40]

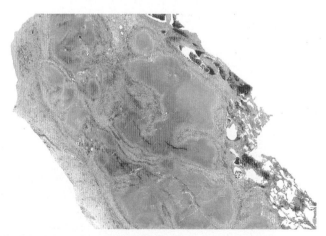

FIGURE 40.6 ▲ Pleural tuberculosis. There is zonal necrosis at the interface between the pleura and lung, with surrounding granulomatous inflammation.

Clinical Features

The clinicopathologic spectrum of infections due to nontubercu-lous mycobacteria includes cavitary disease, opportunistic infection, and nodular disease associated with bronchiectasis. The diagnosis of pulmonary infection requires the presence of symptoms, radiologic abnormalities, and exclusion of other potential etiologies, in addition to positive culture.

There are two commonly encountered patterns of pulmonary infec-tions caused by nontuberculous mycobacteria in immunocompetent patients. Upper lobe fibrocavitary disease reminiscent of *M. tuberculo-sis* infection typically occurs in patients with emphysema or fibrosing lung diseases such as silicosis, pneumoconiosis, or prior tuberculosis. The other is a slowly progressing disease in previously normal lungs characterized by nodular opacities accompanied by bronchiectasis. These patients were often older women with pectus excavatum, scolio-sis, and mitral valve prolapse.[41]

A specific form of mycobacterial lung infection in immunocom-petent patients has been termed "*hot tub lung*" because of exposure from contaminated water. These patients typically have symptoms of dyspnea, cough, hypoxia, and fever, with computed tomographic evidence of bilateral patchy ground-glass opacities. Sputum cultures are uniformly positive for atypical mycobacteria (mostly *M. avium-intercellulare*). The reported patients had an excellent prognosis after treatment with antimycobacterial treatment or steroids.[42]

An asymptomatic form of atypical mycobacterial infection is that of the solitary nodule, which reveals granulomatous inflammation at wedge biopsy. These patients generally do well without recurrence, even without treatment.[24]

In immunocompromised patients, especially in AIDS patients, atypical mycobacterium can cause disseminated disease. The factors predisposing to infection are not well understood, but likely are due to an interaction between host defense mechanisms and the load of clini-cal exposure. Disseminated disease is most commonly seen in asso-ciation with profound immunosuppression. In HIV-infected patients, dissemination does not typically occur unless the CD4+ T lymphocyte count is below 50/μL.[43]

Pathologic Findings, Immunocompetent Patients

The histopathologic features of atypical mycobacterial infection are similar to those of tuberculosis (Fig. 40.7). The organisms are identi-cal in appearance and staining characteristics. Localized pulmonary

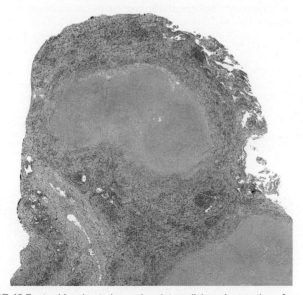

FIGURE 40.7 ▲ *Mycobacterium avium-intercellulare*. A resection of a granuloma with histologic similarities to tuberculous infection.

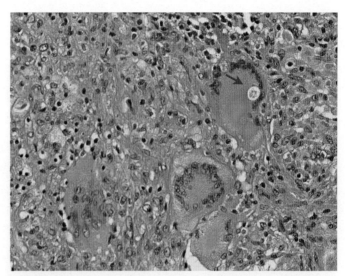

FIGURE 40.8 ▲ *Mycobacterium avium-intercellulare*. There is a necrotizing granuloma with macrophage giant cells, of both foreign body type and Langhans type, one of which shows an inclusion, similar to asteroid body (*arrow*).

nodules show necrotizing granulomas indistinguishable from those caused by *M. tuberculosis*.[24] The granulomas may also mimic those of catscratch disease and sarcoidosis.[27]

All granulomas show multinucleated giant cells (Fig. 40.8), and the majority are multiple histologically. Necrosis is abundant in 75% of cases, and lymphangitic distribution is uncommon. Neutrophils are interspersed within the granulomas in 80%, and eosinophils are rare. Granulomas may occur in vessels walls, but necrotizing vasculitis does not occur. Inclusions, such as asteroid bodies or Schaumann bodies, may be seen in 20% of cases.[24]

In many cases of localized granulomas, there are no organisms noted on acid-fast bacillus stains, in which case a presumed diagnosis of atyp-ical mycobacterial infection is made by culture of the tissue. Histologic studies of atypical mycobacterial infection resulting in "*hot tub lung*" showed abundant nonnecrotizing, bronchiolocentric, granulomas with interstitial inflammation and patchy organizing pneumonia.[42]

Pathologic Findings, Immunosuppressed Patients

Disseminated Infection

Disseminated mycobacterial infection is extensively extrapulmonary, occurring primarily in lymph nodes (hilar, supraclavicular, para-aortic, paratracheal, and mediastinal most frequently) and the gastrointestinal tract. The lung parenchyma is involved in about one-fifth of patients.[44] The histologic features of atypical mycobacterial infection in immuno-compromised patients include necrotizing granulomas and nongranu-lomatous inflammation with sheets of macrophages with necrotizing inflammation.[45] Stains for acid-fast bacilli frequently show abundant organisms.

Pseudotumor

A peculiar form of mycobacterial infection that occurs in immuno-compromised patients with the *mycobacterial spindle cell pseudotumor* (also see Chapter 68). They may involve the lung, in both HIV and transplant patients,[46,47] but more commonly in the lymph nodes, skin, spleen, or bone marrow. Most are caused by nontuberculous mycobac-teria, including *M. avium-intercellulare*, *M. chelonae*, and *M. simiae*, although they may also be caused by *M. tuberculosis*.[46] Histologically, they are proliferations of spindled fibrohistiocytic cells without the formation of epithelioid granulomas (Fig. 40.9). Without staining for acid-fast bacilli, histological distinction from other spindle cell lesions, including Kaposi sarcoma, can be difficult.[47]

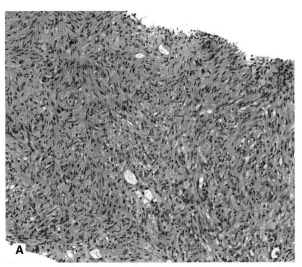
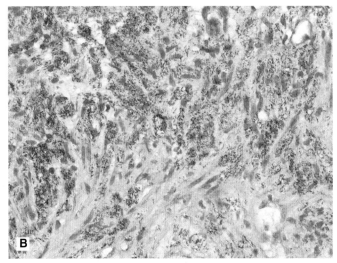

FIGURE 40.9 ▲ *Mycobacterium avium-intracellulare*, immunocompromised patient with lung mass. **A.** Histologically, there is an inflammatory pseudotumor mimicking inflammatory pseudotumor or even leiomyoma. The cells were positive for CD68 indicating macrophage derivation (not shown). **B.** There were numerous acid-fast bacilli (40×).

Practical Points

▶ Biopsy for pulmonary tuberculosis is performed only if sputum culture is negative, and is usually multimodal (bronchoalveolar lavage, ultrasound-guided FNA, transbronchial biopsy).

▶ In transbronchial biopsies to confirm the diagnosis with negative culture, other infections or processes may be found unexpectedly.

▶ Always perform AFB staining in biopsies where there is necrosis or fibrin exudate, because granulomas may be poorly formed or absent, especially in patients who are immunocompromised.

▶ Open lung biopsy is usually performed for localized masses of unknown etiology, which uncommonly turn out to be tuberculosis; in such instances, necrotizing granulomas are far more likely to be nontuberculous mycobacterial infection.

▶ In immunocompromised patients, include mycobacterial pseudotumor in the differential diagnosis of spindle cell tumors with an inflammatory background, and order AFB stains.

REFERENCES

1. LoBue PA, Enarson DA, Thoen TC. Tuberculosis in humans and its epidemiology, diagnosis and treatment in the United States. *Int J Tuberc Lung Dis.* 2010;14:1226–1232.
2. Zumla A, Raviglione M, Hafner R, et al. Tuberculosis. *N Engl J Med.* 2013;368:745–755.
3. Bourbonnais JM, Sirithanakul K, Guzman JA. Fulminant miliary tuberculosis with adult respiratory distress syndrome undiagnosed until autopsy: a report of 2 cases and review of the literature. *J Intensive Care Med.* 2005;20:354–359.
4. Bae KM, Lim SC, Kim HH, et al. The relevance of biopsy in tuberculosis patients without human immunodeficiency virus infection. *Am J Trop Med Hyg.* 2015;92:636–640.
5. Horsburgh CR Jr. Tuberculosis. *Eur Respir Rev.* 2014;23:36–39.
6. Lawn SD, Zumla AI. Tuberculosis. *Lancet.* 2011;378:57–72.
7. DeRiemer K, Rudoy I, Schecter GF, et al. The epidemiology of tuberculosis diagnosed after death in San Francisco, 1986–1995. *Int J Tuberc Lung Dis.* 1999;3:488–493.
8. Schluger NW, Rom WN. The host immune response to tuberculosis. *Am J Respir Crit Care Med.* 1998;157:679–691.
9. Horsburgh CR Jr, Rubin EJ. Clinical practice. Latent tuberculosis infection in the United States. *N Engl J Med.* 2011;364:1441–1448.
10. Collins CH, Grange JM. Tuberculosis acquired in laboratories and necropsy rooms. *Commun Dis Public Health.* 1999;2:161–167.
11. Barrios-Payan J, Saqui-Salces M, Jeyanathan M, et al. Extrapulmonary locations of mycobacterium tuberculosis DNA during latent infection. *J Infect Dis.* 2012;206:1194–1205.
12. Zumla A, James DG. Granulomatous infections: etiology and classification. *Clin Infect Dis.* 1996;23:146–158.
13. Hunter RL, Jagannath C, Actor JK. Pathology of postprimary tuberculosis in humans and mice: contradiction of long-held beliefs. *Tuberculosis (Edinb).* 2007;87:267–278.
14. Alcais A, Fieschi C, Abel L, et al. Tuberculosis in children and adults: two distinct genetic diseases. *J Exp Med.* 2005;202:1617–1621.
15. Falk A, Fuchs GF. Prophylaxis with isoniazid in inactive tuberculosis. A Veterans Administration Cooperative Study XII. *Chest.* 1978;73:44–48.
16. Lee JY, Lee KS, Jung KJ, et al. Pulmonary tuberculosis: CT and pathologic correlation. *J Comput Assist Tomogr.* 2000;24:691–698.
17. Hunter RL. Pathology of post primary tuberculosis of the lung: an illustrated critical review. *Tuberculosis (Edinb).* 2011;91:497–509.
18. Ray S, Talukdar A, Kundu S, et al. Diagnosis and management of miliary tuberculosis: current state and future perspectives. *Ther Clin Risk Manage.* 2013;9:9–26.
19. Agarwal R, Gupta D, Aggarwal AN, et al. Experience with ARDS caused by tuberculosis in a respiratory intensive care unit. *Intensive Care Med.* 2005;31:1284–1287.
20. Di Perri G, Cazzadori A, Vento S, et al. Comparative histopathological study of pulmonary tuberculosis in human immunodeficiency virus-infected and non-infected patients. *Tuber Lung Dis.* 1996;77:244–249.
21. Bravo C, Roldan J, Roman A, et al. Tuberculosis in lung transplant recipients. *Transplantation.* 2005;79:59–64.
22. Boedefeld RL, Eby J, Boedefeld WM II, et al. Fatal Mycobacterium tuberculosis infection in a lung transplant recipient. *J Heart Lung Transplant.* 2008;27:1176–1178.
23. McAdams HP, Erasmus J, Winter JA. Radiologic manifestations of pulmonary tuberculosis. *Radiol Clin North Am.* 1995;33:655–678.
24. Mukhopadhyay S, Wilcox BE, Myers JL, et al. Pulmonary necrotizing granulomas of unknown cause: clinical and pathologic analysis of 131 patients with completely resected nodules. *Chest.* 2013;144:813–824.

25. Alsoub H, Al Alousi FS. Miliary tuberculosis in Qatar: a review of 32 adult cases. *Ann Saudi Med.* 2001;21:16–20.
26. Ulbright TM, Katzenstein AL. Solitary necrotizing granulomas of the lung: differentiating features and etiology. *Am J Surg Pathol.* 1980;4:13–28.
27. Kommareddi S, Abramowsky CR, Swinehart GL, et al. Nontuberculous mycobacterial infections: comparison of the fluorescent auramine-O and Ziehl-Neelsen techniques in tissue diagnosis. *Hum Pathol.* 1984;15:1085–1089.
28. Fukunaga H, Murakami T, Gondo T, et al. Sensitivity of acid-fast staining for Mycobacterium tuberculosis in formalin-fixed tissue. *Am J Respir Crit Care Med.* 2002;166:994–997.
29. Hsiao CH, Lin YT, Lai CC, et al. Identification of nontuberculous mycobacterial infection by IS6110 and hsp65 gene analysis on lung tissues. *Diagn Microbiol Infect Dis.* 2010;68:241–246.
30. Lin SM, Chung FT, Huang CD, et al. Diagnostic value of endobronchial ultrasonography for pulmonary tuberculosis. *J Thorac Cardiovasc Surg.* 2009;138:179–184.
31. Tamura A, Shimada M, Matsui Y, et al. The value of fiberoptic bronchoscopy in culture-positive pulmonary tuberculosis patients whose pre-bronchoscopic sputum specimens were negative both for smear and PCR analyses. *Intern Med.* 2010;49:95–102.
32. Madan K, Mohan A, Ayub II, et al. Initial experience with endobronchial ultrasound-guided transbronchial needle aspiration (EBUS-TBNA) from a tuberculosis endemic population. *J Bronchology Interv Pulmonol.* 2014;21:208–214.
33. Jacomelli M, Silva PR, Rodrigues AJ, et al. Bronchoscopy for the diagnosis of pulmonary tuberculosis in patients with negative sputum smear microscopy results. *J Bras Pneumol.* 2012;38:167–173.
34. Sayar A, Olcmen A, Metin M, et al. Intrathoracic tuberculous lymphadenitis. *Asian Cardiovasc Thorac Ann.* 2000;8:253–255.
35. Dunlap NE, Bass J, Fujiwara P, et al. Diagnostic Standards and Classification of Tuberculosis in Adults and Children. This official statement of the American Thoracic Society and the Centers for Disease Control and Prevention was adopted by the ATS Board of Directors, July 1999. This statement was endorsed by the Council of the Infectious Disease Society of America, September 1999. *Am J Respir Crit Care Med.* 2000;161:1376–1395.
36. Ambrogi MC, Fanucchi O, Korasidis S, et al. Nonintubated thoracoscopic pulmonary nodule resection under spontaneous breathing anesthesia with laryngeal mask. *Innovations (Phila).* 2014;9:276–280.
37. Treasure RL, Seaworth BJ. Current role of surgery in Mycobacterium tuberculosis. *Ann Thorac Surg.* 1995;59:1405–1407; discussion 1408–1409.
38. Olcmen A, Gunluoglu MZ, Demir A, et al. Role and outcome of surgery for pulmonary tuberculosis. *Asian Cardiovasc Thorac Ann.* 2006;14:363–366.
39. Aubry MC. Necrotizing granulomatous inflammation: what does it mean if your special stains are negative? *Mod Pathol.* 2012;25(suppl 1):S31–S38.
40. Shen MC, Lee SS, Huang TS, et al. Clinical significance of isolation of Mycobacterium avium complex from respiratory specimens. *J Formos Med Assoc.* 2010;109:517–523.
41. Iseman MD, Buschman DL, Ackerson LM. Pectus excavatum and scoliosis. Thoracic anomalies associated with pulmonary disease caused by Mycobacterium avium complex. *Am Rev Respir Dis.* 1991;144:914–916.
42. Khoor A, Leslie KO, Tazelaar HD, et al. Diffuse pulmonary disease caused by nontuberculous mycobacteria in immunocompetent people (hot tub lung). *Am J Clin Pathol.* 2001;115:755–762.
43. Johnson MM, Odell JA. Nontuberculous mycobacterial pulmonary infections. *J Thorac Dis.* 2014;6:210–220.
44. Abdel-Dayem HM, Omar WS, Aziz M, et al. Disseminated mycobacterium avium complex. Review of Ga-67 and Tl-201 scans and autopsy findings. *Clin Nucl Med.* 1996;21:547–556.
45. Farhi DC, Mason UG III, Horsburgh CR Jr. Pathologic findings in disseminated Mycobacterium avium-intracellulare infection. A report of 11 cases. *Am J Clin Pathol.* 1986;85:67–72.
46. Philip J, Beasley MB, Dua S. Mycobacterial spindle cell pseudotumor of the lung. *Chest.* 2012;142:783–784.
47. Franco M, Amoroso A, Burke AP, et al. Pulmonary mycobacterial spindle cell pseudotumor in a lung transplant patient: progression without therapy and response to therapy. *Transpl Infect Dis.* 2015;17(3):424–428.

41 Fungal Infections

Brandon T. Larsen, M.D., Ph.D., Allen P. Burke, M.D., and Fabio R. Tavora, M.D., Ph.D.

General

Fungi are eukaryotic organisms that are found ubiquitously in the natural environment. Of the more than 1.5 million known species of fungi, the majority of infections are caused by only a small number of species. These fungi include those that are found throughout the world (e.g., *Aspergillus*, *Candida*) as well as endemic fungi that are limited to a certain geographic region (e.g., *Blastomyces*, *Coccidioides*).

For most pathogenic fungi, the lungs represent the most common site of infection, through inhalation of fungal spores from the environment.[1] Clinical presentation of fungal pneumonia can range from asymptomatic or self-limited infections of little significance to severe invasive or disseminated infections that can be rapidly fatal. The incidence of invasive fungal infections has increased considerably in recent decades, largely due to rising numbers of immunocompromised patients with acquired immunodeficiency syndrome (AIDS) or iatrogenic immunosuppression.

When fungal pneumonia is suspected, diagnosis thereof often requires a combination of histologic evaluation, special stains, cultures, serologic studies, and/or molecular testing. Unfortunately, tissue reactions are nonspecific and cannot be relied upon for classification of the culprit organism. These changes also vary widely depending on the patient's immune status, ranging from robust inflammatory reactions in the immunocompetent to virtually no inflammatory response in the severely immunocompromised. In the lung, fungal infections often incite necrotizing granulomatous inflammation that forms nodules or even large cavitary masses, but poorly formed, nonnecrotizing or miliary granulomas can also be seen. Fungal infections can also produce other patterns of injury, such as diffuse alveolar damage, acute fibrinous injury, foamy alveolar casts, organizing pneumonia, acute bronchopneumonia, or airway disease. When acute lung injury is identified in a biopsy, infection should always be considered, even if organisms are not visible on the initial H&E-stained slide.

In tissue, fungi may appear as unicellular, round to oval yeasts that may display budding and/or as filamentous forms (hyphae) that may or may not be segmented (Table 41.1). When segmentation is observed, true hyphae are distinguished by their parallel walls and discrete perpendicular septa. In contrast, pseudohyphae are formed by budding yeasts that have failed to separate, producing chains of elongated yeast forms with bulging, nonparallel walls that pinch together at the septa, akin to sausage links. These morphologic features can provide important clues to narrow the differential diagnosis, although significant overlap occurs among organisms and definitive classification is often not possible by morphologic evaluation alone.[2] Nevertheless, when fungal organisms are encountered in tissue, a pathologist should provide at least a provisional diagnosis regarding their potential identity, as well as an opinion regarding the significance thereof (invasive infection vs. allergic or saprophytic infection). This can be particularly helpful in immunocompromised patients, for whom rapid diagnosis is essential to initiate antifungal treatment, often before ancillary studies or cultures can be completed.[3]

TABLE 41.1 Histologic Differentiating Features of Fungi That Commonly Infect the Lung

Organism	Size (µM)	Morphology	Mucicarmine	Granulomas	Clinical
Histoplasma	1–5	Oval budding yeast	Negative	Necrotizing	• Acute, usually self-limited • Disseminated (immunocompromised) • Chronic (underlying lung disease, e.g., emphysema)
Coccidioides	30–60 (spherules) 2–5 (endospores)	No budding, thick wall	Negative	Necrotizing, neutrophils early, eosinophils	• Primary (asymptomatic, or self-limited ("valley fever") • Persistent: lung nodules • Disseminated (immunocompromised)
Cryptococcus	2–15	Round, budding yeast, variation, fragmentation, capsule (halo)	Positive; when negative, Fontana-Masson positive	Nonnecrotizing or necrotizing	• Exposure: pigeon droppings • Asymptomatic, mildly symptomatic cavitary lesions • Disseminated (immunocompromised)
Blastomyces	2–30	Round, uniform, budding, thick cell wall	Negative	Necrotizing, neutrophils	• Acute self-limited • Progressive • Chronic/reactivation

Visualization of fungal morphology is aided by special stains, such as Gomori methenamine–silver (GMS), periodic acid–Schiff (PAS), and mucicarmine stains. Some fungi display characteristic morphologic features that can facilitate identification (e.g., the thick mucoid capsule of *Cryptococcus* and the large spherules of *Coccidioides* filled with endospores). However, atypical forms also occur.[4] When morphologic findings are inconclusive, ancillary studies are required. Fungal cultures, antigen detection, and serologic testing are often very helpful. Molecular PCR testing is also useful, particularly when unusual morphology is encountered.

Histoplasmosis

Histoplasmosis is encountered worldwide, but is most common in the Ohio and Mississippi River valleys of the central United States where it is endemic.[5] *Histoplasma capsulatum*, the causative agent, is found in soils contaminated with bird or bat droppings, and infection usually involves inhalation of spores from these soils. Common sites of exposure include farms, chicken coops, construction sites, and caves, although the specific site of exposure remains elusive in most cases.[6]

Clinical Features

Most acute infections with *H. capsulatum* are asymptomatic.[5] When symptoms develop, histoplasmosis usually presents as a mild and self-limited pneumonia. Chest imaging typically shows patchy or nodular infiltrates, often with hilar or mediastinal lymphadenopathy. In more severe cases, infiltrates can be diffuse or miliary, often accompanied by respiratory failure, findings that suggest disseminated infection.[7] Fibrous nodules or cavitary lung masses may develop in chronic infections, particularly in the upper lobes, mimicking chronic tuberculous infection. Cavitary infections can be complicated by bronchopleural fistulae and effusions.[8] Other cases can show significant mediastinal disease with bulky lymphadenopathy that may become calcified. Rare cases are complicated by fibrosing mediastinitis, with compression or obstruction of mediastinal structures.[9]

Pathologic Findings

In tissue, *H. capsulatum* appears as small teardrop-shaped yeasts (2 to 5 µm) with narrow-based budding[10,11] (Fig. 41.1). Organisms are often present in small clusters, either in necrotic areas or filling the cytoplasm of macrophages, although they may also be rare, particularly in old granulomas. When numerous, organisms are visible on H&E-stained sections as punctate dot-like structures within macrophages, but are more easily visible with GMS stains. Rarely, hyphae or pseudohyphae may be formed.[12] Tissue reactions vary widely and may include necrotizing, nonnecrotizing, or old hyalinized and calcified granulomas, as well as larger fibrotic and even cavitary granulomatous masses.[13] In immunocompromised patients, diffuse macrophage infiltrates may dominate the histologic picture, and fibrinopurulent exudates can also be seen.

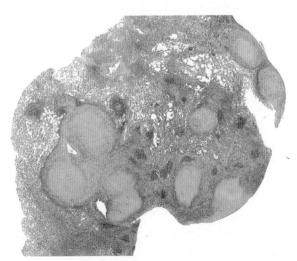

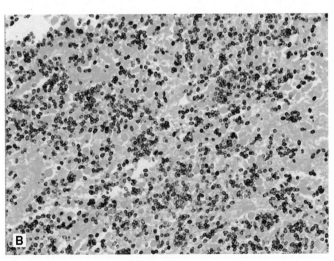

FIGURE 41.1 ▲ Histoplasmosis. **A.** At low magnification, there are multiple necrotizing granulomas. **B.** GMS stain shows small yeast forms with occasional budding.

Treatment

Treatment of histoplasmosis varies depending on the clinical presentation. Most acute pulmonary infections are mild and self-limited and do not require therapy.[6] When infections are more severe or when infections become chronic or cavitating, long-term antifungal therapy is usually employed. Itraconazole is typically used for mild to moderate infections,[14] and amphotericin B is usually required for severe infections.[6,15]

Coccidioidomycosis

Coccidioidomycosis is primarily encountered in lower deserts of the southwestern United States and northwestern Mexico where it is endemic, especially in the states of Arizona, California, and Sonora, but is also found in other isolated pockets in the Western Hemisphere.[16,17] Infection is caused by the dimorphic fungi *Coccidioides immitis* and *C. posadasii*, usually by inhalation of spores that are ubiquitous in desert soils.

Clinical Features

Like histoplasmosis, most acute infections with *Coccidioides* spp. are asymptomatic.[18] When symptoms develop, coccidioidomycosis usually presents as a mild and self-limited pneumonia with patchy or nodular pulmonary infiltrates and is a common cause of community-acquired pneumonia in endemic areas.[19] In more severe cases, infiltrates can be diffuse or miliary, often accompanied by respiratory failure, which may progress to involve extrapulmonary sites, especially bones, joints, and meninges.[20] Chronic infections typically present as a solitary lung nodule, often discovered incidentally on imaging studies performed for other reasons. Less commonly, chronic infections progress to form larger cavitary masses that can be complicated by rupture into the pleural space and empyema.[21,22]

Pathologic Findings

In tissue, *Coccidioides* spp. appear as spherules of widely variable size with a thick refractile wall, including large spherules (40 to 60 μm) filled with endospores, as well as empty or previously ruptured spherules (Fig. 41.2). Organisms may be rare, particularly in old granulomas. Complicating their identification, psammomatous calcification in old granulomas may closely mimic coccidioidal spherules. Fortunately, distinction between spherules and calcification is readily achieved by GMS staining, which only stains organisms. Rarely, septate hyphae may be seen, particularly in the setting of cavitary infection or a bronchopleural fistula.[21] Tissue reactions vary widely based upon the immune status of the patient and may include necrotizing or nonnecrotizing granulomas that may be hyalinized and even calcified. Less commonly, cavitary granulomatous masses can form, sometimes complicated by rupture into the pleural space with acute fibrinous or granulomatous pleuritis.[22] In immunocompromised patients, severe acute bronchopneumonia may occur with innumerable spherules present.

Treatment

Most acute pulmonary coccidioidal infections are mild and self-limited and do not require therapy. When infections are more severe, long-term antifungal therapy is usually employed. Ketoconazole is typically used for mild to moderate infections, and amphotericin B is usually required for severe infections.[20] When cavitary infections are complicated by rupture and empyema, surgical resection with pleural decortication is often required.[22]

Cryptococcosis

Cryptococcosis occurs worldwide. *Cryptococcus neoformans* is the principle causative agent and is found in soils contaminated with guano from pigeons, chickens, and other birds. Infections with *C. gattii* are much less common, but are endemic in the tropics and subtropics, especially Australia and Papua New Guinea, as well as the Pacific Northwest of the United States and British Columbia, Canada.[23,24]

Clinical Features

In immunocompetent patients, cryptococcosis is usually subclinical. In contrast, cryptococcosis in immunocompromised patients is almost always symptomatic. In the setting of severe immunodeficiency, cryptococcosis can result in acute respiratory failure or can disseminate, especially to the central nervous system, an important cause of mortality in patients with human immunodeficiency virus (HIV) infection or a history of organ transplantation.[25]

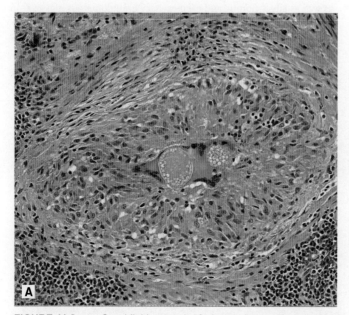
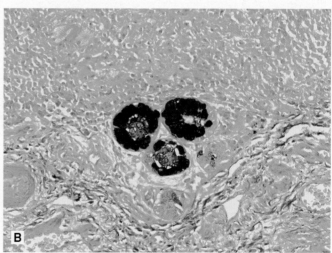

FIGURE 41.2 ▲ Coccidioidomycosis. **A.** A granuloma with macrophage giant cells containing a coccidioidomycosis spherule. The outline of the endospores is visible. **B.** GMS stain shows the larger spherules containing the smaller endospores.

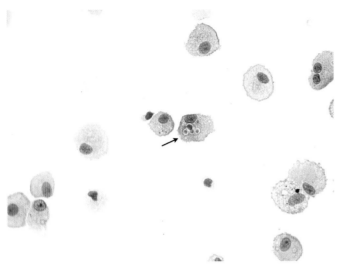

FIGURE 41.3 ▲ Cryptococcosis. In this cytologic smear, the encapsulated yeasts are seen within macrophages (*arrows*).

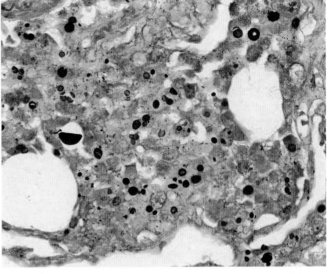

FIGURE 41.4 ▲ Cryptococcosis. There is variation in size and fragmentation of yeast forms (GMS stain).

Pathologic Findings

In tissue, *Cryptococcus* spp. typically appear as small (4 to 7 μm) round yeast forms, surrounded by a halo of clear space due to a thick mucoid capsule (Figs. 41.3 and 41.4). A mucicarmine stain readily highlights the characteristic capsule and is diagnostic when this structure is present, although capsule-deficient forms can also occur.[26–28] Tissue reactions vary widely depending on the immune status of the patient and may include necrotizing or nonnecrotizing granulomas, histiocytic pneumonia, mucoid pneumonia with virtually no inflammatory reaction, or intravascular cryptococcosis with innumerable organisms filling alveolar septal capillaries in the most severely immunocompromised patients[29] (Fig. 41.5).

Treatment

Symptomatic cryptococcosis generally requires chronic antifungal therapy. Fluconazole is typically used for mild to moderate infections. Severe or disseminated infections require aggressive treatment, with an induction regimen including amphotericin B plus flucytosine, followed by consolidation and chronic maintenance therapy with fluconazole.[25]

Blastomycosis

Blastomycosis is endemic in the central and southeastern United States, particularly in the Ohio and Mississippi River valleys. *Blastomyces dermatitidis*, the causative agent, is found in moist soils and decaying organic matter, and infection usually involves inhalation of spores from the environment. Individuals living in or exposed to wooded areas are at increased risk of infection, such as farmers, hunters, and campers.

Clinical Features

Many infections with *Blastomyces* are asymptomatic; when symptoms develop, the lungs are most commonly infected, and patients usually present with nonspecific symptoms that mimic bacterial or viral

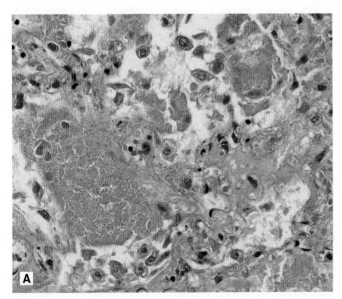

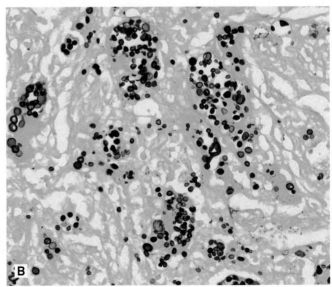

FIGURE 41.5 ▲ Cryptococcosis, disseminated, immunocompromised patient, autopsy lung. **A.** There is a fibrinous exudate within the alveolar spaces. **B.** GMS stain shows yeasts within the exudate. In contrast to pneumocystis, there is variation in yeast size and focal budding.

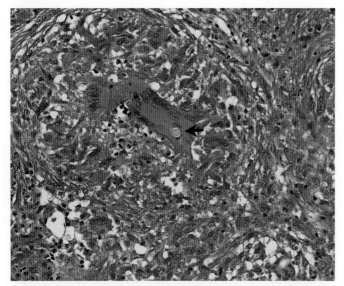

FIGURE 41.6 ▲ Blastomycosis. A yeast is seen in a macrophage giant cell (*arrow*) within a macrophage giant cell in a granuloma.

pneumonia. Radiologic findings vary widely and may include patchy alveolar infiltrates, masses, or miliary infiltrates.[30,31] Extrapulmonary dissemination occurs in ~20% of patients, with the skin being the most common site of involvement.[32]

Pathologic Findings

In tissue, *Blastomyces* typically appear as medium-sized (8 to 15 μm) yeast with thick, refractile, double-contoured walls, with broad-based budding,[33] although larger yeast forms may also be encountered (up to 30 μm), mimicking the spherules of *Coccidioides*[34] (Fig. 41.6). Necrotizing and often suppurative granulomatous inflammation is usually seen, but nonnecrotizing granulomas can also be encountered.

Treatment

Symptomatic blastomycosis generally requires antifungal therapy. Itraconazole is typically used for mild to moderate infections, and aggressive treatment with amphotericin B is usually required for severe infections.[35]

Aspergillosis

Aspergillus spp. are found ubiquitously in nature. Most infections are caused by *A. fumigatus*, although numerous other species are also pathogenic, and aspergillosis remains an important cause of morbidity and mortality in immunocompromised patients.[36] In the lung, aspergillosis is classified into three categories of disease, including saprophytic forms of infection, allergic or hypersensitivity forms, and invasive disease, with the latter including both minimally invasive chronic necrotizing infections and angioinvasive and disseminated disease[37–41] (Table 41.2). In tissue, *Aspergillus* spp. appear as septate hyphae of uniform width, with 45-degree angle dichotomous branching. Although this morphology is characteristic of *Aspergillus* spp., numerous fungal

look-alikes occur, especially *Pseudallescheria*, *Fusarium*, and the zygomycetes (e.g., *Rhizopus*, *Absidia*), as well as *Candida* in some cases and numerous less common molds (e.g., *Scedosporium*, *Acremonium*, *Paecilomyces*).[40] For this reason, definitive classification should be deferred to microbiologic cultures whenever possible.

Saprophytic

Saprophytic infections are characterized by superficial colonization of obstructed bronchi, as in the setting of cystic fibrosis or bronchiectasis, or a preexisting cavitary lesion, as in the setting of tuberculosis, sarcoidosis, or an old abscess, where accumulation of fungal mycelia results in the formation of a fungus ball ("aspergilloma"). Saprophytic infections are generally asymptomatic and do not require treatment,[41] although occasionally patients with a long-standing aspergilloma may develop hemoptysis and require surgical resection.

Allergic

In some cases, superficial colonization of airways by *Aspergillus* spp. induces a complex allergic or hypersensitivity reaction to fungal antigens. Allergic bronchopulmonary aspergillosis (ABPA) typically occurs in patients with chronic asthma or cystic fibrosis and is characterized by eosinophil-rich chronic inflammation of airways, with obstructive plugging of bronchi by allergic mucin. Histologically, allergic mucin is dense and basophilic and contains abundant eosinophils with Charcot-Leyden crystals. Organisms are sometimes seen within allergic mucin, but they do not invade the bronchial wall. Other patterns of disease include eosinophilic pneumonia, bronchocentric granulomatosis, and/or hypersensitivity pneumonitis.[40] Treatment of ABPA aims to limit progressive inflammatory injury and worsening of bronchiectasis; corticosteroids are a mainstay of therapy, often in combination with itraconazole.[41]

Invasive

Invasive aspergillosis is typically seen in the immunocompromised host with neutropenia.[42] In patients who are only mildly immunocompromised, a minimally invasive infection may result in necrotizing pseudomembranous tracheobronchitis, characterized by mucosal erosion, ulceration, and pseudomembrane formation within large airways, often with bronchial obstruction. Other minimally invasive infections result in chronic necrotizing pulmonary aspergillosis (CNPA), characterized by chronic upper lobe–predominant infiltrates and fibrocavitary masses. In severely immunocompromised patients, angioinvasive infection results in vascular obstruction, hemorrhagic pulmonary infarcts, and dissemination to other organs, a devastating condition with a very poor prognosis (Fig. 41.7). Treatment typically includes aggressive antifungal therapy with voriconazole, often in combination with an echinocandin, and reduction in immunosuppression whenever possible.[41]

Paracoccidioidomycosis

Paracoccidioidomycosis, caused by *Paracoccidioides brasiliensis* and *P. lutzii*, primarily occurs in tropical and subtropical regions of South America, especially in Brazil, Venezuela, and Columbia, but is also encountered in parts of Mexico and Central America.[43,44] The disease almost exclusively affects postpubertal men, especially in rural areas, and is rare in women, likely due to a protective effect of female hormones that retard fungal growth.[45]

TABLE 41.2 Pulmonary Manifestations of Aspergillosis

Designation	Type of Infection	Clinical	Pathology
Aspergilloma	Saprophytic	Usually asymptomatic	Fungus ball colonizing preexisting cavity
Allergic bronchopulmonary aspergillosis	Allergic	Asthma, cystic fibrosis	"Allergic" mucin in distended bronchi with few hyphae
Invasive aspergillosis	Opportunistic pathogen in immunocompromised patients	Necrotizing pneumonia	Abundant invasive hyphae with necrosis and infarction

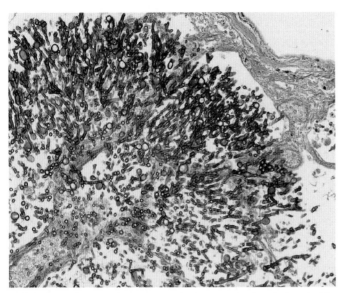

FIGURE 41.7 ▲ Invasive aspergillosis. There are cavitary lesions in this autopsy lung. A high magnification shows septate hyphae (picture insert).

Clinical Features

Paracoccidioidomycosis most commonly presents as a chronic progressive systemic mycosis in middle-aged men that may be confined to the lungs, or may disseminate, especially to the oropharyngeal mucous membranes. Radiologic findings in the lungs are nonspecific and may include infiltrates, nodules, cavitary masses, and/or fibrosis.[46] Less commonly, an acute form of infection occurs in children and adolescents, typically with rapid widespread dissemination, lymphadenopathy, and hepatosplenomegaly.[47]

Pathologic Findings

In tissue, *Paracoccidioides* spp. appear as yeast of widely variable sizes (3 to 60 μm), including large spherical yeast forms surrounded by multiple smaller teardrop-shaped buds with narrow necks ("mariner's wheel" or "ship's wheel"). Fractured cell walls may also be seen. When buds are few, organisms may closely resemble *Histoplasma*, *Blastomyces*, capsule-deficient *Cryptococcus*, or *Coccidioides*, depending on their size. In patients with chronic disease, tissue reactions include necrotizing or nonnecrotizing granulomas, often with interstitial fibrosis. An acute bronchopneumonia pattern is usually seen in young patients.

Treatment

Paracoccidioidomycosis typically requires chronic antifungal treatment with itraconazole or similar azole derivatives and/or a sulfonamide compound. Amphotericin B is typically reserved for severe infections.[48]

Candidiasis

Candida spp. are found ubiquitously in nature and are an important cause of morbidity and mortality in immunocompromised patients. *C. albicans* is the most common species isolated, but numerous others are medically important, especially *C. parapsilosis*, *C. krusei*, *C. glabrata*, and *C. tropicalis*.

Clinical Features

Most clinically significant pulmonary infections occur in immunocompromised patients via hematogenous seeding of the lungs in the setting of fungemia.[49,50] Such infections typically present with miliary nodular infiltrates, often associated with dissemination to other organs, and carry a poor prognosis. Less commonly, aspiration of saprophytic organisms from the oropharynx causes acute candidal bronchopneumonia.[51]

Pathologic Findings

In tissue, *Candida* spp. appear as small (2 to 6 μm) oval budding yeast that stain not only with GMS and PAS but also with a Gram stain (weakly Gram positive). Most species also produce branching pseudohyphae, with the exception of *C. glabrata* that only forms yeast in tissue.[52] Numerous fungal look-alikes occur, especially *Histoplasma* and *Aspergillus*, which must be distinguished from the yeast and pseudohyphae of *Candida*, respectively; the former is distinguished from *Candida* by its intracellular location and lack of Gram staining and the latter by its true hyphae and lack of yeast forms. However, definitive classification should be reserved for microbiologic cultures whenever possible. Tissue reactions generally depend on the mode of acquisition, with hematogenous infections manifesting as necroinflammatory miliary nodules with hemorrhage and aspiration manifesting as airway-centered acute bronchopneumonia, sometimes accompanied by aspirated food or foreign material.

Treatment

Pulmonary candidiasis and other deeply invasive or disseminated forms of infection require prolonged antifungal treatment, typically with an echinocandin, voriconazole, or amphotericin B.[53]

Zygomycosis

Zygomycetes are a class of related organisms that are ubiquitous in nature and that cause serious and often fatal angioinvasive fungal infections. Within this class, organisms of the order Mucorales are usually encountered, from which the alternative term "mucormycosis" is derived. *Absidia* and *Rhizopus* are the most common agents of infection, but *Mucor*, *Rhizomucor*, and numerous others may also cause infection.[54]

Clinical Features

Zygomycosis is a devastating infection with very high mortality rates that usually occurs in immunocompromised patients, especially those with hematologic malignancies and diabetes mellitus with acidosis, and may involve rhinocerebral, pulmonary, gastrointestinal, and/or cutaneous sites. In the lungs, infection may present as nodular infiltrates, lobar consolidation, cavitary masses, and/or hemorrhagic infarcts.

Pathologic Findings

In tissue, zygomycetes appear as broad (6 to 25 μm), thin-walled, pauciseptate hyphae of varying width, with nonparallel walls and random 90-degree-angle branching. Hyphae may display neurotropism as well as angiotropism.[55] When hyphae are of lesser width, they may occasionally mimic *Aspergillus* and other *Aspergillus*-like molds, as well as the pseudohyphae of *Candida* spp. in some cases.

Treatment

Zygomycosis requires immediate treatment including aggressive surgical debridement and intravenous amphotericin B as soon as the diagnosis is suspected.[56] Unfortunately, prognosis is grim even with aggressive therapies, especially with pulmonary involvement.

Miscellaneous
Sporotrichosis

Sporothrix schenckii is found in soils worldwide, and infection is usually limited to the skin and lymphatics after direct inoculation through a puncture wound ("rose gardener's disease"), although dissemination may occur in the immunocompromised host. In the lungs, infection may produce granulomatous nodules or cavitary masses. In tissue, *Sporothrix* appears as very small (2 to 3 μm) oval yeast with narrow-based budding or cigar-shaped forms.[57] Organisms are often rare and may closely mimic *Histoplasma* or *Candida*.

Pseudallescheriasis/Scedosporiosis

Pseudallescheria boydii and the closely related *Scedosporium prolificans* are found worldwide and are emerging causes of disseminated opportunistic infections in immunocompromised hosts.[58] Infection may result in pulmonary infiltrates, consolidation, nodules, cavitary masses, or dissemination. In tissue, *P. boydii* and *S. prolificans* are indistinguishable from *Aspergillus*; definitive diagnosis requires cultures or molecular testing.

Fusariosis

Fusarium spp. are important emerging opportunistic fungi that cause life-threatening invasive infections, occurring almost exclusively in severely immunocompromised patients with hematologic malignancies.[59] Infection usually results in severe pneumonia and dissemination. Portals of entry include the respiratory tract and skin. In tissue, *Fusarium* is indistinguishable from *Aspergillus*; definitive diagnosis requires cultures or molecular techniques.

Penicilliosis

Penicillium marneffei is endemic to Southeast Asia and is a very common opportunistic infection in AIDS in that region, but may also be seen in immunocompromised travelers who have been to Southeast Asia. Patients present with pulmonary infiltrates, with or without dissemination. In tissue, *Penicillium* closely mimics *Histoplasma*, with small (2.5 to 5 μm) yeast filling alveolar macrophages. Clues to the correct diagnosis include the presence of elongated, curved "sausage" forms, short hyphal forms, or yeast with a single transverse septum.[60]

REFERENCES

1. Saubolle MA. Fungal pneumonias. *Semin Respir Infect.* 2000;15:162–177.
2. Watts JC, Chandler FW. Morphologic identification of mycelial pathogens in tissue sections. A caveat. *Am J Clin Pathol.* 1998;109:1–2.
3. Powers CN. Diagnosis of infectious diseases: a cytopathologist's perspective. *Clin Microbiol Rev.* 1998;11:341–365.
4. Kaufman L, Valero G, Padhye AA. Misleading manifestations of *Coccidioides immitis* in vivo. *J Clin Microbiol.* 1998;36:3721–3723.
5. Kauffman CA. Histoplasmosis: a clinical and laboratory update. *Clin Microbiol Rev.* 2007;20:115–132.
6. Wheat LJ, Conces D, Allen SD, et al. Pulmonary histoplasmosis syndromes: recognition, diagnosis, and management. *Semin Respir Crit Care Med.* 2004;25:129–144.
7. Wheat LJ. Improvements in diagnosis of histoplasmosis. *Expert Opin Biol Ther.* 2006;6:1207–1221.
8. Goodwin RA Jr, Owens FT, Snell JD, et al. Chronic pulmonary histoplasmosis. *Medicine (Baltimore).* 1976;55:413–452.
9. Loyd JE, Tillman BF, Atkinson JB, et al. Mediastinal fibrosis complicating histoplasmosis. *Medicine (Baltimore).* 1988;67:295–310.
10. Vanek J, Schwarz J. The gamut of histoplasmosis. *Am J Med.* 1971;50:89–104.
11. Binford CH. Histoplasmosis: tissue reactions and morphologic variations of the fungus. *Am J Clin Pathol.* 1955;25:25–36.
12. Riddell Jt, Kauffman CA, Smith JA, et al. Histoplasma capsulatum endocarditis: multicenter case series with review of current diagnostic techniques and treatment. *Medicine (Baltimore).* 2014;93:186–193.
13. Goodwin RA Jr, Shapiro JL, Thurman GH, et al. Disseminated histoplasmosis: clinical and pathologic correlations. *Medicine (Baltimore).* 1980;59:1–33.
14. Dismukes WE, Bradsher RW Jr, Cloud GC, et al. Itraconazole therapy for blastomycosis and histoplasmosis. NIAID Mycoses Study Group. *Am J Med.* 1992;93:489–497.
15. Wheat LJ, Cloud G, Johnson PC, et al.; Mycoses Study Group of NIAID. Clearance of fungal burden during treatment of disseminated histoplasmosis with liposomal amphotericin B versus itraconazole. *Antimicrob Agents Chemother.* 2001;45:2354–2357.
16. Hector RF, Rutherford GW, Tsang CA, et al. The public health impact of coccidioidomycosis in Arizona and California. *Int J Environ Res Public Health.* 2011;8:1150–1173.
17. McNabb SJ, Jajosky RA, Hall-Baker PA, et al. Summary of notifiable diseases—United States, 2006. *MMWR Morb Mortal Wkly Rep* 2008;55:1–92.
18. Nguyen C, Barker BM, Hoover S, et al. Recent advances in our understanding of the environmental, epidemiological, immunological, and clinical dimensions of coccidioidomycosis. *Clin Microbiol Rev.* 2013;26:505–525.
19. Valdivia L, Nix D, Wright M, et al. Coccidioidomycosis as a common cause of community-acquired pneumonia. *Emerg Infect Dis.* 2006;12:958–962.
20. Galgiani JN, Ampel NM, Blair JE, et al. Coccidioidomycosis. *Clin Infect Dis.* 2005;41:1217–1223.
21. Sobonya RE, Yanes J, Klotz SA. Cavitary pulmonary coccidioidomycosis: pathologic and clinical correlates of disease. *Hum Pathol.* 2014;45:153–159.
22. Shekhel TA, Ricciotti RW, Blair JE, et al. Surgical pathology of pleural coccidioidomycosis: a clinicopathological study of 36 cases. *Hum Pathol.* 2014;45:961–969.
23. Chaturvedi V, Chaturvedi S. *Cryptococcus gattii*: a resurgent fungal pathogen. *Trends Microbiol.* 2011;19:564–571.
24. Harris J, Lockhart S, Chiller T. *Cryptococcus gattii*: where do we go from here? *Med Mycol.* 2012;50:113–129.
25. Perfect JR, Dismukes WE, Dromer F, et al. Clinical practice guidelines for the management of cryptococcal disease: 2010 update by the Infectious Diseases Society of America. *Clin Infect Dis.* 2010;50:291–322.
26. Farmer SG, Komorowski RA. Histologic response to capsule-deficient *Cryptococcus* neoformans. *Arch Pathol.* 1973;96:383–387.
27. Gutierrez F, Fu YS, Lurie H. Cryptococcosis histologically resembling histoplasmosis. A light and electron microscopical study. *Arch Pathol.* 1975;99:347–352.
28. Harding SA, Scheld WM, Feldman PS, et al. Pulmonary infection with capsule-deficient cryptococcus neoformans. *Virchows Arch A Pathol Anat Histol.* 1979;382:113–118.
29. McDonnell JM, Hutchins GM. Pulmonary cryptococcosis. *Hum Pathol.* 1985;16:121–128.
30. Sheflin JR, Campbell JA, Thompson GP. Pulmonary blastomycosis: findings on chest radiographs in 63 patients. *AJR Am J Roentgenol.* 1990;154:1177–1180.
31. Brown LR, Swensen SJ, Van Scoy RE, et al. Roentgenologic features of pulmonary blastomycosis. *Mayo Clin Proc.* 1991;66:29–38.
32. Chapman SW, Lin AC, Hendricks KA, et al. Endemic blastomycosis in Mississippi: epidemiological and clinical studies. *Semin Respir Infect.* 1997;12:219–228.
33. Taxy JB. Blastomycosis: contributions of morphology to diagnosis: a surgical pathology, cytopathology, and autopsy pathology study. *Am J Surg Pathol.* 2007;31:615–623.
34. Hussain Z, Martin A, Youngberg GA. *Blastomyces dermatitidis* with large yeast forms. *Arch Pathol Lab Med.* 2001;125:663–664.
35. Chapman SW, Dismukes WE, Proia LA, et al.; Infectious Diseases Society of America. Clinical practice guidelines for the management of blastomycosis: 2008 update by the Infectious Diseases Society of America. *Clin Infect Dis.* 2008;46:1801–1812.
36. Latge JP. *Aspergillus fumigatus* and aspergillosis. *Clin Microbiol Rev.* 1999;12:310–350.
37. Bosken CH, Myers JL, Greenberger PA, et al. Pathologic features of allergic bronchopulmonary aspergillosis. *Am J Surg Pathol.* 1988;12:216–222.
38. Yousem SA. The histological spectrum of chronic necrotizing forms of pulmonary aspergillosis. *Hum Pathol.* 1997;28:650–656.
39. Denning DW, Riniotis K, Dobrashian R, et al. Chronic cavitary and fibrosing pulmonary and pleural aspergillosis: case series, proposed nomenclature change, and review. *Clin Infect Dis.* 2003; 37(suppl. 3):S265–S280.
40. Kradin RL, Mark EJ. The pathology of pulmonary disorders due to *Aspergillus* spp. *Arch Pathol Lab Med.* 2008;132:606–614.
41. Walsh TJ, Anaissie EJ, Denning DW, et al.; Infectious Diseases Society of America. Treatment of aspergillosis: clinical practice guidelines of the Infectious Diseases Society of America. *Clin Infect Dis.* 2008;46:327–360.
42. Segal BH. Aspergillosis. *N Engl J Med.* 2009;360:1870–1884.
43. Brummer E, Castaneda E, Restrepo A. Paracoccidioidomycosis: an update. *Clin Microbiol Rev.* 1993;6:89–117.
44. Restrepo A. The ecology of *Paracoccidioides brasiliensis*: a puzzle still unsolved. *Sabouraudia.* 1985;23:323–334.
45. Blotta MH, Mamoni RL, Oliveira SJ, et al. Endemic regions of paracoccidioidomycosis in Brazil: a clinical and epidemiologic study of 584 cases in the southeast region. *Am J Trop Med Hyg.* 1999;61:390–394.
46. Barreto MM, Marchiori E, Amorim VB, et al. Thoracic paracoccidioidomycosis: radiographic and CT findings. *Radiographics.* 2012;32:71–84.
47. Pereira RM, Bucaretchi F, Barison Ede M, et al. Paracoccidioidomycosis in children: clinical presentation, follow-up and outcome. *Rev Inst Med Trop Sao Paulo.* 2004;46:127–131.
48. Travassos LR, Taborda CP, Colombo AL. Treatment options for paracoccidioidomycosis and new strategies investigated. *Expert Rev AntiInfect Ther.* 2008;6:251–262.

49. Fridkin SK. The changing face of fungal infections in health care settings. *Clin Infect Dis.* 2005;41:1455–1460.

50. Rose HD, Sheth NK. Pulmonary candidiasis. A clinical and pathological correlation. *Arch Intern Med.* 1978;138:964–965.

51. Masur H, Rosen PP, Armstrong D. Pulmonary disease caused by *Candida* species. *Am J Med.* 1977;63:914–925.

52. Fidel PL Jr, Vazquez JA, Sobel JD. *Candida glabrata*: review of epidemiology, pathogenesis, and clinical disease with comparison to C. albicans. *Clin Microbiol Rev.* 1999;12:80–96.

53. Pappas PG, Kauffman CA, Andes D, et al.; Infectious Diseases Society of America. Clinical practice guidelines for the management of candidiasis: 2009 update by the Infectious Diseases Society of America. *Clin Infect Dis.* 2009;48:503–535.

54. Roden MM, Zaoutis TE, Buchanan WL, et al. Epidemiology and outcome of zygomycosis: a review of 929 reported cases. *Clin Infect Dis.* 2005;41:634–653.

55. Frater JL, Hall GS, Procop GW. Histologic features of zygomycosis: emphasis on perineural invasion and fungal morphology. *Arch Pathol Lab Med.* 2001;125:375–378.

56. Spellberg B, Ibrahim AS. Recent advances in the treatment of mucormycosis. *Curr Infect Dis Rep.* 2010;12:423–429.

57. England DM, Hochholzer L. Primary pulmonary sporotrichosis. Report of eight cases with clinicopathologic review. *Am J Surg Pathol.* 1985;9:193–204.

58. Quan C, Spellberg B. Mucormycosis, pseudallescheriasis, and other uncommon mold infections. *Proc Am Thorac Soc.* 2010;7:210–215.

59. Nucci M, Anaissie E. Fusarium infections in immunocompromised patients. *Clin Microbiol Rev.* 2007;20:695–704.

60. Deng ZL, Connor DH. Progressive disseminated penicilliosis caused by *Penicillium marneffei*. Report of eight cases and differentiation of the causative organism from *Histoplasma capsulatum*. *Am J Clin Pathol.* 1985;84:323–327.

42 Pneumocystis Pneumonia

Allen P. Burke, M.D.

Background

Pneumocystis organisms were first described in rats and guinea pigs in the early 20th century as protozoa related to trypanosomes (reviewed by Catherinot et al.[1]). Pneumocystis was recognized as a fungus relatively recently, based on rRNA sequencing.[2] In the 1950s, the first human infections were identified in malnourished and premature infants and rarely in adults.[3,4] Later, pneumocystis pneumonia (PCP) was a recognized pathogen in immunocompromised children[5,6] and then in adults with HIV disease. The routine use of highly active antiretroviral therapy (HAART) has seen a decline in its incidence,[7] and the primary clinical setting of PCP is no longer AIDS, but immunosuppression secondary to chemotherapy for hematologic malignancies.[8]

Pneumocystis has its own class, order, and family under the phylum Ascomycota. The organism was known as *Pneumocystis carinii* for many years, named after one of the first discoverers of the organism in animals. Although the human species was recommended to be called "jiroveci" (after one of the first discoverers of human infection) as long ago as 1976,[9] only in 2001 was it decided to use the designation *carinii* specifically for one of the animal species of the fungus.[10] The current accepted designation for the human pathogen is "jirovecii" (with two terminal "Is").[1]

Pneumocystis jirovecii is a normal bronchial inhabitant in infants and children, with serologic conversion common at an early age.[1] Although species of pneumocystis are found in diverse reservoirs, including in bats, swine, hens, as well as rats and guinea pigs, no animal reservoir for *P. jirovecii* has been found.[1,11] Most studies have shown 0% to 20% colonization rate in healthy adults, although there is a wide range of sampling and methodology for detection of the organism. Using sensitive polymerase chain reaction (PCR) techniques and tissue concentration methods, the organism has been identified in nearly two-thirds of traumatic and natural deaths in adult lungs.[12] There is an increased incidence of bronchial colonization in chronic lung disease, smoking, HIV, steroid use, and children.[1]

Clinical Settings of Pneumocystis Pneumonia

Before AIDS and the widespread use of immunosuppressive drugs, PCP was a rare disease, reported in only 10 patients per year in the United States, mostly children with immunodeficiency or acute leukemia (Table 42.1).[5]

Although the largest numbers of PCPs were seen in the early years of the AIDS epidemic, the rate of PCP in HIV-infected adults has dropped to 0.3 per 100 person-years in developed countries. This figure represents a more than 10-fold decrease compared to era of HIV therapies before the availability of HAART.[15] Despite the decline in incidence since the beginning of the AIDS epidemic, *P. jirovecii* pneumonia remains the most common cause of respiratory failure in HIV patients even in the HAART era, for which the mortality rate remains around 10%.[16–18] In this group of patients, CD4 as biomarker works well, with a cutoff of 200 cells per μL of blood, or 15% of T cells, a reliable indication for treatment prophylaxis.

Primary immunodeficiency syndromes predispose to PCP, usually those affecting T cells.[6] Most patients are infants under 1 year of age, and two-thirds suffer from severe combined immunodeficiency.[5] The incidence of pneumocystis ranges between one-fourth and one-half of patients prior to bone marrow transplant, depending on whether the infant is on pneumocystis prophylaxis.[6,19,20] PCP is rare in pure B-cell disorders and agammaglobulinemia.[21]

The rate of PCP complicating hematologic and solid malignancies is fairly low, in the range of 1% to 2%. Immunosuppression by steroids especially predisposes to pneumocystis infection, although a large number of drugs have been implicated.

Prior to routine prophylaxis, PCP was relatively common in solid organ transplants, occurring in up to 50% of heart transplant recipients and 10% of kidney and liver transplants. Currently, the rate is closer to 1%, affecting patients who did not receive prophylaxis or who discontinued trimethoprim–sulfamethoxazole.[22] The rate is slightly higher in patients with allogeneic stem cell transplant, and similarly occurs in patients who are no longer on prophylaxis, typically with low CD4 counts or with recurrent malignancy.[23]

Autoimmune connective tissues have a low rate of pneumocystis infection complicating immunosuppression, generally <0.5%. Virtually any condition treated with steroids may predispose to PCP including steatohepatitis.[24]

Clinical and Radiologic Findings

PCP is in the differential diagnosis of an immunocompromised patient with bilateral pulmonary infiltrates, typically with fever and cough. The major clinical diagnostic considerations include other infections, interstitial pneumonia (usually diffuse alveolar damage or organizing pneumonia), drug toxicity, and malignancy (Table 42.2). Serologic screening for 1,3-beta-D-glucan may be useful in diagnosing invasive fungal infection, but is not specific for pneumocystis.[28]

TABLE 42.1   Clinical Settings of Pneumocystis Pneumonia

Cause for Immunosuppression	Features
HIV/AIDS	Rate about 0.3% in patients where HAART is available
	Relatively good rate of treatment response
	Occurs almost exclusively with CD4 counts < 200 μL
	No longer the majority of cases of PCP
Hematologic malignancies	Steroids typically involved
	Cytarabin, vincristine, cyclophosphamide, methotrexate, alemtuzumab, bortezumib[13]
	Rituximab (rarely)
Solid tumors	Treatment for brain tumors/metastasis associated with highest rate of PCP, because of high-dose steroid treatment
Solid organ transplants	Around 1%–2% of patients
	Does not occur while patient on prophylaxis
	Prednisone, tacrolimus, and mycophenolate mofetil
Stem cell transplant	Higher with allogeneic transplants
	Typically during immunosuppression and early after transplant
	Associated with low CD4 count and lymphoma/leukemia relapses
Autoimmune connective tissue diseases	Occurs during immunosuppression, especially steroids
	Granulomatosis with polyangiitis (Wegener's) most frequent
	Rheumatoid arthritis
	Giant cell arteritis (rare)[14]
Primary immunodeficiency	SCID (>2/3 of cases)
	X-linked hyper-IgM syndrome
	Usually infants < 1 y of age
	Rarely primary agammaglobulinemia syndromes

PCP, pneumocystis (jirovecii) pneumonia. Although initially designating "*Pneumocystis carinii* pneumonia," the acronym persists to indicate "pneumocystis [jirovecii] pneumonia"; HAART, highly active antiretroviral therapy; SCID, severe combined immunodeficiency.

On chest radiograph, PCP usually presents with bilateral, diffuse, reticular, or granular opacities. Up to one-fourth of patients have predominantly nodular densities.[29] Chest radiograph may be normal. Chest computed tomography typically shows ground-glass opacities predominating in perihilar regions of lungs.[30] Atypical patterns are more common currently with treatment and prophylaxis and include predominantly upper lobe disease, pneumothorax, and cyst formation (Fig. 42.1). Cyst formation, which may lead to pneumothorax, may reverse with treatment.[31] Other atypical findings include large nodules or areas of consolidation that may cavitate with thick walls. Lymphadenopathy and effusions are infrequent.[30]

Tissue Sampling

Most cases of PCP are diagnosed by cytologic smears. Samples from the lower respiratory tract are more sensitive than nasopharyngeal

TABLE 42.2   Lung Infections in Immunocompromised Patients with Diffuse Lung Infiltrates, Diagnosed by Open Lung Biopsy[19,25–27]

Diagnosis	Approximate Frequency
All infections[a]	10%–74%
Pneumocystis	3%–45%
ARDS/DAD	3%–7%
Organizing pneumonia	3%
Interstitial pneumonitis, NOS	20%–65%
Chemotherapy-related pneumonitis	12%–20%
Recurrent leukemia/lymphoma/solid tumor	10%–20%
Vasculitis/capillaritis	0%–5%
Lipoid pneumonia	0%–5%
Sarcoid	0%–2%
Nondiagnostic	5%

[a]*Legionella, Aspergillus, Nocardia, Haemophilus,* cytomegalovirus, *Candida, Staphylococcus.*
NOS, not otherwise specified; ARDS, acute respiratory distress syndrome; DAD, diffuse alveolar damage.

swabs, and bronchoalveolar lavage specimens have a higher yield than do sputum samples. The sensitivity is somewhat increased using immunologic stains, such as direct immunofluorescence, over Gomori methenamine–silver stains.[32–35] PCR testing may be useful for increasing the sensitivity of nasopharyngeal samples in children with suspected PCP.[32]

In rare instances, bronchoalveolar lavage specimens may be negative, especially in cases of granulomatous disease.[8,36] In such cases, open lung biopsies are required for diagnosis. In older series of immunosuppressed patients with lung infiltrates of unclear etiology, who were subjected to open lung biopsy for definitive diagnosis, an infection was diagnosed in ~50% of patients, with pneumocystis the largest group.[25,26,37] In patients who failed antibiotic treatment, the rate of infection was lower with acute alveolar injury more common than infection.[27] In some cases, the alveolar injury may be sampled at an organizing phase (sometimes called "bronchiolitis obliterans organizing pneumonia" (see Chapter 19).[38]

The need for routine staining of open lung biopsies with acid-fast stains, fungal stain, and Gram stains has been emphasized, on both touch preps of fresh tissue and frozen control samples.[26] In addition, immunohistochemical staining for viruses such as cytomegalovirus is routinely indicated.

Microscopic Findings

In histologic sections, PCP is characterized by a lack of inflammatory response, due to the immunosuppression that predisposes to the organism's proliferation and adhesion to alveolar walls. The organisms are admixed with small amounts of fibrin and impart a typical bubbly or foamy nature to the pink intra-alveolar exudate. The interstitium is typically only mildly thickened by chronic inflammatory cells, although in children, a prominent plasmacytic response may be seen in the alveolar walls.[4] Occasionally, there may be alveolar simplification with loss of alveolar walls and cyst formation, corresponding to computed tomographic findings (Fig. 42.2).

The organisms are identified by special stains (Table 42.3) and have two forms: cysts and trophs. The diagnosis is typically based on identification of cysts by Gomori methenamine–silver staining

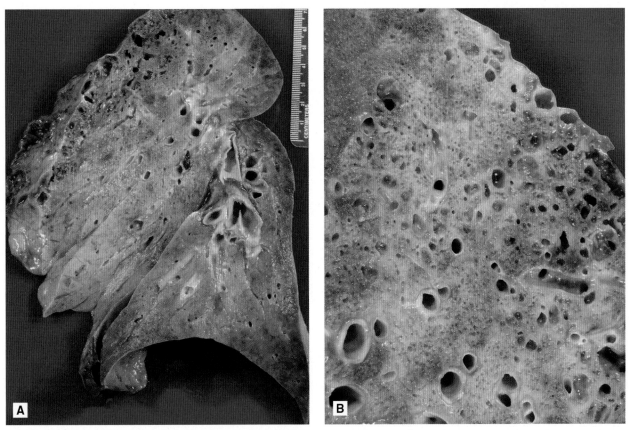

FIGURE 42.1 ▲ Gross lungs, patient with PCP, HIV disease. **A.** There is cystic change in a subpleural location.
B. A higher magnification shows small cysts and interstitial thickening.

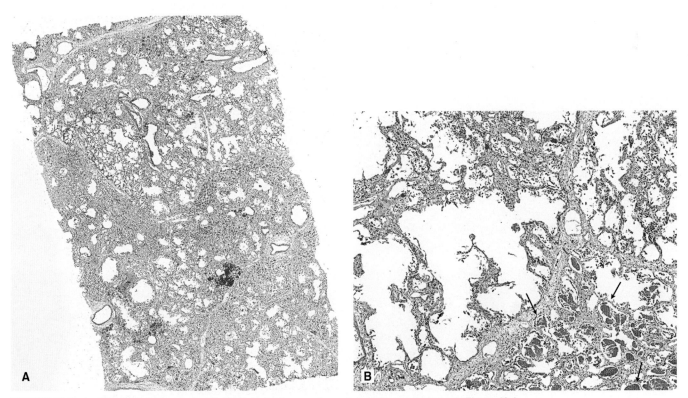

FIGURE 42.2 ▲ Histologic findings, chronic PCP. **A.** A microscopic section of the lungs shown in Figure 42.1
shows interstitial thickening with inflammation and early cystic change. **B.** A higher magnification shows early cysts
and areas with intra-alveolar exudate (*arrows*).

TABLE 42.3 Stains Utilized in Detected Pneumocystis Organisms (Smears)

Cysts	Trophs
Gomori methenamine–silver	Papanicolaou
Cresyl echt violet	Giemsa
Toluidine blue	Gram-Weigert
Calcofluor white	Direct immunofluorescence
Direct immunofluorescence	

(Figs. 42.3 and 42.4), typically in clusters of 2 to 8. They are round, oval, or flat and are 4 to 10 μM in diameter, depending on the method of staining, but typically described as 5 to 6 μM.[39] The cyst may have kidney bean–, double parenthesis–, or comma-shaped areas that stain darker with the silver deposition stains. These "intracystic bodies" are regions of thickened cyst wall, as demonstrated by ultrastructural analysis.[40] Trophic forms are more numerous than cysts, are a fraction of the size, and range from about one-tenth to half the size of the cysts. Immunofluorescent monoclonal antibodies stain for both trophic forms and cysts.

Rarely, pneumocystis infection causes a granulomatous reaction. In cases of granulomatous PCP, the computed tomographic findings are atypical and the bronchoalveolar lavage specimens negative. Histologically, clusters of Gomori methenamine–silver–positive Pneumocystis organisms are seen within granulomas, which are usually well-formed non-necrotizing. Macrophage giant cells, a fibrous rim around the nodule, and eosinophils are common. Foamy exudates typical of intra-alveolar pneumocystis infection are usually absent, but may be seen within necrotizing granulomas and rarely in adjacent parenchyma.[8,36]

Molecular Findings

PCR molecular techniques are used mostly in the research setting and may have application for screening of easily accessible nasopharyngeal

samples.[32] Conventional PCR has a low specificity because it may detect colonization in the absence of infection, but has a high negative predictive value, allowing withdrawal of anti-PCP therapy. Quantitative PCR may allow for cutoff between colonization and infection.[1]

Differential Diagnosis

The histologic differential diagnosis includes other entities that can cause an eosinophilic intra-alveolar exudate, other fungal infections, and exclusion of concomitant infections. The intra-alveolar exudate of pneumocystis is characteristic, but must be confirmed by identifying the organism resulting in the small bubbles, and differentiated from fibrin (which is typically fibrillar), proteinosis (which lacks the foamy nature and typically has granules or clefts), and edema fluid. The cysts of pneumocystis have been described as resembling "crushed ping-pong balls" and are present in aggregates, unlike *Histoplasma* or *Cryptococcus*. *Histoplasma* yeasts are smaller (3 to 5 μM) and may show budding forms, unlike pneumocystis. The yeasts of *Cryptococcus* vary in size, show budding, and have a thick capsule.

Prognosis and Treatment

Treatment for pneumocystis entails both prophylaxis and therapy for symptomatic pneumonitis (Table 42.4). Trimethoprim–sulfamethoxazole is the standard of treatment for lung infections and is more effective in AIDS (about 90% survival) than non–HIV-related disease (50% to 80% survival). Early treatment, especially in non-HIV patients, may decrease need for intubation, emphasizing the need for rapid diagnosis and hospitalization for immunocompromised patients with suspected opportunistic lung infections.[41]

Chemoprophylaxis is used in high-risk patients (e.g., early after transplant, active immunosuppression, and low CD4 counts), usually as aerosolized pentamidine monthly. For patients with autoimmune collagen vascular disease, such as granulomatosis with polyangiitis, or cancer patients, high-dose steroid treatment may lead to a consideration of pneumocystis prophylaxis.

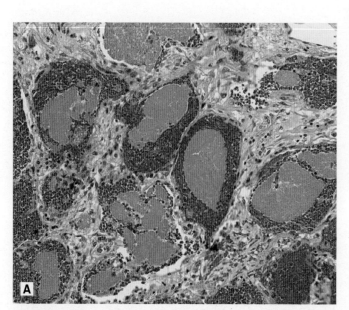
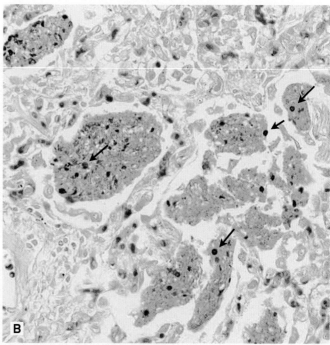

FIGURE 42.3 ▲ Histologic findings, PCP. **A.** A high magnification of a different area of the lung illustrated in Figures 42.1 and 42.2 shows typical foamy exudate. In this case, there is intra-alveolar hemorrhage surrounding the aggregates of organisms. **B.** A Gomori methenamine–silver stain demonstrates the cysts (*arrows*), while much of the fluffy exudate is composed of trophs, which stain weakly or not at all.

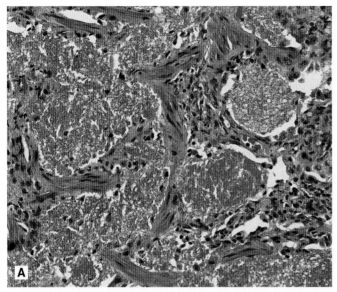 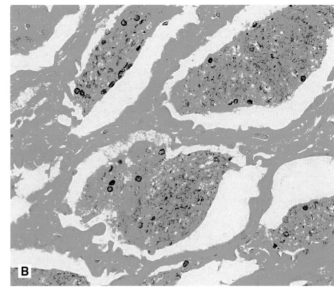

FIGURE 42.4 ▲ Histologic findings, PCP, open lung biopsy. It is unusual to diagnosed PCP on open biopsy, because cytologic examination of bronchoalveolar lavage fluid is less invasive. In this case, however, the patient's first manifestation of HIV disease was lung infiltrates, which were diagnosed before blood count information was available. **A.** There is mild interstitial thickening and foamy intra-alveolar exudates. **B.** GMS stain shows cyst forms and patchy staining of the smaller trophs.

TABLE 42.4 Treatment Regimens for Pneumocystis Pneumonia

Prophylaxis	Pneumonia
Trimethoprim–sulfamethoxazole, intravenous or oral	Trimethoprim–sulfamethoxazole, intravenous or oral
Dapsone, oral	Dapsone + trimethoprim, oral
Dapsone + pyrimethamine, oral	Atovaquone, oral
Atovaquone, oral	Clindamycin + primaquine, oral
Pentamidine, aerosol	Intravenous pentamidine

Catherinot E, Lanternier F, Bougnoux ME, et al. *Pneumocystis jirovecii* pneumonia. *Infect Dis Clin North Am.* 2010;24:107–138.

REFERENCES

1. Catherinot E, Lanternier F, Bougnoux ME, et al. Pneumocystis jirovecii pneumonia. *Infect Dis Clin North Am.* 2010;24:107–138.
2. Edman JC, Kovacs JA, Masur H, et al. Ribosomal RNA sequence shows Pneumocystis carinii to be a member of the fungi. *Nature.* 1988;334:519–522.
3. Vanek J. Parasitic pneumonia caused by Pneumocystis carinii in a 60-year-old woman. *Cas Lek Cesk.* 1952;91:1260–1262.
4. Vanek J, Jirovec O. [Parasitic pneumonia. Interstitial plasma cell pneumonia of premature, caused by Pneumocystis carinii]. *Zentralbl Bakteriol Parasitenkd Infektionskr Hyg.* 1952;158:120–127.
5. Walzer PD, Schultz MG, Western KA, et al. Pneumocystis carinii pneumonia and primary immune deficiency diseases of infancy and childhood. *J Pediatr.* 1973;82:416–422.
6. Leggiadro RJ, Winkelstein JA, Hughes WT. Prevalence of Pneumocystis carinii pneumonitis in severe combined immunodeficiency. *J Pediatr.* 1981;99:96–98.
7. Llibre JM, Revollo B, Vanegas S, et al. Pneumocystis jirovecii pneumonia in HIV-1-infected patients in the late-HAART era in developed countries. *Scand J Infect Dis.* 2013;45:635–644.
8. Harris K, Maroun R, Chalhoub M, et al. Unusual presentation of pneumocystis pneumonia in an immunocompetent patient diagnosed by open lung biopsy. *Heart Lung Circ.* 2012;21:221–224.
9. Frenkel JK. Pneumocystis jiroveci n. sp. from man: morphology, physiology, and immunology in relation to pathology. *Natl Cancer Inst Monogr.* 1976;43:13–30.
10. Stringer JR, Cushion MT, Wakefield AE. New nomenclature for the genus Pneumocystis. *J Eukaryot Microbiol.* 2001;(suppl):184S–189S.
11. Riebold D, Mohr E, Sombetzki M, et al. Pneumocystis species in Brown Leghorn laying hens—a hint for an extra-mammalian reservoir. *Poult Sci.* 2012;91:1813–1818.
12. Ponce CA, Gallo M, Bustamante R, et al. Pneumocystis colonization is highly prevalent in the autopsied lungs of the general population. *Clin Infect Dis.* 2010;50:347–353.
13. Wondergem MJ, Grunberg K, Wittgen BP, et al. Interstitial pneumonitis caused by Pneumocystis jirovecii pneumonia (PCP) during bortezomib treatment. *Histopathology.* 2009;54:631–633.
14. Kermani TA, Ytterberg SR, Warrington KJ. Pneumocystis jiroveci pneumonia in giant cell arteritis: a case series. *Arthritis Care Res (Hoboken).* 2011;63:761–765.
15. Weverling GJ, Mocroft A, Ledergerber B, et al. Discontinuation of Pneumocystis carinii pneumonia prophylaxis after start of highly active antiretroviral therapy in HIV-1 infection. EuroSIDA Study Group. *Lancet.* 1999;353:1293–1298.
16. Powell K, Davis JL, Morris AM, et al. Survival for patients with HIV admitted to the ICU continues to improve in the current era of combination antiretroviral therapy. *Chest.* 2009;135:11–17.
17. Radhi S, Alexander T, Ukwu M, et al. Outcome of HIV-associated pneumocystis pneumonia in hospitalized patients from 2000 through 2003. *BMC Infect Dis.* 2008;8:118.
18. Walzer PD, Evans HE, Copas AJ, et al. Early predictors of mortality from Pneumocystis jirovecii pneumonia in HIV-infected patients: 1985–2006. *Clin Infect Dis.* 2008;46:625–633.
19. Bortin MM, Rimm AA. Severe combined immunodeficiency disease. Characterization of the disease and results of transplantation. *JAMA.* 1977;238:591–600.

20. Lauzon D, Delage G, Brochu P, et al. Pathogens in children with severe combined immune deficiency disease or AIDS. *CMAJ.* 1986;135:33–38.

21. Dittrich AM, Schulze I, Magdorf K, et al. X-linked agammaglobulinaemia and Pneumocystis carinii pneumonia—an unusual coincidence? *Eur J Pediatr.* 2003;162:432–433.

22. Wang EH, Partovi N, Levy RD, et al. Pneumocystis pneumonia in solid organ transplant recipients: not yet an infection of the past. *Transpl Infect Dis.* 2012;14:519–525.

23. De Castro N, Neuville S, Sarfati C, et al. Occurrence of Pneumocystis jiroveci pneumonia after allogeneic stem cell transplantation: a 6-year retrospective study. *Bone Marrow Transplant.* 2005;36:879–883.

24. Faria LC, Ichai P, Saliba F, et al. Pneumocystis pneumonia: an opportunistic infection occurring in patients with severe alcoholic hepatitis. *Eur J Gastroenterol Hepatol.* 2008;20:26–28.

25. Cheson BD, Samlowski WE, Tang TT, et al. Value of open-lung biopsy in 87 immunocompromised patients with pulmonary infiltrates. *Cancer.* 1985;55:453–459.

26. Haverkos HW, Dowling JN, Pasculle AW, et al. Diagnosis of pneumonitis in immunocompromised patients by open lung biopsy. *Cancer.* 1983;52:1093–1097.

27. McKenna RJ, Jr, Mountain CF, McMurtrey MJ. Open lung biopsy in immunocompromised patients. *Chest.* 1984;86:671–674.

28. Onishi A, Sugiyama D, Kogata Y, et al. Diagnostic accuracy of serum 1,3-beta-D-glucan for Pneumocystis jiroveci pneumonia, invasive candidiasis, and invasive aspergillosis: systematic review and meta-analysis. *J Clin Microbiol.* 2012;50:7–15.

29. Torres HA, Chemaly RF, Storey R, et al. Influence of type of cancer and hematopoietic stem cell transplantation on clinical presentation of Pneumocystis jiroveci pneumonia in cancer patients. *Eur J Clin Microbiol Infect Dis.* 2006;25:382–388.

30. Boiselle PM, Crans CA, Jr., Kaplan MA. The changing face of Pneumocystis carinii pneumonia in AIDS patients. *AJR Am J Roentgenol.* 1999;172:1301–1309.

31. Lu CL, Hung CC. Reversible cystic lesions of Pneumocystis jirovecii pneumonia. *Am J Respir Crit Care Med.* 2012;185:e7–e8.

32. Samuel CM, Whitelaw A, Corcoran C, et al. Improved detection of Pneumocystis jirovecii in upper and lower respiratory tract specimens from children with suspected pneumocystis pneumonia using real-time PCR: a prospective study. *BMC Infect Dis.* 2011;11:329.

33. Oren I, Hardak E, Finkelstein R, et al. Polymerase chain reaction-based detection of Pneumocystis jirovecii in bronchoalveolar lavage fluid for the diagnosis of pneumocystis pneumonia. *Am J Med Sci.* 2011;342:182–185.

34. Wang Y, Doucette S, Qian Q, et al. Yield of primary and repeat induced sputum testing for Pneumocystis jiroveci in human immunodeficiency virus-positive and -negative patients. *Arch Pathol Lab Med.* 2007;131:1582–1584.

35. Huang L, Morris A, Limper AH, et al. An Official ATS Workshop Summary: recent advances and future directions in pneumocystis pneumonia (PCP). *Proc Am Thorac Soc.* 2006;3:655–664.

36. Hartel PH, Shilo K, Klassen-Fischer M, et al. Granulomatous reaction to pneumocystis jirovecii: clinicopathologic review of 20 cases. *Am J Surg Pathol.* 2010;34:730–734.

37. Browne MJ, Potter D, Gress J, et al. A randomized trial of open lung biopsy versus empiric antimicrobial therapy in cancer patients with diffuse pulmonary infiltrates. *J Clin Oncol.* 1990;8:222–229.

38. Deeren D, Lammertijn L, Van Dorpe J. Relapsing infiltrates after pneumocystis pneumonia in stem cell transplant patients: think about BOOP! *Acta Clin Belg.* 2010;65:200–201.

39. Harrington BJ. Staining of cysts of Pneumocystis jiroveci (P. carinii) with the fluorescent brighteners Calcofluor White and Uvitex 2B: a review *Labmedicine.com.* 2008;39:731–735.

40. Watts JC, Chandler FW. Pneumocystis carinii pneumonitis. The nature and diagnostic significance of the methenamine silver-positive "intracystic bodies". *Am J Surg Pathol.* 1985;9:744–751.

41. Ainoda Y, Hirai Y, Fujita T, et al. Analysis of clinical features of non-HIV Pneumocystis jirovecii pneumonia. *J Infect Chemother.* 2012;18:722–728.

43 Pulmonary Parasitic Infections

Bobbi S. Pritt, M.D., MSc

Overview

A number of parasites may be found in the human lung, including unicellular protozoa, helminths (worms), and, rarely, arthropods.[1–5] The types of parasites may vary significantly with host exposure, age, gender, and immune status.[1,2,4,5]

Tables 43.1 to 43.4 list the parasites that may infect the lung. The most common protozoan pulmonary diseases worldwide are amebiasis, malaria lung, and toxoplasmosis, while the most common helminthic diseases are dirofilariasis, echinococcosis, paragonimiasis, schistosomiasis, strongyloidiasis, and trichinosis. In addition, three common pulmonary syndromes due to helminths are Loeffler syndrome, tropical pulmonary eosinophilia, and visceral larva migrans.[5,6] The anatomic pathologist may play a role in diagnosing all of these infections, although most are usually detected using traditional laboratory methods such as serology and blood film microscopy.

Protozoa

Lung infection by protozoa is usually a component of systemic or disseminated disease. The protozoa most likely to be encountered by the pathologist are *Entamoeba histolytica* and *Toxoplasma gondii*. The free-living amebae (FLA), *Acanthamoeba* spp. and *Balamuthia mandrillaris*, are only rarely encountered. It is important to note that protozoal infection is not usually accompanied by peripheral eosinophilia, as is common with many helminth infections.

Entamoeba histolytica (Amebiasis)

General

Entamoeba histolytica is a protozoan parasite that inhabits the human intestinal tract and causes locally invasive and disseminated disease.[3,7] Amebiasis is responsible for 40,000 to 100,000 deaths annually, making it the third most common cause of death due to parasitic infection worldwide after malaria and schistosomiasis.[8,9] Humans acquire infection primarily through ingestion of environmentally resistant cysts in fecally contaminated food or water. In the United States, disease is seen primarily in immigrants and travelers from endemic areas. Following ingestion of infectious cysts, trophozoites are released into the intestinal lumen and colonize the colon. Most cases of amebiasis (>90%) are asymptomatic, with only a minority of patients developing clinical manifestations.[3] When present, symptoms commonly include watery or bloody diarrhea, abdominal pain, and dysentery. In rare cases, trophozoites may enter the portal blood supply and disseminate to other organs.[3,10]

Pleuropulmonary disease is the second most common form of extraintestinal amebiasis, after the liver.[8,11] Nearly all cases result from direct extension of a liver or subphrenic abscess across the diaphragm, and thus, the right lung is most commonly affected. Forms of lung involvement include pleuritis, pleural empyema, pulmonary abscess, bronchohepatic fistula, bronchobiliary fistula, lung abscess, and, rarely, superior vena cava syndrome.[8,12] Symptoms may include right upper quadrant pain, pleuritic chest pain, dyspnea, fever, cough, and hemoptysis. Expectoration of thick

TABLE 43.1   Protozoan Parasites of the Human Lung

Parasite/Infection	Infection	Pulmonary Pathology and Manifestations	Geographic Distribution
Acanthamoeba spp. (free-living ameba)	Amebiasis[a]	Bronchial pneumonia: cough, dyspnea, fatigue, fever	Worldwide, profoundly immunocompromised hosts
Babesia species	Babesiosis	Interstitial pneumonia, acute respiratory distress syndrome: cough, dyspnea, fatigue, fever	Temperate climates worldwide including North America, Europe, and Asia where Ixodes spp. ticks present
Balamuthia mandrillaris (free-living ameba)	Amebiasis[a]	Bronchial pneumonia: cough, dyspnea, fatigue, fever	Worldwide, usually immunocompromised hosts
Cryptosporidium spp.	Cryptosporidiosis	Bronchitis, interstitial pneumonia: cough, dyspnea, fatigue, fever	Worldwide, usually immunocompromised hosts
Cystoisospora (Isospora) belli	Cyclosporiasis	Interstitial pneumonia: cough, dyspnea, fatigue, fever	Regions of the tropics and subtropics worldwide
Entamoeba histolytica[b]	Amebiasis[a]	Abscess, bronchohepatic fistula, liver abscess: cough, hemoptysis, chest pain, right upper quadrant pain	Worldwide, settings with poor sanitation
Leishmania spp.	Visceral leishmaniasis	Interstitial pneumonia, usually a component of disseminated disease: cough, dyspnea, fatigue, fever	Regions of the tropics and subtropics worldwide
Plasmodium falciparum[b]	Malaria lung	Pulmonary edema, acute respiratory distress syndrome: cough, dyspnea, severe hypoxia, respiratory failure	Regions of the tropics and subtropics worldwide
Trichomonas tenax	Trichomoniasis	Pneumonia: cough, dyspnea, fatigue, fever	Worldwide, associated with poor oral hygiene
Toxoplasma gondii[b]	Toxoplasmosis	Interstitial pneumonia, bronchiolar exudates, pulmonary edema, cough, dyspnea, tachypnea, +/− fever	Worldwide, profoundly immunocompromised hosts and in neonates
Trypanosoma cruzi	Chagas disease	Interstitial pneumonia, usually a component of disseminated disease: cough, dyspnea, fatigue, +/− fever	Mexico, Central and South America

[a]The term amebiasis may be used to describe infection with any of the parasitic or free-living amebae but is most commonly used to describe infection with Entamoeba histolytica.
[b]Most common parasites causing human disease.
Modified from Procop GW, Neafie RC. Human parasitic pulmonary infections. In: Zander DS, Farver CF, eds. *Pulmonary Pathology*. Philadelphia, PA: Churchill Livingstone; 2008:287–314; Kim K, Weiss LM, Tanowitz HB. Parasitic infections. In: Broaddus VS, Mason RJ, Ernst JD, et al., eds. *Murray and Nadel's Textbook of Respiratory Medicine*. Philadelphia, PA: Elsevier Saunders; 2016:682–698.

TABLE 43.2   Nematode Parasites of the Human Lung

Parasite	Infection	Pulmonary Pathology and Manifestations	Geographic Distribution
Ancylostoma duodenale[a]	Hookworm infection	Loeffler syndrome[b]	Tropics and subtropics worldwide with poor sanitation
Ascaris lumbricoides[a]	Ascariasis	Loeffler syndrome,[b] bronchopneumonia due to larvae, rarely adult worms may migrate to trachea, lung, pulmonary artery, and pleurae	Tropics and subtropics worldwide with poor sanitation
Baylisascaris procyonis	Baylisascariasis, visceral larva migrans	Eosinophilic pneumonia: cough, dyspnea, fatigue, fever	North America where raccoons are found
Brugia species[a]	Filariasis	Tropical pulmonary eosinophilia[c] due to microfilariae, adult worms in pulmonary arteries cause thrombosis and occlusion	Tropics, especially South and Southeast Asia
Dirofilaria immitis and other Dirofilaria species[a]	Dirofilariasis	Pulmonary nodule, lung infarction: cough, hemoptysis, fever, chest pain	Worldwide, including the southeastern United States
Gnathostoma spinigerum	Gnathostomiasis	Bronchitis, pneumonia, cough, hemoptysis, fever, respiratory failure, chest pain, pneumothorax, pleural effusion, expectorated worm	Southeast Asia and Mexico where insufficiently cooked fish, frog, or snake is ingested
Mansonella perstans	Filariasis	Pleural cavity filariasis, microfilariae released into peripheral blood: fever	Parts of Africa, South America
Necator americanus[a]	Hookworm infection	Loeffler syndrome[b]	Regions of the tropics and subtropics worldwide with poor sanitation

TABLE 43.2 Nematode Parasites of the Human Lung (continued)

Parasite	Infection	Pulmonary Pathology and Manifestations	Geographic Distribution
Strongyloides stercoralis[a]	Strongyloidiasis, *Strongyloides* hyperinfection syndrome	Loeffler syndrome,[b] bronchial infiltration, secondary bacterial pneumonia: cough, dyspnea	Tropics and subtropics worldwide with poor sanitation including southeastern United States (Appalachia)
Trichinella spiralis and other *Trichinella* species	Trichinosis, trichinellosis	Pneumonia, respiratory failure, usually a component of disseminated disease: cough, dyspnea	Worldwide, where insufficiently cooked flesh of carnivores (pig, boar, bear, walrus) is consumed
Toxocara canis and *Toxocara cati*[a]	Toxocariasis, visceral larva migrans	Eosinophilic pneumonia; cough, dyspnea, fatigue, fever	Worldwide
Wuchereria bancrofti[a]	Filariasis	Tropical pulmonary eosinophilia[c] due to microfilariae, adult worms in pulmonary arteries cause thrombosis and occlusion	Tropics, especially South and Southeast Asia

[a]Most common parasites causing human disease. Other nematodes have rarely been reported to involve the lung. These include anisakiasis (infection with *Anisakis* spp. and *Pseudoterranova decipiens*) (eosinophilic pleural effusion); angiostrongyliasis (pulmonary artery thrombosis); capillariasis (*Capillaria aerophila*) (bronchial infection); pinworm infection (*Enterobius vermicularis*) (pulmonary nodules, cough, and dyspnea); halicephalobus (*Halicephalobus/Micronema gingivalis* aka *H. deletrix*) (associated with fatal encephalitis); lagochilascariasis (*Lagochilascaris minor*) (pulmonary nodule); and onchocerciasis (*Onchocerca volvulus*); and syngamosis (*Mammomonogamus laryngeus*) (cough, hemoptysis, worms attached to mucosa).
[b]Loeffler syndrome is associated with the pulmonary migration stage of certain intestinal nematodes. It is characterized by self-limited fever, dry cough, wheezing, and peripheral and tissue eosinophilia.
[c]Tropical pulmonary eosinophilia is a syndrome associated with infection with the filarial worms that cause lymphatic filariasis. It is characterized by chronic low-grade fever, nocturnal paroxysmal dry cough and wheezing, high peripheral and tissue eosinophilia. Microfilariae are rarely seen in tissue sections. When present, they are generally within eosinophilic necrotizing granulomas.
Modified from Procop GW, Neafie RC. Human parasitic pulmonary infections. In: Zander DS, Farver CF, eds. *Pulmonary Pathology*. Philadelphia, PA: Churchill Livingstone; 2008:287–314; Kim K, Weiss LM, Tanowitz HB. Parasitic infections. In: Broaddus VS, Mason RJ, Ernst JD, et al., eds. *Murray and Nadel's Textbook of Respiratory Medicine*. Philadelphia, PA: Elsevier Saunders; 2016:682–698.

TABLE 43.3 Cestodes of the Human Lung

Parasite	Infection	Pulmonary Pathology and Manifestations	Geographic Distribution
Echinococcus granulosus[a] and other *Echinococcus multilocularis*	Hydatid cyst; alveolar echinococcosis	Pulmonary cyst; cough, hemoptysis, fever, allergic symptoms, and anaphylaxis with cyst rupture. Pulmonary alveolar echinococcosis is usually spread from the liver	Worldwide, rural sheep-rearing regions and where dogs ingest raw viscera of infected animals
Spirometra spp.	Sparganosis	Pulmonary or pleural nodule, pneumonia: cough, sputum production, fever, chest pain	Worldwide where humans ingest insufficiently cooked frogs and snakes or use frog/snake flesh as a wound poultice
Taenia solium	Cysticercosis	Pulmonary nodules, usually a component of disseminated disease: cough, sputum production	Worldwide where humans ingest insufficiently cooked pork (prerequisite for acquiring the adult tapeworm and shedding infectious eggs into the environment)

[a]Most common cestode to infect the lung.

TABLE 43.4 Trematodes (Flukes) of the Human Lung

Parasite	Infection	Pulmonary Pathology and Manifestations	Geographic Distribution
Alaria spp.	Alariasis	Single case reported of human respiratory involvement: cough, dyspnea, hemoptysis, fatal asphyxia	Parts of Southeast Asia where insufficiently cooked frogs and snakes are consumed
Clinostomum complanatum	Clinostomiasis	Worm attaches to mucosa of the larynx: throat pain and discomfort, tickling sensation	Parts of Japan and Korea where insufficiently cooked freshwater fish is consumed
Fasciola hepatica	Fascioliasis	Eosinophilic pneumonia, usually associated with liver involvement: cough, dyspnea, fatigue, fever, right hypochondrial pain, chest pain, hepatomegaly	Worldwide, sheep and cattle-rearing regions where raw watercress is ingested
Paragonimus species[a]	Paragonimiasis	Cavitary lesions and pleural effusion: cough, hemoptysis, dyspnea, severe chest pain, night sweats	Parts of Southeast Asia, Africa, North, Central and South America where insufficiently cooked crustaceans are ingested
Schistosoma species[a]	Schistosomiasis, Katayama fever	Pulmonary hypertension, cor pulmonale: dyspnea, fatigue, chest pain, pleural effusion, ascites	Parts of Asia, Africa, South America

[a]Most frequent trematodes to affect the lung.

red-brown sputum resembling "anchovy paste" or "chocolate sauce" is indicative of a bronchohepatic fistula.[8,11,13] Risk factors for pleuropulmonary amebiasis include male sex, atrial septal defect, malnutrition, alcoholism, and immunocompromised state.[8,11]

Organisms are not usually microscopically detectable in stool of patients with extraintestinal disease; the ova and parasite (O&P) exam is positive in only 35% of cases.[8] Therefore, serologic detection of parasite-specific IgG class antibodies is the preferred method of diagnosis.[3,7] Microscopic examination of aspirated abscess fluid and sputum and less commonly biopsy of affected organs may also be useful for confirming the diagnosis in conjunction with clinical and radiologic features and serology.[7]

Radiologic Findings

Chest radiographs and CT scans are commonly used for diagnosing and monitoring extraintestinal amebiasis. Common findings include pleural effusion, pneumothorax, and lung abscess. Pleuropulmonary amebiasis due to extension from a hepatic source is commonly associated with hepatomegaly, elevated right hemidiaphragm, right pleural effusion, and basal lung opacity.[8,9,11]

Tissue Sampling

Aspirated pleural fluid, abscess material, or expectorated pus generally contains few microscopically recognizable organisms.[3,11] In these specimens, detection of *E. histolytica* DNA using molecular tests such as polymerase chain reaction (PCR) may be useful for confirming the diagnosis. The sensitivity of identifying trophozoites in abscess material may be increased by examining the very last portion of aspirated fluid since this presumably comes from the abscess edge where trophozoites are more prevalent.[11] Biopsies and tissue sections should also be taken from the edge of an abscess to increase the likelihood of finding microscopically recognizable trophozoites.

Gross and Microscopic Findings

Grossly, amebic abscesses contain yellow-gray to red-brown granular opaque fluid, classically described as resembling "anchovy paste" or "chocolate sauce."[3] Abscesses consist of amorphous necrotic material surrounded by a fibrinous wall and outer rim of edematous host tissue with a mixed inflammatory infiltrate. Neutrophils are generally absent.[3] Trophozoites are found most readily in clumps within the fibrin of the abscess wall and can be recognized using standard H&E-stained sections (Fig. 43.1); they generally measure <35 μm in greatest dimension and have dense bubbly cytoplasm that may contain engulfed erythrocytes and a single eccentrically placed round nucleus measuring 4 to 5 μm in diameter.[3] Nuclei have characteristic finely clumped peripheral chromatin and a tiny dot-like central karyosome (nucleolus). The trophozoite nucleus may not always be present in each plane of section and the central dot-like karyosome is not as distinct in tissue sections as it is seen in standard stool preparations. Trophozoites may be highlighted using PAS, GMS, and Warthin-Starry stains, while the Brown-Hopps tissue Gram stain may accentuate the nuclear karyosome.[3]

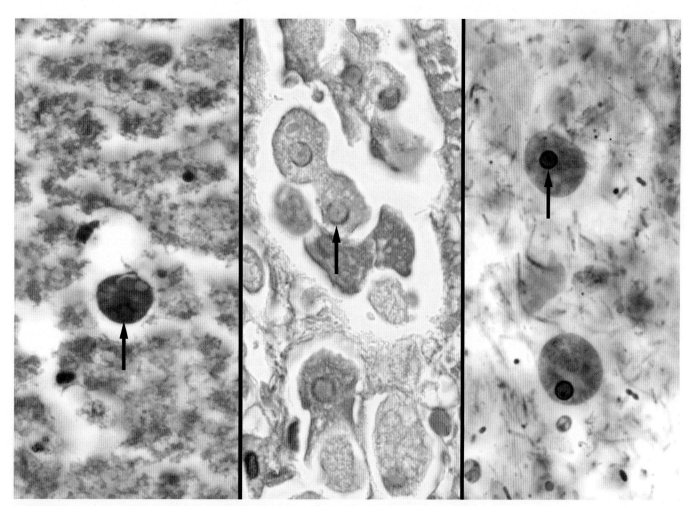

FIGURE 43.1 ▲ In extraintestinal abscesses (left panel, PAS), trophozoites are relatively small with dense cytoplasm and a small nucleus with poorly defined chromatin (*arrow*). The characteristic peripheral chromatin with central karyosome (nucleolus) may be more readily apparent in invasive intestinal disease (*arrow*, central panel) but still is not as well defined as in routine stool preparations (*arrow*, right panel, iron hematoxylin).

Differential Diagnosis

Amebic abscess must be differentiated from other causes of abscess using standard histochemical stains for microorganisms. It is important to correlate the histopathologic findings with the results of bacterial, mycobacterial, and fungal cultures.

The trophozoites of *E. histolytica* may be confused with macrophages or degenerated epithelial cells but can usually be differentiated by their smaller nucleus and characteristic chromatin pattern. Rarely, trophozoites of the FLA, *Acanthamoeba* species and *B. mandrillaris*, may also involve the lung and must be differentiated from trophozoites of *E. histolytica*. The FLA may have both cyst and trophozoite forms in human infection, while only trophozoites are seen with invasive *E. histolytica* infection. Also, the FLA are seen within alveoli rather than within an abscess (Fig. 43.2), and they have a smaller nucleus with large central karyosome.

Treatment and Prognosis

The standard therapy for extraintestinal amebiasis is oral or parenteral metronidazole or other nitroimidazole drug.[8,12] As metronidazole will not effectively kill the intestinal cyst forms, patients are also commonly given paromomycin, iodoquinol, or diloxanide furoate to prevent recurrent disease. Surgical resection is contraindicated.[8,12] Percutaneous needle or catheter aspiration and drainage of amebic lung abscesses is also not routinely indicated but may be performed in patients who do not improve with metronidazole therapy or who pose

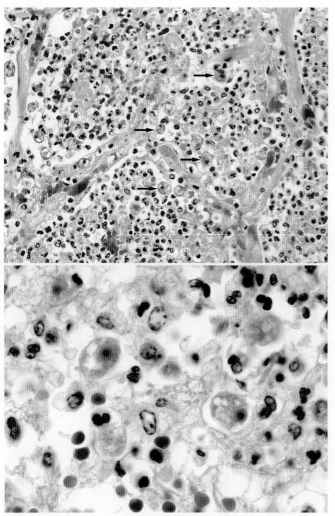

FIGURE 43.2 ▲ Amebic pneumonia due to *Acanthamoeba* sp./*Balamuthia mandrillaris*. Low magnification (**top**) demonstrates multiple trophozoites (*arrows*) within a neutrophilic alveolar infiltrate. At higher magnification (**bottom**), characteristic trophozoites with a small round nucleus and large central karyosome can be appreciated.

a risk for rupture. If untreated, pleuropulmonary amebiasis is usually fatal.

Toxoplasma gondii (Toxoplasmosis)

General

Toxoplasma gondii commonly causes asymptomatic or self-limited infection, but can also cause life-threatening disease in immunocompromised individuals and devastating congenital infections. As many as one-half of the world's population is estimated to be infected.[5] The prevalence in the United States ranges from 3% to 20%, with the highest prevalence found in individuals living in the central and eastern states and among Native Americans.[5]

Humans become infected in a variety of manners including ingestion of tissue cysts in undercooked meat, ingestion of oocysts in contaminated food and water, and transplacental transmission from a newly infected mother to her developing fetus.

Immunocompetent individuals are generally asymptomatic but may experience an acute, self-limited mononucleosis-like illness with or without lymphadenopathy, and occasionally accompanied by pneumonia and myocarditis.[5] Following primary infection, the parasite remains dormant but may reactivate if the patient becomes immunocompromised. In immunocompromised patients, primary or reactivated infection can result in life-threatening disseminated disease involving the brain and multiple other organs including the lung.[14] The brain is the most common site for disseminated disease, but a pulmonary component is seen more than 70% of patients with disseminated disease.[5] Congenital infections can also result in pulmonary involvement. The most common signs and symptoms of pulmonary toxoplasmosis are cough, dyspnea, and fever. If untreated, *Toxoplasma* pneumonia is progressive and fatal.[5]

Diagnosis of pulmonary toxoplasmosis is usually accomplished by testing for *T. gondii*–specific IgM and IgG antibodies. False-positive IgM results are not uncommon, and tests for both IgM and IgG antibodies may be negative in profoundly immunocompromised patients.[14] Detection of *T. gondii* DNA in respiratory specimens provides supportive evidence of infection, while detection of tachyzoites in sputa, BAL, or biopsy is diagnostic of acute toxoplasmosis.[15]

Radiologic Findings

CT scans commonly show diffuse interstitial and alveolar infiltrates.[5] Focal consolidation may also be present, while mediastinal and hilar lymphadenopathy are usually absent.

Gross and Histologic Findings

Lungs may demonstrate regions of hemorrhage and consolidation, particularly in fatal disseminated infections.[5] Areas of gross consolidation are most likely to contain the highest numbers of *T. gondii* parasites.[15]

Early pulmonary involvement is usually characterized by a cellular interstitial pneumonia, edema, alveolar fibrinous exudates, vasculitis, and coagulative necrosis.[15] Acute inflammation (Fig. 43.3) and evidence of diffuse alveolar damage may also be seen. Parasites are most numerous in areas of necrosis and are seen as free and intracellular round, oval, or arc-shaped tachyzoites measuring 2 to 8 μm in greatest dimension.[5] The characteristic arc shape is best appreciated on smears. Tachyzoites can infect any nucleated cell, but are most commonly seen within alveolar epithelial cells and macrophages. They can form free-standing clusters without a surrounding wall (pseudocysts). True tissue cysts with a well-defined cyst wall are less commonly seen during active infection and are the form found in dormant chronic infection.[5,15] Organisms are best appreciated on H&E-stained sections, but can also be seen on a variety of other common histochemical stains. Free tachyzoites do not usually stain with GMS, but cysts and pseudocysts may be GMS positive. Organisms are also negative by PAS and faintly Gram negative using tissue Gram stains such as the Brown and Hopps method.[15]

Toxoplasma gondii is one of the few parasites in which immunohistochemical (IHC) stains are commercially available and widely used in clinical practice. Both cyst and tachyzoite forms are generally highlighted by IHC (Fig. 43.3).

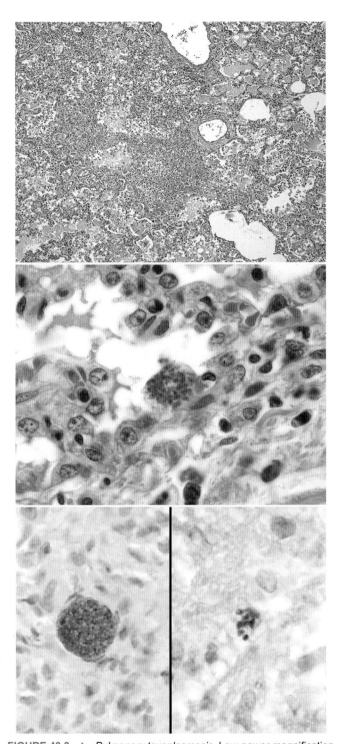

FIGURE 43.3 ▲ *Pulmonary toxoplasmosis*. Low-power magnification (**above**) shows a diffuse alveolar exudates, neutrophilic inflammation, and necrotic foci. At higher magnification, collections of free tachyzoites can be appreciated (**middle**). Immunohistochemistry highlights both cyst (**left**) and tachyzoite (**right**) forms (**bottom**).

PCR is another commonly used ancillary method for supporting the diagnosis of pulmonary toxoplasmosis and can be performed on a variety of specimen types including sputum, respiratory secretions, and tissue (fresh and formalin fixed, paraffin embedded).[15–17]

Differential Diagnosis

A variety of small (1- to 5-μm) microorganisms may be mistaken for *T. gondii* tachyzoites and cysts in tissue sections but can be differentiated through careful evaluation of microscopic features and selective use of IHC or in situ hybridization stains.[15,16]

Treatment and Prognosis

The preferred therapy for pulmonary toxoplasmosis is pyrimethamine plus sulfadoxine, which is active against the replicating tachyzoites but will not eradicate dormant cysts. Immunocompromised patients are at risk for future relapses, and therefore, ongoing prophylaxis is recommended.[17] Unfortunately, the prognosis is poor for patients with disseminated disease and pulmonary involvement.[17]

Pulmonary Malaria

Malaria, including *Plasmodium falciparum* and *vivax*, can result in disseminated infection involving the lung. The primary histologic finding at autopsy is diffuse vascular congestion by erythrocytes laden with malarial pigment, seen in more than one-half of lungs.[18] The primary complication of malaria that contributes to death is acute respiratory distress syndrome[19] (Fig. 43.4), which is thought to be triggered by

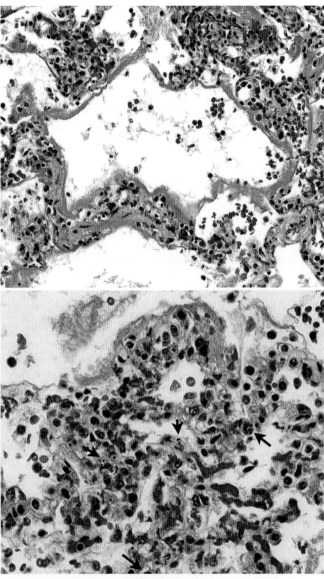

FIGURE 43.4 ▲ Acute respiratory distress syndrome secondary to malaria. The patient diagnosed clinically by blood smear after returning from overseas travel and presented with headache and respiratory failure. Hyaline membranes typical of diffuse alveolar damage are seen (**above**). There are multiple foci of pigment in alveolar lining cells and endothelial cells (*arrows*), **bottom**.

toxic effects of hemozoin pigment, which is present primarily in macrophages and erythrocytes.[20]

Helminths

Helminths are classically divided into three major groups: the nematodes (roundworms), cestodes (tapeworms), and trematodes (flukes). Of these, only *Paragonimus* species preferentially infect the lung. Unlike protozoal infection, helminth infection is commonly associated with eosinophilia. The parasites most commonly encountered and seen in pathology preparations are *Dirofilaria immitis*, *Echinococcus granulosus*, *Paragonimus westermani*, *Schistosoma* spp., *Strongyloides stercoralis*, and the larval form of *Taenia solium* (cysticercosis).[5,6]

Dirofilaria immitis (Dirofilariasis)

General

Pulmonary dirofilariasis is most commonly caused by the roundworm *D. immitis*, otherwise known as the "dog heart worm." Less commonly, *Dirofilaria repens* may involve the lung.[21] Dogs are the natural host for both species, and therefore, infection is seen predominantly in regions where there are numerous stray dogs and where household dogs are not routinely "dewormed."[21,22] In North America, infection is seen predominantly in the Southeastern United States.[23]

Dirofilariasis is a vector-transmitted infection. After being introduced into the skin through the bite of an infected mosquito, *Dirofilaria* spp. larvae enter the bloodstream and travel through the systemic circulation to the heart. From there, they are carried to the pulmonary vasculature where they embolize within small vessels and cause tissue infarction and necrosis.[21] The larvae cannot survive or mature in humans, and therefore, humans are considered accidental, "dead-end" hosts.[21]

Most patients with dirofilariasis are asymptomatic or have only mild symptoms. In these cases, infection is usually discovered when a solitary pulmonary nodule is noted on imaging. When present, symptoms commonly consist of cough, chest pain, and hemoptysis.[21] Peripheral eosinophilia is only present in a minority (~10%) of cases.[24] Definitive diagnosis is made by histopathologic examination of the resected nodule.[21,24] There are currently no commercially available serologic or molecular-based methods for diagnosis.

Radiologic Findings

The classic radiologic finding is a well-circumscribed peripheral solitary nodule measuring up to 4 cm, seen in old, healed disease.[21] In contrast, chest radiography obtained early in infection generally shows localized, patchy opacification and associated pleural effusion. Without surgical intervention, the opacified area will eventually form a solitary nodule. CT scan may reveal central cavitation and calcification is unusual.[25]

Tissue Sampling

Diagnosis has occasionally been made by needle core biopsy, but excision is more likely to reveal the worm, which is needed for definitive diagnosis.[21]

Gross and Histologic Findings

The characteristic dirofilarial nodule consists of a well-defined area of necrosis with surrounding normal lung parenchyma (Fig. 43.5A). One or more slender white-tan worms may be identified within the region of necrosis.[26]

Histologically, degenerating worms are seen in longitudinal and/or cross section within a blood vessel, with a well-defined surrounding region of coagulative necrosis.[21] Worms measure 100 to 350 μm in diameter.[5,26] Surrounding the central region of necrosis is a rim of fibrosis and a chronic inflammation that may be granulomatous or include eosinophils.[21] The features of the worm's externally ridged cuticle, musculature, and internal lateral ridges underlying the lateral

chords (Fig. 43.5B–D) are generally well preserved and allow for definitive identification.

Differential Diagnosis

The appearance of single necrotizing granulomas with eosinophils should prompt the pathologist to consider dirofilariasis, even in the absence of a worm. Deeper sections may be indicated to look for the worm. Identification of roundworm measuring 100 to 350 μm is consistent with a diagnosis of dirofilariasis. Special stains for mycobacteria and fungi are also indicated to rule out other infections.

Treatment and Prognosis

Dirofilaria spp. cannot reproduce in humans and will quickly die in the lung. Therefore, excision is not necessary, other than for the purposes of excluding other causes of pulmonary nodules.[26]

Echinococcus species (Echinococcosis, Hydatid Disease)

General

Human echinococcosis is caused by several cestodes in the genus *Echinococcus*. *Echinococcus granulosus*, the "dog tapeworm" is the cause of cystic hydatid disease, and is by far the most common species to infect humans and the most common species to involve the lung.[6,27] Alveolar echinococcosis is less common in humans and is caused by infection with the larval stage of *Echinococcus multilocularis* and causes a more aggressive disease. Canids are the definitive host for all *Echinococcus* species, whereas humans serve as the intermediate host and become host to the larval parasite form, similar to cysticercosis. There are at least 1 million individuals infected with echinococcosis worldwide. The majority of cases of alveolar echinococcosis, which is relatively uncommon, occur in China.[28]

Humans become infected when accidentally ingesting microscopic eggs that are shed in the stool of infected canids.[6,27] The lung is the second most common organ to be infected after the liver, with involvement reported in 20% to 40% of cases.[6,25] Up to 16% of pulmonary echinococcosis is reported to be associated with concurrent liver disease.[25]

Small, unruptured pulmonary cysts are generally asymptomatic and may be discovered incidentally by imaging.[21] As the cyst increases in size, it may cause symptoms by compressing surrounding structures, even leading to death by asphyxiation, or rupturing into an airway.[6] Cyst rupture usually leads to abrupt onset of cough, fever, and expectoration of "salty tasting fluid" or material resembling "grape skins."[21] Cyst rupture into the pleura can cause hydropneumothorax and empyema. Some patients may experience a hypersensitivity reaction due to systemic release of parasite antigens and may experience pruritus, urticaria, hypotension, and even anaphylaxis.[21]

Diagnosis of pulmonary echinococcosis is based primarily on clinical and radiologic findings in conjunction with positive serology results.[29] Since humans are only infected with the larval tissue form and not the intestinal tapeworm, there is no role for stool ova and parasite exam in diagnosing human infection.

Ultrasound or CT-guided FNA may be useful for confirming the diagnosis by detecting immature tapeworms (protoscoleces) and free hooklets in aspirated cyst fluid. These may also be seen in the sputum in cases of cyst rupture.[21] Biopsy or resection may be performed in cases with an atypical presentation in which echinococcosis is not initially suspected and may be indicated in settings of impending rupture.[27]

Radiologic Findings

Cystic hydatid disease most commonly presents as a solitary, well-circumscribed cyst with an outer fibrous capsule (pericyst) and surrounding compressed pulmonary tissue. Cysts range in size from 1 to 20 cm or more in diameter and may become lobulated. Multiple pulmonary cysts are rare.[21,25] CT may be useful for demonstrating the presence of smaller daughter cysts within the larger cyst.

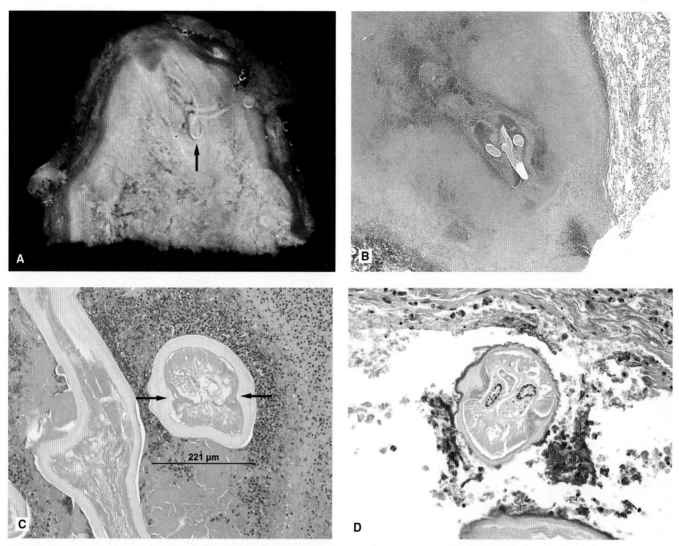

FIGURE 43.5 ▲ Pulmonary dirofilariasis. **A.** Portion of a resected nodule demonstrating a smooth-contoured outer rim of fibrosis with central necrosis. A small partly coiled worm is visible (*arrow*) within the necrotic focus. **B.** At low magnification, longitudinal and cross sections of a dying worm are seen within a well-circumscribed nodule of infarcted lung. **C.** Higher magnification reveals characteristic prominent internal lateral ridges (*arrows*) within the degenerated worm. **D.** A different case of pulmonary dirofilariasis also shows these characteristic internal ridges, which are clearly visible despite the degenerated state of the worm. Smaller external ridges are also present on the outer aspect of the cuticle.

In cases of cyst rupture into an airway, the resultant air entering the cyst may create an air–fluid level that is visible by routine chest radiographs. Over time, the inner parasite-derived layer may detach from the pericyst in partially collapsed cysts and float on the remaining fluid; this resultant appearance on x-ray, ultrasound, or CT is referred to as the "water lily" sign and is considered pathognomonic of a collapsed echinococcal cyst.[21,25]

Pulmonary alveolar echinococcosis is characterized by multiple variably sized cysts that can span two segments of the lung. Lung involvement almost always occurs due to dissemination from a primary hepatic source, and therefore, evidence of liver involvement will also be present on imaging studies.[30]

Gross and Histologic Findings

Early cysts are generally simple fluid-filled structures. Enlarging cysts commonly produce smaller internal delicate-walled brood capsules, which enlarge into daughter cysts, creating the classic "cysts-within-a-cyst" appearance (Fig. 43.6A). Larger lesions are surrounded by the fibrous pericyst measuring up to 3 mm in thickness. Intact cysts

contain clear to cloudy gelatinous fluid and may have a fine gritty consistency due to free-floating hooklets and immature hooked protoscoleces ("hydatid sand"). Eventually, cysts may rupture or collapse and undergo fibrosis. Histologically, the outer parasite cyst wall and each internal daughter cyst are composed of an outer eosinophilic acellular laminated layer (Figs. 43.6B–D and 43.7A–B). Just below the laminated layer is the germinal layer from which the protoscoleces arise. Protoscoleces are ovoid, measure ~100 μm in greatest dimension, and have two circular rows of hooklets and four cup-shaped suckers. Occasionally, protoscoleces will evert so that the hooklets are exposed. Free-floating hooklets measure 15 to 30 μm and are weakly birefringent in cytology preparations.[27]

Ruptured cysts generally trigger an acute and granulomatous host inflammatory reaction that surrounds and infiltrates the cyst structures.[21] Over time, the protoscoleces and germinal layer die and may appear as mummified structures among a granulomatous or fibrotic host response. The presence of the laminated layer should prompt a careful search for protoscoleces and free hooklets. All larval (and adult) cestodes contain small variably sized calcified bodies (calcareous corpuscles); the presence of these bodies should also raise the possibility

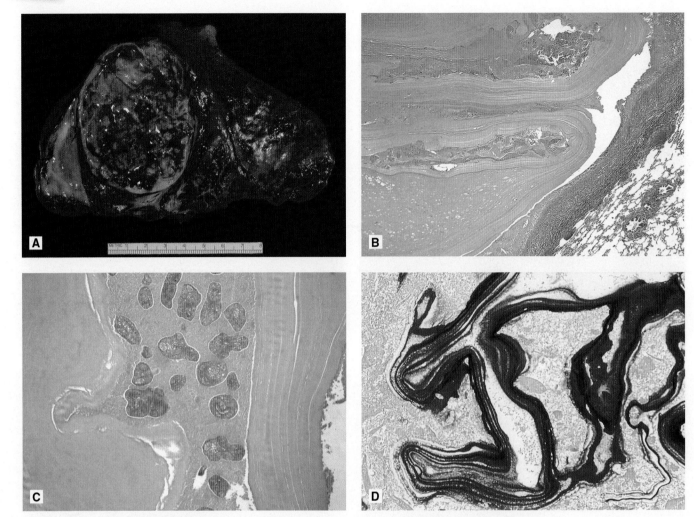

FIGURE 43.6 ▲ Echinococcosis. **A.** A moderately sized pulmonary hydatid cyst with multiple internal collapsed daughter cysts. **B.** At low magnification, a large nodule consisting primarily of collapsed acellular laminated layer material with intervening necrotic eosinophilic debris is seen. **C.** Mummified protoscoleces are also present and confirm the diagnosis of echinococcosis. **D.** PAS staining of *Echinococcus* laminated layers.

of echinococcosis. Hooklets are refractile and weakly birefringent; narrowing the microscope condenser or using polarized light is useful for highlighting rare hooklets within older lesions.

Alveolar hydatid disease does not have a surrounding outer cyst wall to restrict the growth of the parasite. Instead, this form of echinococcosis extends in a tumor-like manner with infiltration of daughter cysts throughout host tissue.[27] The individual cysts are not surrounded by a laminated layer and are instead connected by a cellular stroma (Fig. 43.7D). Protoscoleces are rarely produced.[27]

Differential Diagnosis

Pulmonary echinococcosis is easily diagnosed when characteristic morphologic structures such as protoscoleces and free hooklets are seen. However, the identification can be more challenging in collapsed or old and degenerating cysts where parasite forms are not readily identified. A careful search using low light and a narrowed condenser will highlight free hooklets and facilitate the diagnosis. Hooklets stain deep red using Ziehl-Neelsen, which may help with their identification.[27] In cases in which only the laminated layers are present, GMS and PAS stains can be used to highlight these structures and differentiate them from other similar-appearing structures (Fig. 43.6D).[27] Layered deposition of fibrin can have a similar laminated appearance but does not stain with GMS and PAS.

Treatment and Prognosis

Patients are usually treated by surgical removal of the cyst.[6,21] Injection of a hypertonic saline prior to surgery or use of hypertonic-soaked gauze in the operating field may be used to minimize the consequences of accidental cyst content spillage during the procedure.[6,31] Excision or drainage is usually accompanied by albendazole therapy.[32] The most common side effects of surgery are pleural infection and prolonged air leakage.[31] Less commonly, cystic echinococcosis may recur when cyst contents were spilled during surgery.[31]

Paragonimus species (Paragonimiasis)

General

Paragonimiasis is caused by several species of trematodes (flukes) in the genus *Paragonimus*.[33] Humans acquire infection primarily by ingestion of raw or inadequately cooked crustaceans such as crayfish and crabs; infection is therefore most commonly seen in regions where these foods are routinely eaten.[33,34]

Following ingestion of an infected crustacean, metacercariae penetrate the intestinal wall and migrate to the lungs where they mature and live singly, or in pairs within cystic cavities. Pulmonary symptoms include chronic blood-tinged sputum, chest pain, and fever. Pneumothorax and pleural effusion are potential complications.[33–36]

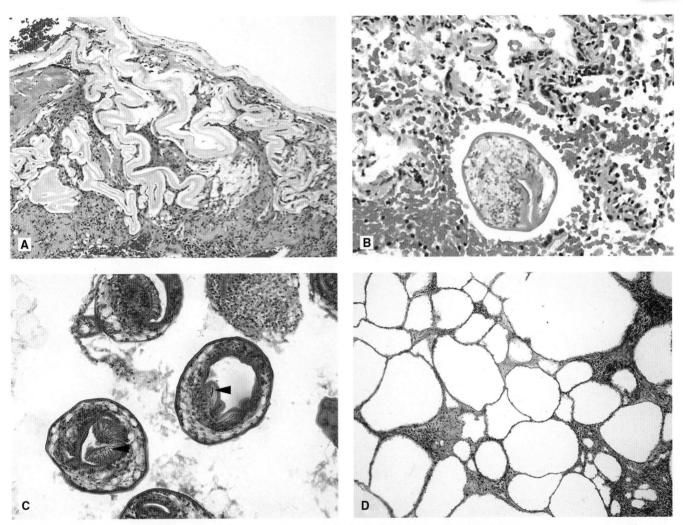

FIGURE 43.7 ▲ Echinococcosis. **A.** Ruptured pulmonary hydatid cyst showing disrupted hyaline membranes. **B.** There are free protoscoleces among a granulomatous host response. **C.** Internal refractile hooklets (*arrowheads*) are clearly seen within the inverted protoscoleces. The condenser is narrowed to emphasize the hooklets. **D.** Alveolar echinococcosis consisting of multiple cysts without outer laminated layers. Each daughter cyst is separated only by parasite-derived stroma. Note the absence of protoscoleces.

Diagnosis is usually based on microscopic identification of *Paragonimus* spp. eggs in sputum, stool, and, less commonly, pleural fluid. Eggs may also be seen in tissue specimens, although FNA and biopsy are rarely used for diagnosis. Serologic testing provides supportive evidence of infection when eggs are not seen by microscopy. Paragonimiasis is clinically similar to tuberculosis and should therefore be considered when individuals fail to improve with standard antituberculosis therapy.[37]

Radiologic Findings

Evidence of migrating larvae may be detected within the first 1 to 2 months of infection as pleural thickening, pleural effusion, patchy infiltrates at the base of the lungs, and pneumothorax. Established pulmonary disease commonly begins as patterns of parenchymal and pleural pneumonia and matures to cyst and nodule formation and eventually fibrosis and calcification.[35,36]

Tissue Sampling

Excision of the entire cystic cavity allows for identification of the adult flukes. Fine needle aspiratory biopsy has also been used for the diagnosis of pulmonary paragonimiasis.[38] In cases with pleural effusion, the aspirated pleural fluid should be examined for eggs.

Gross and Histologic Findings

Lungs commonly contain one or more cystic cavities measuring 1 to 3 cm in diameter, commonly located near or communicating with airways.[21] The cavity wall may be thin or measure up to several millimeters in thickness.[33] Each cavity contains mucinous or necrotic fluid and one or two flukes.[21] Adult flukes are ovoid, red-brown, and measure ~7 to 12 mm in length; they have been described as having a "coffee-bean" or "lemon" shape.[33]

Histologically, flukes within cystic cavities are surrounded by eosinophilic and granulomatous inflammation. Over time, a nonspecific mononuclear infiltrate and fibrosis develop at the periphery of the cavity (Fig. 43.8A).[21] Adult flukes produce large eggs measuring ~90 μm in length; they have a birefringent wall and a shouldered operculum (an opening with outward bumps on either side) (Fig. 43.8B-D).

Differential Diagnosis

Identification of adult flukes or characteristic eggs in pulmonary specimens allows for definitive diagnosis of paragonimiasis. Eggs of *Schistosoma japonicum* may resemble those of *Paragonimus* sp. and can uncommonly be found in the lung; however, they lack an operculum and are not birefringent.[33]

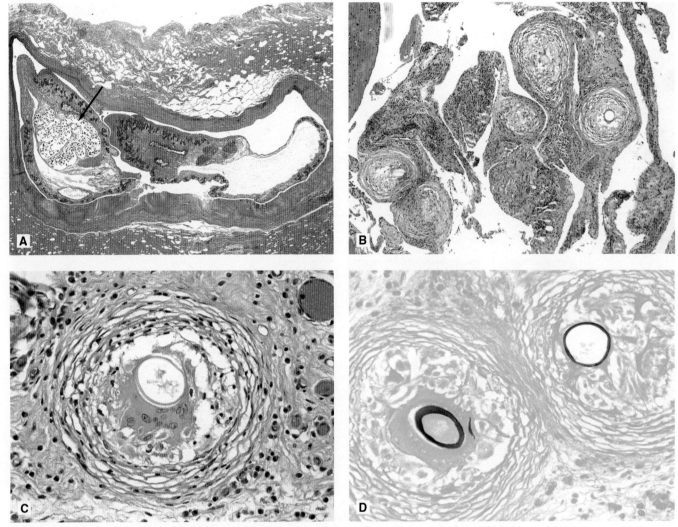

FIGURE 43.8 ▲ Pulmonary paragonimiasis. **A.** Wedge resection of lung demonstrating a cystic cavity with two adult flukes. A uterus containing numerous eggs is readily apparent in one fluke (*arrow*). **B.** There are multiple eggs surrounded by inflammation. **C.** The eggs may be surrounded by granulomas, in this example nonnecrotizing. **D.** The egg walls stain positively with Gomori methenamine–silver impregnation stain.

Treatment and Prognosis

Given the long life of the adult fluke in humans (5 to 20 years), treatment is recommended to minimize the complications of long-standing pulmonary infection.[6] Praziquantel is widely considered to be the drug of choice for paragonimiasis. Triclabendazole and bithionol are alternative therapies.[39]

Schistosoma spp. (Schistosomiasis)

General

Schistosomiasis is caused by several species of trematodes in the genus *Schistosoma*. The WHO estimates that nearly 240 million people worldwide are infected with these parasites.[40] Endemic areas include parts of the Middle East, Africa, Asia, South America, and the Caribbean.[40]

Humans become infected when coming into contact with fresh water containing microscopic swimming parasites (cercariae), which can penetrate intact skin, then migrate through the lungs and liver, and eventually reside in the blood vessels around the bladder or intestine. Pulmonary schistosomiasis can occur when eggs bypass the liver and reach the heart and pulmonary artery, either through the portal blood supply or directly via the inferior vena cava. Eggs usually embed in pulmonary vessel walls and the surrounding lung parenchyma where they can cause blood flow obstruction and, eventually, pulmonary hypertension.[6] Cardiopulmonary involvement is uncommon, occurring in <10% of patients.[41]

Within hours of infection, patients may develop a self-limited maculopapular rash at the site of cercariae penetration.[6] Several weeks later, patients may also experience self-limited immunologically mediated symptoms referred to as Katayama fever, with fever, cough, headache, diarrhea, and wheezing. Lymphadenopathy, hepatosplenomegaly, peripheral eosinophilia, and elevated serum IgE levels are commonly present.[6] Once the infection is well established, patients present with symptoms related to the ongoing deposition of eggs and associated inflammation and fibrosis. Patients with pulmonary schistosomiasis may present with dyspnea and other symptoms of pulmonary hypertension.[21]

Infection is usually diagnosed by microscopic identification of eggs in urine or stool. Since eggs are not shed until 6 weeks after exposure, serologic testing is the test of choice during early infection.[6] Less commonly, diagnosis is made by tissue examination. Confirmation of pulmonary involvement requires detection of eggs in tissue or other respiratory specimens.[6]

Radiologic Findings

Acute disease generally appears as diffuse pulmonary opacities or nodules on chest radiographs; these nodules may have a "ground-glass" halo on CT.[6] Thoracic lymphadenopathy and pleural effusion may also be seen in early disease. Advanced disease is commonly associated with miliary and cavitary lesions, and changes consistent with pulmonary hypertension (e.g., pulmonary artery enlargement).[6] Concomitant liver involvement is almost always present.[42]

Gross and Histologic Findings

Parenchymal nodules and arteriolar thickening may be noted grossly. Histologically, *Schistosoma* eggs lodge in small arterioles (50 to 100 μm) and cause a granulomatous endarteritis.[42] Granulomas surrounding collapsed eggs may also be seen in the lung parenchyma (Fig. 43.9). Changes associated with pulmonary hypertension such as arteriolar medial hypertrophy, endothelial proliferation, and plexiform lesions are common in advanced stage disease.[42] The eggs vary in size and shape depending on the infecting species and may be surrounded by an eosinophilic precipitate forming club-like projections (Splendore-Hoeppli phenomenon).[43] Eggs of the three most common *Schistosoma* species to parasitize humans are shown in Figure 43.9.

Differential Diagnosis

When large eggs are found in respiratory or pleural fluid specimens, the primary considerations are *Schistosoma* and *Paragonimus* infection.

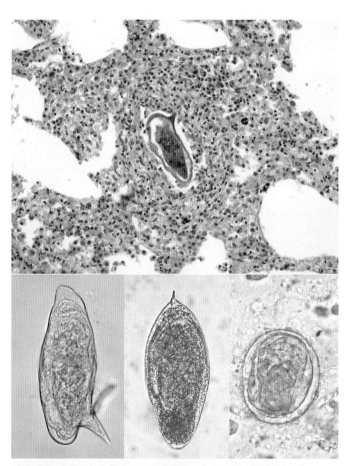

FIGURE 43.9 ▲ Pulmonary schistosomiasis. A careful search reveals an egg with a well-defined lateral spine, consistent with *Schistosoma mansoni* (**top**). From left to right, eggs of *Schistosoma mansoni*, *S. haematobium*, and *S. japonicum* are shown as they appear in unstained wet mount preparation, with lateral, terminal, and rudimentary spines, respectively (**bottom**). (Images from Pritt, B. *Parasitology Benchtop Reference Guide*. Chicago, IL: College of American Pathologists Press; 2014:63, 92; Used with permission.)

Although normally easy to differentiate in cytology preparations, distortion of eggs commonly occurs with histology processing and can make identification more challenging. Helpful differentiating features include the thicker, brightly birefringent walls of *Paragonimus* eggs; in comparison, *Schistosoma* eggs are often thinner and demonstrate only weak birefringence.[42]

Treatment and Prognosis

Praziquantel is the drug of choice for pulmonary schistosomiasis, delivered in one to two doses in a single day. Repeating the treatment in 2 to 6 weeks has been shown to increase the cure rate. Artemisinin may be administered following exposure to decrease the risk of infection.[44]

Strongyloides stercoralis (Strongyloidiasis)

General

Strongyloidiasis is most commonly caused by infection with the nematode *Strongyloides stercoralis*. Infection is endemic in the tropics and subtropics worldwide, including parts of the southeastern United States.[21] Humans become infected when infectious larvae directly penetrate exposed human skin. Larvae enter the soil in feces from infected humans. Unlike other intestinal nematodes, *Strongyloides stercoralis* can also exist as a free-living nematode in the environment.

Initial symptoms include skin irritation and rash at the site of larval penetration. Later when the larvae are migrating through the lungs as part of their normal reproductive cycle, patients may present with dry cough and wheezing (Loeffler syndrome). The intestinal stage of infection may be asymptomatic or present with diarrhea and abdominal discomfort. Life-threatening infection occurs in immunocompromised hosts with hyperinfection syndrome in which larvae are migrating from the intestine to the lungs and other organs in large numbers.[45,46] In this setting, pulmonary symptoms include hemoptysis, dyspnea, and respiratory failure.[21]

Strongyloidiasis is usually diagnosed by finding characteristic larvae in stool or sputum. Serology is a useful adjunctive method for diagnosing strongyloidiasis and has relatively high sensitivity, but false-positive results are common in patients with other roundworm infection.[47] Pulmonary involvement is confirmed by identification of *S. stercoralis* larvae in respiratory specimens (Fig. 43.10).

Radiologic Findings

Chest radiographs and chest CT are usually abnormal in patients with symptomatic pulmonary strongyloidiasis.[25,45] Common findings include diffuse interstitial reticulation, miliary nodules, and, in advanced cases, pleural effusions and features of bronchopneumonia with scattered, segmental, or lobar opacities.[25,45] Migratory opacities may be seen on serial radiographs, much like what is seen with Loeffler syndrome. Evidence of ARDS, pneumonia and pulmonary hemorrhage, with extensive pulmonary opacities, may be seen in severe and fatal cases.[45]

Tissue Sampling

Filariform larvae may be found in sputum, pleural fluid, and other respiratory secretions.[45] Tissue sampling should focus on consolidated regions.

Gross and Histologic Findings

The lungs often show large areas of hemorrhage and consolidation.[48] Larvae may be seen within alveoli without an associated inflammatory response, or in the presence of alveolar hemorrhage and mixed inflammatory infiltrate. Larvae measure 400 to 700 μm in length by 10 to 20 μm in diameter (Fig. 43.10).[5] Secondary bacterial pneumonia is common.

Differential Diagnosis

Strongyloides stercoralis larvae must be differentiated from other larvae such as those of *Ascaris lumbricoides* and hookworm. Examination of

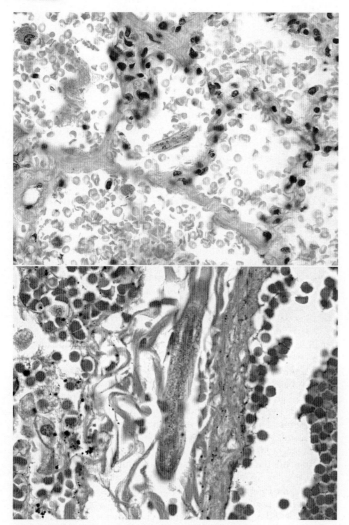

FIGURE 43.10 ▲ Pulmonary strongyloidiasis. Section of *Strongyloides stercoralis* larva within an alveolus (**top**). It is important to not mistake incomplete sections of larvae as foreign bodies. A high magnification demonstrates rows of small nuclei within the larva (**bottom**).

morphologic features such as the tail (notched in *S. stercoralis*) and lateral spines (also known as alae, found with *A. lumbricoides*) is helpful.[48] Stool ova and parasite exam will often demonstrate characteristic eggs (hookworm and *A. lumbricoides*) or larvae (*S. stercoralis*). Rarely, microfilariae of *Wuchereria bancrofti* and *Brugia malayi* may be found in pleural fluid and lung biopsies of patients with tropical pulmonary eosinophilia. Histopathology typically reveals eosinophilic pneumonia and eosinophilic abscesses surrounding rare degenerating microfilariae.[21,49,50] Finally, helminths that cause visceral larva migrans (*Toxocara* species, *Baylisascaris procyonis*) can migrate through the lung and cause eosinophilic abscesses. Like *A. lumbricoides*, they have lateral alae when seen on cross section.[48]

Treatment and Prognosis

Ivermectin is the drug of choice for strongyloidiasis. Albendazole may also be used.[51] The prognosis for patients with pulmonary strongyloidiasis depends on the severity of disease and is worse in immunocompromised patients with hyperinfection.[52]

Taenia solium (Cysticercosis)

General

Cysticercosis is due to infection with the cystic larval form of the pork tapeworm, *T. solium*. In this infection, cysts (cysticerci) form in multiple tissues throughout the body, including skin and soft tissue, the brain

(neurocysticercosis), eye, and lung. Most patients with cysticercosis in the United States are originally from endemic countries.[53] Unlike infection with the adult worm, infection is not acquired through ingestion of pork, but is instead due to ingestion of eggs in fecally contaminated food or water. Following ingestion, the eggs hatch to release parasitic onchospheres, which enter the bloodstream and migrate throughout the body to various organs to form cysticerci.

Clinical presentation varies based on the predominant sites of infection. Neurocysticercosis is one of the most devastating forms of infection and may cause seizures, mental status changes, and death.[53] Thoracic involvement is usually limited to the respiratory muscles but rarely involves the lung parenchyma and pleura. Patients may present with chest pain and dyspnea.[21]

Cysticercosis is usually diagnosed using serologic testing in conjunction with clinical and radiologic findings. The CDC's immunoblot assay using purified *T. solium* antigens is generally considered to be the test of choice for the immunodiagnosis of cysticercosis.[54,55] Identification of cysticerci in tissue biopsy allows for definitive diagnosis and may be useful in cases with atypical clinical or radiologic findings or negative serology results.

Radiologic Findings

Cysticerci are generally seen on chest radiograph as round cysts, 3 to 10 mm in diameter. Older cysts may have a calcified outer shell. On CT, cysts have been described as nodules with fluid attenuation and a visible scolex.[56]

Gross and Histologic Findings

An entire nodule should be excised so that the protoscolex can be identified. An intact cysticercus consists of an invaginated protoscolex with four suckers and refractile hooklets (Fig. 43.11).[53] The protoscolex is attached to an infolded neck region, and the combined structures are surrounded by a thin-walled cyst sometimes referred to as a bladder.[53] Viable cysticerci do not usually invoke a host inflammatory response, but degenerating cysticerci trigger an intense immune response with recruitment of neutrophils, macrophages, and eosinophils.[53] In this setting, the neck region is often the most prominently recognizable feature; occasionally, suckers and hooklets may also be seen. Calcified bodies called calcareous corpuscles are found in the stroma of all cestodes (adult and larval forms) and are a useful supporting histopathologic feature.

Differential Diagnosis

Identification of an invaginated protoscolex within a small cyst is diagnostic of cysticercosis. However, the diagnosis can be particularly challenging in the setting of degenerated or calcified cysts. Correlation with clinical presentation, imaging, and cysticercosis serology is useful for supporting the histopathologic impression. It is also helpful to remember that pulmonary cysticercosis is rare and is usually accompanied by cysts in other organs. Other cestode infections that may resemble cysticercosis include echinococcosis and sparganosis. In contrast to cysticercosis, however, echinococcal cysts can grow to very large sizes (>10 cm) and usually contain multiple protoscoleces, often inside of daughter cysts.[27] Sparganosis differs from both cysticercosis and echinococcosis in that no protoscoleces are seen. Instead, the cestode appears as a single elongated larva with myxoid stroma containing calcareous bodies and smooth muscle fibers.

Treatment and Prognosis

Albendazole is the drug of choice for the treatment of cysticercosis. Praziquantel can also be used, but is not FDA approved for this purpose.[57] Antigen testing is available through the CDC and may be useful for monitoring response to albendazole, since levels drop quickly with successful treatment.

Parasitic Mimics

Detached ciliary tufts (also known as ciliocytophthoria) and degenerated ciliated respiratory epithelial cells are convincing mimics of ciliated or flagellated parasites and are commonly seen in respiratory specimens.[58]

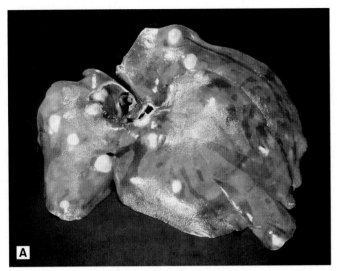

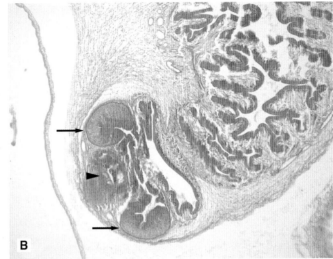

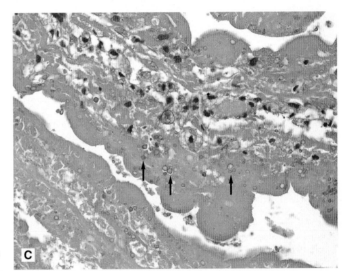

FIGURE 43.11 ▲ Pulmonary cysticercosis. **A.** Lung with numerous cysticerci. (From Temesgen Z, ed. *Mayo Clinic Infectious Diseases Board Review*. New York, NY: Mayo Clinic Scientific Press/Oxford University Press; 2011: 212. Used with permission.) **B.** Intact cysticercus with dense invaginated protoscolex and surrounding fluid-filled cyst. Two of the four suckers (*arrows*) and refractile hooklets (*arrowhead*) are seen. **C.** Degenerated cysticercus with prominent calcareous corpuscles (*arrows*).

Furthermore, ciliated epithelial cells are often motile on unpreserved wet preparations. Fortunately, detached ciliary tufts have key morphologic differences that allow them to be differentiated from true parasites: they are small (measuring only 5 to 15 μm in diameter), the cilia are present in a dense mat and attached to a terminal plate, and the cilia beat in a rhythmic motion without propelling the object forward. Of note, the FLA that infect humans do not have a flagellated form in the human body and therefore should not enter the differential of detached ciliary tufts.

Aspirated food material and inspissated mucus coils (i.e., Curschmann spirals) can be convincing mimics of roundworms in respiratory specimens.[59–61] The pathologist should therefore be familiar with the characteristic features of each that allow them to be differentiated from true parasites.

Certain types of food material such as seeds and nuts are especially reminiscent of parasites since they have internal structures that resemble helminth organs in tissue sections. In contrast to helminths, however, plant material is often composed of multiple small cells with rigid walls; the walls may be pigmented and the cells often contain hyaline globules. Peanuts and lentils are among the most commonly aspirated objects worldwide.[61] The clearly defined thick cuticle, muscle cells, and digestive and reproductive organs of roundworms are lacking. Furthermore, internal structures containing starch are often birefringent with polarized light, unlike nematodes.

Curschmann spirals have been recognized for over 100 years in respiratory specimens from patients with inflammatory conditions such as asthma and chronic bronchitis.[60] Although they have a superficial worm-like quality, they can be differentiated from true worms by their abundant coils, variable diameter, and lack of internal structures.

REFERENCES

1. Cheepsattayakorn A, Cheepsattayakorn R. Parasitic pneumonia and lung involvement. *Biomed Res Int*. 2014;2014:874021.
2. Khemasuwan D, Farver CF, Mehta AC. Parasites of the air passages. *Chest*. 2014;145:883–895.
3. Klassen-Fischer MK, Wear DJ, Neafie RC. Amebiasis. In: Meyers WM, Firpo A, Wear DJ, eds. *Topics on the Pathology of Protozoan and Invasive Arthropod Diseases*. Washington, DC: Armed Forces Institute of Pathology; 2011: 1–15.
4. Kunst H, Mack D, Kon OM, et al. Parasitic infections of the lung: a guide for the respiratory physician. *Thorax*. 2011;66:528–536.
5. Procop GW, Neafie RC. Human parasitic pulmonary infections. In: Zander DS, Farver CF, eds. *Pulmonary Pathology*. Philadelphia, PA: Churchill Livingstone; 2008:287–314.
6. Kim K, Weiss LM, Tanowitz HB. Parasitic infections. In: Broaddus VS, Mason RJ, Ernst JD, et al., eds. *Murray and Nadel's Textbook of Respiratory Medicine*. Philadelphia, PA: Elsevier Saunders; 2016:682–698.
7. Pritt BS, Clark CG. Amebiasis. *Mayo Clin Proc*. 2008;83:1154–1159; quiz 1159–1160.
8. Shamsuzzaman SM, Hashiguchi Y. Thoracic amebiasis. *Clin Chest Med*. 2002;23:479–492.

9. Walsh JA. Problems in recognition and diagnosis of amebiasis: estimation of the global magnitude of morbidity and mortality. *Rev Infect Dis.* 1986;8:228–238.

10. Stanley SL Jr. Amoebiasis. *Lancet.* 2003;361:1025–1034.

11. Lyche KD, Jensen WA. Pleuropulmonary amebiasis. *Semin Respir Infect.* 1997;12:106–112.

12. Lichtenstein A, Kondo AT, Visvesvara GS, et al. Pulmonary amoebiasis presenting as superior vena cava syndrome. *Thorax.* 2005;60:350–352.

13. Stephen SJ, Uragoda CG. Pleuro-pulmonary amoebiasis. A review of 40 cases. *Br J Dis Chest.* 1970;64:96–106.

14. Derouin F, Devergie A, Auber P, et al. Toxoplasmosis in bone marrow-transplant recipients: report of seven cases and review. *Clin Infect Dis.* 1992;15:267–270.

15. Neafie RC, Klassen-Fischer MK, Meyers WM. Toxoplasmosis. In: Meyers WM, Firpo A, Wear DJ, eds. *Topics on the Pathology of Protozoan and Invasive Arthropod Diseases.* Washington, DC: Armed Forces Institute of Pathology; 2011.

16. Vasoo S, Pritt BS. Molecular diagnostics and parasitic disease. *Clin Lab Med.* 2013;33:461–503.

17. Fricker-Hidalgo H, Brion JP, Durand M, et al. Disseminated toxoplasmosis with pulmonary involvement after heart transplantation. *Transpl Infect Dis.* 2005;7:38–40.

18. Menezes RG, Pant S, Kharoshah MA, et al. Autopsy discoveries of death from malaria. *Leg Med (Tokyo).* 2012;14:111–115.

19. Lacerda MV, Fragoso SC, Alecrim MG, et al. Postmortem characterization of patients with clinical diagnosis of Plasmodium vivax malaria: to what extent does this parasite kill? *Clin Infect Dis.* 2012;55:e67–e74.

20. Deroost K, Tyberghein A, Lays N, et al. Hemozoin induces lung inflammation and correlates with malaria-associated acute respiratory distress syndrome. *Am J Respir Cell Mol Biol.* 2013;48:589–600.

21. Fraser R. Protozoal and helminthic pulmonary disease. In: Churg AM, et al., eds. *Thurlbeck's Pathology of the Lung.* New York, NY: Thieme; 2005:315–329.

22. Milanez de Campos JR, Barbas CS, Filomeno LT, et al. Human pulmonary dirofilariasis: analysis of 24 cases from Sao Paulo, Brazil. *Chest.* 1997;112: 729–733.

23. Asimacopoulos PJ, Katras A, Christie B. Pulmonary dirofilariasis. The largest single-hospital experience. *Chest.* 1992;102:851–855.

24. Flieder DB, Moran CA. Pulmonary dirofilariasis: a clinicopathologic study of 41 lesions in 39 patients. *Hum Pathol.* 1999;30:251–256.

25. Palmer PE. Diagnostic imaging in parasitic infections. *Pediatr Clin North Am.* 1985;32:1019–1040.

26. Marty AM, Neafie RC. Dirofilariasis. In: Meyers WM, Neafie RC, Marty AM, et al., eds. *Pathology of Infectious Diseases.* Washington, DC: Armed Forces Institute of Pathology; 2000:275–286.

27. Marty AM, Johnson LK, Neafie RC. Hydatidosis (echinococcosis). In: Meyers WM, Neafie RC, Marty AM, et al., eds. *Pathology of Infectious Diseases.* Washington, DC: Armed Forces Institute of Pathology; 2000:145–164.

28. Torgerson PR, Keller K, Magnotta M, et al. The global burden of alveolar echinococcosis. *PLoS Negl Trop Dis.* 2010;4:e722.

29. Manzano-Roman R, Sanchez-Ovejero C, Hernandez-Gonzalez A, et al. Serological diagnosis and follow-up of human cystic Echinococcosis: a new hope for the future? *Biomed Res Int.* 2015;2015:428205.

30. Ohsaki Y, Sasaki T, Shibukawa K, et al. Radiological findings of alveolar hydatid disease of the lung caused by Echinococcus multilocularis. *Respirology.* 2007;12:458–461.

31. Santivanez SJ, Naquira C, Gavidia CM, et al. Household factors associated with the presence of human hydatid disease in three rural communities of Junin, Peru. *Rev Peru Med Exp Salud Publica.* 2010;27:498–505.

32. Hemphill A, Stadelmann B, Rufener R, et al. Treatment of echinococcosis: albendazole and mebendazole—what else? *Parasite.* 2014;21:70.

33. Marty AM, Neafie RC. Paragonimiasis. In: Meyers WM, Neafie RC, Marty AM, et al., eds. *Pathology of Infectious Diseases.* Washington, DC: Armed Forces Institute of Pathology; 2000:49–68.

34. Narain K, Devi KR, Bhattacharya S, et al. Declining prevalence of pulmonary paragonimiasis following treatment & community education in a remote tribal population of Arunachal Pradesh, India. *Indian J Med Res.* 2015;141:648–652.

35. Kanpittaya J, Sawanyawisuth K, Vannavong A, et al. Different chest radiographic findings of pulmonary paragonimiasis in two endemic countries. *Am J Trop Med Hyg.* 2010;83:924–926.

36. Seon HJ, Kim YI, Lee JH, et al. Differential chest computed tomography findings of pulmonary parasite infestation between the paragonimiasis and nonparagonimiatic parasite infestation. *J Comput Assist Tomogr.* 2015;39:956–961.

37. Lee S, Yu Y, An J, et al. A case of delayed diagnosis of pulmonary paragonimiasis due to improvement after anti-tuberculosis therapy. *Tuberc Respir Dis (Seoul).* 2014;77:178–183.

38. Zarrin-Khameh N, Citron DR, Stager CE, et al. Pulmonary paragonimiasis diagnosed by fine-needle aspiration biopsy. *J Clin Microbiol.* 2008;46:2137–2140.

39. Calvopina M, Guderian RH, Paredes W, et al. Treatment of human pulmonary paragonimiasis with triclabendazole: clinical tolerance and drug efficacy. *Trans R Soc Trop Med Hyg.* 1998;92:566–569.

40. Utzinger J, Raso G, Brooker S, et al. Schistosomiasis and neglected tropical diseases: towards integrated and sustainable control and a word of caution. *Parasitology.* 2009;136:1859–1874.

41. Morris W, Knauer CM. Cardiopulmonary manifestations of schistosomiasis. *Semin Respir Infect.* 1997;12:159–170.

42. Cheever AW, Neafie RC. Schistosomiasis. In: Meyers WM, Neafie RC, Marty AM, et al., eds. *Pathology of Infectious Diseases.* Washington, DC: Armed Forces Institute of Pathology; 2000:23–48.

43. Hussein MR. Mucocutaneous Splendore-Hoeppli phenomenon. *J Cutan Pathol.* 2008;35:979–988.

44. Dong L, Duan W, Chen J, et al. An artemisinin derivative of praziquantel as an orally active antischistosomal agent. *PLoS One.* 2014;9:e112163.

45. Woodring JH, Halfhill H II, Berger R, et al. Clinical and imaging features of pulmonary strongyloidiasis. *South Med J.* 1996;89:10–19.

46. Woodring JH, Halfhill H, II, Reed JC. Pulmonary strongyloidiasis: clinical and imaging features. *AJR Am J Roentgenol.* 1994;162:537–542.

47. Biggs BA, Caruana S, Mihrshahi S, et al. Management of chronic strongyloidiasis in immigrants and refugees: is serologic testing useful? *Am J Trop Med Hyg.* 2009;80:788–791.

48. Meyers WM, Neafie RC, Marty AM. Strongyloidiasis. In: Meyers WM, Neafie RC, Marty AM, et al., eds. *Pathology of Infectious Diseases.* Washington, DC: Armed Forces Institute of Pathology; 2000:341–352.

49. Ong RK, Doyle RL. Tropical pulmonary eosinophilia. *Chest.* 1998;113: 1673–1679.

50. Webb JK, Job CK, Gault EW. Tropical eosinophilia: demonstration of microfilariae in lung, liver, and lymphnodes. *Lancet.* 1960;1:835–842.

51. Luvira V, Watthanakulpanich D, Pittisuttithum P. Management of Strongyloides stercoralis: a puzzling parasite. *Int Health.* 2014;6:273–281.

52. Asdamongkol N, Pornsuriyasak P, Sungkanuparph S. Risk factors for strongyloidiasis hyperinfection and clinical outcomes. *Southeast Asian J Trop Med Public Health.* 2006;37:875–884.

53. Neafie RC, Marty AM, Johnson LK. Taeniasis and cysticercosis. In: Meyers WM, Neafie RC, Marty AM, et al., eds. *Pathology of Infectious Diseases.* Washington, DC: Armed Forces Institute of Pathology; 2000:117–136.

54. Noh J, Rodriguez S, Lee YM, et al. Recombinant protein- and synthetic peptide-based immunoblot test for diagnosis of neurocysticercosis. *J Clin Microbiol.* 2014;52:1429–1434.

55. Levine MZ, Lewis MM, Rodriquez S, et al. Development of an enzyme-linked immunoelectrotransfer blot (EITB) assay using two baculovirus expressed recombinant antigens for diagnosis of Taenia solium taeniasis. *J Parasitol.* 2007;93:409–417.

56. Mamere AE, Muglia VF, Simao GN, et al. Disseminated cysticercosis with pulmonary involvement. *J Thorac Imaging.* 2004;19:109–111.

57. Garcia HH, Gonzales I, Lescano AG, et al. Efficacy of combined antiparasitic therapy with praziquantel and albendazole for neurocysticercosis: a double-blind, randomised controlled trial. *Lancet Infect Dis.* 2014;14:687–695.

58. Khan S, Kumar VA, Venkitachalam A, et al. Detached ciliary tufts masquerading as free-living amoebae. *Int J Infect Dis.* 2015;30:142–143.

59. Antonakopoulos GN, Lambrinaki E, Kyrkou KA. Curschmann's spirals in sputum: histochemical evidence of bronchial gland ductal origin. *Diagn Cytopathol.* 1987;3:291–294.

60. Cenci M, Giovagnoli MR, Alderisio M, et al. Curschmann's spirals in sputum of subjects exposed daily to urban environmental pollution. *Diagn Cytopathol.* 1998;19:349–351.

61. Pritt B, Harmon M, Schwartz M, et al. A tale of three aspirations: foreign bodies in the airway. *J Clin Pathol.* 2003;56:791–794.

44 Centrilobular Emphysema

Allen P. Burke, M.D., and Joseph J. Maleszewski, M.D.

General Features

Emphysema, along with chronic bronchitis, is in a category of disease known collectively as chronic obstructive pulmonary disease. It is characterized by destruction of alveolar septa, which contributes to irreversible airflow obstruction by lost of elastic recoil of peribronchiolar tissue. Emphysema is classified into one of three varieties based on the part of the acinus or lobule that it primarily involves: centriacinar/ centrilobular, panacinar/panlobular, or distal acinar/paraseptal.

Centrilobular emphysema accounts for more than 75% of total cases of emphysema and is defined by abnormal enlargement of airspaces centered on the respiratory bronchiole with eventual coalescence of destroyed lobules within the secondary lobule.[1,2] The enlargement of alveoli into cystic spaces together with small airway obstruction results in air trapping and marked increases in total lung volume.[3]

Pathophysiology

The root cause of centrilobular emphysema is persistent inflammation to noxious environmental stimuli, usually cigarette smoke, with inflammatory-mediated proteolysis. Exposure to coal dust is also a risk factor for the development of emphysema.[4] Cigarette smoking induces emphysema by up-regulation of proteases, including elastases, cathepsins, and proteolytic matrix metalloproteases, secreted by neutrophils and macrophages, which are increased in small airways of smokers.[3] Cigarette smoke also forms reactive oxygen and nitrogen species, which result in direct tissue destruction and increased levels of pro-inflammatory cytokines. Other factors involved in the pathogenesis of emphysema include autoimmunity and viral infections.[5,6]

Although most causes of centrilobular emphysema are environmental, <50% of smokers develop the disease. The risk of chronic bronchitis in smokers is approximately 40% over 30 years,[2] and radiologically defined emphysema is seen in 27% of smokers with more than a 10 pack-year history.[1] Polymorphisms for several genes, including TGFB1, EPHX1, SERPINE2, and ADRB2, are found at increased frequencies in smokers with emphysema, indicating a partial genetic basis.[7]

Clinical Findings

Emphysema is defined by imaging or pathologic findings of alveolar wall destruction, with confirmation of obstruction and increased lung volume by pulmonary function testing. Chronic bronchitis, which is typically also present, is defined by symptoms of chronic cough and sputum production for at least 3 months per year for 2 consecutive years.[2] Symptoms of emphysema are somewhat nonspecific and include dyspnea and exercise intolerance. Other findings include hyperinflation of the lungs with increased total lung capacity, decreased diffusing capacity, and increased peripheral white blood cell counts.[1] Although primarily an obstructive disease, manifest by decreased forced expiratory volume, it has been recently appreciated that approximately 8% of patients with centrilobular emphysema have interstitial findings that may result in a component of restrictive lung disease.[8] This finding reflects the discovery of smoking-related interstitial fibrosis

(see Chapter 18), which is distinct from other types of interstitial lung disease.[9]

Pulmonary hypertension with cor pulmonale occurs relatively commonly in emphysema and occurs at a greater rate than with pulmonary fibrosis.[10] Progression of pulmonary hypertension occurs slowly, unless there is significant hypoxemia.[11] There is likely a direct effect of tobacco smoke on small muscular arteries and arterioles, with alterations in vasoconstriction and vasodilatation, and increased vascular smooth muscle cell proliferation.[3]

Radiologic Findings

Radiologic findings include increased lung volumes and diffuse decreased in lung density, predominantly in the upper lobes.[1] This upper lobe distribution is helpful in discriminating centrilobular emphysema from panlobular and paraseptal forms. By computed tomography, there are focal regions of low attenuation, surrounded by normal lung attenuation, located within the central portion of secondary pulmonary lobules. In advanced stages, there is pruning of vessels with enlarging areas of low attenuation. Pathologic–imaging correlation has shown a high correlation between areas of low attenuation and histologic emphysema.[12]

Tissue Sampling

The pathologic assessment of emphysema is often made as a secondary finding in specimens resected for lung cancer. It can also be seen in specimens removed during lung allotransplantation or in specimens taken for lung reduction surgery. Pulmonary function tests and imaging, rather than histologic assessment, are the mainstays of diagnosis.

Gross Findings

Grossly, emphysematous lungs have a porous or spider web appearance, owing to the destruction of the underlying pulmonary parenchyma (Fig. 44.1). The disease has a very characteristic upper lung zone distribution (Fig. 44.2). The centrilobular distribution can sometimes be difficult to assess by routine visual inspection (Fig. 44.3); however, examining a parasagittal section of lung under water or alcohol can help to demonstrate the pathology and distribution. For research purposes, the tissue loss of emphysema can also be seen by parasagittal sections of the lung, mounted on paper (Gough section) (Fig. 44.3).[13–15] Distention of the airways with fixative is helpful in the overall assessment (both grossly and histologically), but overdistention can result in artifactual changes that resemble emphysema. There have been several methods of quantification of the extent of emphysema, using point-counting methods and, more recently, computerized imaging.[12,15–18]

Parenchymal bullae and pleural blebs are also commonly seen in the setting of emphysema. While some have distinguished between bullae and blebs based on size, the latter usually described as <2 cm and the former >2 cm, the distinction is traditionally based on location.[19] A bleb is thought to represent dissection of air into the visceral pleura, resulting from a rupture alveolus. A bulla, on the other hand, is a coalescence of lost parenchyma resulting in a cyst-like airspace

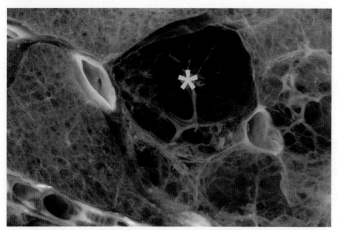

FIGURE 44.1 ▲ Lung explant, patient transplanted for centrilobular emphysema. A high magnification of a different case demonstrates parenchymal loss with widening of the airspaces and a "spider web-like" architecture. The *asterisk* indicates a portion of the lung with bulla formation creating a cyst-like space.

within the alveolated parenchyma (Fig. 44.1). Bullous disease is frequently seen in the apices but does not correlate with the degree of severity of symptoms.[20]

Microscopic Findings

Histologically, centrilobular emphysema is characterized by destruction of alveolar walls with enlargement of airspaces, without fibrosis, in a peribronchiolar distribution (Figs. 44.4 to 44.6). The degree of

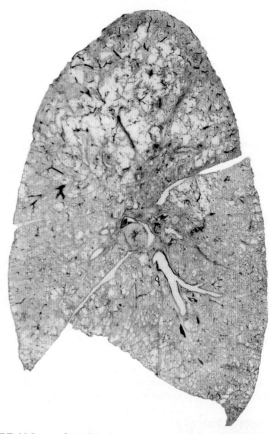

FIGURE 44.3 ▲ Centrilobular emphysema. A Gough section (paper whole mount) demonstrates the upper lung zone distribution of disease.

airspace enlargement can be measured morphometrically using the average interalveolar wall distance and increases with the degree of emphysema.[21] The cyst-like lesions seen in centrilobular emphysema have been measured at a mean diameter of 5 mm.[22] Increased alveolar wall thickness only occurs if there is associated smoking-related fibrosis (also termed airspace enlargement with fibrosis).[22] Small airway

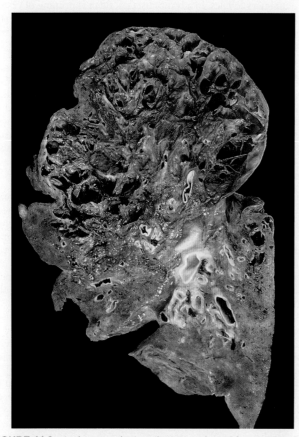

FIGURE 44.2 ▲ Lung explant, patient transplanted for centrilobular emphysema. There is marked airspace loss with gross bullous change in the upper lobe.

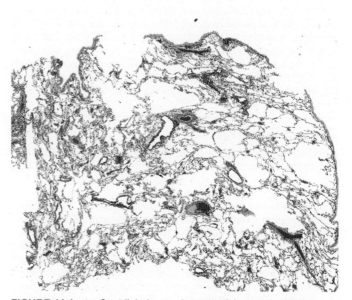

FIGURE 44.4 ▲ Centrilobular emphysema. A low-power photomicrograph shows areas of parenchymal rarefaction with widened airspaces.

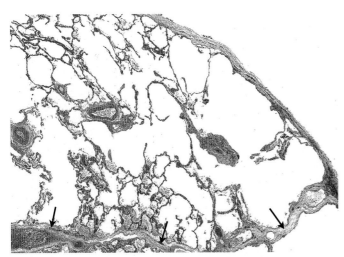

FIGURE 44.5 ▲ Centrilobular emphysema. The areas of airspace enlargement are central and subpleural, with relative sparing at the edge of the lobule at the interlobular septum (*arrows*).

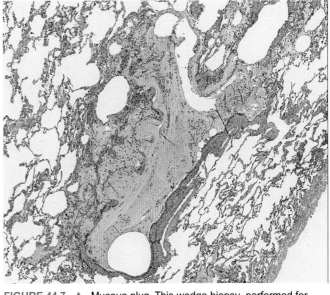

FIGURE 44.7 ▲ Mucous plug. This wedge biopsy, performed for volume reduction, shows pools of mucin in a small airway extending into the alveolar spaces. The emphysema is not particularly evident *in this field*.

thickening reflecting chronic bronchitis is frequently present as well,[21] in addition to increased mucus-secreting goblet cells, another feature of chronic bronchitis (Fig. 44.7).[23] Bullae and blebs can also be identified, microscopically.

There are frequently other histologic findings not directly related to emphysema. These include other smoking-related processes (see Chapter 18), such as respiratory bronchiolitis (Fig. 44.8), smoking-related interstitial fibrosis (Fig. 44.9), and pulmonary Langerhans cell histiocytosis. Non–smoking-related changes that may be present include small airway disease, poorly formed granulomas, foci or organizing pneumonia, and changes related to prior spontaneous pneumothorax.

Prognosis and Treatment

The medical treatment of emphysema is essentially equivalent to that of chronic obstructive lung disease. Stable disease is treated with bronchodilators, corticosteroids, nutritional support, and volume

reduction surgery (bullectomy). The indications for surgical therapy include high trapped lung volumes and bullae >1/3 the hemithorax, general in younger patients with normal diffusing capacities and arterial oxygen tension.[24,25] Histologically, the findings in volume reduction surgeries generally show features of emphysema with bulla formation (Fig. 44.10). Treatment of exacerbations of emphysema include, in addition to that of stable disease, antibiotics and, if necessary, mechanical ventilation. The indications for lung transplant include markedly decreased forced expiratory volumes (<25% expected), increased arterial carbon dioxide tension, and pulmonary hypertension.[26]

The prognosis of emphysema depends on the degree of impairment of gas exchange and extent of airway obstruction. Conditions associated with poor survival in acute exacerbations include congestive heart failure, coronary artery disease, diabetes mellitus, and renal and liver failure.[26]

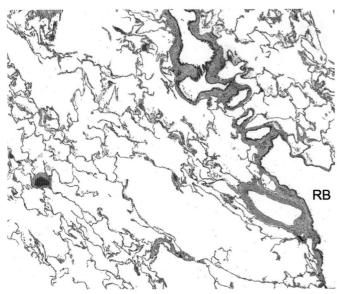

FIGURE 44.6 ▲ Lung explant with airspace enlargement near the bronchovascular bundles and a dilated respiratory bronchiole (RB).

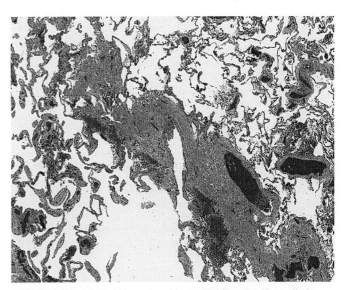

FIGURE 44.8 ▲ Smoking-related interstitial fibrosis. Also called "airspace enlargement with fibrosis," there is patchy dense, relatively acellular fibrosis and mild thickening of the alveolar septa.

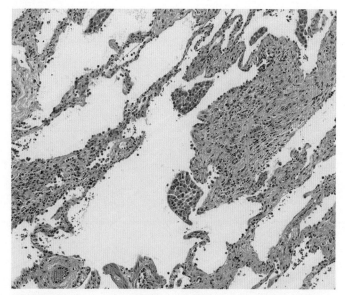

FIGURE 44.9 ▲ Respiratory bronchiolitis. A common finding with emphysema and related to smoking, there are discrete collections of macrophages that contain a fine, granular, golden pigment within the airspaces.

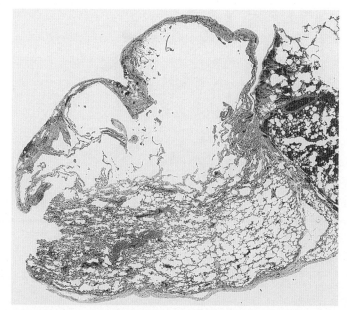

FIGURE 44.10 ▲ Subpleural bulla. This wedge biopsy, performed for volume reduction, shows a markedly enlarged airspace that is large enough to be seen grossly and on imaging. Bullae are caused by loss of alveolar tissue, similar to smaller emphysematous airspaces. There is procedural hemorrhage at the right, bounded by an interlobular septum.

REFERENCES

1. Smith BM, et al. Pulmonary emphysema subtypes on computed tomography: the MESA COPD study. *Am J Med.* 2014;127(1):94e7–9423.
2. Kim V, Criner GJ. Chronic bronchitis and chronic obstructive pulmonary disease. *Am J Respir Crit Care Med.* 2013;187(3):228–237.
3. Wright JL, Churg A. Current concepts in mechanisms of emphysema. *Toxicol Pathol.* 2007;35(1):111–115.
4. Kuempel ED, et al. Contributions of dust exposure and cigarette smoking to emphysema severity in coal miners in the United States. *Am J Respir Crit Care Med.* 2009;180(3):257–264.
5. Tuder RM, Yun JH. It takes two to tango: cigarette smoke partners with viruses to promote emphysema. *J Clin Invest.* 2008;118(8):2689–2693.
6. Voelkel N, Taraseviciene-Stewart L. Emphysema: an autoimmune vascular disease? *Proc Am Thorac Soc.* 2005;2(1):23–25.
7. Kim WJ, et al. Association of COPD candidate genes with computed tomography emphysema and airway phenotypes in severe COPD. *Eur Respir J.* 2011;37(1):39–43.
8. Washko GR, et al. Lung volumes and emphysema in smokers with interstitial lung abnormalities. *N Engl J Med.* 2011;364(10):897–906.
9. Katzenstein AL, et al. Clinically occult interstitial fibrosis in smokers: classification and significance of a surprisingly common finding in lobectomy specimens. *Hum Pathol.* 2010;41(3):316–325.
10. Wright JL, Tazelaar HD, Churg A. Fibrosis with emphysema. *Histopathology.* 2011;58(4):517–524.
11. Kessler R, et al. "Natural history" of pulmonary hypertension in a series of 131 patients with chronic obstructive lung disease. *Am J Respir Crit Care Med.* 2001;164(2):219–224.
12. Hruban RH, et al. High resolution computed tomography of inflation-fixed lungs. Pathologic-radiologic correlation of centrilobular emphysema. *Am Rev Respir Dis.* 1987;136(4):935–940.
13. Thurlbeck WM. Measurement of pulmonary emphysema. *Am Rev Respir Dis.* 1967;95(5):752–764.
14. Saito K, Thurlbeck WM. Measurement of emphysema in autopsy lungs, with emphasis on interlobar differences. *Am J Respir Crit Care Med.* 1995;151(5):1373–1376.
15. Gillooly M, Lamb D, Farrow AS. New automated technique for assessing emphysema on histological sections. *J Clin Pathol.* 1991;44(12):1007–1011.
16. Bankier AA, et al. Pulmonary emphysema: subjective visual grading versus objective quantification with macroscopic morphometry and thin-section CT densitometry. *Radiology.* 1999;211(3):851–858.
17. Bergin C, et al. The diagnosis of emphysema. A computed tomographic-pathologic correlation. *Am Rev Respir Dis.* 1986;133(4):541–546.
18. Foster WL Jr, et al. Centrilobular emphysema: CT-pathologic correlation. *Radiology.* 1986;159(1):27–32.
19. Massie JR Jr, Welchons GA. Pulmonary blebs and bullae. *Ann Surg.* 1954;139(5):624–634.
20. Gould GA, et al. Parenchymal emphysema measured by CT lung density correlates with lung function in patients with bullous disease. *Eur Respir J.* 1993;6(5):698–704.
21. Kim WD, et al. The association between small airway obstruction and emphysema phenotypes in COPD. *Chest.* 2007;131(5):1372–1378.
22. Yamada T, et al. Airspace enlargement with fibrosis shows characteristic histology and immunohistology different from usual interstitial pneumonia, nonspecific interstitial pneumonia and centrilobular emphysema. *Pathol Int.* 2013;63(4):206–213.
23. Innes AL, et al. Epithelial mucin stores are increased in the large airways of smokers with airflow obstruction. *Chest.* 2006;130(4):1102–1108.
24. Geiser T, et al. Outcome after unilateral lung volume reduction surgery in patients with severe emphysema. *Eur J Cardiothorac Surg.* 2001;20(4):674–678.
25. Kim V, et al., Small airway morphometry and improvement in pulmonary function after lung volume reduction surgery. *Am J Respir Crit Care Med.* 2005;171(1):40–47.
26. Celli BR, MacNee W, Force AET. Standards for the diagnosis and treatment of patients with COPD: a summary of the ATS/ERS position paper. *Eur Respir J.* 2004;23(6):932–946.

45 Panlobular Emphysema

Allen P. Burke, M.D., and Joseph J. Maleszewski, M.D.

General Features

Panlobular emphysema is characterized by uniform destruction of the pulmonary acinus. This is in contrast to the centriacinar variety, which begins in the respiratory bronchiole (central portion of the acinus/lobule). Also in distinction from centriacinar emphysema, panacinar emphysema has a predilection for the lower lung zones. It is the least common form of emphysema, estimated at about 5% to 15% of cases.[1]

Pathophysiology

Panacinar emphysema is highly associated with alpha-1 antitrypsin (AAT) deficiency. AAT, synthesized in the liver, is an acute phase reactant of the serpin family of protease inhibitors. Although its best-known function is the inhibition of neutrophil elastase, AAT inhibits a wide range of proteases, leading to its alternate designation "alpha1-protease." The disease is inherited in an autosomal recessive fashion and depends on the inheritance of specific allelic variants.

The gene *SERPINA1* has two codominant alleles, with 75 variations designated by letters reflected by electrophoretic mobility. The most prevalent genotype is PiMM (PI, protease inhibitor; M, allele type). The Pi*Z allele is the most important and strongest genetic variant responsible for decreased plasma AAT levels. The frequency of PiZZ homozygotes, which represent a large proportion of symptomatic patients, is approximately 1 in 2,000 to 1 in 5,000 persons.[2,3] The other genotype responsible for the majority of remaining emphysematous patients is PiSZ, occurring at about half the rate of PiZZ. In directed studies of patients with obstructive lung disease, the proportion of PiSZ or ZZ patients varies widely, from 1% to 3% in patients with some degree of airway obstruction or COPD[4-6] to up to 12% with severe emphysema.[7]

Approximately 3% of North Americans are PI*MZ heterozygotes. PI*MZ heterozygotes are not considered to be at increased risk for emphysema; however, meta-analyses have suggested the possibility of an increased risk in some patients.[8,9]

Because of the lack of cost-effectiveness of population-based screening, and frequent presence of other risk factors, there are little data regarding the actual relative risk of a patient with PiZZ of PiSZ developing emphysema.

The mechanism of AAT deficiency and emphysema lies in its inhibitory effect on serine proteases, such as elastase and proteinase 3 (PR3), and other anti-inflammatory and tissue-protective effects that are independent of protease inhibition. These include interactions with dendritic cells, T-cell regulation, and inhibition of interleukin-1 receptor and IL-10, among others.

The risk for developing emphysema with the genetic background of AAT deficiency is enhanced by risk factors, primarily cigarette smoking.[10]

Clinical Features

Patients with panlobular-predominant emphysema have lower rate of smoking than those with centrilobular emphysema and a lower body mass index. Manifestations are similar, including dyspnea, exercise intolerance, hyperinflation, and lower diffusing capacity.[1] In addition to pulmonary disease, patients with AAT deficiency may have liver dysfunction or cirrhosis as well.

Radiologic Findings

Although there is considerable intraobserver variation among radiologists in assessing emphysema subtypes, there is general agreement that there are diffuse regions of low attenuation involving the entire secondary lobules, with eventual attenuation of peripheral vessels.[1] In contrast to centrilobular emphysema, which involves upper lobes predominantly, there is no variation in the severity between upper and lower lobes. Bulla formation occurs in about one-third of patients but is not a major feature.[11] Computed tomography densitometry is often used as a method of monitoring disease progression.[12]

Gross Findings

At autopsy or explant, specimens should be perfusion fixed by infusing formalin under pressure in the trachea or bronchi. Changes suggestive of tissue loss are present diffusely in all lobes (Fig. 45.1). The panlobular distribution of alveolar septal destruction is difficult to ascertain without special techniques such as paper-mounted whole lung sections.[13]

Microscopic Findings

Histologically, there is diffuse alveolar wall loss (Figs. 45.2 to 45.4). Depending on smoking history, there may be superimposed changes of respiratory bronchiolitis and smoking-related fibrosis, although these are less common than in centrilobular emphysema. There are also frequent secondary findings of organizing pneumonia, scattered granulomas, and patchy interstitial inflammation.

Prognosis and Treatment

Patients with severe panlobular emphysema have markedly decreased survival. The life expectancy for patients who, by pulmonary function

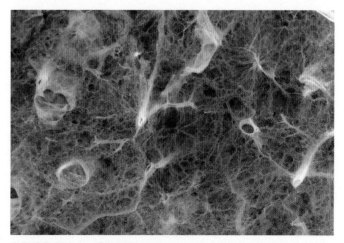

FIGURE 45.1 ▲ Panlobular emphysema, patient with alpha-1 antitrypsin deficiency. Diffuse parenchymal loss can be seen to involve the entire lobule.

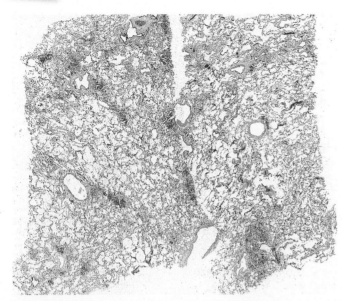

FIGURE 45.2 ▲ Panlobular emphysema, explanted lung in a patient with alpha-1 antitrypsin deficiency, low magnification. There is generalized loss of alveolar septa, although the change is subtle at this magnification.

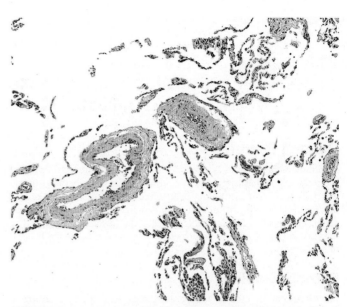

FIGURE 45.4 ▲ Panlobular emphysema, explanted lung. In this field, there is marked loss of alveolar parenchyma.

studies, qualify for lung transplant is 5 years.[14] The most common mechanism of death is respiratory failure.

Treatment for panlobular emphysema includes aggressive treatment of infectious exacerbations,[15] alpha-1 antitrypsin augmentation therapy, and lung transplant. Intravenous infusion of purified human plasma-derived AAT or recombinant AAT has been shown to prolong survival in patients with panlobular emphysema by up to 10 years in nonsmokers.[16] Lung transplantation has been shown to prolong survival of an average of 6 years, compared to controls.[14]

REFERENCES

1. Smith BM, Austin JH, Newell JD Jr, et al. Pulmonary emphysema subtypes on computed tomography: the MESA COPD study. *Am J Med.* 2014;127:94.e7–94. e23.
2. Elzouki AN, Hultcrantz R, Stal P, et al. Increased PiZ gene frequency for alpha 1 antitrypsin in patients with genetic haemochromatosis. *Gut.* 1995;36:922–926.
3. Chorostowska-Wynimko J, Struniawski R, Poplawska B, et al. [The incidence of alpha-1-antitrypsin (A1AT) deficiency alleles in population of Central Poland—preliminary results from newborn screening]. *Pneumonol Alergol Pol.* 2012;80:450–453.
4. Carroll TP, O'Connor CA, Floyd O, et al. The prevalence of alpha-1 antitrypsin deficiency in Ireland. *Respir Res.* 2011;12:91.
5. Molina J, Flor X, Garcia R, et al. The IDDEA project: a strategy for the detection of alpha-1 antitrypsin deficiency in COPD patients in the primary care setting. *Ther Adv Respir Dis.* 2011;5:237–243.
6. Rahaghi FF, Sandhaus RA, Brantly ML, et al. The prevalence of alpha-1 antitrypsin deficiency among patients found to have airflow obstruction. *COPD.* 2012;9:352–358.
7. Stoller JK, Brantly M. The challenge of detecting alpha-1 antitrypsin deficiency. *COPD.* 2013;10(suppl 1):26–34.
8. Hersh CP, Dahl M, Ly NP, et al. Chronic obstructive pulmonary disease in alpha1-antitrypsin PI MZ heterozygotes: a meta-analysis. *Thorax.* 2004;59:843–849.
9. Sorheim IC, Bakke P, Gulsvik A, et al. alpha(1)-Antitrypsin protease inhibitor MZ heterozygosity is associated with airflow obstruction in two large cohorts. *Chest.* 2010;138:1125–1132.
10. Mayer AS, Stoller JK, Vedal S, et al. Risk factors for symptom onset in PI*Z alpha-1 antitrypsin deficiency. *Int J Chron Obstruct Pulmon Dis.* 2006;1:485–492.
11. Guest PJ, Hansell DM. High resolution computed tomography (HRCT) in emphysema associated with alpha-1-antitrypsin deficiency. *Clin Radiol.* 1992;45:260–266.
12. Brebner JA, Stockley RA. Recent advances in alpha-1-antitrypsin deficiency-related lung disease. *Expert Rev Respir Med.* 2013;7:213–229; quiz 230.
13. Leopold JG, Gough J. The centrilobular form of hypertrophic emphysema and its relation to chronic bronchitis. *Thorax.* 1957;12:219–235.
14. Tanash HA, Riise GC, Hansson L, et al. Survival benefit of lung transplantation in individuals with severe alpha1-anti-trypsin deficiency (PiZZ) and emphysema. *J Heart Lung Transplant.* 2011;30:1342–1347.
15. Vijayasaratha K, Stockley RA. Relationship between frequency, length, and treatment outcome of exacerbations to baseline lung function and lung density in alpha-1 antitrypsin-deficient COPD. *Int J Chron Obstruct Pulmon Dis.* 2012;7:789–796.
16. Sclar DA, Evans MA, Robison LM, et al. alpha1-Proteinase inhibitor (human) in the treatment of hereditary emphysema secondary to alpha1-antitrypsin deficiency: number and costs of years of life gained. *Clin Drug Investig.* 2012;32:353–360.

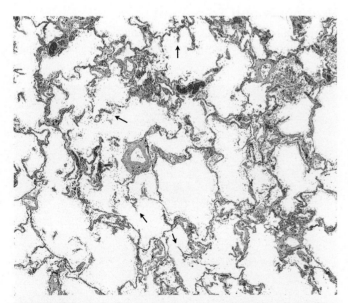

FIGURE 45.3 ▲ Panlobular emphysema, explanted lung in a patient with alpha-1 antitrypsin deficiency, high magnification. The alveolar spaces are enlarged because of destruction of numerous alveolar walls, resulting in ends of alveolar septa within the enlarged spaces (*arrows*). There is no apparent centrilobular distribution. There is no significant interstitial fibrosis.

46 Paraseptal and Interstitial Emphysema

Marie-Christine Aubry, M.D., and Allen P. Burke, M.D.

Paraseptal Emphysema

Definition

Paraseptal (distal acinar) emphysema is the third major subtype of emphysema, after centrilobular (Chapter 44) and panlobular emphysema (Chapter 45). It differs from centrilobular and panlobular emphysema by involving the distal portion of the acinus. Although the pathogenesis of centrilobular and panlobular emphysema is attributed to the imbalance between proteases and antiproteases leading to the destruction of the alveolated lung parenchyma, the pathogenesis of paraseptal emphysema is less certain.[1]

Clinical Findings

Paraseptal emphysema is associated with the formation of apical bullae, a bulla being defined as an enlarged airspace of >1 cm. In isolation, it is seen predominantly in men presenting with a spontaneous pneumothorax and otherwise no increase in symptoms and no airflow limitation.

Most often, paraseptal emphysema is seen in association with centrilobular emphysema in smokers. A small subset (<10%) of smokers with emphysema will have predominantly paraseptal emphysema on computed tomography scans.[2]

Radiologic Findings

Paraseptal emphysema is seen on CT scans as subpleural areas of low attenuation (Fig. 46.1). It is seen predominantly in the upper lung zones. In over 75% of patients with centrilobular emphysema, there is a minor component of paraseptal emphysema.[2]

Gross Findings

The gross findings mimic the radiologic findings. Paraseptal emphysema is usually subpleural, more frequent in the upper lobes (Fig. 46.2). Bullae are typically present in resected specimens. The dilated airspaces are often collapsed and may not be nearly as dramatic as the appearance by computed tomographic scans.

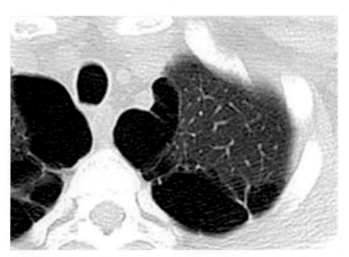

FIGURE 46.1 ▲ CT scan of lung showing subpleural enlarged airspaces with bulla formation in the upper lobes as seen in paraseptal emphysema.

Microscopic Findings

In paraseptal emphysema, the alveolar ducts are enlarged with destruction of distal alveolar septa. Bulla appears often as thin-walled cysts with fibrous wall. The adjacent lung parenchyma appears normal unless there is associated centrilobular emphysema.

Prognosis and Treatment

When in isolation, paraseptal emphysema is not associated with any physiologic abnormality. The main complication is formation of bulla, which may lead to recurrent spontaneous pneumothorax. Treatment includes tube thoracotomy and surgical resection of abnormal lung.[3]

Pulmonary Interstitial Emphysema

Definition

In contrast to the major types of emphysema, pulmonary interstitial emphysema (PIE) is a fundamentally different process in that the formation of the enlarged airspaces is not related to destruction of alveolar septa. In contrast, interstitial emphysema is the result of air dissecting through the alveolar walls into the adjacent interstitial tissues where it forms cystic spaces.

Clinical Findings

PIE is seen primarily in four settings: in neonates with premature lung disease on mechanical ventilation, in adults with centrilobular emphysema, in adults with underlying fibrotic lung disease, and in adults on mechanical ventilation. The major risk factors for the development of PIE in infants are very low birth weight and mechanical ventilation for respiratory distress syndrome. PIE may rarely occur in infants on continuous positive airway pressure (CPAP) who are not mechanically ventilated.[4] Occasional reports describe infants developing PIE in the setting of laryngeal disease or pneumonia in the absence of mechanical ventilation or CPAP.[4] PIE in infants is often associated with pneumothorax or pneumomediastinum.[5]

In adults, incidental interstitial emphysema is a common finding in explants for interstitial lung disease, most frequently usual interstitial pneumonia (see Chapter 17), but is rarely diagnosed radiologically, because of the presence of honeycomb cystic change.[6] An association has been found between a history of previous mechanical ventilation and/or biopsy and the histologic presence of PIE.[6]

In adults on mechanical ventilation, the development of PIE can, in the presence of underlying lung pathology, result in air leak, air block, and secondary infection and may lead to right heart failure and death.[7] There may be extension of the air into perivascular and peribronchial spaces in addition to subpleural areas, in patients with barotrauma,[8] and there may be other air leaks such as pneumothorax and pneumomediastinum.

Radiologic Findings

PIE may be localized or diffuse. Localized PIE (restricted to ≤2 lobes) is characterized by large cysts, whereas diffuse PIE involves all lobes with smaller air cysts.[4] PIE appears as cyst-like radiolucencies or as perivascular linear lucencies. In infants, PIE may resemble congenital pulmonary adenomatoid malformation, bronchogenic cyst, and congenital lobar emphysema.[4]

In adults, in the setting of interstitial lung disease, the most common location is the left upper lobe, and the least common location the right middle lobe.[6]

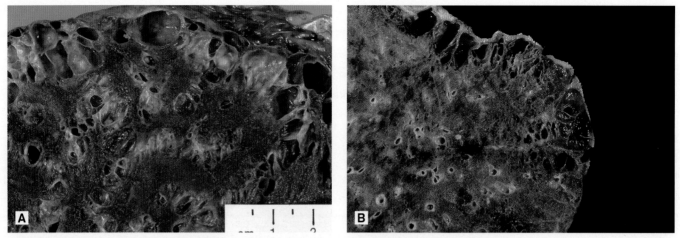

FIGURE 46.2 ▲ **A.** Gross image of paraseptal emphysema with enlarged airspaces located under the pleura and along the interlobular septa. The airspaces are mostly <1 cm. **B.** In contrast, in this gross image, many of the airspaces are >1 cm and constitute bulla. (Gross images courtesy of Dr. Jeffrey Myers.)

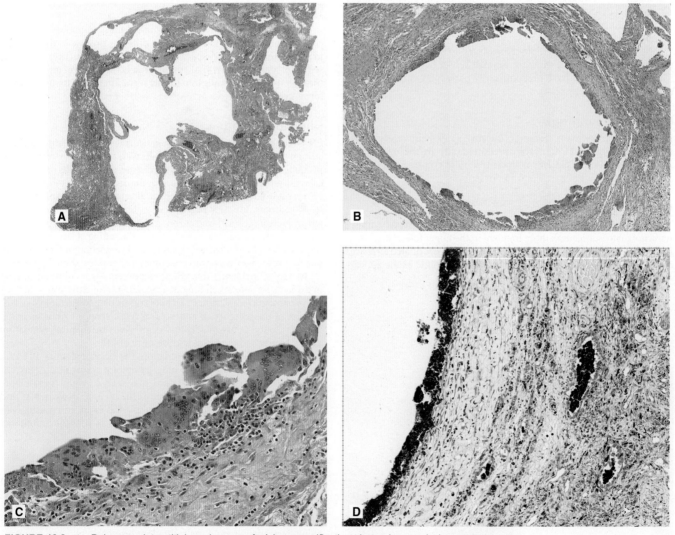

FIGURE 46.3 ▲ Pulmonary interstitial emphysema. **A.** A low magnification photomicrograph demonstrates several enlarged airspaces through the lung resection. **B.** At higher power, this regular, round airspace is surrounded by fibrous tissue of the interstitium and lined by macrophages and multinucleated giant cells. **C.** A higher magnification photomicrograph demonstrates the macrophages and multinucleated giant cells lining the cyst, with underlying collagen. **D.** Immunohistochemical staining for CD68 confirms the nature of the lining cells.

Microscopic Findings

Airspaces around bronchovascular bundles or subpleural spaces are present surrounded by fibrous tissue and recognized by the lining of macrophages with multinucleated giant cells or mesothelial cells (Fig. 46.3). In contrast, enlarged airspaces of the major types of emphysema are bordered by lung tissue or interlobular septa and lined by pneumocytes.

There may be a chronic inflammatory reaction including eosinophils and loose fibrotic reaction mimicking organizing pneumonia.[6] Immunohistochemical staining for CD68 is helpful in delineating the macrophages and giant cells lining the cyst walls.

Prognosis and Treatment

In a review of the published literature, a significant proportion of localized PIE in children eventually require surgical resection. Some cases in infants can be treated conservatively.[5]

In the adult patient who is already in a state of respiratory compromise, PIE with pneumothorax and alteration in cardiovascular dynamics can constitute a terminal event.[7,8]

REFERENCES

1. Kukkonen MK, Tiili E, Vehmas T, et al. Association of genes of protease-antiprotease balance pathway to lung function and emphysema subtypes. *BMC Pulm Med.* 2013;13:36.
2. Smith BM, Austin JH, Newell JD Jr, et al. Pulmonary emphysema subtypes on computed tomography: the MESA COPD study. *Am J Med.* 2014;127:94.e7–94.e23.
3. Jordan KG, Kwong JS, Flint J, et al. Surgically treated pneumothorax. Radiologic and pathologic findings. *Chest.* 1997;111:280–285.
4. Bawa P, Soontarapornchai K, Perenyi A, et al. Development of localized pulmonary interstitial emphysema in a late preterm infant without mechanical ventilation. *Case Rep Pediatr.* 2014;2014:429797.
5. Jassal MS, Benson JE, Mogayzel PJ Jr. Spontaneous resolution of diffuse persistent pulmonary interstitial emphysema. *Pediatr Pulmonol.* 2008;43:615–619.
6. Barcia SM, Kukreja J, Jones KD. Pulmonary interstitial emphysema in adults: a clinicopathologic study of 53 lung explants. *Am J Surg Pathol.* 2014;38:339–45.
7. Unger JM, England DM, Bogust GA. Interstitial emphysema in adults: recognition and prognostic implications. *J Thorac Imaging.* 1989;4:86–94.
8. Sherren PB, Jovaisa T. Pulmonary interstitial emphysema presenting in a woman on the intensive care unit: case report and review of literature. *J Med Case Rep.* 2011;5:236.

SECTION SEVEN
AUTOIMMUNE LUNG DISEASE

47 Pulmonary Capillaritis
Fabio R. Tavora, M.D., Ph.D., and Allen P. Burke, M.D.

Background

Pulmonary vasculitis denotes inflammation of the capillaries of the alveolar septa (small-vessel vasculitis), a condition that often causes diffuse alveolar hemorrhage (DAH).[1,2] Vasculitis involving muscular arteries may occur with granulomatosis with polyangiitis and secondarily with infections, and vasculitis of elastic pulmonary arteries may occur in Takayasu disease and Behçet disease (Chapter 51).[3]

Pulmonary capillaritis is only one cause of DAH (see Chapter 29). While DAH is usually a clinical and radiologic diagnosis, largely based on the finding of blood in the bronchoalveolar lavage, pulmonary capillaritis is by definition diagnosed histologically. In most cases, it is associated with systemic, especially renal disease.[4,5]

The most common entities associated with pulmonary capillaritis are granulomatosis with polyangiitis (Wegener disease) and microscopic polyangiitis (MPA), both discussed in Chapter 48, and anti–glomerular basement membrane (GBM) disease (Chapter 50). Other collagen vascular diseases, especially systemic lupus erythematosus, may manifest as capillaritis. A list of causes of pulmonary capillaritis is presented in Table 47.1.

Pathogenesis

The deposition of immune complexes along the capillary vasculature plays an important role in the pathogenesis of pulmonary capillaritis. Furthermore, a genetic basis is suspected for cases of autoimmune disease–associated DAH, especially in cases of MPA.[6,7] Serum antinuclear cytoplasmic autoantibodies (ANCA) directly activate neutrophils, causing injury to the capillary endothelium, chemotaxis, and release of myeloperoxidase (MPO) that damages the endothelium

TABLE 47.1 Conditions Associated with Pulmonary Capillaritis

Pauci-immune
Microscopic polyangiitis
Granulomatosis with polyangiitis
Idiopathic (isolated) pauci-immune pulmonary capillaritis (IPPC)
Idiopathic (isolated) pauci-immune pulmonary–renal syndrome
Eosinophilic granulomatosis with polyangiitis (Churg-Strauss)
Drug-induced ANCA (hydralazine, PTU)

Immune-complex–mediated and other immunologic disorders
Anti–glomerular basement membrane disease
Systemic lupus erythematosus
Rheumatoid arthritis
IgA nephropathy
Behçet syndrome
Acute allograft rejection
Antiphospholipid syndrome
Inflammatory bowel disease
Autoimmune hepatitis
Juvenile rheumatoid arthritis

resulting in hemorrhage. Increased vascular permeability also contributes to acute hemorrhage.

Clinical Findings

Although most cases of biopsy-proven capillaritis occur in patients with DAH, many patients with DAH have other causes (see Chapter 29).[8] Hypoxemic respiratory failure accompanied by a decline of hemoglobin without hemolysis is suggestive of DAH. The diagnosis is confirmed by bronchoalveolar lavage retrieving bright red fluid, or increasing blood in the fluid, with negative cultures and the appearance of hemosiderin macrophages.

Lung biopsy is generally not recommended for confirmation of the diagnosis, unless there is question about the presence of alveolar hemorrhage and the etiology of interstitial lung process.

It is unknown how often capillaritis is subclinical without causing overt pulmonary hemorrhage. In a series of open lung biopsies for granulomatous lesions of granulomatosis with polyangiitis without DAH, almost one-third showed areas of capillaritis.[9] In an autopsy study of 90 patients with lupus, of the 3 with capillaritis, only 1 had massive DAH.[10] Subclinical hemorrhage in MPA has been hypothesized to result in chronic fibrotic lung disease.[11]

Among patients with MPA, which is frequently associated with capillaritis, the most common symptoms are weight loss, malaise, myalgias, and arthralgias; only 10% develop DAH.[12]

Pulmonary–Renal Syndrome

The term "pulmonary–renal syndrome" is often employed for the concomitant inflammation of glomerular capillaries (glomerulonephritis) and pulmonary capillaritis. Many of the causes of capillaritis can also result in renal disease, notable MPA, granulomatosis with polyangiitis, and anti-GBM disease. Capillaritis is an uncommon manifestation of lupus erythematosus and is even less common in other autoimmune disorders.

Hypertensive renal crisis with or without systemic sclerosis (scleroderma renal crisis) is associated with pulmonary hemorrhage, but renal biopsies demonstrate thrombotic microangiopathy, and there is often clinical evidence of hemolysis; histologic findings in the lung are unknown in this syndrome.[13–15]

Radiologic Findings

Imaging demonstrates alveolar opacities with density ranging from ground glass to consolidation that are typically bilateral, symmetric, diffuse, and depending, sometimes with crazy paving and airspace bronchograms.

Pathologic Findings

The classical pathologic description of pulmonary capillaritis was published in 1985.[1] The features include interstitial red blood cells or hemosiderin, fibrinoid necrosis of capillary walls, fibrin

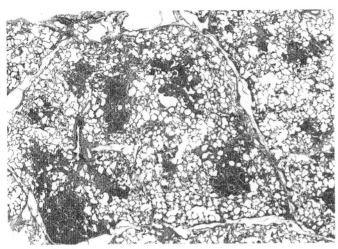

FIGURE 47.1 ▲ Pulmonary capillaritis. Low magnification shows patchy interstitial hemorrhage.

thrombi, neutrophils in the interstitium and within alveoli, and fibrin deposition in the interalveolar septa (Figs. 47.1 and 47.2). Intra-alveolar collections of red blood cells, fibrin, and hemosiderin-laden macrophages, admixed with neutrophils with mild thickening of the interstitium, with neutrophils and lymphocytes, are typical.[5,16]

The role of immunofluorescence in the diagnosis, especially to distinguish pauci-immune from immune-complex–related capillaritis, is not as established as that for glomerulonephritis. Immunohistochemical staining for complement deposition in lung capillaries is difficult, especially on paraffin-embedded material, and is most extensively studied in transplant lung biopsies, in which case it is not generally recommended. If the surgeon requests immunofluorescent study on lung biopsies for complement deposition

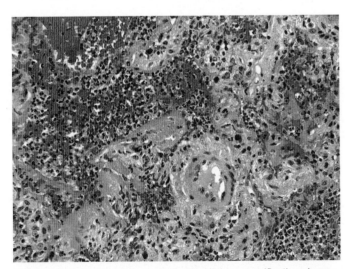

FIGURE 47.2 ▲ Pulmonary capillaritis. Higher magnification shows necrosis of alveolar septa with neutrophils in the septa and alveolar spaces.

(especially in cases without renal biopsy), then one biopsy fragment should be retained for direct immunofluorescence for a panel of complement and immunoglobulins that is generally performed in the renal pathology laboratory. A linear distribution is characteristic of anti-GB disease, similar to the findings in glomeruli. A negative or weak result is consistent with pauci-immune capillaritis, and granular deposits immune-complex–mediated capillaritis. In practice, the immunofluorescent study is performed only after routine light microscopy demonstrates findings suspicious or diagnostic of capillaritis. Otherwise, the tissue can be processed normally for additional light microscopic study.

The diagnosis of capillaritis is usually made by video-assisted thoracoscopic wedge biopsy, although it can be suggested by transbronchial biopsies.[17]

REFERENCES

1. Mark EJ, Ramirez JF. Pulmonary capillaritis and hemorrhage in patients with systemic vasculitis. *Arch Pathol Lab Med.* 1985;109:413–418.
2. Myers JL, Katzenstein AL. Wegener's granulomatosis presenting with massive pulmonary hemorrhage and capillaritis. *Am J Surg Pathol.* 1987;11: 895–898.
3. Fishbein GA, Fishbein MC. Lung vasculitis and alveolar hemorrhage: pathology. *Semin Respir Crit Care Med.* 2011;32:254–263.
4. Jin JJ, Shi JH, Lu WX, et al. [Clinical features of pulmonary involvement in patients with microscopic polyangiitis]. *Zhonghua Jie He He Hu Xi Za Zhi.* 2011;34:339–343.
5. Travis WD, Colby TV, Lombard C, et al. A clinicopathologic study of 34 cases of diffuse pulmonary hemorrhage with lung biopsy confirmation. *Am J Surg Pathol.* 1990;14:1112–1125.
6. Collins CE, Quismorio FP Jr. Pulmonary involvement in microscopic polyangiitis. *Curr Opin Pulm Med.* 2005;11:447–451.
7. Kupfer O, Ridall LA, Hoffman LM, et al. Pulmonary capillaritis in monozygotic twin boys. *Pediatrics.* 2013;132:e1445–e1448.
8. Fullmer JJ, Langston C, Dishop MK, et al. Pulmonary capillaritis in children: a review of eight cases with comparison to other alveolar hemorrhage syndromes. *J Pediatr.* 2005;146:376–381.
9. Travis WD, Hoffman GS, Leavitt RY, et al. Surgical pathology of the lung in Wegener's granulomatosis. Review of 87 open lung biopsies from 67 patients. *Am J Surg Pathol.* 1991;15:315–333.
10. Quadrelli SA, Alvarez C, Arce SC, et al. Pulmonary involvement of systemic lupus erythematosus: analysis of 90 necropsies. *Lupus.* 2009;18:1053–1060.
11. Birnbaum J, Danoff S, Askin FB, et al. Microscopic polyangiitis presenting as a "pulmonary-muscle" syndrome: is subclinical alveolar hemorrhage the mechanism of pulmonary fibrosis? *Arthritis Rheum.* 2007;56: 2065–2071.
12. Agard C, Mouthon L, Mahr A, et al. Microscopic polyangiitis and polyarteritis nodosa: how and when do they start? *Arthritis Rheum.* 2003;49: 709–715.
13. Badwal S, Kotwal J, Varma PP. Unusual case of pulmonary renal syndrome with autopsy findings. *Indian J Pathol Microbiol.* 2013;56:294–296.
14. Abdallah E, Al-Helal B, Al-Rashidi A, et al. ANCA negative pulmonary renal syndrome with pathologic findings of thrombotic microangiopathy. *Arab J Nephrol Transplant.* 2013;6:31–35.
15. Park HS, Hong YA, Chung BH, et al. Malignant hypertension with an unusual presentation mimicking the immune mediated pulmonary renal syndrome. *Yonsei Med J.* 2012;53:1224–1227.
16. Myers JL, Katzenstein AA. Microangiitis in lupus-induced pulmonary hemorrhage. *Am J Clin Pathol.* 1986;85:552–556.
17. Ishiguro T, Takayanagi N, Yamaguchi S, et al. Pulmonary Capillaritis in Wegener's Granulomatosis Detected Via Transbronchial Lung Biopsy. *Intern Med.* 2012;51:905–909.

48 ANCA-Associated Vasculitides: Granulomatosis with Polyangiitis and Microscopic Polyangiitis

Andre C. Teixeira, M.D., Fabio R. Tavora, M.D., Ph.D., and Marie-Christine Aubry, M.D.

Introduction and Terminology

ANCA-associated vasculitides (AAV) are considered necrotizing vasculitides, with few or no immune deposits, predominantly affecting small vessels (capillaries, venules, arterioles, and small arteries), characterized by circulating antibodies, the antineutrophil cytoplasmic antibodies (ANCAs). They are further classified as granulomatosis with polyangiitis (GPA, formerly Wegener granulomatosis [WG]), microscopic polyangiitis (MPA), and eosinophilic granulomatosis with polyangiitis (EGPA, formerly Churg-Strauss syndrome) (Chapter 49).

Since the first descriptions by Godman and Churg,[1,2] vasculitides have been classified by the caliber of the vessel involved. In 1990, the American College of Rheumatology (ACR) criteria assigned a new classification to most patients, but there was an unacceptable degree of overlap between the entities.[3,4] These criteria were amended in 1994 by the Chapel Hill Consensus Conference, which restricted WG to those with granulomatous inflammation, included ANCAs, and introduced MPA as a novel category.[5] A further change to the nomenclature of AAV occurred in 2012, following a second Chapel Hill Consensus Conference.[6] Eponyms were replaced where possible with terms consistent with the known pathophysiology of each condition; hence, WG was renamed GPA.[7]

GPA is defined as a necrotizing granulomatous inflammation of the upper and lower respiratory tract, with necrotizing vasculitis of small- and medium-sized vessels. Necrotizing glomerulonephritis is common, but it is not essential for the diagnosis. According to the current criteria of the ACR, GPA is defined by the presence of at least two of the following four criteria: sinus involvement, lung x-ray showing nodules, a fixed pulmonary infiltrate or cavities, urinary sediment with hematuria or red cell casts, and histologic granulomas within an artery or in the perivascular area of an artery or arteriole. MPA is a necrotizing vasculitis, with few or no immune deposits, predominantly affecting small vessels. Necrotizing arteritis involving small and medium arteries may be present.[8] Necrotizing glomerulonephritis is very common, and pulmonary capillaritis often occurs, but granulomatous inflammation is usually absent.

Etiology and Pathogenesis

The causes of AAV are unknown, and multiple factors play a role in its pathogenesis. AAV have a higher prevalence among the Chinese and Japanese populations.[9] Familial AAV has been described and, while a putative hereditary factor has never been demonstrated, studies have indicated some genes related to disease susceptibility such as SERPINA-1 and PRTN-3.[9,10] Single nucleotide polymorphisms in the major histocompatibility complex have also been reported. Several environmental factors probably related to AAV are deficiency of vitamin D, infections, silica exposure, and cocaine use.[11-13]

AAV is characterized by pauci-immune vascular inflammation, in which immunoglobulin deposition cannot be detected, and circulation of ANCAs is present. The proposed role for ANCA is of indirect recruitment of an autoinflammatory response.[10] There is increasing evidence of other factors involved in AAV pathogenesis, like complement factors and T cells. By indirect immunofluorescence, two well-recognized staining patterns of ANCA tend to show associations with specific diseases. In active GPA, the majority of ANCA demonstrates a cytoplasmic pattern (c-ANCA), although 5% to 20% of ANCA may exhibit a perinuclear pattern (p-ANCA). In MPA, the staining pattern tends to be perinuclear. The target antigen of c-ANCA is antiproteinase 3 (PR3-ANCA), a constituent of the azurophilic granules, and of p-ANCA, antimyeloperoxidase (MPO-ANCA).

Granulomatosis with Polyangiitis

Incidence, Clinical and Radiologic Findings

GPA is approximately twice as common as MPA. The age at diagnosis is between 45 and 60 years, and men and women are affected with similar frequency. The incidence of GPA has been evaluated between 7 and 12 new cases per million inhabitants per year.[14] Constitutional signs (fever, asthenia, weight loss) are frequent (50%) but nonspecific. Sinonasal involvement is the most common manifestation of GPA. Ear, nose, and throat symptoms and signs are present in 70% to 100% of cases at diagnosis. Lung involvement affects 50% to 90% of patients, sometimes associated with tracheal and subglottic stenosis (16%).[15] The most typical form of renal involvement is focal segmental necrotizing glomerulonephritis without deposition of immune complexes. The peripheral nervous system is affected in about one-third of patients, characterized by sensorimotor neuropathy. Other common sites of involvement are skin (10% to 50%), eyes (14% to 60%), heart (<10%), and gastrointestinal tract (5% to 11%). GPA may also be limited to the lungs with no other organ involvement and usually associated with a negative ANCA.[16]

The most common radiologic patterns of GPA include multiple angiocentric nodules or masses, frequently cavitated and associated with signs of hemorrhage as random alveolar opacities and pneumonic condensations. Pulmonary fibrosis and pleural involvement occur less commonly but can be present.

Histopathology

The classic histologic picture of GPA consists of necrotizing granulomatous inflammation accompanied by necrotizing vasculitis. The necrotic areas are usually irregular in contour, so-called geographic, with a basophilic "dirty" appearance due to the nuclear debris of the necrotic neutrophils (Fig. 48.1). The necrotic areas are surrounded by palisading epithelioid histiocytes and typically include multinucleated giant cells (Fig. 48.1). The multinucleated giant cells are often scattered in the inflammatory background. They have a distinctive appearance due to their hyperchromatic nuclei and thus easily recognizable even at low power. Background interstitial fibrosis and nonspecific chronic inflammation are typically present.

Necrotizing vasculitis is recognized by the presence of fibrinoid necrosis and neutrophils involving the media of the vessels. In florid cases, the entire vessel may be involved (Fig. 48.2). However, the vasculitis is most readily recognized when it only partially affects the vessel. Subtle cases of vasculitis may show only necrotic neutrophils in the vessel wall. It is important to identify the vasculitis in the surrounding viable parenchyma to avoid overdiagnosing necrotizing vasculitis as vessels in areas of necrosis will appear necrotic regardless of the etiology of the necrosis. An elastic stain may assist in identifying the vasculitis.

Eosinophils can be present, but they are usually less numerous than neutrophils. Other features commonly present are small micro-abscesses, necrosis of collagen, and organizing pneumonia (OP) at the periphery of the main lesions.[17]

Vasculitis in GPA affects both arteries and veins. Occasionally, capillaries may be predominantly involved by a necrotizing capillaritis. In this setting, patients present with a clinical picture of diffuse alveolar

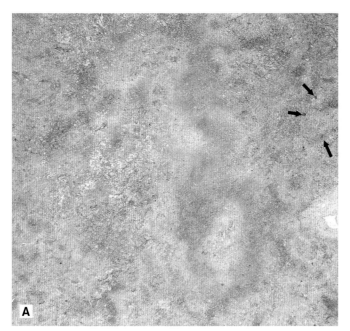

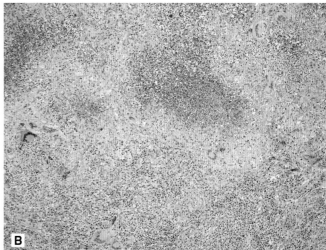

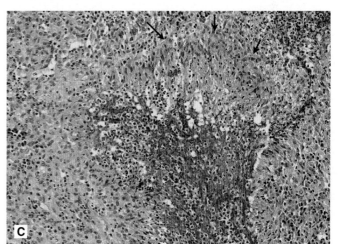

FIGURE 48.1 ▲ Granulomatosis with polyangiitis. **A.** Geographic necrosis, low magnification. The basophilic necrosis is the result of apoptotic neutrophils. Even at low power, dark staining multinucleated giant cells are visible (*arrows*) **B.** Isolated giant cells that do not form distinct granulomas are typical. **C.** There is often palisading of slightly spindled macrophages (*arrows*).

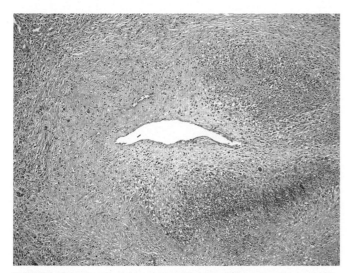

FIGURE 48.2 ▲ Granulomatosis with polyangiitis, necrotizing arteritis. The vessel is nearly all involved by an inflammatory and destructive process. Large areas of necrosis with giant cells replace most of the wall of the vessel.

hemorrhage similar to MPA and the diagnosis of GPA made on the basis of the PR3-ANCA.

GPA may be suspected and even diagnosed in small biopsies, usually transthoracic needle biopsies (Fig. 48.3). The diagnosis is almost never made in transbronchial biopsies due to sampling.

Variants of GPA have been described. They include the bronchocentric variant (Fig. 48.4), OP-like variant (Fig. 48.4), and eosinophilic variant. There is no clinical significance to these variants.

Differential Diagnosis

GPA is typically biopsied in an unusual clinical setting. When classic histologic features are present, GPA can be diagnosed on the basis of morphology alone. The main differential diagnosis is with necrotizing granulomatous inflammation due to infection. Histologically, the necrosis in infectious necrotizing granulomas tends to be more regular and circumscribed in contrast to the irregular, jagged contours of the necrosis in GPA. Although prominent inflammation may be seen in the vessels adjacent to infectious necrotizing granulomas, a true necrotizing vasculitis is not typically present. Identification of microorganisms with microbiologic studies and histochemical stains is critical to the diagnosis. However, the absence of microorganisms does not indicate that the granulomatous inflammation is due to GPA.[18] Finally, lymph node involvement by granulomatous inflammation is absent in GPA.

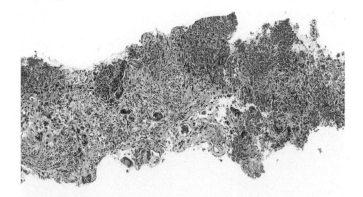

FIGURE 48.3 ▲ Granulomatosis with polyangiitis, core biopsy. "Dirty" suppurative necrosis with scattered hyperchromatic multinucleated giant cells suggests the diagnosis of GPA.

In GPA-eosinophilic variant, the eosinophilic infiltrate may be so prominent as to raise the diagnosis of EGPA (Chapter 49). In GPA-bronchocentric variant, the necrotizing granulomatous inflammation centers upon and destroys bronchioles and needs to be distinguished from bronchocentric granulomatosis (BCG) (Chapter 33). In the OP-like GPA, extensive intraluminal organization is present mimicking OP (Chapter 5); however, the distinctive multinucleated giant cells of GPA are present within the intraluminal fibrosis as well as hemosiderin-laden macrophages. Small suppurative granulomas may also be seen.[19]

Lymphomatoid granulomatosis (Chapter 90) may mimic GPA because of the presence of necrosis and angiocentric inflammation. The angiocentric inflammation contains atypical, neoplastic, lymphocytes.

Rheumatoid nodule can be indistinguishable from the necrotizing granulomatous inflammation of GPA. A true necrotizing vasculitis is not present. Finally, rheumatoid nodules in the lung rarely occur in the absence of rheumatoid nodules of the skin and known history of rheumatoid arthritis.

Prognosis and Treatment

GPA is a serious disease, with a nearly always-fatal outcome in the absence of treatment. Relapses occur frequently. One-quarter of patients relapse within 2 years of the diagnosis.

Current therapeutic strategies consist of glucocorticoids in conjunction with either conventional (azathioprine, methotrexate, and leflunomide) or biologic agents (rituximab, etanercept) for both induction of remission or remission maintenance. Cyclophosphamide in combination with glucocorticoids is the main option for severe AAV. Due to toxicity and side effect profile of long-term treatment, the paradigm in AAV has been to induce remission with cyclophosphamide and then switch to an alternative immunosuppressive therapy after three to 6 months. In patients receiving rituximab or methotrexate as initial induction therapy, these same medications can often be continued to maintain remission.[20,21]

Microscopic Polyangiitis

Incidence, Clinical and Radiologic Findings

The age of onset of MPA ranges from 50 to 60 years old, with a slight male predominance. Fever and weight loss are common symptoms. The kidney is the most commonly affected organ. Other sites of involvement are lungs, joints, heart, and the gastrointestinal and the peripheral nervous systems. Renal involvement in MPA is present in 90% of cases and is usually manifested by microscopic hematuria with cellular casts in combination with proteinuria. Lung involvement is characterized by diffuse alveolar hemorrhage with dyspnea, cough, and hemoptysis. In contrast to GPA, sinonasal manifestations are generally absent.[22,23] ANCA are present in up to 80% of patients and are usually p-ANCA (MPO-ANCA).

MPA manifests as bilateral alveolar consolidations, indicative of alveolar hemorrhages. There are usually no masses or nodules. Pulmonary fibrosis has been described in patients with MPA and is more common than in the setting of GPA.[24]

Histopathology

MPA is mainly characterized by diffuse alveolar hemorrhage with capillaritis (Chapter 47) (Fig. 48.5). The hemorrhage is characterized by alveolar spaces filled with fibrin admixed with red cells. Hemosiderin-laden macrophages are common. The diagnosis of capillaritis is suspected by the focal expansion and disruption of alveolar septa by inflammation, predominantly by neutrophils, often necrotic with nuclear dust. Necrotizing arteritis involving small- and medium-sized arteries can be present. Occasionally, particularly at autopsy, the histologic picture may be complicated by diffuse alveolar damage with hyaline membranes.[25-29]

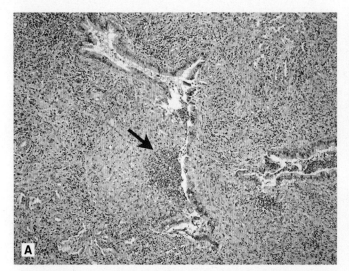
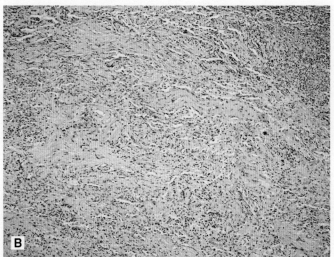

FIGURE 48.4 ▲ **A.** GPA-bronchocentric variant. The bronchial wall is partially replaced by the necrotizing granulomatous inflammation (*arrow*). **B.** GPA-organizing pneumonia-like variant. Organizing pneumonia (OP) dominates the histologic findings, however, hemosiderin-laden macrophages and multinucleated giant cells are admixed. Areas of necrotic neutrophils are also present.

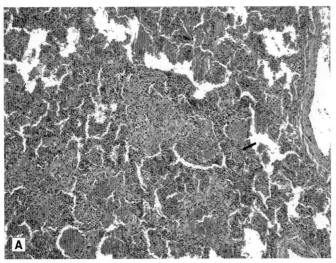
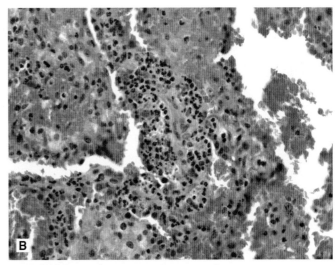

FIGURE 48.5 ▲ Microscopic polyangiitis. **A.** Alveolar hemorrhage dominates the histologic picture. Focally (*arrow*), the alveolar septa are expanded by an inflammatory process. **B.** Capillaritis with expansion of the alveolar septa by neutrophils and eosinophils. Nuclear dust as a result of necrotic neutrophils is present.

Differential Diagnosis

Diffuse alveolar hemorrhage and capillaritis is not specific to MPA and many other etiologies produce the same histologic picture (Chapter 47). The final diagnosis and etiology rely on the clinical history and presentation and serologic tests.

Prognosis and Treatment

MPA's prognosis is reserved without treatment (mortality of 90% after 1 year). The introduction of aggressive immunosuppressive treatment, in particular cyclophosphamide in combination with prednisone, has substantially improved the prognosis. Mortality within first year of disease occurs due to infection or active vasculitis, whereas later in the disease course, mortality is related to cardiovascular disease, malignancy, and infections.

REFERENCES

1. Godman GC, Churg J. Wegener's granulomatosis: pathology and review of the literature. *AMA Arch Pathol.* 1954;58(6):533–553.
2. Mohammad AJ, et al. Incidence and survival rates in Wegener's granulomatosis, microscopic polyangiitis, Churg-Strauss syndrome and polyarteritis nodosa. *Rheumatology (Oxford).* 2009;48(12):1560–1565.
3. Hunder GG, et al. The American College of Rheumatology 1990 criteria for the classification of vasculitis. Introduction. *Arthritis Rheum.* 1990;33(8):1065–1067.
4. Fries JF, et al. The American College of Rheumatology 1990 criteria for the classification of vasculitis. Summary. *Arthritis Rheum.* 1990;33(8):1135–1136.
5. Jennette JC, et al. Nomenclature of systemic vasculitides. Proposal of an international consensus conference. *Arthritis Rheum.* 1994;37(2):187–192.
6. Jennette JC, et al. 2012 Revised International Chapel Hill Consensus Conference nomenclature of vasculitides. *Arthritis Rheum.* 2013;65(1):1–11.
7. Falk RJ, et al. Granulomatosis with polyangiitis (Wegener's): an alternative name for Wegener's granulomatosis. *J Am Soc Nephrol.* 2011;22(4):587–588.
8. Jennette JC. Overview of the 2012 revised International Chapel Hill Consensus Conference nomenclature of vasculitides. *Clin Exp Nephrol.* 2013;17(5):603–606.
9. Bonatti F, et al. Genetic susceptibility to ANCA-associated vasculitis: state of the art. *Front Immunol.* 2014;5:577.
10. McKinney EF, et al. The immunopathology of ANCA-associated vasculitis. *Semin Immunopathol.* 2014;36(4):461–478.
11. Graf J, et al. Purpura, cutaneous necrosis, and antineutrophil cytoplasmic antibodies associated with levamisole-adulterated cocaine. *Arthritis Rheum.* 2011;63(12):3998–4001.
12. Cantorna MT, Mahon BD. Mounting evidence for vitamin D as an environmental factor affecting autoimmune disease prevalence. *Exp Biol Med (Maywood).* 2004;229(11):1136–1142.
13. Hogan SL, et al. Association of silica exposure with anti-neutrophil cytoplasmic autoantibody small-vessel vasculitis: a population-based, case–control study. *Clin J Am Soc Nephrol.* 2007;2(2):290–299.
14. Corral-Gudino L, et al. Differences in the incidence of microscopic polyangiitis and granulomatosis with polyangiitis (Wegener's). Is there a latitudinal gradient? *J Rheumatol.* 2011;38(11):2494–2496.
15. Gomez-Gomez A, et al. Pulmonary manifestations of granulomatosis with polyangiitis. *Reumatol Clin.* 2014;10:288–293.
16. Pagnoux C, et al. Wegener's granulomatosis strictly and persistently localized to one organ is rare: assessment of 16 patients from the French Vasculitis Study Group database. *J Rheumatol.* 2011;38(3):475–478.
17. Travis WD, et al. Surgical pathology of the lung in Wegener's granulomatosis. *Am J Surg Pathol.* 1991;15(4):315–333.
18. Mukhopadhyay S, et al. Pulmonary necrotizing granulomas of unknown cause: clinical and pathologic analysis of 131 patients with completely resected nodules. *Chest.* 2013;144(3):813–824.
19. Uner AH, Rozum-Slota B, Katzenstein AL. Bronchiolitis obliterans-organizing pneumonia (BOOP)-like variant of Wegener's granulomatosis. A clinicopathologic study of 16 cases. *Am J Surg Pathol.* 1996;20(7):794–801.
20. Ozaki T, et al. Large-vessel involvement in granulomatosis with polyangiitis successfully treated with rituximab: a case report and literature review. *Mod Rheumatol.* 2015:1–6.
21. Lembicz M, Batura-Gabryel H, Nowicka A. [Granulomatosis with polyangiitis—clinical picture and review of current treatment options]. *Pneumonol Alergol Pol.* 2014;82(1):61–73.
22. Lally L, Spiera R. Current therapies for ANCA-associated vasculitis. *Annu Rev Med.* 2014;66(1):227–240.
23. Katsuyama T, Sada KE, Makino H. Current concept and epidemiology of systemic vasculitides. *Allergol Int.* 2014;63(4):505–513.
24. Comarmond C, et al. Pulmonary fibrosis in antineutrophil cytoplasmic antibodies (ANCA)-associated vasculitis. *Medicine.* 2014;93(24):318–327.
25. Gaudin PB, et al. The pathologic spectrum of pulmonary lesions in patients with anti-neutrophil cytoplasmic autoantibodies specific for anti-proteinase 3 and anti-myeloperoxidase. *Am J Clin Pathol.* 1995;104(1):7–16.
26. Akikusa B, et al. Six cases of microscopic polyarteritis exhibiting acute interstitial pneumonia. *Pathol Int.* 1995;45(8):580–588.
27. Gal AA, Salinas FF, Staton GW Jr. The clinical and pathological spectrum of antineutrophil cytoplasmic autoantibody-related pulmonary disease. A comparison between perinuclear and cytoplasmic antineutrophil cytoplasmic autoantibodies. *Arch Pathol Lab Med.* 1994;118(12):1209–1214.
28. Wang H, Sun L, Tan W. Clinical features of children with pulmonary microscopic polyangiitis: report of 9 cases. *PLoS One.* 2015;10(4):e0124352.
29. Fishbein GA, Fishbein MC. Lung vasculitis and alveolar hemorrhage: pathology. *Semin Respir Crit Care Med.* 2011;32(3):254–263.

49 Eosinophilic Granulomatosis with Polyangiitis (Churg-Strauss Syndrome)

Allen P. Burke, M.D., and Marie-Christine Aubry, M.D.

Terminology

Eosinophilic granulomatosis with polyangiitis (EGPA), also known as Churg-Strauss syndrome, is a systemic vasculitis that typically involves the lungs.[1] The eponym "Churg-Strauss syndrome" stems from a publication of Jacob Churg and Lotte Strauss in 1951, in which they described 13 patients with pulmonary "periarteritis nodosa," allergic symptoms, peripheral eosinophilia, and eosinophilic vasculitis.[2] The term "Churg-Strauss syndrome" was not applied to the disease until the 1970s.[3,4] In 1985, Andrew Churg clarified the distinction between EGPA and granulomatosis with polyangiitis (GPA) also known as Wegener granulomatosis, two systemic vasculitic syndromes with a granulomatous component, from other granulomatous diseases of the lung such as bronchocentric granulomatosis, lymphomatoid granulomatosis, and necrotizing sarcoidosis.[5] Another term that has been used for Churg-Strauss syndrome is "allergic granulomatosis and angiitis."[4,6,7] The current International Chapel Hill Consensus Conference nomenclature refers to Churg-Strauss syndrome as EGPA, in part because the allergic nature of the disease has been questioned, and for "symmetry" with GPA and microscopic polyangiitis (MPA).[8] Since 30% to 40% of patients with EGPA have antineutrophilic cytoplasmic antibodies (ANCA), it is classified with GPA and MPA as one of the ANCA-associated vasculitides.[8] In the ACR/CHCC (American College of Rheumatology/Chapel Hill Consensus Conference), EGPA is defined as "Eosinophil-rich and necrotizing granulomatous inflammation often involving the respiratory tract, and necrotizing vasculitis predominantly affecting small to medium vessels, and associated with asthma and eosinophilia. ANCA is more frequent when glomerulonephritis is present."[8] This description is "nosologic" or definitional, not to be used for diagnostic criteria.[8]

Etiology

The classic theory asserts that EGPA is an allergic reaction with an exaggerated tissue response resulting in tissue destruction mediated by destructive enzymes within eosinophil granules.[7,9] There may be a genetic component predisposing to the disease, as there has been a reported association with HLA-DRB4 haplotype. Eosinophils show in vitro abnormalities, and humoral immunity is also abnormal, as demonstrated by prominent IgG4 and IgE responses.[9]

Many triggers may be involved in the initial onset of disease, including infection, drugs, and vaccinations.[1] Several reports have documented the progression of asthma to EGPA after leukotriene receptor antagonist treatment,[10] which may represent unmasking of the disease or a reaction to the therapy.

Incidence and Clinical Findings

EGPA is one of the less common vasculitides, and as such a rare disease. Its prevalence ranges from 10.7 to 13 cases per million inhabitants, with an annual incidence of 0.5 to 6.8.[1,9]

As with other vasculitic syndromes, a diagnosis rests on clinical and pathologic findings. A clinical definition without pathologic confirmation includes asthma, blood eosinophilia exceeding 1,500/mm³, and clinical features suggestive of vasculitis involving two or more organs.[11] However, asthma may follow and not precede the vasculitic phase; eosinophilia may fluctuate and disappear, especially after treatment

with corticosteroids; and the clinical manifestations of vasculitis are nonspecific without biopsy confirmation.[1]

The pulmonary manifestations of EGPA include cough, exertional dyspnea, hemoptysis, and chest pain.[12] The division of clinical symptoms into stages (allergic, eosinophilic, and vasculitis) is largely of historic interest as there is no uniform progression of these manifestations.[13]

Extrapulmonary involvement with EGPA is most common in the peripheral nerves and musculoskeletal system, followed by gastrointestinal tract, skin, kidney, central nervous system, and heart. Thrombotic episodes are not uncommon.[14] Multiorgan involvement is typical.[15]

Heart involvement,[16] followed by kidney and lungs,[17] may lead to life-threatening events.

Chest CT scans show bilateral ground-glass opacities and consolidations. Linear opacities, interlobular septal thickening, bronchial dilatation or thickening, and micronodules are not uncommon.[7,12,18]

Serologic Findings

Fewer than one-half of patients show serologic abnormalities, generally perinuclear ANCA (p-ANCA) indirect fluorescence pattern corresponding to the presence of antimyeloperoxidase (MPO) antibodies, as assessed by enzyme-linked immunosorbent assay (ELISA).[19] Antibody levels do not correspond to disease activity. Depending on the series, rheumatoid factor may be positive in almost as high a proportion of patients,[11,20] although antinuclear autoantibodies are generally absent.

Recent data suggest that ANCA positivity separates EGPA into two different clinicopathologic syndromes. Serum autoantibodies are far more common in patients with manifestations of small-vessel vasculitis, especially necrotizing glomerulonephritis, peripheral neuropathy, and pulmonary vasculitis. Patients with cardiac involvement are less likely to have serum ANCA.[1,21]

Microscopic Pathology

EGPA is characterized by a classic triad of eosinophilic pneumonia, granulomatous inflammation, and necrotizing vasculitis. This triad is rarely present in a surgical lung biopsy and the yield in a transbronchial biopsy is even lower[12]; in one report, the diagnosis was made in only 2 of 88 patients.[22] The most common histologic finding is that of an eosinophilic pneumonia (Chapter 26), characterized by airspace accumulation of eosinophils and macrophages (Fig. 49.1). Eosinophilic abscesses and parenchymal necrosis are frequently present and a clue to the diagnosis of EGPA. The granulomatous inflammation, when present, is characterized by palisading histiocytes surrounding areas of necrosis. The vasculitis involves both arteries and veins. Typically, transmural eosinophilic inflammation is present, often with fibrinoid necrosis and with or without granulomatous or giant cell inflammation (Fig. 49.2). Capillaritis is typically not a feature of EGPA.[23,24]

As lung biopsies are often nondiagnostic, skin, nerve, and muscle biopsies are usually performed due to their higher sensitivities (67.4%, 65.7%, and 47.9%, respectively).[22]

Mediastinal lymph node involvement is rare but can be a major or the only manifestation of EGPA.[25–27]

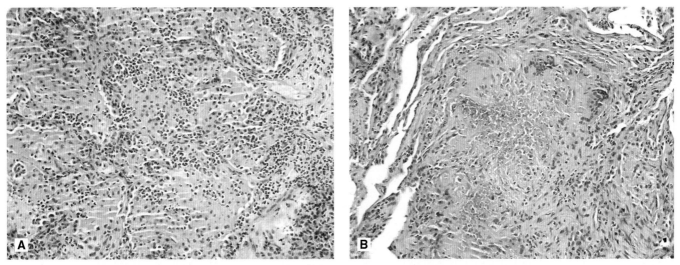

FIGURE 49.1 ▲ **A.** EGPA is characterized by an eosinophilic pneumonia with airspace filling by eosinophils and macrophages (H&E, 200×). **B.** Although not common, necrotizing granulomatous inflammation distinguishes EGPA from simple eosinophilic pneumonia (H&E, 200×).

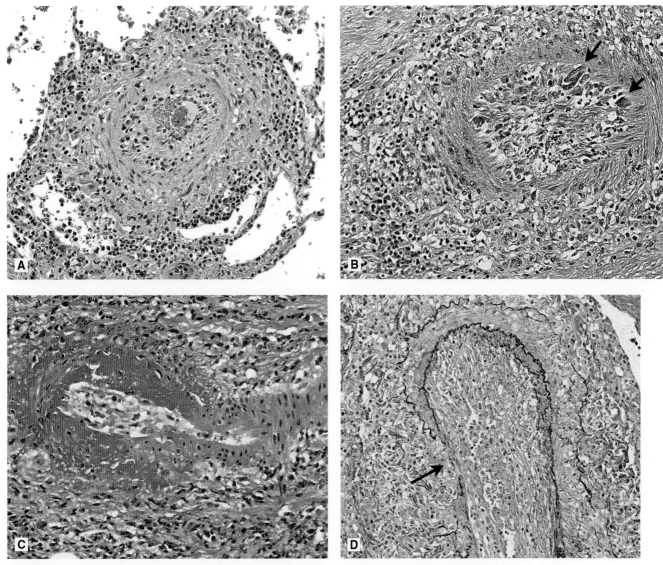

FIGURE 49.2 ▲ **A.** The vasculitis in EGPA is characterized by transmural eosinophilic inflammation, often with intimal thickening and remodeling of the vessel. Multinucleated giant cells **(B)** and fibrinoid necrosis **(C)** confirm the diagnosis of vasculitis. **D.** An elastic stain such as Verhoeff-Van Gieson may be helpful in demonstrating medial destruction (*arrow*).

Differential Diagnosis

The major differential diagnostic considerations are other ANCA vasculitis, especially GPA, with which there may be overlap.[28] Asthma and peripheral eosinophilia are not typically seen in GPA. Furthermore, the serologic finding in GPA is cytoplasmic-ANCA (c-ANCA) directed against proteinase 3. Organs involved also differ. In GPA, the upper respiratory tract is commonly involved and typically not in EGPA. Histologically, GPA shares the presence of necrotizing inflammation and vasculitis. It may even show tissue eosinophilia. But it differs from EGPA by the geographic basaloid ("dirty") necrosis of the granulomatous inflammation. Even when the eosinophils are prominent in GPA, the basaloid necrosis remains comprised of necrotic neutrophils.

EGPA overlaps with hypereosinophilic syndrome (HES), but with a vasculitis component. In general, compared to EGPA, HES patients are less likely to have mononeuritis multiplex, cardiomyopathy, pulmonary manifestations and serum ANCA, and have a higher eosinophil count. Lymphocyte immunophenotyping, clonal T-cell studies, and molecular analyses to detect Fip1-like 1 (FIP1L1) platelet-derived growth factor receptor-alpha (PDGFA) gene fusion are helpful in distinguishing EGPA from lymphoid or myeloid forms of HES.[1]

When EGPA only manifests histologically as eosinophilic pneumonia, it cannot be differentiated from other causes of eosinophilic pneumonia (Chapter 26).

Treatment and Prognosis

The treatment of EGPA is immunosuppressive therapy, primarily glucocorticosteroids.[28] The prognosis and treatment are often measured by a "five-factor" prognostic score, also used for other vasculitic syndromes, such as GPA, MPA, and polyarteritis nodosa. These factors are serum creatinine, proteinuria, gastrointestinal involvement, cardiomyopathy, and central nervous system involvement. Any score above 0 may warrant cyclophosphamide in addition to steroids. Rituximab and mepolizumab (eosinophil-targeted anti-interleukin-5) have also been used in refractory cases.[29]

Prognosis depends partly on extrapulmonary involvement, as assessed by the "five-factor" score.[30] Overall, the 5-year mortality is 8% to 14%, with a relapse-free survival of 57% at 7 years.[19,30] In another study, the 10-year survival rate was even higher (89%), which was comparable to the general population; only cardiac failure resulted in increased mortality in this series.[17]

Bad prognostic signs include age over 65 years; renal, gastrointestinal, or cardiac involvement; presence of anti-MPO antibodies; and eosinophil count below $3,000/mm^3$.[19]

REFERENCES

1. Mouthon L, Dunogue B, Guillevin L. Diagnosis and classification of eosinophilic granulomatosis with polyangiitis (formerly named Churg-Strauss syndrome). *J Autoimmun.* 2014;48–49:99–103.
2. Churg J, Strauss L. Allergic granulomatosis, allergic angiitis, and periarteritis nodosa. *Am J Pathol.* 1951;27(2):277–301.
3. Rosenberg TF, Medsger TA, Jr., DeCicco FA, et al. Allergic granulomatous angiitis (Churg-Strauss syndrome). *J Allergy Clin Immunol.* 1975;55(1):56–67.
4. Chumbley LC, Harrison EG Jr, DeRemee RA. Allergic granulomatosis and angiitis (Churg-Strauss syndrome). Report and analysis of 30 cases. *Mayo Clin Proc.* 1977;52(8):477–484.
5. Churg A. Pulmonary angiitis and granulomatosis revisited. *Hum Pathol.* 1983;14(10):868–883.
6. Masi AT, Hunder GG, Lie JT, et al. The American College of Rheumatology 1990 criteria for the classification of Churg-Strauss syndrome (allergic granulomatosis and angiitis). *Arthritis Rheum.* 1990;33(8):1094–1100.
7. Jeong YJ, Kim KI, Seo IJ, et al. Eosinophilic lung diseases: a clinical, radiologic, and pathologic overview. *Radiographics.* 2007;27(3):617–637; discussion 637–639.
8. Jennette JC, Falk RJ, Bacon PA, et al. 2012 Revised International Chapel Hill Consensus Conference Nomenclature of Vasculitides. *Arthritis Rheum.* 2013;65(1):1–11.
9. Vaglio A, Buzio C, Zwerina J. Eosinophilic granulomatosis with polyangiitis (Churg-Strauss): state of the art. *Allergy.* 2013;68(3):261–273.
10. Wechsler ME, Garpestad E, Flier SR, et al. Pulmonary infiltrates, eosinophilia, and cardiomyopathy following corticosteroid withdrawal in patients with asthma receiving zafirlukast. *JAMA.* 1998;279(6):455–457.
11. Lanham JG, Elkon KB, Pusey CD, et al. Systemic vasculitis with asthma and eosinophilia: a clinical approach to the Churg-Strauss syndrome. *Medicine (Baltimore).* 1984;63(2):65–81.
12. Feng RE, Xu WB, Shi JH, et al. Pathological and high resolution CT findings in Churg-Strauss syndrome. *Chin Med Sci J.* 2011;26(1):1–8.
13. Alberts WM. Pulmonary manifestations of the Churg-Strauss syndrome and related idiopathic small vessel vasculitis syndromes. *Curr Opin Pulm Med.* 2007;13(5):445–450.
14. Whyte AF, Smith WB, Sinkar SN, et al. Clinical and laboratory characteristics of 19 patients with Churg-Strauss syndrome from a single South Australian centre. *Intern Med J.* 2013;43(7):784–790.
15. Choi YH, Im JG, Han BK, et al. Thoracic manifestation of Churg-Strauss syndrome: radiologic and clinical findings. *Chest.* 2000;117(1):117–124.
16. Courand PY, Croisille P, Khouatra C, et al. Churg-Strauss syndrome presenting with acute myocarditis and cardiogenic shock. *Heart Lung Circ.* 2012;21(3):178–181.
17. Moosig F, Bremer JP, Hellmich B, et al. A vasculitis centre based management strategy leads to improved outcome in eosinophilic granulomatosis and polyangiitis (Churg-Strauss, EGPA): monocentric experiences in 150 patients. *Ann Rheum Dis.* 2013;72(6):1011–1017.
18. Szczeklik W, Sokolowska B, Mastalerz L, et al. Pulmonary findings in Churg-Strauss syndrome in chest X-rays and high resolution computed tomography at the time of initial diagnosis. *Clin Rheumatol.* 2010;29(10):1127–1134.
19. Samson M, Puechal X, Devilliers H, et al. Long-term outcomes of 118 patients with eosinophilic granulomatosis with polyangiitis (Churg-Strauss syndrome) enrolled in two prospective trials. *J Autoimmun.* 2013;43:60–69.
20. Yokoyama A, Kohno N, Fujino S, et al. IgG and IgM rheumatoid factor levels parallel interleukin-6 during the vasculitic phase in a patient with Churg-Strauss syndrome. *Intern Med.* 1995;34(7):646–648.
21. Pagnoux C, Guillevin L. Churg-Strauss syndrome: evidence for disease subtypes? *Curr Opin Rheumatol.* 2010;22(1):21–28.
22. Guillevin L, Cohen P, Gayraud M, et al. Churg-Strauss syndrome. Clinical study and long-term follow-up of 96 patients. *Medicine (Baltimore).* 1999;78(1):26–37.
23. Jagadeesh LY, Sangle SR, Verma H, D'Cruz D. Alveolar haemorrhage in eosinophilic granulomatosis and polyangiitis (Churg-Strauss). *Clin Rheumatol.* 2014;33(8):1177–1179.
24. Lai RS, Lin SL, Lai NS, et al. Churg-Strauss syndrome presenting with pulmonary capillaritis and diffuse alveolar hemorrhage. *Scand J Rheumatol.* 1998;27(3):230–232.
25. Churg A, Brallas M, Cronin SR, et al. Formes frustes of Churg-Strauss syndrome. *Chest.* 1995;108(2):320–323.
26. Cualing H, Schroder L, Perme C. Allergic granulomatosis secondary to a limited form of Churg-Strauss syndrome. *Arch Pathol Lab Med.* 2001;125(7):954–957.
27. Casey M, Radel E, Ratech H. Lymph node manifestations of limited Churg-Strauss syndrome. *J Pediatr Hematol Oncol.* 2000;22(5):468–471.
28. Uematsu H, Takata S, Sueishi K, et al. Polyangiitis overlap syndrome of granulomatosis with polyangiitis (Wegener's granulomatosis) and eosinophilic granulomatosis with polyangiitis (Churg-Strauss syndrome). *BMJ Case Rep.* 2014;2014.
29. Mahr A, Moosig F, Neumann T, et al. Eosinophilic granulomatosis with polyangiitis (Churg-Strauss): evolutions in classification, etiopathogenesis, assessment and management. *Curr Opin Rheumatol.* 2014;26(1):16–23.
30. Guillevin L, Pagnoux C, Seror R, et al. The Five-Factor Score revisited: assessment of prognoses of systemic necrotizing vasculitides based on the French Vasculitis Study Group (FVSG) cohort. *Medicine (Baltimore).* 2011;90(1):19–27.

50 Lung Disease in Systemic Autoimmune Disorders

Allen P. Burke, M.D., Seth Kligerman, M.D., and Fabio R. Tavora, M.D., Ph.D.

General Considerations

Virtually, all patterns of lung injury have been associated with rheumatologic lung disease, and none is specific for any given entity (Table 50.1). However, many pathologic diagnoses are more common in some connective tissue disorders than others (Table 50.2). It is important, in general terms, for the pathologist to assess acute changes, such as acute alveolar injury and capillaritis, as well as chronic changes such as the degree of fibrosis, as these features have special importance for short- and long-term prognosis, respectively. In cases of diffuse interstitial lung disease, the presence of pleural inflammation and reactive lymphoid follicles favors autoimmune disease, although these may also occur in idiopathic interstitial pneumonias.

Pulmonary arterial hypertension occurs with increased frequency in patients with autoimmune connective tissue disorders (Table 50.3). In this setting, it is often termed "associated" pulmonary arterial hypertension (see Chapters 62 and 63).

There is often difficulty in establishing a specific diagnosis of connective tissue diseases, as autoantibody levels can fluctuate, along with clinical symptoms. Furthermore, it is not uncommon for lung manifestations to occur at the initial phase of disease or even predate the onset of extrapulmonary symptoms. The concept of undifferentiated connective tissue disease has only relatively recently been developed and is a frequent underlying condition in interstitial lung disease, especially nonspecific interstitial pneumonia (Chapter 17).

Because the treatment of autoimmune diseases is immunosuppression, the primary differential diagnostic consideration, both clinically and pathologically, is an infectious process, which must always be excluded by special stains, especially if fibrin or granulomas are present. Drug reactions are also always a diagnostic consideration. Unlike infections, however, there are no specific tests to prove drug toxicity, which is a diagnosis of exclusion and can only be surmised based on clinical correlation.

Rheumatoid Arthritis

Given the prevalence of rheumatoid arthritis, rheumatoid lung disease is probably the most common "autoimmune lung disorder." Approximately 10% of patients have clinical lung disease, risk factors being advanced age, severe joint symptoms, and male gender.[2] When patients are screened by high-resolution computed tomography, the rate of lung abnormalities is 20% to 44%.[3] It has even been suggested that up to two-thirds of rheumatoid arthritis patients will develop interstitial lung disease.[4]

Clinically, symptoms are variable, including shortness of breath, exercise intolerance, and cough or symptoms related to pleural inflammation. Pulmonary function testing shows obstructive disease, resulting for airway disease; restrictive disease, if there is progression to fibrosis; or a combination of both. There are four major imaging patterns, which correlate to pathologic diagnoses. There are a UIP-like pattern with bilateral subpleural reticulation; an NSIP-like pattern with predominant ground-glass opacities; an inflammatory airway disease pattern with centrilobular branching lines, with or without bronchial dilatation; and an organizing pneumonia pattern with patchy areas of consolidation.[5]

Pathologically, there is a wide range of manifestations of rheumatoid arthritis–interstitial lung disease, although the subacute and chronic phases are most common. Even though organizing pneumonia was classically associated with rheumatoid lung disease, histologic studies show that usual interstitial pneumonia is the most common histopathologic pattern, followed by nonspecific interstitial pneumonia (Fig. 50.1) and then organizing pneumonia.[2] The only specific finding is the presence of rheumatoid nodules, which are uncommon in the lung (Fig. 50.2). *Caplan syndrome*, or rheumatoid pneumoconiosis, is a rare reaction to mineral, coal, or silica dust, manifested by numerous rheumatoid nodules and pulmonary fibrosis in rheumatoid arthritis patients.

Acute lung injury due to diffuse alveolar damage (acute interstitial pneumonia) is an uncommon initial manifestation of rheumatoid lung disease and is similar pathologically and clinically to idiopathic acute interstitial pneumonia. Acute lung injury is more frequently seen as an acute exacerbation of chronic lung disease, sometimes triggered by drug treatment, especially newer immunologic agents.[6–8] Methotrexate-induced pneumonitis is an uncommon complication with nonspecific clinical and histologic findings and is a diagnosis of exclusion.[9]

There are a variety of airway diseases that also occur in rheumatoid lung disease. Bronchiolitis, follicular bronchiolitis, and constrictive bronchiolitis have all been described in rheumatoid arthritis patients.[10,11] Although some degree of airway obstruction and inflammation is common, constrictive bronchiolitis is rare and has a very poor prognosis. It is difficult to ascertain the exact incidence of constrictive (obliterative) bronchiolitis, because of the confusion between organizing pneumonia (bronchiolitis obliterans–organizing pneumonia), which is common, and true obliterative bronchiolitis.[4]

Pulmonary vascular disease is a relatively rare manifestation of rheumatoid arthritis. Pulmonary arterial hypertension is more common in other autoimmune diseases (especially systemic sclerosis).

TABLE 50.1 Pulmonary Pathology in Autoimmune Connective Tissue Disorders

Acute interstitial changes
- Diffuse alveolar damage/acute interstitial pneumonia
- Capillaritis
- Diffuse alveolar hemorrhage

Subacute interstitial changes
- Organizing diffuse alveolar damage
- Organizing pneumonia (OP)
- Nonspecific interstitial pneumonia (NSIP), cellular phase[a]
- Lymphoid (lymphocytic) interstitial pneumonia

Chronic fibrotic changes
- Nonspecific interstitial pneumonia (NSIP), fibrotic phase
- Usual interstitial pneumonia (UIP)

Pulmonary nodules
- Rheumatoid nodules
- Necrobiotic granulomas (Wegener granulomatosis)

Small airway disease
- Bronchiolitis, acute and chronic
- Constrictive (obliterative) bronchiolitis
- Granulomatous bronchiolitis
- Follicular bronchiolitis

Vascular disease
- Pulmonary arterial hypertension
- Thrombosis and thromboembolism
- Capillaritis

[a]An older term, cellular interstitial pneumonia, is not currently in widespread use but describes features of cellular NSIP, Ref.[1]

TABLE 50.2 Frequency and Types of Lung Involvement with Autoimmune Connective Tissue Diseases

Connective Tissue Disease	Frequency of Lung Involvement	Phase of Injury		
		Acute	Subacute	Chronic
Rheumatoid arthritis	20%–40%	Diffuse alveolar damage (uncommon) Capillaritis (rare)	Follicular bronchiolitis Organizing pneumonia (common)	UIP (common) NSIP (less common)
Systemic lupus erythematosus	10%	Capillaritis (rare) Diffuse alveolar damage 1%–4%	Cellular NSIP Organizing pneumonia (uncommon) Lymphoid interstitial pneumonia (uncommon)	NSIP Lymphoid interstitial pneumonia 3%–8%
Mixed connective tissue disease	50% or more	Acute interstitial pneumonia and capillaritis (rare)	Not described	Nonspecific interstitial pneumonia, with rare honeycombing 50% overall, 20% severe
Systemic sclerosis	70% abnormal lung function 90% abnormal computed tomography scans	Diffuse alveolar damage (uncommon) Aspiration may occur due to esophageal involvement. Capillaritis rare	Organizing pneumonia (uncommon)	NSIP common UIP pattern, less common
Polymyositis and dermatomyositis	5%–30% symptomatic involvement 40% abnormal lung scans	Diffuse alveolar damage (5%)	Organizing pneumonia (<5%)	NSIP (40%) UIP (<5%)
Sjögren syndrome	9%–12% clinical involvement 43%–75% abnormal lung scans	Acute interstitial pneumonia (rare)	Follicular bronchiolitis/lymphoid interstitial pneumonia (common)	NSIP (common) UIP (rare)

NSIP, nonspecific interstitial pneumonia; UIP, usual interstitial pneumonia.

Although rheumatoid vasculitis is a relatively common vasculitis, pulmonary involvement is unusual. Small-vessel vasculitis of the lung (capillaritis) is an uncommon cause of diffuse alveolar hemorrhage in patients with rheumatoid arthritis.[12]

Systemic Lupus Erythematosus

Pleural involvement occurs in almost one-half of patients with systemic lupus erythematosus, and effusions occur in 20%.

Acute lupus pneumonitis is diagnosed clinically in ~5% of patients during the course of disease and is manifested by fever, cough, and bibasilar fluffy reticular densities. Acute lung disease is the initial manifestation of lupus in up to 50% of patients.[13] There may be an association with anti-dsDNA and anti-Ro/SSA serum autoantibodies. Histologic findings are variable; an early description a half a century ago described a variety of findings, including acute alveolar injury (diffuse alveolar damage), cellular interstitial inflammation (cellular interstitial pneumonia) resembling cellular NSIP, and arteriolar thrombosis.[14] Some authors associate acute lupus pneumonitis with diffuse alveolar damage and hyaline membranes only and would include cellular interstitial pneumonia as nonspecific interstitial pneumonia of chronic lupus pneumonitis.[1] Capillaritis with pulmonary hemorrhage is also in the spectrum of acute lupus pneumonitis (Fig. 50.3) but is usually clinically designated as diffuse alveolar hemorrhage (as opposed to lupus pneumonitis). The histologic finding of capillaritis is important to note,

as it imparts a bad prognosis and is often treated more aggressively than simple steroid therapy.[13] Because "acute lupus pneumonitis" is a clinical term, it is best avoided as a pathologic diagnosis. Instead, the type or types of lung injury should be noted, with special emphasis on the features of acute alveolar damage and capillaritis. Because the etiology of capillaritis is immune mediated, immunofluorescence for IgG and complement is sometimes a useful adjunct to diagnosis. A linear alveolar basement membrane deposit of IgG is suggestive of anti-GBM disease, and granular endothelial capillary deposition is suggestive of lupus-related capillaritis.

Chronic lupus pneumonitis is a clinical term for chronic interstitial lung disease in lupus patients and includes nonspecific interstitial

TABLE 50.3 Autoimmune Connective Tissue Diseases and Pulmonary Arterial Hypertension

Common (>20% of patients)
    Systemic sclerosis
    Mixed connective tissue disease
Not uncommon (>10% of patients)
    Systemic lupus erythematosus
Uncommon (<10% of patients)
    Dermatomyositis
    Rheumatoid arthritis
    Sjögren syndrome

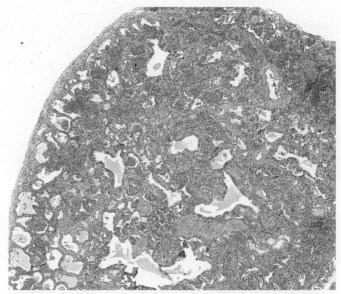

FIGURE 50.1 ▲ Rheumatoid arthritis–associated interstitial lung disease, nonspecific interstitial pneumonia pattern. There is diffuse interstitial thickening with inflammation and fibrosis, without subpleural accentuation or spatial heterogeneity.

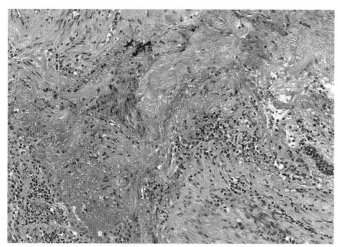

FIGURE 50.2 ▲ Rheumatoid nodule. There is an irregular area of necrotic debris mixed with fibrin, surrounded by acute and chronic inflammatory cells. The remainder of the specimen showed predominantly usual interstitial pneumonia pattern.

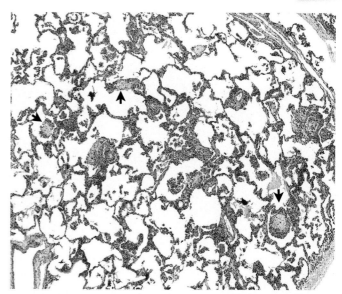

FIGURE 50.4 ▲ Chronic interstitial inflammation with patchy organizing pneumonia, systemic lupus erythematosus. There is patchy interstitial inflammation and small foci of organizing pneumonia (*arrows*).

pneumonia (the most common pattern) and usual interstitial pneumonia. Clinically, it is similar to idiopathic pulmonary fibrosis, with a better prognosis. Organizing pneumonia is a frequent histologic component, especially in combination with nonspecific interstitial pneumonia (Fig. 50.4).

Chronic interstitial lung disease affects 3% to 8% of patients with systemic lupus, with a progressive increase in prevalence with disease duration, and is relatively less common than in other connective tissue disorders.[13] In hospitalized patients with lupus, interstitial lung disease is seen in one-fourth of patients.[15] In addition to usual and nonspecific interstitial pneumonia, lymphoid interstitial pneumonia has been described in occasional patients with lupus, usually in association with Sjögren syndrome. In these cases, the development of lung cysts by computed tomography is typical.[13] Similar to acute lupus pneumonitis, an association between interstitial lung disease and the presence of anti-Ro/SSA autoantibodies has been observed for the chronic form of lung disease.[15]

In an autopsy study, the main pulmonary findings in patients dying with lupus included pleuritis and bacterial infections, including opportunistic infections, and pulmonary thromboembolism.[16] Pulmonary

hemorrhage occurred in one-fourth of patients, but fewer than 5% of the total showed capillaritis. An additional 5% of patient showed pulmonary hypertension with plexiform lesions.[16]

Pulmonary arterial hypertension develops more commonly in lupus patients than in individuals with rheumatoid arthritis, affecting 12% to 28% of patients. It is associated with Raynaud phenomenon, high levels of rheumatoid factor, and anti-RNP autoantibodies.[13,17]

Antiphospholipid Syndrome

The antiphospholipid syndrome is caused by circulating autoantibodies against phospholipid-binding plasma proteins that increase the risk of thrombosis and pregnancy loss. It is most frequently a primary syndrome but may be associated with other autoimmune diseases, most often systemic lupus erythematosus.

The pulmonary manifestations are presented in Table 50.4. The most common manifestation of lung disease in antiphospholipid syndrome is *acute pulmonary embolism*, which may often be the presenting symptom. Recurrent pulmonary emboli may give rise to pulmonary hypertension and *chronic thromboembolic pulmonary hypertension*. The prevalence of pulmonary hypertension in primary antiphospholipid

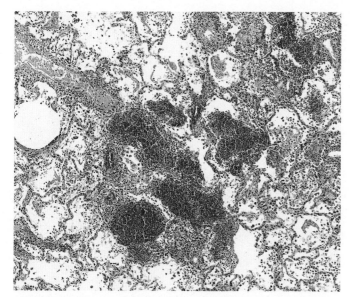

FIGURE 50.3 ▲ Capillaritis, systemic lupus erythematosus. There is patchy hemorrhage. The interstitium is markedly infiltrated by mixed inflammatory cells, including neutrophils.

TABLE 50.4 Pulmonary Involvement in Antiphospholipid Syndrome (Patterns Often Coexist)

Clinical Diagnoses	Pathologic Diagnosis
Pulmonary embolism (acute or recurrent)	Pulmonary embolism Pulmonary infarction
CTEPH	In situ thrombosis, acute, organizing, and recanalized Elastic arteries Small arteries Arterioles
Pulmonary hypertension	Medial hypertrophy, arteries Intimal thickening, arteries, typically eccentric
DAH	Capillaritis
ARDS	Diffuse alveolar damage
CAPS	Intra-alveolar hemorrhage

CTEPH, chronic thromboembolic pulmonary hypertension; DAH, diffuse alveolar hemorrhage; ARDS, acute respiratory distress syndrome; CAPS, catastrophic antiphospholipid syndrome.

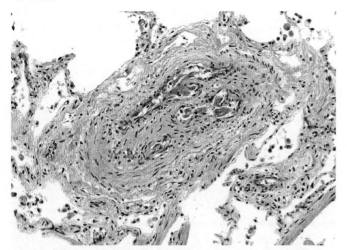

FIGURE 50.5 ▲ Recanalized arterial thrombus, antiphospholipid syndrome, autopsy. There is a small muscular artery with recanalization. The lumen shows superimposed more acute fibrin platelet thrombosis. The patient had widespread small-vessel thrombosis and expired from myocardial ischemia.

syndrome and antiphospholipid syndrome associated with systemic lupus erythematosus has been estimated to be between 1.8% and 3.5%, respectively.[18] Conversely, the prevalence of antiphospholipid autoantibodies in patients with chronic thromboembolic pulmonary hypertension varies between 10% and 20%.[18]

In addition to embolism, in situ thrombosis occurs in various sized arteries, including arterioles, in the lungs of patients with antiphospholipid syndrome. These patients have initially fever, cough, and shortness of breath, with patchy bilateral reticular and ground-glass lung opacities. Biopsies demonstrate acute and organizing thrombi within small arteries and arterioles (Fig. 50.5). Patients may die with widespread thrombotic occlusions at autopsy, progress to right heart failure, or respond to steroid therapy.[18]

Among patients with antiphospholipid syndrome, there is an increased risk for *diffuse alveolar hemorrhage*. Those patients developing diffuse alveolar hemorrhage are more likely to have mitral valve disease, skin disease, central nervous system involvement, and high-titer antiphospholipid levels.[19] Bronchoalveolar lavage fluid is typically bloody, indicative of alveolar hemorrhage. Histologic findings in patients with diffuse alveolar hemorrhage complicating antiphospholipid syndrome include capillaritis, interstitial inflammation, and microthrombi.[20,21] In some cases, histologic findings are limited to intra-alveolar hemorrhage and chronic interstitial inflammation, without microthrombi or capillaritis (so-called bland diffuse alveolar hemorrhage).[20] There is speculation that neutrophils are involved in the mechanism of alveolar injury and hemorrhage.[20] The prognosis of diffuse alveolar hemorrhage complicating antiphospholipid syndrome is poor, with one-third mortality.[21] Treatment includes cyclophosphamide, rituximab, and intravenous gamma globulin.[21]

Some patients with antiphospholipid syndrome and diffuse alveolar hemorrhage have diffuse alveolar damage (clinically *acute respiratory distress syndrome*, ARDS). ARDS with concomitant multiorgan failure in these patients is termed *catastrophic antiphospholipid syndrome* (CAPS). Histologically, there are extensive small-vessel thromboses, intra-alveolar hemorrhage, and diffuse alveolar damage with hyaline membranes. Capillaritis is a variable finding.[18] Mortality is more than 50%, despite treatment with anticoagulation, high-dose steroids, and immunosuppression.[18]

Systemic Sclerosis

Pulmonary involvement in systemic sclerosis centers on pulmonary vascular disease, resulting in pulmonary hypertension, and interstitial fibrosis, typically of the nonspecific interstitial pneumonia pattern. Both pulmonary hypertension and interstitial fibrosis may coexist.

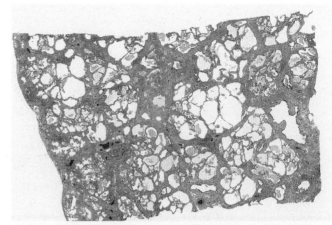

FIGURE 50.6 ▲ Systemic sclerosis, nonspecific interstitial pneumonia, fibrotic type. There is fairly uniform fibrosis affecting the lung diffusely, without subpleural accentuation typical of usual interstitial pneumonia. The pleura is at the left.

Up to 90% of patients with systemic sclerosis show evidence of interstitial fibrosis by high-resolution computed tomographic scans, and up to 50% will have abnormalities on pulmonary function tests. Imaging findings include bibasilar interstitial infiltrates, ground-glass abnormalities (typically > idiopathic pulmonary fibrosis), evidence of pulmonary hypertension, pleural thickening, and esophageal dilatation.

Histologically, fibrosis of scleroderma is relatively uniform, in a nonspecific interstitial pneumonia pattern (Figs. 50.6 and 50.7). In most cases, the type of nonspecific interstitial pneumonia is fibrotic, although in <10% of patients with systemic sclerosis–associated lung disease, the lungs exhibit interstitial lymphocytic infiltrates (cellular nonspecific interstitial pneumonia pattern).[22] In the largest histologic study of surgical lung biopsies, 77% of patients showed a nonspecific interstitial pneumonia pattern (three-fourths of which were fibrotic), the remainder usual interstitial pneumonia or unclassified end-stage fibrosis.[23] There may be bronchiolocentricity with constrictive (obliterative) bronchiolitis, although clinically detected obstructive airway disease is rare in scleroderma patients. Organizing pneumonia and acute lung injury with diffuse alveolar damage are uncommon.

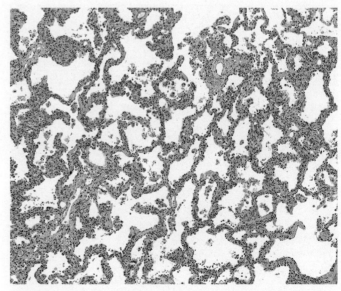

FIGURE 50.7 ▲ Systemic sclerosis, nonspecific interstitial pneumonia, cellular type. There is diffuse thickening of the alveolar septa with chronic inflammation and mild fibrosis.

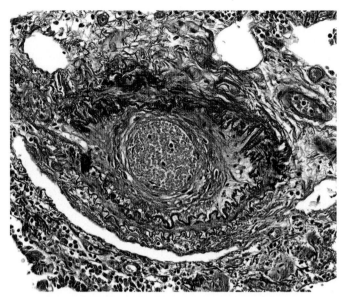

FIGURE 50.8 ▲ Systemic sclerosis, concentric intimal thickening, muscular artery. Pulmonary arterial hypertension is common in systemic sclerosis and is usually histologic manifested as thickened intima. Note discrete internal and external elastic laminae. Elastic van Gieson stain.

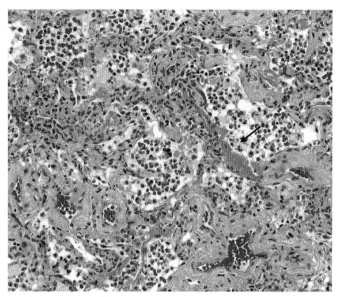

FIGURE 50.9 ▲ Dermatomyositis–polymyositis, diffuse alveolar damage. The alveolar septa are barely discernable, in this acute phase of alveolar injury before proliferation and reaction with type II pneumocytes. There is an early hyaline membrane (*arrow*).

The clinical course of scleroderma-related lung disease is that of progressive decline in lung function, lack of response to immunosuppression, and occasional acute exacerbations.[22] In one study, 10-year survival ranged between 30% and 70%, depending on the histologic pattern of fibrosis, with the presence of increased eosinophils in the bronchoalveolar lavage fluid, a significant negative prognostic finding.[23]

Pulmonary arterial hypertension occurs in 10% to 50% of patients, depending on the method of detection. Pathologically, there is concentric intimal thickening of arteries (Fig. 50.8), with occasional veno-occlusive–like changes in pulmonary veins.[24] Plexiform lesions have been described only rarely.[25] Autopsy studies have shown arterial lesions in up to 50% of patients.

A rare complication of systemic sclerosis is a pulmonary–renal syndrome characterized by diffuse alveolar hemorrhage and acute renal failure. There are three pathologic types: pulmonary–renal syndrome with thrombotic microangiopathy, pulmonary–renal syndrome with small-vessel vasculitis (capillaritis), and D-penicillamine–induced Goodpasture-like syndrome.[26]

Dermatomyositis and Polymyositis

Interstitial lung disease occurs in 30% to 50% of patients with dermatomyositis and polymyositis, which, with inclusion body myositis and overlap syndromes, form the *idiopathic inflammatory myopathies* or *autoimmune inflammatory myopathies*. The distinction between polymyositis and dermatomyositis depends on the presence of skin involvement and characteristic muscle biopsy findings. The two syndromes are generally considered together in context of pulmonary involvement.[27] The frequency of dermatomyositis and polymyositis is approximately equal in series of patients with interstitial lung disease.[28]

Pulmonary disease in polymyositis and dermatomyositis usually presents as antibiotic-resistant community-acquired pneumonia and may be the initial manifestation of polymyositis to dermatomyositis. Chest radiographs and computed tomography usually show bilateral irregular linear opacities involving the lung bases with occasional consolidations. Surgical lung biopsies typically demonstrate nonspecific interstitial pneumonia, followed by organizing diffuse alveolar damage (Fig. 50.9), organizing pneumonia (Fig. 50.10), and uncommonly usual interstitial pneumonia.[29]

In a subset of patients, the presenting illness is more acute and is characterized by diffuse alveolar injury characterized on imaging by ground-glass opacities; in these cases, lung biopsy shows diffuse alveolar damage.[30]

The prognosis of nonspecific interstitial pneumonia in dermatomyositis–polymyositis is good, with a mean survival of 20 years, which is similar to overall survival of patients without lung disease.[30] However, acute alveolar injury with diffuse alveolar damage imparts a dismal prognosis, with a mean survival of < 1 year.[30]

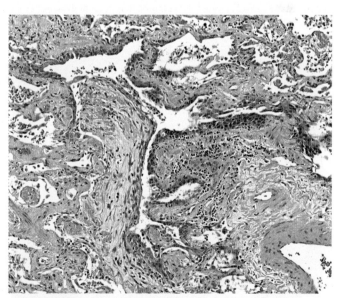

FIGURE 50.10 ▲ Dermatomyositis–polymyositis, organizing pneumonia. There is a plug of loose fibrosis adjacent to the bronchiole. The location near the airway is used as justification for the use of the term "bronchiolitis obliterans–organizing pneumonia (BOOP)." However, there is no obliteration of the airway in the sense that the lumen is intact, and the lesion is not circumferential. Such lesions are the root of the long-standing controversy regarding the terms BOOP, bronchiolitis obliterans, and obliterative bronchiolitis.

Antisynthetase Syndrome

The *antisynthetase syndrome* is the concurrence of fevers, myositis, interstitial lung disease, "mechanic's hands," Raynaud phenomenon, and polyarthritis and is defined by the presence of serum autoantibodies to aminoacyl-transfer RNA synthetases, the most common being anti-Jo-1. It is generally considered a subset of dermatomyositis–polymyositis. "Mechanics' hands" refer to thickened, hyperkeratotic, and fissured skin at the margins of the fingertips. Several studies have shown a higher frequency (from 30% to 70%) of anti-Jo autoantibodies in dermatomyositis–polymyositis patients with lung disease compared to those without.[28–31] The antisynthetase syndrome is more often associated with polymyositis than dermatomyositis and in one study was not associated with malignancy.[28] Muscle biopsies show macrophages and lymphocytes, in contrast to the predominantly lymphocytic infiltrates typical of polymyositis and dermatomyositis.

Lung biopsies demonstrate similar findings to those of dermatomyositis lung disease without antisynthetase syndrome, with nonspecific interstitial pneumonia, with or without areas of organization. Treatment includes glucocorticoids, immunosuppressive agents such as azathioprine or methotrexate, and cyclophosphamide for severe lung disease.[32]

Over one-third of patients with antisynthetase syndrome have concomitant anti-Ro/SSA (anti-Ro52) autoantibodies.[33] The presence of anti-Ro/SSA antibodies in patients with anti-Jo-1 syndrome may predict a worse pulmonary outcome than in those with anti-Jo-1 antibody alone[32,34] and may have increased risk of developing cancer and severe joint involvement.[33]

Sjögren Syndrome

Sjögren syndrome is classified as "primary" or "secondary," the latter referring to sicca syndrome in the presence of other autoimmune disease. Symptomatic lung disease occurs in about 10% of patients with primary Sjögren syndrome, whereas abnormal lung findings are present by high-resolution computed tomography scans in over one-half.[35] Lung disease is more frequent in patients with autoantibodies to SSA/Ro. Acute interstitial pneumonia is rare[36] and may be accompanied by diffuse alveolar hemorrhage. More commonly, there is lymphoid interstitial pneumonia (Fig. 50.11), typically with follicular bronchiolitis and cystic change seen on computed tomography scans. Lymphoid interstitial pneumonia overlaps with features of nonspecific interstitial pneumonia, cellular type, which may demonstrate areas of organizing pneumonia. The nonspecific organizing pneumonia pattern is a common CT finding in Sjögren lung disease. Usual interstitial pneumonia is a less common manifestation of Sjögren-associated interstitial lung disease.

In Sjögren syndrome, similar to other connective tissue disease, lung involvement is more frequent in patients with hypergammaglobulinemia and anti-SSA/Ro antibodies.[35]

The prognosis of interstitial lung disease in patients with Sjögren syndrome is similar regardless of the type, at ~90% over 5 years.[37] The treatment includes steroids, cyclosporine, azathioprine, and cyclophosphamide.

Pulmonary hypertension is a rare complication of Sjögren syndrome and may be secondary to pulmonary arterial and venous hypertension and chronic thromboembolic pulmonary hypertension or secondary to fibrotic lung disease.[35]

Mixed Connective Tissue Disease

The term mixed connective tissue disease is used for patients with combined features of systemic lupus erythematosus, systemic sclerosis, and polymyositis–dermatomyositis, with high serum titers of autoantibodies against uridine-rich small nuclear ribonucleoprotein particles (U1 snRNP). Respiratory involvement is observed in 20% to 80% of patients.[38] Juvenile-onset mixed connective tissue disease is associated with a 25% rate of lung disease, with a characteristic microcystic fine reticular pattern on computed tomography scans.[39]

As in other autoimmune disorders, lung disease in mixed connective tissue disease is clinically assessed as infection, drug reaction, or manifestation of the underlying connective tissue disease and is generally clinically diagnosed. Based on imaging findings in the absence of pathologic data, it is assumed that much of the fibrosis seen in mixed connective tissue disease is likely nonspecific interstitial pneumonia pattern, which may demonstrate areas of ground-glass and fine reticulation in the absence of overt honeycombing. In one cross-sectional study (with histologic information), 52% of patients with mixed connective tissue disease had abnormal high-resolution computed tomography findings, most commonly reticular patterns consistent with lung fibrosis that was severe in 19% of patients.[40] In a different

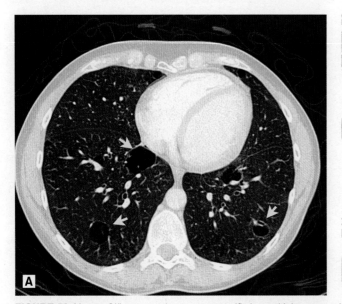

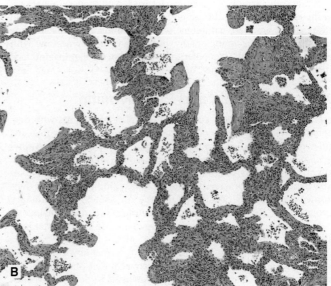

FIGURE 50.11 ▲ Sjögren syndrome, nonspecific interstitial pneumonia, with cyst formation. **A.** High-resolution computed tomographic scans. In addition to diffuse interstitial markings, there are scattered cysts, typical of Sjögren disease (*yellow arrows*) (see Figure 36.7). **B.** There is diffuse thickening of the alveolar septa, primarily by chronic inflammation, with focal fibrosis. There is simplification of the airspaces, possibly explaining the cystic change seen on imaging. The intense interstitial inflammation frequently results in the term "lymphoid (or lymphocytic) interstitial pneumonia" for patients with Sjögren interstitial lung disease.

series, two-thirds of patients with mixed connective tissue disease had computed tomographic abnormalities, most frequently ground-glass opacity, reticular densities consistent with mild fibrosis, and only one patient with subpleural honeycombing.[41] Contrastingly, a study comparing computed tomographic findings across groups of autoimmune connective tissue disorders reported the frequency of ground-glass opacity in mixed connective tissue disease as lower than in other disorders, the frequency of septal thickening higher, and frequency of honeycombing intermediate between systemic sclerosis (highest) and polymyositis–dermatomyositis.[42]

Treatment of interstitial lung disease includes glucocorticosteroids and cyclophosphamide for severe cases, with a low rate of progression of the fibrosis.[41] Patients with severe fibrosis have a decreased survival compared to those with less advanced disease.[40]

Typical of other autoimmune connective tissue disorders, pleural involvement is common, with effusions present in one-half of patients and symptomatic pleuritis in one-fifth.[38]

Pulmonary arterial hypertension is relatively common in mixed connective tissue disease, is a serious complication characterized by a rapidly fatal course, and occurs in about 25% of patients.[43] The histologic features are varied and have been reported primarily in case reports of lung biopsy[43] or autopsy samples. In one pathologic series of biopsies of pulmonary arterial hypertension, mixed connective tissue disease was the most common underlying autoimmune disorder.[44] Histologic findings include concentric intimal thickening of large, medium-sized, and small arteries, medial hypertrophy, organizing thrombi, plexiform arteriopathy, and arteritis.[43–45]

Adult-Onset Still Disease

Lung disease in adult-onset Still disease (AOSD) has not been as extensively characterized. There have been histologically documented reports of organizing pneumonia, interstitial pneumonitis, and organizing diffuse alveolar damage with nonspecific interstitial pneumonia pattern.[46]

Psoriasis

Most psoriatic patients with diffuse lung infiltrates suffer from infections or drug hypersensitivity to methotrexate, retinoids (e.g., acitretin), or monoclonal antibody therapy (e.g., infliximab).[47] There are rare reports of acute interstitial pneumonia and organizing pneumonia presumably not as a reaction to drugs.[48,49]

Undifferentiated Connective Tissue Disease

Undifferentiated connective tissue disease is defined as one or more symptoms of an autoimmune connective tissue disorder, elevated autoantibodies, and lack of fulfillment of clinical and serologic criteria for an established connective tissue disease. Because this group is hard to exactly define, the rate of lung disease is not readily known, especially since many patients with defined connective tissue diseases have lung manifestations prior to development of extrapulmonary symptoms. Interstitial lung disease with a histologic pattern of nonspecific interstitial pneumonia is the most frequent lung finding.[50] In fact, because of the high percentage of autoantibodies and extrapulmonary symptoms in series of patients with nonspecific interstitial pneumonia, it has even been suggested the nonspecific interstitial pneumonia is a manifestation of undifferentiated connective tissue disease (see Chapter 17).[51]

Ankylosing Spondylitis

Ankylosing spondylitis is a common cause of pulmonary apical fibrocystic disease, also termed "fibrobullous disease." Pathologic features of this entity are largely unknown, because of lack of histologic sampling. It is unclear how specific the changes are, which have been described in other conditions such as rheumatoid arthritis and degenerative osteoarthropathy, as the condition is entirely diagnosed by imaging. The bullae may become infected with mycobacteria or fungi, which may require surgical intervention.

Other lung findings in ankylosing spondylitis include interstitial lung disease (largely asymptomatic), emphysema, bronchiectasis, pleuritis, chest wall restriction causing a restrictive lung defect, and spontaneous pneumothorax.[52]

Goodpasture Disease

Antibasement membrane antibody disease (Goodpasture syndrome or disease) is a rare autoimmune disorder defined by the serologic or tissue identification of autoantibodies directed against the carboxyl terminus of the noncollagenous domain of the alpha-3 chain of type IV collagen. The specific epitope is primarily located on alveolar and glomerular basement membranes; autoantibody binding results in rapidly progressive crescentic glomerulonephritis and diffuse alveolar hemorrhage. In about half of patients, there is concomitant alveolar hemorrhage and renal involvement; in most of the remainder, there is glomerulonephritis without alveolar hemorrhage. In a small proportion of cases, alveolar hemorrhage is isolated. The overall incidence of alveolar hemorrhage, which results in hemoptysis, alveolar opacities, anemia, and hypoxemia, ranges from 45% to 67% in patients with Goodpasture disease.

Bronchoalveolar lavage fluid demonstrates blood and hemosiderin macrophages. Histologic sections of lung histopathology show diffuse or multifocal alveolar hemorrhage with numerous red blood cells and hemosiderin-laden macrophages in alveolar spaces. Capillaritis is present in a minority of cases and is generally minimal, with only few interstitial neutrophils.[53] It is always important to retain a lung sample frozen for immunofluorescence in order to evaluate the presence of linear immunoglobulin deposition along alveolar basement membranes. These studies may be in addition to immunofluorescence done on renal biopsies of the same patient, as it is rare to have involvement limited to the lung. In most instances in which lung biopsy is performed, there may be doubt about the underlying diagnosis of Goodpasture syndrome, the main purpose of the biopsy to exclude infections or diffuse acute or organizing alveolar damage. In such instances, lung immunofluorescence is helpful to exclude the diagnosis of anti-GBM disease.

Inflammatory Bowel Disease

There are numerous thoracic manifestations of inflammatory bowel disease, both Crohn disease and ulcerative colitis. Sterile necrotizing granulomas may cause lung nodules in Crohn disease patients and clinically mimic carcinoma.[54] The most common finding in both Crohn and ulcerative colitis is bronchiectasis, caused by chronic infections. Airway stenosis (proximal tracheobronchial fibrosis), organizing pneumonia, pleuritis with effusions and scarring, fistulae, cavitary lesions, and interstitial fibrosis have all been reported as clinical and radiologic findings. A somewhat characteristic lesion with pathologic confirmation is granulomatous bronchiolitis associated with Crohn disease, which has been reported in a handful of patients.[55–57] As is typical of immunosuppressed patients, including those with autoimmune diseases, it may be difficult to distinguish lung involvement from drug reaction.[58] Reports of "bronchiolitis obliterans" in patients with Crohn disease and ulcerative colitis probably include organizing pneumonia as well as constrictive bronchiolitis, as the terms are often confused in clinical reports.

Patients with inflammatory bowel disease have a threefold risk of venous thromboembolism, including pulmonary embolism. There is a weak association between inflammatory bowel disease and other lung diseases, including sarcoidosis, asthma, alpha(1)-antitrypsin deficiency,[59] and granulomatosis with polyangiitis (Wegener granulomatosis).[60]

Autoimmune Liver Disease

Organizing pneumonia may occur in primary sclerosing cholangitis, in association with ulcerative colitis and mesalazine treatment.[61] Primary biliary cirrhosis is also associated with interstitial lung disease, sometimes associated with other autoimmune disorders such as rheumatoid arthritis.[62,63]

REFERENCES

1. Colby TV. Pulmonary pathology in patients with systemic autoimmune diseases. *Clin Chest Med.* 1998;19:587–612, vii.
2. Lee HK, Kim DS, Yoo B, et al. Histopathologic pattern and clinical features of rheumatoid arthritis-associated interstitial lung disease. *Chest.* 2005;127:2019–2027.
3. Mohd Noor N, Mohd Shahrir MS, Shahid MS, et al. Clinical and high resolution computed tomography characteristics of patients with rheumatoid arthritis lung disease. *Int J Rheum Dis.* 2009;12:136–144.
4. Amital A, Shitrit D, Adir Y. The lung in rheumatoid arthritis. *Presse Med.* 2011;40:e31–e48.
5. Tanaka N, Kim JS, Newell JD, et al. Rheumatoid arthritis-related lung diseases: CT findings. *Radiology.* 2004;232:81–91.
6. Hozumi H, Nakamura Y, Johkoh T, et al. Acute exacerbation in rheumatoid arthritis-associated interstitial lung disease: a retrospective case control study. *BMJ Open.* 2013;3:e003132.
7. Hagiwara K, Sato T, Takagi-Kobayashi S, et al. Acute exacerbation of preexisting interstitial lung disease after administration of etanercept for rheumatoid arthritis. *J Rheumatol.* 2007;34:1151–1154.
8. Dias OM, Pereira DA, Baldi BG, et al. Adalimumab-induced acute interstitial lung disease in a patient with rheumatoid arthritis. *J Bras Pneumol.* 2014;40:77–81.
9. Anaya JM, Diethelm L, Ortiz LA, et al. Pulmonary involvement in rheumatoid arthritis. *Semin Arthritis Rheum.* 1995;24:242–254.
10. Aubry MC. Pulmonary Pathology: LC22-1 non-neoplastic pulmonary lymphoid proliferations. *Pathology.* 2014;46(suppl 2):S36–S37.
11. Devouassoux G, Cottin V, Liote H, et al. Characterisation of severe obliterative bronchiolitis in rheumatoid arthritis. *Eur Respir J.* 2009;33:1053–1061.
12. Schwarz MI, Zamora MR, Hodges TN, et al. Isolated pulmonary capillaritis and diffuse alveolar hemorrhage in rheumatoid arthritis and mixed connective tissue disease. *Chest.* 1998;113:1609–1615.
13. Torre O, Harari S. Pleural and pulmonary involvement in systemic lupus erythematosus. *Presse Med.* 2011;40:e19–e29.
14. Matthay RA, Schwarz MI, Petty TL, et al. Pulmonary manifestations of systemic lupus erythematosus: review of twelve cases of acute lupus pneumonitis. *Medicine (Baltimore).* 1975;54:397–409.
15. Boulware DW, Hedgpeth MT. Lupus pneumonitis and anti-SSA(Ro) antibodies. *J Rheumatol.* 1989;16:479–481.
16. Quadrelli SA, Alvarez C, Arce SC, et al. Pulmonary involvement of systemic lupus erythematosus: analysis of 90 necropsies. *Lupus.* 2009;18:1053–1060.
17. Li M, Wang Q, Zhao J, et al. Chinese SLE Treatment and Research group (CSTAR) registry: II. Prevalence and risk factors of pulmonary arterial hypertension in Chinese patients with systemic lupus erythematosus. *Lupus.* 2014;23:1085–1091.
18. Espinosa G, Cervera R, Font J, et al. The lung in the antiphospholipid syndrome. *Ann Rheum Dis.* 2002;61:195–198.
19. Scheiman Elazary A, Cohen MJ, Aamar S, et al. Pulmonary hemorrhage in antiphospholipid antibody syndrome. *J Rheumatol.* 2012;39:1628–1631.
20. Koolaee RM, Moran AM, Shahane A. Diffuse alveolar hemorrhage and Libman-Sacks endocarditis as a manifestation of possible primary antiphospholipid syndrome. *J Clin Rheumatol.* 2013;19:79–83.
21. Cartin-Ceba R, Peikert T, Ashrani A, et al. Primary antiphospholipid syndrome-associated diffuse alveolar hemorrhage. *Arthritis Care Res (Hoboken).* 2014;66:301–310.
22. Herzog EL, Mathur A, Tager AM, et al. Review: interstitial lung disease associated with systemic sclerosis and idiopathic pulmonary fibrosis: how similar and distinct? *Arthritis Rheumatol.* 2014;66:1967–1978.
23. Bouros D, Wells AU, Nicholson AG, et al. Histopathologic subsets of fibrosing alveolitis in patients with systemic sclerosis and their relationship to outcome. *Am J Respir Crit Care Med.* 2002;165:1581–1586.
24. Solomon JJ, Olson AL, Fischer A, et al. Scleroderma lung disease. *Eur Respir Rev.* 2013;22:6–19.
25. Chatterjee S. Pulmonary hypertension in systemic sclerosis. *Semin Arthritis Rheum.* 2011;41:19–37.
26. Naniwa T, Banno S, Sugiura Y, et al. Pulmonary-renal syndrome in systemic sclerosis: a report of three cases and review of the literature. *Mod Rheumatol.* 2007;17:37–44.
27. Fathi M, Lundberg IE, Tornling G. Pulmonary complications of polymyositis and dermatomyositis. *Semin Respir Crit Care Med.* 2007;28:451–458.
28. La Corte R, Lo Mo Naco A, Locaputo A, et al. In patients with antisynthetase syndrome the occurrence of anti-Ro/SSA antibodies causes a more severe interstitial lung disease. *Autoimmunity.* 2006;39:249–253.
29. Douglas WW, Tazelaar HD, Hartman TE, et al. Polymyositis-dermatomyositis-associated interstitial lung disease. *Am J Respir Crit Care Med.* 2001;164:1182–1185.
30. Selva-O'Callaghan A, Labrador-Horrillo M, Munoz-Gall X, et al. Polymyositis/dermatomyositis-associated lung disease: analysis of a series of 81 patients. *Lupus.* 2005;14:534–542.
31. Targoff IN. Update on myositis-specific and myositis-associated autoantibodies. *Curr Opin Rheumatol.* 2000;12:475–481.
32. Chatterjee S, Prayson R, Farver C. Antisynthetase syndrome: not just an inflammatory myopathy. *Cleve Clin J Med.* 2013;80:655–666.
33. Marie I, Hatron PY, Dominique S, et al. Short-term and long-term outcome of anti-Jo1-positive patients with anti-Ro52 antibody. *Semin Arthritis Rheum.* 2012;41:890–899.
34. Conway R, O'Donnell R, Fahy R, et al. Anti-Ro 52 positive dermatomyositis presenting as rapidly progressive interstitial lung disease. *QJM.* 2013;107:593–594.
35. Hatron PY, Tillie-Leblond I, Launay D, et al. Pulmonary manifestations of Sjogren's syndrome. *Presse Med.* 2011;40:e49–e64.
36. Tomita Y, Mori S, Arima N, et al. Rapidly progressive pulmonary fibrosis following the onset of diffuse alveolar hemorrhage in Sjogren's syndrome: an autopsy case report. *Intern Med.* 2012;51:295–299.
37. Enomoto Y, Takemura T, Hagiwara E, et al. Prognostic factors in interstitial lung disease associated with primary Sjogren's syndrome: a retrospective analysis of 33 pathologically-proven cases. *PLoS One.* 2013;8:e73774.
38. Prakash UB. Respiratory complications in mixed connective tissue disease. *Clin Chest Med.* 1998;19:733–746, ix.
39. Aalokken TM, Lilleby V, Soyseth V, et al. Chest abnormalities in juvenile-onset mixed connective tissue disease: assessment with high-resolution computed tomography and pulmonary function tests. *Acta Radiol.* 2009;50:430–436.
40. Gunnarsson R, Aalokken TM, Molberg O, et al. Prevalence and severity of interstitial lung disease in mixed connective tissue disease: a nationwide, cross-sectional study. *Ann Rheum Dis.* 2012;71:1966–1972.
41. Bodolay E, Szekanecz Z, Devenyi K, et al. Evaluation of interstitial lung disease in mixed connective tissue disease (MCTD). *Rheumatology (Oxford).* 2005;44:656–661.
42. Saito Y, Terada M, Takada T, et al. Pulmonary involvement in mixed connective tissue disease: comparison with other collagen vascular diseases using high resolution CT. *J Comput Assist Tomogr.* 2002;26:349–357.
43. Vegh J, Soos G, Csipo I, et al. Pulmonary arterial hypertension in mixed connective tissue disease: successful treatment with Iloprost. *Rheumatol Int.* 2006;26:264–269.
44. Burke AP, Farb A, Virmani R. The pathology of primary pulmonary hypertension. *Mod Pathol.* 1991;4:269–282.
45. Wiener-Kronish JP, Solinger AM, Warnock ML, et al. Severe pulmonary involvement in mixed connective tissue disease. *Am Rev Respir Dis.* 1981;124:499–503.
46. Zhao DB, Dai SM, Liu XP, et al. Interstitial inflammation in visceral organs is a pathologic feature of adult-onset Still's disease. *Rheumatol Int.* 2011;31:923–927.
47. Bale J, Chee P. Acute alveolitis following infliximab therapy for psoriasis. *Australas J Dermatol.* 2013;54:61–63.
48. Abou-Samra T, Constantin JM, Amarger S, et al. Generalized pustular psoriasis complicated by acute respiratory distress syndrome. *Br J Dermatol.* 2004;150:353–356.
49. Penizzotto M, Retegui M, Arrien Zucco MF. [Organizing pneumonia associated with psoriasis]. *Arch Bronconeumol.* 2010;46:210–211.
50. Lunardi F, Balestro E, Nordio B, et al. Undifferentiated connective tissue disease presenting with prevalent interstitial lung disease: case report and review of literature. *Diagn Pathol.* 2011;6:50.
51. Kinder BW, Collard HR, Koth L, et al. Idiopathic nonspecific interstitial pneumonia: lung manifestation of undifferentiated connective tissue disease? *Am J Respir Crit Care Med.* 2007;176:691–697.
52. Quismorio FP Jr. Pulmonary involvement in ankylosing spondylitis. *Curr Opin Pulm Med.* 2006;12:342–345.
53. Lazor R, Bigay-Game L, Cottin V, et al. Alveolar hemorrhage in anti-basement membrane antibody disease: a series of 28 cases. *Medicine (Baltimore).* 2007;86:181–193.
54. Coonar AS, Hwang DM, Darling G. Pulmonary involvement in inflammatory bowel disease. *Ann Thorac Surg.* 2007;84:1748–1750.
55. Agarwal R, Kumar V, Jindal SK. Obstructive granulomatous bronchiolitis obliterans due to Mycobacterium tuberculosis. *Monaldi Arch Chest Dis.* 2005;63:108–110.
56. Trow TK, Morris DG, Miller CR, et al. Granulomatous bronchiolitis of Crohn's disease successfully treated with inhaled budesonide. *Thorax.* 2009;64:546–547.

57. Vandenplas O, Casel S, Delos M, et al. Granulomatous bronchiolitis associated with Crohn's disease. *Am J Respir Crit Care Med*. 1998;158:1676–1679.
58. Haralambou G, Teirstein AS, Gil J, et al. Bronchiolitis obliterans in a patient with ulcerative colitis receiving mesalamine. *Mt Sinai J Med*. 2001;68:384–388.
59. Black H, Mendoza M, Murin S. Thoracic manifestations of inflammatory bowel disease. *Chest*. 2007;131:524–532.
60. Vaszar LT, Orzechowski NM, Specks U, et al. Coexistent pulmonary granulomatosis with polyangiitis (Wegener granulomatosis) and Crohn disease. *Am J Surg Pathol*. 2014;38:354–359.
61. Kevans D, Greene J, Galvin L, et al. Mesalazine-induced bronchiolitis obliterans organizing pneumonia (BOOP) in a patient with ulcerative colitis and primary sclerosing cholangitis. *Inflamm Bowel Dis*. 2011;17: E137–E138.
62. Cavazza A, Rossi G, Corradi D, et al. Cellular non-specific interstitial pneumonia as a pulmonary manifestation of primary biliary cirrhosis. *Pathology*. 2010;42:596–598.
63. Harada M, Hashimoto O, Kumemura H, et al. Bronchiolitis obliterans organizing pneumonia in a patient with primary biliary cirrhosis and rheumatoid arthritis treated with prednisolone. *Hepatol Res*. 2002;23:301.

51 IgG4-Related Lung Disease and Miscellaneous Vasculitis

Eunhee S. Yi, M.D., and Marie-Christine Aubry, M.D.

IgG4-Related Lung Disease

Introduction

IgG4-related disease (IgG4-RD) is a recently recognized fibroinflammatory condition that typically presents as tumefactive lesions involving one or more organs showing dense lymphoplasmacytic infiltrate containing increased IgG4-positive plasma cells, storiform fibrosis, and nonnecrotizing vascular inflammation on histologic examination.[1] IgG4-RD may affect the lung as well as virtually any body site. Pulmonary manifestations of IgG4-RD are varied, with an involvement of not only the lung parenchyma but also the pleura, the mediastinum, and the thoracic lymph nodes. In a cross-sectional study, 16 of 114 patients (14%) with IgG4-RD were found to have lung or pleural involvement, in the presence or absence of other extrapulmonary manifestations such as type I autoimmune pancreatitis (AIP).[2,3]

Clinical Features

Patients with IgG4-RD involving the lung have similar epidemiologic features to those with extrapulmonary disease with an average age of 69 years and male predominance (70% to 80%).[3] Approximately 50% of patients with pulmonary IgG4-RD have respiratory symptoms including cough, dyspnea on exertion, and chest pain, while the remaining patients present with incidentally found radiologic abnormalities in the absence of significant respiratory symptoms.[2,4–6] Constitutional symptoms such as high fever and remarkable weight loss are uncommon. Overall, the clinical manifestations in pulmonary IgG4-RD patients are nonspecific.[2,4–6] No known risk factors such as smoking or inhalation exposure have been identified in these patients.

Radiologic Findings

Patients with pulmonary IgG4-RD reveal various patterns of abnormalities. Four types of intrapulmonary lesions in chest CT scan have been reported[5,7]: (1) thickening of bronchovascular bundles and interlobular septa, (2) solid nodules resembling primary lung cancer, (3) interstitial involvement, and (4) round-shaped ground-glass opacities. The rounded opacities may vary in size from subcentimeter to > 5 cm in diameter. The opacity can manifest as solid or ground-glass attenuation. The margin of the opacity may be smooth or irregular and spiculated. In some patients, patchy consolidation and ground-glass opacities may suggest organizing pneumonia.[5,8–10] In others, reticular opacities and honeycombing may predominate similar to the findings seen in nonspecific interstitial pneumonia or idiopathic pulmonary fibrosis, respectively.[5,11,12] Infiltrates along bronchovascular bundles and interlobular septa may raise the suspicion of sarcoidosis especially when accompanied by thoracic lymphadenopathy.[5] Some patients may present with pleural effusion or nodular lesions involving the pleura.[5,13]

Mediastinal and/or hilar lymphadenopathy is not uncommon and may be seen with or without parenchymal lung involvement.[2,14–18] On 18F-fluorodeoxyglucose–positron emission tomography (FDG-PET) scanning, abnormal FDG uptake can be observed in IgG4-related lung lesions and thus will not help distinguish IgG4-related lung nodule or mass from lung cancer.

Laboratory Abnormalities

Serum IgG4 level is elevated in the majority of patients with pulmonary as well as extrapulmonary IgG4-RD.[2,5,11,17,19] A serum level of IgG4 > 135 mg/dL, the upper normal used in many laboratories, has been reported in 1,586 of 1,883 (84%) of patients in a large-scale study.[19] The mean serum IgG4 level was 760 mg/dL.[19] Sensitivity and specificity of elevated serum IgG4 level with respect to IgG4-RD are not precisely known in pulmonary IgG4-RD or in IgG4-RD in general. It has been well recognized, however, that there is a broad spectrum of diseases that have elevated serum IgG4 level above 135 mg/dL without evidence of IgG4-RD.[20] Thus, one should be aware of the fact that merely elevated serum IgG4 level is neither sufficient nor necessary for the diagnosis of IgG4-RD.

Recent studies have purported that plasmablast concentration in peripheral blood on flow cytometry could be a useful biomarker not only for the initial diagnosis but also for following disease activity of the patients with IgG4-RD.[21,22] By flow cytometry, plasmablast concentration can be measured by gating CD19^low CD38^+CD20^−CD27^+ cells. Concentration of IgG4+ plasmablasts can be also determined by flow cytometry.[21] Additional studies are required, however, before plasmablast concentration by flow cytometry can be widely used as a clinical test.

Mild to moderate eosinophilia is found in 34% of IgG4-RD patients, but this finding is nonspecific. Elevated C-reactive protein (CRP) levels were reported in 23% of cases; even in the setting of multiorgan disease, however, elevations in serum CRP are generally modest and are less pronounced than in erythrocyte sedimentation rate. Polyclonal hypergammaglobulinemia (total serum IgG levels >1,800 mg/dL) was reported in 313 of 510 (61%). Serum IgE level was elevated in 58%.[7,23–28] No specific autoantibody has been described consistently in patients with IgG4-RD, but the presence of nonspecific antibodies prevalent to other immune-mediated conditions is not uncommon; antinuclear antibody (ANA) and rheumatoid factor (RF) are found in nearly 30% and 20%, respectively. Hypocomplementemia is quite common especially in the patients with renal involvement by IgG4-RD.[20]

Treatment and Prognosis

As AIP, the prototype of IgG4-RD, and other extrapancreatic IgG4-RD, IgG4-related lung disease generally responds well to corticosteroid therapy.[4,5,9–11,13,29,30] Although the response to corticosteroid therapy is favorable in most patients with IgG4-related lung disease, long-term follow-up data are currently not available. These patients may develop extrapulmonary lesions in the months and years following their initial diagnosis.[2] Some patients with IgG4-related pulmonary disease may not experience complete resolution of their lung manifestations and have residual radiologic abnormalities. Zen et al.[4] described residual radiologic abnormalities in 3 of their 21 patients with IgG4-related pulmonary and pleural disease after treatment. Association with malignancies has been described in patients with IgG4-RD. These malignancies include malignant lymphoma, pancreatic cancer, and lung cancer, among others.[2,4,16,31] Some suggested that a subset of IgG4-RD may represent a paraneoplastic syndrome.[32]

Histopathology

Histopathologic features associated with pulmonary IgG4-RD are similar to those seen in other sites, characterized by mixed chronic inflammatory infiltrate, fibrosis, nonnecrotizing vascular inflammation, and increased IgG4-positive plasma cells in both the absolute count and the ratio with IgG-positive plasma cells.[2,5,11,13,33] Plasma cells comprise the main cell type in the inflammatory infiltrates (usually >50%), followed by lymphocytes and histiocytes. Eosinophilic infiltration can be prominent. Granulomas are rarely present and are usually small and poorly formed.[4,11] These changes are better appreciated on surgical lung biopsies but can also be identified on small biopsies such as transbronchial and needle biopsies[11,14] On surgical lung biopsies, prominent lymphangitic distribution involving the interlobular septa and visceral pleura is often seen.[11]

The morphologic spectrum of pulmonary IgG4-RD is wide and seemingly more diverse than the characteristic findings of IgG4-RD in general. Most characteristic findings of IgG4-RD in any body site include the following: (1) dense lymphoplasmacytic infiltrate; (2) fibrosis, usually storiform in character; and (3) obliterative phlebitis.[34] Pulmonary IgG4-RD may show some features distinct from those of other sites (Fig. 51.1). Unlike in many other organs, vascular inflammation seen in pulmonary IgG4-RD tends to involve both pulmonary arteries and veins with myointimal lymphoplasmacytic infiltration and variable degree of luminal narrowing. Fibrinoid necrosis of the vessel is not a feature of IgG4-RD as in any other site. Involved lung tissue usually does not reveal conspicuous storiform fibrosis and may show mainly collagen deposition with or without active fibroblastic proliferation.[11]

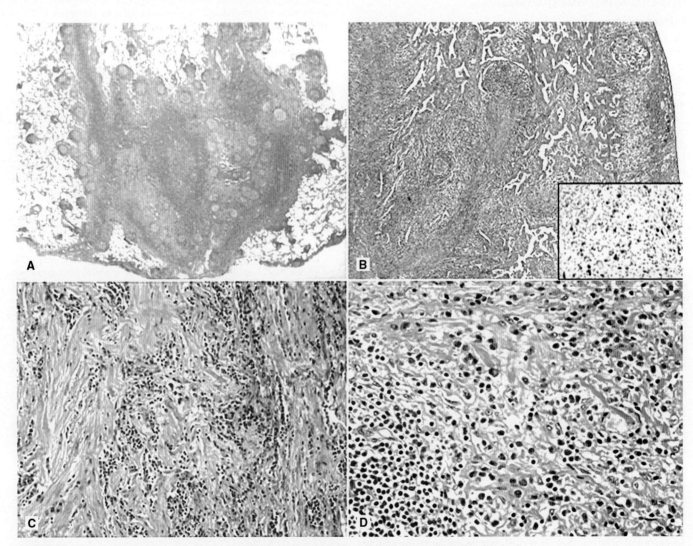

FIGURE 51.1 ▲ Histopathology of pulmonary IgG4-RD. **A.** Mass-like fibroinflammatory process showing prominent lymphoid hyperplasia and interlobular septal involvement resulting in lymphangitic pattern. **B.** Lymphoplasmacytic infiltrates in the visceral pleura as well as in the underlying lung parenchyma with a marked increase in IgG4-positive plasma cells (**inset**, anti-IgG4 staining). **C.** Active fibrosis with plasma cell–rich inflammatory infiltrate; a classic storiform fibrosis is often not very apparent in the IgG4-RD. **D.** Very prominent eosinophilic infiltrate is seen in some IgG4-RD cases.

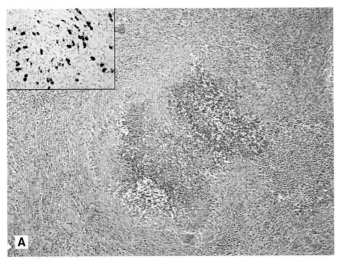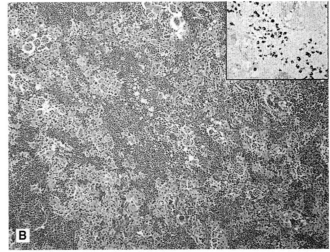

FIGURE 51.2 ▲ Nonspecificity of IgG4 staining. **A.** Increased IgG4-positive plasma cells (**inset**, anti-IgG4 staining) in a case of GPA involving soft tissue near the salivary gland. **B.** Rosai-Dorfman disease (**inset**, anti-IgG4 staining).

The current consensus guideline recommends >20 (in small biopsies) or >50 (surgical lung biopsies) IgG4-positive plasma cells per high-power field in hot spots with the IgG4+/IgG ratio > 40% for both small biopsies and surgical biopsy specimens.[34]

Differential Diagnosis

Many conditions that are not IgG4-RD may show increased IgG4-positive plasma cells both in absolute count and IgG4+/IgG+%, including granulomatosis with polyangiitis (GPA, formerly Wegener granulomatosis) (Fig. 51.2A), eosinophilic granulomatosis with polyangiitis (EPGA, formerly Churg-Strauss syndrome), Rosai-Dorfman disease (Fig. 51.2B), various hematolymphoid and solid organ malignancies, infections, inflammatory bowel disease (IBD), and rheumatoid arthritis, to name a few.[35]

Diagnosis of IgG4-Related Lung Disease

IgG4-RD in the lung can be encountered in the presence or absence of extrapulmonary disease including AIP. In patients who already have an established diagnosis of IgG4-RD, any thoracic abnormalities should raise a concern for pulmonary IgG4-RD. Due to the diversity of thoracic manifestations of IgG4-RD, any nodular or interstitial lung infiltrates, mediastinal or hilar lymphadenopathy, and pleural processes need to be further evaluated. In most cases, tissue biopsy would be needed not only to establish the diagnosis of IgG4-RD but also to exclude a separate process such as lung carcinoma, lymphoma, sarcoidosis, or other distinct disease processes.

In patients without established diagnosis of IgG4-RD, one can easily overlook a possibility of IgG4-related lung disease due to the nonspecific nature of clinical, radiologic, and histopathologic manifestations. It is crucial to consider a possibility of IgG4-RD in unexplained fibroinflammatory diseases with prominent plasma cell infiltrates. IgG4 immunostaining as well as testing serum IgG4 level can aid in the diagnosis, but ultimately, a comprehensive clinical, radiologic, and laboratory correlation along with the histopathologic evaluation would be required in reaching the diagnosis of IgG4-RD.

Miscellaneous Vasculitis

By definition, vasculitis means inflammation of a blood vessel wall. However, a true pulmonary vasculitis generally refers to capillaritis (leukocytoclastic vasculitis in alveolar capillaries) or vasculitis with fibrinoid necrosis involving pulmonary arteries and veins in the setting of idiopathic vasculitis syndromes such as GPA (Wegener granulomatosis) and EGPA (Churg-Strauss syndrome) (Fig. 51.3). Vasculitis associated with GPA and EGPA is covered under the heading of diffuse alveolar hemorrhage in Chapter 29. Pulmonary vascular inflammation with or without necrosis may occur in a broad spectrum of systemic disorders, infection, or iatrogenic injuries caused by radiation and drugs (Fig. 51.4). Vasculitis is often seen in classic sarcoidosis as well as in necrotizing sarcoid granulomatosis (Chapter 22). Pulmonary vasculitis is one of the many manifestations of systemic rheumatologic disorders that are separately discussed in Chapter 50. Also, one should be aware of the fact that any pulmonary vessels in severely inflamed lung tissue will show some inflammatory infiltrates in the walls as a nonspecific change, which could mimic a genuine vasculitis (Fig. 51.5). Occasionally, tumor emboli may masquerade as vasculitis due to admixed inflammatory infiltrate, which result in rapidly progressive pulmonary hypertension associated with thrombotic microangiopathy.[36]

Pulmonary vasculitis has been reported in patients with IBD, especially ulcerative colitis.[37,38] Vasculitis in IBD, however, would be difficult to differentiate from drug reaction since IBD patients are frequently treated with sulfonamides that have been well recognized to cause pulmonary vasculitis. Patients with IBD often show positive serology for p-ANCA, but it does not correlate with activity of IBD or evidence of systemic or pulmonary vasculitis. Coexistent pulmonary GPA and Crohn disease have been recently reported.[38]

A granulomatous arteritis may occasionally be encountered in lung biopsies, in which there are inflammation and scarring not only in the vessel wall but also in the adventitia, resulting in mass lesion (Fig. 51.6). The etiology is unclear, but there may be a relation with IgG4-RD.

Pulmonary vascular inflammation is not uncommon in any type of infection especially when it is severe. Invasion and necrosis of blood vessel walls is a characteristic feature of certain bacterial pneumonias. Vasculitis can also occur in association with necrotizing granulomas caused by fungal or mycobacterial infections, which can mimic GPA. Angioinvasive fungal infection in immunocompromised hosts is a life-threatening condition and often associated with pulmonary infarction. Rarely, pneumocystis pneumonia in AIDS patients can invade blood vessels causing vasculitis as well.

Vascular changes seen in the radiated lung tissue include endothelial necrosis, intimal edema with fibrosis, and medial injury. Foam cell accumulation in the vascular intima and media can be present in some cases. These findings can be reminiscent of pulmonary vasculitis, but clinical correlation should help in differential diagnosis. Drug-induced pulmonary vasculitis is uncommon. It might reflect a localized pulmonary reaction or be part of a systemic vasculitis. Since patients with

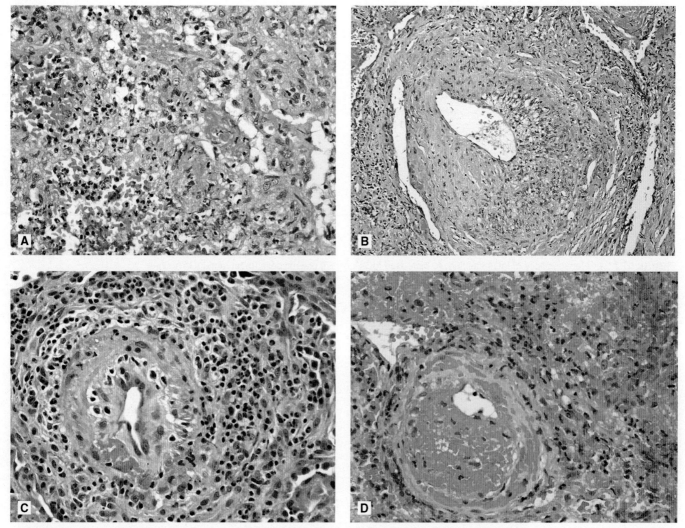

FIGURE 51.3 ▲ True pulmonary vasculitis. **A.** Granulomatosis with polyangiitis. There is capillaritis with acute lung injury. **B.** Granulomatosis with polyangiitis. There is necrotizing arteritis. **C.** Eosinophilic granulomatosis with polyangiitis. Necrotizing vasculitis with eosinophils. **D.** Eosinophilic granulomatosis with polyangiitis. Necrotizing vasculitis with fibrinoid necrosis.

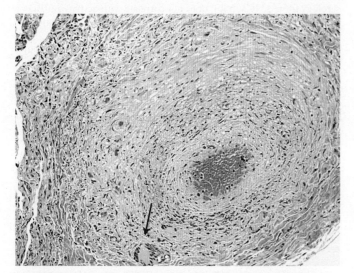

FIGURE 51.4 ▲ Necrotizing vasculitis seen in a case of atypical mycobacterial infection may be similar to that seen in GPA. There is a macrophage giant cell (*arrow*).

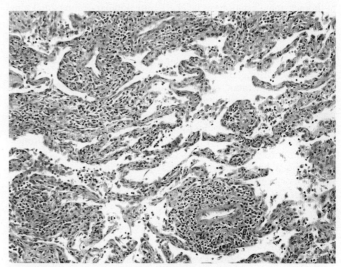

FIGURE 51.5 ▲ Nonspecific vascular inflammation is commonly seen in the lung tissue with marked inflammation.

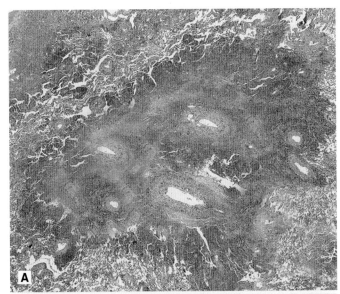

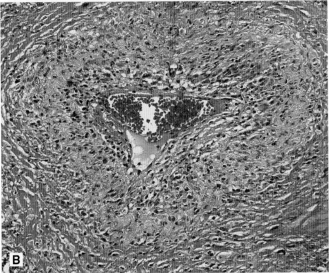

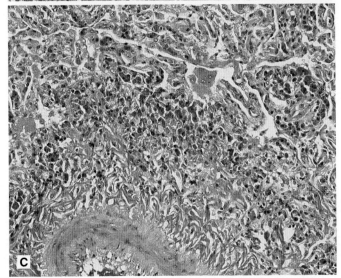

FIGURE 51.6 ▲ Granulomatous arteritis, unclassified. **A.** There is marked perivascular inflammation and scarring forming a mass. **B.** An artery shows granulomatous inflammation in the wall. **C.** There are adventitial giant cells and mixed chronic inflammation with eosinophils, the latter suggesting a possible drug etiology.

drug-induced vasculitis may have a complex clinical picture, it can be difficult to prove that a given drug was the sole cause of the vasculitis. Careful correlation with the history of drug intake, the clinical presentation, and the response to withdrawal of the drug is essential before implicating the drug as the cause of vasculitis. Association with vasculitis has been reported in a variety of drugs including alpha adrenergic nasal sprays, carbamazepine, diphenylhydantoin, allopurinol, cromoglycate, penicillin, nitrofurantoin, propylthiouracil, sulfonamides, procainamide, oral contraceptives, and anti-Tac antibodies.[39] Drug-induced pulmonary vasculitis can closely resemble an idiopathic vasculitis syndrome. The clinical severity may vary from mild to severe disease and may be fatal.[39] Some cases may be self-limited, and others may have a prolonged chronic course. Treatment for drug-induced vasculitis includes discontinuation of the offending drug with steroids or other immunosuppressive agents as needed.

Practical Points

▶ Lung and pleural lesions are seen in ~10% to 20% of patients with IgG4-RD.

▶ Patients with IgG4-related lung disease present with nonspecific respiratory illnesses or incidental radiologic abnormalities without related symptoms.

▶ Unexplained fibroinflammatory lesion with a prominent plasma cell infiltrate should raise a possibility of IgG4-RD.

▶ Elevated serum IgG4 level (>135 mg/dL) and increased IgG4-positive plasma cells in tissue (>20 and >50 per high-power field in small biopsy and surgical biopsy, respectively, with >40% in IgG4+/IgG+ ratio for both specimen types) could be supportive of the diagnosis.

▶ Corticosteroid therapy is generally effective in the treatment of IgG4-related pulmonary disease, but some patients have recurrences or residual radiologic abnormalities.

▶ Pulmonary vasculitis can be associated with not only GPA and EGPA but also many other conditions including systemic rheumatologic disorders, IBD, various infections, radiation injury, and drug reaction, among others.

▶ Clinical correlation is very important to find an underlying cause for potentially effective treatment (e.g., antibiotics for infections, discontinuation of offending drugs for drug-induced vasculitis, etc.).

▶ Nonspecific vascular inflammation can be seen in virtually any lung tissue involved by marked inflammation.

REFERENCES

1. Stone JH, Zen Y, Deshpande V. IgG4-related disease. *N Engl J Med.* 2012;366:539–551.
2. Zen Y, Nakanuma Y. IgG4-related disease: a cross-sectional study of 114 cases. *Am J Surg Pathol.* 2010;34:1812–1819.
3. Yi ES, Sekiguchi H, Peikert T, et al. Pathologic manifestations of Immunoglobulin(Ig)G4-related lung disease. *Semin Diagn Pathol.* 2012;29:219–225.
4. Zen Y, Inoue D, Kitao A, et al. IgG4-related lung and pleural disease: a clinicopathologic study of 21 cases. *Am J Surg Pathol.* 2009;33:1886–1893.
5. Inoue D, Zen Y, Abo H, et al. Immunoglobulin G4-related lung disease: CT findings with pathologic correlations. *Radiology.* 2009;251:260–270.
6. Khosroshahi A, Stone JH. A clinical overview of IgG4-related systemic disease. *Curr Opin Rheumatol.* 2011;23:57–66.

7. Matsui S, Hebisawa A, Sakai F, et al. Immunoglobulin G4-related lung disease: clinicoradiological and pathological features. *Respirology.* 2013;18:480–487.

8. Kobayashi H, Shimokawaji T, Kanoh S, et al. IgG4-positive pulmonary disease. *J Thorac Imaging.* 2007;22:360–362.

9. Hirano K, Kawabe T, Komatsu Y, et al. High-rate pulmonary involvement in autoimmune pancreatitis. *Intern Med J.* 2006;36:58–61.

10. Taniguchi T, Hamasaki A, Okamoto M. A case of suspected lymphocytic hypophysitis and organizing pneumonia during maintenance therapy for autoimmune pancreatitis associated with autoimmune thrombocytopenia. *Endocr J.* 2006;53:563–566.

11. Shrestha B, Sekiguchi H, Colby TV, et al. Distinctive pulmonary histopathology with increased IgG4-positive plasma cells in patients with autoimmune pancreatitis: report of 6 and 12 cases with similar histopathology. *Am J Surg Pathol.* 2009;33:1450–1462.

12. Takato H, Yasui M, Ichikawa Y, et al. Nonspecific interstitial pneumonia with abundant IgG4-positive cells infiltration, which was thought as pulmonary involvement of IgG4-related autoimmune disease. *Intern Med.* 2008;47:291–294.

13. Yamashita K, Haga H, Kobashi Y, et al. Lung involvement in IgG4-related lymphoplasmacytic vasculitis and interstitial fibrosis: report of 3 cases and review of the literature. *Am J Surg Pathol.* 2008;32:1620–1626.

14. Tsushima K, Tanabe T, Yamamoto H, et al. Pulmonary involvement of autoimmune pancreatitis. *Eur J Clin Invest.* 2009;39:714–722.

15. Naitoh I, Nakazawa T, Ohara H, et al. Clinical significance of extrapancreatic lesions in autoimmune pancreatitis. *Pancreas* 2010;39:e1–e5.

16. Cheuk W, Yuen HK, Chu SY, et al. Lymphadenopathy of IgG4-related sclerosing disease. *Am J Surg Pathol.* 2008;32:671–681.

17. Hamano H, Arakura N, Muraki T, et al. Prevalence and distribution of extrapancreatic lesions complicating autoimmune pancreatitis. *J Gastroenterol.* 2006;41:1197–1205.

18. Saegusa H, Momose M, Kawa S, et al. Hilar and pancreatic gallium-67 accumulation is characteristic feature of autoimmune pancreatitis. *Pancreas.* 2003;27:20–25.

19. Brito-Zeron P, Ramos-Casals M, Bosch X, et al. The clinical spectrum of IgG4-related disease. *Autoimmun Rev.* 2014;13:1203–1210.

20. Ryu JH, Horie R, Sekiguchi H, et al. Spectrum of disorders associated with elevated serum IgG4 levels encountered in clinical practice. *Int J Rheumatol.* 2012;2012:232960.

21. Wallace ZS, Mattoo H, Carruthers M, et al. Plasmablasts as a biomarker for IgG4-related disease, independent of serum IgG4 concentrations. *Ann Rheum Dis.* 2015;74:190–195.

22. Mattoo H, Mahajan VS, Della-Torre E, et al. De novo oligoclonal expansions of circulating plasmablasts in active and relapsing IgG4-related disease. *J Allergy Clin Immunol.* 2014;134:679–687.

23. Li Y, Nishihara E, Hirokawa M, et al. Distinct clinical, serological, and sonographic characteristics of hashimoto's thyroiditis based with and without IgG4-positive plasma cells. *J Clin Endocrinol Metab.* 2010;95:1309–1317.

24. Moteki H, Yasuo M, Hamano H, et al. IgG4-related chronic rhinosinusitis: a new clinical entity of nasal disease. *Acta Otolaryngol.* 2011;131:518–526.

25. Sato Y, Takeuchi M, Takata K, et al. Clinicopathologic analysis of IgG4-related skin disease. *Modern Pathol.* 2013;26:523–532.

26. Hirano K, Tada M, Sasahira N, et al. Incidence of malignancies in patients with IgG4-related disease. *Intern Med.* 2014;53:171–176.

27. Sogabe Y, Ohshima K, Azumi A, et al. Location and frequency of lesions in patients with IgG4-related ophthalmic diseases. *Graefe's Arch Clin Exp Ophthalmol.* 2014;252:531–538.

28. Della Torre E, Mattoo H, Mahajan VS, et al. Prevalence of atopy, eosinophilia, and IgE elevation in IgG4-related disease. *Allergy.* 2014;69:269–272.

29. Zen Y, Kitagawa S, Minato H, et al. IgG4-positive plasma cells in inflammatory pseudotumor (plasma cell granuloma) of the lung. *Hum Pathol.* 2005;36:710–717.

30. Hamed G, Tsushima K, Yasuo M, et al. Inflammatory lesions of the lung, submandibular gland, bile duct and prostate in a patient with IgG4-associated multifocal systemic fibrosclerosis. *Respirology.* 2007;12:455–457.

31. Takahashi N, Ghazale AH, Smyrk TC, et al. Possible association between IgG4-associated systemic disease with or without autoimmune pancreatitis and non-Hodgkin lymphoma. *Pancreas.* 2009;38:523–526.

32. Shiokawa M, Kodama Y, Yoshimura K, et al. Risk of cancer in patients with autoimmune pancreatitis. *Am J Gastroenterol.* 2013;108:610–617.

33. Smyrk TC. Pathological features of IgG4-related sclerosing disease. *Curr Opin Rheumatol.* 2011;23:74–79.

34. Deshpande V, Zen Y, Chan JK, et al. Consensus statement on the pathology of IgG4-related disease. *Modern Pathol.* 2012;25:1181–1192.

35. Chang SY, Keogh KA, Lewis JE, et al. IgG4-positive plasma cells in granulomatosis with polyangiitis (Wegener's): a clinicopathologic and immunohistochemical study on 43 granulomatosis with polyangiitis and 20 control cases. *Hum Pathol.* 2013;44:2432–2437.

36. Buser M, Felizeter-Kessler M, Lenggenhager D, et al. Rapidly progressive pulmonary hypertension in a patient with pulmonary tumor thrombotic microangiopathy. *Am J Respir Crit Care Med.* 2015;191:711–712.

37. Levine JB, Lukawski-Trubish D. Extraintestinal considerations in inflammatory bowel disease. *Gastroenterol Clin North Am.* 1995;24:633–646.

38. Vaszar LT, Orzechowski NM, Specks U, et al. Coexistent pulmonary granulomatosis with polyangiitis (Wegener granulomatosis) and Crohn disease. *Am J Surg Pathol.* 2014;38:354–359.

39. Cuellar ML. Drug-induced vasculitis. *Curr Rheumatol Rep.* 2002;4:55–59.

52 Acute Cellular and Antibody-Mediated Rejection of Lung Allografts

Anja C. Roden, M.D., Allen P. Burke, M.D., and Joseph J. Maleszewski, M.D.

Acute Cellular Rejection

Acute cellular rejection occurs due to an immune response of the host to donor antigens. This immune response is an alloimmune T-cell response that triggers T-cell cytotoxicity, T-cell–mediated delayed type II hypersensitivity, and potentiation of the B-cell–mediated antibody response.[1] About one-third of adult lung allograft recipients have at least one episode of acute rejection between discharge and 1-year follow-up.[2] Risk factors for acute rejection include HLA mismatch, type of immunosuppression, infection, and recipient factors including genetic factors and possibly vitamin D deficiency. In adults, acute rejection is most common between ages 18 and 34 years old.[2] Although acute rejection is the cause of death in <3% of patients, it is an adverse prognostic parameter in lung allografts. Therefore, routine surveillance for such is important.

Patients with acute cellular rejection may present with cough and shortness of breath, tremors, and problems with activities of daily lives, or they may be asymptomatic.[3] Imaging studies might show groundglass opacities, interlobular septal thickening, volume loss, nodules, and/or pleural effusion; however, these findings are not specific or sensitive for acute cellular rejection.[4] Lung function in these patients is typically obstructed as manifested by decrease in FEV1 or restricted with reduction in FVC and FEV1.[5] However, the sensitivity and specificity of a decrease in FEV1 for detecting acute cellular rejection are low. Therefore, bronchoscopic biopsy is currently the gold standard for evaluation of acute cellular rejection in lung allografts.

The histopathologic grading of acute cellular rejection has been defined as the "A" grade by the International Society of Heart and Lung Transplantation (ISHLT).[6] The diagnosis of acute cellular rejection requires the exclusion of an infection because of some overlapping morphologic features. Acute cellular rejection is characterized by an infiltrate of mononuclear lymphoid cells around capillaries and small vessels with or without extension into the surrounding interstitium. These lymphoid cells are predominantly of T-cell phenotype. Acute cellular rejection is graded as minimal, mild, moderate, and severe based upon the extent of the lymphocytic infiltrate and the presence or absence of additional findings such as acute lung injury (Table 52.1; Fig. 52.1).

Histologic findings of acute cellular rejection usually involve more than one vessel; however, on occasion, it might be seen only in a single location.[6] Therefore, each H&E level should be carefully reviewed. Furthermore, acute cellular rejection should be recorded even if only one vessel is involved. Foci of acute cellular rejection can be of varying grades, and the highest grade should be recorded. Lymphocytic infiltrates surrounding small vessels in the wall of airways should be regarded as airway inflammation rather than acute cellular rejection. Grades A1 and A2 are considered low-grade rejection; grades A3 and A4 are thought of high-grade rejection.

Acute Small Airway Rejection (Lymphocytic Bronchiolitis)

Acute small airway rejection is characterized by a mononuclear lymphoid cell infiltrate surrounding small airways including terminal and respiratory bronchioles. It is defined as the "B" grade by the

International Society of Heart and Lung Transplantation (Table 52.2; Fig. 52.2).[6] The "R" behind grades B1 and B2 denotes the revised grading in 2007. Inflammation of large airways should be described separately.

Differential Diagnosis of Acute Cellular Rejection and Acute Small Airway Rejection

The diagnosis of acute rejection requires the exclusion of infection, which can morphologically mimic rejection. Specifically, cytomegalovirus or *Pneumocystis jirovecii* infection might present with perivascular lymphocytic infiltrates.[7] Furthermore, features of acute lung injury as seen in high-grade rejection might also mimic an infectious process including viral, bacterial, or fungal infections. Multinucleated giant cells might occur in high-grade acute cellular rejection; however, well-formed granulomas are not a feature of rejection and are suggestive of an infectious process or aspiration. Careful examination of the H&E slides for viral inclusions or foreign body material is important, and the threshold of adding stains for microorganisms should be low.

TABLE 52.1 Histopathologic Grading of Acute Cellular Rejection of Lung Allografts, International Society of Heart and Lung Transplantation (2007)

Grade	Definition	Morphologic Findings
A0	None	No lymphoid infiltrate surrounding vessels
A1	Minimal	Small lymphoid infiltrates surround capillaries or small vessels; usually, only few vessels are involved
A2	Mild	Larger lymphoid infiltrates surround capillaries or small vessels; usually, a larger number of vessels are involved
A3	Moderate	Lymphoid infiltrates surround vessels and extend into the adjacent interstitium. Eosinophils might be present. Subendothelial lymphocytes can occur (i.e., endotheliitis). Morphologic features of acute lung injury might be focally present
A4	Severe	Lymphoid infiltrates surround vessels and extend into the adjacent interstitium; eosinophils and acute lung injury including organizing pneumonia, fibrinous organizing pneumonia, or hyaline membranes are present, which can be accompanied by a nonspecific neutrophilic infiltrate. Endotheliitis is usually identified. The vascular lymphoid infiltrate might be paradoxically diminished

Stewart S, Fishbein MC, Snell GI, et al. Revision of the 1996 working formulation for the standardization of nomenclature in the diagnosis of lung rejection. *J Heart Lung Transplant.* 2007;26:1229–1242.

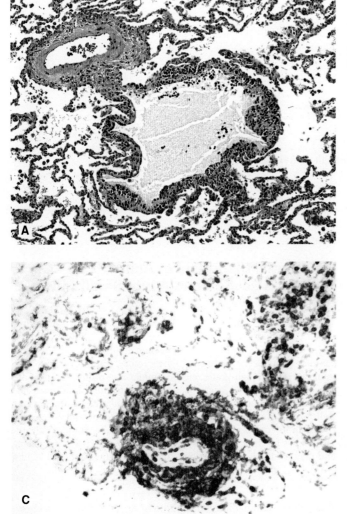

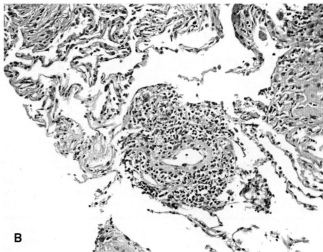

FIGURE 52.1 ▲ Acute cellular rejection. **A.** In low-grade rejection (ISHLT grades A1 and A2), there is perivascular chronic inflammation without extension into surrounding alveolar walls. **B.** There is moderate expansion of the perivascular space (ISHLT grade A2). **C.** Immunohistochemical staining for CD3 highlights T-cell infiltrate.

TABLE 52.2   Histopathologic Grading of Acute Small Airway Rejection of Lung Allografts According to the Most Recent Revision of the International Society of Heart and Lung Transplantation (2007)

Grade	Definition	Morphologic Findings
B0	None	No lymphoid infiltrate surrounding small airways
B1R	Low grade	Submucosal lymphocytic infiltrate, scattered, or circumferential. No intraepithelial component or epithelial damage
B2R	High grade	Marked lymphocytic infiltrate of airway epithelium and wall. Greater number of eosinophils and plasmacytoid cells. Epithelial damage is characterized by necrosis, metaplasia, ulceration, and/or marked intraepithelial lymphocytic infiltration
BX	Ungradable	Due to lack of small airways, infection, tangential cutting, artifact, etc.

"R" indicates revision but does not need to be routinely designated on diagnosis. Stewart S, Fishbein MC, Snell GI, et al. Revision of the 1996 working formulation for the standardization of nomenclature in the diagnosis of lung rejection. *J Heart Lung Transplant.* 2007;26:1229–1242.

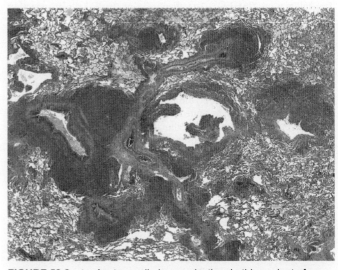

FIGURE 52.2 ▲ Acute small airway rejection. In this explant of a previously transplanted lung, there is marked peribronchiolar inflammation in a patient whose immunosuppression was discontinued prior to retransplant. The differential diagnosis is posttransplant lymphoproliferative disease, which was ruled out by testing for EBV and immunophenotyping of the cellular infiltrate. Ultimately, the findings were attributed to ISHLT grade B2R rejection.

Moreover, serology and molecular studies can help to identify infectious organisms.

Posttransplant lymphoproliferative disorders might also be considered when perivascular and interstitial inflammatory infiltrates are seen (see Chapter 54). Recurrent disease, especially sarcoidosis, should be excluded. In the early posttransplantation period, ischemia/reperfusion injury is a possibility that usually presents with features of acute lung injury.

Antibody-Mediated Rejection

Antibody-mediated rejection (AMR) is thought to be the consequence of the binding of circulating antibodies to antigens. Antigen–antibody complexes activate the complement cascade resulting in graft injury and ultimately graft failure.

Hyperacute rejection is a rare but life-threatening form of rejection to preexisting antibodies that occurs within minutes and a few hours following transplantation.[8] It might be already recognized intraoperatively as the allograft becomes edematous and cyanotic. Morphologically, platelet thrombi, infiltration of neutrophils, fibrin thrombi, necrosis of vessel walls, and features of diffuse alveolar damage might be seen.[8,9]

Most cases of AMR are thought to occur later after transplantation. The diagnosis is challenging because no single feature or marker specific for AMR has been identified yet. Therefore, the true incidence is unknown. Patients clinically might present with graft dysfunction. Circulating donor-specific antibodies can be identified in some patients. Morphologic features of AMR are still debated. It appears that the histopathologic findings in AMR are nonspecific patterns of lung injury that can also be seen in association with other conditions such as severe acute cellular rejection, infection, ischemia/reperfusion injury, and abnormal drug reactions. Recently, the Pathology Council of the International Society of Heart and Lung Transplantation has published guidelines for the diagnosis of AMR emphasizing the importance of a multidisciplinary approach—specifically "triple test."

The triple test includes evaluation for graft dysfunction, circulating donor-specific antibodies, and capillary endothelial complement 4d (C4d) reactivity (by immunohistochemistry or immunofluorescence).[10] C4d is a complement split product, and its capillary endothelial/subendothelial deposition has been suggested as a surrogate marker for AMR in other solid organ allografts including the heart, kidney, and pancreas.[11–13] However, in the lung, the specificity and sensitivity of C4d deposition in AMR are still under investigation.[14] If not performed

TABLE 52.3 Morphologic Features that Should Trigger Staining with C4d

Neutrophilic capillaritis
Neutrophilic septal margination
High-grade acute cellular rejection (□ ISHLT grade A3)
Persistent/recurrent acute cellular rejection (any ISHLT grade A)
Acute lung injury pattern/diffuse alveolar damage
High-grade acute small airway rejection (ISHLT grade B2R)
Persistent low-grade acute small airway rejection (ISHLT grade B1R)
Obliterative bronchiolitis (ISHLT grade C1)
Arteritis in the absence of infection or cellular rejection
Graft dysfunction without morphologic explanation
Any histologic findings in setting of de novo donor-specific antibodies

Modified from Berry G, Burke M, Andersen C, et al. Pathology of pulmonary antibody-mediated rejection: 2012 update from the Pathology Council of the ISHLT. *J Heart Lung Transplant.* 2013;32:14–21.

routinely, morphologic features that should trigger immunostaining with C4d are summarized in Table 52.3 and demonstrated in Figure 52.3.

C4d deposition should only be evaluated in interalveolar septal capillaries.[10] According to the current guidelines, C4d staining can be "strong" (continuous linear endothelial/subendothelial deposition within capillaries) (Fig. 52.4) or "weak" (fainter/weaker C4d deposition with patchy, granular endothelial staining).[10] Multifocal or diffuse C4d deposition (>50% of interalveolar septal capillaries staining) is considered positive. Positive C4d staining should be recorded as "findings suggestive of AMR" with the understanding that the final diagnosis of AMR should only be made after comprehensive clinical, serologic, microbiologic, and pathologic correlation and exclusion of other etiologies.[10] Although focal and <50% of interstitial capillaries staining is currently regarded as negative, its presence should be conveyed to the clinician as serologic testing for donor-specific antibodies, and clinical monitoring might become necessary.

Because C4d deposition occurs due to complement activation, it is not specific to AMR and can also be seen in other processes including reperfusion injury or infection. In addition, C4d in the lung often has a high background staining due to nonspecific binding by serum and elastic laminas of vessels and airways. CD68 immunostaining appears to be of limited diagnostic value due to numerous intravascular macrophages in lung allografts. The experience with C3d is still limited in lung allografts.

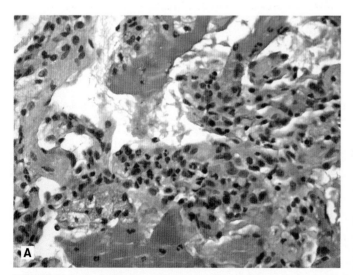

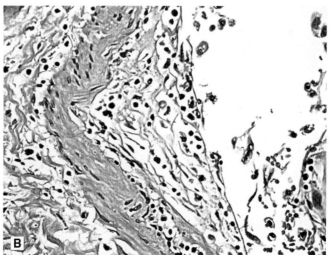

FIGURE 52.3 ▲ Antibody-mediated rejection, histologic clues. **A.** Neutrophils in the capillary walls are a sign of antibody-mediated rejection and warranted immunohistochemical staining for complement. **B.** Inflammation in arteries is another such sign.

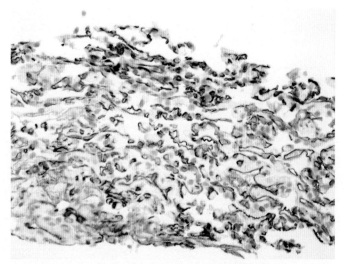

FIGURE 52.4 ▲ Antibody-mediated rejection, anti-C4d immunohisto-chemical stain. There is diffuse and strong capillary deposition of C4d.

REFERENCES

1. McManigle W, Pavlisko EN, Martinu T. Acute cellular and antibody-mediated allograft rejection. *Semin Respir Crit Care Med.* 2013;34:320–335.
2. Christie JD, Edwards LB, Kucheryavaya AY, et al. The Registry of the International Society for Heart and Lung Transplantation: 29th adult lung and heart–lung transplant report—2012. *J Heart Lung Transplant.* 2012;31:1073–1086.
3. De Vito Dabbs A, Hoffman LA, Iacono AT, et al. Are symptom reports useful for differentiating between acute rejection and pulmonary infection after lung transplantation? *Heart Lung.* 2004;33:372–380.
4. Ng YL, Paul N, Patsios D, et al. Imaging of lung transplantation: review. *AJR Am J Roentgenol.* 2009;192:S1–S13, quiz S14–S19.
5. Van Muylem A, Melot C, Antoine M, et al. Role of pulmonary function in the detection of allograft dysfunction after heart–lung transplantation. *Thorax.* 1997;52:643–647.
6. Stewart S, Fishbein MC, Snell GI, et al. Revision of the 1996 working formulation for the standardization of nomenclature in the diagnosis of lung rejection. *J Heart Lung Transplant.* 2007;26:1229–1242.
7. Tazelaar HD. Perivascular inflammation in pulmonary infections: implications for the diagnosis of lung rejection. *J Heart Lung Transplant.* 1991;10:437–441.
8. De Jesus Peixoto Camargo J, Marcantonio Camargo S, Marcelo Schio S, et al. Hyperacute rejection after single lung transplantation: a case report. *Transplant Proc.* 2008;40:867–869.
9. Roden AC, Tazelaar HD. Lung. In: Liapis H, Wang HL, eds. *Pathology of Solid Organ Transplantation.* Heidelberg, Germany: Springer; 2011:171–198.
10. Berry G, Burke M, Andersen C, et al. Pathology of pulmonary antibody-mediated rejection: 2012 update from the Pathology Council of the ISHLT. *J Heart Lung Transplant.* 2013;32:14–21.
11. de Kort H, Munivenkatappa RB, Berger SP, et al. Pancreas allograft biopsies with positive c4d staining and anti-donor antibodies related to worse outcome for patients. *Am J Transplant.* 2010;10:1660–1667.
12. Tan CD, Baldwin WM, III, Rodriguez ER. Update on cardiac transplantation pathology. *Arch Pathol Lab Med.* 2007;131:1169–1191.
13. Herman J, Lerut E, Van Damme-Lombaerts R, et al. Capillary deposition of complement C4d and C3d in pediatric renal allograft biopsies. *Transplantation.* 2005;79:1435–1440.
14. Wallace WD, Weigt SS, Farver CF. Update on pathology of antibody-mediated rejection in the lung allograft. *Curr Opin Organ Transplant.* 2014;19:303–308.

53 Chronic Lung Allograft Dysfunction (Obliterative Bronchiolitis, Chronic Vascular Rejection, and Restrictive Allograft Syndrome)

Anja C. Roden, M.D., Allen P. Burke, M.D., and Joseph J. Maleszewski, M.D.

Chronic Lung Allograft Disease

The current understanding of the different pathologic manifestations ("phenotypes") of chronic rejection of the lung is evolving. From a pathologic standpoint, chronic rejection has been considered to affect either the airways (obliterative bronchiolitis, which is fairly well characterized) or the vessels, especially arteries (chronic vascular rejection).[1]

Similar to the heart, the diagnosis is not generally made on biopsy samples. In contrast to the heart, where chronic rejection is synonymous with chronic allograft vasculopathy, very little is understood or reported on vascular rejection of the lung. Chronic rejection of the lung has, until recently, denoted obliterative bronchiolitis, resulting clinically in bronchiolitis obliterans syndrome. Recently, it has been appreciated that chronic parenchymal lung rejection may have a restrictive component, which is termed restrictive allograft syndrome (RAS). RAS overlaps clinically and pathologically with pleuroparenchymal fibroelastosis (see Chapter 20). Because of the overlap of obstructive and restrictive disease that characterizes chronic rejection of the lung, the general term "chronic lung allograft dysfunction" (CLAD) has been suggested.[2]

Obliterative Bronchiolitis

Constrictive or obliterative bronchiolitis is a form of small airway disease characterized by concentric peribronchiolar fibrosis. The term "obliterative" is preferred in the setting of lung transplantation.[3] A similar histologic process, usually termed constrictive bronchiolitis, occurs in autoimmune syndromes, allogeneic stem cell transplant, and after inhalational lung injury.[4]

Obliterative bronchiolitis represents about one-half of chronic lung rejection and two-thirds of irreversible forms.[2] The risk is 70% at 10 years posttransplant[5,6] and 50% after 5 years.[2] The strongest risk factor for allograft failure due to bronchiolitis obliterans is lymphocytic bronchiolitis (acute small airway rejection, ISHLT grade B1R or B2R) diagnosed by transbronchial biopsy. A patient with a single B2R lesion has a 75% chance of developing bronchiolitis obliterans syndrome in the subsequent 3 years and a 50% chance of dying.[7]

Clinically, pulmonary function tests reveal respiratory obstruction manifest by normal or decreased forced vital capacity (FVC), reduced forced expiratory volume in 1 second (FEV_1), and reduced ratio of FEV_1 to FVC, without significant response to inhaled bronchodilators. Total lung capacity is normal, and air trapping results in

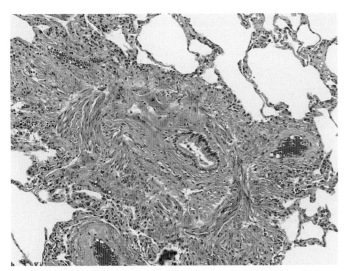

FIGURE 53.1 ▲ Obliterative bronchiolitis. There is concentric peribronchiolar fibrosis. In this example, a small airway remains, as well as the muscular wall of the bronchiole. There is concentric fibrosis between the epithelium and the smooth muscle.

high residual volume.[4] The bronchiolitis obliterans syndrome occurs more frequently in transplant patients with a history of acute cellular rejection, circulating donor-specific antibodies, gastroesophageal reflux disease and microaspiration, and respiratory viral infections. Microvascular insufficiency secondary to the lack of allograft bronchial arteries is also a possible cause.[8] Other risk factors include primary graft dysfunction, lymphocytic bronchiolitis, autoimmunity, and genetic factors.[9]

Obliterative bronchiolitis is the pathologic manifestation of the clinical bronchiolitis obliterans syndrome and is characterized by dense hyaline fibrosis in the bronchiolar submucosa, resulting in partial or complete luminal occlusion (Figs. 53.1 and 53.2). It differs from organizing pneumonia in that loose fibrosis within terminal bronchioles is generally absent, and there is destruction of the respiratory epithelium, initially with reactive changes. Evidence of obstruction in the form of extravasated mucus (mucostasis) and foamy macrophages in the distal airspaces may be present and is sometimes the only manifestation of the disease. Because transbronchial biopsies often fail to sample a large number of small airways, a negative biopsy does not exclude the diagnosis. If present, obliterative bronchiolitis in lung allograft biopsies should be reported as ISHLT grade C1.[1]

Histologic phases of lymphocytic bronchiolitis (grade B rejection) progressing to obliterative bronchiolitis have been described as inflammatory active, fibrotic active, and inactive obliterative bronchiolitis, reflecting the presence of chronic inflammation, scarring, or both.[10] In practice, the use of the term obliterative bronchiolitis is restricted to those biopsies with fibrosis. It is useful, however, to describe the concomitant presence of active inflammation (lymphocytic bronchiolitis or grade B rejection) in biopsies with obliterative bronchiolitis.

Neutrophilic Reversible Allograft Dysfunction

Neutrophilic reversible allograft dysfunction describes a subset of obstructive lung disease in transplant patients that, in contrast to obliterative bronchiolitis, is reversible and is associated with increased neutrophils in the bronchoalveolar lavage. Neutrophilic reversible allograft dysfunction responds to azithromycin, is characterized by small airway thickening (tree-in-bud) changes on computed tomography scans, and has a relatively good prognosis.[10]

The mechanism of action of the macrolide antibiotics is believed to be related to their anti-inflammatory, rather than antimicrobial, activity. The histologic features on transbronchial biopsies are those of lymphocytic bronchiolitis (ISHLT grade B cellular rejection), without significant acute inflammation, despite the cytologic findings of neutrophils in lavage samples. Therefore, neutrophilic reversible allograft dysfunction is strictly a clinical diagnosis to be considered in a patient with evidence of small airway rejection and neutrophils in the lavage specimens.

Although obliterative bronchiolitis may stabilize, it is typically a progressive disease, with a median graft survival of 35 months.[2,6]

Chronic Vascular Rejection

Chronic vascular rejection, previously termed accelerated graft vascular sclerosis,[11] denotes intimal inflammation, predominantly of muscular arteries, with resulting intimal thickening, thrombosis, and occlusion (Fig. 53.3). The inflammatory cells are primarily

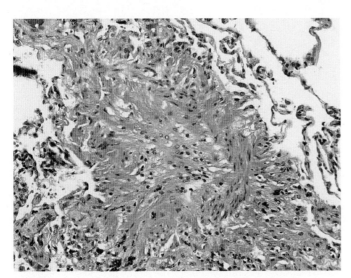

FIGURE 53.2 ▲ Obliterative bronchiolitis. The bronchiole shows end-stage obliteration, without remaining mucosa.

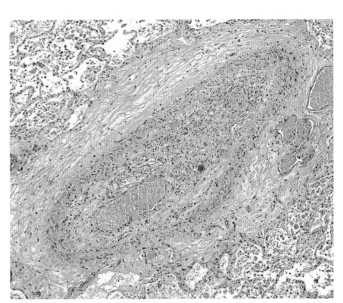

FIGURE 53.3 ▲ Chronic vascular rejection. There is inflammation in the media and organized luminal thrombus.

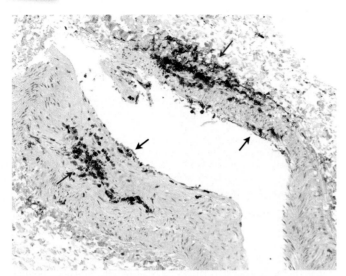

FIGURE 53.4 ▲ Chronic vascular rejection. Immunohistochemical staining for CD3 shows T lymphocytes in the intima (*black arrows*) and adventitia (*brown arrows*).

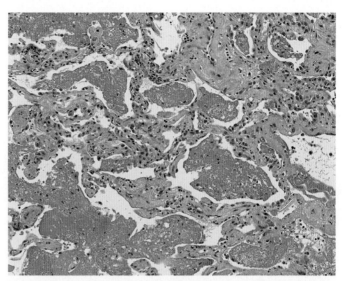

FIGURE 53.6 ▲ Restrictive allograft syndrome. There are areas of acute lung injury with fibrin in dilated airspaces and reactive pneumocytes.

T lymphocytes (Fig. 53.4). The process is similarly histologic to cardiac allograft vasculopathy. "Chronic vascular rejection" has also been designated for acellular hyaline venous sclerosis, which is not inflammatory mediated and which is increased in incidence in older donors. Chronic vascular rejection is infrequently present on lung biopsies but may be diagnosed in wedge biopsies or autopsy material. In fact, according to the ISHLT, grading of chronic vascular rejection is not reported in allograft transbronchial biopsies, probably because of the usually insufficient number of pulmonary arteries and veins in transbronchial biopsies.[1]

Restrictive Allograft Syndrome

Approximately 30% of chronic rejection in lung transplant patients is primarily restrictive, as defined by decreased total lung capacity, decreased FEV_1, and normal ratio of FEV_1 to FVC.[2,12] RAS occurs in about 2% to 3% of lung transplant patients, at a median of 700 days

posttransplant.[12,13] Computed tomographic findings include ground-glass opacities, traction bronchiectasis, architectural distortion with or without hilar retraction, and areas of consolidation.[2] Pathologically, there is upper lobe fibrosis and parenchymal interstitial fibrosis (Fig. 53.5). In almost all cases, there is prominent elastic tissue within the scars, which are most typically subpleural, but may also occur paraseptally and centrally. A characteristic finding is the presence of acute alveolar injury with fibrin, in areas of scarring,[12,14] in a pattern that has been described as acute fibrinous and organizing pneumonia (Fig. 53.6). Concomitant obliterative bronchiolitis is common (Fig. 53.7), as well as areas of organizing pneumonia and chronic vascular rejection. The survival of RAS is worse than other forms of chronic rejection, with a median of 8 months.[2]

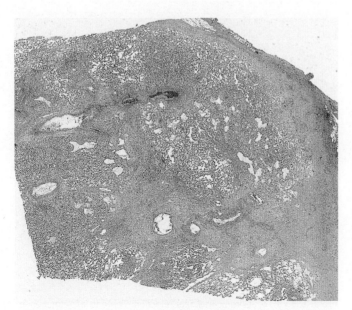

FIGURE 53.5 ▲ Restrictive allograft syndrome. There is interstitial fibrosis, predominantly septal, and subpleural.

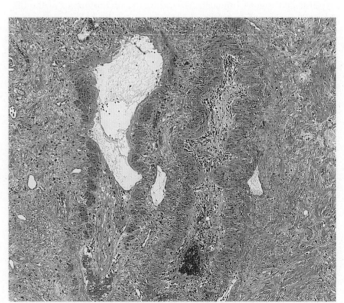

FIGURE 53.7 ▲ Obliterative bronchiolitis and chronic vascular rejection in restrictive allograft syndrome. The airway (**left**) shows denuded epithelium and focal necrosis with fibrosis (**bottom**). The artery of this bronchovascular bundle (**right**) shows diffuse intimal thickening with intimitis.

REFERENCES

1. Stewart S, Fishbein MC, Snell GI, et al. Revision of the 1996 working formulation for the standardization of nomenclature in the diagnosis of lung rejection. *J Heart Lung Transplant.* 2007;26:1229–1242.
2. Verleden SE, de Jong PA, Ruttens D, et al. Functional and computed tomographic evolution and survival of restrictive allograft syndrome after lung transplantation. *J Heart Lung Transplant.* 2014;33:270–277.
3. Meyer KC, Raghu G, Verleden GM, et al. An international ISHLT/ATS/ERS clinical practice guideline: diagnosis and management of bronchiolitis obliterans syndrome. *Eur Respir J.* 2014;44:1479–1503.
4. Barker AF, Bergeron A, Rom WN, et al. Obliterative bronchiolitis. *N Engl J Med.* 2014;370:1820–1828.
5. Benden C, Edwards LB, Kucheryavaya AY, et al. The Registry of the International Society for Heart and Lung Transplantation: fifteenth pediatric lung and heart–lung transplantation report—2012. *J Heart Lung Transplant.* 2012;31:1087–1095.
6. Christie JD, Edwards LB, Kucheryavaya AY, et al. The Registry of the International Society for Heart and Lung Transplantation: 29th adult lung and heart–lung transplant report—2012. *J Heart Lung Transplant.* 2012;31:1073–1086.
7. Glanville AR, Aboyoun CL, Havryk A, et al. Severity of lymphocytic bronchiolitis predicts long-term outcome after lung transplantation. *Am J Respir Crit Care Med.* 2008;177:1033–1040.
8. Dhillon GS, Zamora MR, Roos JE, et al. Lung transplant airway hypoxia: a diathesis to fibrosis? *Am J Respir Crit Care Med.* 2010;182:230–236.
9. Verleden GM, Vos R, Vanaudenaerde B, et al. Current views on chronic rejection after lung transplantation. *Transpl Int.* 2015;28:1131–1139.
10. Vanaudenaerde BM, Meyts I, Vos R, et al. A dichotomy in bronchiolitis obliterans syndrome after lung transplantation revealed by azithromycin therapy. *Eur Respir J.* 2008;32:832–843.
11. Yousem SA, Berry GJ, Cagle PT, et al. Revision of the 1990 working formulation for the classification of pulmonary allograft rejection: Lung Rejection Study Group. *J Heart Lung Transplant.* 1996;15:1–15.
12. Ofek E, Sato M, Saito T, et al. Restrictive allograft syndrome post lung transplantation is characterized by pleuroparenchymal fibroelastosis. *Mod Pathol.* 2013;26:350–356.
13. Pakhale SS, Hadjiliadis D, Howell DN, et al. Upper lobe fibrosis: a novel manifestation of chronic allograft dysfunction in lung transplantation. *J Heart Lung Transplant.* 2005;24:1260–1268.
14. Sato M, Waddell TK, Wagnetz U, et al. Restrictive allograft syndrome (RAS): a novel form of chronic lung allograft dysfunction. *J Heart Lung Transplant.* 2011;30:735–742.

54 Miscellaneous Pathologic Findings in Lung Allografts

Anja C. Roden, M.D., Allen P. Burke, M.D., and Joseph J. Maleszewski, M.D.

Posttransplant Acute Lung Injury (Primary Graft Dysfunction)

Primary graft dysfunction (PGD) is a syndrome that is presumed secondary to ischemia and reperfusion injury. It is characterized by acute lung injury and occurs within the first 72 hours after lung transplantation. PGD is the most common cause of death within 30 days of transplant. There may be a relation between the duration of nonperfusion of the graft (cold ischemic storage) and the respiratory and circulatory conditions of the donor prior to transplant. The clinical findings are similar to hyperacute rejection in patients with preformed antibodies, which are generally a contraindication for transplant, but may be occult. In studies published after the International Society of Heart and Lung Transplantation (ISHLT) Working Group on Primary Graft Dysfunction published a standardized definition and grading system, the reported incidence of severe PGD ranged between 22% and 32% of transplant patients.[1] The mortality and morbidity are high.[2] Furthermore, PGD has been associated with decreased functional status and bronchiolitis obliterans syndrome.[3]

Histologically, PGD manifests as diffuse alveolar damage. Generally, at the time of biopsy, the phase of injury will be organizing, with minimal residual fibrin, thickened interstitium, and reactive endothelial cells (Figs. 54.1 to 54.3). The differential diagnosis includes acute cellular rejection, although interstitial T-cell infiltration is not prominent in cases of organizing alveolar injury, and there are no perivascular aggregates of lymphocytes. If there are areas of severe ischemia with early infarct, there may be hemorrhage and acute interstitial inflammation, which is difficult to distinguish from hyperacute rejection (Fig. 54.4). The organizing features of diffuse alveolar damage, due to any cause but including PGD, are somewhat similar to organizing pneumonia in that there are nests of proliferating fibroblasts. In general, in organizing diffuse alveolar damage, proliferating fibroblasts are within alveolar septa leading to their expansion, while organizing pneumonia is characterized by intra-alveolar and intrabronchiolar polypoid plugs of proliferating fibroblasts (Masson bodies). However, it may be impossible to distinguish organizing pneumonia from organizing diffuse alveolar lung injury on transbronchial biopsy, although the presence of some normal alveoli, without inflammation, edema, or reactive pneumocytes, favors organizing pneumonia.

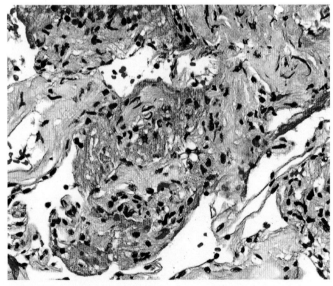

FIGURE 54.1 ▲ Acute and organizing acute alveolar injury (diffuse alveolar damage), allograft transbronchial biopsy. The biopsy was performed 2 weeks after transplant. There is intra-alveolar fibrin, and the interstitium is thickened by edema and sparse fibrosis.

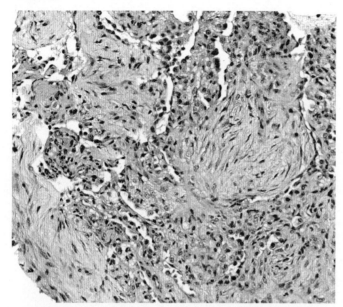

FIGURE 54.2 ▲ Organizing acute alveolar injury (diffuse alveolar damage), allograft transbronchial biopsy. There is organization with loose fibrosis and diffusely thickened inflamed interstitium.

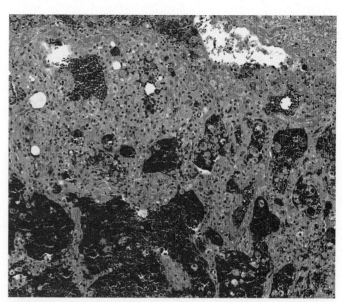

FIGURE 54.4 ▲ Acute infarct, allograft, retransplant. The patient required retransplantation 4 days after transplant for acute graft dysfunction due to ischemia. There is necrosis of the alveolar septa, which are infiltrated by inflammatory cells.

Lung Infections

Infections are common in lung transplant patients and require consideration in the differential of a patient with suspected rejection (Table 54.1). After graft dysfunction, infections are the second most common cause of death in the first month and the most common cause of death between 31 days and 1 year after transplantation in adults.[4] The clinical diagnosis of infection is based largely on culture results. Pathogenicity, titer or colony number, and multiplicity of organisms are important considerations in determining if these organisms are contaminants.

Biopsies are performed in order to exclude acute rejection as a cause for the patient's graft dysfunction. Bacterial infections generally cause acute exudates, with fibrin and acute and chronic inflammatory cells in the alveolar spaces, a pattern that does not resemble cellular- or antibody-mediated rejection. Viral and fungal infections, however, can mimic acute cellular rejection, with interstitial and perivascular infiltrates of T lymphocytes.[5] For this reason, it is impossible to exclude a viral etiology in all histologically diagnosed rejection. Rejection and infection might coexist, which may be suggested in cases of bacterial infections, in which there is both an acute exudate and interstitial T-cell infiltrates suggestive of cellular rejection.

Because cytomegalovirus and pneumocystis are relatively common infections in transplant patients and may be seen readily in biopsy material, it is especially important to exclude these organisms on a routine basis. Immunohistochemical stains for cytomegalovirus (Fig. 54.5) and Gomori methenamine–silver staining for pneumocystis are common diagnostic aids in biopsy samples that complement cytologic preparations of bronchoalveolar lavage fluid. Viral titer quantitation by polymerase chain reaction is of limited benefit in establishing symptomatic infection by cytomegalovirus.[6,7]

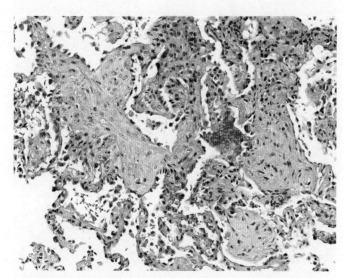

FIGURE 54.3 ▲ Organizing acute alveolar injury (diffuse alveolar damage), allograft transbronchial biopsy. The organization is more focal, with uninvolved relatively thin alveolar septa, although there is diffuse hyperplasia of lining pneumocytes. This pattern overlaps with organizing pneumonia. The clinical history was more consistent with healing acute graft dysfunction (biopsy 4 weeks after transplant).

TABLE 54.1   Findings Other Than Rejection to Consider in Lung Allograft

- Posttransplant acute lung injury (diffuse alveolar damage)
- Infection
- Mesothelium
- Recurrent native disease
- Anastomotic complications (endobronchial biopsy)
- Pulmonary alveolar proteinosis
- Malignancy
- Hemosiderosis
- Organizing pneumonia
- Aspiration
- Bronchus-associated lymphoid tissue
- Posttransplant lymphoproliferative disease
- Large airway inflammation
- Smoker-type respiratory bronchiolitis

Many of these are discussed in Stewart D. International classification of functioning, disability and health. *Can J Occup Ther.* 2007;74 Spec No.:217–220, Ref.[31].

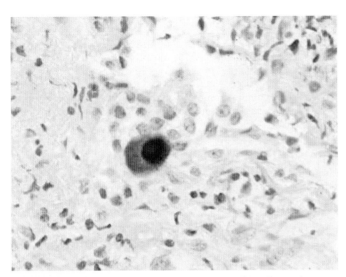

FIGURE 54.5 ▲ Cytomegalovirus pneumonia, allograft transbronchial biopsy. Immunohistochemical staining demonstrates positivity in the cytoplasm and nucleus.

Mesothelium in Transbronchial Biopsies

Although the acquisition of pleural tissue is rare in transbronchial biopsies,[8] it may be somewhat more common in biopsies of allograft lungs, because of the restriction and decreased lung volumes that often occur later in the course of transplant. When reactive, mesothelial cells can mimic carcinoma and necessitate immunohistochemical studies to confirm their origin (Fig. 54.6).

Recurrent Diseases

Of those diseases that commonly lead to transplant, only sarcoidosis often recurs in the allograft lung, without a detriment in survival.[9] Histologic features of recurrent sarcoidosis are identical to native lung disease (Fig. 54.7), and the granulomas appear to be derived from recipient cells.[10,11] Lymphangioleiomyomatosis recurring in donor lungs has also been reported,[12] and, similar to sarcoid, the lesional cells

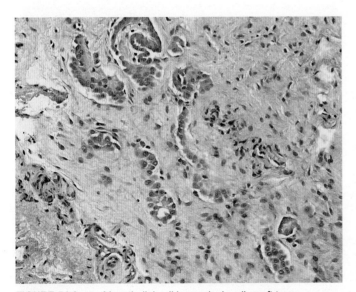

FIGURE 54.6 ▲ Mesothelial cell hyperplasia, allograft transbronchial biopsy. In ~1% to 3% of allograft biopsies, mesothelium is present. When reactive, the appearance may mimic carcinoma. Immunohistochemical stains confirmed mesothelial differentiation (not shown).

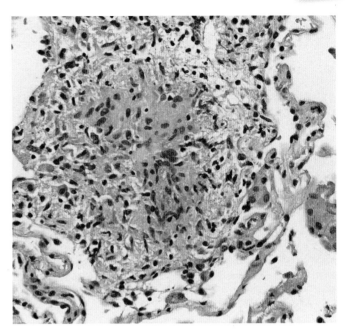

FIGURE 54.7 ▲ Recurrent sarcoidosis, allograft transbronchial biopsy. The patient was transplanted 9 months prior to this biopsy for fibrotic sarcoid lung disease. There is an interstitial granuloma consistent with sarcoidosis. Subsequent biopsies have been negative for granulomas.

have a recipient origin.[13] Other diseases that have been reported to recur in the lung allograft include pulmonary Langerhans cell histiocytosis, giant cell interstitial pneumonia, allergic bronchopulmonary aspergillosis, desquamative interstitial pneumonia, squamous cell and adenocarcinomas, alveolar proteinosis, and panbronchiolitis.

Anastomotic Complications

Airway anastomotic complications occur in ~10% of lung transplant recipients and include strictures, bronchomalacia, and dehiscence.[14] Endobronchial biopsies are often performed at these sites and usually disclose granulation tissue or acellular necrotic material. It is generally recommended to perform fungal stains to exclude fungal organisms. In some cases, invasive fungus derived from donor tissue can result in serious anastomotic complications necessitating retransplantation (Figs. 54.8 and 54.9).

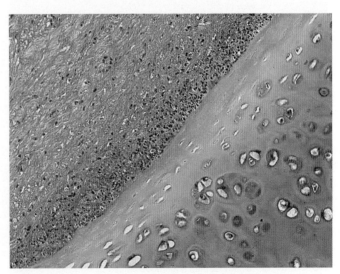

FIGURE 54.8 ▲ Invasive mucormycosis, allograft anastomosis, explant. There is necrotic submucosa, cartilage at the right. The patient required retransplantation 3 weeks after first transplant.

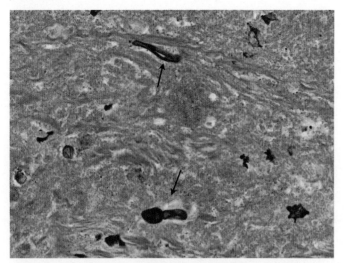

FIGURE 54.9 ▲ Invasive mucormycosis, allograft anastomosis, explant. Gomori methenamine–silver stain shows broad hyphae (*arrows*). Culture confirmed mucor species.

Pulmonary Alveolar Proteinosis

Pulmonary alveolar proteinosis is a rare complication in lung transplant patients and may be precipitated by reperfusion injury, rejection, infection, and abnormal drug reaction.[15-17] A case has also been reported after chemotherapy for acute leukemia developing after lung transplantation.[18]

Malignancies

Malignancies develop in solid organ transplant recipients at twice the rate of the general population. The most common are squamous skin cancers, which, when they occur, result in death in 8% of patients.[19] They may metastasize to the lung and lead to resection (Figs. 54.10 and 54.11). Rarely, pulmonary and extrapulmonary malignancies arising in the donor can also be transmitted to the recipient from contamination of the graft.[20,21]

Hemosiderin Macrophages

Hemosiderin-laden macrophages are present in approximately one-third to one-half of lung transplant biopsies. They have been associated with multiple episodes of rejection,[22] but may also occur in a biopsy of a previously biopsied area and are of little diagnostic significance.

Organizing Pneumonia and Aspiration

Areas of organizing pneumonia in transplant biopsies are not uncommon and may be a manifestation of organized ischemic injury (Fig. 54.3), moderate rejection, infection, aspiration, and as a reaction to drugs, including sirolimus. Therefore, its finding must be considered in context with other abnormalities present on the biopsy in addition to clinical history. The presence of eosinophils may possibly favor a drug reaction, although eosinophils have also been associated with rejection. Viewing the biopsy under polarized light for the detection of foreign material is helpful diagnostically to exclude aspiration (Fig. 54.12). It is debated if the presence of organizing pneumonia within the first year of transplant increases the risk for bronchiolitis obliterans syndrome.[23,24]

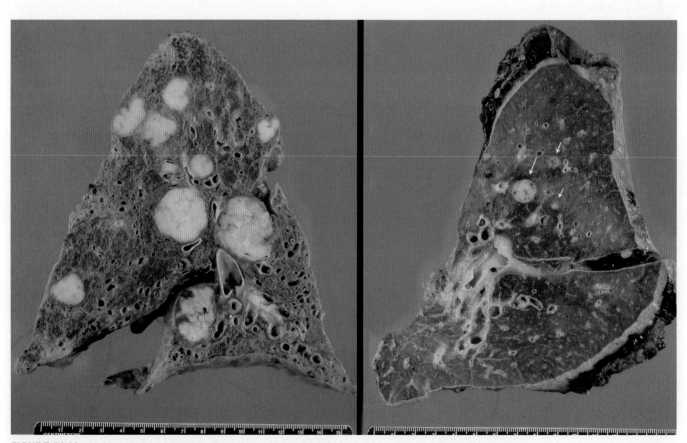

FIGURE 54.10 ▲ Metastatic squamous cell carcinoma, lung allograft. An autopsy showing metastatic squamous cell carcinoma to the native lung with idiopathic pulmonary fibrosis **(left)** and the allograft that had smaller nodules **(right**, *arrows*). The primary site was the facial skin.

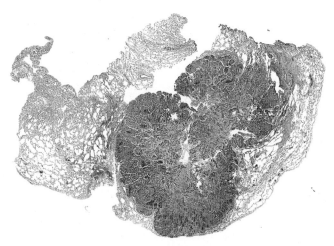

FIGURE 54.11 ▲ Metastatic squamous cell carcinoma, lung allograft. Another patient had a primary squamous cell carcinoma from the skin around the anus (not shown). Surgery was performed for oligometastases resection with wedge lung resection.

Hyperplasia of Bronchus-Associated Lymphoid Tissue

Bronchus-associated lymphoid tissue occurs in ~10% to 20% of lung transplant biopsies and does not appear to be associated with an increased risk of obliterative bronchiolitis or acute cellular rejection.[25] Distinction between reactive lymphoid hyperplasia and acute cellular rejection is made histologically by lack of infiltration of the bronchiolar mucosa and the nodular peribronchiolar configuration of the inflammation. Because histologic features are often distorted on transbronchial specimens, immunohistochemical staining is highly effective in distinguishing CD20-positive follicular hyperplasia from T-cell interstitial and peribronchial infiltrates.

Posttransplant Lymphoproliferative Disease

Posttransplant lymphoproliferative disorders (PTLDs) are derived from recipient cells and often contain Epstein-Barr virus. The incidence of

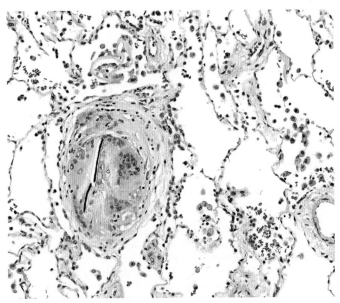

FIGURE 54.12 ▲ Aspiration, explanted lung. The patient had a retransplant for presumed bronchiolitis obliterans syndrome. Pathologically, the small airways were obstructed by granulomas surrounding aspirated plant material.

posttransplant lymphoproliferative disease following lung transplantation ranges from 2% to 6%.[26–28]

In a series of 4,747 patients with solid organ and stem cell/bone marrow transplants, 38 patients (0.8%) developed PTLD, of which 11 occurred in the thorax and 5 in the lung. In the same series, of 83 lung transplant patients, 3 (3.6%) developed thoracic PTLDs, in the mediastinum, donor lung, and native lung, respectively.[27] There were three additional pulmonary PTLDs, in patients who received bone marrow and kidney transplants.[27]

The histologic finding of pulmonary PTLDs is most commonly that of a monomorphic B-cell lymphoma of the diffuse large B-cell type, although polymorphic PTLD and monomorphic B-cell lymphoma of the Burkitt type have also been reported.[29,30]

Histologically, sheets of plasmacytoid or atypical lymphocytes favor lymphoma over rejection, and flow cytometry, molecular studies, and in situ hybridization for Epstein-Barr viral RNA are confirmatory for the diagnosis.

REFERENCES

1. Christie JD, Carby M, Bag R, et al. Report of the ISHLT Working Group on Primary Lung Graft Dysfunction part II: definition. A consensus statement of the International Society for Heart and Lung Transplantation. *J Heart Lung Transplant*. 2005;24:1454–1459.
2. Christie JD, Kotloff RM, Pochettino A, et al. Clinical risk factors for primary graft failure following lung transplantation. *Chest*. 2003;124:1232–1241.
3. Suzuki Y, Cantu E, Christie JD. Primary graft dysfunction. *Semin Respir Crit Care Med*. 2013;34:305–319.
4. Yusen RD, Christie JD, Edwards LB, et al. The Registry of the International Society for Heart and Lung Transplantation: Thirtieth Adult Lung and Heart-Lung Transplant Report—2013; focus theme: age. *J Heart Lung Transplant*. 2013;32:965–978.
5. Tazelaar HD. Perivascular inflammation in pulmonary infections: implications for the diagnosis of lung rejection. *J Heart Lung Transplant*. 1991;10: 437–441.
6. Riise GC, Andersson R, Bergstrom T, et al. Quantification of cytomegalovirus DNA in BAL fluid: a longitudinal study in lung transplant recipients. *Chest*. 2000;118:1653–1660.
7. Zedtwitz-Liebenstein K, Jaksch P, Bauer C, et al. Association of cytomegalovirus DNA concentration in epithelial lining fluid and symptomatic cytomegalovirus infection in lung transplant recipients. *Transplantation*. 2004;77:1897–1899.
8. Bejarano PA, Garcia MT, Ganjei-Azar P. Mesothelial cells in transbronchial biopsies: a rare complication with a potential for a diagnostic pitfall. *Am J Surg Pathol*. 2007;31:914–918.
9. Schultz HH, Andersen CB, Steinbruchel D, et al. Recurrence of sarcoid granulomas in lung transplant recipients is common and does not affect overall survival. *Sarcoidosis Vasc Diffuse Lung Dis*. 2014;31:149–153.
10. Ionescu DN, Hunt JL, Lomago D, et al. Recurrent sarcoidosis in lung transplant allografts: granulomas are of recipient origin. *Diagn Mol Pathol*. 2005;14:140–145.
11. Milman N, Andersen CB, Burton CM, et al. Recurrent sarcoid granulomas in a transplanted lung derive from recipient immune cells. *Eur Respir J*. 2005;26:549–552.
12. Pechet TT, Meyers BF, Guthrie TJ, et al. Lung transplantation for lymphangioleiomyomatosis. *J Heart Lung Transplant*. 2004;23:301–308.
13. Karbowniczek M, Astrinidis A, Balsara BR, et al. Recurrent lymphangiomyomatosis after transplantation: genetic analyses reveal a metastatic mechanism. *Am J Respir Crit Care Med*. 2003;167:976–982.
14. Alvarez A, Algar J, Santos F, et al. Airway complications after lung transplantation: a review of 151 anastomoses. *Eur J Cardiothorac Surg*. 2001;19:381–387.
15. Narotzky S, Kennedy CC, Maldonado F. An unusual cause of respiratory failure in a 25-year-old heart and lung transplant recipient. *Chest*. 2015;147:e185–e188.
16. Yousem SA. Alveolar lipoproteinosis in lung allograft recipients. *Hum Pathol*. 1997;28:1383–1386.
17. Gal AA, Bryan JA, Kanter KR, et al. Cytopathology of pulmonary alveolar proteinosis complicating lung transplantation. *J Heart Lung Transplant*. 2004;23:135–138.

18. Du EZ, Yung GL, Le DT, et al. Severe alveolar proteinosis following chemotherapy for acute myeloid leukemia in a lung allograft recipient. *J Thorac Imaging.* 2001;16:307–309.

19. Buell JF, Hanaway MJ, Thomas M, et al. Skin cancer following transplantation: the Israel Penn International Transplant Tumor Registry experience. *Transplant Proc.* 2005;37:962–963.

20. Armanios MY, Grossman SA, Yang SC, et al. Transmission of glioblastoma multiforme following bilateral lung transplantation from an affected donor: case study and review of the literature. *Neuro Oncol.* 2004;6:259–263.

21. Buell JF, Trofe J, Hanaway MJ, et al. Transmission of donor cancer into cardiothoracic transplant recipients. *Surgery.* 2001;130:660–666; discussion 666–668.

22. Clelland CA, Higenbottam TW, Stewart S, et al. The histological changes in transbronchial biopsy after treatment of acute lung rejection in heart-lung transplants. *J Pathol.* 1990;161:105–112.

23. Milne DS, Gascoigne AD, Ashcroft T, et al. Organizing pneumonia following pulmonary transplantation and the development of obliterative bronchiolitis. *Transplantation.* 1994;57:1757–1762.

24. Siddiqui MT, Garrity ER, Husain AN. Bronchiolitis obliterans organizing pneumonia-like reactions: a nonspecific response or an atypical form of rejection or infection in lung allograft recipients? *Hum Pathol.* 1996;27:714–719.

25. Hasegawa T, Iacono A, Yousem SA. The significance of bronchus-associated lymphoid tissue in human lung transplantation: is there an association with acute and chronic rejection? *Transplantation.* 1999;67:381–385.

26. Angel LF, Cai TH, Sako EY, et al. Posttransplant lymphoproliferative disorders in lung transplant recipients: clinical experience at a single center. *Ann Transplant.* 2000;5:26–30.

27. Halkos ME, Miller JI, Mann KP, et al. Thoracic presentations of posttransplant lymphoproliferative disorders. *Chest.* 2004;126:2013–2020.

28. Levine SM, Angel L, Anzueto A, et al. A low incidence of posttransplant lymphoproliferative disorder in 109 lung transplant recipients. *Chest.* 1999;116:1273–1277.

29. Kirby S, Satoskar A, Brodsky S, et al. Histological spectrum of pulmonary manifestations in kidney transplant recipients on sirolimus inclusive immunosuppressive regimens. *Diagn Pathol.* 2012;7:25.

30. Lucioni M, Capello D, Riboni R, et al. B-cell posttransplant lymphoproliferative disorders in heart and/or lungs recipients: clinical and molecular-histogenetic study of 17 cases from a single institution. *Transplantation.* 2006;82:1013–1023.

31. Stewart D. International classification of functioning, disability and health. *Can J Occup Ther.* 2007;74 Spec No.:217–220.

55 Lung Disease in Bone Marrow Transplant Patients

Fabio R. Tavora, M.D., Ph.D., and Allen P. Burke, M.D.

Graft-Versus-Host Disease

Incidence

Graft-versus-host disease (GVHD) occurs in approximately one-third of patients with allogeneic stem cell transplants and primarily affects the skin, liver, and gastrointestinal tract. Clinically significant pulmonary complications occur in 40% to 60% of all patients, of which nearly one-half have noninfectious causes and are related to GVHD.[1] While less common than in other organ systems, patients with pulmonary GHVD tend to have more severe long-term complications and shorter disease-specific survival. Only a small proportion of patients with clinical pulmonary GHVD undergo biopsy, and histologic descriptions in the literature are few.[2] Although GVHD has been reported after autologous stem cell transplant,[3] the lung as a target organ has yet to be reported.

Stages of Pulmonary GVHD

Traditionally, pulmonary GVHD is synonymous with bronchiolitis obliterans syndrome (BOS), considered a chronic form of GVHD, and histologic similar to chronic lung allograft rejection. Although "acute" GVHD is not applied to a specific pulmonary syndrome, there is evidence that an acute form of pulmonary GVHD may exist. GVHD is a risk factor for the development of idiopathic pneumonia syndrome (IPS), which is a form of acute lung injury. Acute and organizing lung injury may be seen in biopsies of patients with extrapulmonary acute GVHD.[2] Additionally, CT abnormalities have been described in patients with acute GVHD, which correspond to interstitial lung disease with relatively acute patterns of injury.

The concept of "stages" of pulmonary GVHD, which have been described in lung biopsies and imaging studies,[1,2,4,5] is not widespread in the clinical literature.

Acute GVHD: Clinical and Imaging Findings

The diagnostic criteria of acute GVHD-induced lung injury are as follows: (1) patients have manifestations of GVHD in other organs (skin, liver, or gut); (2) patients have abnormal chest high-resolution computed tomography (HRCT) scans; (3) lung injury induced by infection and heart diseases are excluded; and (4) chest HRCT scans are improved after treatment for acute GVHD.[4] Because the clinical concept of acute pulmonary GVHD is not generally accepted, pulmonary function test (PFT) results have not been extensively reported.[6]

The median onset of acute GVHD with pulmonary involvement was 31 days, with a range of 17 to 122 days.[4] Several studies, in fact, reported the incidence acute noninfectious lung injury in the first 120 days after stem cell transplantation to be 3% to 15%.[7]

HRCT findings of acute GVHD include nonclassifiable interstitial pneumonia, ground-glass opacities, reticulation, and crazy pavement pattern.[1,4,8]

Pathologic Findings

The diagnosis of lung involvement with GVHD is generally based on clinical findings of noninfectious lung infiltrates in a patient with documented GVHD of other organs, often with biopsy of the skin, colon, and liver. In the lung, there are no accepted grading systems for GVHD. Because biopsies are seldom performed, it is endorsed that the diagnosis of chronic GVHD/BOS can be done using PFT alone. In fact, the lung score proposed by the 2014 Diagnosis and Staging Working Group report emphasizes clinical symptoms and FEV1 in lung function tests to increase sensitivity, but does not require biopsy diagnosis.[9]

Histologic findings of pulmonary GVHD include acute lung injury, chronic interstitial inflammation, organizing pneumonia, and obliterative bronchiolitis (OB) (Figs. 55.1 to 55.5). Denuded bronchiolar epithelium, regenerating atypical respiratory epithelial cells, and reactive pneumocytes are common.[1,2] Prominent apoptotic debris and a chronic venulitis have also been described.[5]

The distinction between obliterative bronchiolitis and organizing pneumonia should be made, as the former is characteristic of BOS and the latter is a nonspecific pattern of subacute lung injury that does not inevitably scar the airway.[2] A follow-up pathologic study showed that those patients who progressed to BOS showed chronic inflammatory changes, not organizing pneumonia, on prior lung biopsies.[5]

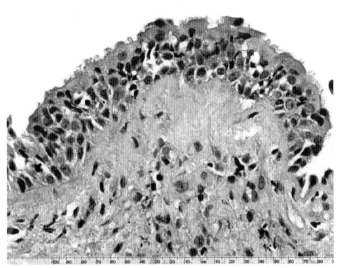

FIGURE 55.1 ▲ GVHD. The respiratory epithelium shows inflammatory infiltrates by mature lymphocytes and apoptotic bodies.

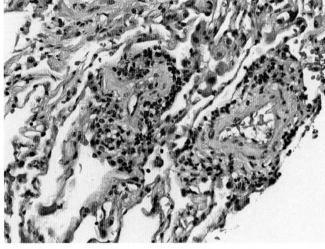

FIGURE 55.3 ▲ GVHD and perivenulitis. Chronic inflammatory infiltrates primarily in the adventitia of veins.

The histopathologic findings in pulmonary GVHD have been grouped in overlapping phases of lung injury. Diffuse alveolar damage (acute lung injury) has been reported in lung biopsies between 4 and 32 months after transplant, organizing pneumonia between 4 and 25 months, interstitial chronic inflammation between 3 and 83 months, and obliterative bronchiolitis between 4 and 110 months.[2,5]

Special Studies

Immunohistochemical staining shows a high proportion of CD8 cells, compared to CD4-positive T lymphocytes, as seen in cutaneous GVHD.[10] There are increased number of overall T cells by CD3 immunostaining in the submucosa and surface epithelium.[5]

Treatment and Prognosis

The prognosis of acute GVHD is not well studied from a clinical standpoint, as most follow-up studies involve the chronic form of disease. In a radiologic series of 17 patients with lung disease and acute GVHD, there were 10 deaths, most from acute GVHD or infections.[4] In another radiologic series, 5 patients with interstitial pneumonia and extrapulmonary GVHD all developed progression with the development of traction bronchiectasis and honeycombing on follow-up CT scans, with a median follow-up period of 22 months.[1]

In a pathologic series of GVHD showing lung injury other than obliterative bronchiolitis, three of three patients with diffuse alveolar damage (DAD) died; one of four patients with organizing pneumonia died, with stabilization in the other patients; and four of seven patients with chronic interstitial inflammation developed BOS.[5] In another series with pathologic documentation, 7 of 17 patients died within 2 years of diagnosis.[2]

Chronic GVHD/Bronchiolitis Obliterans Syndrome

Incidence and Definition

BOS is the best-defined pulmonary manifestation of chronic GVHD. BOS is diagnosed in ~6% of all HCT recipients.[11] Other forms of chronic GVHD are less common, such as chronic interstitial lung disease resembling nonspecific interstitial pneumonia.[1,4]

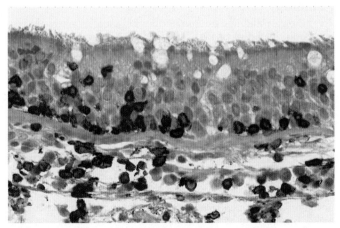

FIGURE 55.2 ▲ GVHD. Immunohistochemical staining for CD3 shows infiltration of T cells in the submucosa and surface epithelium.

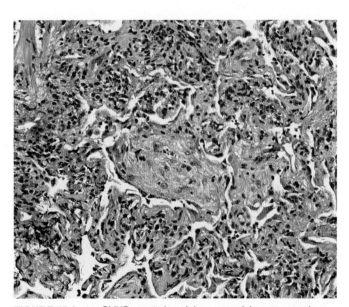

FIGURE 55.4 ▲ GVHD, acute lung injury, organizing pneumonia pattern. A focus of organizing pneumonia in a background of chronic inflammatory infiltrates within alveolar septa.

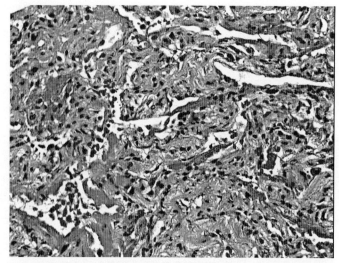

FIGURE 55.5 ▲ GVHD, acute lung injury. Diffuse alveolar injury, with widening of the septa by edema, inflammation, and intra-alveolar fibrin.

Clinical Features

Standardized definitions for the diagnosis of BOS in the setting of stem cell transplantation include decreased FEV1/FVC ratio, decreased FEV1, air trapping demonstrated by increased residual volume, and absence of an infectious etiology.[1,4]

Risk Factors for BOS

The major risk factor for BOS is chronic GVHD. Other factors include the use of methotrexate as GVHD prophylaxis, use of busulfan, use of peripheral blood as the stem cell source, low serum IgG, viral pneumonia within the first 100 days after transplant, and pulmonary dysfunction before transplant.[12]

HRCT Findings

The HRCT findings of BOS include geographic hypoattenuation (mosaicism), air trapping on expiratory views, and a subpleural distribution of findings.

Histologic Features

Histologic findings in biopsies with the clinical syndrome of BOS have shown two distinct histologic patterns: constrictive (obliterative) bronchiolitis and lymphocytic bronchiolitis.[13] OB is a pathologic term that corresponds in many cases to a clinical diagnosis BOS. The absence of findings of OB in a subset of patients with clinical BOS is likely not due to sampling, because of a difference in survival between the two groups.[13]

The histologic features of obliterative bronchiolitis are discussed in Chapters 37 and 53.

Survival

Bronchiolitis obliterans syndrome has been associated with dismal outcomes, with 44% survival at 2 years and 13% survival at 5 years.[14] Survival is greatly affected by a clinical score based on respiratory symptoms, FEV1, and DLCO (diffusion capacity of the lung for carbon monoxide).[14]

In a recent study of patients with clinical BOS subjected to transbronchial lung biopsies, there was a 60% 2-year survival with histologic obliterative bronchiolitis and a 90% 5-year survival with lymphocytic bronchiolitis.[13]

Idiopathic Pneumonia Syndrome

Clinical

Idiopathic pneumonia syndrome (IPS) is a clinical designation that spans heterogeneous pathologic entities. IPS is characterized by widespread alveolar injury on imaging, symptoms and signs of pneumonia, and absence of active lower respiratory tract infection. Infection is aggressive excluded before a diagnosis IPS is rendered, by bronchoalveolar lavage or lung biopsy. Stains and cultures for bacteria, fungi, and viruses, cytology for viral inclusions and *Pneumocystis carinii,* and molecular testing for CMV, respiratory syncytial virus, influenza virus, parainfluenza virus, and adenovirus have been recommended.[15]

There is an association with GVHD, with as many as 64% of patients having grade 2 to 4 extrapulmonary GVHDs.[15]

A recent study using quantitative polymerase chain reaction and galactomannan assay for aspergillus showed that 57% had a detected pathogen essentially excluding a diagnosis of IPS by strict criteria.[16]

Role of Lung Biopsy and Pathologic Findings

The diagnosis of IPS is rarely made or confirmed by tissue biopsy given the significant mortality risks of open lung biopsy in the early transplant period. There are no diagnostic pathologic criteria for the diagnosis, other than of excluding infections.

An autopsy study demonstrated that 28% of patients with a clinical diagnosis of IPS actually had infections, usually fungal; 56% had diffuse alveolar damage; and 16% had acute and organizing pneumonia.[15]

A series of open lung biopsies performed in stem cell transplant recipients who had diffuse infiltrates demonstrated that two-thirds were noninfectious and presumably fit a clinical syndrome of IPS. Of these, the majority showed nonspecific interstitial infiltrates or organizing pneumonia.[17]

Prognosis

The prognosis of IPS is poor, with a 1-year survival rate of <20%.[16]

Diffuse Alveolar Hemorrhage

Incidence

Alveolar hemorrhage is clinically defined as acute onset of alveolar ground-glass opacities, hypoxemia, absence of an infectious etiology, and progressively bloodier alveolar lavage on bronchoscopy (see Chapter 29). The reported incidence of DAH after stem cell transplant ranges from 1% to 5% in autologous transplants and 3% to 7% of allogeneic transplants. The relatively small difference is consistent with the fact that DAH is not thought to be mediated by alloimmunity and is not associated with GVHD, unlike IPS.

Etiology

DAH after stem cell transplant is multifactorial in origin, and the specific etiology is often unknown. It is postulated to be a response to alveolar injury resulting in vascular damage and inflammation from chemotherapy, radiation therapy, immune-mediated events, and occult infections.[18]

Pathology

The histologic findings are nonspecific, and biopsies are rarely performed in the setting of DAH in transplant patients. The pathologic features of DAH are discussed in detail in Chapter 29.

Acute Infections

Role of Biopsy

Lung disease is a major cause of morbidity and mortality following stem cell transplant, is the result of up to 80% of deaths, and caused by infections in about 50% of patients overall. Twenty percent of patients with stem cell transplants develop pulmonary infiltrates, of which 50% are lethal. Of these, one-third of biopsied patients demonstrate infectious processes.

Because the possible etiologies of pulmonary infiltrates in immunocompromised patients are numerous and may coexist, open lung biopsy is sometimes advocated, although no study has shown a positive effect on survival. However, one study showed that biopsy results altered therapy in two-thirds of patients.[17]

Pathologic Findings

The largest study of open lung biopsies in stem cell transplant recipients with diffuse bilateral lung infiltrates showed that 34% were infectious, with CMV the common agent, followed by tuberculosis, pneumocystis, and aspergillosis. Other findings included organizing pneumonia, interstitial inflammation, diffuse alveolar hemorrhage, capillaritis, lymphoma relapse, and posttransplant lymphoproliferative disease.[17]

REFERENCES

1. Song I, Yi CA, Han J, et al. CT findings of late-onset noninfectious pulmonary complications in patients with pathologically proven graft-versus-host disease after allogeneic stem cell transplant. *AJR Am J Roentgenol.* 2012;199:581–587.
2. Yousem SA. The histological spectrum of pulmonary graft-versus-host disease in bone marrow transplant recipients. *Hum Pathol.* 1995;26:668–675.
3. Lee SE, Yoon JH, Shin SH, et al. Skin graft-versus-host disease following autologous stem cell transplantation for multiple myeloma. *Immune Netw.* 2013;13:107–110.
4. Liu QF, Luo XD, Ning J, et al. Association between acute graft versus host disease and lung injury after allogeneic haematopoietic stem cell transplantation. *Hematology.* 2009;14:63–72.
5. Xu L, Drachenberg C, Tavora F, et al. Histologic findings in lung biopsies in patients with suspected graft-versus-host disease. *Hum Pathol.* 2013;44:1233–1240.
6. Madanat-Harjuoja LM, Valjento S, Vettenranta K, et al. Pulmonary function following allogeneic stem cell transplantation in childhood: a retrospective cohort study of 51 patients. *Pediatr Transplant.* 2014;18:617–624.
7. Cooke KR, Yanik G. Acute lung injury after allogeneic stem cell transplantation: is the lung a target of acute graft-versus-host disease? *Bone Marrow Transplant.* 2004;34:753–765.
8. Worthy SA, Flint JD, Muller NL. Pulmonary complications after bone marrow transplantation: high-resolution CT and pathologic findings. *Radiographics.* 1997;17:1359–1371.
9. Jagasia MH, Greinix HT, Arora M, et al. National Institutes of Health Consensus Development Project on Criteria for Clinical Trials in Chronic Graft-versus-Host Disease: I. The 2014 Diagnosis and Staging Working Group report. *Biol Blood Marrow Transplant.* 2015;21:389–401.e1.
10. Soares AB, Faria PR, Magna LA, et al. Chronic GVHD in minor salivary glands and oral mucosa: histopathological and immunohistochemical evaluation of 25 patients. *J Oral Pathol Med.* 2005;34:368–373.
11. Chien JW, Duncan S, Williams KM, et al. Bronchiolitis obliterans syndrome after allogeneic hematopoietic stem cell transplantation-an increasingly recognized manifestation of chronic graft-versus-host disease. *Biol Blood Marrow Transplant.* 2010;16:S106–S114.
12. Gazourian L, Rogers AJ, Ibanga R, et al. Factors associated with bronchiolitis obliterans syndrome and chronic graft-versus-host disease after allogeneic hematopoietic cell transplantation. *Am J Hematol.* 2014;89:404–409.
13. Holbro A, Lehmann T, Girsberger S, et al. Lung histology predicts outcome of bronchiolitis obliterans syndrome after hematopoietic stem cell transplantation. *Biol Blood Marrow Transplant.* 2013;19:973–980.
14. Palmer J, Williams K, Inamoto Y, et al. Pulmonary symptoms measured by the national institutes of health lung score predict overall survival, nonrelapse mortality, and patient-reported outcomes in chronic graft-versus-host disease. *Biol Blood Marrow Transplant.* 2014;20:337–344.
15. Kantrow SP, Hackman RC, Boeckh M, et al. Idiopathic pneumonia syndrome: changing spectrum of lung injury after marrow transplantation. *Transplantation.* 1997;63:1079–1086.
16. Seo S, Renaud C, Kuypers JM, et al. Idiopathic pneumonia syndrome after hematopoietic cell transplantation: evidence of occult infectious etiologies. *Blood.* 2015;125:3789–3797.
17. Wang JY, Chang YL, Lee LN, et al. Diffuse pulmonary infiltrates after bone marrow transplantation: the role of open lung biopsy. *Ann Thorac Surg.* 2004;78:267–272.
18. Majhail NS, Parks K, Defor TE, et al. Diffuse alveolar hemorrhage and infection-associated alveolar hemorrhage following hematopoietic stem cell transplantation: related and high-risk clinical syndromes. *Biol Blood Marrow Transplant.* 2006;12:1038–1046.

56 Asbestos-Related Lung Disease

Michael Lewin-Smith, M.B., B.S., and Allen P. Burke, M.D.

Types of Asbestos

Asbestos is a group of silicates that are defined by the formation of very long, thin fibers. Legally, there are six mineral types of "asbestos," one in the serpentine group of magnesium silicates (chrysotile) and five in the amphibole group (amosite, anthophyllite, actinolite, tremolite, and crocidolite).[1] The last three are noncommercial; sources of exposure for these include rock or gravel or contamination of other mineral mines. The elements (other than silicon) in the amphibole group include combinations of ferrous iron, calcium, and magnesium (Table 56.1).

Chrysotile forms 90% of commercial asbestos and is the least likely to cause tumors and lung fibrosis, because of the relative instability of the fibers in tissues. In North America, most of the amphibole is amosite, whereas in the United Kingdom and Australia, there has been more exposure to crocidolite.

Ferruginous and Asbestos Bodies

When asbestos fibers are inhaled, the alveolar macrophages frequently cover them with an iron–protein–mucopolysaccharide coating, forming "asbestos bodies." "Ferruginous bodies" also include nonasbestos-based bodies ("pseudoasbestos bodies") that have a somewhat different histologic appearance and that are not fibrogenic.[1,2] Currently, the term "ferruginous body" is used preferentially for nonasbestos-containing fibers.[2]

Histochemical stains for iron highlight the ferruginous material along asbestos bodies as well as ferruginous material in nonasbestos-containing ferruginous bodies (Fig. 56.1).

Many asbestos fibers are inhaled and remain uncoated and are not easily visible on routine microscopy. The typical ratio of fibers to bodies is 10–40:1.

In order to prove asbestos origin, the uncoated fiber or core of the asbestos body is analyzed by energy-dispersing x-ray analysis or micro-Raman spectroscopy.[1]

In tissues, asbestos bodies are golden–brown, beaded, or dumbbell shaped with a thin, translucent core (Figs. 56.2 and 56.3). They are typically found embedded within fibrous tissue, but they may occur in alveolar spaces or within the alveolar macrophages near or around bronchioles, often in areas of anthracosis.[2] Pseudoasbestos bodies may have a black core or broad, yellow sheet-like cores and should be distinguished from true asbestos bodies.[2]

Quantification may be accomplished by routine light microscopy (generally per square centimeter of tissue) or by digestion in sodium hypochlorite and filtering. Scanning electron microscopy and especially transmission electron microcopy are the most sensitive techniques for identifying small, uncoated fibers[3] (Fig. 56.4).

To quantify fibers in digested samples, a correction factor of 0.7 is applied to paraffin-embedded sections to compare to wet fixed tissues.[3]

Both asbestos bodies (coated fibers) and uncoated fibers are defined as at least 5μm in length, with the length at least three times the width, and roughly parallel sides.[3]

Lung Disease Caused by Asbestos

Amphiboles are far more potent in the induction of asbestosis, lung cancer, and malignant mesothelioma than chrysotile. There is a long latency between exposure and development of lung disease (typically 10 to 30 years), and there is wide individual variation in susceptibility, for reasons that are not well understood.

Pleural Plaques

In most patients with asbestos-related lung disease, there are parietal pleural plaques or diffuse pleural fibrosis[2] (Fig. 56.5). Patients with pleural plaques have lower amphibole asbestos fiber counts than those with pulmonary asbestosis and are on par with those with mesothelioma.[2]

Among asbestos-exposed individuals, those having radiographic evidence of pleural plaques are at increased risk for lung cancer and pleural mesothelioma, compared to the general population. However, there is no evidence that pleural plaque confers an increased risk of lung cancer or pleural mesothelioma within a population of individuals having the same cumulative asbestos exposure.[4]

Histologically, asbestos plaques have a typical basket-weave acellular appearance (Fig. 56.6).

TABLE 56.1 Types of Asbestosis

Designation	Type	Color	Chemical Formula	Risk for Development of Fibrosis/Neoplasia	Geographic Distribution
Chrysotile	Serpentine	White	$Mg_3(Si_2O_5)(OH)_4$	Low	Canada
Crocidolite	Amphibole	Blue	$Na_2(Fe^{2+})_3(Fe^{3+})_2Si_8O_{22}(OH)_2$	High	Africa, Australia
Amosite	Amphibole	Brown	$(Fe^{2+})_7Si_8O_{22}(OH)_2$	Intermediate	Mined in South Africa
Anthophyllite	Amphibole	Various	$(Mg;Fe^{2+})_7Si_8O_{22}(OH)_2$	Low–intermediate	Mined in Eastern and Southeastern U.S. Finland Japan
Actinolite	Amphibole	Various	$Ca_2(Mg;Fe^{2+})_5Si_8O_{22}(OH)_2$	Intermediate–high	Relatively rare; found in metamorphic rocks; found in New Jersey Meadowlands dump; previously mined in Australia
Tremolite	Amphibole	Various	$Ca_2Mg_5Si_8O_{22}(OH)_2$	High	May contaminate vermiculite mines

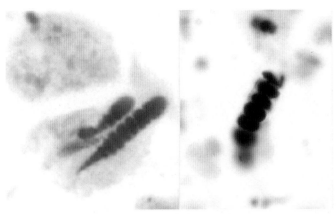

FIGURE 56.1 ▲ Ferruginous bodies, iron stain. There is a beaded appearance **(left)**. The central core is not readily visible in this photograph. The bodies are within a macrophage that contains dusty hemosiderin particles. A definitive diagnosis of asbestos body would require additional testing. Histologic section from an autopsy of a patient with known asbestos exposure **(right)**. The lack of internal structure and beaded appearance are not pathognomonic for asbestosis.

Asbestos-Related Pulmonary Fibrosis (Pulmonary Asbestosis)

Asbestosis is a fibrosing lung disease defined by interstitial and peribronchiolar fibrosis and asbestos bodies. The degree of pulmonary fibrosis is related to the fiber burden in the lung and the type and duration of the exposure.[3]

The minimum criteria necessary for a diagnosis of asbestosis are discrete foci of peribronchiolar fibrosis associated with accumulations of asbestos bodies.[2]

More than 95% of asbestosis cases have more than 2 asbestos bodies per square centimeter of tissue.[3] If there are fewer than 3 bodies found in 5 to 10 sections, an etiology for fibrosis other than asbestosis should be considered. The average rate of asbestos bodies is 2 per cm[2] of lung tissue or greater.[2]

The severity of asbestosis can be graded based on the number of bronchioles involved with fibrosis and distance to which the fibrosis extends into adjacent alveoli. The second and highest grades are interstitial fibrosis extending between two separate airways and honeycomb changes, respectively.[3]

The degree of fibrosis correlates best with uncoated amphibole fibers, followed by ferruginous bodies, in populations with a high exposure to commercial amphiboles.[3]

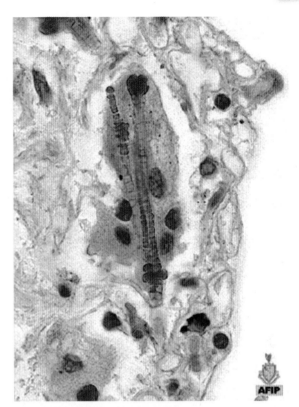

FIGURE 56.3 ▲ Asbestos body, within macrophage. Note typical beaded appearance with *dumbbell shape*. The central core is best appreciated by adjusting the focus.

Erionite, a nonasbestos fiber, is a noncommercial mineral found in Turkey that increases the risk of mesothelioma (see Chapter 97) as well as interstitial lung disease (>15% of the local population).[2]

Chest X-ray may demonstrate interstitial fibrosis and pleural plaques. High-resolution computed tomographic scans show pleural-based intralobular and interlobular lines, ground-glass attenuation, and

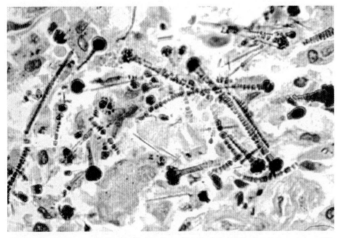

FIGURE 56.2 ▲ Asbestosis bodies. Typical dumbbell appearance with beaded cores. Also, numerous noncoated needle-like fibers are seen.

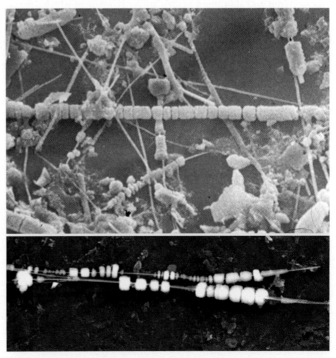

FIGURE 56.4 ▲ Asbestos body, scanning electron microscopy. Note typical beaded appearance.

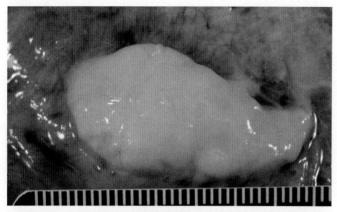

FIGURE 56.5 ▲ Pleural plaque, related to asbestos exposure. There is a firm, *white* raised fibrous nodule that is typically on the parietal pleura.

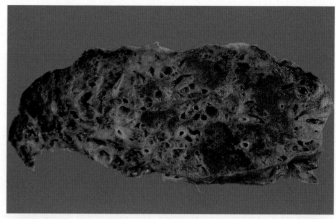

FIGURE 56.7 ▲ Pulmonary asbestosis. There is diffuse fibrosis with cystic change.

honeycombing, features that overlap with usual interstitial pneumonia. Isolated "dot-like" structures in the lower lung periphery correlate with peribronchiolar nodular fibrosis that does not reach the pleural surface.[2]

Grossly, the fibrosis of asbestosis is diffuse, with cystic change with no particular subpleural accentuation, unlike usual interstitial pneumonia (Fig. 56.7). In contrast to usual interstitial pneumonia, the fibrosis in asbestosis is relatively paucicellular, with little inflammation and few fibroblasts (Figs. 56.8 to 56.10). The scarring begins in the centers of the lobules and extends outward, linking adjacent bronchioles, most prominently in a subpleural location. The spatial heterogeneity of the usual interstitial pneumonia is not prominent, and areas resembling the fibrotic variant of nonspecific interstitial pneumonitis are frequent, with fibroblastic foci rare.[2]

Differential Diagnosis of Pulmonary Asbestosis

Mineral dust disease is restricted to small airways, where multifocal peribronchiolar fibrosis is accompanied by macrophages containing silicates, iron and aluminum oxides, and coal, many of which are visible using polarized light.[2]

The distinction between usual interstitial pneumonia or nonspecific interstitial pneumonia and asbestosis rests in part on a history of exposure and the finding of sufficient numbers of asbestos fibers or bodies in lung tissue. Fibroblastic foci are more common in usual interstitial pneumonia than in asbestosis, and inflammation, while typical of idiopathic interstitial pneumonia, is not prominent in the bland fibrosis of asbestosis. Prominent pleural fibrosis is suggestive of asbestosis and usually not prominent in nonspecific or usual interstitial pneumonia.

Carcinomas of the Lung

An association between lung cancer and asbestosis was made in 1949, when lung cancer was reported in 13% of 235 men dying with asbestosis, compared with 1.2% of 6,884 men dying with silicosis.[2] All histologic types have been described, most frequently squamous cell, followed by small cell and adenocarcinomas.[5]

Malignant Mesothelioma (see Chapter 97)

The risk of mesothelioma and pleural plaques is less dose dependent than the risk of development of fibrotic lung disease. The induction of mesothelioma occurs most frequently by fibers that are long (>8 μm) and narrow (<0.25 μm in diameter).[2]

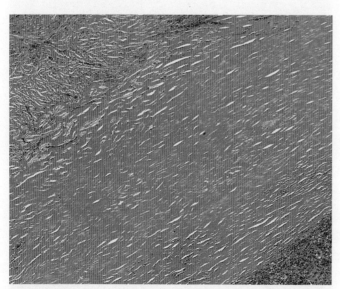

FIGURE 56.6 ▲ Pleural plaque, histologic appearance. The collagen bundles are virtually acellular and have an interdigitating "basket-weave" appearance.

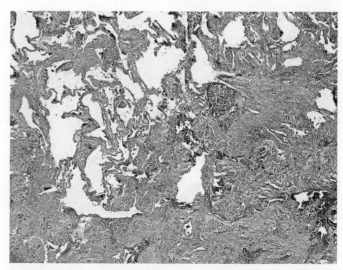

FIGURE 56.8 ▲ Pulmonary asbestosis. There is diffuse fibrosis with areas of loose collagen. The pattern is nonspecific.

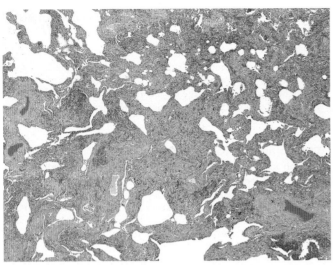

FIGURE 56.9 ▲ Pulmonary asbestosis. There is diffuse interstitial fibrosis with minimal chronic inflammation. The pattern is nonspecific.

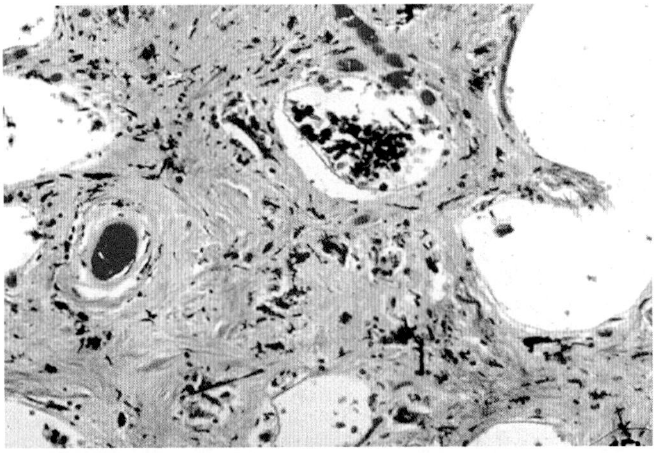

FIGURE 56.10 ▲ Pulmonary asbestosis. The collagen is paucicellular with little inflammation, with abundant asbestos bodies in this case.

Practical Points

▶ The development of fibrotic lung disease is heavily dose dependent, less so for pleural plaques and mesothelioma.

▶ In tissue, most asbestos fibers are uncoated; coated fibers are more readily identified and highlighted by iron stains.

▶ Other iron-coated nonasbestos bodies are called ferruginous bodies and histologically do not have typical central core and dumbbell-shaped or beaded appearance.

▶ Asbestosis is defined by bronchiolocentric pulmonary fibrosis, presence of asbestos bodies, and history of asbestos exposure; end-stage disease is similar to usual interstitial pneumonia, but fibroblast foci are not numerous.

▶ Pleural plaques almost always are present with asbestosis, occur on the parietal pleura, and have a "basket-weave" histologic collagen pattern.

REFERENCES

1. Croce A, Musa M, Allegrina M, et al. Environmental scanning electron microscopy technique to identify asbestos phases inside ferruginous bodies. *Microsc Microanal.* 2013;19:420–424.
2. Roggli VL, Gibbs AR, Attanoos R, et al. Pathology of asbestosis—an update of the diagnostic criteria: report of the asbestosis committee of the college of american pathologists and pulmonary pathology society. *Arch Pathol Lab Med.* 2010;134:462–480.
3. Schneider F, Sporn TA, Roggli VL. Asbestos fiber content of lungs with diffuse interstitial fibrosis: an analytical scanning electron microscopic analysis of 249 cases. *Arch Pathol Lab Med.* 2010;134:457–461.
4. Ameille J, Brochard P, Letourneux M, et al. Asbestos-related cancer risk in patients with asbestosis or pleural plaques. *Rev Mal Respir.* 2011;28:e11–e17.
5. Gurbuz B, Metintas S, Metintas M, et al. Epidemiological features of bronchial carcinoma cases with environmental asbestos exposure. *Tuberk Toraks.* 2004;52:5–13.

57 Silicosis

Marisa Dolhnikoff, M.D., Ph.D., and Fabio R. Tavora, M.D., Ph.D.

Definition

Silicosis is a fibrotic pulmonary disease caused by the inhalation and deposition of crystalline silica particles.[1]

Incidental silicoanthracotic nodules are common in lymph nodes and occasionally lung parenchyma resected for lung cancer and are of no clinical significance. However, the macrophage reaction may result in increased uptake on positron emission tomography scans and cause false-positive results.[2]

Epidemiology and Exposure Risks

Silicosis is the most prevalent occupational disease worldwide and an occupational health concern, especially in developing countries.

As sources of silica are common, disease potential is high. Decreases in incidence largely depend on preventive and control measures. From 1975 to 2007, the proportions of White and Black South African gold mine workers with silicosis increased from 18% to 22% and from 3% to 32%, respectively[3]; in 2013, there were an estimated 11.5 million workers exposed to silica dust in India.[4] A prevalence as high as 54% is reported in Brazilian stone carvers,[5] and high prevalence has also been reported in Chinese pottery workers and tin and tungsten miners.[6] Although the incidence of silicosis has decreased dramatically in the last decades in countries like the United States and in Europe, where appropriate measures have been taken, more than 100,000 US workers are still in high-risk jobs.[7]

The disease is associated to a number of occupational activities, the greatest risk being associated to mining and processing of stone, well drilling, sandblasting, ceramic and glass production, and construction-related activities such as drilling of rock, abrasive blasting of concrete, sawing, hammering, drilling, grinding, and chipping of concrete or masonry.[1]

Silica is a major component of sand, rock, and mineral ores and is the second most common mineral in the earth's crust, next to feldspar. The general term silica refers to silicon dioxide (SiO_2), which occurs naturally in crystalline, amorphous, and glassy states.[8] Crystalline silica, the form of silica that poses the occupational respiratory hazard, is a basic component of soil, sand, granite, and many other minerals. Quartz is the most common form of crystalline silica; cristobalite and tridymite are two other. All three forms may become inhalable size particles when workers chip, cut, drill, or grind objects that contain crystalline silica.

The risk of developing silicosis is related to the concentration of dust-containing silica in workplace air, the percentage of respirable silica in the total dust, the particle size, the nature of the silica (crystalline or noncrystalline), and the duration of the exposure.[9] Silicosis is a progressive disease and may appear many years after exposure to silica ceases.[3]

Exposure to crystalline silica has been also associated with other health effects, including increased susceptibility to tuberculosis, lung cancer, chronic obstructive pulmonary disease, autoimmune diseases, and chronic renal disease.[10]

Pathophysiology

Pulmonary lesions in silicosis are modulated and triggered by the immune system, involving both innate and adaptive immunities. The activation of receptors expressed on the surface of macrophages such as the macrophage receptor with collagenous structure (MARCO) seems to have a crucial role in silica-induced lung injury and apoptosis, as well as in the pulmonary expression of proinflammatory cytokines such as TNF-alpha.[11] Phagocytosis of crystalline silica causes lysosomal damage, activating the NALP3 inflammasome that triggers the inflammatory cascade with subsequent fibrosis.[12] Silica also stimulates the release of chemotactic agents, such as platelet-activating factor (PAF), macrophage inflammatory protein 2 (MIP-2), and cytokine-induced neutrophil chemoattractant (CINC) from alveolar macrophages, inducing a pronounced recruitment of inflammatory cells both in the alveolar walls and on the alveolar epithelial surface.[11,13]

The proinflammatory cytokines released by macrophages and also by neutrophils, mast cells, and B lymphocytes participate in the exaggerated deposition of matrix protein by producing significant levels of profibrotic mediators that stimulate the recruitment and the proliferation of mesenchymal cells as well as regulate neovascularization and reepithelialization of injured tissues. These mediators mainly include fibrogenic cytokines (TNF-alpha, IL-1, and TGF-beta), growth factors such as platelet-derived growth factor (PDGF), the alveolar macrophage form of insulin-like growth factor (IGF), and fibronectin.[11] Silica particles also induce the generation of reactive oxygen species (ROS) directly or by stimulation of cells.[13] The generation of oxidants by silica particles and silica-activated immune cells results in macrophage apoptosis, lung damage, inflammation, and cell transformation. Silica-induced acute inflammation is also accompanied by thrombosis, suggesting that inhaled silica particles may also induce extrapulmonary lesions.[11]

Clinical Forms, Pathology, and Radiologic Presentation

There are three main forms of silicosis, depending on the airborne concentration of respirable crystalline silica: (1) acute silicosis (also referred to as silicoproteinosis), (2) accelerated silicosis, and (3) chronic (or classic) silicosis, the most common form of the disease.[1]

Incidental silicoanthracotic nodules do not form symptomatic lung disease and are not considered a form of silicosis.

Acute Silicosis (Silicoproteinosis)

Acute and accelerated silicosis describe rapidly progressive forms, usually associated with intense silica exposure.[14] Acute silicosis is a rare presentation of silicosis and occurs following a heavy inhalational exposure to silica dusts for a few weeks to 5 years. It most commonly affects sandblasters.[1] Clinically, it may resemble pulmonary alveolar proteinosis (PAP)[15]; besides dyspnea and dry cough, constitutional symptoms can be present, such as fever, fatigue, and weight loss. The clinical course is usually progressive, and respiratory failure and death often occur within a few months.[1]

The pathologic features of acute silicosis differ substantially from the chronic form and resemble those of primary PAP, that is, alveolitis and filling of the airspaces with proteinaceous material that are PAS positive (Fig. 57.1). Minimal collagen deposition and fibrosis can be present.[1,16]

Despite the pathologic similarities, PAP and silicoproteinosis have distinct imaging features. Silicoproteinosis presents with bilateral dependent consolidation often with areas of calcification and/or ground-glass opacities. Bilateral crazy-paving pattern with areas of geographic sparing, characteristic of PAP, is not usually seen in silicoproteinosis.[16,17]

Accelerated Silicosis

Accelerated silicosis shares similar clinical and radiographic findings with chronic silicosis but tends to progress rapidly.[1,18] It appears after more intense exposures to silica dust and is characterized by an earlier onset (usually 5 to 10 years after exposure) than the chronic form (10 to 15 years or more).[19] It can produce symptoms as early as within a year of first exposure, and deaths may occur within 5 years.[20] Due to the improvement in working conditions, accelerated silicosis has become uncommon in developed countries. However, serious health threat still exists, especially in small-scale mining in developing countries.[19] Patients with accelerated silicosis are at a higher risk of developing

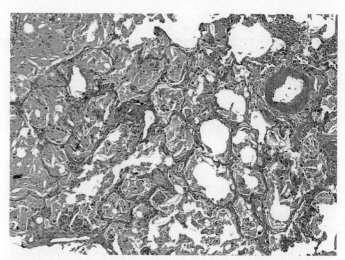

FIGURE 57.1 ▲ Acute silicosis. Alveolar tissue with preserved architecture and homogeneous filling of the airspaces with proteinaceous material.

progressive massive fibrosis (PMF) as well as other complications.[21] The pathologic picture is similar to that of classic silicosis or may show a combination of acute and chronic features, with areas of alveolar proteinosis associated with the presence of silicotic nodules that develop sooner and are more cellular than in chronic silicosis.[18,21] Sequential biopsies may show interstitial inflammation and alveolar proteinosis with minimal fibrosis progressing to diffuse fibrosis within 6 months.[21]

Chronic (Classic) Silicosis

Chronic, classic, or nodular silicosis is the most common form of the disease and occurs after 10 to 20 years of exposure to low concentrations of silica dust.[18] It may be classified as either simple or complicated, according to the radiographic findings. Simple silicosis is defined by a radiographic pattern of small and round opacities, whereas complicated silicosis, or PMF, is characterized by large conglomerate opacities.[16] Individuals with simple silicosis can be asymptomatic and diagnosed incidentally on radiologic examination. Patients might have a cough, which is usually due to chronic bronchitis, and exertional dyspnea may occur if silicosis progresses to PMF, or if it is associated to tuberculosis, lung cancer, or COPD. Impairment of lung function increases with disease progression, even after the patient is no longer exposed.[1,18] Diagnosis of silicosis requires both a history of exposure to crystalline silica, characteristic findings on chest radiographs, and exclusion of other competing diagnoses.[1,22]

Radiology

On chest radiographs, classic silicosis is characterized by multiple nodular well-defined and symmetrically distributed opacities, ranging from 2 to 10 mm in diameter. The nodules are predominantly located in the upper lobes and posterior portions of the lung. Calcification might be seen.[16,18] The computed tomography (CT) shows multiple small nodules diffusely distributed throughout both lungs but usually most numerous in the upper lobes. At thin-section CT, nodules have usually perilymphatic distribution, being observed in centrilobular, paraseptal, and subpleural areas. Rounded subpleural nodules may be confluent and resemble pleural plaques. Hilar and mediastinal lymph node enlargement may precede the parenchymal nodular lesions. Calcification of lymph nodes is common and occurs at the periphery of the node (eggshell calcification).[16,23]

Pathologic Findings

Silicotic nodules are the characteristic feature in chronic silicosis. These nodules measure around 3 mm in diameter in the first phase of the disease, involving hilar lymph nodes and upper lobes. As disease progresses, they may be found in the mid- and basal zones and in the visceral pleura. Grossly, nodules are rounded and firm, ranging from slate gray to dense black (Figs. 57.2 and 57.3). A lymphatic distribution can be seen, that is, nodules tend to be located around small bronchioles and pulmonary arteries, as well as in subpleural and paraseptal spaces. Microscopically, silicotic nodules present as well-demarcated central areas of whorled, mature, hyalinized collagen, with aggregates of dust-laden macrophages at the periphery (Figs. 57.4 to 57.7). Using polarized light microscopy, birefringent particles can be seen within the nodules at the cellular level or in the interstitial tissue. With increasing exposure to silica, the nodules can become confluent, obliterating normal intervening lung parenchyma and resulting in PMF. The lesions may reach many centimeters in diameter and completely efface the upper lobe architecture.[16,18]

Incidental silicotic nodules frequently occur in mediastinal lymph nodes and result in false-positive positron emission tomography scans for metastatic lung disease. The histologic appearance is that of prominent macrophage infiltration of the sinusoids that may mimic sarcoidosis, usually with prominent anthracotic pigment. Polarization of the slide will demonstrate typical silica crystals.

Progressive Massive Fibrosis

Simple classic silicosis can progress to large opacities known as PMF. It represents the expansion and confluence of individual silicotic nodules

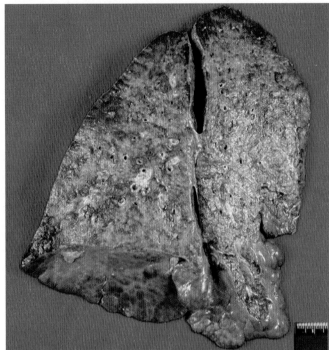
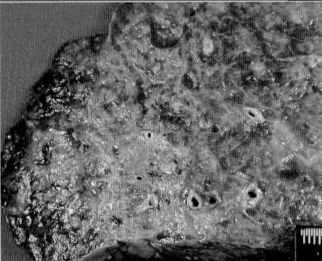

FIGURE 57.2 ▲ Chronic silicosis. Multiple small slate gray coalescent nodules diffusely distributed throughout the lung. Note individual (**right**) and coalescent (**left**) slate gray pulmonary nodules (**bottom**).

and can lead to distortion of the adjacent pulmonary parenchyma, the hila, and the mediastinum. PMF is associated with progressive impairment in lung function, with the development of severe airflow limitation, hypoxemia, and carbon dioxide retention. The scarring associated with PMF results in the contraction of the adjacent lung and the development of cystic spaces or paracicatricial emphysema. The masses, larger than 1 cm by definition, develop slowly over many years and are usually located in the posterior regions of the upper lobes but may also involve the lower lobes. When unilateral masses occur, the differential diagnosis with neoplastic lesions can be difficult.[18,22] Over time, the fibrotic masses can occupy most of both lung fields, and the discrete small rounded opacities may disappear, making the diagnosis of silicosis more difficult.[18] Eggshell-type calcification in hilar and mediastinal lymph nodes is frequent.[24]

Pleural disease in silicosis is more prevalent in advanced disease and can occur as pleural effusion, pleural thickening, and pleural invagination, the latter being associated to PMF.[25]

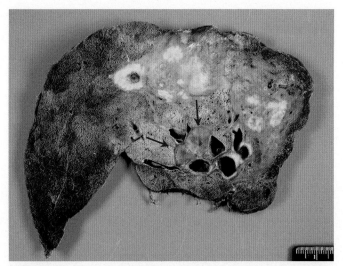

FIGURE 57.3 ▲ Chronic silicosis. Large coalescent nodules partially replace the pulmonary parenchyma. The lymph node is also involved (*arrows*).

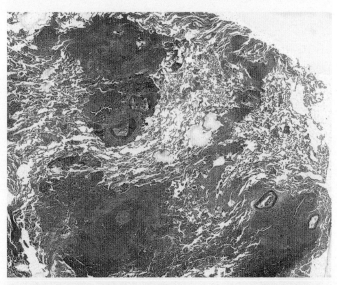

FIGURE 57.4 ▲ Lymphatic distribution of silicotic nodules around small bronchioles and pulmonary arteries.

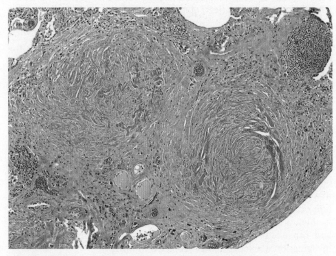

FIGURE 57.5 ▲ High-power view of silicotic nodules composed of a well-demarcated central area of whorled, mature, hyalinized collagen, with dust-laden macrophages at the periphery.

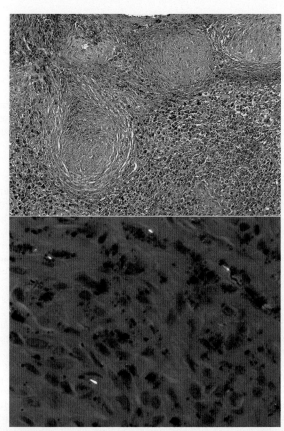

FIGURE 57.6 ▲ Silicotic nodules in hilar lymph nodes associated with intense anthracosis (**top**). Polarization of a silicotic nodule shows birefringent needle-shaped silica particles (**bottom**).

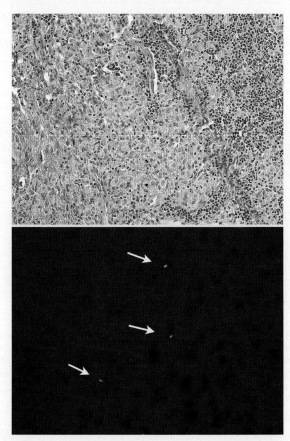

FIGURE 57.7 ▲ Incidental silicoanthracosis, mediastinal lymph node from patients with lung cancer. The macrophages may be plump and mimic sarcoid. At bottom is a higher magnification of the field viewed under polarized light. Arrows show birefringent silica particles.

Pathologic Findings

PMF is characterized by a large conglomerate lesion, composed of multiple foci of central hyalinized collagen and a surrounding rim of pigmented macrophages. Focal necrosis is common in the central portions of the lesion and is occasionally associated with granulomatous inflammation that can resemble tuberculosis infection. Less often, cavitation secondary to ischemic necrosis may occur in the mass. The intervening lung parenchyma shows paracicatricial emphysema.[16]

Silicotuberculosis

There is a clear association between silicosis and tuberculosis (TB). TB rates in individuals with advanced simple silicosis can be threefold higher than in silica workers without silicosis. The risk of developing tuberculosis is proportional to the severity of silicosis and the intensity of the exposure, being considerably higher in patients with acute and accelerated forms of silicosis. Exposure to silica increases the risk of tuberculosis even in the absence of silicosis.[3]

Gold miners in South Africa have among the highest TB incidence rates in the world (3,821/100,000 in 2004).[26] The increased risk of both pulmonary and extrapulmonary TB continues even if exposure ceases.

The prevalence of silica-related TB is also exacerbated by human immunodeficiency virus (HIV) infection.[18]

Silica-induced alterations in the immune response of the lungs, impairment of metabolism and function of pulmonary macrophages, and macrophage apoptosis have been suggested as possible mechanisms involved in the increased risk for tuberculosis in individuals exposed to silica.[27] An excess of surfactant protein A in silicosis seems also to be associated with higher susceptibility to tuberculosis. Surfactant protein A suppresses reactive nitrogen intermediates by alveolar macrophages in response to *Mycobacterium tuberculosis*[28] and allows mycobacteria to enter the alveolar macrophages without triggering cytotoxicity.[27,29]

Active TB superimposed on silicosis should be investigated with imaging and sputum microscopy and culture. The main findings on chest CT are thick-walled cavities, consolidations, a tree-in-bud pattern, nodular image asymmetry, and rapid disease progression.[27] The presence of cavitation in a conglomerate mass of PMF is an indication of associated tuberculosis.[30]

There are very few pathologic series of silicotuberculosis. The diagnosis is often missed clinically.[31] Silicotic nodules demonstrate central necrosis with cavitation, revealing acid-fast organisms on special stains (Fig. 57.8).

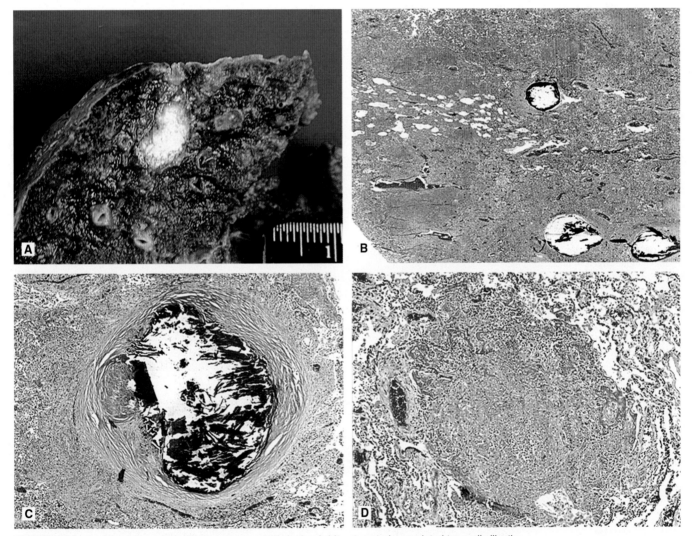

FIGURE 57.8 ▲ Silicotuberculosis. Tuberculous necrotic lesion (white at center) associated to small silicotic nodules (**A**). Multiple calcified silicotic nodules associated to exudative granulomatous lesions (**B**). Calcified silicotic nodule. Note the pigmented macrophages at the periphery (**C**). Exudative granulomatous lesion characterized by necrotic and exudative center and few epithelioid cells at the periphery. Mycobacteria were present at Ziehl-Neelsen staining in this case (**D**).

Practical Points

▶ Silicosis results from inhalation of crystalline silica, usually from occupational exposure. Occupations commonly associated with the entity are mining, foundry work, sandblasting, stonemasonry, and quarry work.

▶ Acute silicosis is usually a rapidly progressive disease that clinically and pathologically resembles PAP. Fibrosis can occur but is usually mild and late in the course.

▶ Accelerated silicosis may show features of both acute and chronic silicosis. This form has become uncommon in the past decade.

▶ Chronic silicosis is the classic form of the disease and can progress to PMF. The nodules follow a lymphatic distribution, and the disease may also involve the pleural with thickening and mass formation.

▶ Patients with silicosis have a high incidence of associated tuberculosis, up to 10-fold.

▶ Pathologists will commonly encounter silica as incidental macrophage reactions in lymph nodes from cancer patients with positive positron emission tomography scans and occasionally as incidental lung nodules, usually with abundant anthracotic pigment (silicoanthracosis).

REFERENCES

1. Leung CC, Yu IT, Chen W. Silicosis. *Lancet.* 2012;379:2008–2018.
2. Koksal D, Demirag F, Bayiz H, et al. The correlation of SUVmax with pathological characteristics of primary tumor and the value of Tumor/Lymph node SUVmax ratio for predicting metastasis to lymph nodes in resected NSCLC patients. *J Cardiothorac Surg.* 2013;8:63.
3. Ross MH, Murray J. Occupational respiratory disease in mining. *Occup Med (Lond).* 2004;54:304–310.
4. Jindal SK. Silicosis in India: past and present. *Curr Opin Pulm Med.* 2013;19:163–168.
5. Antao VC, Pinheiro GA, Kavakama J, et al. High prevalence of silicosis among stone carvers in Brazil. *Am J Ind Med.* 2004;45:194–201.
6. Chen W, Hnizdo E, Chen JQ, et al. Risk of silicosis in cohorts of Chinese tin and tungsten miners, and pottery workers (I): an epidemiological study. *Am J Ind Med.* 2005;48:1–9.
7. 't Mannetje A, Steenland K, Attfield M, et al. Exposure-response analysis and risk assessment for silica and silicosis mortality in a pooled analysis of six cohorts. *Occup Environ Med.* 2002;59:723–728.
8. Raymond LW, Wintermeyer S. Medical surveillance of workers exposed to crystalline silica. *J Occup Environ Med.* 2006;48:95–101.
9. Buchanan D, Miller BG, Soutar CA. Quantitative relations between exposure to respirable quartz and risk of silicosis. *Occup Environ Med.* 2003;60:159–164.
10. Laney AS, Weissman DN. The classic pneumoconioses: new epidemiological and laboratory observations. *Clin Chest Med.* 2012;33:745–758.
11. Huaux F. New developments in the understanding of immunology in silicosis. *Curr Opin Allergy Clin Immunol.* 2007;7:168–173.
12. Cassel SL, Eisenbarth SC, Iyer SS, et al. The Nalp3 inflammasome is essential for the development of silicosis. *Proc Natl Acad Sci USA.* 2008;105:9035–9040.
13. Ding M, Chen F, Shi X, et al. Diseases caused by silica: mechanisms of injury and disease development. *Int Immunopharmacol.* 2002;2:173–182.
14. Beckett W, Abraham J, Backlake M, et al. Adverse effects of crystalline silica exposure. American Thoracic Society Committee of the Scientific Assembly on Environmental and Occupational Health. *Am J Respir Crit Care Med.* 1997;155:761–768.
15. Stafford M, Cappa A, Weyant M, et al. Treatment of acute silicoproteinosis by whole-lung lavage. *Semin Cardiothorac Vasc Anesth.* 2013;17:152–159.
16. Chong S, Lee KS, Chung MJ, et al. Pneumoconiosis: comparison of imaging and pathologic findings. *Radiographics.* 2006;26:59–77.
17. Souza CA, Marchiori E, Goncalves LP, et al. Comparative study of clinical, pathological and HRCT findings of primary alveolar proteinosis and silicoproteinosis. *Eur J Radiol.* 2012;81:371–378.
18. Rees D, Murray J. Silica, silicosis and tuberculosis. *Int J Tuberc Lung Dis.* 2007;11:474–484.
19. Tse LA, Li ZM, Wong TW, et al. High prevalence of accelerated silicosis among gold miners in Jiangxi, China. *Am J Ind Med.* 2007;50:876–880.
20. Jiang CQ, Xiao LW, Lam TH, et al. Accelerated silicosis in workers exposed to agate dust in Guangzhou, China. *Am J Ind Med.* 2001;40:87–91.
21. Hutyrova B, Smolkova P, Nakladalova M, et al. Case of accelerated silicosis in a sandblaster. *Ind Health.* 2015;53:178–183.
22. Marchiori E, Ferreira A, Saez F, et al. Conglomerated masses of silicosis in sandblasters: high-resolution CT findings. *Eur J Radiol.* 2006;59:56–59.
23. Satija B, Kumar S, Ojha UC, et al. Spectrum of high-resolution computed tomography imaging in occupational lung disease. *Indian J Radiol Imaging.* 2013;23:287–296.
24. Gera K, Pilaniya V, Shah A. Silicosis: progressive massive fibrosis with eggshell calcification. *BMJ Case Rep.* 2006;2014.
25. Arakawa H, Honma K, Saito Y, et al. Pleural disease in silicosis: pleural thickening, effusion, and invagination. *Radiology.* 2005;236:685–693.
26. Glynn JR, Murray J, Bester A, et al. Effects of duration of HIV infection and secondary tuberculosis transmission on tuberculosis incidence in the South African gold mines. *AIDS.* 2008;22:1859–1867.
27. Barboza CE, Winter DH, Seiscento M, et al. Tuberculosis and silicosis: epidemiology, diagnosis and chemoprophylaxis. *J Bras Pneumol.* 2008;34:959–966.
28. Pasula R, Wright JR, Kachel DL, et al. Surfactant protein A suppresses reactive nitrogen intermediates by alveolar macrophages in response to Mycobacterium tuberculosis. *J Clin Invest.* 1999;103:483–490.
29. Gold JA, Hoshino Y, Tanaka N, et al. Surfactant protein A modulates the inflammatory response in macrophages during tuberculosis. *Infect Immun.* 2004;72:645–650.
30. Martins P, Marchiori E, Zanetti G, et al. Cavitated conglomerate mass in silicosis indicating associated tuberculosis. *Case Rep Med.* 2010;2010.
31. Tung AH, Ngai JC, Ko FW, et al. Diagnosis of silicotuberculosis by Endobronchial Ultrasound-Guided Transbronchial Needle Aspiration (EBUS-TBNA). *Respirology.* 2013;18:383–384.

58 Miscellaneous Pneumoconioses

Allen P. Burke, M.D.

Background

Pneumoconiosis is defined as a restrictive lung disease resulting from occupational inhalation of dust, usually inorganic particulates. It differs histologically and pathogenetically from hypersensitivity pneumonitis, which may initially have an obstructive component and which results from an immune-mediated reaction to inhaled organic material. Hypersensitivity pneumonitis may also result from occupational exposure, however (see Chapter 23).

Pneumoconioses are characterized histologically by bronchiolocentric aggregates of dust-laden macrophages forming macules or nodules. The macrophages may track along lymphatic routes (bronchovascular bundles, pleural surfaces, and interlobular septa).

TABLE 58.1 Pneumoconioses

	Exposure	Fibrogenicity	Relative Incidence Worldwide	Histologic Findings
Silicosis	SiO$_2$ (silica)	High	Common	Fibrotic nodules with small silica crystals (birefringent, about 5 µM)
Asbestosis	Asbestos (various)	Very high	Common	Peribronchiolar fibrosis progressing to diffuse fibrosis; asbestos bodies
Coal workers' pneumoconiosis (CWP)	Coal dust exposure	Low	Common	Anthracotic macules, fibrotic nodules, and progressive massive fibrosis
Caplan syndrome	Coal or silica, with underlying rheumatoid arthritis	—	Rare	Rheumatoid nodules, with or without anthracotic or silicotic nodules
Cobalt pneumoconiosis	Hard metals (often with tungsten)	Low	Rare	Giant cell interstitial pneumonitis (old term)
Aluminum pneumoconiosis	Aluminum	Low	Rare	Macrophages filled with gray dust, usually not birefringent
Siderosis	Iron	Low	Rare	Peribronchiolar macrophages with iron granules, larger than hemosiderin
Berylliosis	Beryllium	Low	Very rare	Sarcoid-like granulomas
Silicatosis	Inhalation of talc and other silicates	Minimal	Uncommon	Birefringent large (10–100 µM) crystals, rhomboid, with macrophage giant cell reaction

The distinction between pneumoconiosis and hypersensitivity becomes somewhat blurred for some conditions. For example, berylliosis is believed to be an immune-related disease with a sarcoid-like reaction that does not resemble other types of pneumoconiosis.

Epidemiology

Worldwide, pneumoconiosis represents the second leading cause of death among the chronic respiratory diseases (second to chronic obstructive lung disease), resulting in over 250,000 deaths annually.[1] Nearly one-half are caused by silicosis, asbestosis, and coal workers' pneumoconiosis (in descending order). Asbestosis and silicosis are discussed in Chapters 56 and 57, respectively. Other pneumoconioses are relatively uncommon (Table 58.1).

Coal Miners' (Workers') Pneumoconiosis

The prevalence of coal workers' pneumoconiosis has declined to 2% among underground coal miners in the U.S. Appalachia, with a similar rate among aboveground miners.[2] The disease is assessed radiographically and is staged based on the numbers of rounded opacities and presence of consolidation or diffuse fibrosis.

Grossly, there are black-stained nodules or masses that are predominantly centrally located. Histologically, coal dust is present within macrophages or the interstitium, beginning around airways. There may be occasional ferruginous bodies with a black core. The smallest lesion is called a macule (0.5 to 6 mm), which may progress to a fibrotic nodule. Coalescing fibrous nodules are termed *progressive massive fibrosis*, which can result in diffuse interstitial fibrosis.[3]

Caplan Syndrome

Caplan syndrome, or rheumatoid pneumoconiosis, was first identified in coal workers with rheumatoid arthritis and lung nodules and later found in other types of pneumoconiosis, especially silicosis. The opacities range from 0.5 to 5 cm in diameter and, unlike pneumoconiosis, are well defined, numerous, and predominantly peripheral, presumably representing rheumatoid nodules.[4]

There are few histologic descriptions of the pulmonary nodules of Caplan syndrome. Both silicotic nodules and rheumatoid nodules have been documented histologically in the same patient.[5] The precise relationship between the pneumoconiosis and rheumatoid nodules is unknown, but they may represent a chance coincidence, or a predisposition to form rheumatoid nodules when there is inhalation of particulate matter.

Cobalt Pneumoconiosis

Hard metal pneumoconiosis is sometimes used synonymously with cobalt pneumoconiosis.[6] Cobalt is used as a binder in producing hard metals composed of carbon, tungsten, and other elements. The cobalt elicits a fibrotic reaction that initially manifests as inflammatory small airway disease. Workers at risk include machinists and other employees in the metal industry and previously dental technicians.

Symptoms include cough and hemoptysis. Computed tomograms show diffuse bilateral ground-glass attenuation and interstitial linear markings.

Histologically, there are inflammatory bronchiolar infiltrates, peribronchiolar fibrosis with peribronchiolar metaplasia, and macrophages within peribronchiolar alveoli containing tight aggregates of macrophages and giant cells without well-formed granulomas.[7] The multinucleated giant cells are characteristic and led to the former designation *giant cell interstitial pneumonia*.

Other histologic features include type II pneumocyte hyperplasia and a fibrotic reaction that rarely progresses to usual interstitial pneumonia.

Because the cobalt is water soluble and disappears with processing, energy dispersive spectroscopy detects tungsten, which is present in the macrophages. There are typically no particles or refractile material present in histologic sections. Because of the relative specificity of the giant cell reaction, special techniques to detect tungsten are not routinely done.[7]

Cobalt pneumoconiosis is rare, with few case reports in the previous decades.[7,8]

Aluminosis (Aluminum Pneumoconiosis)

Aluminosis is a very rare pneumoconiosis caused by inhalation of aluminum particles. Workers at risk include those involved in bauxite smelting, the use of fine aluminum powder, and aluminum welding, grinding, or polishing. Clinically, patients have exertional dyspnea with dry, nonproductive cough. Pulmonary function tests show initially obstructive or restrictive patterns, progressing to pure restrictive abnormalities. By imaging, there are nodular irregular opacities predominantly in the upper lobes that occasionally progress to pulmonary fibrosis and honeycombing.[9]

Pathologically, there are bronchiolocentric aluminum-laden macrophages with grayish-tan intracytoplasmic dust. Granulomas are usually not present, and if so, are poorly formed. There may by a desquamative interstitial pneumonia (DIP) or proteinosis-like reaction. Birefringent material by polarized light is generally absent, although there may be few birefringent particles or larger particles if there is mixed pneumoconiosis. In advanced stages, there may be extensive pulmonary fibrosis.[10]

Scanning electron microscopy and energy dispersion x-ray analysis will demonstrate on tissue sections aluminum-containing metallic

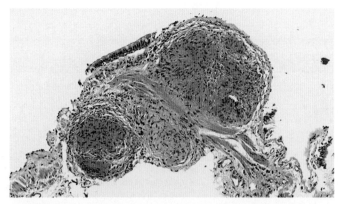

FIGURE 58.1 ▲ Sarcoid-like granuloma in berylliosis exposure. A transbronchial biopsy shows changes indistinguishable from sarcoidosis. There was a history of beryllium exposure. Lymphocyte stimulation test was inconclusive. The diagnosis of berylliosis remained as a possibility but not confirmed.

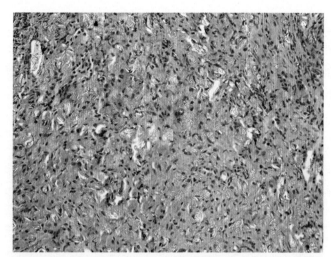

FIGURE 58.2 ▲ Talc nodule. The patient presents with small bilateral masses and one larger one suspicious for malignancy. A history of inhalational illicit drug use was obtained after biopsy results.

particles.[10] The presence of aluminum can also be confirmed by microparticle-induced x-ray emission analysis.[11]

Siderosis

Pulmonary siderosis is rare and occurs secondary to inhalation of iron particles, especially in arc welders. Most patients are asymptomatic. Chest computed tomography scan shows bilateral small nodular opacities, predominantly in the mid- and upper zones.

Histologically, there are clusters of iron-containing macrophages centered on bronchioles. In distinction from hemosiderin macrophages caused by hemorrhage or heart failure, siderotic histiocytes are bronchiolocentric and contain large iron particles with central cores that do not stain with stains for hemosiderin (Prussian blue). Only the peripheral rims are blue with iron stains.

There may be associated peribronchiolar fibrosis, but fibrotic lung disease is rare.[12]

Berylliosis

Berylliosis is a rare, environmental, inflammatory disorder caused by inhalation of beryllium dusts. A human leukocyte antigen class II marker (HLA-DP Glu69) has been found to be strongly associated with the disease.[13] Berylliosis is pathologically indistinguishable from sarcoid (Fig. 58.1), and mediastinal lymph nodes can be involved.[14] It is

not clear that it is possible to distinguish berylliosis from sarcoidosis other than by history of exposure. The role of lymphocyte proliferation testing to beryllium is somewhat controversial but provides supportive evidence of berylliosis if positive.[14]

Silicatosis (Talcosis)

In contrast to pure silica (silicon dioxide, SiO_2; see Chapter 57), *silicates* contain magnesium, potassium, iron, sodium, aluminum, and calcium and are minimally if at all fibrogenic. The most common silicate is talc, which has many potential routes to the upper respiratory tract. Talc is used in the manufacture of illicit drugs and can be inhaled or injected. Talc is occasionally used for pleurodesis to treat malignant effusions.

Talcosis or silicatosis can occasionally occur as a pneumoconiosis, for example, in carpet workers and other occupations such as soapstone sculptors.[15–18] Other silicates that may have occupational uses include mica and kaolin. Inhaling perfumed powders that contain talc and other silicates may also result in silicatosis.[15]

On computed tomography, there are multiple bilateral nodules that may coalesce. Mediastinal lymph nodes are generally normal in size.[15]

Talc and other silicates are easy to identify histologically. They are rhomboid, refractile, and strongly polarizable crystals that elicit a marked macrophage giant cell reaction (Figs. 58.2 and 58.3).

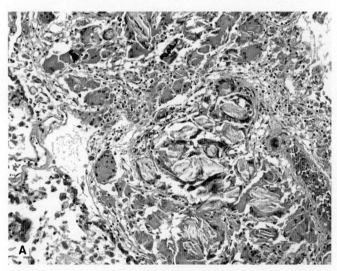

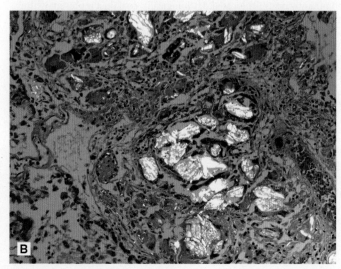

FIGURE 58.3 ▲ Talcosis. **A.** Typical talc crystals with giant cell reaction are present. **B.** Same field is viewed with polarized light. The patient had a history of illicit drug use, both inhalational and intravenous.

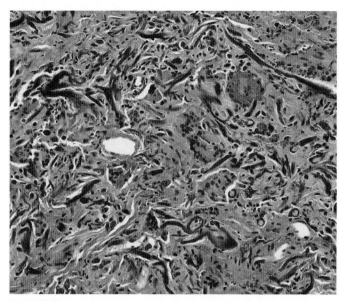

FIGURE 58.4 ▲ Endogenous pneumoconiosis. There is a macrophage reaction to mineralized degenerated elastic tissue. The lesion was an incidental nodule.

The location of the crystals depends on the route of exposure. In the case of inhaled powder, they are present around airways, and in cases of intravenous drug abuse, they are typically centered in vessels. In the case of illicit drug abuse, both routes may occur and the exact site of crystals may be difficult to ascertain if they are extremely numerous.[19]

Endogenous Pneumoconiosis

Endogenous inclusions found in granulomas are in the differential diagnosis of aspirated material, including asteroid and Schaumann (conchoidal) bodies (Fig. 58.4). In addition, large polarizable crystals representing calcium oxalate and calcium carbonate are sometimes present and are a by-product of endogenous cell metabolism. The crystals are often numerous and should not be confused with inhaled or injected substance.[20] Calcification of elastic tissue, especially in patients with renal failure and hypercalcemia, can result in a foreign body giant cell reaction and is a major form of endogenous pneumoconiosis (see Chapter 58).

REFERENCES

1. Naghavi M, Murray CJL, Wang H, et al. Global, regional, and national age-sex specific all-cause and cause-specific mortality for 240 causes of death, 1990–2013: a systematic analysis for the Global Burden of Disease Study 2013. *Lancet*. 2015;385:117–171.
2. Pneumoconiosis and advanced occupational lung disease among surface coal miners—16 states, 2010–2011. *MMWR Morb Mortal Wkly Rep*. 2012;61:431–434.
3. Laney AS, Petsonk EL, Hale JM, et al. Potential determinants of coal workers' pneumoconiosis, advanced pneumoconiosis, and progressive massive fibrosis among underground coal miners in the United States, 2005–2009. *Am J Public Health*. 2012;102 (suppl 2):S279–S283.
4. Caplan A. Certain unusual radiological appearances in the chest of coal-miners suffering from rheumatoid arthritis. *Thorax*. 1953;8:29–37.
5. Arakawa H, Honma K, Shida H, et al. Computed tomography findings of Caplan syndrome. *J Comput Assist Tomogr*. 2003;27:758–760.
6. Moreira MA, Cardoso Ada R, Silva DG, et al. Hard metal pneumoconiosis with spontaneous bilateral pneumothorax. *J Bras Pneumol*. 2010;36:148–151.
7. Enriquez LS, Mohammed TL, Johnson GL, et al. Hard metal pneumoconiosis: a case of giant-cell interstitial pneumonitis in a machinist. *Respir Care*. 2007;52:196–199.
8. Selden A, Sahle W, Johansson L, et al. Three cases of dental technician's pneumoconiosis related to cobalt–chromium–molybdenum dust exposure. *Chest*. 1996;109:837–842.
9. Smolkova P, Nakladalova M. The etiology of occupational pulmonary aluminosis—the past and the present. *Biomed Pap Med Fac Univ Palacky Olomouc Czech Repub*. 2014;158:535–538.
10. Hull MJ, Abraham JL. Aluminum welding fume-induced pneumoconiosis. *Hum Pathol*. 2002;33:819–825.
11. Chino H, Hagiwara E, Sugisaki M, et al. Pulmonary aluminosis diagnosed with in-air microparticle induced X-ray emission analysis of particles. *Intern Med*. 2015;54:2035–2040.
12. McCormick LM, Goddard M, Mahadeva R. Pulmonary fibrosis secondary to siderosis causing symptomatic respiratory disease: a case report. *J Med Case Rep*. 2008;2:257.
13. Amicosante M, Berretta F, Rossman M, et al. Identification of HLA-DRPhebeta47 as the susceptibility marker of hypersensitivity to beryllium in individuals lacking the berylliosis-associated supratypic marker HLA-DPGlubeta69. *Respir Res*. 2005;6:94.
14. Contini S, Mattioli G, Berretta F, et al. Berylliosis in Italy: a case of "sarcoidosis" under the threshold limit value. *Med Lav*. 2006;97:592–596.
15. Szeinuk J, Wilk-Rivard EJ. Case report: silicatosis in a carpet installer. *Environ Health Perspect*. 2007;115:932–935.
16. Nath D, Vaideeswar P, Chaudhary J, et al. "Samosa" pneumoconiosis: a case of pulmonary talcosis uncovered during a medicolegal autopsy. *Am J Forensic Med Pathol*. 2014;35:11–14.
17. Pereira Faria H, de Souza Veiga A, Coutinho Teixeira L, et al. Talcosis in soapstone artisans: high-resolution CT findings in 12 patients. *Clin Radiol*. 2014;69:e136–e139.
18. Shakoor A, Rahatullah A, Shah AA, et al. Pulmonary talcosis 10 years after brief teenage exposure to cosmetic talcum powder. *BMJ Case Rep*. 2011;2011.
19. Altraja A, Jurgenson K, Roosipuu R, et al. Pulmonary intravascular talcosis mimicking miliary tuberculosis in an intravenous drug addict. *BMJ Case Rep*. 2014;2014.
20. El-Zammar OA, Katzenstein AL. Pathological diagnosis of granulomatous lung disease: a review. *Histopathology*. 2007;50:289–310.

59 Drug-Induced Lung Injury

Allen P. Burke, M.D.

Patterns of Lung Injury Associated with Drugs

General Considerations

The diagnosis of drug-induced lung injury is one of exclusion, as the histologic findings are nonspecific, and the manifestations may overlap with underlying rheumatologic disease or radiation treatment. Although there is variability depending on the drug, there is no consistent relationship with exposure, both dose and interval between onset of lung symptoms and onset of therapy. Furthermore, many patients are on multiple medications, and it may be hard to discern the specific toxic agent. A presumed diagnosis is made only when infections, heart disease, and collagen vascular disease are excluded, and the lung findings resolve with cessation of drug. In only rare instances is the diagnosis confirmed by rechallenge with the offending agent to confirm the association between exposure and pulmonary manifestations.

The radiologic findings are generally those of diffuse disease, with symmetric reticular densities, nodules, and ground-glass opacities, depending on the pattern of lung injury. Nodular opacities occur with the organizing pneumonia pattern and with hypersensitivity-like reaction. Rarely, asymmetric large nodules can mimic metastatic tumor.

The major histologic findings are those of acute lung injury, interstitial inflammation, organizing pneumonia, and nonspecific interstitial pneumonia (Table 59.1). Less commonly, there is an eosinophilic pneumonia. Diffuse alveolar hemorrhage is generally diagnosed by the finding of red blood cells in bronchoalveolar lavage fluid and is an uncommon manifestation of drug-induced lung injury (see Chapter 32).

Because tissue sampling is usually performed by transbronchial biopsy, there is limited tissue, and the histologic findings may not be representative. In addition, there is a spectrum of findings spanning acute alveolar injury, chronic interstitial inflammation, and organizing pneumonia, which may represent manifestations of the same process at different phases of injury. Furthermore, nonspecific interstitial pneumonia is difficult to diagnose without open lung biopsy and is often diagnosed on smaller biopsies based on the findings in chronic interstitial inflammation with reactive pneumocytes (a finding that may be present in organizing acute lung injury). Therefore, transbronchial biopsy should exclude an infectious or neoplastic cause for the patient's lung disease and document specific histologic findings that indicate acute lung injury (intra-alveolar fibrin with hyaline membranes) or organizing phase of injury (organizing pneumonia). Interstitial inflammation with or without reactive pneumocytes should be reported as a nonspecific finding, with a comment that correlation with imaging is necessary to suggest a diagnosis of nonspecific interstitial pneumonia. There is little documentation of histologic findings in end-stage fibrotic lung disease due to drugs, but the imaging data in these rare patients suggest a nonclassifiable type of fibrosis that is typical neither of nonspecific interstitial pneumonia nor of usual interstitial pneumonia.

Pulmonary function tests generally show decreased lung volumes and diffusing capacity for carbon monoxide. Treatment is drug cessation with or without prednisone.[1]

Acute Lung Injury (Diffuse Alveolar Damage)

Acute lung injury secondary to drug exposure typically occurs within weeks of treatment and may clinically mimic acute pulmonary edema. The patient typically presents with dyspnea, cough, and decreased diffusing capacity for carbon monoxide, with variable fever. Imaging by computed tomography shows bilateral opacities, usually more prominent in the mid- and lower lung fields, with diffuse, ground glass. Transbronchial biopsies show acute lung injury, with hyaline membranes, thickened alveolar septa with chronic interstitial inflammation, and reactive type II pneumocytes. There may be organization with loose interstitial fibrosis that may overlap with an organizing pneumonia pattern (Figs. 59.1 to 59.3). It is important to document a lack of organisms by stains for acid-fast bacilli, fungi, and bacteria. The acute exudative phase, which occurs during the first week, is characterized by intra-alveolar fibrin and alveolar septal edema, and the later phase by interstitial fibroblasts are reactive alveolar pneumocytes. In reported fatal cases, histologic findings are typically intense interstitial inflammation with early organization.[2,3]

Chronic Interstitial Inflammation

Expansion of interstitium by chronic inflammation is a common finding in drug reactions and overlaps with nonspecific interstitial pneumonia, if there is mild interstitial fibrosis, and organizing diffuse alveolar damage, if there is marked pneumocyte atypia and interstitial edema.[4] Interstitial inflammation is also common in organizing pneumonia and in itself is not a specific pattern of lung injury. If the only finding in a small lung biopsy, concomitant bronchiolar or peribronchiolar inflammation should be noted and a differential diagnosis based on exclusion of other findings and computed tomographic studies presented. There may be scattered eosinophils in the interstitium in drug reactions, as has been reported in organizing pneumonia secondary to nitrofurantoin.[5]

Organizing Pneumonia

Organizing lung injury may form nodules with relatively uninvolved surrounding lung ("organizing pneumonia"), may be seen in diffuse chronic inflammation typical of nonspecific interstitial pneumonia, or may manifest as multiple areas in organizing diffuse alveolar damage. The process is more often interstitial than peribronchiolar, although the term bronchiolitis obliterans organizing pneumonia is often (confusingly) applied.[6] Organizing pneumonia is a common finding in drug toxicity (Figs. 59.4 and 59.5), including that secondary to methotrexate, gemcitabine, amiodarone, penicillamine, and sirolimus.[6–10]

Fibrotic Lung Changes

The most common type of fibrosing lung disease associated with drug toxicity is nonspecific interstitial pneumonia. The histologic features on small biopsy, however, consist of chronic interstitial inflammation, mild interstitial fibrosis, and reactive pneumocyte hyperplasia, which are features that overlap with organizing diffuse alveolar damage and

TABLE 59.1 Histopathologic Features of Lung Drug Toxicity

Histologic Pattern	Common Drugs Implicated	Infrequently Implicated Chemotherapeutic Agents	Infrequently Implicated Nonchemotherapeutic Agents
DAD	Bleomycin Busulfan Carmustine Cyclophosphamide Mitomycin Gold salts	Azathioprine Cytosine arabinoside Gemcitabine Methotrexate Nitrogen mustards Vinblastine Interleukin-2	Amiodarone Overdose (aspirin, NSAIDs, sedatives) Sulfasalazine Interferon-γ
Organizing pneumonia	Bleomycin Methotrexate Amiodarone	Cyclophosphamide Mitomycin C	Amphotericin B Carbamazepine Cocaine Nitrofurantoin Penicillamine Phenytoin Sirolimus Sulfasalazine Ticlopidine
Interstitial lung disease (generally NSIP)	Amiodarone Methotrexate Carmustine	Azathioprine Busulfan Chlorambucil Fludarabine Gemcitabine Gold salts 6-Mercaptopurine Mitomycin C Paclitaxel Tyrosine kinase inhibitors Lenalidomide	Amiodarone Cocaine Gold Methysergide Nitrofurantoin Penicillamine Phenytoin Sirolimus Statins Sulfasalazine Tocainide
Eosinophilic pneumonia (pulmonary infiltrates with eosinophilia)	Antibiotics (β-lactam, sulfa containing) Daptomycin Penicillamine Sulfasalazine Nitrofurantoin Methotrexate NSAIDs	Azathioprine Bleomycin Busulfan Imatinib Procarbazine Taxanes Lenalidomide	Isoniazid Phenytoin Statins
Pulmonary hemorrhage	Anticoagulants Amphotericin B Cytarabine	Mitomycin C Bevacizumab Alemtuzumab	Cocaine Penicillamine Amiodarone

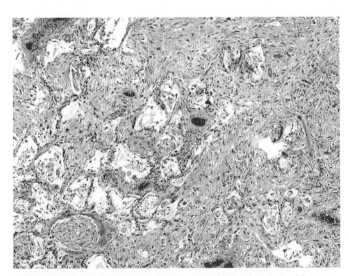

FIGURE 59.1 ▲ Diffuse alveolar damage, organized phase, bleomycin. There is diffuse thickening of the alveolar septa, as well as intra-alveolar involvement, by loose fibrosis and collagen. The patient developed acute lung injury that progressed to diffuse lung fibrosis, precipitated by bleomycin administered for ovarian cancer (immature teratoma).

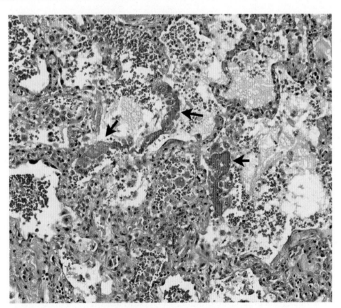

FIGURE 59.2 ▲ Acute lung injury, methotrexate. There is diffuse interstitial inflammation, intra-alveolar edema, and areas of fibrin exudate (*arrows*).

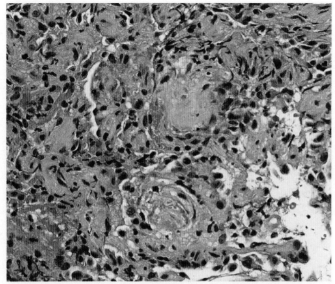

FIGURE 59.3 ▲ Subacute lung injury, methotrexate. There is mild interstitial fibrosis with diffuse hyperplasia of type II pneumocytes, with organizing pneumonia.

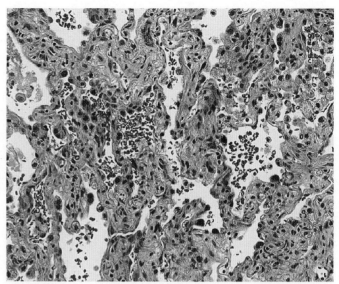

FIGURE 59.5 ▲ Amiodarone toxicity, subacute phase. There is diffuse interstitial thickening with markedly atypical and reactive pneumocytes. In this case, the clinical course, imaging findings, and degree of fibroblastic proliferation in the airways favor organizing diffuse alveolar damage. The vacuolization cannot be appreciated at this magnification.

which may be seen to some extent in organizing pneumonia. In most cases, the diagnosis of nonspecific interstitial pneumonia is made by imaging. More advanced stages of lung fibrosis are uncommon in drug toxicity and have been reported especially in children treated with chemotherapeutic agents such as carmustine.[11] Reports of imaging findings in fibrotic lung disease document dense scars with cystic change and honeycombing, which are not features of nonspecific interstitial pneumonia.[12,13]

Eosinophilic Pneumonia

Eosinophilic pneumonia is a relatively uncommon manifestation of drug toxicity. Conversely, eosinophilic lung disease is caused by drugs

in a relatively small proportion of patients (see Chapter 29). Patients typically present with progressive dyspnea, dry cough, and occasionally fever. Peripheral eosinophilia and elevated serum IgE levels are common. Chest radiographs show homogeneous opacities that typically have a peripheral and upper lobe distribution. Biopsies show findings of eosinophilia pneumonia, namely, intra-alveolar fibrin with interstitial and intra-alveolar eosinophils. Organizing pneumonia is a common additional histologic feature. Beta-lactam antibiotics, those that contain sulfa, and daptomycin are relatively common drugs associated with eosinophilic pneumonia.[14]

Granulomatous Interstitial Lung Disease

Granulomas have been described in the interstitial infiltrates secondary to nitrofurantoin, sulfasalazine, and sirolimus lung toxicity and may be poorly formed, or discrete and well formed, mimicking sarcoidosis.[15–17]

Nodular Lung Disease

Prominent nodules on computed tomographic scans are seen in lung toxicity when the histologic pattern is primarily organizing pneumonia.[18] Less commonly, nodules that can mimic metastatic malignancies on imaging occur as fibrotic masses as a reaction to bleomycin or cyclophosphamide toxicity.[19,20] Inflammatory nodules may be seen in amiodarone toxicity,[21] and Wegener-like necrotizing granulomas have been described as a reaction to sulfasalazine.[22]

Constrictive (Obliterative) Bronchiolitis

Obliterative bronchiolitis is a rare manifestation of drug toxicity. It has been reported in patients taking penicillamine for rheumatoid arthritis or systemic sclerosis, both of which may themselves predispose to constrictive bronchiolitis.[10,23]

Pulmonary Hemorrhage

Anticoagulants, amphotericin B, high-dose cyclophosphamide, mitomycin C, cytarabine, and penicillamine can cause diffuse pulmonary hemorrhage (see Chapter 32). Antiangiogenic drugs, particularly antivascular endothelial growth factor agents, may result in bleeding complications, including in the lung.[24] Bevacizumab is associated with intratumoral hemorrhage, especially those with squamous cell histology.[25]

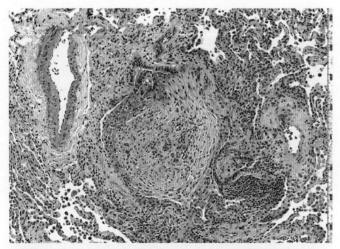

FIGURE 59.4 ▲ Organizing pneumonia with bronchiolocentricity, methotrexate. There is a plug of organizing pneumonia within a bronchiole. The artery is at the left. The patient was on methotrexate for Crohn disease. Although difficult to prove an association, there was suspicion that the lung symptoms were associated with methotrexate, which was withdrawn resulting in clinical improvement. Although the term "bronchiolitis obliterans organizing pneumonia" is often used for this histologic appearance, it should not be confused with obliterative bronchiolitis, which is concentric fibrosis between the mucosal epithelium and smooth muscle layer, eventually resulting in obliteration of the airway.

TABLE 59.2   Patterns of Lung Injury in Methotrexate Toxicity

Histologic Pattern	Frequency
Cellular interstitial inflammation, with or without poorly formed granulomas	Frequent
Reactive pneumocyte hyperplasia	Frequent
DAD	Unusual, may be more common in biopsies exampled
Interstitial fibrosis	Some degree common; established NSIP or UIP pattern rare
Tissue eosinophilia	Occasional
Organizing pneumonia	Uncommon

Specific Drugs Associated with Lung Injury

Methotrexate

The incidence of methotrexate-induced lung injury is difficult to assess, because over 50% of patients who take the drug have rheumatoid arthritis, which itself is associated with interstitial lung disease. If strict criteria for the histologic diagnosis of methotrexate-induced lung injury are used, including resolution of symptoms with drug cessation, then the incidence is <1%.[26]

Methotrexate-induced lung injury has been reported to occur at a wide range of doses, from 2.5 to 1,400 mg per week. There is no clear association with dose, duration of exposure, or clinical severity of rheumatoid arthritis.[27] The pathologic features of methotrexate lung injury are present in Table 59.2. Most typically, there are features of hypersensitivity pneumonitis with cellular interstitial inflammation and poorly formed granulomas, although the histologic reaction may be nonspecific (Figs. 59.2 and 59.3).[12] EBV-associated lymphoproliferative disease has been reported as a rare complication of methotrexate toxicity, with pulmonary involvement in some cases.[28,29]

Antitumor Drugs

Cytotoxic drugs constitute the largest and most important group of agents associated with lung toxicity and are often given in combination. In one series of patients with clinically documented lung toxicity, antitumor drugs accounted for 42% of cases; the remainder were antirheumatic drugs (24%), antiarrhythmic drugs (9%), nonsteroidal anti-inflammatory drugs (6%), and others (19%).[1] The antitumor drugs in this series, in decreasing order of frequency, were gemcitabine, docetaxel and paclitaxel, gefitinib, tegafur (oral 5-fluorouracil analog), pemetrexed, bleomycin, doxorubicin, carboplatin, imatinib, everolimus, and anastrozole.

Computed tomographic findings of lung toxicity secondary to antineoplastic agents are mostly frequently nonspecific interstitial pneumonia (71%), followed by hypersensitivity pneumonitis pattern, diffuse alveolar damage, and organizing pneumonia.[1]

Nucleoside analogs include gemcitabine, 5-fluorouracil, and tegafur. Pulmonary reactions to these drugs include rapidly fatal diffuse alveolar damage, diffuse alveolar injury with resolution, and transient organizing pneumonia.[1,3,6,30]

Cyclophosphamide is associated with lung injury that may progress to pulmonary fibrosis in <1% of patients and is related to dosage and concomitant radiation therapy.[12] Histologic findings include organizing diffuse alveolar damage,[31] interstitial inflammation with organizing pneumonia,[32] and fibrosis with arterial intimal thickening.[33]

Carmustine (BCNU) shows a clear relationship between cumulative dose and lung injury, with an increased risk with concomitant radiation therapy.[11] Carmustine-induced lung injury occurs in 20% to 30% of treated patients overall, but the incidence increases to 50% if the cumulative dose is more than 1.5 g/m²[.34] Lung fibrosis presents on average 14 years after exposure to the drug.[35] Histologic findings include interstitial fibroelastosis and interstitial lymphoplasmacytic

infiltrates.[35] In the past, one-third of children treated for neoplasms of the central nervous system with carmustine developed pulmonary fibrosis, with a high mortality, especially for those treated under the age of 5 years.[11] Acute lung injury has also been reported, especially with combined cyclophosphamide–cisplatin–BCNU therapy.[36]

Paclitaxel and docetaxel, often when administered with other drugs such as trastuzumab or gemcitabine, may result in pulmonary infiltrates, which, on biopsy, show chronic interstitial inflammation.[3,37]

Bleomycin-induced lung injury usually occurs in 3% to 5% of treated patients, although there is an increased risk if the total cumulative dose is more than 450 units and if the drug is given in combination. Bleomycin-related interstitial pneumonia occurs in about 15% of patients with Hodgkin lymphoma treated with adriamycin, bleomycin, vinblastine, and dacarbazine, defined as pulmonary symptoms, bilateral interstitial infiltrates, computed tomography or presence of lung fibrosis, and the absence of infection.[38] Diffuse alveolar damage is the most common manifestation (Fig. 59.1), followed by nonspecific interstitial pneumonia and organizing pneumonia.[12] Bleomycin toxicity can result in lung nodules that histologically are fibrotic scars or organizing pneumonia.[18–20] Eosinophilic pneumonia is a rare toxic effect of bleomycin.[39]

Busulfan rarely causes fatal fibrosis[40] and organizing diffuse alveolar damage.[41]

Monoclonal antibody drugs, including alemtuzumab and bevacizumab, may result in interstitial pneumonitis and pulmonary hemorrhage, which may be fatal.[2,24,25,42] Nilotinib and erlotinib (small molecular tyrosine kinase inhibitors) have been associated with both reversible and irreversible lung injuries.[43–45]

Amiodarone

Amiodarone is a commonly implicated drug in lung toxicity. Pulmonary toxicity occurs in ~5% to 10% of patients, usually within months of starting therapy, and can occur between weeks and decades of treatment (Table 59.3). The prognosis is good, with most patients improving after discontinuation of therapy. A distinctive computed tomographic feature of amiodarone toxicity is the occurrence of focal, homogeneous peripheral opacities with high attenuation. Similar opacities may occur in the liver and spleen.[12]

Interstitial inflammation, nonspecific interstitial pneumonia, and organizing pneumonia patterns (the latter two often coexisting) are the most frequently histologic manifestations of amiodarone toxicity. Pleural inflammation and effusions are common.

A characteristic histologic feature of amiodarone exposure is the presence of fine vacuoles within intra-alveolar macrophages as well as type II pneumocytes[21] (Fig. 59.6). These inclusions are found in macrophages of bronchoalveolar lavage samples of all patients taking the drug, whether or not there is lung injury.[46] Histologically, they are noted only in pneumocytes if they are prominent and atypical in reaction to alveolar damage, usually in the setting of organizing diffuse alveolar

TABLE 59.3   Histopathologic Findings in Amiodarone Toxicity

Histologic Feature	Comments
Diffuse vacuolization, macrophages	Universal finding, with or without lung symptoms
Acute lung injury (diffuse alveolar damage), with vacuolization of reactive pneumocytes as well as macrophages	Uncommon, usually organizing phase
Organizing pneumonia	Common
Interstitial inflammation/nonspecific interstitial pneumonia	Common
Necrotizing nodules composed of vacuolated macrophages, simulating Wegener or other autoimmune disease	Uncommon
Eosinophilic pneumonia	Rare

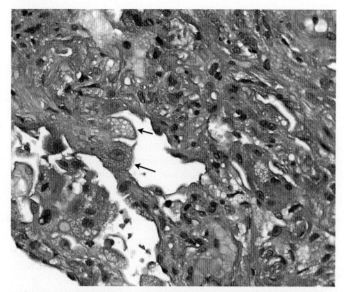

FIGURE 59.6 ▲ Amiodarone toxicity, organizing diffuse alveolar damage. There is diffuse vacuolization of the pneumocytes (*arrows*).

damage or interstitial inflammation with organizing pneumonia. The differential diagnosis includes foamy lipid-laden macrophages seen in postobstructive pneumonia, which should be excluded histologically. The vacuoles of amiodarone are distinctive histologically, with diffuse vacuolization dispersed throughout the cytoplasm, with occasional unilocular spaces that displace the nucleus to the periphery.[21] The finding of vacuolated pneumocytes also excludes lipid macrophages of lipoid pneumonia.

Ultrastructurally, the inclusions are osmiophilic, lamellated, round, whorled, structures. They may be identified by ultrastructure in macrophages and neutrophils in patients exposed to the drug, with or without pulmonary symptoms, and can be sampled by fine-needle aspiration.[9,47]

An unusual form of amiodarone lung toxicity is manifest by multiple nodules that clinically simulate malignancy. Histologically, they are composed of vacuolated macrophages with central necrosis, which may be basophilic, and contain neutrophilic microabscesses, similar to Wegener granulomatosis.[21] Palisading epithelioid macrophages and multinucleated giant cells are absent, however.[21]

More recently, Larsen et al. reported two other rare patterns of amiodarone lung disease: lymphocytic interstitial pneumonia and eosinophilic pneumonia.[48] In addition to interstitial inflammation with vacuolated macrophages, lymphoid hyperplasia with follicular bronchiolitis, features seen in lymphocytic interstitial pneumonia, was the predominant finding in eight and eosinophilic pneumonia in four patients. Two of the eosinophilic pneumonias were acute, with diffuse alveolar damage, and two with acute and organizing pneumonia with interstitial inflammation and eosinophilia.[48]

Nitrofurantoin

Nitrofurantoin is a frequently prescribed drug used to treat urinary tract infections. Nitrofurantoin-induced lung injury is uncommon, but the widespread use of the drug results in a relatively large number of cases. Computed tomographic findings typically show interstitial–alveolar pattern (reticular and ground-glass opacities) in the lung bases, although upper lobe predominance has been reported.[49] Histologically, a variety of patterns occur on transbronchial or open lung biopsy, including granulomatous interstitial inflammation,[15] interstitial inflammation with eosinophils,[50] and organizing pneumonia.[5] Lung fibrosis with honeycomb formation has been reported after prolonged nitrofurantoin use, but causation linking the fibrosis to the drug is difficult to substantiate in individual cases.[13]

Sulfasalazine

Sulfasalazine can occasionally cause lung toxicity such as interstitial pneumonitis and eosinophilic pneumonias. A case of sarcoid-like granulomas attributed to sulfasalazine has been reported.[17]

REFERENCES

1. Tamura M, Saraya T, Fujiwara M, et al. High-resolution computed tomography findings for patients with drug-induced pulmonary toxicity, with special reference to hypersensitivity pneumonitis-like patterns in gemcitabine-induced cases. *Oncologist.* 2013;18:454–459.
2. Creelan B, Ferber A. A fatal case of alemtuzumab-associated interstitial pneumonitis. *Am J Ther.* 2008;15:82–84.
3. Dunsford ML, Mead GM, Bateman AC, et al. Severe pulmonary toxicity in patients treated with a combination of docetaxel and gemcitabine for metastatic transitional cell carcinoma. *Ann Oncol.* 1999;10:943–947.
4. Smith GJ. The histopathology of pulmonary reactions to drugs. *Clin Chest Med.* 1990;11:95–117.
5. Bhullar S, Lele SM, Kraman S. Severe nitrofurantoin lung disease resolving without the use of steroids. *J Postgrad Med.* 2007;53:111–113.
6. Kawsar HI, Spiro TP, Cocco A, et al. BOOP as a rare complication of gemcitabine therapy. *BMJ Case Rep.* 2011;2011.
7. Hsu PC, Lan JL, Hsieh TY, et al. Methotrexate pneumonitis in a patient with rheumatoid arthritis. *J Microbiol Immunol Infect.* 2003;36:137–140.
8. Kirby S, Satoskar A, Brodsky S, et al. Histological spectrum of pulmonary manifestations in kidney transplant recipients on sirolimus inclusive immunosuppressive regimens. *Diagn Pathol.* 2012;7:25.
9. Omeroglu G, Kalugina Y, Ersahin C, et al. Amiodarone lung toxicity in a cardiac transplant candidate initially diagnosed by fine-needle aspiration: cytologic, histologic, and electron microscopic findings. *Diagn Cytopathol.* 2006;34:351–354.
10. Boehler A, Vogt P, Speich R, et al. Bronchiolitis obliterans in a patient with localized scleroderma treated with D-penicillamine. *Eur Respir J.* 1996;9:1317–1319.
11. O'Driscoll BR, Kalra S, Gattamaneni HR, et al. Late carmustine lung fibrosis. Age at treatment may influence severity and survival. *Chest.* 1995;107:1355–1357.
12. Rossi SE, Erasmus JJ, McAdams HP, et al. Pulmonary drug toxicity: radiologic and pathologic manifestations. *Radiographics.* 2000;20:1245–1259.
13. Willcox PA, Maze SS, Sandler M, et al. Pulmonary fibrosis following long-term nitrofurantoin therapy. *S Afr Med J.* 1982;61:714–717.
14. Corona Perez-Cardona PS, Barro Ojeda V, Rodriguez Pardo D, et al. Clinical experience with daptomycin for the treatment of patients with knee and hip periprosthetic joint infections. *J Antimicrob Chemother.* 2012;67:1749–1754.
15. Sakata KK, Larsen BT, Boland JM, et al. Nitrofurantoin-induced granulomatous interstitial pneumonia. *Int J Surg Pathol.* 2013;22:352–357.
16. Molinari L, Rosenbaum T, Aruj P, et al. Sirolimus-associated interstitial pneumonia in four renal transplant recipients. *Chest.* 2014;145:630A.
17. Mohyuddin GR, Sultan F, Zhang K, et al. Sulfasalazine induced lung toxicity masquerading as sarcoidosis—case report and review of the literature. *Sarcoidosis Vasc Diffuse Lung Dis.* 2013;30:226–230.
18. Cohen MB, Austin JH, Smith-Vaniz A, et al. Nodular bleomycin toxicity. *Am J Clin Pathol.* 1989;92:101–104.
19. Ben Arush MW, Roguin A, Zamir E, et al. Bleomycin and cyclophosphamide toxicity simulating metastatic nodules to the lungs in childhood cancer. *Pediatr Hematol Oncol.* 1997;14:381–386.
20. Scharstein R, Johnson JF, Cook BA, et al. Bleomycin nodules mimicking metastatic osteogenic sarcoma. *Am J Pediatr Hematol Oncol.* 1987;9:219–221.
21. Ruangchira-Urai R, Colby TV, Klein J, et al. Nodular amiodarone lung disease. *Am J Surg Pathol.* 2008;32:1654–1660.
22. Salerno SM, Ormseth EJ, Roth BJ, et al. Sulfasalazine pulmonary toxicity in ulcerative colitis mimicking clinical features of Wegener's granulomatosis. *Chest.* 1996;110:556–559.
23. Schlesinger C, Veeraraghavan S, Koss MN. Constructive (obliterative) bronchiolitis. *Curr Opin Pulm Med.* 1998;4:288–293.
24. Elice F, Rodeghiero F. Side effects of anti-angiogenic drugs. *Thromb Res.* 2012;129 (suppl 1):S50–S53.
25. Johnson DH, Fehrenbacher L, Novotny WF, et al. Randomized phase II trial comparing bevacizumab plus carboplatin and paclitaxel with carboplatin and paclitaxel alone in previously untreated locally advanced or metastatic non-small-cell lung cancer. *J Clin Oncol.* 2004;22:2184–2191.

26. Sathi N, Chikura B, Kaushik VV, et al. How common is methotrexate pneumonitis? A large prospective study investigates. *Clin Rheumatol.* 2012;31:79–83.
27. Taniguchi K, Usui Y, Matsuda T, et al. Methotrexate-induced acute lung injury in a patient with rheumatoid arthritis. *Int J Clin Pharmacol Res.* 2005;25:101–105.
28. Ochi N, Yamane H, Yamagishi T, et al. Methotrexate-induced lymphoproliferative disease: Epstein–Barr virus-associated lymphomatoid granulomatosis. *J Clin Oncol.* 2013;31:e348–e350.
29. Yamakawa H, Yoshida M, Katagi H, et al. Pulmonary and retroperitoneal lesions induced by methotrexate-associated lymphoproliferative disorder in a patient with rheumatoid arthritis. *Mod Rheumatol.* 2014.
30. Galvao FH, Pestana JO, Capelozzi VL. Fatal gemcitabine-induced pulmonary toxicity in metastatic gallbladder adenocarcinoma. *Cancer Chemother Pharmacol.* 2010;65:607–610.
31. Fassas A, Gojo I, Rapoport A, et al. Pulmonary toxicity syndrome following CDEP (cyclophosphamide, dexamethasone, etoposide, cisplatin) chemotherapy. *Bone Marrow Transplant.* 2001;28:399–403.
32. Ochoa R, Bejarano PA, Gluck S, et al. Pneumonitis and pulmonary fibrosis in a patient receiving adjuvant docetaxel and cyclophosphamide for stage 3 breast cancer: a case report and literature review. *J Med Case Rep.* 2012;6:413.
33. Segura A, Yuste A, Cercos A, et al. Pulmonary fibrosis induced by cyclophosphamide. *Ann Pharmacother.* 2001;35:894–897.
34. Litam JP, Dail DH, Spitzer G, et al. Early pulmonary toxicity after administration of high-dose BCNU. *Cancer Treat Rep.* 1981;65:39–44.
35. Hasleton PS, O'Driscoll BR, Lynch P, et al. Late BCNU lung: a light and ultrastructural study on the delayed effect of BCNU on the lung parenchyma. *J Pathol.* 1991;164:31–36.
36. Jones RB, Matthes S, Shpall EJ, et al. Acute lung injury following treatment with high-dose cyclophosphamide, cisplatin, and carmustine: pharmacodynamic evaluation of carmustine. *J Natl Cancer Inst.* 1993;85:640–647.
37. Abulkhair O, El Melouk W. Delayed Paclitaxel–trastuzumab-induced interstitial pneumonitis in breast cancer. *Case Rep Oncol.* 2011;4:186–191.
38. Ngeow J, Tan IB, Kanesvaran R, et al. Prognostic impact of bleomycin-induced pneumonitis on the outcome of Hodgkin's lymphoma. *Ann Hematol.* 2011;90:67–72.
39. Hapani S, Chu D, Wu S. Eosinophilic pneumonia associated with bleomycin in a patient with mediastinal seminoma: a case report. *J Med Case Rep.* 2010;4:126.
40. Pearl M. Busulfan lung. *Am J Dis Child.* 1977;131:650–652.
41. Vergnon JM, Boucheron S, Riffat J, et al. Interstitial pneumopathies caused by busulfan. Histologic, developmental and bronchoalveolar lavage analysis of 3 cases. *Rev Med Interne.* 1988;9:377–383.
42. Ikeda S, Sekine A, Kato T, et al. Diffuse alveolar hemorrhage as a fatal adverse effect of bevacizumab: an autopsy case. *Jpn J Clin Oncol.* 2014;44:497–500.
43. Go SI, Lee WS, Lee GW, et al. Nilotinib-induced interstitial lung disease. *Int J Hematol.* 2013;98:361–365.
44. Ren S, Li Y, Li W, et al. Fatal asymmetric interstitial lung disease after erlotinib for lung cancer. *Respiration.* 2012;84:431–435.
45. Kitajima H, Takahashi H, Harada K, et al. Gefitinib-induced interstitial lung disease showing improvement after cessation: disassociation of serum markers. *Respirology.* 2006;11:217–220.
46. Bedrossian CW, Warren CJ, Ohar J, et al. Amiodarone pulmonary toxicity: cytopathology, ultrastructure, and immunocytochemistry. *Ann Diagn Pathol.* 1997;1:47–56.
47. Azzam I, Tov N, Elias N, et al. Amiodarone toxicity presenting as pulmonary mass and peripheral neuropathy: the continuing diagnostic challenge. *Postgrad Med J.* 2006;82:73–75.
48. Larsen BT, Vaszar LT, Colby TV, et al. Lymphoid hyperplasia and eosinophilic pneumonia as histologic manifestations of amiodarone-induced lung toxicity. *Am J Surg Pathol.* 2012;36:509–516.
49. Martins RR, Marchiori E, Viana SL, et al. Chronic eosinophilic pneumonia secondary to long-term use of nitrofurantoin: high-resolution computed tomography findings. *J Bras Pneumol.* 2008;34:181–184.
50. Milic R, Plavec G, Tufegdzic I, et al. Nitrofurantoin-induced immune-mediated lung and liver disease. *Vojnosanit Pregl.* 2012;69:536–540.

60 Radiation-Induced Lung Injury

Allen P. Burke, M.D., and Joseph J. Maleszewksi, M.D.

General

Radiation-induced lung injury is clinically classified into acute radiation pneumonitis, chronic radiation pneumonitis (radiation fibrosis), and sporadic radiation pneumonitis, characterized by migratory pulmonary infiltrates. This process is usually confined to the field of radiation but can spread outside of the irradiated field via a presumed immunologic reaction.[1] The frequency of lung injury is dependent on a number of complex factors.

Factors influencing the incidence and severity include total dose of radiation, rate of delivery of radiation, volume of irradiated lung tissue, history of prior radiation, previous or concomitant chemotherapy, withdrawal of steroid therapy, and pre-existing lung disease.

Patients with a variety of malignancies are at risk for radiation pneumonitis (Table 60.1). In patients with lung cancer, pneumonitis risk is lessened by more localized treatments such as intensity-modulated radiation therapy. Stereotactic radiation therapy is sometimes a primary treatment for peripheral lesions and carries a small risk for radiation pneumonitis. Patients with Hodgkin lymphoma frequently present with mediastinal disease and are especially prone to radiation pneumonitis.[10] The incidence of clinical effects is relatively lower in patients treated for breast cancer.

Treatment with bleomycin, cyclosporine, gemcitabine, cisplatin, and melphalan may enhance the risk, which is dependent on total lung dose.

Patients with relapsed Hodgkin lymphoma who undergo stem cell transplant are particularly susceptible to radiation pneumonitis, because of combined effects of radiation for local disease control and high-dose chemotherapy given during the transplant. Other pulmonary complications, such as obliterative bronchiolitis, are frequent in patients with stem cell transplants, especially those with allogeneic transplants, resulting in a total risk of 11% to 50% for any severe lung complications.[10,12]

Clinical Findings

Acute radiation pneumonitis usually occurs between 2 weeks and 6 months following completion of radiation therapy. Dyspnea, nonproductive cough, and fever are common symptoms. If there is extensive acute alveolar injury, patients develop acute respiratory distress syndrome, which may even progress to death from respiratory failure[13] (Table 60.2). The most common laboratory findings include polymorphonuclear leukocytosis and elevated erythrocyte sedimentation rate.[14]

Chronic radiation pneumonitis is the resultant scarring that develops from organizing diffuse alveolar damage and becomes apparent typically at about 1 year. Patients exhibit signs and symptoms of interstitial lung disease, and pulmonary function tests show restrictive abnormalities.

TABLE 60.1   Selected Conditions with Increased Risk for Radiation Pneumonitis

Condition Treated	Treatment	Approximate Rate of Radiation Pneumonitis, %[a]	Risk Factors	References
Lung cancer	Stereotactic body radiation	10%	Female, smoking history, tumor size, dose[b]	Baker et al.[2] Barriger et al.[3]
Lung cancer	Intensity modulated RT + chemotherapy	10%	Dose, COPD	Shi et al.[4]
Lung cancer	Conventional (3DRT) + chemotherapy	20%	Dose	Hernando et al.[5]
Esophageal cancer	Conventional (3DRT) with or without prior chemotherapy	20%	Dose	Nomura et al.[6] Kumar et al.[7]
Breast cancer	Conventional	<3%	Taxanes (up to 15%)	Taghian et al.[8]
Multiple myeloma	Autologous SCT with TBI[c]	Up to 30%		Chen et al.[9]
Mediastinal HL	Conventional 3DRT	2%–3% up to 30% (older series)	Chemotherapy, dose, older age, dose	Fox et al.[10] Koh et al.[11]
Relapsed or refractory HL	Autologous SCT with TBI (no prior radiation) or without TBI (prior radiation)	21%–23%	Pretransplant radiation, dose	Fox et al.[10] Moskowitz et al.[12]

SBRT, stereotactic body radiation; IMRT, intensity-modulated radiation therapy.
[a]At least grade 2, in most series.
[b]Usually defined as mean lung dose, Gy (MLD), or as volume % of lung volume (excluding tumor) receiving a certain level of radiation in Gy, for example, V20, V30.
[c]Includes high-dose chemotherapy.

Sporadic radiation pneumonitis is a less common manifestation, resembling cryptogenic organizing pneumonia, with most patients experiencing resolution of symptoms without further consequence.[1,15]

Radiologic Findings

Computed tomographic findings of radiation pneumonitis include ground-glass opacities and patchy or homogeneous consolidation, usually confined to lung parenchyma underlying the radiation fields.[16] Findings observed outside of the radiation field are often less severe. Other findings include pleural thickening, loss of lung volume, fibrotic strands, bronchiectasis, and loss of normal lung markings.[16,17]

Gross Findings

The gross findings of acute radiation pneumonitis are indistinguishable from diffuse alveolar damage and may be difficult to ascertain in autopsy specimens. Radiation fibrosis demonstrates dense scars, generally without cysts, that are present in the areas of treatment (Fig. 60.1).

Microscopic Findings

The pathologic features of radiation pneumonitis progress from acute lung injury to interstitial fibrosis that may resemble the fibrotic type of nonspecific interstitial pneumonia. Acute radiation injury appears indistinguishable from diffuse alveolar damage, with hyaline membranes, interstitial edema and inflammation, and reactive type II pneumocytes (Fig. 60.2). A characteristic feature of radiation is the marked enlargement of pneumocytes, endothelial cells, and stromal cells, often with severe atypia (Fig. 60.3). Radiation fibrosis represents organized diffuse alveolar injury with prominent interstitial fibrosis and destruction of alveolar architecture (Fig. 60.4).

The pattern of fibrosis is nonspecific, without formation of subpleural cysts or cystic remodeling as would be seen in usual interstitial pneumonia. At the periphery of the denser scars, there may be areas of diffuse alveolar wall thickening, similar to nonspecific interstitial pneumonia (Fig. 60.5). There may be areas of ossification, which can occur in any type of fibrotic lung disease. Intimal thickening of vessels, especially arteries, is always present (Fig. 60.6). Rarely, radiation can affect primarily veins, resulting in venoocclusive disease.[18]

Sporadic radiation pneumonitis has been shown to exhibit a pattern of organizing pneumonia.[1]

TABLE 60.2   Radiation Therapy Oncology Group Clinical Grading for Radiation Pneumonitis

Grade	Definition
1	Nonproductive cough or dyspnea on exertion
2	Cough requiring narcotic antitussives or dyspnea with minimal exertion
3	Severe cough unresponsive to narcotic antitussives, dyspnea at rest, radiologic evidence of pneumonitis, or need for intermittent oxygen or steroids
4	Continuous oxygen or assisted ventilation
5	Death

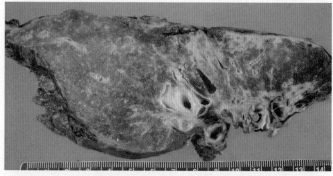

FIGURE 60.1 ▲ Radiation fibrosis, explanted lung. The patient had a history of radiation for Hodgkin lymphoma many years prior to transplant that resulted in respiratory failure due to radiation lung injury. There is fibrosis with restriction of the upper lobe. The scars are present near the hilum and subpleurally.

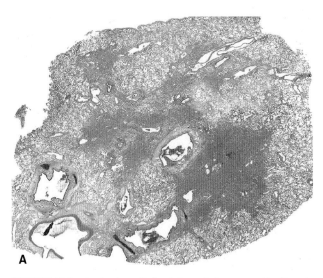

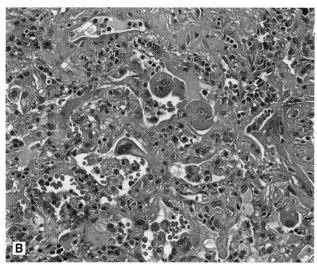

FIGURE 60.2 ▲ Acute radiation injury. **A.** Low magnification shows an irregular area of consolidation. **B.** High magnification demonstrates reactive pneumocytes, thickened interstitium, and intra-alveolar fibrin that is merging into the interstitium.

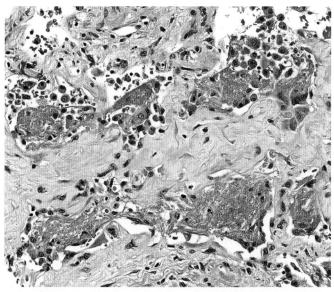

FIGURE 60.3 ▲ Organizing radiation injury. There is loose fibrosis, with atypical stromal cells and intra-alveolar fibrin. The area was adjacent to a lung tumor that had been irradiated prior to resection.

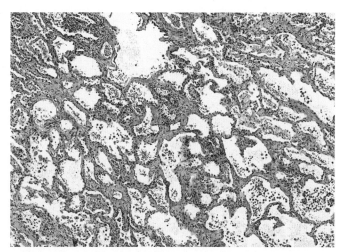

FIGURE 60.5 ▲ Chronic radiation fibrosis. In this field, there is uniform mild interstitial fibrosis with diffuse pneumocyte hyperplasia, at this magnification indistinguishable from idiopathic nonspecific interstitial pneumonia.

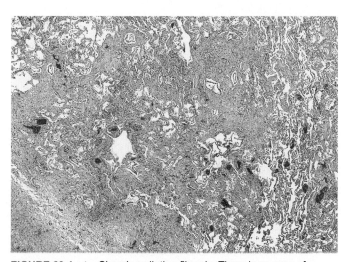

FIGURE 60.4 ▲ Chronic radiation fibrosis. There is an area of uniform fibrosis with residual small airspaces lined by cuboidal pneumocytes. The pattern somewhat resembles nonspecific interstitial pneumonia, but the degree of scarring is unusual for that.

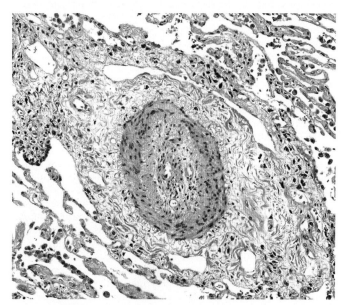

FIGURE 60.6 ▲ Intimal arterial thickening, radiation fibrosis. Intimal damage occurs invariably in radiation damage and progressed to concentric intimal hyperplasia of arteries.

REFERENCES

1. Arbetter KR, Prakash UB, Tazelaar HD, et al. Radiation-induced pneumonitis in the "nonirradiated" lung. *Mayo Clin Proc.* 1999;74:27–36.
2. Baker R, Han G, Sarangkasiri S, et al. Clinical and dosimetric predictors of radiation pneumonitis in a large series of patients treated with stereotactic body radiation therapy to the lung. *Int J Radiat Oncol Biol Phys.* 2013;85:190–195.
3. Barriger RB, Forquer JA, Brabham JG, et al. A dose-volume analysis of radiation pneumonitis in non-small cell lung cancer patients treated with stereotactic body radiation therapy. *Int J Radiat Oncol Biol Phys.* 2012;82:457–462.
4. Shi A, Zhu G, Wu H, et al. Analysis of clinical and dosimetric factors associated with severe acute radiation pneumonitis in patients with locally advanced non-small cell lung cancer treated with concurrent chemotherapy and intensity-modulated radiotherapy. *Radiat Oncol.* 2010;5:35.
5. Hernando ML, Marks LB, Bentel GC, et al. Radiation-induced pulmonary toxicity: a dose-volume histogram analysis in 201 patients with lung cancer. *Int J Radiat Oncol Biol Phys.* 2001;51:650–659.
6. Nomura M, Kodaira T, Furutani K, et al. Predictive factors for radiation pneumonitis in oesophageal cancer patients treated with chemoradiotherapy without prophylactic nodal irradiation. *Br J Radiol.* 2012;85:813–818.
7. Kumar G, Rawat S, Puri A, et al. Analysis of dose-volume parameters predicting radiation pneumonitis in patients with esophageal cancer treated with 3D-conformal radiation therapy or IMRT. *Jpn J Radiol.* 2012;30:18–24.
8. Taghian AG, Assaad SI, Niemierko A, et al. Is a reduction in radiation lung volume and dose necessary with paclitaxel chemotherapy for node-positive breast cancer? *Int J Radiat Oncol Biol Phys.* 2005;62:386–391.
9. Chen CI, Abraham R, Tsang R, et al. Radiation-associated pneumonitis following autologous stem cell transplantation: predictive factors, disease characteristics and treatment outcomes. *Bone Marrow Transplant.* 2001;27:177–182.
10. Fox AM, Dosoretz AP, Mauch PM, et al. Predictive factors for radiation pneumonitis in Hodgkin lymphoma patients receiving combined-modality therapy. *Int J Radiat Oncol Biol Phys.* 2012;83:277–283.
11. Koh ES, Sun A, Tran TH, et al. Clinical dose-volume histogram analysis in predicting radiation pneumonitis in Hodgkin's lymphoma. *Int J Radiat Oncol Biol Phys.* 2006;66:223–228.
12. Moskowitz CH, Nimer SD, Zelenetz AD, et al. A 2-step comprehensive high-dose chemoradiotherapy second-line program for relapsed and refractory Hodgkin disease: analysis by intent to treat and development of a prognostic model. *Blood.* 2001;97:616–623.
13. Movsas B, Raffin TA, Epstein AH, et al. Pulmonary radiation injury. *Chest.* 1997;111:1061–1076.
14. Rosiello RA, Merrill WW. Radiation-induced lung injury. *Clin Chest Med.* 1990;11:65–71.
15. Crestani B, Valeyre D, Roden S, et al. Bronchiolitis obliterans organizing pneumonia syndrome primed by radiation therapy to the breast. The Groupe d'Etudes et de Recherche sur les Maladies Orphelines Pulmonaires (GERM"O"P). *Am J Respir Crit Care Med.* 1998;158:1929–1935.
16. Libshitz HI. Radiation changes in the lung. *Semin Roentgenol.* 1993;28:303–320.
17. Ikezoe J, Takashima S, Morimoto S, et al. CT appearance of acute radiation-induced injury in the lung. *AJR Am J Roentgenol.* 1988;150:765–770.
18. Kramer MR, Estenne M, Berkman N, et al. Radiation-induced pulmonary veno-occlusive disease. *Chest.* 1993;104:1282–1284.

61 Miscellaneous Iatrogenic Lung Disease: Extracorporeal Membrane Oxygenation, Hydrophilic Polymer Embolization, Therapeutic Microsphere Embolization

Allen P. Burke, M.D., and Joseph J. Maleszewski, M.D.

Extracorporeal Membrane Oxygenation

Technical Considerations

First introduced for clinical use in 1972, extracorporeal membrane oxygenation (ECMO) is a form of prolonged cardiopulmonary bypass to treat respiratory and cardiac failure. Since earliest reports of pathologic findings attributable to ECMO published in the 1990s,[1] there have been several technical improvements that have lessened the complication rate. These improvements include the development of more biocompatible materials, more efficient oxygenators, refinements in double lumen cannulas, and smaller, less thrombogenic circuits that decreased turbulence and hemolysis.[2,3]

ECMO was initially used in neonates but is now a common therapy in older children and adults. ECMO circuits consist of cannulas, which are typically double-lumen catheters or surgically placed conduits, an oxygenator, and a centrifugal pump. There are two major configurations (Table 61.1). Venoarterial ECMO provides circulatory support as well as oxygenation. Venovenous ECMO has a lower risk of central nervous injury and mortality but requires adequate biventricular cardiac output. Central venoarterial ECMO requires cannulation of the right atrium and returns blood to the ascending aorta via surgical anastomoses. Peripheral venoarterial ECMO utilizes catheters, inserted in the femoral or internal jugular vein and common femoral artery, and is typically used in children. Central venovenous ECMO involves two cannulas in the right atrium, and peripheral venovenous ECMO drains blood from the femoral or jugular vein and returns it through the internal jugular vein.[4] In autopsies, venovenous or peripheral arteriovenous ECMO is often not readily apparent, especially if the catheters have been removed. Central arteriovenous ECMO is generally used in patients with recent heart surgery and postoperative heart failure and is evident postmortem by synthetic cannulas sutured to the ascending aorta and right atrium, which course outside the chest.

▶ **TABLE 61.1 Types of ECMO Circuits**

Arteriovenous (central)
Surgically placed conduit in right atrium
Blood pumped to oxygenator
Surgically placed conduit in ascending aorta
Oxygenated blood returned to systemic circulation
Arteriovenous (peripheral)
Venous cannula in femoral or jugular vein
Blood directed to oxygenator
Arterial cannula in femoral or carotid artery
Oxygenated blood returned to systemic circulation
Venovenous
Venous cannula in femoral or jugular vein
Blood directed to oxygenator
Venous cannula in femoral or carotid artery
Oxygenated blood returned to systemic circulation

TABLE 61.2 Indications of ECMO in Neonates and Children

Meconium aspiration syndrome
Persistent pulmonary hypertension of the newborn
Sepsis
Acute respiratory distress syndrome
Congenital diaphragmatic hernia
Alveolar capillary dysplasia
Pneumonia
   HSV
   RSV
Congenital heart disease
   TAPVR
   Postoperative heart failure
Pulmonary hypoplasia
Bridge to transplant

TABLE 61.4 Complications of ECMO

Thrombosis
   Deep venous thrombosis
   Heparin-induced thrombocytopenia
Hemorrhage
   Pulmonary
   Central nervous system
   Gastrointestinal
Infections
   Sepsis
   Pneumonia
Central nervous system
   Edema
   Hemorrhage
   Infarction
Pulmonary
   Hemorrhage
   Fibrosis (children)
   Hemothorax
   Effusions
Renal
   Acute renal failure
Gastrointestinal
   Acute pancreatic insufficiency
   Necrotizing enterocolitis
   Mesenteric insufficiency with ischemic bowel

In venovenous ECMO, pulmonary blood flow and pulsatile systemic flow are maintained by native cardiac function, with preserved oxygenation of blood in the left ventricle and aortic root.[3] Venous emboli are filtered by the patient's native lungs. In contrast, venoarterial ECMO, especially peripheral, results in decreased oxygenated blood flow to the left ventricle and aortic root, and there is a greater risk of systemic thromboembolism, ischemic extremities, misdistribution of oxygen, and increased left ventricular wall tension.[2]

Indications for ECMO

In children, there are a variety of respiratory conditions that may necessitate ECMO treatment. Acute respiratory distress syndrome (ARDS) due to prematurity is currently an uncommon indication, as other treatments have become available. More frequent indications include respiratory failure secondary to meconium aspiration syndrome or persistent pulmonary hypertension of the newborn (Table 61.2).

In adults, there are several indications for ECMO (Table 61.3). ECMO may be used as a *bridge to transplant* and may allow some patients to be removed from mechanical ventilation and have relative autonomy in preparation for transplantation. Venovenous ECMO is often sufficient, although acute exacerbations can lead to pulmonary hypertension, right-sided heart failure, and the need for venoarterial ECMO.[5]

Acute pneumonia, especially influenza A (H1N1), can be successfully treated with ECMO. The pandemic in 2009 created a resurgence of interest in venovenous ECMO for the treatment of life-threatening lung infections.[6]

The utility of ECMO in the treatment of *acute respiratory distress syndrome* is unclear, as the mortality remains high even with this therapy. The efficacy and cost of ECMO treatment for ARDS, in comparison to mechanical ventilation, have been reviewed.[7,8] Venovenous ECMO is the preferred method, even if there is transient acute right heart failure secondary to ARDS, since oxygenation of pulmonary artery blood will decrease hypoxia-induced vasoconstriction.[2]

Patients with complicated open heart surgery develop heart failure and are unable to be weaned from bypass at a rate of about 1%. Arteriovenous ECMO, often with aortic balloon pump placement, is an accepted treatment for these patients.[9]

ECMO has been used for cardiopulmonary support for organ donation after neurologic determination of death.[10]

TABLE 61.3 Indications for ECMO in Adults

Pneumonia (especially influenza)
Postoperative heart failure
Acute respiratory distress syndrome
Bridge to transplant

Complications of ECMO

There are several factors that affect the rate of survival and complications following ECMO therapy. These include arteriovenous ECMO, prolonged therapy, need for transfusions, severity of underlying disease, age of patient, prior mechanical ventilation, flow rate, and number of transfusions. The overall mortality is variable depending on these factors, and has been estimated at 43%.[3]

The most common complications of ECMO are bleeding, venous thromboembolism, and infection (Table 61.4). Central nervous system complications and renal failure are more frequent in venoarterial ECMO than venovenous ECMO. An early autopsy study showed that in children with prolonged (>28 days) ECMO treatment, most patients eventually die of complications, which include multiorgan failure, sepsis, renal insufficiency requiring dialysis, pancreatic insufficiency, neurologic complications related to central nervous system thrombosis and hemorrhage, necrotizing enterocolitis, and gastrointestinal bleeding. About two-thirds of these patients will develop lung complications, which include pulmonary hemorrhage, hemothorax, effusions, and chronic fibrotic lung disease.[11]

In adults treated with ECMO for postoperative heart failure, the most common complications are renal failure, followed by cerebral hemorrhage, infection, and lower limb ischemia. There is a high mortality, usually from cardiac failure.[9]

Pulmonary Manifestations of ECMO

Histologic features of chronic lung disease secondary to ECMO have not been fully determined, as underlying conditions likely confound the situation. An early study found that interstitial and intra-alveolar hemorrhage, hyaline membranes, type II pneumocyte hyperplasia, squamous metaplasia, smooth muscle hyperplasia, and reactive respiratory epithelial changes were present in the lungs of children dying after ECMO treatment. However, many of these changes were likely part of the underlying lung disease.[1] More recent studies of open lung biopsies after ECMO therapy have found only recent or remote hemorrhage and have not found that ECMO-related changes confound interpretation of the lung biopsies.[12,13] The histologic manifestations of ECMO-related hemorrhage are hemosiderin-laden macrophages, which are not only in the alveolar spaces but also in the interstitium (Figs. 61.1 and 61.2).

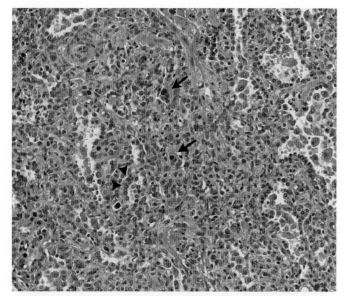

FIGURE 61.1 ▲ Pulmonary hemorrhage, ECMO. The findings are nonspecific. There is diffuse type II pneumocyte hyperplasia (*arrowheads*) and hemosiderin macrophages (*arrows*).

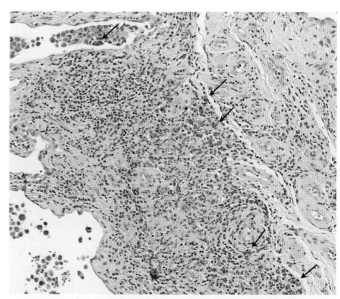

FIGURE 61.2 ▲ Pulmonary hemorrhage, ECMO. There is a sheet of chronic inflammatory cells under the thickened pleura, intermixed with hemosiderin macrophages (*arrows*). The inflammation was likely related to the underlying disease (idiopathic pulmonary fibrosis). Hemorrhage within chronic inflammation, however, is unusual and suggestive of ECMO.

Hydrophilic Polymer Embolization

Etiology

Guidewires and sheaths used for catheter-based interventions are often coated with a hydrophilic polymer for lubrication and ease of insertion. Some of this coating may embolize during the catheterization procedure, entering the pulmonary circulation after venous procedures, and the systemic circulation after arterial punctures.

Clinical Findings

In most cases, pulmonary embolization with hydrophilic polymers cause no clinical symptoms and are incidental findings at autopsy, explant, and, less commonly, transbronchial biopsy.[14] Rarely, embolization may result in pulmonary infarcts and granulomatous arteritis with cavitary lung nodules.[15,16]

Histologic Findings

Hydrophilic gels are basophilic, homogenous linear structures that often coil within the artery (Fig. 61.3). Depending on the time interval between catheterization and tissue acquisition, there may be a tissue response, including foreign body macrophages and thrombosis. Rarely, there may be destruction of the underlying arterial media from this tissue reaction (Fig. 61.4).

Microscopic Pulmonary Embolization of Indwelling Central Venous Catheters

There have been rare reports of tips of indwelling central lines degenerating into small fragments that embolize into the pulmonary circulation with a granulomatous reaction.[17] The diagnosis rests on identification of the specific polymer within granulomas in the lung.

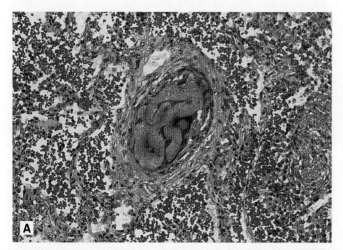
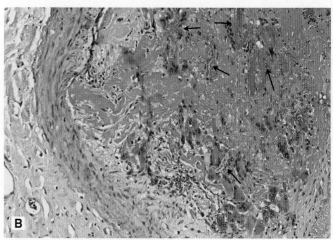

FIGURE 61.3 ▲ Hydrophilic polymer embolization. **A.** A small muscular artery is distended with a coiled fragment of polymer, which is homogeneous, basophilic, and finely granular. The diameter of the material is ~20 μm. **B.** In other areas, there is a foreign body macrophage reaction with thrombosis. The polymer (*arrows*) is surrounded by foreign body macrophages, and there is intervening thrombus. The specimen was an explant in a patient with cystic fibrosis.

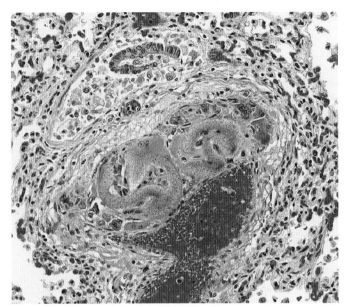

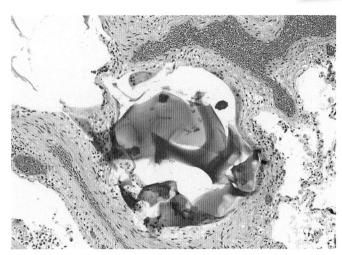

FIGURE 61.5 ▲ Therapeutic polyamide acrylic microsphere embolization. A relatively intact microsphere shows the homogenous eosinophilic round structure. There is a rim of surrounding macrophage foreign body giant cells.

FIGURE 61.4 ▲ Hydrophilic polymer embolization. At autopsy, this small muscular artery was distended and partly occluded by the foreign material, macrophage giant cells, and eccentric organized thrombus. The arterial media is thinned and destroyed by the inflammation.

Bronchial Artery Embolization for Pulmonary Hemorrhage

Composition

Therapeutic embolization with microparticles is frequently accomplished with the use of polyvinyl alcohol particles, Gelfoam, or thrombin, which incite a relatively limited inflammatory reaction. Other spherical agents include those made with collagen, dextran, and trisacryl polymer cross-linked with gelatin.[18] For bronchial artery embolization, polyvinyl alcohol or acrylic polyamide plastic microspheres are most frequently used.[19,20]

Indications

Microspheres are commonly injected into tumors (such as uterine leiomyomas or liver cancers) to induce necrosis preoperatively or as definitive therapy. In the lung, particles are injected into the bronchial arteries to prevent persistent hemoptysis refractory to conventional treatment. Conditions causing severe hemoptysis that are treated by embolization include bronchiectasis, pulmonary hypertension, malignancy, and mycetomas.[19-21]

Histologic Findings

Therapeutic embolization is an incidental finding in bronchial arteries at autopsy, explant, or tumor resection. Polyvinyl alcohol is a particulate substance forming irregular homogenous basophilic particles that lodge within small muscular arteries with intervening thrombus.[22] Polyamide microspheres are round, homogenous eosinophilic bodies that often undergo fragmentation (Fig. 61.5).[18] There may be surrounding infarction.

REFERENCES

1. Chou P, Blei ED, Shen-Schwarz S, et al. Pulmonary changes following extracorporeal membrane oxygenation: autopsy study of 23 cases. *Hum Pathol.* 1993;24:405–412.
2. MacLaren G, Combes A, Bartlett RH. Contemporary extracorporeal membrane oxygenation for adult respiratory failure: life support in the new era. *Intensive Care Med.* 2012;38:210–220.
3. Maslach-Hubbard A, Bratton SL. Extracorporeal membrane oxygenation for pediatric respiratory failure: History, development and current status. *World J Crit Care Med.* 2013;2:29–39.
4. Esper SA, Levy JH, Waters JH, et al. Extracorporeal membrane oxygenation in the adult: a review of anticoagulation monitoring and transfusion. *Anesth Analg.* 2014;118:731–743.
5. Javidfar J, Brodie D, Iribarne A, et al. Extracorporeal membrane oxygenation as a bridge to lung transplantation and recovery. *J Thorac Cardiovasc Surg.* 2012;144:716–721.
6. Davies A, Jones D, Bailey M, et al. Extracorporeal membrane oxygenation for 2009 influenza A(H1N1) acute respiratory distress syndrome: Australia, New Zealand Extracorporeal Membrane Oxygenation Influenza Investigators. *JAMA.* 2009;302:1888–1895.
7. Combes A, Bacchetta M, Brodie D, et al. Extracorporeal membrane oxygenation for respiratory failure in adults. *Curr Opin Crit Care.* 2012;18:99–104.
8. Peek GJ, Mugford M, Tiruvoipati R, et al. Efficacy and economic assessment of conventional ventilatory support versus extracorporeal membrane oxygenation for severe adult respiratory failure (CESAR): a multicentre randomised controlled trial. *Lancet.* 2009;374:1351–1363.
9. Doll N, Kiaii B, Borger M, et al. Five-year results of 219 consecutive patients treated with extracorporeal membrane oxygenation for refractory postoperative cardiogenic shock. *Ann Thorac Surg.* 2004;77:151–157; discussion 157.
10. Magliocca JF, Magee JC, Rowe SA, et al. Extracorporeal support for organ donation after cardiac death effectively expands the donor pool. *J Trauma.* 2005;58:1095–1101; discussion 1101–1102.
11. Gupta P, McDonald R, Chipman CW, et al. 20-year experience of prolonged extracorporeal membrane oxygenation in critically ill children with cardiac or pulmonary failure. *Ann Thorac Surg.* 2012;93:1584–1590.
12. Bond SJ, Lee DJ, Stewart DL, et al. Open lung biopsy in pediatric patients on extracorporeal membrane oxygenation. *J Pediatr Surg.* 1996;31:1376–1378.
13. Sebire NJ, Ramsay AD, Malone M. Histopathological features of open lung biopsies in children treated with extracorporeal membrane oxygenation (ECMO). *Early Hum Dev.* 2005;81:455–460.
14. Mehta RI, Mehta RI, Choi JM, et al. Hydrophilic polymer embolism and associated vasculopathy of the lung: prevalence in a retrospective autopsy study. *Hum Pathol.* 2015;46:191–201.
15. Mehta RI, Mehta RI, Solis OE, et al. Hydrophilic polymer emboli: an under-recognized iatrogenic cause of ischemia and infarct. *Mod Pathol.* 2010;23:921–930.
16. Schipper ME, Stella PR, de Jonge N, et al. Embolization of hydrophilic coating material to small intracardial arteries after multiple percutaneous transluminal angioplasty procedures. *Int J Cardiol.* 2012;155:e45–e46.

17. Baydur A, Koss MN, Sharma OP, et al. Microscopic pulmonary embolisation of an indwelling central venous catheter with granulomatous inflammatory response. *Eur Respir J*. 2005;26:351–353.

18. Murakata LA, Lewin-Smith MR, Specht CS, et al. Characterization of acrylic polyamide plastic embolization particles in vitro and in human tissue sections by light microscopy, infrared microspectroscopy and scanning electron microscopy with energy dispersive X-ray analysis. *Mod Pathol*. 2006;19:922–930.

19. Cantu JA, Safdar Z. Hemoptysis requiring bronchial artery embolization in pulmonary arterial hypertension. *South Med J*. 2010;103:887–891.

20. Corr PD. Bronchial artery embolization for life-threatening hemoptysis using tris-acryl microspheres: short-term result. *Cardiovasc Intervent Radiol*. 2005;28:439–441.

21. Ustunsoz B, Bozlar U, Ors F, et al. Bronchial artery embolization: experience with 10 cases. *Diagn Interv Radiol*. 2006;12:43–46.

22. Siskin GP, Dowling K, Virmani R, et al. Pathologic evaluation of a spherical polyvinyl alcohol embolic agent in a porcine renal model. *J Vasc Interv Radiol*. 2003;14:89–98.

SECTION ELEVEN
VASCULAR LUNG DISEASE

62 Pulmonary Hypertension: Classification and General Histologic Features

Allen P. Burke, M.D., and Joseph J. Maleszewski, M.D.

Definition

Pulmonary hypertension is defined clinically as a mean pulmonary artery pressure of ≥25 mm Hg at rest. The normal mean pulmonary pressure is between 9 and 18 mm Hg, and levels between 18 and 25 are considered borderline and may indicate increased mortality in patients with associated conditions, such as interstitial lung disease. Right heart catheterization is the gold standard for measuring pressures, though echocardiography with Doppler is sometimes used as a surrogate, though the correlations are not particularly good.[1] Pulmonary hypertension is caused by a variety of conditions that originate in the arteries (precapillary), veins (postcapillary), or capillaries.

Classification

The clinical classification of pulmonary hypertension has evolved appreciably over time. Initially, the classification was dichotomous and based on whether or not an identifiable cause for the hypertension was present. The term *primary pulmonary hypertension* was used when no cause for the elevated pressures could be identified, and the term *secondary pulmonary hypertension* was used when a cause was identified. Pulmonary hypertension has been classified according to site of obstruction (precapillary, capillary, or postcapillary).

In 1998, the World Health Organization revamped the clinical classification to better reflect etiology and mechanism.[2] The new classification allows for classification of pulmonary hypertension into five basic groups (Table 62.1). Group 1 (pulmonary arterial hypertension) includes idiopathic pulmonary arterial hypertension, familial pulmonary arterial hypertension, and pulmonary arterial hypertension due to drugs, toxins, connective tissue diseases, infection, portal hypertension, and congenital heart disease. Group 2 (left heart disease) are those cases of pulmonary hypertension owing to underlying structural heart disease (e.g., ischemic heart disease, valvular heart disease, hypertensive heart disease, and cardiomyopathy). Group 3 (lung disease) is pulmonary hypertension caused by lung disease and/or chronic hypoxemia (e.g., chronic obstructive pulmonary disease, interstitial lung disease, obstructive sleep apnea, etc.). Group 4 (thromboembolic disease) is arterial hypertension secondary to chronic thromboembolic occlusion of the pulmonary vessels. Group 5 (multifactorial) is a category reserved for those with unclear mechanisms such as in the setting of metabolic disorders, chronic renal failure, or hemolytic anemia. Pulmonary hypertension in the newborn setting and in pulmonary veno-occlusive disease (PVOD) have been given their own subgrouping (groups 1″ and 1′, respectively).

Although the above classification system is useful and widely used clinically, it is more common for pathologists to group the changes into one that describes the location of the identified histopathologic changes. Recognizing that it is not uncommon to identify changes in the absence of elevated pressures and vice versa, it is important to indicate that identified changes (or lack thereof) should be correlated with pressures for comprehensive interpretation. Precapillary pulmonary hypertension includes those in which arterial changes are identified in the setting of either primary or secondary pulmonary hypertension. Post–capillary-type pulmonary hypertension will include PVOD and pulmonary venous hypertension (owing to left-sided heart disease). Arterial hypertensive changes in the setting of interstitial lung disease occur typically in a background of fibrosis and parenchymal distortion. Thrombotic/embolic changes include those that arise in the setting of thromboembolic disease. Hypertensive changes can also be seen in the setting of sarcoidosis, infection, and other miscellaneous conditions.

Histologic Changes Associated with Precapillary Pulmonary Hypertension

Approach to Histologic Evaluation

Arterial and venous abnormalities are most easily appreciated with the use of elastic stains. Pulmonary arteries travel within the bronchovascular bundles, and are usually near airways. Muscular arteries, unlike veins and systemic arteries, have a distinct internal and external elastic lamina. Elastic arteries are easily distinguished by parallel elastic layers. Pulmonary veins travel within interlobular septa. Bronchial arteries, which supply oxygenated blood to larger airways, originate from the aortic arch and intercostal arteries. Of note, bronchial arteries do not have a distinct external elastic membrane, but rather have a fragmented elastic layer like other systemic arteries. Bronchial arteries are more easily identified in cases of bronchial artery embolization, which is used for patients with intractable hemoptysis (see Chapter 61).

Interpretation and Specificity of Findings

There is a poor correlation between extent of histologic vascular changes and actual arterial pressures measured by catheterization. This discrepancy is likely related to sampling and lack of histologic

TABLE 62.1 World Health Organization Classification of Pulmonary Hypertension[a]

Group	
1	Pulmonary arterial hypertension (idiopathic, heritable, drug/toxin, infection, congenital heart disease, connective tissue disease)
1′	Pulmonary veno-occlusive disease
1″	Persistent pulmonary hypertension of the newborn
2	Left-sided heart disease
3	Interstitial lung disease and chronic hypoxia
4	Pulmonary thromboembolic disease
5	Unclear multifactorial mechanisms (e.g., metabolic, systemic, and hematologic disorders)

[a]Adapted from Simonneau G, Gatzoulis MA, Adatia I, et al. Updated clinical classification of pulmonary hypertension. *J Am Coll Cardiol.* 2013;62(25 suppl):D34–D41.

manifestations of vasoconstriction, which is an important component contributing to increased pulmonary resistance. Therefore, a diagnosis of "pulmonary hypertension" is not appropriate on a surgical pathology report, rather "changes of pulmonary arterial hypertension" with an appropriate comment indicating that necessity of correlation with hemodynamic data. Historical grading systems based on histologic findings (i.e., Heath et al.,[3] which were devised for preoperative evaluation of patients with congenital right-to-left cardiac shunts) are no longer in use.

In general, plexiform lesions are present only in a subset of conditions, including idiopathic pulmonary artery hypertension, familial pulmonary hypertension, and pulmonary arterial hypertension associated with autoimmune connective tissue disorders, congenital right-to-left shunts, portal hypertension, and certain drugs and toxins (e.g., fenfluoramine and monocrotaline). Careful evaluation for such, with a histopathologic diagnosis of "plexogenic pulmonary arteriopathy" can be useful in refining the clinical diagnosis.

The most common condition associated with histologic changes of pulmonary hypertension (other than plexiform lesions) is fibrotic lung disease. Intimal arterial thickening is common in wedge biopsies with interstitial lung disease (over 90%),[4] and patients with idiopathic pulmonary fibrosis demonstrate increased pulmonary arterial pressures in up to one-third of cases.[5]

Muscularization of Arterioles

In general, arterial pulmonary vessels <100 μm in diameter are considered arterioles. They continue to progressively arborize and lose their muscular walls with very little muscle usually identified in vessels <20 μm in diameter. A distinct muscular wall in vessels of this size is abnormal. In infants, vessels even smaller than this can be seen with a muscular wall in cases of abnormal shunts or persistent pulmonary hypertension of the newborn (see Chapter 13).

Muscular Hypertrophy of the Pulmonary Arteries

Muscular (medial) hypertrophy of muscular arteries has been defined as thickening of the muscular arterial wall (distance between the elastic layers) of >10%.[6] The mean medial thickness of normal pulmonary arteries is 5% of the vessel diameter and normally is <8% to 10%. The percentage is calculated from measuring the medial thickness, multiplying by two, and dividing by the external diameter of the vessel. Medial hypertrophy is nonspecific and may be seen in pre- and postcapillary hypertension, interstitial lung disease, and as an incidental

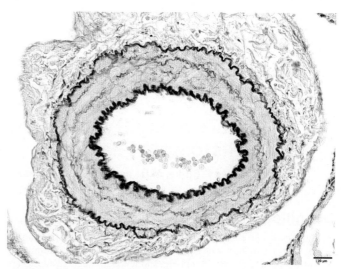

FIGURE 62.1 ▲ Medial hypertrophy (muscular hypertrophy). The artery is markedly thickened due to medial hypertrophy (Verhoeff van-Giesson stain).

finding (usually focally) (Fig. 62.1). It is commonly associated with intimal thickening.

Intimal Thickening, Eccentric

Intimal thickening can be described both by geometry (eccentric vs. concentric), as well as consistency (what forms the intimal tissue). "Eccentric" is defined as noncircumferential intimal thickening (Fig. 62.2); "concentric" refers to circumferential intimal thickening. In general, the eccentric type is generally thought to represent an organized thrombosis. "Cellular" intimal thickening may be eccentric or concentric and is formed mostly of smooth muscle cells, and "acellular" intimal thickening is formed of collagen, may have prominent proteoglycans, and may have depositions (sometimes laminar) of elastic tissue.

Recanalized Thrombus

There is an overlap between eccentric plaque and organized thrombus. If there is recanalization, then there is little doubt as to the thromboembolic etiology of the intimal thickening. The multiple channels in the artery are lined by endothelial cells and have variable amounts of

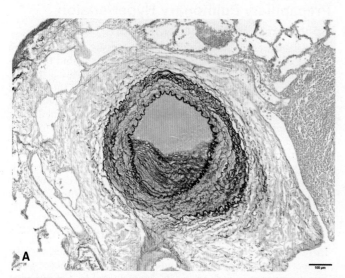

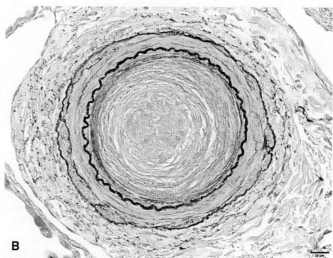

FIGURE 62.2 ▲ Intimal thickening. **A.** Eccentric intimal thickening characterized by a noncircumferential intimal lesion. **B.** Concentric intimal thickening is a circumferential luminal narrowing (Verhoeff van Gieson stains).

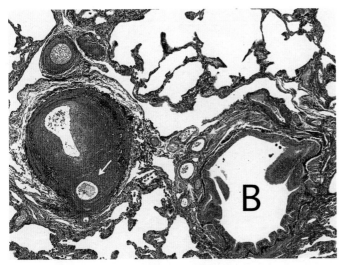

FIGURE 62.3 ▲ Recanalized thrombus, muscular artery. The artery **(left)** is largely occluded by intimal thickening, with one area of neovessel (recanalization) (*white arrow*). The bronchiole is at the right (*B*), and there are associated bronchiolar arterial branches (*yellow arrows*) (Elastic van Gieson).

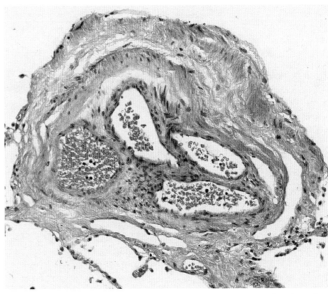

FIGURE 62.5 ▲ Recanalized thrombus. In situ thrombosis of smaller more peripheral pulmonary arteries can result in recanalization.

smooth muscle media. They may be present in elastic arteries, larger proximal muscular arteries (Figs. 62.3 to 62.5), or distal small muscular arteries (Fig. 62.6). As a rule, the more proximal the thrombus, the more likely an embolic etiology. Conversely, the more distal the thrombus, the more likely it arose in situ.

Intimal Thickening, Concentric

Smooth muscle cell–rich intimal thickening is not uncommon in patients with pulmonary arterial hypertension, as well as interstitial lung disease. The lumen may be patent with mild degrees of obstruction (Figs. 62.6 and 62.7) or more severe with near occlusion (Fig. 62.8). Acellular concentric intimal thickening may lead to greater degrees of stenosis and may consist of primarily of collagen (Fig. 62.9) or collagen with proteoglycans (Fig. 62.10) and may show elastosis, typically in cases of plexiform arteriopathy (Fig. 62.11).

Plexiform Lesions

Although rarely reported in other conditions, plexiform lesions are seen in the setting of idiopathic or familial forms of pulmonary hypertension, congenital heart disease, portal hypertension, connective tissue disease, certain infections (e.g., HIV), and drugs/toxins (fenfluramine and denatured rapeseed oil). They are not universally present and may be missed due to sampling if there is limited tissue. Histologically, they occur as medium- to small-sized pre- and intra-acinar muscular arteries with an external diameter of 50 to 400 μm (roughly the size of a glomerulus).[7] They consist of a proliferation of capillary-sized vessels extending outside the artery, sometimes with a connection to the parent vessel imparting and aneurysmal appearance (Fig. 62.12). Distinguishing plexiform lesions from organized/recanalized thrombi can be difficult. The absence of hemosiderin and an aneurysmal outpouching are more characteristic of the former.

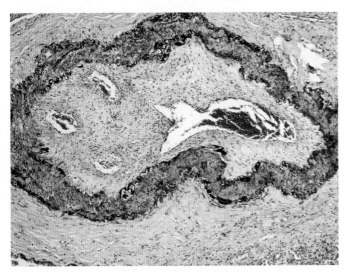

FIGURE 62.4 ▲ Recanalized thrombus. A large muscular artery with some residual elastic layering (transition from elastic artery) shows a recanalized thrombus (Movat pentachrome).

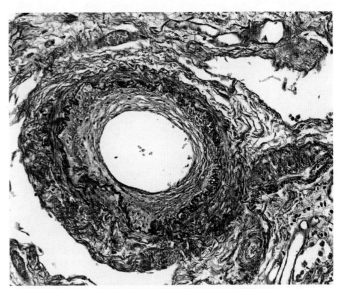

FIGURE 62.6 ▲ Concentric intimal thickening. The artery shows a thin layer of intimal thickening that is concentric. The artery is from an autopsy of a patient dying with scleroderma lung disease.

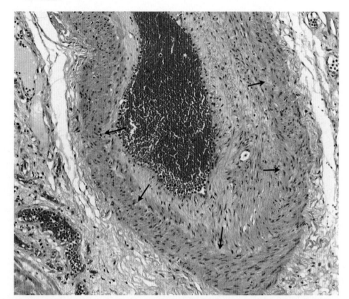

FIGURE 62.7 ▲ Concentric intimal thickening, rich in smooth muscle cells. The neointima can be so rich in smooth muscle cells that it mimics the arterial media. The media–intimal junction is marked by *arrows*.

Arterial Necrosis (Vasculitis)

Necrotizing arteritis can be seen in some cases of pulmonary arterial hypertension, including the plexogenic variety.[8] There is destruction of the media with necrosis and fibrin deposition (Fig. 62.13). These lesions usually occur in association with plexiform lesions and may be causative or represent an early phase of the lesion.

Nonthrombotic Embolism

Microembolism of tumors (so-called tumor thrombotic microangiopathy) may result in progressive pulmonary hypertension and even be the presenting feature of adenocarcinomas of the gastrointestinal tract

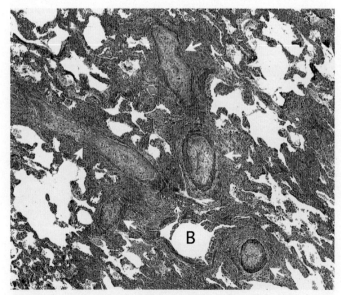

FIGURE 62.8 ▲ Concentric intimal thickening with marked luminal narrowing. The section is from an explanted lung transplanted for Sjögren lung disease. On low magnification, the arteries (*white arrows*) are nearly obliterated. The bronchiole is seen as well (*B*). The patient had signs of pulmonary hypertension as well as interstitial lung disease (nonspecific interstitial pneumonia), and a bilateral lung transplant was necessary because of increased pulmonary arterial pressures (Elastic van Gieson).

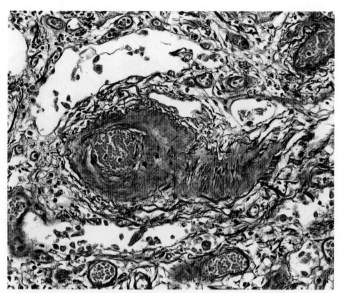

FIGURE 62.9 ▲ Acellular intimal thickening. This small muscular artery shows concentric intimal thickening formed mostly of collagen (Elastic van Gieson). The section is from an autopsy from a patient dying with scleroderma lung disease.

and breast.[9] Histologically, there is diffuse enlargement of muscular pulmonary arteries that are filled with fibrin clot and metastatic tumor microemboli (Fig. 62.14).

Microembolism of foreign material includes self-injected drugs that may contain talc and fillers (such as polyvinylpyrrolidine). There is typically a giant cell reaction with thrombosis (Fig. 62.15).

Histologic Changes Associated with Postcapillary Pulmonary Hypertension

Arterial Changes

All arterial changes present in precapillary causes of pulmonary hypertension may be seen in condition that cause obstruction of pulmonary venous outflow (e.g., heart failure) with the exception of plexiform lesions.

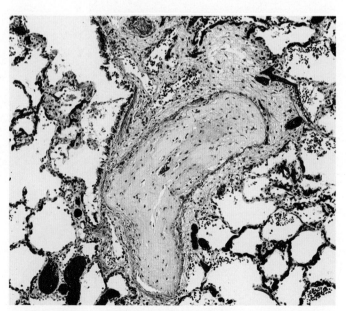

FIGURE 62.10 ▲ Acellular intimal thickening. This small muscular artery is obliterative by proteoglycan-rich collagen with few cells. The section is from an autopsy of a patient dying suddenly with iPAH, plexiform type.

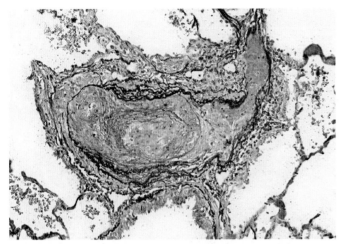

FIGURE 62.11 ▲ Concentric intimal thickening with elastosis. There are indistinct layers of elastic tissue, which is rare as a reactive finding. The section is from an explanted lung from a patient with iPAH, plexiform type.

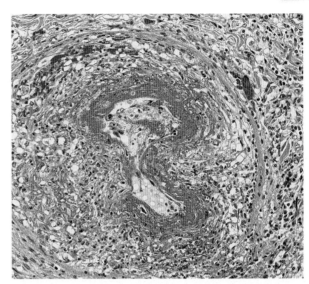

FIGURE 62.13 ▲ Necrotizing arteritis, iPAH. There is circumferential fibrinoid necrosis and adventitial inflammation. Elsewhere there were typical plexiform lesions.

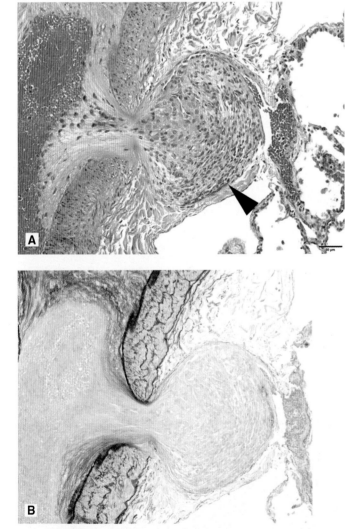

FIGURE 62.12 ▲ Plexiform lesion. There is an interruption of the arterial media with a collection of capillary-sized vessels outside the artery (*arrowhead*). **A.** Hematoxylin–eosin stain. **B.** Verhoeff van Gieson stain.

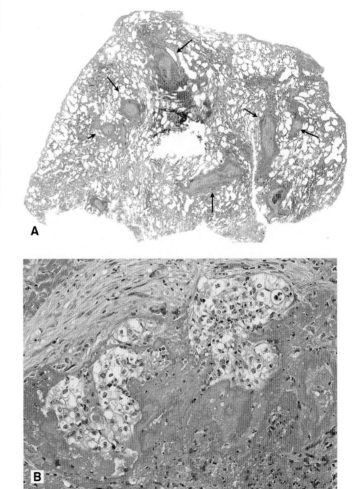

FIGURE 62.14 ▲ Pulmonary tumor microangiopathy, autopsy. **A.** The arteries are diffusely enlarged and occluded (*arrows*). **B.** Higher magnification shows carcinoma within the artery, admixed with thrombus. Clinically, the diagnosis was severe pulmonary hypertensions. The patient had an occult pancreatic primary diagnosed initially at autopsy.

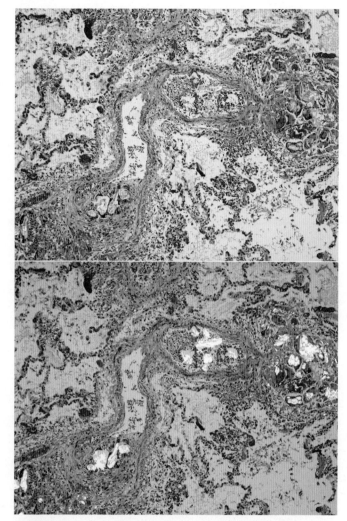

FIGURE 62.15 ▲ Pulmonary talc microembolization. Sections demonstrate intra-arterial accumulations of foreign material and giant cell reaction that are refractile viewed with polarized light **(below)**. The patient was self-injection pain medications through a subcutaneous port and had unexplained pulmonary infiltrates with pulmonary hypertension.

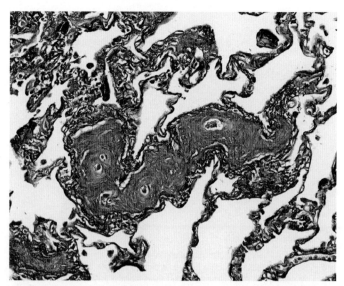

FIGURE 62.17 ▲ Perivenous sclerosis. There is dense collagen surrounding small veins in a branch of an interlobular septum. The patient underwent wedge biopsy and was subsequently found to have significant mitral stenosis.

Septal Edema

Acute elevation of central venous pressure results in edema of the interlobular septa, sometimes with dilatation of the lymphatics (Fig. 62.16A). Changes of chronicity, such as hemosiderin-macrophages (heart failure cells), are frequently seen (Fig. 62.16B).

Venous Sclerosis

Chronic heart failure or mitral valve disease results in scarring of the interlobular septa, with thickening of veins (Fig. 62.17).

Venous Recanalization

Venous recanalization is considered specific for idiopathic pulmonary hypertension (pulmonary veno-occlusive disease). The identification of veins depends on their location in the interlobular septa and not in the bronchovascular bundle.

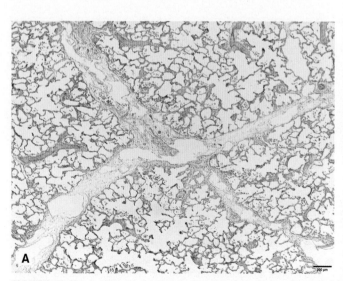

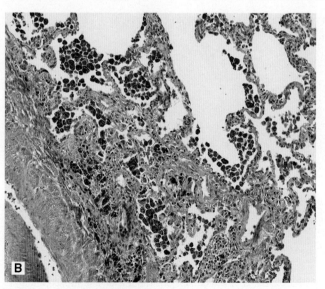

FIGURE 62.16 ▲ Edema, interlobular septum. In acute or chronic left heart failure, there is accumulation of edema fluid, with widening of the interstitium within the interlobular septa, often with lymphatic dilatation (**A**, Verhoeff van Gieson stain). There are typically hemosiderin macrophages resulting from microhemorrhages (**B**).

REFERENCES

1. Fisher MR, Forfia PR, Chamera E, et al. Accuracy of Doppler echocardiography in the hemodynamic assessment of pulmonary hypertension. *Am J Respir Crit Care Med.* 2009;179(7):615–621.
2. Simonneau G, Gatzoulis MA, Adatia I, et al. Updated clinical classification of pulmonary hypertension. *J Am Coll Cardiol.* 2013;62(25 suppl):D34–D41.
3. Heath D, Frederic Helmholz H, Burchell HB, et al. Relation between structural change in the small pulmonary arteries and the immediate reversibility of pulmonary hypertension following closure of ventricular and atrial septal defects. *Circulation.* 1958;18(6):1167–1174.
4. Travis WD, Matsui K, Moss J, et al. Idiopathic nonspecific interstitial pneumonia: prognostic significance of cellular and fibrosing patterns: survival comparison with usual interstitial pneumonia and desquamative interstitial pneumonia. *Am J Surg Pathol.* 2000;24(1):19–33.
5. Lettieri CJ, Nathan SD, Barnett SD, et al. Prevalence and outcomes of pulmonary arterial hypertension in advanced idiopathic pulmonary fibrosis. *Chest.* 2006;129(3):746–752.
6. Edwards WD. Pathology of pulmonary hypertension. *Cardiovasc Clin.* 1988;18(2):321–359.
7. Yi ES, Kim H, Ahn H, et al. Distribution of obstructive intimal lesions and their cellular phenotypes in chronic pulmonary hypertension. A morphometric and immunohistochemical study. *Am J Respir Crit Care Med.* 2000;162(4 Pt 1):1577–1586.
8. Pietra GG. Histopathology of primary pulmonary hypertension. *Chest.* 1994;105(2 suppl):2S–6S.
9. Uruga H, Fujii T, Kurosaki A, et al. Pulmonary tumor thrombotic microangiopathy: a clinical analysis of 30 autopsy cases. *Intern Med.* 2013;52(12):1317–1323.

63 Pulmonary Arterial Hypertension and Pulmonary Venoocclusive Disease

Allen P. Burke, M.D., and Fabio R. Tavora, M.D., Ph.D.

Terminology and Classification

Pulmonary hypertension is classified pathologically by the site of injury into precapillary, capillary, and postcapillary hypertension (Table 63.1). "Pulmonary arterial hypertension" is a term frequently used for precapillary pulmonary hypertension. Rare idiopathic diseases of pulmonary capillaries and veins (capillary hemangiomatosis and pulmonary venoocclusive disease, respectively) are considered subcategories of pulmonary arterial hypertension (PAH) (see Chapter 62), given the clinical overlap, and are therefore considered in this chapter.

Pathogenesis

PAH is frequently idiopathic (idiopathic pulmonary arterial hypertension, or iPAH). A similar clinicopathologic syndrome is seen with chronic increased pulmonary flow, such as in untreated ventricular or atrial septal defects. There are many noncardiac conditions that impart an increased risk for PAH, by mechanisms that are incompletely understood. These include primarily autoimmune connective tissue diseases, liver disease that results in portal hypertension, and drugs and toxins.

The histologic feature that is frequently seen several types PAH is the "plexiform lesion." Although not always present, and often only focal, this lesion is generally absent in secondary pulmonary artery hypertension.

A pathogenetic link across these disorders has been long searched for, in the hopes of developing treatment strategies that are currently ineffective. Processes that have been implicated in the pathogenesis of PAH include vasoconstriction, endothelial dysfunction, smooth muscle cell proliferation, impaired endothelial cell apoptosis, mitochondrial dysfunction, inflammation, angiogenesis, right ventricular cardiomyocyte abnormalities, and metabolic abnormalities.[1]

TABLE 63.1 Causes of Pulmonary Hypertension, Pathologic Classification

Precapillary
Pulmonary arterial hypertension
  Idiopathic
  Associations (autoimmune, liver disease, toxic, etc.)
Embolic
  Recurrent thromboembolism/CTEPH
  Tumor microembolism
Heart disease associated: right to left shunt with reversal (Eisenmenger syndrome)

Postcapillary
Heart disease
  Mitral stenosis
  Mitral insufficiency
  Left heart failure
Idiopathic
  Pulmonary venoocclusive disease
Secondary venous obliteration
Sarcoid involvement of veins

Capillary
Secondary to lung disease and hypoxemia (emphysema, interstitial lung disease, etc.)
Idiopathic (capillary hemangiomatosis)

Clinical Findings

Idiopathic PAH is rare disease, occurring at a rate of about six per million. There is a female/male ratio of 1.7:1 with a mean age at diagnosis of 37 years.[2] By histologic subtype, the mean age was 16 years for primary pulmonary arteritis, and 21 to 34 years for plexogenic pulmonary arteriopathy, primary medial hypertrophy, and pulmonary venoocclusive disease.[3]

Symptoms include shortness of breath and decreased exercise tolerance. Auscultation reveals changes of increased right heart pressures, including systolic clicks and murmurs related to turbulent flow at the pulmonary valve. Increasing right heart failure results in jugular venous distention, pulsatile liver, hepatosplenomegaly, and ascites.

Most cases of PAH are idiopathic. Approximately 10% are familial, and depending on the population studied, 10% to 20% of patients have associations including portal hypertension ("portopulmonary hypertension"), autoimmune connective tissue disorders, and HIV infection.

Radiologic Findings

Chest radiography is abnormal only late in the disease course. The main pulmonary arterial segment is prominent, the central hilar vessels are dilated, and the peripheral vascularity is diminished.

Echocardiography is a good noninvasive tool to measure systolic pulmonary arterial pressure using peak tricuspid regurgitant jet velocity; however, it does not perfectly correlate with the gold standard, right heart catheterization. Mean pulmonary arterial pressures >20 mm Hg are elevated (normal 9 to 18), and values of >40 are considered severe.

Multidetector computed tomography (CT) characterizes both the cardiovascular and parenchymal changes of pulmonary hypertension, which are especially prevalent in PAH associated with connective tissue diseases. An enlarged CT-determined mean pulmonary artery diameter of ≥29 mm has a high sensitivity and specificity for pulmonary hypertension, regardless of cause.[4]

Evaluation of right ventricular function is important for prognosis. By echocardiogram, increased right ventricular volume and decreased ejection fraction are indicative of right heart failure.[4]

Tissue Sampling

The evaluation and diagnosis of pulmonary hypertension is generally made clinically. Wedge biopsy may occasionally be performed in cases of chronic venous hypertension from occult mitral valve disease, because of increased interstitial lung markings (see Chapter 64). PAH is an uncommon indication for lung transplantation, in which case the diagnosis is generally made, and a spectrum of histologic findings found.[5]

Autopsies are sometimes performed on patients with known idiopathic PAH, in which cases the pathologist will encounter the spectrum of vascular changes. The pathologist may initially identify a specific secondary cause, such as tumor microembolization resulting in clinically diagnosed PAH, at autopsy.[6] Rarely, the initial diagnosis is made at forensic autopsy in patients with the initial presentation of sudden cardiac death.[3]

Gross Findings

The primary finding at autopsy or explant in cases of primary pulmonary hypertension is that of dilatation of the proximal pulmonary arteries, including the pulmonary trunk and right and left main arteries. In addition to dilatation, there may be superimposed atherosclerotic change of fibrous plaques, fatty streaks, and calcified plaques.

Microscopic Findings

The pathologic findings of PAH include nonspecific features of intimal thickening, medial hypertrophy, and extension of media into acinar arterioles, all of which may be secondary reaction to localized fibrosis or inflammation of any etiology.[7] There are several grading systems, which are seldom used today, that were initially applied to PAH secondary to cardiac right-to-left shunts (Fig. 63.1). When diffuse, or if accompanied by plexiform lesions, these changes are characteristic of PAH (Figs. 63.2 to 63.4).

Histologic studies focusing on plexiform lesions have shown that the affected arteries in idiopathic PAH are pulmonary (without contribution of bronchial arteries) and most frequently 50 to 100 μm in diameter.[9] Plexiform lesions occur at branch points of axial arteries (so-called supernumerary arteries), interlobular arteries associated with bronchioles, or more distal intra-acinar arterioles (unassociated with airways).[7,10] Arteritis and dilatation lesions are also in the spectrum of PAH with plexiform lesions.[7] Arteritis occurs in about 10% of plexiform arteriopathy and may be the predominant finding (Fig. 63.5).[3,11]

Thrombosis is common, and can be the predominant finding in PAH. When central, thrombi in most patients can be attributed to recurrent thromboembolism (chronic thromboembolic pulmonary hypertension, CTEPH, see Chapter 67). When thrombi are in smaller muscular arteries, usually with recanalization, they are presumed caused by in situ thrombosis. The characteristic lesion of recanalized thrombus in a distal vessel has been described as a "colander lesion."[7] Recanalized thrombi within distal pulmonary arteries <400 μm characterize a form of PAH lacking plexiform lesions termed "primary thrombotic pulmonary hypertension."[3,12] In the WHO classification,

thrombi in distal arteries are included in secondary thromboembolic pulmonary hypertension (Chapter 67).

The frequency of plexiform lesions in pathologic series range from 22% to 73%, depending in part upon inclusion of thromboembolic PAH. Fewer than 10% have primary medial hypertrophy and intimal

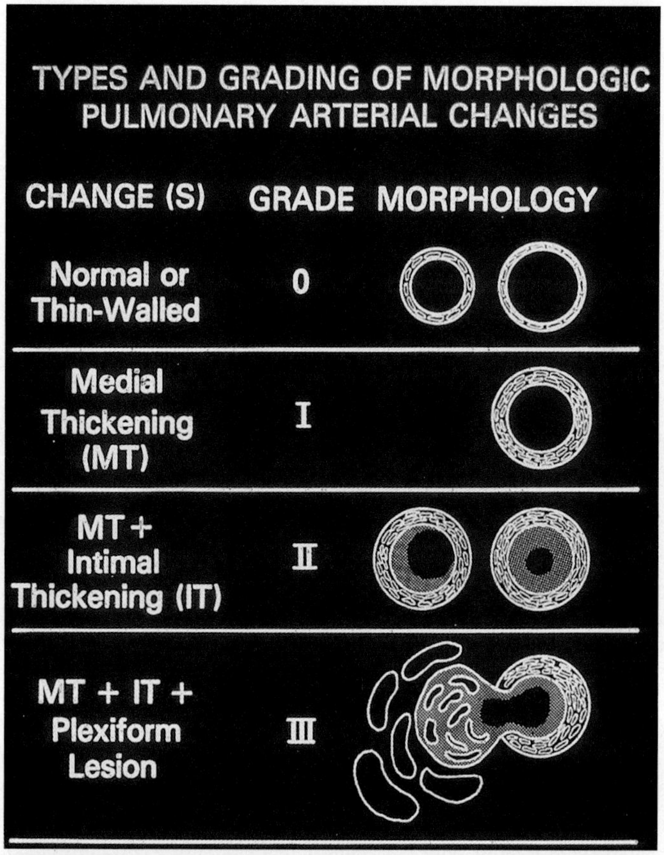

TYPES AND GRADING OF MORPHOLOGIC PULMONARY ARTERIAL CHANGES

CHANGE (S)	GRADE	MORPHOLOGY
Normal or Thin-Walled	0	
Medial Thickening (MT)	I	
MT + Intimal Thickening (IT)	II	
MT + IT + Plexiform Lesion	III	

FIGURE 63.1 ▲ Progression of pulmonary hypertension changes, pulmonary arteries. First, there is medial thickening without intimal proliferation (grade 1), followed by cellular intimal thickening composed of smooth muscle cells (grade 2). Intimal thickening with concentric elastosis (grade 3) usually is accompanied by the formation of plexiform lesions (grade 4) (Reproduced from Frazier AA, Galvin JR, Franks TJ, et al. From the archives of the AFIP: pulmonary vasculature: hypertension and infarction. *Radiographics.* 2000;20:491–524; quiz 530–531, 532., with permission; Ref.[8]).

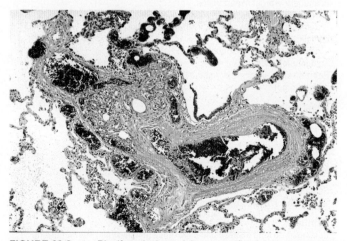

FIGURE 63.2 ▲ Plexiform lesions. A low magnification demonstrates a small muscular artery at a branch point, with a plexiform (sometimes called glomeruloid) lesion emanating from a defect in the muscular wall.

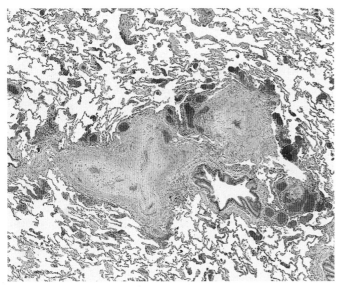

FIGURE 63.3 ▲ Plexiform lesion with diffuse concentric intimal thickening. Adjacent to a plexiform lesion (not shown), diffuse cellular intimal thickening with destruction of the arterial wall is typical of plexiform arteriopathy.

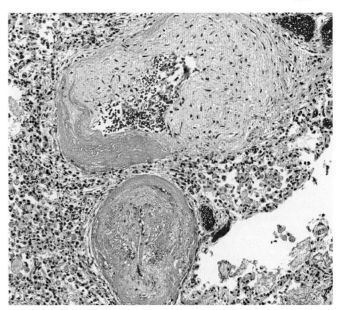

FIGURE 63.5 ▲ Arteritis with fibrinoid necrosis. There is segmental replacement of the arterial wall by fibrinoid material. There were nearby plexiform lesions (not shown).

thickening without plexiform lesions or arteritis.[3,11] Secondary changes of medial hypertrophy and intimal thickening frequently occur in arteries in cases of venous hypertension and venoocclusive disease.[3,11]

Clinical Associations

Among connective tissue disorders, PAH is most commonly associated with systemic sclerosis, usually in women. Between 7% and 26% of patients with scleroderma develop pulmonary hypertension (see Chapter 53). Patients with systemic lupus erythematosus develop PAH with a lower prevalence (0.4% to 14%). PAH develops much less frequently in polymyositis, dermatomyositis, and rheumatoid arthritis, with lower severity and impact. Serum autoantibodies, even in the absence of overt connective tissue diseases, are associated with PAH.[13]

In series of PAH studied pathologically, about 10% of patients have autoimmune rheumatologic disorders without significant fibrotic lung disease. Mixed connective tissue disease is also a relatively common autoimmune disorder seen in patients with PAH.[11] The histologic findings are similar to idiopathic PAH and include thrombotic, intimal thickening, and plexiform histologic patterns.

Because there is frequent interstitial lung disease, patients with connective tissue disease–related PAH tend to show a mild restrictive defect with significantly reduced DLCO (diffusing capacity of the lung for carbon monoxide).

There is long-recognized association between appetite suppressant drugs that increase serotonin release and block serotonin reuptake and PAH. These include aminorex fumarate, fenfluramine, and dexfenfluramine (Fig. 63.6).[2]

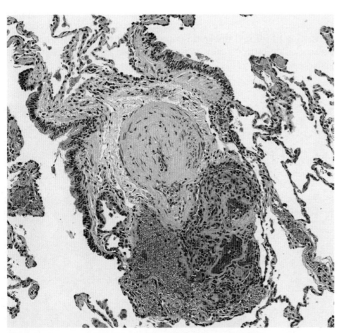

FIGURE 63.4 ▲ Plexiform lesion. The plexiform lesion is often accompanied by dilated capillaries (dilatation lesion).

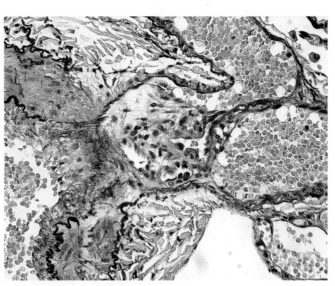

FIGURE 63.6 ▲ Plexiform lesion, elastic stain. The patient died from rapidly progressing pulmonary hypertension after taking phentermine–fenfluramine to lose weight. The junction between the arterial media and the "glomeruloid lesion" to the right is quite abrupt.

Autopsy and clinical studies have shown an association between liver disease, especially cirrhosis and PAH. Hemodynamic studies show a 2% to 6% rate of PAH, with histologic findings of PAH, including plexiform lesions, in 0.73.[2] Slightly over 20% of patients in a pathologic series of PAH had portal hypertension.[11] As with idiopathic PAH and PAH associated with connective tissue disease, a spectrum of pulmonary arterial injury can be shown that correlates poorly with the degree of pulmonary hypertension. Plexogenic arteriopathy, fibrotic intimal thickening, and thrombotic arteriopathy have been described, in diverse types of liver disease include primary biliary cirrhosis, cryptogenic cirrhosis, and cirrhosis caused by alcoholism and viral hepatitis.[5,11]

Although pulmonary hypertension occurs in only 0.5% of patients with HIV, the rate is far higher than the general population. The cause for the link is unknown, and there is no correlation with length of infection or CD4 blood counts.[14] A review from the 1990's showed that 61% of HIV-infected patients with PAH were male; 85% of histologically sampled showed plexiform lesions, and the remaining proximal thrombotic arteriopathy (due to recurrent embolism), distal thrombosis (presumed in situ thrombosis), and venoocclusive disease.[15]

Pulmonary hypertension that develops in patients with ventricular or septal defects that are not operated early is pathologically indistinguishable from primary pulmonary hypertension. Any condition that results in significant right-to-left shunt results in increased pulmonary/systemic flow and predisposes to pulmonary hypertension. Shunts may be classified as pretricuspid (atrial septal defects of any type), simple posttricuspid (ventricular septal defect and patent ductus arteriosus), and complex congenital heart disease. Complex shunts include complete atrioventricular septal defect, truncus arteriosus, transposition of the great arteries with ventricular septal defect, and functional single ventricles with unobstructed blood flow. Shunts begin as systemic-to-pulmonary and, with increased pulmonary vascular resistance, reverse to pulmonary-to-systemic (Eisenmenger syndrome).[16]

Complications

The major pathologic complications of PAH include right ventricular hypertrophy and dilatation and, rarely, pulmonary artery dissection. Hypertrophy of the right ventricle may eventually lead to right-sided chamber dilatation, tricuspid valve incompetency, interventricular septal reversal, and ultimately right ventricular reduced contractility and failure (cor pulmonale) (see Chapter 140).

Genetics

Hereditary transmission of PAH has been reported in ~6% to 10% of patients. In 90% of these individuals, mutations in *BMPR2* have been identified, which have also been found in up to 25% of patients with idiopathic PAH. Another gene in the transforming growth factor beta receptor pathway, activin-like kinase-1, has been implicated in the pathogenesis of familial PAH. These mutations lead to loss of function in the SMAD signaling pathway.[2]

More recently, mutations in the type I receptor *ACVRL1* and the type III receptor *ENG* (both associated with hereditary hemorrhagic telangiectasia), caveolin-1 (*CAV1*), and KCNK3 have been discovered in patients with familial PAH.[17]

Prognosis and Treatment

The most important prognostic indicator in pulmonary hypertension of any cause is the degree of right ventricular failure and remodeling. There is an overall 50% 5-year survival after diagnosis for idiopathic PAH, which is better than that associated with connective tissue disease or HIV.[2]

The primary treatment for PAH is medical therapy with vasodilators phosphodiesterase-5 inhibitors, endothelin receptor antagonists, and prostacyclin analogues.[18]

About 4% of lung and combined heart–lung transplants are for the primary indication of PAH. One-, 3-, 5-, and 10-year survivals have been reported at 66%, 57%, 47%, and 27%, respectively.[19]

Pulmonary Venoocclusive Disease

Pulmonary venoocclusive disease was reported in 1966[20] and later described in detail by Wagenvoort, who considered that the etiology of the venous sclerosis was endothelial injury and venous thrombosis.[21,22] There is no female gender predilection, as with idiopathic PAH and PAH associated with connective tissue disorders. As with idiopathic PAH, symptoms are related to right-sided heart failure. In contrast to PAH, there may be interstitial markings on pulmonary imaging secondary to septal fibrosis.

There are reports of pulmonary venoocclusive disease in patients with immune disorders, including systemic lupus erythematosus, systemic sclerosis, rheumatoid arthritis, Raynaud phenomenon, Hashimoto thyroiditis, and in HIV infection. In a subset of patients, the venous injury is secondary to radiation therapy, chemotherapy, and stem cell transplants.[23]

PVOD is histologically characterized by intimal fibrosis that narrows and occludes the pulmonary veins (Figs. 63.7 and 63.8). Interlobular septa are typically edematous or fibrotic and contain dilated lymphatic spaces. A common problem in diagnosis results from secondary arterial changes, which can include significant intimal and medial thickening, and rarely thrombotic lesions.[11] It has been suggested that the severity of arterial lesions in venoocclusive disease may sometimes blur the distinction between primary arterial and primary venous pulmonary hypertension.[11]

Mutations in eukaryotic initiation factor 2 alpha kinase 4 (*EIF2AK4*) have been linked to both pulmonary venoocclusive disease and pulmonary capillary hemangiomatosis (PCH).[17]

Capillary Hemangiomatosis

PCH was first recognized in 1978 as a form of tumor-like proliferation of pulmonary capillaries.[24] It is quite rare and generally the subject of case reports or small series. PCH has been described in patients with systemic sclerosis, systemic lupus erythematosus, mixed connective tissue disease, and other rheumatologic conditions.[23,25] Computed tomography scans generally demonstrated opacities or centrilobular nodules.

The most distinctive histologic feature of PCH is the proliferation of capillary channels within alveolar walls, with patchy thickening of the alveolar septa. There are frequently secondary arterial changes consisting of intimal thickening and medial hypertrophy. There may be an overlap histologically between PCH and pulmonary venoocclusive disease.[11]

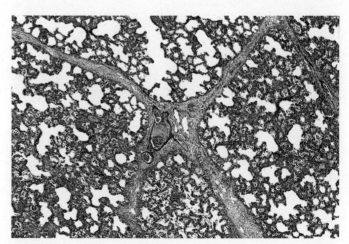

FIGURE 63.7 ▲ Pulmonary venoocclusive disease. There is widening and fibrosis of the interlobular septa.

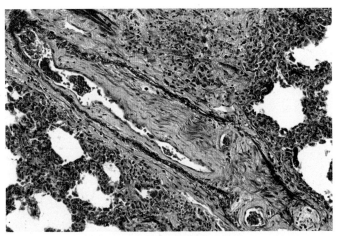

FIGURE 63.8 ▲ Pulmonary venoocclusive disease. There is a recanalized thrombus within the interlobular septum.

REFERENCES

1. Wilkins MR. Pulmonary hypertension: the science behind the disease spectrum. *Eur Respir Rev.* 2012;21:19–26.
2. McLaughlin VV, Archer SL, Badesch DB, et al. ACCF/AHA 2009 expert consensus document on pulmonary hypertension. *J Am Coll Cardiol.* 2009;53: 1573–1619.
3. Bjornsson J, Edwards WD. Primary pulmonary hypertension: a histopathologic study of 80 cases. *Mayo Clin Proc.* 1985;60:16–25.
4. Frazier AA, Burke AP. The imaging of pulmonary hypertension. *Semin Ultrasound CT MR.* 2012;33:535–551.
5. Krowka MJ, Edwards WD. A spectrum of pulmonary vascular pathology in portopulmonary hypertension. *Liver Transpl.* 2000;6:241–242.
6. Lo Priore E, Fusi-Schmidhauser T. When the pathologist is giving the answer: an unusual case of pulmonary hypertension. *Praxis (Bern 1994).* 2014;103: 1081–1083.
7. Pietra GG, Capron F, Stewart S, et al. Pathologic assessment of vasculopathies in pulmonary hypertension. *J Am Coll Cardiol.* 2004;43:25S–32S.
8. Frazier AA, Galvin JR, Franks TJ, et al. From the archives of the AFIP: pulmonary vasculature: hypertension and infarction. *Radiographics.* 2000;20: 491–524; quiz 530–531, 532.
9. Yi ES, Kim H, Ahn H, et al. Distribution of obstructive intimal lesions and their cellular phenotypes in chronic pulmonary hypertension. *Am J Respir Crit Care Med.* 2000;162:1577–1586.
10. Jamison B, Michel R. Different distribution of plexiform lesions in primary and secondary pulmonary hypertension. *Hum Pathol.* 1995;26:987–993.
11. Burke AP, Farb A, Virmani R. The pathology of primary pulmonary hypertension. *Mod Pathol.* 1991;4:269–282.
12. Pietra GG, Edwards WD, Kay JM, et al. Histopathology of primary pulmonary hypertension. A qualitative and quantitative study of pulmonary blood vessels from 58 patients in the National Heart, Lung, and Blood Institute, Primary Pulmonary Hypertension Registry. *Circulation.* 1989;80:1198–1206.
13. Nicolls MR, Taraseviciene-Stewart L, Rai PR, et al. Autoimmunity and pulmonary hypertension: a perspective. *Eur Respir J.* 2005;26:1110–1118.
14. Dai HL, Zhang M, Xiao ZC, et al. Pulmonary arterial hypertension in HIV infection: a concise review. *Heart Lung Circ.* 2014;23:299–302.
15. Mesa RA, Edell ES, Dunn WF, et al. Human immunodeficiency virus infection and pulmonary hypertension: two new cases and a review of 86 reported cases. *Mayo Clin Proc.* 1998;73:37–45.
16. Simonneau G, Robbins IM, Beghetti M, et al. Updated clinical classification of pulmonary hypertension. *J Am Coll Cardiol.* 2009;54:S43–S54.
17. Best DH, Austin ED, Chung WK, et al. Genetics of pulmonary hypertension. *Curr Opin Cardiol.* 2014;29:520–527.
18. Shah SJ. Pulmonary hypertension. *JAMA.* 2012;308:1366–1374.
19. Trulock EP, Edwards LB, Taylor DO, et al. Registry of the International Society for Heart and Lung Transplantation: twenty-third official adult lung and heart–lung transplantation report—2006. *J Heart Lung Transplant.* 2006;25:880–892.
20. Heath D, Segel N, Bishop J. Pulmonary veno-occlusive disease. *Circulation.* 1966;34:242–248.
21. Wagenvoort CA, Wagenvoort N, Takahashi T. Pulmonary veno-occlusive disease: involvement of pulmonary arteries and review of the literature. *Hum Pathol.* 1985;16:1033–1041.
22. Wagenvoort CA, Wagenvoort N. The pathology of pulmonary veno-occlusive disease. *Virchows Arch A Pathol Anat Histol.* 1974;364:69–79.
23. Frazier AA, Franks TJ, Mohammed TL, et al. From the archives of the AFIP: pulmonary veno-occlusive disease and pulmonary capillary hemangiomatosis. *Radiographics.* 2007;27:867–882.
24. Masur Y, Remberger K, Hoefer M. Pulmonary capillary hemangiomatosis as a rare cause of pulmonary hypertension. *Pathol Res Pract.* 1996;192: 290–295; discussion 296–299.
25. Odronic SI, Narula T, Budev M, et al. Pulmonary capillary hemangiomatosis associated with connective tissue disease: a report of 4 cases and review of the literature. *Ann Diagn Pathol.* 2015;19:149–153.

64 Secondary Pulmonary Hypertension

Allen P. Burke, M.D.

General

Pulmonary hypertension secondary to heart and lung diseases is common (Table 64.1) compared to idiopathic and associated pulmonary arterial hypertension, which are relatively rare (Chapter 63). Postcapillary pulmonary hypertension is the result of pulmonary venous hypertension, usually caused by left-sided heart disease. Pulmonary parenchymal diseases, especially chronic obstructive lung disease, are frequent causes of pulmonary hypertension (see Chapter 44) related to hypoxia and destruction of the capillary bed. The most common form of secondary precapillary hypertension is that of recurrent embolism.

Signs and symptoms of secondary pulmonary hypertension are similar to those of primarily pulmonary hypertension but are often less severe. In addition, there are clinical and pathologic features related to the underlying disorder.

In general, plexiform lesions are not considered a feature of secondary pulmonary hypertension. In fact, the reported finding of plexiform lesions in pulmonary hypertension secondary to HIV, schistosomiasis, and sickle cell disease has led to their placement from "secondary" to "associated" pulmonary arterial hypertension, similar to connective tissue diseases and portopulmonary hypertension.[1]

Pulmonary Hypertension Secondary to Heart Disease

Left heart disease probably represents the most frequent cause of pulmonary hypertension.[1] The mechanism involves increased left atrial pressures. In contrast to arterial hypertension, pulmonary, vascular resistance is normal or near normal. Left heart disease that results in pulmonary hypertension includes systolic dysfunction, diastolic dysfunction, and mitral valve disease.

TABLE 64.1 WHO Classification of Secondary Pulmonary Hypertension[1]

General Cause	Specific Cause
Heart disease	Left-sided atrial or ventricular heart disease
	Left-sided valve disease
Lung disease	COPD
	Interstitial lung disease
	Mixed obstructive–restrictive lung disease
	Sleep-disordered breathing
	Alveolar hypoventilation disorders
	Chronic exposure to high altitude
	Developmental disorders
Thrombotic disease	Proximal pulmonary arteries
	Distal pulmonary arteries
	Tumor microembolism
Miscellaneous	Sarcoid
	Langerhans cell histiocytosis
	Compression of lung veins (tumor, lymphadenopathy, sclerosing mediastinitis)

Pathologically, there is edema and fibrosis in the interlobular septa, with thickening of veins (Figs. 64.1 and 64.2). In contrast to pulmonary venoocclusive disease, thrombi are absent in veins. There is typically mild thickening of alveolar walls due to capillary congestion. Intraalveolar edema fluid and scattered hemosiderin macrophages (heart failure cells) are commonly present (Fig. 64.3).

Vascular changes include medial thickening of muscular arteries and eccentric or concentric intimal thickening, which is typically bland and relatively acellular. Concentric rings of elastic tissue and plexiform lesions are not a feature of pulmonary venous hypertension.

Pulmonary Hypertension Related to Lung Disease and/or Hypoxia

The predominant cause of pulmonary hypertension in this category is alveolar hypoxia. This may occur secondary to intrinsic lung disease, especially emphysema and interstitial fibrosis; secondary to impaired control of breathing, as in obstructive sleep apnea; or secondary to residence at high altitude.

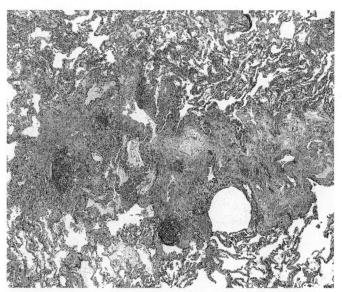

FIGURE 64.2 ▲ Pulmonary venous hypertension, secondary to mitral valve stenosis. In this case, the septal fibrosis is marked.

The degree of pulmonary hypertension with parenchymal lung disease is generally modest, with mean arterial pressures 25 to 35 mm Hg. In patients with chronic obstructive pulmonary disease who underwent right heart catheterization, only 1% had mean arterial pressures over 40 mm Hg.[2] In patients with combined pulmonary fibrosis and emphysema, however, the prevalence of pulmonary hypertension is almost 50%.[3]

There are no reliable histologic changes that predict the degree of pulmonary arterial pressure narrowing in patients with parenchymal lung disease. Nonspecific changes such as intimal thickening and medial hypertrophy are common (Fig. 64.4). As with pulmonary hypertension secondary to heart disease, plexiform lesions, concentric elastosis, and arteritis are absent. In situ thrombosis in distal arteries or proximal thromboemboli are also absent and should raise the possibility of a coagulopathy, such as antiphospholipid syndrome, or thromboembolic disease, respectively.

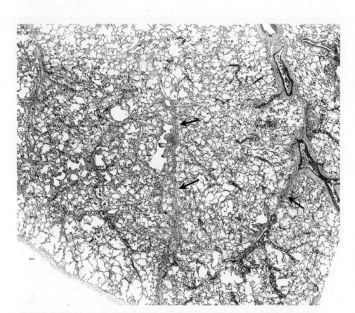

FIGURE 64.1 ▲ Pulmonary venous hypertension, secondary to mitral valve stenosis. Low magnification demonstrates interlobular septal thickening (*arrows*).

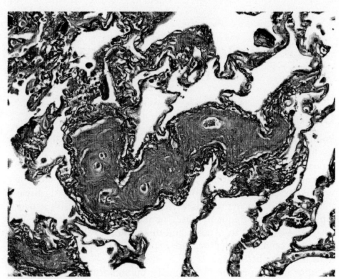

FIGURE 64.3 ▲ Pulmonary venous hypertension, secondary to mitral valve stenosis. Elastic stain demonstrates marked septal fibrosis with sclerotic veins.

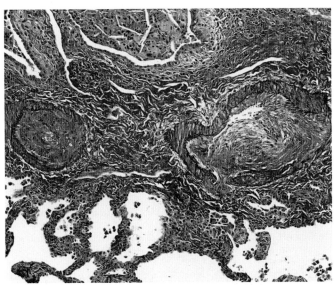

FIGURE 64.4 ▲ Pulmonary arterial thickening, Sjögren syndrome. There is interstitial fibrosis and marked intimal thickening of the arteries (elastic van Gieson). In patients with rheumatologic connective tissue diseases, secondary pulmonary hypertension may occur from fibrosis, as in this case, or be primary, without significant fibrosis and showing the spectrum of histologic changes identical to idiopathic pulmonary arterial hypertension.

Pulmonary hypertension is a recognized complication of sarcoidosis, with a reported prevalence of 1% to 28%.[4,5] Several mechanisms may contribute to the development of pulmonary hypertension, including destruction of the capillary bed, hypoxemia, extrinsic compression of large pulmonary arteries by mediastinal and hilar adenopathy, and granulomatous involvement of veins, mimicking venoocclusive disease, as well as arteries (see Chapter 22)[4,5] (Fig. 64.5).

Pulmonary Langerhans cell histiocytosis (Chapter 24) may cause severe pulmonary hypertension in end stages. Pathologically, there is diffuse pulmonary vasculopathy involving predominantly interlobular pulmonary veins and, to a lesser extent, muscular pulmonary arteries. The changes are nonspecific intimal thickening and muscular hypertrophy present in interstitial lung disease regardless of etiology.[6]

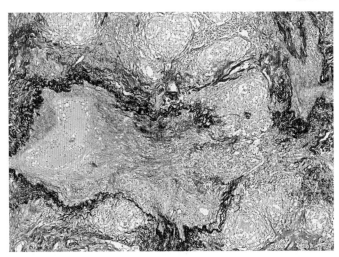

FIGURE 64.5 ▲ Sarcoidosis with vascular involvement. The vein is partly obliterated by granulomas (elastic van Gieson stain). Arteries may also be affected.

Chronic Thromboembolic Pulmonary Hypertension

Chronic thromboembolic pulmonary hypertension (CTEPH) is a frequent cause of pulmonary hypertension and occurs in up to 4% of patients who are diagnosed with acute pulmonary embolus. There is no consensus regarding the division between so-called proximal CTEPH, accessible to pulmonary thromboendarterectomy, and distal CTEPH, which is not accessible to surgery. Thromboembolectomy is the only curative treatment, in which case the pathologist will receive a thrombus that usually shows various stages of organization (Fig. 64.6).

The decision to operate depends on how central the thrombus is, degree of mechanical obstruction assessed by angiography, comorbidities, and the experience of the surgeon in performing a technically challenging procedure. The value of thrombolytic treatment and vasodilator therapy has not been well studied in this group of patients.[1]

Patients with clinically documented CTEPH who have been treated with proximal thromboendarterectomy have been shown pathologically to have the full range of peripheral arterial lesions, including

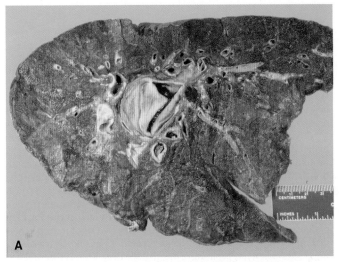

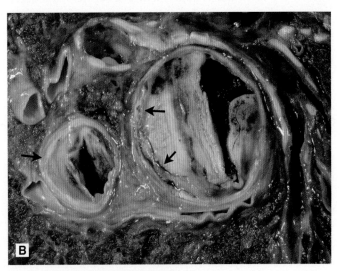

FIGURE 64.6 ▲ Chronic thromboembolic pulmonary hypertension (CTEPH). **A.** Autopsy heart shows layered thrombus in the markedly dilated central main pulmonary artery. The patient did not respond to anticoagulation and was not a surgical candidate. **B.** Higher magnification demonstrates calcified atheromatous plaque (*arrows*), indicative of chronic pulmonary arterial hypertension.

plexiform lesions. Furthermore, plexiform lesions have been demonstrated in some patients, indicating that recurrent embolism may occur in patients with primary pulmonary arteriopathy.[7]

Pulmonary Tumor Thromboembolism, Microscopic Pulmonary Neoplastic Embolism, and Pulmonary Tumor Thrombotic Microangiopathy

Tumors can embolize to the pulmonary circulation in relatively large fragments, even resulting in saddle embolism,[8] or, more commonly, as microscopic microemboli that are surrounded in fibrin thrombi. The latter has been termed "pulmonary tumor thrombotic microangiopathy" and is an unusual cause of pulmonary hypertension. The diagnosis is often missed clinically and made first at autopsy. A variety of tumors may embolize to the lungs, most commonly gastrointestinal adenocarcinomas and breast carcinomas; occasionally, the primary is never identified.[9,10]

Miscellaneous Causes of Pulmonary Hypertension

In areas endemic for the disease, *schistosomiasis* is a relatively common cause of pulmonary hypertension. It was initially believed that the mechanism involved embolic obstruction of pulmonary arteries by *Schistosoma* eggs. Schistosomiasis can have a similar clinical presentation to idiopathic pulmonary hypertension; however, it is associated with portal hypertension and may show plexiform lesions histologically. For these reasons, schistosomiasis is sometimes considered a form of associated pulmonary arterial hypertension, instead of secondary pulmonary hypertension.[1]

The chronic hemolytic anemias, especially sickle cell disease, are also associated with pulmonary arterial hypertension. The incidence of pulmonary hypertension in sickle cell disease ranges from 20% to 63% of patients.[11] A pathologic series showed a high frequency of plexiform lesions.[11] Other histologic findings include medial hypertrophy, fibrotic intimal thickening, and fibroelastotic changes in small arteries and arterioles.

REFERENCES

1. Simonneau G, Robbins IM, Beghetti M, et al. Updated clinical classification of pulmonary hypertension. *J Am Coll Cardiol.* 2009;54:S43–S54.
2. Chaouat A, Bugnet AS, Kadaoui N, et al. Severe pulmonary hypertension and chronic obstructive pulmonary disease. *Am J Respir Crit Care Med.* 2005;172:189–194.
3. Wright JL, Tazelaar HD, Churg A. Fibrosis with emphysema. *Histopathology.* 2011;58:517–524.
4. Shorr AF, Helman DL, Davies DB, et al. Pulmonary hypertension in advanced sarcoidosis: epidemiology and clinical characteristics. *Eur Respir J.* 2005;25:783–788.
5. Nunes H, Humbert M, Capron F, et al. Pulmonary hypertension associated with sarcoidosis: mechanisms, haemodynamics and prognosis. *Thorax.* 2006;61:68–74.
6. Fartoukh M, Humbert M, Capron F, et al. Severe pulmonary hypertension in histiocytosis X. *Am J Respir Crit Care Med.* 2000;161:216–223.
7. Moser KM, Bloor CM. Pulmonary vascular lesions occurring in patients with chronic major vessel thromboembolic pulmonary hypertension. *Chest.* 1993;103:685–692.
8. Wilson MK, Granger EK, Preda VA. Pulmonary hypertension due to isolated metastatic squamous cell carcinoma thromboemboli. *Heart Lung Circ.* 2006;15:143–145.
9. Sancho-Chust JN, Ferreres J, Pineda J, et al. Pulmonary tumor embolism as an initial manifestation of pancreatic adenocarcinoma. *Respir Care.* 2009;54: 1732–1735.
10. Mutlu GM, Factor P. Pulmonary tumor embolism of unknown origin. *Mayo Clin Proc.* 2006;81:721.
11. Haque AK, Gokhale S, Rampy BA, et al. Pulmonary hypertension in sickle cell hemoglobinopathy: a clinicopathologic study of 20 cases. *Hum Pathol.* 2002;33:1037–1043.

65 Pulmonary Embolism and Infarction

Allen P. Burke, M.D., and Joseph J. Maleszewski, M.D.

Thromboembolism

Epidemiology

Precise epidemiologic data for pulmonary embolism (PE) have been difficult to obtain owing to the relatively high incidence of clinically silent disease and variable rates of autopsy. Nevertheless, it is believed responsible for about 1% of hospital admissions, present in up to 30% of hospital-based autopsies, and considered the cause of the death in ~3% to 5% of hospitalized patients.[1] Annual clinical incidence rates estimate that venous thrombosis and PE affect 0.5 to 1.0 per 1,000 individuals in a population.[2] The overall death rate among adults is about 20 per 100,000[3] and has been decreasing.[4]

The rate of PE at autopsy ranges from 15% to 30% and is considered the cause of death in 5% to 12%. The diagnosis is clinically suspected in less than one in five cases, the high incidence possibly due to autopsy selection bias in unexplained sudden death. The rate of PE at autopsy has declined from 20% to 10% over the last several decades.[1,5] The source of emboli includes the lower extremity (70.8%), pelvic veins (4.2%), upper extremity (1.1%), and no source identified (22.6%). The presence of chronic obstructive lung disease has been associated with unidentifiable venous source for pulmonary emboli in a retrospective analysis.[6]

Risk Factors

Venous thrombosis and pulmonary thromboembolism are a spectrum and therefore share many risk factors (Table 65.1). Compared with deep venous thrombosis, PE is more strongly associated with major surgery, trauma, advanced age, myocardial infarction, and chronic heart failure, whereas malignancy and thrombophilia are stronger predictors of deep venous thrombosis.[7]

Over one-third of patients with deep venous thrombosis have a hypercoagulable state, most frequently factor V Leiden (activated protein C resistance, 47%), followed by prothrombin G20210A mutation (25%), multiple abnormalities (10%), protein C deficiency (7%), protein S deficiency (6%), and antithrombin III deficiency (5%).[8] In contrast, the risk of PE is only increased in patients with antithrombin deficiency or with prothrombin abnormality. The lack of risk for PE in patients with factor V Leiden despite the increased risk for deep venous thrombosis (so-called factor V Leiden paradox) has no clear explanation,[9] although it has been suggested that the deep venous thrombi with factor V Leiden are more distal and less likely to embolize.[10]

Less than 1% of surgical patients develop PE, with a higher rate after surgery for trauma and those who do not receive appropriate

TABLE 65.1 Major Causes and Risk Factors for the Development of Pulmonary Embolism

Age	>60
Cardiac conditions	Atrial fibrillation
	Heart failure
Cigarette smoking	
Drugs	Estrogen receptor modulators
	Heparin-induced thrombocytopenia and thrombosis
	Exogenous estrogens
Trauma	Especially extremity or pelvic trauma
Hypercoagulability disorders	Antiphospholipid antibody syndrome
	Antithrombin III deficiency
	Factor V Leiden[a]
	Hereditary fibrinolytic defects
	Hyperhomocysteinemia
	Increase in factor VIII
	Increase in factor XI
	Increase in von Willebrand factor
	Paroxysmal nocturnal hemoglobinuria
	Protein C and S deficiencies
Immobilization	
Indwelling venous catheters	
Malignancy	
Myeloproliferative disease	
Nephrotic syndrome	
Obesity	
Pregnancy and postpartum	
Exacerbation of COPD	
Prior venous thromboembolism	
Sickle cell anemia	
Surgery within past 3 months	

[a]Factor V Leiden increases the risk of deep venous thrombosis but not pulmonary embolism per se, by reasons that are unclear.

prophylaxis.[11] The risk for pulmonary embolism typically peaks 2 to 3 weeks after trauma or surgery but may occur the first day. In 25% of patients, there are no known risk factors.

Among subjects with a malignant neoplasm, patients with pancreatic and gastric cancer, cancer of the large bowel, and women with ovarian cancers had the highest frequency of PE.[12-14] One percent to five percent of cancer patients have unsuspected PE.[15] Atrial fibrillation can be both a predisposing cause as well as an effect of chronic thromboembolic disease, and decreases overall survival.[16]

Systemic lupus erythematosus is associated with an increased risk of both PE and deep venous thrombosis, 13 to 20 times higher than the general population.[17] Exacerbation of chronic obstructive lung disease is associated with an increased risk of PE.[18]

Clinical Findings

Clinically, PE is typically characterized by dyspnea and/or tachypnea. Cough and chest pain are also very common, though also nonspecific. Pleuritic chest pain is seen more commonly in those who have peripheral infarction with irritation of the visceral pleura. Lower extremity swelling can be an indicator of deep venous thrombosis. Fainting, syncope, and hemoptysis are also sometimes seen.[19]

Approximately 25% of patients dying suddenly have visited an emergency facility shortly prior to death, usually for dyspnea or chest pain, without a diagnosis.[20] In an additional one-third of patients dying suddenly, sudden death is the initial manifestation.[20]

Diagnosis

The clinical diagnosis of PE is based on a combination of symptoms, D-dimer levels, lower extremity ultrasound, lung ventilation perfusion scan, and computer tomographic pulmonary angiography.[21,22] D-dimer is a sensitive but not specific test and can be seen in other cardiovascular conditions such as aortic dissection.[23]

Most cases of fatal PE diagnosed at autopsy are diagnosed premortem. PE remains the most important cause of missed clinical diagnoses and major discrepancies between ante- and postmortem assessments.[24-26]

Pathology

From pathologists' perspective, acute pulmonary thromboemboli are most frequently seen in the setting of autopsy. Chronic thromboemboli can be seen either in autopsy or occasionally for thromboendarterectomy. At autopsy, the evaluation of the pulmonary vascular tree should extend from the pulmonary trunk and main pulmonary arteries to lobar and segmental arteries. Features for the autopsy pathologist to consider are the point of origin, final localization, size and age of thromboemboli, the presence or absence of pulmonary infarction, and the underlying cardiac or other conditions. Although saddle emboli are invariably fatal, pulmonary emboli in cases of sudden death may be segmental, only involving lobar arteries.

Grossly, a recent thromboembolus is usually cylindrical and takes the form of the originating vessel (usually a deep vein) and not the pulmonary artery (Figs. 65.1 and 65.2). There is a wide variety of patterns of pulmonary embolism, but there is a predisposition to the right lung and lower lobes, and multiple emboli are the rule.

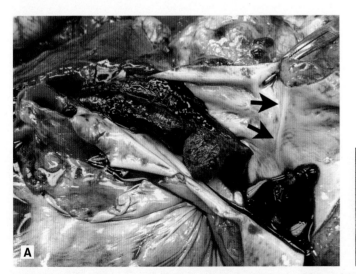
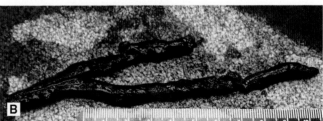

FIGURE 65.1 ▲ Pulmonary embolism, gross. **A.** There is occlusion of the right and left pulmonary arteries at the junction of the pulmonary trunk. The *arrows* point to the flow divider. **B.** The extracted thrombus is branched, indicating origin from venous bifurcation in the legs.

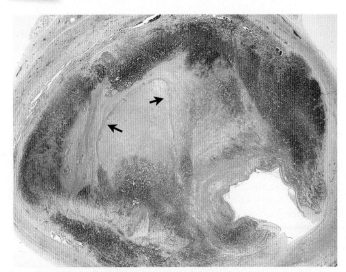

FIGURE 65.2 ▲ Pulmonary embolism. The thrombus appears adherent to the arterial wall. There are lines of Zahn (*arrows*). The entrapped blood (*dark red areas*) and fibrin (*pinker areas*) are somewhat layered out.

TABLE 65.2 Estimated Times of Histologic Findings on Pulmonary Embolism

Time Course	Finding (in Approximate Order of Occurrence)
0–3 days	Lines of Zahn (immediate)
2–7 days	Neutrophil pyknosis
	Macrophage swelling
	Beginning of endothelial overgrowth at edges
	Adherence to vessel wall
	Adventitial hemorrhage
5–14 days	Hemosiderin macrophages
	Surface endothelialization
	Degeneration of white cells
	Degeneration and homogenization of fibrin strands with hyalinization of thrombus
	Fibroblast ingrowth
2–5 weeks	Collagenization with granulation tissue (abundant capillaries) at periphery of thrombus at junction of thrombus with vessel
2–4 months	Increased collagenization, organization throughout the thrombus, with residual fibrin cavities in larger thrombi
5+ months	Disappearance of fibrin, recanalization complete with variable elastic and mature smooth muscle cells

Thromboemboli encountered at autopsy are usually blunt with a smooth surface. Occasionally, impressions from the venous valves can be identified. Unlike postmortem clots, they protrude from the surface of the cut lung and are impacted in the distended artery. Lines of Zahn, a manifestation of blood flow, can be seen grossly and microscopically and confirm the antemortem nature. There is usually attachment to the vascular wall, but care should be taken while grossing the specimen not to dislodge the embolus while removing and dissecting the lung. If possible, sections of the thromboembolus with the attachment to the vessel should be submitted to histology. Obstruction of medium to large arteries may cause pulmonary infarction, which should also be noted and submitted to histology.

Microscopically, the intima contains collagen in all cases, with elastin in two-thirds, hemosiderin in one-half, and atherosclerosis in one-third.[27] Unusual histologic findings in patients with pulmonary thromboendarterectomy include pulmonary artery sarcoma metastatic tumor embolism and isolated pulmonary arteritis.[28]

The pathologist may be asked to estimate the age of the thromboembolic event in autopsy material, which may have clinical and legal implications. The task is especially important in the forensic field. Specific dating of the embolus is, however, impossible based on histologic grounds alone, and in selected cases, an estimate may only be attempted. Early histologic changes include endothelial activation of intima, ingrowth of myofibroblasts, formation of clefts lined by endothelial cells, centripetal ingrowth of capillaries and fibroblasts, deposition of reticulin, and endothelialization of the surface of the clot, while later events are characterized by hemosiderin and collagen deposition and recanalization. Table 65.2 outlines general time lengths on the appearance of histologic findings. Emboli in different vessels can demonstrate various ages, indicating that the patient was sending emboli for some time prior to death. Figures 65.2 to 65.7 show progressive phases of organization, from acute thrombus to organizing and eventually recanalized thrombi.

Septic emboli differ from sterile thromboemboli by the presence of numerous neutrophils and typically the presence of intracellular bacteria, usually within neutrophils and macrophages (Fig. 65.8). The major risk factors for septic pulmonary emboli are intravenous drug use, intravascular indwelling catheter, and purulent skin or soft tissue purulent infection, especially with *Staphylococcus*. In addition to bacteria, septic emboli may also be due to *Candida*, especially in intravenous drug addicts.[29]

Treatment

The treatment of PE relies on removal or lysis of the embolus. In massive PE, defined as a hemodynamically unstable event, thrombolysis is the recommended therapy.[30,31] Embolectomy can also be attempted.[32] In low-risk PE or deep venous thrombosis, subcutaneous low molecular weight heparin or oral anticoagulations may be used.[2,33]

Thromboendarterectomy is performed to treat chronic thromboembolic pulmonary hypertension (see Chapter 67). The procedure differs somewhat from acute embolectomy, in that adherent thrombus must be separated from the media.

Other Embolic Phenomena

Tumor Embolism

Pulmonary tumor emboli occur in two distinct ways, as large emboli, which are usually proximal and may present clinically as acute pulmonary embolism, and secondly as small emboli into the microvasculature that can cause increased pulmonary arterial pressure. While considered an uncommon event in surgical pathology practices, one autopsy study has found pulmonary tumor emboli in more than one-fourth of patients dying from cancer.[34] The diagnosis is often missed premortem.[35] Tumors that are likely to embolize to the proximal pulmonary

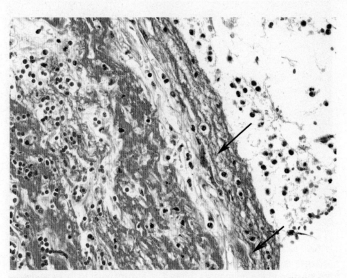

FIGURE 65.3 ▲ Pulmonary embolism, early organization. There is an ingrowth of stromal cells (*arrows*) under the surface fibrin.

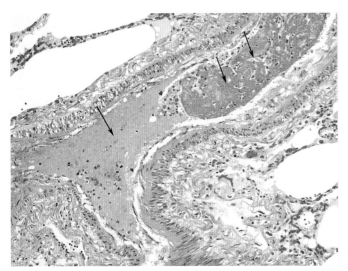

FIGURE 65.4 ▲ Distal pulmonary embolism. There are often emboli in branch vessels in cases of multiple emboli, but they are uncommon in sudden massive saddle emboli. There is a fibrin thrombus with early organization (**top right**, *double arrows*), with postmortem clot in the remaining portion of the artery (*single arrow*).

tree include hepatocellular carcinoma and renal cell carcinoma, but a variety of others have been reported.[13,36–39] Occasionally, intravascular lymphomas can "embolize" and obstruct the pulmonary circulation.[40]

Fat and Tissue Embolism

Bone marrow embolism is common after resuscitation or blunt-force injury and manifests as intact fragments of fat with marrow in distal muscular arteries (Fig. 65.9). Fat embolism is less common and is seen after orthopedic surgery, massive trauma, bone marrow transplant, and liposuction and in patients with pancreatitis or hemoglobinopathies.[41–43] Histologically, there are fat globules distending small arteries and arterioles, extending even into capillaries (Fig. 65.10). A diagnosis can be confirmed by performing fat stains on fixed tissue, mounted for frozen section without processing.

Other sources are liver tissue following trauma and herniated nucleus pulposus.[44–46] There is one report of brain tissue embolizing and "growing" in the pulmonary vasculature in a baby with perinatal brain injury.[47]

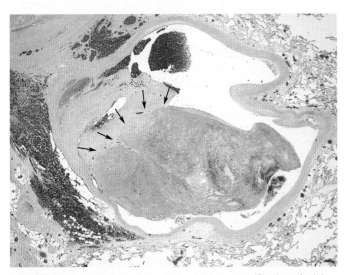

FIGURE 65.5 ▲ Pulmonary embolism. A low magnification of a lobar pulmonary artery shows a subocclusive thrombus. The base of the thrombus **(left)** is old, formed of fibrous tissue; the tip of the thrombus is more recent, composed mostly of fibrin. The junction of the older area and more recent growth of the thrombus is indicated by *arrows*.

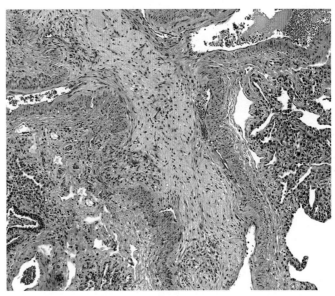

FIGURE 65.6 ▲ Pulmonary embolism, organized. There is no residual fibrin. There is an ingrowth of granulation tissue. Recanalization has not yet occurred.

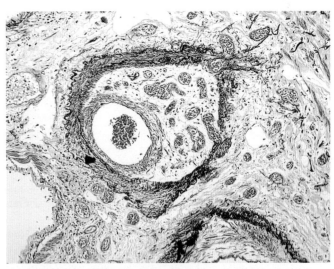

FIGURE 65.7 ▲ Recanalized thrombus. An elastic stain demonstrates a well-formed neomedial layer.

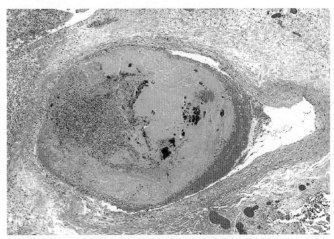

FIGURE 65.8 ▲ Septic embolus. The thrombus contains a mass of neutrophils at the left, and clusters of bacteria are visible toward the right.

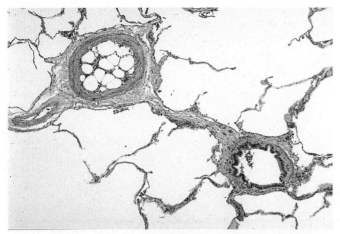

FIGURE 65.9 ▲ Bone marrow embolus. This is a common incidental finding at autopsy if there is resuscitation involving breakage of the ribs. Note the artery **(left)** and accompanying bronchiole **(right)**.

Amniotic Fluid Embolism

Amniotic fluid embolism usually occurs during late pregnancy, often during labor or shortly after, with more than 80% mortality. Approximately 5% of sudden deaths in the peripartum period are due to amniotic fluid embolism.[48] The introduction of amniotic fluid and debris into the pulmonary circulation results in severe hemodynamic disturbance, consisting of transient pulmonary hypertension, profound hypoxia, and left ventricular failure, followed by secondary coagulopathy.[49] Grossly, there are no changes; histologically, there is squamous debris in the peripheral lung arteries.

Embolization of Foreign Material

Embolization of foreign material, including talc, may be seen in peripheral segments in the pulmonary arteries and capillaries of intravenous drug users.[50] Birefringent material is most often seen in lung tissue (94%), followed by the spleen (76%), liver (55%), portal lymph nodes (39%), and bone marrow (24%). There may be a granulomatous reaction in the lungs, and chronic pulmonary hypertension may ensue.

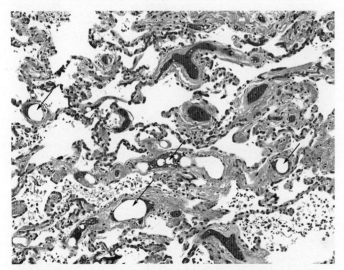

FIGURE 65.10 ▲ Fat embolus. In contrast to bone marrow embolus, fat embolism results in diffuse massive peripheral arterial embolization and sudden death. A high magnification demonstrates globules of fat within an alveolar septal capillary (*arrows*). Often the capillaries are distended with empty vacuoles. Oil red O staining on fixed frozen sections are helpful in confirming the diagnosis (not shown).

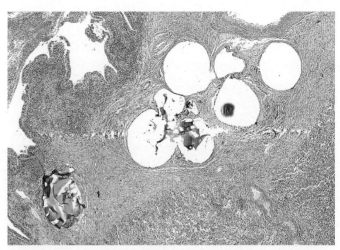

FIGURE 65.11 ▲ Intravascular microbeads, remote therapeutic embolization. The specimen was an explant of a patient with pulmonary arterial hypertension who had been treated with bronchial artery embolization for recurrent hemoptysis.

Therapeutic embolism of beads is performed in cases of intractable hemoptysis, injected into branches of the bronchial arteries via the aorta. The spherical bodies will be seen in bronchial arteries (see Chapter 64) (Fig. 65.11). Hydrophilic polymer embolism may occur as a complication of material that coat catheter sheaths.

Pulmonary Infarction

Pathophysiology

Infarction occurs less commonly in the lung after arterial occlusion than in other organs, such as the heart, kidney, or spleen, largely owing to the dual arterial supply of the lung. Pulmonary and bronchial circulations are connected to one another by several microvascular anastomoses.[51] Bronchial blood flow increases by as much as three times normal in patients with chronic thromboembolic pulmonary hypertension, lessening the risk of infarcts even in these patients.[52]

Following ischemia, first there is damage to the endothelial cells and pneumocytes, resulting in intra-alveolar hemorrhage. Increased vascular permeability leads to extravasation of blood from the bronchial circulation. If the interruption to pulmonary blood flow is permanent and the bronchial supply inadequate, coagulative necrosis and "red" infarction ensue.

Peripheral, rather than central, pulmonary embolism is more likely to result in infarction because the bronchial arteries play a less prominent role in supplying oxygen to the smaller airways. However, computed tomographic angiography has shown that central embolism is also more likely to be present in lungs with infarcts compared to those without, possibly due to the greater overall thrombotic burden in these patients.[53]

Clinical Findings

Clinical findings of lung infarction are similar to those of pulmonary embolism, namely shortness of breath, tachycardia, hypoxia, chest pain, and possibly lower extremity swelling or pain (in a setting of deep vein thrombosis). Among patients with acute pulmonary emboli, pleuritic chest pain is present significantly more frequently in patients with infarction than in those without.[54]

Pulmonary infarcts can undergo cavitation and transform into abscesses, especially if there is acute respiratory distress syndrome.[55,56] Rarely, infarcts can rupture, causing hemothorax.[57] Overall, however, pulmonary embolism–related deaths are not more frequent if there is an infarct, compared to those without infarction, indicating that pulmonary infarction is not a prognostic indicator of recurrence and mortality after pulmonary embolism.[53]

Chronic pulmonary infarcts may be asymptomatic and be detected radiographically as a mass lesion simulating tumor.[58] Peripheral infarcts in patients with lung cancers can simulate metastatic disease, because the surrounding inflammation may result in false-positive positron emission tomographic scans.[59,60]

Radiologic Findings

On chest radiography, pulmonary infarcts appear as a peripheral wedge-shaped opacity (so-called Hampton hump). Small reversible infarcts cause a transient roentgen shadow that resolves in 2 to 4 days, corresponding to resorption of intra-alveolar blood. Irreversible ischemia causes a peripheral scar.[54]

The computed tomographic findings of pulmonary infarction include an area of decreased parenchymal enhancement with a broad pleural base and truncated apex. Features that help distinguish infarcts from pleural-based tumors, scars, or granulomas include central lucencies, a thick vessel leading to the apex of the lesions, and, to a lesser degree, triangular shape.[54,61] Central cavitation caused by infection can confuse the radiologic diagnosis.[55] Computed tomographic angiography typically demonstrates an obstructed artery corresponding to the thromboembolus leading to the infarct.[62]

Pulmonary Infarction Due to Arterial Occlusion

The overwhelming majority of pulmonary infarcts are caused by pulmonary arterial thromboembolism from the peripheral venous circulation. At autopsy, between 10% and 30% of patients with pulmonary embolism have pulmonary infarction.[63] A variety of other conditions can also result in obstruction of pulmonary arteries with infarction (Table 65.3).

There are several risk factors predisposing to infarction in patients with pulmonary embolism (Table 65.4). The most common is heart failure, which increases pulmonary venous pressures and the likelihood of endothelial damage after arterial occlusion. Any condition that impairs bronchial flow, such as lung transplantation, also increases the risk of infarction.[64] The main conditions predisposing to pulmonary infarction are premortem functional status, emboli in more than one lobe, left ventricular failure, and the presence of malignancy including lung cancer.[54,65] In patients with systemic lupus erythematosus, antiphospholipid syndrome increases the risk of infarct after pulmonary embolism.[66]

Tumors may cause pulmonary infarcts by direct vascular invasion, embolism, or direct extension into pulmonary arteries.[60,67] Tumors that directly extend into the pulmonary arterial circulation include those that grow through the vena cava and right heart (e.g., hepatocellular, adrenal cortical, and renal carcinoma), and pulmonary artery intimal sarcomas.[68,69] In leukemic patients, infarcts may occur following leukostasis due to high leukocyte counts, or may be secondary to vascular thrombi.[70]

TABLE 65.3 Causes of Pulmonary Infarcts

Arterial
Thromboembolism
Tumor occlusion
   Tumor embolus
   Tumor extension into pulmonary artery
   Bronchogenic carcinoma with vascular invasion
   Pulmonary artery sarcoma
Invasive fungal infection
In situ thrombosis (hemoglobinopathies, vasculitis, disseminated intravascular coagulation)
Postthoracic surgery
Nonthrombotic embolization
   Devices (e.g., superior vena cava stent)
   Bullets
   Air embolism
High altitude disease

Venous
Postsurgical pulmonary vein obstruction (e.g., transplant)
Left atrial ablation for atrial fibrillation
Tumor obstruction
   Metastatic
   Left atrial myxoma
   Bronchogenic carcinoma

TABLE 65.4 Factors Increasing the Risk for Pulmonary Infarct in Patients with Thromboembolism

- Heart failure
- Malignancy, especially lung cancer
- High embolic burden
- Diminished bronchial flow (shock, hypotension, post lung transplant)
- Vasodilators
- Increased pulmonary venous pressure (other than heart failure)
- Hepatopulmonary syndrome
- Antiphospholipid syndrome

In situ thrombosis and pulmonary infarcts have been described in hematologic conditions such as disseminated intravascular coagulation[71] and hemoglobinopathies, including β-thalassemia[72] and sickle cell disease.[73] Patients with sickle cell disease also have an increased risk for peripheral thrombosis and pulmonary thromboembolism.[74]

Invasive fungal infection, especially aspergillosis, can occlude pulmonary vessels with resulting infarcts.[75,76] Primary arteritis, such as Takayasu disease, Churg-Strauss syndrome (allergic granulomatosis with polyangiitis), and giant cell arteritis, may also predispose to infarction.[77-79]

Pulmonary infarction can be the result of thoracic surgery, with a high morbidity. The cause is often obscure.[80] After transplant surgery, prolonged ischemic time can cause infarction of one or more lung segments. In ~10% of autopsies on patients dying with high altitude sickness, pulmonary infarcts are seen in association with small artery thrombi.[81] Foreign materials may lodge into pulmonary arteries causing pulmonary infarction, including vena cava filters,[82] venous catheter tips,[83] bullets,[84] and embolized air.[85]

Pulmonary Infarction Due to Venous Occlusion

Venous infarction results from severe venous outflow obstruction, usually at the level of the pulmonary veins. Marked congestion results in segmental hypoxia and necrosis, with hemorrhagic infarct (Figs. 65.12 and 65.13). A relatively common cause is obstruction at the pulmonary venous anastomoses following lung transplantation, which removes the bronchial circulation. Postoperative venous infarct is a devastating complication that becomes manifest at 4 to 6 hours and leads to irreversible lung damage requiring retransplantation or resection of the infarcted transplanted lung.[86]

Venous infarction may also occur after left atrial ablation for atrial fibrillation, which typically involves the ostia of the pulmonary veins and may result in delayed obstruction. The radiologic appearance may resemble consolidation. Treatment includes anticoagulation and pulmonary vein angioplasty.[87-89]

Tumors may result in venous infarcts, by occlusion of one or more pulmonary veins. Metastatic sarcoma,[90] left atrial myxomas,[91] and primarily lung tumors have resulted in pulmonary venous infarcts.[92] Rarely, atrial sarcomas may grow into pulmonary veins, resulting in hemorrhagic segmental infarcts (Figs. 65.12 and 65.13).

Pathology

Grossly, a recent lung infarct is a pleural-based, well-demarcated hemorrhagic area (so called red infarcts). Septic emboli are associated with cavitation of an infarct, which may simulate or produce a lung abscess. Older infarcts are more pale, with a rim of hyperemia (Figs. 65.14 and 65.15).

Histologically, the earliest phase of infarction is a localized acute lung injury, manifest by interstitial inflammation, intra-alveolar fibrin, and hemorrhage, without tissue necrosis (Fig. 65.15). The junction with uninvolved lung demonstrates inflammation and granulation tissue (Fig. 65.16). Tissue necrosis ensues if there is inadequate collateral circulation and manifests as coagulative necrosis of the alveolar walls, bronchi, and vessels (Fig. 65.17). Elastic fibers tend to remain intact giving a false impression of elastosis. There is reactive pleuritis of the overlying pleura. There may be evidence of recanalized thrombi in medium-sized arteries adjacent to the infarct (Fig. 65.18). Secondary

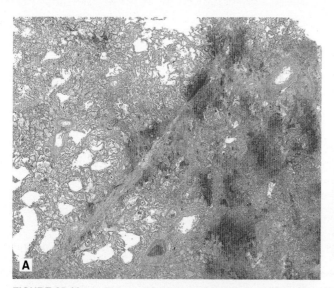
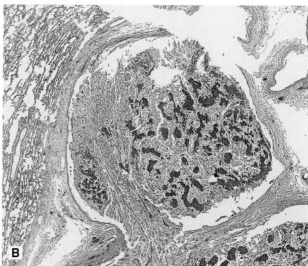

FIGURE 65.12 ▲ Venous infarct secondary to tumor obstruction of left pulmonary veins. **A.** At low magnification, there is patchy hemorrhage and interlobular septal congestion. **B.** The infarct was caused by extension of a left atrial osteosarcoma into the pulmonary vein branches.

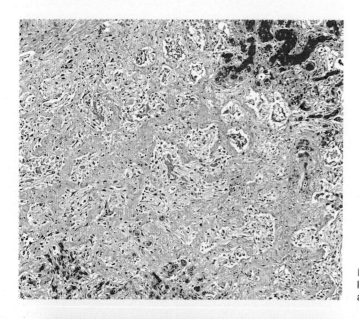

FIGURE 65.13 ▲ Venous infarct secondary to tumor obstruction of left pulmonary veins. In areas, there was chronic infarction with necrotic alveolar septa and fibrosis in the alveolar septa.

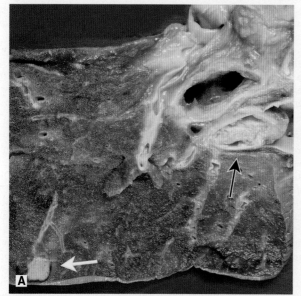
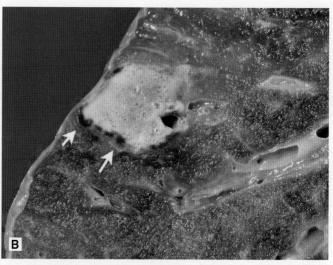

FIGURE 65.14 ▲ Remote pulmonary infarct. **A.** Low magnification demonstrating central thromboembolus (*black arrow*) and peripheral infarct (*white arrow*). **B.** A higher magnification of the infarct at a different level demonstrating the hyperemic border (*arrows*).

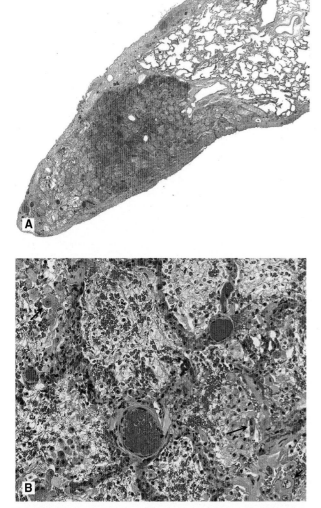

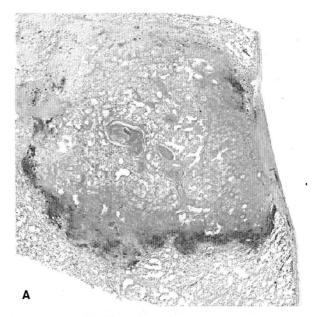

A

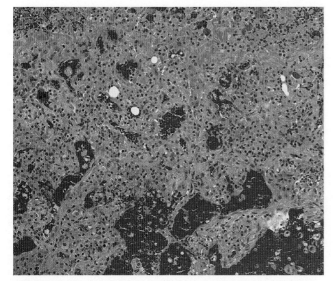

FIGURE 65.15 ▲ Acute pulmonary infarct. **A.** There is a zone of hemorrhage at low magnification. **B.** There is intra-alveolar fibrin and alveolar septal inflammation. There are scattered reactive pneumocytes (*arrows*).

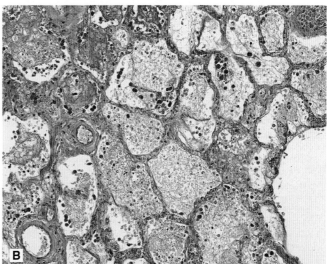

FIGURE 65.17 ▲ Organizing infarct. **A.** Low magnification demonstrates a pale area surrounded by a hyperemic rim. The corresponding gross photograph is shown in Figure 65.14B. **B.** The center of the infarct demonstrates necrosis of alveolar walls and intra-alveolar acellular debris.

FIGURE 65.16 ▲ Periphery of acute infarct. The infarct demonstrates intra-alveolar hemorrhage **(below)** and an accumulation of macrophage and chronic inflammatory cells **(above)**.

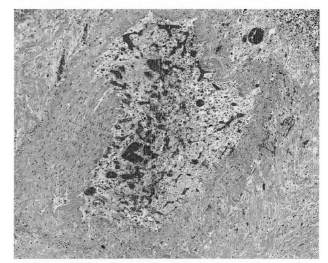

FIGURE 65.18 ▲ Organized recanalized thrombus, periphery of remote infarct. The artery is completely obliterated by an organized, recanalized thrombus. The artery was at the periphery of the infarct shown in Figures 65.1 and 65.4.

infection of an infarcted focus results in lung abscess. As organization ensues, significant squamous metaplasia may be seen and should not be mistaken for neoplasia. In a remote infarct, there is diffuse necrosis, with faint, ghost-like remnants of alveolar architecture present on higher magnification.

REFERENCES

1. Kakkar N, Vasishta RK. Pulmonary embolism in medical patients: an autopsy-based study. *Clin Appl Thromb Hemost.* 2008;14(2):159–167.
2. Torbicki A, et al. Guidelines on the diagnosis and management of acute pulmonary embolism: the Task Force for the Diagnosis and Management of Acute Pulmonary Embolism of the European Society of Cardiology (ESC). *Eur Heart J.* 2008;29(18):2276–2315.
3. Olie V, et al. Time trends in pulmonary embolism mortality in France, 2000–2010. *Thromb Res.* 2015;135(2):334–338.
4. Laribi S, et al. Trends in death attributed to myocardial infarction, heart failure and pulmonary embolism in Europe and Canada over the last decade. *QJM.* 2014;107(10):813–820.
5. Pulido T, et al. Pulmonary embolism as a cause of death in patients with heart disease: an autopsy study. *Chest.* 2006;129(5):1282–1287.
6. Tadlock MD, et al. The origin of fatal pulmonary emboli: a postmortem analysis of 500 deaths from pulmonary embolism in trauma, surgical, and medical patients. *Am J Surg.* 2015;209(6):959–968.
7. Nielsen JD. The incidence of pulmonary embolism during deep vein thrombosis. *Phlebology.* 2013;28(suppl 1):29–33.
8. Rossi E, et al. The risk of symptomatic pulmonary embolism due to proximal deep venous thrombosis differs in patients with different types of inherited thrombophilia. *Thromb Haemost.* 2008;99(6):1030–1034.
9. van Stralen KJ, et al. Mechanisms of the factor V Leiden paradox. *Arterioscler Thromb Vasc Biol.* 2008;28(10):1872–1877.
10. Huisman MV, et al. Factor V Leiden is associated with more distal deep vein thrombosis of the left. *J Thromb Haemost.* 2008;6:544–546.
11. Gudipati S, et al. A cohort study on the incidence and outcome of pulmonary embolism in trauma and orthopedic patients. *BMC Med.* 2014;12:39.
12. Hauch O, et al. Fatal pulmonary embolism associated with surgery. An autopsy study. *Acta Chir Scand.* 1990;156(11–12):747–749.
13. Natsuaki M, et al. Recurrence of pulmonary embolism in young man with retroperitoneal tumor despite insertion of temporary IVC filter. *Circ J.* 2009;73(9):1756–1758.
14. Ito M. Pathology of pulmonary embolism. *Kokyu To Junkan.* 1991;39(6):567–572.
15. van Es N, Bleker SM, Di Nisio M. Cancer-associated unsuspected pulmonary embolism. *Thromb Res.* 2014;133(suppl 2):S172–S178.
16. Barra SN, et al. Atrial fibrillation in acute pulmonary embolism: prognostic considerations. *Emerg Med J.* 2014;31(4):308–312.
17. Chung WS, et al. Systemic lupus erythematosus increases the risks of deep vein thrombosis and pulmonary embolism: a nationwide cohort study. *J Thromb Haemost.* 2014;12(4):452–458.
18. Akpinar EE, et al. Incidence of pulmonary embolism during COPD exacerbation. *J Bras Pneumol.* 2014;40(1):38–45.
19. Miniati M, et al. Clinical presentation of acute pulmonary embolism: survey of 800 cases. *PLoS One.* 2012;7(2):e30891.
20. Shimi M, et al. Sudden death due to pulmonary embolism in north Tunisia: 37 cases study. *Tunis Med.* 2014;92(10):610–614.
21. White RH, Zhou H, Romano PS. Incidence of symptomatic venous thromboembolism after different elective or urgent surgical procedures. *Thromb Haemost.* 2003;90(3):446–455.
22. Goldhaber SZ, Elliott CG. Acute pulmonary embolism: part I: epidemiology, pathophysiology, and diagnosis. *Circulation.* 2003;108(22):2726–2729.
23. Le Gal G, Righini M, Wells PS. D-dimer for pulmonary embolism. *JAMA.* 2015;313(16):1668–1669.
24. Tavora F, et al. Discrepancies in initial death certificate diagnoses in sudden unexpected out-of-hospital deaths: the role of cardiovascular autopsy. *Cardiovasc Pathol.* 2008;17(3):178–182.
25. Kotovicz F, Mauad T, Saldiva PH. Clinico-pathological discrepancies in a general university hospital in Sao Paulo, Brazil. *Clinics (Sao Paulo).* 2008;63(5):581–588.
26. Fares AF, et al. Clinical and pathological discrepancies and cardiovascular findings in 409 consecutive autopsies. *Arq Bras Cardiol.* 2011;97(6):449–455.
27. Blauwet LA, et al. Surgical pathology of pulmonary thromboendarterectomy: a study of 54 cases from 1990 to 2001. *Hum Pathol.* 2003;34(12):1290–1298.
28. Bernard J, Yi ES. Pulmonary thromboendarterectomy: a clinicopathologic study of 200 consecutive pulmonary thromboendarterectomy cases in one institution. *Hum Pathol.* 2007;38(6):871–877.
29. Ye R, et al. Clinical characteristics of septic pulmonary embolism in adults: a systematic review. *Respir Med.* 2014;108(1):1–8.
30. Stein PD, Dalen JE. Thrombolytic therapy for acute pulmonary embolism: when do the benefits exceed the risks? *Am J Med.* 2014;127(11):1031–1032.
31. Chatterjee S, et al. Thrombolysis for pulmonary embolism and risk of all-cause mortality, major bleeding, and intracranial hemorrhage: a meta-analysis. *JAMA.* 2014;311(23):2414–2421.
32. Kilic A, et al. Nationwide outcomes of surgical embolectomy for acute pulmonary embolism. *J Thorac Cardiovasc Surg.* 2013;145(2):373–377.
33. Mandernach MW, Beyth RJ, Rajasekhar A. Apixaban for the prophylaxis and treatment of deep vein thrombosis and pulmonary embolism: an evidence-based review. *Ther Clin Risk Manag.* 2015;11:1273–1282.
34. Winterbauer RH, Elfenbein IB, Ball WC, Jr. Incidence and clinical significance of tumor embolization to the lungs. *Am J Med.* 1968;45(2):271–290.
35. Yao DX, Flieder DB, Hoda SA. Pulmonary tumor thrombotic microangiopathy: an often missed antemortem diagnosis. *Arch Pathol Lab Med.* 2001;125(2):304–305.
36. Shigematsu H, Andou A, Matsuo K. Pulmonary tumor embolism. *J Thorac Oncol.* 2009;4(6):777; author reply 777–778.
37. Rekik S, et al. Myofibroblastic tumor of the right ventricle causing bilateral pulmonary embolism in a 31 year-old woman. *Int J Cardiol.* 2009;131(3):e131–e133.
38. Roberts KE, et al. Pulmonary tumor embolism: a review of the literature. *Am J Med.* 2003;115(3):228–232.
39. Fracasso T, Varchmin-Schultheiss K. Sudden death due to pulmonary embolism from right atrial myxoma. *Int J Legal Med.* 2009;123(2):157–159.
40. Georgin-Lavialle S, et al. Intravascular lymphoma presenting as a specific pulmonary embolism and acute respiratory failure: a case report. *J Med Case Reports.* 2009;3:7253.
41. Kwiatt ME, Seamon MJ. Fat embolism syndrome. *Int J Crit Illn Inj Sci.* 2013;3(1):64–68.
42. Bhalla A, et al. Cerebral fat embolism as a rare possible complication of traumatic pancreatitis. *JOP.* 2003;4(4):155–157.
43. Ballas SK, et al. Postmortem diagnosis of hemoglobin SC disease complicated by fat embolism. *Ann Clin Lab Sci.* 1998;28(3):144–149.
44. Barz H, Majerowitsch B. Myelomalacia caused by embolism of the substantia gelatinosa in the vertebral column and spinal cord arteries. *Zentralbl Allg Pathol.* 1986;131(2):119–125.
45. Mayron R, et al. Tissue-fat pulmonary embolism occurring in a patient with a severe pelvic fracture. *J Emerg Med.* 1985;2(4):251–256.
46. Tozzini S, et al. Pulmonary embolism by liver tissue. *Am J Forensic Med Pathol.* 2004;25(1):87.
47. Tan KL, Hwang WS. Neonatal brain tissue embolism in the lung. *Aust N Z J Med.* 1976;6(2):146–149.
48. Shinagawa S, et al. An autopsy study of 306 cases of maternal death in Japan. *Nippon Sanka Fujinka Gakkai Zasshi.* 1983;35(2):194–200.
49. Lau G. Amniotic fluid embolism as a cause of sudden maternal death. *Med Sci Law.* 1994;34(3):213–220.
50. Kringsholm B, Christoffersen P. The nature and the occurrence of birefringent material in different organs in fatal drug addiction. *Forensic Sci Int.* 1987;34:53–62.
51. Deffebach ME, et al. The bronchial circulation. Small, but a vital attribute of the lung. *Am Rev Respir Dis.* 1987;135(2):463–481.
52. Kauczor HU, et al. Spiral CT of bronchial arteries in chronic thromboembolism. *J Comput Assist Tomogr.* 1994;18(6):855–861.
53. Cha SI, et al. Clinical relevance of pulmonary infarction in patients with pulmonary embolism. *Thromb Res.* 2012;130(3):e1–e5.
54. He H, et al. Pulmonary infarction: spectrum of findings on multidetector helical CT. *J Thorac Imaging.* 2006;21(1):1–7.
55. Libby LS, et al. Pulmonary cavitation following pulmonary infarction. *Medicine (Baltimore).* 1985;64(5):342–348.
56. Redline S, Tomashefski JF, Jr., Altose MD. Cavitating lung infarction after bland pulmonary thromboembolism in patients with the adult respiratory distress syndrome. *Thorax.* 1985;40(12):915–919.

57. Wick MR, Ritter JH, Schuller D. Ruptured pulmonary infarction: a rare, fatal complication of thromboembolic disease. *Mayo Clin Proc.* 2000;75(6):639–642.

58. Erdman S, Vidne B, Levy MJ. Lung pseudotumor caused by pulmonary infarction. *Geriatrics.* 1975;30(5):103–105.

59. Kamel EM, et al. Occult lung infarction may induce false interpretation of 18F-FDG PET in primary staging of pulmonary malignancies. *Eur J Nucl Med Mol Imaging.* 2005;32(6):641–646.

60. Kang CH, et al. Lung metastases manifesting as pulmonary infarction by mucin and tumor embolization: radiographic, high-resolution CT, and pathologic findings. *J Comput Assist Tomogr.* 1999;23(4):644–646.

61. Revel MP, et al. Is it possible to recognize pulmonary infarction on multisection CT images? *Radiology.* 2007;244(3):875–882.

62. Casullo J, Semionov A. Reversed halo sign in acute pulmonary embolism and infarction. *Acta Radiol.* 2013;54(5):505–510.

63. Tsao MS, Schraufnagel D, Wang NS. Pathogenesis of pulmonary infarction. *Am J Med.* 1982;72(4):599–606.

64. Krivokuca I, et al. Pulmonary embolism and pulmonary infarction after lung transplantation. *Clin Appl Thromb Hemost.* 2011;17(4):421–424.

65. Schraufnagel DE, et al. Factors associated with pulmonary infarction. A discriminant analysis study. *Am J Clin Pathol.* 1985;84(1):15–18.

66. Weng CT, et al. A retrospective study of pulmonary infarction in patients with systemic lupus erythematosus from southern Taiwan. *Lupus.* 2011;20(8):876–885.

67. Vaideeswar P. Pure pulmonary arterial tumour embolism—a rare cause of pulmonary infarction. *Indian J Pathol Microbiol.* 2004;47(2):255–257.

68. Ishiguro T, et al. Primary pulmonary artery sarcoma detected with a pulmonary infarction. *Intern Med.* 2007;46(9):601–604.

69. Sawhney S, Burney I, Jain R. Pulmonary infarction: a rare case of adrenal carcinoma. *Sultan Qaboos Univ Med J.* 2007;7(1):55–57.

70. Hildebrand FL, Jr., et al. Pulmonary complications of leukemia. *Chest.* 1990;98(5):1233–1239.

71. Katsumura Y, Ohtsubo K. Incidence of pulmonary thromboembolism, infarction and haemorrhage in disseminated intravascular coagulation: a necroscopic analysis. *Thorax.* 1995;50(2):160–164.

72. Hayashi S, et al. A case of alpha-thalassemia-2 associated with pulmonary infarction. *Lung.* 2006;184(4):223–227.

73. Maggi JC, Nussbaum E. Massive pulmonary infarction in sickle cell anemia. *Pediatr Emerg Care.* 1987;3(1):30–32.

74. Prakash UB. Lungs in hemoglobinopathies, erythrocyte disorders, and hemorrhagic diatheses. *Semin Respir Crit Care Med.* 2005;26(5):527–540.

75. Landonio G, et al. Pulmonary and myocardial infarction secondary to arterial occlusion by *Aspergillus fumigatus* in ANLL. *Haematologica.* 1989;74(5):503–505.

76. Narita J, et al. Pulmonary artery involvement in Takayasu's arteritis with lung infarction and pulmonary aspergillosis. *J Clin Rheumatol.* 2002;8(5):260–264.

77. de Heide LJ, Pieterman H, Hennemann G. Pulmonary infarction caused by giant-cell arteritis of the pulmonary artery. *Neth J Med.* 1995;46(1):36–40.

78. Ikemoto Y, et al. Pulmonary infarction and deep venous thrombosis in a 13-year-old boy with Churg-Strauss syndrome. *Pediatr Int.* 2001;43(4):441–443.

79. Nakamura T, et al. Pulmonary infarction as the initial manifestation of Takayasu's arteritis. *Intern Med.* 2006;45(11):725–728.

80. Manoly I, et al. Pulmonary infarction after repair of type B aortic dissection. *Ann Thorac Surg.* 2012;94(1):e13–e15.

81. Hultgren HN, Wilson R, Kosek JC. Lung pathology in high-altitude pulmonary edema. *Wilderness Environ Med.* 1997;8(4):218–220.

82. Anand G, et al. Superior vena cava stent migration into the pulmonary artery causing fatal pulmonary infarction. *Cardiovasc Intervent Radiol.* 2011;34(suppl 2):S198–S201.

83. Mancano AD, et al. Pulmonary infarction from a fractured and embolized central venous catheter. *Ann Thorac Surg.* 2014;97(6):2198.

84. Duke E, Peterson AA, Erly WK. Migrating bullet: a case of a bullet embolism to the pulmonary artery with secondary pulmonary infarction after gunshot wound to the left globe. *J Emerg Trauma Shock.* 2014;7(1):38–40.

85. Kadokura M, et al. A surgical case of pulmonary adenocarcinoma complicated with pulmonary infarction presenting as an intrapulmonary metastasis. *J Cardiovasc Surg (Torino).* 2007;48(3):389–392.

86. Choong CK, Hu DZ, Huddleston CB. Pulmonary segmental venous infarction after living-donor lobar lung transplantation. *J Thorac Cardiovasc Surg.* 2005;130(3):919–921.

87. Duehmke RM, Fynn SP, Gopalan D. Pulmonary venous infarction following pulmonary vein isolation. *Eur Heart J.* 2008;29(23):2893.

88. Ravenel JG, McAdams HP. Pulmonary venous infarction after radiofrequency ablation for atrial fibrillation. *AJR Am J Roentgenol.* 2002;178(3):664–666.

89. Yataco J, Stoller JK. Pulmonary venous thrombosis and infarction complicating pulmonary venous stenosis following radiofrequency ablation. *Respir Care.* 2004;49(12):1525–1527.

90. Nelson E, Klein JS. Pulmonary infarction resulting from metastatic osteogenic sarcoma with pulmonary venous tumor thrombus. *AJR Am J Roentgenol.* 2000;174(2):531–533.

91. Stevens LH, et al. Left atrial myxoma: pulmonary infarction caused by pulmonary venous occlusion. *Ann Thorac Surg.* 1987;43(2):215–217.

92. Williamson WA, et al. Pulmonary venous infarction secondary to squamous cell carcinoma. *Chest.* 1992;102(3):950–952.

SECTION TWELVE
BENIGN LUNG TUMORS

66 Papillomas

Allen P. Burke, M.D., and Marie-Christine Aubry, M.D.

Squamous Papilloma

General

Squamous cell papilloma is a benign tumor consisting of delicate connective tissue fronds with a squamous epithelial surface.[1-11] Squamous papillomas can be solitary or multiple.[12] In the latter instance, they are frequently associated with respiratory papillomatosis or recurrent laryngeal papillomatosis.

It has been recognized since the 1980s that the lower respiratory tract can be involved with HPV-related papillomas extending from the larynx.[13] The cause is presumed to be exposure to maternal human papillomavirus (HPV) during vaginal birth. Tracheal involvement in recurrent laryngeal papillomatosis occurs in up to 10% of patients, with pulmonary parenchymal involvement in < 2%.[14] Laryngotracheal papillomatosis is synonymous with "respiratory papillomatosis" or "recurrent respiratory papillomatosis."[13-15] Tracheal and bronchial papillomatoses are defined endoscopically by the presence of papillomas at the level of the first tracheal ring and distally. Pulmonary papillomatosis is diagnosed using chest radiographs or computed tomography scans that show multiple rounded, solid, or cystic nodules.[14]

Clinical Features

Solitary Squamous Papilloma

Solitary squamous papilloma is a rare tumor that accounts for <1% of all lung tumors.[1,2,12,16] The tumor has a variety of clinical presentations, including cough, dyspnea, hemoptysis, and recurrent pneumonia.[1,12,16] Solitary squamous papillomas are predominant in male smokers (male-to-female ratio of 3:1) in their sixth decade.[2,16] Bronchial squamous papilloma usually presents as an endobronchial mass in the segmental bronchi with abnormal radiologic findings such as a round tumor shadow, parenchymal infiltrative opacity, atelectasis, and hilar mass on chest x-ray or computed tomography (CT) scan.[16] There are two peculiar features in the clinical history of these lesions: (1) a tendency to spread to multiple sites within the bronchial tree and (2) a substantial potential for malignant transformation.[11] These two characteristics strongly implicate an infectious etiology of SSPs. The clinical behavior closely resembles that of recurrent respiratory papillomatosis and natural history of sinonasal papillomas.[11] HPV appears to play a pathogenetic role in solitary squamous papilloma.[1] The malignant potential of solitary squamous papilloma ranges from 8% to 40%.[16]

Respiratory Papillomatosis

Risks for extension of HPV-related papillomas to the lower airways include tracheotomy for laryngeal stenosis, and early onset of disease, with a mean of 20 months of age.[14] Most children develop laryngeal papillomas by the age of 5, and lung lesions may occur as late as age 30.[13,15] Frequently, there are numerous endoscopic procedures and ablations of upper airway lesions before lung lesions appear.[13] Radiographs and chest computed tomography scans show round

or irregular cysts, usually <5 cm diameter, often with air–fluid levels.[13] These cysts progress to nodules, with a predilection of bilateral lower lobes. Symptoms include respiratory insufficiency and signs of pneumonia, although many lesions are found during screening chest radiographs.[13] Treatment includes interferon, local injection with cidofovir, and antiproliferative drugs.[15] In the largest study of lower respiratory papillomatosis, 48% of patients achieved remission, 23% had persistence into childhood, 16% had persistence into adulthood, and 13% died from respiratory failure or progression to squamous cell carcinoma.[14]

Pathologic Findings

Solitary Squamous Papilloma

Endobronchial solitary squamous papilloma must be distinguished from more aggressive neoplasms. This distinction is particularly important when one encounters this neoplasm in a peripheral location at frozen section. Solitary squamous papilloma can be exophytic or, less frequently, inverted or plaque-like[16,17] (Fig. 66.1). The histologic examination shows papillary lesions composed of fibrovascular interstitium and proliferation of stratified squamous epithelium with orderly maturation from the base to the superficial layer[16] (Fig. 66.2). Typically, the squamous epithelium is bland; however, cell atypia and increased mitotic activity indicative of dysplasia may be seen and

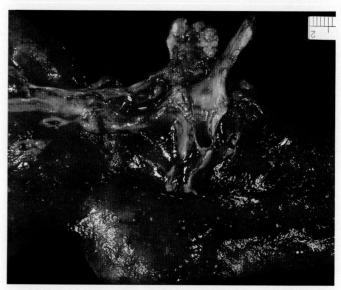

FIGURE 66.1 ▲ Squamous papilloma. Grossly, the tumor forms an exophytic obstructive lesion arising in a large airway. The surface of the tumor is irregular with frond-like projections.

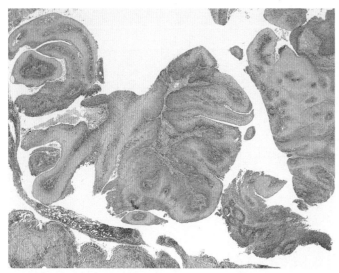

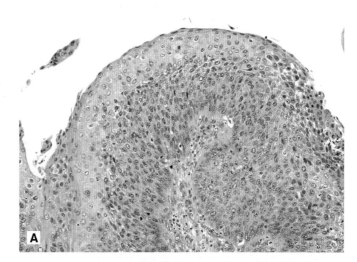

FIGURE 66.2 ▲ Endobronchial squamous papilloma. Histologically, the tumor resembles squamous papillomas of other sites, such as the head and neck.

should be graded accordingly (Fig. 66.3). Endobronchial papillomas, particularly inverted ones, may extend into and replace submucosal glands. This results in small squamous nests in the submucosa and should not be misconstrued as invasion. These squamous nests remain invested of a basal layer. The distinction with a papillary squamous cell carcinoma can be challenging. Papillary squamous cell carcinoma will appear overtly malignant cytologically. Invasion may be difficult to appreciate, but desmoplasia and parenchymal destruction are helpful features when present. Immunohistochemically, p63, p40, CK903, and CK5/6 are diffusely positive, indicative of their squamous differentiation.

There is a strong but not absolute association between solitary squamous papilloma and HPV identification either by characteristic cytopathic changes (i.e., koilocytosis) or by in situ hybridization.[8,9,18] SSPs show an association with HPV type 11 and rarely with type 6, whereas type 16 or 18, sometimes in combination with type 31/33/35, is found in SSPs associated with squamous cell carcinoma.[2,19]

Respiratory Papillomatosis

There are few pathologic studies of pulmonary papillomatosis. At autopsy, the proximal airways have been described as relatively free of disease, with extensive parenchymal nodules.[13] Lesions within the lung parenchyma vary from small clusters of 20 to 30 squamous cells within two or three adjacent alveoli to large cavitating structures that are several centimeters in size. The walls of the cavitating lesions are formed by irregular sheets of nonkeratinizing squamous epithelium.[13]

At surgical resection of lung lesions, there are parenchymal papillomas resembling those of the upper respiratory tract, but an association with a bronchus is not always present (Fig. 66.4). The lesions are squamous cell papillomas, with p16 expression correlating with positive HPV in situ hybridization. Areas of dysplasia or carcinoma need to be carefully excluded.

The most common HPV isolated in pulmonary papillomatosis mirrors that of the larynx, with HPV types 11 and 16 predominating.[14]

Glandular and Mixed Papillomas

General

Solitary endobronchial papillomas are rare neoplasms.[1–11] Only sporadic cases have been documented. The histologic classification

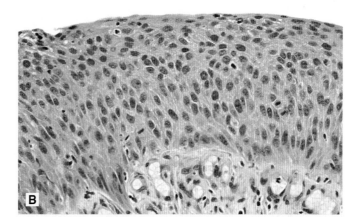

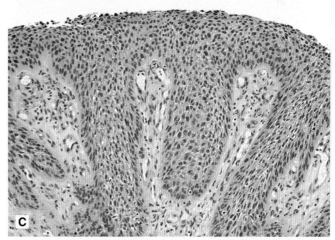

FIGURE 66.3 ▲ Various severity of squamous dysplasia. Mild dysplasia **(A)**, moderate **(B)**, and squamous carcinoma in situ all within a squamous papilloma **(C)**.

of these tumors remains problematic, and little is known about their clinical behavior. Three morphologically distinct histologic types are recognized: (1) squamous cell papillomas (see above), (2) glandular papillomas, and (3) mixed squamous and glandular papillomas.[12]

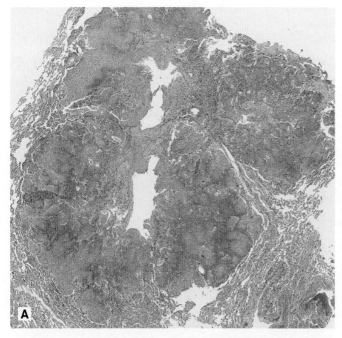

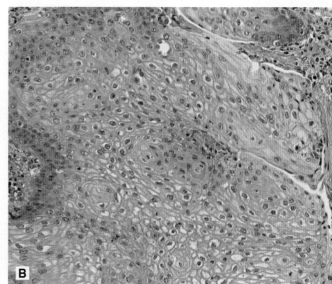

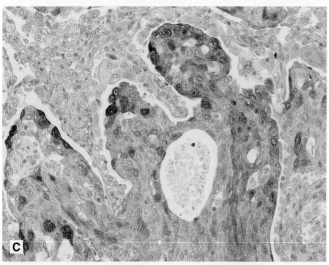

FIGURE 66.4 ▲ Respiratory papillomatosis, lung involvement. **A.** At low magnification, there is a papillary squamous lesion that was resected by open lung biopsy. **B.** Note viral cytopathic changes (koilocytosis). **C.** p16 immunostaining is positive.

Glandular papilloma is a benign tumor lined by ciliated or nonciliated columnar cells, with varying numbers of cuboidal cells and goblet cells.[5,10,12,20]

Mixed squamous and glandular papilloma is a benign tumor showing a mixture of squamous and glandular epithelium.[4,6,7,12,21] One-third of the epithelium should be composed of the second epithelial type.[12]

Clinical Features

Glandular and mixed squamous cell and glandular papilloma (mixed papilloma) of the lung are extremely rare neoplasms.[4–7,10,21] Mixed papillomas are predominantly lesions of male smokers in their sixth decade.[17,22] Glandular papillomas, the rarest of all endobronchial papillomas, are found in an older age group than squamous and mixed papillomas with female predominance, and most patients are nonsmokers.[22]

Glandular and mixed papillomas occur predominantly in the central tracheobronchial tree and may produce obstructive symptoms.[23]

Involvement of the peripheral lung is uncommon.[5] In some cases, solitary papillomas go undetected for years, being detected only by chance.[5,10] It might be difficult to distinguish a glandular papilloma from active inflammation, granulomatous disease, carcinoid, and lung cancer based only on imaging findings.[5,10] Bronchoscopic biopsy or CT-guided needle biopsy is necessary to confirm the diagnosis. Glandular papillomas associated with mucus retention may grow rapidly, mimicking a malignant neoplasm.[10]

Malignant transformation has been reported with the mixed type of solitary papilloma of the lung.[4] The glandular variant has shown no tendency toward local recurrence after local excision and has no apparent malignant potential.[5] Complete surgical resection is currently the standard treatment for this pathology.[5]

Pathologic Findings

Glandular and mixed papilloma present as a well-circumscribed, whitish or yellowish nodular mucous endobronchial or pulmonary mass (with or without cystic changes).[4–7,10,12,21] Microscopic examination of

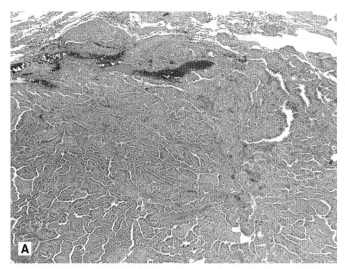
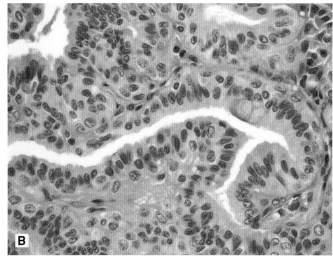

FIGURE 66.5 ▲ Glandular papilloma. **A.** At low power, the diagnostic considerations would be between adenocarcinoma, predominantly papillary, and glandular papilloma. The glandular papilloma is well circumscribed, sharply demarcated from the adjacent normal lung parenchyma. **B.** At high power, the glandular cells lining the papillary fronds contain mucous cell admixed with cylindrical cells. Brush borders and cilia are present.

glandular papilloma shows papillary fronds lined by a stratified columnar epithelium in the lumens of bronchi and bronchioles, with numerous arborizing papillary elements, some of which grow into adjacent alveolar spaces (Fig. 66.5). The stratified columnar epithelium consists of ciliated, mucous, and basal cells.[5,24] Glandular papillomas seldom show necrosis, and the presence of ciliated cells is considered to be an important finding for ruling out peripheral well-differentiated adenocarcinoma.[10,25]

Mixed papilloma shows prominent papillary growth of squamous, transitional, and pseudostratified columnar epithelium. The later consists of ciliated and nonciliated columnar cells and many mucous cells (Fig. 66.6). Cytologic atypia of the squamous epithelium is commonly observed but typically not of the glandular cells.[22]

Immunohistochemically, intracellular mucin is positive for MUC5AC, which is expressed in tracheobronchial goblet cells.[12] Glandular papilloma is TTF-1 positive, cytokeratin-7 positive, and cytokeratin-20 negative on immunostaining.[10]

In mixed papilloma, the pseudostratified columnar epithelium is positive for CK5/6 and CK7 but negative for CK20.[21] Immunopositivity for p40 staining is mostly observed in the basal and squamous cells. TTF-1 and CEA are negative on immunostaining.[21] CAM5.2 and CK19 are diffusely positive in mixed papilloma, indicating that the tumor originates from the columnar epithelium by squamous metaplasia.[12]

Both glandular and mixed papillomas are HPV negative.[22]

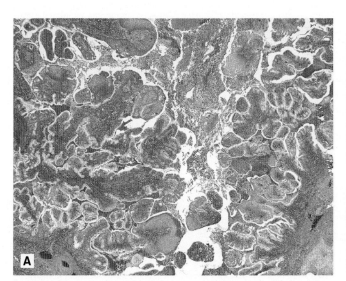
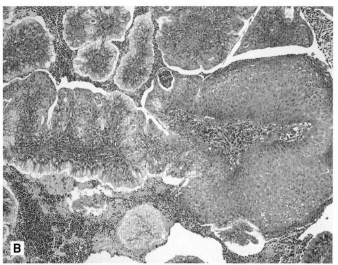

FIGURE 66.6 ▲ Mixed squamous cell and glandular papilloma. **A.** The tumor is composed of papillary fronds lined by a mixture of squamous and glandular epithelium. **B.** The squamous epithelium shows only mild atypia with preserved maturation. Mitosis is limited to the basal layers.

Practical Points

▶ Papillomas are rare benign neoplasms, classified as squamous cell papilloma, glandular papilloma, and mixed squamous cell and glandular papilloma.

▶ Squamous cell papilloma is lined by benign squamous epithelium but can be involved by dysplasia or carcinoma. Squamous cell carcinoma is recognized by its overt cytologic atypia.

▶ Respiratory papillomatosis is characterized by diffuse airway involvement by squamous cell papillomas as a result of HPV infection. HPV infection may also play a role in some solitary squamous cell papillomas.

▶ Glandular papilloma is a benign papillary neoplasm lined by glandular epithelium. The epithelium is composed of a mixture of cell types, columnar, mucous, and ciliated. In contrast, adenocarcinoma typically has a single predominant cell type and is not ciliated.

▶ Mixed papilloma is characterized by a mixture of glandular and squamous epithelium lining papillae.

REFERENCES

1. Cook JR, Hill DA, Humphrey PA, et al. Squamous cell carcinoma arising in recurrent respiratory papillomatosis with pulmonary involvement: emerging common pattern of clinical features and human papillomavirus serotype association. *Mod Pathol.* 2000;13:914–918.
2. Harada H, Miura K, Tsutsui Y, et al. Solitary squamous cell papilloma of the lung in a 40-year-old woman with recurrent laryngeal papillomatosis. *Pathol Int.* 2000;50:431–439.
3. Inoue Y, Oka M, Ishii H, et al. A solitary bronchial papilloma with malignant changes. *Intern Med.* 2001;40:56–60.
4. Kadota K, Haba R, Katsuki N, et al. Cytological findings of mixed squamous cell and glandular papilloma in the lung. *Diagn Cytopathol.* 2010;38:913–917.
5. Kaseda K, Horio H, Harada M, et al. Solitary glandular papilloma of the peripheral lung: a report of two cases. *World J Surg Oncol.* 2014;12:149.
6. Kozu Y, Maniwa T, Ohde Y, et al. A solitary mixed squamous cell and glandular papilloma of the lung. *Ann Thorac Cardiovasc Surg.* 2014;20(suppl):625–628.
7. Lagana SM, Hanna RF, Borczuk AC. Pleomorphic (spindle and squamous cell) carcinoma arising in a peripheral mixed squamous and glandular papilloma in a 70-year-old man. *Arch Pathol Lab Med.* 2011;135:1353–1356.
8. Roglic M, Jukic S, Damjanov I. Cytology of the solitary papilloma of the bronchus. *Acta Cytol.* 1975;19:11–13.
9. Rubel L, Reynolds RE. Cytologic description of squamous cell papilloma of the respiratory tract. *Acta Cytol.* 1979;23:227–231.
10. Suzuki S, Goto T, Emoto K, et al. Rapidly growing glandular papilloma associated with mucus production: a case report. *World J Surg Oncol.* 2014;12:160.
11. Syrjanen K, Syrjanen S. Solitary bronchial squamous cell papilloma—another human papillomavirus (HPV)-associated benign tumor: systematic review and meta-analysis. *Contemp Oncol (Pozn).* 2013;17:427–434.
12. Flieder DB, Nicholson A, Travis WD, et al. Papillomas. In: Travis WD, Brambilla E, Burke AP, et al., eds. *World Health Classification of Tumours. Tumours of the Lung, Pleura, Thymus and Heart.* Lyon, France: IARC Press; 2015:106–109.
13. Kramer SS, Wehunt WD, Stocker JT, et al. Pulmonary manifestations of juvenile laryngotracheal papillomatosis. *AJR Am J Roentgenol.* 1985;144:687–694.
14. Soldatski IL, Onufrieva EK, Steklov AM, et al. Tracheal, bronchial, and pulmonary papillomatosis in children. *Laryngoscope.* 2005;115:1848–1854.
15. Ruan SY, Chen KY, Yang PC. Recurrent respiratory papillomatosis with pulmonary involvement: a case report and review of the literature. *Respirology.* 2009;14:137–140.
16. Kim SR, Park JK, Park SJ, et al. Solitary bronchial squamous papilloma presenting as a plaque-like lesion in a subject with asthma. *Am J Respir Crit Care Med.* 2011;183:555–556.
17. Lang TU, Khalbuss WE, Monaco SE, et al. Solitary tracheobronchial papilloma: cytomorphology and ancillary studies with histologic correlation. *Cytojournal.* 2011;8:6.
18. McNamee CJ, Lien D, Puttagunta L, et al. Solitary squamous papillomas of the bronchus: a case report and literature review. *J Thorac Cardiovasc Surg.* 2003;126:861–863.
19. Popper HH, el-Shabrawi Y, Wockel W, et al. Prognostic importance of human papilloma virus typing in squamous cell papilloma of the bronchus: comparison of in situ hybridization and the polymerase chain reaction. *Hum Pathol.* 1994;25:1191–1197.
20. Spencer H, Dail DH, Arneaud J. Non-invasive bronchial epithelial papillary tumors. *Cancer.* 1980;45:1486–1497.
21. Inamura K, Kumasaka T, Furuta R, et al. Mixed squamous cell and glandular papilloma of the lung: a case study and literature review. *Pathol Int.* 2011;61:252–258.
22. Flieder DB, Koss MN, Nicholson A, et al. Solitary pulmonary papillomas in adults: a clinicopathologic and in situ hybridization study of 14 cases combined with 27 cases in the literature. *Am J Surg Pathol.* 1998;22:1328–1342.
23. Tryfon S, Dramba V, Zoglopitis F, et al. Solitary papillomas of the lower airways: epidemiological, clinical, and therapeutic data during a 22-year period and review of the literature. *J Thorac Oncol.* 2012;7:643–648.
24. Aida S, Ohara I, Shimazaki H, et al. Solitary peripheral ciliated glandular papillomas of the lung: a report of 3 cases. *Am J Surg Pathol.* 2008;32:1489–1494.
25. Emerson LL, Layfield LJ. Solitary peripheral pulmonary papilloma evaluation on frozen section: a potential pitfall for the pathologist. *Pathol Res Pract.* 2012;208:726–729.

67 Pulmonary Adenomas

Allen P. Burke, M.D.

Sclerosing Pneumocytoma (Hemangioma)

Sclerosing pneumocytoma is a distinctive benign tumor of pneumocyte origin. Although the epithelial nature of the tumor has been established for over 25 years,[1] the term "sclerosing hemangioma" is entrenched in the medical literature and appears synonymously with "pneumocytoma" to this day.

Sclerosing pneumocytomas are rare, with few published series of more than 10 patients[2,3]; there appears to be a higher prevalence in China than in Western countries.[4-7] There is a >5:1 female predominance, up to 15:1 in China.[6] The mean or median age was 46 in the two largest series published.[3,4] Most are discovered incidentally, although some patients present with cough or hemoptysis.

Although a predilection for the right middle lobe has been reported,[4] there was no site predilection in the largest study from the United States.[3] Fewer than 5% of sclerosing pneumocytomas are multiple, and when they are, the nodules are usually in the same lobe, as a dominant mass with satellite nodules.[3,5] The typical tumor is peripheral or subpleural. Rare endobronchial[8] or visceral pleural-based tumors have been reported.[3] Sclerosing pneumocytomas are typically well circumscribed, solid, and homogeneous, without cystic areas (only 3% in the largest series).[3] Foci of hemorrhage are seen in about one-fourth of tumors and

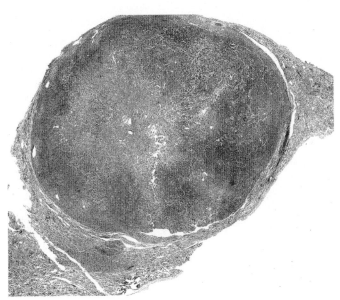

FIGURE 67.1 ▲ Sclerosing pneumocytoma. At low power, the tumor is highly circumscribed. At this magnification, a benign tumor or metastatic lesion is likely.

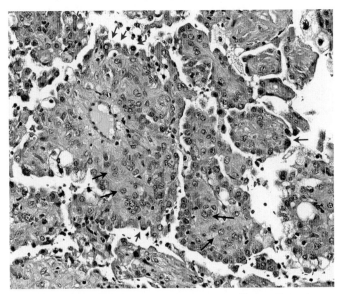

FIGURE 67.3 ▲ Sclerosing pneumocytoma, papillary pattern. A higher magnification of a different example from that shown in the previous figure shows very monotonous cells, with two populations: the lining surface cells (*red arrows*) and the rounded tumor cells within the papillae (*black arrows*). The two cell population and bland cytologic features distinguish this lesion from papillary adenocarcinoma.

correspond to the hemorrhagic histologic pattern. The mean size is 25 to 30 mm, with the largest reported at 8 cm.[6] By computed tomographic scans, most are round, with absent or small spicules and homogenous. There may be calcifications or heterogeneous enhancement, especially in larger tumors. Because of the nonspecificity of computed tomographic findings and positivity on positron emission tomography, many sclerosing pneumocytomas are diagnosed as probably malignancies.[5,7,9]

Histologically, there are two cell types (round and surface) that classically form four overlapping patterns. The most common is the papillary pattern (Figs. 67.1 to 67.3), followed by sclerotic, solid, and hemorrhagic patterns (Figs. 67.4 and 67.5). About one-half of tumors show all four. It is generally believed that the "tumor" cell is the round cell, which is present within the papillary stalks and in the sclerotic and solid areas, and that the cells lining the surfaces of the papillae and tubular structures are reactive ("activated") pneumocytes. The hemorrhagic pattern is characterized by blood-filled spaces lined by

pneumocytes and the sclerotic pattern by small nests of round cells in a dense collagen stroma. The surface cells may show multinucleation and intranuclear inclusions. Entrapped cysts may be lined by reactive pneumocytes or ciliated bronchiolar epithelium that may fill with mucus.[3]

Immunohistochemically and ultrastructurally, the two cell types show divergent characteristics, the surface cells showing features of mature "type II" pneumocytes and the round cells more primitive pneumocytes (sometimes called "pneumoblasts"[10]). The finding of a low proliferative index in the round cells, compared to zero Ki-67 proliferative index in the surface cells, supports this concept,[6] as well as the finding of hepatocyte nuclear factor-3α and nuclear factor-3β within the round cells.[10]

For diagnostic purposes, immunohistochemistry is useful in separating the round cells from the more differentiated, reactive surface cells (Figs. 67.6 to 67.9; Table 67.1). Round cells are negative for

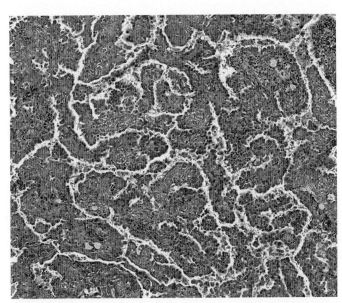

FIGURE 67.2 ▲ Sclerosing pneumocytoma, papillary pattern. At first glance, a papillary adenocarcinoma comes to mind. However, the lining cells are very uniform and not very columnar like those of papillary adenocarcinoma.

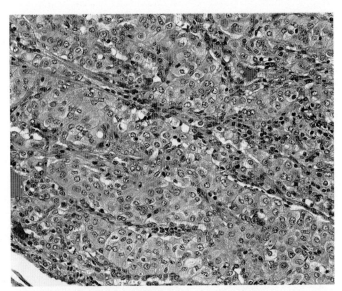

FIGURE 67.4 ▲ Sclerosing pneumocytoma, solid pattern. In this tumor, the solid areas have almost a trabecular appearance mimicking carcinoid. However, most sclerosing pneumocytomas have a distinctive papillary pattern, and negative staining with endocrine markers and strong TTF-1 positivity essentially would exclude an endocrine tumor.

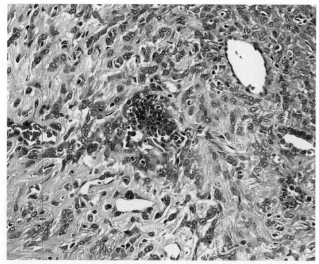

FIGURE 67.5 ▲ Sclerosing pneumocytoma, sclerosing pattern. The sclerosing areas sometimes impart a somewhat spindled appearance, not suggesting an epithelial neoplasm. However, other areas were characteristic, with a papillary growth pattern.

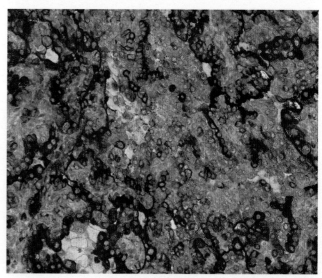

FIGURE 67.8 ▲ Sclerosing pneumocytoma, epithelial membrane antigen. Both cell types express this antigen, surface cells more strongly.

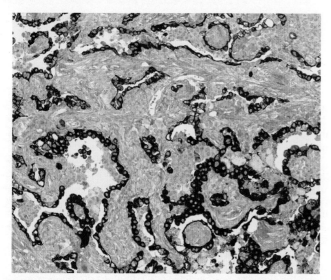

FIGURE 67.6 ▲ Sclerosing pneumocytoma, cytokeratin 7 staining. Only the surface lining cells express cytokeratin 7 staining, and when the rounded cells are positivity, it is usually relatively weak.

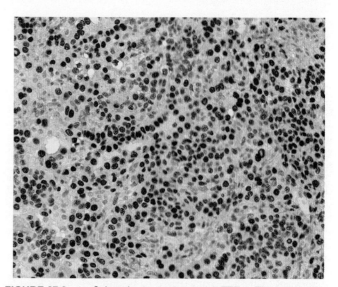

FIGURE 67.9 ▲ Sclerosing pneumocytoma, TTF-1. This marker is expressed equally strongly in both cell populations, which are indistinguishable with this stain. The area was a similar papillary area as shown in the previous three photomicrographs.

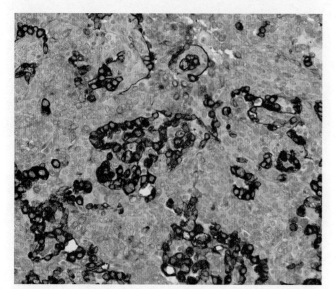

FIGURE 67.7 ▲ Sclerosing pneumocytoma, cam 5.2 (cytokeratin 8/18). There is weak staining of some of the rounded cells and strong staining of the surface cells.

TABLE 67.1 Sclerosing Pneumocytoma[a]

Cell types
Rounded cell (tumor cell)
 AE1/AE3 negative
 Uncommonly cytokeratin 7 or napsin A positive (15%–20%)[a]
 TTF-1 positive
 Vimentin positive
 EMA positive (usually weaker than surface cell)
Surface cell (reactive pneumocyte)
 Pancytokeratin, cytokeratin 7 positive
 TTF-1 positive
 Napsin A positive
 EMA positive (strong)
 Uncommonly vimentin positive (~20%)

Growth patterns
Papillary
Sclerosing
Solid
Hemorrhagic

[a]Distinction from surface cell type indicated in italics.

cytokeratin AE1/AE3 and usually negative (about 80%) for cytokeratin 7 and napsin A. Both populations express TTF-1 and EMA.[3,11,12] Endocrine differentiation with synaptophysin may occur in some tumors, and vimentin is more likely positive in the tumor cells than in the surface cells.[3] In practice, the tumor and reactive cell populations often seem to overlap, but it is generally not difficult to identify that there are two separate cell types.

The clinical behavior of sclerosing pneumocytoma is benign, and there are no reports of recurrence or distant metastasis. However, approximately 5% will demonstrate regional lymph node metastasis,[3,6,13] but follow-up on four patients with regional lymph node involvement showed no progression or recurrence.[14]

The differential diagnosis of sclerosing pneumocytoma is bronchogenic carcinoma, especially papillary adenocarcinoma, metastatic tumor, hamartoma, and carcinoid tumor. In a series from China, where the tumor is relatively common, most sclerosing pneumocytomas were correctly diagnosed on frozen section, although 25% were misdiagnosed as adenocarcinomas or adenosquamous carcinomas.[4] The two biggest clues that the tumor is benign are the circumscription and rounded border (extremely uncommon in primary lung cancers) and monotonous bland histologic features of the tumor (to distinguish from metastasis). On permanent sections, histologic features and immunohistochemical findings readily separate the tumor from hamartoma and carcinoid tumor.

Alveolar Adenoma

Alveolar adenomas are benign tumors of pneumocyte derivation, similar to sclerosing pneumocytoma. However, they have a distinctive histologic appearance and lack the sclerosing or papillary features typical of sclerosing pneumocytoma.

Alveolar adenomas typically present as asymptomatic solitary lung nodules in adults. The reported cases have occurred between the age of 39 and 74. There is no gender predilection, unlike sclerosing pneumocytoma. Avidity with positron emission tomography has been reported.[15] An incidental 1-mm alveolar adenoma was described in a resection specimen for an unrelated lung cancer.[16]

The mean tumor size is somewhat smaller than sclerosing pneumocytoma, reported at 2.2 cm in the largest series.[17] They are well-circumscribed, peripheral nodules that may compress airways resulting in symptoms of cough. The largest alveolar adenoma reported was 10 cm, occurred in the lingula, and compressed adjacent airways, causing dyspnea.

Grossly, alveolar adenomas are soft, multicystic, and mucoid. Histologically, they are well-demarcated tumors composed of cystic spaces lined by cuboidal epithelial cells, which are of pneumocyte origin. The cysts frequently contain eosinophilic proteinaceous material (Fig. 67.10). There is variable thickening of the septa between the cyst

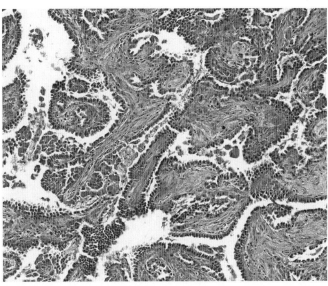

FIGURE 67.11 ▲ Papillary adenoma. There are fibrovascular stalks lined by monomorphous pneumocyte-like epithelial cells. There should be no atypia or mitotic activity, and the lesion should be homogenous and well circumscribed, in contrast to papillary carcinoma.

walls, ranging from thin, alveolar septum–like structures to thick walls with a myxoid stroma rich in spindle cells. Immunohistochemically, the epithelial cells stain with pancytokeratin, cytokeratin AE1/AE2, TTF-1, and surfactant proteins. The stroma is typically formed entirely of fibroblast-like cells, with variable actin staining, although a case with fat and S100-positive cells has been reported,[18] as well as one with CD34-positive stromal cells.[16] The latter finding raises the question if the spindle cells are neoplastic one that has not yet been fully answered. Both epithelial and spindle cells show a low proliferative index.[19]

Miscellaneous Adenomas

Papillary adenomas clinically resemble sclerosing pneumocytomas and alveolar adenomas, in that they are usually asymptomatic solitary lung nodules. There have been only about 25 reported in the literature, and there appears to be a male predominance.[20,21] Histologically, they share features with the papillary type of sclerosing pneumocytoma, but the tumor cells line papillary stalks, and round cells and sclerosis are absent (Fig. 67.11). These tumors are monomorphic papillary proliferations containing fibrovascular cores lined by a single layer of tumor cells that

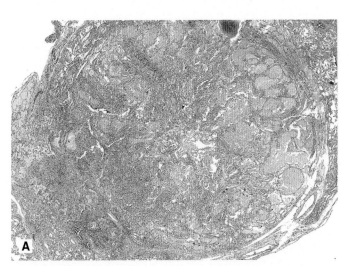

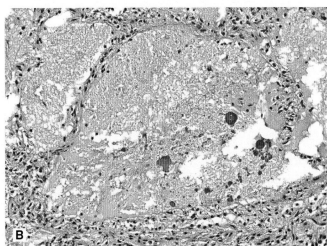

FIGURE 67.10 ▲ Alveolar adenoma. **A.** Low magnification shows a well-circumscribed nodule composed of cysts. **B.** The cysts contain proteinaceous material resembling alveolar proteinosis.

should lack atypia, mitoses, or necrosis. The major differential diagnosis is papillary adenocarcinoma, which differs in that there is tumor heterogeneity, cytologic atypia, and irregular borders. Some tumors diagnosed as papillary adenoma have been described with mitotic activity and p53 expression and may represent a lesion intermediate between adenoma and well-differentiated papillary adenocarcinoma.[20,21]

Pneumocytic adenomyoepithelioma is a recently described benign tumor showing myoepithelial as well as pneumocyte differentiation. Unlike salivary gland tumors, these are believed to derive in part from pneumocytes. The five patients reported were women with single or multiple grossly circumscribed lung nodules.[22] The tumors are biphasic, with epithelial cells lining the inner lining of glandular spaces expressing pneumocyte markers (epithelial membrane antigen, cytokeratin 7, surfactant proteins, and TTF-1) and the stromal spindle cells expressing myoepithelial markers (high molecular weight keratin, smooth muscle actin, S100, calponin, and p63).

Mucus gland adenomas are rare exophytic tumors of the bronchial mucus glands. Histologically, they are composed of mucus-filled cysts, glands, and papillae lined by a mixture of columnar cells, flattened cuboidal cells, goblet cells, oncocytic cells, and clear cells.[23]

Mucinous cystadenoma is an exceedingly rare peripheral lung lesion that has been reported in both males and females, primarily in the sixth and seventh decades.[24]

REFERENCES

1. Satoh Y, Tsuchiya E, Weng SY, et al. Pulmonary sclerosing hemangioma of the lung. A type II pneumocytoma by immunohistochemical and immuno-electron microscopic studies. *Cancer.* 1989;64:1310–1317.
2. Illei PB, Rosai J, Klimstra DS. Expression of thyroid transcription factor-1 and other markers in sclerosing hemangioma of the lung. *Arch Pathol Lab Med.* 2001;125:1335–1339.
3. Devouassoux-Shisheboran M, Hayashi T, Linnoila RI, et al. A clinicopathologic study of 100 cases of pulmonary sclerosing hemangioma with immunohistochemical studies: TTF-1 is expressed in both round and surface cells, suggesting an origin from primitive respiratory epithelium. *Am J Surg Pathol.* 2000;24:906–916.
4. Chen B, Gao J, Chen H, et al. Pulmonary sclerosing hemangioma: a unique epithelial neoplasm of the lung (report of 26 cases). *World J Surg Oncol.* 2013;11:85.
5. Lei Y, Yong D, Jun-Zhong R, et al. Treatment of 28 patients with sclerosing hemangioma (SH) of the lung. *J Cardiothorac Surg.* 2012;7:34.
6. Chan AC, Chan JK. Pulmonary sclerosing hemangioma consistently expresses thyroid transcription factor-1 (TTF-1): a new clue to its histogenesis. *Am J Surg Pathol.* 2000;24:1531–1536.
7. Wang QB, Chen YQ, Shen JJ, et al. Sixteen cases of pulmonary sclerosing haemangioma: CT findings are not definitive for preoperative diagnosis. *Clin Radiol.* 2011;66:708–714.
8. Devouassoux-Shisheboran M, de la Fouchardiere A, Thivolet-Bejui F, et al. Endobronchial variant of sclerosing hemangioma of the lung: histological and cytological features on endobronchial material. *Mod Pathol.* 2004;17:252–257.
9. Kamaleshwaran KK, Rajan F, Mehta S, et al. Multiple pulmonary sclerosing hemangiomas (pneumocytoma) mimicking lung metastasis detected in fluorine-18 fluorodeoxyglucose positron emission tomography/computed tomography. *Indian J Nucl Med.* 2014;29:168–170.
10. Yamazaki K. Type-II pneumocyte differentiation in pulmonary sclerosing hemangioma: ultrastructural differentiation and immunohistochemical distribution of lineage-specific transcription factors (TTF-1, HNF-3 alpha, and HNF-3 beta) and surfactant proteins. *Virchows Arch.* 2004;445:45–53.
11. Rossi G, Cadioli A, Mengoli MC, et al. Napsin A expression in pulmonary sclerosing haemangioma. *Histopathology.* 2012;60:361–363.
12. Schmidt LA, Myers JL, McHugh JB. Napsin A is differentially expressed in sclerosing hemangiomas of the lung. *Arch Pathol Lab Med.* 2012;136:1580–1584.
13. Yano M, Yamakawa Y, Kiriyama M, et al. Sclerosing hemangioma with metastases to multiple nodal stations. *Ann Thorac Surg.* 2002;73:981–983.
14. Miyagawa-Hayashino A, Tazelaar HD, Langel DJ, et al. Pulmonary sclerosing hemangioma with lymph node metastases: report of 4 cases. *Arch Pathol Lab Med.* 2003;127:321–325.
15. Nosotti M, Mendogni P, Rosso L, et al. Alveolar adenoma of the lung: unusual diagnosis of a lesion positive on PET scan. A case report. *J Cardiothorac Surg.* 2012;7:1.
16. Bhavsar T, Uppal G, Travaline JM, et al. An unusual case of a microscopic alveolar adenoma coexisting with lung carcinoma: a case report and review of the literature. *J Med Case Rep.* 2011;5:187.
17. Burke LM, Rush WI, Khoor A, et al. Alveolar adenoma: a histochemical, immunohistochemical, and ultrastructural analysis of 17 cases. *Hum Pathol.* 1999;30:158–167.
18. Cavazza A, Paci M, De Marco L, et al. Alveolar adenoma of the lung: a clinicopathologic, immunohistochemical, and molecular study of an unusual case. *Int J Surg Pathol.* 2004;12:155–159.
19. Sak SD, Koseoglu RD, Demirag F, et al. Alveolar adenoma of the lung. Immunohistochemical and flow cytometric characteristics of two new cases and a review of the literature. *APMIS.* 2007;115:1443–1449.
20. Cornejo KM, Shi M, Akalin A, et al. Pulmonary papillary adenoma: a case report and review of the literature. *J Bronchology Interv Pulmonol.* 2013;20:52–57.
21. Nakano T, Yokose T, Hasegawa C, et al. Papillary adenoma of the lung with a peculiar raw macroscopic feature. *Pathol Int.* 2011;61:475–480.
22. Chang T, Husain AN, Colby T, et al. Pneumocytic adenomyoepithelioma: a distinctive lung tumor with epithelial, myoepithelial, and pneumocytic differentiation. *Am J Surg Pathol.* 2007;31:562–568.
23. England DM, Hochholzer L. Truly benign "bronchial adenoma". Report of 10 cases of mucous gland adenoma with immunohistochemical and ultrastructural findings. *Am J Surg Pathol.* 1995;19:887–899.
24. Gao ZH, Urbanski SJ. The spectrum of pulmonary mucinous cystic neoplasia: a clinicopathologic and immunohistochemical study of ten cases and review of literature. *Am J Clin Pathol.* 2005;124:62–70.

68 Inflammatory Myofibroblastic Tumor

Eunhee S. Yi, M.D., Jennifer M. Boland, M.D., and Marie-Christine Aubry, M.D.

Introduction

Inflammatory myofibroblastic tumor (IMT) is a neoplasm characterized by a proliferation of fibroblasts and myofibroblasts mixed with varying numbers of plasma cells, lymphocytes, macrophages, and other inflammatory cells on histopathologic examination.[1] IMT has formely been known under various other names including plasma cell granuloma, inflammatory pseudotumor (IPT), and xanthomatous pseudotumor.[1] IPT was regarded as an entirely reactive lesion until recently, when it became apparent that some cases represented a true myofibroblastic neoplasm evidenced by a clonal gene rearrangement involving chromosome 2p23, which encodes the *ALK* gene.[2] The term IMT is now preferred to define a true neoplasm, while the term IPT or plasma cell granuloma is used for nonneoplastic fibroinflammatory localized processes, which are not IMT or other specific entities such as IgG4-related disease (see Chapter 51). Under the rubric of IPT, various nonneoplastic processes were included in the past, such as pulmonary nodular lymphoid hyperplasia (also known as pseudolymphoma), postinfectious fibroinflammatory lesions, nodular presentation of organizing pneumonia, and other nonspecific fibroinflammatory processes. The distinction of IMT from these other conditions is very important, and the term IPT should no longer be used to encompass IMT, which is a true neoplasm with somewhat unpredictable biologic behavior; IMTs, especially those in the extrapulmonary sites, have the potential for locally aggressive growth, recurrence, and even distant metastases in rare cases.

Clinical Features

The lung is a relatively common site for IMT, along with abdominal cavity and retroperitoneum.[3–6] Pulmonary IMTs occur most commonly in children and young adults,[5] but the observed age range is quite broad.[3,4] A subset of patients (up to 20%) with IMT will present with a systemic inflammatory syndrome, which may include fever, weight loss, malaise, anemia, thrombocytosis, leukocytosis, elevated sedimentation rate, and hypergammaglobulinemia.[3,5] Patients with pulmonary IMT may also present with localizing symptoms, especially if the tumor is endobronchial, which include cough, dyspnea, and hemoptysis.[4,5]

Radiologic Features

Agrons et al. described the radiographic features in 61 cases of pulmonary IPT, which likely includes both IMT and nonneoplastic conditions.[7] Fifty-two of their 61 patients (85%) had a solitary peripheral nodule or mass, and 11 (18%) patients had extraparenchymal involvement including hilar, mediastinal, and airway invasion. On computed tomography (CT) scan, 12 lesions had heterogeneous attenuation while 5 lesions were homogenous.[7] FDG uptake in IMTs varies from low to high, which may be due to variability in tumor cellularity, biologic behavior of the tumor cells, the composition and proportion of inflammatory cells, and the extent of activation of the inflammatory cells, according to a retrospective study using 18F-FDG–PET/CT scan.[8]

Prognosis and Treatment

The biologic behavior of IMT is unpredictable, and thus, these lesions should be completely excised if possible, and patients should have long-term follow-up to monitor for recurrence or metastasis.[5] While most cases of IMT will be cured by surgical excision, ~25% will show locally aggressive behavior with recurrence. Although rare, distant metastases have occurred to the mediastinum, chest wall, liver, lung, and brain.[3,5] ALK-negative IMTs seem more likely to metastasize, but other histologic features are not reliable predictors of behavior, and thus, all patients should be followed closely.[3,5]

At present, surgery is the principal treatment, although nonsteroidal anti-inflammatory drugs, anti-TNF alpha antibody, corticosteroids, and chemotherapy have been reported in a few cases.[9] There is some evidence that patients with IMTs harboring ALK rearrangements may benefit from the ALK and ROS1 inhibitor crizotinib.[10]

Gross Findings

IMTs are typically lobulated and circumscribed fleshy masses.[3] They vary widely in size (1 to 15 cm) and may be endobronchial or parenchymal.[4,11] Most tumors are solitary, but multiple masses may occur.[5,11] Involvement of the chest wall or mediastinum is rare.[4,11]

Histologic Findings

The neoplastic cells of IMT are the myofibroblasts/fibroblasts, which are usually plump and spindle shaped with indistinct cell borders, and grow in a fascicular pattern (Fig. 68.1).[4,11,12] These cells typically lack cytologic atypia or show only mild atypia.[11] The spindle cell component is admixed and may be partially obscured by mixed chronic inflammatory cells, which typically include prominent plasma cells (Fig. 68.1) with a more variable number of lymphocytes and eosinophils, while neutrophils are infrequent.[3] The morphology may be quite variable depending on the proportion of spindled and inflammatory components, as well as the presence of other secondary changes that can be observed in some cases, including collagen deposition, myxoid change,

and edema.[12] Many IMTs contain characteristic large epithelioid myofibroblasts that resemble ganglion cells, which have vesicular chromatin and prominent red nucleoli.[3] Rare examples of IMT have an entirely epithelioid morphology, which has been associated with a poor prognosis.[13] Atypical histologic features may occur in a subset of IMT, characterized by high cellularity, pleomorphism, necrosis, prominent fascicular or herringbone growth pattern, and brisk mitotic activity.[3]

Ancillary Studies

Spindle cells of IMT are usually positive for smooth muscle actin but variable for desmin and usually negative for myogenin, myoglobin, CD117, and S100 protein, in keeping with a myofibroblastic immunophenotype. Low molecular weight keratin expression is observed in up to one-third of IMTs, which is a potential diagnostic pitfall.[12] ALK is positive in ~40% to 50% of IMT (Fig. 68.1) patients, who are usually younger than 40 years of age, while ALK positivity is much lower in the older patients. p53 positivity is rare and reported in association with recurrence and malignant transformation.[14] The plasma cells are polyclonal.

About half of IMTs show recurrent rearrangement of the ALK gene, resulting in fusion with various partner genes including TPM3 and TPM4, which is in keeping with cytoplasmic ALK protein expression detectable by immunohistochemistry.[3,15] Recently, alternative rearrangements involving the ROS1, RET, and PDGFRβ genes have been noted in IMTs that are negative for ALK rearrangement.[6,16] The EML4–ALK fusion first described in pulmonary adenocarcinoma has also been observed in IMTs.[6] Tumors showing these rearrangements are more common in children and young adults and are uncommon in older adults, similar to ALK protein expression.[3,6] In ambiguous or difficult cases, FISH using an ALK break-apart probe may be useful to support the diagnosis of IMT; FISH testing for ROS1 or RET fusions could also be performed if inhibitors of these tyrosine kinases are being considered therapeutically. However, since not all IMTs harbor these fusions, negativity for these rearrangements does not exclude the diagnosis. A recent study reported that expression of ROS1 protein predicted ROS1 gene rearrangement in IMTs.[17]

Differential Diagnosis

Cellular examples of IMT may be confused with a variety of benign and malignant spindle cell neoplasms (especially malignant fibrous histiocytoma, smooth muscle neoplasms, inflammatory sarcomatoid carcinoma, etc.), but careful attention to the inflammatory background and incorporation of immunohistochemical data and clinical/radiographic features should lead to the correct diagnosis of IMT in most cases. The differential diagnosis of IMT may also vary depending on the degree of inflammatory cell infiltrate in the tumor. The mix of bland spindled cells and inflammation may mimic a reactive process. In fact, it can be quite difficult to differentiate ALK-negative IMT from (nonneoplastic) IPT, especially in older individuals (Fig. 68.2). Inflammatory or infectious processes should be considered, especially in cases where the inflammation partially obscures the myofibroblastic component. Pulmonary IPT generally contains hypocellular fibrosis and mixed chronic inflammatory infiltrate and typically lacks the plump robust myofibroblastic component typical of true IMT. Pulmonary IgG4-related disease may manifest as IPT as in other organs, but the presence of storiform fibrosis, obliterative phlebitis or arteritis, and a marked increase in IgG4-positive plasma cells (typically >50/hpf with >40% in IgG4/IgG ratio) as well as the clinical features are helpful in making the diagnosis of IgG4-related disease (see Chapter 51). It should be noted that a mild to moderate increase in IgG4-positive plasma cells has been noted in some cases of IMT.[18] Thus, increased IgG4-positive cell count alone should not be used to make a diagnosis of IgG4-related disease.

Some IPT or its mimics may be related to an infection or postinfectious sequella. Human herpesvirus or Epstein-Barr virus has been implicated in the pathogenesis of IPT,[19,20] but other studies have failed to confirm this finding.[21–23] Mycobacterial spindle cell pseudotumor (MSP) involving the lung may mimic IPT or IMT[24] (see Chapter 40).

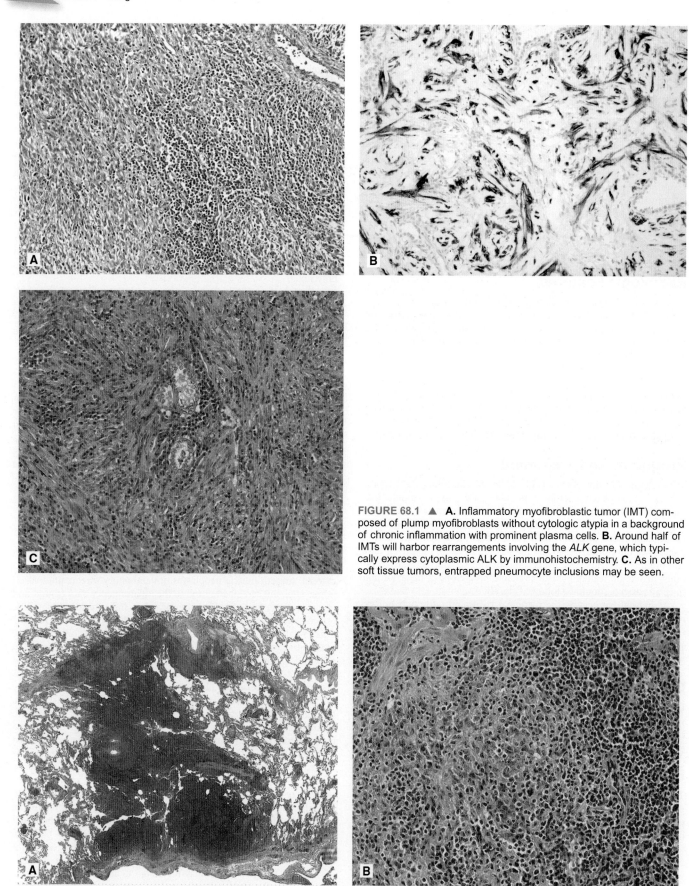

FIGURE 68.1 ▲ **A.** Inflammatory myofibroblastic tumor (IMT) composed of plump myofibroblasts without cytologic atypia in a background of chronic inflammation with prominent plasma cells. **B.** Around half of IMTs will harbor rearrangements involving the *ALK* gene, which typically express cytoplasmic ALK by immunohistochemistry. **C.** As in other soft tissue tumors, entrapped pneumocyte inclusions may be seen.

FIGURE 68.2 ▲ Nonneoplastic inflammatory pseudotumor (plasma cell granuloma) shows a mass lesion that has a less circumscribed outline than IMT **(A)**, and shows a spindle cell proliferation with heavy inflammatory infiltrate including plasma cells, vaguely reminiscent of neoplastic IMT **(B)** (H&E, 20× and 200×, respectively).

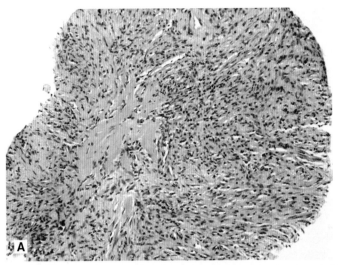
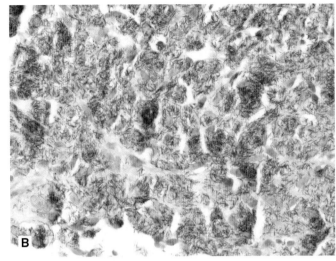

FIGURE 68.3 ▲ Mycobacterial spindle cell pseudotumor may mimic IMT (**A**, H&E, 200×) but is composed of histiocytes containing numerous acid-fast bacilli (**B**, Ziehl-Neelsen staining, 200×).

However, the spindle cells in MSP are histiocytes, not myofibroblasts or fibroblasts, and contain numerous acid-fast bacilli (Fig. 68.3). Therapeutic approaches to MSP will be different from those to IMT or IPT of noninfectious origin for the obvious reasons, and a thorough evaluation to exclude a treatable infection such as MSP is important whenever a histopathologic diagnosis of IMT or IPT is made.

Practical Points

▶ IMT is a true neoplasm that occurs most commonly in children or young adults, with clonal translocation involving 2p23 region encoding *ALK* gene in 40% to 50% of patients.

▶ IMT is usually an indolent neoplasm but may follow an unpredictable or aggressive clinical course.

▶ IPT (also known as plasma cell granuloma) has historically encompassed both nonneoplastic (i.e., pseudotumor) and neoplastic processes, but this term should not be used for true IMT.

▶ Use of the term IPT should be limited to the mass-forming fibroinflammatory conditions that do not fit any currently defined categories such as IgG4-related disease, nodular lymphoid hyperplasia, and organizing pneumonia.

▶ Infection needs to be carefully excluded for an appropriate treatment.

REFERENCES

1. Bahadori M, Liebow AA. Plasma cell granulomas of the lung. *Cancer.* 1973;31(1):191–208.
2. Snyder CS, et al. Clonal changes in inflammatory pseudotumor of the lung: a case report. *Cancer.* 1995;76(9):1545–1549.
3. Coffin CM, Hornick JL, Fletcher CD. Inflammatory myofibroblastic tumor: comparison of clinicopathologic, histologic, and immunohistochemical features including ALK expression in atypical and aggressive cases. *Am J Surg Pathol.* 2007;31(4):509–520.
4. Pettinato G, et al. Inflammatory myofibroblastic tumor (plasma cell granuloma). Clinicopathologic study of 20 cases with immunohistochemical and ultrastructural observations. *Am J Clin Pathol.* 1990;94(5):538–546.
5. Chun YS, et al. Pediatric inflammatory myofibroblastic tumor: anaplastic lymphoma kinase (ALK) expression and prognosis. *Pediatr Blood Cancer.* 2005;45(6):796–801.
6. Antonescu CR, et al. Molecular characterization of inflammatory myofibroblastic tumors with frequent ALK and ROS1 gene fusions and rare novel RET rearrangement. *Am J Surg Pathol.* 2015;39:957–967.
7. Agrons GA, et al. Pulmonary inflammatory pseudotumor: radiologic features. *Radiology.* 1998;206(2):511–518.
8. Dong A, et al. Inflammatory myofibroblastic tumor: FDG PET/CT findings with pathologic correlation. *Clin Nucl Med.* 2014;39(2):113–121.
9. Myers JL, Colby TV. Pathologic manifestations of bronchiolitis, constrictive bronchiolitis, cryptogenic organizing pneumonia, and diffuse panbronchiolitis. *Clin Chest Med.* 1993;14(4):611–622.
10. Butrynski JE, et al. Crizotinib in ALK-rearranged inflammatory myofibroblastic tumor. *N Engl J Med.* 2010;363(18):1727–1733.
11. Travis WD, et al. WHO classification of tumours of the lung, pleura, thymus and heart. In: Bosman FT, et al., eds. *WHO Classification of Tumours.* Lyon: IARC Press; 2015:341.
12. Fletcher CD, et al. Tumors of soft tissue and bone. In: Bosman FT, et al., eds., *WHO Classification.* Lyon, France: IARC Press; 2013:468.
13. Marino-Enriquez A, et al. Epithelioid inflammatory myofibroblastic sarcoma: an aggressive intra-abdominal variant of inflammatory myofibroblastic tumor with nuclear membrane or perinuclear ALK. *Am J Surg Pathol.* 2011;35(1):135–144.
14. Ledet SC, Brown RW, Cagle PT. p53 immunostaining in the differentiation of inflammatory pseudotumor from sarcoma involving the lung. *Mod Pathol.* 1995;8(3):282–286.
15. Lawrence B, et al. TPM3-ALK and TPM4-ALK oncogenes in inflammatory myofibroblastic tumors. *Am J Pathol.* 2000;157(2):377–384.
16. Lovly CM, et al. Inflammatory myofibroblastic tumors harbor multiple potentially actionable kinase fusions. *Cancer Discov.* 2014;4(8):889–895.
17. Hornick JL, et al. Expression of ROS1 predicts ROS1 gene rearrangement in inflammatory myofibroblastic tumors. *Mod Pathol.* 2015;28(5):732–739.
18. Saab ST, et al. IgG4 plasma cells in inflammatory myofibroblastic tumor: inflammatory marker or pathogenic link? *Mod Pathol.* 2011;24(4):606–612.
19. Gomez-Roman JJ, et al. Human herpesvirus-8 genes are expressed in pulmonary inflammatory myofibroblastic tumor (inflammatory pseudotumor). *Am J Surg Pathol.* 2001;25(5):624–629.
20. Kutok JL, et al. Inflammatory pseudotumor of lymph node and spleen: an entity biologically distinct from inflammatory myofibroblastic tumor. *Hum Pathol.* 2001;32(12):1382–1387.
21. Tavora F, et al. Absence of human herpesvirus-8 in pulmonary inflammatory myofibroblastic tumor: immunohistochemical and molecular analysis of 20 cases. *Mod Pathol.* 2007;20(9):995–999.
22. Yamamoto H, et al. Absence of human herpesvirus-8 and Epstein-Barr virus in inflammatory myofibroblastic tumor with anaplastic large cell lymphoma kinase fusion gene. *Pathol Int.* 2006;56(10):584–590.
23. Swain RS, et al. Inflammatory myofibroblastic tumor of the central nervous system and its relationship to inflammatory pseudotumor. *Hum Pathol.* 2008;39(3):410–419.
24. Philip J, Beasley MB, Dua S. Mycobacterial spindle cell pseudotumor of the lung. *Chest.* 2012;142(3):783–784.

69 Hamartoma and Chondroma

Marie-Christine Aubry, M.D., and Fabio R. Tavora, M.D., Ph.D.

General

Hamartoma and chondroma are neoplasms with overlapping histologic features, mainly the presence of cartilage. However, they are distinct and should be separated from each other because of the potential clinical implication of a diagnosis of chondroma. Hamartomas are the most common benign tumor of the lung and are composed of various soft tissue components beyond cartilage, including adipose tissue and smooth muscle, with entrapped reactive bronchiolar epithelium. Hamartomas occur most commonly in older men (reported ratio of ~2:1 and mean age of 65 years).[1] They are typically asymptomatic solitary lesions found during investigation of various medical or surgical conditions or incidentally found during surgical resection of lung cancers.[1,2] In contrast, chondromas are rare benign cartilaginous neoplasms, typically presenting in patients with Carney triad, a rare disorder that includes gastrointestinal stromal tumors, extra-adrenal paragangliomas, and other neoplasms and thus affecting predominantly young women with incidental multiple nodules.[3] Chondromas may also be sporadic, occurring in older men as incidental solitary nodules.[3]

Radiologic Findings

Hamartomas are most commonly peripheral lesions (>90%) but can present as endobronchial lesions. They are distributed evenly in the right and left lung and show no lobe predilection. Hamartomas form well-demarcated lobulated nodules or masses (Fig. 69.1). Imaging by CT scan is often considered diagnostic if popcorn-like calcifications and/or fat density is identified.[4] However, these findings are not always present and have also been described in chondromas. Rare cases of PET-positive hamartomas have been reported.[5]

Chondromas are also evenly distributed among the lobes. They are described as round or lobulated well-circumscribed nodules. These tumors are often calcified, and calcifications are described as central, popcorn-like, or peripheral[3] (Fig. 69.2).

Gross Findings

Hamartomas vary in size with an average size of 1.5 to 2 cm, but tumors over 25 cm have been described and are often referred to as giant hamartoma.[1,2,6] They are well-circumscribed, lobulated, firm lesions that typically shell out from the surrounding lung[1] (Fig. 69.1).

Chondromas range in size between 1 and 9 cm and have an average size of 3 cm. They are described as well circumscribed and bosselated with a gritty cut surface of white color (Fig. 69.2). They are occasionally cystic or hemorrhagic.[3]

Microscopic Findings

Hamartomas are lobulated with entrapped benign bronchiolar epithelium lining the lobules. The lobules are typically composed of a combination of hyaline cartilage, fibromyxoid soft tissue, mature adipose tissue, and smooth muscle[1] (Figs. 69.3 and 69.4). Calcification and ossification of the cartilage may occur. Occasionally, a single soft tissue component predominates, not uncommonly hindering the diagnosis. These hamartomas have been described under other names such as lipomatous hamartoma,[7] adenoleiomyomatous hamartoma,[8] or adenofibroma (Fig. 69.5).[9] Diagnosis of pulmonary hamartoma on fine needle aspiration has been reported, but the features overlap with other biphasic tumors and tissue sample may be required for the correct diagnosis.[10]

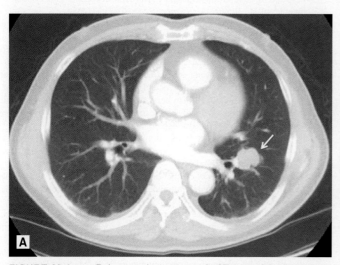
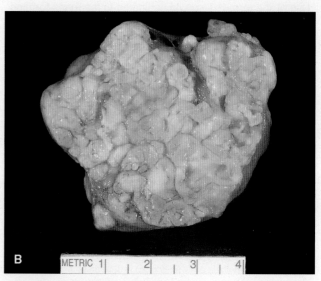

FIGURE 69.1 ▲ Pulmonary hamartoma. **A.** CT scan of the lung shows a well-demarcated lobulated tumor in the left lower lobe. Focally, peripheral calcification is seen. **B.** Gross photograph displaying the typical lobulated, so-called popcorn, appearance of hamartoma. The glistening white appearance indicates predominance of cartilage in this tumor.

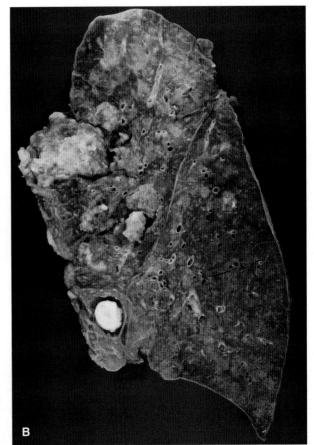

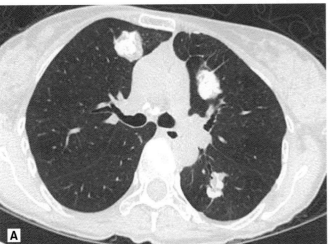

FIGURE 69.2 ▲ Pulmonary chondroma. **A.** Chest CT scan from patient with Carney triad shows multiple partially calcified nodules. **B.** The gross appearance of the chondroma reveals a well-circumscribed mass with a yellow-white gritty cut surface due to the typically calcified and ossified cartilage.

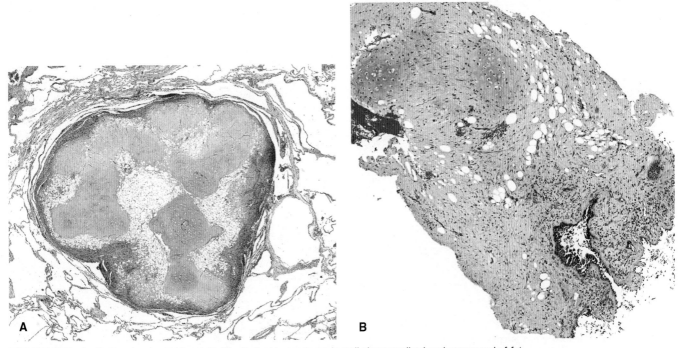

FIGURE 69.3 ▲ Pulmonary hamartoma. **A.** The typical hamartoma is well circumscribed and composed of fat, cartilage, and epithelial cells. **B.** Pulmonary hamartoma may be diagnosed on small biopsies if a combination of various soft tissue components is present as in this case.

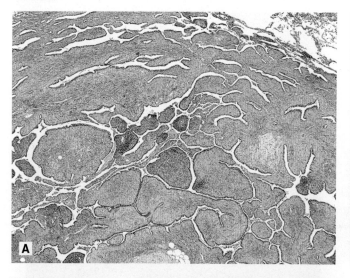

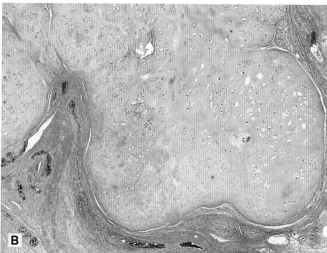

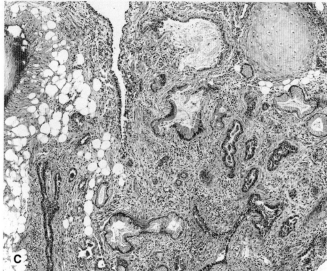

FIGURE 69.4 ▲ Pulmonary hamartoma. **A.** A characteristic histologic feature is the lobulated appearance causing benign airway epithelium to become entrapped between the lobules. This hamartoma is characterized by the predominance of a spindle cell proliferation with mild adipose tissue. **B.** This hamartoma contains predominantly cartilage but retains its characteristic lobulation. **C.** Occasionally, when hamartoma arises in proximity to a large airway, the benign submucosal glands become entrapped and distorted. This feature can occasionally be confused with glandular malignancy.

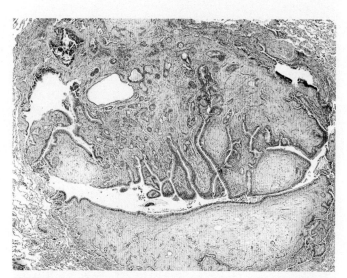

FIGURE 69.5 ▲ Pulmonary hamartoma may be composed predominantly of a proliferation of fibroblasts with entrapped benign epithelium, so-called adenofibroma. The lobulated appearance is apparent at the periphery of the tumor.

Chondromas are distinguished from hamartomas by their lack of lobulation, forming a smooth round nodule separated from the adjacent lung parenchyma by a fibrous pseudocapsule without entrapment of benign epithelium[3] (Fig. 69.6). They are almost exclusively composed of cartilage that is commonly calcified and ossified. The cartilage is often myxoid, moderately cellular with no significant cytologic atypia.[3] Adipose tissue may be present as part of bone marrow within the ossification.

Ancillary Studies

There are no diagnostic ancillary studies in the diagnosis of hamartoma or chondroma. The diagnosis relies on histomorphologic characteristics. By immunohistochemistry, estrogen receptor and progesterone receptor may be expressed primarily in the stromal component. The spindle cells also stain for vimentin, S100 protein, glial fibrillary acid protein, smooth muscle actin, and calponin suggesting incomplete myoepithelial differentiation.[11]

Gains of chromosome 6 and loss of 1q have been reported in chondromas of patients with Carney triad.[12]

Differential Diagnosis

The main differential diagnosis with chondroid hamartoma and chondroma is chondrosarcoma, primary or metastatic. Even a predominantly chondroid hamartoma will have another soft tissue component

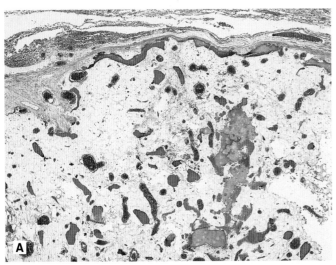
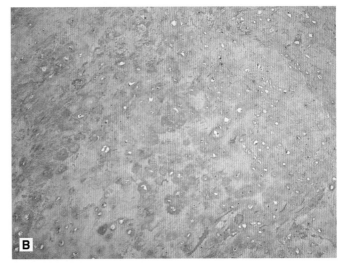

FIGURE 69.6 ▲ Pulmonary chondroma. **A.** The interface between the lung and the chondroma is smooth, not lobulated, demarcated by a fibrous pseudocapsule with no entrapped epithelium. This example of chondroma shows extensive bone metaplasia with bone marrow adipose tissue. **B.** Chondroma is composed of cartilage, which may be hyaline and/or myxoid. Mild cytologic atypia can be seen.

and maintain its lobulated architecture with entrapped epithelium, which makes it readily distinguishable from chondrosarcoma. The distinction of chondroma from chondrosarcoma is more challenging and may not be possible on a small biopsy sample. Typically, chondrosarcoma displays increased cytologic atypia with binucleation and cellularity compared to chondroma.

Prognosis and Predictive Factors

Hamartomas are usually benign and do not recur following resection.[1] There are case reports of malignant transformation of the epithelial and mesenchymal components, including salivary gland–type tumor,[13] well-differentiated liposarcoma, and undifferentiated sarcoma.[14] Hamartomas can be suspected radiologically and be followed in some cases. Cases without the typical radiologic characteristics are usually resected, and frozen section can be performed to avoid large resections such as lobectomies.

Chondromas in Carney triad frequently recur, but no cases of metastasis or related death have been reported.[3]

Practical Points

▶ Hamartomas and chondromas are distinct benign lung neoplasms.

▶ Hamartomas are typically incidental and sporadic, while chondromas are most often diagnosed in Carney triad.

▶ Hamartomas are lobulated mesenchymal neoplasms with entrapped epithelium. The mesenchymal components include cartilage, adipose tissue, and smooth muscle in variable amount. Any soft tissue component may predominate.

▶ In contrast, chondromas are smooth contoured with a pseudocapsule and composed solely of cartilage, which may exhibit osseous metaplasia.

▶ The distinction between chondroid predominant hamartoma, chondroma, and chondrosarcoma is often not possible on a small biopsy specimen.

REFERENCES

1. Gjevre JA, Myers JL, Prakash UB. Pulmonary hamartomas. *Mayo Clin Proc.* 1996;71:14–20.
2. Salminen US. Pulmonary hamartoma. A clinical study of 77 cases in a 21-year period and review of literature. *Eur J Cardiothorac Surg.* 1990;4:15–18.
3. Rodriguez FJ, Aubry MC, Tazelaar HD, et al. Pulmonary chondroma: a tumor associated with Carney triad and different from pulmonary hamartoma. *Am J Surg Pathol.* 2007;31:1844–1853.
4. Siegelman SS, Khouri NF, Scott WW Jr, et al. Pulmonary hamartoma: CT findings. *Radiology.* 1986;160:313–317.
5. Himpe U, Deroose CM, Leyn PD, et al. Unexpected slight fluorodeoxyglucose-uptake on positron emission tomography in a pulmonary hamartoma. *J Thorac Oncol.* 2009;4:107–108.
6. Ganti S, Milton R, Davidson L, et al. Giant pulmonary hamartoma. *J Cardiothorac Surg.* 2006;1:19.
7. Tsitouridis I, Michaelides M, Kyriakou V, et al. Endobronchial lipomatous hamartoma with mediastinal extension. *J Thorac Imaging.* 2010;25:W6–W9.
8. Kara M, Onder S, Firat P, et al. A rare histological presentation of a common lung tumor: adenoleiomyomatous hamartoma. *Acta Chir Belg.* 2012;112:74–76.
9. Kumar R, Desai S, Pai T, et al. Pulmonary adenofibroma: clinicopathological study of 3 cases of a rare benign lung lesion and review of the literature. *Ann Diagn Pathol.* 2014;18:238–243.
10. Vitkovski T, Zeltsman D, Esposito M, et al. Pulmonary adenofibroma: cytologic and clinicopathologic features of a rare benign primary lung lesion. *Diagn Cytopathol.* 2013;41:991–996.
11. Pelosi G, Rosai J, Viale G. Immunoreactivity for sex steroid hormone receptors in pulmonary hamartomas. *Am J Surg Pathol.* 2006;30:819–827.
12. Stratakis CA, Carney JA. The triad of paragangliomas, gastric stromal tumours and pulmonary chondromas (Carney triad), and the dyad of paragangliomas and gastric stromal sarcomas (Carney-Stratakis syndrome): molecular genetics and clinical implications. *J Intern Med.* 2009;266:43–52.
13. Pelosi G, Rodriguez J, Viale G, et al. Salivary gland-type tumors with myoepithelial differentiation arising in pulmonary hamartoma: report of 2 cases of a hitherto unrecognized association. *Am J Surg Pathol.* 2006;30:375–387.
14. Trahan S, Erickson-Johnson MR, Rodriguez F, et al. Formation of the 12q14-q15 amplicon precedes the development of a well-differentiated liposarcoma arising from a nonchondroid pulmonary hamartoma. *Am J Surg Pathol.* 2006;30:1326–1329.

70 Meningothelial-Like Nodule

Allen P. Burke, M.D., and Marie-Christine Aubry, M.D.

General

Meningothelial-like nodules (MLNs) have several designations, including "minute meningothelial-like nodule," "meningothelial nodules," and "chemodectoma." They are quite common as incidental findings and only rarely cause pulmonary symptoms, when diffuse and bilateral in so-called *diffuse pulmonary meningotheliomatosis*.[1] Although they were initially thought to be neuroendocrine and therefore called chemodectoma, subsequent studies confirmed the meningothelial nature of the cells of MLN.[2]

Histogenesis

The cells of MLN share many features with cells of meningiomas, including histologic appearance, ultrastructural finding, and frequent immunohistochemical expression of epithelial membrane antigen and CD56. MLNs have not been reported in children; hence, they are not thought to be congenital. A loss of heterozygosity (LOH) study comparing single MLN to meningiomas found multiple events only in meningiomas. The same study demonstrated that cases of multiple MLNs (meningotheliomatosis) occasionally harbored multiple LOH events, but at a lower rate than meningiomas, suggesting that single MLNs are reactive and that multiple tumors may represent the transition between a reactive and neoplastic proliferation.[3]

Incidence and Clinical Presentation

Meningothelial nodules are common, and many are likely overlooked. The incidence in lung resections for other conditions ranges from 7% to 42%.[4,5] They are twice as common in women as men, without predilection for any lobe. They are increased in frequency in resections for malignancies, especially adenocarcinomas, as opposed to benign conditions,[4] and are also common in lung resections showing infarcts, thromboembolic disease, and respiratory bronchiolitis.[5] They are multiple in over 50% of cases.[5] In rare patients, MLN may be so numerous as to mimic an interstitial lung disease or metastatic malignancy. Indeed, these patients present with shortness of breath with mild restriction on pulmonary function tests and bilateral reticulonodular infiltrates radiologically. This disease manifestation has been called *diffuse pulmonary meningotheliomatosis*.[1]

Microscopic Findings

Histologically, MLNs range in size from 1 to 4 mm and are randomly located throughout the lung. They are composed of monotonous, bland, ovoid to spindle cells that form stellate structures that typically insinuate into alveolar septa (Fig. 70.1). The cells have indistinct cell borders, and the nuclei have a fine chromatin pattern (Fig. 70.2). Occasionally, the tumor cells may form whorls, and pseudonuclear inclusions are seen. No atypia or mitotic activity is appreciated. Immunohistochemically, the cells are positive for CD56, progesterone receptor, and vimentin and negative for keratins, S100 protein, melan-A, chromogranin A, synaptophysin, and TTF-1 (Fig. 70.3).[5,6] Although studies often report a 100% staining for epithelial membrane antigen,[1,6] one group found that only one in three MNL was positive.[3]

Differential Diagnosis

Occasionally, it may be difficult to distinguish an MLN from a *carcinoid tumorlet* (Chapter 81). The latter is more discrete, often in a fibrous background, located centered on a bronchiole. If in doubt,

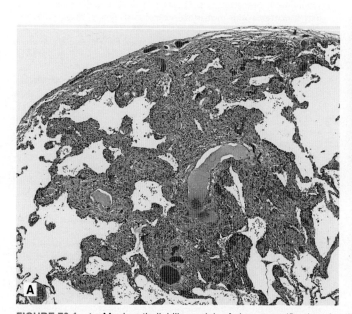
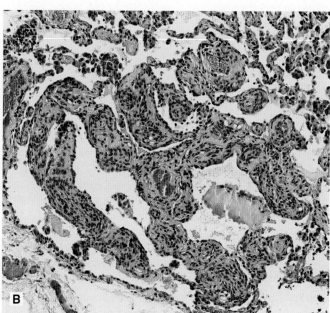

FIGURE 70.1 ▲ Meningothelial-like nodule. **A.** Low magnification showing irregular-shaped nodule with the tumor cells insinuated within alveolar septa. The appearance is often not that of a discrete solid nodule but rather nodular interstitial thickening by the tumor cells. **B.** Another example demonstrating the interstitial growth pattern of most MLN.

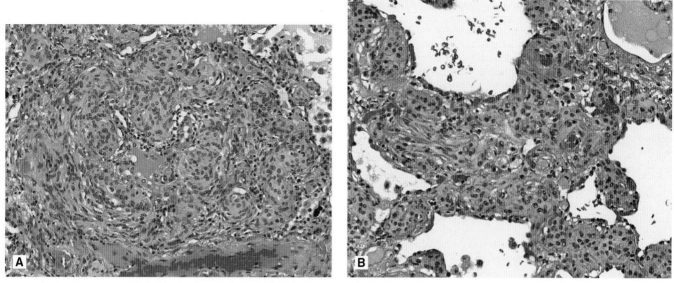

FIGURE 70.2 ▲ Meningothelial-like nodule. **A.** A higher magnification demonstrates bland spindled cells forming whorls reminiscent of meningioma. **B.** The cells have indistinct cell borders, and many of the nuclei contain pseudoinclusions.

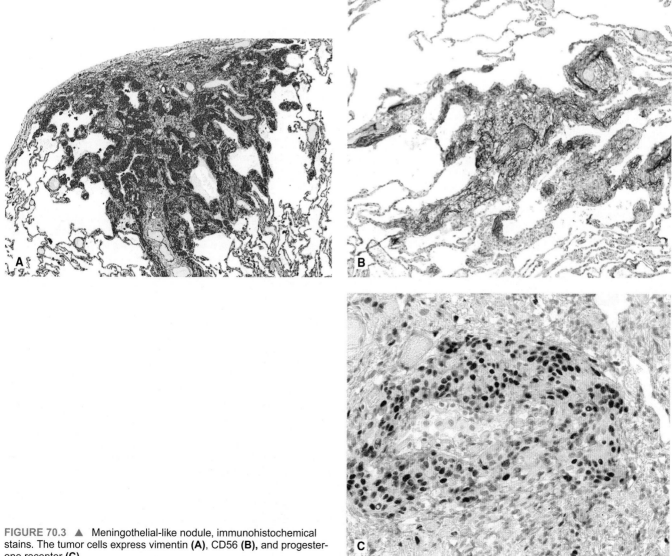

FIGURE 70.3 ▲ Meningothelial-like nodule, immunohistochemical stains. The tumor cells express vimentin **(A)**, CD56 **(B),** and progesterone receptor **(C)**.

positive staining for keratins, chromogranin, and TTF-1 will confirm a diagnosis of carcinoid tumorlet and exclude MLN.

Primary pulmonary meningioma is an extremely rare lesion that is easily distinguished from MLN by a larger size, solid nodule, and histologic features similar to meningeal meningioma[7] (see Chapter 94).

Metastatic meningioma from a meningeal primary could theoretically cause confusion with MLN. Distant metastasis occurs in 0.1% to 0.7% of meningiomas, most commonly to the lung, usually from high-grade tumors. Lung metastases are much larger than MLN, usually 1 to 3 cm,[8,9] and generally occur after resection of the primary meningeal lesion, although presentation as a lung mass has been reported.[10]

REFERENCES

1. Suster S, Moran CA. Diffuse pulmonary meningotheliomatosis. *Am J Surg Pathol.* 2007;31:624–631.
2. Churg AM, Warnock ML. So-called "minute pulmonary chemodectoma": a tumor not related to paragangliomas. *Cancer.* 1976;37:1759–1769.
3. Ionescu DN, Sasatomi E, Aldeeb D, et al. Pulmonary meningothelial-like nodules: a genotypic comparison with meningiomas. *Am J Surg Pathol.* 2004;28:207–214.
4. Mizutani E, Tsuta K, Maeshima AM, et al. Minute pulmonary meningothelial-like nodules: clinicopathologic analysis of 121 patients. *Hum Pathol.* 2009;40:678–682.
5. Mukhopadhyay S, El-Zammar OA, Katzenstein AL. Pulmonary meningothelial-like nodules: new insights into a common but poorly understood entity. *Am J Surg Pathol.* 2009;33:487–495.
6. Niho S, Yokose T, Nishiwaki Y, et al. Immunohistochemical and clonal analysis of minute pulmonary meningothelial-like nodules. *Hum Pathol.* 1999;30:425–429.
7. Weber C, Pautex S, Zulian GB, et al. Primary pulmonary malignant meningioma with lymph node and liver metastasis in a centenary woman, an autopsy case. *Virchows Arch.* 2013;462:481–485.
8. Kanzaki R, Higashiyama M, Fujiwara A, et al. Surgical resection of pulmonary metastases from meningioma: report of a case. *Surg Today.* 2011;41:995–998.
9. Nakayama Y, Horio H, Horiguchi S, et al. Pulmonary and pleural metastases from benign meningeal meningioma: a case report. *Ann Thorac Cardiovasc Surg.* 2014;20(5):410–413.
10. Okiror L, von der Thusen J, Ladas G. Solitary lung meningioma with synchronous brain nodules: clinical and pathological features. *Gen Thorac Cardiovasc Surg.* 2013;61:648–650.

71 PEComatous Tumors

Marie-Christine Aubry, M.D., and Fabio R. Tavora, M.D., Ph.D.

Definition

PEComatous tumors encompass tumors thought to arise from perivascular epithelioid cells (PECs). PECs were first described in 1943 and are cells with variable morphology. The cells may be round to spindled and the cytoplasm variably clear to granular and eosinophilic. Similarly, the immunoprofile may be variable. By definition, PECs are positive for HMB45, melan-A, MART-1, and MITF. Expression of actin, estrogen (ER) and progesterone receptors (PR), and S100 protein tends to vary with the tumor type. In the lung, PEComatous tumors include lymphangioleiomyomatosis (LAM), clear cell tumor, angiomyolipoma, and a rare process often referred to as diffuse PEComatosis.[1–3]

Lymphangioleiomyomatosis

Clinical Findings

LAM constitutes <1% of cases of diffuse parenchymal lung disease. This disease affects predominantly women in reproductive age, with a mean age of 40 years at diagnosis, although it has also been described in postmenopausal women.[4,5] LAM is associated with TSC and affects up to 40% of women with TSC.[5,6] LAM is rarely reported in men, with only four biopsy-proven cases, three of whom likely had TSC.[7]

The most common presenting symptom is progressive dyspnea, followed by cough and hemoptysis.[4,8] Complications associated with LAM include spontaneous pneumothorax in up to 70% of patients and lymphatic obstruction (chylothorax, chyloperitoneum, chylopericardium, and chyluria).[4,5,8] Renal angiomyolipomas occur in 30% to 60% of patients with sporadic LAM[4] and 93% of patients with TSC and LAM. Retroperitoneal and mediastinal lymphangioleiomyomas can also be seen along the lymphatic routes and with nodal involvement.[4,9] Pulmonary function tests often show an obstructive or mixed pattern with increased gas volumes and reduced diffusing capacity, but a third of patients have a restrictive pattern or normal tests.[4,5,10]

Radiologic Findings

Radiologic findings include diffuse bilateral thin-walled cysts usually ranging from 0.2 to 2.0 cm in diameter on high-resolution chest computerized tomography scan (HRCT) (Fig. 71.1). Diffuse bilateral reticular infiltrates are seen in 80% of patients, pneumothorax in 30% to 40% of patients, and pleural effusion in 10% to 20% of patients. Hyperinflation is common.

Gross Findings

Grossly, LAM is characterized by diffuse bilateral cysts usually <2 cm in greatest dimension, but 10 cm in diameter cysts have been reported (Fig. 71.1).

Microscopic Findings

Histologically, thin-walled cysts are distributed throughout the lung. The walls of the cysts are lined by a nodular proliferation of cells (Fig. 71.2). Sometimes, it is difficult to appreciate the bundles of cells, which may appear inconspicuously at the cyst edges. LAM cells are variably round and epithelioid or spindled, with only minimal pleomorphism (Fig. 71.2). Nuclei are oval to cigar shaped, with fine to vesicular chromatin. Mitotic figures are rare. Cytoplasm is eosinophilic and moderately abundant and may show perinuclear vacuoles. LAM cells may infiltrate the blood vessels resulting in accumulation of hemosiderophages. In cases complicated by pneumothorax, the pleura may show reactive eosinophilic pleuritis. Lungs of patients with TSC may also show additional lesions including micronodular pneumocyte hyperplasia (MNPH) (Fig. 71.3), clear cell tumor, angiomyolipoma, and localized angiomyolipoma-like infiltrative lesions.[1,11,12]

The histologic findings of LAM are distinctive enough to confirm the diagnosis on a transbronchial biopsy, although they can be very subtle. Recognizing a smooth muscle cell proliferation distinct from the normal smooth muscle of vessels or airways is key and can be aided by immunostaining these cells with markers such as HMB45 and β-catenin, typically negative in normal smooth muscle.[13]

Ancillary Studies

Immunohistochemical studies show that LAM cells are usually strongly and diffusely reactive with antibodies to smooth muscle actin (SMA), desmin, and vimentin (Fig. 71.4). They can also be reac-

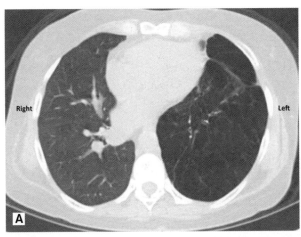
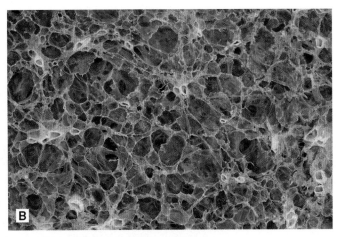

FIGURE 71.1 ▲ Lymphangioleiomyomatosis. **A.** Chest tomography of patient with LAM post single right lung transplantation. The right lung is radiologically normal. In contrast, the left lung shows innumerable thin-walled cysts filled with air. **B.** The gross highlights the numerous thin-walled cysts distributed throughout the lung parenchyma.

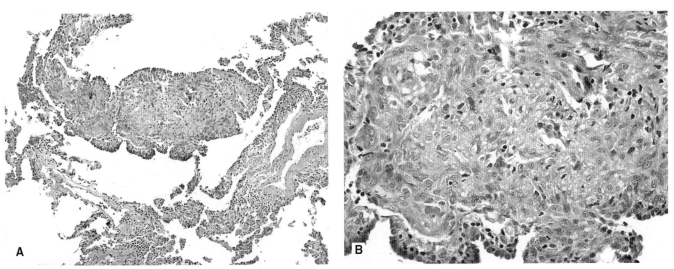

FIGURE 71.2 ▲ Lymphangioleiomyomatosis. **A.** The wall of the cyst contains a cell proliferation of round to oval cells that is morphologically distinct from the normal smooth muscle cells of airways and vessels. **B.** Higher power of LAM cells that are round to spindle shaped with oval nuclei and vesicular chromatin. The cytoplasm is slightly vacuolated.

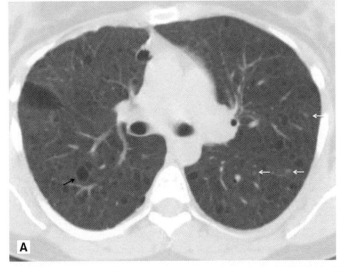
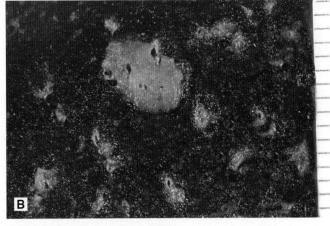

FIGURE 71.3 ▲ Micronodular pneumocyte hyperplasia (MNPH). **A.** Chest CT scan reveals numerous small nodules (*white arrows*) interspersed among the thin-walled cysts (*black arrow*). **B.** The gross examination of a lung wedge resection reveals a well-circumscribed tan nodule (courtesy of Dr. J.L. Myers).

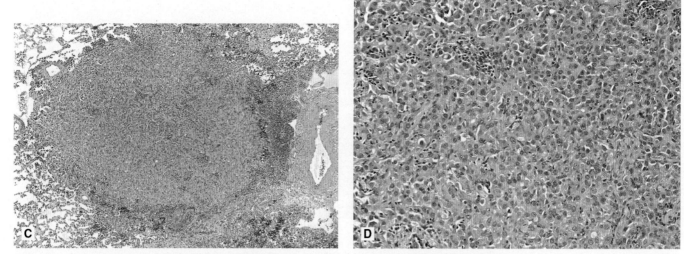

FIGURE 71.3 (*Continued*) ▲ **C.** At low power, MNPH forms well-circumscribed small (typically < 8 mm) nodule, sharply demarcated from the surrounding lung parenchyma. **D.** MNPH is composed of bland small cuboidal cells, often with distinct nucleoli. These cells are pneumocytes and will be positive for TTF-1 and negative for HMB45 and ER/PR.

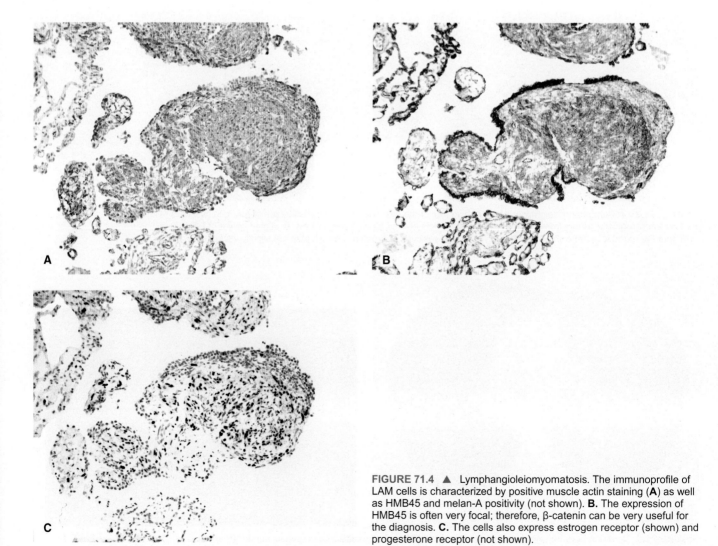

FIGURE 71.4 ▲ Lymphangioleiomyomatosis. The immunoprofile of LAM cells is characterized by positive muscle actin staining (**A**) as well as HMB45 and melan-A positivity (not shown). **B.** The expression of HMB45 is often very focal; therefore, β-catenin can be very useful for the diagnosis. **C.** The cells also express estrogen receptor (shown) and progesterone receptor (not shown).

tive to ER and PR.[14] The distinctive feature is immunoreactivity with HMB45 and MART-1 (melan-A), usually focal in the epithelioid LAM cells. β-catenin and cathepsin-κ are other useful diagnostic markers, shown to be more sensitive than HMB45 and ER/PR, and also specific when compared to entities that may enter the differential diagnosis of cystic lesions such as pulmonary Langerhans cell histiocytosis and emphysema.

Pathogenesis

LAM is considered a low-grade neoplasm with a metastatic behavior, accounting for its spread. Genetic analyses of recurrent LAM in lung transplant patients have demonstrated that LAM cells genetically identical to those in the original LAM cells in the explanted organ can disseminate through the blood and lymphatics.[15,16] Additionally, due to inactivating mutations of either TSC1 or TSC2, the mTOR pathway is abnormally activated in LAM providing the abnormal cells with a significant survival advantage. Accordingly, although LAM cells do not exhibit atypia, the progressive infiltration of lung parenchyma can be considered evidence of metastatic spread. Another postulated mechanism of spread is the formation of clusters of LAM cells that shed into the lymphatic circulation, implant, and proliferate in another site, resulting in new LAM lesions.[17]

Mutations in TSC 1 or TSC 2 genes, which cause deficiency or dysfunction in hamartin and tuberin proteins, respectively, have been linked to both sporadic and tuberous sclerosis complex (TSC)-associated LAM and non-TSC PEComas.[18,19] TSC1 and TSC2 genes have an important role in the regulation of the cell cycle via the mTOR pathway. Mammalian target of rapamycin (mTOR) is a family member of phosphatidylinositol 3-kinase (PI3-kinase). A signaling molecule, Ras homologue enriched in brain (Rheb), found downstream of the tuberin/hamartin complex, activates mTOR. When tuberin and hamartin are deficient or defective, they constitutively activate Rheb and in turn mTOR. The activation of mTOR leads to cell growth and proliferation, which may ultimately result in an overexpression of cathepsin K and lead to the cystic change so common in this disease. This pathway can be targeted by drugs and used in the treatment of LAM.

Treatment and Prognosis

Since LAM occurs mostly in premenopausal women, sex hormones have been assumed to play an important role in the pathogenesis of LAM. Therefore, the therapeutic strategy has mainly relied on hormonal manipulation, mainly progesterone therapy, but also tamoxifen, or oophorectomy, with no clear evidence of effectiveness. A subset of patients may require lung transplantation, but complications are frequent including recurrence of LAM in the allograft. Five-year survival is 65% for LAM lung transplant patients.[8] Promising therapeutic avenues include inhibitors of lymphangiogenesis, angiogenesis, and mTOR pathway, and metalloproteinase, among others.

The natural history of LAM is characterized by progressive respiratory insufficiency with cor pulmonale. The reported rate of progression is quite variable, and, although earlier studies stated average survivals of 3 to 5 years, more recent series suggest longer survival, up to 80% at 10 years.[8] In patients with TSC, death results generally from pulmonary complications.

Differential Diagnosis

The pathologic differential diagnosis includes diseases with cysts and/or nodules. In emphysema, cystic changes are devoid of a true wall and the cysts do not contain smooth muscle. The cysts in Birt-Hogg-Dubé syndrome are true cysts, but they also lack smooth muscle cells (Fig. 71.5).[20] Metastatic endometrial stromal sarcoma (ESS) is well known to mimic LAM. Indeed, metastatic ESS can form cystic lesions with focal proliferation of spindle cells displaying the vascular pattern characteristic of ESS. In contrast to LAM, the spindle cells are uniform with little cytoplasm. These cells can express SMA, ER, and PR; however, they are negative for HMB45. In pulmonary Langerhans cell histiocytosis, the cysts are more irregular and nodules are stellate shaped, centered on airways (Chapter 24). The nodules appear more fibrotic and inflammatory. Langerhans cells are S100 protein, langerin, and CD1a positive. Benign metastasizing leiomyoma is also characterized by a smooth muscle proliferation; however, the smooth muscle cells form solid nodules and are rarely cystic.[21] Entrapped alveolar epithelium is commonly identified, imparting a biphasic appearance to the nodules. Although the cells can express SMA, ER, and PR, they are negative for HMB45.

Clear Cell Tumor

Clinical Findings

Clear cell tumors of the lung are rare, benign neoplasms, usually presenting as an asymptomatic solitary pulmonary nodule.[22] There may be an association with PEComas in other organs, such as the liver.[23] There is no sex predominance. The mean age at onset is in

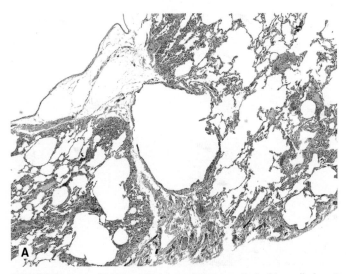
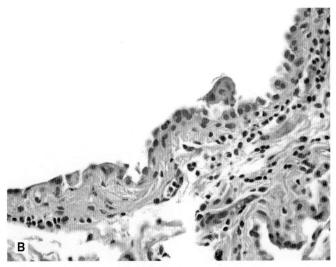

FIGURE 71.5 ▲ Birt-Hogg-Dubé syndrome results in thin-walled cysts of the lung. **A.** At low power, the histologic features may raise the diagnosis of LAM. **B.** However, in BHD syndrome, the cysts are lined by normal benign lung without a spindled cell proliferation (Photographs courtesy of Dr. T.V. Colby).

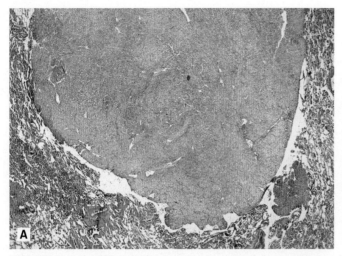
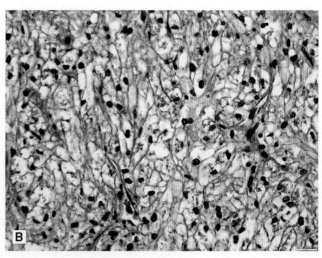

FIGURE 71.6 ▲ Pulmonary clear cell tumor. **A.** On low magnification, the tumor is homogenous and well circumscribed. **B.** The cells are oval with clear cytoplasm. Occasionally, the cytoplasm is more granular. The nuclei are small without significant atypia.

the 5th decade.[24] Symptoms occur in one-third of patients and include cough, fever, sputum, dyspnea, and chest pain.[24] An association with essential thrombocythemia and reactive thrombocytosis has been reported.[22,25] The majority of clear cell tumors are cured by excision. Rarely, they may exhibit a malignant behavior with distant metastasis.

Gross Findings

Grossly, the tumors vary in size and may attain large proportions and infiltrate adjacent structures.[26] The average size is 3.6 cm.[24] There is no specific lobar distribution.[24]

Histologic Findings

Histologically, the tumor is composed of clear to eosinophilic large polygonal cells with a distinct cell border. Nuclei are indented and mildly pleomorphic (Fig. 71.6). There may be a "hemangiopericytoma"-like vascular pattern with thin-walled vascular spaces and sinusoid-type vessels. The diagnosis may be suggested by fine needle aspiration cytology.[27]

Occasional tumors show malignant characteristics, including mitotic activity, nuclear atypia, and necrosis.[28,29]

Ancillary Studies

The clear cytoplasm contains glycogen granules as demonstrated by periodic acid–Schiff staining. Immunohistochemically, clear cell tumors are positive for melanocytic markers (HMB45 and melan-A) and negative for epithelial membrane antigen and cytokeratin. There is generally S100 protein positivity and negativity for smooth muscle markers, in contrast to LAM.

Differential Diagnosis

The differential diagnosis includes other neoplasms characterized by clear or granular eosinophilic cytoplasm such as non–small cell carcinoma with clear cell features, metastatic renal cell carcinoma, carcinoid tumor, and granular cell tumor. These can be easily distinguished from clear cell tumor using ancillary studies.

Angiomyolipoma

Primary angiomyolipoma of the lung is rare, with only nine cases reported.[30] Most patients are women, with asymptomatic, solitary lung nodules. Pulmonary angiomyolipoma may occasionally be associated with renal angiomyolipoma, but there is no clear association with tuberous sclerosis.[30,31] The histologic features are those of renal angiomyolipoma (Fig. 71.7).

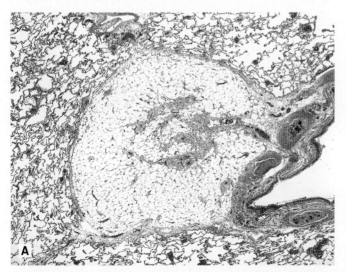
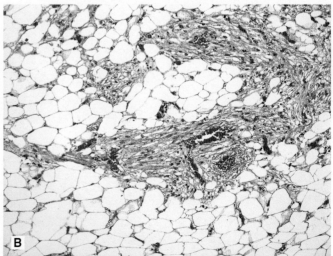

FIGURE 71.7 ▲ Pulmonary angiomyolipoma. **A.** AML arising from bronchus, forming a well-circumscribed nodule. **B.** The tumor is predominantly composed of mature adipose tissue admixed with fascicles of smooth muscles and a few blood vessels (Photographs courtesy of Dr. J.L. Myers).

Diffuse PEComatosis

A rare diffuse lung disease with overlapping features between LAM and clear cell tumor has been described in women as clear cell proliferation of the lung with LAM-like change. These patients present with diffuse cystic changes, but the cells in the walls of the cysts have the morphology and phenotype of clear cells and lack smooth muscle differentiation of LAM.[12] Alternatively, some patients with clinical and radiologic features that are not typical of LAM yet histologically with pulmonary lesions that are fairly typical for LAM have been described. This process has been called diffuse PEComatosis, or "progressive PEComatosis."[32]

REFERENCES

1. Flieder DB, Travis WD. Clear cell "sugar" tumor of the lung: association with lymphangioleiomyomatosis and multifocal micronodular pneumocyte hyperplasia in a patient with tuberous sclerosis. *Am J Surg Pathol.* 1997;21(10):1242–1247.
2. Argani P, Aulmann S, Illei PB, et al. A distinctive subset of PEComas harbors TFE3 gene fusions. *Am J Surg Pathol.* 2010;34(10):1395–1406.
3. Nicholson AG, Henske E, Travis WD. PEComatous tumours. In: Travis WD, et al., eds. *WHO Classification of Tumours of the Lung, Pleura, Mediastinum and Heart.* Lyon, France: IARC Press; 2015:117–118.
4. Chu SC, et al. Comprehensive evaluation of 35 patients with lymphangioleiomyomatosis. *Chest.* 1999;115(4):1041–1052.
5. Ryu JH, et al. The NHLBI lymphangioleiomyomatosis registry: characteristics of 230 patients at enrollment. *Am J Respir Crit Care Med.* 2006;173(1):105–111.
6. Costello LC, Hartman TE, Ryu JH. High frequency of pulmonary lymphangioleiomyomatosis in women with tuberous sclerosis complex. *Mayo Clin Proc.* 2000;75(6):591–594.
7. Schiavina M, et al. Pulmonary lymphangioleiomyomatosis in a karyotypically normal man without tuberous sclerosis complex. *Am J Respir Crit Care Med.* 2007;176(1):96–98.
8. Urban T, et al. Pulmonary lymphangioleiomyomatosis. A study of 69 patients. Groupe d'Etudes et de Recherche sur les Maladies "Orphelines" Pulmonaires (GERM"O"P). *Medicine (Baltimore).* 1999;78(5):321–337.
9. Matsui K, et al. Extrapulmonary lymphangioleiomyomatosis (LAM): clinicopathologic features in 22 cases. *Hum Pathol.* 2000;31(10):1242–1248.
10. Moss J, et al. Prevalence and clinical characteristics of lymphangioleiomyomatosis (LAM) in patients with tuberous sclerosis complex. *Am J Respir Crit Care Med.* 2001;164(4):669–671.
11. Wu K, Tazelaar HD. Pulmonary angiomyolipoma and multifocal micronodular pneumocyte hyperplasia associated with tuberous sclerosis. *Hum Pathol.* 1999;30(10):1266–1268.
12. Pileri SA, et al. Clear-cell proliferation of the lung with lymphangioleiomyomatosis-like change. *Histopathology.* 2004;44(2):156–163.
13. Bonetti F, et al. Transbronchial biopsy in lymphangiomyomatosis of the lung. HMB45 for diagnosis. *Am J Surg Pathol.* 1993;17(11):1092–1102.
14. Ohori NP, et al. Estrogen and progesterone receptors in lymphangioleiomyomatosis, epithelioid hemangioendothelioma, and sclerosing hemangioma of the lung. *Am J Clin Pathol.* 1991;96(4):529–535.
15. Bittmann I, et al. Recurrence of lymphangioleiomyomatosis after single lung transplantation: new insights into pathogenesis. *Hum Pathol.* 2003;34(1):95–98.
16. Karbowniczek M, et al. Recurrent lymphangiomyomatosis after transplantation: genetic analyses reveal a metastatic mechanism. *Am J Respir Crit Care Med.* 2003;167(7):976–982.
17. Kumasaka T, et al. Lymphangiogenesis-mediated shedding of LAM cell clusters as a mechanism for dissemination in lymphangioleiomyomatosis. *Am J Surg Pathol.* 2005;29(10):1356–1366.
18. Strizheva GD, et al. The spectrum of mutations in TSC1 and TSC2 in women with tuberous sclerosis and lymphangioleiomyomatosis. *Am J Respir Crit Care Med.* 2001;163(1):253–258.
19. Carsillo T, Astrinidis A, Henske EP. Mutations in the tuberous sclerosis complex gene TSC2 are a cause of sporadic pulmonary lymphangioleiomyomatosis. *Proc Natl Acad Sci U S A.* 2000;97(11):6085–6090.
20. Butnor KJ, Guinee DG Jr. Pleuropulmonary pathology of Birt-Hogg-Dube syndrome. *Am J Surg Pathol.* 2006;30(3):395–399.
21. Aboualfa K, et al. Benign metastasizing leiomyoma presenting as cystic lung disease: a diagnostic pitfall. *Histopathology.* 2011;59(4):796–799.
22. Sen S, et al. PEComa (clear cell "sugar" tumor) of the lung: a benign tumor that presented with thrombocytosis. *Ann Thorac Surg.* 2009;88(6):2013–2015.
23. Neri S, et al. Multiple perivascular epithelioid cell tumors: clear cell tumor of the lung accompanied by angiomyolipoma of the liver. *Ann Thorac Cardiovasc Surg* 2014;20(suppl):453–456.
24. Chen YB, et al. Clear cell tumor of the lung: a retrospective analysis. *Am J Med Sci.* 2014;347(1):50–53.
25. Yazak V, et al. Lung clear "Sugar" cell tumor and JAK V617F positive essential thrombocythemia: a simple coincidence? *Mediterr J Hematol Infect Dis.* 2013;5(1):e2013021.
26. Kavunkal AM, et al. Large clear cell tumor of the lung mimicking malignant behavior. *Ann Thorac Surg.* 2007;83(1):310–312.
27. Wang GX, et al. Clear cell tumor of the lung: a case report and literature review. *World J Surg Oncol* 2013;11:247.
28. Yan B, Yau EX, Petersson F. Clear cell 'sugar' tumour of the lung with malignant histological features and melanin pigmentation—the first reported case. *Histopathology.* 2011;58(3):498–500.
29. Ye T, et al. Malignant clear cell sugar tumor of the lung: patient case report. *J Clin Oncol.* 2010;28(31):e626–e628.
30. Hino H, et al. Angiomyolipoma in the lung detected 15 years after a nephrectomy for renal angiomyolipoma. *Ann Thorac Surg.* 2010;89(1):298–300.
31. Marcheix B, et al. Pulmonary angiomyolipoma. *Ann Thorac Surg.* 2006;82(4):1504–1506.
32. Lawson K, et al. Successful treatment of progressive diffuse PEComatosis. *Eur Respir J.* 2012;40(6):1578–1580.

72 Carcinomas of the Lung: Classification and Genetics

Allen P. Burke, M.D., and Fabio R. Tavora, M.D., Ph.D.

Classification

General

The classification of lung carcinomas is presented in Table 72.1, which conforms to the latest World Health Organization approach.[1]

The most frequent subtype of lung carcinoma is adenocarcinoma, which is steadily increasing in proportion to other tumors (Fig. 72.1). Currently, it is more than twice as common in women as small cell or squamous cell carcinomas, which are about equal in incidence. In men, squamous carcinomas are still relatively frequent, accounting for 30% of tumors, but ten percentage points behind adenocarcinoma.

There has been a marked shift in frequency of histologic types. In the latter part of the last century, squamous carcinomas were more than twice as common in men than adenocarcinomas, and lung cancers were relatively infrequent in women. Today, there are few gender differences in rates of lung cancer by type, except that squamous carcinomas are relatively infrequent in women.[2]

Incidence

Lung cancer is one of the most common tumors and has a high rate of mortality. There are ~55/100,000 new cases annually, with 45/100,000 deaths yearly (http://seer.cancer.gov/statfacts/html/lungb.html). The rate of lung cancer diagnosis and deaths is on the decline, from a peak of 70/100,000 and 60/100,000 per year, respectively, in the early 1990s.

Adenocarcinomas

Adenocarcinomas are classified on the basis of cell type, namely nonmucinous, derived from pneumocyte-like cells, which generally express TTF-1, and mucinous adenocarcinomas. Nonmucinous adenocarcinomas are typically classified by growth pattern. These include acinar (the term used for tubular or glandular growth), papillary, micropapillary, and solid growth patterns.

One pattern that is included in the classification is the lepidic, or in situ growth pattern, which sets lung carcinomas apart from classification of other cancers. A previous term that came to designate "in situ" carcinoma without invasion, namely, "bronchioloalveolar carcinoma," has been abandoned in favor of the term "adenocarcinoma in situ."

TABLE 72.1 Classification of Carcinomas of the Lung

Adenocarcinomas	Lepidic adenocarcinoma
	Acinar adenocarcinoma
	Papillary adenocarcinoma
	Micropapillary adenocarcinoma
	Solid adenocarcinoma
	Invasive mucinous adenocarcinoma
	Mixed invasive mucinous and nonmucinous adenocarcinoma
	Colloid adenocarcinoma
	Fetal adenocarcinoma
	Enteric adenocarcinoma
	Minimally invasive adenocarcinoma
	Nonmucinous
	Mucinous
Squamous cell carcinoma	Keratinizing squamous cell carcinoma
	Nonkeratinizing squamous cell carcinoma
	Basaloid squamous cell carcinoma
Neuroendocrine carcinomas	Small cell carcinoma
	Combined small cell carcinoma
	Large cell neuroendocrine carcinoma
	Combined large cell neuroendocrine carcinoma
	Carcinoid tumors
	Typical carcinoid tumor
	Atypical carcinoid tumor
Large cell carcinomas	
Adenosquamous carcinoma	
Sarcomatoid carcinoma	Pleomorphic carcinoma
	Spindle cell carcinoma
	Giant cell carcinoma
Carcinosarcoma	
Pulmonary blastoma	
Lymphoepithelioma-like carcinoma	
Salivary gland-type tumors	Mucoepidermoid carcinoma
	Adenoid cystic carcinoma
	Epithelial–myoepithelial carcinoma
	Pleomorphic adenoma

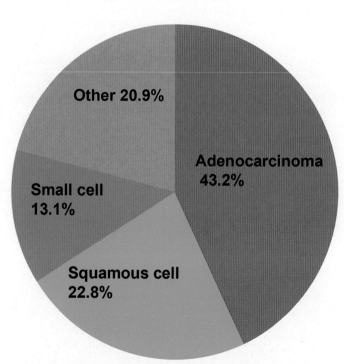

FIGURE 72.1 ▲ Approximate frequency of subtypes of carcinomas of the lung. (Adapted from SEER data, http://seer.cancer.gov/statfacts/html/lungb.html.)

Other 20.9%
Adenocarcinoma 43.2%
Small cell 13.1%
Squamous cell 22.8%

Adenocarcinomas with predominantly in situ growth are now designated "lepidic predominant adenocarcinoma" or "minimally invasive adenocarcinoma," if the invasive component is <5 mm (see Chapter 74 for details).

Mucinous adenocarcinomas of the lung are heterogeneous and have growth patterns that generally mimic that of nonmucinous tumors. They have a propensity for in situ growth and multiplicity and may demonstrate features that resemble colloid carcinomas of the colon and appendix, in which case colonic markers may be expressed. Their molecular profile is distinct from that of nonmucinous carcinoma and is characterized by *KRAS* mutations (see Chapter 76).

Squamous Cell Carcinomas

Squamous cell carcinomas are similar to their counterparts in other organ sites and are very strongly associated with cigarette smoking. "Basaloid" carcinomas were previously separated from conventional squamous carcinomas, because of their relatively poor prognosis. However, they are now considered a variant of squamous carcinoma. In the WHO classification, lymphoepithelial-like carcinomas have a separate classification. In this book, they are considered in the chapter on squamous carcinoma, as they often express similar markers immunohistochemically.

Small Cell Carcinomas

In the most recent classification of lung tumors, small cell carcinomas are considered in the same overall framework as large cell neuroendocrine carcinomas and carcinoid tumors (see Chapter 79). Like squamous carcinomas, they are strongly associated with smoking. Their histologic features and biologic behavior are well known and studied. Occasionally, adenocarcinomas with EGFR mutations (that usually occur in nonsmokers) may acquire resistance to EGFR TKI drugs and recur with endocrine differentiation and resemble small cell carcinomas. Rarely, small cell carcinomas arise de novo in patients who have never smoked.

Neuroendocrine Carcinomas

In the lung, the term "carcinoid tumor" is still used for low-grade neuroendocrine carcinomas. The distinction between carcinoid and atypical carcinoid tumor is still made based on light microscopic features (i.e., mitotic counting).

Large cell neuroendocrine carcinoma is now relatively firmly established as a specific clinicopathologic entity that clinically behaves similar to small cell carcinoma, but has a different histologic appearance. It is defined by both histologic and immunohistochemical features.

Large Cell Carcinomas

The last relatively large group of lung cancers that is controversial and not well defined is that of "large cell carcinoma." Its use as term is no longer applied to large cell neuroendocrine carcinoma and is also not applied to small biopsy samples (see Chapter 82). Currently, it denotes a poorly differentiated tumor without small cell, neuroendocrine, or sarcomatoid features that is presumably either a primitive squamous or adenocarcinoma. Molecular studies have demonstrated that most "large cell carcinomas" are likely poorly differentiated adenocarcinomas that do not express classic adenocarcinoma markers.

Combined Carcinomas

Another area of potential difficulty is terminology for carcinomas with varied histologic types. The most common combined carcinoma is adenosquamous carcinoma (Chapter 83), followed by combined small cell carcinoma (with adeno- or squamous carcinoma). These diagnoses are generally straightforward with adequate tissue sampling, unless the squamous component lacks keratinization and is poorly differentiated. Combined large cell neuroendocrine with small cell carcinoma is generally considered small cell carcinoma for treatment purposes. Areas of undifferentiated, nonsarcomatoid tumors (large cell carcinoma) are usually not separated into a combined category.

Sarcomatoid Carcinomas

The classification of carcinomas with spindling involves poorly differentiated tumors, spans a large range of histologic patterns, and rests on convention. In this book, we have adhered fairly closely to the WHO (Chapter 85). Pleomorphic carcinoma is applied to combined spindle and adeno- or squamous carcinoma. Spindle cell carcinoma is reserved for tumors that lack differentiated areas and carcinosarcoma to combined tumors with heterologous elements. Highly pleomorphic tumors with giant cells are given the designation "giant cell carcinoma" and often have areas of other high-grade histology.

Genetics of Lung Carcinomas

General

Lung cancers, both squamous and adenocarcinomas, have high numbers of mutations per genome among human cancers, second only to melanoma (Fig. 72.2). A recent Cancer Genome Atlas on lung adenocarcinomas (using messenger RNA, microRNA, DNA sequencing,

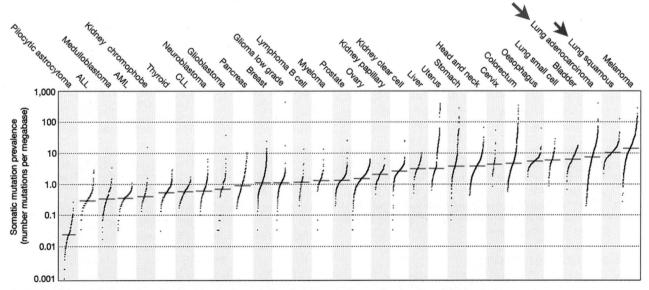

FIGURE 72.2 ▲ Relative frequencies of somatic mutations in human cancers. Carcinomas of the lung are near the top of the list (*arrows*). (Reproduced from Alexandrov LB, Nik-Zainal S, Wedge DC, et al. Signatures of mutational processes in human cancer. *Nature.* 2013;500:415–421, with permission.)

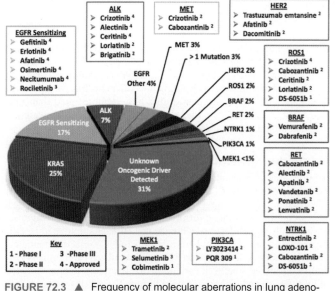

FIGURE 72.3 ▲ Frequency of molecular aberrations in lung adeno-carcinomas and current available therapeutic agents. EGFR, epidermal growth factor receptor; ALK, anaplastic lymphoma receptor tyrosine kinase; MET, mesenchymal-to-epithelial transition factor; HER2, ERBB2 receptor tyrosine kinase 2; ROS1, ROS proto-oncogene 1, receptor tyrosine kinase; BRAF, B-Raf proto-oncogene, serine/threonine kinase; RET, ret proto-oncogene; NTRK1, neurotrophic tyrosine kinase receptor type 1; PIK3A, phosphatidylinositol-4,5-bisphosphate 3-kinase catalytic subunit alpha; MEK1, mitogen-activated protein kinase kinase 1; KRAS, Kirsten rat sarcoma viral oncogene homolog. Reproduced with permission, Tsao AS, Scagliotti GV, Bunn PA Jr, et al. Scientific advances in lung cancer 2015. *J Thorac Oncol.* 2016;11(5):613–638. doi: 10.1016/j.jtho.

copy number analysis, methylation and proteomic analyses) revealed that the most common mutations are in the tumor suppressor gene TP53 (46%) and in the oncogenes *KRAS (33%)* and *EGFR (15%)* (Fig. 72.3).[3] In squamous cell carcinomas of the lung, one can rarely identify mutations in drug targets such as EGFR and ALK. In these tumors, TP53 mutations are also prevalent (80%), followed by *CDCKN2A* (15%), *PIK3CA* (16%), and *PTEN* (8%).[4]

The list of identified mutations is ever increasing, lowering the percentage of tumors with no identifiable driver mutation. These recent discoveries have played an enormous role in identifying new potential therapeutic targets.[5]

EGFR and EML4–ALK fusion are the most common mutations identified for directed therapies. Guidelines for tissue acquisition and testing for these two mutations have been published (see Tables 72.2 to 72.4).[6]

Mutations that occur only rarely may nevertheless be used for directed treatment. Because of their low frequency, they are not amenable to screening molecular testing or targeted diagnostic approaches. Next-generation sequencing (NGS) methods are applied to advanced tumors refractory to conventional treatments in order to find these mutations, which include ROS1, *RET*, *PTEN*, and *BRAF*. NGS, with its diminishing cost and turnaround time, also plays a role in identifying de novo mutations in cases of drug resistance and new drivers in the progression of some tumors.[7]

Immunotherapy is a newer type of chemotherapy that targets tumor antigens that decrease immune surveillance by the host and thereby activate tumor-specific immune response.

Case Selection for Testing

Many tissue samples received in the anatomic pathology laboratory to render a diagnosis of lung cancer are small. Genetic testing may be requested on product of transbronchial biopsies, transthoracic core biopsies, fine needle aspirations, or other cytology methods, from the primary tumor or mediastinal lymph nodes. This scenario reinforces the important role of the surgical pathologist in selecting cases for molecular testing, preserving tissue from the block, and trying to maximize information that can be gathered from the small tissue samples.

First and foremost, the distinction between small cell and non–small cell lung cancer is based on morphology with the help of a limited panel of immunohistochemistry (limited with the aim to conserve tissue for molecular testing). According to the current recommendations, all adenocarcinomas, mixed tumors with adenocarcinoma component, or non–small cell carcinomas that cannot be further classified should be forwarded to molecular testing. Cytology specimens and samples from metastatic sites are also suitable for testing. Cell block preparations are preferred. Although there are many potential algorithms

TABLE 72.2 CAP Guidelines for Genetic Testing of Lung Cancers (Patient Selection)

Question	Guidelines
Which patients should be tested for EGFR and ALK?	• All adenocarcinomas regardless of clinical status (gender, smoking, etc.) • All combined carcinomas that have an adeno-carcinoma component • Other tumors are not to be tested when there is adequate sample • Small biopsy samples may be tested even without adenocarcinoma histology if clinically indicated (e.g., young age, no smoking history) • Metastatic or primary tumors are acceptable for testing • Multiple tumors should be tested separately if possible
When should tumors be tested for EGFR and ALK?	At the time of diagnosis for stage IV disease Optional for stage I, II, and III disease (to be determined by multidisciplinary approach) Tissues should be prioritized for EGFR–ALK testing, with minimal IHC staining for diagnosis
How rapid should testing be available?	2 weeks Specimen should be sent within 3 working days of biopsy with finalized diagnosis for outside testing

TABLE 72.3 CAP Guidelines for Performance of EGFR Testing

Question	Guidelines
Specimen processing	PPFE, frozen, or alcohol fixed Avoid decalcification and fixatives with heavy metals Cell blocks are preferred over cytologic smears
Specimen adequacy	Individual laboratories prepare guidelines for cancer cell content, DNA quality depending on validated assay Individual pathologists have guidelines in assessing cancer cell/tumor content
Methodology	Any validated test (e.g., PCR/sequencing) Those that can detect mutations ≥ 10% tumor content are favored over those that can detect mutations ≥ 50% tumor content All mutations that comprise ≥1% of known EGFR mutations should be detected IHC and FISH are not recommended
Role of KRAS analysis	KRAS mutation testing is not recommended as a sole determinant of EGFR TKI therapy
Requirement for testing recurrent tumors with acquired EGFR TKI resistance	Tests should be able to detect the secondary EGFR T790M mutation in as few as 5% of cells

TABLE 72.4   CAP Guidelines for Performance of ALK Testing

Laboratories should use an ALK FISH assay using dual-labeled break-apart probes for selecting patients for ALK TKI therapy.

ALK immunohistochemistry, if carefully validated, may be considered as a screening methodology to select specimens for ALK FISH testing.

A pathologist should be involved in the selection of sections for *ALK* FISH testing, by assessing tumor architecture, cytology, and specimen quality.

A pathologist should participate in the interpretation of ALK FISH slides, either by performing the analysis directly or by reviewing the interpretations of cytogeneticists or technologists with specialized training in solid tumor FISH analysis.

that can be followed, testing for EGFR and ALK are usually the first choices (see below), and these tests can be done reflexive or upon clinician request should be decided by a multiprofessional team in each institution.

It is the role of the pathologist to choose the best paraffin block for further testing, assess tumor content and viability and extent of necrotic material, and, in some cases, help in identifying or dissecting tumor-rich areas that will yield better DNA content. With more advanced techniques, high-throughput analysis will require less tissue, but preanalytical variables such as adequate fixation, storage, and tissue processing may play a role in the final results, and it is paramount that care should be taken from the biopsy procurement to the final tissue archiving in order to maximize tissue quality.

EGFR Mutations

Tyrosine kinase inhibitor (TKI) sensitizing mutations in *EGFR* occur in 10% to 15% of adenocarcinomas of Caucasians and in 50% of Asians. They occur more often in young female nonsmokers. Since 2004, with the discovery of EGFR gene mutations linked to clinical response with tyrosine kinase inhibitors (gefitinib and erlotinib), personalized cancer treatment revolutionized the approach to diagnosis and treatment in lung carcinomas.

Epidermal growth factor receptor (EGFR, or ERBB1) is a cell surface protein kinase belonging to the ErbB transmembrane growth factor receptor family. Ligand binding by epidermal growth factor triggers dimerization with ERBB2 (HER2/neu), ERBB3, and ERBB4, triggering tyrosine autophosphorylation in the cytoplasmic kinase domain and activation of downstream PI3K/AKT/mTOR and RAS/RAF/MAPK pathways. Most mutations occur in exons 19 (45%), 21 (40% to 45%), 18 (5%), and 20 (<1%).[6,8]

There have been several studies that correlate histologic subtyping with the presence of EGFR mutations, with a moderate association of presence of mutations with acinar predominant, lepidic predominant, and micropapillary adenocarcinomas.[9,10] Solid-predominant tumors are less likely to harbor EGFR mutations, and have an association with KRAS.[7,11]

Testing can be performed on formalin-fixed paraffin-embedded tissues by dioxy (Sanger) sequencing, pyrosequencing, or more sensitive methods such as ARMS, other allele-specific real-time PCR, SNaPshot, PNA Clamp, and PCT/fluorescent RFLP.

First-generation drugs that are currently in use against EGFR-mutated adenocarcinomas include gefitinib, erlotinib, and afatinib.[6,8] with second-generation inhibitors being pan-HER inhibitors (neratinib, dacomitinib, afatinib) reserved usually for resistant tumors. There are also new drugs being developed to address specific EGFR T790M-mutated tumors, and also other compounds that can target dual targets such as EGFR/ALK and EGFR/VEGF.[12,13]Resistance to EGFR may develop, and recurrent tumors may show alterations in histologic features. TKI resistance has been explained by several biologic phenomena that include de novo mutations (especially in the T790M locus); mesenchymal–epithelial transition; activation of additional

signaling pathways such as Met, HER2, CRKL, and KRAS; and finally the transformation into small cell neuroendocrine lung cancer.[14]

ALK-1 TK Rearrangement

The second most common targeted therapy against lung adenocarcinomas is that directed against tumors harboring tyrosine kinase fusions involving ALK1, which lead to aberrant activation of downstream signaling pathways MAPK and PI3K–AKT. These occur in 5% to 7% of tumors and have been diagnosed by break-apart FISH assays, but currently, new immunohistochemical techniques have been applied and show good sensitivity for either screening or diagnostic methods.

ALK1 is present on chromosome 2p23, and the most common rearrangement in lung tumors is to EML4 (2p21) representing a paracentric inversion. Other fusion partners include TFG, KIF5B, KLC1, and STRN.

ALK1-mutated tumors are susceptible to small molecule agents such as crizotinib and ceritinib, with more drugs in development (e.g., alectinib).[15] The overall response to target drugs in patient who harbor the translocation is more than 70%. Patients with ALK1 translocation lung cancers are usually young (mean 51 years), often (65%) never smokers, and typically have malignant pleural effusions (70%). Signet ring, mucinous, and cribriform patterns are typical histologically.[16]

FISH is the standard method to diagnose ALK translocations. Other tests have been used, such as real-time PCR, which can result in false positives by not detecting non-EML4 fusions such as TGF-ALK and KIF5B-ALK. Immunohistochemical staining for ALK is an acceptable screening test, due to its high sensitivity, provided that the stain is validated in the laboratory against standard FISH, and positive results confirmed by FISH. Emerging clinical trials that accept ALK immunohistochemistry as inclusion criteria generally accept the Ventana assay.[17]

Currently, it is recommended that ALK testing should be performed at the same time of EGFR analysis or in cases with negative EGFR mutation results, depending on the institution's algorithm.

Mutations in Squamous Cell Carcinoma

In the past, driver mutations in squamous cell carcinoma have been limited, but now, several targets mainly involving the fibroblast growth receptor (FGFR) family and the PI3K/*AKT* pathway have been discovered.

FGFR1 has been shown to be amplified commonly in SCC, with an association with poor prognosis and increase in proliferation rate.[18–20] Currently, there are several ongoing clinical trials testing drugs that target FGFR with promising results in advanced stage tumors, alone or in combination with conventional platinum-based chemotherapy.[18,21]

The PI3K/*AKT* family plays an important role in cell proliferation and growth, activating the AKT/MTOR pathway. There is an inverse inhibitor role of the tumor suppressor gene PTEN. It is estimated that more than 40% of SCC hold mutations or amplifications in the PI3K/AKT pathway genes and 15% PTEN alterations.[22,23] In this scenario, PI3K inhibitors, MTOR inhibitors, and AKT inhibitors are being tested in patients with squamous cell carcinoma.

Targeted Therapies for Less Common Mutations

NGS involves spatial separation of individual DNAs with sequencing in parallel and allows for computerized comprehensive assessment of multiple genes in relatively small samples, including formalin-fixed paraffin-embedded samples. NGS is generally used to detect low-frequency target-based mutations in patients with advanced lung cancer. Although currently target therapies may not be available for some of the identifiable mutations, ever-going studies may find drugs for these tumors.

ROS1 6q22

The ROS1 gene encodes a tyrosine kinase receptor from the insulin receptor family. The first ROS1 rearrangement was identified in lung cancer in 2007, and it is believed to be present in about 1.5% to 2%

of lung adenocarcinomas. The demographics are similar to ALK translocation patients, predominantly found in younger patients with adenocarcinoma morphology, with a mild or no history of smoking. Rare cases of ROS1 mutations have been identified in squamous cell carcinomas.[24]

In patients with mutated ROS1, crizotinib seems to be a very effective option, with other agents being identified and tested. As in other mutations, acquired resistance exists in ROS1-mutated tumors. EGFR pathway activation is one of the proposed mechanisms.[25] FISH is the standard method for the detection of ROS1alterations, with RT-PCR and immunohistochemistry being viable alternatives.[26]

PIK3CA

The phosphatidylinositol 3-kinase (PI3K)–AKT–mTOR pathway is one of the most common altered pathways in human carcinomas.[27] Mutations and amplifications are found in 2% and 12% to 16% respectively, and are even higher in squamous cell carcinomas. PIK3CA mutations in lung adenocarcinoma often coexist with another oncogenic mutations, such as an EGFR or KRAS mutation, or in the setting of acquired EGFR TKI resistance.[28] PI3K tyrosine kinase inhibitors are being currently tested with promising results.

BRAF

BRAF mutations occur in fewer than 2% of lung cancers, with half the cases showing the classic V600E mutation that is usually identified in melanoma and other tumors. The BRAF[V600] mutation in lung adenocarcinomas is associated with women, nonsmokers, and micropapillary histology, whereas other mutations (within exons 11 and 15) are typically seen in male smokers.[29]

BRAF mutations lead to MAPK pathway activation and are mutually exclusive to EGFR and KRAS mutations. Adenocarcinomas with BRAF mutations have shown susceptibility to vemurafenib, and BRAF-mutated tumors may also show response to MEK inhibition. Ongoing trials in BRAF-mutated lung adenocarcinoma investigate BRAF, MEK, and AKT inhibitors.[27]

MET

MET is a tyrosine kinase receptor for the hepatocyte growth factor (HGF) that may be overexpressed, amplified, mutated, or rearranged in lung carcinomas (~4%). MET protein overexpression and increased MET gene number have been identified as poor prognostic factors in lung adenocarcinomas.[30] Mutations in the MET exon 14 RNA splice acceptor and donor sites lead to exon skipping and decreased turnover of aberrant MET protein, resulting in increased expression by immunohistochemistry. Small molecule agents such as crizotinib and cabozantinib have been used in patients whose tumors harbor genetic alterations in MET.[31]

Splice amplification in MET is associated with acquired resistance of EGFR tyrosine kinase inhibitors.

MET aberrations are identified by increased gene copy number (FISH), protein immunohistochemistry, or mutational analysis. Overexpression of MET assessed by immunohistochemical staining shows that 35% to 54% of adenocarcinomas stain positively, which is associated with a poor prognosis. A higher rate (about 70%) of EGFR-positive lung adenocarcinomas tumors also coexpresses MET. Met positivity tumor is defined as ≥50% of tumor cells with moderate or strong membranous or cytoplasmic staining.[32] Tumors with met amplification or mutations may respond to onartuzumab and tivantinib.

HER2

The HER2 oncogene, also known as c-erbB-2, HER2/neu, or p185neu, is located in the chromosomal region 17q11.2-q12. The dimerization of HER2 with EGFR can activate the downstream signaling pathways involving PI3K/AKT/mTOR and RAS/RAF/MAPK.

In NSLC, although overexpression by immunohistochemistry can be detected in 15% to 20% of cases, amplification of HER (as detected by ISH) can be found in only 2% to 4% of patients. Only 1% to 4% show mutations by NGS with no clear association with HER2 amplification.[33] HER2-positive lung cancers are more frequent in women, Asians, and nonsmokers.

Agents that may be effective in the treatment of HER2 lung adenocarcinomas include afatinib, neratinib, dacomitinib, and trastuzumab.[34-36]

Ret 10q11.2

RET (rearranged during transfection) is a receptor tyrosine kinase that is detected in about 1.5% of NSLC, with predilection for young, light, or never smokers and adenocarcinoma histology. The tumors are usually poorly differentiated or show signet ring features. Diagnosis is usually performed by FISH or anchored multiplex PCR.

The ALK inhibitor alectinib has shown antitumor activity against RET translocated NSLC. Other drugs such as cabozantinib (c-Met, VEGFR2 inhibitor) and vandetanib (VEGFR, EGFR, RET inhibitor) are also being tested.

Other Genomic Alterations

Several low percentage genomic alterations are reported in lung cancer, and the list increases with the advances in molecular techniques. MEK1 mutations occur in 1% or less of NSCLC, mostly in adenocarcinomas. NTRIK1 fusions have been described in 3% of tumors in never smokers, with some variant showing oncogenic potential and targetable sites. PTEN loss with AKT overexpression occurs in one-third of lung tumors, more commonly in squamous cell carcinomas.[5,7,27,37]

Common Mutations Not Associated with Targeted Therapies

KRAS

KRAS is one of the first well-described human oncogenes and one of the most common drivers in lung adenocarcinomas, present in about 20% to 30% of tumors and about 5% of squamous cell cancer.[7] However, despite being common and easily identifiable, direct targeting of KRAS in lung tumors has been unsuccessful to date. KRAS mutations are associated with mucinous adenocarcinomas and generally preclude mutations in EGFR and ALK. In addition, the presence of KRAS mutations (while it may predict lack of response to target therapies of other sites) has not been associated with prognostic and predictive of response to adjuvant chemotherapy.[38] Currently, there are several clinical trials in place with several drugs for KRAS-mutated lung cancer. Due to the high prevalence of KRAS mutations, targeting the downstream signaling pathways may be effective in these tumors. MAPK, MEK, and PI3K are obvious targets, with some other clinical trials looking into these options for safety and efficacy.

Immunotherapy

In the past years, immunotherapy has been a hot subject as a new approach to cancer targeting, in blocking immune checkpoints and achieving T-cell response and antitumor activity. The main checkpoints are cytotoxic T-lymphocyte–associated antigen-4 (CTLA-4), programmed cell death protein 1 (PD1), and programmed death ligand 1 (PD-L1).[39] Immunotherapies stimulate or modulate the host immune system to mount an attack against a tumor, changing the microenvironment and increasing susceptibility of conventional chemotherapy, which is usually used in association.

PD1 and PDL1 antibodies are used to blockade the checkpoints, the former targeting T cells and the latter antigen-presenting cells and tumor cells. It suggested that tumor cells used PD-1 pathway to evade immune detect.[14] Several ongoing studies are attempting to use immunotherapy in naive tumors as well as in tumors with acquired resistance to TKIs. Some preliminary studies that assessed PDL1 expression by immunohistochemistry have shown prediction of response to PD1 antibody therapy. However, there are no published guidelines in reporting PDL1 expression, and more studies are needed to prove its power in predicting therapy.[40,41]

REFERENCES

1. Travis WD, Brambilla E, Burke AP, et al. *WHO Classification of Tumours of the Lung, Pleura, Thymus and Heart.* 5th ed. Lyon, France: IARC Press; 2015.

2. Meza R, Meernik C, Jeon J, et al. Lung cancer incidence trends by gender, race and histology in the United States, 1973–2010. *PLoS One.* 2015;10:e0121323.

3. Cancer Genome Atlas Research N. Comprehensive molecular profiling of lung adenocarcinoma. *Nature.* 2014;511:543–550.

4. Cancer Genome Atlas Research N. Comprehensive genomic characterization of squamous cell lung cancers. *Nature.* 2012;489:519–525.

5. Khoo C, Rogers TM, Fellowes A, et al. Molecular methods for somatic mutation testing in lung adenocarcinoma: EGFR and beyond. *Transl Lung Cancer Res.* 2015;4:126–141.

6. Lindeman NI, Cagle PT, Beasley MB, et al. Molecular testing guideline for selection of lung cancer patients for EGFR and ALK tyrosine kinase inhibitors: guideline from the College of American Pathologists, International Association for the Study of Lung Cancer, and Association for Molecular Pathology. *J Thorac Oncol.* 2013;8:823–859.

7. Richer AL, Friel JM, Carson VM, et al. Genomic profiling toward precision medicine in non-small cell lung cancer: getting beyond EGFR. *Pharmgenomics Pers Med.* 2015;8:63–79.

8. Leighl NB, Rekhtman N, Biermann WA, et al. Molecular testing for selection of patients with lung cancer for epidermal growth factor receptor and anaplastic lymphoma kinase tyrosine kinase inhibitors: American Society of Clinical Oncology endorsement of the College of American Pathologists/International Association for the study of lung cancer/association for molecular pathology guideline. *J Clin Oncol.* 2014;32:3673–3679.

9. Villa C, Cagle PT, Johnson M, et al. Correlation of EGFR mutation status with predominant histologic subtype of adenocarcinoma according to the new lung adenocarcinoma classification of the International Association for the Study of Lung Cancer/American Thoracic Society/European Respiratory Society. *Arch Pathol Lab Med.* 2014;138:1353–1357.

10. Kadota K, Yeh YC, D'Angelo SP, et al. Associations between mutations and histologic patterns of mucin in lung adenocarcinoma: invasive mucinous pattern and extracellular mucin are associated with KRAS mutation. *Am J Surg Pathol.* 2014;38:1118–1127.

11. Sun Y, Yu X, Shi X, et al. Correlation of survival and EGFR mutation with predominant histologic subtype according to the new lung adenocarcinoma classification in stage IB patients. *World J Surg Oncol.* 2014;12:148.

12. Yu HA, Riely GJ. Second-generation epidermal growth factor receptor tyrosine kinase inhibitors in lung cancers. *J Natl Compr Canc Netw.* 2013;11:161–169.

13. Stasi I and Cappuzzo F. Second generation tyrosine kinase inhibitors for the treatment of metastatic non-small-cell lung cancer. *Transl Respir Med.* 2014;2:2.

14. Xu M, Xie Y, Ni S, et al. The latest therapeutic strategies after resistance to first generation epidermal growth factor receptor tyrosine kinase inhibitors (EGFR TKIs) in patients with non-small cell lung cancer (NSCLC). *Ann Transl Med.* 2015;3:96.

15. Mologni L. Expanding the portfolio of anti-ALK weapons. *Transl Lung Cancer Res.* 2015;4:5–7.

16. Solomon BJ, Mok T, Kim DW, et al. First-line crizotinib versus chemotherapy in ALK-positive lung cancer. *N Engl J Med.* 2014;371:2167–2177.

17. Wynes MW, Sholl LM, Dietel M, et al. An international interpretation study using the ALK IHC antibody D5F3 and a sensitive detection kit demonstrates high concordance between ALK IHC and ALK FISH and between evaluators. *J Thorac Oncol.* 2014;9:631–638.

18. Weiss J, Sos ML, Seidel D, et al. Frequent and focal FGFR1 amplification associates with therapeutically tractable FGFR1 dependency in squamous cell lung cancer. *Sci Transl Med.* 2010;2:62ra93.

19. Jiang T, Gao G, Fan G, et al. FGFR1 amplification in lung squamous cell carcinoma: a systematic review with meta-analysis. *Lung Cancer.* 2015;87:1–7.

20. Boehm D, von Massenhausen A, Perner S. Analysis of receptor tyrosine kinase gene amplification on the example of FGFR1. *Methods Mol Biol.* 2015;1233:67–79.

21. Gavine PR, Mooney L, Kilgour E, et al. AZD4547: an orally bioavailable, potent, and selective inhibitor of the fibroblast growth factor receptor tyrosine kinase family. *Cancer Res.* 2012;72:2045–2056.

22. Beck JT, Ismail A, Tolomeo C. Targeting the phosphatidylinositol 3-kinase (PI3K)/AKT/mammalian target of rapamycin (mTOR) pathway: an emerging treatment strategy for squamous cell lung carcinoma. *Cancer Treat Rev.* 2014;40:980–989.

23. Sun Z, Wang Z, Liu X, et al. New development of inhibitors targeting the PI3K/AKT/mTOR pathway in personalized treatment of non-small-cell lung cancer. *Anticancer Drugs.* 2015;26:1–14.

24. Davies KD, Le AT, Theodoro MF, et al. Identifying and targeting ROS1 gene fusions in non-small cell lung cancer. *Clin Cancer Res.* 2012;18:4570–4579.

25. Davies KD, Mahale S, Astling DP, et al. Resistance to ROS1 inhibition mediated by EGFR pathway activation in non-small cell lung cancer. *PLoS One.* 2013;8:e82236.

26. Lee SE, Lee B, Hong M, et al. Comprehensive analysis of RET and ROS1 rearrangement in lung adenocarcinoma. *Mod Pathol.* 2015;28:468–479.

27. Rothschild SI. Targeted therapies in non-small cell lung cancer-beyond EGFR and ALK. *Cancers (Basel).* 2015;7:930–949.

28. Chaft JE, Arcila ME, Paik PK, et al. Coexistence of PIK3CA and other oncogene mutations in lung adenocarcinoma-rationale for comprehensive mutation profiling. *Mol Cancer Ther.* 2012;11:485–491.

29. Marchetti A, Felicioni L, Malatesta S, et al. Clinical features and outcome of patients with non-small-cell lung cancer harboring BRAF mutations. *J Clin Oncol.* 2011;29:3574–3579.

30. Finocchiaro G, Toschi L, Gianoncelli L, et al. Prognostic and predictive value of MET deregulation in non-small cell lung cancer. *Ann Transl Med.* 2015;3:83.

31. Paik PK, Drilon A, Fan PD, et al. Response to MET inhibitors in patients with stage IV lung adenocarcinomas harboring MET mutations causing exon 14 skipping. *Cancer Discov.* 2015;5:842–849.

32. Spigel DR, Edelman MJ, Mok T, et al. Treatment rationale study design for the MetLung trial: a randomized, double-blind phase III study of onartuzumab (MetMAb) in combination with erlotinib versus erlotinib alone in patients who have received standard chemotherapy for stage IIIB or IV Met-positive non-small-cell lung cancer. *Clin Lung Cancer.* 2012;13:500–504.

33. Arcila ME, Chaft JE, Nafa K, et al. Prevalence, clinicopathologic associations, and molecular spectrum of ERBB2 (HER2) tyrosine kinase mutations in lung adenocarcinomas. *Clin Cancer Res.* 2012;18:4910–4918.

34. Liu HQ, Wang DM, Qu H, et al. Preparation and characterization of specific monoclonal antibodies against HER2. *Xi Bao Yu Fen Zi Mian Yi Xue Za Zhi.* 2010;26:456–458.

35. Reis H, Herold T, Ting S, et al. HER2 expression and markers of phosphoinositide-3-kinase pathway activation define a favorable subgroup of metastatic pulmonary adenocarcinomas. *Lung Cancer.* 2015;88:34–41.

36. Suzuki M, Shiraishi K, Yoshida A, et al. HER2 gene mutations in non-small cell lung carcinomas: concurrence with Her2 gene amplification and Her2 protein expression and phosphorylation. *Lung Cancer.* 2015;87:14–22.

37. Sherwood JL, Muller S, Orr MC, et al. Panel based MALDI-TOF tumour profiling is a sensitive method for detecting mutations in clinical non small cell lung cancer tumour. *PLoS One.* 2014;9:e100566.

38. Shepherd FA, Domerg C, Hainaut P, et al. Pooled analysis of the prognostic and predictive effects of KRAS mutation status and KRAS mutation subtype in early-stage resected non-small-cell lung cancer in four trials of adjuvant chemotherapy. *J Clin Oncol.* 2013;31:2173–2181.

39. Pardoll DM. The blockade of immune checkpoints in cancer immunotherapy. *Nat Rev Cancer.* 2012;12:252–264.

40. Yang CY, Lin MW, Chang YL, et al. Programmed cell death-ligand 1 expression in surgically resected stage I pulmonary adenocarcinoma and its correlation with driver mutations and clinical outcomes. *Eur J Cancer.* 2014;50:1361–1369.

41. Kerr KM, Tsao MS, Nicholson AG, et al. Programmed death-ligand 1 immunohistochemistry in lung cancer: in what state is this art? *J Thorac Oncol.* 2015;10:985–989.

42. Alexandrov LB, Nik-Zainal S, Wedge DC, et al. Signatures of mutational processes in human cancer. *Nature.* 2013;500:415–421.

43. Cardarella S, Ortiz TM, Joshi VA, et al. The introduction of systematic genomic testing for patients with non-small-cell lung cancer. *J Thorac Oncol.* 2012;7:1767–1774.

73 Staging of Lung Cancer

Andre L. Moreira, M.D., Fabio R. Tavora, M.D., Ph.D., and Marie-Christine Aubry, M.D.

Introduction

Staging of lung cancer currently follows the eighth edition of the American Joint Committee on Cancer (AJCC) cancer stage manual. The seventh edition as published in 2002[1-3] is at the time of this writing being replaced by the eighth edition as proposed by the International Association for the Study of Lung Cancer (IASLC) in association with AJCC and the International Union Against Cancer (UICC).

The IASLC stage committee evaluated over 80,000 cases of lung cancer obtained from multiple centers in twenty countries and four continents. This large study provided a robust validation of the system and proposed changes from the previous editions. The current staging system is also based on the TNM system, where T stands for the size and local extent of the tumor, N stands for the extent of nodal metastasis, and M for the presence or absence of metastasis. The TNM staging system is the most important prognostic marker for patients with lung cancer. It is also an important guide for patient management.

In a very simplified way, patients with stage one are treated with surgery alone. Patients with stages two and three receive adjuvant therapy after excision of the carcinoma; patients with lung cancer within stage three can also be candidates for neoadjuvant therapy followed by resection of residual tumor. Patients with stage four are treated predominantly with chemotherapy and are not usually surgical candidates.

The staging system can be clinical or pathologic. The pathologic stage is based on the examination of excised tumor or the presence of local or distant metastasis by biopsy material including cytology specimens. Pathologic stage should be preceded by the letter p, therefore pTNM. The clinical staging is composed of radiographic, nuclear medicine, and surgical information that is not always available to the pathologist during the time of examination of the excised specimen. The final stage should be done by the treating physician and incorporates the information obtained by the pathologic and clinical TNM.

Compared to the seventh edition of the cancer staging manual, the changes in the eighth edition are predominately seen on the size of tumor (T). pT1a (mi) has been added for minimally invasive carcinomas. pT1a is currently ≤1 cm (previously ≤2 cm). pT1b is now ≤ 2 cm (previously ≤3 cm). pT1c has been added for tumors between 2 cm and 3 cm. pT2a designates tumors 3 to 4 cm, pT2b 4 cm to 5 cm, pT3 5 cm to 7 cm, and pT4 tumors ≥ 7 cm. Other features override size. If there is involvement of the main bronchus without involving the carina, visceral pleural invasion, or obstructive pneumonitis that extends to the hilum, tumors ≤ 3 cm are designated pT2a tumors. pT3 tumors include tumors < 5 cm that invade the chest wall, phrenic nerve, parietal pericardium, or associated separate tumor nodule(s) seen grossly or by imaging in the same lobe (satellite nodules). pT4 tumors include those < 7 cm involving the diaphragm, mediastinum, heart, great vessels, trachea, recurrent laryngeal nerve, esophagus, vertebral body, carina, or tumor nodules in a different ipsilateral lobe.

Modifications in the T Category

The key changes in the current staging system occurred in T category. In the seventh AJCC edition, T1 was subclassified as T1a and T1b according to tumor size.[1] In the eighth edition, there are three stages, T1a–c, <1, 1 to 2, and 2 to 3 cm (see above). Similar changes occurred in T2 tumors. In the seventh AJCC edition, T2a are tumors larger than 3 cm but smaller than 5 cm, and T2b are larger than five centimeters but <7 cm in greatest dimension; the corresponding sizes have been changed to 3 to 4 and 4 to 5 cm. As previously, a T1 tumor can be upgraded to T2 if pleural invasion is identified, if located within 2 cm of the carina, or if associated with atelectasis or obstructive pneumonitis.

The designation of T3 is used for tumors that measure more than 5 cm in the eighth edition, as compared to 5 cm previously, or tumors of any size with direct involvement of the chest wall or any other structure such as mediastinal pleura or pericardium.

T4 tumors are tumors now > 7 cm (previously of any size) or that invade the mediastinum, heart, great vessels, trachea, recurrent laryngeal nerve, esophagus, vertebral body, and carina. Patients with tumor nodules showing the same morphologic characteristics in a different ipsilateral lobe from that of the main primary tumor are still designated as T4. The analysis of survival data shows that patients with ipsilateral lung nodules with the same morphology behave as stage IIIB and not as stage IV if these satellite nodules were to be considered metastatic sites.[4]

Problems with the Determination of T Category

Assessment of Tumor Size

One of the most important problems with the T category is the accurate determination of the size of the tumor.[5-8] The tumor size can be overestimated when it is accompanied by a prominent reactive process assumed to represent the true dimensions of the neoplastic process. Examples of these reactive processes are obstructive pneumonia, organizing pneumonia, and even scars. These overestimations can be done during the pathologic examination of the excised specimen, but tumor size can also be overestimated radiographically. In most cases, these discrepancies become irrelevant when there is a good correlation between gross and radiographic measurements. In case of a large discrepancy, the microscopic measurement of the tumor is adequate, especially when obstructive pneumonia or an extensive area of organizing pneumonia is diagnosed under the microscope. A microscopic measurement of the tumor should be indicated in the report with an explanation about the discrepancy between macroscopic and microscopic size determination.

Differences between measurements in fresh or formalin-fixed tissue have also been reported.[6,9,10] However, eventhough the discrepancy may be small, it could lead to reporting a T2a tumor as a T1b. In reality, the survival curves for T2a and T1b are not significantly different when tumor size is the only prognostic indicator.[9]

On the other hand, the tumor size can be underestimated, which is more commonly seen when an adenocarcinoma with a predominant lepidic component is present. In these cases, the gross measurements are often determined by the invasive component of the tumor that forms a solid mass due to desmoplastic reaction or tumor growth. This is particularly important in the setting of the new classification where adenocarcinoma in situ and minimally invasive adenocarcinomas are diagnosed based on the size of the invasive component.

Lepidic or papillary patterns of growth may resemble normal lung tissue and are often difficult to see grossly during specimen evaluation of fresh tissue. Awareness of the radiographic image of the tumor and radiographic size estimation is an important aspect of gross examination to ensure that appropriate numbers of sections are taken and all components of an adenocarcinoma are sampled. Lepidic growth pattern is often described radiographically as ground-glass opacities, whereas invasive components are often described as solid.[11] There is currently discussion in the thoracic pathology literature on tumor size determination for adenocarcinoma with a prominent or exclusive lepidic component.[11-15] The lepidic component is largely believed to represent in situ carcinoma, and as with other organs, it has been suggested that it should not be included in total tumor size estimate.[1] However, as this chapter is being written, there is no consensus on this issue; the total size of the tumor including the in situ component currently remains included in the pathologic tumor size (pT).

Assessing Distance from Carina

The relationship of the tumor with anatomic structures such as the distance from the carina is an important determinant of the T category because it is independent of tumor size; however, this spatial relationship cannot be determined by the examination of a lobectomy or pneumonectomy specimen. Thus, refinement of the T classification should be done in conjunction and in consultation with the surgeon.

Assessing Invasion into Adjacent Organs

Another problem that may emerge for an accurate determination of T category by pathologists is invasion into adjacent organs. Often, adjacent organ involvement by tumor is dealt by surgeons at the time of excision; in most cases, the pathologist receives a separate additional specimen-labeled pericardial biopsy or soft tissue nodule in the ascending aorta, for example. These separate materials, if positive, can modify the T determination and should be incorporated into the final pathologic stage for the specimen. In another scenario, a fragment of pericardium or pleura may be attached to the main specimen. The role of the pathologist is to determine if the tumor invades into these structures or is simply adhered, which is important for an accurate determination of the pT category.

Determination of Pleural Invasion

Pleural invasion is an important modifier of the T category; its presence upgrades a pT1 to a pT2 tumor. However, it is not always easy to determine if a tumor invades the pleura or not on H&E-stained slides alone. Disruption of the pleura by collapse of the underlying structures, elastotic scars, and subpleural fibrosis can render that determination almost impossible on H&E alone. Pleura invasion is defined as the presence of carcinoma beyond the external elastic layer of the visceral pleura.[16-18] Pushing of the tumor to the elastic layer is not considered as an evidence of invasion (PL0) (Fig. 73.1). Most often, an elastic stain is necessary to help the pathologist evaluate pleural invasion.[16-18]

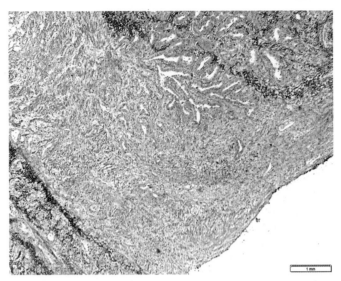

FIGURE 73.2 ▲ Elastic stain showing fibrosis and invagination of the pleura with tumor cells above the external elastic layer (PL1). The invasion of tumor cells through the pleura was not evident in the H&E-stained sections.

Evaluation of elastic stain poses yet another set of pitfalls. Very often, the stain has a suboptimal technical quality, which impairs interpretation. Even with a good quality stain, the elastic fibers of the pleura may not have a continuous layer. In addition, there are multiple variations in the elastic layers of the normal pleura.[6]

The determination of PL1 (Fig. 73.2) is used to indicate that there is pleural invasion through the external elastic layer as indicated above; PL2 is used to designate tumor that invades through the pleura and is seen on the pleural surface (Fig. 73.3). The presence of PL1 or PL2 upstages a tumor to at least pT2a. PL3 is used to designate a tumor that invades the parietal pleura or chest wall. The presence of PL3 upstages a tumor to pT3.[19]

Presence of Multiple Nodules

The presence of multiple nodules in the same lobe or ipsilateral lobes is an important feature for the determination of T category in the

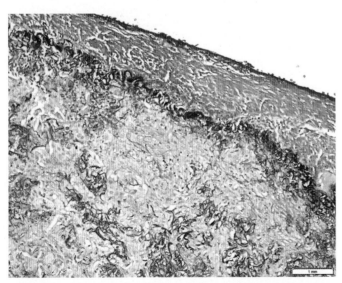

FIGURE 73.1 ▲ Elastic stain showing tumor cells approaching the external elastic layer, but not penetrating through (PL0). There is no evidence of pleural invasion.

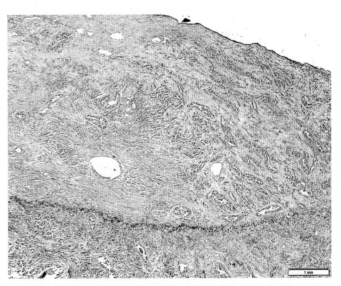

FIGURE 73.3 ▲ Elastic stain showing tumor cells invading through the pleura reaching the pleural surface (PL2). In this image, it appears that the elastic layer is intact, but the tumor has invaded the pleura to grow above the represented elastic layer.

pathologic stage as seen above. However, one of the main difficulties rests in deciding whether the separate nodules are indeed satellite tumor nodules or whether they represent separate primaries in patients with multifocal disease. This differential diagnosis has become an important and difficult feature in pulmonary pathology.

Martini and Melamed[20] were the first to address the issue of multiple pulmonary tumor nodules and tried to separate synchronous or metachronous primaries from intrapulmonary metastatic disease in excised specimens. In the original publication, it was stated that tumor with different morphology represents separate (synchronous or metachronous) carcinomas. The presence of lymphovascular invasion or lymph node metastasis was favored to indicate metastatic disease if the tumors shared the same histology.

In that first scheme, however, different histologic features meant adenocarcinoma versus squamous cell carcinoma. In the case of adenocarcinomas that are well known to be histologically heterogeneous, often presenting with multiple histologic growth patterns, the proposed Martini and Melamed scheme is less reliable.

The current classification of lung carcinomas by the World Health Organization (WHO) recognizes five growth patterns: lepidic, acinar, papillary, solid, and micropapillary.[21] Other variants such as cribriform and complex glands have been described[22,23] but are not recognized by the WHO at this time. The current WHO classification also proposes that a pulmonary adenocarcinoma should be classified by its predominant pattern.[21,24] However, simple determination of the predominant pattern is often inadequate for the determination of separate primaries or metastatic disease. It is known that high-grade components such as solid, micropapillary, and cribriform patterns can be overexpressed at the metastatic site.[23,25] Therefore, when dealing with multifocal adenocarcinoma, it is possible to encounter a situation where one tumor is predominantly papillary, whereas the other is predominantly solid. The simple determination of the predominant pattern may not be helpful if both tumors share the same or similar growth patterns heterogeneity. In these cases, it is important to look at all the histologic patterns of the tumors as well as the cytologic characteristics to determine whether they represent the same tumor with intrapulmonary spread (pT3 or pT4) or multifocal adenocarcinomas. Separate primaries should be staged individually, which changes patient management. In most cases, even a careful histologic evaluation cannot be used to determine with certainty if a tumor represents separate primaries or tumor spread. In these situations, molecular evaluation of the nodules can be helpful. Somatic mutational profile has been proposed as a tool to distinguish independent primaries from metastasis; however, because of their commonality, some mutations may be shared between independent primaries. Alternatively, somatic genomic rearrangements have proven to be more unique and therefore potentially more accurate for this purpose.[26–29]

N Category

The current (eighth) staging manual makes no changes in pN staging (pN1 = ipsilateral hilar or peribronchial, all with number designations 10 or greater; pN2 = ipsilateral mediastinal or carinal nodes, all with number designations 9 or less; pN3 = contralateral mediastinal or peribronchial or any scalene or supraclavicular lymph node involvement). The direct invasion of a lymph node by a tumor should be counted as lymph node metastasis (pN1). The same is true for a peribronchial or hilar lymph node that is completely replaced by tumor. In the latter case, the finding of a round tumor mass separated from the invasive carcinoma with no evidence of remaining lymph node tissue should also be counted as a metastatic lymph node pN1. Metastatic disease to other, nonregional lymph nodes should be considered as M1.

Isolated tumor cells in lymph nodes are a rare finding in pulmonary pathology. They are better described in other organ systems. Isolated tumor cells are defined as isolated or small clusters of cells (<0.2 cm) seen in the subcapsular space of a lymph node without evidence of invasion or desmoplastic reaction.[1] There are few studies to support the

evidence of isolated tumor cells as having an impact on tumor biology; therefore, the presence of isolated tumor cells do not constitute at this moment an evidence of regional lymph node metastasis, but their presence can be indicated by the denomination pN0 (i+).[30,31]

Although extranodal extension has been shown to impart an unfavorable prognosis, it does not affect N staging.[32]

M (Metastatic) Disease

Tumors with direct invasion to the visceral pleura are classified as T2[2,5,20]; however, the presence of discontinuous tumor nodules or implants in the pleura or pericardium is classified as M1a.[30,33] A positive pleural or pericardium effusion by cytology also qualifies for the designation of M1a. In patients with recurrent effusions but with negative cytology, M0 is the correct classification, thus reinforcing the concept that tissue diagnosis is paramount for confirmation of metastatic disease. In a patient with cancer, other comorbidities may exist that can be the cause of pleural/pericardial effusion.

The term M1b is a designation used exclusively for distant metastasis. It is recommended that all sites of metastatic disease be biopsied to document disease spread. The term M1c is being proposed for multiple, as opposed to single distant metastases.

Neuroendocrine Tumors

Contrary to previous editions, it is now recommended that small cell carcinoma and carcinoid tumors (typical and atypical carcinoids) should be staged similarly to non–small cell lung cancers.[1,18,34]

Although carcinoid tumors have a better survival curve as compared to non–small cell carcinomas, the TNM classification still offers significant prognostic indication for tumors in more advanced stage. Most carcinoid tumors, either typical or atypical carcinoids, are rarely larger than 3 cm; therefore, there is no significant difference between survival curves of tumors in stages 1 and 2, but the presence of lymph node metastasis (N) or distant metastasis (M) heralds a significant difference in prognosis. The inclusion of these tumors in the TNM classification offers a reproducible and uniform staging classification and guides therapeutic decisions as well.

For small cell carcinomas, the previously used terminology of limited or extensive disease should be discontinued.

REFERENCES

1. Edge S, Byrd DR, Compton CC, et al. *AJCC Cancer Staging Manual.* 7th ed. New York: Springer; 2010.
2. Goldstraw P, Crowley J, Chansky K, et al. The IASLC Lung Cancer Staging Project: proposals for the revision of the TNM stage groupings in the forthcoming (seventh) edition of the TNM Classification of malignant tumours. *J Thorac Oncol.* 2007;2:706–714.
3. Rusch VW, Crowley J, Giroux DJ, et al. The IASLC Lung Cancer Staging Project: proposals for the revision of the N descriptors in the forthcoming seventh edition of the TNM classification for lung cancer. *J Thorac Oncol.* 2007;2:603–612.
4. Rami-Porta R, Ball D, Crowley J, et al. The IASLC Lung Cancer Staging Project: proposals for the revision of the T descriptors in the forthcoming (seventh) edition of the TNM classification for lung cancer. *J Thorac Oncol.* 2007;2:593–602.
5. Flieder DB. Commonly encountered difficulties in pathologic staging of lung cancer. *Arch Pathol Lab Med.* 2007;131:1016–1026.
6. Jones KD. An update on lung cancer staging. *Adv Anat Pathol.* 2010;17:33–37.
7. Marchevsky AM. Problems in pathologic staging of lung cancer. *Arch Pathol Lab Med.* 2006;130:292–302.
8. Sica GL, Gal AA. Lung cancer staging: pathology issues. *Semin Diagn Pathol.* 2012;29:116–126.
9. Hsu PK, Huang HC, Hsieh CC, et al. Effect of formalin fixation on tumor size determination in stage I non-small cell lung cancer. *Ann Thorac Surg.* 2007;84:1825–1829.
10. Travis WD, Committee IS. Reporting lung cancer pathology specimens. Impact of the anticipated 7th Edition TNM classification based on recommendations of the IASLC Staging Committee. *Histopathology.* 2009;54:3–11.

11. Austin SE, Hegele RA. Clinical implications of direct-to-consumer genetic testing for cardiovascular disease risk. *Can J Cardiol.* 2011;27:682–684.

12. Borczuk AC, Qian F, Kazeros A, et al. Invasive size is an independent predictor of survival in pulmonary adenocarcinoma. *Am J Surg Pathol.* 2009;33:462–469.

13. Sakao Y, Nakazono T, Tomimitsu S, et al. Lung adenocarcinoma can be subtyped according to tumor dimension by computed tomography mediastinal-window setting. Additional size criteria for clinical T1 adenocarcinoma. *Eur J Cardiothorac Surg.* 2004;26:1211–1215.

14. Suzuki K, Koike T, Asakawa T, et al. A prospective radiological study of thin-section computed tomography to predict pathological noninvasiveness in peripheral clinical IA lung cancer (Japan Clinical Oncology Group 0201). *J Thorac Oncol.* 2011;6:751–756.

15. Yoshizawa A, Motoi N, Riely GJ, et al. Impact of proposed IASLC/ATS/ERS classification of lung adenocarcinoma: prognostic subgroups and implications for further revision of staging based on analysis of 514 stage I cases. *Mod Pathol.* 2011;24:653–664.

16. Butnor KJ, Cooper K. Visceral pleural invasion in lung cancer: recognizing histologic parameters that impact staging and prognosis. *Adv Anat Pathol.* 2005;12:1–6.

17. Butnor KJ, Travis WD. Recent advances in our understanding of lung cancer visceral pleural invasion and other forms of minimal invasion: implications for the next TNM classification. *Eur J Cardiothorac Surg.* 2013;43:309–311.

18. Travis WD, Brambilla E, Rami-Porta R, et al. Visceral pleural invasion: pathologic criteria and use of elastic stains: proposal for the 7th edition of the TNM classification for lung cancer. *J Thorac Oncol.* 2008;3:1384–1390.

19. Yoshida J, Nagai K, Asamura H, et al. Visceral pleura invasion impact on non-small cell lung cancer patient survival: its implications for the forthcoming TNM staging based on a large-scale nation-wide database. *J Thorac Oncol.* 2009;4:959–963.

20. Martini N, Melamed MR. Multiple primary lung cancers. *J Thorac Cardiovasc Surg.* 1975;70:606–612.

21. Travis WD, Brambilla E, Noguchi M, et al. International association for the study of lung cancer/American thoracic society/European respiratory society international multidisciplinary classification of lung adenocarcinoma. *J Thorac Oncol.* 2011;6:244–285.

22. Moreira AL, Joubert P, Downey RJ, et al. Cribriform and fused glands are patterns of high-grade pulmonary adenocarcinoma. *Hum Pathol.* 2014;45:213–220.

23. Xu L, Tavora F, Burke A. Histologic features associated with metastatic potential in invasive adenocarcinomas of the lung. *Am J Surg Pathol.* 2013;37:1100–1108.

24. Travis WD. The 2015 WHO classification of lung tumors. *Pathologe.* 2014;35(suppl 2):188.

25. Sica G, Yoshizawa A, Sima CS, et al. A grading system of lung adenocarcinomas based on histologic pattern is predictive of disease recurrence in stage I tumors. *Am J Surg Pathol.* 2010;34:1155–1162.

26. Finley CJ, Bendzsak A, Tomlinson G, et al. The effect of regionalization on outcome in pulmonary lobectomy: a Canadian national study. *J Thorac Cardiovasc Surg.* 2010;140:757–763.

27. Girard N, Deshpande C, Lau C, et al. Comprehensive histologic assessment helps to differentiate multiple lung primary nonsmall cell carcinomas from metastases. *Am J Surg Pathol.* 2009;33:1752–1764.

28. Girard N, Ostrovnaya I, Lau C, et al. Genomic and mutational profiling to assess clonal relationships between multiple non-small cell lung cancers. *Clin Cancer Res.* 2009;15:5184–5190.

29. Murphy SJ, Aubry MC, Harris FR, et al. Identification of independent primary tumors and intrapulmonary metastases using DNA rearrangements in non-small-cell lung cancer. *J Clin Oncol.* 2014;32:4050–4058.

30. Coello MC, Luketich JD, Litle VR, et al. Prognostic significance of micrometastasis in non-small-cell lung cancer. *Clin Lung Cancer.* 2004;5:214–225.

31. Hermanek P, Hutter RV, Sobin LH, et al. International Union Against Cancer. Classification of isolated tumor cells and micrometastasis. *Cancer.* 1999;86:2668–2673.

32. Lee YC, Wu CT, Kuo SW, et al. Significance of extranodal extension of regional lymph nodes in surgically resected non-small cell lung cancer. *Chest.* 2007;131:993–999.

33. Postmus PE, Brambilla E, Chansky K, et al. The IASLC Lung Cancer Staging Project: proposals for revision of the M descriptors in the forthcoming (seventh) edition of the TNM classification of lung cancer. *J Thorac Oncol.* 2007;2:686–693.

34. Shepherd FA, Crowley J, Van Houtte P, et al. The International Association for the Study of Lung Cancer lung cancer staging project: proposals regarding the clinical staging of small cell lung cancer in the forthcoming (seventh) edition of the tumor, node, metastasis classification for lung cancer. *J Thorac Oncol.* 2007;2:1067–1077.

74 Atypical Adenomatous Hyperplasia, Adenocarcinoma In Situ, and Minimally Invasive Adenocarcinoma (Nonmucinous)

Fabio R. Tavora, M.D., Ph.D., Allen P. Burke, M.D., and Marie-Christine Aubry, M.D.

Introduction

The concept of precursor lesions to adenocarcinomas of the lung has been debated since the 1960s[1] and later addressed by several authors who proposed a stepwise process analogous to the adenoma–carcinoma sequence in the colon.[2–4] Noninvasive lesions include *atypical adenomatous hyperplasia* (AAH), which is considered a precursor lesion but not malignant (similar to an adenoma in the gastrointestinal tract), and *adenocarcinoma in situ* (AIS), which is a noninvasive carcinoma with the histologic features of malignancy. A third lesion, *minimally invasive adenocarcinoma* (MIA), has recently been designated as a lesion composed primarily of adenocarcinoma with lepidic growth and with a degree of invasion that is insufficient to result in a significant risk for metastatic disease.

AAH, by definition, is a nonmucinous proliferation. Mucinous AIS and mucinous MIA are genetically distinct from their nonmucinous counterparts and are considered in Chapter 76. "AIS" and "MIA" when used in this chapter are presumed to denote the nonmucinous (most common) type.

Atypical Adenomatous Hyperplasia

Background

AAH is considered the precursor lesion to pulmonary adenocarcinoma based on epidemiologic, morphologic, immunohistochemical, and, more recently, molecular studies.[3,5–10] The current belief clearly states a direct relationship of AAH as a precursor to well-differentiated adenocarcinomas. This concept has grown in importance in the past two decades with advances in imaging and screening protocols for patients at risk that have led to an increase in the detection of early lesions such as AAH.[6,11–13]

Radiologic Findings

AAH is found as an incidental lesion on high-resolution CT scans, often in patients with other invasive adenocarcinomas. Recent advances in radiologic techniques have helped increase detection radiologically, generally in the periphery, with a predilection to upper lobes.[13] The classic radiologic description of AAH is an oval pure ground-glass

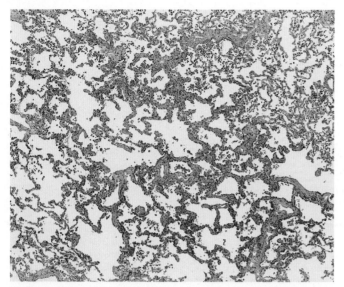

FIGURE 74.1 ▲ AAH, low power. Note slightly thickened septa with a monotonous proliferation of mildly atypical cells.

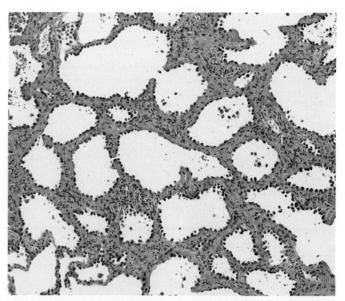

FIGURE 74.2 ▲ AAH, high power. Note cytologic features of AAH: monotonous proliferation of mildly atypical cells with thickened alveolar septa. A space is present between the nuclei.

opacity without any central solid component on CT scan,[14,15] which is similar to the description of AIS (formerly bronchioloalveolar carcinoma). The detection of ground-glass opacities has increased in the past 5 years, due to screening of a high-risk population, and pathologic sampling of these peripheral nodules is also on the rise.[16,17] Radiologic characteristics such as sphericity, nodule size, and internal air bronchogram may be features that help distinguish between AAH and AIS.[18–21]

Incidence

AAH is usually found incidentally in surgical specimens of patients with lung cancer.[3,20,22] Several reports have identified an incidence of AAH in specimens of lung adenocarcinomas separate from the main tumors in 5% to 20% of cases.[2,19,22,23] On imaging, AAH is found up to 30% of patients with nodules of invasive adenocarcinoma.[19]

Gross Features

Grossly, AAH lesions are not detected, but can be appreciated as poorly defined tan or gray nodules close to the pleura. AAH has also been detected in random sections of normal lung parenchyma.[24]

Histologic Features

AAH is pathologically characterized by a small (<0.5 cm) proliferation of mildly atypical cells resembling type II pneumocytes or Clara cells, in a lepidic growth, spreading along the alveolar septa. The alveolar septa are mildly thickened but without loss of the normal lung architecture (Fig. 74.1). Mitoses are rare to absent. Cytologically, the cells

are mildly atypical with increased nuclear size and nuclear to cytoplasmic ratio. The atypia is less pronounced than in AIS. The cell proliferation appears monotonous, and a gap is present between the cells (Fig. 74.2). Multiple lesions of AAH can be seen in the same sample of invasive tumors.

AAH should be distinguished from reactive pneumocyte hyperplasia and from AIS (Table 74.1). Typically, pneumocyte hyperplasia appears less monotonous that AAH and usually is in reaction to another process occurring in the lung such as fibrosis and inflammation. In AIS, the cell proliferation loses the space in between the cells, leading to nuclear crowding and overlapping. Although classification of AAH into low and high grade has been reported, it is not recommended in the current WHO classification.[25]

Molecular Findings

AAH has been reported to harbor driver mutations such as KRAS and EGFR, supporting the notion that AAH is a direct precursor lesion of lung adenocarcinoma. However, mitochondrial DNA sequencing and loss of heterozygosity analysis have shown a lack of correlation between AAH and associated adenocarcinomas,[9,26] suggesting that AAH is not always a precursor, but a smoking-induced low-grade neoplastic lesion.

EGFR mutations are found in as few as 3%[8] to about one-third of AAH[27] and are less common than in AIS.[8,28] Concordance of EGFR and KRAS mutations between AAH and associated carcinomas is seen in 63% to 75% of tumors.[10]

TABLE 74.1 Pathologic Characteristics of Preinvasive and Minimally Invasive Lepidic Pulmonary Lesions

Lesions	Size	Invasive Focus	Architecture	Cellular Characteristics
Atypical adenomatous hyperplasia	<5 mm	None	Slightly thickened alveolar walls, well demarcated from adjacent lung. Homogeneous growth pattern with little to absent inflammation and no fibrosis	Mildly atypical cells with little variation in size and shape
Adenocarcinoma in situ	<30 mm	None	Thickened alveolar walls	Moderate to severe nuclear atypia, anisocytosis, macronucleoli, atypical mitoses
Minimally invasive adenocarcinoma	<30 mm	Invasive focus <5 mm	Similar to AIS, with invasion into stroma that is commonly central and resembles scar, with angulated glands, solid growth, and stromal reaction	Similar to AIS

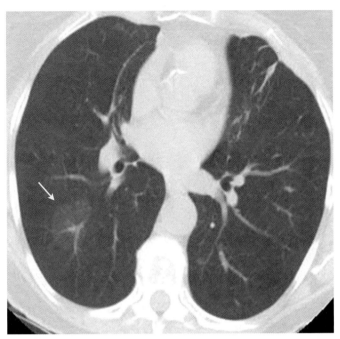

FIGURE 74.3 ▲ CT scan of AIS showing a pure ground-glass opacity in the right lung (*arrow*).

Mutations in the KRAS gene have been found in up to 33% of AAH, a higher rate than AIS or invasive carcinomas.[29]

Adenocarcinoma In Situ (Nonmucinous)

Background

The term AIS was officially proposed in the 2011 IASLC/ATS/ERS classification of adenocarcinomas and the 2015 WHO Classification of Lung Tumors to replace the term "bronchioloalveolar carcinoma."[30,31] It is defined as an adenocarcinoma <3 cm in size with neoplastic cells growing along the preexisting alveolar septa (the definition of pure lepidic growth) with no stromal, vascular, or pleural invasion. Recently, alveolar space invasion ("spread through alveolar spaces") has been added as

a feature that excludes the diagnosis.[31] Nonmucinous AIS is far more common than mucinous AIS, as mucinous lesions are generally larger and contain invasive elements that exclude an in situ designation.[31]

Clinical and Radiologic Findings

Patients typically are asymptomatic, and AIS is an incidental finding on imaging. The CT findings of AIS are similar if not identical to AAH and consist of a mostly pure ground-glass opacity (Fig. 74.3). Rarely, the opacity may be subsolid. The lesions of AIS are typically larger with less smooth borders than those of AAH.

Pathologic Features

Grossly, AIS lesions are tan-white, poorly defined nodules, difficult to distinguish from normal surrounding lung.

Histologically, as with AAH, the neoplastic cell appear monotonous, growing along intact alveolar septa. The nuclei are enlarged with mild cytologic atypia. The cells show nuclear overlapping and tufting, features absent in AAH (Fig. 74.4). AIS appears sharply demarcated from the adjacent normal lung (Fig. 74.4). Alveolar septal thickening with fibrosis and/or elastosis is common in AIS. And in fact, occasionally, the fibrosis and elastosis may result in a central scar, distorting the normal architecture. This leads to the neoplastic cells to form acinar structures entrapped in the scar. Distinguishing this from true invasion may be challenging. With invasion, the acinar structures become small and irregular with angled shape and are associated with a fibroblastic proliferation representing desmoplasia (Fig. 74.5). If in doubt and the area suspected of invasion is ≤5 mm, a diagnosis of MIA may be more appropriate. The clinical outcome is similar for AIS and MIA. Papillary or micropapillary structures should be absent as they are indicative of invasion.[32–35]

Because AIS is defined by the absence of invasion, whether pleural, vascular, or stromal, the diagnosis requires thorough examination of a resected tumor. On a small biopsy, including transbronchial and transthoracic needle specimens, if the adenocarcinoma shows a pure lepidic growth pattern, a diagnosis of adenocarcinoma with lepidic pattern should be made with a comment that an invasive component cannot be excluded (Fig. 74.6). A diagnosis of AIS or MIA should not be made on such small specimens (Table 74.2).

Molecular Findings

Hypermethylation has been described in several genes associated with adenocarcinoma oncogenesis, including *2C35*, *EYA4*, *HOXA1*,

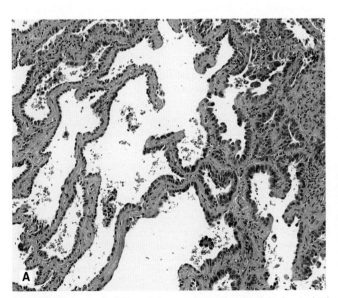

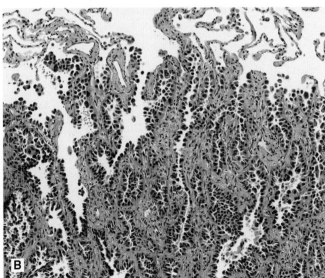

FIGURE 74.4 ▲ **A.** AIS contains more prominent cytologic atypia than AAH as well as nuclear overlapping. **B.** The AIS abruptly transitions into the adjacent normal lung.

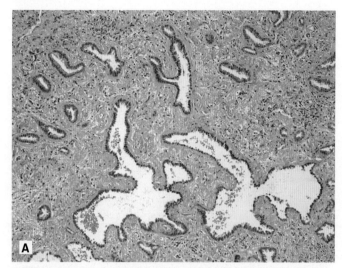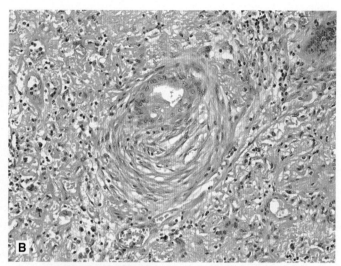

FIGURE 74.5 ▲ A. AIS with scar. The acinar structures are overall large and the stroma shows no desmoplasia. **B.** In contrast, early invasion with the acinar structure is small and associated with desmoplasia. This finding would exclude the diagnosis of AIS.

HOXA11, NEUROD1, NEUROD2, and *TMEFF2* in cases of AIS.[36] In a Japanese series, the *KRAS* gene was mutated in 12% of cases, with EGFR mutations in 51%.[29] Other studies have found a lower rate of somatic EGFR mutations, with an incidence of 11%.[8]

Minimally Invasive Adenocarcinoma (Nonmucinous)

Definition

MIA is defined as adenocarcinoma 3 cm and less with stromal invasion of 5 mm or less. This amount of invasion defines an adenocarcinoma with limited to no metastatic potential. Initially, a central scar of 6 mm or greater was proposed to diagnose an invasive adenocarcinoma.[37] Subsequently, an area of 5 mm of tumor invasion or greater was shown to be a relevant cutoff to separate tumors with and without malignant potential.[35,38–40]

Radiologic Findings

Nodules of MIA may also show pure ground-glass opacities in CT scan, but solid areas representing invasion and increased attenuation can also be seen. A recent study of 52 MIA showed that most cases appeared as pure or part-solid ground-glass nodules, with frequent interval growth at follow-up at a higher rate than seen in AIS.[41]

Histologic Findings

AIS and MIA share similar architectural and cytologic features, except for foci of invasion ≤ 5 mm in MIA. Invasion is defined by any patterns that are not lepidic, including acinar, papillary, micropapillary, solid patterns, and single cells in a desmoplastic stroma (Fig. 74.7). Lymphatic invasion, invasion of airspaces, necrosis, and pleural invasion exclude the diagnosis of MIA.[31] The focus of invasion is measured along its largest dimension. If multiple, the largest focus of invasion is used. Another way that has been suggested is to estimate the percentage of invasion, add the percentages, and then multiply by the overall tumor diameter in mm. If the result is ≤5 mm, then a diagnosis of MIA should be rendered.

The differential diagnosis between AIS, MIA, and lepidic predominant AD can be very challenging and interobserver variation with only moderate level of agreement has been reported. The distinction between AIS and MIA does not appear to be critical because both have a similar excellent prognosis. However, lepidic adenocarcinoma is associated with increased risk of recurrence and metastasis.[34,35,42] Therefore, it is best not to underestimate the degree of invasion.[43]

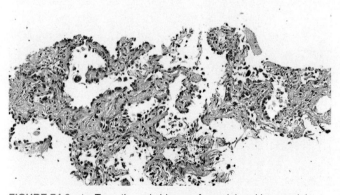

FIGURE 74.6 ▲ Transthoracic biopsy of a peripheral lung nodule showing a well-differentiated adenocarcinoma with exclusive lepidic growth. Although in the sample there is no evidence of stromal or vascular invasion, a comment should be added that an invasive focus cannot be excluded in an eventual resected specimen.

TABLE 74.2 Terminology to be Used in Biopsy Material and in Resected Specimens

Resected Specimen Terminology	Small Biopsy Terminology	Notes
Atypical adenomatous hyperplasia	Not addressed	Usually not resected by itself and found adjacent to invasive lesions
Adenocarcinoma in situ	Adenocarcinoma with lepidic pattern	In biopsy material, add a comment that an invasive component cannot be excluded
Minimally invasive adenocarcinoma	Adenocarcinoma with lepidic pattern	Not advised to attempt to measure extent of invasion in biopsy and a comment can be added similar to the above

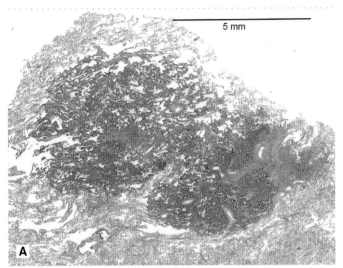
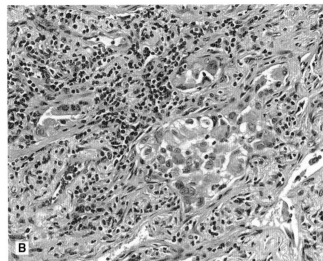

FIGURE 74.7 ▲ MIA. **A.** Low magnification shows a tumor measuring about 1 cm, which is predominantly in situ. Focal fibrosis is seen raising concern for invasion. **B.** High magnification shows invasion with solid growth.

Treatment and Prognosis

The reported prognosis of AIS and MIA is 100% disease-free and recurrence-free survival if entirely resected. Currently, the standard of care for AIS and MIA is surgical resection with lobectomy. Considering the excellent prognosis of AIS and MIA, sublobar resection may be a valid option. However, results of clinical trials assessing sublobar resection (segmentectomy or wedge resection) as a viable oncologic procedure have not yet been published.

REFERENCES

1. Meyer EC, Liebow AA. Relationship of interstitial pneumonia honeycombing and atypical epithelial proliferation to cancer of the lung. *Cancer.* 1965;18:322–351.
2. Carey FA, Wallace WA, Fergusson RJ, et al. Alveolar atypical hyperplasia in association with primary pulmonary adenocarcinoma: a clinicopathological study of 10 cases. *Thorax.* 1992;47:1041–1043.
3. Kitamura H, Kameda Y, Ito T, et al. Atypical adenomatous hyperplasia of the lung. Implications for the pathogenesis of peripheral lung adenocarcinoma. *Am J Clin Pathol.* 1999;111:610–622.
4. Miller RR, Nelems B, Evans KG, et al. Glandular neoplasia of the lung. A proposed analogy to colonic tumors. *Cancer.* 1988;61:1009–1014.
5. Weng S, Tsuchiya E, Satoh Y, et al. Multiple atypical adenomatous hyperplasia of type II pneumonocytes and bronchiolo-alveolar carcinoma. *Histopathology.* 1990;16:101–103.
6. Sone S, Takashima S, Li F, et al. Mass screening for lung cancer with mobile spiral computed tomography scanner. *Lancet.* 1998;351:1242–1245.
7. Sone S, Li F, Yang ZG, et al. Results of three-year mass screening programme for lung cancer using mobile low-dose spiral computed tomography scanner. *Br J Cancer.* 2001;84:25–32.
8. Yoshida Y, Shibata T, Kokubu A, et al. Mutations of the epidermal growth factor receptor gene in atypical adenomatous hyperplasia and bronchioloalveolar carcinoma of the lung. *Lung Cancer.* 2005;50:1–8.
9. Morandi L, Asioli S, Cavazza A, et al. Genetic relationship among atypical adenomatous hyperplasia, bronchioloalveolar carcinoma and adenocarcinoma of the lung. *Lung Cancer.* 2007;56:35–42.
10. Sartori G, Cavazza A, Bertolini F, et al. A subset of lung adenocarcinomas and atypical adenomatous hyperplasia-associated foci are genotypically related: an EGFR, HER2, and K-ras mutational analysis. *Am J Clin Pathol.* 2008;129:202–210.
11. Weichert W, Warth A. Early lung cancer with lepidic pattern: adenocarcinoma in situ, minimally invasive adenocarcinoma, and lepidic predominant adenocarcinoma. *Curr Opin Pulm Med.* 2014;20:309–316.
12. Zhang H, Duan J, Li ZJ, et al. Analysis on minimally invasive diagnosis and treatment of 49 cases with solitary nodular ground-glass opacity. *J Thorac Dis.* 2014;6:1452–1457.
13. Nakahara R, Yokose T, Nagai K, et al. Atypical adenomatous hyperplasia of the lung: a clinicopathological study of 118 cases including cases with multiple atypical adenomatous hyperplasia. *Thorax.* 2001;56:302–305.
14. Truong MT, Ko JP, Rossi SE, et al. Update in the evaluation of the solitary pulmonary nodule. *Radiographics.* 2014;34:1658–1679.
15. Kaneko M, Eguchi K, Ohmatsu H, et al. Peripheral lung cancer: screening and detection with low-dose spiral CT versus radiography. *Radiology.* 1996;201:798–802.
16. Braillon A. Bronchioalveolar lung cancer: screening and overdiagnosis. *J Clin Oncol.* 2014;32:3575.
17. Gierada DS, Pinsky P, Nath H, et al. Projected outcomes using different nodule sizes to define a positive CT lung cancer screening examination. *J Natl Cancer Inst.* 2014;106.
18. Oda S, Awai K, Liu D, et al. Ground-glass opacities on thin-section helical CT: differentiation between bronchioloalveolar carcinoma and atypical adenomatous hyperplasia. *AJR Am J Roentgenol.* 2008;190:1363–1368.
19. Chapman AD, Kerr KM. The association between atypical adenomatous hyperplasia and primary lung cancer. *Br J Cancer.* 2000;83:632–636.
20. Liu LH, Liu M, Wei R, et al. CT findings of persistent pure ground glass opacity: can we predict the invasiveness? *Asian Pac J Cancer Prev.* 2015;16:1925–1928.
21. Gu B, Burt BM, Merritt RE, et al. A dominant adenocarcinoma with multifocal ground glass lesions does not behave as advanced disease. *Ann Thorac Surg.* 2013;96:411–418.
22. Koga T, Hashimoto S, Sugio K, et al. Lung adenocarcinoma with bronchioloalveolar carcinoma component is frequently associated with foci of high-grade atypical adenomatous hyperplasia. *Am J Clin Pathol.* 2002;117:464–470.
23. Nakanishi K. Alveolar epithelial hyperplasia and adenocarcinoma of the lung. *Arch Pathol Lab Med.* 1990;114:363–368.
24. Mori M, Rao SK, Popper HH, et al. Atypical adenomatous hyperplasia of the lung: a probable forerunner in the development of adenocarcinoma of the lung. *Mod Pathol.* 2001;14:72–84.
25. Kitamura H, Kameda Y, Nakamura N, et al. Atypical adenomatous hyperplasia and bronchoalveolar lung carcinoma. Analysis by morphometry and the expressions of p53 and carcinoembryonic antigen. *Am J Surg Pathol.* 1996;20:553–562.
26. Gradowski JF, Mantha GS, Hunt JL, et al. Molecular alterations in atypical adenomatous hyperplasia occurring in benign and cancer-bearing lungs. *Diagn Mol Pathol.* 2007;16:87–90.
27. Noguchi M, Yatabe Y, Brambilla E, et al. Preinvasive lesions. Atypical adenomatous hyperplasia. Adenocarcinoma in situ. In: Travis WD, et al., eds. *WHO Classification of Tumours of the Lung, Pleura, Thymus and Heart.* Lyon, France: IARC Press; 2015:46–50.
28. Pastorino U, Calabro E, Tamborini E, et al. Prolonged remission of disseminated atypical adenomatous hyperplasia under gefitinib. *J Thorac Oncol.* 2009;4:266–267.

29. Sakamoto H, Shimizu J, Horio Y, et al. Disproportionate representation of KRAS gene mutation in atypical adenomatous hyperplasia, but even distribution of EGFR gene mutation from preinvasive to invasive adenocarcinomas. *J Pathol.* 2007;212:287–294.

30. Travis WD, Brambilla E, Noguchi M, et al. International association for the study of lung cancer/american thoracic society/european respiratory society international multidisciplinary classification of lung adenocarcinoma. *J Thorac Oncol.* 2011;6:244–285.

31. Travis WD, Noguchi M, Yatabe Y, et al. Minimally invasive adenocarcinoma. In: Travis WD, et al., eds. *WHO Classification of Tumours of the Lung, Pleura, Thymus and Heart.* Lyon, France: IARC Press; 2015:44–46.

32. Schmidt L, Myers J. Bronchioloalveolar carcinoma and the significance of invasion: predicting biologic behavior. *Arch Pathol Lab Med.* 2010;134:1450–1454.

33. Xu L, Tavora F, Burke A. 'Bronchioloalveolar carcinoma': is the term really dead? A critical review of a new classification system for pulmonary adenocarcinomas. *Pathology.* 2012;44:497–505.

34. Maeshima AM, Niki T, Maeshima A, et al. Modified scar grade: a prognostic indicator in small peripheral lung adenocarcinoma. *Cancer.* 2002;95:2546–2554.

35. Terasaki H, Niki T, Matsuno Y, et al. Lung adenocarcinoma with mixed bronchioloalveolar and invasive components: clinicopathological features, subclassification by extent of invasive foci, and immunohistochemical characterization. *Am J Surg Pathol.* 2003;27:937–951.

36. Selamat SA, Galler JS, Joshi AD, et al. DNA methylation changes in atypical adenomatous hyperplasia, adenocarcinoma in situ, and lung adenocarcinoma. *PLoS One.* 2011;6:e21443.

37. Suzuki K, Yokose T, Yoshida J, et al. Prognostic significance of the size of central fibrosis in peripheral adenocarcinoma of the lung. *Ann Thorac Surg.* 2000;69:893–897.

38. Borczuk AC. Assessment of invasion in lung adenocarcinoma classification, including adenocarcinoma in situ and minimally invasive adenocarcinoma. *Mod Pathol.* 2012;25(suppl 1):S1–S10.

39. Borczuk AC, Qian F, Kazeros A, et al. Invasive size is an independent predictor of survival in pulmonary adenocarcinoma. *Am J Surg Pathol.* 2009;33:462–469.

40. Xu L, Tavora F, Battafarano R, et al. Adenocarcinomas with prominent lepidic spread: retrospective review applying new classification of the American Thoracic Society. *Am J Surg Pathol.* 2012;36:273–282.

41. Lee SM, Goo JM, Lee KH, et al. CT findings of minimally invasive adenocarcinoma (MIA) of the lung and comparison of solid portion measurement methods at CT in 52 patients. *Eur Radiol.* 2015.

42. Xu L, Tavora F, Burke A. Histologic features associated with metastatic potential in invasive adenocarcinomas of the lung. *Am J Surg Pathol.* 2013;37:1100–1108.

43. Kadota K, Villena-Vargas J, Yoshizawa A, et al. Prognostic significance of adenocarcinoma in situ, minimally invasive adenocarcinoma, and nonmucinous lepidic predominant invasive adenocarcinoma of the lung in patients with stage I disease. *Am J Surg Pathol.* 2014;38:448–460.

75 Adenocarcinoma, Nonmucinous

Allen P. Burke, M.D., Fabio R. Tavora, M.D., Ph.D., and Haresh Mani, M.D.

Classification

The majority of adenocarcinomas of the lung are derived from cells localized to the bronchoalveolar duct junction that differentiate to Clara cells or pneumocytes.[1] Expression profiles have classified adenocarcinomas into so-called terminal respiratory unit type and nonterminal respiratory type, roughly corresponding to nonmucinous and mucinous adenocarcinomas, respectively.[2] TTF-1 expression is localized to pneumocytes and terminal respiratory cells and is the hallmark of nonmucinous adenocarcinomas, although a small proportion of nonmucinous tumors cannot express this antigen and are of uncertain histogenesis.

Nonmucinous adenocarcinomas are further subclassified based on growth patterns; the predominant type is used as a modifier, and the tumor checklist should provide an estimate as to the proportions (in percentages) of the other subtypes present.

Clinical and Incidence

The overall proportion of lung cancers that are adenocarcinomas is increasing and is now over 40%, with squamous and small cell constituting the majority of the remainder.[3] There is no longer a male predilection, as the rates of smoking are no longer gender biased. Adenocarcinomas represent the largest group of carcinomas in patients who have never smoked, now constituting over 10% of cases.[4] Lung cancer in the never smokers affects women more often than men and is more likely to harbor epidermal growth factor receptor (EGFR) mutations.

Radiologic Findings

Invasive adenocarcinomas are typically peripheral nodules, which have irregular, spiculated borders. Cavitation, as is commonly seen in squamous carcinomas, does not occur. Those tumors with an in situ (lepidic) growth pattern will show a corresponding ground-glass component on high-resolution computed tomography scans.[5] Similar to histopathologic assessment, solid tumors by computed tomographic scans show a significantly greater rate of lymphatic, vascular, and pleural invasion and lymph node metastasis compared with tumors with ground-glass (in situ) component.[6]

Tissue Sampling

Adenocarcinomas of the lung are often diagnosed on cytologic samples or small biopsies. Patients with advanced disease are usually treated without resection; therefore, proper diagnosis of these samples is critical to treat advanced stage patients, and a nonspecific diagnosis such as "non–small cell lung cancer" is not sufficient (see Chapter 72). Features important to note on wedge biopsies, segmentectomies, or lobectomies include invasion into the pleura, distance of tumor from margin, and size of invasive tumor. Wedge biopsy may be performed for intraoperative confirmation of malignancy and invasion >5 mm, by frozen section, after which completion lobectomy is performed. Mediastinoscopy is often performed prior to wedge resection if there are enlarged level II or level III lymph nodes, which will be sent for frozen section to rule out metastatic disease. In general, disease spread to these nodes will preclude surgery for the primary tumor, and the surgery will be terminated.

Peripheral adenocarcinomas may occasionally be treated with neoadjuvant chemoradiation prior to tumor resection. In these cases, it is important to state the degree of treatment effect, preferably as a percentage tumor necrosis or fibrosis.

Gross Findings

Adenocarcinomas of the lung are usually peripheral nodules with irregular borders (Fig. 75.1), which often have central scarring, which may retract the pleural surface (Fig. 75.2).

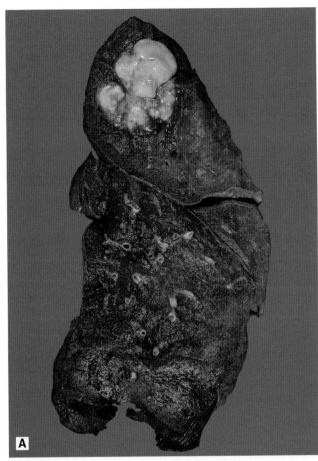

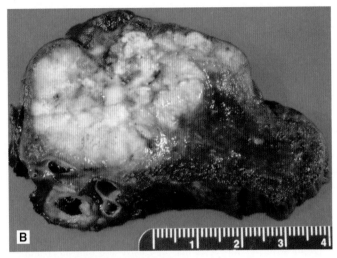

FIGURE 75.1 ▲ Gross features, adenocarcinomas of the lung. **A.** Adenocarcinoma, left upper lobe, autopsy specimen. There are irregular margins, and the tumor is solid and noncavitary. **B.** A higher magnification of a different tumor shows anthracosis and gritty fleshy appearance.

Microscopic Findings

Well-differentiated adenocarcinomas generally have a peripheral in situ (lepidic) component and typically have a central scar that is rich in elastic tissue (Fig. 75.3). Poorly differentiated tumors are less likely to have abundant fibrosis and more likely to show pleural, lymphatic, and large-vessel invasion. A desmoplastic reaction to tumor invasion

occurs occasionally, but is less common than squamous carcinomas. Necrosis is not uncommon in higher-grade tumors, but central cavitation, as occurs in squamous carcinoma, is exceptionally rare.

There are five predominant histologic patterns of nonmucinous adenocarcinomas of the lung: in situ (lepidic), acinar, papillary, micropapillary, and solid. The cribriform pattern is usually considered

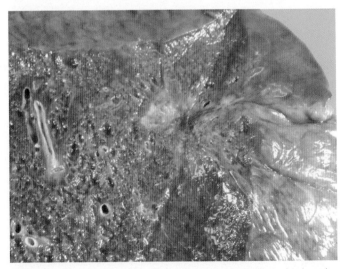

FIGURE 75.2 ▲ Peripheral adenocarcinoma, scar. There is pleural puckering.

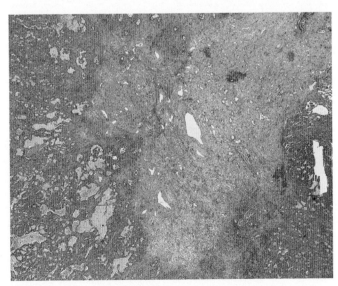

FIGURE 75.3 ▲ Peripheral adenocarcinoma. The scar is formed largely of grayish-blue elastotic fibrosis.

a subset of the solid pattern, but is sometimes separated out, as it has a prognosis intermediate between solid and acinar. The tumor is generally diagnosed by the predominant pattern, and other types described as percent growth. The frequencies of the individual tumor patterns vary by series and country, with papillary carcinoma common in Japan.[7] Otherwise, most series place acinar predominant as the most common type, followed by solid, lepidic predominant, and papillary, with micropapillary having a relatively wide range, depending on the series.[8-10]

It is well known that over 90% of lung adenocarcinomas have more than one pattern (hence the abandonment of the term "mixed" subtype, which was previously applied to most tumors). In one series, 93% were mixed with >1 pattern, 46% had >2 patterns, 20% had >3 patterns, and 3% had >4 patterns.[10] Tumors with solid growth have a higher proportion of this pattern overall, with micropapillary pattern usually representing a relatively small portion of the tumor.

Vascular invasion may manifest as lymphatic, arterial, and venous invasion. Relatively recently, spread through alveolar spaces (tumor islands, or intra-alveolar tumor nests) has been recognized as a type of invasion.[11]

An alternative classification of lung adenocarcinomas considers lepidic and acinar as "alveolar," retains a papillary classification, and refers to solid and other types of invasive growth as "destructive."[12]

Lepidic Predominant

Because all lung adenocarcinomas are designated based on the predominant pattern, the term "lepidic predominant" is synonymous with "lepidic adenocarcinoma," and the terms are used interchangeably.[10,13] "Predominant" generally signifies >50% of the tumor, although some have used the percent surrounding edge of the adenocarcinoma with in situ growth pattern.[14] The histologic features of this pattern are identical with nonmucinous adenocarcinoma in situ or the lepidic areas in minimally invasive adenocarcinoma (see previous chapter).

The invasive areas of lepidic-predominant tumors usually have extensive areas of acinar growth. The border separating the invasive and noninvasive (in situ) areas may be elusive and difficult to pinpoint.[14] The distinction between acinar and lepidic is based on absence of underlying alveolar architecture in the former and the recognition of intact alveolar septa in the latter. Less commonly, the invasive components are higher grade, such as micropapillary, solid, and cribriform.

Acinar

Acinar adenocarcinoma is composed of glands or tubules that are either closely packed (Fig. 75.4) or separated by fibrous or elastotic

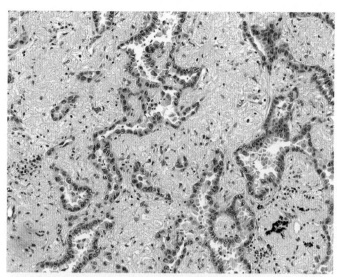

FIGURE 75.5 ▲ Acinar adenocarcinoma. In this example, the acinar structures are separated by elastotic stroma.

stroma (Fig. 75.5). Tumor cells with prominent snouts that resemble Clara cells are common in well-differentiated tumors (Fig. 75.6). Acinar adenocarcinomas with higher cytoplasmic grade (mitotic activity, nuclear pleomorphism) are more likely to have invasive cribriform or solid areas, as well as vascular invasion.

Papillary

Classic papillary adenocarcinomas are composed of fibrovascular cores lined by columnar or cuboidal cells, sometimes with apical snouts ("Clara cell" morphology) (Fig. 75.7). Often, there is a combination of acinar and papillary growth, with smaller papillary projections within somewhat cystically dilated acini. As with other types, pure papillary tumors are uncommon and often accompanied by acinar or micropapillary areas.

Cribriform

Cribriform adenocarcinoma ranges from fairly large cystic spaces within dilated acini to patterns that merge with solid, having only

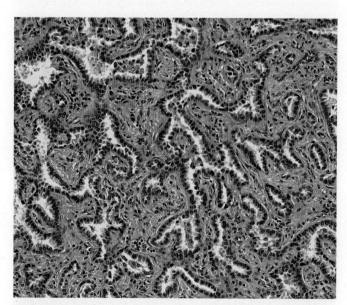

FIGURE 75.4 ▲ Acinar adenocarcinoma. This pattern may be difficult to distinguish from adenocarcinoma in situ, but an intact alveolar architecture is absent.

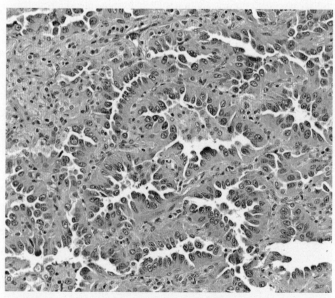

FIGURE 75.6 ▲ Acinar adenocarcinoma. There is minimal scarring. The tumor cells have a characteristic hobnail appearance (Clara cell differentiation).

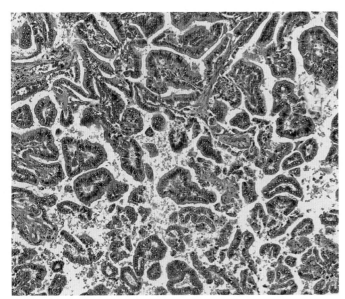

FIGURE 75.7 ▲ Adenocarcinoma, papillary type. The tumor has vascular cores.

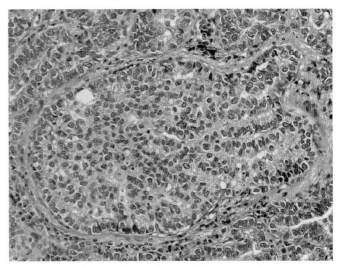

FIGURE 75.8 ▲ Adenocarcinoma, solid type. Adenocarcinoma with cribriforming is generally considered a solid subtype.

inconspicuous glandular areas (Fig. 75.8). When there is "dirty necrosis" within the irregular and variously sized cribriform glands, the term "enteric" is often applied, especially when the cribriform spaces have an appearance of garlands (a term seemingly reserved for enteric adenocarcinoma in this setting). Enteric carcinoma is discussed further in Chapter 77.

Solid

Like cribriform adenocarcinoma, solid adenocarcinoma is also a heterogeneous group, ranging on one end to tumors that show no evidence of differentiation other than TTF-1 positivity, to distinct cribriform adenocarcinoma (Fig. 75.9). When mucin vacuoles are evident by light microscopy or mucin stains (mucicarmine or periodic acid–Schiff [PSA]), then adenocarcinoma can be diagnosed without

immunohistochemical stains (Fig. 75.10). Somewhat arbitrarily, it has been recommended that intracellular mucin should be present in at least five tumor cells in each of two high-power fields, seen on PAS or mucicarmine stains, if there are no clear glandular areas.[15]

Micropapillary

Micropapillary adenocarcinoma is similar to that seen in other organs, such as the bladder, breast, and ovary. The papillary tufts form florets that lack fibrovascular cores, resulting in inverted polarity, with mucinous brush border along the membrane segment facing the outer periphery of the papillary cluster. Micropapillary adenocarcinoma may occur within stroma (stromal invasion), lymphatics, or alveolar spaces (Fig. 75.11).[16] With aerogenous spread, the clusters appear detached in the alveolar spaces as rings and cribriform glandular structures. In all three patterns, the tumor cells are small and cuboidal with minimal nuclear atypia, and lymphatic invasion is frequent. Psammoma bodies may be present.

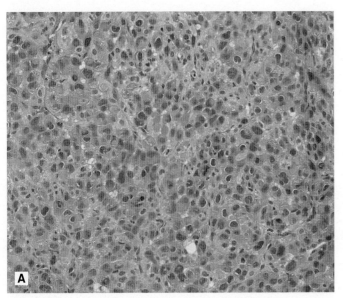

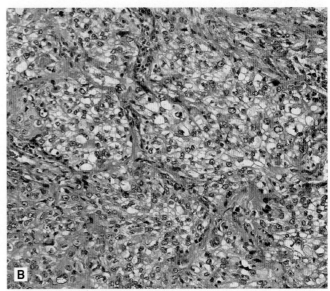

FIGURE 75.9 ▲ Adenocarcinoma, solid type. There is no gland formation or vacuoles. **A.** The cells have an eosinophilic cytoplasm. The diagnosis of adenocarcinoma is based on TTF-1 positivity (not shown). **B.** Solid adenocarcinoma may demonstrate clear areas, a nonspecific feature.

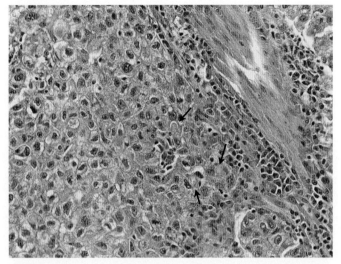

FIGURE 75.10 ▲ Adenocarcinoma, solid type. There are focal mucin vacuoles (*arrows*).

Tumor Islands

The presence of tumor islands (also known as "spread through alveolar spaces,"[11] "aerogenous spread,"[16] and "small cluster invasion")[17] is typically associated with micropapillary adenocarcinoma. They have also been described in solid and mucinous adenocarcinomas and infrequently in lepidic or acinar growth patterns. Tumor islands have been associated with smokers and higher nuclear grade.[18]

Immunohistochemical Findings

Thyroid Transcription Factor-1

Thyroid transcription factor-1 (TTF-1) is the most frequently applied immunohistochemical marker for nonmucinous adenocarcinoma and has even been found to have prognostic significance.[19] There are many reports of the sensitivity and specificity of this marker, with a range of results. A study of tissue microarrays demonstrated a sensitivity of 86%,[20] very similar to a sensitivity of 88% in resected specimens.[21] These values are higher than a recent meta-analysis showing a sensitivity (combined with napsin-A) of only 76%.[22] Importantly, the subtype of adenocarcinoma affects the rate of TTF-1 positivity

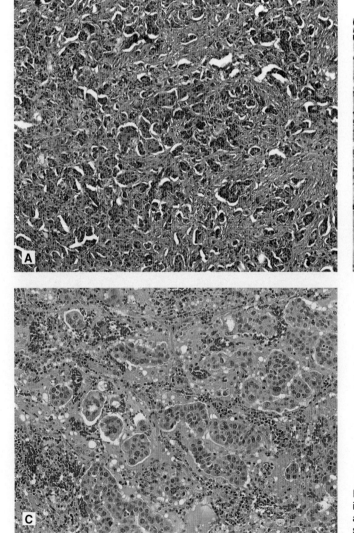

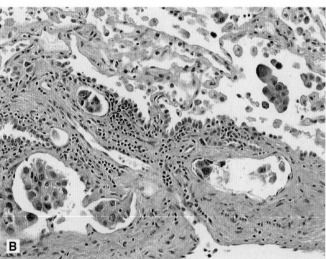

FIGURE 75.11 ▲ Adenocarcinoma, micropapillary type. **A.** The tumor invades the stroma. **B.** The micropapillary structures invade lymphatics and airspaces. **C.** The tumor invades airspaces (spread through alveolar spaces).

TABLE 75.1 Histologic Patterns of Adenocarcinoma: Frequency of Predominance, TTF-1 Expression, Mutational Correlation, and Prognostic Import

Pattern	% As Predominant Pattern	TTF-1 Staining, % Positive	Associated Mutations	Prognostic Significance
Lepidic (in situ)	5%–10%	>95%	EGFR	Good
Acinar	30%–65%	>95%	EGFR	Good to intermediate
Papillary	5%–10%[a]	>95%	EGFR	Intermediate
Micropapillary	0%–20%	90%–95%	EGFR	Poor
Solid	25%–24%	69%–85%	ALK-1, KRAS	Poor
Mucinous	15%–20%	50%–60%	KRAS	Intermediate

[a]Higher in Japanese series.

(Table 75.1). Virtually all nonmucinous lepidic-predominant and papillary adenocarcinomas are TTF-1 positive, compared to 94% of acinar-predominant adenocarcinoma, 93% of patients with micropapillary-predominant adenocarcinoma, and 86% of solid-predominant adenocarcinoma.[19] Another study found that in solid adenocarcinomas, any nuclear TTF-1 expression was present in 69% of tumors.[23] The subgroup with the lowest rate (50% to 60%) is mucinous adenocarcinoma (see subsequent Chapter 76). TTF-1 positivity is most helpful in differential diagnosis of tumors with a solid growth pattern (Fig. 75.12).

Typically, any degree of positivity (>1%) is used as a positive result, although some series use a 10% cutoff.[24–26] It is generally considered that TTF-1 positivity excludes the diagnosis of squamous carcinoma, although some series report a very low rate of positivity for squamous carcinoma.[27] In the majority of positive tumors, the extent of tumor staining is more than half of the tumor area, with only 7% of tumors showing focal positivity (<50%).[21]

Napsin-A

Napsin-A expression correlates well with TTF-1, with a similar sensitivity and specificity (around 90%, depending on subtype).[20] In contrast to nuclear staining of TTF-1, napsin-A is seen as cytoplasmic granules (Fig. 75.13).[26] The advantage in using napsin-A is that it has a higher specificity than TTF-1, being negative in neuroendocrine carcinomas.[28]

Squamous Markers and Use of Panels

The most common differential diagnostic problem, especially on small biopsy specimens, is to distinguish poorly differentiated adenocarcinoma from squamous cell carcinoma. This situation occurs when there are no glandular, papillary, or cribriform structures, and keratinization and intercellular bridges are absent. The rate of positivity of squamous markers in lung adenocarcinoma varies by the antibody used, as well as tumor subtype. The most specific markers for squamous carcinoma are cytokeratin 5/6 and p40, present in only 5% to 20% of adenocarcinomas.[20,21,27,29] However, p40 is a more sensitive squamous marker, essentially 100%, and is therefore the preferred marker. p63 is not as specific for squamous (expressed in 15% to 30% of adenocarcinomas)[29] and has been essentially replaced by p40 to identify squamous carcinomas of the lung.[30] p40 has the additional advantage of a very low rate staining small cell carcinomas (and lower than p63),[31] which may occasional form a differential diagnosis in small biopsies.

The use of multiple antibodies adds to the discriminating value of immunohistochemistry in distinguishing squamous from adenocarcinoma. In general, at least one squamous marker (p40 preferred) and TTF-1 (adenocarcinoma marker) are used, often in conjunction with endocrine markers, if small cell or large cell neuroendocrine carcinoma is in the differential diagnosis based on routine stains. The addition of napsin-A may improve specificity (being negative in endocrine carcinomas),[20] and cytokeratin 7, being negative in 63% to 80% squamous carcinomas, has been recommended for use in a panel.[27,29] When saving tissue with limited sampling is paramount, in case of molecular study, a panel of two stains (TTF-1 or mucicarmine and p40) is recommended, if on light microscopy the differential diagnosis is solid adenocarcinoma and nonkeratinizing squamous carcinoma.[32]

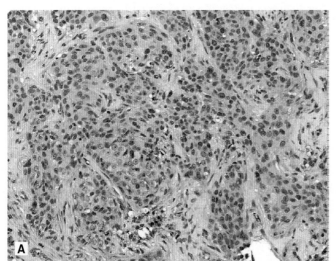
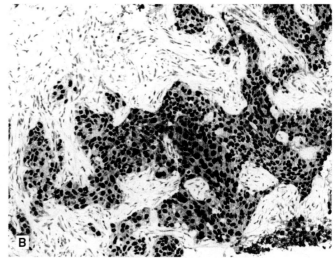

FIGURE 75.12 ▲ Adenocarcinoma, solid type. **A.** The morphology is that of "large cell" carcinoma. **B.** TTF-1 immunostaining confirms adenocarcinoma.

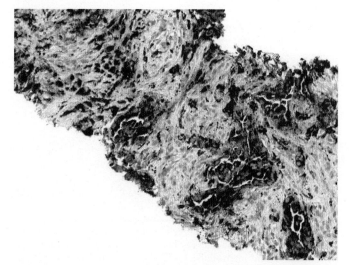

FIGURE 75.13 ▲ Adenocarcinoma, solid type. Immunohistochemical staining for napsin-A confirms adenocarcinoma in this core biopsy.

Differential from Metastatic Disease

The most useful information in distinguishing primary from metastatic adenocarcinoma of the lung is clinical, namely, imaging findings, multiplicity, mediastinal disease, and history of a known extrapulmonary primary. The addition of napsin-A may be helpful in a panel to establish the lung as the primary site.[24] In cases of nonmucinous carcinoma, there may occasionally be a question of metastatic colon or prostatic adenocarcinoma, in which case relevant stains (cytokeratins 7 and 20, CDX2, and prostatic markers) may be useful. CDX2 has been described to be essentially absent in pulmonary adenocarcinomas not enriched for colloid or enteric types,[33] but has also been reported in up to 10% of unselected adenocarcinomas of the lung.[34] In occasional cases, lung metastases from the breast may be difficult to discern from a primary lung tumor, although breast cancers typically spread to lymph nodes and pleura. In any case, antibodies to breast-specific antigens (such as GATA3) and steroid markers may be useful if there is a question of breast primary. Mucinous adenocarcinomas are notoriously difficult to distinguish from metastases, especially from the pancreas, because of great overlap of immunohistochemical markers. Napsin-A, for example, has been shown to be unreliable to distinguish primary from secondary mucinous tumors of the lung.[35] In such cases, clinical and imaging findings are especially crucial in determining site of origin.

Molecular Alterations (See Chapter 72)

Epidermal Growth Factor Receptor

Approximately 10% to 20% of non–small cell lung cancers, primarily adenocarcinomas, respond to treatment with EGFR tyrosine kinase inhibitors, such as gefitinib and erlotinib.[36] Responsive tumors are most common in nonsmokers, women, and Asians.[7] Specific missense and in-frame deletion mutations in the kinase domain of EGFR are found in over 80% of these tumors.[36,37] The mutations result in up-regulation of receptor, selectively enhancing ligand-dependent activation of the AKT/STAT survival pathways.[38] Mutational status is generally determined by polymerase chain reaction sequencing of target exons 18, 19, and 21 from paraffin-embedded tissue sections.

There is a significant correlation between histologic type and EGFR mutational status. Those subtypes with an increased frequency of EGFR mutations include papillary,[39] micropapillary,[7] acinar,[8] and lepidic-predominant tumors,[40] indicating a propensity for better differentiated tumors.

There is some evidence that underlying germline mutations in EGFR may play a role, in addition to superimposed somatic tumor mutations, in familial adenocarcinoma.[38]

Anaplastic Lymphoma Kinase-1 Gene Rearrangements

Three to seven percent of non–small cell lung cancers (mostly adenocarcinomas) harbor anaplastic lymphoma kinase-1 (ALK-1) rearrangements, which are associated with never or light smoking history, frequent nodal metastasis, higher stage of disease at diagnosis, and an absence of EGFR mutations.[41,42] The mRNA fusion product of ALK-1 and echinoderm microtubule-associated protein-like-4 (EML4) is detected primarily by in situ hybridization (fluorescent or chromogenic). The ALK-1 gene rearrangement has been described in a wide range of growth patterns, including papillary, acinar, and lepidic[43]; solid growth pattern and invasive tumors[44]; and micropapillary and acinar-predominant adenocarcinomas.[39] A high rate of ALK-1 gene rearrangement has been described in signet ring adenocarcinomas, a variant of solid adenocarcinoma.[45]

Identification ALK-positive patients is clinically important as ALK rearrangements are associated with sensitivity to the tyrosine kinase inhibitor crizotinib. After initial response, delayed resistance is common and not associated with secondary EGFR or KRAS mutations, although additional ALK mutations or amplification may occur in these patients.[41]

KRAS, BRAF, NRAF, and ERBB2 Mutations

KRAS mutations are present in ~10% of adenocarcinomas of the lung[7,46,47] and are associated with poorly differentiated adenocarcinomas[8] and those with mucinous phenotype.[39,40] In a series of 95 solid adenocarcinomas, 38% demonstrated *KRAS* mutations, and one demonstrated *ALK-1* rearrangement, while none harbored *EGFR* mutations.[23]

BRAF mutations occur in 2% of adenocarcinomas and squamous carcinomas of the lung and, unlike melanoma, do not involve amino acid V599.[47] Activating mutations of BRAF may play a role in up-regulation and increased gene expression of MEK and ERK1/2.[47]

NRAS mutations occur in only 1% of lung adenocarcinomas, but up to 18% of large cell-neuroendocrine carcinomas.[47]

Increased her2-neu expression from mutations in *ERBB2* occurs in 10% of lung adenocarcinomas, although, unlike in breast cancer, ERBB2 inhibitors have not been shown to be effective treatment.[48]

Multiple Adenocarcinomas

Unlike other types of lung cancers, adenocarcinomas have a relatively high rate of multiplicity, especially if there is a lepidic component. A separate tumor is defined as one that is grossly visible, as multiplicity does not apply to microscopic satellite foci. Up to 14% of lung cancers that have an in situ component seen as ground-glass opacities on computed tomographic scans are multiple.[49] In fact, the original definition of "bronchioloalveolar carcinoma" included multiplicity as a defining feature.[50]

There are no standardized rules for the treatment of patients with synchronous primary nodules,[46] although lung-sparing surgery with avoidance of lobectomy and pneumonectomy is recommended.[49] For staging purposes, it is important to distinguish intraparenchymal metastasis, which significantly increases the "T" stage, from multiple primaries. Forty years ago, Martini and Melamed defined a second distinct pulmonary malignancy either if histologic appearance differs from those of the index tumor or if the tumors are in different lobes or segments, with no intervening lymph node deposits or metastasis.[51] Histologic features such as divergent morphology of predominant tumor growth pattern (or significant difference in proportions of subtypes) and absence of vascular invasion favor synchronous primaries, which are staged according to the most advanced lesion.[52,53] The presence of carcinoma in situ (lepidic growth pattern) increases the likelihood of a separate primary, as molecular analysis of multiple tumors with a lepidic component showed different EGFR or KRAS mutational profiles, suggesting that they were independent events.[46] Areas of atypical adenomatous hyperplasia are not uncommon in specimens resected with multiple primary lesions, which is another feature of multiple primary tumors.

Histologic evaluation other than predominant tumor pattern may also be helpful in determining recurrence versus second primary. These include cytologic features, patterns of stroma (collagen, desmoplasia, inflammation, lymphoid hyperplasia), necrosis, presence of intra-alveolar tumor islands, clear cell or signet ring features, and fetal patterns.[52] The addition of these features decreases the proportion of tumors misclassified by Martini-Melamed criteria, which can be as high as 18% of cases.[53]

A related problem occurs with metachronous adenocarcinomas, in distinguishing recurrence of the same biologic tumor, from a new second primary unrelated to the first. For recurrences outside the lung, it is usually straightforward to assume a metastasis from the previously resected tumor, provided that there is no new lung mass on imaging, no second extrapulmonary primary, or if the metastatic deposit has histologic features similar to the original lesion. If there is a new adenocarcinoma in the lung, it may be difficult and arbitrary to make the distinction between local recurrence and second primary, but a similar approach (combination of Martini-Melamed criteria with additional histologic findings) is used as that for synchronous tumors, with the added stipulation that after 2 years of diagnosis of the primary tumor, the new lesion is considered a second primary.[52,53]

Prognosis and Grading

The prognosis of adenocarcinoma of the lung varies widely and depends primarily on stage, with minimally invasive lesions having essentially 100% disease-related survival, and high-grade and advanced stage tumors with a median survival of months.

Histologically, both architectural and cytologic features are associated with prognosis. Two recent studies reported 5-year disease-free survival rates by predominant growth pattern as 100% for adenocarcinoma in situ and minimally invasive adenocarcinoma, 93% to 94% for lepidic-predominant adenocarcinoma, 89% for invasive mucinous adenocarcinoma, 67% to 70% for acinar adenocarcinoma, 67% to 74% for papillary adenocarcinoma, 43% to 58% for solid adenocarcinoma, and 0% to 62% for micropapillary adenocarcinoma.[23,39,40] The high rate of disparity in micropapillary may reflect the relative rarity of this subtype as a predominant pattern.

Many studies have supported the concept that ≤5 mm of invasion is equivalent prognostically with adenocarcinoma in situ[54] with a 5-year survival approaching 100%. Recurrent lepidic-predominant adenocarcinoma, which generally has a good prognosis, is associated with sublobar resection with close margins, minor micropapillary component, and lymphatic or vascular invasion.[13]

The association between micropapillary growth and poor survival has been repeatedly demonstrated.[13,55–57]

The cribriform growth pattern is generally considered a subset of solid, as the prognosis is worse than acinar or papillary predominant, and comparable to solid or micropapillary.[58]

Addition of cytologic features (nucleolar enlargement, mitotic activity, and necrosis) to predominant growth pattern has been shown to increase the association between tumor grade and metastasis, both lymph node and distant.[9] Lymphatic invasion has been shown to impact prognosis in the absence of lymph node metastasis.[59]

The prognosis of lung adenocarcinomas with tumor islands has been shown to be poor independent of other histologic finding.[18] Absence of TTF-1 expression was found to be an independent predictor of disease recurrence.[19]

REFERENCES

1. Giangreco A, Reynolds SD, Stripp BR. Terminal bronchioles harbor a unique airway stem cell population that localizes to the bronchoalveolar duct junction. *Am J Pathol.* 2002;161:173–182.
2. Takeuchi T, Tomida S, Yatabe Y, et al. Expression profile-defined classification of lung adenocarcinoma shows close relationship with underlying major genetic changes and clinicopathologic behaviors. *J Clin Oncol.* 2006;24:1679–1688.
3. Devesa SS, Bray F, Vizcaino AP, et al. International lung cancer trends by histologic type: male:female differences diminishing and adenocarcinoma rates rising. *Int J Cancer.* 2005;117:294–299.
4. Subramanian J, Govindan R. Lung cancer in never smokers: a review. *J Clin Oncol.* 2007;25:561–570.
5. Nakamura S, Fukui T, Taniguchi T, et al. Prognostic impact of tumor size eliminating the ground glass opacity component: modified clinical T descriptors of the tumor, node, metastasis classification of lung cancer. *J Thorac Oncol.* 2013;8:1551–1557.
6. Tsutani Y, Miyata Y, Yamanaka T, et al. Solid tumors versus mixed tumors with a ground-glass opacity component in patients with clinical stage IA lung adenocarcinoma: prognostic comparison using high-resolution computed tomography findings. *J Thorac Cardiovasc Surg.* 2013;146: 17–23.
7. Motoi N, Szoke J, Riely GJ, et al. Lung adenocarcinoma: modification of the 2004 WHO mixed subtype to include the major histologic subtype suggests correlations between papillary and micropapillary adenocarcinoma subtypes, EGFR mutations and gene expression analysis. *Am J Surg Pathol.* 2008;32:810–827.
8. Russell PA, Barnett SA, Walkiewicz M, et al. Correlation of mutation status and survival with predominant histologic subtype according to the new IASLC/ATS/ERS lung adenocarcinoma classification in stage III (N2) patients. *J Thorac Oncol.* 2013;8:461–468.
9. Xu L, Tavora F, Burke A. Histologic features associated with metastatic potential in invasive adenocarcinomas of the lung. *Am J Surg Pathol.* 2013;37:1100–1108.
10. Warth A, Muley T, Meister M, et al. The novel histologic International Association for the Study of Lung Cancer/American Thoracic Society/European Respiratory Society classification system of lung adenocarcinoma is a stage-independent predictor of survival. *J Clin Oncol.* 2012;30: 1438–1446.
11. Travis WD, Brambilla E, Noguchi M, et al. Diagnosis of lung adenocarcinoma in resected specimens: implications of the 2011 International Association for the Study of Lung Cancer/American Thoracic Society/European Respiratory Society classification. *Arch Pathol Lab Med.* 2013;137:685–705.
12. Sardari Nia P, Van Marck E, Weyler J, et al. Prognostic value of a biologic classification of non-small-cell lung cancer into the growth patterns along with other clinical, pathological and immunohistochemical factors. *Eur J Cardiothorac Surg.* 2010;38:628–636.
13. Kadota K, Villena-Vargas J, Yoshizawa A, et al. Prognostic significance of adenocarcinoma in situ, minimally invasive adenocarcinoma, and nonmucinous lepidic predominant invasive adenocarcinoma of the lung in patients with stage I disease. *Am J Surg Pathol.* 2014;38:448–460.
14. Xu L, Tavora F, Burke A. 'Bronchioloalveolar carcinoma': is the term really dead? A critical review of a new classification system for pulmonary adenocarcinomas. *Pathology.* 2012;44:497–505.
15. Travis WD, Brambilla E, Muller-Hermelink HK, et al. *Pathology and Genetics. Tumours of the Lung, Pleura, Thymus and Heart.* Lyon, France: IARC Press; 2004.
16. Ohe M, Yokose T, Sakuma Y, et al. Stromal micropapillary component as a novel unfavorable prognostic factor of lung adenocarcinoma. *Diagn Pathol.* 2012;7:3.
17. Kawakami T, Nabeshima K, Hamasaki M, et al. Small cluster invasion: a possible link between micropapillary pattern and lymph node metastasis in pT1 lung adenocarcinomas. *Virchows Arch.* 2009;454:61–70.
18. Onozato ML, Kovach AE, Yeap BY, et al. Tumor islands in resected early-stage lung adenocarcinomas are associated with unique clinicopathologic and molecular characteristics and worse prognosis. *Am J Surg Pathol.* 2013;37:287–294.
19. Kadota K, Nitadori J, Sarkaria IS, et al. Thyroid transcription factor-1 expression is an independent predictor of recurrence and correlates with the IASLC/ATS/ERS histologic classification in patients with stage I lung adenocarcinoma. *Cancer.* 2013;119:931–938.
20. Ao MH, Zhang H, Sakowski L, et al. The utility of a novel triple marker (combination of TTF1, napsin A, and p40) in the subclassification of non-small cell lung cancer. *Hum Pathol.* 2014;45:926–934.
21. Rekhtman N, Ang DC, Sima CS, et al. Immunohistochemical algorithm for differentiation of lung adenocarcinoma and squamous cell carcinoma based on large series of whole-tissue sections with validation in small specimens. *Mod Pathol.* 2011;24:1348–1359.

22. Li L, Li X, Yin J, et al. The high diagnostic accuracy of combined test of thyroid transcription factor 1 and Napsin A to distinguish between lung adenocarcinoma and squamous cell carcinoma: a meta-analysis. *PLoS One*. 2014;9:e100837.

23. Hwang DH, Szeto DP, Perry AS, et al. Pulmonary large cell carcinoma lacking squamous differentiation is clinicopathologically indistinguishable from solid-subtype adenocarcinoma. *Arch Pathol Lab Med*. 2014;138:626–635.

24. Zhang P, Han YP, Huang L, et al. Value of napsin A and thyroid transcription factor-1 in the identification of primary lung adenocarcinoma. *Oncol Lett*. 2010;1:899–903.

25. Tacha D, Yu C, Bremer R, et al. A 6-antibody panel for the classification of lung adenocarcinoma versus squamous cell carcinoma. *Appl Immunohistochem Mol Morphol*. 2012;20:201–207.

26. Collins BT. Endobronchial ultrasound fine-needle aspiration biopsy of pulmonary non-small cell carcinoma with subclassification by immunohistochemistry panel. *Cancer Cytopathol*. 2013;121:146–154.

27. Warth A, Muley T, Herpel E, et al. Large-scale comparative analyses of immunomarkers for diagnostic subtyping of non-small-cell lung cancer biopsies. *Histopathology*. 2012;61:1017–1025.

28. Zhang C, Schmidt LA, Hatanaka K, et al. Evaluation of napsin A, TTF-1, p63, p40, and CK5/6 immunohistochemical stains in pulmonary neuroendocrine tumors. *Am J Clin Pathol*. 2014;142:320–324.

29. Terry J, Leung S, Laskin J, et al. Optimal immunohistochemical markers for distinguishing lung adenocarcinomas from squamous cell carcinomas in small tumor samples. *Am J Surg Pathol*. 2010;34:1805–1811.

30. Bishop JA, Teruya-Feldstein J, Westra WH, et al. p40 (DeltaNp63) is superior to p63 for the diagnosis of pulmonary squamous cell carcinoma. *Mod Pathol*. 2012;25:405–415.

31. Tatsumori T, Tsuta K, Masai K, et al. p40 is the best marker for diagnosing pulmonary squamous cell carcinoma: comparison with p63, cytokeratin 5/6, desmocollin-3, and sox2. *Appl Immunohistochem Mol Morphol*. 2014;22:377–382.

32. Travis WD, Brambilla E, Noguchi M, et al. Diagnosis of lung cancer in small biopsies and cytology: implications of the 2011 International Association for the Study of Lung Cancer/American Thoracic Society/European Respiratory Society classification. *Arch Pathol Lab Med*. 2013;137:668–684.

33. Kim JH, Choi YD, Lee JS, et al. Utility of thyroid transcription factor-1 and CDX-2 in determining the primary site of metastatic adenocarcinomas in serous effusions. *Acta Cytol*. 2010;54:277–282.

34. Cowan ML, Li QK, Illei PB. CDX-2 Expression in primary lung adenocarcinoma. *Appl Immunohistochem Mol Morphol*. 2016;24:16–19.

35. Heymann JJ, Hoda RS, Scognamiglio T. Polyclonal napsin A expression: a potential diagnostic pitfall in distinguishing primary from metastatic mucinous tumors in the lung. *Arch Pathol Lab Med*. 2014;138:1067–1071.

36. Lynch TJ, Bell DW, Sordella R, et al. Activating mutations in the epidermal growth factor receptor underlying responsiveness of non-small-cell lung cancer to gefitinib. *N Engl J Med*. 2004;350:2129–2139.

37. Paez JG, Janne PA, Lee JC, et al. EGFR mutations in lung cancer: correlation with clinical response to gefitinib therapy. *Science*. 2004;304:1497–1500.

38. Bell DW, Gore I, Okimoto RA, et al. Inherited susceptibility to lung cancer may be associated with the T790M drug resistance mutation in EGFR. *Nat Genet*. 2005;37:1315–1316.

39. Tsuta K, Kawago M, Inoue E, et al. The utility of the proposed IASLC/ATS/ERS lung adenocarcinoma subtypes for disease prognosis and correlation of driver gene alterations. *Lung Cancer*. 2013;81:371–376.

40. Yoshizawa A, Sumiyoshi S, Sonobe M, et al. Validation of the IASLC/ATS/ERS lung adenocarcinoma classification for prognosis and association with EGFR and KRAS gene mutations: analysis of 440 Japanese patients. *J Thorac Oncol*. 2013;8:52–61.

41. Gainor JF, Varghese AM, Ou SH, et al. ALK rearrangements are mutually exclusive with mutations in EGFR or KRAS: an analysis of 1,683 patients with non-small cell lung cancer. *Clin Cancer Res*. 2013;19:4273–4281.

42. Soda M, Choi YL, Enomoto M, et al. Identification of the transforming EML4-ALK fusion gene in non-small-cell lung cancer. *Nature*. 2007;448:561–566.

43. Inamura K, Takeuchi K, Togashi Y, et al. EML4-ALK fusion is linked to histological characteristics in a subset of lung cancers. *J Thorac Oncol*. 2008;3:13–17.

44. Kim H, Jang SJ, Chung DH, et al. A comprehensive comparative analysis of the histomorphological features of ALK-rearranged lung adenocarcinoma based on driver oncogene mutations: frequent expression of epithelial-mesenchymal transition markers than other genotype. *PLoS One*. 2013;8:e76999.

45. Yoshida A, Tsuta K, Watanabe S, et al. Frequent ALK rearrangement and TTF-1/p63 co-expression in lung adenocarcinoma with signet-ring cell component. *Lung Cancer*. 2011;72:309–315.

46. Chung JH, Choe G, Jheon S, et al. Epidermal growth factor receptor mutation and pathologic-radiologic correlation between multiple lung nodules with ground-glass opacity differentiates multicentric origin from intrapulmonary spread. *J Thorac Oncol*. 2009;4:1490–1495.

47. Brose MS, Volpe P, Feldman M, et al. BRAF and RAS mutations in human lung cancer and melanoma. *Cancer Res*. 2002;62:6997–7000.

48. Stephens P, Hunter C, Bignell G, et al. Lung cancer: intragenic ERBB2 kinase mutations in tumours. *Nature*. 2004;431:525–526.

49. Trousse D, Barlesi F, Loundou A, et al. Synchronous multiple primary lung cancer: an increasing clinical occurrence requiring multidisciplinary management. *J Thorac Cardiovasc Surg*. 2007;133:1193–1200.

50. Liebow AA. Bronchiolo-alveolar carcinoma. *Adv Intern Med*. 1960;10:329–358.

51. Martini N, Melamed MR. Multiple primary lung cancers. *J Thorac Cardiovasc Surg*. 1975;70:606–612.

52. Girard N, Deshpande C, Lau C, et al. Comprehensive histologic assessment helps to differentiate multiple lung primary nonsmall cell carcinomas from metastases. *Am J Surg Pathol*. 2009;33:1752–1764.

53. Girard N, Ostrovnaya I, Lau C, et al. Genomic and mutational profiling to assess clonal relationships between multiple non-small cell lung cancers. *Clin Cancer Res*. 2009;15:5184–5190.

54. Borczuk AC, Qian F, Kazeros A, et al. Invasive size is an independent predictor of survival in pulmonary adenocarcinoma. *Am J Surg Pathol*. 2009;33:462–469.

55. Russell PA, Wainer Z, Wright GM, et al. Does lung adenocarcinoma subtype predict patient survival?: a clinicopathologic study based on the new International Association for the Study of Lung Cancer/American Thoracic Society/European Respiratory Society international multidisciplinary lung adenocarcinoma classification. *J Thorac Oncol*. 2011;6:1496–1504.

56. Nitadori J, Bograd AJ, Kadota K, et al. Impact of micropapillary histologic subtype in selecting limited resection vs lobectomy for lung adenocarcinoma of 2cm or smaller. *J Natl Cancer Inst*. 2013;105:1212–1220.

57. Cha MJ, Lee HY, Lee KS, et al. Micropapillary and solid subtypes of invasive lung adenocarcinoma: clinical predictors of histopathology and outcome. *J Thorac Cardiovasc Surg*. 2014;147:921–928e2.

58. Kadota K, Yeh YC, Sima CS, et al. The cribriform pattern identifies a subset of acinar predominant tumors with poor prognosis in patients with stage I lung adenocarcinoma: a conceptual proposal to classify cribriform predominant tumors as a distinct histologic subtype. *Mod Pathol*. 2014;27:690–700.

59. Nentwich MF, Bohn BA, Uzunoglu FG, et al. Lymphatic invasion predicts survival in patients with early node-negative non-small cell lung cancer. *J Thorac Cardiovasc Surg*. 2013;146:781–787.

76 Mucinous Adenocarcinoma

Allen P. Burke, M.D., and Adina Paulk, M.D.

Introduction and Terminology

The classification of mucinous adenocarcinomas of the lung is complicated and has been described as "difficult and somewhat arbitrary"[1] as well as "controversial."[2] The difficulties stem from the fact that many mucinous carcinomas show mixed patterns (including so-called enteric; see Chapter 77), and there is a variable in situ or lepidic component, a feature that in lung cancers has long caused confusion. Furthermore, mucin takes many forms, including intracellular (in goblet, columnar, and signet ring cells) as well as extracellular, often entrapping small tumor nests (a feature characterizing "colloid" carcinoma).

A general concept maintains that there are two cell types of origin for lung adenocarcinomas: pneumocytes with either type II pneumocyte or Clara cell morphology[3] or a mucin-producing cell corresponding to bronchial goblet cells (see chapter 75).[4] It is generally recognized as well that mucinous adenocarcinomas are TTF-1 negative, although there are many mixed tumors with a subpopulation of TTF-1 positive non–mucin-secreting cells.

For purposes of this chapter, only adenocarcinomas with extensive extracellular mucin are considered. Solid adenocarcinomas with prominent intracellular mucin vacuoles or signet ring morphology are considered as solid (nonmucinous) adenocarcinomas and for the most part are TTF-1 positive.[4,5]

In contrast to nonmucinous carcinomas, mucinous adenocarcinomas of the lung are not often entirely in situ. Because few data exist for large noninvasive tumors, any mucinous adenocarcinoma >3 cm with an in situ (lepidic) growth pattern is considered invasive by the World Health Organization classification[6] (Table 76.1).

Mucinous Adenocarcinoma In Situ and Minimally Invasive Adenocarcinoma

Definition

Mucinous adenocarcinoma in situ is 3 cm or smaller and is composed entirely of lepidic growth.[6] Minimally invasive adenocarcinoma allows only 5 mm of invasive growth, without lymphatic invasion or necrosis. In practice, mucinous adenocarcinoma in situ and minimally invasive mucinous adenocarcinoma are rare, because any detached intra-alveolar tumor cells or multiplicity (other than clearly separate primaries) exclude the diagnosis and indicate invasive adenocarcinoma.[6] These features (so-called spread through alveolar spaces or aerogenous spread and multiplicity) are more common in mucinous as compared to nonmucinous in situ adenocarcinomas.

Microscopic Findings

Unlike nonmucinous adenocarcinomas, the lepidic spread of mucinous adenocarcinoma in situ is characterized by completely normal alveolar septa without any fibrotic thickening (Fig. 76.1). The tumor cells are more often columnar than goblet, follow the contours of the alveolar septa, and show uniform polarity, apical intracellular mucin (as nuclei are parallel and basally located), and a fine brush border (Fig. 76.2). Alternatively (and in mixed mucinous and nonmucinous tumors), cells may be more cuboidal, with variable numbers of goblet cells (Figs. 76.3 and 76.4). The alveolar spaces are typically filled with mucin and scattered inflammatory cells. By definition, there are no detached intra-alveolar tumor cell clusters in pure adenocarcinoma in situ or minimally invasive adenocarcinoma, and the lesion is single. If there is an invasive component, it is by definition <5 mm (minimally invasive adenocarcinoma) and consists entirely of acinar, solid, or papillary growth without necrosis or lymphatic invasion.

Immunohistochemical Findings

Mucinous adenocarcinoma in situ is typically TTF-1 negative[5] although older reports using the term "bronchioloalveolar carcinoma" have shown up to a 30% positivity rate.[1,4] It is often difficult to distinguish tumor cell nuclei from native pneumocytes lining the alveolar spaces, especially if the tumor nuclei are compressed toward the cell base (goblet cell morphology). Other pneumocyte-related antigens

TABLE 76.1 Histologic Features of Mucinous Adenocarcinomas of the Lung

Term	Synonyms (Obsolete)	Defining Features	Absent Features	Immunohistochemical Findings
Mucinous adenocarcinoma in situ (AIS)	Mucinous bronchioloalveolar carcinoma (BAC)	Mucin-secreting cells lining relatively intact alveolar walls	Tissue invasion Necrosis Intra-alveolar tumor clusters Size >3 cm Necrosis Multiplicity	TTF-1 negative or focally positive (<1/3) CK7 positive CK20 positive (about 50%) CDX2 negative
Minimally invasive mucinous adenocarcinoma	Mucinous BAC, mixed pattern (BAC + invasive part)	Same as AIS Acinar invasion <5 mm	Same as AIS	
Mucinous adenocarcinoma	Mucinous BAC, mixed pattern BAC + (invasive part)	Predominant mucin-forming cells, usually in situ component	Colloid adenocarcinoma	TTF-1 somewhat more likely to be focally positive than noninvasive tumors CK7 positive CK20 positive (50%) CDX2 negative
Colloid adenocarcinoma	Mucinous adenocarcinoma Cystadenocarcinoma			TTF-1 usually positive CK20, CDX2 positive in TTF-1 negative subpopulation CK7 positive

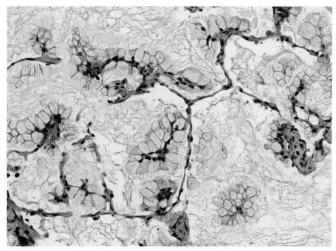

FIGURE 76.1 ▲ Mucinous adenocarcinoma in situ. The alveolar septa are typically thin and normal in appearance.

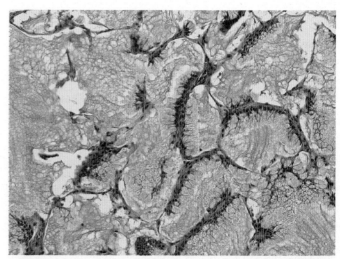

FIGURE 76.3 ▲ Mucinous adenocarcinoma in situ, goblet cell predominance. The lepidic component may have a predominance of goblet cells, with flattened basal nuclei. The tumor cell apices seem to be extruding mucin into the alveolar spaces.

such as napsin-A and surfactant proteins (such as SP1) are negative as well.[1] Expression of MUC5A5 (secreted tracheobronchial mucin) is present, and MUC2 (secreted intestinal mucin) is absent.[4] Mucinous adenocarcinoma in situ is negative for CDX2.[1]

Prognosis and Treatment

Mucinous adenocarcinoma in situ is cured with resection, without risk for metastasis, based on reports combining mucinous and nonmucinous tumors.[6,7]

Invasive Mucinous Adenocarcinoma

Terminology

The term "mucinous adenocarcinoma" or "invasive mucinous adenocarcinoma" is currently considered a "variant" of adenocarcinoma by the International Association for the Study of Lung Cancer, American Thoracic Society, and European Respiratory Society (and hence the World Health Organization).[6] Because the term replaced the previous "mucinous bronchioloalveolar carcinoma," it presumably denotes the presence of a prominent in situ component. However, prior to the

abolition of "bronchioloalveolar carcinoma," the term was usually used interchangeably with "colloid carcinoma."[1] Mucinous adenocarcinomas without a predominant lepidic growth and that do not fit the criteria for colloid carcinoma do exist; however, these do not have a comfortable niche in the current WHO schema, and will also be considered here.

For historical reasons, the "patterns" of carcinoma growth (solid, acinar, papillary, and micropapillary) have not been applied to the invasive areas of mucinous adenocarcinomas, along with adenocarcinomas of other "variant" histology.[6,8] However, each of these patterns occurs in mucinous adenocarcinomas, as well as in mixed mucinous and nonmucinous adenocarcinomas. To be considered mucinous, it is generally accepted that the predominant component (>50%) of the tumor be composed of goblet or columnar cells with intracytoplasmic mucin; tumors with lesser degrees of mucinous differentiation are included under conventional adenocarcinoma and typed by growth pattern.[6,8]

The term "cystadenocarcinoma" has also been abandoned and is now considered a synonym for or variant of colloid carcinoma.[6]

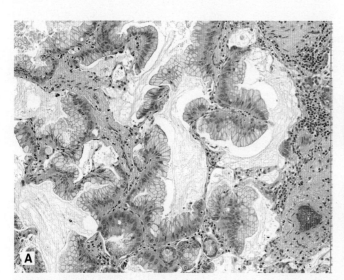

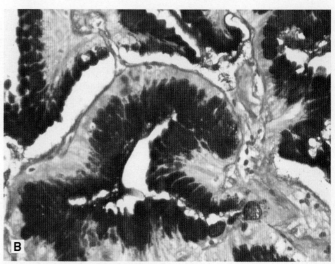

FIGURE 76.2 ▲ Mucinous adenocarcinoma in situ, columnar cells. The lining cells are often columnar, with pseudostratified parallel nuclei at the base. **A.** Routine stain showing apical mucin vacuoles and intra-alveolar mucin. **B.** A periodic acid–Schiff stain demonstrates diffuse cytoplasmic mucin, with apparent basal sparing because of the nuclei.

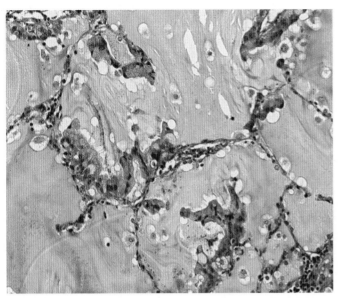

FIGURE 76.4 ▲ Mucinous adenocarcinoma in situ, cuboidal cell predominance. The cells are rounded with scattered signet ring–appearing cells.

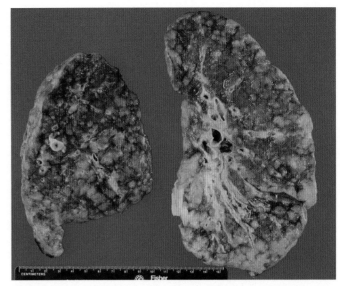

FIGURE 76.5 ▲ Mucinous adenocarcinoma, multifocal. The pneumonitic spread of mucinous adenocarcinoma may result in multiple consolidations.

Incidence

Mucinous adenocarcinomas account for between 2.4%[8,9] and 10% of invasive lung adenocarcinomas.[10,11] Adenocarcinomas with a minor mucinous component constituted 7% in one series.[8]

Radiologic Findings

The radiographic findings of mucinous adenocarcinoma are generally similar to lepidic-predominant adenocarcinomas that are nonmucinous, and vary considerably. There are most commonly single or multiple ground-glass opacities with areas of solid attenuation that correspond to invasive tumor.[12] The "pneumonic" form can spread rapidly due to aerogenous metastases and result in diffuse consolidation and has been described in mucinous as well as nonmucinous lepidic-predominant adenocarcinomas.[13,14]

For mucinous and nonmucinous adenocarcinomas with a large in situ (lepidic) component, positron emission tomography (PET) is of limited use in distinguishing adenocarcinoma from reactive nodules.[15,16] In one series, the average standard uptake value (SUV) by PET was only 2.69 for invasive mucinous adenocarcinoma, which overlapped with benign nodules and noninvasive mucinous tumors.[17]

Clinical Findings

Mucinous adenocarcinoma typically presents as a solitary lung nodule and rarely as a rapidly advancing pneumonia.[13] There is a slight female predominance, with an average age at initial diagnosis of 60 to 65 years. There is a weaker association between smoking and mucinous adenocarcinomas than with lepidic-predominant and other nonmucinous adenocarcinomas.[18]

Tissue Sampling

It is recommended that adenocarcinomas with a predominant lepidic growth pattern be completely sampled to assess for invasive areas. Mucinous adenocarcinomas are typically excised by wedge resection, and if there is invasion of size >3 cm, completion lobectomy is typically performed. The pathologist may be called on frozen section to determine the presence of invasion in order to guide further resection of the lobe or segment.

Gross Findings

Mucinous adenocarcinomas are typically peripheral nodules that, on rare occasions, form coalescing consolidations from diffuse aerogenous spread (Fig. 76.5). They are relatively well circumscribed, gray-white, and soft with gelatinous and occasionally pseudocystic centers. Necrosis and hemorrhage are absent.[1]

Microscopic Findings

Mucinous adenocarcinomas usually show mixed in situ and invasive areas, although some tumors lack lepidic growth. Multifocality, both gross and microscopic, is common. The in situ components are identical to those in noninvasive or minimally invasive tumors. The invasive components are most frequently acinar, followed by papillary and solid components (Fig. 76.6). The solid areas may contain abundant signet ring cells. Nests of aerogenous spread through alveolar spaces are frequent, although lymphatic invasion as often seen with micropapillary carcinoma is not seen (Fig. 76.7).

The invading acini in mucinous adenocarcinomas often form large cyst-like spaces with a surrounding desmoplastic stroma (features of so-called mucinous cystadenocarcinoma). There may be irregular cribriform spaces at the periphery of these cysts, with "garland" formation similar to enteric adenocarcinoma. However, "dirty necrosis" is usually absent (Fig. 76.8).

The cells lining the cysts are typically columnar and contain intracytoplasmic mucin throughout the cytoplasm. Mucin stains often show an apical mucin distribution, because of the basal location of the nuclei. Less frequently, there are goblet cells, with a rounded mucin vacuole that compresses the nucleus toward the cell base. These may be interspersed with cuboidal cells with minimal mucin, or columnar mucin-secreting cells. Sometimes, most of the lining cells have histologic features of pneumocytes (with corresponding immunohistochemical findings) with a minority of tumor cells secreting mucin that fills the cysts and alveolar spaces.

Immunohistochemical Stains

Mucinous adenocarcinomas of the lung are virtually always positive for cytokeratin 7, with frequent weak staining of cytokeratin 20 (up to 90% of cases in one series).[1] The rate of TTF-1 positivity, which is typically focal, is around 30%[1,4] and often is expressed in non–mucin-forming cells (Fig. 76.9). CDX2 is negative in most reported series.[1]

Molecular Findings

Mutations in epidermal growth factor receptor gene (EGFR) occur less often in mucinous adenocarcinomas than in nonmucinous

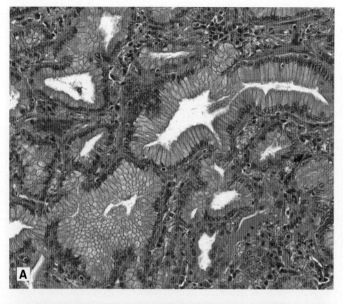

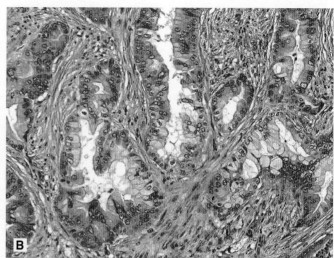

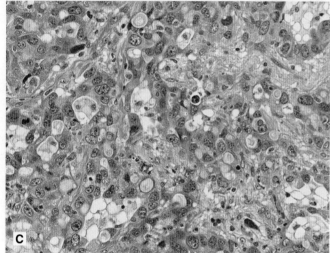

FIGURE 76.6 ▲ Mucinous adenocarcinoma, invasive components. **A.** The infiltrating tumor forms acini with columnar cells. **B.** Acinar invasion may be accompanied by a desmoplastic response, mimicking enteric carcinoma, but there is no dirty necrosis. **C.** Invasive mucinous adenocarcinoma, with areas of solid signet ring cell growth. The mucinous areas are not shown.

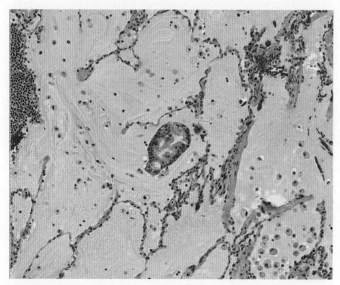

FIGURE 76.7 ▲ Intra-alveolar cell clusters. Also known as spread through alveolar spaces, this is indicative of invasion and precludes a diagnosis of in situ or minimally invasive adenocarcinoma. In mucinous tumors, the cells may float within otherwise acellular mucin.

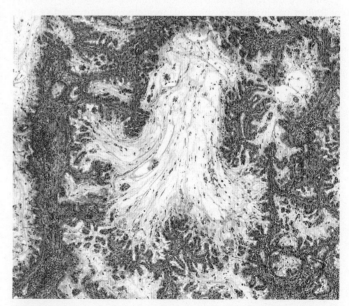

FIGURE 76.8 ▲ Invasive mucinous adenocarcinoma, with cystic dilatation. The invasive acinar structures can occasionally be cystically dilated, similar to so-called cystadenocarcinoma.

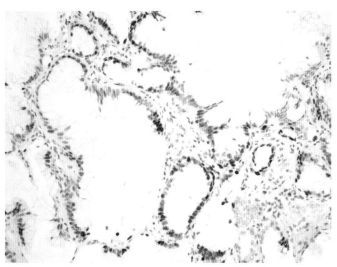

FIGURE 76.9 ▲ Mucinous adenocarcinoma, TTF-1 staining. This tumor shows numerous positive cells. The corresponding hematoxylin–eosin stain is shown in Figure 76.2A.

lepidic-predominant adenocarcinomas, at a rate of 0% to 15%.[11,18,19] In contrast, mutations in KRAS are much more frequent, occurring in 63% to 86% of tumors.[11,18,19]

Recently, a novel somatic gene fusion, CD74-NRG1, was found in 4 of 102 adenocarcinomas of the lung with negative mutational analysis; all were of the mucinous phenotype.[20]

Prognosis and Treatment

The prognosis of mucinous adenocarcinoma is dependent on the extent and type of invasive component, similar to nonmucinous lepidic-predominant adenocarcinomas.[9,21] One series showed better survival rates than invasive nonmucinous adenocarcinomas, with a median 88-month disease-free survival.[8] A different study with incomplete histologic data showed a median survival of only 17 months, however.[22] Compared to other types of adenocarcinoma, mucinous tumors showed a relatively high rate of distant metastasis, but a relatively low rate of nodal metastasis, in a third study.[10]

There are few data regarding response to chemotherapy for mucinous adenocarcinoma, as many references combine mucinous and nonmucinous tumors under the previous designation of "bronchioloalveolar carcinoma." Tyrosine kinase inhibitors are relatively effective in treating lepidic-predominant adenocarcinomas in general[22] but are likely to be relatively ineffective in mucinous adenocarcinomas due to a low rate of EGFR mutations. Because the genetics are different, it is likely that current targeted therapy for mucinous adenocarcinoma will differ from therapy for nonmucinous tumors. One series of 16 mucinous "bronchioloalveolar carcinomas" showed a response to paclitaxel infusion in three cases.[22] Two mucinous adenocarcinomas showed a high sensitivity to combination therapy with cisplatin, pemetrexed, and bevacizumab.[23]

Colloid Adenocarcinoma

Definition

Although forming a spectrum with mucinous adenocarcinomas, colloid carcinomas form mucin pools that either distend alveolar spaces or infiltrate stromal soft tissue and have a minimal in situ component. Confusingly, colloid carcinomas were previously termed "mucinous adenocarcinoma," which is now used for mucinous carcinomas, typically with a prominent in situ component, without colloid features (previously bronchioloalveolar carcinoma). Another obsolete term, which has been replaced by colloid adenocarcinoma, is "mucinous cystadenocarcinoma," which was used for lung adenocarcinomas with copious mucin production resembling their counterparts in the ovary, pancreas, and breast.

Incidence

Colloid carcinomas are rare, with an incidence in one series of 13 in 5,427 adenocarcinomas of the lung (0.24%).[1]

Gross

Colloid carcinomas are well-circumscribed, unencapsulated peripheral nodules with a gelatinous consistency. The center may be filled with a substance resembling strawberry jelly macroscopically.[24] There is no necrosis or hemorrhage, and the size ranges from 1.5 to 5.5 cm.[1] There may be punctuate calcifications on cut surface.[25]

Histologic Features

Colloid carcinomas are very similar in appearance to mucinous adenocarcinomas of the gastrointestinal tract, with large areas of acellular mucin in which float single cells, nests, or tubules of adenocarcinoma. The intraalveolar tumor clusters may have a prominent signet ring component. The in situ component is minimal and characteristically lines relatively small portions of the alveolar walls, without encircling them like in situ mucinous adenocarcinoma. Another distinguishing feature from mucinous adenocarcinoma is the cell type, which is typically cuboidal, not columnar, with a mixed population of more stratified mucin-forming cells (Fig. 76.10).

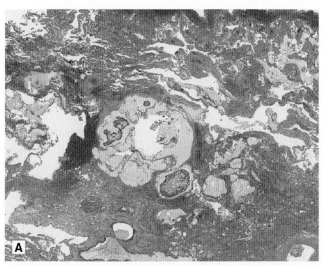

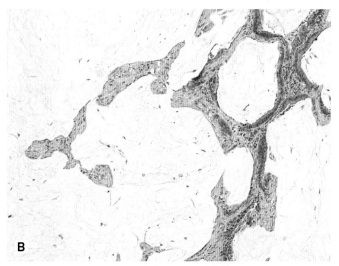

FIGURE 76.10 ▲ Colloid carcinoma. **A.** The tumor is composed mostly of acellular mucin, with tumor nests floating within. **B.** The alveolar spaces tend to be lined partially and not encircling the entire alveolar spaces as in mucinous adenocarcinoma in situ.

The invasive component of colloid carcinoma is predominantly the intra-alveolar tumor (spread through alveolar spaces). However, a minor component of stromal invasion may occur, with acinar, solid, or cribriform patterns.

Immunohistochemically, colloid carcinomas are typically TTF-1 positive in a focal pattern, coexpress CK20 and CK7, and generally stain with anti-CDX2, unlike mucinous adenocarcinomas. There is often a dual cell population, one expressing TTF-1 and lacking CDX2 and mucin-secreting cells with converse staining.[1]

Course

The course of colloid adenocarcinomas is variable but generally indolent; fewer than one-fifth of patients have an aggressive course.[1,25] Although not fully studied, metastatic disease is likely related to the proportion of invasive tumor. Nodal disease is uncommon. In one series, 11 of 13 patients were alive and well with a median follow-up of 26 months.[1]

REFERENCES

1. Rossi G, Murer B, Cavazza A, et al. Primary mucinous (so-called colloid) carcinomas of the lung: a clinicopathologic and immunohistochemical study with special reference to CDX-2 homeobox gene and MUC2 expression. *Am J Surg Pathol.* 2004;28:442–452.
2. Yousem SA. Pulmonary intestinal-type adenocarcinoma does not show enteric differentiation by immunohistochemical study. *Mod Pathol.* 2005;18: 816–821.
3. Travis WD, Brambilla E, Noguchi M, et al. International association for the study of lung cancer/American Thoracic Society/European Respiratory Society International Multidisciplinary Classification of lung adenocarcinoma. *J Thorac Oncol.* 2011;6:244–285.
4. Tsuta K, Ishii G, Nitadori J, et al. Comparison of the immunophenotypes of signet-ring cell carcinoma, solid adenocarcinoma with mucin production, and mucinous bronchioloalveolar carcinoma of the lung characterized by the presence of cytoplasmic mucin. *J Pathol.* 2006;209:78–87.
5. Wu J, Chu PG, Jiang Z, et al. Napsin A expression in primary mucin-producing adenocarcinomas of the lung: an immunohistochemical study. *Am J Clin Pathol.* 2013;139:160–166.
6. Travis WD, Brambilla E, Noguchi M, et al. Diagnosis of lung adenocarcinoma in resected specimens: implications of the 2011 International Association for the Study of Lung Cancer/American Thoracic Society/European Respiratory Society classification. *Arch Pathol Lab Med.* 2013;137:685–705.
7. Xu L, Tavora F, Battafarano R, et al. Adenocarcinomas with prominent lepidic spread: retrospective review applying new classification of the American Thoracic Society. *Am J Surg Pathol.* 2012;36:273–282.
8. Warth A, Muley T, Meister M, et al. The novel histologic International Association for the Study of Lung Cancer/American Thoracic Society/European Respiratory Society classification system of lung adenocarcinoma is a stage-independent predictor of survival. *J Clin Oncol.* 2012;30: 1438–1446.
9. Borczuk AC, Qian F, Kazeros A, et al. Invasive size is an independent predictor of survival in pulmonary adenocarcinoma. *Am J Surg Pathol.* 2009;33:462–469.
10. Xu L, Tavora F, Burke A. Histologic features associated with metastatic potential in invasive adenocarcinomas of the lung. *Am J Surg Pathol.* 2013;37:1100–1108.
11. Hata A, Katakami N, Fujita S, et al. Frequency of EGFR and KRAS mutations in Japanese patients with lung adenocarcinoma with features of the mucinous subtype of bronchioloalveolar carcinoma. *J Thorac Oncol.* 2010;5:1197–1200.
12. Gandara DR, Aberle D, Lau D, et al. Radiographic imaging of bronchioloalveolar carcinoma: screening, patterns of presentation and response assessment. *J Thorac Oncol.* 2006;1:S20–S26.
13. Garfield DH and Franklin W. Dramatic response to pemetrexed in a patient with pneumonic-type mucinous bronchioloalveolar carcinoma. *J Thorac Oncol.* 2011;6:397–398.
14. Tanaka J, Tajima S, Ito R, et al. A case of non-small cell lung carcinoma dying of acute respiratory failure due to aerogenous metastasis. *Nihon Kokyuki Gakkai Zasshi.* 2009;47:652–657.
15. Chun EJ, Lee HJ, Kang WJ, et al. Differentiation between malignancy and inflammation in pulmonary ground-glass nodules: the feasibility of integrated (18)F-FDG PET/CT. *Lung Cancer.* 2009;65:180–186.
16. Usuda K, Sagawa M, Motono N, et al. Diagnostic performance of diffusion weighted imaging of malignant and benign pulmonary nodules and masses: comparison with positron emission tomography. *Asian Pac J Cancer Prev.* 2014;15:4629–4635.
17. Shim SS, Han J. FDG-PET/CT imaging in assessing mucin-producing non-small cell lung cancer with pathologic correlation. *Ann Nucl Med.* 2010;24:357–362.
18. Kakegawa S, Shimizu K, Sugano M, et al. Clinicopathological features of lung adenocarcinoma with KRAS mutations. *Cancer.* 2011;117:4257–4266.
19. Finberg KE, Sequist LV, Joshi VA, et al. Mucinous differentiation correlates with absence of EGFR mutation and presence of KRAS mutation in lung adenocarcinomas with bronchioloalveolar features. *J Mol Diagn.* 2007;9: 320–326.
20. Fernandez-Cuesta L, Plenker D, Osada H, et al. CD74-NRG1 fusions in lung adenocarcinoma. *Cancer Discov.* 2014;4:415–422.
21. Sakao Y, Miyamoto H, Sakuraba M, et al. Prognostic significance of a histologic subtype in small adenocarcinoma of the lung: the impact of nonbronchioloalveolar carcinoma components. *Ann Thorac Surg.* 2007;83:209–214.
22. West HL, Franklin WA, McCoy J, et al. Gefitinib therapy in advanced bronchioloalveolar carcinoma: Southwest Oncology Group Study S0126. *J Clin Oncol.* 2006;24:1807–1813.
23. Yamakawa H, Takayanagi N, Ishiguro T, et al. A favorable response to cisplatin, pemetrexed and bevacizumab in two cases of invasive mucinous adenocarcinoma formerly known as pneumonic-type mucinous bronchioloalveolar carcinoma. *Intern Med.* 2013;52:2781–2784.
24. Okimasa S, Kurimoto N. Mucinous (colloid) adenocarcinoma. *Jpn J Thorac Cardiovasc Surg.* 2005;53:305–308.
25. Murai T, Hara M, Ozawa Y, et al. Mucinous colloid adenocarcinoma of the lung with lymph node metastasis showing numerous punctate calcifications. *Clin Imaging.* 2011;35:151–155.

77 Fetal and Enteric Carcinoma

Marie-Christine Aubry, M.D.

General Overview

In addition to mucinous and colloid carcinomas, "variants" of adenocarcinomas according to the WHO include fetal and enteric carcinomas. Fetal carcinomas overlap with pulmonary blastomas, which are classified as a subtype of sarcomatoid carcinoma and are biphasic tumors with a fetal adenocarcinoma component and a malignant-appearing immature stroma (see Chapter 85). Fetal adenocarcinomas lack the malignant stromal component.

Enteric adenocarcinoma is a term applied to primary lung tumors that histologically resemble colorectal carcinomas and can be confused with metastatic colorectal carcinoma to the lung.

Fetal Adenocarcinoma

Clinical

The clinical characteristics of fetal adenocarcinomas vary by their histologic subtype. Fetal adenocarcinomas that are low grade, with homogenous histologic findings, are typically seen in young to middle-aged females with a modest or no smoking history. High-grade fetal adenocarcinomas present at a mean age in years in the low 60s and occur mostly in male smokers.

High-grade fetal adenocarcinomas account for <0.5% of adenocarcinomas of the lung.[1] Low-grade fetal adenocarcinomas are rare tumors and are less common than the high-grade variant. It was initially described in 1984 as "well-differentiated adenocarcinoma simulating fetal tubules"[2] and later in 1994 as "pulmonary endodermal tumor resembling fetal lung."[3]

Microscopic Findings in Low-Grade Fetal Adenocarcinoma

Well-differentiated fetal adenocarcinoma is composed of glycogen-rich glands and tubules that resemble fetal lung at 10 to 15 weeks of gestation.[2,4] The tumor cells are cuboidal to columnar cells, with minimal atypia, and are arranged in complex structures and small rosettes, with apical cytoplasmic vacuoles (Fig. 77.1). Squamous morules are common. Areas of necrosis may occur but are less frequent than in high-grade tumors.

The intervening stroma is scant and composed of benign spindled myofibroblastic cells. The presence of immature cellular stroma, with or without heterologous elements, warrants a designation of pulmonary blastoma (Chapter 85).[4,5]

Periodic acid–Schiff (PAS) staining demonstrates glycogen within the cytoplasm of the cells. Mucicarmine and PAS staining with diastase are negative.

Microscopic Finings in High-Grade Fetal Adenocarcinoma

High-grade fetal adenocarcinomas have, in addition to fetal lung–like areas, prominent nuclear atypia, a lack of morules, and a transition to conventional adenocarcinoma (Fig. 77.2). The term "blastomatoid variant of carcinosarcoma" is sometimes used for tumors with high-grade fetal lung–like epithelium and malignant spindled cell component (see Chapter 85).[5]

High-grade fetal adenocarcinomas show complex glandular, cribriform, and papillary structures, columnar cells with clear cytoplasm, supranuclear or subnuclear vacuoles, pseudostratified nuclei, and prominent nuclear atypia (Fig. 77.2). There are flat apical borders, absence of morules, and membranous or nuclear staining for β-catenin.[1]

The amount of tumor resembling fetal adenocarcinoma is quite variable. At least 5% of a given tumor must have areas typical of the entity according to published reports.[1,5] However, the WHO requires 50%.[6]

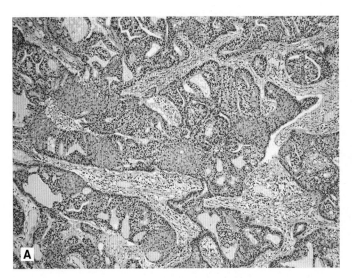

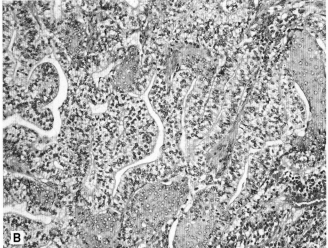

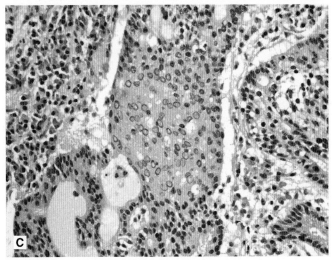

FIGURE 77.1 ▲ Fetal adenocarcinoma, low grade. **A.** The tumor is composed of glands that are often configured in a cribriform pattern. Several morules are present. The stroma is composed of benign spindle cells in a myxoid background. **B.** The glands are lined by columnar cells with a clear cytoplasm. The cell atypia is minimal. **C.** The morules are solid with polygonal cells containing eosinophilic cytoplasm. The main characteristic is the optically clear nuclei.

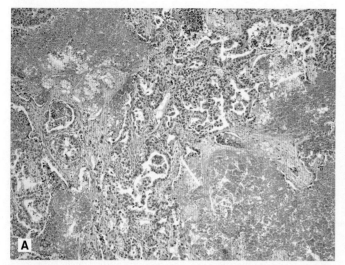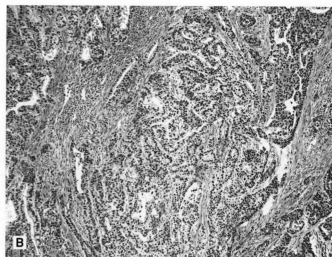

FIGURE 77.2 ▲ Fetal adenocarcinoma, high grade. **A.** In this photomicrograph, the tumor resembles a more typical adenocarcinoma with areas of necrosis and higher cytologic atypia. **B.** Areas typical of low-grade fetal adenocarcinoma are also seen.

The other nonfetal adenocarcinoma areas include virtually all patterns of typical adenocarcinomas of the lung, including acinar, lepidic, and papillary. Areas of hepatoid growth, clear cell adenocarcinoma, and large cell neuroendocrine carcinoma are common in high-grade fetal adenocarcinomas.[1,5]

Immunohistochemical Stains

Low-grade fetal adenocarcinomas show immunoreactivity for low molecular weight cytokeratins, carcinoembryonic antigen, TTF-1, and focal positivity for epithelial membrane antigen. β-Catenin positivity is seen in the nuclei of morules and can be a useful marker in the differential diagnosis. This finding is typically absent in high-grade tumors. Neuroendocrine markers (chromogranin and synaptophysin) are commonly positive. Estrogen and progesterone receptors, desmin, and S100 protein are usually negative.[4] In high-grade tumors, there may be expression of alpha-fetoprotein, glypican-3, and SALL4. Synaptophysin, chromogranin, TTF-1, CDX2, and p53 are also commonly positive.[5]

Molecular Findings

Low-grade adenocarcinoma of fetal lung type is characterized by β-catenin gene (*CTNNB1*) mutations leading to aberrant β-catenin expression both in the nucleus and in the cytoplasm.[5,6]

High-grade tumors may occasionally harbor EGFR and KRAS mutations.[5]

Differential Diagnosis

The lack of pleomorphism and growth pattern of well-differentiated fetal adenocarcinoma may suggest carcinoid tumor. As fetal adenocarcinoma may express neuroendocrine markers, the presence of morules with β-catenin expression favors fetal adenocarcinoma.[4]

The morphology of the glands along with the morules raises the possibility of metastatic endometrial carcinoma. Using TTF-1 and estrogen receptor immunostains will assist with the differential diagnosis.

Prognosis and Treatment

The prognosis of well-differentiated adenocarcinoma is good, with a mortality of only 15%.[7] The outcome of high-grade fetal adenocarcinoma is more similar to that of typical adenocarcinoma of the lung.[1,5]

Enteric Adenocarcinoma

Clinical

Pulmonary adenocarcinomas with enteric features constitute nearly 3% of lung adenocarcinomas. The mean age is 50 years, and there is no gender predilection.[8]

Gross Findings

Enteric adenocarcinomas are gray–white on cut surface with dot-like or geographic necrosis.[9]

Microscopic Findings

In 1991, Tsao and Fraser reported the first case enteric adenocarcinoma primary to the lung and described a tumor with absorptive cells with brush borders, goblet cells, Paneth cells, and neuroendocrine cells.[10] The cellular features that impart a "colonic" or "enteric" appearance include tall columnar cells, brush borders, large vesicular nuclei, and eosinophilic cytoplasm. Architectural features include papillary structures, preservation of nuclear polarity, nuclear palisading, large irregular glands with necrotic "dirty" debris, and a "garland" growth pattern (Fig. 77.3). Similar to other adenocarcinomas of the lung, a central elastotic scar may be present.[8,11,12]

Immunohistochemical Findings

Most reports of enteric adenocarcinomas document an immunohistochemical profile similar to that of primary lung adenocarcinomas, with diffuse cytokeratin 7 positivity and variable TTF-1 expression. In contrast to nonenteric type of lung adenocarcinoma, staining for CDX2, cytokeratin 20, villin, and Muc2 have been reported, but it is usually

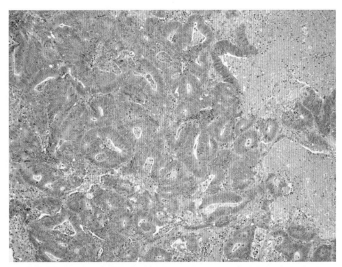

FIGURE 77.3 ▲ Enteric adenocarcinoma. There are large gland-like spaces with cribriform glands and necrosis. Immunohistochemical staining (TTF-1, cytokeratin 7, and cytokeratin 20) confirmed pulmonary origin (not shown).

patchy.[8,9,11] And in contrast to colorectal cancers, staining for cytokeratin 7 is typically strong and diffuse. The focal expression of CDX2 and cytokeratin 20 does occur in other primary lung adenocarcinomas, specifically the colloid type (see Chapter 76).

There have been two reports of putative primary lung adenocarcinomas with entirely colonic immunohistochemical profile (absent cytokeratin 7, positive cytokeratin 20), which were histologically indistinguishable from metastatic colonic adenocarcinoma.[12,13] In these cases, clinical follow-up or autopsy confirmed the absence of a colorectal primary tumor.

Molecular Findings

There are few data on molecular findings in pulmonary adenocarcinoma with enteric differentiation. EGFR and KRAS have been found to be wild type in the few reported cases.[8]

Differential Diagnosis

The differential diagnosis is with metastatic colonic adenocarcinoma. In most cases, immunohistochemical staining is confirmatory of a lung primary. In cases of pancreatic metastasis, documentation of a second lung primary can be especially difficult, because there are no immunohistochemical stains that reliably separate pancreatic versus pulmonary adenocarcinoma.

REFERENCES

1. Suzuki M, Yazawa T, Ota S, et al. High-grade fetal adenocarcinoma of the lung is a tumour with a fetal phenotype that shows diverse differentiation, including high-grade neuroendocrine carcinoma: a clinicopathological, immunohistochemical and mutational study of 20 cases. *Histopathology.* 2015.
2. Kodama T, Shimosato Y, Watanabe S, et al. Six cases of well-differentiated adenocarcinoma simulating fetal lung tubules in pseudoglandular stage. Comparison with pulmonary blastoma. *Am J Surg Pathol.* 1984;8: 735–744.
3. Nakatani Y, Kitamura H, Inayama Y, et al. Pulmonary endodermal tumor resembling fetal lung. The optically clear nucleus is rich in biotin. *Am J Surg Pathol.* 1994;18:637–642.
4. Sheehan KM, Curran J, Kay EW, et al. Well differentiated fetal adenocarcinoma of the lung in a 29 year old woman. *J Clin Pathol.* 2003;56: 478–479.
5. Morita S, Yoshida A, Goto A, et al. High-grade lung adenocarcinoma with fetal lung-like morphology: clinicopathologic, immunohistochemical, and molecular analyses of 17 cases. *Am J Surg Pathol.* 2013;37:924–932.
6. Travis WD, Yatabe Y, Brambilla E, et al. Variants of adenocarcinoma. In: Travis WD, et al., eds. *WHO Classification of Tumours of the Lung, Pleura, Mediastinum and Heart.* Lyon, France: IARC Press; 2015: 38–43.
7. Nakatani Y, Kitamura H, Inayama Y, et al. Pulmonary adenocarcinomas of the fetal lung type: a clinicopathologic study indicating differences in histology, epidemiology, and natural history of low-grade and high-grade forms. *Am J Surg Pathol.* 1998;22:399–411.
8. Wang CX, Liu B, Wang YF, et al. Pulmonary enteric adenocarcinoma: a study of the clinicopathologic and molecular status of nine cases. *Int J Clin Exp Pathol.* 2014;7:1266–1274.
9. Inamura K, Satoh Y, Okumura S, et al. Pulmonary adenocarcinomas with enteric differentiation: histologic and immunohistochemical characteristics compared with metastatic colorectal cancers and usual pulmonary adenocarcinomas. *Am J Surg Pathol.* 2005;29:660–665.
10. Tsao MS; Fraser RS. Primary pulmonary adenocarcinoma with enteric differentiation. *Cancer.* 1991;68:1754–1757.
11. Yousem SA. Pulmonary intestinal-type adenocarcinoma does not show enteric differentiation by immunohistochemical study. *Mod Pathol.* 2005;18: 816–821.
12. Laszlo T, Lacza A, Toth D, et al. Pulmonary enteric adenocarcinoma indistinguishable morphologically and immunohistologically from metastatic colorectal carcinoma. *Histopathology.* 2014;65:283–287.
13. Hatanaka K, Tsuta K, Watanabe K, et al. Primary pulmonary adenocarcinoma with enteric differentiation resembling metastatic colorectal carcinoma: a report of the second case negative for cytokeratin 7. *Pathol Res Pract.* 2011;207:188–191.

78 Squamous Cell, Basaloid, and Lymphoepithelial-Like Carcinoma

Andre L. Moreira, M.D., Fabio R. Tavora, M.D., Ph.D., and Allen P. Burke, M.D.

Invasive Squamous Cell Carcinoma

Epidemiology

Between 1977 and 1986, squamous cell carcinoma accounted for more than 30% of lung cancers, a rate that has decreased to <20% because of a decrease in cigarette smoking.[1] Approximately 224,000 new lung cancers (of all types) were predicted to occur in the United States in 2014,[2] indicating about 45,000 that are of the squamous type. Although there is a nearly equal gender distribution for all lung cancers,[2] there is still a male predominance in most series of squamous carcinomas of the lung.[3]

TABLE 78.1 Rate of Positivity, Pulmonary Squamous Cell Carcinomas, Selected Immunohistochemical Markers

Antibody	Resected Tumors	TMA Samples	Peripheral Tumors (TMA)	Central Tumors (TMA)
p63	100%[2,3,4,5]	100%[6] 94%[7] 95%[12]	71%[1]	65%[1]
p40 (δNp63)[a]	100%[d]	100%[6] 81%[7]		
Cytokeratin 7	20%–60%[2,3]		40%[1]	4.7%[1]
TTF-1	0%[2,3] 3% (focal)[d]	0[6] 0%[12] 2%[12]	5%[1]	0%[1]
Napsin-A	0%[2]	2%[12]		
Cytokeratin 5/6	73%–100%[2,3,4]	53%[12]	85%[1]	90%[1]
34βE12 (CK903)	100%[2,4]	—	—	—
p16				
All tumors	10%[9]; 21%[13]; 63%[8]			
HPV+[b]	71%[8]–100%[9,11]			
HPV–	0[10]; 6%[9]; 18%[11]; 21%[13]; 62%[8]			
p53		—	—	—
All tumors	53%[8]			
HPV+	76%[8]			
HPV–	50%[8]			

1. Saijo et al. (2006).[10]
2. Mukhopadhyay and Katzenstein (2011).[11]
3. Pelosi et al. (2011).[12]
4. Rekhtman et al. (2011).[13]
5. Bishop et al. (2012).[14]
6. Nonaka (2012).[15]
7. Ao et al. (2014).[16]
8. Fan et al. (2015) Cytoplasmic OR nuclear staining.[17]
9. Gatta et al. (2012) Nuclear AND cytoplasmic staining.[18]
10. van Boerdink Nuclear OR cytoplasmic >70% of tumor.[7]
11. Yanagawa et al. (2013) Nuclear only, > 10%.[6]
12. Whithaus et al. (2012); TTF-1 stained 2% of squamous carcinoma using one antibody (Leica) and 0% using another (Dao).[19]
13. Bishop et al. (2012); strong and diffuse cytoplasmic and nuclear staining in >70% of tumor cells.[14]
TMA, tissue microarray.
[a]Preferred because of greatest specificity for squamous differentiation.
[b]By in situ hybridization and/or polymerase chain reaction, primarily metastatic tumors.

Risk Factors

Similar to small cell carcinoma, squamous cell carcinoma is highly related to degree of exposure to cigarettes, especially to tar in the smoke.[4] A man who smokes more than 30 cigarettes a day is 103.5 times more likely to develop squamous carcinoma of the lung than is a nonsmoker.[5] Occupational agents that increase the likelihood of lung cancer, including squamous carcinoma, include asbestos and arsenic.[4] The association between human papillomavirus infection and squamous lung carcinoma is weak, at least in Western populations.[6,7]

Radiologic Findings

Although two-thirds of all squamous carcinomas are central, squamous cell carcinomas that are surgically resected are slightly more likely to be peripheral.[8,9] On computed tomography scans, they are less often spiculated, less often have internal air bronchograms, and are more likely to have heterogeneous enhancement and cavitation, as compared to pulmonary adenocarcinomas.[9]

Gross Findings and Staging

Central squamous carcinomas usually arise in a main or lobar bronchus (Table 78.1). These tumors may form intraluminal polypoid masses or endobronchial papillary tumors (Fig. 78.1).[20] Uncommonly, they spread superficially and are limited to the bronchial wall, in which case they are classified as T1a, regardless of size and whether or not they extend to the main bronchus.[21] Squamous cell carcinoma typically infiltrates adjacent structures through direct invasion. On cut surface, they are firm and gritty, and there may be focal carbon pigment deposits in the center. Cavitation occurs in about 20% of tumors, typically those

that attain a large size (Fig. 78.2). Postobstructive changes, including endogenous lipid pneumonia, are common in central lesions.

Microscopic Findings

Well-differentiated squamous carcinomas typically have intracellular bridges and foci of keratinization and form sheets of cells

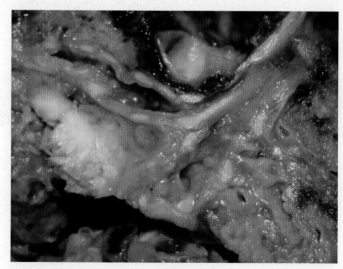

FIGURE 78.1 ▲ Squamous cell carcinoma. The tumor distorts the bronchial surface and invades the adjacent lung.

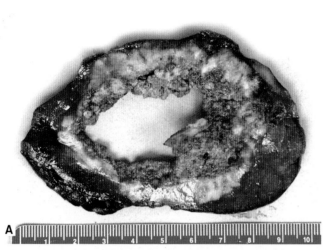
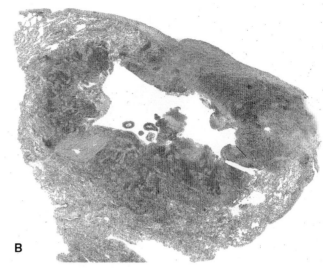

FIGURE 78.2 ▲ Squamous cell carcinoma. Approximately 20% of tumors, especially those that are central, form cavitary masses. **A.** Gross photograph. **B.** Corresponding histologic section.

without glandular structures or mucin vacuoles (Figs. 78.3 and 78.4). Nonkeratinizing, poorly differentiated tumors may have a basaloid appearance (see below) or resemble adenocarcinomas with a solid growth pattern, in which case immunohistochemical stains are necessary for a definitive diagnosis. Proximal tumors tend to have a papillary or endophytic growth pattern (Fig. 78.5). Peripheral tumors grow in two overlapping patterns: one that respects alveolar architecture, filling alveolar spaces (Fig. 78.6), and one that is accompanied by fibrosis, with a pushing, destructive edge (Fig. 78.7).[8,22] Peripheral tumors are more likely to have vascular (Fig. 78.8) and pleural invasion and less likely to be associated with squamous metaplasia in adjacent bronchi than proximal tumors.[10] There may be large areas of cytoplasmic clearing due to intracytoplasmic glycogen (Fig. 78.9), a nonspecific finding that is common in both squamous and adenocarcinoma. Squamous carcinomas may grow along alveolar walls, a pattern that is often confused with adenosquamous carcinoma. This growth pattern has been termed "endoalveolar growth" or "invasion along alveolar walls" and is seen in up to 20% of squamous carcinomas.[23,24]

Pathologic studies of early squamous carcinomas that are occult on chest x-ray and detected by screening show that they progress from in situ lesions to mucosal, muscular, cartilaginous, and extrabronchial invasion.[25] Infiltration of the bronchial wall is of two types: one extensive bronchiolar spread without extending through the cartilage and the other penetrating deeply into the wall, presumably advancing within a short period.[25]

There is no standardized grading of squamous carcinomas, although the proportion of tumor with keratinization or intracellular bridges is a useful grading tool (Fig. 78.10). Well-differentiated tumors show more than 50% keratinization with intracellular bridges; moderately differentiated tumors have less than one-half; and poorly differentiated tumors have minimal if any keratinization.[11]

Immunohistochemical Stains

As in other sites, a variety of markers (p63, p40, cytokeratin 5/6, cytokeratin 903/34βE12) are used to identify squamous differentiation in lung carcinomas (Table 78.1). Cytokeratin 903, although highly sensi-

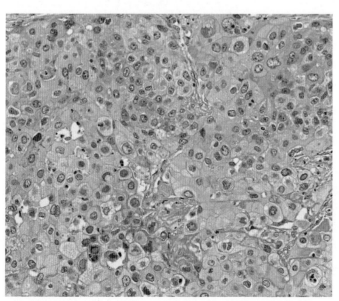

FIGURE 78.3 ▲ Squamous cell carcinoma. Tumor forms cohesive sheets with scattered dyskeratotic cells.

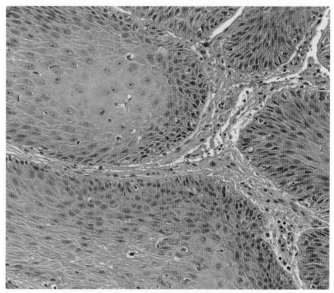

FIGURE 78.4 ▲ Squamous cell carcinoma. In well-differentiated tumors, intercellular bridges may be evident.

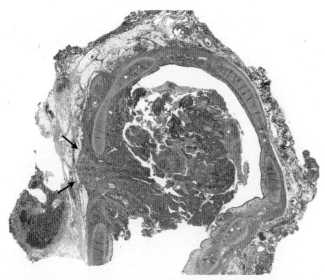

FIGURE 78.5 ▲ Squamous cell carcinoma. Proximal tumors may grow predominantly within the bronchial lumen. There is almost invariably invasion into the wall of the airway (*arrows*).

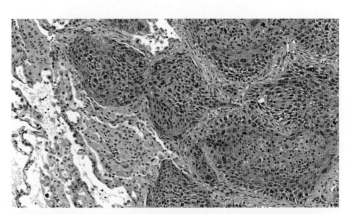

FIGURE 78.6 ▲ Squamous cell carcinoma. The periphery of the tumor may grow with preservation of the alveolar architecture.

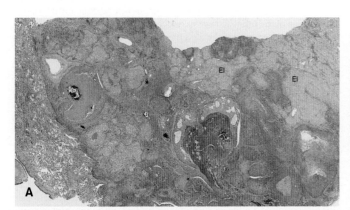

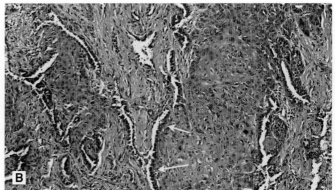

FIGURE 78.7 ▲ Squamous cell carcinoma. More commonly, there is destructive pushing growth. **A.** Note areas of elastotic scar (El) and areas of keratinization. **B.** In another area, at the edge of the tumor, there was focal residual alveolar lining with reactive pneumocytes (*arrow*).

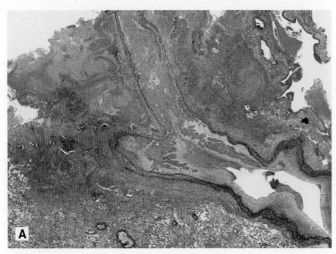

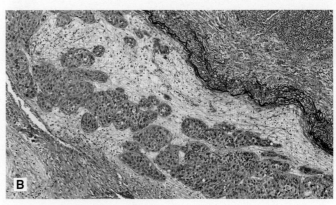

FIGURE 78.8 ▲ Squamous cell carcinoma with arterial invasion. Arterial invasion may be present (elastic van Gieson staining). **A.** Low magnification. **B.** Higher magnification showing the media of the muscular artery.

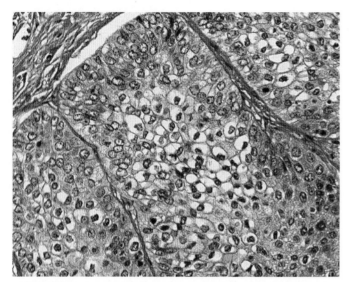

FIGURE 78.9 ▲ Squamous cell carcinoma with clear cell change. Areas of cytoplasmic clearing are not uncommon.

TABLE 78.2 Rates of Positivity of Selected Squamous Markers in Pulmonary Adenocarcinomas

	Adenocarcinoma (All Types)	Adenocarcinoma, Enriched for Poorly Differentiated
p40 (δNp63)	0% (any)[5]	0% (diffuse)[4]
	10%[6]	3% (any)[4]
p63	11% (diffuse)[5]	4% (diffuse)[3,4]
	20%[6]	10%[1]
	25% (any)[5]	15%[7]
	33% (diffuse)[2]	31% (any)[4]
	47% (any)[2]	32% (any)[3]
Cytokeratin 5/6	5%[2]	0%[1]
	20%[6]	3% (diffuse)[3]
		18% (any)[3]
34βE12		45% (diffuse)[3]
		60%[1]
		83% (any)[3]

[1] Mukhopadhyay and Katzenstein (2011).
[2] Pelosi et al. (2011).
[3] Rekhtman et al. (2011).
[4] Bishop et al. (2012).
[5] Nonaka (2012) (tissue microarray).
[6] Ao et al. (2014) (tissue microarray).
[7] Hwang (2014).

tive, lacks specificity (Table 78.2). δNp63 (p40) is of similar sensitivity as p63, but more specific, as it is less likely expressed in adenocarcinomas and neuroendocrine carcinomas than p63.[26] For this reason, it has largely replaced p40 in distinguishing poorly differentiated squamous from adenocarcinomas of the lung. Cytokeratin 5/6 is nearly as sensitive and specific as p40 and is often used in panels that include other markers in the distinction between squamous and other carcinomas of the lung.[11-13]

Cytokeratin 7 expression is not specific for adenocarcinoma, is seen in a significant number of squamous carcinomas, and has been shown to be more common in peripheral than central tumors.[10] Reports of p16 expression in squamous carcinomas of the lung are hampered by variation in defining positive staining, with results ranging from essentially none to over 50%.[6,7,17,18]

Differential Diagnosis

Invasive keratinizing squamous carcinomas pose little difficulty in diagnosis. In the case of poorly differentiated nonkeratinizing tumors,

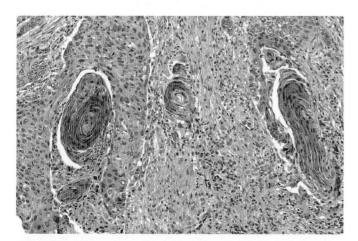

FIGURE 78.10 ▲ Squamous cell carcinoma, with keratinization. There are two prominent areas of keratin pearl formation. The degree of keratinization may be used as a grading system.

solid adenocarcinoma is usually easily excluded by the presence of diffuse staining for one or more of the squamous markers (p40, cytokeratin 5/6, or cytokeratin 34bE12) in the absence of TTF-1 or napsin-A (Fig. 78.11).[13]

The differential diagnosis of nonkeratinizing squamous carcinomas with basaloid features is primarily that of large cell neuroendocrine carcinoma or occasionally small cell carcinoma (see Basaloid Carcinoma). In smaller samples, the distinction among nonkeratinizing squamous carcinoma, solid adenocarcinoma, and neuroendocrine tumors is often more difficult, a problem confounded by the need to preserve tissue for potential molecular study (see Chapter 86).

Peripheral squamous carcinomas with an intra-alveolar spread, with relatively intact alveolar walls, can form a nested growth pattern that may be confused with endocrine tumors.[22] The less common endoalveolar growth pattern (growth along alveolar walls without filling them) is often confused with adenosquamous or adenocarcinomas. Endoalveolar squamous carcinoma is distinguished by characteristic immunohistochemical staining with TTF-1 showing preserved pneumocytes toward the alveolar spaces and p40 (or other squamous marker) positivity in the malignant cells deep to them (Fig. 78.12).

Molecular Findings

Although squamous carcinomas have a relatively high rate of exonic mutations compared to other cancers,[27] targeted treatment for molecular alterations lags behind that of adenocarcinomas. Mutations in TP53 are especially common in DNA extracted from squamous carcinomas, as well as genes involving HLA-A class I major histocompatibility antigen, phosphatidylinositol-3-OH kinase pathway genes, and NFE2L2, KEAP1, CDKN2A, and RB1.[27] Amplification of SOX2 and PDGFRA has been reported in squamous carcinoma cell lines.[28,29]

Differentiating Second Lung Primary Versus Metastatic Disease in Patients with Known Squamous Carcinomas of the Head and Neck

Because cigarette smoking is a risk factor for both squamous carcinomas of the head and neck as well as the lung, it is not uncommon to encounter lung tumors in patients with prior cancers of the oral mucosa, larynx, or pharynx. Metastatic disease tends to result in multiple lung lesions in patients with advanced primary tumors, although

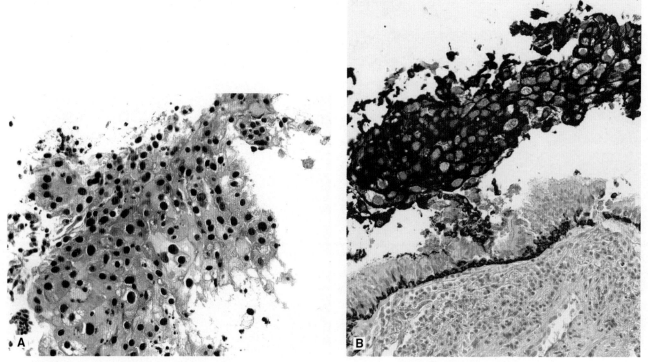

FIGURE 78.11 ▲ Squamous cell carcinoma, positive for cytokeratin 5/6. **A.** The hematoxylin eosin slide shows non–small cell carcinoma small biopsy. **B.** There is diffuse positivity for cytokeratin 5/6, essentially pathognomonic for squamous differentiation if seen to this degree and extent. Note the positivity in the basal layer of the airway.

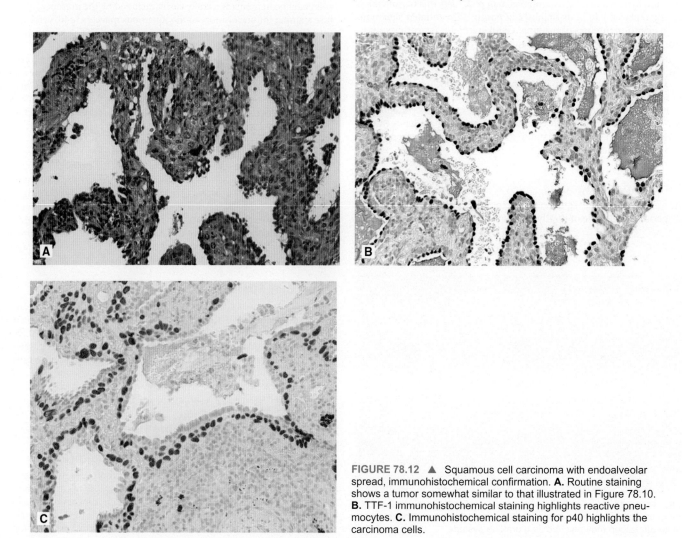

FIGURE 78.12 ▲ Squamous cell carcinoma with endoalveolar spread, immunohistochemical confirmation. **A.** Routine staining shows a tumor somewhat similar to that illustrated in Figure 78.10. **B.** TTF-1 immunohistochemical staining highlights reactive pneumocytes. **C.** Immunohistochemical staining for p40 highlights the carcinoma cells.

TABLE 78.3 Methods of Determining Squamous Lung Primary in Patients with Previous Squamous Carcinoma in the Head and Neck

Parameter	Criterion	Interpretation	Reliability
Spread of ENT tumor	Stage I or II	Second primary	Moderate
	Stage III or IV	Metastasis	Moderate
	Local recurrence at time of lung tumor	Metastasis	Moderate
Lung tumor imaging	Central	Second primary	Moderate
	Multiple	Metastasis	Moderate/good
	Single	Second primary	Poor/moderate
Time of occurrence of lung lesion	>3 y	Second primary	Poor/moderate
Histology	Discordant (keratinizing vs. basaloid, well vs. poorly differentiated)	Second primary	Moderate
Immunohistochemical staining	p53, divergent[a]	Second primary	Good; useful in < half of tumors
	P16, divergent[a]	Second primary	Moderate; useful in <20% of tumors
Molecular testing	Concordant mutational analysis and/or LOH	Metastasis	Good
	Discordant mutational analysis and/or LOH	Second primary	Good

[a]Percent of tumor cells with p53 expression varying by >50.

the clinical distinction is not reliable in all cases; metastases can occur up to 8 years after the primary tumor is treated.[14] Histologic comparison may be helpful, as ENT carcinomas vary from keratinizing to non-keratinizing types (especially in the oropharynx)[30] (Table 78.3).

Typing for human papillomavirus (HPV) by in situ hybridization or polymerase chain reaction may be helpful to establish a second lung primary. However, a high proportion (43% to 80%) of primary ENT carcinomas are negative, limiting the usefulness of this test in many patients.[14,31] A positive result is indicative of metastatic disease, because primary lung cancers rarely, if ever, harbor HPV, at least in developed countries.[7,14,32,33] The rate of HPV in Asian patients with squamous lung cancers is about 10%.[33] The likelihood of HPV positivity in metastatic squamous carcinomas to the lung varies by location in the head and neck, with no or few positive tumors in the larynx or oral cavity and a high rate in the oropharynx (up to 40%).[14]

Immunohistochemical staining may help in establishing a second primary if there is discordant expression, but no marker is helpful for confirming metastasis, as there is overlap for all antigens tested this far. p16 is not considered a surrogate for HPV infection and is present in about 20% of primary lung cancers, including adenocarcinomas, if defined strictly as nuclear and cytoplasmic positivity in more than two-thirds of the tumor.[14] Immunohistochemical staining for p53 has shown discordant results between ENT and lung squamous carcinomas supporting a diagnosis of second primary in up to one-third of patients.[34]

Molecular testing including mutational analysis and loss of heterozygosity has been used as an investigational tool to distinguish second primary squamous carcinomas of the lung from metastatic lesions. For example, the presence of specific *TP53* mutations in one or both tumors allowed this distinction in 38% of patients.[34] Analysis of loss of heterozygosity allows the distinction in 81% to 98% of tumor pairs.[30,35,36] In over one-third of tumors, the molecular analysis was at odds with the clinical determination.[30]

Prognosis and Treatment

Although the prognosis of adenocarcinomas has improved over the last decades, there has been no similar improvement in squamous carcinomas, in part because of lack of gene-targeted therapies. In addition, squamous carcinomas are more likely to result in life-threatening hemorrhage than adenocarcinomas after treatment with anti-VEGF (bevacizumab) and small molecule inhibitors (motesanib, sunitinib, sorafenib), restricting their use for tumors of squamous histology.[37] The reason for the increased risk for hemorrhage after treatment for squamous carcinomas is not known, but central location and proximity to major blood vessels may play a role in this association.[37]

Squamous Dysplasia and Carcinoma In Situ

General

Noninvasive neoplastic squamous lesions progress from low-grade dysplasia to moderate dysplasia, severe dysplasia, and carcinoma in situ. Severe dysplasia is sometimes reported separately from carcinoma in situ.[38] In other studies, severe dysplasia and carcinoma in situ are combined.[39]

Incidence

Among heavy smokers, bronchoscopy screening has shown that nearly 2% of patients harbor squamous carcinoma in situ, with an additional 20% of patients showing squamous dysplasia.[40]

Clinical Findings

There is a marked male predominance, and most patients are heavy cigarette smokers.[41,42] About one-third of patients have prior or concurrent invasive lung cancers.[41] Bronchoscopically, intraepithelial squamous neoplasia appears as a flat or slightly raised patch, often with increased vascularity. In addition to conventional white-light illumination, blue light (autofluorescence) imaging, narrow band imaging, and laser-induced fluorescence endoscopy have been used to increase the detection of small intraepithelial lesions.[43–46]

Histologic Findings

Preinvasive squamous lesions form a continuum from squamous metaplasia to in situ carcinoma. In general, dysplasia is characterized by nuclear pleomorphism, decrease in orderly maturation, and mitotic activity (Fig. 78.13). Carcinoma in situ is diagnosed when there is disorganization of the entire thickness and mitotic figures and apoptotic cells are present throughout (see Table 78.4) (Fig. 78.14). In many cases, there is adjacent invasive tumor. Severe dysplasia and carcinoma in situ are considered synonymous by some[48] and separate by others,[49] with severe dysplasia still possessing some degree, at least focally, of maturation toward the surface. One study found better reproducibility with a four-tiered system (low-, intermediate-, and high-grade dysplasia and carcinoma in situ) than a three-tiered one (metaplastic/low grade, moderate dysplasia, and high grade/CIS).[50]

Prognosis and Treatment

The progression rate of bronchial squamous dysplasia to invasive carcinoma is low, but high-grade dysplastic lesions are likely to persist. In a meta-analysis of 8 studies that included patients with and without treatment and with variable follow-up, McDaniel et al. found that

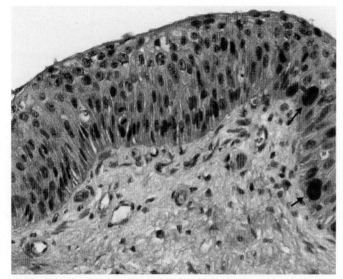

FIGURE 78.13 ▲ Squamous dysplasia. There are scattered enlarged nuclei with dispersed chromatin (*arrows*). Polarity and partial surface maturation is preserved.

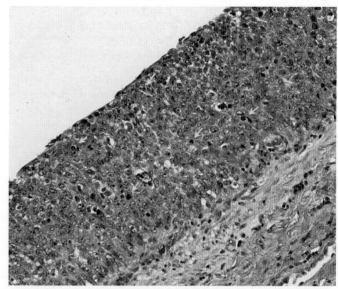

FIGURE 78.14 ▲ Squamous carcinoma in situ. The entire thickness is replaced by malignant-appearing squamous cells. There is no preservation of polarity. There are mitotic figures and apoptotic cells randomly throughout, including near the surface (*arrows*).

5% of mild to moderate dysplasia progressed to higher-grade lesions, and only one of 371 (0.3%) developed invasive carcinoma. In the same meta-analysis, 10 of 87 (11%) of severe dysplasia progressed to carcinoma in situ, but only 2 (2%) developed invasive carcinoma. Only in the group of carcinoma in situ (or those studies that combined severe dysplasia with carcinoma in situ) was there a significant risk for developing invasive disease (24/126, 19%).

A study of McCaughan et al., using a two-tiered system (low-grade dysplasia and high-grade dysplasia including carcinoma in situ), also found that low-grade dysplasia was indolent and that 8 of 10 high-grade dysplasia or carcinoma in situ developed invasive carcinomas. However, of these 8 patients, only 2 had carcinomas clearly at the same site, and one was alive and well at last follow-up. This study demonstrates that high-grade in situ lesions are often a marker of invasive cancers that coexist or develop adjacent or elsewhere in the bronchial tree.[39]

The treatment of preinvasive squamous neoplasia of the bronchus includes photodynamic therapy,[51] electrocautery, argon plasma coagulation, cryotherapy, laser, and intraluminal radiation therapy (brachytherapy).[42]

Immunohistochemistry

In severe dysplasia and carcinoma in situ, a higher number of suprabasal cells express EGFR, Ki 67, and p53 in the suprabasal area, as compared to lower-grade lesions.[49,52,53] In practice, the diagnosis of intraepithelial squamous lesions is generally made by histologic evaluation alone, however.

Genetics

Genetic alterations occur with increased frequency in carcinoma in situ compared to lower grades of dysplasia. These include loss of heterozygosity in chromosomes 3p[38] and 9p[54] and chromosome 3q amplification, associated with amplification of SOX2 and PIK3CA.[39] Less commonly, there is loss of heterozygosity on chromosomes 5q, 17p (17p13; TP53 gene), and 13q (13q14; retinoblastoma gene). Genetic alterations may be present in histologically normal or metaplastic mucosa as well as those showing dysplasia, but are generally absent in nonsmokers.[54]

Basaloid Carcinoma

The cardinal histopathologic features distinguishing this tumor from other non–small cell lung cancers are a lobular growth pattern of small cells with moderately hyperchromatic nuclei, with no prominent nucleoli,

TABLE 78.4 Histologic Features of Bronchial Squamous Intraepithelial Neoplasia

	Anisocytosis and Pleomorphism	Maturation	Mitoses and Apoptotic Debris	Nucleoli	Nuclei	Cell Size
Mild dysplasia	Mild	Preserved, with superficial flattening	Absent	Absent	Oval or round, finely granular chromatin	Mild increase
Moderate dysplasia	Moderate	Expanded basal zone, superficial flattening	Mostly in basal third	Absent or inconspicuous	Irregular, finely granular chromatin	Mild increase
Severe dysplasia	Marked	Absence of maturation, with superficial flattening	Mostly in basal two-thirds	Usually present	Markedly irregular, Coarse chromatin	Increased, with variation
Carcinoma in situ	Marked	Absence maturation or polarity, little or no superficial flattening, scattered dyskeratotic cells throughout	Throughout	Usually present	Markedly irregular, coarse chromatin	Increased, with variation

Adapted from Travis WD. Pathology of lung cancer. *Clin Chest Med.* 2011;*32*:669–692, Ref.[47]

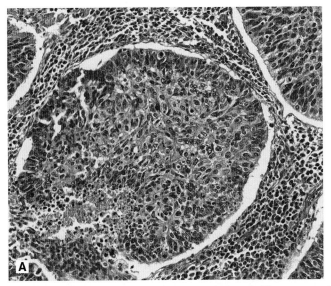
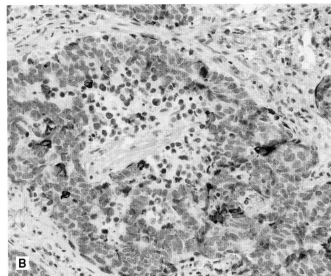

FIGURE 78.15 ▲ Basaloid squamous carcinoma. **A.** There are nests of tumor cells with peripheral palisading. **B.** Many cells express cytokeratin 903 (34βE12).

and with scant cytoplasm, a high mitotic rate, and peripheral palisading (Fig. 78.15). One study showed that basaloid carcinoma was present in a pure form in 19 cases and the other 19 tumors were of a mixed type.[55]

Basaloid tumors display a specific mRNA expression profile, encoding factors controlling the cell cycle, transcription, chromatin, and splicing, with prevalent expression in germline and stem cells, while genes related to squamous differentiation are underexpressed. From this signature, a recent study derived a 2-genes (SOX4, IVL) immunohistochemistry-based predictor that discriminated basaloid tumors (pure and mixed) from nonbasaloid tumors with 94% accuracy in an independent series. The pure basaloid tumors are also distinguished through unsupervised analyses. The corresponding molecular subtype was found in 8 independent public datasets and was shown to be associated with a very poor survival as compared with other SCCs.[24]

Lymphoepithelial-Like Carcinoma

General

Lymphoepithelial-like carcinoma is a variant of squamous carcinoma, which is classified by histologic features and by the intratumoral presence of Epstein-Barr viral RNA. Like their counterparts in the head and neck, lymphoepithelial-like carcinomas occur almost exclusively in East Asians, and most series are of Chinese patients. The first case of a pulmonary lymphoepithelioma-like carcinoma was reported in 1987 in a nonsmoker of Asian descent.[56] The first series followed in 1995, reporting patients from Hong Kong, most of whom were nonsmokers.[57] In southern China, 0.9% of lung cancers show lymphoepithelioma-like histologic features, over 90% of which are demonstrated to harbor evidence of EBV.[58] In this same series, none of the carcinomas without typical histologic features demonstrated the presence of EBV RNA, indicating a high specificity of histologic findings for the diagnosis.[58]

Gross Findings

Grossly, lymphoepithelial-like carcinomas are usually peripheral nodules, although diffuse pneumonitic-like spread may rarely occur.[57] Tumors may be of any size, reportedly from 1.2 to 11.0 cm.[59]

Histologic Findings, Including Immunohistochemistry and In Situ Hybridization

Histologically, lymphoepithelial-like carcinoma is characterized by anastomosing islands and sheets, composed of syncytial epithelioid

cells with vesicular nuclei and prominent nucleoli[57] (Fig. 78.16). Rarely, there may be granulomatous reaction[58] or amyloid stroma.[59] Immunohistochemically, tumors express squamous markers, including CK 5/6, p40, and p63.[60]

The neoplastic cells contain Epstein-Barr virus (EBV) as demonstrated by in situ hybridization for EBV-encoded small nuclear RNAs (EBER).[57] By World Health Organization criteria, the detection of EBV is considered a requirement for diagnosis. Immunohistochemical detection of EBV latent membrane protein-1 and viral capsid antigen is variable, generally fewer than half.[58,59]

Genetics

Molecular alterations are found in a minority of tumors. *EGFR* has been found to be exclusively wild type,[61] although in a different report, one-fifth of tumors harbored EGFR mutations, the majority in exon 21.[60] Up to 7% of tumors have been found to have mutations in the p53 gene.

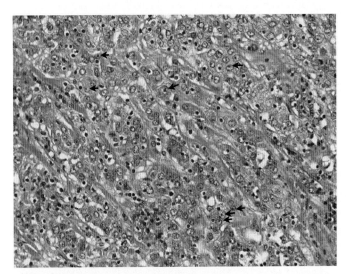

FIGURE 78.16 ▲ Lymphoepithelial-like carcinoma. Tumor cells lack borders and nuclei are large and vesicular (*arrows*). There is a diffuse lymphocytic infiltrate.

Prognosis

The prognosis of lymphoepithelial-like carcinoma is variable, and 1/3 of patients have metastatic disease at the time of diagnosis.[57] In general, the prognosis is better than that of other poorly differentiated lung carcinomas, with a 2-year and 5-year overall survival rate of 88% and 62%, respectively.[61] The survival rate compared to other lung carcinomas is better in stages II, III, and IV.[62]

REFERENCES

1. Molina JR, Yang P, Cassivi SD, et al. Non-small cell lung cancer: epidemiology, risk factors, treatment, and survivorship. *Mayo Clin Proc.* 2008;83:584–594.
2. Siegel R, Ma J, Zou Z, et al. Cancer statistics, 2014. *CA Cancer J Clin.* 2014;64:9–29.
3. Brcic L, Sherer CK, Shuai Y, et al. Morphologic and clinicopathologic features of lung squamous cell carcinomas expressing Sox2. *Am J Clin Pathol.* 2012;138:712–718.
4. Park SK, Cho LY, Yang JJ, et al. Lung cancer risk and cigarette smoking, lung tuberculosis according to histologic type and gender in a population based case-control study. *Lung Cancer.* 2010;68:20–26.
5. Pesch B, Kendzia B, Gustavsson P, et al. Cigarette smoking and lung cancer—relative risk estimates for the major histological types from a pooled analysis of case-control studies. *Int J Cancer.* 2012;131:1210–1219.
6. Yanagawa N, Wang A, Kohler D, et al. Human papilloma virus genome is rare in North American non-small cell lung carcinoma patients. *Lung Cancer.* 2013;79:215–220.
7. van Boerdonk RA, Daniels JM, Bloemena E, et al. High-risk human papillomavirus-positive lung cancer: molecular evidence for a pattern of pulmonary metastasis. *J Thorac Oncol.* 2013;8:711–718.
8. Funai K, Yokose T, Ishii G, et al. Clinicopathologic characteristics of peripheral squamous cell carcinoma of the lung. *Am J Surg Pathol.* 2003;27:978–984.
9. Koenigkam Santos M, Muley T, Warth A, et al. Morphological computed tomography features of surgically resectable pulmonary squamous cell carcinomas: impact on prognosis and comparison with adenocarcinomas. *Eur J Radiol.* 2014;83:1275–1281.
10. Saijo T, Ishii G, Nagai K, et al. Differences in clinicopathological and biological features between central-type and peripheral-type squamous cell carcinoma of the lung. *Lung Cancer.* 2006;52:37–45.
11. Mukhopadhyay S, Katzenstein AL. Subclassification of non-small cell lung carcinomas lacking morphologic differentiation on biopsy specimens: utility of an immunohistochemical panel containing TTF-1, napsin A, p63, and CK5/6. *Am J Surg Pathol.* 2011;35:15–25.
12. Pelosi G, Rossi G, Bianchi F, et al. Immunohistochemistry by means of widely agreed-upon markers (cytokeratins 5/6 and 7, p63, thyroid transcription factor-1, and vimentin) on small biopsies of non-small cell lung cancer effectively parallels the corresponding profiling and eventual diagnoses on surgical specimens. *J Thorac Oncol.* 2011;6:1039–1049.
13. Rekhtman N, Ang DC, Sima CS, et al. Immunohistochemical algorithm for differentiation of lung adenocarcinoma and squamous cell carcinoma based on large series of whole-tissue sections with validation in small specimens. *Mod Pathol.* 2011;24:1348–1359.
14. Bishop JA, Ogawa T, Chang X, et al. HPV analysis in distinguishing second primary tumors from lung metastases in patients with head and neck squamous cell carcinoma. *Am J Surg Pathol.* 2012;36:142–148.
15. Nonaka D. A study of DeltaNp63 expression in lung non-small cell carcinomas. *Am J Surg Pathol.* 2012;36:895–899.
16. Ao MH, Zhang H, Sakowski L, et al. The utility of a novel triple marker (combination of TTF1, napsin A, and p40) in the subclassification of non-small cell lung cancer. *Hum Pathol.* 2014;45:926–934.
17. Fan X, Yu K, Wu J, et al. Correlation between squamous cell carcinoma of the lung and human papillomavirus infection and the relationship to expression of p53 and p16. *Tumour Biol.* 2015;36:3043–3049.
18. Gatta LB, Balzarini P, Tironi A, et al. Human papillomavirus DNA and p16 gene in squamous cell lung carcinoma. *Anticancer Res.* 2012;32:3085–3089.
19. Whithaus K, Fukuoka J, Prihoda TJ, et al. Evaluation of napsin A, cytokeratin 5/6, p63, and thyroid transcription factor 1 in adenocarcinoma versus squamous cell carcinoma of the lung. *Arch Pathol Lab Med.* 2012;136:155–162.
20. Dulmet-Brender E, Jaubert F, Huchon G. Exophytic endobronchial epidermoid carcinoma. *Cancer.* 1986;57:1358–1364.
21. Edge SB, Compton CC. The American Joint Committee on Cancer: the 7th edition of the AJCC cancer staging manual and the future of TNM. *Ann Surg Oncol.* 2010;17:1471–1474.
22. Yousem SA. Peripheral squamous cell carcinoma of lung: patterns of growth with particular focus on airspace filling. *Hum Pathol.* 2009;40:861–867.
23. Nakanishi K, Kawai T, Suzuki M, et al. Bronchogenic squamous cell carcinomas with invasion along alveolar walls. *Histopathology.* 1996;29:363–368.
24. Brambilla C, Laffaire J, Lantuejoul S, et al. Lung squamous cell carcinomas with basaloid histology represent a specific molecular entity. *Clin Cancer Res.* 2014;20:5777–5786.
25. Nagamoto N, Saito Y, Imai T, et al. Roentgenographically occult bronchogenic squamous cell carcinoma: location in the bronchi, depth of invasion and length of axial involvement of the bronchus. *Tohoku J Exp Med.* 1986;148:241–256.
26. Butnor KJ, Burchette JL. p40 (DeltaNp63) and keratin 34betaE12 provide greater diagnostic accuracy than p63 in the evaluation of small cell lung carcinoma in small biopsy samples. *Hum Pathol.* 2013;44:1479–1486.
27. Cancer Genome Atlas Research N. Comprehensive genomic characterization of squamous cell lung cancers. *Nature.* 2012;489:519–525.
28. Bass AJ, Watanabe H, Mermel CH, et al. SOX2 is an amplified lineage-survival oncogene in lung and esophageal squamous cell carcinomas. *Nat Genet.* 2009;41:1238–1242.
29. McDermott U, Ames RY, Iafrate AJ, et al. Ligand-dependent platelet-derived growth factor receptor (PDGFR)-alpha activation sensitizes rare lung cancer and sarcoma cells to PDGFR kinase inhibitors. *Cancer Res.* 2009;69:3937–3946.
30. Geurts TW, Nederlof PM, van den Brekel MW, et al. Pulmonary squamous cell carcinoma following head and neck squamous cell carcinoma: metastasis or second primary? *Clin Cancer Res.* 2005;11:6608–6614.
31. Weichert W, Schewe C, Denkert C, et al. Molecular HPV typing as a diagnostic tool to discriminate primary from metastatic squamous cell carcinoma of the lung. *Am J Surg Pathol.* 2009;33:513–520.
32. Koshiol J, Rotunno M, Gillison ML, et al. Assessment of human papillomavirus in lung tumor tissue. *J Natl Cancer Inst.* 2011;103:501–507.
33. Srinivasan M, Taioli E, Ragin CC. Human papillomavirus type 16 and 18 in primary lung cancers—a meta-analysis. *Carcinogenesis.* 2009;30:1722–1728.
34. Geurts TW, van Velthuysen ML, Broekman F, et al. Differential diagnosis of pulmonary carcinoma following head and neck cancer by genetic analysis. *Clin Cancer Res.* 2009;15:980–985.
35. van der Sijp JR, van Meerbeeck JP, Maat AP, et al. Determination of the molecular relationship between multiple tumors within one patient is of clinical importance. *J Clin Oncol.* 2002;20:1105–1114.
36. Leong PP, Rezai B, Koch WM, et al. Distinguishing second primary tumors from lung metastases in patients with head and neck squamous cell carcinoma. *J Natl Cancer Inst.* 1998;90:972–977.
37. Piperdi B, Merla A, Perez-Soler R. Targeting angiogenesis in squamous non-small cell lung cancer. *Drugs.* 2014;74:403–413.
38. Ishizumi T, McWilliams A, MacAulay C, et al. Natural history of bronchial preinvasive lesions. *Cancer Metastasis Rev.* 2010;29:5–14.
39. McCaughan F, Pole JC, Bankier AT, et al. Progressive 3q amplification consistently targets SOX2 in preinvasive squamous lung cancer. *Am J Respir Crit Care Med.* 2010;182:83–91.
40. Lam S, leRiche JC, Zheng Y, et al. Sex-related differences in bronchial epithelial changes associated with tobacco smoking. *J Natl Cancer Inst.* 1999;91:691–696.
41. Bota S, Auliac JB, Paris C, et al. Follow-up of bronchial precancerous lesions and carcinoma in situ using fluorescence endoscopy. *Am J Respir Crit Care Med.* 2001;164:1688–1693.
42. Daniels JM, Sutedja TG. Detection and minimally invasive treatment of early squamous lung cancer. *Ther Adv Med Oncol.* 2013;5:235–248.
43. Herth FJ, Eberhardt R, Anantham D, et al. Narrow-band imaging bronchoscopy increases the specificity of bronchoscopic early lung cancer detection. *J Thorac Oncol.* 2009;4:1060–1065.
44. Shibuya K, Nakajima T, Fujiwara T, et al. Narrow band imaging with high-resolution bronchovideoscopy: a new approach for visualizing angiogenesis in squamous cell carcinoma of the lung. *Lung Cancer.* 2010;69:194–202.
45. Hirsch FR, Prindiville SA, Miller YE, et al. Fluorescence versus white-light bronchoscopy for detection of preneoplastic lesions: a randomized study. *J Natl Cancer Inst.* 2001;93:1385–1391.
46. Moro-Sibilot D, Jeanmart M, Lantuejoul S, et al. Cigarette smoking, pre-

invasive bronchial lesions, and autofluorescence bronchoscopy. *Chest.* 2002;122:1902–1908.

47. Travis WD. Pathology of lung cancer. *Clin Chest Med.* 2011;32:669–692.
48. Jeremy George P, Banerjee AK, Read CA, et al. Surveillance for the detection of early lung cancer in patients with bronchial dysplasia. *Thorax.* 2007;62:43–50.
49. Breuer RH, Pasic A, Smit EF, et al. The natural course of preneoplastic lesions in bronchial epithelium. *Clin Cancer Res.* 2005;11:537–543.
50. Nicholson AG, Perry LJ, Cury PM, et al. Reproducibility of the WHO/IASLC grading system for pre-invasive squamous lesions of the bronchus: a study of inter-observer and intra-observer variation. *Histopathology.* 2001;38:202–208.
51. Kato H, Okunaka T, Shimatani H. Photodynamic therapy for early stage bronchogenic carcinoma. *J Clin Laser Med Surg.* 1996;14:235–238.
52. Merrick DT, Kittelson J, Winterhalder R, et al. Analysis of c-ErbB1/epidermal growth factor receptor and c-ErbB2/HER-2 expression in bronchial dysplasia: evaluation of potential targets for chemoprevention of lung cancer. *Clin Cancer Res.* 2006;12:2281–2288.
53. Sousa V, Espirito Santo J, Silva M, et al. EGFR/erB-1, HER2/erB-2, CK7, LP34, Ki67 and P53 expression in preneoplastic lesions of bronchial epithelium: an immunohistochemical and genetic study. *Virchows Arch.* 2011;458:571–581.
54. Wistuba, II, Lam S, Behrens C, et al. Molecular damage in the bronchial epithelium of current and former smokers. *J Natl Cancer Inst.* 1997;89:1366–1373.
55. Brambilla E, Moro D, Veale D, et al. Basal cell (basaloid) carcinoma of the lung: a new morphologic and phenotypic entity with separate prognostic significance. *Hum Pathol.* 1992;23:993–1003.
56. Begin LR, Eskandari J, Joncas J, et al. Epstein-Barr virus related lymphoepithelioma-like carcinoma of lung. *J Surg Oncol.* 1987;36:280–283.
57. Chan JK, Hui PK, Tsang WY, et al. Primary lymphoepithelioma-like carcinoma of the lung. A clinicopathologic study of 11 cases. *Cancer.* 1995;76:413–422.
58. Han AJ, Xiong M, Zong YS. Association of Epstein-Barr virus with lymphoepithelioma-like carcinoma of the lung in southern China. *Am J Clin Pathol.* 2000;114:220–226.
59. Chang YL, Wu CT, Shih JY, et al. New aspects in clinicopathologic and oncogene studies of 23 pulmonary lymphoepithelioma-like carcinomas. *Am J Surg Pathol.* 2002;26:715–723.
60. Chang YL, Wu CT, Shih JY, et al. Unique p53 and epidermal growth factor receptor gene mutation status in 46 pulmonary lymphoepithelioma-like carcinomas. *Cancer Sci.* 2011;102:282–287.
61. Liang Y, Wang L, Zhu Y, et al. Primary pulmonary lymphoepithelioma-like carcinoma: fifty-two patients with long-term follow-up. *Cancer.* 2012;118:4748–4758.
62. Han AJ, Xiong M, Gu YY, et al. Lymphoepithelioma-like carcinoma of the lung with a better prognosis. A clinicopathologic study of 32 cases. *Am J Clin Pathol.* 2001;115:841–850.

79 Small Cell Carcinoma

Allen P. Burke, M.D.

Definition and Terminology

Small cell lung carcinoma (SCLC) is a high-grade, highly proliferative carcinoma with characteristic histologic features and frequent endocrine differentiation. It is most common in the lung, but occurs in virtually every organ that may develop epithelial malignancy. The term "small cell carcinoma" is the preferred term for carcinomas with areas of classic morphology. Although 5% to 7% of cases may be difficult to separate from non–small cell carcinoma on routine microscopy, the use of "intermediate" or "gray-zone" categories has been discouraged.[1] The term "combined small cell carcinoma" is used if there are areas of other carcinoma types.

Epidemiology

The proportion of lung cancers that are small cell lung carcinomas has declined over the past several decades, from about 20% in the late 1990s to 15% of primary lung cancers today; this is attributed to the concurrent decrease in smoking. Small cell carcinoma is more highly associated with smoking than are adenocarcinomas, as 98% of small cell cancer patients are smokers.[2] The relative risk for a man smoking >30 cigarettes daily is 111.3 times that of a nonsmoker compared to 103.5 for squamous carcinoma and 21.9 for adenocarcinoma.[3] The decrease in rate of small cell carcinoma has been proportionately less in women and nonwhites.[4,5]

There is no gender bias for small cell carcinoma. A high proportion of patients (60%) present with advanced disease (stage IV).[4]

Staging

Staging of small cell carcinoma is similar to that of other lung carcinomas.[6] Because of the high proportion of advanced stages, a simplified system of limited (combined stages I to III) and extensive (stage IV) is sometimes used.[4]

Radiologic Findings

Small cell lung cancers are central lesions, most presenting with hilar or mediastinal lymph node metastases. Only 5% occur as a peripheral solitary coin lesion.[7] The mass is often lobulated and is less frequently endobronchial than squamous carcinomas and only rarely cavitary. Compared to other primary lung cancers, invasion of hilar vessels and of the superior vena cava is relatively common.

Tissue Sampling

Almost all patients with small cell carcinoma are diagnosed on cytologic preparations, which include smears and cell blocks, on which immunohistochemical preparations can be done. Only 3.5% of cancer resections of the lung reveal pure small cell carcinoma.[8] Because small cell carcinomas are usually central lesions with positive lymph node disease, diagnostic procedures include, in addition to endoscopic or transbronchial biopsy, needle aspiration cytology from either pulmonary endoscopy (endobronchial ultrasound [EBUS] guided) or esophageal endoscopy (endoscopic ultrasound [EUS] guided). In addition to establishing a diagnosis, lymph node biopsy by these techniques also confirms clinical staging by CT and/or PET/CT scans.

Gross Findings

Small cell carcinoma typically has a tan, homogeneous, soft to rubbery cut surface, often with necrotic areas. Cavitation and hemorrhage are not generally present.

Microscopic Findings

Small cell carcinoma is defined by histologic features present on hematoxylin–eosin stains (Table 79.1). Although immunohistochemical stains are often very helpful, their results can be misleading, because

TABLE 79.1   Cytologic Features Distinguishing Small Cell from Large Cell Neuroendocrine Carcinoma

Feature	Small Cell Carcinoma	Large Cell Neuroendocrine Carcinoma
Cell size	<24 microns	≥25 microns
Nuclear/ cytoplasmic ratio	High	Variable, usually intermediate
Nucleoli	Faint, inconspicuous	Present
Chromatin	Granular, without significant clearing	Variable, with areas of clearing frequent
Nuclear molding	Frequent	Inconspicuous
Cell shape	Small round, fusiform, oval	Polygonal

some tumors fail to express any markers other than pan-cytokeratin, and expression is often patchy. On routine stains, cells are small, generally under 25 microns in diameter, round, oval, or slightly spindled, with finely granular nuclear chromatin, scant cytoplasm, and inconspicuous nucleoli (Figs. 79.1 to 79.3). There is no clear definition of "inconspicuous," although plainly eosinophilic nucleoli should be absent or only occasional. Typically, there is nuclear molding (Figs. 79.4 and 79.5). Necrosis is common, and mitotic activity is high, with at least one per high-powered (40×) field (Figs. 79.6 and 79.7). Mitotic figures may be difficult to identify on cytologic samples, however, and the presence of apoptotic debris is a reasonable substitute, unless Ki 67 staining is performed, which should show a proliferative index of at least 50%. Multinucleated cells with minimal cytoplasm may be interspersed among otherwise typical small cell carcinoma (Fig. 79.8). Growth patterns of neuroendocrine differentiation including rosettes, peripheral palisading, organoid nesting, and trabeculae may occur in small cell carcinoma (Fig. 79.9) and do not exclude the diagnosis provided that cytologic features typical of small cell carcinoma are present. If there are prominent nucleoli and larger cells, then these features define large cell neuroendocrine carcinoma. When present in at least 5% to 10% of cells, then the diagnosis is combined small cell and large cell neuroendocrine carcinoma.

Crush artifact, especially on cytologic samples, is very common and often necessitates immunohistochemical staining for further characterization. Encrustation of vessel walls by basophilic degenerated nuclear debris from necrotic tumor cells may be seen and is termed the "Azzopardi effect."[1]

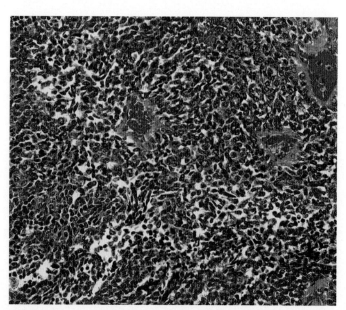

FIGURE 79.2 ▲ Small cell carcinoma. There is typical small fusiform "oat cell" morphology in this case, with barely discernable cytoplasm and dispersed nuclei without nucleoli.

Neuroendocrine architectural patterns are especially frequent in resected specimens. Other histologic findings in wedge biopsies or lobectomies that differ from small samples include relatively infrequent crush artifact, slightly larger cell size, occasional prominent nucleoli, and vesicular nuclear chromatin.[9]

Immunohistochemical Stains

Endocrine Markers

In contrast to large cell neuroendocrine carcinomas, there is often spotty staining for endocrine markers in small cell carcinoma, with 10% expression generally considered positive.[10] Because of the focal nature of staining, there is a wide range in the reported rate of positivity for endocrine markers (Table 79.2).

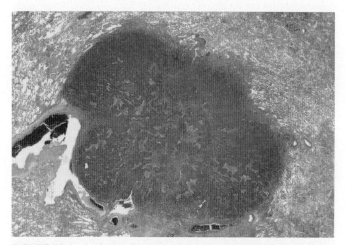

FIGURE 79.1 ▲ Small cell carcinoma. Low magnification demonstrating relatively circumscribed homogeneous cellular tumor.

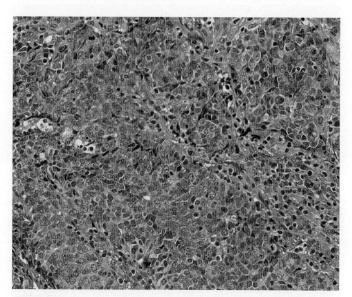

FIGURE 79.3 ▲ Small cell carcinoma. In this tumor, there are slightly larger cells with some cytoplasm, but dispersed nuclear chromatin and inconspicuous nucleoli are typical.

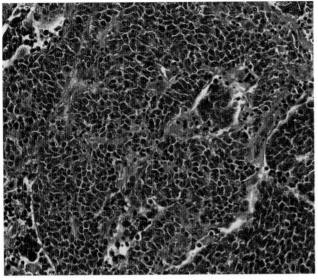

FIGURE 79.4 ▲ Small cell carcinoma. In this example, nuclear molding is prominent, and there is a slightly organoid growth pattern.

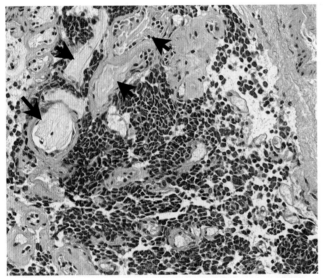

FIGURE 79.5 ▲ Small cell carcinoma. This tumor has the typical small, ovoid cellular structure and invades among mucous glands (*arrows*) in the bronchial wall.

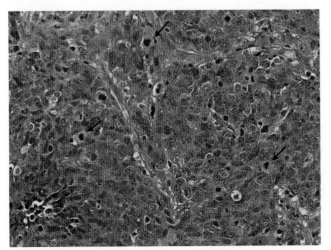

FIGURE 79.6 ▲ Small cell carcinoma. Small cell carcinoma typically has several mitotic figures (*arrows*) per high-powered 40× field, but these may be difficult to identify on cytology specimens or needle biopsies.

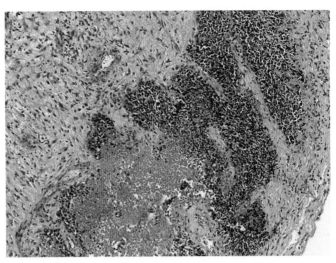

FIGURE 79.7 ▲ Small cell carcinoma. Necrosis is typical in small cell carcinoma, in which cell outlines are still visible.

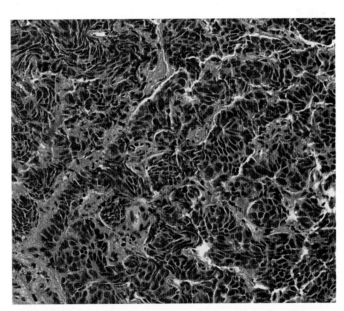

FIGURE 79.8 ▲ Small cell carcinoma. Endocrine growth patterns are particularly common in resected specimens, but may also be seen in biopsies, such as this one, which shows trabecular growth with ribbons.

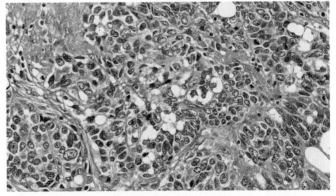

FIGURE 79.9 ▲ Small cell carcinoma. Crush artifact renders diagnosis difficult and may mimic lymphoid lesions, low-grade endocrine tumors, and other high-grade carcinomas. This area is a different one sampled from the tumor shown in Figure 79.8, where there was no crush artifact.

TABLE 79.2 Immunohistochemical Findings in Pulmonary Small Cell Carcinoma

Antibody	Positivity Rates
Chromogranin A	45%–60%, often patchy
Synaptophysin	60%–90%
Neural cell adhesion molecule (CD56)	60%–90%
Positive for any endocrine marker	90%–95%
TTF-1	70%–95%, may be patchy
p63	14%–24%
p40	1%–2%
Cytokeratin 5/6	1%–2%
34βE12 (K903)	10%
Cytokeratin 7	50%
Cytokeratin 20	<10%
Ki 67	100% > 50% proliferative index (most >70%)
CD117	75%

Chromogranin A is considered the most specific neuroendocrine marker. It is present within neuroendocrine granules, imparting a granular cytoplasmic staining (Fig. 79.10). Rates of positivity in small cell carcinomas of the lung vary from 45% to 60% with higher rates in resected specimens.[10,11] The most common neuropeptide found in the granules is bombesin, present in 45% of tumors.[11] *Synaptophysin* and *CD56 (neural cell adhesion molecule)* show membranous cytoplasmic positivity and are detected in approximately two-thirds of resected tumors (Fig. 79.10).[10] However, in other studies of biopsy material, CD56 has been reported to be present in over 90% of tumors.[12–14] Leu-7 (CD57), an endocrine marker currently not in widespread use, is positive in about one-third of tumors.[11] On small biopsies, up to two-thirds of tumors are negative for both chromogranin and synaptophysin, and in 5% to 10% of tumors, all three markers are negative.[10,12–14] Despite the frequency with which small cell carcinoma shows only focal or absent staining, it is important to remember that small cell carcinomas can stain diffusely and strongly with all three neuroendocrine markers.[1]

Squamous Markers and Cytokeratins

Immunohistochemical localization for p63 is found in 14% to 24% of small cell carcinoma of the lung.[10,15] In contrast, only 1% to 2% of small cell carcinomas express p40, cytokeratin 5/6, or desmocollin.[15,16] About 10% express 34βE12 or K903.[10,17] Approximately 50% of tumors stain with cytokeratin 7, and fewer than 10% with cytokeratin 20, occasionally in a dot-like pattern. It is extremely unusual for small cell carcinoma to lack expression of all cytokeratins.[1]

Adenocarcinoma Markers

Expression of TTF-1 is found in 70% to 95% of small cell lung cancers (Fig. 79.11), but staining can be patchy.[1,18] There is a small increase in the rate of positivity with clone SPT24 as compared to clone 8G7G3/1.[19] Napsin-A has been negative in tumors tested.[16]

Virtually all small cell carcinomas express Ber-EP4.[11]

Ki 67 and CD117

SCLC show a high proliferation rate by Ki 67 (Fig. 79.12), averaging 80%; in one series, all tumors had a proliferative index of >70%.[10] CD117 (c-kit) is found in about 75% of SCLCs[20,21] but is not specific and lacks diagnostic usefulness.

Molecular Findings

Molecular alterations have not yet resulted in targeted therapy for small cell carcinoma, unlike for adenocarcinoma of the lung. Increased insulin-like growth factor 1 receptor protein expression and gene copy number occurs in small cell cancers, but monoclonal therapy has not yet shown efficacy.[22]

Small cell carcinoma, similar to large cell neuroendocrine carcinoma, has a high frequency of loss of heterozygosity (LOH) for 3p, RB, 5q21, 9p, and p53[1] as well as alterations in the P16INK4/cyclin D1/Rb pathway. Correspondingly, there is frequently loss of expression of retinoblastoma protein (Rb).[23,24] SOX2 is a frequently amplified gene in small cell lung cancer.[25]

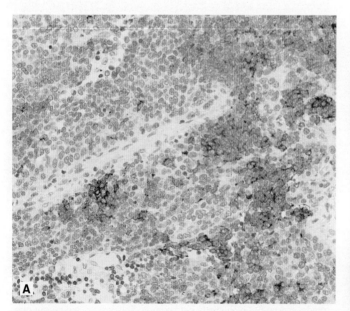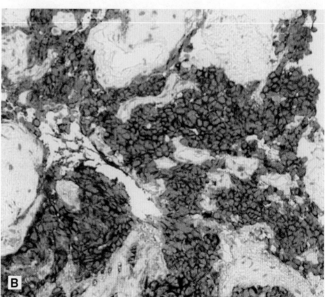

FIGURE 79.10 ▲ Small cell carcinoma, endocrine markers. **A.** Chromogranin typically shows granular cytoplasmic staining that is often focal or patchy. **B.** Synaptophysin staining is cytoplasmic and is more likely diffuse as in this case, but may also be patchy or even negative. In this case, there was extensive crush artifact, and the immunohistochemical stain documented tumor cells and cytoplasmic borders and endocrine differentiation.

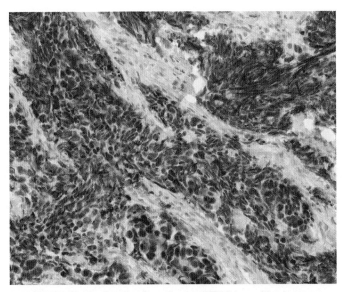

FIGURE 79.11 ▲ Small cell carcinoma. TTF-1 is positive in more than 90% of cases and in this example was strong and diffuse.

Small Cell Carcinoma in Nonsmokers and Transformed Small Cell Carcinoma

Only 3% of patients with SCLCs are never-smokers.[26] These are a heterogeneous group of tumors. Approximately one-fifth occur as transformation to small cell carcinoma after acquired resistance to epidermal growth factor receptor tyrosine kinase inhibitors. The remainder are de novo small cell cancers, which may harbor *EGFR*, *p53*, *RB1*, and other mutations.[2]

Combined Small Cell Carcinoma

"Combined small cell carcinoma" denotes an additional component that consists of any of the histologic types of non–small cell carcinoma,

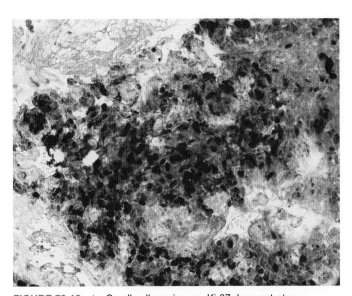

FIGURE 79.12 ▲ Small cell carcinoma. Ki 67 demonstrates increased proliferative index, with virtual 100% nuclear staining, as in this case, not unusual. This area also showed extensive crush artifact, in which mitotic figures could not be identified, and the Ki 67 was very helpful in ascertaining the diagnosis. Most small cell carcinomas show at least 70% proliferation index.

namely, adenocarcinoma, squamous cell carcinoma, large cell carcinoma (not otherwise specified), large cell neuroendocrine carcinoma, or pleomorphic carcinoma. In general, any squamous or glandular component warrants the term "combined," and at least 5%[27] or 10%[9] of large cell neuroendocrine component has been suggested as a requirement for the term. In surgical resections, over 25% of small cell carcinomas show another component, most frequently large cell carcinoma.[9] In series including biopsies, the rate is lower, at around 5%.[27] The overall rate of combined small cell carcinoma in surgically resected lung carcinomas of all types is 1%.[8] The presence of adenocarcinoma and squamous carcinoma in combined tumors generally indicates features that can be diagnosed on light microscopy, namely, gland formation and keratinization, respectively. Occasionally, the squamous component is nonkeratinizing, but there is a sharp demarcation between areas expressing endocrine markers and those expressing squamous markers, without overlap.

The distinction between large cell and large cell neuroendocrine carcinoma as a combined component of small cell carcinoma is difficult, and not possible on biopsies. For this reason, the diagnosis of small cell carcinoma should be made in small tissue samples if there is a significant portion of tumor with small cell morphology, also if there are areas of both small cell and large cell morphology without adenocarcinoma or squamous cell carcinoma. In larger samples, the distinction between large cell (not otherwise specified) and large cell neuroendocrine carcinoma is based on endocrine growth patterns and immunohistochemical expression of endocrine marker(s). The determination of large cell is very open to interpretation, however, as tumor cells appear larger because they are better fixed.[1] In the largest series of combined tumors, it was difficult to determine expression of endocrine markers in the large cell component of mixed small cell carcinoma.[9] In this series, neuroendocrine markers were expressed in both components in the majority of combined small and large cell carcinomas, based on a lack of both histologic and immunohistochemical evidences for neuroendocrine differentiation in the large cell component.[9] The distinction between palisading (indicative of neuroendocrine growth pattern) and basaloid squamous carcinoma on routine microscopy can be arbitrary, and requires immunohistochemical confirmation.

Differential Diagnosis

Large Cell Neuroendocrine Carcinoma

The distinction between small cell carcinoma and large cell neuroendocrine carcinoma is based on histologic features. Favoring small cell carcinoma are smaller cell size (smaller than 3× the diameter of a lymphocyte), high nuclear/cytoplasmic ratio, granular chromatin with absent nucleoli (or "faint," "inconspicuous," or "not prominent") nuclear molding, fusiform shape, and nuclear smearing artifact. Favoring large-cell neuroendocrine carcinoma are a polygonal cell shape, prominent nucleoli, and lower nuclear/cytoplasmic ratio.

Although immunohistochemistry is generally not helpful in the distinction between these two tumors, a recent study showed that CDX2 and VIL1 were more likely expressed in large cell neuroendocrine carcinoma and BAI3 in small cell carcinoma.[28]

Lymphoma

In biopsy samples, it may be difficult to distinguish lymphoma from small cell carcinoma. Staining for pancytokeratin such as AE1/AE3 helps to demonstrate that the tumor is a carcinoma rather than a lymphoid lesion, and CD20 staining will be present in the majority of lymphomas that occur in the mediastinum.

Basaloid and Nonkeratinizing Squamous Carcinoma

The distinction between basaloid nonkeratinizing squamous carcinoma and the palisading of neuroendocrine carcinoma can be very difficult.[10] Neuroendocrine (diffuse CD56 or synaptophysin positivity)

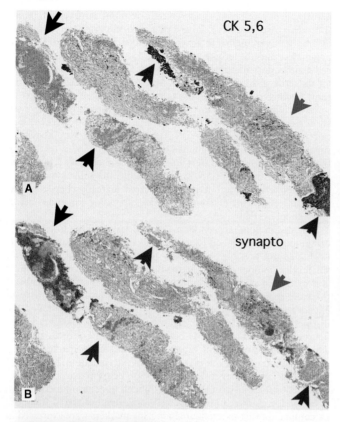

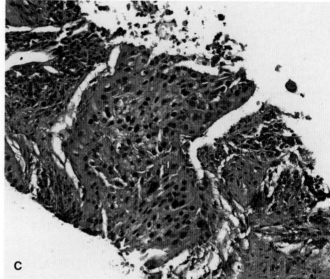

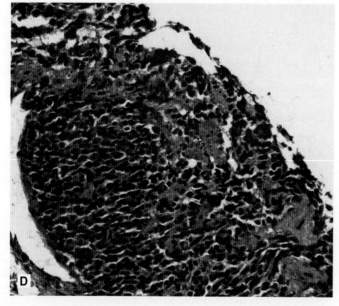

FIGURE 79.13 ▲ Combined small cell carcinoma and squamous carcinoma. **A.** Low magnification of core biopsies stained with cytokeratin 5/6 shows areas of strong staining (*red arrows*) corresponding to squamous carcinoma. Other foci (*black arrows*) represent small cell carcinoma, without staining. Other areas with spotty staining were a mixture of small cell and squamous carcinoma (*blue arrows*). **B.** Corresponding neural cell adhesion molecule (CD56) staining shows diffuse positivity in the small cell regions (*black arrows*), no staining in the squamous areas (*red arrows*), and spotty staining in the more mixed areas (*blue arrows*). **C.** A higher magnification of the squamous cell carcinoma area illustrated in **(A)** and **(B)**. **D.** A higher magnification of the small cell carcinoma area, with extensive crush artifact.

and squamous markers (p40 or cytokeratin 5/6) are very helpful to make this differential diagnosis, although mixed tumors do occur (Figs. 79.13 and 79.14). If all markers are negative, then the diagnosis of neuroendocrine carcinoma (not otherwise specified) is warranted. The light microscopic features favoring small cell carcinoma include streaming, rosettes, and nesting, whereas desmoplasia favors basaloid squamous carcinoma.

Carcinoid Tumor: Typical and Atypical

Overdiagnosis of carcinoid tumor as small cell carcinoma in small biopsies occurs relatively frequently, because of crush artifact and

difficulty in identifying mitotic figures. Evaluation of tumor cell proliferation by Ki 67 (MIB1)-labeling index demonstrates >70% of nuclear staining in small cell carcinomas,[29,30] whereas in atypical and typical carcinoid tumors, the expression is always <50%.[31]

Metastatic Small Cell Carcinoma

Metastatic small cell carcinoma from nonpulmonary sites may not be possible to distinguish from those that are primary in the lung, because TTF-1 expression frequently occurs in nonpulmonary small cell cancers. In general, however, Merkel cell carcinoma arising in the skin is usually negative for TTF-1 and frequently expresses cytokeratin 20 in a dot-like pattern.[18]

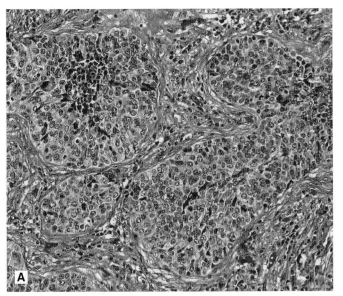
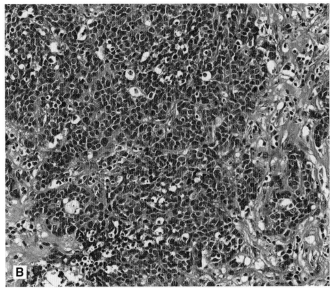

FIGURE 79.14 ▲ Small cell carcinoma with areas of basaloid carcinoma. **A.** This area resembles basaloid squamous carcinoma, with relatively abundant cytoplasm, and scattered nucleoli. Immunohistochemical stains were positive in this area for p63 and high molecular weight cytokeratin with absent endocrine staining (not shown). **B.** Another area showing typical small cell carcinoma, which expressed diffusely CD56 (not shown) but were negative for squamous and other endocrine markers.

Prognosis and Treatment

The treatment of small cell carcinoma consists primarily of chemo- and radiation therapy, with combination therapy more often used in earlier stage disease. Median survival is only about 1 year, and 5-year survival is <5%.[2,4,27] Those rare patients with stage 1 disease have a much better survival, around 40% at 5 years, which is far lower than other carcinoma types at the same stage.[10] Unfortunately, there has been little improvement in survival over the last two decades.[4] Screening with computed tomography scans may identify more early-stage cases and decrease the number of deaths from the disease.[7]

There may be relatively good survival in patients with small cell carcinomas with low neuroendocrine marker expression.[10]

Combined small cell carcinomas have a somewhat better prognosis than does typical small cell carcinoma, but 5-year survival is rare even for this subgroup.[8]

REFERENCES

1. Travis WD. Update on small cell carcinoma and its differentiation from squamous cell carcinoma and other non-small cell carcinomas. *Mod Pathol.* 2012;25(suppl 1):S18–S30.
2. Varghese AM, Zakowski MF, Yu HA, et al. Small-cell lung cancers in patients who never smoked cigarettes. *J Thorac Oncol.* 2014;9:892–896.
3. Pesch B, Kendzia B, Gustavsson P, et al. Cigarette smoking and lung cancer—relative risk estimates for the major histological types from a pooled analysis of case-control studies. *Int J Cancer.* 2012;131:1210–1219.
4. Gaspar LE, McNamara EJ, Gay EG, et al. Small-cell lung cancer: prognostic factors and changing treatment over 15 years. *Clin Lung Cancer.* 2012;13:115–122.
5. Riaz SP, Luchtenborg M, Coupland VH, et al. Trends in incidence of small cell lung cancer and all lung cancer. *Lung Cancer.* 2012;75:280–284.
6. Shepherd FA, Crowley J, Van Houtte P, et al. The International Association for the Study of Lung Cancer lung cancer staging project: proposals regarding the clinical staging of small cell lung cancer in the forthcoming (seventh) edition of the tumor, node, metastasis classification for lung cancer. *J Thorac Oncol.* 2007;2:1067–1077.
7. Austin JH, Yip R, D'Souza BM, et al. Small-cell carcinoma of the lung detected by CT screening: stage distribution and curability. *Lung Cancer.* 2012;76:339–343.
8. Hage R, Elbers JR, Brutel de la Riviere A, et al. Surgery for combined type small cell lung carcinoma. *Thorax.* 1998;53:450–453.
9. Nicholson SA, Beasley MB, Brambilla E, et al. Small cell lung carcinoma (SCLC): a clinicopathologic study of 100 cases with surgical specimens. *Am J Surg Pathol.* 2002;26:1184–1197.
10. Hamanaka W, Motoi N, Ishikawa S, et al. A subset of small cell lung cancer with low neuroendocrine expression and good prognosis: a comparison study of surgical and inoperable cases with biopsy. *Hum Pathol.* 2014;45:1045–1056.
11. Guinee DG, Jr, Fishback NF, Koss MN, et al. The spectrum of immunohistochemical staining of small-cell lung carcinoma in specimens from transbronchial and open-lung biopsies. *Am J Clin Pathol.* 1994;102:406–414.
12. Bobos M, Hytiroglou P, Kostopoulos I, et al. Immunohistochemical distinction between merkel cell carcinoma and small cell carcinoma of the lung. *Am J Dermatopathol.* 2006;28:99–104.
13. Hiroshima K, Iyoda A, Shida T, et al. Distinction of pulmonary large cell neuroendocrine carcinoma from small cell lung carcinoma: a morphological, immunohistochemical, and molecular analysis. *Mod Pathol.* 2006;19:1358–1368.
14. Kontogianni K, Nicholson AG, Butcher D, et al. CD56: a useful tool for the diagnosis of small cell lung carcinomas on biopsies with extensive crush artefact. *J Clin Pathol.* 2005;58:978–980.
15. Tatsumori T, Tsuta K, Masai K, et al. p40 is the best marker for diagnosing pulmonary squamous cell carcinoma: comparison with p63, cytokeratin 5/6, desmocollin-3, and sox2. *Appl Immunohistochem Mol Morphol.* 2014;22:377–382.
16. Masai K, Tsuta K, Kawago M, et al. Expression of squamous cell carcinoma markers and adenocarcinoma markers in primary pulmonary neuroendocrine carcinomas. *Appl Immunohistochem Mol Morphol.* 2013;21:292–297.
17. Sturm N, Rossi G, Lantuejoul S, et al. 34BetaE12 expression along the whole spectrum of neuroendocrine proliferations of the lung, from neuroendocrine cell hyperplasia to small cell carcinoma. *Histopathology.* 2003;42:156–166.
18. Kaufmann O, Dietel M. Expression of thyroid transcription factor-1 in pulmonary and extrapulmonary small cell carcinomas and other neuroendocrine carcinomas of various primary sites. *Histopathology.* 2000;36:415–420.
19. La Rosa S, Chiaravalli AM, Placidi C, et al. TTF1 expression in normal lung neuroendocrine cells and related tumors: immunohistochemical study comparing two different monoclonal antibodies. *Virchows Arch.* 2010;457:497–507.
20. Lopez-Martin A, Ballestin C, Garcia-Carbonero R, et al. Prognostic value of KIT expression in small cell lung cancer. *Lung Cancer.* 2007;56:405–413.

21. Pelosi G, Masullo M, Leon ME, et al. CD117 immunoreactivity in high-grade neuroendocrine tumors of the lung: a comparative study of 39 large-cell neuroendocrine carcinomas and 27 surgically resected small-cell carcinomas. *Virchows Arch.* 2004;445:449–455.
22. Martinez P, Sales Fidalgo PA, Felip E. Ganitumab for the treatment of small-cell lung cancer. *Expert Opin Investig Drugs.* 2014;23:1423–1432.
23. Beasley MB, Lantuejoul S, Abbondanzo S, et al. The P16/cyclin D1/Rb pathway in neuroendocrine tumors of the lung. *Hum Pathol.* 2003;34:136–142.
24. Dosaka-Akita H, Cagle PT, Hiroumi H, et al. Differential retinoblastoma and p16(INK4A) protein expression in neuroendocrine tumors of the lung. *Cancer.* 2000;88:550–556.
25. Rudin CM, Durinck S, Stawiski EW, et al. Comprehensive genomic analysis identifies SOX2 as a frequently amplified gene in small-cell lung cancer. *Nat Genet.* 2012;44:1111–1116.
26. Ou SH, Ziogas A, Zell JA. Prognostic factors for survival in extensive stage small cell lung cancer (ED-SCLC): the importance of smoking history, socioeconomic and marital statuses, and ethnicity. *J Thorac Oncol.* 2009;4:37–43.
27. Babakoohi S, Fu P, Yang M, et al. Combined SCLC clinical and pathologic characteristics. *Clin Lung Cancer.* 2013;14:113–119.
28. Bari MF, Brown H, Nicholson AG, et al. BAI3, CDX2 and VIL1: a panel of three antibodies to distinguish small cell from large cell neuroendocrine lung carcinomas. *Histopathology.* 2014;64:547–556.
29. Pelosi G, Rodriguez J, Viale G, et al. Typical and atypical pulmonary carcinoid tumor overdiagnosed as small-cell carcinoma on biopsy specimens: a major pitfall in the management of lung cancer patients. *Am J Surg Pathol.* 2005;29:179–187.
30. Lin O, Olgac S, Green I, et al. Immunohistochemical staining of cytologic smears with MIB-1 helps distinguish low-grade from high-grade neuroendocrine neoplasms. *Am J Clin Pathol.* 2003;120:209–216.
31. Liu SZ, Staats PN, Goicochea L, et al. Automated quantification of Ki-67 proliferative index of excised neuroendocrine tumors of the lung. *Diagn Pathol.* 2014;9:174.

80 Large Cell Neuroendocrine Carcinoma

Allen P. Burke, M.D., and Fabio R. Tavora, M.D., Ph.D.

General

"Large cell neuroendocrine carcinoma" was once considered a type of "large cell carcinoma," a term that is in decline, as subsets of that designation are currently being redefined by immunohistochemical profiles (see Chapter 82). For example, basaloid carcinoma, a previous subset of "large cell carcinoma," is now considered a form of squamous carcinoma, provided that squamous markers are confirmed immunohistochemically. The current term "large cell neuroendocrine carcinoma" encompasses tumors that demonstrate neuroendocrine histologic features and immunohistochemical confirmation of diffuse endocrine differentiation.

Clinical and Imaging Findings

The overall incidence of large cell neuroendocrine carcinoma is increasing, probably due to better awareness. It now accounts for 1% to 3% of lung cancers.[1,2]

In contrast to small cell carcinoma, large cell neuroendocrine carcinoma is usually (80% of cases) peripheral.[3] Dyspnea, chest pain, cough, hemoptysis, and symptoms related to postobstructive pneumonia are common symptoms.

Unlike small cell carcinoma, bulky enlargement of intrathoracic lymph nodes is uncommon.[4] Pleural effusions and cavitation are not common.[4] Central inhomogeneous enhancement occurs in larger tumors.[5]

Gross Findings

Large cell neuroendocrine carcinomas are typically 3 to 4 cm[6–9] and are most frequent in the periphery (84%) and the upper lobes (63%).[5,10] Similar to small cell carcinoma, cavitation is rare, and the cut surface is usually homogenous and soft, because of the relative infrequency of fibrosis typical of adenocarcinomas.

Microscopic Findings

By definition, large cell neuroendocrine carcinoma shows "neuroendocrine" morphology, in the form of nesting, trabecular growth, or rosettes (Figs. 80.1 to 80.4). These are features that may also be seen in small cell carcinoma. Solid nests frequently form cribriform patterns with peripheral palisading (Figs. 80.2 and 80.4). In contrast to small cell carcinoma, cells are generally large, with moderate or abundant and, in areas, prominent nucleoli. Similar to small cell carcinomas, mitotic counts are >10 per 10 high-powered fields (by definition, in distinction from atypical carcinoid). The proliferation index is >50%, usually more than 75%.[11] Zonal or punctate necrosis is typical (Fig. 80.3B).

Immunohistochemical Findings

Unlike small cell carcinoma, the diagnosis of large cell neuroendocrine carcinoma requires immunohistochemical confirmation of diffuse staining (>10% of the tumor) with neuroendocrine markers.[11,12]

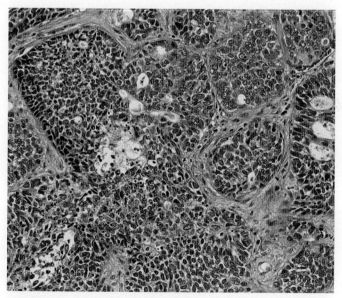

FIGURE 80.1 ▲ Large cell neuroendocrine carcinoma. The tumor is composed of rounded sheets of polygonal cells with nuclear clearing, abundant cytoplasm, and rosette-like glands.

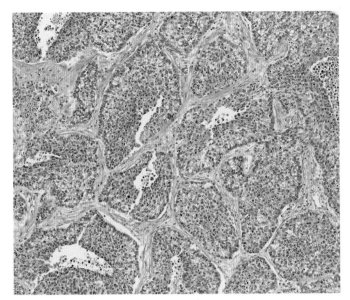

FIGURE 80.2 ▲ Large cell neuroendocrine carcinoma. In this tumor, peripheral palisading is especially prominent.

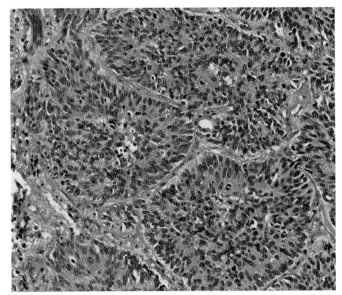

FIGURE 80.4 ▲ Large cell neuroendocrine carcinoma. In this tumor, the abundant cytoplasm is typical of large cell neuroendocrine carcinoma, although the nuclear features (dispersed chromatin, inconspicuous nucleoli) are more reminiscent of small cell carcinoma.

Chromogranin A stains 80% to 85% of large cell neuroendocrine marker and is the most specific for endocrine differentiation (Fig. 80.5). The most sensitive (and least specific) marker is neural cell adhesion molecule (CD56), which stains 92% to 100% of tumors (Fig. 80.6). Synaptophysin is expressed in 50% to 60% of large cell neuroendocrine carcinoma (Fig. 80.7).[6,10,12–15] Fewer large cell neuroendocrine carcinomas (about one-half) express TTF-1 than small cell carcinomas (Fig. 80.8). Therefore, this marker is of limited diagnostic use.[10,13,16] Ki-67 is helpful, especially in small biopsies, to distinguish large cell neuroendocrine carcinoma from atypical carcinoid (Fig. 80.9). Atypical carcinoid tumors generally have a proliferation rate of <30%, whereas large cell carcinomas have a proliferative index of more than 60%.[11] Napsin A has not been described in large cell neuroendocrine carcinoma.[13]

Large cell neuroendocrine carcinomas express cytokeratin 7[12,13,15] but generally do not express high molecular weight forms such as CK5/6[17] or cytokeratin 903 (34βE12).[18,19] It must be remembered that p63 is less specific than p40 for squamous differentiation and may be seen in over 10% of large cell neuroendocrine carcinomas,[20,21] while p40 is seen in fewer than 5%.[21] More than 70% of large cell neuroendocrine carcinomas express CD117,[22] which has been associated with a relatively poor prognosis.[23]

Differential Diagnosis

Large cell neuroendocrine carcinoma must be distinguished from small cell carcinomas, basaloid or nonkeratinizing squamous carcinomas,

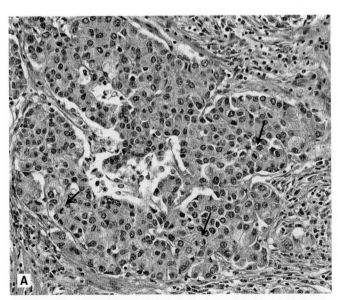
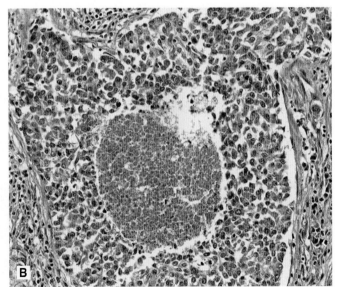

FIGURE 80.3 ▲ Large cell neuroendocrine carcinoma, carcinoid-like appearance. **A.** There are abundant mitotic figures (*arrows*), which distinguish this tumor from atypical carcinoid. **B.** Another distinguishing feature is the presence of central necrosis.

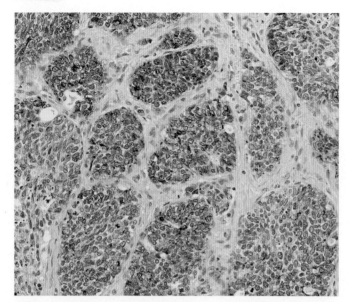

FIGURE 80.5 ▲ Large cell neuroendocrine carcinoma, chromo-granin immunohistochemical staining. Chromogranin staining is typical patchy and confined to the cytoplasm.

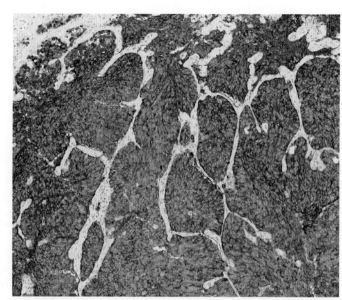

FIGURE 80.7 ▲ Large cell neuroendocrine carcinoma, synaptophy-sin. This particular tumor shows diffuse cytoplasmic and membranous staining.

solid-type adenocarcinomas, and atypical carcinoid tumors. There are no immunohistochemical studies that separate large cell neuroendocrine carcinoma from small cell carcinoma, which is a diagnosis based on light microscopy (see this chapter). Histologic features that favor large cell over small include cell size > 25 microns, abundant cytoplasm, nucleoli and nuclear clearing, and polygonal cell shape. Nuclear molding is more common in small cell carcinoma but may be somewhat prominent in large cell neuroendocrine carcinoma. Combined small cell and large cell neuroendocrine carcinoma is the most common type of combined small cell carcinoma and should be considered if there is at least 10% of the tumor that resembles small cell carcinoma by light microscopy. Basaloid squamous carcinoma should be excluded by immunohistochemical stains (positivity for p40 and negativity for endocrine markers CD56, chromogranin, and synaptophysin).

Similarly, solid adenocarcinoma should be excluded by lack of cribriform areas and lack of expression of endocrine markers; TTF-1 is not helpful in this distinction. Atypical carcinoids may be difficult to distinguish from large cell neuroendocrine carcinoma, and if there is limited sampling precluding a reliable mitotic count, then immunohistochemical staining for Ki-67 may be helpful.[11]

Prognosis and Treatment

Large cell neuroendocrine carcinoma is essentially as aggressive as small cell carcinoma and has a similar tendency for widespread metastases, including the lung, regional and distant lymph nodes, liver, brain, and skeleton.[24,25] The prognosis is worse than other types of non–small cell carcinoma, even for patients with stage I disease,

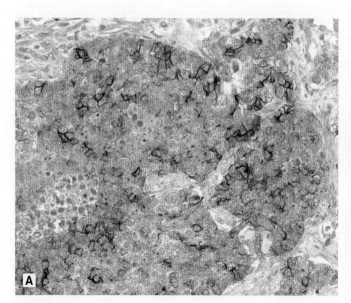

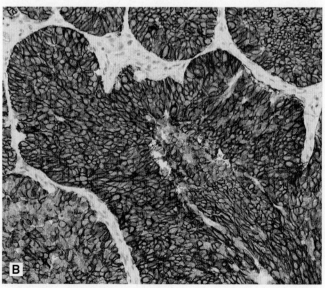

FIGURE 80.6 ▲ Large cell neuroendocrine carcinoma, CD56 immunohistochemical staining. **A.** There is patchy staining. **B.** In this case, staining is diffuse and involves cell membranes as well as cytoplasm, unlike chromogranin.

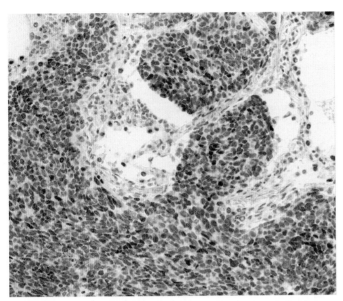

FIGURE 80.8 ▲ Large cell neuroendocrine carcinoma, TTF-1 immunohistochemical stain. In this stain, the impression is that of small cell carcinoma. However, some areas had histologic features more of large cell carcinoma (same tumor as that shown in Fig. 80.1).

who have a 5-year survival of only 33%.[25-27] Overall median disease-free survival is only 10 months.[11] Over one-third of patients have stage IV disease, with the most common distal sites representing the liver (47%), bone (32%), and brain (23%). Although the clinical features and survival resemble small cell carcinoma, the frequency of surgical resection and adjuvant chemotherapy more resembled non–small cell carcinoma.[1]

The role of chemoradiation therapy in early-stage disease is not yet established. Systemic chemotherapy for unresectable large cell neuroendocrine carcinoma may result in tumor response, and patients may benefit more from a small cell–based chemotherapy than for non–small cell tumor regimens.[27]

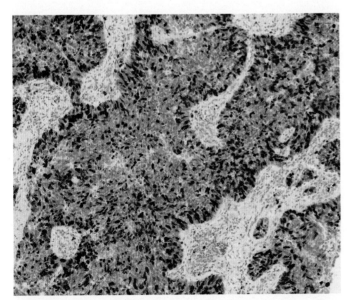

FIGURE 80.9 ▲ Large cell neuroendocrine carcinoma, Ki-67 immunohistochemical stain. There is a high proliferative rate, similar to small cell carcinoma.

REFERENCES

1. Derks JL, Hendriks LE, Buikhuisen WA, et al. Clinical features of large cell neuroendocrine carcinoma: a population-based overview. *Eur Respir J.* 2015.
2. Fasano M, Della Corte CM, Papaccio F, et al. Pulmonary large-cell neuroendocrine carcinoma: from epidemiology to therapy. *J Thorac Oncol.* 2015;10:1133–1141.
3. Lee KW, Lee Y, Oh SW, et al. Large cell neuroendocrine carcinoma of the lung: CT and FDG PET findings. *Eur J Radiol.* 2015;84:2332–2338.
4. Akata S, Okada S, Maeda J, et al. Computed tomographic findings of large cell neuroendocrine carcinoma of the lung. *Clin Imaging.* 2007;31:379–384.
5. Oshiro Y, Kusumoto M, Matsuno Y, et al. CT findings of surgically resected large cell neuroendocrine carcinoma of the lung in 38 patients. *AJR Am J Roentgenol.* 2004;182:87–91.
6. Travis WD. Advances in neuroendocrine lung tumors. *Ann Oncol.* 2010;21(suppl 7):vii65–vii71.
7. Iyoda A, Hiroshima K, Toyozaki T, et al. Clinical characterization of pulmonary large cell neuroendocrine carcinoma and large cell carcinoma with neuroendocrine morphology. *Cancer.* 2001;91:1992–2000.
8. Yeh YC, Chou TY. Pulmonary neuroendocrine tumors: study of 90 cases focusing on clinicopathological characteristics, immunophenotype, preoperative biopsy, and frozen section diagnoses. *J Surg Oncol.* 2014;109: 280–286.
9. den Bakker MA, Thunnissen FB. Neuroendocrine tumours—challenges in the diagnosis and classification of pulmonary neuroendocrine tumours. *J Clin Pathol.* 2013;66:862–869.
10. Rossi G, Marchioni A, Milani M, et al. TTF-1, cytokeratin 7, 34betaE12, and CD56/NCAM immunostaining in the subclassification of large cell carcinomas of the lung. *Am J Clin Pathol.* 2004;122:884–893.
11. Liu SZ, Staats PN, Goicochea L, et al. Automated quantification of Ki-67 proliferative index of excised neuroendocrine tumors of the lung. *Diagn Pathol.* 2014;9:174.
12. Travis WD, Linnoila RI, Tsokos MG, et al. Neuroendocrine tumors of the lung with proposed criteria for large-cell neuroendocrine carcinoma. An ultrastructural, immunohistochemical, and flow cytometric study of 35 cases. *Am J Surg Pathol.* 1991;15:529–553.
13. Rossi G, Mengoli MC, Cavazza A, et al. Large cell carcinoma of the lung: clinically oriented classification integrating immunohistochemistry and molecular biology. *Virchows Arch.* 2014;464:61–68.
14. Iyoda A, Travis WD, Sarkaria IS, et al. Expression profiling and identification of potential molecular targets for therapy in pulmonary large-cell neuroendocrine carcinoma. *Exp Ther Med.* 2011;2:1041–1045.
15. Travis WD, Rush W, Flieder DB, et al. Survival analysis of 200 pulmonary neuroendocrine tumors with clarification of criteria for atypical carcinoid and its separation from typical carcinoid. *Am J Surg Pathol.* 1998;22:934–944.
16. Sturm N, Rossi G, Lantuejoul S, et al. Expression of thyroid transcription factor-1 in the spectrum of neuroendocrine cell lung proliferations with special interest in carcinoids. *Hum Pathol.* 2002;33:175–182.
17. Nitadori J, Ishii G, Tsuta K, et al. Immunohistochemical differential diagnosis between large cell neuroendocrine carcinoma and small cell carcinoma by tissue microarray analysis with a large antibody panel. *Am J Clin Pathol.* 2006;125:682–692.
18. Sturm N, Rossi G, Lantuejoul S, et al. 34BetaE12 expression along the whole spectrum of neuroendocrine proliferations of the lung, from neuroendocrine cell hyperplasia to small cell carcinoma. *Histopathology.* 2003;42:156–166.
19. Sturm N, Lantuejoul S, Laverriere MH, et al. Thyroid transcription factor 1 and cytokeratins 1, 5, 10, 14 (34betaE12) expression in basaloid and large-cell neuroendocrine carcinomas of the lung. *Hum Pathol.* 2001;32:918–925.
20. Pelosi G, Pasini F, Olsen Stenholm C, et al. p63 immunoreactivity in lung cancer: yet another player in the development of squamous cell carcinomas? *J Pathol.* 2002;198:100–109.
21. Tatsumori T, Tsuta K, Masai K, et al. p40 is the best marker for diagnosing pulmonary squamous cell carcinoma: comparison with p63, cytokeratin 5/6, desmocollin-3, and sox2. *Appl Immunohistochem Mol Morphol.* 2014;22:377–382.
22. Pelosi G, Masullo M, Leon ME, et al. CD117 immunoreactivity in high-grade neuroendocrine tumors of the lung: a comparative study of 39 large-cell neuroendocrine carcinomas and 27 surgically resected small-cell carcinomas. *Virchows Arch.* 2004;445:449–455.
23. Casali C, Stefani A, Rossi G, et al. The prognostic role of c-kit protein expression in resected large cell neuroendocrine carcinoma of the lung. *Ann Thorac Surg.* 2004;77:247–252; discussion 252–253.

24. Gollard R, Jhatakia S, Elliott M, et al. Large cell/neuroendocrine carcinoma. *Lung Cancer.* 2010;69:13–18.
25. Battafarano RJ, Fernandez FG, Ritter J, et al. Large cell neuroendocrine carcinoma: an aggressive form of non-small cell lung cancer. *J Thorac Cardiovasc Surg.* 2005;130:166–172.
26. Fernandez FG, Battafarano RJ. Large-cell neuroendocrine carcinoma of the lung. *Cancer Control.* 2006;13:270–275.
27. Rossi G, Cavazza A, Marchioni A, et al. Role of chemotherapy and the receptor tyrosine kinases KIT, PDGFRalpha, PDGFRbeta, and Met in large-cell neuroendocrine carcinoma of the lung. *J Clin Oncol.* 2005;23:8774–8785.

81 Diffuse Idiopathic Pulmonary Neuroendocrine Cell Hyperplasia and Carcinoid Tumor

Fabio R. Tavora, M.D., Ph.D., Allen P. Burke, M.D., and Marie-Christine Aubry, M.D.

Classification of Pulmonary Neuroendocrine Tumors

Neuroendocrine tumors of the lung are divided into four categories: typical carcinoid (TC), atypical carcinoid (AC), large cell neuroendocrine carcinoma (LCNEC) (Chapter 80), and small cell carcinoma (SCLC) (Chapter 79). Diffuse idiopathic pulmonary neuroendocrine cell hyperplasia (DIPNECH) is considered a preinvasive lesion in the WHO classification of tumors of the lung.

The terminology of neuroendocrine tumors in the different organ systems varies, and there is some debate if the lung classification should also follow a classification of the gastrointestinal system, which separates the lesions into well, moderately, and poorly differentiated tumors, based on mitotic count and Ki-67 labeling index.[1–3] However, the current WHO classification of tumors of the lung maintains the classification scheme of TC, AC, SCLC, and LCNEC.

Low- and intermediate-grade lesions (TC and AC) usually bear close resemblance to normal cells and show architecture and cytologic patterns of nonneoplastic cells and positivity for neurosecretory proteins. High-grade lesions (poorly differentiated carcinomas) are classified in the lung by the current WHO into SCLC and LCNEC. These tumors also express neuroendocrine markers, albeit less intensely, and also show reminiscence of neuroendocrine morphology.

Regardless of the classification used in the various organs, prognostic stratification is clinically relevant and reproducible among pathologists. Some evidence suggests that TC and AC, although variably aggressive, are genetically different from the high-grade lesions, which are uniformly aggressive.[2,4,5] In the lung, SCLC exhibits marked sensitivity to platinum-based chemotherapy, whereas lower-grade lesions are unresponsive to these regimens.[6]

Carcinoid Tumors

Incidence

TC and AC tumors are rare and account for ~1% to 2% of all lung carcinomas.[7–9] The estimated incidence of carcinoid tumors ranges from 0.1 per 100,000 to 1.5 per 100,000, with 70% to 90% being TC.[9] About 30% of carcinoid tumors in the body occur in the lung, second only to the tubular gastrointestinal system.[10]

Clinical and Radiologic Features

Carcinoid tumors occur in patients younger than high-grade lesions (mean age for carcinoid 45 to 50 years) with no predilection for sex or smoking history.[1] Carcinoid tumors are the most common lung tumor seen in children. Carcinoid tumors can occur in the setting of familial syndromes, especially MEN1. Association with carcinoid syndrome is rare in lung tumors, occurring in <2% of the lesions.[11] Cushing syndrome occurs more commonly, in up to 4% of patients, typically with peripheral TC. Other rare endocrine syndromes reported with carcinoid tumors include acromegaly and elevated parathyroid hormone.

Approximately 75% of carcinoid tumors are central in location, growing along the tracheobronchial tree, with invasion into the adjacent lung parenchyma or with an endoluminal growth. Therefore, patients often present with symptoms of obstruction including dyspnea, productive cough, wheezing, hemoptysis, and recurrent pneumonia. Peripheral tumors are usually discovered incidentally.

Radiologically, central carcinoid tumors present with atelectasis or obstructive pneumonia. Peripheral carcinoid tumors are well circumscribed with demarcated, rounded contours. Uptake on positron emission tomography (PET) tends to be lower in carcinoid tumors compared to other malignant carcinomas of the lung and usually lower in TC compared to AC. Octreotide imaging is often weak in pulmonary carcinoid tumors, compared to abdominal carcinoid tumors, because many do not have somatostatin receptors.

Gross Pathologic Findings

Grossly, these lesions are usually tan colored, well circumscribed, and round and may be pedunculated measuring a few centimeters.[12] Central tumors with endoluminal obstruction are commonly associated with obstructive pneumonia. Localized bronchiectasis may also be seen (Fig. 81.1).

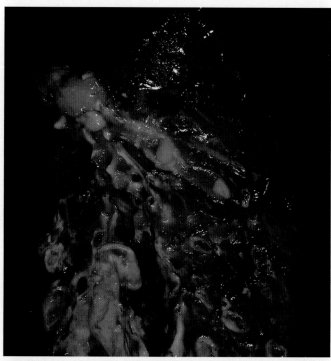

FIGURE 81.1 ▲ Typical carcinoid tumor, gross appearance. The tumor obstructs the lobar bronchus and has resulted in obstructive pneumonia with golden consolidation of the lung parenchyma and marked bronchiectasis.

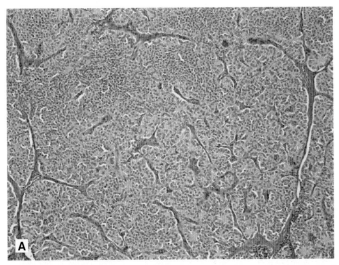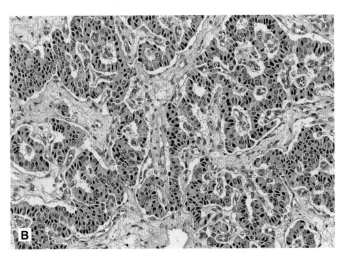

FIGURE 81.2 ▲ Typical carcinoid. **A.** Organoid-nested morphology. **B.** Trabecular and pseudoglandular growth patterns.

Histologic Features

The overall morphology of TC and AC is similar to low- and intermediate-grade neuroendocrine tumors of other organs. The two most common growth patterns are organoid and trabecular (Fig. 81.2), but a heterogeneous mix of growth patterns can be easily seen in most lesions, with papillary formations, spindle cell change, and pseudoglandular growth among the most common (Fig. 81.2). While the tumor cells are usually bland, of small to intermediate size, scattered larger cells with striking pleomorphism is sometimes seen. These changes do not alter the diagnosis to AC category, although AC may show more prominent nucleoli and nuclear pleomorphism. The cell morphology in carcinoid tumors can be quite variable and may cause diagnostic challenges. Indeed, carcinoid tumor cells may have predominantly clear cytoplasm as seen in PEComa (Chapter 71) or metastasis from renal cell carcinoma, or abundant granular eosinophilic cytoplasm reminiscent of an oncocytoma (Fig. 81.3). Carcinoid tumors may have a prominent spindle cell morphology, typically in peripheral lesions (Fig. 81.3). Stromal hyalinization including bone formation (Fig. 81.4), mucinous background (Fig. 81.4), and amyloid has also been described.

The morphologic distinction between the TC and AC is based on only two features: mitotic count and necrosis.[13,14] According to the current WHO classification, TC should measure more than 0.5 cm in size, contain < 2 mitoses per 2 mm^2 (~10 high-powered fields), and lack necrosis. ACs have 2 to 10 mitoses per 2 mm^2 and/or foci of necrosis (Fig. 81.5). The necrosis is usually punctuate and focal in the tumor. Because of the importance of mitotic count to distinguish these two lesions, the WHO recommends that mitoses should be counted in the areas of highest activity, but if the cutoff of 2 or 10 is neared, at least three sets of 2 mm^2 should be counted and the mean used for determining the mitotic rate, rather than the single highest rate. Furthermore, distinguishing typical from AC tumor may not be possible on a small biopsy specimen due to sampling.

Immunohistochemistry

Immunohistochemical studies have classically been used to confirm the diagnosis of neuroendocrine carcinomas. In most cases of carcinoids, the morphology is obvious and precludes the absolute need for confirmatory studies, especially if it fits the clinical scenario.

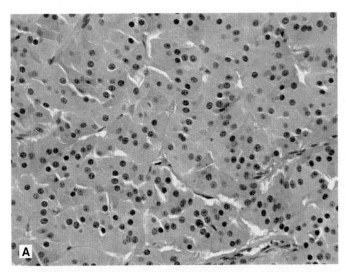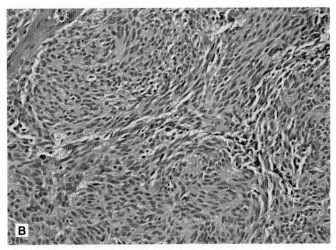

FIGURE 81.3 ▲ Typical carcinoid. **A.** Cells contain abundant granular cytoplasm with oncocytic features. **B.** Spindle cell morphology usually seen in peripheral carcinoid tumor.

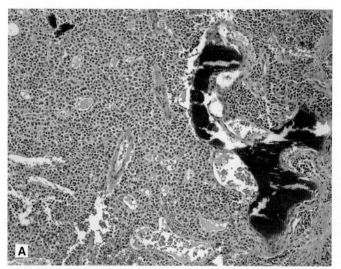

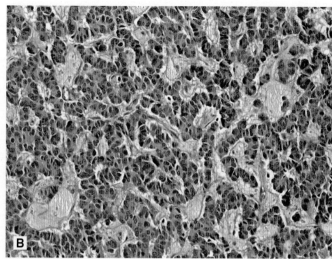

FIGURE 81.4 ▲ Typical carcinoid. **A.** Presence of osseous metaplasia. **B.** Classic cellular morphology and growth pattern in a mucinous background.

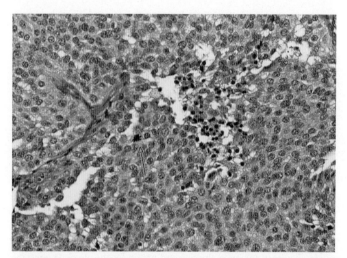

FIGURE 81.5 ▲ Atypical carcinoid tumor. There is punctate necrosis and mitosis (*arrow*).

Most carcinoid tumors are positive for keratins, such as CK7, CK8, CK18, and other commercially available cocktails. CK20 positivity is uncommon. High molecular weight cytokeratins are usually negative. There is a distinctive pattern of positivity of intermediate filaments in neuroendocrine tumors, which is punctate and cytoplasmic, sometimes referred to as dot like or paranuclear.

When needed, neuroendocrine differentiation can be proved using three antibodies: chromogranin, CD56, and synaptophysin, with virtually 100% of tumors staining diffusely with at least one of these markers (Fig. 81.6). Other markers that can be positive in lung carcinoids, but should be used with care due to low sensitivity and specificity, include CD57, CD99, neuron-specific enolase, PGP9.5, CD117, and PAX5. The tumors can also express peptides such as calcitonin, gastrin, and adrenocorticotropic hormone, but because the staining does not correlate with hormonal production, their usefulness for the diagnosis is debatable, and therefore, they are not recommended.

A low proliferation rate by Ki-67 is expected for TCs, with several cutoffs proposed, including 4%, 7%, 10%, and 20%.[7,15–17] ACs have a proliferative rate usually below 40%.

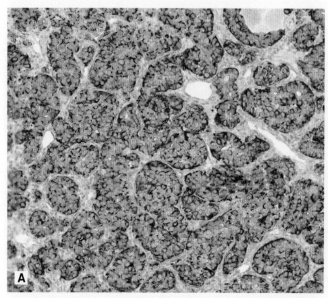

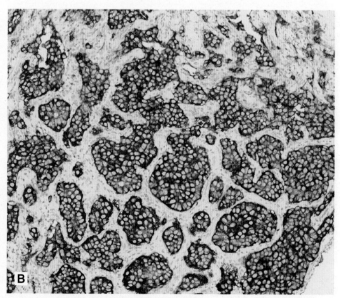

FIGURE 81.6 ▲ Atypical carcinoid tumor. Strong and diffuse staining with chromogranin **(A)** and synaptophysin **(B)**.

TTF-1 positivity is variable in TCs and ACs and ranges from 0%[18,19] to 27%.[20] Carcinoid tumorlets and peripheral spindle cell carcinoids have the highest rate of positivity, especially the former.[20] TTF-1 is not expressed in extrapulmonary carcinoids, so it is a specific, although insensitive, marker for pulmonary origin.[20]

Prognosis and Treatment

Although carcinoid tumors have excellent prognosis, they can metastasize. As with other non–small cell carcinomas, prognosis depends on the TNM staging and surgical resectability as these tumors are much less responsive to chemo- and radiation therapy. The majority of TC present at an early stage with lymph metastasis occurring in < 15% of patients. The overall survival at 5 years is >90% for resected TC. The 5-year overall survival for AC is lower, ranging between 61% and 88%. Patients with AC presents more often with lymph node metastasis (35% to 65%).[21] Late metastases are also known to occur.[1]

Differential Diagnosis

The main differential diagnoses of pulmonary carcinoid tumors are with metastatic carcinoid from other primary sites. Typically, metastatic carcinoid tumors will present with multiple nodules with hematogenous and lymphangitic spread. TTF-1 although not sensitive is specific from pulmonary carcinoid tumors.

ACs may be hard to distinguish from LCNECs, which may show overlapping morphologic features, such as peripheral palisading, rosette formation, and cells with conspicuous nucleoli. However, the degree of cell atypia and mitotic rate is greater in LCNEC. There are rare examples of morphologic "bland" carcinoid tumors with high mitotic rate of > 10 mitosis per 2 mm^2, and the current recommendation is to classify these as LCNEC, although the exact prognosis of such tumors remains unclear.

For small biopsy samples, the major pitfall is with higher-grade neuroendocrine carcinomas such as SCLC. Indeed, in small biopsies, the crushing artifact, a common phenomenon in neuroendocrine tumors, may lead to an erroneous diagnosis of SCLC because the cells will appear hyperchromatic and nuclei molded.[15] The absence of cell necrosis and mitosis should raise a concern about the diagnosis of SCLC, but these morphologic features may also be difficult to appreciate on a crushed specimen. Immunostaining for Ki-67 (Mib1) is useful in this situation as SCLC typically have high labeling index, above 50%.[15]

Carcinoid tumors in cytology specimens are sometimes hard to distinguish from other non–small cell carcinoma lesions and also from lymphoproliferative disorders. These samples usually show a moderately cellular specimen with discohesive cells and occasional rosettes. Bare nuclei or spindle-shaped cells can also be visualized.

Central carcinoid tumors enter the differential diagnosis of other low-grade neoplasms with a predilection for large airways such as salivary gland–type tumors (Chapter 84) and unusual mesenchymal tumors such as glomangioma. Furthermore, paraganglioma also needs to be distinguished from carcinoid tumors. The existence of primary pulmonary paraganglioma remains disputed because carcinoid tumors may rarely be keratin negative and are known to have S100 protein–positive sustentacular cells, although there are rare convincing reports in the literature.[22] But, metastatic paraganglioma from another primary site should always be ruled out.

Spindle cell carcinoid needs to be distinguished from low-grade mesenchymal lesions such as inflammatory myofibroblastic tumor (Chapter 68) and solitary fibrous tumor (Chapter 96).

DIPNECH

Definition

DIPNECH is defined as a proliferation of neuroendocrine cells in the lung that may be confined to the mucosa of the airways, that may invade beyond the basal lamina forming carcinoid tumorlets, and/or that may develop into carcinoid tumors. Chronic inflammation and fibrosis of the airways, occasionally resulting in constrictive bronchiolitis, are often present. Because carcinoid tumors are part of the spectrum of DIPNECH, DIPNECH is considered a preinvasive lesion. However, DIPNECH has only been associated with peripheral carcinoid tumors and, therefore, seems unlikely to be the precursor lesion for all carcinoid tumors.

Clinical and Radiologic Presentation

DIPNECH develops predominantly in middle-aged women (average age 60 to 65 years), most of which are never smokers.[23,24] There appear to be three types of clinical presentations[9,20]: (1) Most patients are asymptomatic and are found to have incidental multiple small lung nodules. These patients commonly have a history or suspected history of malignancy, and the new discovery of multiple lung nodules raises a clinical concern for metastatic disease. Pulmonary function tests are often normal or show mild obstruction. (2) The second most common clinical presentation is of an airway disease. These patients present with cough, dyspnea, wheezing, and breathlessness, often of >5 years duration.[25] They often have a diagnosis of asthma or chronic obstructive pulmonary disease.[26] These patients are more likely to have constrictive bronchiolitis as part of their DIPNECH syndrome and show mixed physiology or moderate to severe obstruction on pulmonary function tests.[27,28] (3) The rarest presentation is of an endocrine syndrome, such as acromegaly, Cushing syndrome, and MEN1.[1]

Radiologic features on high-resolution CT scan vary with the clinical presentations. The presence and number of nodules are more prominent in patients with incidental DIPNECH. The nodules are small usually 6 to 10 mm, round, and well circumscribed. Patients with airway disease are more likely to show air trapping with mosaicism and airway abnormalities such as wall thickening and dilatation.[20]

Histologic Features

The histologic findings reflect the spectrum of DIPNECH. The easiest recognizable lesion is the carcinoid tumorlet. Although carcinoid tumorlets are common incidental and clinically insignificant findings,[4] they should prompt the pathologist to assess for more subtle findings of neuroendocrine hyperplasia and constrictive bronchiolitis of DIPNECH.

By definition, carcinoid tumorlets measure <5 mm in greatest dimension, and morphologically, they are identical to TC tumors. They are centered on small airways, often with a fibrotic stroma, which results in luminal occlusion (Fig. 81.7). Mitosis and necrosis are typically absent.

Neuroendocrine cell proliferation can be more subtle and easier to observe with a neuroendocrine immunostain. These cells appear oval to round and contain a round nucleus with finely granular chromatin. The cytoplasm is often clear to pale eosinophilic. The proliferation typically starts in the basal layer and raises the glandular cells of the mucosa (Fig. 81.8). The proliferation may be linear or form nodular aggregates within the basal membrane. Once the proliferation invades beyond the basal membrane, it is considered invasive.

Prognosis and Treatment

The overall prognosis for DIPNECH is usually good with many patients experiencing stable disease. Progression of symptoms due to the obliterative bronchiolitis may occur and require treatment with steroids or even lung transplantation. Increase in the number or size of tumor nodules may be seen. Rarely, the disease may progress with the development of regional and distant metastasis. In these patients, treatment with somatostatin analogs may be considered.[29]

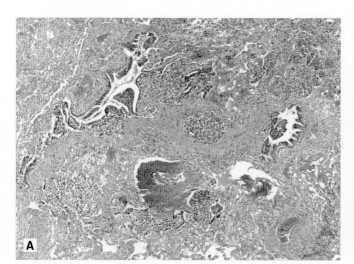

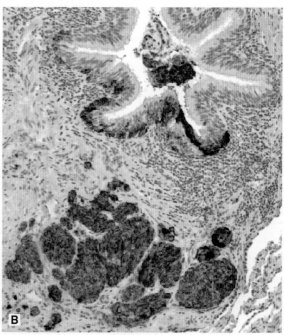

FIGURE 81.7 ▲ **A.** Carcinoid tumorlet arising from neuroendocrine cell hyperplasia in adjacent airway. **B.** The chromogranin immunostain highlights the neuroendocrine cell proliferation.

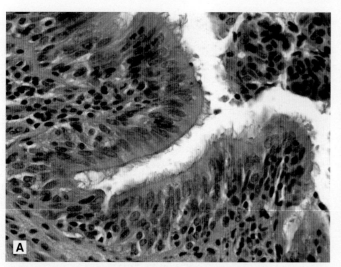

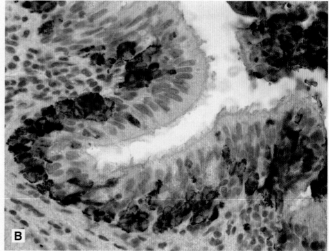

FIGURE 81.8 ▲ **A.** Neuroendocrine cell hyperplasia characterized by cells with clear cytoplasm and small nuclei in the basal layer and best seen with chromogranin **(B)**.

REFERENCES

1. Rekhtman N. Neuroendocrine tumors of the lung: an update. *Arch Pathol Lab Med.* 2010;134:1628–1638.

2. Klimstra DS, Beltran H, Lilenbaum R, et al. The spectrum of neuroendocrine tumors: histologic classification, unique features and areas of overlap. *Am Soc Clin Oncol Educ Book.* 2015;35:92–103.

3. Klimstra DS, Modlin IR, Coppola D, et al. The pathologic classification of neuroendocrine tumors: a review of nomenclature, grading, and staging systems. *Pancreas.* 2010;39:707–712.

4. Travis WD. Advances in neuroendocrine lung tumors. *Ann Oncol.* 2010;21(suppl 7):vii65–vii71.

5. Travis WD. Pathology and diagnosis of neuroendocrine tumors: lung neuroendocrine. *Thorac Surg Clin.* 2014;24:257–266.

6. Fasano M, Della Corte CM, et al. Pulmonary large-cell neuroendocrine carcinoma: from epidemiology to therapy. *J Thorac Oncol.* 2015;10(8):1133–1141.

7. Liu SZ, Staats PN, Goicochea L, et al. Automated quantification of Ki-67 proliferative index of excised neuroendocrine tumors of the lung. *Diagn Pathol.* 2014;9:174.

8. Garcia-Yuste M, Matilla JM, Cueto A, et al. Typical and atypical carcinoid tumours: analysis of the experience of the Spanish Multi-centric Study of Neuroendocrine Tumours of the Lung. *Eur J Cardiothorac Surg.* 2007;31:192–197.

9. Beasley MB, Brambilla E, Chirieac LR, et al. Carcinoid tumors. In: Travis WD, et al., eds. *WHO Classification of Tumours of the Lung, Pleura, Mediastinum and Heart.* Lyon, France: IARC Press; 2015:73–77.

10. Gustafsson BI, Kidd M, Modlin IM. Neuroendocrine tumors of the diffuse neuroendocrine system. *Curr Opin Oncol.* 2008;20:1–12.

11. McCaughan BC, Martini N, Bains MS. Bronchial carcinoids. Review of 124 cases. *J Thorac Cardiovasc Surg.* 1985;89:8–17.

12. Carretta A, Ceresoli GL, Arrigoni G, et al. Diagnostic and therapeutic management of neuroendocrine lung tumors: a clinical study of 44 cases. *Lung Cancer.* 2000;29:217–225.

13. Travis WD. Lung tumours with neuroendocrine differentiation. *Eur J Cancer.* 2009;45(suppl 1):251–266.

14. Tang LH, Gonen M, Hedvat C, et al. Objective quantification of the Ki67 proliferative index in neuroendocrine tumors of the gastroenteropancreatic system: a comparison of digital image analysis with manual methods. *Am J Surg Pathol.* 2012;36:1761–1770.

15. Pelosi G, Rodriguez J, Viale G, et al. Typical and atypical pulmonary carcinoid tumor overdiagnosed as small-cell carcinoma on biopsy specimens: a major pitfall in the management of lung cancer patients. *Am J Surg Pathol.* 2005;29:179–187.

16. Aslan DL, Gulbahce HE, Pambuccian SE, et al. Ki-67 immunoreactivity in the differential diagnosis of pulmonary neuroendocrine neoplasms in specimens with extensive crush artifact. *Am J Clin Pathol.* 2005;123:874–878.

17. Grimaldi F, Muser D, Beltrami CA, et al. Partitioning of bronchopulmonary carcinoids in two different prognostic categories by ki-67 score. *Front Endocrinol.* 2011;2:20.

18. Sturm N, Rossi G, Lantuejoul S, et al. Expression of thyroid transcription factor-1 in the spectrum of neuroendocrine cell lung proliferations with special interest in carcinoids. *Hum Pathol.* 2002;33:175–182.

19. Rugge M, Fassan M, Clemente R, et al. Bronchopulmonary carcinoid: phenotype and long-term outcome in a single-institution series of Italian patients. *Clin Cancer Res.* 2008;14:149–154.

20. Du EZ, Goldstraw P, Zacharias J, et al. TTF-1 expression is specific for lung primary in typical and atypical carcinoids: TTF-1-positive carcinoids are predominantly in peripheral location. *Hum Pathol.* 2004;35:825–831.

21. Fink G, Krelbaum T, Yellin A, et al. Pulmonary carcinoid: presentation, diagnosis, and outcome in 142 cases in Israel and review of 640 cases from the literature. *Chest.* 2001;119:1647–1651.

22. Aubertine CL, Flieder DB. Primary paraganglioma of the lung. *Ann Diagn Pathol.* 2004;8:237–241.

23. Aubry MC, Thomas CF, Jr, Jett JR, et al. Significance of multiple carcinoid tumors and tumorlets in surgical lung specimens: analysis of 28 patients. *Chest.* 2007;131:1635–1643.

24. Kim Y, Choi YD, Kim BJ, et al. Multiple peripheral typical carcinoid tumors of the lung: associated with sclerosing hemangiomas. *Diagn Pathol.* 2013;8:97.

25. Gorshtein A, Gross DJ, Barak D, et al. Diffuse idiopathic pulmonary neuroendocrine cell hyperplasia and the associated lung neuroendocrine tumors: clinical experience with a rare entity. *Cancer.* 2012;118:612–619.

26. Carr LL, Chung JH, Duarte Achcar R, et al. The clinical course of diffuse idiopathic pulmonary neuroendocrine cell hyperplasia. *Chest.* 2015;147:415–422.

27. Ge Y, Eltorky MA, Ernst RD, et al. Diffuse idiopathic pulmonary neuroendocrine cell hyperplasia. *Ann Diagn Pathol.* 2007;11:122–126.

28. Oba H, Nishida K, Takeuchi S, et al. Diffuse idiopathic pulmonary neuroendocrine cell hyperplasia with a central and peripheral carcinoid and multiple tumorlets: a case report emphasizing the role of neuropeptide hormones and human gonadotropin-alpha. *Endocr Pathol.* 2013;24:220–228.

29. Davies SJ, Gosney JR, Hansell DM, et al. Diffuse idiopathic pulmonary neuroendocrine cell hyperplasia: an under-recognised spectrum of disease. *Thorax.* 2007;62:248–252.

82 Large Cell Carcinoma

Allen P. Burke, M.D., and Borislav A. Alexiev, M.D.

General

Large cell carcinoma, once a relatively large proportion of lung carcinomas, has now greatly dropped in frequency, as immunohistochemical typing has reassigned many of the previous subsets. Currently, large cell carcinoma is defined as lacking immunohistochemical differentiation of squamous cell or adenocarcinoma, as well as lacking histologic features of other carcinoma types. Among the subtypes of large cell carcinoma previously recognized by the World Health Organization, large-cell neuroendocrine carcinoma, basaloid carcinoma, and lymphoepithelial-like carcinoma have been reassigned as separate entities in the newer classification system. Basaloid carcinomas are therefore discussed with squamous cell carcinomas, as

well as lymphoepithelial-like carcinoma (see Chapter 78). Large-cell neuroendocrine carcinoma is a separate entity within the spectrum of neuroendocrine carcinomas (see Chapter 80). The "rhabdoid" and "clear cell" subtypes are now considered histologic variations that may occur in defined histologic types of non–small cell lung carcinoma (especially adenocarcinoma and squamous carcinoma) (Tables 82.1 and 82.2).

The rationale behind narrowing the scope of "large cell carcinoma" lies largely in the realization that molecular classification of many histologically undifferentiated carcinomas corresponds to immunohistochemical profiles.[1–4] Although "large cell carcinoma" now denotes absence of immunohistochemical evidence of differentiation ("large cell carcinoma with null phenotype" or "large cell undifferentiated

TABLE 82.1 Terminology of Poorly Differentiated Lung Carcinomas

Old Designation	Current Designation	Distinguishing Features
Adenocarcinoma, solid growth pattern	Adenocarcinoma, solid growth pattern	Histologic features (not small cell or LCNEC) *and* mucin vacuoles *or* TTF-1 *or* napsin-A expression
Large cell carcinoma, basaloid type	Basaloid carcinoma (variant of squamous cell)	Histologic features *and* IHC evidence of squamous differentiation
Large cell carcinoma, neuroendocrine type	Large-cell neuroendocrine carcinoma	Endocrine histologic features *and* endocrine differentiation (by IHC)
Rhabdoid carcinoma	None[a]	Light microscopic features
Clear cell carcinoma	None[b]	Light microscopic features
Large cell carcinoma, null type	Large cell carcinoma Large cell undifferentiated carcinoma	Histologic features (not small cell or LCNEC) *and* absence of histologic features of sarcomatoid carcinoma *and* absence of IHC evidence of adeno- or squamous carcinoma
Lymphoepithelioma	Lymphoepithelial-like carcinoma[c]	Histologic features *and* ISH positivity for EBER

IHC, immunohistochemistry; EBER, EBV-encoded small nuclear RNAs.

[a]Now a descriptive designation; diagnosis is based on areas of differentiation (adenocarcinoma, squamous carcinoma, etc.), or if all rhabdoid without evidence of specific differentiation, then "large cell carcinoma, rhabdoid type."

[b]Also a descriptive designation; diagnosis is based on adenocarcinoma or squamous carcinoma differentiation or rarely large cell (undifferentiated).

[c]Variably classified separately (e.g., WHO) or as a variant of squamous cell carcinoma.

TABLE 82.2   Immunohistochemical Staining of Undifferentiated Lung Carcinomas

	Antibody	Note
Squamous differentiation	p40	Preferred
	p63	Less specific than p40
	Cytokeratin 5/6	Less specific than p40
	Desmocollin-3	Not in wide use
	Cytokeratin 903 (34βE12)	Lacks sensitivity and specificity
Adenocarcinoma differentiation	TTF-1	Preferred
	Napsin-A	Occasionally positivity in TTF-1–negative tumors
	Cytokeratin 7	Not specific

carcinoma"), it must be noted that "large cell carcinoma" is still occasionally applied to TTF-1–positive tumors.[5]

Tissue Sampling

Because "large cell carcinoma" is a diagnosis of exclusion, it should not be made on small biopsy samples, including cell blocks or cytologic preparations. To conserve tissue for molecular studies, the term "non–small cell carcinoma," with modifiers favoring squamous or adenocarcinoma, is preferred, after utilizing only a small panel of immunohistochemical stains (usually TTF-1 and p40; see Chapter 86).

Incidence

The frequency of large cell carcinoma is difficult to determine, as it is based on negativity for TTF-1 and squamous markers. There is variation in published reports regarding the type of squamous marker used (p63, p40, cytokeratin 5/6, desmocollin-3, among others) as well as threshold for positivity. One series of tumor resections found that only 0.4% of lung carcinomas were large cell,[1] which compared to over 9% in a series of microarray samples.[6] Among undifferentiated or poorly differentiated tumors, there is a range of 2% to 31% of tumors that do not show evidence of squamous or adenocarcinoma by immunohistochemical study,[1–3,5–8] again the higher numbers representing series of small tissue samples.

Clinical Findings

Large cell carcinomas are typically peripheral lesions that may present at any stage. Most patients are smokers, and the mean tumor size is 3 cm. Mean age at presentation is 62 years, and there is no gender predilection.[1]

Microscopic Findings

Large cell carcinoma is composed of sheets of cohesive cells that have ample cytoplasm but do not form nests or cords and usually lack palisading or basaloid features (Figs. 82.1 and 82.2). Typically, nuclei show various degrees of anaplasia with nuclear clearing and prominent nucleoli. There may be rhabdoid differentiation (Fig. 82.2). By definition, there are no glandular or cribriform structures; if present to any significant degree in a tumor, then the "large cell" area is considered solid growth of adenocarcinoma. Mucicarmine or PAS stains demonstrate an absence of mucin vacuoles or fewer than 5 in 2 high-powered fields[5] (Fig. 82.3). If there is a basaloid pattern or nests with peripheral palisading, then squamous and neuroendocrine differentiation (respectively) must be especially excluded by immunohistochemical staining (Fig. 82.4). Large cell areas frequently can combine with spindle cell or giant-cell areas, in which case the term "pleomorphic carcinoma" is used (Fig. 82.5).

In the series of Rekhtman et al.,[1] in which resected carcinomas were classified as large cell based on absence of TTF-1 and p40 staining, and lack of endocrine features, 10% had basaloid, rhabdoid, or focal pleomorphic areas (respectively), and 5% clear cell areas.

Immunohistochemical Findings

By definition, large cell carcinoma implies "large cell undifferentiated" carcinoma and is negative for adenocarcinoma and squamous cell markers. This simplest paradigm is to limit immunohistochemical staining to TTF-1 and p40 in solid undifferentiated tumors without glands or mucin vacuoles and assign a diagnosis of large cell carcinoma based on negativity for both markers.[1] A cutoff of 10% for squamous markers and any staining for TTF-1 are often used thresholds for positivity.[1] By expanding staining to a more comprehensive panel, including napsin-A for adenocarcinoma and cytokeratin 5/6, p63, cytokeratin 903 (34βE12), and desmocollin-3 for squamous carcinoma, a smaller proportion of tumors remain that qualify as "large cell carcinoma."[2,3] For example, a diagnosis of large cell carcinoma may

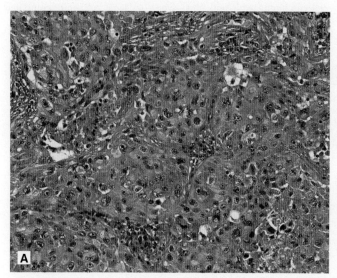
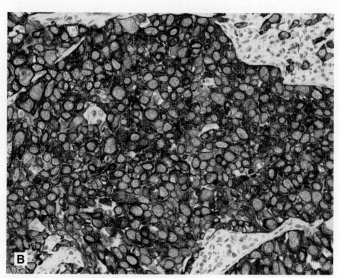

FIGURE 82.1 ▲ Large cell carcinoma. **A.** The tumor is composed of pleomorphic epithelioid cells, which are large, have prominent nucleoli, and are cohesive. **B.** Cytokeratin 7 immunohistochemical stain is positive, which is not considered specific enough for the designation of adenocarcinoma. In this case, immunohistochemical stains for p40, napsin-A, and TTF-1 were negative (not shown).

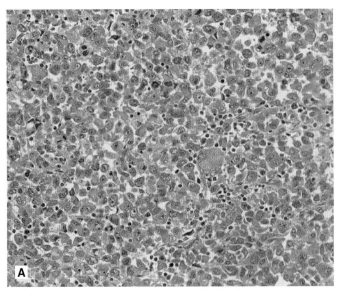
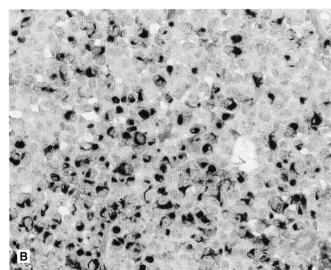

FIGURE 82.2 ▲ Large cell carcinoma. **A.** On routine stains, there are rhabdoid features, characterized by rounded areas of pink cytoplasm. **B.** A cytokeratin 8/18 immunohistochemical stain shows focal positivity. Immunohistochemical stains for TTF-1, p40, and napsin-A were negative (not shown).

been assigned if only one or no squamous marker is positive, focally or weakly, in addition to TTF-1 and napsin-A negativity.[3] Cytokeratin 7 is insufficiently specific for adenocarcinoma, being frequently expressed in nonkeratinizing squamous carcinomas, to be considered an adenocarcinoma marker.[2,3] A large panel is of course not recommended for use in small biopsies, in order to preserve tissue for molecular studies. Although napsin-A is generally positive only in tumors that are TTF-1 positive, there are occasional reports of significant numbers of napsin-A–positive, TTF-1–negative adenocarcinomas.[2,3] Two percent to 5% of undifferentiated tumors coexpress TTF-1 and p40 (Fig. 82.6), in which case, a diagnosis of poorly differentiated adenocarcinoma is favored, based on evaluation of resection specimens.[1,3,9] A similar proportion of undifferentiated adenocarcinomas coexpress TTF-1 and p63 or cytokeratin 5/6.[2] The immunohistochemical profile of poorly differentiated lung carcinomas is in a state of evolution, and the group "large cell" is likely to eventually disappear. Most if not all large cell

carcinomas lacking squamous markers, TTF-1, and napsin-A express cytokeratin 7, suggesting that they lean toward adenocarcinomatous differentiation.[2]

The rate of neuroendocrine marker positivity in large cell undifferentiated carcinoma is unclear, as studies previously included large-cell neuroendocrine carcinoma as a subset of large cell carcinoma. It is not recommended to perform immunohistochemical staining for chromogranin, synaptophysin, and CD56 on undifferentiated carcinomas without endocrine morphology. Rarely, undifferentiated tumors with endocrine features fail to express endocrine markers by immunohistochemistry and are considered large cell (undifferentiated) carcinomas.

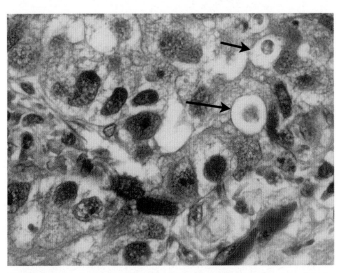

FIGURE 82.3 ▲ Differential diagnosis of large cell carcinoma: Poorly differentiated adenocarcinoma. Mucin vacuoles (*arrows*) can be seen on hematoxylin and eosin. Mucicarmine or PAS diastase (not shown) facilitates their identification.

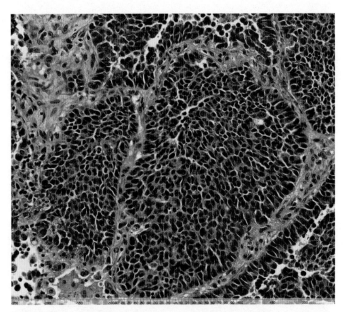

FIGURE 82.4 ▲ Differential diagnosis of small cell carcinoma: Poorly differentiated squamous carcinoma, basaloid type. Nested areas of tumor with peripheral cells having the appearance of basal cells (relatively scant cytoplasm) identify basaloid carcinoma. Confirmation of the diagnosis depends on identification of squamous markers by immunohistochemical staining (not shown).

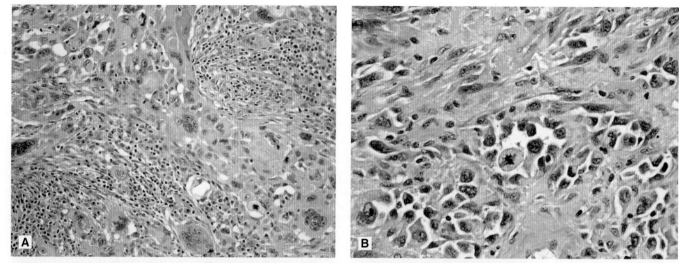

FIGURE 82.5 ▲ Differential diagnosis of large cell carcinoma: Pleomorphic carcinoma. Areas of sarcomatoid pattern often coexist with large cell (undifferentiated) carcinoma. **A.** Areas of tumor giant cells ("giant-cell carcinoma") were present in an otherwise large cell carcinoma (not shown). **B.** The same tumor had areas of spindling with pleomorphic cells.

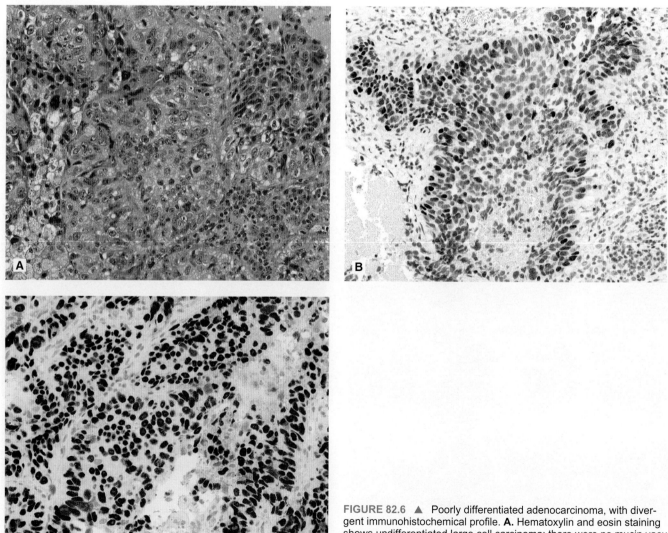

FIGURE 82.6 ▲ Poorly differentiated adenocarcinoma, with divergent immunohistochemical profile. **A.** Hematoxylin and eosin staining shows undifferentiated large cell carcinoma; there were no mucin vacuoles. **B.** TTF-1 immunohistochemical staining is positive in large areas, indicating an adenocarcinoma. **C.** p40 immunohistochemical staining is positive as well; coexpression of these two markers is uncommon.

Molecular Findings

As noted above, histologically undifferentiated carcinomas that express TTF-1 are more likely to harbor *KRAS, ALK, BRAF, EGFR,* and *MAP2K1* mutations than those that express squamous markers and are therefore considered adenocarcinomas.[1] Undifferentiated carcinomas with null phenotype (large cell carcinomas) have been reported to lack known mutations.[6] Rekhtman et al.,[1] in contrast, found mutations in *KRAS* in 25% and for *BRAF* in 5% of large cell (undifferentiated) carcinomas, possibly because their panel of immunohistochemical markers was restricted to only two antibodies.

Differential Diagnosis

In small biopsy samples, the differential diagnosis of carcinomas with equivocal or negative staining for TTF-1 and squamous markers includes both adenocarcinoma and squamous carcinoma, with lack of sampling of more differentiated areas. Studies of resected carcinomas "enriched" for poorly differentiated ones have shown that 98% of squamous carcinomas show >50% staining with p40[10] and that 94% of adenocarcinomas show >50% staining with TTF-1, suggesting that the sampling problem is not significant, especially for squamous carcinomas. However, Barbareschi et al. showed that 3 of 14 resected nonkeratinizing poorly differentiated squamous carcinomas (21%) were only focally positive for p40.[3]

Small cell carcinoma is in the differential diagnosis in small biopsy samples and should be excluded by histologic features and, if necessary, immunohistochemical staining for endocrine markers and Ki 67. Large cell carcinoma is often a component of pleomorphic carcinoma. Basaloid carcinoma is differentiated from large cell (undifferentiated) carcinoma based on presence of squamous differentiated by p40 expression, although occasional basaloid tumors may show divergent expression of endocrine and squamous markers (see Chapter 78). Large-cell neuroendocrine carcinoma is distinguished from large cell undifferentiated carcinoma primarily based on histologic features; on small biopsy samples, immunohistochemical confirmation of endocrine differentiation may be necessary.

Prognosis and Treatment

The prognosis of large cell carcinoma is poor. Rekhtman et al.[1] found a 5-year disease-free and overall survival of only 9% and 12%, respectively.

REFERENCES

1. Rekhtman N, Tafe LJ, Chaft JE, et al. Distinct profile of driver mutations and clinical features in immunomarker-defined subsets of pulmonary large-cell carcinoma. *Mod Pathol.* 2013;26:511–522.
2. Rossi G, Mengoli MC, Cavazza A, et al. Large cell carcinoma of the lung: clinically oriented classification integrating immunohistochemistry and molecular biology. *Virchows Arch.* 2014;464:61–68.
3. Barbareschi M, Cantaloni C, Del Vescovo V, et al. Heterogeneity of large cell carcinoma of the lung: an immunophenotypic and miRNA-based analysis. *Am J Clin Pathol.* 2011;136:773–782.
4. Büttner R, Wolf J, Thomas RK. A genomics-based classification of human lung tumors. *Sci Transl Med.* 2013;5:209ra153.
5. Hwang DH, Szeto DP, Perry AS, et al. Pulmonary large cell carcinoma lacking squamous differentiation is clinicopathologically indistinguishable from solid-subtype adenocarcinoma. *Arch Pathol Lab Med.* 2014;138:626–635.
6. Thunnissen E, Boers E, Heideman DA, et al. Correlation of immunohistochemical staining p63 and TTF-1 with EGFR and K-ras mutational spectrum and diagnostic reproducibility in non small cell lung carcinoma. *Virchows Arch.* 2012;461:629–638.
7. Mukhopadhyay S, Katzenstein AL. Subclassification of non-small cell lung carcinomas lacking morphologic differentiation on biopsy specimens: utility of an immunohistochemical panel containing TTF-1, napsin A, p63, and CK5/6. *Am J Surg Pathol.* 2011;35:15–25.
8. Pardo J, Martinez-Penuela AM, Sola JJ, et al. Large cell carcinoma of the lung: an endangered species? *Appl Immunohistochem Mol Morphol.* 2009;17:383–392.
9. Rekhtman N, Ang DC, Sima CS, et al. Immunohistochemical algorithm for differentiation of lung adenocarcinoma and squamous cell carcinoma based on large series of whole-tissue sections with validation in small specimens. *Mod Pathol.* 2011;24:1348–1359.
10. Bishop JA, Teruya-Feldstein J, Westra WH, et al. p40 (DeltaNp63) is superior to p63 for the diagnosis of pulmonary squamous cell carcinoma. *Mod Pathol.* 2012;25:405–415.

83 Adenosquamous Carcinoma

Marie-Christine Aubry, M.D., and Allen P. Burke, M.D.

General

Adenosquamous carcinoma is composed of an adenocarcinoma and squamous cell carcinoma component comprising at least 10% of the whole tumor.[1-3] Various hypotheses for the pathogenesis of adenosquamous carcinomas include primarily adenocarcinomas with squamous differentiation, collision tumors, a variant of high-grade mucoepidermoid carcinoma, or tumors of pluripotential undifferentiated cell origin.[4]

Adenosquamous carcinomas represent between 1.1% and 2.2% of resected lung cancers.[5-8]

Clinical

There is a male predominance of 2 to 4:1. The mean age at presentation is 60 to 70 years, and about 80% are smokers.[5,7,9] The rate of smoking is lower in patients with a well-differentiated adenocarcinoma component.[10]

Radiologic Findings

Adenosquamous carcinomas form ill-defined (38%), lobulated (32%), or spiculated (19%) masses. Fewer than 10% show ground-glass areas.[8] Pleural indentation indicative of likely pleural invasion is seen in one-third of tumors.[8]

Gross Findings

Adenosquamous carcinomas are generally larger than adenocarcinomas or squamous carcinomas and are solid, irregular masses with variable necrosis.[9] About four of five tumors are peripheral.[11]

Microscopic Findings

Adenosquamous cell carcinoma morphologically shows two distinct cell population. The adenocarcinoma is acinar, papillary, or lepidic or a combination of these, in ~75% of tumors (Fig. 83.1). In about 25% of cases, the adenocarcinoma is solid comprised of only large cells or cribriform. If entirely solid, it is confirmed as adenocarcinoma by immunohistochemical staining for TTF-1.[10] By definition, the squamous component shows keratinization or intercellular bridges.

Adenosquamous carcinomas are more likely than other non–small cell carcinomas to have lymphatic, blood vessel, and visceral pleural invasion (11%, 20%, and 30%, respectively).[9]

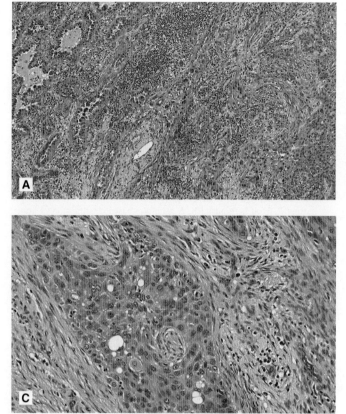

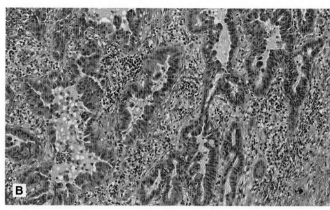

FIGURE 83.1 ▲ Adenosquamous carcinoma. **A.** Low-power photomicrograph showing both the adenocarcinoma and squamous component, which is on the right. **B.** A high magnification of the adeno-carcinoma component shows a well-differentiated carcinoma with an acinar pattern. **C.** The squamous component shows individual cell keratinization and intercellular bridges.

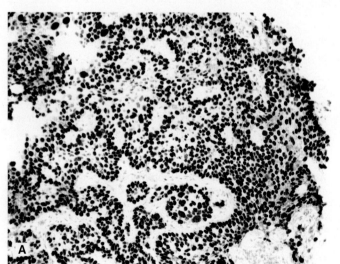

Immunohistochemistry

Immunohistochemistry is not necessary if the two population of cells, adenocarcinoma and squamous cell carcinoma, are morphologically recognizable by regular H&E. But in cases where the adenocarcinoma component is solid and the squamous cell carcinoma nonkeratinizing and higher grade, performing TTF-1 and p40 assists with the diagnosis. As with morphology, the immunoprofile reveals two distinct population of cells, one that is TTF-1 positive and a separate that is p40 positive. Rarely, TTF-1–positive cells may be seen in squamous

cell carcinoma and p40 in adenocarcinoma. This does not constitute an adenosquamous cell carcinoma (Fig. 83.2).

Molecular Findings

Comparative transcriptome analysis has shown that adenosquamous carcinoma is a mix of adeno- and squamous cell carcinoma, but exhibiting molecular specificities in neuroendocrine differentiation and *ERK* proliferation pathways, suggesting a somewhat unique molecular profile.[1] Next-generation sequencing has also shown that expression of

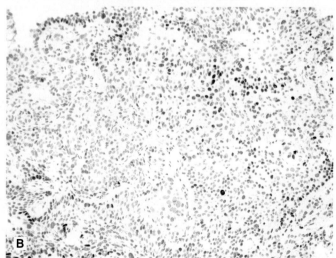

FIGURE 83.2 ▲ Squamous cell carcinoma with focal TTF-1 positivity. **A.** p40 is diffusely positive in all the cells. **B.** TTF-1 is focally positive in both entrapped pneumocytes and rare tumor cells. This represents focal nonspecific staining of TTF-1 in a squamous cell carcinoma and not a distinct component of adenocarcinoma.

classifier miR-205 was intermediate between that of adenocarcinoma and squamous cell carcinoma, indicating a possible transitional stage between these tumor types.[12]

EGFR mutations and mutations in the PI3K signaling pathway are more frequent than expected compared to adenocarcinomas in Caucasians (about 30%), whereas *KRAS* mutations are less frequent.[6,12] In Asians, 22% to 24% of Japanese patients with adenosquamous carcinomas had EGFR mutations, most frequently deletions in exon 19.[7,13] A similar proportion (32%) was found in a study from China.[10] The rate is higher in adenosquamous carcinomas with a well-differentiated adenocarcinoma component, as compared to squamous predominant or tumors with a solid adenocarcinoma component.[10]

Other genomic abnormalities described in adenosquamous carcinomas include RET and ALK rearrangements and mutations in AKT1 and HER2. The rate of RET mutations is higher in those with a solid adenocarcinoma component.[10]

Most studies have not separated the histologic patterns for mutational analysis. Wang et al. showed that most mutations were present in both adeno- and squamous carcinoma areas subjected to microdissection and that in a minority, KRAS, HER2, and EGFR mutations were found only in the adenocarcinoma component.[10]

A case report showed an ALK1 fusion in both the primary adenocarcinoma and metastatic squamous carcinoma in a patient with presumed pulmonary adenosquamous carcinoma.[14]

Differential Diagnosis

The main differential diagnosis is high-grade mucoepidermoid carcinoma (Chapter 84). This differential is typically considered when the TTF-1 is negative in the glandular component. The distinction between a high-grade mucoepidermoid carcinoma and adenosquamous cell carcinoma is not always possible, but the recommended criteria for the diagnosis of mucoepidermoid carcinoma include (1) airway location and endobronchial exophytic component, (2) no squamous carcinoma in situ, (3) lack of individual cell keratinization and squamous pearl formation, and (4) areas of transition from a lower-grade MEC (see Chapter 84).[15] Furthermore, mucoepidermoid carcinoma can be positive for smooth muscle actin and S100 protein, usually negative in non–small cell carcinoma.[16] Also, as in the head and neck, rearrangement of MAML2 by FISH can be detected in pulmonary mucoepidermoid carcinoma.[17]

Entrapped pneumocytes in a squamous cell carcinoma or squamous metaplasia in entrapped small airways of an adenocarcinoma also needs to be differentiated from an adenosquamous cell carcinoma.

In small biopsies, there is always the possibility that one component of the tumor is missed and becomes manifest only on tumor resection or metastasis.[14] Furthermore, it is well documented that a metastasis from an adenosquamous cell carcinoma may be comprised solely of the squamous or adenocarcinoma component.[18]

Prognosis and Treatment

Adenosquamous carcinomas are more aggressive than adenocarcinomas and squamous carcinomas. The reported 5-year survival rates vary widely and range from 15% to 23%[5,19] to between 30% and 54%.[2,7-9]

Favorable prognostic factors include EGFR mutations[7] and lack of expression of PIK3CA and survivin as determined by immunohistochemistry.[20]

REFERENCES

1. Bastide K, Ugolin N, Levalois C, et al. Are adenosquamous lung carcinomas a simple mix of adenocarcinomas and squamous cell carcinomas, or more complex at the molecular level? *Lung Cancer.* 2010;68:1–9.
2. Shimoji M, Nakajima T, Yamatani C, et al. A clinicopathological and immunohistological re-evaluation of adenosquamous carcinoma of the lung. *Pathol Int.* 2011;61:717–722.
3. Yatabe Y, Brambilla E, Rekhtman N, et al. Adenosquamous carcinoma. In: *WHO Classification of Tumours of the Lung, Pleura, Mediastinum and Heart.* Travis WD, et al., eds. Lyon, France: IARC Press; 2015:86–89.
4. Yamatani C, Abe M, Shimoji M, et al. Pulmonary adenosquamous carcinoma with mucoepidermoid carcinoma-like component with characteristic p63 staining pattern: either a novel subtype originating from bronchial epithelium or variant mucoepidermoid carcinoma. *Lung Cancer.* 2014;84: 45–50.
5. Filosso PL, Ruffini E, Asioli S, et al. Adenosquamous lung carcinomas: a histologic subtype with poor prognosis. *Lung Cancer.* 2011;74:25–29.
6. Powrozek T, Krawczyk P, Ramlau R, et al. EGFR gene mutations in patients with adenosquamous lung carcinoma. *Asia Pac J Clin Oncol.* 2014;10:340–345.
7. Shiozawa T, Ishii G, Goto K, et al. Clinicopathological characteristics of EGFR mutated adenosquamous carcinoma of the lung. *Pathol Int.* 2013;63: 77–84.
8. Watanabe Y, Tsuta K, Kusumoto M, et al. Clinicopathologic features and computed tomographic findings of 52 surgically resected adenosquamous carcinomas of the lung. *Ann Thorac Surg.* 2014;97:245–251.
9. Mordant P, Grand B, Cazes A, et al. Adenosquamous carcinoma of the lung: surgical management, pathologic characteristics, and prognostic implications. *Ann Thorac Surg.* 2013;95:1189–1195.
10. Wang R, Pan Y, Li C, et al. Analysis of major known driver mutations and prognosis in resected adenosquamous lung carcinomas. *J Thorac Oncol.* 2014;9:760–768.
11. Lee Y, Chung JH, Kim SE, et al. Adenosquamous carcinoma of the lung: CT, FDG PET, and clinicopathologic findings. *Clin Nucl Med.* 2014;39: 107–112.
12. Vassella E, Langsch S, Dettmer MS, et al. Molecular profiling of lung adenosquamous carcinoma: hybrid or genuine type? *Oncotarget.* 2015;6:23905–23916.
13. Morodomi Y, Okamoto T, Takenoyama M, et al. Clinical significance of detecting somatic gene mutations in surgically resected adenosquamous cell carcinoma of the lung in Japanese patients. *Ann Surg Oncol.* 2015;22(8):2593–2598.
14. Chaft JE, Rekhtman N, Ladanyi M, et al. ALK-rearranged lung cancer: adenosquamous lung cancer masquerading as pure squamous carcinoma. *J Thorac Oncol.* 2012;7:768–769.
15. Yousem SA, Hochholzer L. Mucoepidermoid tumors of the lung. *Cancer.* 1987;60:1346–1352.
16. Moran CA, Suster S. Mucoepidermoid carcinomas of the thymus. A clinicopathologic study of six cases. *Am J Surg Pathol.* 1995;19:826–834.
17. Roden AC, Garcia JJ, Wehrs RN, et al. Histopathologic, immunophenotypic and cytogenetic features of pulmonary mucoepidermoid carcinoma. *Mod Pathol.* 2014;27:1479–1488.
18. Takamori S, Noguchi M, Morinaga S, et al. Clinicopathologic characteristics of adenosquamous carcinoma of the lung. *Cancer.* 1991;67:649–654.
19. Maeda H, Matsumura A, Kawabata T, et al. Adenosquamous carcinoma of the lung: surgical results as compared with squamous cell and adenocarcinoma cases. *Eur J Cardiothorac Surg.* 2012;41:357–361.
20. Yu S, Zhang Z, Zhang B, et al. Clinical significance of PIK3CA and survivin in primary adenosquamous lung carcinoma. *Med Oncol.* 2014;31:983.

84 Salivary Gland–Type Tumors of the Lung

Marie-Christine Aubry, M.D., and Allen P. Burke, M.D.

General

Salivary gland–type tumors of the lung are rare tumors with a reported frequency of 0.1% to 0.2% of all primary lung tumors. They are thought to arise from the submucosal glands of the bronchi and are morphologically identical to their salivary gland counterparts. Mucoepidermoid carcinoma (MEC) and adenoid cystic carcinoma (ACC) are the most common type of salivary gland–type tumors of the lung,[1–3] followed by epithelial–myoepithelial carcinoma (EMC).[1,4–6] Pleomorphic adenoma, carcinoma ex pleomorphic adenoma, and acinic cell carcinoma have also rarely been described.[7,8]

Salivary gland–type tumors usually occur in adults, in their fourth to sixth decade, but they are also reported in children, particularly MEC.[1,4,9,10] There is no gender predilection.[1,4,9,10] Causal relationship with cigarette smoking is controversial, but in one series, nearly half of patients with MEC and 70% of patients with ACC were former or current smokers.[1] Because of their location, patients often present with symptoms of airway involvement and obstruction such as cough, hemoptysis, wheezing, and obstructive pneumonia.[1,3,9–11]

These tumors typically arise in the tracheobronchial tree, forming central endobronchial polypoid tumors[1,12] (Fig. 84.1). Size is variable, ranging between 0.5 and 6.0 cm. These tumors are usually well circumscribed with smooth contours. On cut section, the tumors are gray–white, tan, and variably solid–cystic. MEC and pleomorphic adenoma often appear mucoid. These tumors are readily identified on CT scan as endobronchial masses but can also manifest as circumferential thickening of the airway or thick-walled cyst[13] (Fig. 84.1). Obstructive pneumonia or atelectasis is a common finding, seen in up to 50% of patients.[13,14] Punctate calcifications and secondary localized bronchiectasis are additional findings.[13,14] These tumors are usually PET avid, and thus, PET/CT is useful for detection of metastasis.[13,15,16]

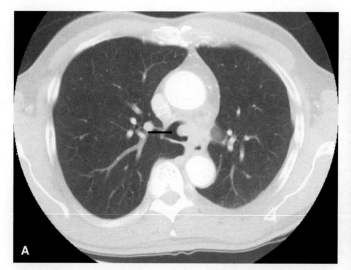

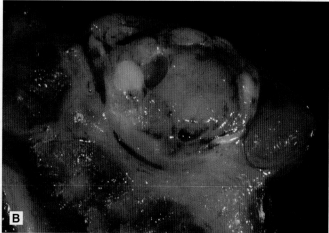

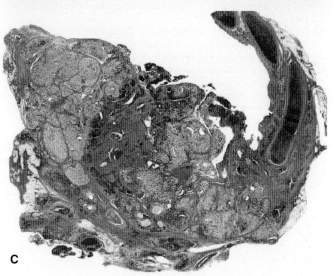

FIGURE 84.1 ▲ A. Chest tomography of adenoid cystic carcinoma (ACC) showing a polypoid mass arising in the lower trachea (*black arrow*). B. Gross photograph of an ACC forming an endobronchial mass occluding the lumen. C. Lowest histologic magnification showing involvement of the lumen and bronchial wall by the ACC.

Distinguishing primary salivary gland–type tumors of the lung from primary salivary gland metastasis is important as lung is a favored site of metastasis for these tumors and can occur many years after the initial diagnosis. The presence of peripheral or multiple nodules should lead to a thorough search for a primary salivary gland tumor.

Surgery is the treatment of choice, usually lobectomy, followed by tracheal or sleeve resection based on the airway involved.[1,3,4,10] Lymph node sampling is recommended for high-grade MEC and ACC. As in the salivary glands, ACC often tracks along nerve bundles, and resection margins are not uncommonly positive.[1,3,4] Adjuvant chemotherapy or radiation may be offered for incompletely resected or advanced-stage disease.[4,9,17] There are rare case reports of EGFR TKI response in MEC.[18,19] KIT kinase inhibitor, imatinib, has been used in the treatment of ACC with rare reports of moderate sustained response.[20]

Mucoepidermoid Carcinoma

Clinical

MEC tends to occur at a younger age compared to other salivary gland–type tumors and low-grade MEC occurring in younger patients compared to high-grade MEC.[4,9,10] MEC rarely presents with locoregional lymph node involvement or distant metastasis, usually seen in high-grade tumors (2% to 15%).[1,3,4] Long-term survival for MEC is good, with reported 3-year survival of 94% and 5 and 10 years of 87%, although reported survival for high-grade MEC, more advanced stage, or incompletely resected is lower (66% at 4 years).[1,9,10]

Pathologic Findings

Histologically, MEC is defined by the presence of mucous cells admixed with squamous-, clear-, and intermediate-type cells in various proportions[9,12] (Fig. 84.2). The intermediate cells are often predominant and range in size from small basaloid in appearance to larger polygonal cells with more abundant eosinophilic cytoplasm. The mucous cells by definition contain intracytoplasmic mucin, which may occasionally be only appreciated with a mucin stain and may line cystic glands. The squamous cells can be single or form small nests, and typically nonkeratinizing. In some cases, oncocytic cells may predominate.[9] Occasionally, the stroma may be dense, hyalinized, and amyloid like with calcifications.[9,12]

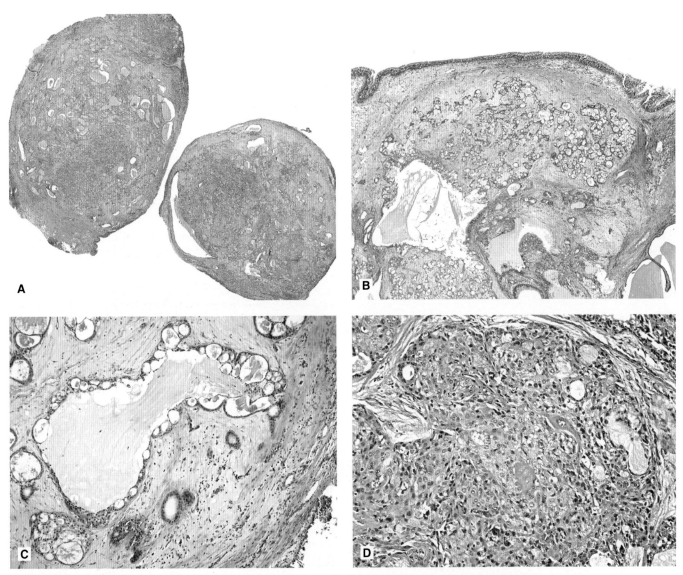

FIGURE 84.2 ▲ A. Lowest magnification shows circumscribed growth. B. Low-grade mucoepidermoid carcinoma growing under the bronchial wall mucosa and demonstrating a cystic glandular pattern. C. The tumor is mostly comprised of mucous cells forming small glands or lining large mucinous cysts. D. Area of squamous-type cells admixed with the mucous cells.

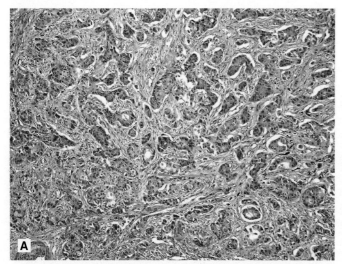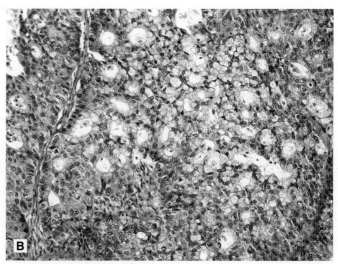

FIGURE 84.3 ▲ **A.** High-grade mucoepidermoid carcinoma showing invasive glandular proliferation with increased cell atypia. **B.** The mucous cells admixed with intermediate cells form solid nests.

Although different grading systems have been applied to pulmonary MEC, MEC is generally classified as low and high grade. Low-grade MEC is characterized by a dominant, cystic glandular component with near absent atypia and mitosis[1,9] (Fig. 84.2). Occasionally, the tumor may exhibit papillary architecture.[9] Although high-grade MEC may share architectural similarities with low-grade MEC, they are more often comprised of solid intermediate and epidermoid cells with significant cell atypia and increased mitotic activity[9] (Fig. 84.3). A mucin stain, such as mucicarmine or periodic acid–Schiff stains, may be helpful in cases where the mucinous/glandular component is inconspicuous.[12]

Differential Diagnosis

Low-grade MEC can be confused with mucous gland adenoma, especially in a small biopsy, and will be distinguished by the presence of intermediate and squamous cells.

Immunohistochemistry may be useful in the differential diagnosis of primary pulmonary adenocarcinoma (Table 84.1). MEC is negative for TTF-1[21] and should show areas of squamous differentiation. More importantly, high-grade MEC needs to be distinguished from adenosquamous carcinoma. Recommended criteria for diagnosing MEC in this context are (1) airway location and endobronchial exophytic component, (2) no squamous carcinoma in situ, (3) lack of individual cell keratinization and squamous pearl formation, and (4) areas of transition from a lower-grade MEC.[9] MEC is variably positive for smooth muscle actin and S100 protein, usually negative in non–small cell carcinoma.[12]

Genetics

Reciprocal translocations including t(11;19)(q14-21;p12) and t(11;19)(q21;p13), identical to those described in MEC of salivary gland tumors, are present in pulmonary MEC.[22] The t(11;19)(q21;p13) encodes for a fusion product MEC translocated 1 mastermind-like 2 (*MECT1–MAML2*) detectable by FISH.[3,23] Another translocation involving chromosome 11 has been reported, t(1;11)(p22;q13), associated with overexpression of cyclin D1.[24] Although not entirely sensitive (reported in 38% to 81% of salivary MEC), these translocations are specific enough to assist with the differential diagnosis.[3,23,25]

In most series, epidermal growth factor receptor (EGFR) mutations are considered nonexistent or extremely rare in MEC.[10,25–27] However, in one series, two of five pulmonary MEC showed a mutation in exon 21 (L858R),[18] predictive of response to EGFR tyrosine kinase inhibitor, while in another series, mutation in exon 21 (L861Q) was found in 25% of studied tumors.[28] Interestingly, there are case reports of MEC showing tyrosine kinase inhibitor response even in the absence of any EGFR mutation.[18,19] The proposed mechanism for these cases is the presence of *MECT1–MAML2*, which may confer susceptibility to tyrosine kinase inhibitor response.[29]

Adenoid Cystic Carcinoma

Clinical

ACC usually presents at a higher stage than MEC and more likely to develop distant metastasis.[1,3] ACC also has a worse prognosis similar to other non–small cell carcinomas, with reported 3-, 5-, and 10-year survival rates of 82%, 70% to 84%, and 63% to 70%.[1,30] The factors that are prognostic and influence survival include tumor size, tumor site, surgical treatment, and positive margins.[1,30] Indeed, tumors > 4 cm, located in the trachea, have worse outcome.[30] Importantly, the complete surgical resection of ACC offers the best chances at survival[1,30] with 5-year survival of resected tumors of up to 100% versus 54% without surgery.[1,30]

Pathologic Findings

As in the salivary gland, ACC of the lung shows all three typical growth patterns: tubular, cribriform, and solid (Fig. 84.4). In the lung, ACC is

TABLE 84.1   Distinguishing Features Between High-Grade Mucoepidermoid Carcinoma and Adenosquamous Carcinoma of the Lung

	Mucoepidermoid Carcinoma	Adenosquamous Carcinoma
Location	Exophytic, endobronchial, or endotracheal	Parenchymal
Squamous carcinoma—in situ	Absent	May be present
Individual cell keratinization and squamous pearls	Absent	Present in squamous areas with distinct separation from adeno-carcinoma areas
Areas of low-grade mucoepidermoid carcinoma	May be present	Absent
TTF-1 expression	Absent	Often present in glandular areas
S100 and smooth muscle actin expression	Usually present	Usually absent

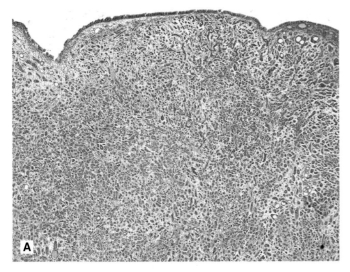

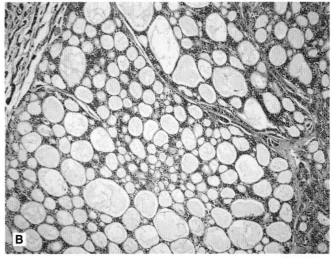

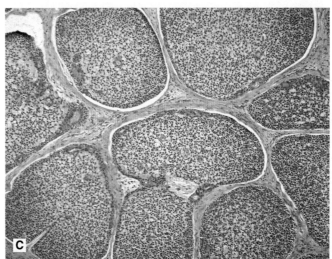

FIGURE 84.4 ▲ Adenoid cystic carcinoma displays three typical growth pattern. **A.** Tubular. **B.** Cribriform. **C.** Solid.

most commonly cribriform.[20,31,32] The tumor cells form nests with sharply outlined lumens containing dense hyaline material (Fig. 84.5). The periphery of the nests often displays prominent palisading. The cells are small, with scant amphophilic cytoplasm and the nuclei are round and vesicular. The solid pattern is similar except with the absence of the lumens.

Tubular ACC is characterized by gland-like structures, lined by a ductal cell layer surrounded by myoepithelial cells (Fig. 84.6). Perineural invasion is common (Fig. 84.5). By immunohistochemistry, the ductal cells express keratin, CEA, and EMA. The myoepithelial cells will express keratin, S100 protein, smooth muscle actin, calponin, and p63[31,32] (Fig. 84.6).

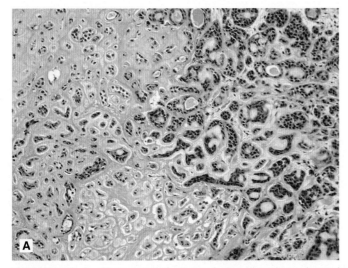

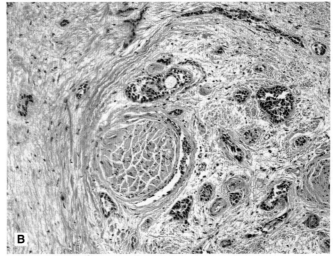

FIGURE 84.5 ▲ Characteristic features of adenoid cystic carcinoma include (**A**) dense basal membrane-like stroma in which the nests of cells are embedded and (**B**) perineural invasion.

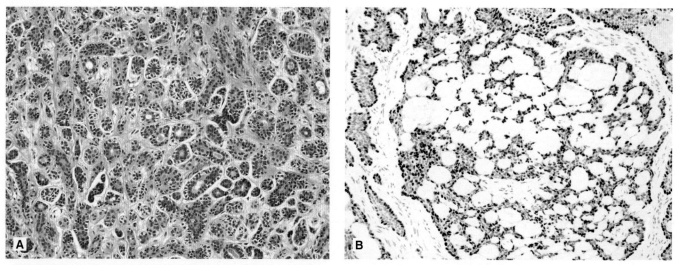

FIGURE 84.6 ▲ **A.** Tubules lined by ductal cells surrounded by myoepithelial cells. **B.** The myoepithelial cells are positive for p63 (anti-p63).

In contrast to PA, GFAP is usually negative.[31] ACC of the lung commonly expresses c-kit, but no mutations have been identified.[20] Expression of c-kit is not specific to ACC of the lung as it is commonly expressed in small cell lung carcinoma and also reportedly positive in EMC.

Epithelial–Myoepithelial Carcinoma

Clinical

EMC has also been called adenomyoepithelioma of the lung. The term "myoepithelial carcinoma" should be reserved for monophasic tumor. Locoregional disease almost never occurs with a single report of lymph node (N1) metastasis.[6] Disease-free survival is not clearly known because the majority of series have only short follow-up with often < 3 years with no report of recurrence or distant metastasis.[1,4–6] However, in one recent series of seven EMC, one recurrence was documented with the OS and DFS of 3 and 5 years reported as 100% and 85.7%.[3]

Pathologic Findings

EMC are typically well circumscribed with pushing margins. They are comprised of bilayered tubules admixed with a solid cellular

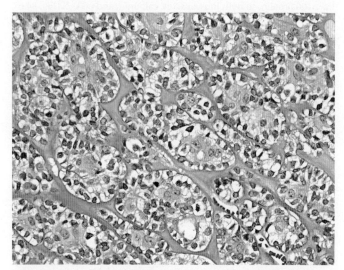

FIGURE 84.7 ▲ Epithelial–myoepithelial carcinoma. The outer myoepithelial cells are characterized by clear cytoplasm with dark nuclei. The epithelial cells are larger, containing abundant eosinophilic cytoplasm. There is no significant cell atypia or mitosis.

proliferation in variable proportions.[6] The tubules are lined by an inner epithelial cell layer, which is cuboidal with eosinophilic cytoplasm and centrally located nuclei. The outer layer is myoepithelial often with abundant clear cytoplasm (Fig. 84.7). The solid component may be comprised of spindle cells forming fascicles or sheets of clear cells embedded in a hyaline stroma. The cells lack cytologic atypia and mitoses are rare.[6] By immunohistochemistry, the tubules have an inner epithelial layer, which is positive for keratins and epithelial membrane antigen, and an outer myoepithelial layer, which is positive for S100 protein, smooth muscle actin, calponin, and p63.[6] The spindle or clear cells of a solid proliferation are also myoepithelial with similar immunoprofile. TTF-1 is generally reported as negative in the ductal epithelial cells although there is a report of TTF-1 expression in these cells.[33] c-Kit expression has also been reported.[34]

Differential Diagnosis

EMC may be confused with other salivary gland–type tumors such as PA and ACC. PAs also have ducts and a myoepithelial cell proliferation, but in contrast to EMC, PA contains a chondroid or myxochondroid stroma.[6] The tubular pattern of ACC can be confused with EMC, but ACC typically is infiltrative with perineural invasion and a more classic cribriform architecture is often present. Tumors with abundant clear cells such as clear cell tumor of the lung or clear cell carcinoma of the lung or kidney enter the differential diagnosis. Clear cell tumor of the lung stains for HMB45 and melan-A and clear cell carcinomas of the lung or kidney typically do not exhibit myoepithelial differentiation.[6]

Pleomorphic Adenoma and Carcinoma Ex Pleomorphic Adenoma

In the lung, pleomorphic adenoma and carcinoma ex pleomorphic adenoma are extremely rare with fewer than 20 cases reported. As with primary salivary gland pleomorphic adenomas, pulmonary tumors have a mixed morphology but differ histologically by rarely displaying cartilage.[31] Furthermore, the epithelial component is less ductal and more solid and myoepithelial, resembling cellular pleomorphic adenoma.[31] Immunophenotypically, the tumor cells express keratin, S100 protein, smooth muscle actin, and GFAP, the latter being useful in distinguishing pleomorphic adenoma from more common salivary gland tumors such as ACC.[7] Histologic criteria for carcinoma ex-PA of the lung have been better defined in a recent small series of five cases.[8] In all cases, focal benign pleomorphic adenoma could be identified. In contrast to primary salivary gland carcinoma ex pleomorphic adenoma, the malignant component shows predominantly myoepithelial differentiation and not adenocarcinoma or salivary duct carcinoma. In contrast to pleomorphic adenoma, carcinoma ex pleomorphic adenoma appears more infiltrative and displays necrosis and increased mitotic activity.[7] Furthermore, these tumors have been shown to have a more aggressive clinical behavior with patients having died due to disease.[8]

Acinic Cell Carcinoma

Acinic cell carcinoma of the lung is exceedingly rare. Unlike other salivary gland tumors, there is no invariable association with a proximal bronchus.[35] Acinic cell carcinoma is a low-grade malignancy rarely presenting with lymph node metastasis and with a single reported case of recurrence following surgical resection.[35–37] Histologically, acinic cell carcinomas are comprised of solid nests or sheets of cells, with occasionally acinar or microcystic architecture. The cells are polygonal with an abundant granular basophilic to clear cytoplasm that is PAS positive.[35,36] The nuclei are often eccentric and hyperchromatic. By immunohistochemistry, the tumor cells are positive for CAM5.2 and EMA.[35] The main differential diagnosis is with carcinoid tumor and clear cell tumor of the lung. In contrast to carcinoid tumors, acinic cell carcinomas are negative for chromogranin and synaptophysin. Similar to clear cell tumors of the lung, acinic cell carcinomas are positive for PAS, but in contrast, they are negative for HMB45 and positive for pan-cytokeratin.[36]

Practical Points

▶ Salivary gland–type tumors of the lung are rare and metastasis from a primary salivary gland should be considered and ruled out.

▶ Salivary gland–type tumors of the lung can occur at any age and usually present with symptoms of obstruction due to its endobronchial growth in large airways.

▶ MECs and ACCs are the two most common types of salivary gland tumors.

▶ Salivary gland–type tumors of the lung are morphologically, immunophenotypically, and cytogenetically similar to their salivary gland counterparts.

REFERENCES

1. Molina JR, Aubry MC, Lewis JE, et al. Primary salivary gland-type lung cancer: spectrum of clinical presentation, histopathologic and prognostic factors. *Cancer.* 2007;110:2253–2259.
2. Wu J, Zhao SH, Guo AT, et al. CT characteristics of primary salivary gland-type lung cancer. *Zhonghua Zhong Liu Za Zhi.* 2011;33:313–315.
3. Zhu F, Liu Z, Hou Y, et al. Primary salivary gland-type lung cancer: clinicopathological analysis of 88 cases from China. *J Thorac Oncol.* 2013;8:1578–1584.
4. Kang DY, Yoon YS, Kim HK, et al. Primary salivary gland-type lung cancer: surgical outcomes. *Lung Cancer.* 2011;72:250–254.
5. Doganay L, Bilgi S, Ozdil A, et al. Epithelial–myoepithelial carcinoma of the lung. A case report and review of the literature. *Arch Pathol Lab Med.* 2003;127:e177–e180.
6. Nguyen CV, Suster S, Moran CA. Pulmonary epithelial–myoepithelial carcinoma: a clinicopathologic and immunohistochemical study of 5 cases. *Hum Pathol.* 2009;40:366–373.
7. Moran CA, Suster S, Askin FB, et al. Benign and malignant salivary gland-type mixed tumors of the lung. Clinicopathologic and immunohistochemical study of eight cases. *Cancer.* 1994;73:2481–2490.
8. Weissferdt A, Moran CA. Pulmonary salivary gland-type tumors with features of malignant mixed tumor (carcinoma ex pleomorphic adenoma): a clinicopathologic study of five cases. *Am J Clin Pathol.* 2011;136:793–798.
9. Yousem SA, Hochholzer L. Mucoepidermoid tumors of the lung. *Cancer.* 1987;60:1346–1352.
10. Xi JJ, Jiang W, Lu SH, et al. Primary pulmonary mucoepidermoid carcinoma: an analysis of 21 cases. *World J Surg Oncol.* 2012;10:232.
11. Li N, Xu L, Zhao H, et al. A comparison of the demographics, clinical features, and survival of patients with adenoid cystic carcinoma of major and minor salivary glands versus less common sites within the Surveillance, Epidemiology, and End Results registry. *Cancer.* 2012;118:3945–3953.
12. Moran CA. Primary salivary gland-type tumors of the lung. *Semin Diagn Pathol.* 1995;12:106–122.
13. Li X, Zhang W, Wu X, et al. Mucoepidermoid carcinoma of the lung: common findings and unusual appearances on CT. *Clin Imaging.* 2012;36:8–13.
14. Kim TS, Lee KS, Han J, et al. Mucoepidermoid carcinoma of the tracheobronchial tree: radiographic and CT findings in 12 patients. *Radiology.* 1999;212:643–648.
15. Ishizumi T, Tateishi U, Watanabe S, et al. F-18 FDG PET/CT imaging of low-grade mucoepidermoid carcinoma of the bronchus. *Ann Nucl Med.* 2007;21:299–302.
16. Elnayal A, Moran CA, Fox PS, et al. Primary salivary gland-type lung cancer: imaging and clinical predictors of outcome. *AJR Am J Roentgenol.* 2013;201:W57–W63.
17. Kanematsu T, Yohena T, Uehara T, et al. Treatment outcome of resected and nonresected primary adenoid cystic carcinoma of the lung. *Ann Thorac Cardiovasc Surg.* 2002;8:74–77.
18. Han SW, Kim HP, Jeon YK, et al. Mucoepidermoid carcinoma of lung: potential target of EGFR-directed treatment. *Lung Cancer.* 2008;61:30–34.
19. Rossi G, Sartori G, Cavazza A, et al. Mucoepidermoid carcinoma of the lung, response to EGFR inhibitors, EGFR and K-RAS mutations, and differential diagnosis. *Lung Cancer.* 2009;63:159–160.
20. Aubry MC, Heinrich MC, Molina J, et al. Primary adenoid cystic carcinoma of the lung: absence of KIT mutations. *Cancer.* 2007;110:2507–2510.
21. Shilo K, Foss RD, Franks TJ, et al. Pulmonary mucoepidermoid carcinoma with prominent tumor-associated lymphoid proliferation. *Am J Surg Pathol.* 2005;29:407–411.
22. Johansson M, Mandahl N, Johansson L, et al. Translocation 11;19 in a mucoepidermoid tumor of the lung. *Cancer Genet Cytogenet.* 1995;80:85–86.
23. Duarte-Achcar R, Nikiforova MN, Dacic S, et al. Mammalian mastermind like 2 11q21 gene rearrangement in bronchopulmonary mucoepidermoid carcinoma. *Hum Pathol.* 2009;40:854–860.
24. Barrett W, Heaps LS, Diaz S, et al. Mucoepidermoid carcinoma of the bronchus in a 15-year-old girl with complex cytogenetic rearrangement involving 11q and over-expression of cyclin D1. *Med Pediatr Oncol.* 2002;39:49–51.
25. Clauditz TS, Gontarewicz A, Wang CJ, et al. 11q21 rearrangement is a frequent and highly specific genetic alteration in mucoepidermoid carcinoma. *Diagn Mol Pathol.* 2012;21:134–137.
26. Dahse R, Driemel O, Schwarz S, et al. Epidermal growth factor receptor kinase domain mutations are rare in salivary gland carcinomas. *Br J Cancer.* 2009;100:623–625.
27. Macarenco RS, Uphoff TS, Gilmer HF, et al. Salivary gland-type lung carcinomas: an EGFR immunohistochemical, molecular genetic, and mutational analysis study. *Mod Pathol.* 2008;21:1168–1175.
28. Yu Y, Song Z, Gao H, et al. EGFR L861Q mutation is a frequent feature of pulmonary mucoepidermoid carcinoma. *J Cancer Res Clin Oncol.* 2012;138:1421–1425.
29. O'Neill ID. t(11;19) translocation and CRTC1–MAML2 fusion oncogene in mucoepidermoid carcinoma. *Oral Oncol.* 2009;45:2–9.
30. Lee JH, Jung EJ, Jeon K, et al. Treatment outcomes of patients with adenoid cystic carcinoma of the airway. *Lung Cancer.* 2011;72:244–249.
31. Moran CA, Suster S, Koss MN. Primary adenoid cystic carcinoma of the lung. A clinicopathologic and immunohistochemical study of 16 cases. *Cancer.* 1994;73:1390–1397.
32. Albers E, Lawrie T, Harrell JH, et al. Tracheobronchial adenoid cystic carcinoma: a clinicopathologic study of 14 cases. *Chest.* 2004;125:1160–1165.
33. Munoz G, Felipo F, Marquina I, et al. Epithelial–myoepithelial tumour of the lung: a case report referring to its molecular histogenesis. *Diagn Pathol.* 2011;6:71.
34. Ru K, Srivastava A, Tischler AS. Bronchial epithelial–myoepithelial carcinoma. *Arch Pathol Lab Med.* 2004;128:92–94.
35. Moran CA, Suster S, Koss MN. Acinic cell carcinoma of the lung ("Fechner tumor"). A clinicopathologic, immunohistochemical, and ultrastructural study of five cases. *Am J Surg Pathol.* 1992;16:1039–1050.
36. Lee HY, Mancer K, Koong HN. Primary acinic cell carcinoma of the lung with lymph node metastasis. *Arch Pathol Lab Med.* 2003;127:e216–e219.
37. Chuah KL, Yap WM, Tan HW, et al. Recurrence of pulmonary acinic cell carcinoma. *Arch Pathol Lab Med.* 2006;130:932–933.

85 Sarcomatoid Carcinoma

Fabio R. Tavora, M.D., Ph.D., Marie-Christine Aubry, M.D., and Allen P. Burke, M.D.

Terminology

Sarcomatoid carcinoma of the lung designates a poorly differentiated and aggressive neoplasm with both carcinoma and mesenchymal differentiation. The epithelial component can be adenocarcinoma, squamous cell carcinoma, or undifferentiated non–small cell carcinoma (i.e., large cell carcinoma). The mesenchymal component is characterized morphologically by spindle cell, giant cell, or sarcoma with heterologous elements such as rhabdomyosarcoma, chondrosarcoma, and osteosarcoma.

If the mesenchymal component is either spindle cell or giant cell, the tumor is designated as pleomorphic carcinoma, while tumors with chondro-, osteo-, or rhabdomyosarcomatous elements are called carcinosarcomas. If a tumor is composed almost entirely by spindle cell or giant cell with no differentiated carcinomatous components, the tumors can be classified as spindle cell carcinoma and giant-cell carcinoma, respectively.

Small cell and large-cell neuroendocrine carcinomas with undifferentiated spindled areas are extremely rare.[1,2]

The 2015 WHO classification of lung tumors recommends that at least 10% of each component (epithelial and mesenchymal) should be present in order to make the diagnosis.[3]

A third subtype of sarcomatoid carcinoma is pulmonary blastoma, defined as a biphasic tumor with components of fetal adenocarcinoma and primitive mesenchymal stroma. Pleuropulmonary blastoma is covered in Chapter 96 and fetal adenocarcinoma in Chapter 77.

Although debated over years, it is now accepted that sarcomatoid carcinomas, including carcinosarcoma, are clonal tumors arising from an epithelial origin.[4,5]

Incidence

Approximately 0.5% of lung tumors are sarcomatoid carcinomas and, of those, only about 5% are carcinosarcomas.[6–15] Pulmonary blastomas are even less common, accounting for <0.1% of lung tumors.[3,16]

Clinical Presentation

Sarcomatoid carcinomas occur in an older population compared to other conventional non–small cell carcinomas, mainly male smokers.[6,9,15,17] Symptoms are similar to other tumors and include cough, hemoptysis, and thoracic pain. The clinical behavior of these tumors is aggressive with a short overall survival rate, even for early-stage tumors, and a high rate of regional and distant metastases.[6,9,15,18] Metastases to unusual sites such as the small intestine have been reported.[19]

Patients with pulmonary blastomas are typically adults, with an average age of 40.[20] Over 80% of patients have a smoking history. They usually present as a large chest mass causing pain, hemoptysis, cough, and dyspnea. The tumor may be an incidental finding in up to 40% of patients.[21]

Pulmonary blastomas are quite aggressive and often metastasize to the central nervous system, as well as unusual locations, such as spleen and axilla.[22–24] Mean survival is 33 months, with a poor response to chemotherapeutic agents.[20]

Radiologic Findings

Sarcomatoid carcinomas have a predilection for the upper lobes, the majority being peripheral.[7,9,17] Tumors are usually large (more than 5 cm). Some studies suggest a high frequency of pleural involvement and chest wall invasion. The CT scan features are not different from other non–small cell carcinomas. Sarcomatoid carcinomas form nodular masses, lobulated or spiculated, and frequently contain central necrosis. Peritumoral areas of ground-glass attenuation are common.[7]

The location of the tumor seems to be dictated by the epithelial component with adenocarcinomas with giant or spindle cell more commonly in the periphery and squamous cell carcinomas with spindle cell with the predilection of a central location. Because carcinosarcomas are more commonly associated with squamous or adenosquamous carcinomas, these lesions are more common centrally. Tumors with large cell carcinoma component also tend to be peripheral with associated tumor necrosis.

Microscopic Findings (Table 85.1)

Pleomorphic, Spindle Cell, and Giant-Cell Carcinomas

The epithelial component is most commonly adenocarcinoma (30% to 70%), followed by squamous cell carcinoma (10% to 25%) and large cell carcinoma (40%) (Figs. 85.1 and 85.2).[3] The epithelial component can be admixed with the sarcomatous elements or be sharply demarcated from those. Carcinomas may be composed

TABLE 85.1   Morphologic Features Sarcomatoid Carcinoma Subtypes

Histologic Type	Epithelial Component	Mesenchymal Component	Immunohistochemistry
Pleomorphic carcinoma	Adenocarcinoma, squamous cell carcinoma, large cell carcinoma, and adenosquamous carcinoma	Spindle cell or giant cell with at least 10% of the tumor	CK, EMA, and CEA + Vimentin + Actin +/– TTF-1 +/–
Spindle cell carcinoma	No distinct epithelial component	Spindle cell	CK, EMA, and CEA +/– Vimentin + Actin + TTF-1 –/+
Giant-cell carcinoma	No distinct epithelial component	Giant cell	CK, EMA, and CEA +/– Vimentin + Actin + TTF-1 –

TABLE 85.1 Morphologic Features Sarcomatoid Carcinoma Subtypes (continued)

Histologic Type	Epithelial Component	Mesenchymal Component	Immunohistochemistry
Carcinosarcoma	Adenocarcinoma, squamous cell carcinoma, large cell carcinoma, and adenosquamous carcinoma	Rhabdomyosarcoma, osteosarcoma, chondrosarcoma, and liposarcoma	CK, EMA, and CEA +/– Vimentin + Actin +/– TTF-1 – Desmin + in rhabdomyosarcoma S100 + in chondrosarcoma
Pulmonary blastoma	Fetal adenocarcinoma usually with low-grade features	Primitive mesenchymal stroma with occasional rhabdomyosarcomatous or osteosarcomatous differentiation	CK, EMA, and CEA +/– Vimentin + Actin + TTF-1 + Chromogranin + Desmin + in rhabdomyosarcoma S100 + in chondrosarcoma β-catenin +

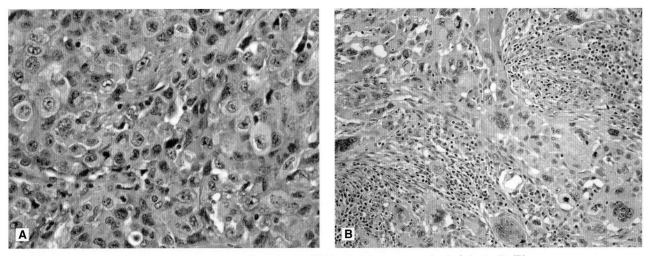

FIGURE 85.1 ▲ Pleomorphic carcinoma. Large cell carcinoma **(A)** blends into area comprised of giant cells **(B)**.

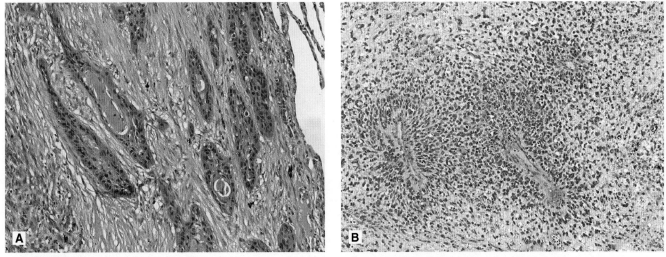

FIGURE 85.2 ▲ Pleomorphic carcinoma. Squamous cell carcinoma **(A)** and sarcomatoid blastoma-like cells **(B)**.

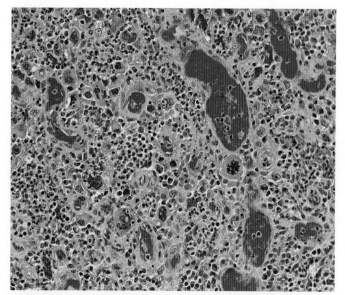

FIGURE 85.3 ▲ Giant-cell carcinoma. All the sampled tissue of this tumor showed pleomorphic cells with abundant giant cells. Emperipolesis of neutrophils is present.

entirely of spindle cells or bizarre multinucleated cells (Figs. 85.3 and 85.4). Malignant spindle cells and giant cells present in a morphologic continuum with undifferentiated epithelial cells arranged in solid sheets, in fascicles, or in a storiform pattern. Emperipolesis of leukocytes is common within malignant giant cells. The stroma is desmoplastic, myxoid, or fibrous. Vascular invasion is very common.

Carcinosarcomas

Carcinosarcomas are tumors with a mixture of non–small cell carcinoma with sarcoma containing heterologous elements, namely, malignant bone (osteosarcoma), cartilage (chondrosarcoma) (Fig. 85.5), or malignant skeletal muscle (rhabdomyosarcoma). Different from pleomorphic carcinomas, the epithelial component of carcinosarcomas is most commonly squamous cell carcinomas (46%) followed by adenocarcinomas (31%) and adenosquamous carcinoma (19%). Areas of undifferentiated non–small cell carcinoma are common. The sarcoma component is most commonly rhabdomyosarcoma, followed by osteosarcoma admixed

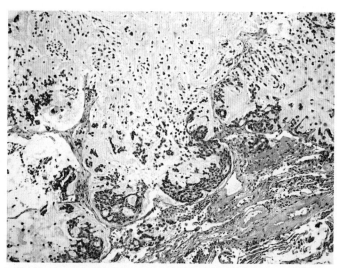

FIGURE 85.5 ▲ Carcinosarcoma comprised of an adenocarcinoma and chondrosarcoma.

with chondrosarcoma, and solely osteosarcoma.[18] Rare cases of liposarcoma or angiosarcoma components have been reported.[16,17] The pathology report should list all components present.

Pulmonary Blastoma

Classic pulmonary blastomas are biphasic tumors composed of a primitive epithelial component—fetal adenocarcinoma—that is usually low grade in appearance, and primitive mesenchymal stroma. The latter may contain foci of rhabdomyosarcoma, osteosarcoma, and chondrosarcoma as well.

Histologically, the fetal adenocarcinoma component is characterized by tubules lined by pseudostratified columnar cells with round bland nuclei and abundant clear cytoplasm, which resemble airway epithelia in fetal lungs (see Chapter 77) (Fig. 85.6). In some areas, the carcinoma may show high-grade features mimicking acinar adenocarcinoma. Morules and clusters of neuroendocrine cells are common. The mesenchymal component is composed of oval cells with high nuclear/cytoplasmic ratio with a myxoid background. Rare unusual components including teratoma, seminoma, embryonal carcinoma, and melanoma have all been described within pulmonary blastomas.

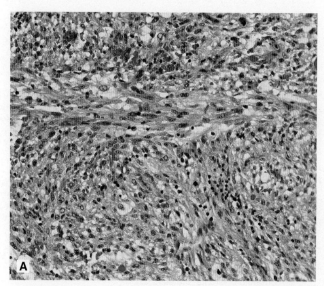
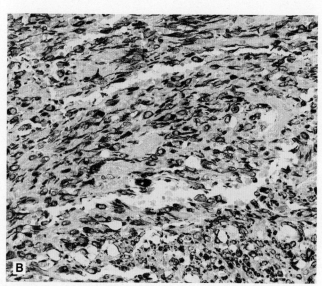

FIGURE 85.4 ▲ Spindle cell carcinoma. **A.** The tumor is entirely comprised of malignant spindle cells. **B.** Immunohistochemical staining for cytokeratin 8/18 is positive indicative of its epithelial nature.

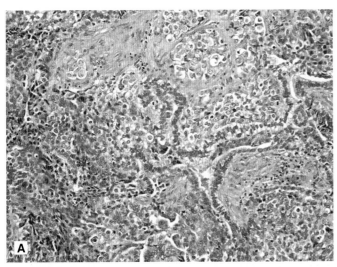 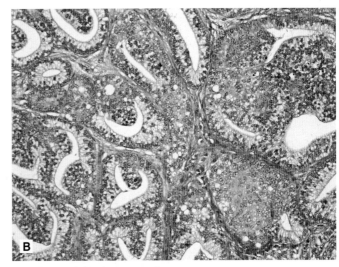

FIGURE 85.6 ▲ Pulmonary blastoma. **A.** This biphasic tumor is comprised of low-grade fetal adenocarcinoma and primitive mesenchyme. In this case, rhabdomyoblastic differentiation was identified. **B.** Fetal adenocarcinoma is characterized by glands and tubules lined by columnar cells with abundant clear cytoplasm resembling fetal airways. Morules are seen in this case.

Immunohistochemistry and Genetic Profile

Pathologic diagnosis of sarcomatoid carcinomas can be done by light microscopy alone, with the morphologic features showing clear epithelial and mesenchymal components. However, in most cases, immunohistochemical studies are helpful in identifying each component and highlighting the cellular histogenesis.

In poorly differentiated tumors with spindle and giant-cell predominance, keratin antibodies or epithelial membrane antigen (EMA) serves to establish the epithelial nature of the tumors and virtually exclude most sarcomas, melanoma, and large cell lymphoma. In some cases, multiple keratin cocktails need to be used in order to get positive results, and positivity may be restricted to better-differentiated areas or be very focal. Even with multiple keratin stains, there may be biopsies with undifferentiated sarcomatoid-appearing cells that do not convincingly express any epithelial marker. In such cases, if other malignancies are excluded, carcinoma is typically favored despite lack of immunohistochemical confirmation, because of the exquisite rarity of primary parenchymal sarcomas of the lung.

Adenocarcinoma components may express TTF-1 and napsin, whereas the squamous cell carcinoma components may express p40, p63, 34betaE12, and other high molecular weight cytokeratins.

Spindle and giant cells may express TTF-1. In fact, TTF-1 positivity occurs in up to 55% of tumors composed exclusively of giant or spindle cells[9] (Figs. 85.7 and 85.8).

In pleomorphic carcinomas, giant tumor cells may stain for human chorionic gonadotropin but should not be confused with a germ-cell tumor from the lung or mediastinum.[17] The mesenchymal component of the tumor is usually positive for vimentin and variably positive for actin and CD34.[15,16]

If the tumor meets the criteria for carcinosarcoma, the sarcomatous component specifically stains as their counterparts in soft tissue. In a large series of carcinosarcomas, keratin cocktails stained the epithelial component in every case and the sarcomatous component in about 28% of cases.[18]

The epithelial component of pulmonary blastoma (fetal-like adenocarcinoma) is positive for TTF-1 and other epithelial markers (CEA, EMA, and keratins), while the mesenchymal component is positive

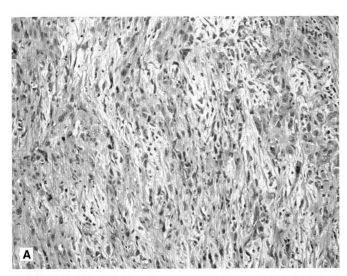 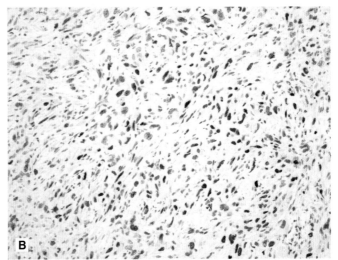

FIGURE 85.7 ▲ Spindle cell carcinoma. **A.** The routine stain shows a pleomorphic population of mostly spindled cells. **B.** Immunohistochemical staining for TTF-1 is positive in the tumor cells assisting with the diagnosis of carcinoma.

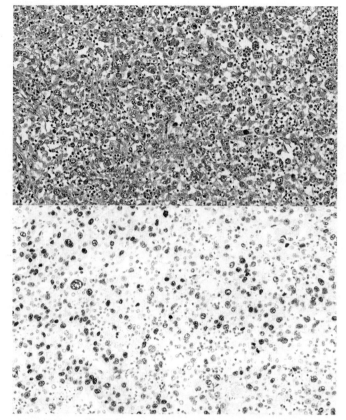

FIGURE 85.8 ▲ Giant-cell carcinoma. The tumor is TTF-1 positive (below).

for vimentin and actin. If a rhabdomyosarcoma component is suspected, desmin and myogenin help to establish the diagnosis. Focal positivity for neuroendocrine markers, including chromogranin and synaptophysin, occurs in the epithelial component. A characteristic feature is the accumulation of β-catenin in the nuclei and cytoplasm of the tumor cells, including the morules.[25]

With the increased importance of genetic testing in non–small cell carcinomas largely to use targeted therapies, several studies have recently focused on the genetic profile of sarcomatoid carcinomas. Mutations in *TP53* are common, as well as aberrant chromosomal gains in multiple loci. *EGFR* and *KRAS* mutation rates are similar to poorly differentiated non–small cell carcinomas and reflect the epithelial component of the tumor, ethnicity, and smoking history.[5,16,26,27] In carcinosarcomas, *EGFR* mutations are extremely rare. ALK-positive sarcomatoid carcinomas have been reported.[28] Pulmonary blastoma's genetic profile has shown mutations in the *CTNNB1* (β-catenin) gene, which activates the Wnt pathway. Rare reports of *EGFR*-mutated pulmonary blastomas also exist.[29]

REFERENCES

1. Goto T, Maeshima A, Kato R. Combined large cell neuroendocrine carcinoma and spindle cell carcinoma of the lung. *Jpn J Clin Oncol.* 2011;41:797–802.
2. Khalifa M, Hruby G, Ehrlich L, et al. Combined large cell neuroendocrine carcinoma and spindle cell carcinoma of the lung. *Ann Diagn Pathol.* 2001;5:240–245.
3. Kerr KM, Pelosi G, Austin JHM, et al. Pleomorphic, spindle cell and giant cell carcinoma. In: Travis WD, et al., eds. *WHO Classification of Tumours of the Lung, Pleura, Thymus and Heart.* Lyon, France: IARP Press; 2015: 88–90.
4. Dacic S, Finkelstein SD, Sasatomi E, et al. Molecular pathogenesis of pulmonary carcinosarcoma as determined by microdissection-based allelotyping. *Am J Surg Pathol.* 2002;26:510–516.
5. Toyokawa G, Takenoyama M, Taguchi K, et al. The first case of lung carcinosarcoma harboring in-frame deletions at exon19 in the EGFR gene. *Lung Cancer.* 2013;81:491–494.
6. Mochizuki T, Ishii G, Nagai K, et al. Pleomorphic carcinoma of the lung: clinicopathologic characteristics of 70 cases. *Am J Surg Pathol.* 2008;32:1727–1735.
7. Kim TS, Han J, Lee KS, et al. CT findings of surgically resected pleomorphic carcinoma of the lung in 30 patients. *AJR Am J Roentgenol.* 2005;185:120–125.
8. Fishback NF, Travis WD, Moran CA, et al. Pleomorphic (spindle/giant cell) carcinoma of the lung. A clinicopathologic correlation of 78 cases. *Cancer.* 1994;73:2936–2945.
9. Rossi G, Cavazza A, Sturm N, et al. Pulmonary carcinomas with pleomorphic, sarcomatoid, or sarcomatous elements: a clinicopathologic and immunohistochemical study of 75 cases. *Am J Surg Pathol.* 2003;27:311–324.
10. Terzi A, Gorla A, Piubello Q, et al. Biphasic sarcomatoid carcinoma of the lung: report of 5 cases and review of the literature. *Eur J Surg Oncol.* 1997;23:457.
11. Venissac N, Pop D, Lassalle S, et al. Sarcomatoid lung cancer (spindle/giant cells): an aggressive disease? *J Thorac Cardiovasc Surg.* 2007;134:619–623.
12. Pelosi G, Fraggetta F, Nappi O, et al. Pleomorphic carcinomas of the lung show a selective distribution of gene products involved in cell differentiation, cell cycle control, tumor growth, and tumor cell motility: a clinicopathologic and immunohistochemical study of 31 cases. *Am J Surg Pathol.* 2003;27:1203–1215.
13. Ro JY, Chen JL, Lee JS, et al. Sarcomatoid carcinoma of the lung. Immunohistochemical and ultrastructural studies of 14 cases. *Cancer.* 1992;69:376–386.
14. Nakajima M, Kasai T, Hashimoto H, et al. Sarcomatoid carcinoma of the lung: a clinicopathologic study of 37 cases. *Cancer.* 1999;86:608–616.
15. Chang YL, Lee YC, Shih JY, et al. Pulmonary pleomorphic (spindle) cell carcinoma: peculiar clinicopathologic manifestations different from ordinary non-small cell carcinoma. *Lung Cancer.* 2001;34:91–97.
16. Travis WD. Sarcomatoid neoplasms of the lung and pleura. *Arch Pathol Lab Med.* 2010;134:1645–1658.
17. Pelosi G, Sonzogni A, De Pas T, et al. Review article: pulmonary sarcomatoid carcinomas: a practical overview. *Int J Surg Pathol.* 2010;18:103–120.
18. Koss MN, Hochholzer L, Frommelt RA. Carcinosarcomas of the lung: a clinicopathologic study of 66 patients. *Am J Surg Pathol.* 1999;23: 1514–1526.
19. Burnette RE, Ballard BR. Metastatic pleomorphic carcinoma of lung presenting as abdominal pain. *J Natl Med Assoc.* 2004;96:1657–1660.
20. Smyth RJ, Fabre A, Dodd JD, et al. Pulmonary blastoma: a case report and review of the literature. *BMC Res Notes.* 2014;7:294.
21. Magistrelli P, D'Ambra L, Berti S, et al. Adult pulmonary blastoma: Report of an unusual malignant lung tumor. *World J Clin Oncol.* 2014;5:1113–1116.
22. Sakata S, Saeki S, Hirooka S, et al. A case of biphasic pulmonary blastoma treated with carboplatin and paclitaxel plus bevacizumab. *Case Rep Oncol Med.* 2015;2015:842621.
23. Xiu Y, Jiang L, Liu W. Classic biphasic pulmonary blastoma with brain and axillary metastases: a case report and molecular analysis and review of literature. *Int J Clin Exp Pathol.* 2015;8:983–988.
24. Kawasaki K, Yamamoto K, Suzuki Y, et al. Surgery and radiation therapy for brain metastases from classic biphasic pulmonary blastoma. *BMJ Case Rep.* 2014;2014.
25. Nakatani Y, Miyagi Y, Takemura T, et al. Aberrant nuclear/cytoplasmic localization and gene mutation of beta-catenin in classic pulmonary blastoma: beta-catenin immunostaining is useful for distinguishing between classic pulmonary blastoma and a blastomatoid variant of carcinosarcoma. *Am J Surg Pathol.* 2004;28:921–927.
26. Giroux Leprieur E, Antoine M, Vieira T, et al. Clinical and molecular features in patients with advanced non-small-cell lung carcinoma refractory to first-line platinum-based chemotherapy. *Lung Cancer.* 2013;79:167–172.
27. Pelosi G, Gasparini P, Cavazza A, et al. Multiparametric molecular characterization of pulmonary sarcomatoid carcinoma reveals a nonrandom amplification of anaplastic lymphoma kinase (ALK) gene. *Lung Cancer.* 2012;77:507–514.
28. Maruyama R, Matsumura F, Shibata Y, et al. Detection of ALK rearrangement in an octogenarian patient with pleomorphic carcinoma of the lung. *Gen Thorac Cardiovasc Surg.* 2014.
29. Macher-Goeppinger S, Penzel R, Roth W, et al. Expression and mutation analysis of EGFR, c-KIT, and beta-catenin in pulmonary blastoma. *J Clin Pathol.* 2011;64:349–353.

86 The Evaluation of Small Biopsies for Lung Cancer

Andre L. Moreira, M.D.

Background

The majority of patients with lung cancer present with advanced disease stage at diagnosis, and small biopsy including cytology is often the only specimen available for diagnosis. Because therapy for lung cancer is highly influenced by disease stage and tumor characteristics, the importance of small biopsy has grown significantly in patients with non–small cell lung cancer (NSCLC) due to the shift to personalized therapy.[1,2] The discoveries of activating mutations in pulmonary adenocarcinomas, and histology-based recommendation to chemotherapeutic drugs in NSCLC, brought many new challenges to pathologists who are now required to subclassify NSCLC in small biopsy material and triage for molecular tests.[3–5]

In response to this challenge, the International Association for the Study of Lung Cancer (IASLC), the American Thoracic Society (ATS), and the European Respiratory Society (ERS) joined force to reevaluate the histologic classification of lung cancer.[6] The proposed changes by the IASLC/ERS/ATS now constitute the recommendations of the 2015 World Health Organization (WHO) classification of lung carcinomas.[7]

Tumor Classification in Small Biopsy and Cytology

Traditionally, there have been four major histologic types of lung cancer: small cell lung carcinoma (SCLC), adenocarcinoma, squamous cell carcinoma, and large cell carcinoma; the latter three categories were often grouped as non–small cell lung carcinoma (NSCLC) in biopsy specimens. Until the last decade or so, there was no need to further subclassify NSCLC, because all these entities were similarly managed clinically.

Squamous cell carcinoma and adenocarcinoma are practically the only histologic subtypes of NSCLC that can be diagnosed in small biopsy and cytologic specimens. The diagnosis of large cell carcinoma cannot be established with certainty in small biopsy material, because the entity is defined as a poorly differentiated carcinoma without histologic evidence of adenocarcinoma (gland formation) or squamous cell carcinoma (keratinization). Therefore, the diagnosis of large cell carcinoma still requires the examination of a resected tumor to exclude differentiation features.[8] Small cell carcinoma and large cell neuroendocrine carcinoma are often diagnosed in small biopsy.[9–11]

The criteria for the diagnosis of adenocarcinoma in a small biopsy are determined by the identification of specific histologic patterns such as lepidic, acinar, papillary, and micropapillary (Fig. 86.1). In biopsies where the only pattern present is lepidic, it is recommended that the nomenclature of "adenocarcinoma with lepidic pattern" be used. The reason for this recommendation is that a biopsy with only lepidic pattern may correspond in a subsequent excision to an adenocarcinoma in situ (AIS), minimally invasive adenocarcinoma (MIA), and a lepidic component of an invasive adenocarcinoma. AIS and MIA should not be diagnosed in a biopsy specimen. These two entities require examination of the entire tumor to exclude an invasive pattern, as well as lymphatic and pleural invasion. The presence of adenocarcinoma patterns in a small biopsy should be sufficient for the diagnosis without the need for further ancillary studies, unless metastatic disease is suspected.[8,12]

The two hallmarks for the diagnosis of squamous cell carcinoma are keratinization and intercellular bridge (Fig. 86.2). Due to the number of advances in therapy for adenocarcinoma, a diagnosis of squamous cell carcinoma in a poorly differentiated NSCLC without proper documentation of squamous cell differentiation can potentially deprive a patient of appropriate and efficient therapy.

A tumor composed of solid pattern without any other histologic differentiating pattern should have evidence of differentiation confirmed by immunohistochemical stains (IHC). In cases of poorly differentiated NSCLC (nonkeratinizing squamous cell carcinoma or adenocarcinoma

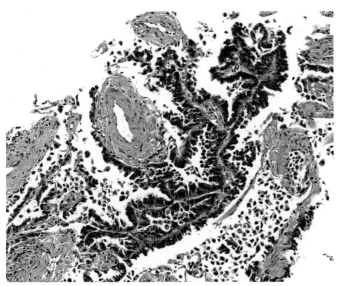

FIGURE 86.1 ▲ Core biopsy of a lung nodule showing an adenocarcinoma with lepidic growth pattern. The identification of lepidic, acinar, papillary, and micropapillary patterns in biopsy specimens are enough for the diagnosis of adenocarcinoma.

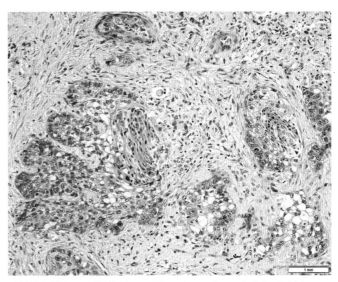

FIGURE 86.2 ▲ Squamous cell carcinoma in an endobronchial biopsy. The presence of keratinization and intracellular bridges (not seen at this magnification) is diagnostic of this entity.

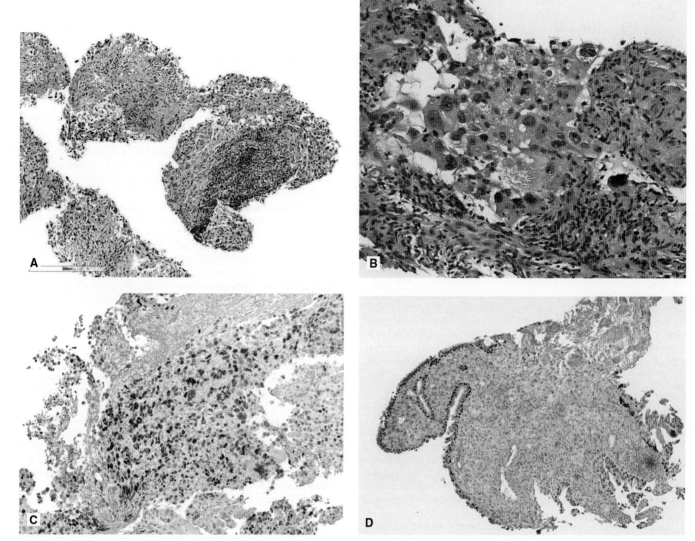

FIGURE 86.3 ▲ Adenocarcinoma with squamoid features (glassy cells). **A.** There is no clear keratinization. **B.** Higher magnification shows abundant cytoplasm. **C.** Immunohistochemical stains showed that the tumor cells were positive for TTF-1. **D.** Immunohistochemical staining is negative for p40.

with solid pattern), when IHC must be used for tumor classification, the current WHO classification recommends the use of the term NSCLC, followed by "favor adenocarcinoma," when IHC favor glandular differentiation; NSCLC, favor squamous cell carcinoma, when the immunoprofile favors a squamous cell carcinoma; and NSCLC-not otherwise specified (NOS), when there is not enough material for IHC or the immunoprofile is equivocal (Fig. 86.3; Table 86.1).[8]

One important pitfall of solid pattern in small biopsy is that a solid-type adenocarcinoma can show squamoid features such as nested appearance and glassy eosinophilic cytoplasm (Fig. 86.3), although there is no clear keratinization or presence of intracellular bridges. This can be seen either on cytology or on small biopsy material and can be confused with squamous cell carcinoma. Knowledge of this pitfall can greatly reduce misclassification of NSCLC.

As demonstrated by Rekhtman et al.,[13] a subclassification of NSCLC into adenocarcinoma and squamous cell carcinoma in cytology specimens can be achieved in ~93% of the cases using cytomorphologic criteria only.[13–15] However, the subclassification of NSCLC can be a problem in paucicellular specimens and in poorly differentiated carcinomas where no clear histologic differentiation is present. In these situations, morphologic features cannot make the distinction between adenocarcinoma and squamous cell carcinoma alone.

The histologic patterns of acinar, papillary, micropapillary, solid, and lepidic can be seen in small biopsy specimens but may be difficult to recognize in cytologic material.[16–18] In the latter, a cell block preparation may be very helpful in identifying histologic patterns of adenocarcinoma that cannot be recognized on smears.[16] In cytology, the determination of predominant type or subtyping of adenocarcinoma is not feasible.[16–19] Rudomina et al. showed that the presence of acini structures in cytology preparations had a predictive value of 94% when correlated with the presence of acinar pattern in resection specimens.[18] Acinar is the most common pattern in adenocarcinomas seen in resected specimens.[20,21] However, the presence of papillary clusters with fibrovascular cores had a predictive value of 75%, and the presence of micropapillary tufts had a predictive value of 64% for micropapillary pattern on excised specimens. The authors found no cytologic features that correlated with solid pattern. Rodriguez et al. demonstrated that in ~40% of cases, an acinar or papillary type can be attributed in cytology material, but there are no reliable cytomorphologic features that correlate with a solid or micropapillary type adenocarcinoma.[17] The latter are important histologic patterns that are associated with poor prognosis. Therefore, as of the writing of this chapter, subtyping of adenocarcinomas in cytology materials is not recommended.

TABLE 86.1 Classification of Non–Small Cell Carcinoma with Solid Growth Patterns

NSCLC	IHC	Pitfall
Favor adenocarcinoma	TTF-1+[a]/p40–	Neuroendocrine tumors Metastatic carcinoma[b]
Favor squamous cell carcinoma	TTF-1–/p40+	Metastatic squamous cell carcinoma from other organ Metastatic urothelial carcinoma
NOS	TTF-1–/p40–	Add napsin A and keratin 5/6
	TTF-1+/p40+[c]	Metastatic carcinoma Entrapped pneumocytes may be TTF-1 positive; residual basal cells may be p40 positive
Favor adenosquamous carcinoma	TTF-1+/p40+	In different cell populations[c]

[a]Focal or diffuse staining for TTF-1.
[b]Metastatic carcinomas from the breast, urothelium, and uterus have been reported to stain positive for TTF-1, mostly with clone SPT24.
[c]Double positive for TTF-1 and p40 in the same cells do not constitute evidence for adenosquamous carcinoma. If staining for TTF is more prominent, then "favor adenocarcinoma" may be used, as "NSCLC NOS" is often considered equivalent to adenocarcinoma for treatment purposes (see text).

Use of a Minimal Panel of IHC

There have been many studies to identify the best panel of stains to be used for the classification of adenocarcinoma and squamous cell carcinoma in small biopsy material.[22–25] Considering the need to save tissue for molecular studies that are indicated in adenocarcinomas, a consensus for the use of a minimal panel has been recommended by the IASLC/ATS/ERS classification and adopted by the WHO.[12] This minimal panel of antibodies includes two markers, TTF-1 (thyroid transcription factor-1) and p63 or p40 (an isoform of p63 that seems to be more specific than p63 for squamous carcinoma). Up to 20% to 30% of lung adenocarcinomas, including those positive for TTF-1, can be positive for p63 but are virtually negative for p40.[26,27]

Several studies have shown that TTF-1 is a good marker for adenocarcinomas of the lung,[22–25] although not specific, because TTF-1 positivity can be seen in tumors of the thyroid gland and in neuroendocrine tumors.[11] In the latter cases, histologic features of these tumors are helpful in establishing the diagnosis. However, when the only clinical possibility is an NSCLC, any staining for TTF-1, either focal or diffuse, is a good indication of adenocarcinoma differentiation. In contrast, NSCLCs that show a strong and diffuse positivity for p63 or p40 and negative reactivity for TTF-1 should be classified as NSCLC,favor squamous cell carcinoma. One of the pitfalls of this minimal panel is the fact that focal positivity for TTF-1 has been reported in squamous cell carcinoma, which can be seen with certain clones of the antibody.[23] Therefore, knowledge of the clone used and its sensitivity and specificity is critical when using the minimal panel of IHC to avoid misclassification. In cases of TTF-1 focal positivity in squamous cell carcinoma, p63/p40 will show their characteristics strong and diffuse positivity in this tumor type, which may help raise suspicion for the correct diagnosis.

Pitfalls of the Biopsy Classification

Although this proposition seems straightforward, there are still some difficulties in classifying tumors that defies this binary approach. For instances, what to do with tumors that show reactivity for both markers or are negative for both markers? The 2015 WHO classification recommends that these tumors should be classified as NSCLC-NOS; thus a specific subtype cannot be determined in the biopsy specimen with certainty.[8] In the case of a double-negative tumor or a carcinoma with ambiguous immunophenotype based on the two markers, other markers such as napsin-1 (positive in adenocarcinoma) and keratin 5/6

(a marker for squamous cell carcinoma when the stain is strong and diffuse) can be added to the panel.

It is imperative to correlate the findings with clinical history. In a patient with previous history of malignancy or a patient with disseminated disease with a tumor of unknown origin, additional IHC stains should be added to the panel to rule out metastatic carcinoma as well as nonepithelial tumor such as melanoma, sarcoma, and lymphoma. Awareness of the limitations of the two-antibody panel, clinical pitfalls, source, specificity, and sensitivity of the clone of antibodies used is essential to avoid misclassification of lung tumors.[28–30]

Studies that evaluated the immunophenotype of adenocarcinomas and squamous cell carcinomas in resection specimens using the binary model of immunoreactivity (TTF-1/p63) have demonstrated that adenocarcinomas have great variability in their staining pattern,[23] whereas squamous cell carcinomas are more homogenous with universal strong and diffuse expression of p63 and/or p40 with negative stain for TTF-1. Therefore, it can be concluded that a negative stain for p63/p40 tends to exclude the diagnosis of squamous cell carcinoma.[23,26,27] In addition, tumors that are double positive (TTF-1+/p63+ or p40+) or double negative (TTF-1–/p63– or p40–) have the same pattern of mutation as do other adenocarcinomas that follow the more common immunoreactivity pattern (TTF-1+/p63– or p40–).[31]

Adenosquamous carcinoma is a rare tumor that can show positivity for both TTF-1 and p40; however, the positive stains cluster with different populations of the tumor and appear to be mutually exclusive, that is, the adenocarcinoma component marks for TTF-1 and the squamous cell carcinoma component marks for p40. In cases like this, a comment can be made that the tumor could represent an adenosquamous carcinoma but that diagnosis requires a resection specimen.[32] Double positivity for TTF-1 and p40 in the same cells does not constitute evidence for adenosquamous carcinoma differentiation.

For practical purposes, the diagnosis of an NSCLC-favor adenocarcinoma or NSCLC-NOS in a small biopsy material should be regarded as equivalent to the diagnosis of adenocarcinoma for therapeutic decision and/or triage for molecular studies.

In patients with a resectable tumor, the diagnosis of NSCLC-NOS in a small biopsy may correlate with the diagnosis in a resected specimen of an adenocarcinoma with a predominant solid pattern, or a large cell carcinoma, if no definite differentiation is identified after examination of the entire tumor.[33,34] In reality, the proposed classification for small biopsy material gives the pathologists some leeway on how to address evolving concepts, such as large cell carcinoma as a histologic independent entity and uncertainties on diagnosis due to sampling issues.[35,36]

Critics of this biopsy classification have pointed out that the use of the term "favor" adenocarcinoma or a squamous cell carcinoma can generate concern and confusion among treating physicians because the term "favor" may be interpreted as doubt about the diagnosis. One possible scenario is that clinicians faced with the diagnosis of NSCLC-favor adenocarcinoma may be reluctant to treat the patient appropriately with drugs that can be used in adenocarcinomas because there is a concern that there might be an underlining squamous cell carcinoma in the biopsy. Therefore, in order to apply this terminology, there must be clear communication with the treating physician on what the diagnosis implies.

Another concern for the term of "NSCLC favor" is triaging of cases for molecular diagnostic tests. This important issue has been addressed by the recent molecular testing guidelines for pulmonary adenocarcinoma recommended by the College of American Pathologists (CAP), IASLC, and Association for Molecular Pathology (AMP).[37,38] In order to reduce the chances of missing a targetable mutation, all tumors with diagnosis of NSCLC-NOS or NSCLC-favor adenocarcinoma in a small biopsy material should be submitted for molecular tests. Only tumors with the histologic diagnosis of squamous cell carcinoma and NSCLC-favor squamous cell carcinoma (diffuse and strong nuclear stain for p63 or p40) should not be sent routinely for molecular diagnostic tests.[37,38]

Alternatively, the diagnosis of adenocarcinoma can be rendered in the cases of NSCLC-favor adenocarcinoma (no histologic evidence of gland formation and IHC profile of TTF-1+/ p63–/p40–) and

NSCLC-NOS (no histologic evidence of gland formation and double-negative immunoreactivity profile of TTF-1-/p63- or p40) based on the variability of reactivity patterns seen in adenocarcinoma,[23] the molecular profile similarities to that of adenocarcinoma, and the levels of confidence of the pathologists rendering the diagnosis.[31]

Another pitfall for biopsy diagnosis of NSCLC is a tumor composed of spindled cells. In these situations, the differential diagnosis includes a sarcomatoid carcinoma, sarcomatoid mesothelioma, and a true sarcoma. The minimal panel of IHC cannot be used in these situations. The diagnostic panel of IHC must include keratin markers, mesothelial markers, and sarcoma markers. The absence of keratin expression is rare in sarcomatoid carcinoma and mesotheliomas. In these cases, a sarcoma diagnosis should be entertained. Primary sarcomas of the lungs are extremely rare, and metastatic sarcomas are more commonly found. Therefore, review of past and current clinical history is imperative to reach the correct diagnosis.

Differentiation between a sarcomatoid carcinoma and sarcomatoid mesothelioma can be extremely difficult, because expression of more specific differentiation markers such a calretinin, D2-40, and WT-1 can be lost in sarcomatoid mesotheliomas, as well as TTF-1 and p63/p40 can be lost in sarcomatoid carcinomas of the lung. In the instance when only keratin is positive, correlation with location of the mass may offer an indication of diagnosis, although it cannot be reached with certainty in a small biopsy.

REFERENCES

1. Campos-Parra AD, Aviles A, Contreras-Reyes S, et al. Relevance of the novel IASLC/ATS/ERS classification of lung adenocarcinoma in advanced disease. *Eur Respir J.* 2014;43:1439–1447.
2. Moreira AL, Thornton RH. Personalized medicine for non-small-cell lung cancer: implications of recent advances in tissue acquisition for molecular and histologic testing. *Clin Lung Cancer.* 2012;13:334–339.
3. Hirsch FR, Spreafico A, Novello S, et al. The prognostic and predictive role of histology in advanced non-small cell lung cancer: a literature review. *J Thorac Oncol.* 2008;3:1468–1481.
4. Travis WD, Rekhtman N. Pathological diagnosis and classification of lung cancer in small biopsies and cytology: strategic management of tissue for molecular testing. *Semin Respir Crit Care Med.* 2011;32:22–31.
5. Travis WD, Rekhtman N, Riley GJ, et al. Pathologic diagnosis of advanced lung cancer based on small biopsies and cytology: a paradigm shift. *J Thorac Oncol.* 2010;5:411–414.
6. Travis WD, Brambilla E, Van Schil P, et al. Paradigm shifts in lung cancer as defined in the new IASLC/ATS/ERS lung adenocarcinoma classification. *Eur Respir J.* 2011;38:239–243.
7. Yatabe Y, Kosaka T, Takahashi T, et al. EGFR mutation is specific for terminal respiratory unit type adenocarcinoma. *Am J Surg Pathol.* 2005;29:633–639.
8. 8. Yatabe Y, Brambilla E, Nicholson A, et al. Rationale for classification in small biopsies and cytology. In: Travis WD, et al., eds. *WHO Classification of Tumours of the Lung, Pleura, Mediastinum and Heart.* Lyon, France: IARC Press; 2015:16–17.
9. Aslan DL, Gulbahce HE, Pambuccian SE, et al. Ki-67 immunoreactivity in the differential diagnosis of pulmonary neuroendocrine neoplasms in specimens with extensive crush artifact. *Am J Clin Pathol.* 2005;123:874–878.
10. Lin O, Olgac S, Green I, et al. Immunohistochemical staining of cytologic smears with MIB-1 helps distinguish low-grade from high-grade neuroendocrine neoplasms. *Am J Clin Pathol.* 2003;120:209–216.
11. Rekhtman N. Neuroendocrine tumors of the lung: an update. *Arch Pathol Lab Med.* 2010;134:1628–1638.
12. Travis WD, Brambilla E, Noguchi M, et al. International Association for the Study of Lung Cancer/American Thoracic Society/European Respiratory Society International Multidisciplinary Classification of Lung Adenocarcinoma. *J Thorac Oncol.* 2011;6:244–285.
13. Rekhtman N, Brandt SM, Sigel CS, et al. Suitability of thoracic cytology for new therapeutic paradigms in non-small cell lung carcinoma: high accuracy of tumor subtyping and feasibility of EGFR and KRAS molecular testing. *J Thorac Oncol.* 2011;6:451–458.
14. da Cunha Santos G, Lai SW, Saieg MA, et al. Cyto-histologic agreement in pathologic subtyping of non small cell lung carcinoma: review of 602 fine needle aspirates with follow-up surgical specimens over a nine year period and analysis of factors underlying failure to subtype. *Lung Cancer.* 2012;77:501–506.
15. Sigel CS, Moreira AL, Travis WD, et al. Subtyping of non-small cell lung carcinoma: a comparison of small biopsy and cytology specimens. *J Thorac Oncol.* 2011;6:1849–1856.
16. Loukeris K, Vazquez MF, Sica G, et al. Cytological cell blocks: Predictors of squamous cell carcinoma and adenocarcinoma subtypes. *Diagn Cytopathol.* 2012;40:380–387.
17. Rodriguez EF, Monaco SE, Dacic S. Cytologic subtyping of lung adenocarcinoma by using the proposed International Association for the Study of Lung Cancer/American Thoracic Society/European Respiratory Society (IASLC/ATS/ERS) adenocarcinoma classification. *Cancer Cytopathol.* 2013;121:629–637.
18. Rudomina DE, Lin O, Moreira AL. Cytologic diagnosis of pulmonary adenocarcinoma with micropapillary pattern: does it correlate with the histologic findings? *Diagn Cytopathol.* 2009;37:333–339.
19. Moreira AL. Subtyping of pulmonary adenocarcinoma in cytologic specimens: the next challenge. *Cancer Cytopathol.* 2013;121:601–604.
20. Sica G, Yoshizawa A, Sima CS, et al. A grading system of lung adenocarcinomas based on histologic pattern is predictive of disease recurrence in stage I tumors. *Am J Surg Pathol.* 2010;34:1155–1162.
21. Yoshizawa A, Motoi N, Riely GJ, et al. Impact of proposed IASLC/ATS/ERS classification of lung adenocarcinoma: prognostic subgroups and implications for further revision of staging based on analysis of 514 stage I cases. *Mod Pathol.* 2011;24:653–664.
22. Loo PS, Thomas SC, Nicolson MC, et al. Subtyping of undifferentiated non-small cell carcinomas in bronchial biopsy specimens. *J Thorac Oncol.* 2010;5:442–447.
23. Rekhtman N, Ang DC, Sima CS, et al. Immunohistochemical algorithm for differentiation of lung adenocarcinoma and squamous cell carcinoma based on large series of whole-tissue sections with validation in small specimens. *Mod Pathol.* 2011;24:1348–1359.
24. Righi L, Graziano P, Fornari A, et al. Immunohistochemical subtyping of nonsmall cell lung cancer not otherwise specified in fine-needle aspiration cytology: a retrospective study of 103 cases with surgical correlation. *Cancer.* 2011;117:3416–3423.
25. Mukhopadhyay S, Katzenstein AL. Subclassification of non-small cell lung carcinomas lacking morphologic differentiation on biopsy specimens: Utility of an immunohistochemical panel containing TTF-1, napsin A, p63, and CK5/6. *Am J Surg Pathol.* 2011;35:15–25.
26. Bishop JA, Teruya-Feldstein J, Westra WH, et al. p40 (DeltaNp63) is superior to p63 for the diagnosis of pulmonary squamous cell carcinoma. *Mod Pathol.* 2012;25:405–415.
27. Pelosi G, Fabbri A, Bianchi F, et al. DeltaNp63 (p40) and thyroid transcription factor-1 immunoreactivity on small biopsies or cellblocks for typing non-small cell lung cancer: a novel two-hit, sparing-material approach. *J Thorac Oncol.* 2012;7:281–290.
28. Kashima K, Hashimoto H, Nishida H, et al. Significant expression of thyroid transcription factor-1 in pulmonary squamous cell carcinoma detected by SPT24 monoclonal antibody and CSA-II system. *Appl Immunohistochem Mol Morphol.* 2014;22:119–124.
29. Matoso A, Sıngh K, Jacob R, et al. Comparison of thyroid transcription factor-1 expression by 2 monoclonal antibodies in pulmonary and nonpulmonary primary tumors. *Appl Immunohistochem Mol Morphol.* 2010;18:142–149.
30. Ordonez NG. Value of thyroid transcription factor-1 immunostaining in tumor diagnosis: a review and update. *Appl Immunohistochem Mol Morphol.* 2012;20:429–444.
31. Rekhtman N, Tafe LJ, Chaft JE, et al. Distinct profile of driver mutations and clinical features in immunomarker-defined subsets of pulmonary large-cell carcinoma. *Mod Pathol.* 2013;26:511–522.
32. Rao N. Adenosquamous carcinoma. *Semin Diagn Pathol.* 2014;31:271–277.
33. Kadota K, Nitadori J, Rekhtman N, et al. Reevaluation and reclassification of resected lung carcinomas originally diagnosed as squamous cell carcinoma using immunohistochemical analysis. *Am J Surg Pathol.* 2015;39:1170–1180.
34. Zachara-Szczakowski S, Verdun T, Churg A. Accuracy of classifying poorly differentiated non-small cell lung carcinoma biopsies with commonly used lung carcinoma markers. *Hum Pathol.* 2015;46:776–782.

35. Pelosi G, Barbareschi M, Cavazza A, et al. Large cell carcinoma of the lung: a tumor in search of an author. A clinically oriented critical reappraisal. *Lung Cancer.* 2015;87:226–231.
36. Sholl LM. Large-cell carcinoma of the lung: a diagnostic category redefined by immunohistochemistry and genomics. *Curr Opin Pulm Med.* 2014;20:324–331.
37. Lindeman NI, Cagle PT, Beasley MB, et al. Molecular testing guideline for selection of lung cancer patients for EGFR and ALK tyrosine

kinase inhibitors: guideline from the College of American Pathologists, International Association for the Study of Lung Cancer, and Association for Molecular Pathology. *J Thorac Oncol.* 2013;8:823–859.
38. Lindeman NI, Cagle PT, Beasley MB, et al. Molecular testing guideline for selection of lung cancer patients for EGFR and ALK tyrosine kinase inhibitors: guideline from the College of American Pathologists, International Association for the Study of Lung Cancer, and Association for Molecular Pathology. *J Mol Diagn.* 2013;15:415–453.

87 Non–Small Cell Lung Carcinoma Evaluation of Pleural and Vascular Invasion, Resection Margins, and Treatment Effect

Allen Burke, M.D., Fabio Tavora, M.D., Ph.D., and Borislav A. Alexiev, M.D.

Pleural Invasion

Histologic Assessment

Invasion into the pleura is a routine assessment for non–small cell lung carcinomas, which is required for tumor staging (see Chapter 73). The extent of invasion has been classified into fibrous tissue under the pleura without invasion of the elastic tissue (PL0), invasion of visceral pleural elastic tissue (PL1), invasion of parietal pleura (PL2), and invasion through parietal pleura (PL3). PL1 or PL2 denotes pT2 stage, and PL3 is equivalent to chest wall invasion (pT3).[1] Therefore, the distinction between invasion of visceral and parietal pleura, which is difficult, is not necessary. When there is chest wall invasion, there is typically resection of ribs (Fig. 87.1).

Invasion into the pleura is often suspected grossly by retraction of the surface.[2] Invasion into the chest wall is generally evident upon reading the operative note and will result in chest wall fat or rib resection. In these cases, it is important to ink the specimen in order to obtain chest wall margins. If the pleura is intact and no chest wall has been removed, inking the pleural surface is unnecessary and may interfere with the microscopic evaluation of tumor invasion. It is important in this context to remember that the visceral pleura is not a surgical margin and that parietal pleura is resected only if there is chest wall invasion.

Use of Elastic Stains

Elastic stains highlight the pleural elastic tissue, which is helpful in assessing invasion, as penetration of the elastic layer is considered the basis for upstaging the tumor to pT2. The elastic lamina appears as a

black serpentine band of interconnecting fibers beneath the mesothelial layer. The pleural visceral layer is usually accentuated in areas of invasion, with a fibroblastic reaction and reaction of the elastic layer into the lung parenchyma[3] (Figs. 87.2 and 87.3).

Taube et al. demonstrated that 17% of adenocarcinomas and 26% of squamous carcinomas that were judged as negative for pleural invasion on hematoxylin–eosin staining were upstaged from pT1 to pT2 tumors after review of elastic stains (Movat pentachrome stains).[3] These findings have led to the recommendation that all pT1 tumors that abut the pleura microscopically be stained for elastic tissue, Verhoeff elastic van Gieson stain, elastin hematoxylin and eosin, Weigert elastic stain, or Movat pentachrome stains.[1]

Adenocarcinoma in situ or minimally invasive adenocarcinomas by definition do not invade the pleura. Also by definition, the lepidic growth pattern of adenocarcinomas does not invade the pleural elastic tissue.[3]

Prognostic Implications

Overall, pleural invasion is identified in about 25% of resected lung cancers[1] although in some series the number is far higher.[4] Over half of lung tumors that have grossly puckered pleural surfaces show pleural invasion histologically using elastic stains.[2] Pleural invasion is associated tumor size >3 cm, higher tumor grade, vascular invasion,

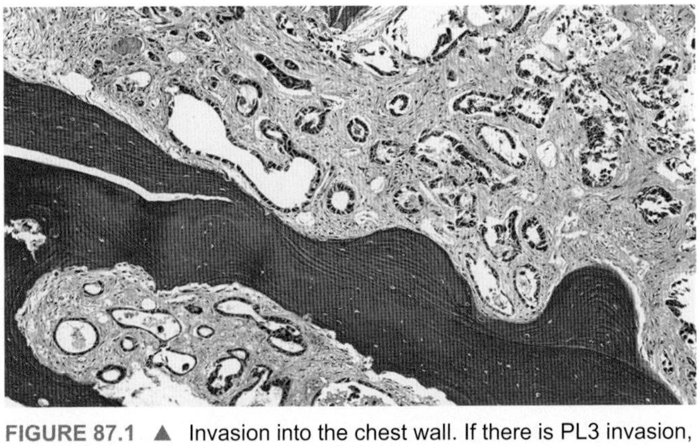

FIGURE 87.1 ▲ Invasion into the chest wall. If there is PL3 invasion, portions of the chest wall (fat, fascia, skeletal muscle or bone) will be removed, necessitating additional margin evaluation. In this case, tumor invaded the bone.

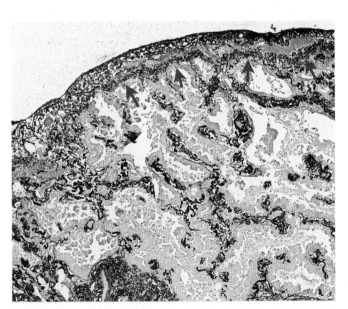

FIGURE 87.2 ▲ No pleural invasion, elastic stain. The elastic layer is intact (*arrows*). The tumor cells are pale tan-brown and barely visible.

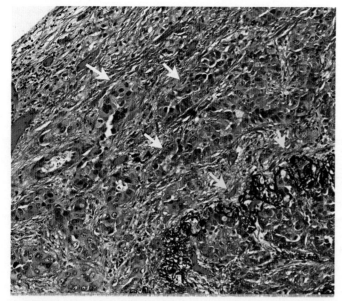

FIGURE 87.3 ▲ With elastic staining, tumor can be seen outside the elastic layer of the pleura (*arrows*).

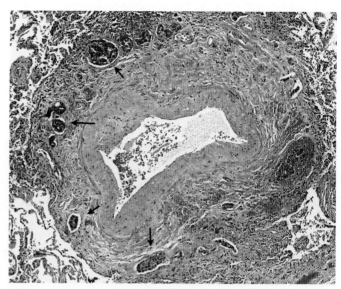

FIGURE 87.4 ▲ Lymphatic invasion. This often occurs around arteries or airways. In this case, the lymphatic surrounds an artery and is filled with adenocarcinoma (*arrows*).

mediastinal lymph node metastasis, extranodal involvement, and higher stage.[2] In one study, the 5-year survival of patients with and without pleural invasion was 57.9% and 83.0%, respectively, justifying its use in pathologic staging.[2] Another study showed that visceral pleural and lymphovascular invasion were poor prognostic factors and that perineural invasion had no effect on survival.[4]

Nitadori et al. showed that pleural invasion in peripheral adenocarcinomas ≤2 cm did not affect survival or risk of recurrence, but affected both survival and recurrence only in tumors that were 2 to 3 cm.[5] Current guidelines, however, still recommend grouping all tumors <3 cm as stage pT2a if there is pleural involvement.

Lymphovascular Invasion

General

The acronym "LVI" was initially applied to "lymphatic vessel invasion" and did not denote blood vessel invasion.[6] Currently, however, LVI frequently refers to "lymphovascular invasion," a term that the College of American Pathologists (CAP) uses for both blood vessel and lymphatic invasion. A synonym is "angiolymphatic invasion," which combines blood vessel and lymphatic invasion.[7] The term "lymphatic permeation" is sometimes used for lymphatic invasion, and "vascular invasion" generally denotes blood vessel invasion.[8]

In the current CAP checklist, the type of invasion (blood vessel vs. lymphatic) is not specified. Lymphatic or blood vessel invasion does not affect the stage of the tumor, unlike pleural invasion.

Lymphatic Invasion

Lymphatic invasion occurs in 13% to 59% of non–small cell lung carcinomas. There is no association with squamous or adenocarcinoma subtypes.[6–9] Lymphatics most frequently are seen surrounding arteries (Fig. 87.4) or airways.

Lymphatic invasion is more frequent in tumors with lymph node metastases and advanced stage, but not with the presence of distant metastasis.[6] There is a weakly significant association with blood vessel invasion.[7] In conjunction with blood vessel invasion, there is an association with size between 2 and 3 cm, standard uptake value (SUV) on positron emission tomography (PET) scans, pleural invasion, and large cell undifferentiated histology.[7]

Studies from the late 1990s showed a higher risk of recurrence and death from disease when lymphatic invasion was present, independent of stage.[6,9] More recent studies have confirmed an association with

poor prognosis and that the impact on survival is additive with blood vessel invasion.[4,7] A significant independent affect on survival was only found for adenocarcinoma, and not squamous carcinoma, in one of these studies.[7] Lymphatic invasion was associated with poorer overall survival especially in early-stage, node-negative tumors.[10]

Arterial and Venous Invasion (Blood Vessel Invasion)

Often overlooked by practicing pathologists, arterial and venous invasion is seen in a high proportion of resected lung cancers, between 29% and 48% of tumors.[8,11–15] Interestingly, most of the publications do not make a distinction between arteries and veins, although most illustrated examples are clearly arteries (Fig. 87.5). Venous invasion occurs as well, but is less frequent in the authors' experience (Fig. 87.6).

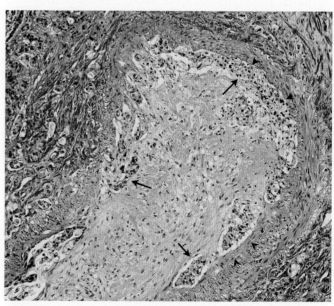

FIGURE 87.5 ▲ Arterial invasion. This poorly differentiated adenocarcinoma (*arrows*) is within the internal elastic lamina (*arrowheads*). The artery is obliterated by fibrous tissue.

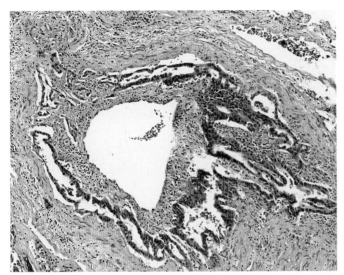

FIGURE 87.6 ▲ Venous invasion. This vein has extensive adenocarcinoma mostly within the adventitia.

Blood vessel invasion in resected non–small cell lung carcinomas is associated with smoking, adenocarcinoma histologic type, lymphatic invasion, large size, and pleural invasion.[14]

Prognostic Implications of Blood Vessel Invasion

Two early studies in the 1990s showed that there was no difference on prognosis by blood vessel invasion.[6,9] Many other recent ones have, however, shown a strong association between blood vessel invasion and prognosis for non–small cell carcinomas of the lung. Kessler et al. showed blood vessel invasion to be the strongest independent factor affecting survival in a series of resected lung tumors.[13] Bodendorf et al. showed a 37% versus 56% 5-year survival for tumors with and without blood vessel invasion, respectively, although the effect on survival was only significant for adenocarcinomas.[11] Kato et al. also showed an adverse correlation between survival and blood vessel invasion that was increased when lymphatic invasion was included and that was significant also only for adenocarcinomas.[7] Gabor et al. showed a striking difference in survival based on the presence of blood vessel invasion, on a relatively small group of 72 non–small cell carcinomas.[12] Khan et al. showed that blood vessel invasion was an independent predictor of mortality, as did Shoji et al.,[16] who showed a relative risk for death of 4.6 compared to patients without blood vessel invasion. Other groups reported similar findings.[14,15]

A more recent study analyzed the prognostic affect of blood vessel invasion on separate histologic subtypes of non–small cell lung carcinomas. Usui et al. showed that there was a significant detrimental impact of blood vessel invasion on adenocarcinomas with predominant lepidic, papillary, and acinar growth patterns, but not for solid predominant tumors. In squamous carcinomas, they found that tumor invasion of blood vessels larger than 1 mm was associated with distant metastasis and cavitary formation.[8]

Evaluation of Resection Margins

General

Peripheral wedge resections contain a parenchymal margin, which is represented by the tissue at the staple line. In most cases, wedge resections are performed for benign disease or are sampled to rule out malignancy by frozen section. If frozen section is positive, in the majority of cases, a completion lobectomy or segmentectomy is performed, and the true margin is represented in the subsequent resection.

Lobectomy and pneumonectomy specimens contain bronchial and vascular margins and, depending on the completeness of the interlobar fissures, may also contain parenchymal margins with staple lines.

When tumors extend into the mediastinum or chest wall, part of the specimen contains additional margins that should be designated by the surgeon, usually with sutures or diagrams, for appropriate handling by the pathologist. When portions of the chest wall are excised, the visceral pleura is adherent to the parietal pleura, and the surface of the specimen should be inked. Note that the visceral pleura is not a margin and that inking is unnecessary if the parietal pleura is not involved and the tumor is not adherent to it.

Evaluation of Stapled Margins

If there is lung-sparing surgery, and a tumor is wedged out without completion lobectomy, it may happen that the pathologist will be asked for margins along a staple line. Gross estimation of distance of tumor to margins by palpation overestimates the actual distance by 11 mm.[17] If the staple line is removed, then about 2 to 3 mm of the true distance to margin is not estimated. This method is acceptable only if the margin is clearly negative, in which case an additional 2 to 3 mm can be added to the distance from the margin in the pathology report.

Because of time restraints, it is usually impossible to attempt to remove the staples individually, which is the "gold standard" for margin assessment in this circumstance. There are two other options. First, the pathologist can prepare a cytologic preparation by scraping the surface of the staples with a slide and staining it by rapid staining techniques or hematoxylin–eosin. This needs to be done obviously before any cut is made into the wedge biopsy. Secondly, a portion of the staple line can be removed in an area deemed closest to the palpated tumor, and a cut perpendicular to the staple line through the exposed area is made.

The cytologic method has been validated in several studies.[18,19] Discussion with the surgeons is key to agree on a method that is mutually acceptable.

It has been shown that 45% of negative margins (as assessed by cutting away individual sutures) show adenocarcinoma in the completion lobectomy.[17] The mean margin distance with positive resection was 0.7 mm, with eighty percent <2 mm. These data suggest that at least 2 mm is a requirement for true negative margins assessed intraoperatively. Clinical data show that margin distance significantly impacts local recurrence, with a "1-cm rule" decreasing recurrence rate by half, compared to smaller margin distances.[20]

Two processes affected wedge resection margin distances: stapling-induced parenchymal stretching, resulting in overestimation of pleural surface-based distances, and microscopic extension of adenocarcinoma beyond the gross perimeter of the neoplasm.[17]

Evaluation of Treatment Effect

Histologic Evaluation

In some patients, neoadjuvant chemo-/radiation therapy is administered prior to surgical excision. In such cases, in addition to standard surgical pathology reporting (with a "y" before "pT" indicating prior treatment), the amount of viable tumor has to be estimated.

The simplest method is to estimate the percentage of tumor that is viable, compared to necrotic tumor or reactive fibrosis. An estimate of the area of viable tumor is also recommended, in mm^2.

The histologic appearance of dead tumor varies depending on time interval between treatment and surgery. In the first days, there are ghost-like outlines of cells that are barely discernable as tumor; these may persistent in the center of the treated area for several weeks. After one to two weeks, there is granulation tissue and fibrotic reaction that typically contains abundant hemosiderin, and there may be residual necrotic areas (Fig. 87.7). In contrast to tumor-related scar, which is usually high in elastic tissue and devoid of hemosiderin, posttreatment fibrosis is relatively cellular, with abundant fibroblasts and macrophages (Fig. 87.8).

Histologic components of tumor necrosis include cholesterol clefts, foreign body giant cells, and stromal hyalinosis. Treatment effects on the cells themselves include bizarre nuclei and marked cellular

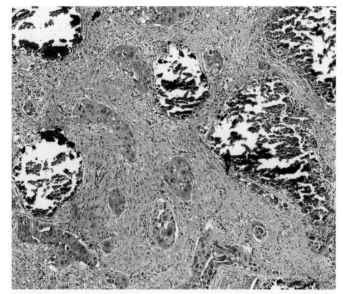

FIGURE 87.7 ▲ Treatment effect, with necrosis and fibrosis. In this tumor, there is early fibrosis around residual viable tumor nests and also around some necrotic nonviable calcified nests. In this field, treatment effect would be about 50%.

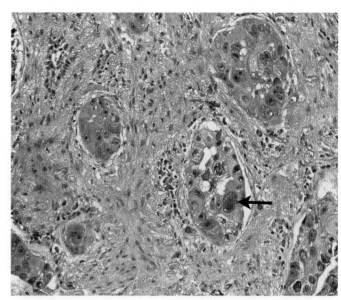

FIGURE 87.9 ▲ Treatment effect on viable tumor cells. Tumor cells with treatment effect show marked enlargement of nuclei and cytoplasm, often with vacuolization (*arrow*). Note that not all cells are equally affected.

enlargement with vacuolization (Fig. 87.9). Tumor cells with apparent treatment effect are still considered potentially viable and are not included as dead tumor.[21]

Prognostic Implications

Postoperative survival is greatly affected by area of residual tumor. Approximately 10% to 20% of tumors will show no residual tumor at all, a finding associated with a relatively good prognosis.[21] Any residual viable tumor is a bad prognostic sign, especially if there is

pleural invasion, with survival measured in months.[21] A cutoff of 400 mm^2 of residual tumor provides a statistically significant difference in survival among patients without complete response, although absence of any residual tumor is the most important prognostic finding.[21]

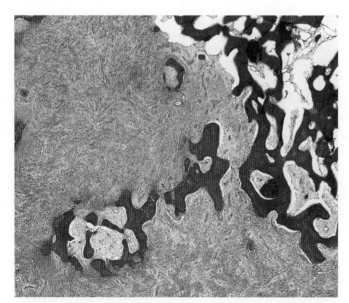

FIGURE 87.8 ▲ Treatment effect, with fibrosis. In this case, fibrosis within the bone suggests prior bone invasion, although radiation fibrosis could not be completely excluded. Staging prior to neoadjuvant chemotherapy had documented chest wall invasion. Posttreatment staging would indicate downstaging in this example as there is no viable tumor in the chest wall.

Practical Points

▶ Pleural invasion is often suggested by gross puckering or retraction of the pleura.

▶ The visceral pleura is not a margin and does not need to be inked.

▶ If there is involvement of the parietal pleura, then there is involvement of the chest wall and the chest wall margin needs to be inked and evaluated.

▶ Elastic stains have been recommended for all carcinomas that are contiguous with the pleura histologically.

▶ Arterial and venous invasion is often overlooked, is highly associated with prognosis, and can be better seen by elastic stains.

▶ Wedge biopsies for determination of malignancy are generally followed by completion surgery (lobectomy or segmentectomy) and are not typically subjected to margin assessment.

▶ When necessary, margins at the staple line can be assessed cytologically obviating the need for staple removal during frozen section.

▶ Assessment for tumor viability after neoadjuvant chemotherapy has important prognostic implications, the most important being no residual viable tumor (100% treatment effect).

REFERENCES

1. Travis WD, et al. Visceral pleural invasion: pathologic criteria and use of elastic stains: proposal for the 7th edition of the TNM classification for lung cancer. *J Thorac Oncol.* 2008;3(12):1384–1390.
2. Chang YL, et al. The significance of visceral pleural surface invasion in 321 cases of non-small cell lung cancers with pleural retraction. *Ann Surg Oncol.* 2012;19(9):3057–3064.
3. Taube JM, et al. Impact of elastic staining on the staging of peripheral lung cancers. *Am J Surg Pathol.* 2007;31(6):953–956.
4. Yilmaz A, et al. Clinical impact of visceral pleural, lymphovascular and perineural invasion in completely resected non-small cell lung cancer. *Eur J Cardiothorac Surg.* 2011;40(3):664–670.
5. Nitadori J, et al. Visceral pleural invasion does not affect recurrence or overall survival among patients with lung adenocarcinoma </= 2 cm: a proposal to reclassify T1 lung adenocarcinoma. *Chest.* 2013;144(5):1622–1631.
6. Brechot JM, et al. Blood vessel and lymphatic vessel invasion in resected nonsmall cell lung carcinoma. Correlation with TNM stage and disease free and overall survival. *Cancer.* 1996;78(10):2111–2118.
7. Kato T, et al. Angiolymphatic invasion exerts a strong impact on surgical outcomes for stage I lung adenocarcinoma, but not non-adenocarcinoma. *Lung Cancer.* 2012;77(2):394–400.
8. Usui S, et al. Differences in the prognostic implications of vascular invasion between lung adenocarcinoma and squamous cell carcinoma. *Lung Cancer.* 2013;82(3):407–412.
9. Roberts TE, et al. Vascular invasion in non-small cell lung carcinoma. *J Clin Pathol.* 1992;45(7):591–593.
10. Nentwich MF, et al. Lymphatic invasion predicts survival in patients with early node-negative non-small cell lung cancer. *J Thorac Cardiovasc Surg.* 2013;146(4):781–787.
11. Bodendorf MO, et al. Prognostic value and therapeutic consequences of vascular invasion in non-small cell lung carcinoma. *Lung Cancer.* 2009;64(1):71–78.
12. Gabor S, et al. Invasion of blood vessels as significant prognostic factor in radically resected T1-3N0M0 non-small-cell lung cancer. *Eur J Cardiothorac Surg.* 2004;25(3):439–442.
13. Kessler R, et al. Blood vessel invasion is a major prognostic factor in resected non-small cell lung cancer. *Ann Thorac Surg.* 1996;62(5):1489–1493.
14. Kudo Y, et al. Proposal on incorporating blood vessel invasion into the T classification parts as a practical staging system for stage I non-small cell lung cancer. *Lung Cancer.* 2013;81(2):187–193.
15. Tsuchiya T, et al. Stage IA non-small cell lung cancer: vessel invasion is a poor prognostic factor and a new target of adjuvant chemotherapy. *Lung Cancer.* 2007;56(3):341–348.
16. Shoji F, et al. Prognostic significance of intratumoral blood vessel invasion in pathologic stage IA non-small cell lung cancer. *Ann Thorac Surg.* 2010;89(3):864–869.
17. Goldstein NS, et al. Wedge resection margin distances and residual adenocarcinoma in lobectomy specimens. *Am J Clin Pathol.* 2003;120(5):720–724.
18. Sawabata N, et al. Cytologic examination of surgical margin of excised malignant pulmonary tumor: methods and early results. *J Thorac Cardiovasc Surg.* 1999;117(3):618–619.
19. Sawabata N, et al. Cytologically malignant margin without continuous pulmonary tumor lesion: cases of wedge resection, segmentectomy and lobectomy. *Interact Cardiovasc Thorac Surg.* 2008;7(6):1044–1048.
20. El-Sherif A, et al. Margin and local recurrence after sublobar resection of non-small cell lung cancer. *Ann Surg Oncol.* 2007;14(8):2400–2405.
21. Yamane Y, et al. A novel histopathological evaluation method predicting the outcome of non-small cell lung cancer treated by neoadjuvant therapy: the prognostic importance of the area of residual tumor. *J Thorac Oncol.* 2010;5(1):49–55.

88 Primary Extranodal Marginal Zone Lymphoma

Cleto D. Nogueira, M.D., Fabio R. Tavora, M.D., Ph.D., and Rima Koka, M.D., Ph.D.

Introduction

Primary lymphoma of the lung is rare, accounting for ~3.5% of all extranodal lymphomas and <0.5% of malignant lung tumors.[1-3] The most common type is the extranodal marginal zone lymphoma (MZL) of mucosa-associated lymphoid tissue (MALT), accounting for more than 75% of lung lymphomas.[4,5] The terms "bronchus-associated lymphoid tissue (BALT) lymphoma" and "MALT lymphoma" are used interchangeably in the lung for extranodal MZL.

Organized lymphoid tissue is not normally present in the lung. BALT is stimulated by chronic inflammatory conditions such as autoimmune disorders, smoking, and infections.[6] BALT is distinct from intrapulmonary lymph nodes, which are usually peripheral nodules incidentally found on imaging or in lung resections for unrelated conditions and which are not associated with the development of lymphoma.

Clinical Presentation

MALT lymphoma tends to affect adults with ages ranging from late 20s to late 80s with a mean age of 65. About half are asymptomatic and the lesions are discovered incidentally.[7] There seems to be no association with tobacco exposure.[8]

When present, symptoms include cough, chest pain, weight loss, dyspnea, or hemoptysis. Fever and night sweats are uncommon, reported in <15% of cases. A serum monoclonal gammopathy is found in up to 43% of patients.[7] There is a slight female predominance in several studies, and most patients present in clinical stages I and II (>85%).[7]

The staging system most frequently used is a modified Ann Arbor system for extranodal (E) lymphomas. Stage IE is confined to the lung; stage II 1E involves hilar lymph nodes; stage II 2E involves mediastinal lymph nodes; stage II 2EW involves chest wall or diaphragm; stage IIIE involves abdominal lymph nodes; and stage IVE indicates extralymphatic extrapulmonary involvement.[2]

There is a well-known association between BALT lymphomas and autoimmune disorders, including Sjögren syndrome and rheumatoid arthritis, although the mechanisms underlying the relationship are unclear.[9] In one of the largest series of BALT lymphomas, only 10% of the patients had an autoimmune disease at presentation.[2] In other studies, autoimmune diseases have been reported in up to 30% of patients.[7]

Radiologic Findings

The most common presentation on routine chest radiology is a solitary, noncalcified nodule or airspace consolidation with or without air bronchogram. However, many reports of bilateral disease have also occurred, which confirm the heterogeneous presentation of BALT lymphomas. Diffuse infiltrates with a lymphangitic appearance, diffuse interstitial lung disease, nodular patterns, bronchiectasis, lobar pneumonia patterns, and ground-glass opacities have all been reported.[1,10,11] The majority of the lesions have a high standardized uptake value (SUV) on positron emission tomography (PET) scans.[1,10]

Tissue Sampling

The diagnosis of BALT lymphoma is made most commonly by VATS (video-assisted thoracoscopy), CT-guided transthoracic biopsy, or transbronchial biopsy. The diagnosis can be suspected, suggested, and rarely confirmed with bronchoalveolar lavage. Cytology specimens procured by fine needle aspiration may yield a diagnosis especially when coupled with flow cytometry and cell block preparations for immunohistochemistry (IHC) so that clonality can be established.[12] In some instances, patients undergo lobectomies, segmentectomies, or even pneumonectomies for the resection of nodular lesions before the diagnosis of BALT lymphoma can be made.[2,8,10,13]

Gross Findings

BALT lymphomas cause yellow-white nodules with a consistency similar to that of nodal lymphomas. Cystic change is rare and associated with coexistent amyloidosis.[3] Mediastinal lymph nodes may be enlarged and are involved histologically in less than half of cases.[7]

Microscopic Findings

BALT lymphomas are distributed in a lymphangitic pattern, typically along bronchovascular bundles, interlobular septa, and visceral pleura. The lymphangitic infiltrates coalesce into masses that extend into the pulmonary parenchyma (Fig. 88.1). Occasionally, the tumor

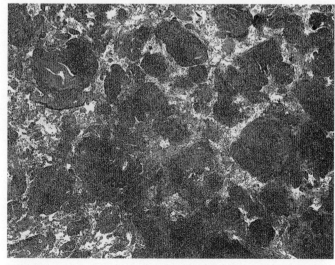

FIGURE 88.1 ▲ Primary marginal zone lymphoma, lung. In this example, there is peribronchial lymphoid proliferation that extends into the lung parenchyma.

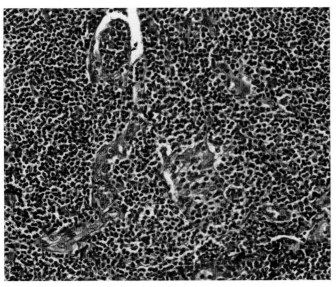

FIGURE 88.2 ▲ Primary marginal zone lymphoma, lung. The tumor cells are small, round lymphocytes.

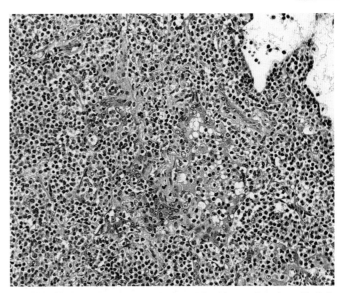

FIGURE 88.4 ▲ Primary marginal zone lymphoma, lymphoepithelial lesion. The tumor cells are infiltrating nests of pneumocytes.

is a single dominant mass. Prominent collagen sclerosis is common and occasionally obscures the lymphoid infiltrate. Vascular invasion is also often noted, while amyloid deposition occurs in fewer than 10% of tumors.[7]

Tumor cells are small lymphocytes with round nuclei, distinctly clumped chromatin, and scant cytoplasm growing in sheets or along the bronchiolar epithelium (Fig. 88.2). They tend to be cytologically indistinguishable from mature lymphocytes, which makes diagnosis on a morphologic basis alone challenging. Clusters of monocytoid B cells, which have abundant pale cytoplasm, are often seen. Plasmacytoid differentiation, often with Dutcher bodies, is common. Nucleoli of tumor cells are usually inconspicuous. The neoplastic infiltrates usually surround reactive lymphoid follicles (Fig. 88.3), and there may be follicular colonization by tumor cells in some cases. Lymphoepithelial lesions are typical (Fig. 88.4) but are not a requirement for the diagnosis. Airways are usually spared. The presence of granulomas is common and may confound the diagnosis in small biopsies.

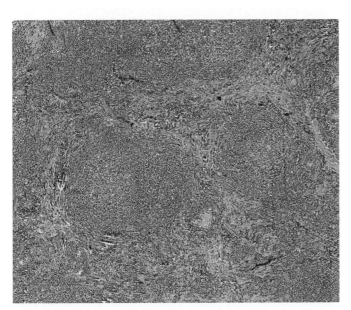

FIGURE 88.3 ▲ Primary marginal zone lymphoma, lung. Nodules of lymphocytes with expanded marginal zones are common.

The morphologic differential diagnoses include lymphoid interstitial pneumonia, nodular lymphoid hyperplasia, bronchiolar folliculitis, and other types of lymphoma (Table 88.1). Distinguishing reactive processes from BALT lymphoma can be challenging on a small biopsy, and establishing clonality through the use of ancillary studies is a requirement. Although use of flow cytometry is ideal for this purpose, in cases with plasmacytic differentiation, IHC can provide a means to assess clonality among the neoplastic plasma cells. When neither flow nor IHC can provide evidence of clonality, molecular methods such as immunoglobulin gene rearrangement studies can be utilized. Whenever sheets of large lymphoid cells are present amidst the lower-grade lesion, the possibility of transformation to diffuse large B-cell lymphoma (DLBCL) from the underlying low-grade MZL should be considered.[7] A more recently described entity of MZL with increased large cells highlights the heterogeneous nature of MZL. This designation should be reserved for those cases in which there is a prominent population of large centroblast- or immunoblast-like cells, which fail to form the large clusters or sheets required for a diagnosis of DLBCL. The precise percentage of large, blastic cells required to meet this diagnosis is not well established. However, an arbitrary percentage of 20% has been applied.[14] Additionally, Ki 67 is higher in this subtype of MZL and tends to preferentially highlight the larger cells. The significance of this subtype is that it may portend a more aggressive clinical course and an increased likelihood of transformation to large cell lymphoma. Proposals for a grading scheme similar to that of follicular lymphoma have been made and may be implemented in the future.[14]

Ancillary Testing and Genetic Profile

The neoplastic cells express B-cell markers (CD20, PAX5, or CD79a) (Table 88.2). There is coexpression of CD43 in ~70% of tumors. The neoplastic cells also typically express BCL-2. Most cases will show light chain restriction for lambda or kappa (Fig. 88.5) along with either IgM or IgA. They generally do not express CD10 and CD5, which help exclude other small cell lymphomas such as follicular lymphoma, chronic lymphocytic leukemia/small lymphocytic lymphoma, and mantle cell lymphoma. The proliferation index, as assessed by Ki 67, is usually low (<20%). The most common genetic aberrations, found in approximately 40% of BALT lymphomas, are t(11:18)(q21:q21) and t(14:18)(q32;q21) involving the *MALT1* gene.

In cases where flow cytometry and IHC cannot be reliably performed, PCR analysis for immunoglobulin heavy-chain gene rearrangements

TABLE 88.1   Pathologic and Radiologic Features of BALT Lymphoma and Other Lymphoproliferative Disorders in the Lung

Entity	Clinical Presentation	CT Features	Pathologic Features
BALT lymphoma	Asymptomatic (50%) Cough and dyspnea	Nodular consolidations, ground-glass attenuation, single or multiple. Rarely cyst or tree-in-bud appearance	Mass lesion with tracking along lymphatic routes; conspicuous *lymphoepithelial lesions*; germinal centers colonized by monocytoid B cells; monoclonal plasmacytoid cells with *Dutcher bodies* frequent May have *amyloid* stroma May have collagenous sclerosis
Follicular bronchiolitis[a]	Nonspecific; recurrent infections, association with autoimmune diseases; cough, dyspnea	Diffuse small airways involvement; nodules of 1–3 mm in diameter. Bronchiectasis may occur.	Peribronchiolar lymphoid hyperplasia with germinal centers that appear normal, with tingible body macrophages Inconspicuous lymphoepithelial lesions
Lymphoid interstitial pneumonia[a]	Common association with autoimmune diseases; cough, dyspnea, weight loss, fever, chest pain, and arthralgias	Diffuse interstitial involvement with ground-glass opacities, bronchovascular thickening, and scattered thin-walled cysts	Diffuse lymphoid hyperplasia along lymphatic routes
Nodular lymphoid hyperplasia[b]	Solitary mass in adults, sometimes in the setting of prior pneumonia, usually asymptomatic	Solitary mass, may be similar to BALT lymphoma	Localized mass with variable destruction of lung parenchyma composed of normal-appearing germinal centers and inconspicuous or absent lymphoepithelial lesions; Dutcher bodies absent; polyclonal by molecular studies
Lymphomatoid granulomatosis	Pleural effusion in 30% of cases. Also, cough, chest pain, and dyspnea common. Central nervous system (ataxia, dementia, cranial nerve palsy) and cutaneous (macular rashes, nodules) signs and symptoms may occur.	Bilateral nodules or masses with a peribronchovascular distribution. Masses may coalesce or be cavitated.	Nodules with central necrosis Mixed vasocentric infiltrate Few neutrophils, eosinophils, macrophage giant cells Absent hyaline sclerosis or lymphoepithelial lesions ***EBV*** identified by IHC/ISH
Diffuse large B-cell lymphoma	Symptoms are common: cough, hemoptysis, and dyspnea. Compression of mediastinal structures may occur with hilar involvement.	Nodule or mass with cavitation, with rare pleural involvement	Monotonous proliferation of B cells, similar in appearance to nodal DLBCL

[a]Often considered part of a spectrum.
[b]Many reported cases likely represent localized marginal zone lymphomas; this diagnosis is only rarely reported currently.

may show clonal immunoglobulin gene rearrangements. However, these results must always be interpreted in the context of the clinical scenario and morphologic and immunohistochemical findings because the sensitivity and specificity of these studies are not high enough to be fully reliant upon their results alone. It is of particular importance that reactive lymphoid proliferations occasionally produce dominant clones, which can be misinterpreted on molecular studies.[15]

Treatment and Prognosis

Treatment includes, either surgery alone or surgery in conjunction with chemotherapy, immunotherapy and radiation therapy. In one study, a majority of patients who had low-stage disease were treated with surgery alone.[7] The tumors are usually indolent and systemic therapies and/or surgery result in a complete response with 5-year disease-free survival in more than 65% of patients.[2,8,11] Some tumors recur within a few months. It is estimated that about one-fourth of cases may have evidence of extrapulmonary involvement. Combination therapies with newer targeted agents such as rituximab have been successfully used.[2,9,11,16]

Transformation of BALT lymphoma into DLBCL has been rarely reported.[17] However, areas of large B-cell lymphoma may be present in up to 20% of tumors at initial diagnosis. These mixed tumors are treated similarly to nodal DLBCL but, in one series, had a similar prognosis to pure MALT lymphomas.[7]

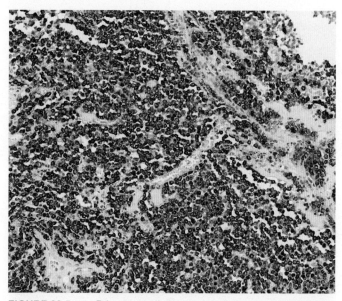

FIGURE 88.5 ▲ Primary marginal zone lymphoma, kappa light chain restriction. In situ hybridization for kappa light chains shows light chain restriction.

TABLE 88.2   Immunohistochemical Findings in BALT Lymphoma

- CD20, PAX5, or CD79a *positive* with coexpression of CD43 in 70% of cases
- BCL-2 typically *positive*
- Usually, CD10, bcl-6, cyclin D1, and CD5 *negative* (rare CD5+ cases)
- Ki 67 proliferative index *low* (<20%)

REFERENCES

1. Bae YA, Lee KS, Han J, et al. Marginal zone B-cell lymphoma of bronchus-associated lymphoid tissue: imaging findings in 21 patients. *Chest.* 2008;133:433–440.

2. Sammassimo S, Pruneri G, Andreola G, et al. A retrospective international study on primary extranodal marginal zone lymphoma of the lung (BALT lymphoma) on behalf of International Extranodal Lymphoma Study Group (IELSG). *Hematol Oncol.* 2015. *In Press.*

3. Nicholson AG, Jaffe E, Guinee D. Lymphohistiocytic tumours. In: Travis WD, et al., eds. *WHO Classification of Tumours of the Lung, Pleura, Mediastinum and Heart.* Lyon, France: IARC Press; 2015:134–136.

4. Harris NL, Jaffe ES, Stein H, et al. A revised European-American classification of lymphoid neoplasms: a proposal from the International Lymphoma Study Group. *Blood.* 1994;84:1361–1392.

5. Isaacson PG, Spencer J. Malignant lymphoma of mucosa-associated lymphoid tissue. *Histopathology.* 1987;11:445–462.

6. Gould SJ Isaacson PG. Bronchus-associated lymphoid tissue (BALT) in human fetal and infant lung. *J Pathol.* 1993;169:229–234.

7. Kurtin PJ, Myers JL, Adlakha H, et al. Pathologic and clinical features of primary pulmonary extranodal marginal zone B-cell lymphoma of MALT type. *Am J Surg Pathol.* 2001;25:997–1008.

8. Imai H, Sunaga N, Kaira K, et al. Clinicopathological features of patients with bronchial-associated lymphoid tissue lymphoma. *Intern Med.* 2009;48:301–306.

9. Oikonomou A, Astrinakis E, Kotsianidis I, et al. Synchronous BALT lymphoma and squamous cell carcinoma of the lung: coincidence or linkage? *Case Rep Oncol Med.* 2013;2013:420393.

10. Kocaturk CI, Seyhan EC, Gunluoglu MZ, et al. Primary pulmonary non-Hodgkin's lymphoma: ten cases with a review of the literature. *Tuberk Toraks.* 2012;60:246–253.

11. Zinzani PL, Pellegrini C, Gandolfi L, et al. Extranodal marginal zone B-cell lymphoma of the lung: experience with fludarabine and mitoxantrone-containing regimens. *Hematol Oncol.* 2013;31:183–188.

12. Chhieng DC. Cytology of bronchial associated lymphoid tissue lymphoma. *Diagn Cytopathol.* 2008;36:723–728.

13. Yoon RG, Kim MY, Song JW, et al. Primary endobronchial marginal zone B-cell lymphoma of bronchus-associated lymphoid tissue: CT findings in 7 patients. *Korean J Radiol.* 2013;14:366–374.

14. Kaur P. Nodal marginal zone lymphoma with increased large cells: myth versus entity. *Arch Pathol Lab Med.* 2011;135:964–966.

15. van Dongen JJ, Langerak AW, Bruggemann M, et al. Design and standardization of PCR primers and protocols for detection of clonal immunoglobulin and T-cell receptor gene recombinations in suspect lymphoproliferations: report of the BIOMED-2 Concerted Action BMH4-CT98-3936. *Leukemia.* 2003;17:2257–2317.

16. Stefanovic A, Morgensztern D, Fong T, et al. Pulmonary marginal zone lymphoma: a single centre experience and review of the SEER database. *Leuk Lymphoma.* 2008;49:1311–1320.

17. Swarup R. Bronchus-associated lymphoid tissue lymphoma stage IV with subsequent histologic transformation to an aggressive lymphoma: a case report. *J Med Case Reports.* 2011;5:455.

89 Diffuse Large B-Cell Lymphoma

Rima Koka, M.D., Ph.D., and Amy Duffield, M.D., Ph.D.

Clinical Characteristics

Diffuse large B-cell lymphoma (DLBCL) is a name given to a heterogeneous group of aggressive mature B-cell malignancies. DLBCLs have an increased propensity to arise in extranodal sites as compared to other B-cell lymphomas. While ~25% of non-Hodgkin lymphomas present with primary involvement of an extranodal site, lung involvement is relatively rare with only 3% presenting primary in the lung and secondary involvement reported to be ~7%.[1–3] DLBCLs have a propensity for extranodal involvement with ~40% occurring in extranodal sites, the majority of which involve the gastrointestinal tract. Primary lung DLBCL is exceedingly rare, and nearly all cases of DLBCL found in the lung represent secondary involvement.[1]

Because pulmonary involvement by DLBCL likely represents secondary involvement by an aggressive lymphoma, the clinical findings are similar to those seen in other patients with advanced-stage disease.[1] The signs and symptoms of the disease are highly variable and depend on the growth rate of the neoplasm, organs involved, and presence of associated mass effects.[4]

Tissue Sampling

The diagnosis of DLBCL can often be made on a core biopsy of the mass. In the setting of secondary involvement of lung in a patient with a history of lymphoma, limited immunohistochemical studies can be employed. However, in the case of a primary diagnosis, multiple immunohistochemical and in situ hybridization studies may be required for further subclassification of the neoplasm to provide information about prognosis or therapeutic options, necessitating a larger biopsy. Furthermore, if sufficient tissue is obtained, then submission of a portion of fresh tissue for flow cytometric analysis may aid in the diagnosis.

Pathologic Findings

The subclassification of DLBCLs can be based on morphology, immunophenotypic differences, and clinical characteristics of the patients. Although in some cases further subclassification may not be clinically meaningful, if distinctions can be reliably made using one or more of the above criteria, then an effort should be made to distinguish between the distinct categories described in the World Health Organization's classification of tumors of hematopoietic and lymphoid tissues (Table 89.1). When a large cell lymphoma cannot be specifically classified as one of these distinct entities, the preferred diagnosis becomes DLBCL, not otherwise specified (DLBCL, NOS). In lymph nodes, DLBCL, NOS, typically leads to diffuse effacement of nodal architecture and replacement of the normal node with atypical cells. The cell morphologies can vary, and three distinct variants have been described. Clinically, the distinction between the morphologic variants is unimportant; however, the appreciation of the morphologic spectrum of DLBCL, NOS, may be important for making an accurate diagnosis. The most common morphologic variant is the centroblastic variant in which the cells are intermediate to large and have oval to round, vesicular nuclei with a finely distributed chromatin pattern (Fig. 89.1). There may be up to four nucleoli, and the scant cytoplasm is amphophilic to basophilic. Cells of the immunoblastic variant have a highly prominent central nucleolus and a fair amount of basophilic cytoplasm. Recognition of the anaplastic variant can be of particular importance because it can be confused with a poorly differentiated

TABLE 89.1   Classification of Large B-Cell Lymphomas

	Clinical Features	Morphologic Characteristics and Variants	Immunohistochemical Features	EBV Status	Prognosis
DLBCL, NOS	Highly variable	Centroblastic Immunoblastic Anaplastic	Germinal center B-cell–like Non–germinal center B-cell–like	Negative	Good
EBV-positive DLBCL of the elderly	Age >50	Hodgkin-like cells may be seen; frequent necrosis	Commonly MUM-1 positive. CD20 may be lacking if plasmablastic or immunoblastic.	Positive	Poor
T-cell/histiocyte-rich large B-cell lymphoma	Often present with fever, malaise, and hepatosplenomegaly	Dispersed large B cells among numerous T cells and histiocytes	BCL-6 with absent follicular dendritic networks (FDC) and lacking IgD-positive mantle cells[a]	If positive, classify as EBV-positive DLBCL of the elderly	Poor
DLBCL associated with chronic inflammation	Involve body cavities, such as pleural cavity, in the context of prolonged inflammation	Mass with diffuse proliferation of large B cells of immunoblastic morphology	If plasmablastic variant, loss of CD20 with expression of MUM-1 and CD138	Positive	Poor
Lymphomatoid granulomatosis	Often associated with immunodeficiency	Angiocentric and angiodestructive polymorphous lymphoid infiltrate Grade 1: Polymorphous without atypia Grade 2: Occasional large cells in polymorphous background Grade 3: Aggregates of large cells		Positive	Variable; often correlates with grade
Primary mediastinal large B-cell lymphoma	Often present with large mediastinal mass with involvement of secondary structures	Sheets of large B cells with clear cytoplasm separated by delicate collagen fibers	MUM-1 and CD23 frequently expressed while BCL-2 and BCL-6 are variable. CD30 is present in many cases but has a heterogeneous pattern of staining.	Negative	Good
Intravascular large B-cell lymphoma	Symptoms related to involved organ. B symptoms are common.	Atypical lymphoid cells restricted to lumina of small or intermediate-sized vessels	MUM-1 is commonly expressed. Small proportion expresses CD5 or CD10	Negative	Poor; those with only cutaneous involvement have better prognosis
ALK-positive large cell lymphoma	Mostly involves lymph nodes but may present as mediastinal mass	Cells of immunoblastic or plasmablastic differentiation	Strongly positive for ALK-1 and CD138. CD30 is negative (unlike ALCL)[b]. CD20 may be weak or negative.	Negative	Poor
Primary effusion lymphoma	Associated with immunodeficiency. History of recurrent effusions with no evidence of lymphadenopathy or organomegaly	Cells of immunoblastic or plasmablastic differentiation	Lack CD19, CD20, and CD79a. Often express CD138	Positive (Coinfection with HHV-8 also found)	Poor

[a]If present, nodular lymphocyte–predominant Hodgkin lymphoma must be considered.
[b]ALCL, anaplastic large cell lymphoma.

carcinoma (Fig. 89.2). The cells are highly pleomorphic and have bizarre nuclear contours and may also resemble cells of Hodgkin lymphoma and anaplastic large cell lymphoma.

The use of immunohistochemical studies is critically important to the diagnosis of DLBCL. The establishment of B-cell lineage requires demonstration of B-cell markers such as CD19, CD20, CD22, CD79a, or PAX-5. If patient has a history of B-cell lymphoma and is on anti-CD20 therapies, expression of CD20 may be weak or absent on the neoplastic cells. Therefore, the use of more than one B-cell–specific antibody may be necessary in such cases. Use of T-cell markers CD3 and CD5 will help delineate whether the neoplastic population aberrantly expresses CD5. In such cases, cyclin D1 may be indicated to exclude the blastoid or pleomorphic variants of mantle cell lymphoma. Ki 67 is useful to identify the proliferative potential of the neoplasm. DLBCL typically demonstrates a proliferative index of >40%.

Immunophenotypic subgrouping of DLBCL, NOS, into germinal center–type and non–germinal center–like subgroups may be required depending on the practice environment. However, similar to the morphologic variants, the clinical significance of this distinction is unclear as various studies have produced conflicting results as to the prognostic utility of this subclassification.[5] Germinal center cell–type DLBCL is defined as cases with CD10 expression by >30% of neoplastic cells with or without concurrent expression of BCL-6. In cases that lack CD10 expression, presence of IRF4/MUM-1 in >30% of cells or lack of expression of all three of these proteins leads to the designation of non–germinal center cell–like DLBCL.[6]

In addition to DLBCL, NOS, there are several other large B-cell lymphomas that may secondarily involve the lung. Those that are classified as distinct entities in the WHO need to be considered in the diagnosis of large B-cell lymphomas involving the lung (Table 89.1). The entity that is of particular interest is EBV-positive DLBCL of the elderly. Seventy percent of these patients present with extranodal disease, with frequent lung involvement.[7]

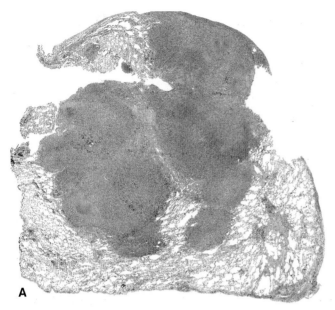

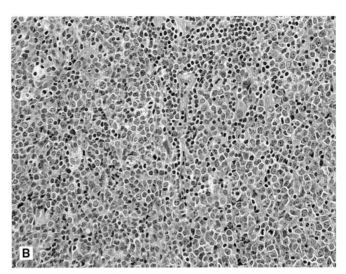

FIGURE 89.1 ▲ Typical histology of diffuse large B-cell lymphoma, not otherwise specified. **A.** Low magnification shows coalescing nodules. **B.** There is a population of moderate to large cells with prominent nucleoli and eosinophilic cytoplasm.

In addition, there are three subtypes of LBCL, which, while rare, have a particular affinity for the lung. They are lymphomatoid granulomatosis, DLBCL associated with chronic inflammation (DLBCL-CI), and primary effusion lymphoma (PEL). Lymphomatoid granulomatosis is an EBV-drive lymphoproliferative disorder, which often affects the lung and brain in a characteristically angiocentric and angiodestructive pattern. This entity will be discussed in detail in Chapter 90. DLBCL-CI occurs in body cavities that have been chronically exposed to inflammation. The most common location is the pleural cavity, and these cases are referred to as pyothorax-associated lymphoma (PAL). This lymphoma is strongly associated with EBV. In contrast to PEL, which is also an EBV-associated lymphoma that often affects the pleural cavity, PAL is a mass-forming lymphoma. Furthermore, PEL is associated with both EBV and human herpes virus 8 (HHV-8) and tends to express plasma cell markers but lack characteristic B-cell antigens.

The other subtypes to consider are primary mediastinal large B-cell lymphoma (see Chapter 127), T-cell/histiocyte-rich large B-cell lymphoma, intravascular large B-cell lymphoma, and ALK-positive large B-cell lymphoma. The morphologic and immunohistochemical characteristics of these entities are described in Table 89.1.

Because DLBCL represents an entity that results from clonal proliferation of B cells, in diagnostically challenging cases, tissue may be submitted for gene rearrangement studies. This polymerase chain reaction (PCR)-based assay relies on the demonstration of the immunoglobulin gene rearrangements that result in an amplicon of the same size in a significant proportion of the B cells in the tissue. This finding raises the likelihood that there is a clonal proliferation of B cells within the tested sample. Recent advances in molecular technologies will soon allow for sequencing of the immunoglobulin gene and will increase the specificity of rearrangement studies.

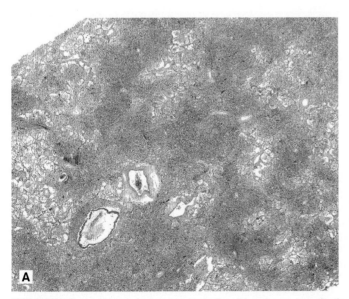

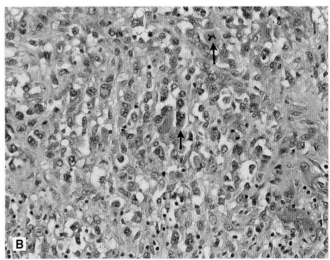

FIGURE 89.2 ▲ Primary pulmonary large B-cell lymphoma, anaplastic variant. **A.** Low magnification shows masses of lymphoma replacing the lung parenchyma. **B.** The lymphoma cells are large and irregular, with atypical mitotic figures (*arrows*).

Differential Diagnosis

The primary differential diagnoses for DLBCL are Burkitt lymphoma and blastoid/pleomorphic mantle cell lymphoma. High-grade variants of mantle cell lymphoma may be readily excluded with immunostaining for CD5 and cyclin D1. Burkitt lymphoma is a malignancy of intermediate-sized B cells, which are highly monomorphic and may appear to have neuroendocrine-like finely dispersed chromatin. The characteristic immunophenotype of Burkitt lymphoma is that of germinal center phenotype B cells; CD10 and BCL-6 are typically expressed while BCL-2 expression is classically absent. Furthermore, the proliferative index in Burkitt lymphoma is extremely high, approaching 100% in most cases. In cases where morphology is suggestive of Burkitt lymphoma but immunophenotype is not consistent with such a diagnosis, the diagnosis of B-cell lymphoma, unclassifiable, with features intermediate between DLBCL and Burkitt lymphoma, can be made. In these rare cases, fluorescence in situ hybridization (FISH) studies for rearrangements involving MYC, BCL-2, and BCL-6 may be necessary to exclude the possibility of a "double-hit" lymphoma in which two or more of these genes will be involved in chromosomal translocations.

In small needle biopsies, it can also be difficult to differentiate between DLBCL and Grade 3B follicular lymphoma. In tissue that has a germinal center phenotype and a vaguely nodular appearance, immunostains for CD21 and/or CD23 can be utilized to assess for the underlying follicular dendritic meshworks characteristic of follicular lymphoma. The distinction may not be critical for clinical care of the patient, and if it is not possible to distinguish between DLBCL and Grade 3B FL, then a diagnosis of "large B-cell lymphoma" can be rendered.

Prognosis and Treatment

The International Prognostic Index (IPI) is a valuable tool to risk-stratify patients based on various clinical parameters.[8] Unfavorable variables include age > 60, poor performance status, advanced stage, involvement of two or more extranodal sites, and high serum LDH. The use of anti-CD20 monoclonal antibody, rituximab in combination with the CHOP regimen (cyclophosphamide, doxorubicin, vincristine sulfate, prednisone), is the standard first-line therapy of most subtypes of DLBCL.[9–11] While there can be significant prognostic differences in certain subtypes of DLBCL, overall, a 5-year progression-free survival of 70% to 80% has been shown in DLBCL, NOS patients who have been treated with R-CHOP.[10,12]

REFERENCES

1. Mian M, Wasle I, Gritsch S, et al. B cell lymphoma with lung involvement: what is it about? *Acta Haematol.* 2015;133:221–225.
2. Rosenberg SA, Diamond HD, Jaslowitz B, et al. Lymphosarcoma: a review of 1269 cases. *Medicine (Baltimore).* 1961;40:31–84.
3. Zucca E, Cavalli F. Extranodal lymphomas. *Ann Oncol.* 2000;11(Suppl 3): 219–222.
4. Armitage JO, Weisenburger DD. New approach to classifying non-Hodgkin's lymphomas: clinical features of the major histologic subtypes. Non-Hodgkin's Lymphoma Classification Project. *J Clin Oncol.* 1998;16:2780–2795.
5. Nyman H, Adde M, Karjalainen-Lindsberg ML, et al. Prognostic impact of immunohistochemically defined germinal center phenotype in diffuse large B-cell lymphoma patients treated with immunochemotherapy. *Blood.* 2007;109:4930–4935.
6. Colomo L, Lopez-Guillermo A, Perales M, et al. Clinical impact of the differentiation profile assessed by immunophenotyping in patients with diffuse large B-cell lymphoma. *Blood.* 2003;101:78–84.
7. Oyama T, Yamamoto K, Asano N, et al. Age-related EBV-associated B-cell lymphoproliferative disorders constitute a distinct clinicopathologic group: a study of 96 patients. *Clin Cancer Res.* 2007;13:5124–5132.
8. Bishton MJ, Hughes S, Richardson F, et al. Delineating outcomes of patients with diffuse large B cell lymphoma using the National Comprehensive Cancer Network-International Prognostic Index and Positron Emission Tomography-defined Remission Status; a population-based analysis. *Br J Haematol.* 2016;172:246–254.
9. Coiffier B. Rituximab therapy in malignant lymphoma. *Oncogene.* 2007;26: 3603–3613.
10. Feugier P, Van Hoof A, Sebban C, et al. Long-term results of the R-CHOP study in the treatment of elderly patients with diffuse large B-cell lymphoma: a study by the Groupe d'Etude des Lymphomes de l'Adulte. *J Clin Oncol.* 2005;23:4117–4126.
11. Pfreundschuh M, Trumper L, Osterborg A, et al. CHOP-like chemotherapy plus rituximab versus CHOP-like chemotherapy alone in young patients with good-prognosis diffuse large-B-cell lymphoma: a randomised controlled trial by the MabThera International Trial (MInT) Group. *Lancet Oncol.* 2006;7:379–391.
12. Liu D, Shimonov J, Primanneni S, et al. t(8;14;18): a 3-way chromosome translocation in two patients with Burkitt's lymphoma/leukemia. *Mol Cancer.* 2007;6:35.

90 Lymphomatoid Granulomatosis

Allen P. Burke, M.D.

Terminology

Lymphomatoid granulomatosis (LyG) was first described in 1972 and survives as a distinct clinicopathologic entity today. Initially considered a proliferation that had features of both Wegener granulomatosis (currently granulomatosis with polyangiitis) and lymphoma, most cases of LyG are now considered a T cell–rich, EBV-related B-cell lymphoma.[1–4]

Diagnostic Criteria

All cases of LyG have a mixed population of atypical B lymphocytes and typical small T lymphocytes, which may predominate. Vascular invasion (angiocentricity) is a requirement for diagnosis. It is still debated if the presence of EBV by in situ hybridization is essential for the diagnosis, because sampling may preclude identification of these cells if they are not numerous or if the sample is small.[1–3]

Although skin and nervous system involvement are common, it is debated if LyG can occur without lung involvement. Series of pathologically documented LyG show no case without lung involvement.[4] The relatively high frequency of the development of nodal lymphoma in earlier studies has been questioned, as they were reported prior to the era of molecular diagnostics,[2] and recent series show no case with nodal lymphoma.[4]

Clinical Findings

Men are more frequently involved than are women, at a rate of about 2:1. The mean age at presentation is between 40 and 50 years, although there is a wide range. The skin and central nervous system are involved in about 1/3 to ½ of patients. Other sites of involvement include the upper respiratory tract, kidney, gastrointestinal tract, eye, adrenal gland, and liver.[4]

Fever and cough are the most common pulmonary symptoms.

Immune disorders and other malignancies have been reported in association with LyG in about 5% of patients.[2]

Radiologic Findings

Chest x-ray and computed tomographic scans show parenchymal lesions that are usually multiple and predominate in the lower lobes. Cavitation may be seen by computed tomography but is not present on chest x-ray.[3]

Microscopic Findings

LyG is characterized by a mixed cell infiltrate of small lymphocytes, large immunoblast-like lymphocytes that type as B cells, macrophages, and plasma cells. Neutrophils and eosinophils are scarce or absent. The infiltrate invariably invades the wall of small and medium-sized arteries, generally without fibrinoid necrosis (Figs. 90.1 to 90.3). Granulomas are absent in the lung, although they have been described in cutaneous disease. Necrosis is common but apoptosis, as often seen in granulomatosis with polyangiitis, is inconspicuous or absent.

Immunohistochemical and Molecular Findings

CD20 immunohistochemical staining is critical in identifying the atypical B cells, which are few in low-grade lesions and more numerous, forming small nests, in higher-grade tumors. Sheets of atypical cells are absent.[4]

CD30 staining is variable in tumor cells, and CD15 is negative. The background lymphocytes are CD3 positive, with a predominance of CD4-positive over CD8-positive cells. The cells in the arterial walls are generally benign CD3-positive lymphocytes.[4]

In situ hybridization or EBV (EBER) is positive in higher-grade lesions (Fig. 90.4). On biopsies, low-grade tumors may not show any positive cells, but EBV genome is detected by polymerase chain reaction.[4]

Light chain restriction occurs in about one-third of cases.[2]

Immunoglobulin gene rearrangements are present in up to 50% of cases, and T-cell receptor gene rearrangements occur in <10%. The significance of the latter finding is unclear, as currently all cases of LyG are considered by some as B-cell proliferations.[4]

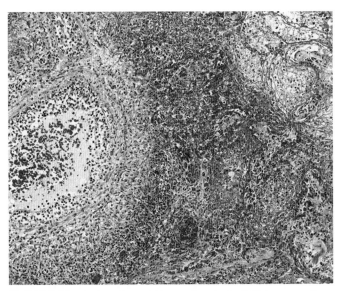

FIGURE 90.2 ▲ Lymphomatoid granulomatosis. A higher magnification of Figure 90.1 demonstrates necrosis surrounding an infiltrated small muscular artery.

Grading

Grading is based on the number of cells containing EBV genome and recommended by the WHO,[3] and a requirement for certain treatment protocols. Fewer than 5 EBER-positive cells per high-power field (hpf) (0 to 5) constitute grade 1; 5 to 50 EBER-positive cells grade 2; and >50 EBER-positive cells grade 3. Grade 1 tumors frequently have no positivity on small biopsy samples and the diagnosis is based on PCR testing for EBV and histologic findings.[4]

Differential Diagnosis

From a practical standpoint, a lymphoid lesion in the lung, which raises the possibility of lymphoma by histologic appearance, requires expert hematopathologic evaluation with current immunohistochemical panels or, in the case of angiocentric lesions, consultation with a pathologist familiar with LyG.

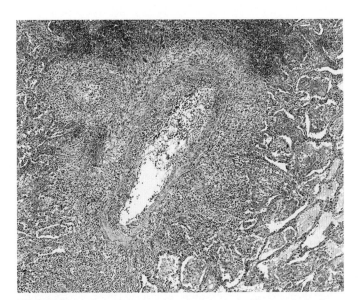

FIGURE 90.1 ▲ Lymphomatoid granulomatosis. There is typically involvement of small to medium-sized arteries.

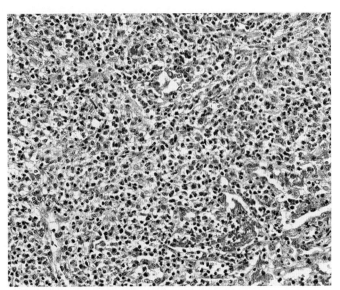

FIGURE 90.3 ▲ Lymphomatoid granulomatosis. The infiltrate is polymorphous. Without immunohistochemical stains, the atypical B cells may not be discernable.

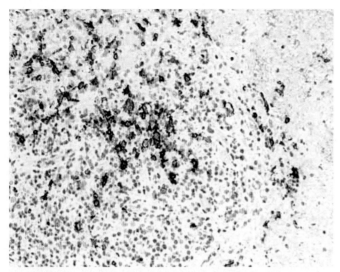

FIGURE 90.4 ▲ Lymphomatoid granulomatosis, in situ hybridization for EBER. There are scattered positive cells, which correspond to atypical B cells. (Reproduced from Colby TV. Current histological diagnosis of lymphomatoid granulomatosis. *Mod Pathol.* 2012;25(suppl 1): S39–S42, with permission.)

The most difficult differential diagnosis is the distinction between LyG and EBV-associated posttransplant lymphoproliferative disease. Posttransplant lymphoproliferative disorders may mimic the histologic findings of LyG, and some authorities hesitate to make a diagnosis of LyG in transplant patients.[2] However, LyG has been reported in immunosuppressed patients with rheumatoid arthritis and Crohn disease, as well as common variable immunodeficiency.[4]

Other EBV-related lymphomas, such as NK/T-cell lymphomas, are also EBV related and angiocentric. NK/T-cell lymphoma, in contrast to LyG, is characterized by apoptotic necrosis, and the atypical cells do not express B-cell markers.

Other entities in the differential diagnosis include Hodgkin lymphoma, which is typically composed of a polymorphous cell population, and granulomatosis with polyangiitis. These entities can typically be distinguished based on histologic and immunohistochemical findings. Hodgkin lymphoma of the lung is rare and should demonstrate Reed-Sternberg cells. The necrosis of granulomatosis with polyangiitis differs markedly from that of LyG, with the presence of abundant neutrophils; there are frequent giant cells and poorly formed granulomas, unlike LyG; and EBV-positive cells are absent.

Prognosis and Treatment

Historically, the prognosis of LyG is poor, with survival rates of 25% to 50% after 1 to 2 years and a median survival of 14 months.[2] A National Cancer Institute protocol, separating patients by grade, has resulted in somewhat better outcomes. Patients with LYG grades 1 and 2 were treated with interferon α and grade 3 with DA-EPOCH-R (dose-adjusted etoposide, prednisone, vincristine, cyclophosphamide, doxorubicin, and rituximab, DA-EPOCH-R).[4]

REFERENCES

1. Colby TV. Current histological diagnosis of lymphomatoid granulomatosis. *Mod Pathol.* 2012;25(suppl 1):S39–S42.
2. Katzenstein AL, Doxtader E, Narendra S. Lymphomatoid granulomatosis: insights gained over 4 decades. *Am J Surg Pathol.* 2010;34:e35–e48.
3. Nicholson AG, Jaffe E, Guinee D, Lymphohistiocytic tumours. In: Travis WD, et al. eds. *WHO Classification of Tumours of the Lung, Pleura, Mediastinum and Heart.* Lyon, France: IARC Press; 2015:134–136.
4. Song JY, Pittaluga S, Dunleavy K, et al. Lymphomatoid granulomatosis—a single institute experience: pathologic findings and clinical correlations. *Am J Surg Pathol.* 2015;39:141–156.

91 Hodgkin Lymphoma

Rima Koka, M.D., Ph.D., and Amy Duffield, M.D., Ph.D.

General

The two distinct branches of Hodgkin lymphoma are nodular lymphocyte–predominant Hodgkin lymphoma (NLPHL) and classical Hodgkin lymphoma (CHL). While NLPHL occurs primarily in males within the 30- to 50-year age group, CHL has a bimodal age distribution with the first peak occurring at 15 to 35 years of age and the second peak occurring around the seventh decade of life. There is a slight male predominance in CHL. A common presenting complaint is peripheral lymphadenopathy, although the nodular sclerosis subtype of CHL is often associated with mediastinal involvement as well. B symptoms, including fever, drenching night sweats, and significant weight loss, are seen in up to 40% of patients.[1]

Secondary pulmonary involvement, typically presenting as an extension of disease originating in mediastinal and hilar lymph nodes, has been shown to occur in 6% to 12% of patients and is usually the classic nodular sclerosing type.[1] Multinodular involvement of the lung is uncommon and indicative of stage IV disease.

Primary pulmonary Hodgkin lymphoma (PPHL) is rare and is thought to arise directly from lung-associated lymphoid tissue.[2] Common presenting symptoms included dry cough, fever, or chest pain.[3] Due to the nonspecific nature of these symptoms, a delay in diagnosis and treatment may occur.[3,4] Most cases are classical nodular sclerosing type,[2,3,5–8] with a few cases of mixed cellularity; other subtypes have not been described as primary in the lung.[4]

Pathologic Findings

The morphologic features of CHL vary based on the subtype, which include nodular sclerosing (NSCHL), mixed cellularity (MCCHL), lymphocyte-rich (LRCHL), and lymphocyte-depleted (LDCHL) Hodgkin lymphoma.

NSCHL, which represents the most common variant of PPHL (60% to 70%), is characterized by large bands of fibrosis, which divide the tissue in nodules[9] (Fig. 91.1). Within the nodules, there are variable numbers of Reed-Sternberg (RS) cells and Hodgkin cells in a mixed inflammatory background (Fig. 91.2). RS cells have two or more nuclear lobes, each with pale chromatin and a prominent eosinophilic nucleolus, as well as abundant, slightly basophilic cytoplasm. Hodgkin cells are mononuclear variants of the classic RS cells (Fig. 91.3). In NSCHL, the RS cells often demonstrate cytoplasmic retraction, which makes them appear to reside within lacunae, and these cells are accordingly referred to as lacunar cells.

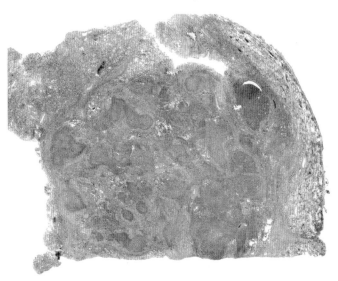

FIGURE 91.1 ▲ Classic Hodgkin lymphoma, nodular sclerosing variant. Wide bands of fibrosis dividing inflammatory cells into nodules.

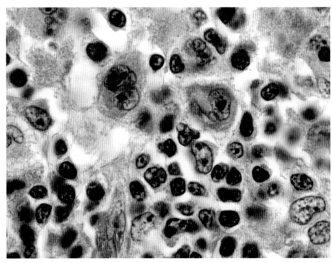

FIGURE 91.3 ▲ Classic Hodgkin lymphoma, nodular sclerosing variant. A high-power view of Reed-Sternberg cells is shown.

Of note, NSCHL may be associated with necrosis and granulomatous inflammation, which may be confused with an infectious process in the lung, especially in limited samples, which may not include readily identifiable Hodgkin and RS cells. The background inflammatory cells in this subtype are typically a mixture of lymphocytes, histiocytes, and eosinophils.

MCCHL is also characterized by an inflammatory background rich in eosinophils, plasma cells, neutrophils, and lymphocytes; granulomas may also be present. LDCHL is an extremely rare subtype of CHL that has been associated with HIV infection. In these cases, RS cells predominate over the background lymphocytes, and this entity may be confused with anaplastic large cell lymphoma (ALCL) or a sarcomatous neoplasm.

LRCHL often has the nodular appearance of NLPHL and has similar follicular dendritic cell networks underlying the nodules. The distinction between NLPHL and LRCHL rests on the immunophenotype of the neoplastic cells. While the histologic subtypes of CHL have varied morphologies on hematoxylin and eosin–stained sections, the immunophenotype of the RS cells in most of these cases is the same.

RS cells invariably express CD30 and dim nuclear Pax-5, and most also coexpress CD15. Despite the fact that the RS cells stain with the B-cell marker Pax-5, they are negative or only weakly positive for CD20. The frequency of association with Epstein-Barr virus (EBV) is dependent on the histologic subtype, with MCCHL being the most commonly associated, followed by LRCHL and NSCHL.[10] Most cases of LDCHL, which occur in the setting of HIV, are also positive for EBV.

Differential Diagnosis

The differential diagnosis of CHL includes ALCL, as the neoplastic cells of both of these entities strongly express CD30. The neoplastic cells of ALCL are of T-cell lineage and tend to be present in larger numbers than would be expected in CHL. While ALCL can lack expression of CD3, the neoplastic cells typically express at least a few T-cell markers including CD2, CD5, CD7, CD4, CD8, and/or TIA-1. Dim expression of PAX-5, which is a fairly B lineage–specific marker, strongly favors CHL over ALCL.

Treatment and Prognosis

In the case of secondary involvement of lung by Hodgkin lymphoma, direct extension into lung parenchyma is classified as stage II disease while noncontiguous extralymphatic involvement of lung is classified as stage IV. While stage II disease still has a relatively good prognosis, stage IV disease does not. Additional unfavorable prognostic factors include age > 45, male gender, anemia, low serum albumin, leukocytosis, and presence of B symptoms, of which fever and weight loss are associated with lower survival rates.[9,10]

REFERENCES

1. Laurent C, Do C, Gourraud PA, et al. Prevalence of common non-Hodgkin lymphomas and subtypes of Hodgkin lymphoma by nodal site of involvement: a systematic retrospective review of 938 cases. *Medicine (Baltimore).* 2015;94:e987.
2. Saraya T, Fujino T, Suzuki A, et al. Hodgkin lymphoma with rapidly destructive, cavity-forming lung disease. *J Clin Oncol.* 2013;31:e211–e214.
3. Cooksley N, Judge DJ, Brown J. Primary pulmonary Hodgkin's lymphoma and a review of the literature since 2006. *BMJ Case Rep.* 2014;2014.
4. Rodriguez J, Tirabosco R, Pizzolitto S, et al. Hodgkin lymphoma presenting with exclusive or preponderant pulmonary involvement: a clinicopathologic study of 5 new cases. *Ann Diagn Pathol.* 2006;10:83–88.

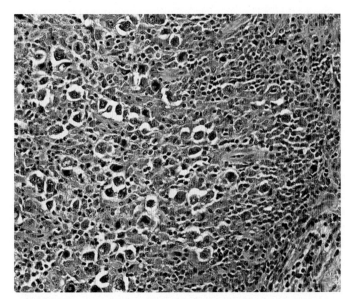

FIGURE 91.2 ▲ Classic Hodgkin lymphoma, nodular sclerosing variant. Numerous Reed-Sternberg and Hodgkin cells in a mixed inflammatory background.

5. Fratoni S, Abruzzese E, Niscola P, et al. Primary pulmonary Hodgkin lymphoma simulating a mediastinal tumour: an uncommon occurrence. *Mediterr J Hematol Infect Dis.* 2013;5:e2013013.

6. Urasinski T, Kamienska E, Gawlikowska-Sroka A, et al. Pediatric pulmonary Hodgkin lymphoma: analysis of 10 years data from a single center. *Eur J Med Res.* 2010;15(suppl 2):206–210.

7. Homma M, Yamochi-Onizuka T, Shiozawa E, et al. Primary pulmonary classical Hodgkin lymphoma with two recurrences in the mediastinum: a case report. *J Clin Exp Hematop.* 2010;50:151–157.

8. Bieliauskas S, Reyes-Trocchia A, Krasan GP, et al. Hodgkin lymphoma presenting as multiple cavitary pulmonary nodules with associated mediastinal adenopathy and neck mass. *J Pediatr Hematol Oncol.* 2009;31:730–733.

9. Moccia AA, Donaldson J, Chhanabhai M, et al. International Prognostic Score in advanced-stage Hodgkin's lymphoma: altered utility in the modern era. *J Clin Oncol.* 2012;30:3383–3388.

10. Hasenclever D, Diehl V. A prognostic score for advanced Hodgkin's disease. International Prognostic Factors Project on Advanced Hodgkin's Disease. *N Engl J Med.* 1998;339:1506–1514.

92 Histiocytic Tumor Proliferations of the Lung

Marie-Christine Aubry, M.D., Allen P. Burke, M.D., and Rima Koka, M.D., Ph.D.

Overview

The differential diagnosis of histiocytic proliferations of the lung is broad (Table 92.1). The main consideration for neoplastic histiocytic proliferations include Rosai-Dorfman disease (RDD), Erdheim-Chester disease (ECD), Langerhans cell histiocytosis (LCH), and other histiocytic and dendritic cell neoplasms. These neoplasms are rare and less common than nonneoplastic proliferations of histiocytes.

Rosai-Dorfman Disease

Clinical

RDD, previously known as sinus histiocytosis with massive lymphadenopathy, is a disease that primarily involves lymph nodes, especially of the neck.[1,2] Most patients present with lymphadenopathy and systemic symptoms of fever and weight loss. Extranodal manifestations occur in 43% of patients, while in 23%, there is no lymph node disease.[3] Pulmonary involvement is uncommon and has been reported in only 2% of patients.[4]

Pulmonary manifestations include an incidental mass, either with or without systemic symptoms resulting from lymph node involvement,[3,5] stridor secondary to airway compression,[6] cough, and syncope.[4,7] Pulmonary artery involvement has been reported.[4,7]

The prognosis for RDD in general is excellent; however, patients with lung involvement may develop progressive disease, resulting in their death.[2]

Radiologic Findings

The imaging findings are variable and include parenchymal nodules, pleural thickening, and pleural effusions.[1,2]

TABLE 92.1 Histiocytic Proliferations of the Lung

(1) Histiocytic neoplasms
   (i) Pulmonary Langerhans cell histiocytosis and sarcoma
   (ii) Erdheim-Chester disease
   (iii) Rosai-Dorfman disease
   (iv) Histiocytic sarcomas
   (v) Interdigitating dendritic cell sarcoma
   (vi) Follicular dendritic cell sarcoma
(2) Nonneoplastic histiocytic lesions
   (i) Storage diseases
      (a) Gaucher disease
      (b) Niemann-Pick disease
      (c) Fabry disease
   (ii) Infections
      (a) Malakoplakia
      (b) Whipple disease
   (iii) Crystal-storing histiocytosis

Microscopic Findings

Histologic findings are those of extrapulmonary lesions. The infiltrates may be nodular (Fig. 92.1) or interstitial, composed of abundant macrophages with large pale cytoplasm, in a background of small lymphocytes, plasma cells, and variable fibrosis. The distinguishing feature of RDD is emperipolesis which is characterized by lymphocytes or neutrophils in the cytoplasm of the macrophages (Fig. 92.1).

Immunohistochemically, the macrophages are typically positive for CD68, CD14, and S100 protein. They are usually negative for CD1a and other dendritic markers such as CD21 and CD35, helpful findings for the differential diagnosis (Table 92.2). IgG4 plasma cells may be prominent, underscoring the lack of specificity of this finding.[5,8,9]

Differential Diagnosis

The differential diagnosis includes other monocytic and histiocytic diseases such as LCH, ECD (see below), IgG4-related diseases (Chapter 51), and lymphomas, particularly Hodgkin lymphoma.

Langerhans Cell Histiocytosis and Sarcoma

General

LCH is a clonal neoplastic disorder seen primarily in children and young adults. LCH is classified according to the sites of involvement. The disease may be localized to one organ, most commonly bone; it may involve multiple sites in one organ system or involve multiple organs (such as diseases previously known as Hand-Schüller-Christian disease or Letterer-Siwe disease). Rarely, the Langerhans cell proliferation may be highly aggressive and the morphology of the Langerhans cells may be overtly malignant warranting a diagnosis of Langerhans cell sarcoma.

Pulmonary Langerhans cell histiocytosis (PLCH) (Chapter 24) differs from most LCH and yet has some overlapping features. Indeed, some adults with PLCH have been described to have co-occurring diabetes insipidus, bone lesions, and skin involvement.[10–12] Like LCH, BRAF mutation is present but only in a subset of cases.[13–15] In contrast to other LCH, PLCH is strongly linked to cigarette smoking.[1] In fact, patients with PLCH and bone lesions have seen their bone lesions regress with smoking cessation.[16]

Clinical

LCH occurs predominantly in children, adolescents, and young adults. The lungs are involved in fewer than 5% of children over 2 years with multiorgan LCH and fewer than 25% of children under 2 years.[17] LCH in children is never isolated to the lungs,[17] although an adolescent with disease limited to nails and lung has been reported.[18] In children with significant pulmonary disease, multisystem involvement is invariably present.[19]

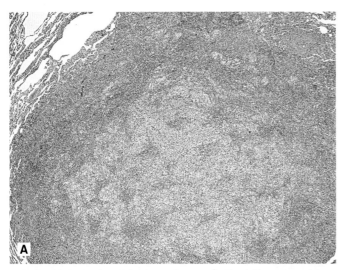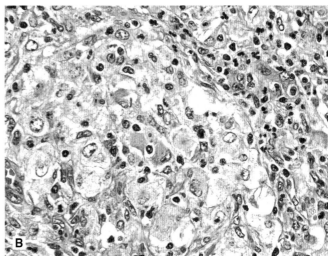

FIGURE 92.1 ▲ Rosai-Dorfman disease. **A.** The infiltrate is nodular, composed mostly of histiocytes with abundant pale eosinophilic cytoplasm admixed with various inflammatory cells including lymphocytes, plasma cells, neutrophils, and eosinophils. **B.** The histiocytes show emperipolesis characterized by intact inflammatory cells within the cytoplasm of the histiocytes.

The self-limited congenital form of LCH that involves the skin[20] only rarely involves the lungs.[21]

Although lung involvement is considered a "risk organ," lung lesions generally result primarily in pneumothorax and do not significantly reduce survival.[17] Other "risk organs" include the liver, spleen, and bone marrow, with multiple "risk" organ involvement imparting a poor prognosis. Most frequent "nonrisk" organs are bones, skin, and pituitary gland, the last resulting in diabetes insipidus.

Langerhans cell sarcoma is mainly a disease of the adult. Although skin and soft tissue are most commonly involved, multiorgan involvement may occur. In a review of the world literature, lung involvement occurred in 2 of 28 reported cases.[22]

Microscopic Findings

Pulmonary lesions in systemic LCH demonstrate nodular proliferations of Langerhans cells and are more monotonous than PLCH (Fig. 92.2). They are not typically fibrotic or stellate. Eosinophils are frequent, and the immunohistochemical profile is that of normal Langerhans cells. *BRAFV600E* mutation can be detected in over a third of cases and confirmed with immunohistochemistry.[14]

Prognosis and Treatment

Childhood LCH is treated with systemic chemotherapy, including prednisone and vinblastine, if there is multifocal bone and risk organ

involvement (including lung involvement). Prognosis is good if there is response to treatment. If there is reactivation of disease, which occurs in less than one-third of patients, the majority of patients die of disease.[17] Intrapleural bleomycin and talc pleurodesis may be performed if the lung involvement results in pneumothorax.[18]

Erdheim-Chester Disease

Background

ECD is a rare non–Langerhans cell histiocytosis that is characterized by bilateral symmetrical sclerotic bone lesions involving the metaphysis and diaphysis of long bones.

Clinical

Almost all patients with ECD have classic bony involvement, typically symmetric bilateral osteosclerotic lesions of the distal long bones.

Extraskeletal manifestations include central nervous system, cardiovascular, retroperitoneal, adrenal, and pulmonary involvement. As with LCH, involvement of the pituitary gland results in diabetes insipidus. Other characteristic features include exophthalmos and xanthelasma.[23]

About two-thirds of patients have lung involvement, as identified by computed tomographic scans, typically involving both the parenchyma and pleura. Less than one-half of those patients have

TABLE 92.2 Immunohistochemical Features of Histiocytic Lesions

	Langerhans Cell Histiocytosis	Erdheim-Chester Disease	Rosai-Dorfman Disease	Interdigitating Dendritic Cell Sarcoma	Follicular Dendritic Cell Sarcoma
CD1a	++	–	–	–	–
CD14	–	++	++	–	–
CD68	+/–	++	++	+/–	+/–
CD163	–	++	++	–	+/–
HLA DR	++	–	+	+	+
Factor XIIIA	–	++	–	–	–
Langerin	++	–	–	–	–
Fascin	–	++	+	++	–
S100	+	–	–	++	+/–
Lysozyme	–	–	++	+/–	–
CD21, CD23, CD35	–	–	–	–	++

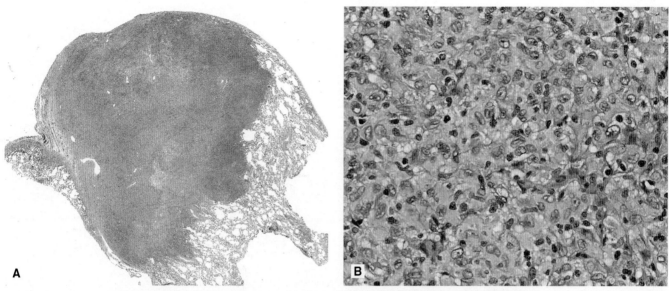

FIGURE 92.2 ▲ Systemic Langerhans cell histiocytosis involving lung in a 16-year-old nonsmoker with multiple lymph node involvement. **A.** Low magnification shows a nodular lung lesion. **B.** High magnification shows an infiltrate composed predominantly of histiocytes with reniform-shaped nuclei and nuclear grooving.

pulmonary symptoms, related to parenchymal involvement or pleural effusions.[23] Symptoms related to pulmonary involvement may be due to infiltration of the lungs or to pulmonary edema secondary to cardiac disease.

The age of onset of patients with pulmonary ECD ranges from 6 to 71 years. Males outnumber females by a 2:1 ratio. The diagnosis is often missed initially, with a range of 0 to 25 years between onset of symptoms and pathologic diagnosis. Typically, diagnosis rests on radiologic features, with confirmation of histologic findings by biopsy of retroperitoneum, skin, pericardium, central nervous system, or kidney.[23]

Radiologic Findings

Pulmonary imaging studies may show changes of congestive heart failure, lymphangitic linear densities, pleural thickening, and effusions.[2] Mediastinal infiltration is common. Poorly defined centrilobular nodular opacities and lung cysts are rarely seen.

Tissue Sampling

The clinical diagnosis of ECD is rarely made by lung biopsy.[23] However, there should be an index of suspicion for the disease if there are interstitial infiltrates of bland mononuclear cells, including macrophages, in open lung biopsies.

Bronchoalveolar Lavage Findings

These include foamy macrophages, siderophages, and typical double-contoured histiocytes.[23]

Microscopic Findings

At low power, ECD has a distinctive lymphangitic distribution with fibrosis and infiltration of foamy "xanthomatous" histiocytes (Fig. 92.3), with abundant cytoplasm and Touton-like multinucleated giant cells. There is minimal involvement of the alveolated lung parenchyma.[1] There is a variable admixture of lymphocytes and eosinophils.

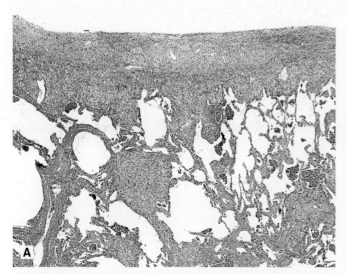
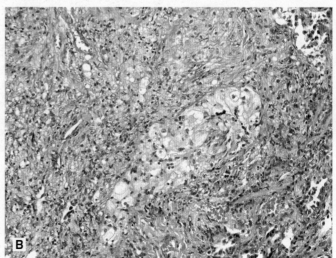

FIGURE 92.3 ▲ Erdheim-Chester disease. **A.** A low-power photomicrograph shows the lymphangitic distribution of the infiltrate with thickening of the pleural and interlobular septa. **B.** The thickening is the result of fibrosis admixed with histiocytes, many of which are foamy, and other inflammatory cells.

Immunohistochemical Stains

ECD macrophages express CD68 and are negative for CD1a. S100 expression is variable (Table 92.2). *BRAFV600E* mutation can be detected in over half of cases and confirmed with immunohistochemistry.[14] Both the foamy histiocytes and the Touton giant cells stain for BRAF.

Prognosis and Treatment

The very long-term prognosis of the disease is poor, but pulmonary involvement is not a major prognostic factor. There is no clear response of ECD lesions to corticosteroids and interferon.[23] The 10-year survival is 70%.[23]

Differential Diagnosis

Because ECD has an exquisite lymphangitic distribution at low magnification, other processes with such distribution enter the differential diagnosis. These processes include sarcoidosis and lymphangitic carcinomatosis. Lymphangitic carcinomatosis is easily ruled out based on the cellularity and cell atypia. Sarcoidosis, when composed of well-formed granulomas, is also easily diagnosed. However, sarcoidosis may become fibrotic with only residual multinucleated giant cells embedded in the fibrosis. These giant cells are not Touton-like as in ECD, and no foamy histiocytes are present.

Malignant Histiocytic Tumors

Histiocytic Sarcoma

Histiocytic sarcomas are rare, and pulmonary involvement is extremely rare.[24] Cells are discohesive and large, with a round or oval nucleus, with frequent multinucleation (Fig. 92.4). Cells are positive for one or more histiocytic markers and negative for dendritic cell markers as well as melanoma and carcinoma markers.[24]

Interdigitating Dendritic Cell Sarcoma

Likewise extremely rare to occur in the lung, interdigitating dendritic cell sarcoma is characterized by polymorphic cells with abundant cytoplasm, multiple nuclei, notched nuclei, and reactive inflammation (Fig. 92.5). The cells form fascicles with a storiform pattern.[25] Immunohistochemical stains show interdigitating dendritic cell makers, including fascin, S100 protein, and CD68.

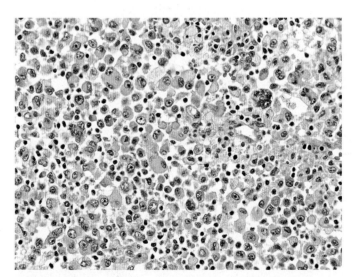

FIGURE 92.4 ▲ Histiocytic sarcoma. The cell proliferation is discohesive. The cells are large with abundant eosinophilic cytoplasm. The nuclei are mostly round with a vesicular cytoplasm and prominent nucleoli. Some cells are multinucleated. The differential diagnosis is broad and confirmed by immunohistochemistry with these cells staining for one of the histiocytic markers (CD68, CD163, or lysozyme).

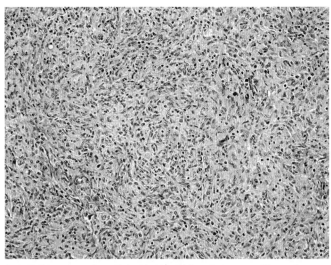

FIGURE 92.5 ▲ Interdigitating dendritic cell sarcoma. The cells contain abundant eosinophilic cytoplasm. The nuclei have irregular contours. The cells form loose fascicles in a storiform pattern.

Follicular Dendritic Cell Sarcoma

Follicular dendritic cell sarcomas may involve the bronchus or lung parenchyma as a mass. Cells show ill-defined borders and pale cytoplasm and are spindled, resembling a soft tissue sarcoma (Fig. 92.6). Immunohistochemically, tumor cells express S100 protein and at least one follicular dendritic cell marker (CD21, C23, and CD35).[26]

Reactive Histiocytic Lesions

General

A variety of reactive conditions may produce a macrophage reaction in the lung. These include the following list (Table 92.3):
- Respiratory bronchiolitis RB (Chapter 18)
- Desquamative interstitial pneumonia (Chapter 18)
- Congenital surfactant deficiency (Chapter 15)
- Infections, especially immunocompromised patients (Chapters 41 and 43)

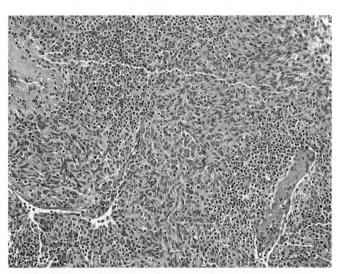

FIGURE 92.6 ▲ Follicular dendritic cell sarcoma. The cells are spindled in well-formed fascicles resembling a soft tissue sarcoma. Small lymphocytes are sprinkled in the background.

TABLE 92.3   Types of Macrophages and Cytoplasmic Characteristics in Reactive Lung Lesions

Content of Macrophage	Appearance	Distribution	Cause
Dust filled	Fine, brown pigment	Intra-alveolar macrophages, often cohesive	Smoking
Anthracosis	Dense black particles	Macrophages with clear or eosinophilic cytoplasm, interstitium, lymph nodes	Occupational exposure, smoking
Silica crystals	Minute, weakly birefringent	Macrophages with eosinophilic cytoplasm, interstitium, lymph nodes, usually with anthracosis, only fibrosis in later stages	Occupational
Hemosiderin	Yellow-brown coarse birefringent granules	Intra-alveolar macrophages, discohesive, may be interstitial	Hemorrhage
Foamy (lipid)	Bubbly clear cytoplasm	Intra-alveolar or interstitium	Obstruction, drug
Large vacuoles	Lipid vacuoles	Intra-alveolar, interstitium	Exogenous lipids

- Lipid pneumonia, endogenous and exogenous (Chapter 25)
- Diffuse panbronchiolitis (Chapter 36)
- Eosinophilic pneumonia (Chapter 26)
- Amiodarone and other drugs (Chapter 59)

Pneumoconioses

The pneumoconiosis are discussed in Chapters 56 to 58 and are caused by inhaled dusts, such as coal, silica, silicates, asbestos, synthetic fibers, organic dusts, aluminum, beryllium, and iron. Any nodular aggregates of macrophages occurring in the interstitium around vessels in a lymphatic distribution should be viewed under polarized light.[1]

Cobalt pneumoconiosis is a specific disease that can cause a desquamative interstitial pneumonia-like reaction with giant cells (previously termed giant cell interstitial pneumonia). The cobalt is lost in tissue processing, and there is no polarizable material to be seen. The diagnosis rests on the identification of tungsten, which usually accompanies the cobalt, by mass spectroscopy or other techniques.

Storage Diseases

The sphingolipidoses, including Fabry, Niemann-Pick, and Gaucher disease, may cause intra-alveolar and interstitial foamy macrophage infiltrates. The diagnosis is rarely based on lung histology, which may mimic postobstructive pneumonia.[1]

Specific Infections with a Primarily Histiocytic Response

Malakoplakia, when it involves the lung, is usually caused by *Rhodococcus equi* infection. Rarely, chronic pneumonia with *Pasteurella multocida*, *Escherichia coli*, and *Acinetobacter* may cause malakoplakia in the lung. The macrophages contain abundant eosinophilic cytoplasm and Michaelis-Gutmann bodies that contain calcium.

Whipple disease, caused by infection with *Tropheryma whippelii*, typically involves the gastrointestinal tract and joints but rarely involves the lung. There are nodular aggregates of macrophages along lymphatic routes, especially peribronchiolar, that contain the typical PAS-positive organisms.

Mycobacterial infections in immunocompromised hosts can result in sheets of bland macrophages that may spindle and form pseudotumors (see Chapter 40).

Cryptococcal pneumonia and *Histoplasma capsulatum* infection in immunocompromised patients is also associated with a marked inflammatory infiltrate of bland, eosinophilic, and vacuolated macrophages.

Crystal-Storing Histiocytosis (Histiocytoma)

Usually seen with lymphoproliferative disorders such as multiple myeloma, low-grade B-cell lymphomas, and monoclonal gammopathy, crystal-storing histiocytosis may result in discrete pulmonary nodules.[27,28] Histologically, there are aggregates of macrophages containing abundant eosinophilic elongated crystals (Fig. 92.7). Careful exclusion of lymphoma or other lymphoproliferative disease is important.

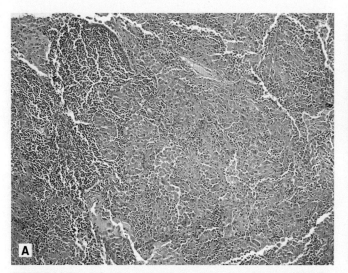 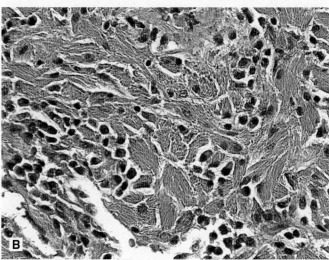

FIGURE 92.7 ▲ Crystal-storing histiocytosis associated with MALT lymphoma. **A.** Sheets of histiocytes are admixed with clusters of bland mildly atypical lymphocytes. **B.** The cytoplasmic crystals are best appreciated without the condenser at high magnification.

REFERENCES

1. Wang C-W, Colby TV. Histiocytic lesions and proliferations in the lung. *Sem Diagn Pathol.* 2007;24:162–182.
2. Nagarjun Rao R, Moran CA, Suster S. Histiocytic disorders of the lung. *Adv Anat Pathol.* 2010;17:12–22.
3. Ji H, Zhang B, Tian D, et al. Rosai-Dorfman disease of the lung. *Respir Care.* 2012;57:1679–1681.
4. Morsolini M, Nicola M, Paulli M, et al. Primary pulmonary artery Rosai-Dorfman disease mimicking sarcoma. *J Thorac Cardiovasc Surg.* 2013;146:e57–e59.
5. Roberts SS, Attanoos RL. IgG4+ Rosai-Dorfman disease of the lung. *Histopathology.* 2010;56:662–664.
6. Walters DM, Dunnington GH, Dustin SM, et al. Rosai-Dorfman disease presenting as a pulmonary artery mass. *Ann Thorac Surg.* 2010;89:300–302.
7. Rehman T, deBoisblanc BP, Kantrow SP. Extranodal Rosai-Dorfman disease involving the pulmonary artery. *Eur J Cardiothorac Surg.* 2013;44:964.
8. de Jong WK, Kluin PM, Groen HM. Overlapping immunoglobulin G4-related disease and Rosai-Dorfman disease mimicking lung cancer. *Eur Respir Rev.* 2012;21:365–367.
9. El-Kersh K, Perez RL, Guardiola J. Pulmonary IgG4+ Rosai-Dorfman disease. *BMJ Case Rep.* 2013;2013.
10. Elia D, Torre O, Cassandro R, et al. Pulmonary Langerhans cell histiocytosis: a comprehensive analysis of 40 patients and literature review. *Eur J Intern Med.* 2015;26:351–356.
11. Thomas G, Dixon RK, Zimrin A, et al. Pulmonary Langerhans cell histiocytosis with systemic features. *Am J Med.* 2015;128:e7–e9.
12. Choi JE, Lee HR, Ohn JH, et al. Adult multisystem Langerhans cell histiocytosis presenting with central diabetes insipidus successfully treated with chemotherapy. *Endocrinol Metab (Seoul).* 2014;29:394–399.
13. Yousem SA, Dacic S, Nikiforov YE, et al. Pulmonary Langerhans cell histiocytosis: profiling of multifocal tumors using next-generation sequencing identifies concordant occurrence of BRAF V600E mutations. *Chest.* 2013;143:1679–1684.
14. Haroche J, Charlotte F, Arnaud L, et al. High prevalence of BRAF V600E mutations in Erdheim-Chester disease but not in other non-Langerhans cell histiocytoses. *Blood.* 2012;120:2700–2703.
15. Roden AC, Hu X, Kip S, et al. BRAF V600E expression in Langerhans cell histiocytosis: clinical and immunohistochemical study on 25 pulmonary and 54 extrapulmonary cases. *Am J Surg Pathol.* 2014;38:548–551.
16. Routy B, Hoang J, Gruber J. Pulmonary Langerhans cell histiocytosis with lytic bone involvement in an adult smoker: regression following smoking cessation. *Case Rep Hematol.* 2015;2015:201536.
17. Kamath S, Arkader A, Jubran RF. Outcomes of children younger than 24 months with Langerhans cell histiocytosis and bone involvement: a report from a single institution. *J Pediatr Orthop.* 2014;34:825–830.
18. Yazc N, Yalcn B, Ciftci AO, et al. Langerhans cell histiocytosis with involvement of nails and lungs in an adolescent. *J Pediatr Hematol Oncol.* 2008;30:77–80.
19. Asilsoy S, Yazici N, Demir S, et al. A different cause for respiratory disorder in children: cases with pulmonary Langerhans cell histiocytosis. *Clin Respir J.* 2015. *In Press.*
20. Aggarwal V, Seth A, Jain M, et al. Congenital Langerhans cell histiocytosis with skin and lung involvement: spontaneous regression. *Indian J Pediatr.* 2010;77:811–812.
21. Chunharas A, Pabunruang W, Hongeng S. Congenital self-healing Langerhans cell histiocytosis with pulmonary involvement: spontaneous regression. *J Med Assoc Thai.* 2002;85(suppl 4):S1309–S1313.
22. Zwerdling T, Won E, Shane L, et al. Langerhans cell sarcoma: case report and review of world literature. *J Pediatr Hematol Oncol.* 2014;36:419–425.
23. Arnaud L, Pierre I, Beigelman-Aubry C, et al. Pulmonary involvement in Erdheim-Chester disease: a single-center study of thirty-four patients and a review of the literature. *Arthritis Rheum.* 2010;62:3504–3512.
24. Tomita S, Ogura G, Inomoto C, et al. Histiocytic sarcoma originating in the lung in a 16-year-old male. *J Clin Exp Hematopathol.* 2015;55:45–49.
25. Radović S, Dorić M, Zuo H, et al. Interdigitating dendritic cell sarcoma of the liver and lung. *Bosn J Basic Med Sci.* 2012;12:203–210.
26. Hollingsworth J, Cooper W, Nicoll KD, et al. Follicular dendritic cell sarcoma of the lung. *Pathology.* 2011;43:67–69.
27. Kawano N, Beppu K, Oyama M, et al. Successful surgical treatment for pulmonary crystal-storing histiocytosis following the onset of gastric non-hodgkin lymphoma. *J Clin Exp Hematop.* 2013;53:241–245.
28. Zhang C, Myers JL. Crystal-storing histiocytosis complicating primary pulmonary marginal zone lymphoma of mucosa-associated lymphoid tissue. *Arch Pathol Lab Med.* 2013;137:1199–1204.

93 Pulmonary Sarcomas

Jennifer M. Boland, M.D., Eunhee S. Yi, M.D., Fabio R. Tavora, M.D., Ph.D. and Allen P. Burke, M.D.

Overview and Terminology

Pulmonary sarcomas are rare, and comprise tumors that arise from the parenchyma and those that occur within the pulmonary arteries (intimal sarcomas). Parenchymal sarcomas are most frequently, synovial sarcomas, epithelioid hemangioendotheliomas (EHEs) leiomyosarcomas, and malignant peripheral nerve sheath tumors.[1] Other sarcomas that have rarely been reported to involve the lung include undifferentiated pleomorphic sarcoma (previously malignant fibrous histiocytoma),[2] liposarcoma,[3,4] and rhabdomyosarcoma.[5,6]

Although there is overlap, mesenchymal tumors that more frequently involve the pleura than the parenchyma, including solitary fibrous tumor, synovial sarcoma, and angiosarcoma, are presented in Chapter 96.

Pleuropulmonary blastoma (PPB) and primary pulmonary myxoid sarcoma (PPMS) are rare sarcomas unique to the lung parenchyma and are also discussed in this chapter.

Leiomyosarcoma

Pulmonary leiomyosarcoma is rare and is diagnosed only after a metastatic tumor from an occult primary site is excluded. These tumors occur in adults of both sexes, but there may be a male predominance.[1] Parenchymal leiomyosarcoma should be considered separately from intimal sarcomas with leiomyosarcomatous differentiation and those rare tumors that arise in the bronchi.[7] The diagnosis can be obtained by surgical resection or endobronchial ultrasound-guided needle biopsy.[8]

Grossly, parenchymal leiomyosarcomas are large, fleshy tumors that are typically larger than 10 cm.[1] Histologically, pulmonary leiomyosarcomas are similar to those arising in soft tissue (Fig. 93.1). Prognosis is poor,[1] although long-term survival has been reported.[9]

Epithelioid Hemangioendothelioma

In the lung, EHE formerly went by the name intravascular bronchioloalveolar tumor (IVBAT), but this term is outdated and should no longer be used.[10]

Clinical Findings

Pulmonary EHE has a predilection for adult females and tends to involve the lung in a multifocal fashion (multiple bilateral nodules < 2 cm, often pleural based).[11,12] The observed age range is wide, spanning children to the elderly, but most patients are middle aged (third to fifth decade of life). Clinical and radiographic findings may suggest metastatic disease involving the lung or old granulomatous disease. However, unusual presentations have been well documented, including a solitary pulmonary nodule, diffuse pleural thickening simulating mesothelioma, and lymphatic distribution mimicking lymphangitic carcinoma.[13] The three most commonly observed radiographic patterns include multiple pulmonary nodules, multiple pulmonary reticulonodular opacities, or diffuse infiltrative pleural thickening.[14] Most patients are asymptomatic at the time of presentation, but some will have localizing symptoms such as cough, dyspnea, hemoptysis, pain, or pleural effusion.[11]

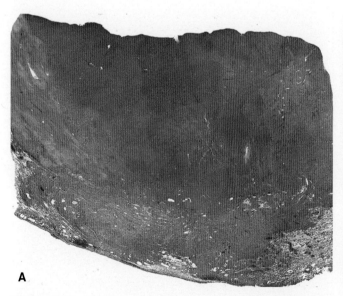

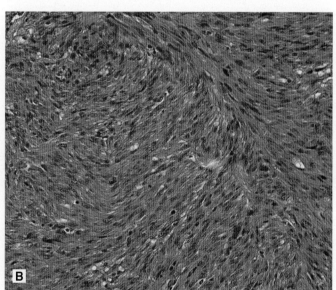

FIGURE 93.1 ▲ Pulmonary leiomyosarcoma. **A.** Low magnification demonstrates a cellular tumor near the pleural surface. **B.** Higher magnification shows typical features of leiomyosarcoma, including fascicles of spindle cells with eosinophilic cytoplasm and cigar-shaped nuclei. This case is relatively low grade. The diagnosis was confirmed by immunohistochemical staining for desmin (not shown). There was no other tumor on extensive imaging evaluation in this middle-aged male, who presented with hemoptysis.

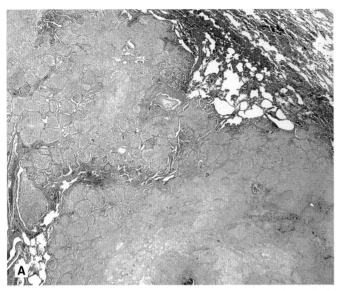
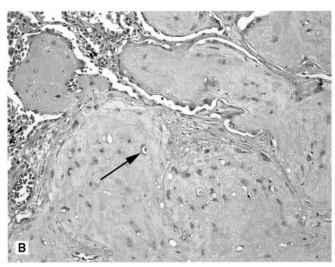

FIGURE 93.2 ▲ Pulmonary epithelioid hemangioendothelioma. **A.** A low magnification photomicrograph shows a well-demarcated hyalinized nodule with central necrosis and prominent micropolypoid growth into alveolar spaces at the periphery. **B.** Cords of bland endothelial cells with frequent cytoplasmic vacuoles are present, embedded in a myxohyaline matrix. Some of the vacuoles contain fragmented erythrocytes (*arrow*).

Pathologic Features

Pulmonary EHE usually appear as circumscribed firm gray-white nodules that may have a chondroid or mucoid cut surface. Some tumors with extensive pleural involvement may alternatively show diffuse pleural thickening.[10] Whether cases of EHE presenting bilaterally in the lungs without an obviously primary site elsewhere may represent metastases from an occult primary remains unclear.[10]

The nodules of pulmonary EHE often have central hyalinization or necrosis with accentuation of cellularity at the periphery of the nodule. The tumor is often associated with vascular structures (arteries, veins, or lymphatics) and often shows intravascular growth. The pleura is often involved and diffusely thickened. The combination of vascular and pleural involvement leads to a lymphangitic growth pattern in many cases.

Bland epithelioid endothelial cells grow in chains and cords and are dispersed in a myxohyaline or myxochondroid matrix (Figs. 93.2 to 93.5). Scattered EHE cells will have intracytoplasmic vacuoles/vascular

lumens, which may contain an erythrocyte (often fragmented), but EHE cells typically do not form extracellular vascular structures.[15] Intranuclear cytoplasmic inclusions have also been noted frequently in EHE.[10] In the lung, EHE tends to show a "micropolypoid" growth pattern, showing protrusion into bronchioles and alveolar spaces, often with little or no apparent reactive response in the alveolar septa. Most "classic" EHEs have bland, low-grade cytology, but some examples may show atypical/intermediate-grade features including moderate pleomorphism, increased cellularity, and necrosis, which may correlate with a more aggressive behavior.[10]

EHEs typically express a variety of vascular endothelial markers including CD31, ERG, Fli1, and CD34, but CD31 and ERG may be the most sensitive for pulmonary EHE.[10] EHEs also commonly express low molecular weight cytokeratin or EMA (25% to 40% of cases), which is a potential diagnostic pitfall.[10] EHEs have recently been discovered to harbor a recurrent t(1;3)(p36;q23–25), resulting in the *WWTR1–CAMTA1* fusion gene in the majority of cases.[10,16,17]

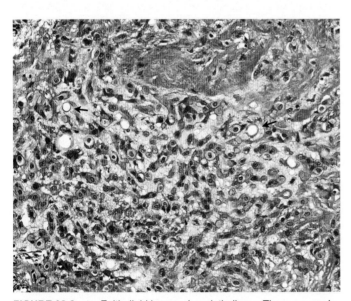
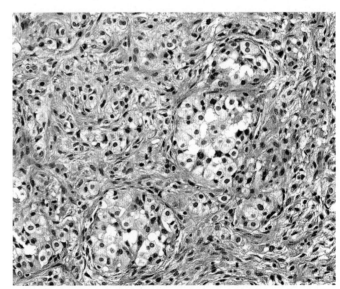

FIGURE 93.3 ▲ Epithelioid hemangioendothelioma. There are cords of cells with abundant pink cytoplasm and occasional vacuoles (*arrows*).

FIGURE 93.4 ▲ Epithelioid hemangioendothelioma. A nested pattern resembling carcinoid tumor may occur.

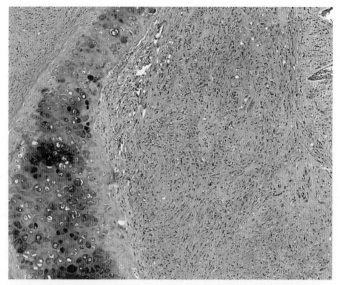

FIGURE 93.5 ▲ Epithelioid hemangioendothelioma. The cords of tumor are present in a prominent proteoglycan matrix and invade in and around a bronchus. Vacuoles are barely discernable at this magnification.

Some EHEs seem to lack this fusion gene, so negative genetic testing, which is not necessary in typical cases, does not exclude the diagnosis.[10]

Prognosis

EHE is generally an indolent tumor, but distant metastases will occur in around 20% to 30% of cases, and 5-year survival is around 60%.[18] Patients with pulmonary EHE who present with clinical symptoms or with extensive involvement of bronchioles, vascular structures, and pleura seem to have a worse outcome.[10] Proposed criteria for classifying a thoracic EHE as intermediate grade/high risk include increased mitotic rate (>1/mm²), necrosis, and moderate nuclear pleomorphism.[10]

Pleuropulmonary Blastoma

PPB is a very rare malignant primitive embryonal tumor of infancy and childhood.[19,20] PPB should not be confused with the similarly named pulmonary blastoma, which is a subtype of sarcomatoid carcinoma (see Chapter 85), and has completely distinct clinical and pathologic characteristics. Despite the name, the earliest phase of PPB is thought to arise in the lung parenchyma and subsequently grow toward the pleural surfaces. For this reason, PPBs are considered primary tumors of the lung parenchyma.

Incidence and Clinical Features

The vast majority of PPBs occur in children under 5 years, although older children can rarely be affected and rare cases have been observed even into young adulthood.[20,21] PPBs should be subtyped based on gross and microscopic proportions of cystic and solid components, as types 1 to 3: type 1 is entirely cystic, type 2 is solid and cystic, while type 3 is entirely solid.[22] The average age seems to correlate with the subtype of PPB, with type 1 patients presenting at the youngest age (average 8 months) and type 3 patients presenting at an older average age (average 41 months).[20,21] Infants with type 1 and 2 lesions often present in respiratory distress, and pneumothorax is also common at presentation due to the cystic nature of the mass.[21] Children with type 2 and 3 PPB may present with localizing symptoms including cough, chest pain, and dyspnea.[23] Imaging studies reveal a lung mass or consolidation, which may have a multiloculated cystic component.[21] Most tumors are

confined to the lung but may rarely extend to involve the mediastinum or chest wall, and some will be multifocal.[24]

Gross Pathology

The cystic component of PPB (if present) is characterized by large thin-walled multiloculated cysts that may collapse upon sectioning.[20,25] The solid components may form nodules, plaques, or polypoid projections in an otherwise cystic lesion.[20] The solid component may vary in appearance from firm and rubbery to soft and gelatinous.[20] In cystic lesions, the specimen should be closely examined for any solid areas, which should be liberally sampled. Some lesions may appear relatively circumscribed, while others infiltrate the surrounding parenchyma.[20]

Microscopic Findings

The cystic spaces of PPB are lined by flattened to cuboidal metaplastic (nonneoplastic) respiratory epithelium, which is often attenuated and may be ciliated.[20,21] Within the septa of the cysts, careful examination typically reveals primitive mesenchymal cells, which show small round blue cell or rhabdomyoblastic morphology.[26] These cells often form a cambium layer below the metaplastic epithelium (Fig. 93.6), but they may be quite subtle and rare in some cases, so any case showing the characteristic large cysts lined by metaplastic epithelium should be carefully examined and liberally sampled. The solid component of PPB is frankly sarcomatous and has a diverse morphology. Observed patterns may be mixed, and often include small round blue cells/blastema, rhabdomyoblastic cells resembling embryonal rhabdomyosarcoma, and/or high-grade spindle cell sarcoma.[20,21] Embryonal (immature) or malignant-appearing cartilage is present in about half of PPBs and is a very helpful morphologic feature to suggest the diagnosis when identified.[20] The proportion of observed cystic and solid components should be used to subtype PPBs. Type 1 PPBs are entirely cystic but still have identifiable primitive cells, type 2 is cystic and solid, and type 3 is completely solid.[20,21] It seems that the immature cells of PPBs may regress completely (PPB-R), leaving only the cystic spaces lined by attenuated epithelium with fibrous septa, without any identifiable primitive cells.[21] Tumors with the typical architecture but with no identifiable residual primitive cells should be categorized as PPB-R.[21]

Special Studies and Genetics

PPB can show a rhabdomyoblastic immunophenotype in some cases, with expression of desmin and myogenin/MyoD-1.[20,27] Otherwise, immunostaining profile is generally nonspecific and often not necessary if the typical morphology is observed. PPBs are associated with germline mutations in the *DICER* gene in about 40% to 66% of children who present with this tumor.[21,28] In about one-quarter of PPB patients, these germline mutations are inherited (familial).[28] While PPB is the classic tumor associated with *DICER*-mutated kindreds and the index tumor type which lead to discovery of this syndrome, many other tumor types have subsequently been identified, including Wilms tumor, embryonal rhabdomyosarcoma and Ewing sarcoma of the uterine cervix, cystic nephroma, teratoma, Sertoli-Leydig cell tumor, and several types of primitive neurologic tumors including medulloblastoma, among others.[21,28,29]

Differential Diagnosis

Congenital pulmonary airway malformation (CPAM), particularly type 1 CPAM, may show some overlapping architectural features with PPB, but the lining cells are typically taller columnar to cuboidal respiratory-type (bronchial) epithelium with sawtoothing of the epithelium, as opposed to the attenuated pneumocyte-like or cuboidal lining of PPB. Lesions classically described as type IV CPAM have extensive morphologic overlap with PPB but lack the primitive cell component, and in fact likely represent regressed PPB (see Chapter 11).[21]

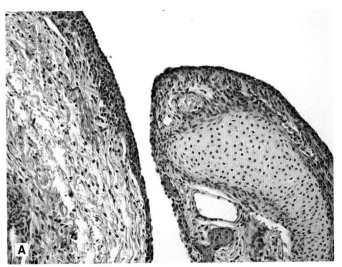

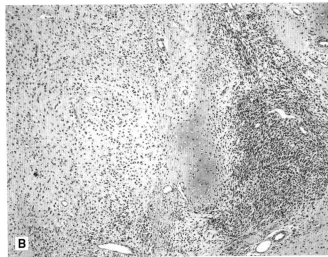

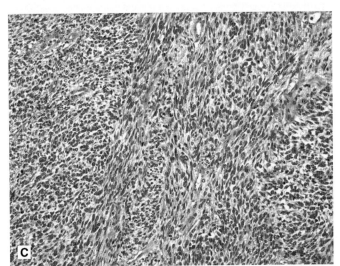

FIGURE 93.6 ▲ Pleuropulmonary blastoma showing nonneoplastic epithelial cells lining thin fibrous septa, which contain primitive small round blue mesenchymal cells forming a cambium layer, and nodules of immature cartilage **(A)**. Solid areas are composed of primitive round cells, malignant spindled cells, and immature cartilage **(B)**. Other areas show high-grade spindle cell sarcoma **(C)**.

Fetal lung interstitial tumor (FLIT) is another tumefactive lesion of infancy, which may be solid and microcystic. However, in contrast to the primitive small round blue cells observed in PPB, the immature mesenchymal cells of FLIT are located in the interstitium of immature-appearing lung (resembling fetal lung at 20 to 24 weeks, inappropriately immature for gestational age) and are polygonal with moderate clear cytoplasm, resembling the cells observed in pulmonary interstitial glycogenosis (PIG).[30]

Congenital peribronchial myofibroblastic tumor (CPMT) may be considered in the differential diagnosis of PPB. CPMTs generally form solid masses in infants and can be recognized by the typical fascicles of proliferating myofibroblasts located exquisitely along bronchovascular bundles, sometimes admixed with malformed cartilage plates, and frequent involvement of the pleural surface[31].

Cystic synovial sarcoma could also be considered in the differential diagnosis, when immunostaining for EMA, keratin, and TLE1 may be helpful, and testing for the fusions characteristic of synovial sarcoma can be performed to confirm the diagnosis (see Chapter 96).

Prognosis

It seems that PPBs show an orderly tumor progression,[28] starting as type 1 cystic lesions: some may regress, some remain stable, and a subset progress to overgrowth of the primitive component and development of frank sarcoma.[21] The outcome of patients with PPB depends on the extent of the solid component.[21] Patients with type 1 PPB have excellent prognosis (80% to 90% 5-year disease-free survival), while

those with type 2 or 3 PPBs can experience distant metastases and death from disease, with a 5-year disease-free survival of <50%.[20,21]

Primary Pulmonary Myxoid Sarcoma

PPMS is a recently described translocation-associated sarcoma occurring exclusively in the lung, nearly always related to a bronchus.[32]

Incidence and Clinical Features

PPMS is a rare entity with the body of literature composed of small series and case reports.[32,33] It affects adults and may have a female predilection.[32] Patients often present with symptoms of bronchial irritation or obstruction, including cough, hemoptysis, postobstructive pneumonia, or bronchiectasis.[32,33]

Gross Pathology

PPMS typically forms a lobulated, well-circumscribed mass, which may be gelatinous, and is most commonly endobronchial.[32] Most tumors measure < 4 cm.[32,33]

Microscopic Findings

PPMS resembles extraskeletal myxoid chondrosarcoma. There are lobulated tumor nodules containing stellate, spindled, and polygonal stromal cells arranged in strands and cords, associated with a myxoid matrix (Fig. 93.7).[32] The degree of atypia is variable, but most PPMS

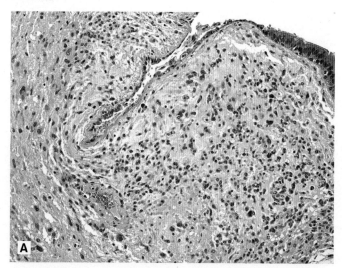 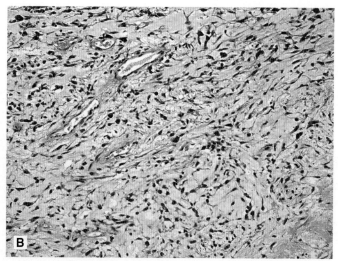

FIGURE 93.7 ▲ Primary pulmonary myxoid sarcoma with *EWSR1–CREB1* fusion forming an endobronchial mass, characterized by epithelioid **(A)** to delicate spindle-shaped cells **(B)** showing mild nuclear atypia, arranged in nests and cords in a myxoid matrix.

appear quite low grade, with mild to moderate atypia and a low mitotic rate. Foci of epithelioid change, necrosis, and nuclear pleomorphism can occur in some cases, but these features are not reliably associated with more aggressive behavior.[32]

Special Studies

Focal immunohistochemical expression of EMA is sometimes observed,[32,33] but generally, the tumor cells are negative for other markers, including keratin, S100 protein, muscle and vascular markers. PPMS has a recurrent *EWRSR1–CREB1* fusion in around 80% of cases.[32] It should be noted that *EWSR1* is commonly rearranged in a variety of soft tissue tumors with varying morphologic features, some of which have been described to form endobronchial masses (including angiomatoid fibrous histiocytoma and Ewing sarcoma). *EWSR1* can also be rearranged in metastatic extraskeletal myxoid chondrosarcoma, so careful staging should be performed.

Prognosis

The behavior of PPMS is unpredictable, with a minority of patients experiencing distant metastases.[32] Metastatic sites observed to date have included brain and kidney.[32] Aggressive behavior does not seem to be reliably predicted by atypical morphologic features,[32] and thus, all patients should have long-term follow-up to monitor for recurrence or metastasis.

Malignant Peripheral Nerve Sheath Tumor

Terminology

MPNSTs are sarcomas with neural/Schwann cell differentiation, typically supported by focal S100 protein expression, evolution from a preexisting neurofibroma, or occurrence in patients with neurofibromatosis type 1 (NF-1).[15]

Incidence and Clinical Features

MPNST are very rare in the pulmonary parenchyma.[34,35] Although many MPNSTs occur in the sporadic setting, they have a strong association with neurofibromatosis type 1 (NF-1).[15]

Gross Pathology

Most examples have been large pleural- or hilar-based masses.[34,35]

Microscopic Findings

The morphology of MPNST can be quite variable, but the most typical pattern is that of a monomorphic spindle cell sarcoma with

fascicular growth, often resembling monophasic synovial sarcoma.[15] Areas of rhabdomyoblastic differentiation can be encountered (malignant Triton tumor), and some tumors will show pleomorphism.[15,35] MPNSTs often show alternating areas of hyper- and hypocellularity. Especially in patients with NF-1, MPNST may arise from a preexisting neurofibroma.[15]

Special Studies

MPNSTs typically show only focal expression of S100.[15] Diffuse S100 expression should lead to consideration of other entities in the differential diagnosis (malignant melanoma, cellular schwannoma, etc.).[15] MPNSTs often show biallelic loss of the *NF1* gene and are usually karyotypically complex.[15]

Prognosis

Pulmonary MPNSTs typically show aggressive behavior typical of most high-grade sarcomas, and prognosis is often poor even with multimodality therapy.[34,35]

Pulmonary Artery (Intimal) Sarcoma

Terminology

Pulmonary artery sarcoma arises from the arterial intima of elastic pulmonary arteries and grows predominantly within the arterial lumen. There are a variety of histologic types that generally conform to variants of soft tissue sarcomas. Because it derives from the intima, the term "intimal sarcoma" is often used, as is the case for aortic sarcomas. There is debate whether the term "intima" should be used for a histologic subtype (as in recent clinical reports)[36] or to simply designate the site of origin.[37] Pulmonary artery sarcomas share histologic features with aortic intimal sarcomas and endocardial-based sarcomas of the left atrium.

Incidence

Pulmonary artery intimal sarcoma is rare, but more common than primary parenchymal sarcomas of the lung. Pulmonary artery intimal sarcomas represent 1% to 4% of pulmonary thromboendarterectomy specimens from patients with chronic thromboembolic pulmonary hypertension.[38]

Clinical Findings

The average age is 56 years (range 26 to 78 years) with an equal sex distribution.[36,39–43] Patients are typically misdiagnosed on clinical grounds as acute or chronic pulmonary embolism. Clinical manifestations include chest or back pain, cough, hemoptysis, weight loss, malaise, syncope, fever, and rarely sudden death.

Radiologic Findings

On computed tomography (CT), intimal sarcomas present as a lobulated enhancing mass in the central arteries causing filling defects with occlusion and expansion of the entire lumen. The findings are generally distinct from those of pulmonary embolism.[44]

Gross Pathologic Features

Pulmonary intimal sarcoma occurs in the proximal elastic arteries, from the level of the pulmonary valve to the lobar branches. Occasionally, they occur on the pulmonary valve itself.[45] Most cases have bilateral involvement, although one side is usually dominant, allowing pneumonectomy as treatment in some patients.[39]

Typically, pulmonary intimal sarcomas are gelatinous soft masses that fill the arteries (Fig. 93.8). Distal extension may show smooth tapering of the mass. The cut surface is soft, with fibrotic or firm foci if the tumor has an osteosarcomatous or chondrosarcomatous component. Hemorrhage and necrosis are common in high-grade intimal sarcomas. Often, the entire tumor is intraluminal and can be shelled out by endarterectomy.

Microscopic Features

The histologic patterns of pulmonary intimal sarcoma are diverse.[39,41–43] The largest group comprises undifferentiated pleomorphic sarcomas, followed by low-grade spindle cell sarcomas with a myxoid background (myxofibrosarcoma) (Fig. 93.9). About one in six pulmonary artery sarcomas show heterologous elements in the form of osteo- or chondrosarcoma. Less common histologic patterns include rhabdomyosarcoma, leiomyosarcoma, undifferentiated sarcoma with epithelioid or round cell features, synovial sarcoma, EHE, and angiosarcoma.[39,41–43]

A rare histologic subtype is low-grade inflammatory myofibroblastic sarcoma, which is characterized by a relative lack of cellularity, a variable inflammatory and myxoid background, lack of pleomorphism or significant mitotic activity, and myofibroblastic cellular appearance ("tissue culture" growth). This subtype reportedly has a good prognosis.

Immunohistochemical studies are not particular helpful to diagnose pulmonary artery sarcomas, other than to identify smooth muscle, skeletal muscle, or endothelial differentiation.

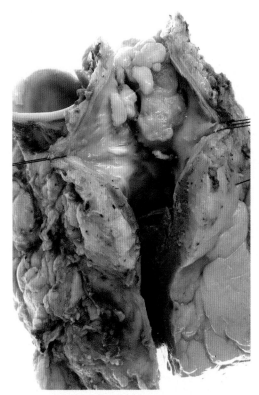

FIGURE 93.8 ▲ Pulmonary artery sarcoma, gross specimen from cardiac explant. The tumor extends into the pulmonary outflow tract. (Reproduced with permission from Burke A, Tavora F, Maleszewski JJ, et al. Tumors of the heart and great vessels, Atlas of tumor pathology. *Am Registry Pathol.* 2015:400)

Molecular Features

Six examined tumors were positive for *MDM2*. In the CGH analysis, gains and amplifications in the 12q13–14 region were found in six of eight tumors.[46] *MDM2* amplification frequently occurs, often coexisting with amplification of *PDGFRA*.[40]

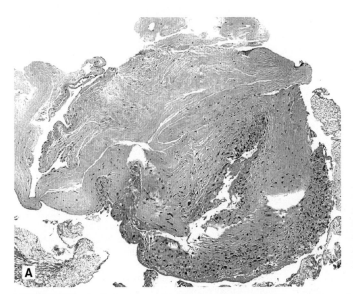

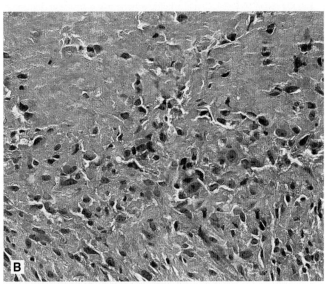

FIGURE 93.9 ▲ Pulmonary artery sarcoma, embolectomy specimen. **A.** The tumor is intermixed with organizing thrombus and can occasionally be overlooked as reactive endothelium. **B.** The tumor cells show pleomorphism and are mixed within fibrin. Immunohistochemical stains are nonspecific and, in this case, showed positivity only for vimentin, with negative staining with cytokeratins, smooth muscle actin, desmin, and CD31 (not shown).

Treatment and Prognosis

Pulmonary intimal sarcomas are treated by endarterectomy, endarterectomy and pneumonectomy, or pneumonectomy alone. The main pulmonary artery may need to have a graft reconstruction procedure. Approximately 70% of patients have tumors that can be excised.[36]

Chemotherapy is usually administered to patients with inoperable disease and often as adjuvant treatment to patients with complete resections. Regimens include vincristine, ifosfamide, and doxorubicin and pegylated liposomal doxorubicin hydrochloride. Radiation therapy is also an option for pulmonary parenchymal metastases.

Pulmonary artery sarcoma has a poor prognosis, although long-term survival has been reported. There is a 17-month median survival, with a 1-, 3-, and 5-year survival rate of 63%, 29%, and 22%, respectively.[36,39] Survival is dependent on completeness of excision and not histologic grade.

REFERENCES

1. Attanoos RL, Appleton MA, Gibbs AR. Primary sarcomas of the lung: a clinicopathological and immunohistochemical study of 14 cases. *Histopathology.* 1996;29:29–36.

2. Patel DP, Gandhi YS, Sommers KE, et al. Primary pulmonary malignant fibrous histiocytoma. *Case Rep Pulmonol.* 2015;2015:381276.

3. Achir A, Ouadnouni Y, Smahi M, et al. Primary pulmonary liposarcoma—a case report. *Thorac Cardiovasc Surg.* 2009;57:119–120.

4. Son C, Choi PJ, Roh MS. Primary pulmonary myxoid liposarcoma with translocation t(12;16)(q13;p11) in a young female patient: a brief case report. *Korean J Pathol.* 2012;46:392–394.

5. Ji GY, Mao H. Primary pulmonary rhabdomyosarcoma in an adult: a case report and review of the literature. *J Zhejiang Univ Sci B.* 2013;14:859–865.

6. Guo Y, Xie D, Yan J, et al. Primary pulmonary rhabdomyosarcoma with brain metastases in a child: a case report with medico-legal implications. *J Forensic Leg Med.* 2013;20:720–723.

7. Luthra M, Khan H, Suhail MF, et al. Primary pulmonary leiomyosarcoma—a case report. *Arch Bronconeumol.* 2012;48:476–478.

8. Nath D, Arava S, Joshi P, et al. Primary pulmonary leiomyosarcoma of lung: an unusual entity with brief review. *Indian J Pathol Microbiol.* 2015;58:338–340.

9. Shen W, Chen J, Wei S, et al. Primary pulmonary leiomyosarcoma. *J Chin Med Assoc.* 2014;77:49–51.

10. Anderson T, Zhang L, Hameed M, et al. Thoracic epithelioid malignant vascular tumors: a clinicopathologic study of 52 cases with emphasis on pathologic grading and molecular studies of WWTR1–CAMTA1 fusions. *Am J Surg Pathol.* 2015;39:132–139.

11. Lau K, Massad M, Pollak C, et al. Clinical patterns and outcome in epithelioid hemangioendothelioma with or without pulmonary involvement: insights from an internet registry in the study of a rare cancer. *Chest.* 2011;140:1312–1318.

12. Dail DH, Liebow AA, Gmelich JT, et al. Intravascular, bronchiolar, and alveolar tumor of the lung (IVBAT). An analysis of twenty cases of a peculiar sclerosing endothelial tumor. *Cancer.* 1983;51:452–464.

13. Yousem SA, Hochholzer L. Unusual thoracic manifestations of epithelioid hemangioendothelioma. *Arch Pathol Lab Med.* 1987;111:459–463.

14. Kim EA, Lele SM, Lackner RP. Primary pleural epithelioid hemangioendothelioma. *Ann Thorac Surg.* 2011;91:301–302.

15. Fletcher CD. The evolving classification of soft tissue tumours—an update based on the new 2013 WHO classification. *Histopathology.* 2014;64:2–11.

16. Errani C, Zhang L, Sung YS, et al. A novel WWTR1–CAMTA1 gene fusion is a consistent abnormality in epithelioid hemangioendothelioma of different anatomic sites. *Genes Chromosomes Cancer.* 2011;50:644–653.

17. Tanas MR, Sboner A, Oliveira AM, et al. Identification of a disease-defining gene fusion in epithelioid hemangioendothelioma. *Sci Transl Med.* 2011;3: 98ra82.

18. Shao J, Zhang J. Clinicopathological characteristics of pulmonary epithelioid hemangioendothelioma: a report of four cases and review of the literature. *Oncol Lett.* 2014;8:2517–2522.

19. Priest JR, Hill DA, Williams GM, et al. Type I pleuropulmonary blastoma: a report from the International Pleuropulmonary Blastoma Registry. *J Clin Oncol.* 2006;24:4492–4498.

20. Priest JR, McDermott MB, Bhatia S, et al. Pleuropulmonary blastoma: a clinicopathologic study of 50 cases. *Cancer.* 1997;80:147–161.

21. Messinger YH, Stewart DR, Priest JR, et al. Pleuropulmonary blastoma: a report on 350 central pathology-confirmed pleuropulmonary blastoma cases by the International Pleuropulmonary Blastoma Registry. *Cancer.* 2015;121:276–285.

22. Castro A, Franzonello C, Leonardi S, et al. Type III pleuropulmonary blastoma in a 7-month-old female baby with impending respiratory failure: a case report. *J Med Case Rep.* 2014;8:221.

23. Orazi C, Inserra A, Schingo PM, et al. Pleuropulmonary blastoma, a distinctive neoplasm of childhood: report of three cases. *Pediatr Radiol.* 2007;37:337–344.

24. Picaud JC, Levrey H, Bouvier R, et al. Bilateral cystic pleuropulmonary blastoma in early infancy. *J Pediatr.* 2000;136:834–836.

25. Onoda T, Kanno M, Sato H, et al. Identification of novel ALK rearrangement A2M-ALK in a neonate with fetal lung interstitial tumor. *Genes Chromosomes Cancer.* 2014;53:865–874.

26. Granata C, Gambini C, Carlini C, et al. Pleuropulmonary blastoma. *Eur J Pediatr Surg.* 2001;11:271–273.

27. Ekmekci S, Aysal A, Olgun N, et al. Pleuropulmonary blastoma: a case report. *Turk Patoloji Derg.* 2015;31:68–71.

28. Hill DA, Ivanovich J, Priest JR, et al. DICER1 mutations in familial pleuropulmonary blastoma. *Science.* 2009;325:965.

29. Foulkes WD, Bahubeshi A, Hamel N, et al. Extending the phenotypes associated with DICER1 mutations. *Hum Mutat.* 2011;32:1381–1384.

30. Dishop MK, McKay EM, Kreiger PA, et al. Fetal lung interstitial tumor (FLIT): a proposed newly recognized lung tumor of infancy to be differentiated from cystic pleuropulmonary blastoma and other developmental pulmonary lesions. *Am J Surg Pathol.* 2010;34:1762–1772.

31. McGinnis M, Jacobs G, el-Naggar A, et al. Congenital peribronchial myofibroblastic tumor (so-called "congenital leiomyosarcoma"). A distinct neonatal lung lesion associated with nonimmune hydrops fetalis. *Mod Pathol.* 1993;6:487–492.

32. Thway K, Nicholson AG, Lawson K, et al. Primary pulmonary myxoid sarcoma with EWSR1–CREB1 fusion: a new tumor entity. *Am J Surg Pathol.* 2011;35:1722–1732.

33. Smith SC, Palanisamy N, Betz BL, et al. At the intersection of primary pulmonary myxoid sarcoma and pulmonary angiomatoid fibrous histiocytoma: observations from three new cases. *Histopathology.* 2014;65:144–146.

34. Boland JM, Colby TV, Folpe AL. Intrathoracic peripheral nerve sheath tumors—a clinicopathological study of 75 cases. *Hum Pathol.* 2015;46:419–425.

35. Kamran SC, Shinagare AB, Howard SA, et al. Intrathoracic malignant peripheral nerve sheath tumors: imaging features and implications for management. *Radiol Oncol.* 2013;47:230–238.

36. Wong HH, Gounaris I, McCormack A, et al. Presentation and management of pulmonary artery sarcoma. *Clin Sarcoma Res.* 2015;5:3.

37. Maleszewski JJ, Tavora F, Burke AP. Do "intimal" sarcomas of the heart exist? *Am J Surg Pathol.* 2014;38:1158–1159.

38. Bernard J, Yi ES. Pulmonary thromboendarterectomy: a clinicopathologic study of 200 consecutive pulmonary thromboendarterectomy cases in one institution. *Hum Pathol.* 2007;38:871–877.

39. Mussot S, Ghigna MR, Mercier O, et al. Retrospective institutional study of 31 patients treated for pulmonary artery sarcoma. *Eur J Cardiothorac Surg.* 2013;43:787–793.

40. Dewaele B, Floris G, Finalet-Ferreiro J, et al. Coactivated platelet-derived growth factor receptor {alpha} and epidermal growth factor receptor are potential therapeutic targets in intimal sarcoma. *Cancer Res.* 2010;70:7304–7314.

41. Tavora F, Miettinen M, Fanburg-Smith J, et al. Pulmonary artery sarcoma: a histologic and follow-up study with emphasis on a subset of low-grade myofibroblastic sarcomas with a good long-term follow-up. *Am J Surg Pathol.* 2008;32:1751–1761.

42. Maruo A, Okita Y, Okada K, et al. Surgical experience for the pulmonary artery sarcoma. *Ann Thorac Surg.* 2006;82:2014–2016.

43. Yi JE, Tazelaar HD, Burke A, et al. Pulmonary artery sarcoma. In: Travis WD, et al., eds. *Tumours of the Lung, Pleura, Thymus and Heart.* Lyon, France: International Agency for Research on Cancer; 2004:109–110.

44. Khawar MU, Bhardwaj B, Bhardwaj H. Pulmonary artery sarcoma: not every filling defect is a pulmonary thromboembolism. *J Thorac Oncol.* 2015;10: 218–219.

45. Scheidl S, Taghavi S, Reiter U, et al. Intimal sarcoma of the pulmonary valve. *Ann Thorac Surg.* 2010;89:e25–e27.

46. Bode-Lesniewska B, Zhao J, Speel EJ, et al. Gains of 12q13–14 and overexpression of MDM2 are frequent findings in intimal sarcomas of the pulmonary artery. *Virchows Arch.* 2001;438:57–65.

94 Metastases to the Lung and Pleura

Marie-Christine Aubry, M.D., and Allen P. Burke, M.D.

General

Metastasis to the lung is the most common pulmonary malignancy, with incidence ranging from 30% to 55%. In autopsy series, the lung is the third most common site, after lymph nodes and liver.[1] Carcinomas are the major source of metastases to both lung and pleura, especially from the gastrointestinal tract, breast, and head and neck, followed by sarcoma and melanoma. In surgically resected tumors, slow-growing tumors are preferentially represented, including salivary gland tumors, renal cell carcinomas, and soft tissue sarcomas.[2] The most common tumor to metastasize to the pleura is lung carcinoma, through direct extension or through seeding resulting in a malignant effusion.

Metastatic disease of the lungs can occur by different mechanisms (Table 94.1). Direct extension of tumor usually occurs from a contiguous neoplasm and mostly seen with primary thymic, esophageal, or thyroid neoplasms. Rarely, direct extension to the lung occurs via the vasculature, such as with renal cell carcinoma or germ cell tumor. True metastases can be defined as viable tumor cells transported from one site to another. They occur due to tumor spread via the vasculature, commonly the pulmonary arteries but also the lymphatic vessels and bronchial arteries. The embolized tumor cells often grow through the vasculature into the surrounding lung parenchyma, forming nodules. In some instances, the tumor cells remain confined to the vasculature and spread diffusely through the vascular channels, including lymphatic vessels. Metastases via bronchial arteries are thought to be much less common and perhaps result in endobronchial metastasis.

TABLE 94.1 Clinical and Radiologic Features of Various Metastatic Mechanisms

Metastatic Mechanisms	Common Associated Primary Tumors
Nodules	
Macronodular	Sarcomas and metastatic gastrointestinal carcinomas
Micronodular (miliary)	Medullary carcinoma of thyroid, prostate, and pancreas and melanoma
Solitary	Renal cell, breast, colon, and urothelial carcinoma, melanoma, and osteosarcoma
Cavitary	Head and neck squamous cell carcinoma and colon carcinoma
Calcified	Papillary thyroid carcinoma and mucinous colon carcinoma
Cystic +/− pneumothorax	Sarcoma, e.g., endometrial stroma sarcoma and leiomyosarcoma
Lymphangitic carcinomatosis with interstitial thickening	Breast, gastric, pancreas, and prostate carcinoma
	Lymphoma
Endobronchial mass with airway obstruction	Breast, renal cell, and colon carcinoma
	Melanoma and sarcoma
Pulmonary hypertension and infarct	Renal cell, gastric, and hepatocellular carcinoma
	Vascular sarcoma and choriocarcinoma
Diffuse alveolar hemorrhage	Angiosarcoma and choriocarcinoma
Pleural effusion	Breast, ovarian, and gastric carcinoma
	Lymphoma
Direct invasion	Thyroid, thymic, and esophageal neoplasms
Aerogenous spread	Mucinous lung adenocarcinoma

Occasionally, tumor cells can be released into the pleural space and transported by the pleural fluid to a site of implantation. Tumor dissemination through the airspace is poorly understood and probably rare but thought to occur in some subtypes of lung cancer that metastasize to the lung without evidence of vascular or lymphatic spread.

Clinical and Radiologic Features

As metastases occur through different mechanisms, each route is usually associated with characteristic clinical, radiologic, and pathologic features, although overlap is frequent (Table 94.1).[1]

Parenchymal Nodules

The most common manifestation of metastatic disease to the lung consists of multiple nodules. The majority of patients with multiple metastatic tumor nodules have a previous or current history of malignancy. Patients are usually asymptomatic. Common symptoms include cough, hemoptysis, and wheezing. Chest pain occurs as a result of extension into pleura and chest wall. Although uncommon, cystic lung disease, occasionally presenting with spontaneous pneumothorax, may be the first manifestation of metastatic disease, usually from sarcomas.

CT scan is the most sensitive imaging modality to assess patients with multiple lung nodules, but because up to 60% of metastases are reported as 0.5 cm or less, the burden of metastatic disease can be underestimated. Also, CT scan is not entirely specific because granulomas or other benign processes also present as solid nodules. Metastatic tumor nodules are usually multiple, ranging in size from hardly visible to large masses capable of occupying an entire lung, with an average size of 1.0 to 2.0 cm. Mediastinal and hilar nodes are usually not enlarged. Pulmonary metastases are most commonly found peripherally, in the lower lobes. Rarely, the deposits are minute and numerous representing a miliary pattern. This *miliary pattern* has been described with medullary carcinoma of the thyroid, malignant melanoma, and prostatic carcinoma, among others. *Cavitation* has been reported in 4% of metastasis and occurs less commonly than with primary lung cancer. It has been described in metastatic squamous cell carcinoma, mainly from the head and neck or cervix; adenocarcinoma of the colon; and osteosarcoma. *Calcification* of metastatic lesions is rare and occurs in neoplasm with matrix production such as osteosarcoma or chondrosarcoma. It has also been described in neoplasms with psammoma bodies such as papillary carcinoma of the thyroid or through dystrophic calcification of mucin in mucinous adenocarcinomas from colon or other primary site. When calcified metastatic lesions are small, they can mimic benign lesions such as calcified granulomas.

Metastatic neoplasm presenting as a solitary nodule is uncommon, accounting for 1% to 5% of all lung metastasis and 2% to 10% of solitary pulmonary nodules. Neoplasms most likely to result in solitary metastasis are carcinoma of the colon, kidney, and breast; sarcomas, particularly osteosarcoma; and malignant melanoma.

Interstitial Thickening

Lymphangitic spread is an uncommon pattern of metastasis disease. It may mimic interstitial lung disease clinically and radiologically. This pattern can be seen with any primary tumors, but the most common include breast, stomach, pancreas, and prostate. Symptoms include dyspnea, typically with an insidious onset yet rapid progression over weeks.

The CT scan appearance is characterized by smooth to nodular thickening of the interlobular septa and peribronchovascular interstitium usually with preservation of the underlying lung parenchyma. The thickening is usually asymmetric. Associated pleural effusion is present in up to 30% of patients and hilar or mediastinal enlargement in up to 40%.

Pulmonary Hypertension and Infarct

Tumor involvement of pulmonary vessels is commonly seen at autopsy, often the cause of death. Most common primary sites resulting in tumor emboli include carcinoma of the stomach, pancreas, breast, and liver and choriocarcinoma. Patients are often asymptomatic. The most common symptom is dyspnea. Patients may develop subacute pulmonary hypertension with signs of cor pulmonale.[3] If the tumor emboli have resulted in infarcts, pleuritic chest pain, hemoptysis, or even sudden death can occur.

Radiologically, these lesions are difficult if impossible to diagnose. Indirect findings of pulmonary hypertension such as dilatation of the central pulmonary arteries and right ventricle can be identified, as well as infarcts. A ventilation–perfusion scan or CT scan with contrast may be helpful in identifying large tumor embolism.

Airway Obstruction

Neoplastic infiltration of the tracheal and main bronchial wall is a common finding at autopsy (19% to 51%), usually as the result of direct extension from parenchymal tumor or nodal metastasis. Metastasis presenting as a distinct, usually solitary, endobronchial mass is uncommon, between 2% and 4% of cases. The most common neoplasms resulting in an endobronchial mass are melanoma, sarcomas, and carcinomas from breast and kidney.[4] Symptoms consist of dyspnea, wheeze, persistent cough, and hemoptysis. Occasionally, expectoration of tumor fragment can occur.

Radiologic findings are those of partial or complete bronchial obstruction with air trapping, atelectasis, or obstructive pneumonia.

Pleural Effusion

The most common cause of exudative pleural effusion is malignancy, with gastric, breast, and ovarian carcinoma and lymphoma the most common primaries leading to pleural effusions.[2] Usually, the effusion occurs on the same side as the primary lesion and bilateral effusions are commonly associated with hepatic metastases. Several explanations for pleural effusions in the setting of cancer have been postulated[5]: (1) Tumor involvement of mediastinal lymph nodes may contribute to pleural fluid accumulation. (2) Direct invasion of pleura results in inflammation, angiogenesis, and vascular leakage with the result of an exudative effusion.[6] Not all pleural effusions are considered malignant. In patients with lung cancer, an exudate effusion (proteinaceous with a low pH) may be presumptive evidence of metastasis even with negative cytology,[6] although documentation of malignant cells by cytologic or surgical pathologic examination is usually a requirement to confirm malignancy.[7] The reported incidence of positive cytologic examination in patients with malignant pleural effusion ranges between 35% and 85%. The highest diagnostic yield is with a thoracoscopic biopsy (91%), followed by ultrasound- or computed tomographic–guided biopsy (76%).

Diffuse Pulmonary Hemorrhage

Diffuse pulmonary hemorrhage (DPH) is an uncommon and unrecognized manifestation of neoplasm. Symptoms and signs of hemoptysis, anemia, and pulmonary alveolar infiltrates are similar to those seen in patients with nonneoplastic causes of DPH, although in patients with neoplasms, radiologic infiltrates will often be described as nodular, surrounded by ground-glass infiltrates.

Metastatic angiosarcoma is the most common neoplasm responsible for DPH. Other neoplasms reported to cause DPH include vascular neoplasms such as Kaposi sarcoma and epithelioid hemangioendothelioma and metastatic choriocarcinoma.

Pathologic Features

Gross

Parenchymal nodules are usually well circumscribed and of variable size. In cavitary nodules, the size of the cavity is often variable, ranging from < 1.0 cm to over 6.0 cm, and the walls are shaggy and thick, measuring between 0.3 and 2.5 cm. Blood, necrotic material, and rarely fungus ball can be identified within the cavity. In cystic metastasis, the wall is usually very thin, <0.3 cm and smooth and the cavity filled with air.

Lymphangitic carcinomatosis is characterized by thickening of the interlobular septa, peribronchovascular, and subpleural connective tissue. The thickening can be linear or nodular and is variable, from slight to obvious thickening of up to 1 cm.

Tumor emboli are usually not visible grossly unless larger, segmental arteries are involved. The appearance of tumor emboli is usually different from thromboemboli, with tumor emboli displaying a more solid, gritty or myxoid texture with white-beige color. Tumor emboli may be associated with an infarct.

Endobronchial metastasis can result in concentric narrowing of the airway or form a polypoid endobronchial mass.

Pleural metastases can vary widely from scattered small nodules to diffuse thickening with a solid rim of the pleura, mimicking mesothelioma.

The gross appearance of neoplasms presenting as DPH can vary with tumor type. In cases of metastatic angiosarcoma or Kaposi sarcoma, multiple subpleural and parenchymal hemorrhagic nodules are typically seen.

Microscopic Findings

Macronodular metastases are typically sharply demarcated "cannonball lesions" (Fig. 94.1), a contrasting feature with primary lung carcinoma. Occasionally, metastases may be cystic rather than solid (Fig. 94.2). Rarely, the growth pattern is lepidic, along intact lung architecture, mimicking a lepidic adenocarcinoma (Fig. 94.3). This growth pattern is seen mainly in mucinous adenocarcinoma of the colon and pancreaticobiliary system.[1,2,8]

In lymphangitic carcinomatosis, the neoplastic cells are usually easily identified within the lymphatic spaces but also form cords and

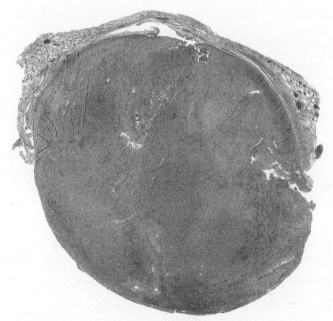

FIGURE 94.1 ▲ Metastatic synovial sarcoma. The lesion is round and well circumscribed, sharply demarcated from the adjacent benign lung.

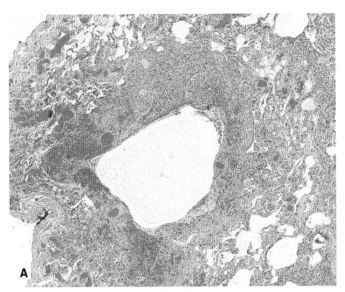
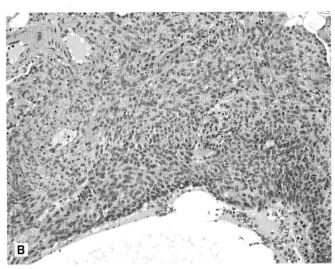

FIGURE 94.2 ▲ Metastatic endometrial stroma sarcoma, detected 11 years after initial surgery. **A.** A low-power photomicrograph shows a cystic lesion. **B.** At higher power, the cells are oval to spindled with scant cytoplasm. Small capillaries are identified. The immunostains demonstrated positive CD10 and ER, and negative for HMB45, supporting a diagnosis of endometrial stromal sarcoma.

clusters within the interstitium, usually associated with a desmoplastic reaction. Occasionally, the desmoplastic reaction is so prominent as to conceal the neoplastic cells, and the clue is the growth pattern along the lymphatic pathways (Fig. 94.4).

Tumor emboli are most often identified only histologically within small-sized arteries and arterioles. Rarely, diffuse alveolar–septal capillary involvement is present. The tumor cells form small clusters with or without associated recent or organized thrombus within vascular spaces (Fig. 94.5).

With endobronchial metastases, the tumor cells are often present within the submucosal lymphatics. Infiltration of the bronchial wall with mucosal replacement from a contiguous mass is commonly seen.

Pleural metastases are typically easy to identify and diagnose (Fig. 94.6). However, they may be associated with a prominent

fibrinous exudate and reactive mesothelial proliferation, both epithelial and spindled (Fig. 94.7), that may overshadow the metastasis.

In DPH, the hemorrhage, characterized by intra-alveolar fibrin admixed with red cells and hemosiderin-laden macrophages, often overshadows the other patterns of metastatic disease, usually lymphangitic and intravascular metastasis (Fig. 94.8).

Treatment and Prognosis

Treatment and prognosis will vary depending on tumor type and extent of metastatic disease, that is, widespread versus limited to the lung. Pulmonary metastases are usually, in up to 85% of patients, the manifestation of widespread disease and thus not amenable to surgery. Metastasectomy, usually with by video-assisted thoracoscopy, is increasingly performed, but several guidelines are followed. The procedure is considered curative and thus reserved for metastasis limited to the lung and completely resectable. Malignancy needs to be ruled out in any pleural or pericardial effusions. Because cytology alone may be falsely negative (up to 60% of cases in some series), a negative result warrants a biopsy. The primary tumor should be controlled before considering curative resection of metastasis. The patient must be able to tolerate the surgery without any significant increase in short- and long-term morbidity and mortality due to associated comorbid factors. And finally, any alternative therapy superior to surgery should be considered, for example, chemotherapy for nonseminomatous germ-cell tumors. When these guidelines are followed, survival rates as high as 60% have been reported following metastasectomy.[9,10]

The prognosis for pleural metastasis is poor, with only 30% survival at 6 months. Primary lung and gastrointestinal sites are also independent predictors of mortality.[11] Treatment includes draining, systemic chemotherapy, and chemical pleurodesis.

Differential Diagnosis

Although recognizing pulmonary metastasis is usually straightforward in patients with known history presenting with multiple nodules, difficulty in diagnosing pulmonary metastasis can arise due to uncommon clinical, radiologic, and histologic manifestations.

Clinicians and/or pathologist may be unaware of a prior diagnosis of malignancy, especially when the malignancy has occurred many years, as much as 30 years, previously. This is well recognized in tumors with good prognosis and thought to be cured, such as with endometrial

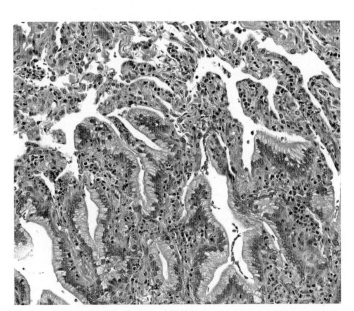

FIGURE 94.3 ▲ Metastatic pancreatic adenocarcinoma. The tumor shows lepidic growth mimicking a primary mucinous adenocarcinoma. The cells are more stratified, columnar, and cytologically atypical than the more typical mucinous adenocarcinoma of the lung.

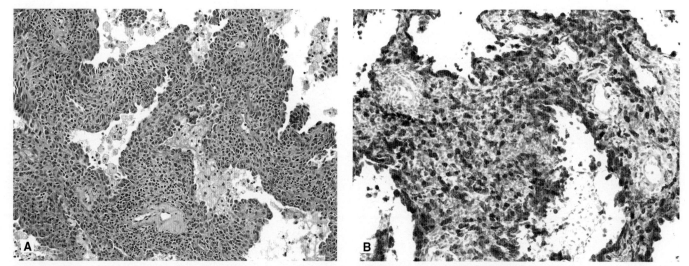

FIGURE 94.4 ▲ Metastatic malignant melanoma. **A.** The tumor nodule shows a prominent lepidic growth pattern suggestive of a well-differentiated primary lung adenocarcinoma. However, the tumor cells lining the alveolar septa show prominent cytologic atypia and form small surface nodules. Furthermore, similar cells are present within the thickened alveolar septa. **B.** Melan-A confirms the diagnosis of malignant melanoma.

stromal sarcoma, stage I carcinoma of colon or kidney, and salivary gland tumors.

Prior misdiagnosis can also be misleading, emphasizing the need to review previous surgical specimens, even of apparently benign tumors.

The metastasis can be the first manifestation of an unrecognized primary. Furthermore, an unusual presentation such as spontaneous pneumothorax, pulmonary hypertension, or DPH may compound the issues. Thus, malignancy should routinely be included in our differential diagnosis even of apparently nonneoplastic disease.

There may be significant morphologic overlap between lung carcinomas and metastasis from other sites. Comparing the morphologic features of the metastasis with the known primary is useful in most cases. However, occasionally, the morphology may be similar between two primaries or the material on the known primary not available for comparison. In these instances, ancillary studies may be helpful but, again, overlap may be seen between the immunoprofiles of lung primaries and primaries from other sites.

For example, TTF-1 (clone STP24) positivity has been reported in several nonlung or thyroid primaries, including breast, gastrointestinal,

and endometrial primaries. Therefore, using a different clone of TTF-1 (8G7G3/1), which is more specific, is important in this clinical setting.

Although CDX2 is considered a marker for gastrointestinal and pancreaticobiliary primaries, it is positive in a subset of primary lung adenocarcinoma, typically mucinous or enteric types. Furthermore, these lung adenocarcinomas will express CK20 along with CK7 and be negative for TTF-1. In this scenario, clinical and radiologic correlation to rule out a nonlung primary is necessary.

Estrogen receptor may be positive in lung adenocarcinoma of women. S100 protein and GATA3 are often positive in breast carcinoma and less so in lung carcinoma. Specific markers for breast carcinoma such GCDFP15 and mammaglobin may be useful although not very sensitive.

Prostatic carcinoma metastatic to the lung can be quite deceptive in mimicking a primary lung tumor. Immunohistochemical stains are very helpful in establishing a primary prostatic tumor, especially prostate-specific membrane antigen and prostatic acid phosphatase.

Lung primary carcinomas exhibit clear cell changes and thus mimic metastatic renal cell carcinoma. Usually, tumor cells in renal cell carcinoma are more nested, invested by a rich capillary network, not seen in lung carcinoma. Furthermore, Pax-8 is a sensitive marker that is not expressed in carcinomas of the lung.[12]

Lung primary carcinomas may be hepatoid and thus have overlapping features with metastatic hepatocellular carcinoma. Furthermore, lung carcinoma can be positive for Her-Par1 immunostain. However, arginase-1 immunostaining has not been reported in lung cancer.

Rarely, mucinous adenocarcinomas of the gastrointestinal or pancreaticobiliary tract can metastasize to the lung with a lepidic growth pattern.[8] Metastases with lepidic growth can be recognized by their greater degree of cytologic, and in addition, they may show cribriform pattern and necrosis focally or angiolymphatic invasion.

Distinguishing primary versus metastatic squamous carcinoma from the head and neck may be difficult. Identifying in situ carcinoma supports a primary lung origin. Histologic correlation with the primary tumor, including degree of keratinization and basaloid features, is helpful. In situ hybridization for HPV may be helpful if positive because primary squamous cell carcinoma is usually negative. p16 immunohistochemistry cannot be used as a surrogate of HPV in the lung setting because many primary lung carcinomas are p16 positive.[13] Distinguishing primary squamous cell carcinoma from metastatic urothelial carcinoma is also challenging. Urothelial carcinomas are typically positive for GATA3 and uroplakin, markers not usually expressed in primary lung carcinomas.

FIGURE 94.5 ▲ Embolic carcinoma metastasis. Metastatic carcinoma resulting in organized thrombus.

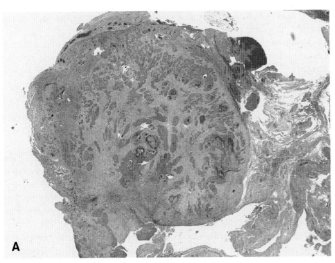 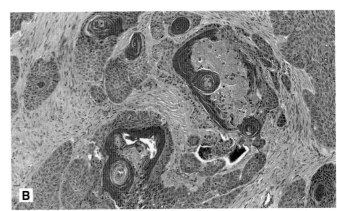

FIGURE 94.6 ▲ Metastatic squamous carcinoma, pleura. **A.** Low magnification shows thickened pleura. **B.** High magnification shows keratinizing squamous carcinoma. The primary site was uterine cervix.

Metastatic sarcoma needs to be distinguished from sarcomatoid carcinomas of the lung. Patients with metastatic sarcomas are typically younger adults and children. Furthermore, in almost all instances of resection, there is known prior history of extrapulmonary sarcoma, and therefore, the diagnosis is generally straightforward. Occasionally, there is prior chemotherapy and radiation, and treatment effect may alter the morphology.[8,14] Keratin staining may be focally positive in many sarcomas; therefore, the specific subtype of the sarcoma may need to be confirmed with immunostains or molecular studies specific to the sarcoma.

Metastatic carcinoma can be distinguished from malignant mesothelioma (Chapter 97) using a variety of immunohistochemical stains. Markers for reactive mesothelial cells include high molecular weight cytokeratins (e.g., cytokeratin 5/6) calretinin, WT-1, and D2-40 (podoplanin) (Table 94.2). Adenocarcinomas of the lung are positive for B72.3, ber-EP4, MOC31, BG-8, and carcinoembryonic antigen, all of which may be expressed at a low rate in benign or malignant mesothelial proliferations.[15] Adenocarcinomas of the lung are usually negative (85%) for cytokeratin 5/6, and mesothelial lesions are almost always negative for BerEp4.[16] WT1 is another useful marker, as nuclear positivity is typical of mesothelial proliferations and is negative in adenocarcinomas of the lung and breast; however, it is positive in tumors of müllerian origin and therefore should be used with caution in woman for whom the differential diagnosis includes a metastasis from the gynecologic tract.

Tissue-specific markers other than TTF-1 are helpful in determining primary site. GATA-3 is especially helpful in determining breast or urothelial origin, as this marker is generally not expressed in lung tumors.[17]

Although comparing the morphologic features of a metastasis to known primary may be helpful in confirming the diagnosis or distinguishing it from a new primary, changes in the morphologic appearance may occur in a metastasis making proper identification of the lesion difficult. For example, metastatic malignant melanoma is often amelanotic or can assume a spindle cell growth pattern, experience stromal hyalinization, or contain osteoclast-like giant cells. Some tumors undergo what is called the "maturation effect," as an inherent property of the tumor, a result of host–tissue interaction, or a treatment effect. This is common in sarcomas, germ-cell tumors, and childhood malignancies such as Wilms tumor or neuroblastoma. Metastatic osteosarcoma can become heavily collagenized resulting in a paucicellular nodule, resembling a scar. Metastatic germ cell tumors often take the form of mature teratoma. Some metastasis displays prominent histologic feature not well demonstrated in

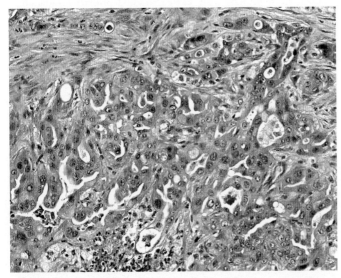 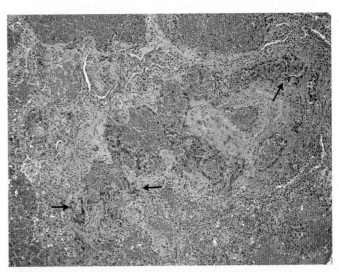

FIGURE 94.7 ▲ Metastatic breast carcinoma. This nest of malignant cells is embedded in a prominent reactive spindled cell proliferation. These cells are commonly reactive mesothelial cells, which may also be positive for keratin.

FIGURE 94.8 ▲ Metastatic angiosarcoma from cardiac primary. In a background of diffuse alveolar hemorrhage, atypical cells (*arrows*) are forming vascular channels.

TABLE 94.2 Immunohistochemical Profile, Metastatic Adenocarcinoma to the Pleura Versus Mesothelial Proliferation ["Mesothelial" Markers Are in Bold; "Adenocarcinoma" Markers in Italics].

	Epithelioid Mesothelioma/ Reactive Mesothelial Hyperplasia	Metastatic Adenocarcinomas
D2-40 (podoplanin)	90%–100%	0%–7%
Calretinin	70%–96%	2%–33%
Cytokeratin 5/6	50%–85%	9%–41%
WT-1	70%–99%	4%–16%
HBME/ mesothelioma cell/mesothelin	77%–100%	30%–60%
p63/p40	50%/7%	15%/2%
Ber-Ep4	5%–20%	72%–80%
MOC-31	2%–10%	90%
B72.3	2%–7%	64%–80%
CEA, monoclonal	2%–7%	59%
Lewis BG-8	3%–7%	90%
TTF-1	0	40%–90% (highest in lung, depending on histologic type)

the primary tumor, such as sex cord–like differentiation in endometrial stromal sarcoma or sarcomatoid differentiation in renal cell carcinoma.

Tumors That Can Be Metastatic or Primary

Neoplasms such as malignant melanoma, thymoma, germ cell tumors, and meningioma can be primary tumors of the lung and often described as tumors of ectopic origin. However, because these tumors most often represent metastatic disease, a primary site always needs to be ruled out clinically.

Malignant Melanoma

Melanomas frequently metastasize to the lung.[18] In a small proportion of patients, no primary is identified. The criteria for primary pulmonary melanoma are based purely on clinical criteria and include exclusion of previous and synchronous cutaneous, ocular, or other mucosal melanomas.[19] Most patients are adults, with a mean age in the sixth decade.[19]

Primary lung melanomas are central or peripheral tumors, predominantly in the lower lobes. Histologically, primary and metastatic malignant melanomas are similar and share all morphologic variations such as spindled or amelanotic features. Primary malignant melanoma may have a pagetoid or lepidic growth. Nevoid-like nests that appear benign may also be present.[19] Immunohistochemistry, using a combination of S100 protein, HMB45, melan-A, and SOX10, is usually necessary to confirm the diagnosis.

Primary malignant melanoma of the lung has a better prognosis than does metastatic melanoma.[20–22] Excision of metastatic melanoma deposits has been shown to extend survival from a mean of 7 to 19 months.[18]

Thymoma

Thymomas typically metastasize to the pleural and pericardial surfaces. Intraparenchymal lung metastases are not infrequent but usually with concomitant pleural involvement.[23] Primary thymoma of the lung is rare, with fewer than 40 reported cases.[24] They are believed to arise from ectopic thymic rests.

Clinically, primary lung thymomas may cause no symptoms, result in cough or hemoptysis, or manifest as symptoms of myasthenia gravis.[19] They may arise in any lobe, with a predilection for upper lobes. The histologic and immunophenotypic features are those of primary lesions in the thymus, with all types reported in approximately equal

rate (types A, AB, B1, B2, and B3). Spindle cell thymomas may entrap normal lung with pneumocyte or bronchiolar inclusions.[24]

Prognosis for primary pulmonary thymoma is good, unless there is incomplete resection or if there is myasthenia gravis that persists after surgery.[25]

Germ Cell Tumors

Primary germ cell tumors of the lung are rare. The criteria for pulmonary origin are exclusion of a gonadal or other extragonadal primary site, and origin entirely within the lung, excluding mediastinal primary.[26]

All reported intrapulmonary germ cell tumors are teratomas.[19] The majority of patients are in the second to fourth decade, with a range of 10 months to 68 years. The left upper lobe is the most common site.[19] Symptoms are usually nonspecific. However, rarely coughing up hair (trichoptysis) may occur, indicating either primary pulmonary teratoma or erosion by mediastinal teratoma into a bronchus.[27,28]

Grossly, the tumors are cystic. Histologically, pulmonary teratomas are generally mature and infrequently contain immature elements.[19] Rarely, other germ cell tumor components, such as seminoma, will be present.

The lung is the most common organ involved in metastases from testicular germ cell tumors. Among patients with retroperitoneal lymph node disease, 38% of patients have lung metastases, followed by the mediastinum (13%) and liver (3%).[29] Most patients are children or young adults. Metastatic germ cell tumors are rarely excised prior to treatment with systemic chemotherapy. Therefore, the histologic appearance of persistent nodules is typically mature teratoma.

Immunohistochemical stains may occasionally be useful to distinguish primary lung carcinoma from germ-cell tumors other than teratoma. The current recommendation by the International Society of Urological Pathology in distinguishing germ cell tumor from carcinoma is to perform SALL4, OCT4, and EMA or if SALL4 unavailable to use OCT4, glypican-3, EMA, and CK7. However, glypican-3 as well as other markers, such as placental-like alkaline phosphatase, human chorionic gonadotropin, and alpha-fetoprotein, lack specificity and can be positive in lung carcinomas.

Meningioma

Metastatic meningioma to the lungs is rare. Metastatic meningiomas are often high grade, and there is typically a history of central nervous system tumor. However, a seemingly primary lung meningioma may uncover a silent primary in the central nervous system.[30]

Primary pulmonary meningioma is even rarer than metastatic meningioma to the lung[19] (Fig. 94.9). Extradural primary meningiomas

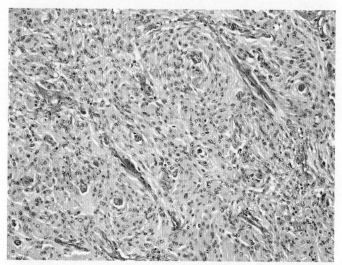

FIGURE 94.9 ▲ Meningioma, lung. A well-circumscribed nodule comprised of bland oval cells with nuclear pseudoinclusions in a typical whorled pattern.

may occur in the head and neck, lung, mediastinum, retroperitoneum, and pelvis and are generally benign.[31] There is a slight female predominance and the median age of 57 years.[19]

Primary pulmonary meningiomas range from 4 mm to 6 cm in diameter. They are histologically and immunophenotypically identical to their dural counterpart. They are typically low grade with only rare reports of anaplastic and chordoid subtypes. The differential diagnosis includes spindle cell thymoma, solitary fibrous tumor, and synovial sarcoma if mitotically active.[19]

REFERENCES

1. Pelosi G, et al. Metastases to the lung. In: Travis WD, et al., eds. *WHO Classification of Tumours of the Lung, Pleura, Thymus and Heart.* Lyon, France: IARC Press; 2015:148–151.
2. Xu L, Burke AP. Pulmonary oligometastases: histological features and difficulties in determining site of origin. *Int J Surg Pathol.* 2012;20(6):577–588.
3. Chinen K, et al. Pulmonary tumor thrombotic microangiopathy caused by an ovarian cancer expressing tissue factor and vascular endothelial growth factor. *Pathol Res Pract.* 2009;205(1):63–68.
4. Coriat R, et al. Endobronchial metastases from colorectal adenocarcinomas: clinical and endoscopic characteristics and patient prognosis. *Oncology.* 2007;73(5–6):395–400.
5. Agalioti T, Giannou AD, Stathopoulos GT. Pleural involvement in lung cancer. *J Thorac Dis.* 2015;7(6):1021–1030.
6. Ryu JS, et al. Prognostic impact of minimal pleural effusion in non-small-cell lung cancer. *J Clin Oncol.* 2014;32(9):960–967.
7. Escayola C, et al. The impact of pleural disease on the management of advanced ovarian cancer. *Gynecol Oncol.* 2015;138(1):216–220.
8. Xu L, Burke A. Pulmonary metastasis from a low grade mucinous appendiceal neoplasm. *Pathology.* 2013;45(2):186–188.
9. Meimarakis G, et al. Resection of pulmonary metastases from colon and rectal cancer: factors to predict survival differ regarding to the origin of the primary tumor. *Ann Surg Oncol.* 2014;21(8):2563–2572.
10. Welter S, et al. Growth patterns of lung metastases from sarcoma: prognostic and surgical implications from histology. *Interact Cardiovasc Thorac Surg.* 2012;15(4):612–617.
11. Abrao FC, et al. Prognostic factors of 30-day mortality after palliative procedures in patients with malignant pleural effusion. *Ann Surg Oncol.* 2015;22(12):4083–4088.
12. Ozcan A, et al. PAX 8 expression in non-neoplastic tissues, primary tumors, and metastatic tumors: a comprehensive immunohistochemical study. *Mod Pathol.* 2011;24(6):751–764.
13. Chang SY, et al. Detection of human papillomavirus in non-small cell carcinoma of the lung. *Hum Pathol.* 2015;46(11):1592–1597.
14. Welter S, et al. Growth patterns of lung metastases from sarcomas. *Virchows Arch.* 2011;459(2):213–219.
15. Kushitani K, et al. Immunohistochemical marker panels for distinguishing between epithelioid mesothelioma and lung adenocarcinoma. *Pathol Int.* 2007;57(4):190–199.
16. Szczepulska-Wojcik E, Langfort R, Roszkowski-Sliz K. A comparative evaluation of immunohistochemical markers for the differential diagnosis between malignant mesothelioma, non-small cell carcinoma involving the pleura, and benign reactive mesothelial cell proliferation. *Pneumonol Alergol Pol.* 2007;75(1):57–69.
17. Miettinen M, et al. GATA3: a multispecific but potentially useful marker in surgical pathology: a systematic analysis of 2500 epithelial and nonepithelial tumors. *Am J Surg Pathol.* 2014;38(1):13–22.
18. Petersen RP, et al. Improved survival with pulmonary metastasectomy: an analysis of 1720 patients with pulmonary metastatic melanoma. *J Thorac Cardiovasc Surg.* 2007;133(1):104–110.
19. Duhig E, Nicholson AG. Tumours of ectopic origin. In: Travis WD, et al., eds. *WHO Classification of Tumours of the Lung, Pleura, Thymus and Heart.* Lyon, France: IARC Press; 2015:144–147.
20. Mahowald MK, et al. Long-term survival after pneumonectomy for primary pulmonary malignant melanoma. *Ann Thorac Surg.* 2015;99(4):1428–1430.
21. dos Santos CL, et al. Primary pulmonary melanoma: the unexpected tumour. *BMJ Case Rep.* 2013;2013.
22. Gong L, et al. Primary pulmonary malignant melanoma: a clinicopathologic study of two cases. *Diagn Pathol.* 2012;7:123.
23. Hanna N, et al. High-dose carboplatin with etoposide in patients with recurrent thymoma: the Indiana University experience. *Bone Marrow Transplant.* 2001;28(5):435–438.
24. Katsura M, et al. Primary intrapulmonary thymoma. *Gen Thorac Cardiovasc Surg.* 2015;63(1):56–59.
25. Myers PO, et al. Primary intrapulmonary thymoma: a systematic review. *Eur J Surg Oncol.* 2007;33(10):1137–1141.
26. Rana SS, et al. Intrapulmonary teratoma: an exceptional disease. *Ann Thorac Surg.* 2007;83(3):1194–1196.
27. Kang HS, et al. Intrapulmonary teratoma presenting with trichoptysis. *J Thorac Oncol.* 2013;8(1):126–127.
28. Guibert N, et al. Mediastinal teratoma and trichoptysis. *Ann Thorac Surg.* 2011;92(1):351–353.
29. Raggi D, et al. Prognostic reclassification of patients with intermediate-risk metastatic germ cell tumors: implications for clinical practice, trial design, and molecular interrogation. *Urol Oncol.* 2015;33(7):332; e19–24.
30. Chiarelli M, et al. An incidental pulmonary meningioma revealing an intracranial meningioma: primary or secondary lesion? *Ann Thorac Surg.* 2015;99(4):e83–e84.
31. Weber C, et al. Primary pulmonary malignant meningioma with lymph node and liver metastasis in a centenary woman, an autopsy case. *Virchows Arch.* 2013;462(4):481–485.

95 Nonneoplastic Diseases of the Pleura

Allen P. Burke, M.D., and Marie-Christine Aubry, M.D.

Infections of the Pleura

Bacterial Infection and Empyema

Definition

Clinically, empyema is defined by the presence of microorganisms in pleural fluid, Gram stain, or culture; pleural pH < 7.2 associated with radiographic features of empyema; or frank pus in the pleural space at the time of thoracoscopy.[1] The pathologic definition is that of purulent inflammation within the pleural cavity.

Etiology and Stages

Empyema is caused by infected parapneumonic effusions, which begin as sterile fluid collections. The first phase is the exudative phase, with free-flowing, nonviscous fluid, which overlaps with parapneumonic effusion; the second is the fibrinopurulent phase (Fig. 95.1), with viscous fluid, loculations, and pleural peels; and finally there is the organizing phase, with fibrosis (Figs. 95.2 and 95.3).[2] The causative organism or organisms are generally that of the adjacent pneumonia and reflect the clinical setting (Chapter 38).

Empyema may also result from hematogenous or direct spread of bacterial infections caused by osteomyelitis, subdiaphragmatic abscesses, surgery, trauma, and gastropleural fistulas, in which cases causative organisms are varied.[2-5]

Incidence

Pneumonias that result in either effusions or empyema occur in about 1 in 1,000 children.[6] Community-acquired pneumonia in adults is complicated by empyema in 0.7% of patients.[1] Patients who are immunocompromised are at increased risk for empyema following pneumonia.[7-9]

Organisms

Most commonly, an empyema develops from similar pathogens that cause a pneumonia.[2] In community-acquired pneumonias, streptococci are the most frequent causes of pneumonia and empyema, with a propensity for pneumonias caused by *Streptococcus viridans* group. Less common organisms include *Staphylococcus aureus*, *Pseudomonas aeruginosa*, *Haemophilus influenzae*, and *Mycoplasma pneumoniae*.[7,10,11] In immunocompromised patients, the bacterial etiology can be quite diverse and includes more frequent Gram-negative rods.[9]

Bacteria are isolated from blood, sputum, or pleural fluid. Because many pleural samples are culture negative, molecular studies are useful in determining the organism and species and serotype of streptococcus.[10]

Spontaneous Bacterial Empyema

Spontaneous bacterial empyema denotes bacterial infection of a previously sterile pleural effusion, in the absence of contiguous pneumonia. It usually occurs in patients with cirrhosis, at a rate of 1% to 2%.[12]

Prognosis and Treatment

The in-hospital mortality rate for patients with empyema is 4% to 15%.[1]

Approximately 40% of patients require surgical intervention, in the form of pleural decortication, obliteration of the pleural space with muscle flaps or omentum flaps, or by thoracoplasty.[13] If only a chest tube is placed, tissue is generally not sampled, but fluid is obtained for microbiologic and cytologic analysis.[6]

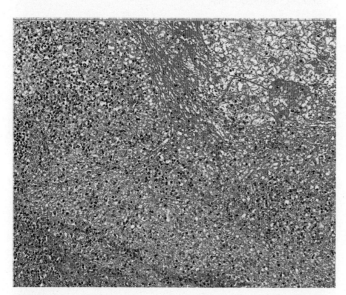

FIGURE 95.1 ▲ Empyema, early stage. There is a fibrinopurulent exudate with abundant neutrophils.

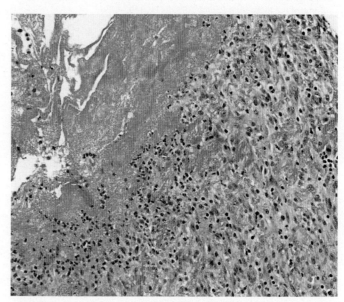

FIGURE 95.2 ▲ Empyema, organizing stage, pleural decortication. There is granulation tissue with abundant fibrin.

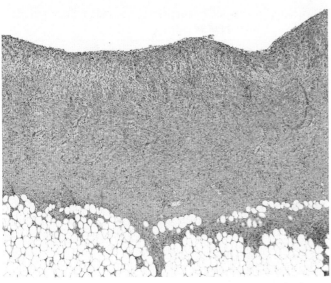

FIGURE 95.3 ▲ Empyema, organized stage, pleural decortication. There is granulation tissue and fibrosis, without residual fibrin.

Gross Findings

Grossly, empyema cavities are generally seen at autopsy at relatively advanced stages and consist of loculated masses with hemorrhagic fluid and frank pus that are generally within the pleural cavity. There may be adjacent abscesses within the lung parenchyma.

Microscopic Findings

Histologically, the findings that are seen in pleural decortications or pleural "peels" include fibrinous pleuritis, acute and chronic inflammation, and granulation tissue. In later stages, there is pleural fibrosis (Fig. 95.4). Occasionally, there is reactive mesothelial hyperplasia that rarely raises the concern for malignancy.

Fungal Pleural Infections

Fungal empyema is rare in community-acquired pneumonia.[1] *Candida* is the most frequent species isolated, typically in mixed bacterial

infections, and may be seen in spread from adjacent osteomyelitis, abscesses, or fistulas.[2,3,5]

Mycobacterial Infections and Empyema Necessitatis

Chronic cavitary tuberculosis frequently involves the pleural cavity. *Empyema necessitatis* is a rare form of empyema in which the pleural infection spreads outside of the pleural space into soft tissues of the chest wall and is usually caused by *Mycobacterium tuberculosis*. Computerized tomographic imaging will reveal a loculated fluid collection extending beyond the thoracic cage to involve the chest wall[8] Rarely, *Actinomyces israelii*, streptococcus, *Mucor*, and staphylococcus pneumonia can cause empyema necessitatis.[8,14]

Chronic tuberculous empyema may increase the risk for serosal cavity lymphomas or "pyothorax-related" lymphomas that include EBV-related B-cell lymphomas and T-cell non-Hodgkin lymphoma.[15,16]

Nocardial infection can occasionally result in a granulomatous pleuritis.[17]

Noninfectious Pleuritis

Chronic Pleuritis

Inflammatory conditions of the pleura characterized by a predominantly lymphocytic infiltrate include tuberculous infection, viral infections, autoimmune disorders (particularly Sjögren syndrome), and postsurgical conditions including coronary bypass surgery.[18] Other etiologic factors include uremia,[19] radiation therapy,[20] and drugs, including methotrexate and monoclonal antibodies.[21,22]

Idiopathic lymphocytic pleuritis is a rare form of diffuse pleural inflammation characterized by extensive lymphocytic infiltration for which no cause is found.[18] It can develop into a chronic fibrosing process (Fig. 95.4).[23,24]

Chronic pleuritis has also been reported in IgG4-related disease.[25,26]

The treatment of noninfectious pleuritis includes steroids and azathioprine.[24]

Eosinophilic Pleuritis

Eosinophilic pleuritis, in addition to accompanying parasitic infection, has been reported as a hypersensitivity reaction to methotrexate and propylthiouracil[21,27] (Fig. 95.5). It is also a common histologic finding following pneumothorax.

Spontaneous Pneumothorax

Etiology

Pneumothorax, or air in the pleural cavity, is classified as nonspontaneous (i.e., iatrogenic and traumatic) or spontaneous. Spontaneous pneumothorax is designated as primary (no identified cause or idiopathic)

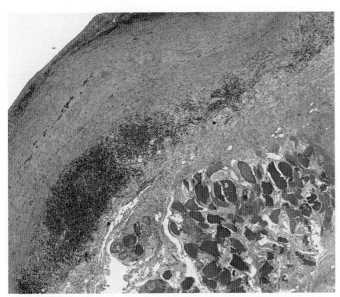

FIGURE 95.4 ▲ Chronic fibrosing pleuritis. There is dense scarring with reactive lymphoid hyperplasia at the junction of the parietal pleura and chest wall.

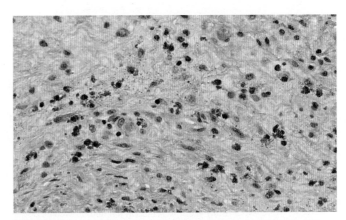

FIGURE 95.5 ▲ Eosinophilic pleuritis, secondary to methotrexate. There are numerous and degranulating eosinophils within the pleura.

and secondary to underlying lung disease. "Catamenial" refers to pneumothorax linked to the menstrual cycle.[28]

Incidence

The incidence of spontaneous pneumothorax has been estimated at 7.4 to 18 per 100,000 per year in men and 1.2 to 6 per 100,000 per year in women.[28]

Clinical Findings

In children, almost two-thirds of spontaneous pneumothorax is idiopathic. The remainder are caused by cystic fibrosis, infections, congenital lung cysts, and infection.[29] Idiopathic spontaneous pneumothorax typically affects young males aged 16 to 25 years.[30] There is a weak association with smoking and asthma.

In adults, spontaneous pneumothorax is associated with a variety of parenchymal lung diseases, most frequently emphysema (Table 95.1). In a subset of patients, the bullae causing the spontaneous pneumothorax may be so large as to cause compression of the adjacent lung. This is referred to as giant bullous emphysema or vanishing lung syndrome. These bullae usually arise in the background of distal emphysema but can also be seen with centrilobular emphysema.[32]

Treatment

The initial treatment of spontaneous pneumothorax is percutaneous aspiration and chest tube placement.[28] Pneumothorax that is refractory to chest tube drainage may require surgical intervention for closure of the leak. Indications for surgical intervention include recurrence and failure of chest tube treatment.[33] Surgery is required in children in more than one-third of patients.[29] Refractory leaks may be treated with pleurodesis, for example, with talc. Patients who require surgical therapy may undergo wedge resection, bullectomy, or pleural decortication.

Histologic Findings

Histologic findings can be divided into those related to pneumothorax, changes secondary to pneumothorax, and finally, underlying lung diseases that may have led to pneumothorax.

In the first category are blebs and bullae from distal emphysema, which result in the air leak by rupturing (Fig. 95.6).

In the second category are a variety of reactive changes to the pleura and lung parenchyma, with mesothelial inflammation and proliferation, fibrous and smooth muscle cell reaction, pneumocyte reactions, and vascular changes (Fig. 95.7). Fibroblastic lesions that mimic organizing pneumonia are especially frequent in idiopathic pneumothorax.[30] Placental transmogrification has been described in patients with

TABLE 95.1	Causes and Associations, Secondary Spontaneous Pneumothorax

Emphysema (Chapter 44–46)
   Distal emphysema
   Centrilobular emphysema
   Panlobular emphysema
Pleural blebs
Congenital cysts (Chapter 12)
Asthma (Chapter 33)
Cystic fibrosis (Chapter 32)
Respiratory bronchiolitis (Chapter 19)
Hypersensitivity pneumonia (Chapter 24)
Usual interstitial pneumonia (Chapter 18)
Lymphocytic interstitial pneumonia (Chapter 21)
Pulmonary infarction (Chapter 65)
Infections
   Pneumocystis jiroveci pneumonia (Chapter 42)
   Tuberculosis or other organisms causing cavitary nodules (Chapter 40)
   Whooping cough
Systemic or congenital disease
   Birt-Hogg-Dube syndrome
   Connective tissue disorders (Marfan, Ehlers-Danlos)
   Endometriosis
   Sarcoidosis (Chapter 23)
Neoplasms
   Lymphangioleiomyomatosis (Chapter 71)
   Pulmonary Langerhans cell histiocytosis (Chapter 25)
   Pleuropulmonary blastoma
   Mesothelioma (Chapter 97)
   Metastatic carcinoma (with cavitation)
   Primary pleural sarcoma and metastatic sarcomas[31] (Chapter 94)

severe bullous emphysema. Papillary structures lined by reactive pneumocytes are present within the bullous changes and mimic the appearance of chorionic villi (Fig. 95.8).[34]

In the third and last category are underlying lung conditions that may have predisposed to pneumothorax such as emphysema, respiratory bronchiolitis, interstitial lung disease, acute pneumonia, and hypersensitivity pneumonia (Table 95.1).

In some cases of recurrent pneumothorax, evidence of prior pleurodesis, with talc crystals and a foreign body reaction, may be encountered (Fig. 95.9).

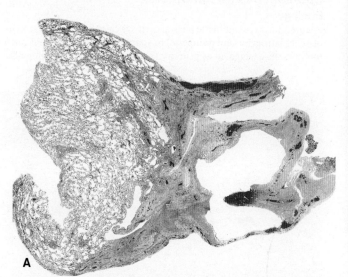
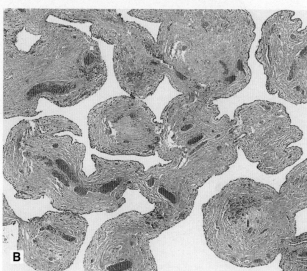

FIGURE 95.6 ▲ Pleural bleb. **A.** A bleb is defined as a collection of air within the visceral pleura. The pleura is thickened by fibrosis. The underlying lung parenchyma is relatively normal except for some subpleural fibrosis below the bleb. **B.** The thickened pleural is lined by reactive mesothelial cells.

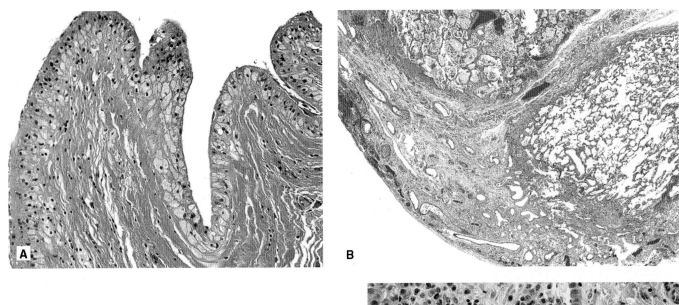

FIGURE 95.7 ▲ Spontaneous pneumothorax, reactive changes. **A.** Foamy macrophages lining a bleb. Foreign body giant cell reaction can also be seen (not illustrate in this image). **B.** Vascularized adhesions and fibrotic areas in the pleura and interlobular septa. **C.** Mesothelial hyperplasia and inflammation composed predominantly of eosinophils representing eosinophilic pleuritic.

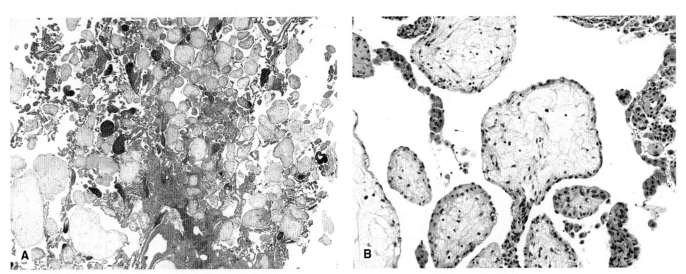

FIGURE 95.8 ▲ Bullous emphysema with placental transmogrification. **A.** The low-power photomicrograph shows the presence of numerous papillary structures filling the enlarged airspaces. **B.** At high power, the papillary structures are lined by reactive pneumocytes. The cores are edematous and contain capillaries.

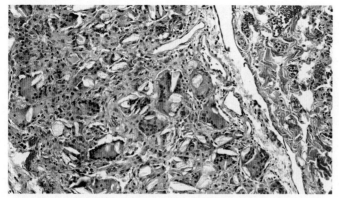

FIGURE 95.9 ▲ Talc crystals in the pleural space. The patient had undergone talc pleurodesis for recurrent pneumothorax.

Differential Diagnosis

The role of the pathologist in the interpretation of specimens obtained for the treatment of spontaneous pneumothorax involves identification of reactive changes as insignificant and in not overlooking an underlying specific etiology.

Reactive pneumocyte hyperplasia can be marked in patients with pneumothorax and mimic adenocarcinoma.[35] The correct diagnosis is possible if all clinical and histologic features are put into context, such as young age, reactive changes that are typical of pneumothorax, and the clinical setting, including the fact that adenocarcinomas rarely present as air leak.

Reactive mesothelial hyperplasia may be marked and may possibly be confused with malignant mesothelioma. Mesothelial hyperplasia is most prominent on the epithelial surface and does not exhibit the invasiveness of a malignant mesothelioma (Chapter 97).

Reactive smooth muscle hyperplasia may form nodules that may superficially resemble lymphangioleiomyomatosis (LAM).[33] Although LAM is frequently complicated by pneumothorax, the diagnosis is rarely made initially on pathologic evaluation but rather by typical radiologic features (Chapter 71). If in doubt in a young female patient, appropriate immunohistochemical stains such as HMB45 can be performed.

Although rare, cystic synovial sarcoma of the pleura and pleuropulmonary blastoma are causes of spontaneous pneumothorax that should be considered if the histologic features are not typical of a reactive process.

REFERENCES

1. Ahmed RA, Marrie TJ, Huang JQ. Thoracic empyema in patients with community-acquired pneumonia. *Am J Med.* 2006;119(10):877–883.
2. Yager NM, et al. A rare case of empyema. Answer: transformation of CLL into diffuse large B-cell lymphoma, also known as Richter syndrome. *Chest.* 2013;144(1):350–353.
3. Guarner J, et al. Unusual empyema. *J Clin Microbiol.* 2013;51(7):2017, 2473.
4. Jari S, et al. Spinal osteomyelitis presenting with a life-threatening pleural empyema. *Spine (Phila Pa 1976).* 1996;21(23):2806–2808.
5. Held J, et al. Photo quiz: mysterious objects in a pleural biopsy sample from a patient with recurrent pleural empyema. *J Clin Microbiol.* 2015;53(7):2005, 2393.
6. Lin TY, et al. Etiology of empyema thoracis and parapneumonic pleural effusion in Taiwanese children and adolescents younger than 18 years of age. *Pediatr Infect Dis J.* 2013;32(4):419–421.
7. Baracaldo R, et al. Empyema caused by *Mycoplasma salivarium. J Clin Microbiol.* 2012;50(5):1805–1806.
8. Bhaskar N, Jagana R, Johnson LG. Nontuberculous empyema necessitatis. *Am J Respir Crit Care Med.* 2013;188(8):e65–e66.
9. Cardile AP, et al. Treatment of KPC-2 Enterobacter cloacae empyema with cefepime and levofloxacin. *Diagn Microbiol Infect Dis.* 2014;78(2):199–200.
10. Lin Q, et al. Eosinophilic pleural effusion due to Spirometra mansoni spargana: a case report and review of the literature. *Int J Infect Dis.* 2015;34:96–98.
11. Mohanty S, et al. Bacteraemic Haemophilus influenzae type B pneumonia complicated with empyema—report of a case and review of literature. *J Commun Dis.* 2013;45(1–2):95–100.
12. Makhlouf HA, et al. Spontaneous bacterial empyema in patients with liver cirrhosis in Upper Egypt: prevalence and causative organisms. *Hepatol Int.* 2013;7(1):274–279.
13. Guerra M, et al. Surgery for thoracic empyema: personal experience and current highlights. *Rev Port Cir Cardiotorac Vasc.* 2012;19(1):21–26.
14. Mizell KN, Patterson KV, Carter JE. Empyema necessitatis due to methicillin-resistant *Staphylococcus aureus*: case report and review of the literature. *J Clin Microbiol.* 2008;46(10):3534–3536.
15. Yun JS, et al. Diffuse large B-cell lymphoma arising from chronic tuberculous empyema. *Korean J Thorac Cardiovasc Surg.* 2015;48(1):82–85.
16. Santini M, et al. A surgical case of pyothorax-associated lymphoma of T-cell origin arising from the chest wall in chronic empyema. *Ann Thorac Surg.* 2009;88(2):642–645.
17. Wada R, et al. Chronic granulomatous pleuritis caused by nocardia: PCR based diagnosis by nocardial 16S rDNA in pathological specimens. *J Clin Pathol.* 2003;56(12):966–969.
18. O'Donnell DH, et al. Idiopathic lymphocytic pleuritis: radiographic and high-resolution CT appearances and changes in response to therapy in two adults. *Clin Imaging.* 2010;34(3):226–230.
19. Rashid-Farokhi F, et al. Uremic pleuritis in chronic hemodialysis patients. *Hemodial Int.* 2013;17(1):94–100.
20. Fentanes de Torres E, Guevara E. Pleuritis by radiation: reports of two cases. *Acta Cytol.* 1981;25(4):427–429.
21. Cudzilo C, et al. Methotrexate-induced pleuropericarditis and eosinophilic pleural effusion. *J Bronchol Interv Pulmonol.* 2014;21(1):90–92.
22. Elkayam O, et al. Tocilizumab in adult-onset Still's disease: the Israeli experience. *J Rheumatol.* 2014;41(2):244–247.
23. Gartmann J. Chronic fibrosing idiopathic pleuritis. A study of 14 patients with histological examination of the decorticated pleura. *Schweiz Med Wochenschr.* 1971;101(38):1367–1373.
24. O'Connor TM, et al. Immunosuppressant-responsive idiopathic lymphocytic pleuritis. *Respiration.* 2005;72(2):202–204.
25. Yamamoto H, et al. IgG4-related pleural disease diagnosed by a re-evaluation of chronic bilateral pleuritis in a patient who experienced occasional acute left bacterial pleuritis. *Intern Med.* 2011;50(8):893–897.
26. Ishida M. et al. Concomitant occurrence of IgG4-related pleuritis and periaortitis: a case report with review of the literature. *Int J Clin Exp Pathol.* 2014;7(2):808–814.
27. Middleton KL, Santella R, Couser Jr, JI. Eosinophilic pleuritis due to propylthiouracil. *Chest.* 1993;103(3):955–956.
28. Aguinagalde B, et al. Percutaneous aspiration versus tube drainage for spontaneous pneumothorax: systematic review and meta-analysis. *Eur J Cardiothorac Surg.* 2010;37(5):1129–1135.
29. Wilcox DT, et al. Spontaneous pneumothorax: a single-institution, 12-year experience in patients under 16 years of age. *J Pediatr Surg.* 1995;30(10):1452–1454.
30. Belchis DA, Shekitka K, Gocke CD. A unique, histopathologic lesion in a subset of patients with spontaneous pneumothorax. *Arch Pathol Lab Med.* 2012;136(12):1522–1527.
31. Fayda M, et al. Spontaneous pneumothorax in children with osteosarcoma: report of three cases and review of the literature. *Acta Chir Belg.* 2012;112(5):378–381.
32. Sharma N, et al. Vanishing lung syndrome (giant bullous emphysema): CT findings in 7 patients and a literature review. *J Thorac Imaging.* 2009;24(3):227–230.
33. Schneider F, et al. Approach to lung biopsies from patients with pneumothorax. *Arch Pathol Lab Med.* 2014;138(2):257–265.
34. Fidler ME, et al. Placental transmogrification of the lung, a histologic variant of giant bullous emphysema. Clinicopathological study of three further cases. *Am J Surg Pathol.* 1995;19(5):563–570.
35. Shilo K, et al. Exuberant type 2 pneumocyte hyperplasia associated with spontaneous pneumothorax: secondary reactive change mimicking adenocarcinoma. *Mod Pathol.* 2007;20(3):352–356.

96 Mesenchymal Tumors of the Pleura

Adina Paulk, M.D., Allen P. Burke, M.D., Juliana Magalhães Cavalcante, M.D., and Fabio R. Tavora, M.D., Ph.D.

Solitary Fibrous Tumor

Terminology

Solitary fibrous tumor (SFT), previously called localized fibrous tumor,[1] is a low-grade mesenchymal neoplasm. Tumors that were previously called hemangiopericytomas are now considered SFTs, except those in the meninges, which still retain the designation. The term "hemangio-pericytoma-like" is still frequently used to describe the characteristic tumor vasculature of these lesions.

Clinical Findings

SFT occurs in adults, most frequently in the sixth decade, but has been reported in patients from their teens to their nineties.[1] There is no gender predilection. SFT represents <5% of primary pleural neoplasms, with an estimated incidence of 2.8 cases per 100,000 individuals.[2]

Many SFTs are asymptomatic and discovered incidentally. Larger tumors cause symptoms of cough, dyspnea, and chest pain. Occasionally, patients become hypoglycemic related to tumor production of an insulin-like growth factor.[3]

Radiologic Findings

On imaging, SFTs are usually sharply demarcated pleural-based soft tissue masses with no chest wall abnormality. Occasionally, they are diagnosed within the parenchyma without pleural attachment.[4] Positron emission tomography (PET) usually shows increased avidity in malignant versus benign tumors, although there is overlap.[5]

Gross Findings

SFTs are well-circumscribed, solid gray, homogenous masses, frequently pedunculated, and are often >10 cm (so-called giant SFTS). Cystic necrosis, hemorrhage, and calcification are occasionally present (Fig. 96.1).

Most SFTs are attached to the pleura, either the visceral or parietal surfaces, more frequently on the visceral pleura. In ~3% of cases, no pleural attachment can be identified and the tumor is surrounded by lung parenchyma.[1,4]

Microscopic Findings and Differential Diagnosis

SFTs have a distinctive morphology, with uniform fibroblastic spindle cells, varying cellularity (cellular and paucicellular areas), variable fibrosis, and branching "hemangiopericytoma-like" or "staghorn" vessels (Figs. 96.2 and 96.3). The differential diagnosis includes synovial sarcoma, which is usually more cellular and mitotically active and lacks background fibrosis, and fibromatosis, which generally occurs in the soft tissue of the chest wall. Occasionally, growth into the lung parenchyma can result in nests and papillae of hyperplastic pneumocytes, mimicking sclerosing pneumocytoma (Fig. 96.4).

Immunohistochemical and Molecular Findings

The large majority of lesions are CD34 positive (Fig. 96.5), but this is nonspecific, and occasional SFTs do not express this marker. Positive staining for Bcl2 and CD99 is also nonspecific (expressed, e.g., in some synovial sarcomas) but can be helpful in evaluating small biopsies.[6] Much more specific is STAT6, which is positive in >95% of cases.[7]

Criteria for Malignancy

The classic study of England et al. determined that a cutoff of >4 mitotic figures per 10 high-powered fields separated benign tumors (without any recurrence on follow-up) to aggressive neoplasms, 65% of which recurred.[1] This criterion is still used, with a variation of 2 mm^2 instead of 10 HPF.[2] Using this criterion, ~10% of SFTs are malignant.

Although recurrences are common in malignant SFT, distant metastases occur rarely.[1,4,6] A single series showed a relatively high rate

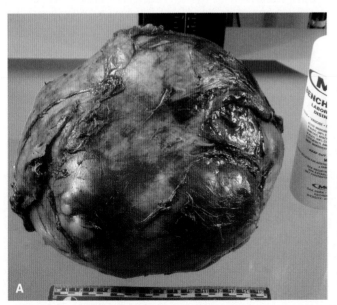
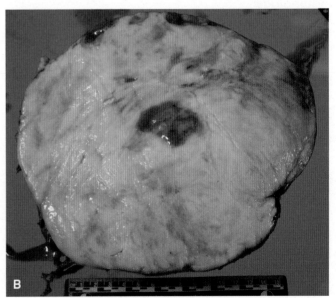

FIGURE 96.1 ▲ Solitary fibrous tumor, gross. **A.** The tumor is over 10 cm in size and partly covered by pleura. **B.** On cut section, there may be areas of cystic change with necrosis.

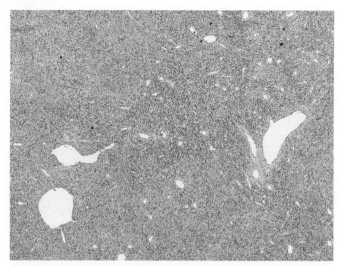

FIGURE 96.2 ▲ Solitary fibrous tumor. The "hemangiopericytoma-like" vascular pattern is evident.

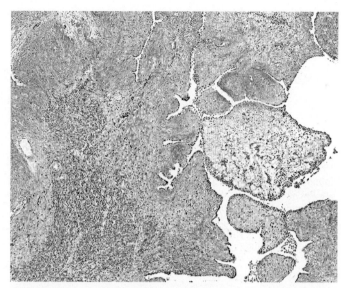

FIGURE 96.4 ▲ Solitary fibrous tumor. There can be areas of dense collagen, and, when invading the lung parenchyma, pneumocyte inclusions or papillae can be seen that are TTF-1 positive (not shown).

of distant metastasis.[8] The histologic appearance of malignant lesions include, in addition to increased mitotic activity, increased cellularity, hemorrhage, necrosis,[1] and areas with the appearance of sarcoma.[9]

Recurrences have shown decrease in CD34 expression, and malignant SFTs are more likely to be p53 and p16 positive than benign SFT.[6,10,11] Ki 67 has been reported as increased as would be expected in high-grade tumors (Fig. 96.6).[6,11] Ki 67 index did not correlate with recurrence in one study, which did show a correlation between recurrence and p16 expression.[6]

A three-tiered grading system has been proposed for SFT of the lung.[4] Low-grade SFT has <4 mitoses per 10 HPF (corresponding to "benign" SFT), intermediate has grade 5 to 10 mitotic figures per 10 HPF with increased cellularity, and high-grade tumors show undifferentiated pleomorphic sarcoma (Fig. 96.6). Another study suggested a grading system based on bad prognostic factors (parietal pleura vs. visceral pleural, sessile vs. pedunculated, >10 cm vs. <10 cm, necrosis, and mitotic figures >4 per HPF).[12]

A single malignant SFT with heterologous elements (osteosarcoma) has been described.[13]

Fibromatosis
Terminology
Fibromatoses are relatively rare tumors derived from fascial or musculoaponeurotic structures. The term "desmoid tumor" is synonymous and favored by surgeons.

Clinical Findings
Approximately one-third of fibromatoses occur on the trunk, usually the chest wall, breast, or axilla.[14–16] Most patients are young or middle-aged adults with visible subcutaneous swelling that frequently invades bone on imaging.[17] A history of prior surgery or trauma is elicited in 10% to 20% of patients.[15] Occasionally, chest wall or mediastinal fibromatoses can involve the pleura or lung, mimicking a primary lung or pleural tumor.[18–20]

Primary pleural fibromatoses are uncommon and usually arise on the parietal pleura. The largest series comprises four cases.[21] Patients ranged from 16 to 66 years, and in two patients (50%), there was an antecedent history of trauma.[21]

Two pleural fibromatoses have been described at prior thoracotomy site for segmentectomy or lobectomy.[22,23]

Gross and Microscopic Findings
Pleural fibromatosis are typically large (mean 12.5 cm) and exhibit a bosselated, firm, white, cut surface.[21] Fibromatoses of the chest wall can reach giant proportions.[24]

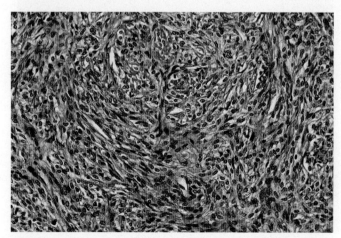

FIGURE 96.3 ▲ Solitary fibrous tumor. Highest magnification demonstrates collagen encircling individual tumor cells.

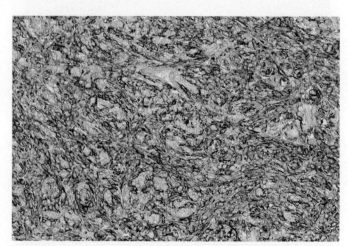

FIGURE 96.5 ▲ Solitary fibrous tumor. CD34 is usually diffusely positive but is not as sensitive or specific as is STAT6.

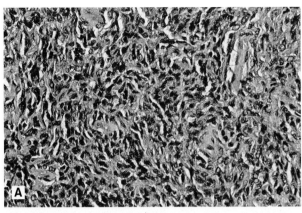
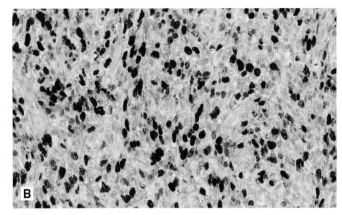

FIGURE 96.6 ▲ Malignant solitary fibrous tumor. **A.** There is increased cellularity and cellular pleomorphism. The appearance is similar to undifferentiated pleomorphic sarcoma. **B.** Immunohistochemical staining for Ki 67 shows a high proliferative rate.

The histologic features of intrathoracic desmoid tumors are similar to those of desmoid tumors elsewhere in the body (Figs. 96.7 and 96.8). Pleural fibromatosis infiltrates the adjacent fat and skeletal muscle (Fig. 96.9). Tumor cells are immunoreactive for vimentin, desmin, smooth muscle actin, and muscle-specific actin, express β-catenin, and are negative for neural markers such as S100 protein and CD34.

A report has described mesothelial rests in axillary lymph nodes draining a chest wall fibromatosis.[25]

Differential Diagnosis

Desmoid tumor should be considered in the differential of localized fibrous tumor of the pleura and neurogenic tumors of the chest wall adjacent to the thoracic spine. The diagnosis is generally made easily by histologic examination. Immunohistochemical stains are helpful to exclude neural tumors (positive for S100 protein, negative for β-catenin) and SFT (positive for CD34, stat6, and negative for β-catenin).

Prognosis and Treatment

Complete resection with wide margins is the standard of care for fibromatoses, regardless of site. Recurrences occur in one-third of tumors in all sites. Because fewer than one-half of patients with positive margins experience recurrence, overly aggressive surgery is to be avoided.

Factors associated with recurrence include tumor size larger than 5 cm, extra-abdominal tumor location, and incomplete resection.[15] Residual disease can remain stable for up to 1 year.[21]

Treatment of nonresectable tumors includes radiation therapy, steroid injection,[26] antiestrogens, aromatase inhibitors,[27] antiprogesterone drugs,[28] and tranilast.[29]

The majority of chest wall fibromatoses can be completely excised, with a low rate of recurrence (17%).[17]

Pleuropulmonary Synovial Sarcoma

Introduction

Synovial sarcoma (SS) is a malignant soft tissue tumor of uncertain differentiation and may be monophasic or biphasic, with epithelial and mesenchymal components. SS of the lung typically involves the pleura with extension into the parenchyma (pleuropulmonary synovial sarcoma), with 75% of tumors showing a pleural base by computed tomography scanning.[30] Pleuropulmonary synovial sarcoma is uncommon; there were fewer than 100 cases reported up until 2007.[30]

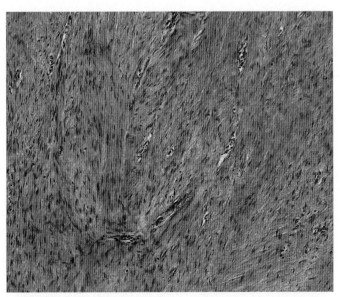

FIGURE 96.7 ▲ Pleural fibromatosis. An intermediate magnification shows dense fascicles of collagen with a low density of parallel-oriented fibroblasts. There are fairly regularly spaced thin-walled vessels.

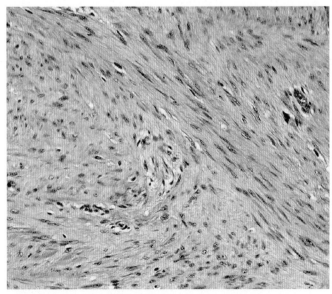

FIGURE 96.8 ▲ Pleural fibromatosis. A higher magnification shows bland fibroblasts and collagen.

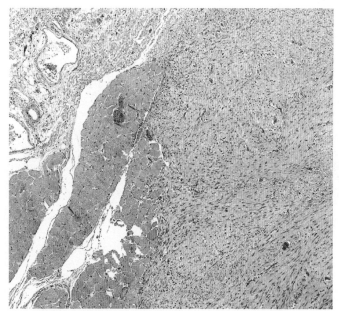

FIGURE 96.9 ▲ Pleural fibromatosis. The tumor is infiltrating skeletal muscle, at the left.

Clinical Features

The mean age range at presentation is 42 to 47 years (overall age range, 9 to 77 years).[30,31] There is no gender predilection.[30–33] Typical signs and symptoms include chest pain (24% to 80%), dyspnea (8% to 36%), cough (8% to 33%), and hemoptysis (20% to 25%).[34] Pleural SS can be aggressive with almost half of patients dead of disease (with a mean of 18 months).[34]

Gross Findings

SS are virtually always single tumors without satellite nodules.[30] They can have a pseudocapsule, causing them to be well demarcated from the surrounding tissues. The tumors may grow on a pedicle. They are usually large tumors with a mean size of 13 cm (range 4 to 21 cm).[30,35] Cut surface of the tumor can show cystic degenerative changes; papillary, hemorrhagic areas; and necrosis.[32,36,37] Occasionally, the cysts can mimic blebs of pneumothorax.[38]

Microscopic Findings

SS of the pleura and lung is most commonly monophasic, 58% in one series[30] (Fig. 96.10). Monophasic SS is composed solely of the spindle cell component, with relatively uniform cells with elongated nuclei, slightly basophilic cytoplasm, and indistinct cell borders. Tumors show dense cellularity, with interlacing fascicles, often with hyalinized eosinophilic stroma. A hemangiopericytoma-like vascular pattern is present in 80% of tumors.[30] Other features include entrapped pneumocyte nests (38%), calcification (17%), myxoid change (50%), and Verocay-like bodies (12%).[30] The mesenchymal cells may occasionally resemble small round cell tumors with minimal spindling (Fig. 96.11).

Biphasic SS comprises both epithelial and spindle cell components. The spindle cell component is similar to that in monophasic tumors.[39,40]

Epithelial areas may contain cleft-like glandular spaces with scattered tubulopapillary differentiation or solid sheets.[39,40] The proportions of the spindle cell and epithelial components vary widely (22). The cells are cuboidal with moderate eosinophilic cytoplasm, round nuclei with granular chromatin, and occasional nucleoli. Mucoid secretions are commonly seen. The cells contain scant cytoplasm with oval nuclei.

Mitotic activity varies greatly (5 to 25/10 HPF). Calcification and mast cell infiltrates may be seen.[30] Approximately two-thirds of pleuro-pulmonary synovial sarcomas are grade 2 by the FNCLCC (Fédération Nationale des Centers de Lutte Contre le Cancer).

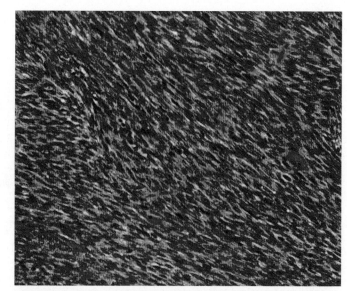

FIGURE 96.10 ▲ Synovial sarcoma, monophasic spindle cell type. There is a monotonous highly cellular spindle cell proliferation.

In the cystic variant, the cells between cysts are spindled and the cysts are lined by epithelioid cells (Fig. 96.12).[38]

Immunohistochemical Findings

Pleuropulmonary SS demonstrates pancytokeratin staining in two-thirds of cases, and more than 50% express EMA, cytokeratin-7, calretinin, and cytokeratin 5/6.[30] The spindled cells are typically positive for CD56 and Bcl-2 (100% in one series).[30] CD99 is present in more than 80% of tumors.

TLE-1 is currently the most specific marker in the differential diagnosis of cases of SS.[41] Another immunohistochemical marker is SYT protein, the gene product resulting from unique synovial sarcoma t(X; 18) translocation and SYT-SSX fusion gene.[42]

Cytogenetic and Molecular Genetic Findings

SS have the specific translocation t(X;18)(p11;q11), regardless of subtype and topography. This translocation involves the fusion of the *SS18*

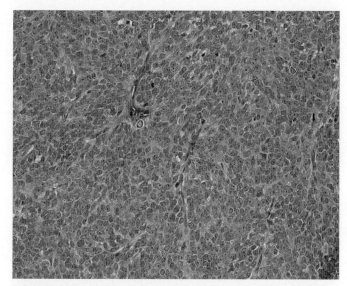

FIGURE 96.11 ▲ Synovial sarcoma, pleura, small round cell type. Higher magnification shows a highly cellular undifferentiated tumor, which in this focus shows little spindling. Diagnosis of this tumor was confirmed by molecular testing.

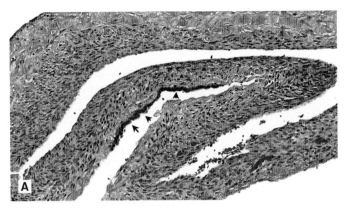
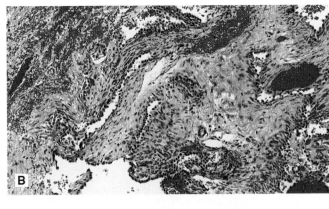
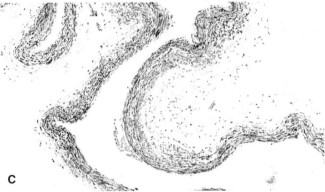
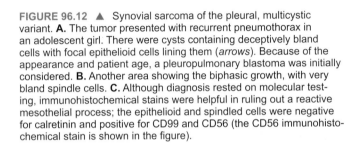

FIGURE 96.12 ▲ Synovial sarcoma of the pleural, multicystic variant. **A.** The tumor presented with recurrent pneumothorax in an adolescent girl. There were cysts containing deceptively bland cells with focal epithelioid cells lining them (*arrows*). Because of the appearance and patient age, a pleuropulmonary blastoma was initially considered. **B.** Another area showing the biphasic growth, with very bland spindle cells. **C.** Although diagnosis rested on molecular testing, immunohistochemical stains were helpful in ruling out a reactive mesothelial process; the epithelioid and spindled cells were negative for calretinin and positive for CD99 and CD56 (the CD56 immunohistochemical stain is shown in the figure).

(also known as *SYT*) gene on chromosome 18 and either the *SSX1* or *SSX2* gene on the *X* chromosome (both at Xp11) or, rarely, with *SSX4* (also at Xp11) (36,The f37). Proximally two-thirds of synovial sarcomas harbor an *SS18-SSX1* fusion and one-third reveal an *SS18-SSX2* fusion. Over 90% of pleuropulmonary SS exhibit the translocation.[30]

Differential Diagnosis

Synovial sarcoma of the pleura must be distinguished from SFT, mesothelioma, metastatic sarcoma, and, in the case of the cystic variant, pleuropulmonary blastoma. The most helpful tools are immunohistochemical staining (especially epithelial markers, TLE1 and CD56) and cytogenetic testing for the translocation, which is readily available on formalin-fixed paraffin-embedded tissues.

Primary Pleural Angiosarcoma
Terminology

Hemangioendotheliomas and *angiosarcomas* are mesenchymal tumors of endothelial origin, rarely arising primary to the pleura. Most epithelioid hemangioendotheliomas of the lung are parenchymal (see Chapter 93), whereas pleural angiosarcoma is more common than parenchymal angiosarcoma. Angiosarcomas that show epithelioid differentiation may be referred to as *epithelioid angiosarcomas* (EAS).[43]

Incidence and Epidemiology

While pleural involvement by primary or metastatic pulmonary angiosarcoma is well documented,[44] primary pleural angiosarcomas are rare and even rarer within the lung parenchyma.[45,46] The average age tends to be slightly older than that of EHE (with a mean age of 57 to 59 years in series),[47–49] with a striking male predominance (male:female ratio ranging from 4:1 to 15:1).[47,49]

Etiology

Some authors have reported an association with tuberculous pyothorax; this has been found exclusively in Japanese patients.[47,50,51] However,

etiology is essentially unknown: case reports of Western patients have described tumors arising in the setting of asbestos and radiation exposure[50,52,53]; however, likely due to the rarity of these tumors, no strong association has been identified.

Clinical Findings

Like EHE, presenting symptoms are not specific: pleural effusions, recurrent hemothorax, chest pain, and dyspnea are commonly reported.[54] As blood-filled cysts are sometimes present, hemoptysis is more commonly seen in angiosarcomas than in EHE and may also be an indicator of poorer outcome.[49,55] Massive hemothorax on presentation has also been reported in a number of cases.[47,48,53,56–59]

Radiologic Findings

Typical radiographic findings include pleural thickening and diffuse opacity with advanced lesions, overlapping largely with mesotheliomas or pleural involvement by pulmonary carcinomas.[60] Computed tomography (CT) findings may mimic mesothelioma showing lobulated, heterogeneously enhancing pleural masses with irregular margins.[61,62] Mass lesions have been found in roughly 50% of patients.[48] PET scans may be useful to define the extent of disease and typically show homogenous fluorodeoxyglucose (FDG)-avid lesions.[61]

Microscopic Findings

Angiosarcomas are sometimes classified as either *classical* or *epithelioid* variants, based on the predominant pattern; however, most tumors show a mixed morphologic picture. The classical pattern is that of irregular anastomosing vascular channels lined by atypical-appearing endothelial cells that form papillations or intraluminal buds. However, tumors may also show solid sheets of spindled cells without clearly identifiable vascular channels, but spindled cells with amphophilic to slightly eosinophilic cytoplasm, prominent nucleoli, and vesicular nuclei.[61,63] The term *epithelioid angiosarcoma* describes a predominant pattern of large round or polygonal cells with abundant eosinophilic cytoplasm amidst vasoformative, slit-like channels,

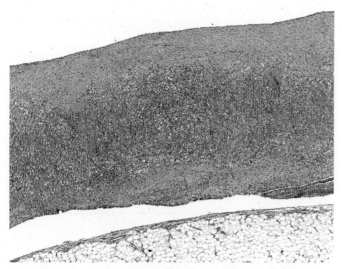

FIGURE 96.13 ▲ Pleural angiosarcoma. There is diffuse pleural thickening.

which often contain degenerated or fragments of erythrocytes. Many tumors contain a mix of patterns (Figs. 96.13 and 96.14).[63]

There are no standardized criteria differentiating EAS from lower-grade epithelioid hemangioendotheliomas histologically. However, in addition to a gene fusion product recently identified in EHE (see *Epithelioid Angiosarcoma*), increased mitoses, cytologic atypia, and necrosis in the absence of a hyalinized or myxoid stroma suggest a diagnosis of EAS over EHE.

Although no longer necessary today due to the availability of immunohistochemical markers, historically, electron microscopy has been used to demonstrate pinocytotic vesicles, prominent basal lamina, and Weibel-Palade bodies, confirming the vascular differentiation.

Immunohistochemical Stains

Like epithelioid hemangioendotheliomas, the vast majority of angiosarcomas (92%) show staining for at least one endothelial marker (including factor VIII, CD31, CD34, or D2-40),with CD31, Fli-1, and ERG considered the most reliable and specific markers (Fig. 96.15).[48,64] Approximately 50% of EAS and 9% of nonepithelioid variants show immunoreactivity to pancytokeratin.[64] Cam5.2, CK18, CK7, and CK8 may be expressed, but positivity is typically patchy or focal.[48,63] WT-1 may be positive.

Prognosis

Prognosis for pleural angiosarcomas is very poor, survival typically lasting only weeks or months after presentation. Hemoptysis at presentation may be a poor prognostic indicator.[49]

Surgery or chemotherapy may be indicated for palliative reasons. Vascular embolization is sometimes used to decrease vascularity for control of bleeding or preoperatively.[48,53]

Epithelioid Hemangioendothelioma of the Pleura

EHE arising primary to the pleura are very rare with only 27 cases reported in the literature to date.[65] In contradistinction to primary pulmonary tumors, which are characteristically seen in asymptomatic women, the typical patient is male (male:female ratio of 2.375), often symptomatic at presentation, and with an average age of 44 years.[66]

Patients are typically symptomatic at presentation. The most commonly reported symptoms are nonspecific and include pleuritic chest pain, dyspnea, and dry cough.[53,59,66]

Histologic features of EHE are similar to those in the lung parenchyma and include short strands, nests, or cords of epithelioid to spindle-shaped cells with abundant eosinophilic cytoplasm, typically lacking in well-formed vascular channels (Fig. 96.16). Vasoformative features are only typically evident in the form of intracytoplasmic lumina (sometimes called "blister cells"), which may contain degenerated or intact erythrocytes.[49,53,67]

Immunohistochemical Stains

Immunoreactivity for vascular markers (such as CD34, CD31, factor VIII, Fli-1, and ERG) confirms the endothelial origin of tumors, with CD31, Fli-1, and ERG reported as the most sensitive and specific marker. Roughly one-third of tumors will show reactivity for at least one cytokeratin marker such as pancytokeratin, Cam5.2, CK7, and CK18. WT-1 may be positive, which may obscure the distinction with mesothelioma. However, calretinin and CK5/6 are negative. In a large series, D2-40 expression was seen in over 50% of tumors.[49]

The smaller subset of tumors associated with a YAP1-TFE3 gene fusion are also immunoreactive to TFE antibody.

The prognosis for primary pleural EHE is universally poor, with a mean survival from onset of symptoms of 9.6 months[53,66,68] due to distant metastasis and local invasion. Symptoms at presentation, lymphangitic spread of tumor, peripheral lymphadenopathy, and hepatic metastases are poor prognostic indicators.[53,65]

There is no consensus regarding optimum treatment; chemotherapy with carboplatin and etoposide has been a reportedly used regimen.[66]

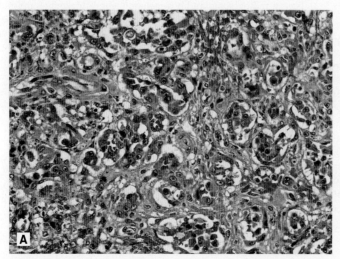
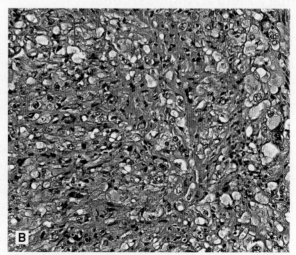

FIGURE 96.14 ▲ Pleural angiosarcoma. **A.** Nests of tumor cells forming poorly formed vascular channels. The differential diagnosis is adenocarcinoma. **B.** An epithelioid variant mimicking angiosarcoma or mesothelioma.

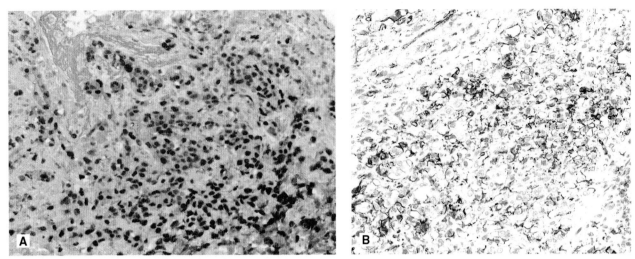

FIGURE 96.15 ▲ Pleural angiosarcoma, immunohistochemical markers. **A.** ERG oncoprotein shows nuclear positivity confirming the diagnosis of angiosarcoma in Figure 96.14A. **B.** CD31 immunohistochemical staining also confirms the diagnosis of angiosarcoma seen in Figure 96.14B.

Differential Diagnosis

The overlap in clinical and radiographic findings as well as the rarity of primary pleural vascular tumors may lead to an erroneous diagnosis of mesothelioma, and the diagnosis may be further obscured by a biphasic spindled and epithelioid histologic picture and occasional positivity for WT-1.[48,69] However, identification of vasoformative features or focal or negative cytokeratin staining should prompt staining for endothelial markers such as CD31, ERG, and Fli-1. While intracytoplasmic lumina may be seen in mesothelioma or vascular tumors, degenerated erythrocytes should only be present in vascular tumors. Mesothelial markers CK5/6 and calretinin are consistently negative in EHE and angiosarcomas, whereas CD31 in most series is specific to vascular tumors.[48,69,70] D2-40 positivity is positive in approximately half of EHE cases and a minority of angiosarcomas.[49]

Intracytoplasmic lumina may be mistaken for mucin vacuoles of metastatic adenocarcinoma, particularly as metastatic carcinoma involving the pleura is far more common than primary pleural vascular tumors. Essentially, the possibility of an EHE must be considered in cases of focal

or spotty cytokeratin staining and what could be vasoformative features. While at least one cytokeratin marker may be positive in a significant proportion of EHE and angiosarcomas,[48,49] positive endothelial staining (CD31, Fli-1, or ERG) would confirm the correct diagnosis.

REFERENCES

1. England DM, Hochholzer L, McCarthy MJ. Localized benign and malignant fibrous tumors of the pleura. A clinicopathologic review of 223 cases. *Am J Surg Pathol.* 1989;13:640–658.
2. Fletcher CDM, Gibbs A. Solitary fibrous tumor. In: Travis WD, et al., eds. *WHO Classification of Tumours of the Lung, Pleura, Mediastinum and Heart.* Lyon, France: IARC Press; 2015:178–179.
3. Otake S, Kikkawa T, Takizawa M, et al. Hypoglycemia observed on continuous glucose monitoring associated with IGF-2-producing solitary fibrous tumor. *J Clin Endocrinol Metab.* 2015;100:2519–2524.
4. Rao N, Colby TV, Falconieri G, et al. Intrapulmonary solitary fibrous tumors: clinicopathologic and immunohistochemical study of 24 cases. *Am J Surg Pathol.* 2013;37:155–166.
5. Lococo F, Cafarotti S, Treglia G. Is 18F-FDG-PET/CT really able to differentiate between malignant and benign solitary fibrous tumor of the pleura? *Clin Imaging.* 2013;37:976.
6. Liu CC, Wang HW, Li FY, et al. Solitary fibrous tumors of the pleura: clinicopathological characteristics, immunohistochemical profiles, and surgical outcomes with long-term follow-up. *Thorac Cardiovasc Surg.* 2008;56:291–297.
7. Mohajeri A, Tayebwa J, Collin A, et al. Comprehensive genetic analysis identifies a pathognomonic NAB2/STAT6 fusion gene, nonrandom secondary genomic imbalances, and a characteristic gene expression profile in solitary fibrous tumor. *Genes Chromosomes Cancer.* 2013;52:873–886.
8. Sung SH, Chang JW, Kim J, et al. Solitary fibrous tumors of the pleura: surgical outcome and clinical course. *Ann Thorac Surg.* 2005;79:303–307.
9. Hanau CA, Miettinen M. Solitary fibrous tumor: histological and immunohistochemical spectrum of benign and malignant variants presenting at different sites. *Hum Pathol.* 1995;26:440–449.
10. Yokoi T, Tsuzuki T, Yatabe Y, et al. Solitary fibrous tumour: significance of p53 and CD34 immunoreactivity in its malignant transformation. *Histopathology.* 1998;32:423–432.
11. Hiraoka K, Morikawa T, Ohbuchi T, et al. Solitary fibrous tumors of the pleura: clinicopathological and immunohistochemical examination. *Interact Cardiovasc Thorac Surg.* 2003;2:61–64.
12. Tapias LF, Mino-Kenudson M, Lee H, et al. Risk factor analysis for the recurrence of resected solitary fibrous tumours of the pleura: a 33-year experience and proposal for a scoring system. *Eur J Cardiothorac Surg.* 2013;44:111–117.
13. Thway K, Hayes A, Ieremia E, et al. Heterologous osteosarcomatous and rhabdomyosarcomatous elements in dedifferentiated solitary fibrous tumor: further support for the concept of dedifferentiation in solitary fibrous tumor. *Ann Diagn Pathol.* 2013;17:457–463.

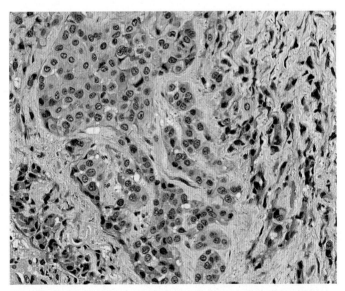

FIGURE 96.16 ▲ Pleural epithelioid hemangioendothelioma. The tumor is deceptively epithelioid in appearance. The differential diagnosis includes carcinoid and metastatic carcinoma. The diagnosis was confirmed by immunohistochemical positivity for endothelial markers (not shown).

14. Mullen JT, Delaney TF, Kobayashi WK, et al. Desmoid tumor: analysis of prognostic factors and outcomes in a surgical series. *Ann Surg Oncol.* 2012;19:4028–4035.

15. Zeng WG, Zhou ZX, Liang JW, et al. Prognostic factors for desmoid tumor: a surgical series of 233 patients at a single institution. *Tumour Biol.* 2014;35:7513–7521.

16. Lee SH, Lee HK, Song JS, et al. Chest wall fibromatosis in the axilla. *Arch Plast Surg.* 2012;39:175–177.

17. Zehani-Kassar A, Ayadi-Kaddour A, Marghli A, et al. Desmoid-type chest wall fibromatosis. A six cases series. *Orthop Traumatol Surg Res.* 2011;97:102–107.

18. Aggarwal D, Dalal U, Mohapatra PR, et al. Intra-thoracic desmoid tumor. *Lung India.* 2012;29:160–162.

19. Dalal AK, Singal R, Dalal U, et al. An unusual case of chest wall desmoid tumor. *Indian J Surg.* 2010;72:336–338.

20. Xie Y, Xie K, Gou Q, et al. Recurrent desmoid tumor of the mediastinum: a case report. *Oncol Lett.* 2014;8:2276–2278.

21. Wilson RW, Gallateau-Salle F, Moran CA. Desmoid tumors of the pleura: a clinicopathologic mimic of localized fibrous tumor. *Mod Pathol.* 1999;12:9–14.

22. Endo T, Endo S, Yamamoto S, et al. Intrathoracic desmoid tumor arising at a distance from thoracotomy sites after thoracoscopic segmentectomy: report of a case. *J Thorac Dis.* 2015;7:E81–E84.

23. Miwa K, Kubouchi Y, Wakahara M, et al. Desmoid tumor requiring differentiation from port-site relapse after surgery for lung cancer. *Asian J Endosc Surg.* 2014;7:182–184.

24. Yamamoto T, Rino Y, Adachi H, et al. Giant desmoid tumor of the chest wall. *J Thorac Oncol.* 2011;6:393–394.

25. Moonim MT, Herbert A, Lucas SB. Benign metastasizing mesothelial cells in an axillary lymph node secondary to a chest wall fibromatosis. *Histopathology.* 2006;48:303–305.

26. Rhee SJ, Paik SH, Shin HK, et al. Treatment of a recurrent chest wall desmoid tumor using a CT-guided steroid injection. *Korean J Radiol.* 2012;13:342–344.

27. Debled M, Le Loarer F, Callonnec F, et al. Complete response to exemestane in a patient with a desmoid tumor. *Future Oncol.* 2012;8:483–486.

28. Halevy A, Samuk I, Halpern Z, et al. Mifepristone (RU486), a pure anti-progesterone drug, in combination with vinblastine for the treatment of progesterone receptor-positive desmoid tumor. *Tech Coloproctol.* 2010;14:265–267.

29. Goto T, Nemoto T, Ogura K, et al. Successful treatment of desmoid tumor of the chest wall with tranilast: a case report. *J Med Case Rep.* 2010;4:384.

30. Hartel PH, Fanburg-Smith JC, Frazier AA, et al. Primary pulmonary and mediastinal synovial sarcoma: a clinicopathologic study of 60 cases and comparison with five prior series. *Mod Pathol.* 2007;20:760–769.

31. Tajima S, Takahashi T, Itaya T, et al. Cystic synovial sarcoma of the pleura mimicking a cystic thymoma: a case report illustrating the role of decreased INI-1 expression in differential diagnosis. *Int J Clin Exp Pathol.* 2015;8:3262–3269.

32. Falkenstern-Ge RF, Kimmich M, Grabner A, et al. Primary pulmonary synovial sarcoma: a rare primary pulmonary tumor. *Lung.* 2014;192:211–214.

33. Colwell AS, D'Cunha J, Vargas SO, et al. Synovial sarcoma of the pleura: a clinical and pathologic study of three cases. *J Thorac Cardiovasc Surg.* 2002;124:828–832.

34. Mirzoyan M, Muslimani A, Setrakian S, et al. Primary pleuropulmonary synovial sarcoma. *Clin Lung Cancer.* 2008;9:257–261.

35. Kim GH, Kim MY, Koo HJ, et al. Primary pulmonary synovial sarcoma in a tertiary referral center: clinical characteristics, CT, and 18F-FDG PET findings, with pathologic correlations. *Medicine (Baltimore).* 2015;94:e1392.

36. Kang MK, Cho KH, Lee YH, et al. Primary synovial sarcoma of the parietal pleura: a case report. *Korean J Thorac Cardiovasc Surg.* 2013;46:159–161.

37. Loscertales J, Trivino A, Gallardo G, et al. Primary monophasic synovial sarcoma of the pleura: diagnosis and treatment. *Interact Cardiovasc Thorac Surg.* 2011;12:885–887.

38. Cummings NM, Desai S, Thway K, et al. Cystic primary pulmonary synovial sarcoma presenting as recurrent pneumothorax: report of 4 cases. *Am J Surg Pathol.* 2010;34:1176–1179.

39. Cappello F and Barnes L. Synovial sarcoma and malignant mesothelioma of the pleura: review, differential diagnosis and possible role of apoptosis. *Pathology.* 2001;33:142–148.

40. Jawahar DA, Vuletin JC, Gorecki P, et al. Primary biphasic synovial sarcoma of the pleura. *Respir Med.* 1997;91:568–570.

41. Jagdis A, Rubin BP, Tubbs RR, et al. Prospective evaluation of TLE1 as a diagnostic immunohistochemical marker in synovial sarcoma. *Am J Surg Pathol.* 2009;33:1743–1751.

42. He R, Patel RM, Alkan S, et al. Immunostaining for SYT protein discriminates synovial sarcoma from other soft tissue tumors: analysis of 146 cases. *Mod Pathol.* 2007;20:522–528.

43. Alexiou C, Clelland CA, Robinson D, et al. Primary angiosarcomas of the chest wall and pleura. *Eur J Cardiothorac Surg.* 1998;14:523–526.

44. Pandit SA, Fiedler PN, Westcott JL. Primary angiosarcoma of the lung. *Ann Diagn Pathol.* 2005;9:302–304.

45. Shimabukuro I, Yatera K, Noguchi S, et al. Primary pulmonary angiosarcoma presenting with hemoptysis and ground-glass opacity: a case report and literature review. *Tohoku J Exp Med.* 2015;237:273–278.

46. Tanaka H, Yorita K, Takahashi N, et al. Primary pulmonary angiosarcoma: a case report. *Pathol Int.* 2015;65:554–557.

47. Dainese E, Pozzi B, Milani M, et al. Primary pleural epithelioid angiosarcoma. A case report and review of the literature. *Pathol Res Pract.* 2010;206:415–419.

48. Kao YC, Chow JM, Wang KM, et al. Primary pleural angiosarcoma as a mimicker of mesothelioma: a case report **VS**. *Diagn Pathol.* 2011;6:130.

49. Anderson T, Zhang L, Hameed M, et al. Thoracic epithelioid malignant vascular tumors: a clinicopathologic study of 52 cases with emphasis on pathologic grading and molecular studies of WWTR1–CAMTA1 fusions. *Am J Surg Pathol.* 2015;39:132–139.

50. Zhang PJ, Livolsi VA, Brooks JJ. Malignant epithelioid vascular tumors of the pleura: report of a series and literature review. *Hum Pathol.* 2000;31:29–34.

51. Aozasa K, Naka N, Tomita Y, et al. Angiosarcoma developing from chronic pyothorax. *Mod Pathol.* 1994;7:906–911.

52. Kimura M, Ito H, Furuta T, et al. Pyothorax-associated angiosarcoma of the pleura with metastasis to the brain. *Pathol Int.* 2003;53:547–551.

53. Crotty EJ, McAdams HP, Erasmus JJ, et al. Epithelioid hemangioendothelioma of the pleura: clinical and radiologic features. *AJR Am J Roentgenol.* 2000;175:1545–1549.

54. Kurtz JE, Serra S, Duclos B, et al. Diffuse primary angiosarcoma of the pleura: a case report and review of the literature. *Sarcoma.* 2004;8:103–106.

55. Baisi A, Raveglia F, De Simone M, et al. Primary multifocal angiosarcoma of the pleura. *Interact Cardiovasc Thorac Surg.* 2011;12:1069–1070.

56. Pramesh CS, Madur BP, Raina S, et al. Angiosarcoma of the pleura. *Ann Thorac Cardiovasc Surg.* 2004;10:187–190.

57. Bocchino M, Barra E, Lassandro F, et al. Primary pleural haemangioendothelioma in an Italian female patient: a case report and review of the literature. *Monaldi Arch Chest Dis.* 2010;73:135–139.

58. Chen CY, Wu YC, Chou TY, et al. Pleural angiosarcoma mimicking pleural haematoma. *Interact Cardiovasc Thorac Surg.* 2013;17:886–888.

59. Lazarus A, Fuhrer G, Malekiani C, et al. Primary pleural epithelioid hemangioendothelioma (EHE)—two cases and review of the literature. *Clin Respir J.* 2011;5:e1–e5.

60. Lorentziadis M, Sourlas A. Primary de novo angiosarcoma of the pleura. *Ann Thorac Surg.* 2012;93:996–998.

61. Abu-Zaid A, Mohammed S. Primary pleural angiosarcoma in a 63-year-old gentleman. *Case Rep Pulmonol.* 2013;2013:974567.

62. Del Frate C, Mortele K, Zanardi R, et al. Pseudomesotheliomatous angiosarcoma of the chest wall and pleura. *J Thorac Imaging.* 2003;18:200–203.

63. Antonescu C. Malignant vascular tumors—an update. *Mod Pathol.* 2014;27 Suppl 1:S30–S38.

64. Rao P, Lahat G, Arnold C, et al. Angiosarcoma: a tissue microarray study with diagnostic implications. *Am J Dermatopathol.* 2013;35:432–437.

65. Wethasinghe J, Sood J, Walmsley R, et al. Primary pleural epithelioid hemangioendothelioma mimicking as a posterior mediastinal tumor. *Respirol Case Rep.* 2015;3:75–77.

66. Salijevska J, Watson R, Clifford A, et al. Pleural epithelioid hemangioendothelioma: literature summary and novel case report. *J Clin Med Res.* 2015;7:566–570.

67. Shao J, Zhang J. Clinicopathological characteristics of pulmonary epithelioid hemangioendothelioma: a report of four cases and review of the literature. *Oncol Lett.* 2014;8:2517–2522.

68. Kim EA, Lele SM, Lackner RP. Primary pleural epithelioid hemangioendothelioma. *Ann Thorac Surg.* 2011;91:301–302.

69. Attanoos RL, Suvarna SK, Rhead E, et al. Malignant vascular tumours of the pleura in "asbestos" workers and endothelial differentiation in malignant mesothelioma. *Thorax.* 2000;55:860–863.

70. De Young BR, Frierson Jr HF, Ly MN, et al. CD31 immunoreactivity in carcinomas and mesotheliomas. *Am J Clin Pathol.* 1998;110:374–377.

97 Mesothelioma of the Pleura
Allen P. Burke, M.D.

Terminology

The majority of mesothelial neoplasms of the pleura are malignant mesotheliomas. To distinguish the typical diffuse form from the rare localized form, the modifier "diffuse" is often placed before "malignant mesothelioma." Low-grade or benign mesothelial neoplasms, which are relatively more common in the peritoneum and exceedingly rare in the pleura, include "well-differentiated papillary" and "multicystic mesotheliomas" and are considered separately.

The most important prognostic pathologic feature is the presence of sarcomatoid differentiation. For this reason, the diagnosis should always include the amount of sarcomatoid change or specifically indicate its absence.

Diffuse Malignant Mesothelioma

Epidemiology

Although they may occur in children, the vast majority of pleural mesotheliomas are seen in adults, usually over 60 years at the time of diagnosis. There is a male predominance of about 4:1. In North America, the rate in men is 23 cases per million per year. Mesotheliomas account for only 1% of malignant pleural effusions.[1]

Asbestos Exposure

In North America, up to 80% to 90% of mesotheliomas in men are related to asbestos exposure. The link between asbestosis and mesothelioma is weaker in women, who account for a relatively small proportion of cases.[2]

Of the types of asbestos, amphibole asbestos (amosite and crocidolite) is two to three orders of magnitude more carcinogenic than is chrysotile asbestos. It has been proposed that contamination of chrysotile by the amphibole fiber tremolite accounts for its carcinogenicity.[3]

The most common thoracic manifestation of asbestos exposure is the pleural plaque, which increases the risk for the development of mesothelioma by nine times over the general population (See Chapter 56).[4]

Erionite Exposure

Erionite is a type of zeolite, a nonasbestos fiber that has similar commercial properties as amphibole asbestos. In the Cappadocia region of Turkey, where there is nonindustrial exposure to erionite-containing rock, the incidence of mesothelioma is extraordinarily high.[3]

Other Risk Factors

Other risk factors for the development of pleural mesotheliomas include radiation and genetics (*BAP1* germline mutations).

Clinical Findings

The manifestations of pleural mesotheliomas are usually related to pleural effusions. Systemic symptoms such as weight loss and fever are common. Because the tumors are initially relatively slow growing, patients can be asymptomatic for a prolonged period, and effusions may be initially diagnosed as negative, because of the low sensitivity of cytologic diagnosis.[5]

Radiologic Findings

Mesotheliomas manifest on imaging as pleural effusions, often with nodules or plaques.

Computed tomography effectively demonstrates the extent of primary tumor, intrathoracic lymphadenopathy, and extrathoracic spread. Thoracic magnetic resonance imaging is particularly useful for identifying invasion of the chest wall, mediastinum, and diaphragm. Positron emission tomography can accurately demonstrate intrathoracic and extrathoracic lymphadenopathy and metastatic disease.[6]

Spread of Disease

The initial spread of mesothelioma is over the parietal pleural surfaces, the typical site of pleural plaques, with direct extension to the visceral pleura, interlobar fissures, and subsequently the chest wall, lung parenchyma, and surrounding structures. Lymphatic dissemination is unusual, and more common in the epithelioid histologic type.

Approximately 10% of pleural mesotheliomas are associated with peritoneal mesotheliomas.

Distant hematogenous metastases are common in late-stage disease, including unusual sites such as soft tissue of the extremities and even gingiva.[7,8] Autopsies of patients dying with pleural mesothelioma show extrapleural dissemination in almost 90% patients, with tumor spread to lymph nodes in 53%, followed by liver (32%), spleen (11%), thyroid (7%), and brain (3%).[9]

Pathologic Staging

Accurate pathologic staging can be difficult on video-assisted thoracic biopsies. Pathologic T1 stage indicates ipsilateral parietal involvement with (1b) or without (1a) visceral involvement. Pathologic stage T2 adds confluent visceral pleural tumor including fissure, diaphragm, or lung parenchyma. Pathologic stage T3 involves endothoracic fascia, mediastinal fat, chest wall, or nontransmural pericardium. Pathologic stage T4 indicates any of the following: multifocal soft tissue spread, rib involvement, transmural diaphragmatic spread, transmural pericardial involvement or heart involvement, positive pericardial cytology, esophageal invasion, contralateral pleura involvement, spinal involvement, or invasion of the brachial plexus.

Gross Findings

Pleural mesotheliomas cause confluent nodules and masses on the parietal and visceral surfaces, usually obliterating the pleural space and interlobar fissures, eventually encasing the lung (Fig. 97.1). In late stages, the pleura may be several centimeters thick. The consistency

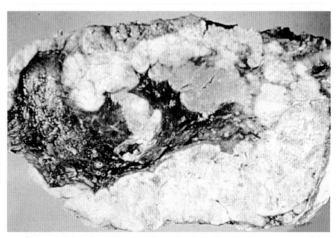

FIGURE 97.1 ▲ Pleural diffuse malignant mesothelioma, gross findings. There is an irregular white-tan tumor encasing the lung.

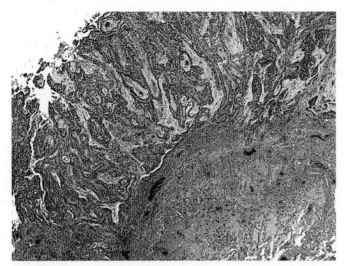

FIGURE 97.2 ▲ Epithelioid mesothelioma, tubulopapillary. There is minimal invasion into the stroma.

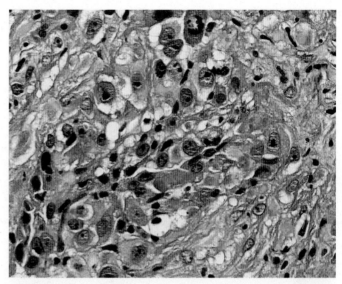

FIGURE 97.4 ▲ Epithelioid mesothelioma, solid growth pattern. The tumor cells at high magnification show large nuclei and nucleoli and variation in size. These are some features of so-called pleomorphic (epithelioid) mesothelioma.

varies according to histologic type; epithelioid tumors are gray-white and soft, often with softer cystic areas containing mucoid-like material. Sarcomatoid tumors are more likely firm, with the appearance of fibromatosis or sarcoma.

Malignant mesothelioma is rarely entirely intraparenchymal, forming miliary nodules.[10]

Epithelioid Mesothelioma, Histologic Findings

The common pattern of growth is tubulopapillary, with anastomosing papillary projects on the pleural surface that form tubules in the stroma (Figs. 97.2 and 97.3). There are frequently solid areas that are associated with nuclear pleomorphism and mitotic activity (Fig. 97.4). Tumor infiltrating into stroma, fat, fascia, muscle, and lung parenchyma represents progressive invasive growth (Fig. 97.5).

A large variety of growth patterns, in addition to tubulopapillary and solid, have been described, but there is little impact on immunohistochemical results, and they are usually intermixed with

more typical mesothelioma. These include trabecular, micropapillary, nested, adenomatoid (microcystic), clear cell, and signet ring patterns.[11-14] The trabecular or nested growth patterns can often have an "endocrine" appearance.

It is not uncommon to have, in the solid growth pattern, areas of tumor with abundant pink cytoplasm resembling decidua; there are no strict criteria for this designation, however.[15] Similar to the deciduoid growth pattern are tumor cells with rhabdoid features.[11]

Malignant mesothelioma with a heavy lymphoid infiltrate obscuring the polygonal neoplastic cells can mimic malignant lymphoma or lymphoepithelioma-like carcinoma and is sometimes designated "lymphohistiocytoid mesothelioma."[16] A clear distinction from more typical mesotheliomas that have a lymphocytic response is not always possible.

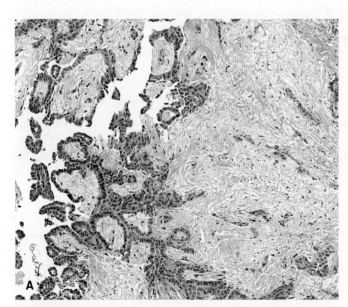
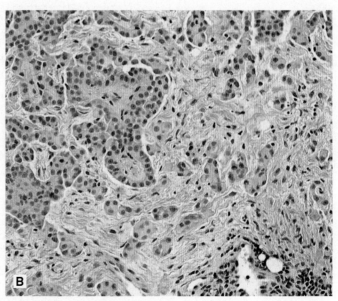

FIGURE 97.3 ▲ Epithelioid mesothelioma, tubulopapillary, invasive. **A.** There is little pleomorphism, but the tumor cells are invading the stroma as cords and nests, with surface papillae evident at the left. **B.** The tumor often invades as tubular structures.

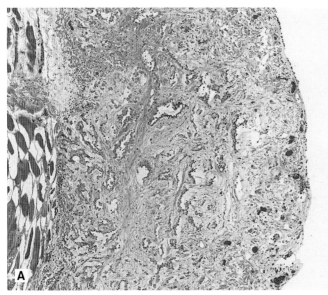
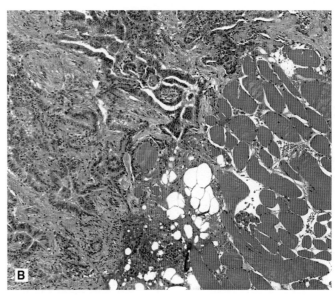

FIGURE 97.5 ▲ Epithelioid mesothelioma, invasive. **A.** The tumor invades stroma but does not involve skeletal muscle of the diaphragm (**left**). **B.** In this field, there is superficial invasion of the skeletal muscle fibers.

A myxoid background is common in the papillary structures and is conspicuous in 5% to 10% of cases (Fig. 97.6A). Rarely, tumor nests or papillae may be seen floating in a myxoid matrix, simulating mucinous carcinoma, with nests of cytologically bland, often vacuolated epithelioid cells (Fig. 97.6B).

One subset of mesotheliomas is intermediate between epithelioid and sarcomatoid mesothelioma. So-called pleomorphic mesotheliomas resemble sarcomas, with large, discohesive cells that vary in size and shape, have abundant cytoplasm and irregular nuclei, usually have prominent nucleoli, and have all characteristics of "sarcomatoid" mesothelioma except cellular spindling. Most often, these tumors show areas of sarcomatoid differentiation and are thus designated biphasic, although rare examples of pure "pleomorphic" types have been described, in the absence of significant cellular elongation. It is likely that these tumors should be best considered sarcomatoid, because the prognosis is similar.[17]

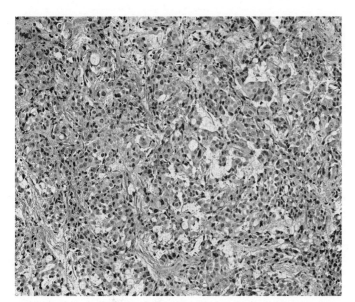

FIGURE 97.6 ▲ Epithelioid mesothelioma, myxoid background. This epithelioid mesothelioma with a solid growth pattern has a focal myxoid stroma. The degree of myxoid background is variable and in some tumors can be quite extensive.

Biphasic and Sarcomatoid Mesothelioma, Histologic Findings

Diffuse biphasic malignant mesothelioma is a mesothelioma showing at least 10% each of epithelioid and sarcomatoid patterns. Because there may be areas of pleomorphism without cellular and nuclear spindling, the distinction is not always precise.

Sarcomatoid mesotheliomas account for <10%, biphasic for 10% to 15%, and desmoplastic for <2% of all mesotheliomas in most series.[3] In the United Kingdom, a rate of nearly double that has been reported for biphasic and sarcomatoid mesotheliomas.[18]

Spindled cells arranged in fascicles or haphazard arrays characterize sarcomatoid mesotheliomas (Fig. 97.7). They often are higher-stage tumors, involving the adipose tissue of the parietal pleura, or extend into the adjacent lung parenchyma.

Mesothelioma with heterologous elements is rare. Types of sarcoma are most often osteosarcoma, followed by chondrosarcoma (often mixed with osteosarcoma) and rhabdomyosarcoma.[19]

Desmoplastic Mesothelioma

A subset of sarcomatoid is the "desmoplastic" mesothelioma, which is characterized by dense collagenized tissue with few interspersed malignant cells. The term is used if more than one-half of the tumor is composed of the desmoplastic pattern. The collagen background lacks the loose fibrosis that is typical of a "desmoplastic reaction," which can occur in otherwise typical mesotheliomas and which occurs frequently in carcinomas.

The importance to the recognition of desmoplastic mesothelioma, which has a poor prognosis similar to that of other sarcomatoid mesotheliomas, lies in the difficulty making the diagnosis, especially in small biopsies. Invasion into fat is the only reliable criterion for diagnosis; other helpful criteria include bland necrosis and areas of typical sarcomatoid mesothelioma (Fig. 97.8).

Mucin Stains

The mucin that is elaborated by mesothelioma is positive for Alcian blue and sensitive to hyaluronidase. Neutral mucin is not usually present, as evidenced by mucicarmine stain of periodic acid–Schiff with diastase, but exceptions make these stains of little general use in the differential diagnosis between mesothelioma and carcinoma.

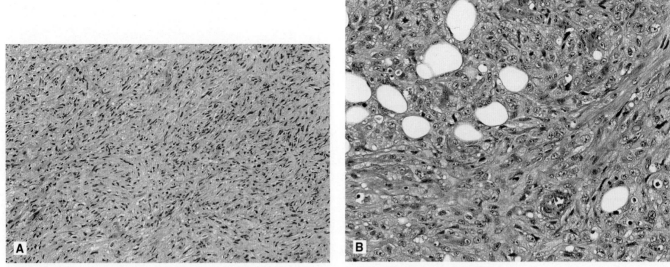

FIGURE 97.7 ▲ Sarcomatoid mesothelioma. **A.** The tumors are spindled, with relatively mild pleomorphism. **B.** In this example, there is more pleomorphism and less spindling (overlap with pleomorphic mesothelioma).

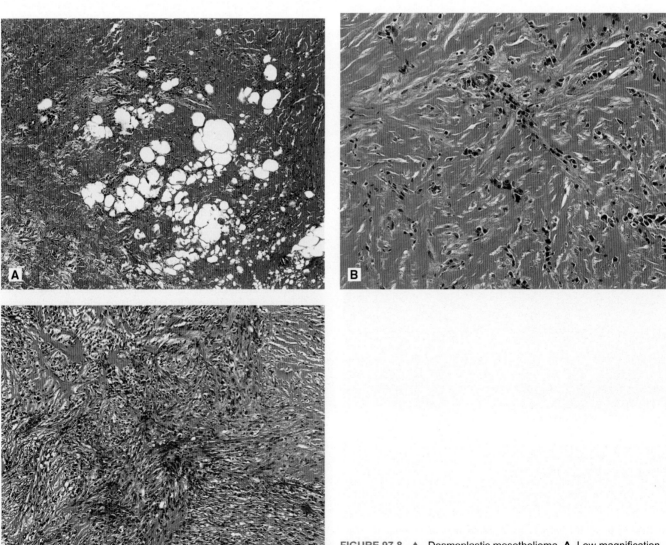

FIGURE 97.8 ▲ Desmoplastic mesothelioma. **A.** Low magnification of what appears to be largely acellular bland fibrous tissue invading fat. **B.** A higher magnification shows scattered atypical spindle cells. **C.** Another area confirms sarcomatoid mesothelioma.

TABLE 97.1 Immunohistochemical Markers and Pleural Mesothelioma, Epithelioid Type

	% Positive in Mesothelioma
Mesothelial markers[a]	
D2-40	90%–100%
Calretinin (cytoplasmic, nuclear)	70%–96% (nuclear and cytoplasmic)
WT1 (nuclear)	70%–99%
Cytokeratin 5/6	50%–85%
GLUT-1	50% (epithelioid), 75% (sarcomatoid), negative in reactive mesothelial hyperplasia
Carcinoma markers[b]	
TTF-1 (nuclear)	0 (nuclear positivity)
Napsin A	0
MOC-31	2%–10%
Carcinoembryonic antigen	<5%
B72.3	2%–7%
Ber-EP4	5%–20%
Cytokeratin 7	78%
Blood group 8 (Lewis)	3%–7%
p40	7%, usually focal
Pax-8[c]	0
Pax-2[c]	0
CA-IX[c]	0

[a]Specificity varies depending on the differential diagnostic consideration. Of the mesothelioma markers listed, only WT1 is negative in >99% of lung carcinomas, both squamous and adenocarcinomas. Squamous carcinomas of the lung often express D2-40, calretinin, and cytokeratin 5/6. Adenocarcinomas of the lung express cytokeratin 5/6 in 2% to 20% of tumors, usually focally.
[b]To be chosen depending on the possible primary site of metastatic carcinoma, most often lung. CD15 is sometimes included as an adenocarcinoma marker, but it is variably positive in mesotheliomas depending on the antigen. MOC-31 and berEP4 are positive in >80% of lung carcinomas, adenocarcinomas, and squamous carcinomas.
[c]Sensitive markers for renal cell carcinoma.
Staining is cytoplasmic unless otherwise stated.

Immunohistochemical Findings

There are a large number of antigens that are commonly expressed in mesothelial cells and mesothelial neoplasms and a similar number that are more commonly expressed in carcinomas (Table 97.1). Because each situation is different, there is no single panel that is recommended for the diagnosis of mesothelioma, but the use of multiple immunohistochemical stains is generally recommended.[3]

The most common mesothelial markers used in immunohistochemistry are calretinin, D2-40 (clone of podoplanin), and WT-1 (Fig. 97.9 to 97.11). None stains 100% of mesotheliomas, although D2-40 has

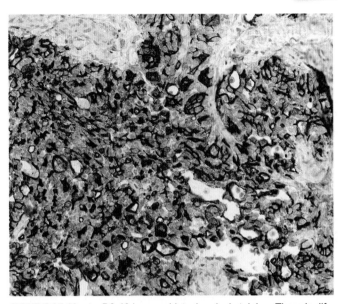

FIGURE 97.10 ▲ D2-40 immunohistochemical staining. There is diffuse cytoplasmic staining. D2-40 is one of the most sensitive mesothelial markers.

probably the highest sensitivity. Other markers, such as mesothelin, which is used as a biomarker, and mesothelial cell (HBME) are not particularly specific and are generally not recommended in diagnostic panels.[20–22]

High molecular weight cytokeratins (e.g., cytokeratin 5/6) are frequently expressed in mesotheliomas but are nonspecific, as they are also present in basal cells and squamous carcinomas. They are helpful, however, in the distinction between mesotheliomas and adenocarcinomas (Table 97.1).

GLUT-1 is a specific but not highly sensitive marker to distinguish malignant from benign mesothelial proliferations. It is expressed in one-half of epithelioid and three-quarters of sarcomatoid mesotheliomas but is absent in reactive mesothelial hyperplasia.[23]

Sarcomatoid mesotheliomas express mesothelial markers at a lower rate than do epithelioid mesotheliomas, although they are generally positive for cytokeratin 7 and pancytokeratin (Fig. 97.12).[17] The differential diagnosis versus adenocarcinoma is therefore more difficult and requires absence of adenocarcinoma marker expression and clinical and imaging information.

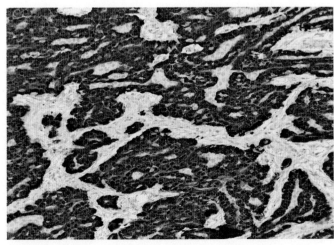

FIGURE 97.9 ▲ Calretinin immunohistochemical staining. There is cytoplasmic and nuclear staining.

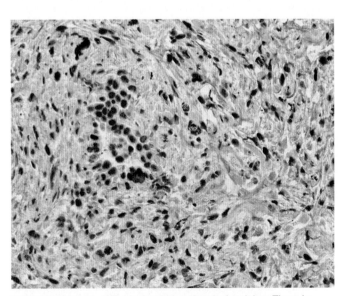

FIGURE 97.11 ▲ WT-1 immunohistochemical staining. There is nuclear staining in both epithelioid and sarcomatoid areas.

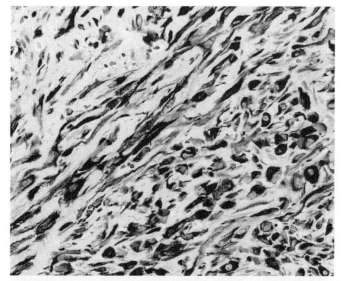

FIGURE 97.12 ▲ Pancytokeratin immunohistochemical staining, sarcomatoid mesothelioma. There is diffuse cytoplasmic positivity in this area.

Because sarcomatoid mesotheliomas show a lower rate of positivity for epithelial markers than does the epithelioid subtype, multiple immunohistochemical stains are important, especially the use of broad-spectrum cytokeratin stains such as AE1/AE3 and cytokeratin 8/18. Of the mesothelial markers, D2-40 is the most likely to be expressed in the spindled areas.[19,24]

Cytokeratin negativity may be encountered in 5% of sarcomatoid malignant mesotheliomas and in 10% of tumors with heterologous elements.[3]

Grading

There is no accepted grading for pleural mesotheliomas, although it is generally known that epithelioid tumors have the best prognosis, followed by biphasic and sarcomatoid tumors. A high mitotic rate and p16 loss by immunohistochemistry were associated with increased risk of death in one series.[25]

Differential Diagnosis: Mesothelioma Versus Reactive Mesothelial Hyperplasia

In most instances, reactive mesothelial hyperplasia is a relatively limited proliferation of mesothelial cells and does not form large sheets or aggregates or irregular invasive growth. In the acute phase, pleuritis can show markedly atypical mesothelial cells that are usually accompanied by fibrinous exudate, acute inflammation, and reactive stromal fibroblasts that do not form solid bundles. Chronic phases of pleural inflammation may show tubules and small papillary projections, but the growths are generally linear and orderly. The distinction between reactive mesothelial hyperplasia and chronic fibrous pleuritis does not rest on degree of atypia, because tubulopapillary mesotheliomas may be generally quite bland despite an invasive growth pattern, which is the key to differential diagnosis. Invasion into fat is considered unequivocal evidence, although artifactual spaces in reactive pleuritis can mimic fat (see Chapter 95).

Immunohistochemical testing is relatively little used in the differential diagnosis between mesothelioma and reactive mesothelial hyperplasia. Epithelial membrane antigen (EMA), p53, and IMP3 are more often expressed in mesotheliomas than reactive mesothelial proliferations, although there is overlap in the case of EMA.[11] GLUT-1 is probably the best marker in distinguishing the two when positive, as it is negative in reactive mesothelial cells and positive in one-half of epithelioid and three-quarters of sarcomatoid mesothelioma.[23] Desmin is more often expressed in reactive mesothelial cells than mesothelioma.[26]

Immunohistochemical staining for p16 (nuclear and cytoplasmic staining) is more diffuse in mesotheliomas than reactive hyperplasia but can occur in 15% of reactive proliferations, limiting diagnostic usefulness. More helpful is the molecular detection of p16/CDKN2A by fluorescent in situ hybridization, which is very specific for malignancy but lacks sensitivity (50% to 60%), which is higher in sarcomatoid than epithelioid mesothelioma.[27,28]

Differential Diagnosis: Epithelioid Mesothelioma Versus Carcinoma

The gross and imaging findings are generally distinct, as most lung adenocarcinomas for parenchymal nodules and mesotheliomas are pleural based. In cases where the clinical distinction is difficult, and in order to exclude pleural-based adenocarcinomas, immunohistochemical testing is necessary. In general, at least two mesothelial markers should be positive, and most adenocarcinomas negative or only focally so (Table 97.1). It is not rare that an otherwise typical mesothelioma may lack one marker (e.g., cytokeratin 5/6 or calretinin) but express the other markers (e.g., D2-40 and WT-1).

Specific metastatic carcinomas, such as renal cell carcinomas, are easily excluded by staining for Pax-8 or kidney-specific cadherin (CA-IX), which are never expressed by mesotheliomas.[29]

Differential Diagnosis: Sarcomatoid Mesothelioma Versus Sarcoma Versus Sarcomatoid Carcinoma

The diagnosis of purely sarcomatoid mesothelioma is difficult, as cytokeratin positivity may be patchy, and not all mesothelioma markers are positive. Clinical and imaging is helpful in establishing a pleural-based tumor. One study showed that D2-40 is the most sensitive mesothelial marker for sarcomatoid mesothelioma, thereby aiding in the distinction from spindle cell carcinoma.[24]

In the distinction from sarcomatoid carcinoma, sampling to exclude areas of differentiated carcinoma is helpful in excluding mesothelioma.

Both pleural-based sarcomatoid carcinomas and sarcomas are quite rare. Synovial sarcoma shows far less pleomorphism typically than does sarcomatoid mesothelioma and can be diagnosed by cytogenetic study (see Chapter 96).

Differential Diagnosis: Mesothelioma Versus Epithelioid Angiosarcoma

Even though both are rare tumors, they may look quite similar histologically.[30] Luckily, expression of CD31 and flt-1 and especially nuclear staining for ERG establish a diagnosis of angiosarcoma and rule out mesothelioma.[31]

Mesothelial Inclusions in Lymph Nodes Versus Metastatic Mesothelioma

Florid mesothelial proliferations have been reported in lymph nodes of patients with recurrent pleuritis without evidence of malignant mesothelioma. They typically involve the subcapsular sinuses without destruction of lymph node architecture.[32,33]

Metastatic mesotheliomas to lymph nodes generally result in effacement of the architecture or diffuse sinusoidal infiltration (Fig. 97.13).

Prognosis and Treatment

There have been limited improvements in overall survival of pleural mesotheliomas over the decades.[34] The average survival is only 15 months.[35] Factors indicating favorable outcome include young age, female gender, low stage, good performance status, and epithelioid morphology. There is some evidence that a myxoid background is also a favorable prognostic sign.[3]

Treatment for pleural mesothelioma includes surgery and chemotherapy. There are two types of surgery for malignant pleural mesothelioma. Extrapleural pneumonectomy involves en bloc resection of the lung, pleura, pericardium, and diaphragm. Pleurectomy/decortication or "total pleurectomy" is a lung-sparing surgery that removes only parietal and visceral pleura.[36] If the diaphragm or pericardium requires resection (without pneumonectomy), the term "radical pleurectomy/decortication" is sometimes used.[37]

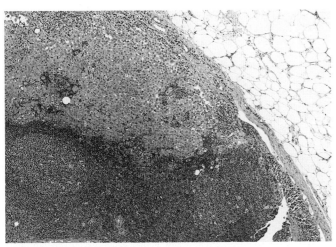

FIGURE 97.13 ▲ Metastatic mesothelioma, hilar lymph node. The tumor expands the subcapsular sinus and, unlike a benign rest, infiltrates the lymph node parenchyma.

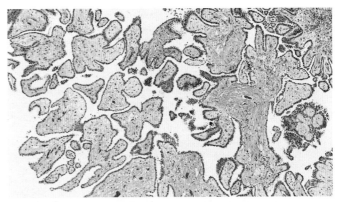

FIGURE 97.14 ▲ Well-differentiated papillary mesothelioma. The cores are vascularized, there are no detached papillary clusters, and the lining cells are bland and flattened.

Pemetrexed and platinum combination chemotherapy has become the cornerstone of therapy for patients with unresectable disease because the combination is associated with improved survival and quality of life in treated patients.[38] Currently, immune therapy, including mesothelin-targeted strategies, and anti-PD-1 and anti-CTLA-4 monoclonal treatments are under investigation.[39,40]

Uncommon Variants

Localized Malignant Mesothelioma

Localized malignant mesothelioma is a rare tumor that grossly appears as a distinctly localized nodular lesion. It shows no gross or microscopic evidence of diffuse pleural spread but has the microscopic and immunohistochemical features of diffuse malignant mesothelioma.[41–43]

There are few studies with follow-up, but it is likely that localized malignant mesothelioma has a better prognosis than does the diffuse form of disease.[42]

Well-Differentiated Papillary Mesothelioma of the Pleura

Well-differentiated papillary mesothelioma is a rare tumor of young women that is relatively localized or involves the peritoneal mesothelial surfaces diffusely. It is characterized histologically by papillae with vascular, myxoid cores covered by a single layer of flattened or cuboidal bland epithelioid cells. Most cases occur in the peritoneum, although there are rare reports of pleural tumors.[44]

In the pleura, there is no gender predilection, and the mean age is 60 years with an asbestos exposure rate of about 50%.[45] The mean survival is 7 years, as opposed to <1 year for diffuse malignant mesothelioma.[45]

The tumors are noninvasive, with stout papillary formations with myxoid cores, lined by bland, flattened, epithelioid cells (Fig. 97.14). Macrophages may be present in the cores of the papillae. The nuclei are round, small, and devoid of atypia and mitoses. In contrast to tubulopapillary malignant mesothelioma, the papillae have stroma and vessels; cells are flattened; and detached cellular clusters without cores are absent or rare. Although true invasion does not occur, nests of adenomatoid-appearing tumor may involve the stroma.[44,46]

Well-Differentiated Multicystic Mesothelioma of the Pleura

Multicystic mesothelioma is a controversial entity that involves the peritoneum and is considered either a benign or low-grade malignant process. There are rare reports of similar tumors in the pleura.[47]

REFERENCES

1. Neumann V, Loseke S, Nowak D, et al. Malignant pleural mesothelioma: incidence, etiology, diagnosis, treatment, and occupational health. *Dtsch Arztebl Int.* 2013;110:319–326.
2. Strauchen JA. Rarity of malignant mesothelioma prior to the widespread commercial introduction of asbestos: the Mount Sinai autopsy experience 1883–1910. *Am J Ind Med.* 2011;54:467–469.
3. Galateau-Salle F, Churg A, Roggli V, et al. Epithelioid malignant mesothelioma. In: Travis WD, et al., eds. *WHO Classification of Tumours of the Lung, Pleura, Mediastinum and Heart.* Lyon, France: IARC Press; 2015: 156–164.
4. Pairon JC, Laurent F, Rinaldo M, et al. Pleural plaques and the risk of pleural mesothelioma. *J Natl Cancer Inst.* 2013;105:293–301.
5. Lovrenski A, Panjkovic M, Tegeltija D, et al. The role of cytological evaluation of pleural fluid in diagnosing malignant mesothelioma. *Med Pregl.* 2012;65:5–8.
6. Nickell LT, Jr., Lichtenberger JP, 3rd, Khorashadi L, et al. Multimodality imaging for characterization, classification, and staging of malignant pleural mesothelioma. *Radiographics.* 2014;34:1692–1706.
7. Tertemiz KC, Ozgen Alpaydin A, Gurel D, et al. Multiple distant metastases in a case of malignant pleural mesothelioma. *Respir Med Case Rep.* 2014;13:16–18.
8. Bille A, Platania M, Pelosi G, et al. Gingival metastasis as first sign of multiorgan dissemination of epithelioid malignant mesothelioma. *J Thorac Oncol.* 2014;9:1226–1229.
9. Finn RS, Brims FJ, Gandhi A, et al. Postmortem findings of malignant pleural mesothelioma: a two-center study of 318 patients. *Chest.* 2012;142:1267–1273.
10. Hida T, Hamasaki M, Matsumoto S, et al. Diffuse intrapulmonary malignant mesothelioma presenting with miliary pulmonary nodules: a case report. *Pathol Int.* 2015;65:318–323.
11. Husain AN, Colby T, Ordonez N, et al. Guidelines for pathologic diagnosis of malignant mesothelioma: 2012 update of the consensus statement from the International Mesothelioma Interest Group. *Arch Pathol Lab Med.* 2013;137:647–667.
12. Kawai T, Kawashima K, Serizawa H, et al. Adenomatoid mesothelioma with intranuclear inclusion bodies: a case report with cytological and histological findings. *Diagn Cytopathol.* 2014;42:436–440.
13. Weissferdt A, Kalhor N, Suster S. Malignant mesothelioma with prominent adenomatoid features: a clinicopathologic and immunohistochemical study of 10 cases. *Ann Diagn Pathol.* 2011;15:25–29.
14. Ordonez NG. Mesothelioma with signet-ring cell features: report of 23 cases. *Mod Pathol.* 2013;26:370–384.
15. Ordonez NG. Deciduoid mesothelioma: report of 21 cases with review of the literature. *Mod Pathol.* 2012;25:1481–1495.
16. Tresserra F, Castella M, Fabra G, et al. Lymphohistiocytoid mesothelioma of the pleura: a case report with cytological findings. *Diagn Cytopathol.* 2013;41:546–549.
17. Ordonez NG. Pleomorphic mesothelioma: report of 10 cases. *Mod Pathol.* 2012;25:1011–1022.

18. Beckett P, Edwards J, Fennell D, et al. Demographics, management and survival of patients with malignant pleural mesothelioma in the National Lung Cancer Audit in England and Wales. *Lung Cancer.* 2015;88:344–348.

19. Klebe S, Mahar A, Henderson DW, et al. Malignant mesothelioma with heterologous elements: clinicopathological correlation of 27 cases and literature review. *Mod Pathol.* 2008;21:1084–1094.

20. Gumurdulu D, Zeren EH, Cagle PT, et al. Specificity of MOC-31 and HBME-1 immunohistochemistry in the differential diagnosis of adenocarcinoma and malignant mesothelioma: a study on environmental malignant mesothelioma cases from Turkish villages. *Pathol Oncol Res.* 2002;8:188–193.

21. Creaney J, Dick IM, and Robinson BW. Comparison of mesothelin and fibulin-3 in pleural fluid and serum as markers in malignant mesothelioma. *Curr Opin Pulm Med.* 2015;21:352–356.

22. Ordonez NG. Value of mesothelin immunostaining in the diagnosis of mesothelioma. *Mod Pathol.* 2003;16:192–197.

23. Husain AN, Mirza MK, Gibbs A, et al. How useful is GLUT-1 in differentiating mesothelial hyperplasia and fibrosing pleuritis from epithelioid and sarcomatoid mesotheliomas? An international collaborative study. *Lung Cancer.* 2014;83:324–328.

24. Chirieac LR, Pinkus GS, Pinkus JL, et al. The immunohistochemical characterization of sarcomatoid malignant mesothelioma of the pleura. *Am J Cancer Res.* 2011;1:14–24.

25. Borczuk AC, Taub RN, Hesdorffer M, et al. P16 loss and mitotic activity predict poor survival in patients with peritoneal malignant mesothelioma. *Clin Cancer Res.* 2005;11:3303–3308.

26. Henderson DW, Reid G, Kao SC, et al. Challenges and controversies in the diagnosis of mesothelioma: Part 1. Cytology-only diagnosis, biopsies, immunohistochemistry, discrimination between mesothelioma and reactive mesothelial hyperplasia, and biomarkers. *J Clin Pathol.* 2013;66:847–853.

27. Chung CT, Santos Gda C, Hwang DM, et al. FISH assay development for the detection of p16/CDKN2A deletion in malignant pleural mesothelioma. *J Clin Pathol.* 2010;63:630–634.

28. Hwang H, Tse C, Rodriguez S, et al. p16 FISH deletion in surface epithelial mesothelial proliferations is predictive of underlying invasive mesothelioma. *Am J Surg Pathol.* 2014;38:681–688.

29. Ordonez NG. Value of PAX8, PAX2, napsin A, carbonic anhydrase IX, and claudin-4 immunostaining in distinguishing pleural epithelioid mesothelioma from metastatic renal cell carcinoma. *Mod Pathol.* 2013;26:1132–1143.

30. Kao YC, Chow JM, Wang KM, et al. Primary pleural angiosarcoma as a mimicker of mesothelioma: a case report **VS**. *Diagn Pathol* 2011;6:130.

31. Fan C, Liu Y, Lin X, et al. Epithelioid angiosarcoma at chest wall which needs to be carefully distinguished from malignant mesothelioma: report of a rare case. *Int J Clin Exp Pathol.* 2014;7:9056–9060.

32. Argani P and Rosai J. Hyperplastic mesothelial cells in lymph nodes: report of six cases of a benign process that can stimulate metastatic involvement by mesothelioma or carcinoma. *Hum Pathol.* 1998;29:339–346.

33. Kim HS, Yoon G, Lee YY, et al. Mesothelial cell inclusions in pelvic and para-aortic lymph nodes: a clinicopathologic analysis. *Int J Clin Exp Pathol.* 2015;8:5318–5326.

34. Musk AW, Olsen N, Alfonso H, et al. Predicting survival in malignant mesothelioma. *Eur Respir J.* 2011;38:1420–1424.

35. Ahn S, Choi IH, Han J, et al. Pleural mesothelioma: an institutional experience of 66 cases. *Korean J Pathol.* 2014;48:91–99.

36. Hasegawa S. Extrapleural pneumonectomy or pleurectomy/decortication for malignant pleural mesothelioma. *Gen Thorac Cardiovasc Surg.* 2014;62:516–521.

37. Rice D, Rusch V, Pass H, et al. Recommendations for uniform definitions of surgical techniques for malignant pleural mesothelioma: a consensus report of the international association for the study of lung cancer international staging committee and the international mesothelioma interest group. *J Thorac Oncol.* 2011;6:1304–1312.

38. Ai J, Stevenson JP. Current issues in malignant pleural mesothelioma evaluation and management. *Oncologist.* 2014;19:975–984.

39. Antoniu SA, Dimofte G, and Ungureanu D. Immune therapies for malignant mesothelioma. *Expert Rev Anticancer Ther.* 2014;14:965–973.

40. Kurz S and Grohe C. Malignant pleural mesothelioma: new aspects of medical therapy. *Pneumologie.* 2014;68:329–335.

41. Hayashi H, Notohara K, Yoshioka H, et al. Localized malignant pleural mesothelioma showing a thoracic mass and metastasizing to the stomach. *Intern Med.* 2010;49:671–675.

42. Takahashi H, Harada M, Maehara S, et al. Localized malignant mesothelioma of the pleura. *Ann Thorac Cardiovasc Surg.* 2007;13:262–266.

43. Hirano H, Takeda S, Sawabata Y, et al. Localized pleural malignant mesothelioma. *Pathol Int.* 2003;53:616–621.

44. Chen X, Sheng W, and Wang J. Well-differentiated papillary mesothelioma: a clinicopathological and immunohistochemical study of 18 cases with additional observation. *Histopathology.* 2013;62:805–813.

45. Galateau-Salle F, Vignaud JM, Burke L, et al. Well-differentiated papillary mesothelioma of the pleura: a series of 24 cases. *Am J Surg Pathol.* 2004;28:534–540.

46. Costanzo L, Scarlata S, Perrone G, et al. Malignant transformation of well-differentiated papillary mesothelioma 13 years after the diagnosis: a case report. *Clin Respir J.* 2014;8:124–129.

47. Agarwal S, Mullick S, Gupta K, et al. Pleural multicystic mesothelial proliferation: a mimicker of benign peritoneal mesothelioma. *Indian J Pathol Microbiol.* 2013;56:476–477.

SECTION ONE
THYMOMAS

98 Thymomas: Classification and Staging

Borislav A. Alexiev, M.D., Anja C. Roden, M.D., and Allen P. Burke, M.D.

Terminology

Thymomas are neoplasms arising from or exhibiting organotypic (thymus-like) architectural features, regardless of the presence and relative numbers of nonneoplastic lymphocytes.[1] Although the prognosis of thymomas is in general good, these tumors are considered malignant as they can metastasize and recur.

Incidence and Clinical

The overall incidence of thymoma in the United States is 0.13 to 0.15 per 100,000 person-years.[2] They represent 50% of all tumors of the anterior mediastinum.[3]

Thymoma is exceedingly uncommon in children and young adults, rises in incidence in middle age, and peaks in the seventh decade of life.[4] Thymoma incidence is especially high among Asians and Pacific Islanders in the United States.[4]

While many patients are asymptomatic, others may exhibit symptoms due to local complications (chest pain, superior vena cava syndrome, cough, dyspnea, and wheezing due to compression/obstruction of adjacent organs), as well as systemic symptoms (fever or weight loss). The neoplasms often manifest clinically by causing autoimmune diseases, in particular myasthenia gravis. In fact, 15% of patients with myasthenia gravis develop a thymoma. Thymoma patients have an increased risk of additional extrathymic malignancies, in particular non-Hodgkin lymphoma.[4,5]

Classification

The histologic typing of thymomas is complex and remains a challenge for surgical pathologists due to the various existing classification schemes that are in clinical use (Table 98.1).[6,7] The first practical histopathologic categorization of thymoma was proposed in 1961 by Bernatz et al.[8] These authors divided thymomas based on their relative proportion of epithelial cells to lymphocytes and on the shape of the epithelial cells.[8] Their classification recognized four basic histopathologic variants: thymoma of predominantly lymphocytic type, epithelial type, mixed type, and spindle cell type.[8]

An additional approach to the classification of thymoma was introduced in 1985. It was proposed by Marino and Müller-Hermelink based on the premise that thymoma represents a neoplastic proliferation of cells that are derived from the cortex or the medulla of the thymus or from a combination thereof.[9] These authors thus classified thymoma into cortical, medullary, and mixed types.[9] This classification subsequently was modified by Kirchner and Müller-Hermelink to include two additional categories, the predominantly cortical thymoma (later renamed "organoid") and the well-differentiated thymic carcinoma.[10]

In 1999, the World Health Organization (WHO) devised five thymoma entities (type A, AB, B1, B2, B3 thymomas) and the more heterogeneous group of thymic carcinomas (collectively called type C thymomas).[11,12] There are two major types of thymoma depending on whether the neoplastic epithelial cells and their nuclei have spindle or oval shape and are uniformly bland (type A) or whether the cells have a round or polygonal appearance (type B).[1] Type A thymomas contain few or no intratumoral immature T cells. The type B thymomas are further subdivided on the basis of the extent of the infiltrate of immature T cells and the degree of atypia of the neoplastic epithelial cells into three subtypes: B1 (richest in immature T cells, areas of medullary differentiation), B2, and B3 (richest in epithelial cells). Thymomas combining type A with B1 or B2 features are designated type AB.

Thymomas of A, AB, and B1 to three types exhibit organotypic (thymus-like) architectural features. These tumors have not been observed in organs other than the thymus, though they may arise from heterotopic thymic tissue.

Thymic carcinomas (obsolete designation is "type C thymoma") exhibit clear-cut cytologic atypia, lack the lobulated architecture of thymomas, shows desmoplastic stromal reaction, and, in contrast to B thymomas, lack immature T lymphocytes. They are indistinguishable from extrathymic carcinomas, that is, they demonstrate morphologic features that are encountered also in organs other than the thymus.

Numerous studies demonstrated that the WHO classification is a prognostic factor.[12–18] However, reproducibility is an issue, particularly for those who may not encounter many thymomas in routine practice.[6,7,19] Suster and Moran proposed a simplified schema in 1999, which essentially condensed thymic epithelial tumors into three histologic groups based on architectural morphology and epithelial cytology: thymoma, atypical thymoma, and thymic carcinoma.[17,20,21] The Suster-Moran "thymoma" includes WHO subtypes A, AB, B1, and B2, whereas "atypical thymoma" corresponds to WHO subtype B3. This simplified scheme has been shown to have good reproducibility and, more importantly, carries adequate prognostic power with regard to survival and recurrence.[6,18]

For the sake of uniformity and clinical implications, it is recommended that either the WHO or the Suster-Moran nomenclature (or both) be parenthetically added to the report if another classification system is being used.[6]

Genetic Findings

The most frequent genetic alterations in thymomas affect chromosome 6q25.2–25.3. In type A thymomas, genetic alterations other than on chromosome 6 are rare.[1] In type AB thymoma, deletion of chromosome 6 with or without formation of ring chromosome 6 as well as complex multiple chromosomal aberrations have been identified.[22] Genetic alterations in type AB thymomas have been described as intermediate between those of type A and those of type B.[23] A few type A and AB thymomas with a clinically benign course may show genetic imbalances (e.g., on chromosome 8p11.21) that are associated with a poor prognosis if encountered in type B2 and B3 thymomas or thymic squamous cell carcinomas.[22]

Cytogenetic data involving alterations at chromosomes 5q21–22, 7p15, and 8p11 show that type B2 thymomas are genetically related to type B3 thymomas, in line with the frequent histologic observation of combinations of type B2 and B3 areas in the same tumor.[22]

TABLE 98.1   Comparison of Major Histologic Classifications of Thymoma

Bernatz et al. (1961)[8]	Kirchner et al. (1989)[10]	Suster and Moran (1999)[21]	Ströbel et al. (2015)[1,a]
Spindle cell	Medullary	Thymoma	Type A thymoma
	Mixed	Thymoma	Type AB thymoma
Lymphocyte rich	Predominantly cortical	Thymoma	Type B1
Mixed epithelial cell and lymphocyte	Cortical	Thymoma	Type B2
Epithelial cell rich	Well-differentiated thymic carcinoma	Atypical thymoma	Type B3
	High-grade thymic carcinoma	Thymic carcinoma	Thymic carcinoma

[a]There are other variants in the WHO classification, such as micronodular thymoma with lymphoid stroma and metaplastic, sclerosing, and microscopic thymoma.

In type B3 thymoma, the most frequent recurrent gains of chromosomal material were on chromosomes 1q (69%) and Xq (19%), while the most frequent recurrent losses were observed for the whole or parts of chromosome 6 (38%) and for 13q (31%).[22] The combined losses at chromosomal regions 5q21–22 (APC), 13q14.3 (RB), and 17p13.1 (p53) were unique to a subset of more invasive type B3 thymomas.[22]

Staging

No TNM protocol has been officially authorized by the American Joint Committee on Cancer (AJCC) or the International Union Against Cancer (UICC) for the staging of thymomas. A proposed staging for the 8th edition is presented in Table 98.2 along with the Koga-Masaoka scheme.[24,25] The new TNM proposal drops consideration of

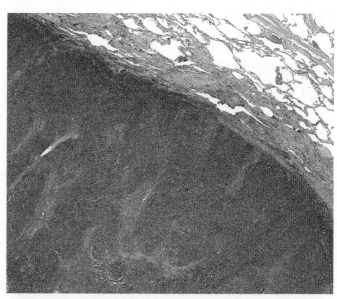

FIGURE 98.1 ▲ Thymoma, extension into the pleura. The tumor abuts lung parenchyma indicating pleural invasion and transcapsular invasion including invasion of submesothelial fibrous layer. This finding indicates involvement of mediastinal pleura (pT1b).

capsular invasion or invasion into fat as a factor in staging, due to poor reproducibility and because this distinction had no impact on clinical outcome in the study of the ITMIOG database of over 10,000 patients with thymic epithelial neoplasms.[24] The scheme developed by Masaoka for thymoma and revised by Koga was frequently used for staging (Table 98.2).[25–27] Recently, Moran et al. proposed a new staging system that offers better stratification and improved histologic definitions for proper staging of cases of thymoma (Table 98.2).[28] Both systems include invasion into adjacent organs as a major discriminator (Figs. 98.1 and 98.2).

TABLE 98.2   Thymoma and Thymic Carcinoma Staging[a]

Stage	Modified Masaoka Staging	Proposed Moran Staging	Proposed IASLC/ITMIG Staging[b]
		Definition	
0[c]		Encapsulated tumor	
I	Macroscopically completely encapsulated Microscopically no capsular invasion	Invasive tumor into perithymic adipose tissue	T1 N0 M0
II	Complete transmural (transcapsular) invasion A. Microscopic transcapsular invasion only B. Macroscopic invasion into extracapsular soft tissue, or tumor grossly adherent to mediastinal pleura or pericardium w/o invasion through these structures	Direct invasion A. Innominate vein, mediastinal pleura, lung B. Pericardium C. Great vessels (aorta, superior vena cava), heart	T2 N0 M0
III	Macroscopic invasion into neighboring organs A. Invasion spares the great vessels B. Invasion includes the great vessels	Metastatic disease A. Intrathoracic structures, e.g., lymph nodes, diaphragm B. Extrathoracic invasion	a. T3 N0 M0 b. T4 N0 M0
IV	Locally advanced thoracic disease or metastasis A. Pleural or pericardial dissemination B. Lymphovascular metastasis		a. T any N1 M0 T any N0,1 M1a b. T any N2 M0,1a T any N any M1b

[a]Reproduced with permission, Roden AC, Yi ES, Jenkins SM, et al. Reproducibility of three histologic classifications and three staging systems for thymic epithelial neoplasms and its effect on prognosis. Am J Surg Pathol. 2015;39(suppl 1):427–441.
[b]T descriptors: T1, (a) encapsulated or unencapsulated, with or without extension into mediastinal fat, (b) extension into mediastinal pleura; T2, involvement of pericardium; T3, involvement of lung, brachiocephalic vein, superior vena cava, chest wall, phrenic nerve, and hilar (extrapericardial) pulmonary vessels; T4, involvement of the aorta, arch vessels, main pulmonary artery, myocardium, trachea, or esophagus. A tumor is classified according to the highest T level of involvement that is present with or without any invasion of structures of lower T levels.
N descriptors: N0, no nodal involvement; N1, anterior (perithymic) nodes; N2, deep intrathoracic or cervical nodes.
M descriptors: M0, no metastatic pleural, pericardial, or distant sites; M1a, separate pleural or pericardial nodule(s); M1b, pulmonary intraparenchymal nodule or distant organ metastasis.
Involvement must be pathologically proven in pathologic staging.
[c]Stage 0 is not used in the Masaoka or proposed IASLC/ITMIG Staging

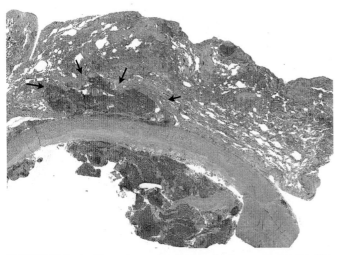

FIGURE 98.2 ▲ Thymoma, extension into the lung parenchyma. The tumor is on both sides of the thickening fibrotic pleura and invades the lung parenchyma (*arrows*). This finding indicates invasion into adjacent organs (see Table 98.2) (pT3).

The major difference between the two systems is the designation of stage IV for pleural metastases (alternatively called "implants" in the Koga-Masaoka system), which is not recognized in the stages of Moran et al., who require skeletal muscle invasion into the diaphragm for the designation of pleural metastasis (Fig. 98.3).[28]

Treatment and Prognosis

Thymomas can be challenging to manage because of local invasion of mediastinal structures and high recurrence rates. Surgery is the mainstay of treatment, and complete resection is associated with the best prognosis.[29–32] Although practices vary, neoadjuvant chemotherapy is often used to improve resectability. Extended resections following neoadjuvant treatment have been safely performed for locally advanced tumors.[29]

The histologic subtype based on the WHO classification is closely related to the tumor stage.[16] Staging is the most important prognostic indicator, whereas gender and myasthenia gravis are not significantly prognostic.[13,33–35] The proportion of tumors in an advanced stage

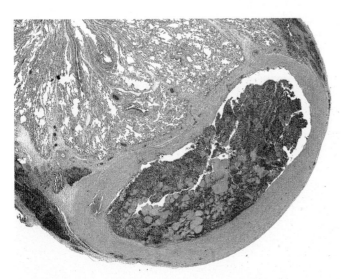

FIGURE 98.3 ▲ Thymoma, "drop metastasis" (pM1a). "Implants" or pleural metastases (dissemination in stage IV Masaoka staging) are not included in Moran et al.'s staging system, which requires invasion into diaphragm to indicate metastatic disease as opposed to an implant (Reference[25]). Invasion into the pleura is seen at the edge of the metastasis/implant.

gradually increases from type A to type B3.[16] In regard to the prognosis of each histologic subtype, patients with type A and AB thymoma have good prognoses, with no thymoma-related deaths.[16] In contrast, the prognoses of patients with type B thymoma tend to gradually worsen from B1 to B3.[16]

REFERENCES

1. Ströbel P, Marx A, Badve S, et al. Type A thymoma, including atypical variant. In: Travis WD, et al., eds. *WHO Classification of Tumours of the Lung, Pleura, Mediastinum and Heart.* Lyon, France: IARC Press; 2015:187–192.
2. Engels EA, Pfeiffer RM. Malignant thymoma in the United States: demographic patterns in incidence and associations with subsequent malignancies. *Int J Cancer.* 2003;105:546–551.
3. Stremmel C, Dango S, Thiemann U, et al. Thymoma—incidence, classification and therapy. *Dtsch Med Wochenschr.* 2007;132:2090–2095.
4. Engels EA. Epidemiology of thymoma and associated malignancies. *J Thorac Oncol.* 2010;5:S260–S265.
5. Weksler B, Nason KS, Mackey D, et al. Thymomas and extrathymic cancers. *Ann Thorac Surg.* 2012;93:884–888.
6. Weydert JA, De Young BR, Leslie KO, et al. Recommendations for the reporting of surgically resected thymic epithelial tumors. *Am J Clin Pathol.* 2009;132:10–15.
7. Weydert JA, De Young BR, Leslie KO, et al. Recommendations for the reporting of surgically resected thymic epithelial tumors. *Hum Pathol.* 2009;40:918–923.
8. Bernatz PE, Harrison EG, Clagett OT. Thymoma: a clinicopathologic study. *J Thorac Cardiovasc Surg.* 1961;42:424–444.
9. Marino M, Muller-Hermelink HK. Thymoma and thymic carcinoma. Relation of thymoma epithelial cells to the cortical and medullary differentiation of thymus. *Virchows Arch A Pathol Anat Histopathol.* 1985;407:119–149.
10. Kirchner T, Schalke B, Marx A, et al. Evaluation of prognostic features in thymic epithelial tumors. *Thymus.* 1989;14:195–203.
11. Okumura M, Ohta M, Miyoshi S, et al. Oncological significance of WHO histological thymoma classification. A clinical study based on 286 patients. *Jpn J Thorac Cardiovasc Surg.* 2002;50:189–194.
12. Okumura M, Ohta M, Tateyama H, et al. The World Health Organization histologic classification system reflects the oncologic behavior of thymoma: a clinical study of 273 patients. *Cancer.* 2002;94:624–632.
13. Chen G, Marx A, Chen WH, et al. New WHO histologic classification predicts prognosis of thymic epithelial tumors: a clinicopathologic study of 200 thymoma cases from China. *Cancer.* 2002;95:420–429.
14. Kondo K, Yoshizawa K, Tsuyuguchi M, et al. WHO histologic classification is a prognostic indicator in thymoma. *Ann Thorac Surg.* 2004;77:1183–1188.
15. Marchevsky AM, Gupta R, Casadio C, et al. World Health Organization classification of thymomas provides significant prognostic information for selected stage III patients: evidence from an international thymoma study group. *Hum Pathol.* 2010;41:1413–1421.
16. Nakagawa K, Asamura H, Matsuno Y, et al. Thymoma: a clinicopathologic study based on the new World Health Organization classification. *J Thorac Cardiovasc Surg.* 2003;126:1134–1140.
17. Rena O, Papalia E, Maggi G, et al. World Health Organization histologic classification: an independent prognostic factor in resected thymomas. *Lung Cancer.* 2005;50:59–66.
18. Roden AC, Yi ES, Jenkins SM, et al. Modified Masaoka stage and size are independent prognostic predictors in thymoma and modified Masaoka stage is superior to histopathologic classifications. *J Thorac Oncol.* 2015;10:691–700.
19. Roden AC, Yi ES, Jenkins SM, et al. Reproducibility of 3 histologic classifications and 3 staging systems for thymic epithelial neoplasms and its effect on prognosis. *Am J Surg Pathol.* 2015;39:427–441.
20. Sonobe S, Miyamoto H, Izumi H, et al. Clinical usefulness of the WHO histological classification of thymoma. *Ann Thorac Cardiovasc Surg.* 2005;11:367–373.
21. Suster S, Moran CA. Thymoma, atypical thymoma, and thymic carcinoma. A novel conceptual approach to the classification of thymic epithelial neoplasms. *Am J Clin Pathol.* 1999;111:826–833.
22. Strobel P, Marino M, Feuchtenberger M, et al. Micronodular thymoma: an epithelial tumour with abnormal chemokine expression setting the stage for lymphoma development. *J Pathol.* 2005;207:72–82.
23. Inoue M, Starostik P, Zettl A, et al. Correlating genetic aberrations with World Health Organization-defined histology and stage across the spectrum of thymomas. *Cancer Res.* 2003;63:3708–3715.

24. Detterbeck FC, Stratton K, Giroux D, et al. The IASLC/ITMIG Thymic Epithelial Tumors Staging Project: proposal for an evidence-based stage classification system for the forthcoming (8th) edition of the TNM classification of malignant tumors. *J Thorac Oncol.* 2014;9:S65–S72.

25. Koga K, Matsuno Y, Noguchi M, et al. A review of 79 thymomas: modification of staging system and reappraisal of conventional division into invasive and non-invasive thymoma. *Pathol Int.* 1994;44:359–367.

26. Masaoka A, Monden Y, Nakahara K, et al. Follow-up study of thymomas with special reference to their clinical stages. *Cancer.* 1981;48:2485–2492.

27. Yamakawa Y, Masaoka A, Hashimoto T, et al. A tentative tumor-node-metastasis classification of thymoma. *Cancer.* 1991;68:1984–1987.

28. Moran CA, Walsh G, Suster S, et al. Thymomas II: a clinicopathologic correlation of 250 cases with a proposed staging system with emphasis on pathologic assessment. *Am J Clin Pathol.* 2012;137:451–461.

29. Ahmad U, Huang J. Current readings: the most influential and recent studies involving surgical management of thymoma. *Semin Thorac Cardiovasc Surg.* 2013;25:144–149.

30. Rajan A, Giaccone G. Treatment of advanced thymoma and thymic carcinoma. *Curr Treat Options Oncol.* 2008;9:277–287.

31. Wright CD, Kessler KA. Surgical treatment of thymic tumors. *Semin Thorac Cardiovasc Surg.* 2005;17:20–26.

32. Wright CD, Wain JC, Wong DR, et al. Predictors of recurrence in thymic tumors: importance of invasion, World Health Organization histology, and size. *J Thorac Cardiovasc Surg.* 2005;130:1413–1421.

33. Chalabreysse L, Roy P, Cordier JF, et al. Correlation of the WHO schema for the classification of thymic epithelial neoplasms with prognosis: a retrospective study of 90 tumors. *Am J Surg Pathol.* 2002;26:1605–1611.

34. Kim HK, Choi YS, Kim J, et al. Type B thymoma: is prognosis predicted only by World Health Organization classification? *J Thorac Cardiovasc Surg.* 2010;139:1431–1435 e1.

35. Quintanilla-Martinez L, Wilkins EW, Jr., Ferry JA, et al. Thymoma—morphologic subclassification correlates with invasiveness and immunohistologic features: a study of 122 cases. *Hum Pathol.* 1993;24:958–969.

99 Type A Thymoma (Spindle Cell or Medullary Thymoma)

Borislav A. Alexiev, M.D., and Anja C. Roden, M.D.

Terminology

Type A thymoma is an organotypic thymic epithelial neoplasm composed of bland spindle/oval epithelial tumor cells with few or no lymphocytes. Alternate designations include spindle cell or medullary thymoma (see Chapter 99). The tumor has been postulated to derive from the normal thymic medullary epithelial cells.[1]

Incidence and Clinical Presentation

Type A thymoma is a relatively uncommon type of thymoma and corresponds to 4% to 19% of all thymomas.[1,2] No consistent gender predilection has been reported. The age at manifestation ranges from 32 to 83 years, with a mean age of 61 years.[1] Type A thymoma may have an associated autoimmune disorder, including but not limited to myasthenia gravis (4% to 24%), Good syndrome, and pure red cell aplasia.[3,4] Patients with type A thymoma may experience symptoms caused by compression of the surrounding organs by an expansive mass. These problems may take the form of superior vena cava syndrome, dysphagia, cough, or chest pain. Some patients with type A thymoma have no symptoms at all, and the tumor can be detected for an unrelated problem as an enlarged mediastinal area or mass by x-ray, CT, or MRI.

Gross Pathology

Grossly, type A thymoma is usually well circumscribed and encapsulated (Fig. 99.1). The cut surface is tan white and shows vague lobulation with less distinct dissecting white fibrous bands than is seen in other types. Cystic change or calcification of the capsule may be seen. Type A thymomas, just like any other histologic variant of thymoma, have a similar potential to become invasive tumors (capsular invasion) capable of spreading locally or outside of the thoracic cavity.[5]

Microscopic Pathology

Histologically, the main morphologic growth pattern is that of a spindle cellular proliferation arranged in short fascicles of spindle- and/or oval-shaped cells with elongated nuclei, dispersed chromatin, and inconspicuous nucleoli (Figs. 99.2 and 99.3). The tumor cells can form a variety of histologic structures.[1] They are arranged in solid sheets without any particular pattern or in a storiform pattern. The tumor cells can form cysts of various sizes, glandular structures, glomeruloid bodies, rosettes with or without a central lumen, hemangioma-like papillary projections in cystic spaces, or meningioma-like whorls. Thin-walled branching vessels in the background may impart a hemangiopericytoma-like appearance. Mitoses are seldom found, but lobular infarcts can occur. Type A thymomas often have few or no lymphocytes and show neither distinct lobules nor dissecting fibrous bands or prominent perivascular spaces as seen in other types of thymoma. Occasional cases may display atypical features (mild to moderate atypia, increased mitotic figures, focal necrosis, "atypical type A thymoma") somewhat resembling B3 thymoma, except for the fact that the tumor cells are spindled instead of round/polygonal and lack intratumoral cortical immature T lymphocytes.[6]

Special Studies

The immunoprofile of type A thymoma remains one of the most controversial questions in the literature. Different studies have generated conflicting results related to antigen expression due to differences in

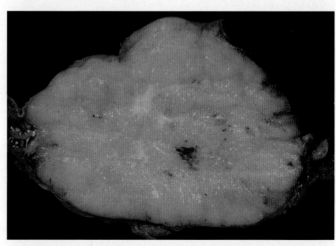

FIGURE 99.1 ▲ Spindle cell (type A) thymoma. Encapsulated thymomas without macroscopic evidence of invasion.

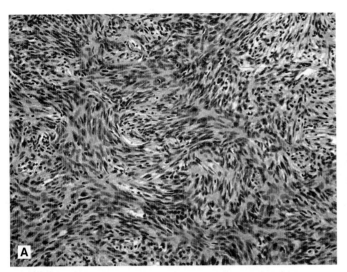
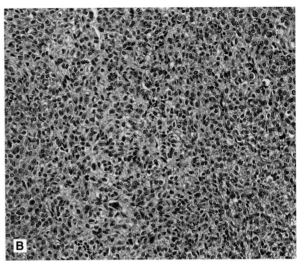

FIGURE 99.2 ▲ Type A thymoma. **A.** Note spindle cellular proliferation arranged in fascicles. **B.** In this example, the cells are more oval. By definition, the cells are bland with few background immature lymphocytes.

detection systems and antibodies used. The tumor cells, similar to normal medullary thymocytes, are strongly positive for EMA (epithelial membrane antigen) (Fig. 99.4), CK8/18, and vimentin. Other cytokeratins of different molecular weights and p63 show variable expression.[7] CD20-positive tumor cells may be detected focally.[8] There is no expression of CD5, and BCL-2, CD57, and CK5/6 are variable and focal.[9,10] Basement membrane–like deposits as demonstrated by antilaminin and anti–type IV collagen antibodies surround most tumor cells. P53 protein and Ki 67 show only low or no expression. The few intratumoral lymphocytes express mature T-cell markers, CD3 and CD5 (Fig. 99.5). Cortical immature T cells (TdT, CD1a, and CD99+), seen in B1, B2, and B3 thymomas, might be absent in type A (Fig. 99.6).[8]

Type A thymoma has been found to have t(15;22)(p11;q11) or a partial loss of the short arm of chromosome 6.[9] The most frequent aberration seen was loss of heterozygosity (LOH) in the region 6q23.3–25.5.[11]

Differential Diagnosis

Type A thymoma may resemble the spindle cell variant of B3 thymoma. In type A thymoma, the degree of atypia is lower, and perivascular spaces with epithelial palisades are absent. In contrast to B3 thymoma, type A thymoma is strongly positive for EMA. CK5/6 shows only low expression or none. Cortical immature T cells, positive for TdT, CD1a, and CD99, as commonly seen in the B3 types of thymoma, might be absent or sparse.[8] Type A thymoma with rosette formation may resemble a well-differentiated neuroendocrine tumor. Unlike type A thymoma, well-differentiated neuroendocrine tumors demonstrated a characteristic "salt and pepper" chromatin pattern and strongly express neuroendocrine markers (synaptophysin, chromogranin, CD56).

Treatment and Prognosis

Surgery is the mainstay of treatment, and complete resection is associated with the best prognosis.[12–14]

Type A thymomas are usually early Masaoka stage tumors.[4] The overall survival of patients with type A thymoma has been reported to reach 100% at 5 and 10 years, even though ~20% of them have stage II or stage III disease.[11,15] Only exceptional case reports of local recurrence or distant metastasis have been documented.[11,16] Rarely, type A thymoma can undergo malignant transformation into thymic carcinoma.[17] The association with myasthenia gravis has been reported to have either a positive effect or no effect on prognosis.[15,18]

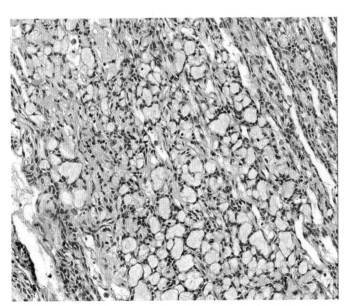

FIGURE 99.3 ▲ Type A thymoma. Microcystic change is frequent.

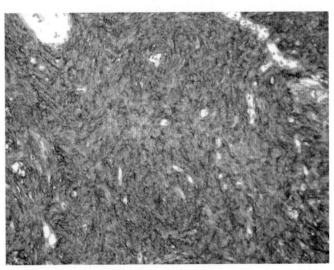

FIGURE 99.4 ▲ Type A thymoma. Note strong EMA expression in neoplastic cells (anti-EMA, ×200).

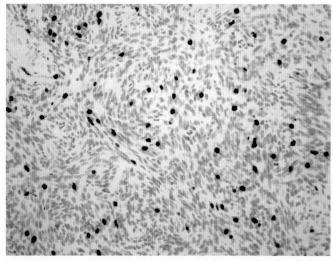

FIGURE 99.5 ▲ Type A thymoma. Note rare CD3-positive intratumoral T cells (anti-CD3, ×200).

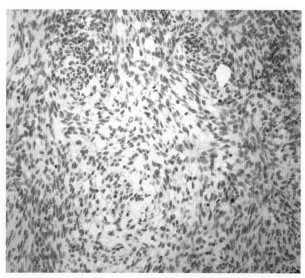

FIGURE 99.6 ▲ Type A thymoma. Note negative TdT stain for intratumoral cortical immature T cells (anti-TdT, ×200).

REFERENCES

1. Ströbel P, Marx A, Badve S, et al. Type A thymoma, including atypical variant. In: Travis WD, et al., eds. *WHO Classification of Tumours of the Lung, Pleura, Mediastinum and Heart.* Lyon, France: IARC Press; 2015:187–192.
2. Ruffini E, Filosso PL, Lausi P, et al. Recurrence of thymoma. *Eur J Cardiothorac Surg.* 2011;40:900–901.
3. Kelleher P, Misbah SA. What is Good's syndrome? Immunological abnormalities in patients with thymoma. *J Clin Pathol.* 2003;56:12–16.
4. Ruffini E, Filosso PL, Mossetti C, et al. Thymoma: inter-relationships among World Health Organization histology, Masaoka staging and myasthenia gravis and their independent prognostic significance: a single-centre experience. *Eur J Cardiothorac Surg.* 2011;40:146–153.
5. Moran CA, Kalhor N, Suster S. Invasive spindle cell thymomas (WHO Type A): a clinicopathologic correlation of 41 cases. *Am J Clin Pathol.* 2010;134:793–798.
6. Nonaka D, Rosai J. Is there a spectrum of cytologic atypia in type a thymomas analogous to that seen in type B thymomas? A pilot study of 13 cases. *Am J Surg Pathol.* 2012;36:889–894.
7. Weissferdt A, Hernandez JC, Kalhor N, et al. Spindle cell thymomas: an immunohistochemical study of 30 cases. *Appl Immunohistochem Mol Morphol.* 2011;19:329–335.
8. Alexiev BA, Drachenberg CB, Burke AP. Thymomas: a cytological and immunohistochemical study, with emphasis on lymphoid and neuroendocrine markers. *Diagn Pathol.* 2007;2:13.
9. Dal Cin P, De Wolf-Peeters C, Deneffe G, et al. Thymoma with a t(15;22) (p11;q11). *Cancer Genet Cytogenet.* 1996;89:181–183.
10. Tateyama H, Eimoto T, Tada T, et al. Immunoreactivity of a new CD5 antibody with normal epithelium and malignant tumors including thymic carcinoma. *Am J Clin Pathol.* 1999;111:235–240.
11. Muller-Hermelink HK, Marx A. Pathological aspects of malignant and benign thymic disorders. *Ann Med.* 1999;31(Suppl 2):5–14.
12. Ahmad U, Huang J. Current readings: the most influential and recent studies involving surgical management of thymoma. *Semin Thorac Cardiovasc Surg.* 2013;25:144–149.
13. Rajan A, Giaccone G. Treatment of advanced thymoma and thymic carcinoma. *Curr Treat Options Oncol.* 2008;9:277–287.
14. Wright CD, Kessler KA. Surgical treatment of thymic tumors. *Semin Thorac Cardiovasc Surg.* 2005;17:20–26.
15. Okumura M, Ohta M, Tateyama H, et al. The World Health Organization histologic classification system reflects the oncologic behavior of thymoma: a clinical study of 273 patients. *Cancer.* 2002;94:624–632.
16. Pan CC, Chen WY, Chiang H. Spindle cell and mixed spindle/lymphocytic thymomas: an integrated clinicopathologic and immunohistochemical study of 81 cases. *Am J Surg Pathol.* 2001;25:111–120.
17. Kuo TT, Chan JK. Thymic carcinoma arising in thymoma is associated with alterations in immunohistochemical profile. *Am J Surg Pathol.* 1998;22:1474–1481.
18. Chalabreysse L, Roy P, Cordier JF, et al. Correlation of the WHO schema for the classification of thymic epithelial neoplasms with prognosis: a retrospective study of 90 tumors. *Am J Surg Pathol.* 2002;26:1605–1611.

100 Type B1 Thymoma (Lymphocyte-Rich or Predominantly Cortical Thymoma)

Borislav A. Alexiev, M.D., and Fabio R. Tavora, M.D., Ph.D.

Terminology

Type B1 thymoma is an organotypic thymic epithelial neoplasm composed predominantly of areas resembling thymic cortex with epithelial cells scattered in a prominent population of immature lymphocytes, and areas of medullary differentiation, with or without Hassall corpuscles. The postulated cell of origin is a thymic epithelial cell capable of differentiating toward both cortical and medullary type.[1]

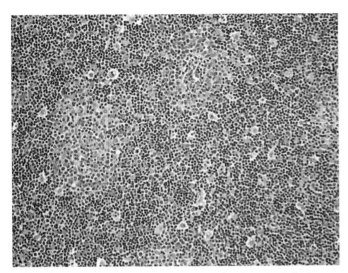

FIGURE 100.1 ▲ Type B1 thymoma. Note the densely packed population of small lymphocytes with pale areas of medullary differentiation (H&E, ×100).

FIGURE 100.3 ▲ Type B1 thymoma. Note the pale areas of medullary differentiation composed of loosely packed lymphocytes (H&E, ×40).

Incidence and Clinical

B1 thymoma is a relatively rare tumor of the adult age (mean of 41 to 47 years) with no significant difference in the distribution of genders. B1 thymoma accounts for 4% to 26% of all thymomas and is often diagnosed because of associated immunologic diseases such as myasthenia gravis (18% to 56% of the cases).[2-6] Patients with type B1 thymoma may experience symptoms caused by compression of the surrounding organs by an expansive mass. Some patients with type B1 thymoma have no symptoms at all, and the tumor can be detected for an unrelated problem as an enlarged mediastinal area or mass by x-ray, CT, or MRI.

Gross Pathology

Grossly, B1 thymoma is usually a well-defined or encapsulated grayish mass. Thick fibrous capsule and septa can be present, as well as cystic spaces or small hemorrhagic and necrotic areas.

Microscopic Pathology

Histologically, B1 thymoma closely resembles normal thymic cortex with interspersed medullary foci.[1,7] The tumors may grow in expansile sheets or display a highly organoid lobular architecture. Unlike the normal thymus, the lobules are of varying sizes and separated by thin or thick acellular fibrous septa. The neoplastic epithelial component is relatively inconspicuous and appears as interspersed oval cells with pale round nuclei and small nucleoli, although some cells may be large and occasionally have conspicuous nucleoli (Figs. 100.1 and 100.2). Long dendritic processes may be visible, best seen on keratin stains. The epithelial cells are dispersed and usually do not form cellular groupings. The lymphoid component is a densely packed population of small lymphocytes with clumped chromatin. Tangible-body macrophages may be scattered throughout giving rise to a starry-sky appearance. Perivascular spaces are not as frequent as in the other B thymomas. Cystic spaces and areas of necrosis, when present, are usually small. Pale areas of medullary differentiation are always present, composed of more loosely packed lymphocytes (Fig. 100.3). Hassall corpuscles may be seen but are less numerous than in normal medulla. They range from poorly formed epithelial groupings to large structures with prominent keratinized centers.

Special Studies

The neoplastic cells strongly express a CK5/6 (Fig. 100.4), CK903, and p63 pattern similar to normal cortical thymocytes. Focal positivity for

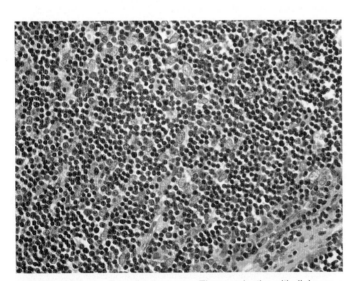

FIGURE 100.2 ▲ Type B1 thymoma. The neoplastic epithelial component is relatively inconspicuous and appears as interspersed oval cells with pale round nuclei and small nucleoli (H&E, ×400).

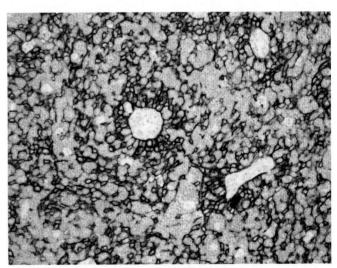

FIGURE 100.4 ▲ Type B1 thymoma. Note the strong CK5/6 expression in neoplastic cells (anti-CK5/6, ×200).

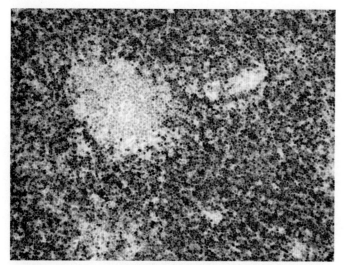

FIGURE 100.5 ▲ Type B1 thymoma. Note numerous TdT-positive intratumoral T cells (anti-TdT, ×200).

CK8/18 and CK7 may also be observed. The proliferative index (Ki-67) is low.[8,9] EMA, CK20, CD20, CD117, and CD5 stains are negative in tumor cells.[10] Admixed lymphocytes demonstrate a cortical immature T-cell immunoprofile (TdT+, CD1a+, CD99+, CD3+, CD4+, CD8+, CD5+) (Fig. 100.5) with high proliferation (Ki 67) rate.[10] In contrast, lymphocytes in the medullary islands are mostly mature T cells (TdT–, CD1a–, CD99–) and B cells (CD20+) (Fig. 100.6).[10]

Differential Diagnosis

Type B1 thymoma is distinguishable from the normal noninvoluted thymus mainly based on architectural differences, including the large excess of cortical areas compared to small areas resembling the thymic medulla, fewer Hassall corpuscles, less regular lobulation, and a thick fibrous capsule or irregular fibrous septa.[7] Similar to type B1 thymoma, B2 thymoma is also lymphocyte rich, but the epithelial cells are large and polygonal and exhibit large vesicular nuclei with prominent nucleoli. In addition, the medullary islands are less prominent than in B1 thymomas. Last but not least, B1 thymoma with a high predominance of immature T lymphocytes may simulate T lymphoblastic lymphoma. The presence of a prominent CK5/6 meshwork and low CDK6 expression in T lymphocytes favor B1 thymoma.

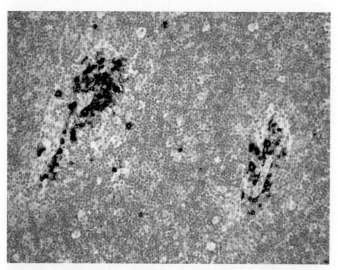

FIGURE 100.6 ▲ Type B1 thymoma. Note CD20-positive B cells in medullary islands (anti-CD20, ×200).

Treatment and Prognosis

Surgery is the mainstay of treatment, and complete resection is associated with the best prognosis.[11–13] Extended resections following neoadjuvant treatment have been safely performed for locally advanced tumors.[11,14]

Staging is the most important prognostic indicator, whereas age, gender, and myasthenia gravis are not significant prognostic parameters.[4,5,15,16] B1 thymoma is considered to have a low-grade malignant potential being completely encapsulated (stage I) in about 53% to 58% of the cases or invading only the mediastinal fat (stage II) in another 24% to 27% of the cases.[4,15] Less frequently, it can invade the pleura, pericardium, great vessels, or adjacent organs; metastases are exceedingly rare.[4,6,15,16] The 5- and 10-year survivals for type B1 thymoma are 100% and 86%, respectively. The tumor is slightly more aggressive than A and AB thymomas, but less malignant than B2 and B3 thymomas and thymic carcinomas.[17]

REFERENCES

1. den Bakker MA, Marx A, Ströbel P, et al. Type B1 thymoma. In: Travis WD, et al., eds. *WHO Classification of Tumours of the Lung, Pleura, Mediastinum and Heart.* Lyon, France: IARC Press; 2015:196–198.
2. Kim HK, Choi YS, Kim J, et al. Type B thymoma: is prognosis predicted only by World Health Organization classification? *J Thorac Cardiovasc Surg.* 2010;139:1431–1435 e1.
3. Ruffini E, Filosso PL, Mossetti C, et al. Thymoma: inter-relationships among World Health Organization histology, Masaoka staging and myasthenia gravis and their independent prognostic significance: a single-centre experience. *Eur J Cardiothorac Surg.* 2011;40:146–153.
4. Chalabreysse L, Roy P, Cordier JF, et al. Correlation of the WHO schema for the classification of thymic epithelial neoplasms with prognosis: a retrospective study of 90 tumors. *Am J Surg Pathol.* 2002;26:1605–1611.
5. Kelleher P, Misbah SA. What is Good's syndrome? Immunological abnormalities in patients with thymoma. *J Clin Pathol.* 2003;56:12–16.
6. Okumura M, Ohta M, Miyoshi S, et al. Oncological significance of WHO histological thymoma classification. A clinical study based on 286 patients. *Jpn J Thorac Cardiovasc Surg.* 2002;50:189–194.
7. Roden AC, Yi ES, Jenkins SM, et al. Reproducibility of 3 histologic classifications and 3 staging systems for thymic epithelial neoplasms and its effect on prognosis. *Am J Surg Pathol.* 2015;39:427–441.
8. Comin CE, Messerini L, Novelli L, et al. KI-67 antigen expression predicts survival and correlates with histologic subtype in the WHO classification of thymic epithelial tumors. *Int J Surg Pathol.* 2004;12:395–400.
9. Hiroshima K, Iyoda A, Toyozaki T, et al. Proliferative activity and apoptosis in thymic epithelial neoplasms. *Mod Pathol.* 2002;15:1326–1332.
10. Alexiev BA, Drachenberg CB, Burke AP. Thymomas: a cytological and immunohistochemical study, with emphasis on lymphoid and neuroendocrine markers. *Diagn Pathol.* 2007;2:13.
11. Ahmad U, Huang J. Current readings: The most influential and recent studies involving surgical management of thymoma. *Semin Thorac Cardiovasc Surg.* 2013;25:144–149.
12. Rajan A, Giaccone G. Treatment of advanced thymoma and thymic carcinoma. *Curr Treat Options Oncol.* 2008;9:277–287.
13. Wright CD, Wain JC, Wong DR, et al. Predictors of recurrence in thymic tumors: importance of invasion, World Health Organization histology, and size. *J Thorac Cardiovasc Surg.* 2005;130:1413–1421.
14. Wright CD, Kessler KA. Surgical treatment of thymic tumors. *Semin Thorac Cardiovasc Surg.* 2005;17:20–26.
15. Chen G, Marx A, Chen WH, et al. New WHO histologic classification predicts prognosis of thymic epithelial tumors: a clinicopathologic study of 200 thymoma cases from China. *Cancer.* 2002;95:420–429.
16. Quintanilla-Martinez L, Wilkins EW, Jr., Ferry JA, et al. Thymoma—morphologic subclassification correlates with invasiveness and immunohistologic features: a study of 122 cases. *Hum Pathol.* 1993;24:958–969.
17. Nakagawa K, Asamura H, Matsuno Y, et al. Thymoma: a clinicopathologic study based on the new World Health Organization classification. *J Thorac Cardiovasc Surg.* 2003;126:1134–1140.

101 Type B2 Thymoma (Lymphoepithelial or Cortical Thymoma)

Borislav A. Alexiev, M.D., and Fabio R. Tavora, M.D., Ph.D.

Terminology

Type B2 thymoma is an organotypic thymic epithelial neoplasm composed of large, polygonal tumor cells that are arranged in a loose network and exhibit large vesicular nuclei with prominent large nucleoli, closely resembling the predominant epithelial cells of the normal thymic cortex.[1] A background population of immature T cells is always present and usually outnumbers the neoplastic epithelial cells.[2] The postulated cell of origin is a thymic epithelial cell capable of differentiating toward cortical-type epithelial cells.[2]

Incidence and Clinical

Type B2 thymoma accounts for ~18% to 42% of all thymomas and depends on the study cited.[3,4] Patients' ages range from 13 to 79 years, with a mean of 47 to 50 years.[3-5] There is no consistent gender predominance.[6,7]

The most frequent manifestations are symptoms of myasthenia gravis in 30% to 82% of cases.[3,4,6,8,9] Rare complications are hypogammaglobulinemia (Good syndrome) and pure red cell anaplasia.[10] Patients with type B2 thymoma may experience symptoms caused by compression of the surrounding organs by an expansive mass. These problems may take the form of superior vena cava syndrome, dysphagia, cough, or chest pain. Some patients with type B2 thymoma have no symptoms at all, and the tumor can be detected for an unrelated problem as an enlarged mediastinal area or mass by x-ray, CT, or MRI.

Gross Pathology

Grossly, type B2 thymomas are encapsulated or vaguely circumscribed.[9] The cut surface is soft or firm and exhibits a tan nodular/lobular architecture. There may be cystic changes, hemorrhage, and fibrosis.[2] The tumor can invade mediastinal fat or adjacent organs.

Microscopic Pathology

Histologically, B2 thymoma demonstrates a coarse lobular architecture with irregular septa (Fig. 101.1), somewhat resembling the lobular architecture of the normal thymic cortex. The neoplastic cell component consists of a prominent large polygonal epithelial cell population with vesicular nuclei and prominent nucleoli admixed with numerous lymphocytes (Figs. 101.1 and 101.2). The neoplastic epithelial cells form a delicate loose network, forming palisades around perivascular spaces and along septa. The tumor lacks extensive areas of virtually pure epithelial cells or pure lymphocytes. This type of thymoma resembles type B1 thymoma in its predominance of lymphocytes, but foci of medullary differentiation are less conspicuous or absent. Lymphocytes may outnumber the epithelial cells but do not obscure them. Lymphoid follicles in perivascular spaces or septa are more frequent in myasthenia gravis–associated cases.

Special Studies

The neoplastic cells strongly express a CK5/6, CK903, and p63 pattern similar to normal cortical thymocytes (Fig. 101.3). Focal positivity for CK8/18 and CK7 may also be observed.[2] Epithelial membrane antigen (EMA), CK20, CD20, CD117, and CD5 stains are negative in tumor cells.[11] Admixed intratumoral lymphocytes demonstrate a cortical immature T-cell immunoprofile: TdT+, CD1a+, CD99+, CD3+, CD4+, CD8+, and CD5+ with high proliferation rate (Figs. 101.4 and 101.5).[12] Lymphocytes in rare medullary islands are mostly mature T cells: CD3+, CD5+, CD1a-, CD99-, TdT-, and significantly less proliferative.[5,6,13,14]

More than 80% of B2 thymomas are aneuploid and share recurrent genetic alterations at chromosomes 5q (adenomatous polyposis coli locus), 7p, 8p,13q (retinoblastoma locus), and 17p (p53) with a subset of type B3 thymomas.[15,16]

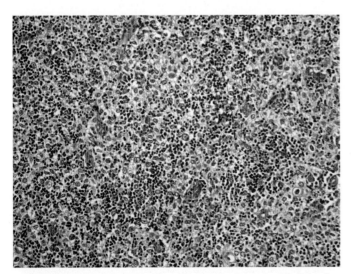

FIGURE 101.1 ▲ Type B2 thymoma. Note prominent epithelial cell population admixed with numerous intratumoral lymphocytes (H&E, ×200).

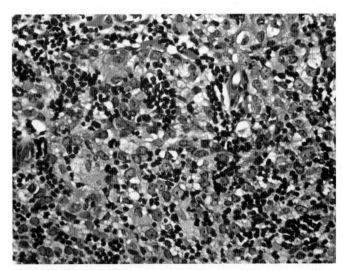

FIGURE 101.2 ▲ Type B2 thymoma. Note large polygonal epithelial cells with vesicular nuclei and prominent nucleoli admixed with numerous intratumoral lymphocytes (H&E, ×400).

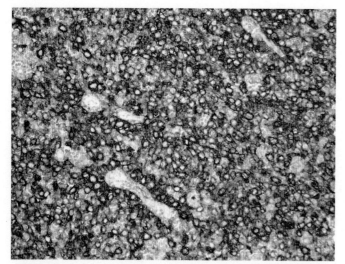

FIGURE 101.3 ▲ Type B2 thymoma. Note strong CK5/6 expression in neoplastic cells (anti-CK5/6, ×200).

Differential Diagnosis

B1 thymoma is also lymphocyte rich, but epithelial cells are inconspicuous, smaller, and less numerous than in B2 thymomas.[2] In addition, the nuclei and nucleoli are smaller and the medullary islands are more prominent than in B2 thymomas.[2] B3 thymoma, in contrast to B2 thymoma, is relatively lymphocyte poor. Neoplastic epithelial cells form confluent sheets and solid areas with a small but distinctive population of intraepithelial immature T cells. The neoplastic cells are usually slightly smaller than those of B2 thymoma, with irregular nuclear membranes, smaller nucleoli, nuclear grooves, and less vesicular chromatin. T lymphoblastic lymphoma may exhibit the same immunophenotype of lymphoid cells as those of B2 thymomas. However, the epithelial network is destroyed (negative CK5/6), and lymphoblasts usually infiltrate beyond the epithelial compartment into the thymic septa and mediastinal fat. Very high CDK6 expression is a distinguishing feature of T lymphoblastic lymphoma.[2]

Treatment and Prognosis

Surgery is the mainstay of treatment, and complete resection is associated with the best prognosis.[17–20] Although practices vary, neoadjuvant chemotherapy is often used to improve resectability. Extended

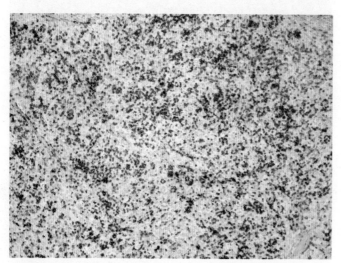

FIGURE 101.4 ▲ Type B2 thymoma. Note CD3-positive intratumoral T cells (anti-CD3, ×200).

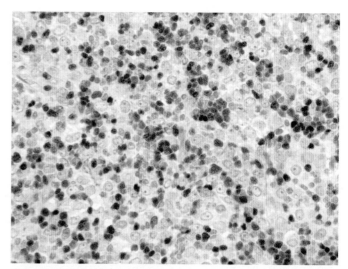

FIGURE 101.5 ▲ Type B2 thymoma. Note numerous TdT-positive intratumoral T cells (anti-TdT, ×400).

resections following neoadjuvant treatment have been safely performed for locally advanced tumors.[17]

Type B2 thymoma is a tumor of moderate malignancy, with higher malignant potential than A, AB, and B1 thymoma, but appears to be slightly less aggressive than type B3 thymoma.[21] It is often invasive, thus nonresectable at presentation in 5% to 15% of cases. Recurrences, even after complete resection, are reported in 5% to 9% and metastases in up to 11%.[7–9] Reported 10-year survival rates range between 50% and 100%.[4,7–9,22] Staging is the most important prognostic indicator, whereas age, gender, and myasthenia gravis are not significant prognostic parameters.[3–5] In regard to the prognosis, the 5- and 10-year survivals for type B2 thymoma are 85% and 85%, respectively.[21]

REFERENCES

1. Roden AC, Yi ES, Jenkins SM, et al. Reproducibility of 3 histologic classifications and 3 staging systems for thymic epithelial neoplasms and its effect on prognosis. *Am J Surg Pathol.* 2015;39:427–441.
2. Marchevsky AM, Marx A, Ströbel P, et al. Type B2 thymoma. In: Travis WD, et al., eds. *WHO Classification of Tumours of the Lung, Pleura, Mediastinum and Heart.* Lyon, France: IARC Press; 2015:199–201.
3. Chalabreysse L, Roy P, Cordier JF, et al. Correlation of the WHO schema for the classification of thymic epithelial neoplasms with prognosis: a retrospective study of 90 tumors. *Am J Surg Pathol.* 2002;26:1605–1611.
4. Chen G, Marx A, Chen WH, et al. New WHO histologic classification predicts prognosis of thymic epithelial tumors: a clinicopathologic study of 200 thymoma cases from China. *Cancer.* 2002;95:420–429.
5. Hattori H, Tateyama H, Tada T, et al. PE-35-related antigen expression and CD1a-positive lymphocytes in thymoma subtypes based on Muller-Hermelink classification. An immunohistochemical study using catalyzed signal amplification. *Virchows Arch.* 2000;436:20–27.
6. Kirchner T, Schalke B, Marx A, et al. Evaluation of prognostic features in thymic epithelial tumors. *Thymus.* 1989;14:195–203.
7. Okumura M, Ohta M, Tateyama H, et al. The World Health Organization histologic classification system reflects the oncologic behavior of thymoma: a clinical study of 273 patients. *Cancer.* 2002;94:624–632.
8. Okumura M, Ohta M, Miyoshi S, et al. Oncological significance of WHO histological thymoma classification. A clinical study based on 286 patients. *Jpn J Thorac Cardiovasc Surg.* 2002;50:189–194.
9. Quintanilla-Martinez L, Wilkins EW Jr, Ferry JA, et al. Thymoma—morphologic subclassification correlates with invasiveness and immunohistologic features: a study of 122 cases. *Hum Pathol.* 1993;24:958–969.
10. Kelleher P, Misbah SA. What is Good's syndrome? Immunological abnormalities in patients with thymoma. *J Clin Pathol.* 2003;56:12–16.
11. Alexiev BA, Drachenberg CB, Burke AP. Thymomas: a cytological and immunohistochemical study, with emphasis on lymphoid and neuroendocrine markers. *Diagn Pathol.* 2007;2:13.

12. Chan JK, Tsang WY, Seneviratne S, et al. The MIC2 antibody 013. Practical application for the study of thymic epithelial tumors. *Am J Surg Pathol.* 1995;19:1115–1123.
13. Moran CA, Kalhor N, Suster S. Invasive spindle cell thymomas (WHO Type A): a clinicopathologic correlation of 41 cases. *Am J Clin Pathol.* 2010;134:793–798.
14. Chilosi M, Doglioni C, Yan Z, et al. Differential expression of cyclin-dependent kinase 6 in cortical thymocytes and T-cell lymphoblastic lymphoma/leukemia. *Am J Pathol.* 1998;152:209–217.
15. Inoue M, Starostik P, Zettl A, et al. Correlating genetic aberrations with World Health Organization-defined histology and stage across the spectrum of thymomas. *Cancer Res.* 2003;63:3708–3715.
16. Gschwendtner A, Fend F, Hoffmann Y, et al. DNA-ploidy analysis correlates with the histogenetic classification of thymic epithelial tumours. *J Pathol.* 1999;189:576–580.
17. Ahmad U, Huang J. Current readings: The most influential and recent studies involving surgical management of thymoma. *Semin Thorac Cardiovasc Surg.* 2013;25:144–149.
18. Rajan A, Giaccone G. Treatment of advanced thymoma and thymic carcinoma. *Curr Treat Options Oncol.* 2008;9:277–287.
19. Wright CD, Kessler KA. Surgical treatment of thymic tumors. *Semin Thorac Cardiovasc Surg.* 2005;17:20–26.
20. Wright CD, Wain JC, Wong DR, et al. Predictors of recurrence in thymic tumors: importance of invasion, World Health Organization histology, and size. *J Thorac Cardiovasc Surg.* 2005;130:1413–1421.
21. Nakagawa K, Asamura H, Matsuno Y, et al. Thymoma: a clinicopathologic study based on the new World Health Organization classification. *J Thorac Cardiovasc Surg.* 2003;126:1134–1140.
22. Pan CC, Chen WY, Chiang H. Spindle cell and mixed spindle/lymphocytic thymomas: an integrated clinicopathologic and immunohistochemical study of 81 cases. *Am J Surg Pathol.* 2001;25:111–120.

102 Type B3 Thymoma (Epithelial-Rich, Cortical, Atypical)

Borislav A. Alexiev, M.D., and Anja C. Roden, M.D.

Terminology

Type B3 thymoma is an organotypic thymic epithelial tumor predominantly composed of medium-sized round or polygonal cells with slight atypia. The epithelial cells are mixed with a minor component of intraepithelial lymphocytes, resulting in a sheet-like growth of epithelial cells. The postulated cell of origin is a thymic epithelial cell capable of differentiating toward a less differentiated cortical-type epithelial cell than in B2 thymoma.[1]

Incidence and Clinical

Type B3 thymomas account for ~7% to 31% of all thymomas, the range reflecting imprecision in distinction from other B thymomas or thymic carcinoma. Patients' ages range from 14 to 78 years, with a mean of 45 to 50 years. There is no consistent gender predominance.[2–9]

The most frequent manifestations are symptoms of myasthenia gravis in 27% to 77% of cases.[2–9] Rare complications are hypogammaglobulinemia (Good syndrome) and pure red cell anaplasia.[6,7,10] Patients with type B3 thymoma may experience symptoms caused by compression of the surrounding organs by an expansive mass, including but not limited to superior vena cava syndrome, dysphagia, cough, or chest pain. Some patients with type B3 thymoma have no symptoms at all, and the tumor can be detected for an unrelated problem as an enlarged mediastinal area or mass by x-ray, CT, or MR imaging.

Gross Pathology

Grossly, type B3 thymomas are usually not encapsulated but show a vaguely infiltrative border with extension into mediastinal fat or adjacent organs (Fig. 102.1).[1] The cut surface is typically firm and exhibits gray to white nodules separated by white fibrous septa.[1] Soft yellow or red foci, cyst formation, or hard calcified regions indicative of regressive changes may be observed.

Microscopic Pathology

Histologically, B3 thymoma demonstrates a lobular growth pattern with irregular septa, somewhat resembling the lobular architecture of the normal thymic cortex. The neoplastic cell component consists of sheets of medium-sized polygonal epithelial cells with eosinophilic to clear cytoplasm admixed with a minor component of lymphocytes (Figs. 102.2 and 102.3). In some type B3 thymomas, immature T lymphocytes might be absent. Foci of medullary differentiation are absent. The nuclei are round or elongated, often folded or grooved,

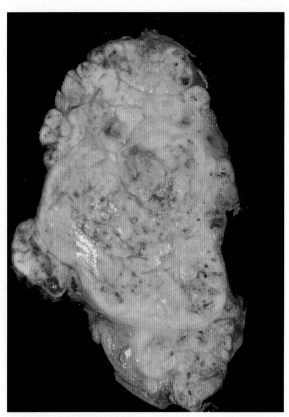

FIGURE 102.1 ▲ B3 thymoma with macroscopic evidence of invasion.

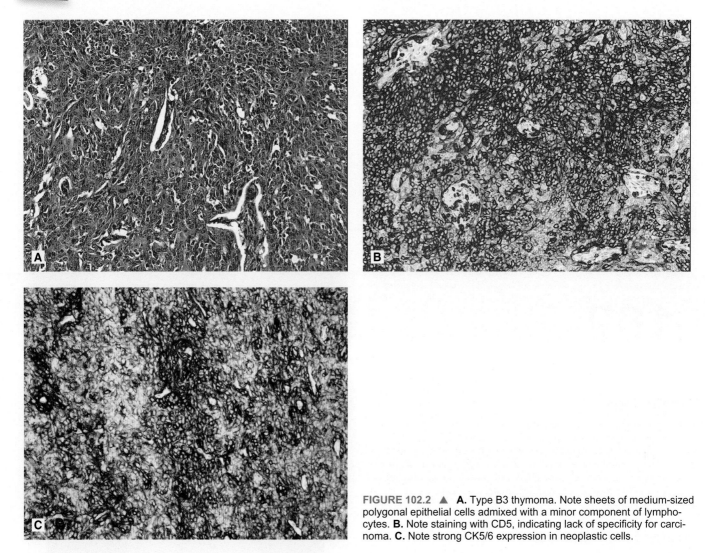

FIGURE 102.2 ▲ **A.** Type B3 thymoma. Note sheets of medium-sized polygonal epithelial cells admixed with a minor component of lymphocytes. **B.** Note staining with CD5, indicating lack of specificity for carcinoma. **C.** Note strong CK5/6 expression in neoplastic cells.

and characteristically smaller with less prominent nucleoli than in B2 thymoma (Figs. 102.2 and 102.3). The neoplastic epithelial cells might form palisades around perivascular spaces and along septa. Small foci of keratinization mimicking Hassall corpuscles may be present.

In a minority of cases, tumor cells with round nuclei and prominent nucleoli resembling those of type B2 thymomas may be observed. Clear cell changes, spindle cell formation, and occasionally giant cells may also occur. Mitoses are rare.

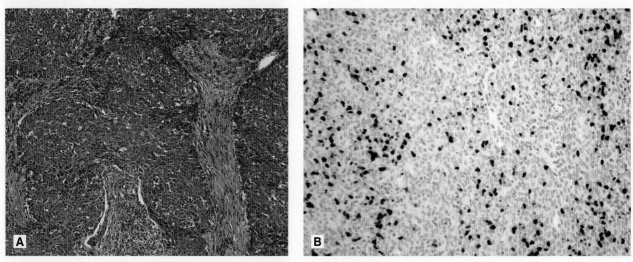

FIGURE 102.3 ▲ Type B3 thymoma. **A.** On low magnification, the tumor grows as sheets and is generally recognizable as an epithelial neoplasm. **B.** Note TdT-positive intratumoral T cells (anti-TdT, ×200).

Special Studies

The neoplastic cells strongly express CK5/6, CK903, and p63 similar to normal cortical thymocytes.[11,12] Focal weak EMA and occasional strong CD5 positivity may also be observed, in contrast to B2 thymomas[11] (Fig. 102.2B, C). CK20, CD20, MUC1, and CD117 stains are negative in these tumors.[13] If present, admixed scattered intratumoral lymphocytes demonstrate a cortical immature T-cell immunoprofile: TdT+ (Fig. 102.3B), CD1a+, CD99+, CD3+, CD4+, CD8+, and CD5+ with high proliferation rate.[14]

Virtually 100% of B3 thymomas are aneuploid by DNA cytometry and share recurrent genetic alterations at chromosomes 5q, 7p, 8p, 13q, and 17p with type B2 thymomas.[12,15,16]

Differential Diagnosis

Type A thymoma may resemble the spindle cell variant of B3 thymoma. In type A thymoma, the degree of atypia is lower, and perivascular spaces with epithelial palisades are absent. In contrast to A thymoma, type B3 thymoma is strongly positive for CK5/6. EMA shows only low expression or is absent in type B3 thymoma. Scattered cortical immature T cells, positive for TdT, CD1a, and CD99, as commonly seen in the B3 types of thymoma, are often absent in type A thymoma.[9] Low-grade squamous cell carcinoma of the thymus shows more pronounced squamous differentiation, usually with readily detectable intercellular bridges, and is characterized by a distorted architecture and presence of desmoplastic stromal reaction. Immature intraepithelial T lymphocytes are absent in thymic carcinoma. Also, immunolabeling for Ki-67 proliferation index may be helpful in distinguishing carcinoma from thymoma.[17]

Treatment and Prognosis

Surgery is the mainstay of treatment, and complete resection is associated with the best prognosis.[18–20] Although practices vary, neoadjuvant chemotherapy is often used to improve resectability. Extended resections following neoadjuvant treatment have been safely performed for locally advanced tumors.[18]

Type B3 thymoma is a tumor of moderate malignancy, with higher malignant potential than A, AB, and B1 thymoma.[5,9,21,22] Some have shown that patients with type B3 thymomas have worse prognosis than do those with type B2 thymomas, whereas others have reported no significant difference in survival between these two groups.[2,3,6,21,23] The tumor is less aggressive than thymic carcinoma. B3 thymoma is often invasive and thus nonresectable at presentation. Recurrences, even after complete resection, and metastases are reported.[21,24] Staging is the most important prognostic indicator, whereas age, gender, and myasthenia gravis are not significant prognostic parameters.[2,3,24–26]

REFERENCES

1. Marx A, Ströbel P, Badve S, et al. Type B3 thymoma. In: Travis WD, et al., eds. *WHO Classification of Tumours of the Lung, Pleura, Mediastinum and Heart.* Lyon, France: IARC Press; 2015:202–204.
2. Chalabreysse L, Roy P, Cordier JF, et al. Correlation of the WHO schema for the classification of thymic epithelial neoplasms with prognosis: a retrospective study of 90 tumors. *Am J Surg Pathol.* 2002;26:1605–1611.
3. Chen G, Marx A, Chen WH, et al. New WHO histologic classification predicts prognosis of thymic epithelial tumors: a clinicopathologic study of 200 thymoma cases from China. *Cancer.* 2002;95:420–429.
4. Kim HK, Choi YS, Kim J, et al. Type B thymoma: is prognosis predicted only by World Health Organization classification? *J Thorac Cardiovasc Surg.* 2010;139:1431–1435e1.
5. Kirchner T, Schalke B, Marx A, et al. Evaluation of prognostic features in thymic epithelial tumors. *Thymus.* 1989;14:195–203.
6. Okumura M, Ohta M, Miyoshi S, et al. Oncological significance of WHO histological thymoma classification. A clinical study based on 286 patients. *Jpn J Thorac Cardiovasc Surg.* 2002;50:189–194.
7. Okumura M, Ohta M, Tateyama H, et al. The World Health Organization histologic classification system reflects the oncologic behavior of thymoma: a clinical study of 273 patients. *Cancer.* 2002;94:624–632.
8. Pan CC, Chen WY, Chiang H. Spindle cell and mixed spindle/lymphocytic thymomas: an integrated clinicopathologic and immunohistochemical study of 81 cases. *Am J Surg Pathol.* 2001;25:111–120.
9. Quintanilla-Martinez L, Wilkins EW Jr, Ferry JA, et al. Thymoma—morphologic subclassification correlates with invasiveness and immunohistologic features: a study of 122 cases. *Hum Pathol.* 1993;24:958–969.
10. Kelleher P, Misbah SA. What is Good's syndrome? Immunological abnormalities in patients with thymoma. *J Clin Pathol.* 2003;56:12–16.
11. Alexiev BA, Drachenberg CB, Burke AP. Thymomas: a cytological and immunohistochemical study, with emphasis on lymphoid and neuroendocrine markers. *Diagn Pathol.* 2007;2:13.
12. Weissferdt A, Hernandez JC, Kalhor N, et al. Spindle cell thymomas: an immunohistochemical study of 30 cases. *Appl Immunohistochem Mol Morphol.* 2011;19:329–335.
13. Kaira K, Murakami H, Serizawa M, et al. MUC1 expression in thymic epithelial tumors: MUC1 may be useful marker as differential diagnosis between type B3 thymoma and thymic carcinoma. *Virchows Arch.* 2011;458:615–620.
14. Kojika M, Ishii G, Yoshida J, et al. Immunohistochemical differential diagnosis between thymic carcinoma and type B3 thymoma: diagnostic utility of hypoxic marker, GLUT-1, in thymic epithelial neoplasms. *Mod Pathol.* 2009;22:1341–1350.
15. Gschwendtner A, Fend F, Hoffmann Y, et al. DNA-ploidy analysis correlates with the histogenetic classification of thymic epithelial tumours. *J Pathol.* 1999;189:576–580.
16. Inoue M, Starostik P, Zettl A, et al. Correlating genetic aberrations with World Health Organization-defined histology and stage across the spectrum of thymomas. *Cancer Res.* 2003;63:3708–3715.
17. Roden AC, Yi ES, Jenkins SM, et al. Diagnostic significance of cell kinetic parameters in World Health Organization type A and B3 thymomas and thymic carcinomas. *Hum Pathol.* 2015;46:17–25.
18. Ahmad U, Huang J. Current readings: the most influential and recent studies involving surgical management of thymoma. *Semin Thorac Cardiovasc Surg.* 2013;25:144–149.
19. Rajan A, Giaccone G. Treatment of advanced thymoma and thymic carcinoma. *Curr Treat Options Oncol.* 2008;9:277–287.
20. Wright CD, Wain JC, Wong DR, et al. Predictors of recurrence in thymic tumors: importance of invasion, World Health Organization histology, and size. *J Thorac Cardiovasc Surg.* 2005;130:1413–1421.
21. Nakagawa K, Asamura H, Matsuno Y, et al. Thymoma: a clinicopathologic study based on the new World Health Organization classification. *J Thorac Cardiovasc Surg.* 2003;126:1134–1140.
22. Roden AC, Yi ES, Jenkins SM, et al. Modified Masaoka stage and size are independent prognostic predictors in thymoma and modified Masaoka stage is superior to histopathologic classifications. *J Thorac Oncol.* 2015;10:691–700.
23. Strobel P, Bauer A, Puppe B, et al. Tumor recurrence and survival in patients treated for thymomas and thymic squamous cell carcinomas: a retrospective analysis. *J Clin Oncol.* 2004;22:1501–1509.
24. Kondo K, Yoshizawa K, Tsuyuguchi M, et al. WHO histologic classification is a prognostic indicator in thymoma. *Ann Thorac Surg.* 2004;77:1183–1188.
25. Moran CA, Walsh G, Suster S, et al. Thymomas II: a clinicopathologic correlation of 250 cases with a proposed staging system with emphasis on pathologic assessment. *Am J Clin Pathol.* 2012;137:451–461.
26. Ruffini E, Filosso PL, Mossetti C, et al. Thymoma: inter-relationships among World Health Organization histology, Masaoka staging and myasthenia gravis and their independent prognostic significance: a single-centre experience. *Eur J Cardiothorac Surg.* 2011;40:146–153.

103 Type AB Thymoma (Mixed Thymoma)

Borislav A. Alexiev, M.D., and Anja C. Roden, M.D.

Terminology

Type AB thymoma is an organotypical thymic epithelial neoplasm composed of a mixture of a lymphocyte-poor type A thymoma component and more lymphocyte-rich type B areas.[1] There is a great variation in the proportion of the two components, and while usually both components are present in most sections, either type A or type B areas can be scanty. The cellular origin of the type A component, like in type A thymoma, has been postulated to derive from or differentiate toward thymic medullary epithelial cells.[2,3] The type B component ultrastructurally resembles epithelial cells at the corticomedullary junction but is similar to thymic subcapsular epithelial cells in expression of CK14; thus, its normal counterpart is uncertain.[1,4]

Incidence and Clinical

Type AB thymoma is either the most or the second most common type of thymoma and accounts for 15% to 43% of all thymomas.[1] The patients' ages range from 29 to 82 years. A slight male predominance has been noted in most reports.[1]

The clinical presentation is similar to that of type A thymoma. Approximately 14% of type AB thymomas are associated with myasthenia gravis.[5–7] Paraneoplastic pure red cell aplasia has also been reported.[8] Other tumors manifest by local symptoms or can be asymptomatic and are found incidentally upon x-ray, CT, or MR imaging examination.

Gross Pathology

Grossly, type AB thymoma is usually encapsulated and the cut surface shows multiple tan-colored nodules of various sizes separated by white fibrous bands.

Microscopic Pathology

Histologically, type AB thymoma shows a nodular growth pattern with diffuse areas and is composed of a variable mixture of a lymphocyte-poor type A thymoma component and lymphocyte-rich type B areas (Figs. 103.1 and 103.2). A type B3 thymoma component is not part of

AB thymoma. All histologic features of type A thymoma can be seen in the type A component. The tumor cells in the type B component are composed predominantly of small polygonal epithelial cells with small round, oval, or spindle pale nuclei showing dispersed chromatin and inconspicuous nucleoli (Fig. 103.3).[9] In contrast to type B2 thymoma, large epithelial cells with prominent nucleoli and vesicular nuclei and nucleoli are uncommon.[9] The type A and type B–like components either form discrete separate nodules or intermix together.[2] The type A component in the latter areas may form bundles of elongated fibroblast-like spindle cells. Type B areas harbor lymphocytes in variable numbers, and medullary differentiation is rarely observed. In particular, Hassall corpuscles are absent. There is a great variation in the proportion of both components, and in particular, type A areas can be extremely scanty to almost absent.[2,9]

Special Studies

The immunoprofile of type AB thymoma is essentially similar to those of type A thymoma (EMA+, vimentin+), except that the epithelial cells in type B areas are usually strongly CK5/6+ and CK14+ (Figs. 103.4 and 103.5).[10,11] CD20+ tumor cells can be seen in both type A and type B areas. In contrast to type A thymoma areas, the type B components are negative or only weakly positive for EMA. Ki-67 expression is low or absent.[1] There is no expression of CD5 in epithelial cells.[10] The lymphocytes in the type A component/foci of medullary differentiation are distinctively CD3+ and CD5+ mature T cells. B cells are usually absent. In the lymphocyte-rich areas (type B component), associated lymphocytes are immature T cells positive for CD3, CD5, TdT, CD1a, and CD99 (Fig. 103.6).[10]

Deletion of chromosome 6 with or without formation of ring chromosome 6 has been found in type AB thymoma.[12] In addition, recurrent allelic imbalances have been described in individual cases.[13] Loss of heterozygosity at 5q21-22 (APC), as seen in type B thymoma, has been detected in a minority of type AB thymoma.[13]

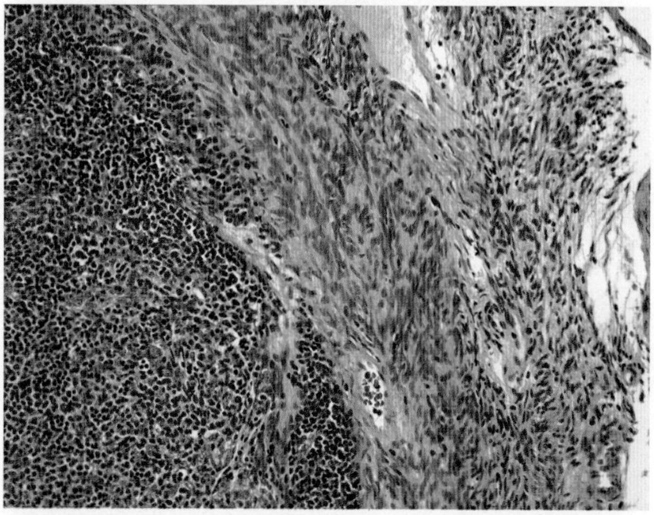

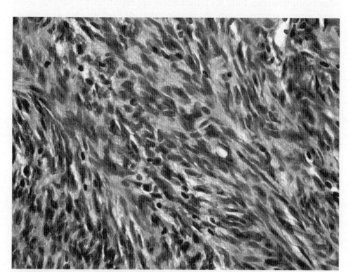

FIGURE 103.1 ▲ Type AB thymoma. Note lymphocyte-poor type A and lymphocyte-rich type B components (H&E, ×100).

FIGURE 103.2 ▲ Type AB thymoma. Note proliferation of spindle and/or oval epithelial tumor cells arranged in fascicles in lymphocyte-poor type A component (H&E, ×400).

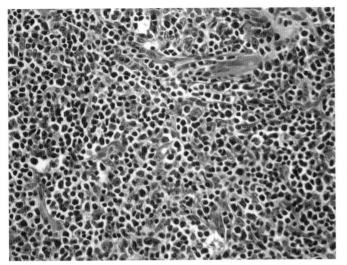

FIGURE 103.3 ▲ Type AB thymoma. Note polygonal epithelial tumor cells with small round, oval, or spindle nuclei and inconspicuous nucleoli in lymphocyte-rich type B component (H&E, ×400).

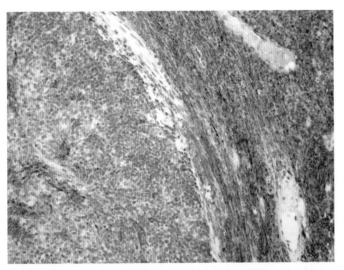

FIGURE 103.4 ▲ Type AB thymoma. Note strong EMA expression in type A component. Tumor cells in type B component are only focally positive (anti-EMA, ×200).

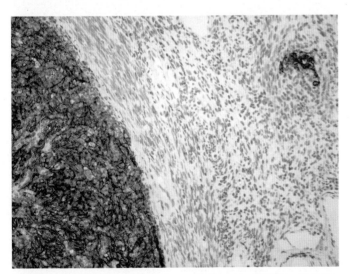

FIGURE 103.5 ▲ Type AB thymoma. Note strong CK5/6 expression in type B component. Tumor cells in type A component are only weekly positive (anti-CK5/6, ×200).

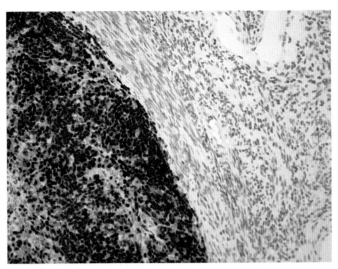

FIGURE 103.6 ▲ Type AB thymoma. The lymphocytes in the type B component are distinctively TdT-positive immature T cells. Immature T cells are absent in type A component (anti-TdT, ×200).

Differential Diagnosis

Conventional AB type thymomas should be differentiated from micronodular thymoma (MNT). In contrast to type AB and other organotypic thymomas, the lymphocytic-rich areas in MNT do not contain epithelium (negative CK5/6) and stromal lymphocytes are mostly mature B and T cells with a predominant cell population of B lymphocytes.[14]

Treatment and Prognosis

Surgery is the mainstay of treatment, and complete resection is associated with the best prognosis.[15–17]

Recurrence and metastasis are exceptionally rare.[18–20] The overall survival rate of patients with type AB thymoma is 80% to 100% at 5 years and 10 years.[4,5]

REFERENCES

1. Ströbel P, Marx A, Badve S, et al. Type AB thymoma. In: Travis WD, et al., eds. *WHO Classification of Tumours of the Lung, Pleura, Mediastinum and Heart*. Lyon, France: IARC Press; 2015:193–195.
2. Muller-Hermelink HK, Marx A. Pathological aspects of malignant and benign thymic disorders. *Ann Med.* 1999;31(suppl 2):5–14.
3. Muller-Hermelink HK, Marx A. Thymoma. *Curr Opin Oncol.* 2000;12:426–433.
4. Kirchner T, Schalke B, Marx A, et al. Evaluation of prognostic features in thymic epithelial tumors. *Thymus.* 1989;14:195–203.
5. Chen G, Marx A, Chen WH, et al. New WHO histologic classification predicts prognosis of thymic epithelial tumors: a clinicopathologic study of 200 thymoma cases from China. *Cancer.* 2002;95:420–429.
6. Nakagawa K, Asamura H, Matsuno Y, et al. Thymoma: a clinicopathologic study based on the new World Health Organization classification. *J Thorac Cardiovasc Surg.* 2003;126:1134–1140.
7. Pan CC, Chen WY, Chiang H. Spindle cell and mixed spindle/lymphocytic thymomas: an integrated clinicopathologic and immunohistochemical study of 81 cases. *Am J Surg Pathol.* 2001;25:111–120.
8. Kelleher P, Misbah SA. What is Good's syndrome? Immunological abnormalities in patients with thymoma. *J Clin Pathol.* 2003;56:12–16.
9. Kuo TT. Cytokeratin profiles of the thymus and thymomas: histogenetic correlations and proposal for a histological classification of thymomas. *Histopathology.* 2000;36:403–414.
10. Alexiev BA, Drachenberg CB, Burke AP. Thymomas: a cytological and immunohistochemical study, with emphasis on lymphoid and neuroendocrine markers. *Diagn Pathol.* 2007;2:13.

11. Kuo T, Lo SK. Immunohistochemical metallothionein expression in thymoma: correlation with histological types and cellular origin. *Histopathology.* 1997;30:243–248.

12. Van den Berghe I, Debiec-Rychter M, Proot L, et al. Ring chromosome 6 may represent a cytogenetic subgroup in benign thymoma. *Cancer Genet Cytogenet.* 2002;137:75–77.

13. Inoue M, Starostik P, Zettl A, et al. Correlating genetic aberrations with World Health Organization-defined histology and stage across the spectrum of thymomas. *Cancer Res.* 2003;63:3708–3715.

14. Kim HK, Choi YS, Kim J, et al. Type B thymoma: is prognosis predicted only by World Health Organization classification? *J Thorac Cardiovasc Surg.* 2010;139:1431–1435.e1.

15. Kondo K, Yoshizawa K, Tsuyuguchi M, et al. WHO histologic classification is a prognostic indicator in thymoma. *Ann Thorac Surg.* 2004;77:1183–1188.

16. Rajan A, Giaccone G. Treatment of advanced thymoma and thymic carcinoma. *Curr Treat Options Oncol.* 2008;9:277–287.

17. Wright CD, Wain JC, Wong DR, et al. Predictors of recurrence in thymic tumors: importance of invasion, World Health Organization histology, and size. *J Thorac Cardiovasc Surg.* 2005;130:1413–1421.

18. Koga K, Matsuno Y, Noguchi M, et al. A review of 79 thymomas: modification of staging system and reappraisal of conventional division into invasive and non-invasive thymoma. *Pathol Int.* 1994;44:359–367.

19. Moran CA, Walsh G, Suster S, et al. Thymomas II: a clinicopathologic correlation of 250 cases with a proposed staging system with emphasis on pathologic assessment. *Am J Clin Pathol.* 2012;137:451–461.

20. Ruffini E, Filosso PL, Lausi P, et al. Recurrence of thymoma. *Eur J Cardiothorac Surg.* 2011;40:900–901.

104 Micronodular Thymoma with Lymphoid Stroma

Borislav A. Alexiev, M.D., and Anja C. Roden, M.D.

Terminology

Micronodular thymoma (MNT) is an organotypical thymic epithelial neoplasm characterized by multiple, discrete epithelial nodules separated by an abundant lymphocytic stroma that usually contains prominent germinal centers.[1] The epithelial component is similar to type A thymoma.

Incidence and Clinical

MNT is an uncommon entity and corresponds to1% to 5% of all thymomas.[1] The age at manifestation ranges from 45 to 95 years. There is no sex predilection.[1]

MNT is rarely (<5%) associated with paraneoplastic myasthenia gravis. Other autoimmune phenomena that are common in other thymoma types have not been reported. Clinical features usually are related to the size and local extension of the tumor. MNT can be asymptomatic and is found incidentally upon x-ray, CT, or MRI examination.[1]

Gross Pathology

Grossly, MNT is usually encapsulated, and the cut surface shows multiple tan-colored nodules of various sizes separated by white fibrous bands and cystic changes.

Microscopic Pathology

Histologically, MNT shows a micronodular growth pattern.[1–7] Multiple, discrete epithelial nodules are separated by an abundant lymphocytic stroma that may contain lymphoid follicles with prominent germinal centers (Fig. 104.1). There are a variable number of mature plasma cells. The epithelial nodules are composed of slender or plump spindle cells with bland-looking oval nuclei and inconspicuous nucleoli (Fig. 104.2). Micro- and macrocystic areas, particularly in subcapsular localization, are common. There are no Hassall corpuscles or perivascular spaces. Mitotic activity is

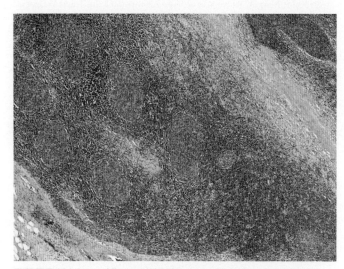

FIGURE 104.1 ▲ Micronodular thymoma. Note discrete epithelial nodules are separated by an abundant lymphocytic stroma.

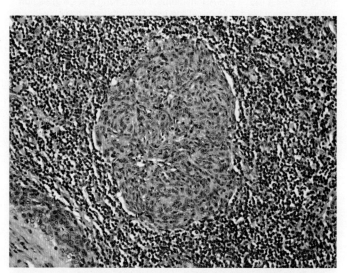

FIGURE 104.2 ▲ Micronodular thymoma. Epithelial nodules are composed of slender or plump spindle cells with bland-looking oval nuclei and inconspicuous nucleoli.

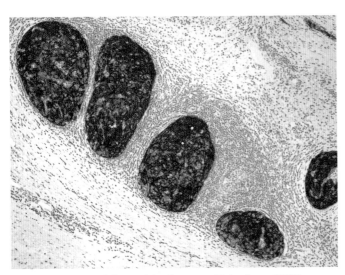

FIGURE 104.3 ▲ Micronodular thymoma. Note strong CK5/6 expression (anti-CK5/6).

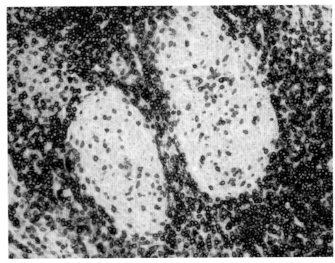

FIGURE 104.5 ▲ Micronodular thymoma. Note strong CD3 expression in lymphocytic stroma (anti-CD3).

absent or minimal. The epithelial nodules contain few interspersed lymphocytes.

MNTs have been described in a multilocular thymic cyst.[8] A case of ectopic MNT in the neck near the parotid gland has been reported.[9]

Special Studies

Immunohistochemically, neoplastic epithelial cells in MNT are strongly positive for CK5/6 (Fig. 104.3), EMA, and CD57 and focally for CK7. CK20, vimentin, and CD5 are all negative.[2,6,7,10] The stroma is composed of large lymphocytic aggregates containing predominantly B lymphocytes (CD20+) (Fig. 104.4) and mature T cells (CD3+, CD5+) (Fig. 104.5). The B cells frequently form follicles with or without germinal centers with a well-developed network of follicular dendritic cells and a population of CD57+ T cells. Immature T cells are restricted to a narrow band surrounding the epithelial cell nodules (Fig. 104.6). Intratumoral lymphocytes are scarce. In rare cases, intratumoral

immature T lymphocytes may be numerous and express CD3, CD5, CD1a, CD99, and TdT, with high Ki-67 proliferation index (>80%). Plasma cells are usually polyclonal.

No specific chromosome abnormalities are described for MNTs.

Differential Diagnosis

MNT should be differentiated from conventional AB-type thymoma. In contrast to type AB and other organotypic thymomas, the lymphocytic-rich areas in MNT do not contain epithelium (negative CK5/6), and stromal lymphocytes are mostly mature B and T cells with a predominant cell population of B lymphocytes.

Treatment and Prognosis

Surgery is the mainstay of treatment. MNT usually presents at Masaoka stage I or II. There have been no reports on recurrences, metastasis, or tumor-related deaths.

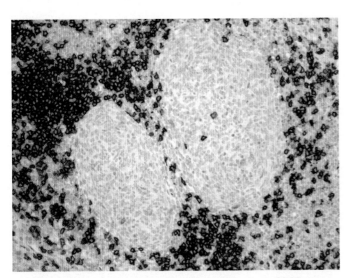

FIGURE 104.4 ▲ Micronodular thymoma. Note strong CD20 expression in lymphocytic stroma (anti-CD20).

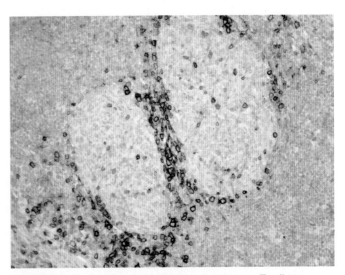

FIGURE 104.6 ▲ Micronodular thymoma. Immature T cells are restricted to a narrow band surrounding the epithelial cell nodules. Intratumoral lymphocytes are scarce (anti-CD99).

REFERENCES

1. Tateyama H, Marx A, Ströbel P, et al. Micronodular thymoma with lymphoid stroma. In: Travis WD, et al., eds. *WHO Classification of Tumours of the Lung, Pleura, Mediastinum and Heart*. Lyon, France: IARC Press; 2015:205–206.
2. Ishikawa Y, Tateyama H, Yoshida M, et al. Micronodular thymoma with lymphoid stroma: an immunohistochemical study of the distribution of Langerhans cells and mature dendritic cells in six patients. *Histopathology*. 2015;66:300–307.
3. Mneimneh WS, Gokmen-Polar Y, Kesler KA, et al. Micronodular thymic neoplasms: case series and literature review with emphasis on the spectrum of differentiation. *Mod Pathol*. 2015;28(11):1415–1427.
4. Strobel P, Marino M, Feuchtenberger M, et al. Micronodular thymoma: an epithelial tumour with abnormal chemokine expression setting the stage for lymphoma development. *J Pathol*. 2005;207:72–82.
5. Ströbel P, Marino M, Feuchtenberger M, et al. Micronodular thymoma: an epithelial tumour with abnormal chemokine expression setting the stage for lymphoma development. *J Pathol*. 2005;207:72–82.
6. Suster S, Moran CA. Micronodular thymoma with lymphoid B-cell hyperplasia: clinicopathologic and immunohistochemical study of eighteen cases of a distinctive morphologic variant of thymic epithelial neoplasm. *Am J Surg Pathol*. 1999;23:955–962.
7. Weissferdt A, Moran CA. Micronodular thymic carcinoma with lymphoid hyperplasia: a clinicopathological and immunohistochemical study of five cases. *Mod Pathol*. 2012;25:993–999.
8. Kim NR, Lee JI, Ha SY. Micronodular thymoma with lymphoid stroma in a multilocular thymic cyst: a case study. *Korean J Pathol*. 2013;47: 392–394.
9. Mende S, Moschopulos M, Marx A, et al. Ectopic micronodular thymoma with lymphoid stroma. *Virchows Arch*. 2004;444:397–379.
10. Alexiev BA, Drachenberg CB, Burke AP. Thymomas: a cytological and immunohistochemical study, with emphasis on lymphoid and neuroendocrine markers. *Diagn Pathol*. 2007;2:13.

105 Miscellaneous Thymomas

Borislav A. Alexiev, M.D., Anja C. Roden, M.D., and Fabio R. Tavora, M.D., Ph.D.

Metaplastic Thymoma (Biphasic Thymoma, Thymoma with Pseudosarcomatous Stroma)

Terminology

Metaplastic thymoma is a biphasic tumor of the thymus in which anastomosing islands of epithelial cells are intermingled with bland-looking spindle cells.[1-6] The spindle cell component is considered a mesenchymal metaplasia of tumor cells, rather than a stromal reaction.[2,4]

Incidence and Clinical

Metaplastic thymoma is a rare tumor that occurs in adult patients of both genders. The age at manifestation ranges from 28 to 71 years (mean, 50.9 years), and the tumor tends to prevail in men.[4,6]

The tumors manifest by local symptoms or can be asymptomatic and are found incidentally upon x-ray, CT, or MRI examination. The

majority of patients have no myasthenia gravis or other paraneoplastic syndromes.[5] A recent report describes symptoms of myasthenia gravis with positive serum titer for antiacetylcholine receptor antibody in a patient with metaplastic thymoma.[1]

Gross Pathology

Grossly, metaplastic thymomas are well circumscribed to encapsulated but can exhibit invasive buds. The cut surfaces are homogeneous, rubbery, and gray to white without evident necrosis.[3,5]

Microscopic Pathology

Microscopically, metaplastic thymoma is characterized by a biphasic pattern composed of epithelial components and spindle cells, sometimes with a narrow rim of residual thymic tissue incorporated in its peripheral portion (Fig. 105.1).[1-6] Occasional cases can show invasion of the surrounding tissues. In contrast to conventional

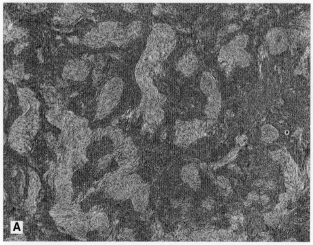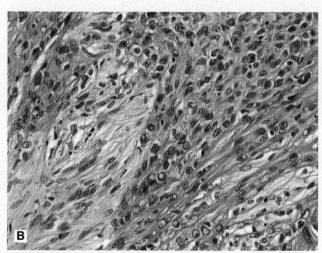

FIGURE 105.1 ▲ Metaplastic thymoma. **A.** A biphasic growth pattern is seen with anastomosing epithelial areas separated by paler-staining stroma. **B.** Higher magnification shows epithelial and stromal cells.

thymomas, metaplastic thymoma does not show a lobulated growth pattern. The epithelial areas consist of anastomosing cords and islands or broad trabeculae of cohesive neoplastic cells. Focal epithelial areas may exhibit whorled squamoid configuration or abortive formation of Hassall corpuscles. The epithelial cells are polygonal, ovoid, or round, with oval nuclei and fairly abundant eosinophilic cytoplasm. Some epithelial cells show the presence of prominent nuclear grooves or nuclear pseudoinclusions. In some areas, the epithelial cells display overt cytologic atypia with large vesicular nuclei, large hyperchromatic nuclei, and multinucleation. Despite the nuclear atypia, mitotic figures are rare. The spindle cell components demonstrate a short fascicular or storiform growth pattern. They are always bland appearing and often mitotically inactive, with fine nuclear chromatin and slender bipolar cell processes. The spindle cell components may show sharp delineation or gradual merging with the epithelial islands. While both the epithelial and spindle cell components are readily recognizable in most cases, some cases show marked predominance of one component to the exclusion of the other in some or most areas. A diagnosis of such cases can be difficult without extensive sampling to identify the typical biphasic pattern. Lymphocytes are usually sparse, but some cases can exhibit a light infiltrate of small lymphocytes and plasma cells. There can be scattered foci of stromal calcification.

Special Studies

Immunohistochemically, the epithelial cells show strong staining for cytokeratin and p63 and variable staining for Epithelial membrane antigen (EMA), and they do not show cell membrane staining for CD5.[1,2,4-6] The spindle cells lack expression of cytokeratin and E-cadherin but show expression of mesenchymal markers (vimentin).[2] CD20 is negative in tumor cells. Proliferative fraction (Ki-67 index) is low (<5%). The T lymphocytes within the tumor proper usually exhibit a mature immunophenotype.

Comparative genomic hybridization and microsatellite studies on a limited number of cases have shown no evident genetic abnormalities, excluding the most common amplifications on chromosome 1q and loss of heterozygosity on chromosome 6 previously identified in types A and B3 thymoma and thymic carcinoma.[2]

Differential Diagnosis

The most important differential diagnostic consideration is sarcomatoid carcinoma.[5] The latter often shows prominent coagulative necrosis, significant cytologic atypia, and readily identified mitotic figures.

Treatment and Prognosis

Surgery is the mainstay of treatment, and complete resection is associated with the best prognosis.[5,7-11]

The majority of metaplastic thymoma presents as Masaoka stage I and follows a benign clinical course[5]; however, Yoneda and colleagues described a patient in whom local recurrence developed at 14 months and who died within 6 years.[6] There has been a report of sarcomatoid carcinoma arising in metaplastic thymoma.[3]

Sclerosing Thymoma ("Ancient" Thymoma)
Terminology

Sclerosing thymoma is a form of conventional thymoma with extensive areas of hyalinized fibroconnective tissue.[5,12-15]

Incidence and Clinical

Sclerosing thymoma is an uncommon entity and corresponds to 1% to 2% of all thymomas.[13-15] These tumors manifest by local symptoms or can be asymptomatic and are found incidentally upon x-ray, CT, or MRI examination. Sclerosing thymomas may be associated on rare occasions to myasthenia gravis.[13,15]

Gross Pathology

Grossly, the tumors are light tan and solid, without areas of hemorrhage or necrosis.

Microscopic Pathology

Microscopically, the main tumor feature is extensive areas of hyalinized fibroconnective tissue constituting about 85% to 90% of the tumor mass (Fig. 105.2). Focal areas of conventional thymoma are present in all tumors.[15] Calcifications might also be identified.

Differential Diagnosis

In view of the prominent hyalinized or sclerotic material present in these thymomas, several considerations might enter the differential diagnosis. These lesions include sclerosing mediastinitis, solitary fibrous tumors, and lymphoma with prominent sclerosis.[15] In all these alternatives, the diagnosis cannot be reached if the only areas sampled correspond to hyalinized material. Sclerosing mediastinitis may show focal areas of inflammatory change. One important aspect of sclerosing mediastinitis is the absence of the dual cell population (epithelial cells and lymphocytes) seen in thymomas.[13,15] The presence of focal areas of spindle epithelial cells is not a component of sclerosing mediastinitis. In cases of solitary fibrous tumor, even though the tumor may show hypocellular areas, the tumor will also show hypercellular areas with a hemangiopericytic pattern or other patterns associated with other types of sarcomas. In addition, immunohistochemical studies for cytokeratin would be negative. Last, in cases of lymphoma with prominent sclerosis, the tumor will lack diffuse keratin-positive epithelial cells within an immature T-cell component.[13,15]

Microscopic Thymoma
Terminology

Microscopic thymoma is the term applied to usually multifocal epithelial proliferations (<1 mm in diameter) that preferentially occur in thymuses without a macroscopically evident tumor.[5,16-20] Microscopic thymoma may arise in cortical or medullary thymic compartment.

The role of microscopic thymoma as an incipient thymoma or precursor of thymoma has not been proven.[16] For several authors, microscopic thymoma should be renamed "nodular hyperplasia of the thymic epithelium"[18], based on the morphologic differences between microscopic thymoma and conventional thymoma with lack of lobulation, immature T cells, perivascular spaces, medullary differentiation, and capsule.[17] In opposition to this, multifocality of microscopic thymoma and description of microscopic thymoma adjacent to conventional thymoma argues for a precursor lesion.[20]

Incidence and Clinical

Microscopic thymoma preferentially occurs in myasthenia gravis–associated thymuses. Respective epithelial nodules occur at lower frequency in nonmyasthenic control thymuses.

Microscopic Pathology

Histologically, microscopic thymoma shows marked heterogeneity and can be composed of bland-looking or more pleomorphic, polygonal, or plump spindle cells, usually without intraepithelial immature T cells (Figs. 105.3 and 105.4).

Differential Diagnosis

Microscopic thymoma is a diagnosis of exclusion, eliminating purely epithelial clusters, which are smaller, unencapsulated, and multifocal and described in involuted thymuses or in congenital immunodeficiency conditions. Furthermore, two cases of a new entity called microthymoma have been described.[17] It differs from conventional thymoma only by its size, <1 cm in diameter, but exhibits the typical

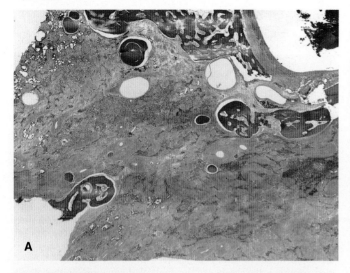

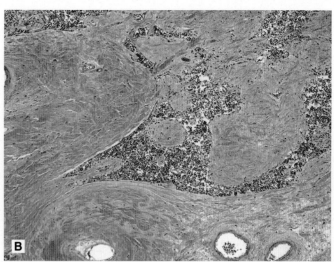

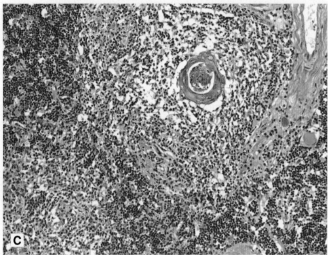

FIGURE 105.2 ▲ Sclerosing thymoma. **A.** Low magnification demonstrates fibrotic tumor with ossification and focal cellular areas. **B.** A higher magnification shows broad collagen bands encasing thymic lymphoid tissue. **C.** There may be Hassall corpuscles within the tumor.

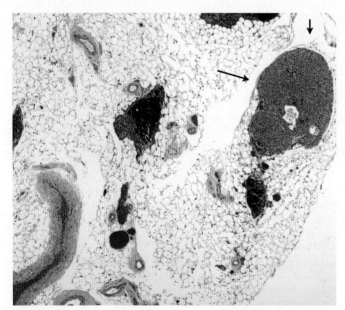

FIGURE 105.3 ▲ Microscopic thymoma. *Arrows* point to a cluster or epithelioid cells in fat.

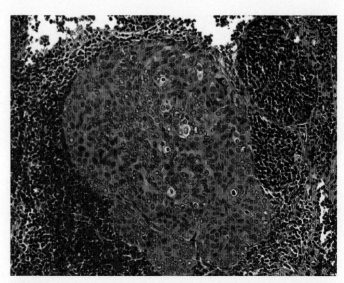

FIGURE 105.4 ▲ Microscopic thymoma. A different example shows a nodule of epithelioid cells with adjacent lymphocytic nodules of the thymus.

histologic features of conventional thymoma. The authors proposed the term microthymoma to distinguish it from the nodular hyperplasia of thymic epithelium, so-called microscopic thymoma.[17]

REFERENCES

1. Kang G, Yoon N, Han J, et al. Metaplastic thymoma: report of 4 cases. *Korean J Pathol.* 2012;46:92–95.

2. Liu B, Rao Q, Zhu Y, et al. Metaplastic thymoma of the mediastinum. A clinicopathologic, immunohistochemical, and genetic analysis. *Am J Clin Pathol.* 2012;137:261–269.

3. Moritani S, Ichihara S, Mukai K, et al. Sarcomatoid carcinoma of the thymus arising in metaplastic thymoma. *Histopathology.* 2008;52:409–411.

4. Suster S, Moran CA, Chan JK. Thymoma with pseudosarcomatous stroma: report of an unusual histologic variant of thymic epithelial neoplasm that may simulate carcinosarcoma. *Am J Surg Pathol.* 1997;21:1316–1323.

5. Travis WD, Brambilla E, Burke AP, et al., eds. *WHO Classification of Tumours of the Lung, Pleura, Thymus, and Heart.* 4th ed. Lyon, France: IARC Press; 2015.

6. Yoneda S, Marx A, Heimann S, et al. Low-grade metaplastic carcinoma of the thymus. *Histopathology.* 1999;35:19–30.

7. Ahmad U, Huang J. Current readings: the most influential and recent studies involving surgical management of thymoma. *Semin Thorac Cardiovasc Surg.* 2013;25:144–149.

8. Ishikawa Y, Kato K, Taniguchi T, et al. Imaging of a case of metaplastic thymoma on 18F-FDG PET/CT. *Clin Nucl Med.* 2013;38:e463–e464.

9. Rajan A, Giaccone G. Treatment of advanced thymoma and thymic carcinoma. *Curr Treat Options Oncol.* 2008;9:277–287.

10. Wright CD, Kessler KA. Surgical treatment of thymic tumors. *Semin Thorac Cardiovasc Surg.* 2005;17:20–26.

11. Wright CD, Wain JC, Wong DR, et al. Predictors of recurrence in thymic tumors: importance of invasion, World Health Organization histology, and size. *J Thorac Cardiovasc Surg.* 2005;130:1413–1421.

12. Kim YH, Ishii G, Naito Y, et al. [A resected case of sclerosing thymoma]. *Nihon Kokyuki Gakkai Zasshi.* 2006;44:420–423.

13. Kuo T. Sclerosing thymoma—a possible phenomenon of regression. *Histopathology.* 1994;25:289–291.

14. Moran CA, Suster S. On the histologic heterogeneity of thymic epithelial neoplasms. Impact of sampling in subtyping and classification of thymomas. *Am J Clin Pathol.* 2000;114:760–766.

15. Moran CA, Suster S. "Ancient" (sclerosing) thymomas: a clinicopathologic study of 10 cases. *Am J Clin Pathol.* 2004;121:867–871.

16. Chalabreysse L, Orsini A, Vial C, et al. Microscopic thymoma. *Interact Cardiovasc Thorac Surg.* 2007;6:133–135.

17. Cheuk W, Tsang WY, Chan JK. Microthymoma: definition of the entity and distinction from nodular hyperplasia of the thymic epithelium (so-called microscopic thymoma). *Am J Surg Pathol.* 2005;29:415–419.

18. Cornea R, Lazar E, Dema A, et al. A nodular hyperplasia of the thymic epithelium (so-called microscopic thymoma). *Rom J Morphol Embryol.* 2009;50:729–731.

19. Mori T, Nomori H, Ikeda K, et al. Microscopic-sized "microthymoma" in patients with myasthenia gravis. *Chest.* 2007;131:847–849.

20. Pescarmona E, Rosati S, Pisacane A, et al. Microscopic thymoma: histological evidence of multifocal cortical and medullary origin. *Histopathology.* 1992;20:263–266.

THYMIC CARCINOMAS AND NEUROENDOCRINE TUMORS

106 Thymic Carcinomas

Borislav A. Alexiev, M.D., Anja C. Roden, M.D., and Allen P. Burke, M.D.

Classification

Thymic carcinomas are a heterogeneous group of malignant epithelial tumors with diverse morphology that resemble carcinomas encountered outside the thymus (Table 106.1).[1] Thymic carcinomas represent a small group of thymic epithelial tumors.[2-4] In the database of the International Thymic Malignancy Interest Group, 14% of all thymic tumors are thymic carcinomas.[5]

Squamous cell carcinomas are the most common thymic carcinoma, representing 41% to 79% in more recent larger series with histologic data.[5-11]

There is a wide variation in the frequency of remaining subtypes. Undifferentiated carcinomas are often the second most frequent,[6,7,10,11] but only represent 3% in the largest series.[5] The other types include lymphoepithelioma like, mucoepidermoid, basaloid, clear cell, sarcomatoid, and adenocarcinomas (including papillary and mucinous). Basaloid carcinomas are sometimes included as a subset of squamous cell carcinomas.[11]

Neuroendocrine carcinomas are generally classified separately from thymic carcinomas and include typical and atypical carcinoids and small cell and large cell neuroendocrine carcinomas. Neuroendocrine carcinomas, when included in series of other thymic malignancies, constitute about 7%[7] and carcinoid tumors up to 15%.[10] The somewhat arbitrary classification is also reflected in the consideration by some of mucoepidermoid carcinomas as distinct from thymic carcinomas.[11] Other salivary gland–type carcinomas, such as adenoid cystic carcinoma, rarely arise in the thymus.[12]

There are rare reports of nuclear protein in testis (NUT) carcinoma and hepatoid carcinoma of the thymus.[13,14]

Clinical Features

The mean age at presentation is about 60 years, although children and adolescents may be affected.[5,6,8,15] There is a slight male predominance. From one-third to three-quarters of patients present with advanced disease (Masaoka stage 3 or 4).[5,6,8,9,15]

Paraneoplastic syndromes occur in 9% of patients, most of which are represented by myasthenia gravis. Twelve percent of patients have prior malignancies.[5]

Staging

The staging system most frequently used for thymic carcinomas is the staging schema of Masaoka et al. for thymoma (see Chapter 98). No TNM protocol has been officially authorized by the American Joint Committee on Cancer (AJCC) or the International Union Against Cancer (UICC) for the staging of thymic epithelial neoplasms. A tentative staging for thymic carcinoma and other malignant thymic epithelial tumors appeared in the UICC TNM Supplement.[16] The eighth edition will merge the staging of thymoma and thymic carcinoma (see Chapter 98, Table 106.2). In this schema, T1a tumors are confined to the mediastinum without adjacent organ involvement; T1b tumors involve the mediastinal pleura; T2 tumors involve the pericardium; T3 tumors invade the lung, brachiocephalic vein, superior vena cava,

phrenic nerve, chest wall, or extrapericardial pulmonary artery or veins; and T4 tumors invade the aorta, arch vessels, intrapericardial pulmonary artery, myocardium, trachea, or esophagus.

For N staging, N1 lymph nodes are those in the anterior mediastinum, N2 in other mediastinal lymph nodes, and N3 in scalene or supraclavicular (or distant) lymph nodes.

Gross Pathologic Features

Thymic carcinomas are generally large; the mean size in one series was reported at 7 cm.[15] They typically infiltrate surrounding structures, resulting in incomplete resections in over one-half of surgical resections.[15]

Histologic Features

The histologic findings depend on the individual tumor types. In general, the architecture is distorted and desmoplastic stromal reaction is present. There is often a dense fibrocollagenous stroma, but there are no areas resembling type B3 thymoma ("organotypic" findings).[11]

Thymic carcinomas are sometimes classified into low-grade (squamous cell carcinoma, mucoepidermoid carcinoma, and basaloid carcinoma) and high-grade tumors (lymphoepithelioma-like carcinoma, small cell carcinoma, undifferentiated carcinoma, sarcomatoid carcinoma, and clear cell carcinoma).[17]

NUT carcinomas are usually of undifferentiated morphology and might show an abrupt squamous differentiation.

Immunohistochemical Findings

Immunohistochemical findings depend on histologic type. There is an often-stated generalization that thymic carcinomas frequently express CD5, in contrast to thymoma. However, CD5 is positive in fewer than 20% of thymic carcinomas, and CD5 may be expressed in thymomas,

TABLE 106.1 Classification of Thymic Carcinomas

Squamous cell carcinoma (40%–80%)
Basaloid carcinoma (3%–6%)
Mucoepidermoid carcinoma (1%–8%)
Lymphoepithelioma-like carcinoma (4%–6%)
Sarcomatoid carcinoma (1%–3%)
Clear cell carcinoma (1%–3%)
Adenocarcinoma, including mucinous and papillary (0%–6%)
Undifferentiated carcinoma (1%–27%)[a]
Carcinoid tumor (typical and atypical)[b]
Large cell neuroendocrine carcinoma (pure or combined with others)[b]
Small cell carcinoma (pure or combined with others)[b]
Others (<1%)
    Combined thymic carcinoma, including adenosquamous
    NUT carcinoma
    Hepatoid carcinoma

[a]Including rare rhabdoid variants.
[b]Neuroendocrine carcinomas including carcinoids are usually considered separately and constitute about 10% of thymic epithelial malignancies.

especially type B3, which is the main differential consideration.[11,18] Furthermore, CD5 is nonspecific and may be expressed in adenocarcinomas and mesothelial proliferations.[11]

TTF-1 and CD30 are negative in thymic carcinomas, although primary adenocarcinomas of the thymus are rare, and the histologic features generally do not overlap with embryonal carcinoma, limiting the diagnostic usefulness of these findings.[11] Pax8 has been shown to be positive in more than 75% of thymic carcinomas, forming the third leg of frequently positive tumors (with renal cell carcinoma and carcinomas of müllerian origin).[11] NUT carcinomas typically can be diagnosed using the NUT immunostain, which has a specificity of 100% and sensitivity of 87% for these tumors.[19] CD5 and CD117 immunohistochemical staining may be helpful, when positive, to distinguish thymic carcinomas, including squamous type, from metastatic carcinomas from the lung.[19,20]

Prognosis

The prognosis of thymic carcinoma is relatively poor, with 5-year survival ranging from 30% to 66%.[6,8,9,11,15] Factors associated with decreased survival include higher stage, lymph node involvement, incomplete resection, male sex, and lack of administration of chemo- or radiation therapy.[5,6,8,11,15]

About 50% of patients with thymic carcinoma develop metastatic disease (Masaoka stage IV, or N1 or M1 disease). About half of these patients have lymph node metastasis (N1, perithymic, or N2, deep thoracic or cervical) and the remainder distant metastases (M1a pleural or pericardial and M1b pulmonary or other distant organs). Distant organ metastases include the lung (70%), followed by the liver, bone, and other viscera.[6]

REFERENCES

1. Ströbel P, Marx A, Zettl A, et al. Thymoma and thymic carcinoma: an update of the WHO Classification 2004. *Surg Today.* 2005;35:805–811.
2. Huang J, Rizk NP, Travis WD, et al. Comparison of patterns of relapse in thymic carcinoma and thymoma. *J Thorac Cardiovasc Surg.* 2009;138:26–31.
3. Thomas de Montpreville V, Ghigna MR, Lacroix L, et al. Thymic carcinomas: clinicopathologic study of 37 cases from a single institution. *Virchows Arch.* 2013;462:307–313.
4. Venuta F, Anile M, Diso D, et al. Thymoma and thymic carcinoma. *Eur J Cardiothorac Surg.* 2010;37:13–25.
5. Ahmad U, Yao X, Detterbeck F, et al. Thymic carcinoma outcomes and prognosis: results of an international analysis. *J Thorac Cardiovasc Surg.* 2015;149:95–100, 101e1–2.
6. Litvak AM, Woo K, Hayes S, et al. Clinical characteristics and outcomes for patients with thymic carcinoma: evaluation of Masaoka staging. *J Thorac Oncol.* 2014;9:1810–1815.
7. Mao Y, Wu S. Treatment and survival analyses of completely resected thymic carcinoma patients. *Onco Targets Ther.* 2015;8:2503–2507.
8. Ruffini E, Detterbeck F, Van Raemdonck D, et al. Thymic carcinoma: a cohort study of patients from the European society of thoracic surgeons database. *J Thorac Oncol.* 2014;9:541–548.
9. Song Z, Zhang Y. Outcomes after surgical resection of thymic carcinoma: a study from a single tertiary referral centre. *Eur J Surg Oncol.* 2014;40:1523–1527.
10. Wang S, Wang Z, Liu X, et al. Prognostic factors of patients with thymic carcinoma after surgery: a retrospective analysis of 58 cases. *World J Surg.* 2014;38:2032–2038.
11. Weissferdt A, Moran CA. Thymic carcinoma, part 1: a clinicopathologic and immunohistochemical study of 65 cases. *Am J Clin Pathol.* 2012;138:103–114.
12. Banki F, Khalil K, Kott MM, et al. Adenoid cystic carcinoma of the thymus gland: a rare tumor. *Ann Thorac Surg.* 2010;90:e56–e58.
13. Franke A, Strobel P, Fackeldey V, et al. Hepatoid thymic carcinoma: report of a case. *Am J Surg Pathol.* 2004;28:250–256.
14. Gokmen-Polar Y, Cano OD, Kesler KA, et al. NUT midline carcinomas in the thymic region. *Mod Pathol.* 2014;27:1649–1656.
15. Weksler B, Dhupar R, Parikh V, et al. Thymic carcinoma: a multivariate analysis of factors predictive of survival in 290 patients. *Ann Thorac Surg.* 2013;95:299–303.
16. International Union against Cancer (UICC). *TNM Supplement: A Commentary on Uniform Use.* 3rd ed. New York, NY: Wiley-Liss; 2003.
17. Wu JX, Chen HQ, Shao LD, et al. Long-term follow-up and prognostic factors for advanced thymic carcinoma. *Medicine (Baltimore).* 2014;93:e324.
18. Alexiev BA, Drachenberg CB, Burke AP. Thymomas: a cytological and immunohistochemical study, with emphasis on lymphoid and neuroendocrine markers. *Diagn Pathol.* 2007;2:13.
19. Haack H, Johnson LA, Fry CJ, et al. Diagnosis of NUT midline carcinoma using a NUT-specific monoclonal antibody. *Am J Surg Pathol.* 2009;33:984–991.
20. Asirvatham JR, Esposito MJ, and Bhuiya TA. Role of PAX-8, CD5, and CD117 in distinguishing thymic carcinoma from poorly differentiated lung carcinoma. *Appl Immunohistochem Mol Morphol.* 2014;22:372–376.

107 Squamous Cell Carcinoma

Borislav A. Alexiev, M.D., and Fabio R. Tavora, M.D., Ph.D.

Terminology

Thymic squamous cell carcinoma shows features of squamous cell carcinoma as seen in other organs, with or without clear-cut evidence of keratinization in routinely stained sections.[1] In contrast to thymomas of the B categories, thymic carcinomas lack immature T lymphocytes. Thymic squamous cell carcinomas may be derived from thymic epithelial stem cells.[1] Some cases of thymic squamous cell carcinoma are thought to arise from preexisting thymomas based on the observation of combined thymic epithelial tumors that harbor squamous cell carcinoma and conventional (usually B3) thymoma components.[2–4] Well-differentiated squamous cell carcinoma may rarely occur in a thymic cyst.[5,6]

Incidence and Clinical

Squamous cell carcinoma is the most frequent subtype of thymic carcinoma, and the frequency is higher in Asia (90%) than in the West (30%).[1] Most cases occur at middle age, and the male-to-female ratio varies from 1 to 2.3.[1] The most frequent symptom is chest pain. Other symptoms are cough, fatigue, fever, anorexia, weight loss, and superior vena cava syndrome. There have been no reports of myasthenia gravis or pure red cell aplasia, but paraneoplastic polymyositis or hypercalcemia can occur.[7]

Gross Pathology

Macroscopically, squamous cell carcinomas usually lack encapsulation or internal fibrous septation that is common in thymomas. They are firm to hard with frequent foci of necrosis and hemorrhage.[1]

Microscopic Pathology

Histologically, squamous cell carcinoma is composed of large polyhedral cells with eosinophilic cytoplasm, hyperchromatic or vesicular nuclei, prominent nucleoli arranged in nests, and cords separated by

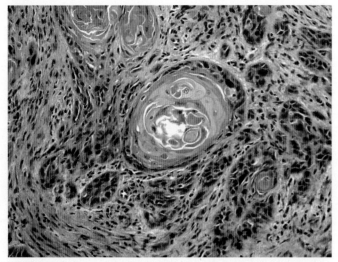

FIGURE 107.1 ▲ Squamous cell carcinoma, well differentiated. Note keratin pearls.

broad zones of fibrous stroma. The neoplasm shows clear-cut cytologic atypia and evidence of keratinization and/or intercellular bridges (Figs. 107.1 and 107.2).[1,8] Foci of spontaneous necrosis are frequently seen, as is the invasion of intratumoral blood vessels. Lymphocytes, when present, are mature and usually admixed with plasma cells. The tumor is sometimes predominantly cystic.[9]

Special Studies

Immunohistochemically, most thymic squamous cell carcinomas are immunoreactive to CK5/6, CK903, p63, CD5, CD70, and CD117. Thymomas are negative to CD5 except for some cases of type B3.[10] Squamous cell carcinomas of other organs are negative to CD5, and thus, this marker is quite useful to confirm the thymic origin of squamous cell carcinoma in the anterior mediastinum.[5] In contrast to undifferentiated thymic carcinomas, there is expression of at least one squamous marker, such as p63 (p40) or CK5/6, with p40 showing the highest specificity.

Neuroendocrine markers (chromogranin, synaptophysin, or CD56/NCAM) alone or in combination are positive in two-thirds of thymic squamous cell carcinomas in focal or dispersed distribution.[11] Some of the neoplastic cells show positivity for human chorionic gonadotropin or adrenocorticotropic hormone.[11] Infiltration of immature T cells (CD1a+, TdT+, CD99+) as seen in B thymomas is not observed in thymic carcinomas.[12]

Primary thymic squamous cell carcinoma and type B3 thymoma partially share genetic aberrations. In primary thymic squamous cell carcinoma, loss of chromosomes 16q, 6, 3p, and 17p and gain of 1q, 17q, and 18 are frequently observed.[13]

Differential Diagnosis

The possibility of lung squamous cell carcinoma showing a prominent extrapulmonary growth is sometimes difficult to exclude. Immunohistochemical evidence (CD5, CD70, and CD117 positivity) may support the thymic origin of the neoplastic squamous cells.[14] In contrast to B3 thymoma, squamous cell carcinoma of the thymus shows more pronounced squamous differentiation, usually with readily detectable intercellular bridges. Significant numbers of immature intraepithelial T lymphocytes (CD1a+, TdT+, CD99+) as seen in B3 thymoma are absent.[10,14] Well-differentiated squamous cell carcinoma with cystic changes needs to be differentiated from the reactive squamous cell proliferations found in thymic cysts.

Treatment and Prognosis

Treatment of choice is radical surgery and postoperative radiotherapy, because of relatively high radiosensitivity.[8] However, thymic squamous cell carcinoma commonly presents with locally advanced disease or with distant metastatic disease, precluding resection as a therapeutic option.[15]

The prognosis of squamous cell carcinomas is largely dependent on tumor stage and grade. They have a better prognosis than other types of thymic carcinomas with the exception of basaloid carcinoma.[1]

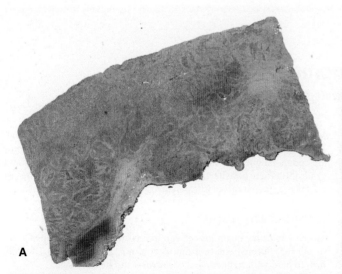

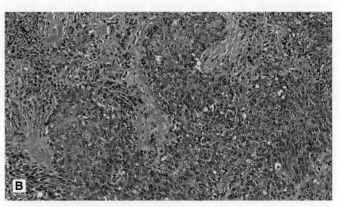

FIGURE 107.2 ▲ Thymic squamous cell carcinoma, poorly differentiated. **A.** A low magnification demonstrates an invasive cellular neoplasm involving the deep margin (*black ink*). **B.** A high magnification demonstrates sheets of squamoid cells without keratinization or intercellular bridges. p63 and high molecular weight cytokeratin staining were positive (not shown). Thymic-related lymphocytes were not present in significant numbers in the tumor (not shown).

REFERENCES

1. Chan JKC, Ströbel P, Marx A, et al. Squamous cell carcinoma. In: Travis WD, et al., eds. *WHO Classification of Tumours of the Lung, Pleura, Mediastinum and Heart. Lyon, France*: IARC Press; 2015:212–216.
2. Chalabreysse L, Roy P, Cordier JF, et al. Correlation of the WHO schema for the classification of thymic epithelial neoplasms with prognosis: a retrospective study of 90 tumors. *Am J Surg Pathol.* 2002;26:1605–1611.
3. Okumura M, Miyoshi S, Fujii Y, et al. Clinical and functional significance of WHO classification on human thymic epithelial neoplasms: a study of 146 consecutive tumors. *Am J Surg Pathol.* 2001;25:103–110.
4. Weissferdt A, Moran CA. Thymic carcinoma associated with multilocular thymic cyst: a clinicopathologic study of 7 cases. *Am J Surg Pathol.* 2011;35:1074–1079.
5. Dorfman DM, Shahsafaei A, Chan JK. Thymic carcinomas, but not thymomas and carcinomas of other sites, show CD5 immunoreactivity. *Am J Surg Pathol.* 1997;21:936–940.
6. Wick MR, Scheithauer BW, Weiland LH, et al. Primary thymic carcinomas. *Am J Surg Pathol.* 1982;6:613–630.
7. Negron-Soto JM, Cascade PN. Squamous cell carcinoma of the thymus with paraneoplastic hypercalcemia. *Clin Imaging.* 1995;19:122–124.
8. Shimosato Y, Kameya T, Nagai K, et al. Squamous cell carcinoma of the thymus. An analysis of eight cases. *Am J Surg Pathol.* 1977;1:109–121.
9. Weissferdt A, Kalhor N, Moran CA. Cystic well-differentiated squamous cell carcinoma of the thymus: a clinicopathological and immunohistochemical study of six cases. *Histopathology.* 2016;68:333–338.
10. Alexiev BA, Drachenberg CB, Burke AP. Thymomas: a cytological and immunohistochemical study, with emphasis on lymphoid and neuroendocrine markers. *Diagn Pathol.* 2007;2:13.
11. Hishima T, Fukayama M, Hayashi Y, et al. Neuroendocrine differentiation in thymic epithelial tumors with special reference to thymic carcinoma and atypical thymoma. *Hum Pathol.* 1998;29:330–338.
12. Sato Y, Watanabe S, Mukai K, et al. An immunohistochemical study of thymic epithelial tumors. II. Lymphoid component. *Am J Surg Pathol.* 1986;10:862–870.
13. Zettl A, Ströbel P, Wagner K, et al. Recurrent genetic aberrations in thymoma ad thymic carcinoma. *Am J Pathol.* 2000;157:257–266.
14. Strobel P, Marx A, Zettl A, et al. Thymoma and thymic carcinoma: an update of the WHO Classification 2004. *Surg Today.* 2005;35:805–811.
15. Okereke IC, Kesler KA, Freeman RK, et al. Thymic carcinoma: outcomes after surgical resection. *Ann Thorac Surg.* 2012;93:1668–1672.

108 Basaloid Carcinoma of the Thymus

Borislav A. Alexiev, M.D., and Allen P. Burke, M.D.

Terminology

Thymic basaloid carcinoma is a rare subtype of thymic carcinoma, with < 40 cases published in the literature, mostly in the form of individual case reports.[1-5] The tumor is composed of compact lobules of neoplastic cells with peripheral palisading and a basophilic staining pattern due to a high nuclear-to-cytoplasmic ratio. Basaloid carcinoma shows a remarkable tendency to originate in multilocular thymic cysts.[6]

Incidence and Clinical

Most cases occur in the fifth decade of life with a male-to-female ratio of 5:1.[7] The symptoms are nonspecific. Patients may show symptoms related to a mediastinal mass, for example, chest pain or dyspnea on exertion.[8] In asymptomatic patients, the tumor may be detected as an incidental finding on radiographic imaging.[8] No paraneoplastic autoimmune phenomena such as myasthenia gravis are observed.[7]

Gross Pathology

Grossly, thymic basaloid carcinomas are mostly well-circumscribed, gray to tan masses surrounded by a thin fibrous capsule with focal hemorrhage and cyst formation. In about 60% of reported cases, basaloid carcinomas were found as a mural nodule in a multilocular thymic cyst and/or showed cystic changes in the tumor.[7,8]

Microscopic Pathology

Microscopically, thymic basaloid carcinoma is composed of monotonous, small- to medium-sized, columnar, round to oval, or vaguely spindled tumor cells with high nuclear-to-cytoplasmic ratios, hyperchromatic round to oval nuclei with inconspicuous nucleoli, scant amount of amphophilic cytoplasm, and indistinct cytoplasmic borders (Fig. 108.1).[7,8] The cells are haphazardly arranged in trabeculae, anastomosing cords, islands, and nests, and typically show prominent palisading at the periphery.[7,8] Occasionally, focal keratinization in the center of the cell nests is noted. Perivascular spaces can be prominent. Mitoses are frequent. There may be areas with numerous poorly formed glands lined by basaloid tumor cells containing pink, amorphous basement membrane–like material.[7,8] The multilocular thymic cyst frequently associated with thymic basaloid carcinoma is lined by benign-appearing squamous epithelium, which may imperceptibly blend with the basaloid tumor cells.[7]

Special Studies

On immunohistochemistry, thymic basaloid carcinomas express pancytokeratin, EMA, CD117, p63, and p53.[7,8] As other thymic carcinomas, they can express CD5.[7,8] Basaloid carcinomas are negative for TTF-1, S100, and neuroendocrine markers and show multiple gains and losses of chromosomal material, among them gain of chromosome 1q and losses of chromosomes 6 and 13. These abnormalities strongly overlap with those previously found in thymic squamous cell carcinomas.[7,8]

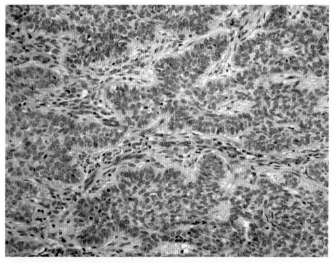

FIGURE 108.1 ▲ Basaloid carcinoma. The histologic findings are similar to basaloid or basal cell carcinomas in other sites (H&E, ×200).

Differential Diagnosis

Neuroendocrine carcinomas may histologically mimic basaloid carcinoma. However, in those cases, the neoplastic cells are positive for neuroendocrine markers. Furthermore, a mediastinal metastasis of a basaloid carcinoma of other primary location needs to be excluded. Immunohistochemical evidence (CD5 positivity) may support the thymic origin of the neoplastic basaloid cells.

Treatment and Prognosis

Treatment of choice is radical surgery.[2] However, much about this tumor remains unknown, and more case reports will help to design better treatments in the future.[1]

Thymic basaloid carcinoma, although previously regarded as a low-grade neoplasm,[9] has shown that it is capable of aggressive behavior and significant mortality.[1,4,8]

Practical Points

▸ Basaloid carcinomas are <5% of thymic carcinomas, which are 20% of thymic epithelial neoplasms.

▸ Solid or cystic, well-circumscribed mass.

▸ Nests of basaloid cells with peripheral palisading.

▸ Cysts frequent, lined by basaloid cells, containing amorphous material.

▸ Amorphous basement membrane material may occur in tumor nests.

▸ Sclerotic stroma.

▸ Abrupt transition to keratinizing squamous carcinoma in up to 50% of tumors.

REFERENCES

1. Suemitsu R, Takeo S, Momosaki S, et al. Thymic basaloid carcinoma with aggressive invasion of the lung and pericardium: report of a case. *Surg Today.* 2011;41:986–988.
2. Sakakura N, Tateyama H, Usami N, et al. Thymic basaloid carcinoma with pleural dissemination that developed after a curative resection: report of a case. *Surg Today.* 2010;40:1073–1078.
3. Posligua L, Ylagan L. Fine-needle aspiration cytology of thymic basaloid carcinoma: case studies and review of the literature. *Diagn Cytopathol.* 2006;34:358–366.
4. Matsuo T, Hayashida R, Kobayashi K, et al. Thymic basaloid carcinoma with hepatic metastasis. *Ann Thorac Surg.* 2002;74:579–582.
5. Kawashima O, Kamiyoshihara M, Sakata S, et al. Basaloid carcinoma of the thymus. *Ann Thorac Surg.* 1999;68:1863–1865.
6. Weissferdt A, Moran CA. Thymic carcinoma associated with multilocular thymic cyst: a clinicopathologic study of 7 cases. *Am J Surg Pathol.* 2011;35:1074–1079.
7. Papotti M, Ströbel P, Marx A, et al. Basaloid carcinoma. In: Travis WD, et al., eds. *WHO Classification of Tumours of the Lung, Pleura, Mediastinum and Heart.* Lyon, France: IARC Press; 2015:216–217.
8. Brown JG, Familiari U, Papotti M, et al. Thymic basaloid carcinoma: a clinicopathologic study of 12 cases, with a general discussion of basaloid carcinoma and its relationship with adenoid cystic carcinoma. *Am J Surg Pathol.* 2009;33:1113–1124.
9. Suster S, Rosai J. Thymic carcinoma. A clinicopathologic study of 60 cases. *Cancer.* 1991;67:1025–1032.

109 Mucoepidermoid Carcinoma

Borislav A. Alexiev, M.D., and Fabio R. Tavora, M.D., Ph.D.

Terminology

Thymic mucoepidermoid carcinoma is a rare morphologic variant of primary thymic carcinoma characterized by the presence of squamous cells, mucus-producing cells, and cells of intermediate type.[1–7] The neoplasm closely resembles mucoepidermoid carcinomas of other organs and may be associated with multilocular thymic cysts.[4,5,7]

Incidence and Clinical

Thymic mucoepidermoid carcinoma comprises ~2% of published thymic carcinoma cases.[1] It tends to occur mostly in middle-aged individuals with a male-to-female ratio of 1.5:1.[2] Mucoepidermoid carcinomas are not associated with myasthenia gravis except in rare instances.[8] The initial manifestations include respiratory symptoms and weight loss. Some patients may be asymptomatic.[4]

Gross Pathology

Grossly, thymic mucoepidermoid carcinomas demonstrate a combination of solid and cystic areas in various proportions.[2–5,9] The cut surface is white–tan, nodular, and cystic, with fibrous bands and focal mucinous appearance.

Microscopic Pathology

The histologic features of these thymic tumors are similar to those occurring in the salivary glands. They are composed of variably sized cysts as well as sheets, lobules, and nests of cells. The cells are a combination of squamoid, mucinous, and intermediate cells in variable proportion (Fig. 109.1).[2–5,9] Gland-like spaces lined by mucin-secreting epithelium may occur, as well as cytoplasmic clearing.

Mucoepidermoid carcinoma of the thymus has been graded similar to salivary mucoepidermoid carcinomas, into well-differentiated, moderately differentiated, and poorly differentiated tumors, or into a two-tiered system.[4,5] There have been several grading systems of salivary gland mucoepidermoid carcinomas that are based on poor prognostic features of mitotic activity, cellular pleomorphism, solid growth (lack of cystic change), necrosis, and perineural invasion.[10,11] Poorly differentiated mucoepidermoid carcinomas may be difficult to distinguish from adenosquamous carcinoma, an even rare thymic tumor.

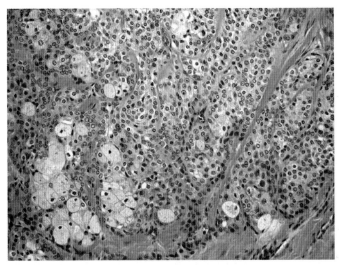

FIGURE 109.1 ▲ Mucoepidermoid carcinoma (H&E, ×200).

Special Studies

Immunohistochemically, mucoepidermoid carcinomas of the thymus are similar to those of salivary glands, with squamous and intermediate cells expressing high molecular weight cytokeratins (CK5/6, CK903) and mucin-producing cells expressing MUC-2. In contrast to other thymic carcinomas, CD5 is negative.[4] Tumor-infiltrating lymphocytes are mostly mature T and B cells (negative for TdT, CD99, and CD1a), in distinction from thymoma.[4,5]

Thymic mucoepidermoid carcinomas have cytogenetic similarities to cases of mucoepidermoid carcinoma arising from other anatomical sites. Translocation t(11;19)(q21;p13) involving the MECT1 and MAML2 genes has been suggested as a diagnostic marker in these tumors.[12,13]

Treatment and Prognosis

Treatment of choice is radical surgery and postoperative radiotherapy. Chemotherapy, including cisplatin, irinotecan, and vinorelbine, has been used with variable success for patients with recurrent or pleural disease.[14,15] Prognosis is dependent on stage and grade of tumor.[4,5] There are no large series of thymic mucoepidermoid carcinomas, although deaths due to disease are reported.[15] In one smaller one, one-third of patients died, all with advanced-stage tumors at the time of diagnosis.[5] High-grade tumors frequently spread to the pericardium, lung, and myocardium. Distant metastases, such as to the skeleton, are rare.[16]

REFERENCES

1. Matsuno Y, Chan JKC, Detterbeck F, et al. Mucoepidermoid carcinoma. In: Travis WD, et al., eds. *WHO Classification of Tumours of the Lung, Pleura, Mediastinum and Heart*. Lyon, France: IARC Press; 2015:218–219.
2. Yasuda M, Yasukawa T, Ozaki D, et al. Mucoepidermoid carcinoma of the thymus. *Jpn J Thorac Cardiovasc Surg*. 2006;54:23–26.
3. Stefanou D, Goussia AC, Arkoumani E, et al. Mucoepidermoid carcinoma of the thymus: a case presentation and a literature review. *Pathol Res Pract*. 2004;200:567–573.
4. Nonaka D, Klimstra D, Rosai J. Thymic mucoepidermoid carcinomas: a clinicopathologic study of 10 cases and review of the literature. *Am J Surg Pathol*. 2004;28:1526–1531.
5. Moran CA, Suster S. Mucoepidermoid carcinomas of the thymus. A clinicopathologic study of six cases. *Am J Surg Pathol*. 1995;19:826–834.
6. Brightman I, Morgan JA, Kunze WP, et al. Primary mucoepidermoid carcinoma of the thymus—a rare cause of mediastinal tumour. *Thorac Cardiovasc Surg*. 1992;40:90–91.
7. Tanaka M, Shimobara R, Matsubara O, et al. Mucoepidermoid carcinoma of the thymic region. *Acta Pathol Jpn*. 1982;32:703–712.
8. Woo WL, Panagiotopoulos N, Gvinianidze L, et al. Primary mucoepidermoid carcinoma of the thymus presenting with myasthenia gravis. *J Thorac Dis*. 2014;6:E223–E225.
9. Kim GD, Kim HW, Oh JT, et al. Mucoepidermoid carcinoma of the thymus: a case report. *J Korean Med Sci*. 2004;19:601–603.
10. Goode RK, Auclair PL, Ellis GL. Mucoepidermoid carcinoma of the major salivary glands: clinical and histopathologic analysis of 234 cases with evaluation of grading criteria. *Cancer*. 1998;82:1217–1224.
11. Auclair PL, Goode RK, Ellis GL. Mucoepidermoid carcinoma of intraoral salivary glands. Evaluation and application of grading criteria in 143 cases. *Cancer*. 1992;69:2021–2030.
12. Prieto-Granada CN, Inagaki H, Mueller J. Thymic mucoepidermoid carcinoma: report of a case with CTRC1/3-MALM2 molecular studies. *Int J Surg Pathol*. 2015;23:277–283.
13. Roden AC, Erickson-Johnson MR, Yi ES, et al. Analysis of MAML2 rearrangement in mucoepidermoid carcinoma of the thymus. *Hum Pathol*. 2013;44:2799–2805.
14. Fuse ET, Kamimura M, Takeda Y, et al. Response of a thymic mucoepidermoid carcinoma to combination chemotherapy with cisplatin and irinotecan: a case report. *Lung Cancer*. 2008;59:403–406.
15. Noda T, Higashiyama M, Oda K, et al. Mucoepidermoid carcinoma of the thymus treated by multimodality therapy: a case report. *Ann Thorac Cardiovasc Surg*. 2006;12:273–278.
16. Tanaka T, Morishita Y, Mori Y, et al. Fine needle aspiration cytology of mucoepidermoid carcinoma of the thymus. *Cytopathology*. 1990;1:49–53.

110 Lymphoepithelioma-Like Carcinoma

Borislav A. Alexiev, M.D., and Allen P. Burke, M.D.

Terminology

Lymphoepithelioma-like carcinoma (LELC) of the thymus is a primary thymic carcinoma characterized by a syncytial growth of undifferentiated carcinoma cells accompanied by a lymphoplasmacytic infiltration similar to undifferentiated carcinoma of the nasopharynx.[1–4] Although a requirement for LELC of the lung, thymic LELC may or may not be associated with Epstein-Barr virus (EBV). Thymic LELC presumably arises from thymic epithelial cells.[5]

Incidence and Clinical

Thymic LELC is a rare tumor. It represents from 4% to 6% of thymic carcinomas.[6–12]

Thymic LELC occurs twice more commonly in male than female patients.[5] The patient's age ranges from 4 to 76 years with a median of 41 years.[5]

Patients typically present with signs and symptoms caused by compression of mediastinal organs, but some patients are asymptomatic and incidentally found to have an anterior mediastinal mass upon

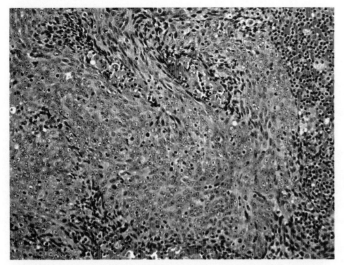

FIGURE 110.1 ▲ Lymphoepithelioma-like carcinoma (H&E, ×200).

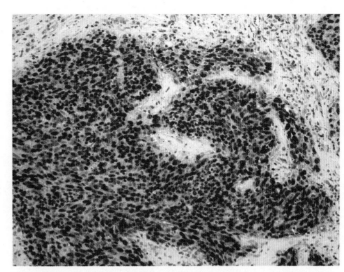

FIGURE 110.2 ▲ Lymphoepithelioma-like carcinoma (EBER, ×200).

imaging examination. Superior vena cava syndrome is seen in patients with more advanced disease.[13] There is no association with myasthenia gravis, but polymyositis, nephritic syndrome, and hypertrophic pulmonary osteoarthropathy have been reported.[1,2,14]

Gross Pathology

Grossly, the tumor is usually incompletely encapsulated, solid, and yellow–white with areas of necrosis and hemorrhage.

Microscopic Pathology

Histologically, the tumor is composed of nests or anastomosing cords of syncytial-appearing carcinoma cells in a lymphoplasmacytic stroma (Fig. 110.1).[5] The tumor cells have large vesicular nuclei with open chromatin and one or more distinct eosinophilic nucleoli and show indistinct cytoplasmic membranes. The nuclei are unevenly crowded and may appear to be overlapping. Lymphocytes and plasma cells are not only present in the stroma but also infiltrate the tumor islands, breaking them up into tiny clusters or single cells and obscuring the epithelial nature of the tumor. Mitotic activity is variable but is often pronounced. Foci of tumor necrosis are usually observed.

Special Studies

Immunohistochemically, the tumor cells show strong staining for pancytokeratin (AE1/AE3) and high molecular weight cytokeratins (CK5/6 and CK903). In most cases, the tumor exhibits strong nuclear staining for p63. CK7 and CK20 are negative. CD5 may be expressed focally or not at all.[15] The carcinoma cells also commonly express BCL-2.[15] The majority of lymphoid cells are mature T cells (CD3+, CD5+, CD1a–, CD99–, and TdT–).[15] Smaller numbers of B cells are present in the stroma and among the carcinoma cells. Plasma cells that are present are polyclonal.[5]

The majority of thymic LELC show association with EBV as demonstrated by EBER in situ hybridization or DNA analysis (Fig. 110.2).[5] EBV is almost always positive in thymic LELC occurring in children and young adults, while EBV positivity rate is lower in adults over the age of 30 years. The association with EBV is not related to geographic or ethnic factors.[5]

Differential Diagnosis

The histopathologic appearances of LELC may overlap with those of poorly differentiated squamous cell carcinoma with a lymphoplasmacytic stroma.[5] The differential diagnosis with germ cell tumors, particularly seminomas, can be difficult but important for treatment.

Treatment and Prognosis

Thymic LELC commonly presents with locally advanced disease or with distant metastatic disease, precluding resection as a therapeutic option. Patients with metastatic disease are initially treated with concurrent chemoradiotherapy followed by systemic chemotherapy.[14]

Thymic LELC is a highly malignant neoplasm with a poor prognosis.[15,16] The estimated average survival is 15 to 16 months, and the 2-year survival rate is 18%.[16] The presence or absence of EBV does not seem to have prognostic significance.[5]

REFERENCES

1. Kilis-Pstrusinska K, Medynska A, Zwolinska D, et al. Lymphoepithelioma-like thymic carcinoma in a 16-year-old boy with nephrotic syndrome—a case report. *Pediatr Nephrol.* 2008;23:1001–1003.
2. Koppula BR, Pipavath S, Lewis DH. Epstein-Barr virus (EBV) associated lymphoepithelioma-like thymic carcinoma associated with paraneoplastic syndrome of polymyositis: a rare tumor with rare association. *Clin Nucl Med.* 2009;34:686–688.
3. Sadat K, Singh A, Rao S, et al. Thymic lymphoepithelioma-like carcinoma mimicking primary tumor of the lung. *Compr Ther.* 2009;35:115–119.
4. Sekihara K, Okuma Y, Kawamoto H, et al. Clinical outcome of thymic lymphoepithelioma-like carcinoma: case report of a 14-year-old male. *Oncol Lett.* 2014;8:2183–2186.
5. Chan JKC, Chalabreysse L, Detterbeck F, et al. Lymphoepithelioma-like carcinoma. In: Travis WD, et al., eds. *WHO Classification of Tumours of the Lung, Pleura, Mediastinum and Heart.* Lyon, France: IARC Press; 2015: 220–222.
6. Ahmad U, Yao X, Detterbeck F, et al. Thymic carcinoma outcomes and prognosis: results of an international analysis. *J Thorac Cardiovasc Surg.* 2015;149:95–100, 101 e1–2.
7. Litvak AM, Woo K, Hayes S, et al. Clinical characteristics and outcomes for patients with thymic carcinoma: evaluation of Masaoka staging. *J Thorac Oncol.* 2014;9:1810–1815.
8. Mao Y, Wu S. Treatment and survival analyses of completely resected thymic carcinoma patients. *Onco Targets Ther.* 2015;8:2503–2507.
9. Ruffini E, Detterbeck F, Van Raemdonck D, et al. Thymic carcinoma: a cohort study of patients from the European society of thoracic surgeons database. *J Thorac Oncol.* 2014;9:541–548.
10. Song Z, Zhang Y. Outcomes after surgical resection of thymic carcinoma: a study from a single tertiary referral centre. *Eur J Surg Oncol.* 2014;40: 1523–1527.
11. Wang S, Wang Z, Liu X, et al. Prognostic factors of patients with thymic carcinoma after surgery: a retrospective analysis of 58 cases. *World J Surg.* 2014;38:2032–2038.

12. Weissferdt A, Moran CA. Thymic carcinoma, part 1: a clinicopathologic and immunohistochemical study of 65 cases. *Am J Clin Pathol.* 2012;138:103–114.

13. Tseng YL, Wang ST, Wu MH, et al. Thymic carcinoma: involvement of great vessels indicates poor prognosis. *Ann Thorac Surg.* 2003;76:1041–1045.

14. Inoue Y, True LD, Martins RG. Thymic carcinoma associated with paraneoplastic polymyositis. *J Clin Oncol.* 2009;27:e33–e34.

15. Chalabreysse L, Etienne-Mastroianni B, Adeleine P, et al. Thymic carcinoma: a clinicopathological and immunohistological study of 19 cases. *Histopathology.* 2004;44:367–374.

16. Nicolato A, Ferraresi P, Bontempini L, et al. Multiple brain metastases from "lymphoepithelioma-like" thymic carcinoma: a combined stereotactic-radiosurgical approach. *Surg Neurol.* 2001;55:232–234.

111 Miscellaneous Carcinomas of the Thymus

Borislav Alexiev, M.D., and Fabio R. Tavora, M.D., Ph.D.

Undifferentiated Thymic Carcinoma

Undifferentiated thymic carcinoma represents between 1% and 27% of thymic carcinomas.[1-7] By definition, these tumors do not fit the criteria for diagnosis of other described subtypes and are undifferentiated carcinomas with solid growth that express at least one epithelial marker (Fig. 111.1).

Distinction from poorly differentiated squamous carcinoma rests on lack of expression of squamous specific markers, such as p40, p63, or cytokeratin 5/6. Distinction from small cell carcinoma rests on histologic features (lack of nuclear molding, stippled chromatin) and lack of diffuse endocrine marker positivity (CD56, synaptophysin, or chromogranin). Rare thymic tumors with rhabdoid features are usually considered as a type of undifferentiated carcinoma or are sometimes considered separately.[7]

Sarcomatoid Carcinoma

Terminology

Sarcomatoid carcinoma is a thymic carcinoma in which part or the entire tumor resembles soft tissue sarcoma morphologically.[8-15] The sarcomatoid component may arise from metaplasia of the carcinomatous component, wherein the tumor cells often gradually lose epithelial characteristics and simultaneously acquire mesenchymal or mesenchymal-like features. Alternatively, the tumor is derived from primitive cells with multidirectional differentiation.

Incidence and Clinical

Sarcomatoid carcinoma is uncommon and accounts for only up to 7% of all thymic carcinomas.[15] It is a tumor of late adulthood, predominantly fourth to eighth decades. No consistent gender predilection has been reported.

The patients present with cough, dyspnea, dysphagia, chest pain, weight loss, or superior vena cava syndrome.[8-14] Imaging studies reveal the presence of an anterior mediastinal mass.

Gross Pathology

Grossly, the tumor is unencapsulated, often with infiltrative borders. The cut surfaces show whitish or grayish fleshy tumor with variable extent of necrosis and hemorrhage.[15]

Microscopic Pathology

Histologically, sarcomatoid carcinoma is an infiltrative tumor often with large areas of coagulative necrosis. It shows intimate intermingling of carcinomatous and sarcomatoid components (Fig. 111.2), but the carcinomatous component can be subtle or demonstrable only by immunohistochemistry or electron microscopy in some cases.[15] The carcinomatous component usually comprises cohesive clusters and sheets of poorly differentiated epithelial cells with significant nuclear pleomorphism.[8-14] The sarcomatoid component frequently comprises fascicles and storiform arrays of discohesive spindle tumor cells with

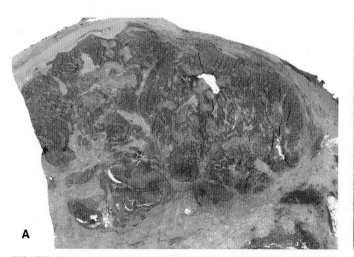

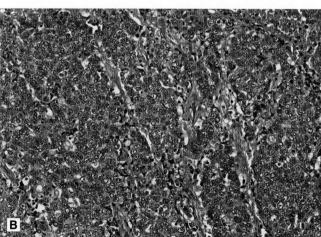

A

B

FIGURE 111.1 ▲ Undifferentiated thymic carcinoma. **A.** Low magnification shows infiltrative tumor with no residual thymus tissue. **B.** Higher magnification shows undifferentiated carcinoma. Immunohistochemical stains for squamous markers (p63, cytokeratin 5/6) were negative (not shown).

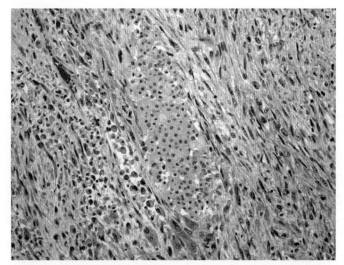

FIGURE 111.2 ▲ Sarcomatoid carcinoma, thymus. Note spindling and focal nests of epithelioid cells.

pleomorphic nuclei, coarse chromatin, distinct nucleoli, and frequent mitotic figures. Heterologous elements may be observed, most commonly rhabdomyosarcomatous and occasionally osteosarcomatous; the term "carcinosarcoma" is sometimes applied for such cases.[15]

Special Studies

Immunohistochemically, the carcinomatous component expresses epithelial markers such as cytokeratin and EMA. In the sarcomatoid areas, cytokeratin-positive tumor cells range from abundant to scanty or even absent.[15] Variable expression of myeloid markers (e.g., desmin, actin, myogenin, myoD1, myoglobin) is seen in the rhabdomyosarcomatous component.[8,13,15] The cases studied for CD5 have been negative for this marker.[15] Only rare tumors have been examined ultrastructurally, but desmosome-like junctions have been described in the spindle cell area of one case.[8]

Only one case has been studied by cytogenetics, with identification of a complex chromosomal abnormality including der(16)t(1;16)(q12;q12.1).[8] This chromosomal translocation has also been previously reported in a case of thymic squamous cell carcinoma, suggesting a pathogenetic relationship with thymic squamous cell carcinoma in at least some cases.

Differential Diagnosis

Sarcomatoid carcinoma may resemble metaplastic thymoma. The former often shows prominent coagulative necrosis, significant cytologic atypia, and readily identified mitotic figures. In a tumor where only sarcomatoid component is identified despite extensive sampling, distinction from a sarcoma depends on the demonstration of epithelial differentiation in at least some tumor cells by immunohistochemistry (cytokeratin, EMA) or electron microscopy. Sarcomatoid carcinoma predominated by rhabdomyosarcomatous component may have been confused with mediastinal rhabdomyosarcoma. The latter sarcoma more commonly affects children and young adults.[15] Although rhabdomyosarcoma can express cytokeratin, the positive tumor cells coexpress myeloid markers, whereas at least some tumor cells in sarcomatoid carcinoma express cytokeratin only.[8,13]

Treatment and Prognosis

Sarcomatoid carcinoma is an aggressive tumor, with frequent invasion of the adjacent pleura, lung, pericardium, and the major blood vessels in the mediastinum. Metastases to mediastinal lymph nodes and parenchymal organs (especially the lungs) are common. Most patients are dying of disease despite aggressive multimodality therapy.[15]

Clear Cell Carcinoma

Terminology

Clear cell carcinoma is a thymic carcinoma predominantly or exclusively composed of cells with optically clear cytoplasm.[15]

Incidence and Clinical

Clear cell carcinomas constitute only 3% of all thymic carcinomas.[16] The age range of the reported cases is 33 to 84 years, and the tumor tends to prevail in men (male to female ratio, 1:6).[15] The patients usually presented with signs and symptoms caused by compression of mediastinal organs, but some patients are asymptomatic and incidentally found to have an anterior mediastinal mass upon imaging examination. There are no associated paraneoplastic autoimmune phenomena.[15]

Gross Pathology

The tumors may appear encapsulated and noninfiltrative, or may extensively infiltrate the surrounding tissues.[15] The cut surface shows solid or cystic tumor with or without hemorrhage and focal necrosis.

Microscopic Pathology

Microscopically, the tumors are composed of cells with clear cytoplasm and rather bland nuclear features and show a lobular, nested, or occasionally sheet-like growth pattern (Fig. 111.3).[15–25] Tumor cells are rather monotonous and polyhedral and usually display slight cellular pleomorphism with round to oval, vesicular nuclei, moderate nuclear atypia, finely dispersed chromatin, and small discernible nucleoli. They have abundant lucent, mostly clear to granular, sometimes faintly eosinophilic, cytoplasm. The stroma is fibrotic and lacks the sinusoidal vasculature characteristic of metastatic clear cell carcinoma of the kidney. Rarely, a few scattered intratumoral lymphocytes, minute foci of squamous differentiation, and focal necrosis are observed. Clear cell carcinomas commonly exhibit an infiltrative growth, with tumor extending into the surrounding mediastinal fat and remnant thymus.

Special Studies

Cytoplasmic glycogen is demonstrable in the majority of cases, whereas mucin is absent. The tumor cells are uniformly immunoreactive for low and high molecular weight keratins and are reactive for EMA in 22% of cases.[19] As in other types of thymic carcinomas, a subgroup of clear cell carcinomas may express CD5.[15] They are negative for PLAP, vimentin, carcinoembryonic antigen (CEA), and S100[15,19] and do not contain a population of immature (CD1a- or CD99-positive) T lymphocytes.[15]

Differential Diagnosis

The differential diagnosis includes mediastinal seminoma, parathyroid carcinoma, malignant melanoma, and metastatic clear cell carcinoma. The diagnosis of primary thymic carcinoma depends on the exclusion of other primary sites clinically, particularly lung and kidney, and the demonstration of positivity for keratins and negativity for placental alkaline phosphatase.[19] Furthermore, thymoma with clear cell features must be differentiated from clear cell carcinoma. Clear cell features are common only in WHO type B3 thymomas, and they are almost always focal.[15] While the conventional B3 areas harbor at least few CD1a+ and CD99+ immature T cells, they may be absent in the clear cell areas. Significant PAS positivity, necrosis, increased proliferative activity, desmoplastic stroma, and TP53 overexpression are typically absent in clear cell foci of WHO B3 thymomas.[15]

Treatment and Prognosis

Clear cell carcinomas are highly malignant, aggressive mediastinal neoplasms with frequent local recurrences and metastases. Most patients are dying of disease despite aggressive multimodality therapy.[15,19]

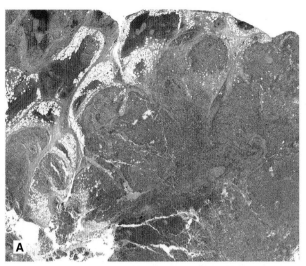
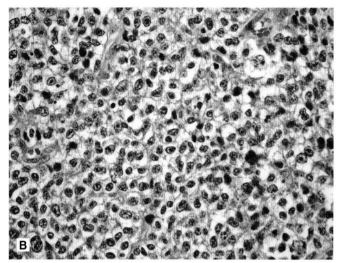

FIGURE 111.3 ▲ Clear cell carcinoma, thymus. **A.** Low magnification shows partial replacement of the thymus. **B.** High magnification shows carcinoma with clear cytoplasm.

Thymic Adenocarcinoma

Terminology

Adenocarcinoma is a primary thymic carcinoma characterized by glandular, papillary, tubulopapillary, or mucinous differentiation.[26–38] The exact origin of thymic adenocarcinoma is not clear. Thymic adenocarcinomas associated with thymic cysts or thymomas have been described.[26,32,33,38] Thymic epithelial cells do have a potential for glandular differentiation, as exemplified by the appearance of ciliated or mucin-secreting cells in cystic and noncystic Hassall corpuscles in response to space-occupying lesions and inflammation, and frequent presence of tubulopapillary structures in type A thymomas.[26]

Incidence and Clinical

The most common morphologic subtypes are papillary carcinoma and mucinous adenocarcinoma.[31] Conventional adenocarcinoma (not otherwise specified) and tubulopapillary carcinoma are extremely rare. Primary thymic adenocarcinomas occur over a wide age range (mean 50 years) with slight male predominance, comparable with the entire group of thymic carcinomas.[26]

Gross Pathology

Macroscopically, the tumors are cystic or solid and white to yellowish-white. Areas with a gelatinous appearance may be present.

Microscopic Pathology

Papillary and mucinous adenocarcinomas are the most common histologic subtype and can show low-grade or high-grade cytology.[26] Thymic papillary adenocarcinoma exhibits a papillary architecture.[27,28,31–33,37,38] Focal areas of solid, tubular, and tubular–papillary morphology are seen as well. Most of the papillae are composed of a monolayer of cuboidal or columnar cells with abundant clear or eosinophilic cytoplasm supported by a thin, somewhat edematous, vascular core. The nuclei are round or ovoid with membrane irregularities and grooves. The chromatin is vesicular. The nucleoli are sometimes prominent. Numerous psammoma bodies are present.[27,28,31–33,37,38] Thymic mucinous adenocarcinoma exhibits features of mucinous (colloid) carcinoma, being composed of islands, strips, or micropapillae of tall columnar cells with eosinophilic granular cytoplasm and apical snout-like features floating in large pools of extracellular mucin (Fig. 111.4).[26,29,30,34,35] Mitoses and occasional areas of coagulative necrosis are observed in all adenocarcinoma subtypes. In some areas, invasive growth of the tumor into the adhesive extrathymic tissues (i.e., mediastinal fat, pleura, and lung) accompanied by dense collagenous stroma is seen.

Special Studies

Immunohistochemically, thymic adenocarcinomas are positive for cytokeratins AE1/AE3, CAM 5.2, CK7, CEA, Ber-EP4, and calretinin.[31–33] Positivity for CD5 is also noted.[26] In mucinous adenocarcinoma, tumor cells and extracellular mucin are strongly positive for MUC5AC and partially positive for MUC6, suggesting that this tumor produces the gastric-type mucin.[35] Thymic adenocarcinomas are negative for markers for pulmonary, thyroid, germ cell, neuroendocrine, squamous cell, and/or large intestine differentiation. Stromal-infiltrating lymphocytes are negative for TdT, CD1a, and/or CD99.[35] The HLA-DRB5 locus in chromosomal region 6p21.32 is homozygously deleted, showing similar genetic aberrations with other thymic epithelial tumors.[31]

Differential Diagnosis

Papillary thyroid carcinoma (either metastatic to mediastinal nodes or arising from a mediastinal thyroid gland) is clearly an important differential diagnosis. Features against this alternative are the absence

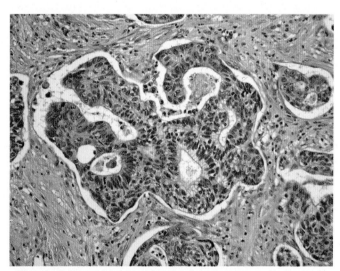

FIGURE 111.4 ▲ Adenocarcinoma, thymus. Note extracellular mucin and focal necrosis.

of the nuclear features characteristic of papillary thyroid carcinoma (i.e., vesicular or ground-glass appearance, nuclear grooves, and pseudoinclusions), the lack of immunoreactivity for thyroglobulin or TTF1, and the presence of a conventional type of thymoma or normal thymic tissue in intimate connection with the tumor.[27,28,32,33,37,38] The possibility of adenocarcinoma arising from mediastinal germ cells and representing a type of teratoma should also be considered; however, the absence of other teratomatous elements makes this highly unlikely.[26]

Because malignant mesothelioma usually shows a tubulopapillary pattern of growth and expresses calretinin, it must also be considered in the differential diagnosis. However, a true malignant mesothelioma presenting as a localized tumor mass in the mediastinum would be exceedingly rare.[35] Furthermore, immunohistochemical demonstration of CEA and BerEP4 strongly supports a diagnosis of adenocarcinoma. The immunohistochemical positivity for CD5 provides other supporting evidence that we are dealing with a primary thymic carcinoma but not with a secondary carcinoma derived from other organs. Pulmonary mucin-rich neoplasms (invasive mucinous adenocarcinoma or colloid carcinoma) involving the thymus show at least one immunohistologic marker of enteric differentiation (CDX-2, CK20, or MUC2).[36] Consistent positivity for TTF1 in approximately half the cases helps in the distinction from primary thymic adenocarcinoma.[36] Thymic mucinous adenocarcinomas, similar to gastric carcinomas, are positive for MUC5AC and MUC6.[35] Other kinds of primary thymic tumors with abundant mucin, such as carcinoid with prominent mucinous stroma and mucoepidermoid carcinoma, should also be considered as differential diagnosis.[35] The carcinoid with prominent mucinous stroma demonstrates a conventional neuroendocrine morphology such as an organoid pattern and delicate fibrovascular septa and immunoreactivity for pan-neuroendocrine markers. For a tumor to be diagnosed as mucoepidermoid carcinoma, both a squamous component and the mucin-producing components should be present. Positive staining for CD5 provides further support for thymic origin.

Treatment and Prognosis

The thymic adenocarcinoma is locally invasive and can metastasize to lymph nodes or other distant sites. The limited available data indicate that the clinical outcome is highly variable, with some patients apparently cured by surgical excision and some dying from the tumor.[26]

Carcinoma with t(15;19) Translocation

Terminology

Carcinoma with translocation t(15;19)(q13:p13.1) is a rare, aggressive, and lethal carcinoma of unknown histogenesis arising in the mediastinum and other midline organs of young people. The tumor is characterized by a chromosomal rearrangement in the nuclear protein in testis (NUT) gene.[15,39-44]

Incidence and Clinical

Carcinomas with t(15;19) are rare. In a series of 148 thymic epithelial tumors (37 carcinomas and 111 thymomas), only one thymic carcinoma (2.7% of thymic carcinomas or 0.68% of thymic epithelial tumors) was found positive for NUT expression and rearrangement.[43] The tumors have been reported primarily in younger individuals (age range: 5 to 34 years), particularly females (F:M ratio =5:1).[43] Aggressive local invasiveness is characteristic. Pleural effusions and superior vena cava syndrome are common. Metastases are common and may involve the lymph nodes, lung, bone, skin, and soft tissue.[15,39-44]

Gross Pathology

Grossly, the tumors are ill-defined with a white-tan gritty cut surface and patchy necrotic, hemorrhagic, and fibrotic areas.

Microscopic Pathology

Histologic features are remarkable for syncytial sheets of very discohesive undifferentiated cells with scant cytoplasm and prominent central nucleoli with frequent mitoses, cell necrosis, and percolating lymphocytes giving a lymphoepithelioma-like appearance.[15,43] Focal squamous differentiation is common, but not always seen, whereas glandular differentiation has only been reported once.[15]

Special Studies

The tumors consistently react, at least focally, with pan-cytokeratin markers. Inconsistent and usually focal positivity occurs for vimentin, EMA, and CEA. CD30, CD45, PLAP, HMB45, S100, and neuroendocrine markers are negative.[15,39-44] These tumors are characterized by rearrangement of the NUT gene on chromosome 15q14, which in most cases fuses to the bromodomain containing 4 (BRD4) gene on chromosome 19 p13.1 through reciprocal t(15;19) translocation, resulting in constitutive BRD4–NUT fusion protein expression.[15,39-43] Nuclear overexpression of the resulting BRD4–NUT fusion protein is detectable by immunohistochemical staining.

Differential Diagnosis

This lesion must be distinguished from t(15;19)-negative carcinomas, particularly lymphoepithelioma-like, poorly differentiated squamous cell, mucoepidermoid, and undifferentiated carcinoma. Care must be taken not to confuse the discohesive, undifferentiated round cells of t(15;19)-positive carcinoma with large cell lymphoma or germ cell tumor.

Treatment and Prognosis

All cases reported so far (in sites other than the mediastinum) followed an extremely aggressive clinical course.[15,39-43] Data of the rare thymic variant are scarce, but the prognosis is presumed poor.

REFERENCES

1. Ahmad U, Yao X, Detterbeck F, et al. Thymic carcinoma outcomes and prognosis: results of an international analysis. *J Thorac Cardiovasc Surg.* 2015;149:95–100, 101 e1–e2.
2. Litvak AM, Woo K, Hayes S, et al. Clinical characteristics and outcomes for patients with thymic carcinoma: evaluation of Masaoka staging. *J Thorac Oncol.* 2014;9:1810–1815.
3. Mao Y, Wu S. Treatment and survival analyses of completely resected thymic carcinoma patients. *Onco Targets Ther.* 2015;8:2503–2507.
4. Ruffini E, Detterbeck F, Van Raemdonck D, et al. Thymic carcinoma: a cohort study of patients from the European society of thoracic surgeons database. *J Thorac Oncol.* 2014;9:541–548.
5. Song Z, Zhang Y. Outcomes after surgical resection of thymic carcinoma: a study from a single tertiary referral centre. *Eur J Surg Oncol.* 2014;40:1523–1527.
6. Wang S, Wang Z, Liu X, et al. Prognostic factors of patients with thymic carcinoma after surgery: a retrospective analysis of 58 cases. *World J Surg.* 2014;38:2032–2038.
7. Weissferdt A, Moran CA. Thymic carcinoma, part 1: a clinicopathologic and immunohistochemical study of 65 cases. *Am J Clin Pathol.* 2012;138:103–114.
8. Eimoto T, Kitaoka M, Ogawa H, et al. Thymic sarcomatoid carcinoma with skeletal muscle differentiation: report of two cases, one with cytogenetic analysis. *Histopathology.* 2002;40:46–57.
9. Liu YG, Sun KK, Sui XZ, et al. Thymic carcinosarcoma consisting of sarcomatous and adenosquamous carcinomatous component. *Chin Med J (Engl).* 2012;125:4154–4155.
10. Lu HS, Gan MF, Zhou T, et al. Sarcomatoid thymic carcinoma arising in metaplastic thymoma: a case report. *Int J Surg Pathol.* 2011;19:677–680.
11. Morita M, Kakimoto S, Isoda K, et al. [A case of thymic carcinoma, sarcomatoid type]. *Kyobu Geka.* 1992;45:371–374.
12. Nishimura M, Kodama T, Nishiyama H, et al. A case of sarcomatoid carcinoma of the thymus. *Pathol Int.* 1997;47:260–263.

13. Okudela K, Nakamura N, Sano J, et al. Thymic carcinosarcoma consisting of squamous cell carcinomatous and embryonal rhabdomyosarcomatous components. Report of a case and review of the literature. *Pathol Res Pract.* 2001;197:205–210.

14. Suarez Vilela D, Salas Valien JS, Gonzalez Moran MA, et al. Thymic carcinosarcoma associated with a spindle cell thymoma: an immunohistochemical study. *Histopathology.* 1992;21:263–268.

15. Thomas de Montpréville V, Chan JK, Detterbeck F, et al. In: Travis WD, et al., eds. *WHO Classification of Tumours of the Lung, Pleura, Thymus, and Heart.* Lyon, France: IARC Press; 2015:232–233.

16. Suster S, Rosai J. Thymic carcinoma. A clinicopathologic study of 60 cases. *Cancer.* 1991;67:1025–1032.

17. Chalabreysse L, Etienne-Mastroianni B, Adeleine P, et al. Thymic carcinoma: a clinicopathological and immunohistological study of 19 cases. *Histopathology.* 2004;44:367–374.

18. Dorfman DM, Shahsafaei A, Chan JK. Thymic carcinomas, but not thymomas and carcinomas of other sites, show CD5 immunoreactivity. *Am J Surg Pathol.* 1997;21:936–940.

19. Hasserjian RP, Klimstra DS, Rosai J. Carcinoma of the thymus with clear-cell features. Report of eight cases and review of the literature. *Am J Surg Pathol.* 1995;19:835–841.

20. Nakano T, Endo S, Tsubochi H, et al. Thymic clear cell carcinoma. *Gen Thorac Cardiovasc Surg.* 2010;58:98–100.

21. Okuda M, Huang CL, Haba R, et al. Clear cell carcinoma originating from ectopic thymus. *Gen Thorac Cardiovasc Surg.* 2009;57:269–271.

22. Ritter JH, Wick MR. Primary carcinomas of the thymus gland. *Semin Diagn Pathol.* 1999;16:18–31.

23. Snover DC, Levine GD, Rosai J. Thymic carcinoma. Five distinctive histological variants. *Am J Surg Pathol.* 1982;6:451–470.

24. Stephens M, Khalil J, Gibbs AR. Primary clear cell carcinoma of the thymus gland. *Histopathology.* 1987;11:763–765.

25. Truong LD, Mody DR, Cagle PT, et al. Thymic carcinoma. A clinicopathologic study of 13 cases. *Am J Surg Pathol.* 1990;14:151–166.

26. Choi WW, Lui YH, Lau WH, et al. Adenocarcinoma of the thymus: report of two cases, including a previously undescribed mucinous subtype. *Am J Surg Pathol.* 2003;27:124–130.

27. Furtado A, Nogueira R, Ferreira D, et al. Papillary adenocarcinoma of the thymus: case report and review of the literature. *Int J Surg Pathol.* 2010;18:530–533.

28. Hosaka Y, Tsuchida M, Umezu H, et al. Primary thymic adenocarcinoma coexisting with type AB thymoma: a rare case with long-term survival. *Gen Thorac Cardiovasc Surg.* 2010;58:488–491; discussion 491–492.

29. Kapur P, Rakheja D, Bastasch M, et al. Primary mucinous adenocarcinoma of the thymus: a case report and review of the literature. *Arch Pathol Lab Med.* 2006;130:201–204.

30. Maeda D, Ota S, Ikeda S, et al. Mucinous adenocarcinoma of the thymus: a distinct variant of thymic carcinoma. *Lung Cancer.* 2009;64:22–27.

31. Maghbool M, Ramzi M, Nagel I, et al. Primary adenocarcinoma of the thymus: an immunohistochemical and molecular study with review of the literature. *BMC Clin Pathol.* 2013;13:17.

32. Matsuno Y, Morozumi N, Hirohashi S, et al. Papillary carcinoma of the thymus: report of four cases of a new microscopic type of thymic carcinoma. *Am J Surg Pathol.* 1998;22:873–880.

33. Morikawa H, Tanaka T, Hamaji M, et al. Papillary adenocarcinoma developed in a thymic cyst. *Gen Thorac Cardiovasc Surg.* 2010;58:295–297.

34. Ra SH, Fishbein MC, Baruch-Oren T, et al. Mucinous adenocarcinomas of the thymus: report of 2 cases and review of the literature. *Am J Surg Pathol.* 2007;31:1330–1336.

35. Takahashi F, Tsuta K, Matsuno Y, et al. Adenocarcinoma of the thymus: mucinous subtype. *Hum Pathol.* 2005;36:219–223.

36. Travis WD, Brambilla E, Noguchi M, et al. Diagnosis of lung adenocarcinoma in resected specimens: implications of the 2011 International Association for the Study of Lung Cancer/American Thoracic Society/European Respiratory Society classification. *Arch Pathol Lab Med.* 2013;137:685–705.

37. Yoshino M, Hiroshima K, Motohashi S, et al. Papillary carcinoma of the thymus gland. *Ann Thorac Surg.* 2005;80:741–742.

38. Zaitlin N, Rozenman J, Yellin A. Papillary adenocarcinoma in a thymic cyst: a pitfall of thoracoscopic excision. *Ann Thorac Surg.* 2003;76:1279–1281.

39. Evans AG, French CA, Cameron MJ, et al. Pathologic characteristics of NUT midline carcinoma arising in the mediastinum. *Am J Surg Pathol.* 2012;36:1222–1227.

40. Kubonishi I, Takehara N, Iwata J, et al. Novel t(15;19)(q15;p13) chromosome abnormality in a thymic carcinoma. *Cancer Res.* 1991;51:3327–3328.

41. Kuzume T, Kubonishi I, Takeuchi S, et al. Establishment and characterization of a thymic carcinoma cell line (Ty-82) carrying t(15;19)(q15;p13) chromosome abnormality. *Int J Cancer.* 1992;50:259–264.

42. Lee AC, Kwong YI, Fu KH, et al. Disseminated mediastinal carcinoma with chromosomal translocation (15;19). A distinctive clinicopathologic syndrome. *Cancer.* 1993;72:2273–2276.

43. Petrini P, French CA, Rajan A, et al. NUT rearrangement is uncommon in human thymic epithelial tumors. *J Thorac Oncol.* 2012;7:744–750.

44. Toretsky JA, Jenson J, Sun CC, et al. Translocation (11;15;19): a highly specific chromosome rearrangement associated with poorly differentiated thymic carcinoma in young patients. *Am J Clin Oncol.* 2003;26:300–306.

112 Thymic Neuroendocrine Carcinomas/Tumors

Borislav A. Alexiev, M.D., Anja C. Roden, M.D., and Allen P. Burke, M.D.

The histopathologic classification of primary neuroendocrine tumors (NETs) of the mediastinum is similar to that of NETs of other organs. There are two classifications. One follows that of the lung (carcinoid, atypical carcinoid, large cell neuroendocrine carcinoma, and small cell carcinoma).[1] The other is similar to that used in the gastrointestinal tract (well-differentiated NET/carcinoma, moderately differentiated neuroendocrine carcinoma, and poorly differentiated neuroendocrine carcinoma).[2] There are advantages to both systems. The rationale for considering all these tumors as carcinomas is the observation that all mediastinal carcinoids bear a significant risk for recurrence, metastasis, and tumor-associated death. However, carcinoids are treated far differently from small cell carcinoma, which is a clinically distinct entity. Not all small cell carcinomas show demonstrable neuroendocrine differentiation, which may justify a category for them separate from large cell neuroendocrine carcinoma (see Chapter 85, Section 1).

Terminology

Thymic epithelial tumors that are predominantly or exclusively composed of neuroendocrine cells are classified as neuroendocrine carcinomas of the thymus. They have to be distinguished (1) from otherwise typical thymic carcinomas, which may contain scattered or groups of neuroendocrine cells, and (2) from nonepithelial neurogenic tumors, particularly paragangliomas.[1]

Typical (classic) carcinoid (well-differentiated NET/NEC, low grade) is a well-differentiated NET composed of polygonal cells with granular cytoplasm arranged in ribbons, festoons, solid nests, and rosette-like glands. Tumors have <2 mitoses per 10 HPF, and necrosis is absent.

Atypical carcinoid (well-differentiated NET/NEC, intermediate grade) is defined as a well-differentiated NET with (1) mitotic rate of 2 to 10 per 10 HPFs and/or (2) necrosis.

Large-cell neuroendocrine carcinoma (poorly differentiated NET/ NEC, high grade): A high-grade thymic tumor composed of large cells with neuroendocrine morphology such as palisading, trabeculae, nesting, or rosette-like features; necrosis that is usually extensive; a high mitotic rate (mitotic rate of >10 per 10 HPF); and either neurosecretory granules by electron microscopy or positive neuroendocrine immunohistochemical markers.

Small cell carcinoma, neuroendocrine type (poorly differentiated NET/NEC, high grade) is a high-grade thymic tumor consisting of small cells (<3 lymphocytes) with scant cytoplasm, ill-defined cell borders, finely granular nuclear chromatin, and absent or inconspicuous nucleoli. The cells are round, oval, or spindle shaped, and nuclear molding and crush artifact with nuclear streaming and incrustation of vessels is prominent. High mitotic rate, apoptotic bodies, and large areas of geographic necrosis are typical. A variant is a combined small cell carcinoma with squamous cell carcinoma or adenocarcinoma.

Incidence and Clinical Presentation

Primary thymic neuroendocrine carcinomas are rare and account for no more than 5% of all mediastinal tumors.[3] Thymic NETs are mainly tumors of adults (mean age 52 years), but have also been rarely observed in children.[4] There is a male preponderance (73%).[4] Whites constituted the highest proportion of patients accounting for 83% of cases.[4] In contrast to histologic similar tumors in the lung, there is no established role of smoking.

In one series of thymectomies performed in patients without myasthenia gravis, 12.5% of tumors were found to be epithelial thymic malignancies, one-half of which were carcinoid tumors.[5]

Thymic neuroendocrine carcinomas exhibit local symptoms (chest pain, cough, dyspnea, or superior vena cava syndrome).[1] About 25% of patients have a family history of MEN1.[6,7] MEN1-associated thymic NETs/NECs have all been carcinoids and occurred almost only in male adults. No high-grade NETs/NECs have been reported in the setting of MEN1 syndrome. Paraneoplastic manifestations include Cushing syndrome, hypercalcemia (resulting either from tumor production of PTHrP or from primary hyperparathyroidism in MEN1 patients), acromegaly, and inappropriate production of antidiuretic hormone or atrial natriuretic peptide.[6-11] Paraneoplastic autoimmune disorders, such as the Lambert-Eaton and myasthenic syndromes, and carcinoid syndrome are very rare (<1%).[1]

Gross Pathology

Well-differentiated (carcinoids) and poorly differentiated thymic neuroendocrine carcinomas are virtually identical macroscopically. The majority of tumors is unencapsulated and can appear either circumscribed or grossly invasive. They are gray-white and firm on cut section, can have a gritty consistency, and usually lack the characteristic lobulated growth pattern of thymomas. Foci of hemorrhage and necrosis are apparent in 70% of cases. Calcifications are frequent.[1]

Microscopic Pathology

Typical carcinoids (well-differentiated NETs/carcinomas) are devoid of necrotic areas and exhibit a low mitotic rate (<2 mitoses per 10 HPFs). The tumor cells are uniform and polygonal, with relatively small, round nuclei, finely granular chromatin, and pale eosinophilic cytoplasm. Most tumors (>50%) show trabecular and rosetting growth patterns, but a number of other patterns, such as ribbons, festoons, solid nests, glandular structures, and nuclear palisading, are also common. A delicate "endocrine tumor–type" vasculature between the nests and trabeculae is characteristic. Lymphovascular invasion is frequent.

Between 60% and 70% of thymic NETs are atypical carcinoids.[2] Atypical carcinoid is defined as a well-differentiated neuroendocrine carcinoma, intermediate grade with (1) mitotic rate of 2 to 10 per 10 HPFs, and/or (2) focal necrosis (Figs. 112.1 and 112.2). Usually, both increased mitotic activity and necrosis are present. Similar to

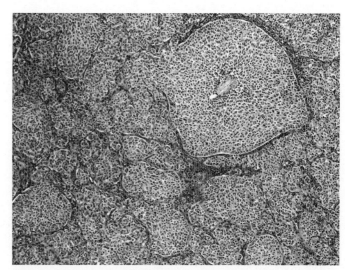

FIGURE 112.1 ▲ Atypical carcinoid (well-differentiated neuroendocrine carcinoma, intermediate grade). Note solid nests and delicate "endocrine tumor-type" vasculature.

their lung counterparts, the upper limit of mitoses in atypical carcinoid is defined as 10 mitoses per 10 HPFs; tumors exceeding that cutoff are classified as high-grade neuroendocrine carcinomas, subtyped as small cell or large cell neuroendocrine carcinomas.

In addition to the different growth patterns, there are a number of recognized variants that can belong to both the typical and the atypical carcinoid categories. These carcinoid variants include spindle cell,[12-14] pigmented,[12,15] oncocytic,[9] mucinous,[16,17] and angiomatoid variants.[15] Large cell neuroendocrine carcinoma of the thymus is defined by high mitotic rate (>10 per 10 HPFs) and extensive necrosis, with neuroendocrine (carcinoid-like) architecture at low-power magnification. Higher magnification shows prominent nucleoli, vesicular rather than finely granular chromatin, abundant cytoplasm, and evident cell membranes (Fig. 112.3). Cells are usually larger than those of small cell carcinoma, but similar to small cell carcinoma, there is significant size variability.

The defining features of small cell carcinoma of the thymus are the same as those of the lung (see Chapter 85, Section 1). Thymic small cell carcinomas are rare and are usually included in series of thymic nonneuroendocrine carcinomas.[18,19] The key defining feature

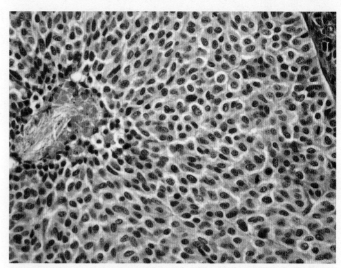

FIGURE 112.2 ▲ Atypical carcinoid (well-differentiated neuroendocrine carcinoma, intermediate grade). Note focal necrosis and mitoses.

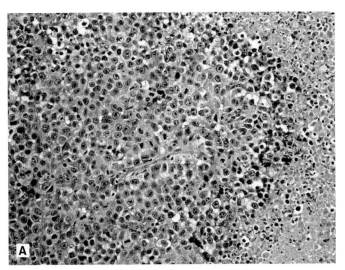
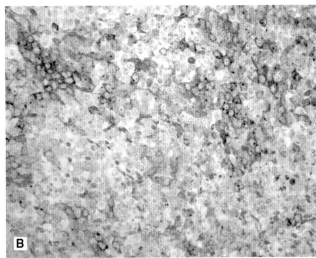

FIGURE 112.3 ▲ Large cell neuroendocrine carcinoma, thymus (high-grade neuroendocrine carcinoma). **A.** There is nuclear clearing with prominent nucleoli, and necrosis is seen at the right. **B.** There is diffuse expression of synaptophysin (immunohistochemical antisynaptophysin staining).

is nuclear appearance, which includes finely granular, dark chromatin, lack of prominent nucleoli, nuclear molding, spindling (fusiform cells), and crush artifact with nuclear streaming and incrustation of vessels (Azzopardi phenomenon). Other defining features are scant cytoplasm and indistinct cell borders. High mitotic rate (>10 per 10 HPFs), apoptotic bodies, and large areas of geographic necrosis are typically present.

Special Studies

Thymic NETs are immunoreactive for keratins (AE1/AE3, CAM5.2), often showing a dot-like staining especially in small cell carcinoma. Neuroendocrine markers such as synaptophysin, chromogranin, and CD56 are usually strongly expressed, especially in lower grade tumors (carcinoids and atypical carcinoids) (Figs. 112.4 and 112.5).[20] Staining in small cell carcinomas is generally more patchy (Fig. 112.6). CD5 is generally negative.[1]

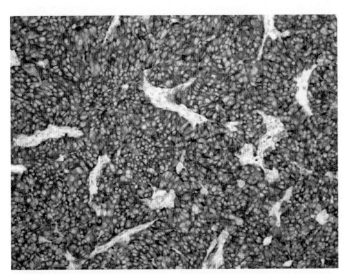

FIGURE 112.4 ▲ Atypical carcinoid (well-differentiated neuroendocrine carcinoma, intermediate grade). Note strong synaptophysin expression (antisynaptophysin).

Thymic carcinoid tumors have been shown to express somatostatin, adrenocorticotropic hormone (especially in association with Cushing syndrome), and occasionally serotonin.[21]

One study demonstrated that well- and moderately differentiated thymic neuroendocrine carcinomas (typical and atypical carcinoids) were positive for PAX8 in 43% and TTF-1 in 8% of tumors.[2]

Comparative genomic hybridization (CGH) analysis of NETs demonstrated gains of chromosomal material on regions X, 7, 8, 11q, 18, and 20p and losses on 3, 6, 9q, 13q, and 11q.[22] These CGH data show a degree of overlap with chromosomal imbalances commonly observed in advanced thymomas.[23]

Differential Diagnosis

The most important considerations in the differential diagnosis of thymic NETs include metastatic neuroendocrine carcinomas, paragangliomas, or ectopic parathyroid adenomas. In cases of metastatic tumors, a precise clinical history and radiologic evaluation are important to properly assess the origin of the tumor. Immunohistochemical detection of TTF-1 expression might be helpful in distinguishing high-grade neuroendocrine carcinomas of the lung from their thymic counterparts, since most thymic tumors are TTF-1 negative, while pulmonary neuroendocrine carcinomas (especially small cell) are almost always TTF-1 positive.

In paragangliomas, the histopathologic characteristic is that these tumors will show a similar growth pattern as low-grade neuroendocrine carcinoma; however, paragangliomas will display negative staining for keratin. In parathyroid adenomas, the presence of prominent clear cells (chief cells) admixed with oncocytic cells may lead to the correct interpretation. In addition, the use of periodic acid–Schiff stain to determine the presence of glycogen and immunohistochemical studies for parathyroid hormone will be helpful in this setting.[3]

Spindle cell carcinoids can resemble other spindle cell tumors of the thymus, including type A thymoma and synovial sarcoma, which are also cytokeratin positive but lack neuroendocrine differentiation, such as chromogranin or synaptophysin expression.[12,13]

The mucinous carcinoid variant can resemble metastatic mucinous carcinoma, such as from the gastrointestinal tract or breast.[24] The angiomatoid variant resembles hemangioma with large blood-filled cystic spaces, but these spaces are lined by polygonal tumor cells and not endothelium.[15] The diagnosis of small cell carcinoma with negative

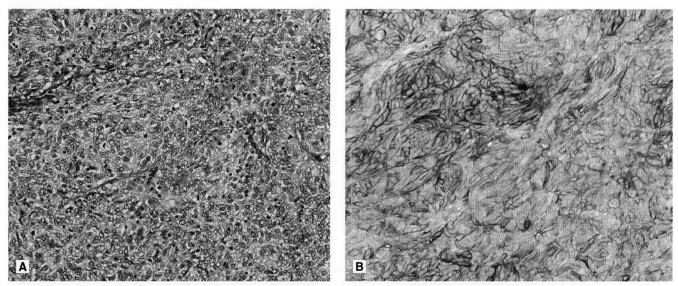

FIGURE 112.5 ▲ Large-cell neuroendocrine carcinoma, thymus. **A.** There is a vague rosette-like pattern with some spindling. **B.** Immunohistochemical staining with antisynaptophysin demonstrates diffuse cytoplasmic predominantly membranous staining.

keratin should be made with great caution after exclusion of lymphoma and primitive neuroectodermal tumor.

Thymic NETs can be admixed with thymoma or different subtypes of thymic carcinoma and have been reported as components of teratomas of the thymus (so-called somatic-type malignancy).[25,26]

Treatment and Prognosis

The prognosis of thymic NETs is linked to the degree of differentiation of these tumors. In the classic paper on thymic carcinoids by Wick and Scheithauer[21] 3 of 12 patients died of disease, 7 had no evident disease at follow-up, and 2 had persistent disease. In the study of Gaur et al.,[4] the median survival was 78, 43, and 23 months for low-grade

(carcinoid), intermediate-grade (atypical carcinoid), and high-grade neuroendocrine carcinomas of the thymus, respectively. In another study, the overall 3-, 5-, and 10-year survival for all three groups combined was 89%, 79%, and 41%, respectively, with complete resection and low Ki-67 index imparting a good prognosis.[27] These two features are highly associated with grade and stage, respectively. Distant metastatic sites include the lung, brain, liver, kidney, bone, adrenal, skin, and pancreas.[27]

The optimal treatment of thymic NETs is controversial. In addition to surgery, chemotherapy with temozolomide and platinum-based therapy has been used with some success.[27] Radiation therapy is also used to control local tumor recurrence when surgical excision is incomplete.[4]

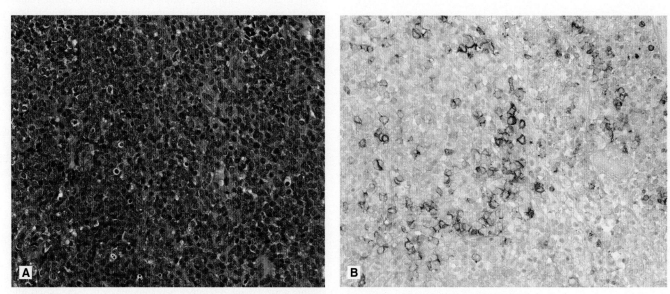

FIGURE 112.6 ▲ Small cell carcinoma, thymus. **A.** The tumor cells are small with inconspicuous nucleoli and little cytoplasm. **B.** There is patchy CD56 (NCAM) staining by immunohistochemistry.

REFERENCES

1. Ströbel P, Marx A, Chan JKC, et al. Thymic neuroendocrine tumors. In: Travis WD, et al., eds. *WHO Classification of Tumours of the Lung, Pleura, Mediastinum and Heart*. Lyon, France: IARC Press; 2015:234–243.

2. Weissferdt A, Tang X, Wistuba, II, et al. Comparative immunohistochemical analysis of pulmonary and thymic neuroendocrine carcinomas using PAX8 and TTF-1. *Mod Pathol*. 2013;26:1554–1560.

3. Moran CA, Suster S. Neuroendocrine carcinomas (carcinoid, atypical carcinoid, small cell carcinoma, and large cell neuroendocrine carcinoma): current concepts. *Hematol Oncol Clin North Am*. 2007;21:395–407; vii.

4. Gaur P, Leary C, Yao JC. Thymic neuroendocrine tumors: a SEER database analysis of 160 patients. *Ann Surg*. 2010;251:1117–1121.

5. Ackman JB, Verzosa S, Kovach AE, et al. High rate of unnecessary thymectomy and its cause. Can computed tomography distinguish thymoma, lymphoma, thymic hyperplasia, and thymic cysts? *Eur J Radiol*. 2015;84:524–533.

6. Lim LC, Tan MH, Eng C, et al. Thymic carcinoid in multiple endocrine neoplasia 1: genotype-phenotype correlation and prevention. *J Intern Med*. 2006;259:428–432.

7. Teh BT, Zedenius J, Kytola S, et al. Thymic carcinoids in multiple endocrine neoplasia type 1. *Ann Surg*. 1998;228:99–105.

8. de Perrot M, Spiliopoulos A, Fischer S, et al. Neuroendocrine carcinoma (carcinoid) of the thymus associated with Cushing's syndrome. *Ann Thorac Surg*. 2002;73:675–681.

9. Yamaji I, Iimura O, Mito T, et al. An ectopic, ACTH producing, oncocytic carcinoid tumor of the thymus: report of a case. *Jpn J Med*. 1984;23:62–66.

10. Saito T, Kimoto M, Nakai S, et al. Ectopic ACTH syndrome associated with large cell neuroendocrine carcinoma of the thymus. *Intern Med*. 2011;50:1471–1475.

11. Hekimgil M, Hamulu F, Cagirici U, et al. Small cell neuroendocrine carcinoma of the thymus complicated by Cushing's syndrome. Report of a 58-year-old woman with a 3-year history of hypertension. *Pathol Res Pract*. 2001;197:129–133.

12. Levine GD, Rosai J. A spindle cell variant of thymic carcinoid tumor. A clinical, histologic, and fine structural study with emphasis on its distinction from spindle cell thymoma. *Arch Pathol Lab Med*. 1976;100:293–300.

13. Moran CA, Suster S. Spindle-cell neuroendocrine carcinomas of the thymus (spindle-cell thymic carcinoid): a clinicopathologic and immunohistochemical study of seven cases. *Mod Pathol*. 1999;12:587–591.

14. Dusenbery D. Spindle-cell thymic carcinoid occurring in multiple endocrine neoplasia I: fine-needle aspiration findings in a case. *Diagn Cytopathol*. 1996;15:439–441.

15. Moran CA, Suster S. Angiomatoid neuroendocrine carcinoma of the thymus: report of a distinctive morphological variant of neuroendocrine tumor of the thymus resembling a vascular neoplasm. *Hum Pathol*. 1999;30:635–639.

16. Gao Z, Kahn L, Bhuiya T. Thymic carcinoid with mucinous stroma: a rare variant of carcinoid with an aggressive clinical course. *Ann Diagn Pathol*. 2006;10:114–116.

17. Suster S, Moran CA. Thymic carcinoid with prominent mucinous stroma. Report of a distinctive morphologic variant of thymic neuroendocrine neoplasm. *Am J Surg Pathol*. 1995;19:1277–1285.

18. Truong LD, Mody DR, Cagle PT, et al. Thymic carcinoma. A clinicopathologic study of 13 cases. *Am J Surg Pathol*. 1990;14:151–166.

19. Zhang Z, Cui Y, Li B, et al. Thymic carcinoma (report of 14 cases). *Chin Med Sci J*. 1997;12:252–255.

20. Moran CA, Suster S. Neuroendocrine carcinomas (carcinoid tumor) of the thymus. A clinicopathologic analysis of 80 cases. *Am J Clin Pathol*. 2000;114:100–110.

21. Wick MR, Scheithauer BW. Thymic carcinoid. A histologic, immunohistochemical, and ultrastructural study of 12 cases. *Cancer*. 1984;53:475–484.

22. Pan CC, Jong YJ, Chen YJ. Comparative genomic hybridization analysis of thymic neuroendocrine tumors. *Mod Pathol*. 2005;18:358–364.

23. Rieker RJ, Aulmann S, Penzel R, et al. Chromosomal imbalances in sporadic neuroendocrine tumours of the thymus. *Cancer Lett*. 2005;223:169–174.

24. Ohchi T, Tanaka H, Shibuya Y, et al. Thymic carcinoid with mucinous stroma: a case report. *Respir Med*. 1998;92:880–882.

25. Schaefer IM, Zardo P, Freermann S, et al. Neuroendocrine carcinoma in a mediastinal teratoma as a rare variant of somatic-type malignancy. *Virchows Arch*. 2013;463:731–735.

26. Lancaster KJ, Liang CY, Myers JC, et al. Goblet cell carcinoid arising in a mature teratoma of the mediastinum. *Am J Surg Pathol*. 1997;21:109–113.

27. Crona J, Bjorklund P, Welin S, et al. Treatment, prognostic markers and survival in thymic neuroendocrine tumours. a study from a single tertiary referral centre. *Lung Cancer*. 2013;79:289–293.

113 Thymic Cysts

Borislav A. Alexiev, M.D., and Allen P. Burke, M.D.

Terminology

Thymic cysts are relatively rare benign lesions. They comprise approximately two-thirds of anterior mediastinal cysts, but only 5% of all mediastinal cysts.[1,2] Other cystic lesions in the mediastinum include bronchogenic cysts, cystic teratomas, hydatid cysts, enteric cysts, and lymphangiomas.

Thymic cysts are commonly classified as either congenital or acquired. Congenital thymic cyst is considered to arise as a congenital defect due to persistence of embryonal remnants.[3] A relative high proportion of congenital ectopic thymic cysts are diagnosed in the neck, where they are easily detected.[4,5]

Congenital thymic cysts are usually unilocular and lack inflammatory processes.[6-8] In contrast, acquired cysts are always multilocular and accompanied by inflammation.[3,9-14] Multilocular cysts most likely result from the cystic transformation of medullary duct epithelium–derived structures (including Hassall corpuscles) induced by an acquired inflammatory process.[3]

Incidence and Clinical

Thymic cysts comprise 3% of published anterior mediastinal masses and 15% of mediastinal cysts.[3,12] Congenital cysts are more common in children.[6,15] Acquired thymic cysts occur in middle-aged and older adults, with a male predominance.[3,10,14] Thymic cysts are most often asymptomatic and discovered incidentally on routine chest x-ray.[3,12] Patients may also present with acute symptoms of chest pain or discomfort, sometimes associated with dyspnea.[3]

Thymic cysts associated with inflammatory conditions such as Sjögren syndrome and HIV, similar to salivary gland cystic lesions, have been described.[9-11,16]

Cysts may also be a prominent component of thymic epithelial tumors, both thymomas and carcinomas.[3,17-19]

Gross Pathology

Congenital cysts are predominantly unilocular, filled with a clear watery fluid, and with smooth and gray-white inner surfaces.[8] On cut section, the acquired cysts show multiloculated cavities with thick gray walls and are filled with turbid yellow fluid.[3,10,11]

Microscopic Pathology

Microscopically, the congenital cysts are lined by a cuboidal and low cylindrical nonciliated epithelium with normal-appearing thymic tissue in the cyst wall (Fig. 113.1). Acquired cysts are characterized by several cystic spaces separated by various thick walls with dense lymphoid tissue containing large reactive germinal centers and intense mixed acute and chronic inflammation (Fig. 113.2).[3,10,11] The inner cyst walls are lined by flattened cuboidal epithelia in some portions. Columnar epithelial cells with focal cilia are rarely observed. The cyst lining is continuous with thymic lobules in the wall. Other areas show extensive cholesterol granuloma formation with foreign body–type giant cells.

Special Studies

Immunohistochemical studies demonstrate thymic epithelial cells (CK5/6+) and immature T cells (TdT+, CD1a+, CD99+) in the cyst walls.

Differential Diagnosis

It is difficult to distinguish nonneoplastic congenital and acquired thymic cysts from thymoma undergoing extensive cystic degeneration.[17]

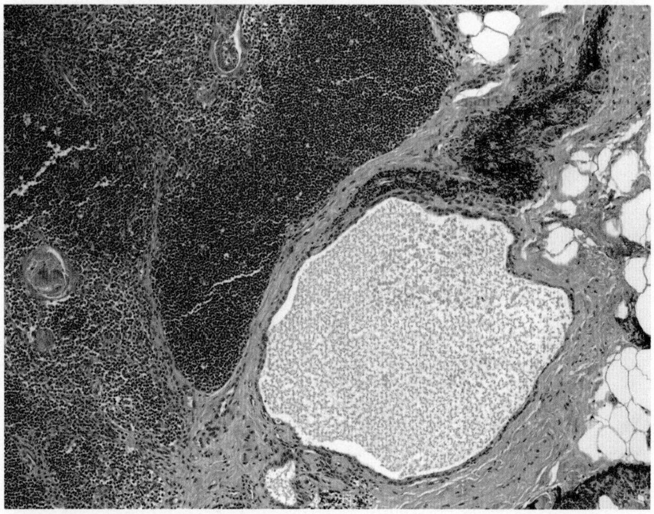

FIGURE 113.1 ▲ Congenital unilocular thymic cyst. Note normal-appearing thymic tissue in the cyst wall and lack of inflammation (H&E, ×40).

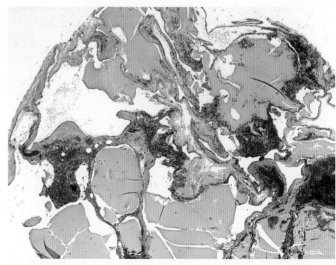

FIGURE 113.2 ▲ Acquired multilocular thymic cyst (H&E, ×40).

In this context, the complete absence of epithelial lining within the cystic wall is an important pathologic feature of cystic thymoma.[3,17] Pericardial cysts are typically adjacent to the diaphragm and are lined by mesothelial cells, and bronchogenic cysts are lined by respiratory-type epithelium, typically with a muscular wall.

Treatment and Prognosis

Thymic cysts are generally cured by surgical excision.[1,2]

REFERENCES

1. Gochi F, Omasa M, Yamada T, et al. Factors affecting the preoperative diagnosis of anterior mediastinal cysts. *Gen Thorac Cardiovasc Surg.* 2015;63:349–353.
2. Aydin Y, Ogul H, Turkyilmaz A, et al. Surgical treatment of mediastinal cysts: report on 29 cases. *Acta Chir Belg.* 2012;112:281–286.
3. Suster S, Rosai J. Multilocular thymic cyst: an acquired reactive process. Study of 18 cases. *Am J Surg Pathol.* 1991;15:388–398.
4. Michalopoulos N, Papavramidis TS, Karayannopoulou G, et al. Cervical thymic cysts in adults. *Thyroid.* 2011;21:987–992.
5. De Caluwe D, Ahmed M, Puri P. Cervical thymic cysts. *Pediatr Surg Int.* 2002;18:477–479.
6. Eifinger F, Ernestus K, Benz-Bohm G, et al. True thymic hyperplasia associated with severe thymic cyst bleeding in a newborn: case report and review of the literature. *Ann Diagn Pathol.* 2007;11:358–362.
7. Kitami A, Kamio Y, Uematsu S, et al. Thymoma with intracystic dissemination arising in a unilocular thymic cyst. *Gen Thorac Cardiovasc Surg.* 2007;55:281–283.
8. Scharifker D. True thymic hyperplasia associated with a unilocular thymic cyst: an unusual combination not previously reported. *Ann Diagn Pathol.* 2006;10:32–35.
9. Avila NA, Mueller BU, Carrasquillo JA, et al. Multilocular thymic cysts: imaging features in children with human immunodeficiency virus infection. *Radiology.* 1996;201:130–134.
10. Izumi H, Nobukawa B, Takahashi K, et al. Multilocular thymic cyst associated with follicular hyperplasia: clinicopathologic study of 4 resected cases. *Hum Pathol.* 2005;36:841–844.
11. Kondo K, Miyoshi T, Sakiyama S, et al. Multilocular thymic cyst associated with Sjogren's syndrome. *Ann Thorac Surg.* 2001;72:1367–1369.
12. Le Pimpec-Barthes F, Cazes A, Bagan P, et al. [Mediastinal cysts: clinical approach and treatment]. *Rev Pneumol Clin.* 2010;66:52–62.
13. Saito Y, Uragami T, Satake A, et al. [Multilocular thymic cyst]. *Kyobu Geka.* 2009;62:227–230.
14. Suster S, Barbuto D, Carlson G, et al. Multilocular thymic cysts with pseudoepitheliomatous hyperplasia. *Hum Pathol.* 1991;22:455–460.
15. Tollefsen I, Yoo M, Bland JD, et al. Thymic cyst: is a correct preoperative diagnosis possible? Report of a case and review of the literature. *Eur J Pediatr.* 2001;160:620–622.
16. Minato H, Kinoshita E, Nakada S, et al. Thymic lymphoid hyperplasia with multilocular thymic cysts diagnosed before the Sjogren syndrome diagnosis. *Diagn Pathol.* 2015;10:103.
17. Honda S, Morikawa T, Sasaki F, et al. Cystic thymoma in a child: a rare case and review of the literature. *Pediatr Surg Int.* 2007;23:1015–1017.
18. Ascani S, Carloni A, Agostinelli C, et al. Thymoma arising in the wall of a thymic cyst. *Pathologica.* 2008;100:476–477.
19. Sugio K, Ondo K, Yamaguchi M, et al. Thymoma arising in a thymic cyst. *Ann Thorac Cardiovasc Surg.* 2000;6:329–331.

114 Thymic Hyperplasia

Borislav A. Alexiev, M.D., and Allen P. Burke, M.D.

Terminology

Most thymic hyperplasia is the result of *reactive lymphoid hyperplasia*, frequently in the setting of autoimmune disease, notably myasthenia gravis. Reactive thymic hyperplasia has also been described with other abnormalities, especially Graves disease,[1,2] sarcoidosis,[3] Castleman disease,[4] and Beckwith-Wiedemann syndrome[5] (Table 114.1). Reactive thymic hyperplasia may also occur in patients without known autoimmune disease.[11]

True thymic hyperplasia is defined as an increase in size and weight of the thymus gland, which by definition maintains a normal histologic architecture. True thymic hyperplasia without any other disease (idiopathic) is a rare disorder, with only a handful of well-documented examples in the literature.[5]

The normal range of thymic mass is age dependent.[12,13] In general, any weight over 15 g is abnormal in older adults, and a weight over 35 g is abnormal in children and young adults. When the weight exceeds 100 g, the term "massive" thymic hyperplasia is used.

Enlargement of the thymus gland may occur as a rebound phenomenon after recovery from severe stress, after administration of steroids, and after treatment of malignant tumors[14–16] (Table 114.2).

Gross Pathology

In cases of true thymic hyperplasia, the thymus is massively and uniformly enlarged, and the parenchyma is whitish-yellow with hemorrhagic areas.[17] In cases of reactive thymic hyperplasia, there are no discerning gross features, although the presence of cysts, firm areas, and necrosis should be documented and sampled, to rule out malignancy. It is also recommended to weigh the gland, in addition to providing standard measurements.

Microscopic Pathology

In true thymic hyperplasia, histologic examination reveals a normal thymic architecture with well-defined cortical and medullary areas (Fig. 114.1).[17–20] In the cortical areas, macrophages with phagocytized nuclear debris (starry sky macrophages) could be observed, suggesting acute cortical involution. Other types of involutional change observed in infants (lymphocyte depletion) are not seen.[21]

TABLE 114.1 Conditions Associated with Thymic Hyperplasia

- Myasthenia gravis
- Graves disease
- Castleman disease[4]
- Beckwith-Wiedemann syndrome[5]
- Sjögren syndrome[6]
- Celiac disease[7]
- Antiphospholipid syndrome[8]
- Systemic sclerosis[9]
- Multiple sclerosis[10]
- Autoimmune hemolytic anemia[10]
- Systemic lupus erythematosus[10]
- Ulcerative colitis[10]
- Sarcoidosis[3]

TABLE 114.2   Differential Diagnosis of Thymic Hyperplasia and Mimickers

	Incidence	Associations	Pathology Findings
True thymic hyperplasia	Rare	None, usually children	Normal architecture, including Hassall corpuscles, degenerative changes of hemorrhage, vascular proliferation
Reactive thymic hyperplasia	Common	Autoimmune disorders (see Table 114.1)	B-cell follicular hyperplasia with follicular dendritic cells and germinal centers
B-cell–rich thymoma	Uncommon	Myasthenia gravis	Thymus-like expansion of neoplastic epithelial cells admixed with immature T cells, replacing normal architecture
Micronodular thymoma	Rare	Myasthenia gravis (uncommon)	Thymoma with large areas of reactive B-cell follicles
Rebound thymic hyperplasia	Rare	Chemotherapy, stress	Few reports; normal thymic architecture with increased size

In reactive lymphoid hyperplasia, seen most frequently in patients with myasthenia gravis, there are B-cell lymphoid follicles with follicular dendritic cells, and often, there are germinal centers with tingible body macrophages. The frequency of finding germinal centers depends on the number of sections studied.[22]

Rarely, thymic hyperplasia may be associated with lymphoepithelial-like lesions that may contain reactive B-cell follicles. These patients did not have underlying myasthenia or autoimmune disease.[11]

The histologic findings of rebound thymic hyperplasia after stress or chemotherapy are not well studied. Reports have demonstrated normal thymic architecture with Hassall corpuscles, despite symptomatic enlargement of the gland.[14,15]

Special Studies

In true thymic hyperplasia, immunohistochemistry reveals normal distribution of CD20-positive B lymphocytes (Fig. 114.2) and CD3-positive T lymphocytes with immature CD99 (Fig. 114.3) and CD1a-positive T cells in the cortex.[23] Pan-cytokeratin immunostaining demonstrates thymic epithelial cells in the cortex, in distinction from lymphoid proliferative disease. The morphologic appearance of the lymphoid cells and the types of cells present and flow cytometric analysis are crucial for excluding morphologically similar entities, especially Hodgkin lymphoma, especially on small biopsy samples.[18]

The Thymus in Myasthenia Gravis

The most frequent finding in thymectomies for myasthenia gravies is hyperplasia, occurring in 40% to 90% of cases (Figs. 114.4 and 114.5).[24–27] There is an especially high rate of thymic hyperplasia reported in ocular myasthenia gravis.[26] Postoperative thymectomy remission rates are highest when hyperplasia is the histologic diagnosis (40%).[28] The benefit of thymectomy remains controversial in patients with myasthenia, however.[28]

Thymomas are found in 10% to 30% of patients with myasthenia gravis (65/326)[24,25,27] and are usually of the lymphoid-rich type (B subsets).

In the remainder of patients (usually <1/3), the thymus is normal (Fig. 114.6).[24,25,27] Other findings that are not uncommon in thymectomies performed in patients for myasthenia gravis include thymic cysts, and ectopic thymic tissue in extrathymic fat.[25]

Hyperplasia in Patients Without Myasthenia Gravis

Patients with enlarged thymuses in the absence of myasthenia gravis may undergo thymectomy in order to rule out malignancy. In a series of nonmyasthenic patients, thymic pathology included hyperplasia in 8% of thymic glands; these patients were not reported to have other autoimmune diseases.[29] The most common fining was thymoma (34%), followed by lymphoma (24%), cysts (11%), hyperplasia (8%), carcinoma (7%), carcinoid (67%), sarcoma (2%), and normal thymus (2%).[29]

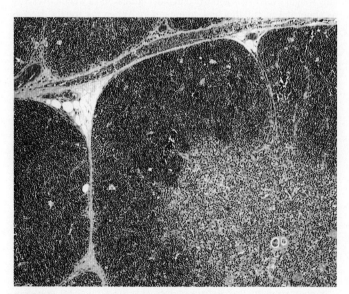

FIGURE 114.1 ▲ True thymic hyperplasia. Note normal histologic architecture (H&E, ×40).

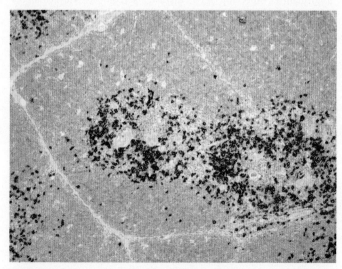

FIGURE 114.2 ▲ True thymic hyperplasia. Note normal distribution of CD20-positive B lymphocytes (anti-CD20, ×40).

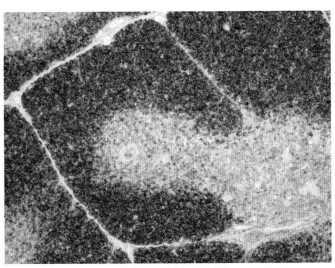

FIGURE 114.3 ▲ True thymic hyperplasia. Note normal distribution of CD99-positive immature T lymphocytes (anti-CD99, ×40).

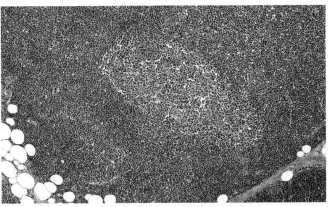

FIGURE 114.5 ▲ Thymic hyperplasia, myasthenia gravis. A higher magnification shows a germinal center.

The patients operated in this series for reactive thymic hyperplasia were considered to be unnecessary operations, other than to exclude a tumor.[29] In general, treatment of substantial thymic hyperplasia depends on the age of the patient and clinical symptoms. The recommended strategy is to closely follow symptomatic patients during a trial of corticosteroids and, in case of poor response, to perform surgery (thymectomy) if the thymus enlarges further or elicits severe symptoms.[12] Recognizing the association between thymic hyperplasia and endocrine abnormalities, and existence of the benign course/regression after treatment of the primary disease may be useful for avoiding unnecessary surgical procedure.[3,30,31]

Differential Diagnosis

The major differential diagnosis of thymic hyperplasia is lymphocyte-rich thymoma, especially types B1 and B2. Replacement of the thymic architecture by tumor is pathognomonic for thymoma, with obliteration of normal fat areas around the corticomedullary structures.

Pan-cytokeratin stains demonstrate highlight tumor cells and distinguish thymoma from hyperplasia or lymphoma (Figs. 114.7 and 114.8). Micronodular thymoma can be especially difficult to distinguish from reactive nodular hyperplasia, because of the reactive follicles, but the identification of the epithelial malignant component allows for the diagnosis.[32]

Hodgkin lymphoma is especially common in the mediastinum and should always be excluded by an appropriate panel of immunohistochemical stains in small biopsies or if there is any suspicion for lymphoma.

T-cell lymphoblastic lymphoma, lymphocyte-rich B1 thymoma, and thymic hyperplasia could all demonstrate large numbers of CD3-positive T cells that would be expected to express surface CD1a and cytoplasmic TdT, with coexpression of surface CD4 and CD8.[18] Lymphoblastic lymphoma on aspirate smears and tissue sections shows a relatively monomorphous population of small-to-medium–sized individual cells with a high nuclear–cytoplasmic ratio, identical to the L2 subtype of blasts seen in acute lymphoblastic leukemia.[18]

True thymic hyperplasia must be differentiated from lymphoid follicular hyperplasia.[33,34] In lymphoid follicular hyperplasia, the perivascular spaces are expanded by B cells forming follicles and germinal centers. In the medulla, the numbers of interdigitating dendritic cells are also increased.[33,34]

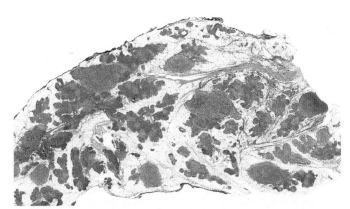

FIGURE 114.4 ▲ Thymic hyperplasia, myasthenia gravis. There are more solid areas corresponding to B-cell lymphoid hyperplasia. The preservation of overall architecture with intervening fat rules out thymoma.

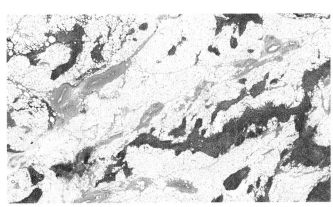

FIGURE 114.6 ▲ Normal thymus, myasthenia gravis. Approximately one-third of thymus glands will be normal. The extent of sectioning has some impact on the rate of detection of lymphoid follicles.

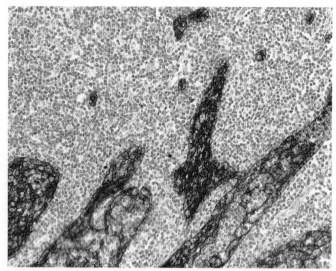

FIGURE 114.7 ▲ Thymic hyperplasia, pan-cytokeratin stain. The cortex and medulla are distinct.

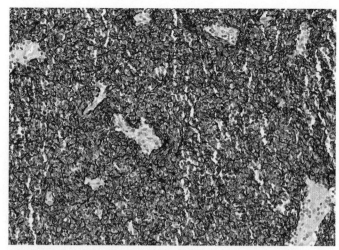

FIGURE 114.8 ▲ Thymoma, pan-cytokeratin staining. There is diffuse infiltration by tumor cells.

REFERENCES

1. Dalla Costa M, Mangano FA, Betterle C. Thymic hyperplasia in patients with Graves' disease. *J Endocrinol Invest.* 2014;37:1175–1179.
2. Hamzaoui AA, Klii RR, Salem RR, et al. Thymic hyperplasia in a patient with Graves' disease. *Int Arch Med.* 2012;5:6.
3. Pardo-Mindan FJ, Crisci CD, Serrano M, et al. Immunological aspects of sarcoidosis associated with true thymic hyperplasia. *Allergol Immunopathol (Madr).* 1980;8:91–96.
4. Kojima M, Shimizu K, Kaneko Y, et al. Lymphoid hyperplasia of the thymus showing Castleman's disease in a patient with myasthenia gravis. *Rheumatol Int.* 2012;32:3695–3697.
5. Sayed S, Sharma V, McBride CA, et al. Massive thymic hyperplasia in a neonate with Beckwith-Wiedemann syndrome. *J Paediatr Child Health.* 2016;52:90–92.
6. Minato H, Kinoshita E, Nakada S, et al. Thymic lymphoid hyperplasia with multilocular thymic cysts diagnosed before the Sjogren syndrome diagnosis. *Diagn Pathol.* 2015;10:103.
7. Innico G, Frassetti N, Coppola B, et al. Autoimmune polyglandular syndrome in a woman of 51 years. *Eur Rev Med Pharmacol Sci.* 2014;18:1717–1719.
8. Carragoso A, Faria B, Silva JR, et al. [Thymus hyperplasia in a patient with antiphospholipid syndrome]. *Acta Reumatol Port.* 2009;34:251–255.
9. Ferri C, Colaci M, Battolla L, et al. Thymus alterations and systemic sclerosis. *Rheumatology (Oxford).* 2006;45:72–75.
10. Sherer Y, Bardayan Y, Shoenfeld Y. Thymoma, thymic hyperplasia, thymectomy and autoimmune diseases (Review). *Int J Oncol.* 1997;10:939–943.
11. Weissferdt A, Moran CA. Thymic hyperplasia with lymphoepithelial sialadenitis (LESA)-like features: a clinicopathologic and immunohistochemical study of 4 cases. *Am J Clin Pathol.* 2012;138:816–822.
12. Kendall MD, Johnson HR, Singh J. The weight of the human thymus gland at necropsy. *J Anat.* 1980;131:483–497.
13. Steinmann G. Changes in the human thymus during aging. In: Müller-Hermelink HK, ed. *The Human Thymus: Histophysiology and Pathology.* Berlin: Springer-Verlag; 1986:43–88.
14. Feldges A, Wagner HP, Bubeck B, et al. Recurrent mediastinal mass in a child with Hodgkin's disease following successful therapy: a diagnostic challenge. *Pediatr Surg Int.* 1997;12:613–617.
15. Miniero R, Busca A, Leonardo E, et al. Rebound thymic hyperplasia following high dose chemotherapy and allogeneic BMT. *Bone Marrow Transplant.* 1993;11:67–70.
16. Priola AM, Priola SM, Ciccone G, et al. Differentiation of rebound and lymphoid thymic hyperplasia from anterior mediastinal tumors with dual-echo chemical-shift MR imaging in adulthood: reliability of the chemical-shift ratio and signal intensity index. *Radiology.* 2015;274:238–249.
17. Pilozzi E, Del Prete F, De Dominicis C, et al. True thymic hyperplasia associated with thymic hemorrhage in an adult patient. *Pathol Res Pract.* 2010;206:331–333.
18. Hoerl HD, Wojtowycz M, Gallagher HA, et al. Cytologic diagnosis of true thymic hyperplasia by combined radiologic imaging and aspiration cytology: a case report including flow cytometric analysis. *Diagn Cytopathol.* 2000;23:417–421.
19. Hofmann WJ, Moller P, Otto HF. Thymic hyperplasia. I. True thymic hyperplasia. Review of the literature. *Klin Wochenschr.* 1987;65:49–52.
20. Tan Z, Ying LY, Zhang ZW, et al. True thymic hyperplasia in an infant. *J Pediatr Surg.* 2010;45:1711–1713.
21. Agapitos E, Kavantzas N, Mavrogeorgis A, et al. Perinatal death and thymus gland. *Arch Anat Cytol Pathol.* 1994;42:163–170.
22. Grody WW, Jobst S, Keesey J, et al. Pathologic evaluation of thymic hyperplasia in myasthenia gravis and Lambert-Eaton myasthenic syndrome. *Arch Pathol Lab Med.* 1986;110:843–846.
23. Eifinger F, Ernestus K, Benz-Bohm G, et al. True thymic hyperplasia associated with severe thymic cyst bleeding in a newborn: case report and review of the literature. *Ann Diagn Pathol.* 2007;11:358–362.
24. Keijzers M, de Baets M, Hochstenbag M, et al. Robotic thymectomy in patients with myasthenia gravis: neurological and surgical outcomes. *Eur J Cardiothorac Surg.* 2015;48:40–45.
25. Marulli G, Schiavon M, Perissinotto E, et al. Surgical and neurologic outcomes after robotic thymectomy in 100 consecutive patients with myasthenia gravis. *J Thorac Cardiovasc Surg.* 2013;145:730–735; discussion 735–736.
26. Liu Z, Feng H, Yeung SC, et al. Extended transsternal thymectomy for the treatment of ocular myasthenia gravis. *Ann Thorac Surg.* 2011;92:1993–1999.
27. Tsinzerling N, Lefvert AK, Matell G, et al. Myasthenia gravis: a long term follow-up study of Swedish patients with specific reference to thymic histology. *J Neurol Neurosurg Psychiatry.* 2007;78:1109–1112.
28. Diaz A, Black E, Dunning J. Is thymectomy in non-thymomatous myasthenia gravis of any benefit? *Interact Cardiovasc Thorac Surg.* 2014;18:381–389.
29. Ackman JB, Verzosa S, Kovach AE, et al. High rate of unnecessary thymectomy and its cause. Can computed tomography distinguish thymoma, lymphoma, thymic hyperplasia, and thymic cysts? *Eur J Radiol.* 2015;84:524–533.
30. Yamanaka K, Nakayama H, Watanabe K, et al. Anterior mediastinal mass in a patient with Graves' disease. *Ann Thorac Surg.* 2006;81:1904–1906.
31. Wiersbowsky-Schmeel A, Helpap B, Totovic V, et al. Thymus in myasthenia gravis: a light and electron microscopic study of a case with thymic follicular hyperplasia. *Pathol Res Pract.* 1984;178:323–331.
32. Weissferdt A, Moran CA. Micronodular thymic carcinoma with lymphoid hyperplasia: a clinicopathological and immunohistochemical study of five cases. *Mod Pathol.* 2012;25:993–999.
33. Hohlfeld R, Wekerle H. Reflections on the "intrathymic pathogenesis" of myasthenia gravis. *J Neuroimmunol.* 2008;201–202:21–27.
34. Marx A, Wilisch A, Schultz A, et al. Pathogenesis of myasthenia gravis. *Virchows Arch.* 1997;430:355–364.

SECTION FOUR
NON-NEOPLASTIC LESIONS OF THE MEDIASTINUM

115 Bronchogenic Cysts

Borislav A. Alexiev, M.D., Fabio R. Tavora, M.D., Ph.D., and Allen P. Burke, M.D.

Definition

Bronchogenic cysts are uncommon congenital anomalies of foregut origin resulting from abnormal ventral budding or branching of the tracheobronchial tree during embryologic development.[1-5] The location of the cyst depends on the embryologic stage of development at which the anomaly occurs. Cysts forming in earliest development occur detached from the airways within the mediastinum. Those forming later are present along the tracheobronchial tree or within the lung parenchyma.

Incidence and Clinical

About one-third of bronchogenic cysts are diagnosed in children, as early as 1 day of age. The others are detected in adults, with a mean age of 41 years and a male-to-female ratio of 1:2.[3]

Bronchogenic cysts account for 50% to 60% of all mediastinal cysts.[2] They may occur in any part of the mediastinum, but most are found in a subcarinal location, in the posterior mediastinum, or in the middle mediastinum in a paratracheal location. Less than 20% occur in the superior or anterior mediastinum[6] (Table 115.1).

In the majority of patients (50% to 75%), there are no clinical symptoms, and the lesions are found incidentally by chest imaging.[4,7] The chief complaint is chest pain. In children, symptoms are somewhat more common and include cough, dyspnea, infection, and hemoptysis.

On imaging, including radiographs and computed tomographic scans, bronchogenic cysts are homogeneous, sharply circumscribed water-density shadows.[3] Malignant transformation occurs occasionally.[8,9]

Gross Pathology

Bronchogenic cysts are unilocular, typically measuring from 4 to 5 cm. The outer surface is tan, smooth, and glistening. The inner lining of the cyst is smooth, without papillary projections. The cyst contents vary in color and texture; they are white, yellow, pale yellow, or brown in color and liquid, sticky and creamy, or mucinous in texture.[4] Occasional tumors become infected, resulted in purulent contents.

Microscopic Pathology

Histopathologic examination shows in all cases a ciliated columnar mucosal lining, sometimes pseudostratified, with rare areas of squamous metaplasia.[4,6,10] The typical bronchogenic cyst has a fairly well-formed structure resembling a bronchus, with bronchial glands, a discrete muscle layer, and sometimes nerves (Fig. 115.1). Chronic inflammatory cells often infiltrate the submucosal layer. Nests of cartilage resembling bronchial cartilage are observed in approximately half of the cases.[4] Rarely, pancreatic tissue is present, and nests of thymic tissue may also occur (Fig. 115.2A). There are frequent areas of fibrosis and degeneration, consisting of collections of foam cells, cholesterol crystals, and microcalcifications (Fig. 115.2B).

Special Studies

The epithelial lining is typically CK7 positive and TTF1 and CDX2 negative. Immunostains for PAX8 and ER are negative in ciliated columnar mucosal lining (see Differential Diagnosis).

Differential Diagnosis

The distinction between bronchogenic and esophageal cysts is difficult.[10] The lining of esophageal duplications reflects its embryologic development and therefore may be ciliated or nonciliated columnar, squamous, or a mixture of these types. When ciliated columnar epithelium is seen in a cyst, the presence of cartilage or respiratory glands indicates bronchogenic differentiation; and the presence of two smooth muscle layers, which recapitulates the esophageal muscular coat, indicates esophageal differentiation.[10] When confronted with a cyst lined by ciliated columnar epithelium and no additional distinguishing features (Fig. 115.3), "foregut cyst" is an appropriate designation.[10]

A mediastinal müllerian cyst is a newly established entity that should be included in the differential diagnosis of posterior mediastinal bronchogenic cysts.[11-15] Under light microscopy, a ciliated cyst of müllerian origin is not very different from a bronchogenic cyst. In this context, distribution and configuration of ciliated cells could be similar to that in bronchogenic cysts. Moreover, apocrine-like secretary cells somehow resemble Clara cells. Absence of goblet cells, any types of glands, and cartilages would be helpful discriminating features. Immunohistochemical detection of PAX8 and ER may be useful for the diagnosis in difficult cases, such as bronchogenic cysts without cartilage.[11-15]

Mediastinal teratoma may be in the differential diagnosis in rare cases of pancreatic heterotopia present in the cyst wall. Unlike bronchogenic cysts, teratomas are typically multilocular, with disorganized cystic spaces and irregular areas of cartilage when present.

Treatment and Prognosis

Complete surgical resection is recommended for all bronchogenic cysts to establish diagnosis, alleviate symptoms, and prevent complication.[2]

TABLE 115.1 Clinicopathologic Characteristics of Bronchogenic Cysts

Location, overall	Mediastinum	60%–80%
	Lung	20%–40%
Mediastinal location	Posterior/subcarinal	50%–70%
	Middle	20%–40%
	Superior	10%
	Anterior	Uncommon
Histologic findings	Ciliated epithelium	100%
	Cartilage	50%
	Submucosal glands	40%
	Smooth muscle wall	40%
	Degenerative changes	50%–60%
	Purulent inflammation	10%
	Pancreatic tissue	<1%

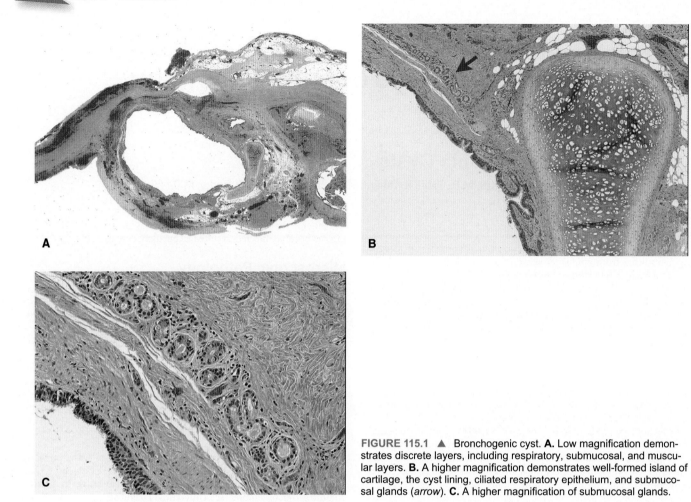

FIGURE 115.1 ▲ Bronchogenic cyst. **A.** Low magnification demonstrates discrete layers, including respiratory, submucosal, and muscular layers. **B.** A higher magnification demonstrates well-formed island of cartilage, the cyst lining, ciliated respiratory epithelium, and submucosal glands (*arrow*). **C.** A higher magnification of submucosal glands.

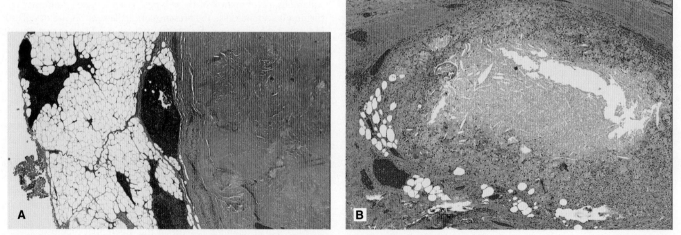

FIGURE 115.2 ▲ Bronchogenic cyst, nonspecific findings. **A.** There may be thymic tissue adjacent to the cyst. **B.** Areas of fibrosis and degeneration are not uncommon. There is a collection of degenerating foamy macrophages.

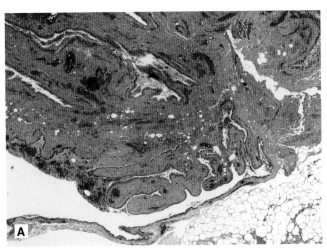
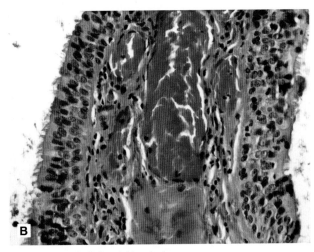

FIGURE 115.3 ▲ Mediastinal foregut cyst lined by columnar epithelium. No additional distinguishing features (cartilage, intestinal mucosa, bronchial glands, and/or muscle tissue) are seen. **A.** Low magnification. **B.** Higher magnification with ciliated columnar epithelium.

Practical Points

▶ Bronchogenic cysts are unilocular cysts located in the mediastinum along the tracheobronchial tree or within the lung parenchyma.

▶ The epithelial lining is ciliated columnar and usually overlying other bronchiolar wall elements such as smooth muscle, mucous glands, and cartilage.

▶ The main differential diagnoses include esophageal duplication cysts, mediastinal müllerian cysts, and teratoma.

▶ Bronchogenic cysts may become infected with purulent material. Complete surgical resection is recommended.

REFERENCES

1. Esme H, Eren S, Sezer M, et al. Primary mediastinal cysts: clinical evaluation and surgical results of 32 cases. *Tex Heart Inst J.* 2011;38:371–374.
2. Le Pimpec-Barthes F, Cazes A, Bagan P, et al. [Mediastinal cysts: clinical approach and treatment]. *Rev Pneumol Clin.* 2010;66:52–62.
3. Limaiem F, Ayadi-Kaddour A, Djilani H, et al. Pulmonary and mediastinal bronchogenic cysts: a clinicopathologic study of 33 cases. *Lung.* 2008;186:55–61.
4. Muramatsu T, Shimamura M, Furuichi M, et al. Thoracoscopic resection of mediastinal bronchogenic cysts in adults. *Asian J Surg.* 2011;34:11–14.
5. Zambudio AR, Lanzas JT, Calvo MJ, et al. Non-neoplastic mediastinal cysts. *Eur J Cardiothorac Surg.* 2002;22:712–716.
6. Kim JH, Goo JM, Lee HJ, et al. Cystic tumors in the anterior mediastinum. Radiologic-pathological correlation. *J Comput Assist Tomogr.* 2003;27:714–723.
7. Cuypers P, De Leyn P, Cappelle L, et al. Bronchogenic cysts: a review of 20 cases. *Eur J Cardiothorac Surg.* 1996;10:393–396.
8. Servais E, Paul S, Port JL, et al. Carcinoid tumor nested within a bronchogenic cyst. *J Thorac Cardiovasc Surg.* 2008;136:227–228.
9. Tsai JH, Lee JM, Lin MC, et al. Carcinoid tumor arising in a thymic bronchogenic cyst associated with thymic follicular hyperplasia. *Pathol Int.* 2012;62:49–54.
10. Harvell JD, Macho JR, Klein HZ. Isolated intra-abdominal esophageal cyst. Case report and review of the literature. *Am J Surg Pathol.* 1996;20:476–479.
11. Hattori H. Ciliated cyst of probable mullerian origin arising in the posterior mediastinum. *Virchows Arch.* 2005;446:82–84.
12. Hattori H. High prevalence of estrogen and progesterone receptor expression in mediastinal cysts situated in the posterior mediastinum. *Chest.* 2005;128:3388–3390.
13. Kobayashi S, Inoue T, Karube Y, et al. A case of Mullerian cyst arising in posterior mediastinum. *Ann Thorac Cardiovasc Surg.* 2012;18:39–41.
14. Simmons M, Duckworth LV, Scherer K, et al. Mullerian cysts of the posterior mediastinum: report of two cases and review of the literature. *J Thorac Dis.* 2013;5:E8–E10.
15. Thomas-de-Montpreville V, Dulmet E. Cysts of the posterior mediastinum showing mullerian differentiation (Hattori cysts). *Ann Diagn Pathol.* 2007;11:417–420.

116 Thoracic Duplication Cysts of the Alimentary Tract

Borislav A. Alexiev, M.D., and Allen P. Burke, M.D.

Terminology

Esophageal and enteric duplication cysts are foregut-derived developmental anomalies most commonly encountered in the mediastinum and rarely in the abdomen.[1-8] The duplication of the hollow structures of the digestive tract manifests three essential points: (1) attachment to at least one point of the alimentary tract, (2) epithelium resembling some part of the alimentary tract, and (3) well-developed coat of smooth muscle (double-layered smooth muscle wall).[7,9,10]

Intramural esophageal cysts result from defects in the tubulation process and are not associated with vertebral anomalies.[7] In contrast, enteric cysts are usually separate from the esophagus and lie in the posterior mediastinum. They are commonly associated with vertebral anomalies and are part of split notochord syndrome.[1,9]

Incidence and Clinical

Among alimentary tract duplication cysts, 20% occur in the mediastinum.[9] The majority of duplications are found in children, the frequency being almost triple to that found in adults.[9] The commonest mode of presentation in the neonatal period is respiratory distress. In adults, they can be discovered as an incidental finding on chest radiograph. About two-thirds of alimentary tract cysts are right sided.[7]

Gross Pathology

Intramural esophageal and enteric cysts are unilocular. The lesions are thin walled and translucent, with a tan, smooth, and glistening outer surface. The inner lining of the cyst is smooth, without papillary projections. The cysts contain pink serous or yellow-gray mucinous fluid.

Microscopic Pathology

Intramural esophageal cysts contain at least two types of epithelium, including ciliated or nonciliated columnar, squamous, or a mixture of these types, heterotopic lung tissue, thyroid stroma, ganglia, and two smooth muscle layers.[6,7,10–12] Heterotopic gastric mucosa and well-differentiated lymphoid aggregates resembling Peyer patches are rarely observed.

Enteric cysts have variable types of epithelium, the most common being gastric or duodenal type, and a double-layered smooth muscle wall, which resembles that of the intestine.[1,9,11,13] Respiratory-type epithelium is frequently observed. Ectopic mucosa representing any part of intestine, thymic, or pancreatic tissue can be found.[1,11] Cartilage is never found in the wall of alimentary tract duplication cysts.[1,9,11,13]

Special Studies

Immunostains for PAX8 and ER are negative in cyst epithelial lining (see differential diagnosis).

Differential Diagnosis

The distinction between alimentary tract duplication cysts and bronchogenic cysts can be challenging.[10] When ciliated columnar epithelium is seen in a cyst, the presence of cartilage or respiratory glands indicates bronchogenic differentiation, and the presence of two smooth muscle layers, which recapitulates the intestinal tract muscular coat, indicates alimentary tract differentiation. When confronted with a cyst lined by ciliated columnar epithelium and no additional distinguishing features, "foregut cyst" is an appropriate designation.[10]

A mediastinal mullerian cyst should be included in the differential diagnosis of posterior mediastinal enteric cyst.[1,5,10,14–16] In mullerian cysts, distribution and configuration of ciliated cells could be similar to that in alimentary tract duplication cyst. Absence of goblet cells and vertebral anomalies would be a helpful discriminating feature.[1,9]

Immunohistochemical detection of PAX8 and ER may be useful for the diagnosis in difficult cases.[1,5,10,14–16] Apart from the developmental mediastinal cysts, differential diagnosis includes neoplasms such as mature cystic teratoma.[1] This tumor becomes clinically apparent during early adult life and contains numerous sebaceous glands and hair follicles. The absence of these features in histologically examined specimens excludes this diagnosis.

Treatment and Prognosis

Surgery for mediastinal cysts is associated with low morbidity and mortality rates and a very low recurrence rate.[17,18] It offers a definitive diagnosis and cure, avoiding the higher morbidity and mortality risks associated with conservative observation.

REFERENCES

1. Anagnostou E, Soubasi V, Agakidou E, et al. Mediastinal gastroenteric cyst in a neonate containing respiratory-type epithelium and pancreatic tissue. *Pediatr Pulmonol.* 2009;44:1240–1243.
2. Ermis B, Yildirim M, Numanoglu V, et al. Mediastinal enteric cyst: an unusual cause of neonatal respiratory distress. *J Pediatr.* 2010;157:692.
3. Hussain N, Wahab S, Javed A, et al. Mediastinal enteric cyst. *J Pak Med Assoc.* 2014;64:1084–1086.
4. Prasad A, Sarin YK, Ramji S, et al. Mediastinal enteric duplication cyst containing aberrant pancreas. *Indian J Pediatr.* 2002;69:961–962.
5. Simmons M, Duckworth LV, Scherer K, et al. Mullerian cysts of the posterior mediastinum: report of two cases and review of the literature. *J Thorac Dis.* 2013;5:E8–E10.
6. Hajjar W, El-Madany Y, Ashour M, et al. Life threatening complications caused by bronchogenic and oesophageal duplication cysts in a child. *J Cardiovasc Surg (Torino).* 2003;44:135–137.
7. Nazem M, Amouee AB, Eidy M, et al. Duplication of cervical oesophagus: a case report and review of literatures. *Afr J Paediatr Surg.* 2010;7:203–205.
8. Zambudio AR, Lanzas JT, Calvo MJ, et al. Non-neoplastic mediastinal cysts. *Eur J Cardiothorac Surg.* 2002;22:712–716.
9. Birmole BJ, Kulkarni BK, Vaidya AS, et al. Intrathoracic enteric foregut duplication cyst. *J Postgrad Med.* 1994;40:228–230.
10. Harvell JD, Macho JR, Klein HZ. Isolated intra-abdominal esophageal cyst. Case report and review of the literature. *Am J Surg Pathol.* 1996;20:476–479.
11. Ildstad ST, Tollerud DJ, Weiss RG, et al. Duplications of the alimentary tract. Clinical characteristics, preferred treatment, and associated malformations. *Ann Surg.* 1988;208:184–189.
12. Ribet M, Gosselin B, Watine O, et al. [Congenital cysts of the esophageal wall with a respiratory type mucosa]. *Ann Chir.* 1989;43:692–698.
13. Dubrava J, Koren J, Pospisilova V. Mediastinal foregut duplication cyst of enteric type containing a persistent thymus, imitating a pericardial cyst. *Bratisl Lek Listy.* 2013;114:480–483.
14. Hattori H. Ciliated cyst of probable mullerian origin arising in the posterior mediastinum. *Virchows Arch.* 2005;446:82–84.
15. Hattori H. High prevalence of estrogen and progesterone receptor expression in mediastinal cysts situated in the posterior mediastinum. *Chest.* 2005;128:3388–3390.
16. Thomas-de-Montpreville V, Dulmet E. Cysts of the posterior mediastinum showing mullerian differentiation (Hattori cysts). *Ann Diagn Pathol.* 2007;11:417–420.
17. Le Pimpec-Barthes F, Cazes A, Bagan P, et al. [Mediastinal cysts: clinical approach and treatment]. *Rev Pneumol Clin.* 2010;66:52–62.
18. Limaiem F, Ayadi-Kaddour A, Djilani H, et al. Pulmonary and mediastinal bronchogenic cysts: a clinicopathologic study of 33 cases. *Lung.* 2008;186:55–61.

117 Ectopic Thymus, Parathyroid, and Thyroid

Borislav A. Alexiev, M.D., and Fabio R. Tavora, M.D., Ph.D.

Ectopic Thymus

Most cases (80% to 90%) of ectopic thymus present as an asymptomatic mass in the neck (84%), typically on the left side (68%), and may be are quite often associated with congenital heart disease.[1] Heterotopic thymic tissue is more frequent in males and usually occurs between the age of 1 and 13 years.[2,3] Ectopic retropharyngeal and intrathyroidal thymus is a rare occurrence.[1,4,5] The occurrence of aberrant thymus in the posterior mediastinum is very uncommon. It is usually positioned on the right side.[3]

Ectopic thymus is generally asymptomatic,[6] and rarely results in a palpable mass.[4]

Ectopic Parathyroid

The prevalence of ectopic parathyroid glands is about 2% to 43% in anatomical series and 14% to 16% in patients with primary and secondary hyperparathyroidism.[7] Ectopic inferior parathyroids are most frequently found in the anterior mediastinum, in association with the thymus (38%) or the thyroid gland (18%), while the most common position for ectopic superior parathyroids is the tracheoesophageal groove and retroesophageal region (31%).[7,8] Uncommon mediastinal sites include the aortic arch and tracheal bifurcation.[9]

Ectopic Thyroid

Most of the cases with ectopic mediastinal thyroid are known to develop in the anterosuperior mediastinum, the so-called cervicomediastinal region.[10] The posterior mediastinum is an atypical localization for the occurrence of ectopic thyroid.[11] The incidence of mediastinal goiter varies from 0.16% to 3.3%.[11]

Ectopic thyroid tissue, like its normal counterpart, may also undergo transformation to hyperplasia or even neoplasms. True ectopic malignant tumors are rare.[12,13]

Routine diagnostic evaluation includes a thorough history, physical examination, blood work, ultrasound of the neck, and chest x-ray.

CT, MRI, and preoperative technetium (99mTc) sestamibi (MIBI) scans can help in the diagnosis of ectopic lesions.

Microscopic Pathology

Histologic examination of ectopic thymus, parathyroid, and thyroid shows features identical to those observed in normal tissue (Fig. 117.1), including benign and malignant lesions, in the orthotopic glands.

Special Studies

Stains for CK5/6 and immature T cells are strongly positive in ectopic thymus. The diagnosis of ectopic thyroid and/or parathyroid tissue is supported by a positive staining for thyroglobulin and TTF1, and parathyroid hormone (PTH), respectively.

Differential Diagnosis

The differential diagnosis of ectopic mediastinal lesions most commonly focuses on benign cysts, lymphoma, inflammatory lymphadenopathy, and mediastinal neoplasia (primary and metastatic).

Treatment and Prognosis

The primary therapeutic approach in cervical thymic ectopia is surgery.[2,6,14] In the neonate, the presence of mediastinal thymus should be documented prior to excision of the cervical mass because of the important role of the thymus in the development of the immune system.[14] Radioguided minimally invasive parathyroidectomy after successful localization, assisted by rapid PTH measurement postoperatively, significantly improves surgical outcomes in patients with ectopic parathyroid adenomas.[7] Surgical resection for ectopic thyroid localized in the mediastinum is recommended when obstructive symptoms occur in relation to its mass effect, such as tracheal, esophageal, or superior vena cava compression.[11,15,16] Prognosis after removal of benign ectopic thymus, parathyroid, and thyroid is excellent.

REFERENCES

1. Gimm O, Krause U, Wessel H, et al. Ectopic intrathyroidal thymus diagnosed as a solid thyroid lesion: case report and review of the literature. *J Pediatr Surg.* 1997;32:1241–1243.
2. Clark JJ, Johnson SM. Solid cervical ectopic thymus in an infant. *J Pediatr Surg.* 2009;44:e19–e21.
3. Jiang L, Sun B, Zheng Y, et al. Posterior mediastinal thymus: case report and literature review. *Iran J Pediatr.* 2011;21:404–408.
4. Lignitz S, Musholt TJ, Kreft A, et al. Intrathyroidal thymic tissue surrounding an intrathyroidal parathyroid gland, the cause of a solitary thyroid nodule in a 6-year-old boy. *Thyroid.* 2008;18:1125–1130.
5. Schramm JC, Perry DA, Sewell RK. Retropharyngeal thymus and parathyroid gland: a case report. *Int J Pediatr Otorhinolaryngol.* 2014;78: 163–165.
6. Saggese D, Ceroni Compadretti G, Cartaroni C. Cervical ectopic thymus: a case report and review of the literature. *Int J Pediatr Otorhinolaryngol.* 2002;66:77–80.
7. Noussios G, Anagnostis P, Natsis K. Ectopic parathyroid glands and their anatomical, clinical and surgical implications. *Exp Clin Endocrinol Diab.* 2012;120:604–610.

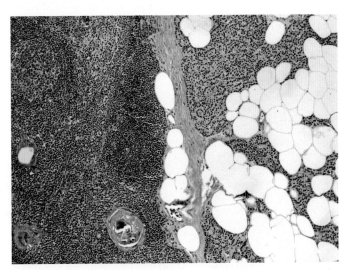

FIGURE 117.1 ▲ Ectopic intrathymic parathyroid gland. Note thymic tissue at left, and parathyroid at right.

8. Roy M, Mazeh H, Chen H, et al. Incidence and localization of ectopic parathyroid adenomas in previously unexplored patients. *World J Surg.* 2013;37:102–106.

9. Onoda N, Ishikawa T, Nishiyama N, et al. Focused approach to ectopic mediastinal parathyroid surgery assisted by radio-guided navigation. *Surg Today.* 2014;44:533–539.

10. Triggiani V, Giagulli VA, Licchelli B, et al. Ectopic thyroid gland: description of a case and review of the literature. *Endocr Metab Immune Disord Drug Targets.* 2013;13:275–281.

11. Demirhan R, Onan B, Oz K, et al. Posterior mediastinal ectopic thyroid: an unusual cause for dysphagia. *Ann Thorac Surg.* 2009;88:656–659.

12. Dominguez-Malagon H, Guerrero-Medrano J, Suster S. Ectopic poorly differentiated (insular) carcinoma of the thyroid. Report of a case presenting as an anterior mediastinal mass. *Am J Clin Pathol.* 1995;104:408–412.

13. Shah BC, Ravichand CS, Juluri S, et al. Ectopic thyroid cancer. *Ann Thorac Cardiovasc Surg.* 2007;13:122–124.

14. Baek CH, Ryu JS, Yun JB, et al. Aberrant cervical thymus: a case report and review of literature. *Int J Pediatr Otorhinolaryngol.* 1997;41:215–222.

15. Guimaraes MJ, Valente CM, Santos L, et al. Ectopic thyroid in the anterior mediastinum. *J Bras Pneumol.* 2009;35:383–387.

16. Pilavaki M, Kostopoulos G, Asimaki A, et al. Imaging of ectopic intrathoracic multinodular goiter with pathologic correlation: a case report. *Cases J.* 2009;2:8554.

118 Mediastinitis

Borislav A. Alexiev, M.D., and Allen P. Burke, M.D.

Terminology

Mediastinitis is defined as acute or chronic inflammation of the mediastinal structures.[1–7] Two broad categories of acute mediastinitis are acute necrotizing mediastinitis and poststernotomy mediastinitis.[8] Chronic mediastinitis has been arbitrarily subdivided into two categories: (1) granulomatous mediastinitis and (2) fibrosing or sclerosing mediastinitis.[8]

Incidence and Clinical

Poststernotomy mediastinitis has an incidence of 0.4% to 5% and a mortality of 16.5% to 47%.[1] The most frequent pathogen is *Staphylococcus aureus*.[1] Esophageal perforation, usually iatrogenic, is the second most frequent cause of acute mediastinitis, produced by common oropharyngeal flora, with a mortality rate of 20% to 60%, depending on the time of diagnosis.[1] The third most frequent cause is descending necrotizing mediastinitis, the origin being an oral caries in 60% and beta-hemolytic streptococcus the causative agent in 71.5% of cases.[1]

Fibrosing (sclerosing) mediastinitis is a rare disorder characterized by the invasive proliferation of fibrous tissue within the mediastinum.[2,4,9,10] Many (and perhaps most) cases in the United States are thought to be caused by an abnormal immunologic response to *Histoplasma capsulatum* infection.[3,11,12] Additional infectious triggers implicated in the pathogenesis of fibrosing (sclerosing) mediastinitis include other fungal and mycobacterial organisms associated with granulomatous mediastinitis.[5,6]

Fibrosing (sclerosing) mediastinitis may be associated sarcoidosis,[13] rheumatoid arthritis,[13] radiotherapy for Hodgkin disease,[13] and mast cell activation disease.[11] Finally, there are rare immune-mediated (idiopathic) and drug-induced (e.g., methysergide) cases of fibrosing (sclerosing) mediastinitis.[6] There is overlap between IgG4-related disease and fibrosing mediastinitis, both clinically and histologically.[6] Interestingly, patients with idiopathic immune-mediated fibrosing (sclerosing) mediastinitis frequently have other disease manifestations such as retroperitoneal fibrosis or Riedel thyroiditis, all of which have been associated with the IgG4-related disease spectrum.[6]

Fibrosing (sclerosing) mediastinitis frequently results in the compression of vital mediastinal structures and has been associated with substantial morbidity and mortality.[4–6] There are two types of fibrosing (sclerosing) mediastinitis: focal and diffuse.[3] CT and MR imaging play a vital role in the diagnosis and management of mediastinitis.[3]

Gross Pathology

The macroscopic features of acute mediastinitis are nonspecific. The serosal surfaces appear dull and are focally or diffusely covered by fibrin and/or yellow-tan purulent and hemorrhagic material. Focal fibrosing (sclerosing) mediastinitis may present as a white-tan, localized, calcified lesion. The diffuse type manifests as a diffusely infiltrating, often noncalcified white-tan mass that affects multiple mediastinal compartments.

Microscopic Pathology

Histologically, acute mediastinitis is characterized by fibrinopurulent exudate, with or without necrosis. The morphologic features of granulomatous mediastinal lesions are identical to those observed in the lung. Fibrosing (sclerosing) mediastinitis is characterized by an inflammatory fibrosing/sclerosing process that shows three distinctive histologic patterns.[4] On the basis of the histologic pattern, it is subdivided into three distinct groups (stages).[4] Stage I demonstrates edematous fibromyxoid tissue with numerous spindle cells, eosinophils, mast cells, lymphocytes, plasma cells, and thin-walled blood vessels (Fig. 118.1);

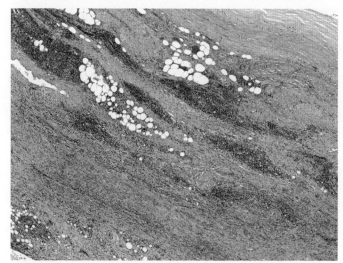

FIGURE 118.1 ▲ Fibrosing mediastinitis. Note diffuse chronic inflammation.

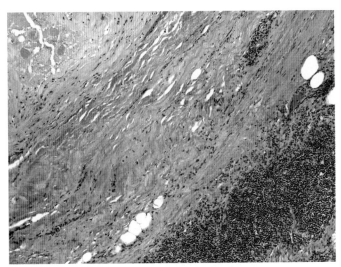

FIGURE 118.2 ▲ Fibrosing mediastinitis. Note marked fibrosis.

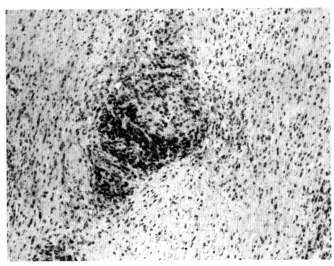

FIGURE 118.4 ▲ Fibrosing mediastinitis. Note prominent T lymphocytic component. (Anti-CD3).

stage II shows thick glassy bands of haphazardly arranged collagen with focal interstitial spindle cells, lymphocytes, and plasma cells; and stage III is characterized by dense acellular collagen with scattered lymphoid follicles and occasional dystrophic calcification (Fig. 118.2).

Special Studies

Special stains for acid-fast bacilli and fungi are positive in tuberculosis and fungal-associated granulomatous mediastinal infection. In fibrosing (sclerosing) mediastinitis, immunohistochemical studies show mixed inflammatory infiltrates with large numbers of B (CD20+) and T (CD3+) lymphocytes (Figs. 118.3 and 118.4).[5] Increased numbers of tissue-infiltrating IgG4-positive plasma cells suggest a diagnosis of IgG-4 related disease. However, they are nonspecific, and have also been found in post-infectious cases of sclerosing mediastinitis.[6]

Differential Diagnosis

In view of the prominent fibrosis/sclerosis present in fibrosing (sclerosing) mediastinitis, several considerations might enter the differential diagnosis. These lesions include sclerosing thymoma, solitary fibrous tumors, and lymphoma with prominent sclerosis.[14,15] In all these alternatives, the diagnosis cannot be reached if the only areas sampled correspond to sclerotic material. One important aspect of fibrosing

(sclerosing) mediastinitis is the absence of the dual cell population (epithelial cells and lymphocytes) seen in thymomas.[15] The presence of focal areas of spindle epithelial cells is not a component of fibrosing (sclerosing) mediastinitis. In cases of solitary fibrous tumor, even though the tumor may show hypocellular areas, the tumor will also show hypercellular areas, which might show a hemangiopericytic pattern or other patterns associated with other types of sarcomas.[15] Histologic features that favor IgG4-related disease include storiform cell-rich fibrosis entrapping lymphoid aggregates an nerves, lymphoid infiltrate with prominent plasma cells, and obliterative phlebitis or arteritis, in addition to IgG4-positive plasma cells. Last, in cases of lymphoma with prominent sclerosis, the tumor will show areas of more immature lymphoid component rather than the mixed inflammatory infiltrate of fibrosing (sclerosing) mediastinitis.[15]

Treatment and Prognosis

In cases of acute mediastinitis, treatment should always be directed toward the primary pathology and the clinical presentation.[8] The worst postsurgical prognostic factor is septic shock.[1] In chronic cases, surgical treatment is only palliative.[8]

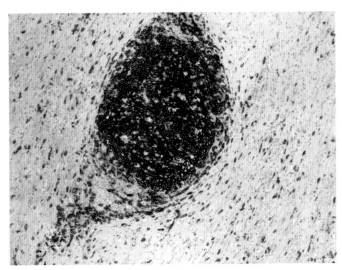

FIGURE 118.3 ▲ Fibrosing mediastinitis. Note prominent B lymphocytic component. (Anti-CD20).

REFERENCES

1. Martinez Vallina P, Espinosa Jimenez D, Hernandez Perez L, et al. [Mediastinitis]. *Arch Bronconeumol.* 2011;47(Suppl 8):32–36.
2. Bays S, Rajakaruna C, Sheffield E, et al. Fibrosing mediastinitis as a cause of superior vena cava syndrome. *Eur J Cardiothorac Surg.* 2004;26:453–455.
3. Rossi SE, McAdams HP, Rosado-de-Christenson ML, et al. Fibrosing mediastinitis. *Radiographics.* 2001;21:737–757.
4. Flieder DB, Suster S, Moran CA. Idiopathic fibroinflammatory (fibrosing/sclerosing) lesions of the mediastinum: a study of 30 cases with emphasis on morphologic heterogeneity. *Mod Pathol.* 1999;12:257–264.
5. Peikert T, Colby TV, Midthun DE, et al. Fibrosing mediastinitis: clinical presentation, therapeutic outcomes, and adaptive immune response. *Medicine (Baltimore).* 2011;90:412–423.
6. Peikert T, Shrestha B, Aubry MC, et al. Histopathologic Overlap between Fibrosing Mediastinitis and IgG4-Related Disease. *Int J Rheumatol.* 2012; 2012:207056.
7. Endo S, Murayama F, Hasegawa T, et al. Guideline of surgical management based on diffusion of descending necrotizing mediastinitis. *Jpn J Thorac Cardiovasc Surg.* 1999;47:14–19.
8. Athanassiadi KA. Infections of the mediastinum. *Thorac Surg Clin.* 2009;19: 37–45, vi.
9. Kalweit G, Huwer H, Straub U, et al. Mediastinal compression syndromes due to idiopathic fibrosing mediastinitis—report of three cases and review of the literature. *Thorac Cardiovasc Surg.* 1996;44:105–109.

10. Kojima S, Sumiyoshi M, Suwa S, et al. Superior vena cava syndrome due to fibrosing mediastinitis histologically identical to xanthogranulomatous pyelonephritis. *Intern Med.* 2003;42:56–59.
11. Afrin LB. Sclerosing mediastinitis and mast cell activation syndrome. *Pathol Res Pract.* 2012;208:181–185.
12. Harman M, Sayarlioglu M, Arslan H, et al. Fibrosing mediastinitis and thrombosis of superior vena cava associated with Behcet's disease. *Eur J Radiol.* 2003;48:209–212.
13. Devaraj A, Griffin N, Nicholson AG, et al. Computed tomography findings in fibrosing mediastinitis. *Clin Radiol.* 2007;62:781–786.
14. Kuo T. Sclerosing thymoma—a possible phenomenon of regression. *Histopathology.* 1994;25:289–291.
15. Moran CA, Suster S. "Ancient" (sclerosing) thymomas: a clinicopathologic study of 10 cases. *Am J Clin Pathol.* 2004;121:867–871.

119 Mediastinal Germ Cell Tumors: Classification and Overview

Anja C. Roden, M.D., Borislav A. Alexiev, M.D., and Allen P. Burke, M.D.

Background

The terminology used for mediastinal germ cell tumors is similar to that of germ cell tumors of the gonads.[1] They have been categorized for therapeutic purposes (in ascending order of aggressive behavior) into teratomas, pure seminomas, and malignant nonseminomatous germ cell tumors (embryonal carcinoma, yolk sac tumor, choriocarcinoma, and mixed germ cell tumors)[1–18] (Tables 119.1 and 119.2).

Pure teratomas composed of mature elements are often classified as "benign" mediastinal germ cell tumors because of lack of metastatic potential. Overall teratomas are the most common single histologic subtype.[14]

Germ cell tumor with somatic-type malignancy contains one or more components of non–germ cell malignant tumor, which may be a sarcoma or a carcinoma.[1,8–10] Germ cell tumors with somatic malignancy have been classified into two clinical and pathologic types: those induced by chemotherapy or irradiation and naturally occurring somatic malignancy.[1] They have also been classified as somatic malignancies with solid-type carcinoma, and somatic-type hematologic malignancies.[1]

Teratomas of the mediastinum are frequently subclassified as immature or mature, based on the presence of fetal-type tissue, especially in children.[2,15] In contrast to ovarian teratomas, mediastinal teratomas with immature elements that do not contain mixed components (most often embryonal carcinoma) are rare. Therefore, although sometimes considered malignant, pure immature teratomas of the mediastinum are not usually graded, as is the case with ovarian teratomas (see Chapter 121).

Pathogenesis

The occurrence of extragonadal germ cell tumors in the mediastinum is explained on the basis of migration of the primitive germ cells during embryonic life from the wall of the yolk sac to the primitive gonad.[20] However, since thymic epithelial stem cells and their plasticity have only partially been characterized, a somatic stem cell derivation of at least some mediastinal germ cell tumors has not been excluded to date.

The only established risk factor for mediastinal nonseminomatous germ cell tumor development is Klinefelter syndrome (reported risk 50 to several hundredfold).[21] Apart from the well-established association between hematologic malignancies and mediastinal nonseminomatous germ cell tumors, the frequency of other neoplasms is not increased in patients with mediastinal germ cell tumors, arguing against a role of common cancer susceptibility genes in the development of mediastinal germ cell tumors.[1]

The risk for the development of metachronous testicular cancer is low in mediastinal germ cell tumors. Intratubular germ cell neoplasia of the testis is a rare accompanying finding in mediastinal germ cell tumors, in contrast to germ cell tumors arising in the retroperitoneum.[22,23]

Incidence

Primary mediastinal germ cell tumors account for ~10% to 20% of all neoplasms of the mediastinum.[24] Mediastinal germ cell tumors account for up to 16% of mediastinal neoplasms in adults and for 19% to 25% of mediastinal tumors in children.[1]

Demographics

Mediastinal germ cell tumors occur at all ages (0 to 79 years), though there is a bimodal age distribution, with a distinct peak in infancy. The occurrence of mediastinal germ cell tumors is similar between different races. In contrast, the annual incidence rates for testicular germ cell tumors are strikingly different between Caucasians and Africans and Asians.[1]

Clinical Findings

The large majority of primary mediastinal germ cell tumors arise in the anterior mediastinum, within or adjacent to the thymus, but teratomas and yolk sac tumors have also been described in the posterior mediastinum.[1–18]

TABLE 119.1 Mediastinal Germ Cell Tumors in Children <15 Years

	Frequency	Prognosis
Teratoma, mature and immature	60%	Excellent
Yolk sac tumor	30%	Variable
Seminoma	<10%[a]	Good
Embryonal carcinoma	<10%[a]	Poor
Choriocarcinoma	<10%[a]	Poor
Mixed germ cell tumor	25%[a]	Poor

Based on series of germ cell tumors in children.[2,14,15]
[a]All >5–10 years of age, and in boys.

TABLE 119.2 Mediastinal Germ Cell Tumors in Adults[4–6,11,13,19]

	Frequency	Prognosis
Teratoma, mature and immature	60%–70%	Excellent
Mixed germ cell tumor	20%	Poor
Seminoma	10%	Good
Yolk sac tumor (pure)	2%–10%	—[a]
Embryonal carcinoma (pure)	<5%	—[a]
Choriocarcinoma	<5%	Poor
Mixed germ cell tumor with somatic solid or hematologic malignancy	<5%	Poor

[a]Few data on prognosis, but presumably similar to mixed germ cell tumors.

Presenting symptoms of germ cell tumors are related to the local mass lesion and comprise chest pain, respiratory distress, cough, hoarseness, and the superior vena cava syndrome. Fever and formation of multilocular thymic cysts result from local inflammatory reactions that frequently accompany germ cell tumors and are most prominent in seminomas.[1]

Precocious puberty due to increased beta–human chorionic gonadotropin levels can accompany mediastinal germ cell tumors.[25,26] Paraneoplastic autoimmune diseases, particularly myasthenia gravis, are virtually nonexistent in patients with mediastinal germ cell tumors.

An almost unique complication of mediastinal germ cell tumors as compared to other extragonadal or testicular germ cell tumors is the development of hematologic malignancies. Hematologic malignancies occur in 2% to 6% of germ cell tumors, are clonally related to the germ cell tumors, and develop independently of chemotherapy.[27,28]

Germ Cell Tumors in Prepubertal Children

The majority of mediastinal germ cell tumors in infants and young children are teratomas and yolk sac tumors. There is a striking difference in gender predilection between prepubertal and postpubertal mediastinal germ cell tumors. In children, there is a slight male predominance, with all malignant germ cell tumors in prepubertal girls representing yolk sac tumor. In adults, there is an overwhelming predominance of men, with the exception of pure teratoma, which in some series has an equal proportion of women.[13]

In prepubertal boys over age of 5 years, there is a more diverse group of tumors that may occur, including seminoma and mixed germ cell tumors in addition to yolk sac tumor and teratoma.[14]

Histologic Findings and Differential Diagnosis

Histologic features of mediastinal germ cell tumors are similar to their gonadal counterparts. Furthermore, mediastinal germ cell tumors typically show immunoreactivity patterns identical to their gonadal counterparts. Because mediastinal tumors are often sampled by mediastinoscopic biopsy, the differential diagnosis with other more common lesions, such as thymoma and thymic carcinoma, can be problematic. Stem cell markers such as SALL4 and OCT3/4 are often expressed in malignant germ cell tumors but are negative in thymic epithelial tumors.[29,30] Stem cell markers and glypican3, a marker most commonly expressed in yolk sac tumor, may also be present in nonthymic carcinomas, however.

Prognosis

The behavior of pediatric germ cell tumors is distinct from that of adult mediastinal germ cell tumors. Within the pediatric age range, prognosis is worse with increasing age.[1]

Pure mediastinal teratomas have an excellent prognosis after complete resection in all age groups.

Seminomas show a favorable response to radiotherapy and cisplatin-based chemotherapies, and their excellent prognosis (~90% survival) is not different from the prognosis of seminomas in other locations.[31]

Nonseminomatous malignant germ cell tumors of the mediastinum often present with advanced disease and do not respond as well to chemotherapy as their gonadal counterparts.[4,13] The overall clinical outcome for primary mediastinal germ cell tumors is worse than that for gonadal germ cell tumors, partly because the tumors are far advanced at the time of diagnosis.[4,13] Nonseminomatous histology, the presence of nonpulmonary visceral metastases, primary mediastinal germ cell tumor location, and elevated beta–human chorionic gonadotropin are independent prognostic factors for shorter survival.[32]

Clinical and pathologic staging is very important in the prognosis of mediastinal germ cell tumors.[4,5,11,13] Unfortunately, there is not an officially recognized UICC-TNM staging protocol for mediastinal germ cell tumors. The WHO recommends using a modification of the AJCC TNM staging of soft tissue tumors. In this system, T1 lesions are confined to mediastinum and mediastinal fat, with a 5-cm cutoff dividing T1a and T1b tumors. T2 tumors invade contiguous organs or are accompanied by a malignant effusion and are similarly divided into T2a and T2b by the 5-cm division. T3 tumors invade the pericardium; pleura, thoracic wall; great vessels; or lung, and T4 tumors demonstrate pleural or pericardial dissemination. N1 nodes refer to those in the anterior mediastinum, N2 nodes refer to other mediastinal nodes, and N3 nodes encompass scalene or supraclavicular lymph nodes.

Moran and Suster proposed a staging system for mediastinal germ cell tumors in 1997.[18] Their recommendation was to treat tumors exclusively confined to the mediastinum without infiltration of adjacent structures (stage I) conservatively, with surgery alone or with surgery and an added modality based on the histology of the tumor. Lesions of advanced stage that showed infiltration into adjacent structures (II) or intrathoracic metastases (IIIa) would require more aggressive treatment with curative intent, whereas palliative treatment was the choice in tumors with extrathoracic metastasis (IIIb).

Treatment

In general, treatment is surgical for teratomas, chemotherapy for seminoma, and neoadjuvant chemotherapy followed by resection of remaining tumor for germ cell tumors containing yolk sac tumor, embryonal carcinoma, or choriocarcinoma. In assessing posttreatment resection specimens, there may be no residual malignant tumor (100% necrosis with or without teratoma) in approximately two-thirds of cases, residual germ cell tumor (excluding teratoma) in one-third of cases, and progression to somatic malignancy in a few patients. Persistence of malignant germ cell tumor (excluding teratoma) or progression to somatic malignancy imparts a poor prognosis.[11]

REFERENCES

1. Moreira AL, Chan JKC, Looijenga LHJ, et al. Germ cell tumours of the mediastinum. In: Travis WD, et al., eds. *WHO Classification of Tumours of the Lung, Pleura, Thymus, and Heart.* Lyon, France: IARC Press; 2015:244–259.
2. Yalcin B, Demir HA, Tanyel FC, et al. Mediastinal germ cell tumors in childhood. *Pediatr Hematol Oncol.* 2012;29:633–642.
3. Tian L, Liu LZ, Cui CY, et al. CT findings of primary non-teratomatous germ cell tumors of the mediastinum—a report of 15 cases. *Eur J Radiol.* 2012;81:1057–1061.
4. Rodney AJ, Tannir NM, Siefker-Radtke AO, et al. Survival outcomes for men with mediastinal germ-cell tumors: the University of Texas M. D. Anderson Cancer Center experience. *Urol Oncol.* 2012;30:879–885.
5. Sarkaria IS, Bains MS, Sood S, et al. Resection of primary mediastinal nonseminomatous germ cell tumors: a 28-year experience at memorial sloan-kettering cancer center. *J Thorac Oncol.* 2011;6:1236–1241.
6. Rivera C, Arame A, Jougon J, et al. Prognostic factors in patients with primary mediastinal germ cell tumors, a surgical multicenter retrospective study. *Interact Cardiovasc Thorac Surg.* 2010;11:585 589.
7. Karangelis D, Kalafati G, Liouras V, et al. Germ cell tumors of the mediastinum. *Interact Cardiovasc Thorac Surg.* 2010;11:829.
8. Contreras AL, Punar M, Tamboli P, et al. Mediastinal germ cell tumors with an angiosarcomatous component: a report of 12 cases. *Hum Pathol.* 2010;41:832–837.
9. Asakura K, Izumi Y, Ikeda T, et al. Mediastinal germ cell tumor with somatic-type malignancy: report of 5 stage I/II cases. *Ann Thorac Surg.* 2010;90:1014–1016.
10. Pelosi G, Sonzogni A, Solli P, et al. Differentiating neuroblastoma arising in mediastinal germ cell tumour. *Histopathology.* 2008;53:350–352.
11. Kesler KA, Rieger KM, Hammoud ZT, et al. A 25-year single institution experience with surgery for primary mediastinal nonseminomatous germ cell tumors. *Ann Thorac Surg.* 2008;85:371–378.
12. Kesler KA, Einhorn LH. Mediastinal germ cell tumors. *Ann Thorac Surg.* 2007;83:1915.
13. Takeda S, Miyoshi S, Ohta M, et al. Primary germ cell tumors in the mediastinum: a 50-year experience at a single Japanese institution. *Cancer.* 2003;97:367–376.
14. Billmire D, Vinocur C, Rescorla F, et al. Malignant mediastinal germ cell tumors: an intergroup study. *J Pediatr Surg.* 2001;36:18–24.

15. Schneider DT, Calaminus G, Reinhard H, et al. Primary mediastinal germ cell tumors in children and adolescents: results of the German cooperative protocols MAKEI 83/86, 89, and 96. *J Clin Oncol.* 2000;18:832–839.

16. Moran CA, Suster S, Przygodzki RM, et al. Primary germ cell tumors of the mediastinum: II. Mediastinal seminomas—a clinicopathologic and immunohistochemical study of 120 cases. *Cancer.* 1997;80:691–698.

17. Moran CA, Suster S, Koss MN. Primary germ cell tumors of the mediastinum: III. Yolk sac tumor, embryonal carcinoma, choriocarcinoma, and combined nonteratomatous germ cell tumors of the mediastinum—a clinicopathologic and immunohistochemical study of 64 cases. *Cancer.* 1997;80:699–707.

18. Moran CA, Suster S. Primary germ cell tumors of the mediastinum: I. Analysis of 322 cases with special emphasis on teratomatous lesions and a proposal for histopathologic classification and clinical staging. *Cancer.* 1997;80:681–690.

19. Moran CA, Suster S. Germ-cell tumors of the mediastinum. *Adv Anat Pathol.* 1998;5:1–15.

20. Chaganti RS, Rodriguez E, Mathew S. Origin of adult male mediastinal germ-cell tumours. *Lancet.* 1994;343:1130–1132.

21. Hasle H, Jacobsen BB. Origin of male mediastinal germ-cell tumours. *Lancet.* 1995;345:1046.

22. Hailemariam S, Engeler DS, Bannwart F, et al. Primary mediastinal germ cell tumor with intratubular germ cell neoplasia of the testis—further support for germ cell origin of these tumors: a case report. *Cancer.* 1997;79:1031–1036.

23. Lee KC. Primary mediastinal germ cell tumor with intratubular germ cell neoplasia of the testis—further support for germ cell origin of these tumors: a case report. *Cancer.* 1997;80:1007–1008.

24. Couto WJ, Gross JL, Deheinzelin D, et al. [Primary mediastinal germ cell tumors]. *Rev Assoc Med Bras.* 2006;52:182–186.

25. Bebb GG, Grannis FW Jr, Paz IB, et al. Mediastinal germ cell tumor in a child with precocious puberty and Klinefelter syndrome. *Ann Thorac Surg.* 1998;66:547–548.

26. Schwabe J, Calaminus G, Vorhoff W, et al. Sexual precocity and recurrent beta-human chorionic gonadotropin upsurges preceding the diagnosis of a malignant mediastinal germ-cell tumor in a 9-year-old boy. *Ann Oncol.* 2002;13:975–977.

27. DeMent SH, Eggleston JC, Spivak JL. Association between mediastinal germ cell tumors and hematologic malignancies. Report of two cases and review of the literature. *Am J Surg Pathol.* 1985;9:23–30.

28. Irie J, Kawai K, Ueno Y, et al. Malignant germ cell tumor of the anterior mediastinum with leukemia-like infiltration. *Acta Pathol Jpn.* 1985;35:1561–1570.

29. Liu A, Cheng L, Du J, et al. Diagnostic utility of novel stem cell markers SALL4, OCT4, NANOG, SOX2, UTF1, and TCL1 in primary mediastinal germ cell tumors. *Am J Surg Pathol.* 2010;34:697–706.

30. Jung SM, Chu PH, Shiu TF, et al. Expression of OCT4 in the primary germ cell tumors and thymoma in the mediastinum. *Appl Immunohistochem Mol Morphol.* 2006;14:273–275.

31. Hartmann JT, Nichols CR, Droz JP, et al. Prognostic variables for response and outcome in patients with extragonadal germ-cell tumors. *Ann Oncol.* 2002;13:1017–1028.

32. Bokemeyer C, Nichols CR, Droz JP, et al. Extragonadal germ cell tumors of the mediastinum and retroperitoneum: results from an international analysis. *J Clin Oncol.* 2002;20:1864–1873.

120 Seminoma

Borislav A. Alexiev, M.D., Anja C. Roden, M.D., and Allen P. Burke, M.D.

Incidence and Clinical

Mediastinal seminoma may be pure, or associated with mixed germ cell tumors. The reported frequency of pure seminomas among primary mediastinal germ cell tumors ranges from 3% to 39%, ranking seminoma second in frequency following teratoma.[1–7] Seminoma also forms a component in 5% to 20% of mediastinal mixed germ cell tumors.[3,8]

With the exception of single cases,[9] all reported mediastinal seminomas have occurred in adolescent boys or men.[1–6] The age ranges from 13 to 79 years, with approximately two-thirds of the cases occurring in the third and fourth decade.[1–6]

In contrast to patients with retroperitoneal seminomas, intratubular germ cell neoplasia of the testis rarely if ever occurs in association with mediastinal germ cell tumors. There are rare reports of intratubular germ cell testicular neoplasia occurring in patients with mediastinal mixed germ cell tumors.[10–12]

Presenting symptoms of mediastinal seminomas are related to the local mass effect and comprise chest pain, respiratory distress, cough, hoarseness, and the superior vena cava syndrome.[1–6] Fever and formation of multilocular thymic cysts may result from local inflammatory reactions.[13]

Mediastinal seminomas occur in patients with Down syndrome[14] and may present with anti-Ma2 encephalitis, a paraneoplastic disorder characterized by limbic, diencephalic, and/or brainstem dysfunction.[15]

Gross Pathology

Macroscopically, mediastinal seminomas are well-circumscribed, fleshy tumors with a homogeneous, slightly lobulated to multinodular, tan-gray or pale cut surface.[16] Hemorrhage and yellowish foci of necrosis may be observed. Thymic seminomas may present as a multilocular cystic lesion showing small focal areas of induration within the cyst walls.[13]

Microscopic Pathology

Mediastinal seminoma is a primitive germ cell tumor composed of fairly uniform round or polygonal cells with distinct cell borders, and a round nucleus with one or more prominent nucleoli, resembling primordial germ cells.[17] The histologic and immunohistochemical features are presented in Table 120.1. The cytoplasm of the tumor cells is usually clear reflecting the glycogen and lipid content. Less commonly, the tumor cells have an eosinophilic cytoplasm. The tumors typically grow in confluent multinodular clusters, sheets, cords, strands, or irregular lobules (Fig. 120.1). Between the tumor cell aggregates, delicate fibrous septa associated with a prominent inflammatory infiltrate of small mature lymphocytes, plasma cells, and eosinophils are observed. Occasionally, lymphoid aggregates with germinal centers are present. Granulomatous reaction and fibrosis are common and occasionally so extensive that the neoplasm is obscured. The seminoma cells may be arranged in a nested pseudoglandular/alveolar, cribriform, or tubular pattern with sparse lymphocytes. Syncytiotrophoblastic cells have only rarely been reported in mediastinal seminoma, in one series seen in one of 23 cases.[18] Necrosis occurs in 35% of tumors, and mitotic figures are not uncommon (mean 4 per 10 HPF).[18]

Mediastinal seminomas with prominent cystic changes occur in fewer than 10% of tumors. Cysts are characteristically lined by squamous or cuboidal epithelium showing severe chronic inflammation with areas of cholesterol cleft granulomas, lymphoid follicular hyperplasia, and scattered foci of residual thymic parenchyma within the walls of the cysts.[13,18] Careful examination reveals areas of seminoma that distinguishes these tumors from thymic cysts.[13,18]

Mediastinal seminoma with florid lymphoid hyperplasia has been reported.[19]

TABLE 120.1 Mediastinal Seminomas, Histologic and Immunohistochemical Features

	Approximate Frequency
Histologic Finding	
Lymphocytic infiltrate	100% (50% diffuse)
Fibrous stroma or septa	90%
Granulomatous inflammation	75%
Cystic change	10%
Cellular pleomorphism with anaplasia	40%
Syncytiotrophoblasts	5%
Small foci of yolk sac tumor or embryonal carcinoma[a]	5%–10%
Small foci of teratoma	5%
Immunohistochemical Findings	
SALL4 (nuclear)	90%–100%
OCT4 (nuclear)	90%–100%
CD117 (c-kit)	70%
Placental-like alkaline phosphatase	40%–50%
Low molecular weight cytokeratin	50%–60%
PAX-8 (nuclear)	5%–10%
Human chorionic gonadotropin	5% (scattered ells)
High molecular weight cytokeratin	0
CD30	0
Alpha-fetoprotein	0
Glypican-3	0

[a]If significant components are present (>5%), then a diagnosis of mixed germ cell tumor is appropriate for therapeutic considerations.

Ancillary Studies

Mediastinal seminomas have been the subject of multiple studies with immunohistochemical markers.[16,18,20–23] The most sensitive markers are OCT4 and SALL4, which are positive in tumor cell nuclei in over 90% of cases[21,23,24] (Fig. 120.2). Placental-like alkaline phosphatase is usually expressed but is not specific (Fig. 120.3). Membranous expression of c-kit (CD117) is not as sensitive (~70%) and placental-like alkaline phosphatase even less so (about 40%).[18,21,25]

Mediastinal seminomas frequently show focal positivity with antibodies to CAM 5.2 and other low molecular weight keratins, which

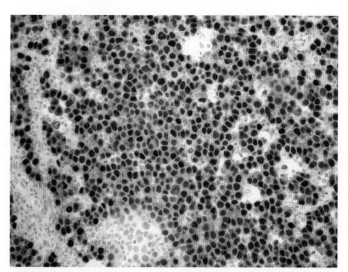

FIGURE 120.2 ▲ Mediastinal seminoma. Note positive staining for OCT4.

may lead to challenges in the distinction from thymic epithelial neoplasms.[18,23] Occasional staining with PAX-8 has also been reported, which may also cause confusion with thymic epithelial tumors.[23]

There may be scattered cells positive for human chorionic gonadotrophic (HCG) in 5% of mediastinal seminomas.[16] Immunostains for CD30, CEA, EMA, CK5/6, GATA-3, SOX2, glypican-3, and alpha-fetoprotein are negative.[22,23]

The vast majority of mediastinal seminomas harbor chromosome 12p abnormalities (12p amplification, isochromosome 12p).[18]

Treatment and Prognosis

Seminomas are extremely sensitive to both chemotherapy and radiation and are primarily treated nonsurgically.[1,2,4–6] Clinical staging and pathologic staging of mediastinal seminomas are important parameters that can be useful in determining the clinical outcomes of patients with these tumors. Tumor invasion into adjacent organs, superior vena cava syndrome, and CNS and liver metastases represent markers of increased morbidity and mortality.[1,2,4–6,26] Patients >37 years of age have worse outcomes than do younger individuals.[16] The 5-year overall survival rate of patients with seminomas is 87.7%.[27]

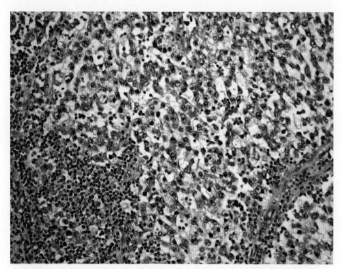

FIGURE 120.1 ▲ Mediastinal seminoma. The tumor is composed of sheets of round or polygonal cells with distinct cell membrane and clear or eosinophilic cytoplasm. Note pronounced infiltration of lymphocytes.

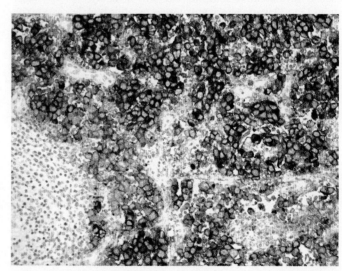

FIGURE 120.3 ▲ Mediastinal seminoma. Note positive staining for PLAP.

REFERENCES

1. Chan AT, Ho S, Yim AP, et al. Primary mediastinal malignant germ cell tumour. Single institution experience in Chinese patients and correlation with specific alpha-fetoprotein bends. *Acta Oncol.* 1996;35:221–227.
2. Hartmann JT, Nichols CR, Droz JP, et al. Prognostic variables for response and outcome in patients with extragonadal germ-cell tumors. *Ann Oncol.* 2002;13:1017–1028.
3. Moran CA, Suster S. Primary germ cell tumors of the mediastinum: I. Analysis of 322 cases with special emphasis on teratomatous lesions and a proposal for histopathologic classification and clinical staging. *Cancer.* 1997;80:681–690.
4. Rivera C, Arame A, Jougon J, et al. Prognostic factors in patients with primary mediastinal germ cell tumors, a surgical multicenter retrospective study. *Interact Cardiovasc Thorac Surg.* 2010;11:585–589.
5. Rodney AJ, Tannir NM, Siefker-Radtke AO, et al. Survival outcomes for men with mediastinal germ-cell tumors: the University of Texas M. D. Anderson Cancer Center experience. *Urol Oncol.* 2012;30:879–885.
6. Takeda S, Miyoshi S, Ohta M, et al. Primary germ cell tumors in the mediastinum: a 50-year experience at a single Japanese institution. *Cancer.* 2003;97:367–376.
7. Chang CC, Chang YL, Lee JM, et al. 18 Years surgical experience with mediastinal mature teratoma. *J Formos Med Assoc.* 2010;109:287–292.
8. Kesler KA, Rieger KM, Hammoud ZT, et al. A 25-year single institution experience with surgery for primary mediastinal nonseminomatous germ cell tumors. *Ann Thorac Surg.* 2008;85:371–378.
9. Brown K, Collins JD, Batra P, et al. Mediastinal germ cell tumor in a young woman. *Med Pediatr Oncol.* 1989;17:164–167.
10. Bohle A, Studer UE, Sonntag RW, et al. Primary or secondary extragonadal germ cell tumors? *J Urol.* 1986;135:939–943.
11. Daugaard G, Rorth M, von der Maase H, et al. Management of extragonadal germ-cell tumors and the significance of bilateral testicular biopsies. *Ann Oncol.* 1992;3:283–289.
12. Hailemariam S, Engeler DS, Bannwart F, et al. Primary mediastinal germ cell tumor with intratubular germ cell neoplasia of the testis—further support for germ cell origin of these tumors: a case report. *Cancer.* 1997;79:1031–1036.
13. Moran CA, Suster S. Mediastinal seminomas with prominent cystic changes. A clinicopathologic study of 10 cases. *Am J Surg Pathol.* 1995;19:1047–1053.
14. Ishida M, Hodohara K, Okabe H. Mediastinal seminoma occurring in Down syndrome. *J Pediatr Hematol Oncol.* 2012;34:387–388.
15. Bosemani T, Huisman TA, Poretti A. Anti-Ma2-associated paraneoplastic encephalitis in a male adolescent with mediastinal seminoma. *Pediatr Neurol.* 2014;50:433–434.
16. Moran CA, Suster S, Przygodzki RM, et al. Primary germ cell tumors of the mediastinum: II. Mediastinal seminomas—a clinicopathologic and immunohistochemical study of 120 cases. *Cancer.* 1997;80:691–698.
17. Moreira AL, Chan JKC, Looijenga LHJ, et al. Germ cell tumours of the mediastinum. In: Travis WD, et al., eds. *WHO Classification of Tumours of the Lung, Pleura, Thymus, and Heart.* Lyon, France: IARC Press; 2015:244–259.
18. Sung MT, Maclennan GT, Lopez-Beltran A, et al. Primary mediastinal seminoma: a comprehensive assessment integrated with histology, immunohistochemistry, and fluorescence in situ hybridization for chromosome 12p abnormalities in 23 cases. *Am J Surg Pathol.* 2008;32:146–155.
19. Weissferdt A, Moran CA. Mediastinal seminoma with florid follicular lymphoid hyperplasia: a clinicopathological and immunohistochemical study of six cases. *Virchows Arch.* 2015;466:209–215.
20. Jung SM, Chu PH, Shiu TF, et al. Expression of OCT4 in the primary germ cell tumors and thymoma in the mediastinum. *Appl Immunohistochem Mol Morphol.* 2006;14:273–275.
21. Liu A, Cheng L, Du J, et al. Diagnostic utility of novel stem cell markers SALL4, OCT4, NANOG, SOX2, UTF1, and TCL1 in primary mediastinal germ cell tumors. *Am J Surg Pathol.* 2010;34:697–706.
22. Suster S, Moran CA, Dominguez-Malagon H, et al. Germ cell tumors of the mediastinum and testis: a comparative immunohistochemical study of 120 cases. *Hum Pathol.* 1998;29:737–742.
23. Weissferdt A, Rodriguez-Canales J, Liu H, et al. Primary mediastinal seminomas: a comprehensive immunohistochemical study with a focus on novel markers. *Hum Pathol.* 2015;46:376–383.
24. Iwamoto N, Ishida M, Yoshida K, et al. Mediastinal seminoma: a case report with special emphasis on SALL4 as a new immunocytochemical marker. *Diagn Cytopathol.* 2013;41:821–824.
25. Kwon MS. Aspiration cytology of mediastinal seminoma: report of a case with emphasis on the diagnostic role of aspiration cytology, cell block and immunocytochemistry. *Acta Cytol.* 2005;49:669–672.
26. Knapp RH, Hurt RD, Payne WS, et al. Malignant germ cell tumors of the mediastinum. *J Thorac Cardiovasc Surg.* 1985;89:82–89.
27. Liu Y, Wang Z, Peng ZM, et al. Management of the primary malignant mediastinal germ cell tumors: experience with 54 patients. *Diagn Pathol.* 2014;9:33.

121 Mediastinal Teratoma

Borislav A. Alexiev, M.D., and Allen P. Burke, M.D.

Terminology

Mediastinal teratoma is a germ cell tumor that is composed of mature and/or immature somatic tissues derived from two or three germinal layers (ectoderm, endoderm, and mesoderm). The WHO classification of germ cell tumors distinguishes mature and immature teratomas as well as teratomas with somatic-type malignancy.[1]

Mature teratoma is a tumor composed exclusively of mature, adult-type tissues. *Dermoid cyst* is a variant that is common in the ovary and rare in the mediastinum and testis, consisting of one or more large cysts lined predominantly by keratinizing squamous epithelium with skin appendages and usually hair.[2] Monodermal teratomas analogous to struma ovarii have not been described in the mediastinum.

Teratomatous component is the term used to describe differentiated somatic tissues associated with a seminoma, embryonal carcinoma, yolk sac tumor, or choriocarcinoma. The teratomatous component of mixed germ cell tumors is very often immature.[1]

The terms "malignant teratoma" and "teratocarcinoma" are obsolete and were used to indicate teratoma with mixed germ cell elements, namely, those that result in elevations of serum tumors markers (α-fetoprotein or β-human chorionic gonadotropin) (so-called secreting tumors).

Incidence

Among teratomas of all sites, up to 27% occur in the mediastinum in adults, and 4% to 13% in children.[3-5] Mediastinal teratomas account for 7% to 9.3% of mediastinal tumors.[4] Approximately 43% to 70% of all mediastinal germ cell tumors[6] contain teratoma and include mature teratoma (63%), immature teratoma (4%), and teratoma with other malignant components (33%).[7,8] In a recent series of mediastinal germ cell tumors, 73% were mature teratomas, 1% immature teratoma, 1% teratoma with somatic malignancy, and the remainder mixed germ cell tumors (22%) and seminomas (3%).[9]

TABLE 121.1   Clinicopathologic Characteristics of Pure Mediastinal Teratomas

Age Range	Proportion of Germ Cell Tumors	M:F	Proportion That Are Histologically Mature	Biologic Behavior
<1 year	100%	2:1	50%–70%	Benign
1–10 years	30%–50%[a]	1:1	70%–90%	Benign
10+ years	50%–70%	1:1.5	95%	Benign if mature Malignant if immature

[a]Remainder predominantly yolk sac tumors or mixed teratomas and yolk sac tumors; in girls in this age, most are pure yolk sac tumors, but in boys, many are mixed.

More than 80% of mature teratomas occur in the anterior mediastinum, 3% to 8% in the posterior mediastinum, and 2% in the middle mediastinum, while 13% to 15% involve multiple mediastinal compartments.[10–12]

Clinical Findings

Pure teratomas are found in both sexes, most frequently during the neonatal period and infancy[13] (Table 121.1). Overall, there is an equal sex distribution or a slight female preponderance (M:F = 1:1.4), but there may be a slight male predominance in infants and young children.[4,12] A strong female predominance has been reported in China in adult teratomas.[9]

The mean age of adults is 28 years (range 18 to 60).[1] In children, teratoma is the predominant mediastinal tumor during the first year and has also been detected in fetuses.[4] The proportion of immature teratomas (up to 40%) is much higher in the first year of life than at older age (~4% to 6%).[4]

Mediastinal teratomas, particularly those in adults, are asymptomatic in up to 53% of cases and are frequently discovered incidentally on chest radiography performed for other reasons.[4,14] Most common initial complaints are dyspnea, cough, anorexia, fatigue, fever, and chest pain.[4,12] Patients with mediastinal teratomas that contain pancreatic tissue have more presenting symptoms (pleural effusions, cardiac tamponade) due to the occurrence of rupture than do those whose tumors were without pancreatic tissue.[9,15,16]

In newborns, these tumors are immature and present with respiratory distress and may reach large sizes.[17,18] Perforation of a mediastinal teratoma is rare but is always symptomatic.[19]

Serum markers (α-fetoprotein and β-human chorionic gonadotropin) are negative in pure teratomas and are helpful in preoperative diagnosis.[9]

Gross Pathology

Mature mediastinal teratomas are usually encapsulated masses and show multilocular cystic structures in almost 90% of cases.[8] The cut surface is variegated, showing cystic spaces with fluid or grumous materials, hair, fat, flecks of cartilage, and rarely teeth or bone. Immature teratomas are often very large and solid.[20] They exhibit a soft to fleshy consistency or are extensively fibrous or cartilaginous. Hemorrhage and necrosis can be present.

Microscopic Pathology

Mature teratomas are characterized by a haphazard admixture of organoid mature tissues derived from 2 or 3 germinal layers (Figs. 121.1 and 121.2; Table 121.2). Skin and cutaneous appendages are consistent constituents and form cyst linings. Bronchial, neural, gastrointestinal, smooth muscle, and adipose tissue components are very frequent (>80%), while skeletal muscle, bone, and cartilage are less common. Salivary gland, prostate, liver, and melanocytes are even less frequent; thyroid tissue has not been reported. Pancreatic tissue is typical of mediastinal teratomas and found in up to 60% of cases, but is rare or absent in teratomas of other sites.[16]

Immature teratomas are characterized by embryonic or fetal tissues derived from the various germinal layers, such as immature glands lined by tall columnar epithelial cells, fetal lung, immature cartilage and bone, rhabdomyoblasts, and blastema-like stromal cells.

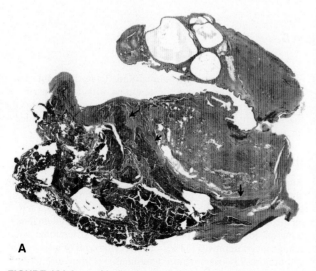
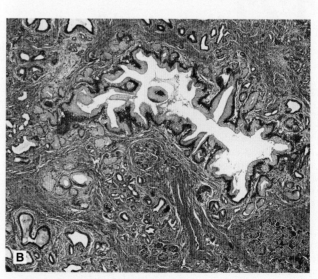

FIGURE 121.1 ▲ Mediastinal mature teratoma. **A.** Low magnification with residual thymus (*arrows*). **B.** High magnification showing gastrointestinal tissue.

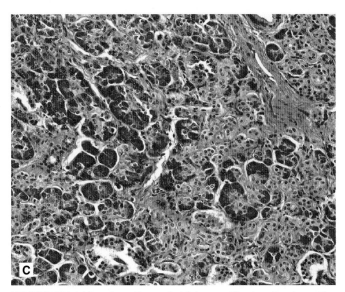

FIGURE 121.1 (Continued) ▲ **C.** High magnification showing salivary gland tissue.

The most common immature components are neuroectodermal tissues (Fig. 121.3), with neuroepithelial cells forming tubules, rosettes, or retinal anlage. By definition, pure immature teratoma should not harbor a morphologically malignant component.

Teratomas with somatic-type malignancy are characterized by a proliferation of markedly atypical (malignant) cells that resemble a malignancy that occurs in normal tissues (see Chapter 126). The somatic malignancy can be intermingled with the germ cell tumor component or forms an expansile nodular proliferation of atypical cells, often with increased mitotic rate and necrosis.[21] Embryonal rhabdomyosarcoma is the single most frequent somatic-type malignancy. Adenocarcinoma, neuroendocrine carcinoma, and hematologic malignancies arising from mediastinal teratomas have also been reported.[22–25]

Pediatric teratomas are graded as follows: grade 0, all component tissues are well differentiated; grade 1, <10% microscopic foci contain immature tissues; grade 2, 10% to 50% of immature tissue; and grade 3, >50% of immature tissue.[5] Immature teratomas, especially grade 3 teratomas, do not occur as pure tumors in the mediastinum and are mixed with other germ cell tumor components.

TABLE 121.2 Histologic Findings in Mature Teratomas of the Mediastinum[9]

Skin	100%
Cartilage	47%
Pancreas	37%
Gastrointestinal	35%
Cartilage	32%
Neural tissue	23%
Fat	14%
Bone	11%
Salivary gland	7%
Hepatic, urothelial	2%–3%
Enamel, sweat gland, breast, müllerian, fallopian tube, thyroid	1%

Adapted from Table 2, Chang CC, Chang YL, Lee JM, et al. 18 Years surgical experience with mediastinal mature teratoma. *J Formos Med Assoc.* 2010;109:287–292, Ref. [9]

Special Studies

The differentiated elements express the immunophenotype expected for that specific cell type. Pure teratomas are negative for placental-like alkaline phosphatase (PLAP) β-human chorionic gonadotropin, and CD30. AFP is usually negative, although liver cells and immature neuroepithelium in teratomas may express AFP.

In contrast to malignant mediastinal GCTs, pure mature and immature teratomas analyzed and reported to date in patients over 8 years of age do not show recurrent genetic gains and losses.[26] Immature teratomas in older children and adults with nonteratomatous components may show gain of 12p (isochromosome 12p) similar to malignant germ cell tumors in other sites.[26] Mature teratoma can be associated with classical (47, XXY) and, very rarely, mosaic Klinefelter syndrome.[27]

Differential Diagnosis

The main differential diagnosis is mixed germ cell tumor with a teratomatous component. Immature teratoma may be difficult to distinguish from teratoma with somatic-type malignancy; the latter usually shows frank cytologic atypia and invasiveness that are absent in pure immature teratomas (see Chapter 29).

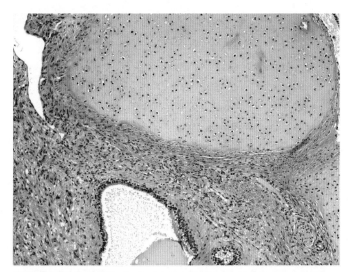

FIGURE 121.2 ▲ Mediastinal mature teratoma. Note mature cartilage.

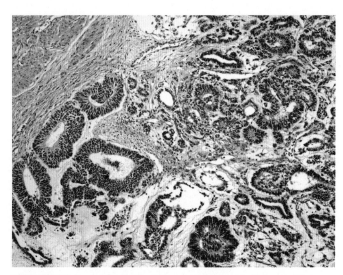

FIGURE 121.3 ▲ Mediastinal immature teratoma. Note primitive neuroepithelium consisting of small hyperchromatic cells arranged in rosettes.

Prognosis

Mature and most immature mediastinal teratomas are benign tumors.[1] Histologic grading is of no prognostic significance in children, in whom pure teratomas are uniformly benign regardless of grade.[4] All immature teratomas of the mediastinum in children and adolescents showed no progression in another series.[26] The largest series did not report any recurrence or metastasis for pure teratomas of the mediastinum at any age.[8]

There are occasional reports of recurrence but no deaths in mediastinal teratomas in children. In one series of mediastinal teratomas in children, 1 of 14 tumors relapsed, with mature histology; all immature teratomas had no progression.[5] One series reported a relapse of a pure immature teratoma of the mediastinum with subsequent long-term survival.[12]

In adults, pure teratomas of the mediastinum are virtually always mature with a benign outcome.[28] In two series, 6% to 7% of patients with adult mediastinal germ cell tumors were reported to have immature teratomas, but no specifics were given, and it is unclear if there were other mixed elements because the samples were biopsies.[29,30]

In general, the finding of immaturity in an adult mediastinal teratoma strongly suggests a mixed, especially yolk sac tumor component, and serologic findings of α-fetoprotein and β-chorionic gonadotrophin are very important.

Incomplete resection and female gender are important risk factors for relapse or death, more so than immature teratoma histology.[5] The prognosis is poor in the cases of tumor rupture.[14,22] Management of mediastinal teratomas is surgical.[4,5,9] No adjuvant therapy is needed for mature teratomas.[12] Immature teratomas must be under close follow-up for recurrences.[12] The prognosis of patients with mature teratoma with somatic-type malignancy, which is completely resected without exposure of the malignant component, seems to be excellent.[22] The effect of adjuvant therapy for recurring teratoma with somatic-type malignancy is uncertain.

REFERENCES

1. Moreira AL, Chan JKC, Looijenga LHJ, et al. Germ cell tumours of the mediastinum. In: Travis WD, et al., eds. *WHO Classification of Tumours of the Lung, Pleura, Thymus, and Heart.* Lyon, France: IARC Press; 2015: 244–259.
2. Singh J, Singh H, Vijayvergiya R, et al. Acquired supravalvular pulmonary stenosis due to extrinsic compression by a mediastinal dermoid cyst. *Eur J Cardiothorac Surg.* 2014;45:576–578.
3. Kooijman CD. Immature teratomas in children. *Histopathology.* 1988;12:491–502.
4. Schneider DT, Calaminus G, Reinhard H, et al. Primary mediastinal germ cell tumors in children and adolescents: results of the German cooperative protocols MAKEI 83/86, 89, and 96. *J Clin Oncol.* 2000;18:832–839.
5. Lo Curto M, D'Angelo P, Cecchetto G, et al. Mature and immature teratomas: results of the first paediatric Italian study. *Pediatr Surg Int.* 2007;23:315–322.
6. Dulmet EM, Macchiarini P, Suc B, et al. Germ cell tumors of the mediastinum. A 30-year experience. *Cancer.* 1993;72:1894–1901.
7. McKenney JK, Heerema-McKenney A, Rouse RV. Extragonadal germ cell tumors: a review with emphasis on pathologic features, clinical prognostic variables, and differential diagnostic considerations. *Adv Anat Pathol.* 2007;14:69–92.
8. Moran CA, Suster S. Primary germ cell tumors of the mediastinum: I. Analysis of 322 cases with special emphasis on teratomatous lesions and a proposal for histopathologic classification and clinical staging. *Cancer.* 1997;80:681–690.
9. Chang CC, Chang YL, Lee JM, et al. 18 Years surgical experience with mediastinal mature teratoma. *J Formos Med Assoc.* 2010;109:287–292.
10. Karl SR, Dunn J. Posterior mediastinal teratomas. *J Pediatr Surg.* 1985;20:508–510.
11. Ogata S, Okusa Y, Ogawa T, et al. Mature cystic teratoma in the posterior mediastinum. *Can J Surg.* 2009;52:E73–E74.
12. Yalcin B, Demir HA, Tanyel FC, et al. Mediastinal germ cell tumors in childhood. *Pediatr Hematol Oncol.* 2012;29:633–642.
13. Schneider DT, Calaminus G, Koch S, et al. Epidemiologic analysis of 1,442 children and adolescents registered in the German germ cell tumor protocols. *Pediatr Blood Cancer.* 2004;42:169–175.
14. Serraj M, Lakranbi M, Ghalimi J, et al. Mediastinal mature teratoma with complex rupture into the lung, bronchus and skin: a case report. *World J Surg Oncol.* 2013;11:125.
15. Chang YL, Wu CT, Lee YC. Mediastinal and retroperitoneal teratoma with focal gastrointestinal adenocarcinoma. *J Thorac Oncol.* 2006;1:729–731.
16. Weichert W, Koch M, Schmidt B, et al. Mature mediastinal teratoma with subtotal unidirectional pancreatic differentiation. *Pathol Res Pract.* 2010;206:346–348.
17. Paradies G, Zullino F, Orofino A, et al. Mediastinal teratomas in children. Case reports and review of the literature. *Ann Ital Chir.* 2013;84: 395–403.
18. Simoncic M, Kopriva S, Zupancic Z, et al. Mediastinal teratoma with hydrops fetalis in a newborn and development of chronic respiratory insufficiency. *Radiol Oncol.* 2014;48:397–402.
19. Hirata J, Ohya M. Cardiac tamponade following traumatic rupture of a mediastinal mature teratoma. *BMJ Case Rep.* 2013;2013. pii: bcr2013200176.
20. Taniyama K, Ohta S, Suzuki H, et al. Alpha-fetoprotein-producing immature mediastinal teratoma showing rapid and massive recurrent growth in an adult. *Acta Pathol Jpn.* 1992;42:911–915.
21. Ryu YJ, Yoo SH, Jung MJ, et al. Embryonal rhabdomyosarcoma arising from a mediastinal teratoma: an unusual case report. *J Korean Med Sci.* 2013;28:476–479.
22. Kim JY, Lee CH, Park WY, et al. Adenocarcinoma with sarcomatous dedifferentiation arising from mature cystic teratoma of the anterior mediastinum. *Pathol Res Pract.* 2012;208:741–745.
23. Schaefer IM, Zardo P, Freermann S, et al. Neuroendocrine carcinoma in a mediastinal teratoma as a rare variant of somatic-type malignancy. *Virchows Arch.* 2013;463:731–735.
24. Takanashi Y, Tajima S, Takahashi T, et al. Mediastinal mature teratoma with complete gastrointestinal and bronchial walls. *Respirol Case Rep.* 2015;3:89–91.
25. Saito A, Watanabe K, Kusakabe T, et al. Mediastinal mature teratoma with coexistence of angiosarcoma, granulocytic sarcoma and a hematopoietic region in the tumor: a rare case of association between hematological malignancy and mediastinal germ cell tumor. *Pathol Int.* 1998;48: 749–753.
26. Schneider DT, Schuster AE, Fritsch MK, et al. Genetic analysis of mediastinal nonseminomatous germ cell tumors in children and adolescents. *Genes Chromosomes Cancer.* 2002;34:115–125.
27. Lachman MF, Kim K, Koo BC. Mediastinal teratoma associated with Klinefelter's syndrome. *Arch Pathol Lab Med.* 1986;110:1067–1071.
28. Takeda S, Miyoshi S, Ohta M, et al. Primary germ cell tumors in the mediastinum: a 50-year experience at a single Japanese institution. *Cancer.* 2003;97: 367–376.
29. Rivera C, Arame A, Jougon J, et al. Prognostic factors in patients with primary mediastinal germ cell tumors, a surgical multicenter retrospective study. *Interact Cardiovasc Thorac Surg.* 2010;11:585–589.
30. Sarkaria IS, Bains MS, Sood S, et al. Resection of primary mediastinal nonseminomatous germ cell tumors: a 28-year experience at memorial sloan-kettering cancer center. *J Thorac Oncol.* 2011;6:1236–1241.

122 Yolk Sac Tumor (Endodermal Sinus Tumor)

Borislav A. Alexiev, M.D., and Anja C. Roden, M.D.

Terminology

Mediastinal yolk sac tumor (YST) is a neoplasm characterized by numerous patterns that recapitulate the yolk sac, allantois, and extraembryonic mesenchyme.

Incidence and Clinical Features

YST of the mediastinum is uncommon. Most patients are young, and the great majority of tumors are found in the anterior mediastinum.[1–3] The neoplasm presents in two distinct age groups. In infants and young children, YST is virtually the only malignant GCT (germ cell tumors) histologic subtype seen and there is a strong predominance of females (F:M, 4:1).[4] The age at presentation ranges from the newborn period to 7 years of age, with over 75% of these patients presenting within the first 3 years of life.[5] Like other mediastinal malignant GCTs in postpubertal patients, YST presents exclusively in males. The age at presentation in postpubertal patients ranges from 14 to 63 years.

YSTs are often seen as one element within a mixed GCT.[3] Patients with mediastinal YST often present with chest pain, dyspnea, chills, fever, and superior vena cava syndrome.[3,4,6] Regardless of the age, alpha fetoprotein (AFP) levels are elevated in over 90% of cases.[3] An almost unique complication of mediastinal YSTs as compared to other extragonadal or testicular YSTs is the development of hematologic malignancies.[7,8] Formation of multilocular thymic cysts results from local inflammatory reactions.[9]

Gross Pathology

Macroscopically, pure YSTs are solid and soft, and the cut surface is typically pale gray or gray-white and somewhat gelatinous or mucoid.[3] The tumors often show hemorrhage and necrosis.

Microscopic Pathology

The histologic appearance is the same, regardless of patient age, and resembles YST of the gonads. A number of different histologic patterns have been described: microcystic (reticular) (Figs. 122.1 to 122.3), macrocystic, glandular–alveolar, endodermal sinus (pseudopapillary), myxomatous, hepatoid, enteric, polyvesicular vitelline, and solid[10–12] (Fig. 122.4). There may be prominent spindling.[13] The majority of YSTs show more than one histologic subtype, and the different subtypes often merge subtly from one to another. The reticular or microcystic variant is the most common histologic subtype and is characterized by a loose network of spaces and channels with small cystic spaces lined by flattened or cuboidal cells with scant cytoplasm, which may contain pale eosinophilic secretion. The nuclei vary in size but generally are small. Mitotic activity is typically brisk. A variant of the microcystic pattern is the myxomatous pattern in which the epithelial-like cells are separated by abundant myxomatous stroma. The endodermal sinus pattern has a pseudopapillary appearance and typically shows numerous Schiller-Duval bodies. These are glomeruloid structures with a central blood vessel covered by an inner rim of tumor cells, surrounded by a capsule lined by an outer (parietal) rim of tumor cells. Although characteristic of YST, Schiller-Duvall bodies are present in only 50% to 75% of YST.[3] The polyvesicular vitelline pattern is composed of compact connective tissue stroma containing cysts lined by cuboidal to flat tumor cells. The solid pattern is uncommon and consists of nodular aggregates of medium-sized polygonal tumor cells with clear cytoplasm and large nuclei. Hepatoid and enteric variants are other less common forms of YST.[3,14] The hepatoid pattern contains cells with abundant eosinophilic cytoplasm resembling fetal or adult liver.[3,14] The enteric and endometrioid patterns show glandular features resembling the fetal human gut and endometrial glands, respectively, and have generally been reported in gonadal sites.[15,16] Hyaline globules are commonly present in YST. However, hyaline droplets may also be

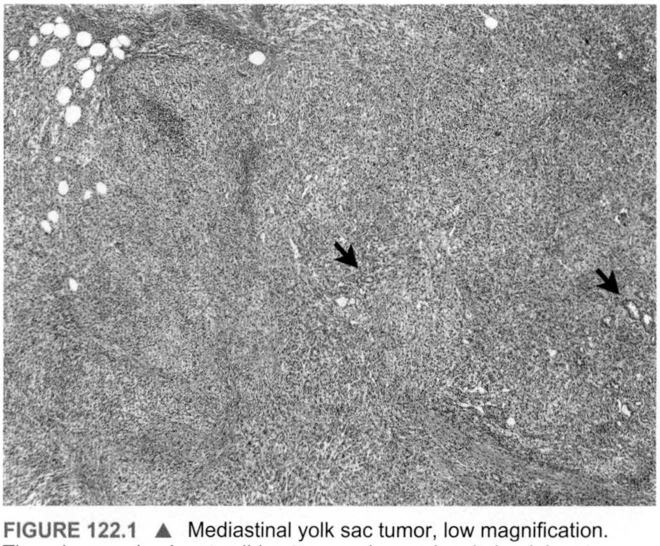

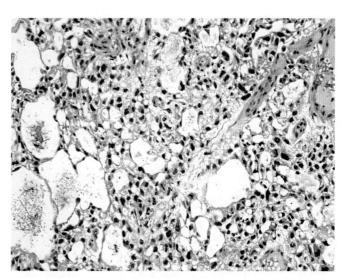

FIGURE 122.1 ▲ Mediastinal yolk sac tumor, low magnification. There is a predominant solid pattern and occasional glandular structures (*arrows*).

FIGURE 122.2 ▲ Mediastinal yolk tumor, in an elderly man. The case is unusual due to the age of the patient. The pattern is microcystic (reticular). An initial core biopsy of the mediastinum was nondiagnostic (not shown).

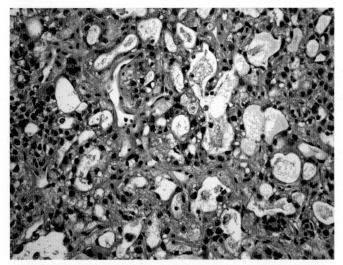

FIGURE 122.3 ▲ A different tumor showing cystic spaces that are lined by small cuboidal and flattened cells.

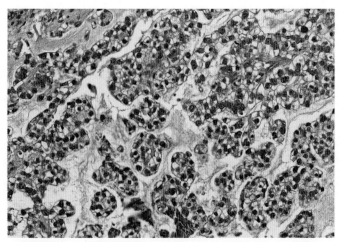

FIGURE 122.4 ▲ Mediastinal yolk sac tumor with pseudopapillary growth with hepatoid cytologic features.

found in a minority of embryonal carcinomas, as well as in some other epithelial tumors. Similar to seminomas, YST can be associated with cystic changes in the thymus.

Ancillary Studies

Hyaline globules are composed of a variety of proteins and are PAS positive, resistant to diastase digestion. By immunohistochemistry, the droplets may be positive for α-fetoprotein as well as alpha-1-antitrypsin.[17] Strong positivity for α-fetoprotein is helpful in the diagnosis of YST. However, the reaction may also be variable, and only about two-thirds of YST express α-fetoprotein. Therefore, negative staining does not exclude the diagnosis.[3,18] Moreover, α-fetoprotein can be expressed occasionally in lung carcinomas, specifically hepatoid lung adenocarcinomas, and therefore is not an entirely specific marker in that location.[19] SALL4 is a more sensitive marker than AFP for YST (Fig. 122.5A), but this marker is also expressed in seminomas among other tumors. It can be diffusely positive in fewer than 10% of carcinomas.[20,21] Almost all YSTs express glypican-3. However, this marker is not specific for YST as it is also expressed in choriocarcinoma, hepatocellular carcinoma, and some squamous cell carcinoma and adenocarcinoma of the lung (Fig. 122.5B).[18,22] YST also shows strong positive

staining with low molecular weight cytokeratin (Fig. 122.5C) and may show some staining with CD30 and CD117 (Fig. 122.5D).[18] Staining for α-fetoprotein tends to be patchy (Fig. 122.5E). In contrast to seminomas and/or embryonal carcinomas, YSTs are negative for OCT4.[20]

Prepubertal YST demonstrate the same recurrent genetic abnormalities described in infantile sacral and testicular YST, including loss of the short arm of chromosome 1 (in particular the 1p36 region), loss of the long arm of chromosome 6, and gain of the long arm of chromosomes 1, and 20, and the complete chromosome 22.[3] In contrast, mediastinal YSTs following puberty are aneuploid and often harbor the isochromosome 12p characteristic of testicular malignant GCTs in the same age group.[3]

Overall, there is no single immunohistochemical or cytogenetic marker that is specific for YST in the mediastinum. Therefore, a panel of immunohistochemical stains might be performed, and the results should be interpreted in the context of morphology and possibly serology.

Differential Diagnosis

The enteric and endometrioid patterns show glandular features resembling the fetal human gut and endometrial glands, respectively. If these patterns are seen within an immature teratoma, it may be difficult to determine whether they represent immature fetal tissue or YST.

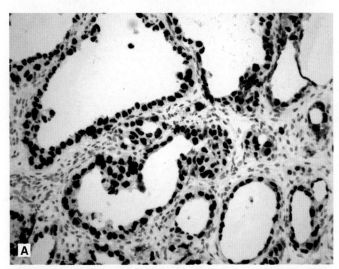

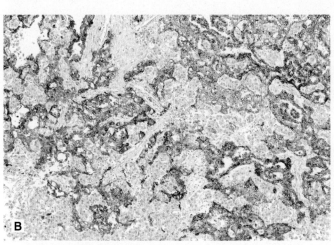

FIGURE 122.5 ▲ Mediastinal yolk sac tumor, immunohistochemical stains. **A.** Note positive nuclear staining for SALL4. **B.** Note cytoplasmic positivity for glypican-3.

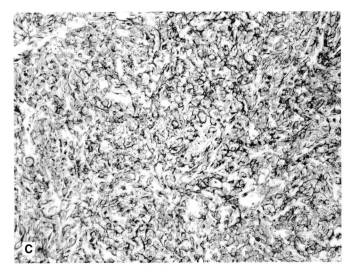

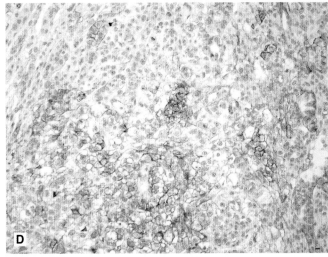

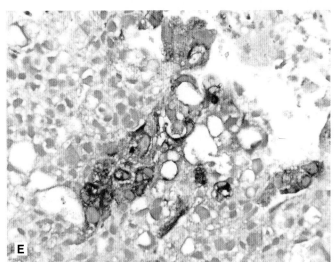

FIGURE 122.5 *(Continued)* ▲ **C.** There is diffuse positivity for keratin AE1/AE. **D.** There is focal positivity for CD117. **E.** There is focal positivity for α-fetoprotein.

Fortunately, these unusual patterns of YST are usually accompanied by other more common patterns. The solid pattern is uncommon and may be difficult to distinguish from embryonal carcinoma or seminoma. However, the cells of YST are smaller and less pleomorphic and usually retain their AFP positivity.

Treatment and Prognosis

Treatment of YSTs includes surgical resection and cisplatin-based chemotherapy. In children < 15 years, the overall survival is nearly 90%.[23–25] In patients > 15 years, the prognosis is less favorable, with 5-year survival rates of under 50%.[3] Pure YST histology is a favorable prognostic sign, along with lack of metastasis, complete resection, normalization of tumor markers, and complete necrosis (100% treatment effect histologically) in resected tumors treated with neoadjuvant chemotherapy.[26]

REFERENCES

1. Konishi T, Fujino S, Chino Y, et al. Posterior mediastinal endodermal sinus (yolk sac) tumor in a female patient. *Ann Thorac Surg.* 1994;58:244–245.
2. Moran CA, Suster S, Koss MN. Primary germ cell tumors of the mediastinum: III. Yolk sac tumor, embryonal carcinoma, choriocarcinoma, and combined nonteratomatous germ cell tumors of the mediastinum—a clinicopathologic and immunohistochemical study of 64 cases. *Cancer.* 1997;80:699–707.
3. Marx A, Moreira AL, Chan JKC, et al. Yolk sac tumour. In: Travis WD, et al., eds. *WHO Classification of Tumours of the Lung, Pleura, Thymus and Heart.* Lyon, France: CRC Press; 2015.
4. Schneider DT, Schuster AE, Fritsch MK, et al. Genetic analysis of mediastinal nonseminomatous germ cell tumors in children and adolescents. *Genes Chromosomes Cancer.* 2002;34:115–125.
5. Schneider DT, Calaminus G, Reinhard H, et al. Primary mediastinal germ cell tumors in children and adolescents: results of the German cooperative protocols MAKEI 83/86, 89, and 96. *J Clin Oncol.* 2000;18:832–839.
6. Takeda S, Miyoshi S, Ohta M, et al. Primary germ cell tumors in the mediastinum: a 50-year experience at a single Japanese institution. *Cancer.* 2003;97:367–376.
7. Chaudary IU, Bojal SA, Attia A, et al. Mediastinal endodermal sinus tumor associated with fatal hemophagocytic syndrome. *Hematol Oncol Stem Cell Ther.* 2011;4:138–141.
8. Govender D, Pillay SV. Mediastinal immature teratoma with yolk sac tumor and myelomonocytic leukemia associated with Klinefelter's syndrome. *Int J Surg Pathol.* 2002;10:157–162.
9. Moran CA, Suster S. Mediastinal yolk sac tumors associated with prominent multilocular cystic changes of thymic epithelium: a clinicopathologic and immunohistochemical study of five cases. *Mod Pathol.* 1997;10:800–803.
10. Kurman RJ, Norris HJ. Endodermal sinus tumor of the ovary: a clinical and pathologic analysis of 71 cases. *Cancer.* 1976;38:2404–2419.
11. Teilum G. Endodermal sinus tumors of the ovary and testis. Comparative morphogenesis of the so-called mesoephroma ovarii (Schiller) and extra-embryonic (yolk sac-allantoic) structures of the rat's placenta. *Cancer.* 1959;12:1092–1105.
12. Ulbright TM. Germ cell tumors of the gonads: a selective review emphasizing problems in differential diagnosis, newly appreciated, and controversial issues. *Mod Pathol.* 2005;18(suppl 2):S61–S79.

13. Moran CA, Suster S. Yolk sac tumors of the mediastinum with prominent spindle cell features: a clinicopathologic study of three cases. *Am J Surg Pathol.* 1997;21:1173–1177.

14. Moran CA, Suster S. Hepatoid yolk sac tumors of the mediastinum: a clinicopathologic and immunohistochemical study of four cases. *Am J Surg Pathol.* 1997;21:1210–1214.

15. Clement PB, Young RH, Scully RE. Endometrioid-like variant of ovarian yolk sac tumor. A clinicopathological analysis of eight cases. *Am J Surg Pathol.* 1987;11:767–778.

16. Cohen MB, Friend DS, Molnar JJ, et al. Gonadal endodermal sinus (yolk sac) tumor with pure intestinal differentiation: a new histologic type. *Pathol Res Pract.* 1987;182:609–616.

17. Palmer PE, Safaii H, Wolfe HJ. Alpha1-antitrypsin and alpha-fetoprotein. Protein markers in endodermal sinus (yolk sac) tumors. *Am J Clin Pathol.* 1976;65:575–582.

18. Kao CS, Idrees MT, Young RH, et al. Solid pattern yolk sac tumor: a morphologic and immunohistochemical study of 52 cases. *Am J Surg Pathol.* 2012;36:360–367.

19. Haninger DM, Kloecker GH, Bousamra Ii M, et al. Hepatoid adenocarcinoma of the lung: report of five cases and review of the literature. *Mod Pathol.* 2014;27:535–542.

20. Cao D, Guo S, Allan RW, et al. SALL4 is a novel sensitive and specific marker of ovarian primitive germ cell tumors and is particularly useful in distinguishing yolk sac tumor from clear cell carcinoma. *Am J Surg Pathol.* 2009;33:894–904.

21. Liu A, Cheng L, Du J, et al. Diagnostic utility of novel stem cell markers SALL4, OCT4, NANOG, SOX2, UTF1, and TCL1 in primary mediastinal germ cell tumors. *Am J Surg Pathol.* 2010;34:697–706.

22. Zynger DL, Everton MJ, Dimov ND, et al. Expression of glypican 3 in ovarian and extragonadal germ cell tumors. *Am J Clin Pathol.* 2008;130: 224–230.

23. Billmire D, Vinocur C, Rescorla F, et al. Malignant mediastinal germ cell tumors: an intergroup study. *J Pediatr Surg.* 2001;36:18–24.

24. De Backer A, Madern GC, Pieters R, et al. Influence of tumor site and histology on long-term survival in 193 children with extracranial germ cell tumors. *Eur J Pediatr Surg.* 2008;18:1–6.

25. Sudour-Bonnange H, Orbach D, Kalfa N, et al. Germ cell tumors in atypical locations: experience of the TGM 95 SFCE trial. *J Pediatr Hematol Oncol.* 2014;36:646–648.

26. Rodney AJ, Tannir NM, Siefker-Radtke AO, et al. Survival outcomes for men with mediastinal germ-cell tumors: the University of Texas M. D. Anderson Cancer Center experience. *Urol Oncol.* 2012;30:879–885.

123 Embryonal Carcinoma

Borislav A. Alexiev, M.D., and Anja C. Roden, M.D.

Background

Mediastinal embryonal carcinoma is a germ cell tumor composed of large primitive cells of epithelial appearance with abundant clear or granular cytoplasm, resembling cells of the embryonic germ disk and growing in solid, papillary, and glandular patterns.[1]

Incidence and Clinical

Embryonal carcinoma of the mediastinum is a tumor of young males (M/F ratio, >10:1).[2,3] It occurs in pure form or as a component in mixed germ cell tumors at about equal frequencies.[4] Embryonal carcinomas (pure or mixed) account for up to 12% of all mediastinal germ cell tumors.[2,4] Between 0% and 26% of nonseminomatous malignant germ cell tumors of the mediastinum are pure embryonal carcinoma, depending on the series.[4–7] The mean age of adult patients is 27 years (range: 18 to 67 years).[2,8]

Pure embryonal carcinoma does not occur in the mediastinum of children.[9] Embryonal carcinoma as part of a mixed germ cell tumor occurs after age 5 in boys.[9–11] Embryonal carcinoma is commonly associated with teratoma (56%), choriocarcinoma (22%), or seminoma (22%).[2,3] The association with yolk sac tumor (YST) is the most common combined form of mixed germ cell tumor in adults[4] and is also not uncommon in children, sometimes with seminoma or choriocarcinoma.[9]

A minority of patients with mediastinal embryonal carcinoma show features of Klinefelter syndrome similar to other germ cell tumors.[12]

Patients present with thoracic or shoulder pain, respiratory distress, hoarseness, cough, fever, and superior vena cava syndrome.[3] Gynecomastia is uncommon. A quarter of patients have pulmonary metastasis at presentation, and virtually all patients exhibit increased serum α-fetoprotein (AFP) levels, while β-hCG levels are elevated in cases with a choriocarcinoma component.[1]

Gross Pathology

Embryonal carcinomas present as large tumors with invasion of the surrounding organs and structures. Grossly, the cut surface often reveals large areas of necrosis and hemorrhage. Viable tumor tissue is soft, fleshy, and gray or white to pink or tan. In mixed germ cell tumors, cystic spaces may be conspicuous.

Microscopic Pathology

Pure embryonal carcinomas show a more solid growth pattern than do other nonseminomatous germ cell tumors. Embryonal carcinomas form sheets, tubules, or vague papillary structures composed of large polygonal or columnar cells (Fig. 123.1). The nuclei are large, round or oval, and often vesicular and can be hyperchromatic or have a light chromatin. They can be crowded and overlapping.

Prominent single or multiple nucleoli are common. The cell borders are often indistinct, especially in the solid areas. The cytoplasm is often amphophilic but can be basophilic, eosinophilic, pale, or clear.[1] As in seminoma, scattered single cells or small groups of syncytiotrophoblasts can occur in embryonal carcinoma. Mitoses are numerous and often atypical. Extensive necrosis can occur and is particularly prominent in embryonal carcinomas combined with YST. The stroma is usually scant in viable tumor areas but fibrotic adjacent to areas with regressive changes. Scattered lymphocytes and a granulomatous reaction are uncommon.

In mixed germ cell tumors, the embryonal carcinoma component may be combined with a YST, teratoma, seminoma, choriocarcinoma, or combinations of these germ cell tumors, and uncommonly somatic-type malignancies.[13]

Special Studies

OCT4, SALL4, and CD30 are expressed in 85% to 100% of pure embryonal carcinoma or embryonal carcinoma components of mixed germ cell tumor (Figs. 123.2 and 123.3), while other germ cell tumors (with the exception of rare cases of seminomas and YSTs and other nonhematopoietic neoplasms) are CD30 negative.[14–18] There is distinct cell membrane staining by CD30 with variable cytoplasmic positivity. However, CD30 is expressed in some lymphomas such as mediastinal large B-cell

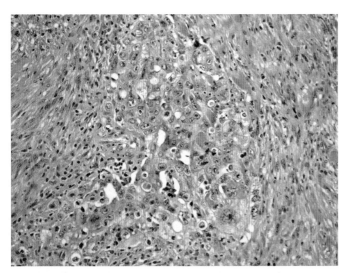

FIGURE 123.1 ▲ Mediastinal embryonal carcinoma. Note syncytial growth pattern, gland-like structures, and marked cytologic atypia.

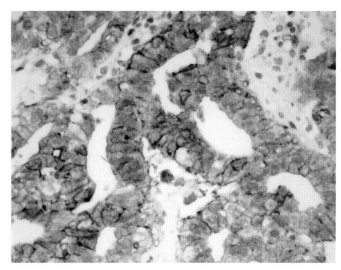

FIGURE 123.3 ▲ Mediastinal embryonal carcinoma. Note positive membranous staining for CD30 (anti-CD30).

lymphoma or Hodgkin lymphoma, which need to be excluded. In addition, embryonal carcinomas are uniformly and strongly reactive with antibodies to low molecular weight cytokeratins, while epithelial membrane antigen (EMA), carcinoembryonic antigen (CEA), and vimentin are usually negative. AFP and placental-like alkaline phosphatase (PLAP) can occur in scattered tumor cells or small foci in about 30% of cases.[18] One-third of cases show β-hCG expression in scattered syncytiotrophoblastic cells.

The genetic changes that have been described in mediastinal embryonal carcinoma are the same as those reported in their testicular counterparts and demonstrate the isochromosome 12p characteristic of postpubertal malignant germ cell tumors at all sites.[1]

Differential Diagnosis

When syncytiotrophoblast areas are extensive, embryonal carcinoma can mimic choriocarcinoma.[4] However, a biphasic pattern produced by a mixture of syncytiotrophoblasts and cytotrophoblasts is lacking, and pure embryonal carcinomas lack the extensive β-hCG immunoreactivity of choriocarcinoma.[4] YSTs can be distinguished from embryonal carcinoma by a more varied growth pattern (most commonly microcystic and reticular), smaller cell size, presence of Schiller-Duval

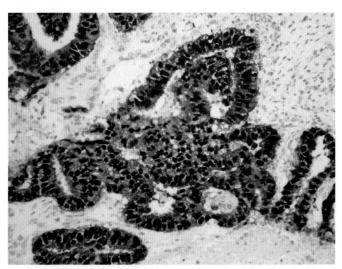

FIGURE 123.2 ▲ Mediastinal embryonal carcinoma. Note positive staining for OCT4 (anti-OCT4).

bodies, and lack of CD30 expression.[1] Embryonal carcinoma can be distinguished from seminoma by showing a greater degree of nuclear pleomorphism, at least focal gland formation, strong staining for cytokeratin and CD30, and usual lack of CD117 expression.[18] Mediastinal metastasis from large cell carcinoma of the lung can be a morphologic mimic.[4] Metastasis to the mediastinum from a testicular embryonal carcinoma or mixed germ cell tumor[1] has to be excluded.

Treatment and Prognosis

There are no reports focusing on the prognostic factors of mediastinal embryonal carcinoma. However, since embryonal carcinoma histology has not been shown to be an adverse prognostic factor in several large clinical studies,[19,20] it is likely that the prognostic factors described for nonseminomatous germ cell tumors apply to embryonal carcinoma. Nonseminomatous histology, presence of extramediastinal disease, and primary mediastinal germ cell tumor location are independent prognostic factors for shorter survival.[21,22]

Analysis of data and results from recent series suggest that the long-term survival rate of ~50% in adult patients with mediastinal embryonal carcinoma after cisplatin-based chemotherapy was very similar to the rates published for large series of adult nonseminomatous germ cell tumors.[3,19,21] Similar conclusions appear justified for children with embryonal carcinoma, although 5-year survival rates are significantly better (>80%) than are those for adults.[9,11,22]

REFERENCES

1. Moreira AL, Chan JKC, Looijenga LHJ, et al. Germ cell tumours of the mediastinum. In: Travis WD, et al., eds. *WHO Classification of Tumours of the Lung, Pleura, Thymus, and Heart.* Lyon, France: IARC Press; 2015:244–259.
2. Knapp RH, Hurt RD, Payne WS, et al. Malignant germ cell tumors of the mediastinum. *J Thorac Cardiovasc Surg.* 1985;89:82–89.
3. Takeda S, Miyoshi S, Ohta M, et al. Primary germ cell tumors in the mediastinum: a 50-year experience at a single Japanese institution. *Cancer.* 2003;97:367–376.
4. Moran CA, Suster S, Koss MN. Primary germ cell tumors of the mediastinum: III. Yolk sac tumor, embryonal carcinoma, choriocarcinoma, and combined nonteratomatous germ cell tumors of the mediastinum—a clinicopathologic and immunohistochemical study of 64 cases. *Cancer.* 1997;80:699–707.
5. Kesler KA, Rieger KM, Hammoud ZT, et al. A 25-year single institution experience with surgery for primary mediastinal nonseminomatous germ cell tumors. *Ann Thorac Surg.* 2008;85:371–378.
6. Rivera C, Arame A, Jougon J, et al. Prognostic factors in patients with primary mediastinal germ cell tumors, a surgical multicenter retrospective study. *Interact Cardiovasc Thorac Surg.* 2010;11:585–589.

7. Rodney AJ, Tannir NM, Siefker-Radtke AO, et al. Survival outcomes for men with mediastinal germ-cell tumors: the University of Texas M. D. Anderson Cancer Center experience. *Urol Oncol.* 2012;30:879–885.
8. Moran CA, Suster S. Primary germ cell tumors of the mediastinum: I. Analysis of 322 cases with special emphasis on teratomatous lesions and a proposal for histopathologic classification and clinical staging. *Cancer.* 1997;80:681–690.
9. Schneider DT, Calaminus G, Reinhard H, et al. Primary mediastinal germ cell tumors in children and adolescents: results of the German cooperative protocols MAKEI 83/86, 89, and 96. *J Clin Oncol.* 2000;18:832–839.
10. Billmire D, Vinocur C, Rescorla F, et al. Malignant mediastinal germ cell tumors: an intergroup study. *J Pediatr Surg.* 2001;36:18–24.
11. Schneider DT, Calaminus G, Koch S, et al. Epidemiologic analysis of 1,442 children and adolescents registered in the German germ cell tumor protocols. *Pediatr Blood Cancer.* 2004;42:169–175.
12. McNeil MM, Leong AS, Sage RE. Primary mediastinal embryonal carcinoma in association with Klinefelter's syndrome. *Cancer.* 1981;47:343–345.
13. Manivel C, Wick MR, Abenoza P, et al. The occurrence of sarcomatous components in primary mediastinal germ cell tumors. *Am J Surg Pathol.* 1986;10:711–717.
14. Iwamoto N, Ishida M, Yoshida K, et al. Mediastinal seminoma: a case report with special emphasis on SALL4 as a new immunocytochemical marker. *Diagn Cytopathol.* 2013;41:821–824.
15. Jung SM, Chu PH, Shiu TF, et al. Expression of OCT4 in the primary germ cell tumors and thymoma in the mediastinum. *Appl Immunohistochem Mol Morphol.* 2006;14:273–275.
16. Liu A, Cheng L, Du J, et al. Diagnostic utility of novel stem cell markers SALL4, OCT4, NANOG, SOX2, UTF1, and TCL1 in primary mediastinal germ cell tumors. *Am J Surg Pathol.* 2010;34:697–706.
17. Sung MT, Maclennan GT, Lopez-Beltran A, et al. Primary mediastinal seminoma: a comprehensive assessment integrated with histology, immunohistochemistry, and fluorescence in situ hybridization for chromosome 12p abnormalities in 23 cases. *Am J Surg Pathol.* 2008;32:146–155.
18. Suster S, Moran CA, Dominguez-Malagon H, et al. Germ cell tumors of the mediastinum and testis: a comparative immunohistochemical study of 120 cases. *Hum Pathol.* 1998;29:737–742.
19. Bokemeyer C, Nichols CR, Droz JP, et al. Extragonadal germ cell tumors of the mediastinum and retroperitoneum: results from an international analysis. *J Clin Oncol.* 2002;20:1864–1873.
20. Wright CD, Kesler KA, Nichols CR, et al. Primary mediastinal nonseminomatous germ cell tumors. Results of a multimodality approach. *J Thorac Cardiovasc Surg.* 1990;99:210–217.
21. Nichols CR, Saxman S, Williams SD, et al. Primary mediastinal nonseminomatous germ cell tumors. A modern single institution experience. *Cancer.* 1990;65:1641–1646.
22. Schneider BP, Kesler KA, Brooks JA, et al. Outcome of patients with residual germ cell or non-germ cell malignancy after resection of primary mediastinal nonseminomatous germ cell cancer. *J Clin Oncol.* 2004;22:1195–1200.

124 Choriocarcinoma

Borislav A. Alexiev, M.D., Fabio R. Tavora, M.D., Ph.D., and Allen P. Burke, M.D.

Terminology

Choriocarcinoma is a highly malignant neoplasm composed of syncytiotrophoblasts, cytotrophoblasts, and variably intermediate trophoblast cells. Mediastinal choriocarcinomas are morphologically indistinguishable from their gonadal or uterine counterparts.

Incidence and Clinical

Pure mediastinal choriocarcinomas are exceedingly rare and virtually nonexistent in children.[1-10] The tumor occurs almost exclusively in young males. Only 2.5% to 5% of mediastinal GCTs are pure choriocarcinoma.[11-15]

The patients' ages range from 17 to 63 (most commonly the third decade of life).[2,7,9] At diagnosis, mediastinal choriocarcinomas are mostly large anterior mediastinal masses. The patients present with symptoms due to the mediastinal mass, such as chest pain, dyspnea, cough, and superior vena cava syndrome. Patients may show gynecomastia due to elevated beta-hCG levels.[2,7,9] Mediastinal choriocarcinomas are highly aggressive neoplasms with early hematogenous dissemination. Metastatic disease to the lungs, liver, kidney, spleen, brain, heart, adrenals, and bone has been observed.[9,10]

Gross Pathology

Choriocarcinomas most commonly present as a hemorrhagic mass that may be surrounded by a discernible rim of white to tan tumor tissue.

Microscopic Pathology

Choriocarcinoma consists of an admixture of syncytiotrophoblasts, cytotrophoblasts, and intermediate trophoblasts[11] (Fig. 124.1). The syncytiotrophoblasts are usually multinucleated with several, large,

irregularly shaped, hyperchromatic nuclei and deeply staining eosinophilic or amphophilic cytoplasm. The cytotrophoblasts have pale to clear cytoplasm with a single, irregularly shaped nucleus and prominent nucleoli. Intermediate trophoblasts are larger than cytotrophoblasts and have a single nucleus with prominent nucleoli and eosinophilic to clear cytoplasm. These cellular components are arranged in varying patterns, usually in an extensively hemorrhagic and necrotic background. Most commonly, they are admixed in a more or less random fashion. In some examples, the syncytiotrophoblasts "cap" nests of cytotrophoblasts in a pattern that is reminiscent of the architecture seen in immature placental villi. Vascular invasion is commonly identified.

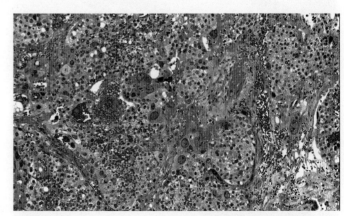

FIGURE 124.1 ▲ Choriocarcinoma of the mediastinum. Note syncytiotrophoblasts and smaller, rounded cytotrophoblasts with background of hemorrhage.

Special Studies

All of the cell types express pancytokeratin CAM5.2 and AE1/AE3, whereas they are negative for AFP, CEA, CD30, and vimentin.[11] Placental alkaline phosphatase (PLAP) shows patchy immunostaining in rare cases. The syncytiotrophoblasts additionally express beta-hCG and inhibin, while the cytotrophoblasts are variably positive for human placental lactogen.[9,11]

The genetic changes that have been described in mediastinal choriocarcinoma are the same as those reported in the testis and demonstrate the isochromosome i(12p) characteristic of postpubertal malignant GCTs at all sites.[16] Such tumors are most commonly aneuploid.

Differential Diagnosis

Apart from metastasis of an extramediastinal choriocarcinoma, the differential diagnoses include mediastinal mixed GCT and mediastinal metastasis from a carcinoma with choriocarcinoma-like features/dedifferentiation.

Treatment and Prognosis

The prognosis of primary mediastinal choriocarcinoma is very poor despite the introduction of combination chemotherapy.[3,9] In most of the reported cases, patients died of disseminated disease shortly after diagnosis (average survival time 1 to 2 months).[9,17] Treatment involves intensive therapy with etoposide and cisplatin-containing agents, which may result in remission.[1]

REFERENCES

1. Zhang F, Zhang W, Shi H, et al. Primary choriocarcinoma of the posterior mediastinum in a male: a case report and review of the literature. *Oncol Lett.* 2014;8:739–741.
2. Gaude GS, Patil P, Malur PR, et al. Primary mediastinal choriocarcinoma. *South Asian J Cancer.* 2013;2:79.
3. Dasanu CA, Shimanovsky A, Jain K, et al. Mediastinal choriocarcinoma presenting with syncope. *Conn Med.* 2013;77:473–475.
4. Lam S, Rizkalla K, Hsia CC. Mediastinal choriocarcinoma masquerading as relapsed Hodgkin lymphoma. *Case Rep Oncol.* 2011;4:512–516.
5. Bachmann J, Ernestus K, Werner T, et al. Detection of primary choriocarcinoma in the mediastinum by F-18 FDG positron emission tomography. *Clin Nucl Med.* 2007;32:663–665.
6. Yun EJ, Chung JY, Han HS. Primary mediastinal choriocarcinoma. *Int J Gynaecol Obstet.* 2005;88:158–159.
7. Shen HH, Zhang GS, Xu F. Primary choriocarcinoma in the anterior mediastinum in a man: a case report and review of the literatures. *Chin Med J (Engl).* 2004;117:1743–1745.
8. Yamashita S, Ohyama C, Nakagawa H, et al. Primary choriocarcinoma in the posterior mediastinum. *J Urol.* 2002;167:1789.
9. Moran CA, Suster S. Primary mediastinal choriocarcinomas: a clinicopathologic and immunohistochemical study of eight cases. *Am J Surg Pathol.* 1997;21:1007–1012.
10. Kathuria S, Jablokow VR. Primary choriocarcinoma of mediastinum with immunohistochemical study and review of the literature. *J Surg Oncol.* 1987;34:39–42.
11. Moreira AL, Chan JKC, Looijenga LHJ, et al. Germ cell tumours of the mediastinum. In: Travis WD, et al., eds. *WHO Classification of Tumours of the Lung, Pleura, Thymus, and Heart.* Lyon, France: IARC Press; 2015:244–259.
12. Kesler KA, Rieger KM, Hammoud ZT, et al. A 25-year single institution experience with surgery for primary mediastinal nonseminomatous germ cell tumors. *Ann Thorac Surg.* 2008;85:371–378.
13. Takeda S, Miyoshi S, Ohta M, et al. Primary germ cell tumors in the mediastinum: a 50-year experience at a single Japanese institution. *Cancer.* 2003;97:367–376.
14. Nichols CR, Saxman S, Williams SD, et al. Primary mediastinal nonseminomatous germ cell tumors. A modern single institution experience. *Cancer.* 1990;65:1641–1646.
15. Knapp RH, Hurt RD, Payne WS, et al. Malignant germ cell tumors of the mediastinum. *J Thorac Cardiovasc Surg.* 1985;89:82–89.
16. Chaganti RS, Rodriguez E, Mathew S. Origin of adult male mediastinal germ-cell tumours. *Lancet.* 1994;343:1130–1132.
17. Dulmet EM, Macchiarini P, Suc B, et al. Germ cell tumors of the mediastinum. A 30-year experience. *Cancer.* 1993;72:1894–1901.

125 Mixed Germ Cell Tumors

Borislav A. Alexiev, M.D., and Allen P. Burke, M.D.

Background

Mixed germ cell tumors (GCT) are composed of more than one type of GCT element and are malignant.[1] Virtually any combination of elements may be present; common combinations include teratoma, embryonal carcinoma, and yolk sac tumor, with or without seminoma. The presence of syncytiotrophoblasts with seminoma in the absence of other tumor types does not define a mixed GCT. However, other than with pure seminoma, the presence of syncytiotrophoblasts always indicates the presence of mixed elements.

Incidence and Clinical

In children, mixed GCTs account for about 20% of mediastinum GCTs, and yolk sac tumor with mature or immature teratoma is the characteristic constellation. Among children <8 years of age, some authors report a preponderance of females, while virtually all adolescent patients >8 years with mixed GCTs are males.[2–4] After the onset of puberty, mixed GCTs can be associated with Klinefelter syndrome.[5,6]

In adults, mixed GCTs account for 13% to 25% of all mediastinal GCTs, second only to teratomas (40% to 60%).[7–12] Virtually all adult patients are male. Most patients present with general and local symptoms identical to those in other mediastinal GCT: chest pain, cough, dyspnea, hoarseness, superior vena cava syndrome, and cardiac tamponade.[12] Most cases (~90%) show elevated serum tumor marker levels.[13] Raised AFP (~80%) is strongly correlated with a yolk sac tumor component, although teratomatous hepatoid cells and teratomatous neuroepithelium can also produce small amounts of AFP.[1] Increased beta-hCG (~30%) levels occur in mixed GCTs with a choriocarcinoma component or with syncytiotrophoblast cells.[14]

Gross Pathology

The tumors are often poorly circumscribed or frankly infiltrative, and show a variegated cut surface because of their different components. Cystic spaces usually indicate presence of a teratomatous component. Foci of hemorrhage and necrosis are common.

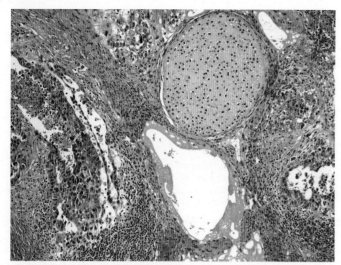

FIGURE 125.1 ▲ Mediastinal mixed GCT. Note teratoma and embryonal carcinoma components.

Microscopic Pathology

The various types of germ cell can occur in any combination, and their appearances are identical to those occurring in pure form (Fig. 125.1). The most common mixtures in adult mediastinal mixed GCTs are teratoma + seminoma, yolk sac tumor, or embryonal carcinoma, embryonal carcinoma + seminoma, yolk sac tumor + seminoma, embryonal carcinoma + seminoma, and embryonal carcinoma + choriocarcinoma.[8,15] In children, various combinations have been reported, including yolk sac tumor + embryonal carcinoma, yolk sac tumor + embryonal carcinoma + choriocarcinoma, yolk sac tumor + embryonal carcinoma + seminoma, yolk sac tumor + embryonal carcinoma + teratoma, yolk sac tumor + teratoma, and embryonal carcinoma + seminoma.[3] The diagnosis should be complemented by listing each component and its approximate proportion.

The histology of metastases usually reflects the histology of the primary GCTs or one of its components; however, other germ cell components and somatic-type malignancies may occur, particularly after chemotherapy.[16] Radiation and chemotherapy may produce the necrosis with inflammatory response, including xanthogranuloma, stromal fibrosis with cellular atypia, and cystic changes. Viable tumor may show loss of marker production (negative staining for AFP or hCG).[1]

Evaluation of Posttreatment Specimens

The treatment of mediastinal mixed GCTs is generally neoadjuvant chemotherapy followed by surgical resection. For this reason, pathologists generally receive only small biopsy samples prior to treatment, as the preoperative diagnosis is suggested by imaging and elevated serum tumor markers.

The resection specimens will often manifest treatment effect or the presence of teratomatous transformation. During or following chemotherapy, 10% to 20% of patients exhibit tumor enlargement. This phenomenon can be due to (a) chemotherapy-resistant GCT components, (b) development of somatic-type malignancies, and (c) the "growing teratoma syndrome."[16] Growing teratoma syndrome is a complication of mixed GCTs defined by (1) an increase in tumor size during or after chemotherapy, (2) normalization of serum tumor markers, and (3) identification exclusively of mature teratoma on histologic analysis of the resected tumor specimen.[16]

In the pathologic evaluation of resection specimens that are posttreatment (neoadjuvant chemotherapy), there is evidence of mature teratoma (growing teratoma syndrome) in about one-third of tumors; one-third show only necrosis; and one-third to one-half show residual

TABLE 125.1   Treatment of Mediastinal GCTs

Tumor Type	Treatment
Teratoma	Surgery
Seminoma	Chemotherapy
Mixed GCTs, embryonal carcinoma, and yolk sac tumor	Neoadjuvant chemotherapy and surgical resection
Histologic findings after neoadjuvant treatment	• 100% necrosis or scar with hemosiderin (best) • Mature teratoma (benign)(growing teratoma syndrome) • Residual mixed GCT (bad prognosis) • Residual mixed GCT with somatic malignancy (hematologic or solid type)

malignant germ cell tumor (GCT), one-half of which contain areas of somatic malignancy.[7,11] It is important for the pathologist to specify into which group the patient's tissue falls, as the prognosis is best if there is only teratoma or necrosis.[7,11] (Table 125.1).

Tumor Spread

Most mixed GCTs of the mediastinum exhibit extensive infiltration into mediastinal structures and adjacent organs. Rates of metastasis at time of diagnosis vary widely in different reports, from 20% to >80%.[3,7,12,14,15] Metastasis to lung is the most common, followed by metastasis to pleura, lymph node, liver, bone and brain being reported.[3,7,12,14,15]

Genetic Studies

In children <8 years old, i(12p) does not occur, and gain of the X chromosome and trisomy 21 are rare findings. Instead, gain of 1q, 3, and 20q and loss of 1p, 4q, and 6q are common in yolk sac tumor; teratomatous elements show no chromosomal abnormalities.

In adults and children >8 years old, the most common recurrent abnormalities of mediastinal mixed GCTs are a gain of chromosome locus12p and sex chromosomal abnormalities (often associated with Klinefelter syndrome). Additional recurrent changes include gain of chromosome 21 and loss of chromosome 13. These abnormalities are also encountered in the mature teratoma component and/or somatic-type malignant components of mixed GCTs, while pure teratomas are typically devoid of genetic imbalances.[5,17–19]

Treatment and Prognosis

In adults, about 40% of patients can envisage long-term survival with modern therapy that includes cisplatin-based chemotherapy followed by surgical resection of residual masses.[7,12] Tumor stage; metastasis to brain, liver, and bone; and elevated beta-hCG levels might be major risk factors for mixed GCTs. In children, mixed GCTs usually harbor only yolk sac tumor and teratomatous components and their prognosis is not different from the prognosis of pure yolk sac tumor, suggesting that 5-year overall survival rates of >80% can be achieved with modern therapies.[1] Among patients who show normalization of tumor markers and a residual tumor mass, completeness of resection is the most important prognostic factor in adults and children.[3,14,20] In addition, postchemotherapy histology has a bearing on prognosis: complete lack of viable tumor cells is associated with a 90% disease-free survival rate, while the rate drops to 60% if viable teratoma, including the growing teratoma syndrome, is encountered.[21] Viable nonteratomatous GCT or somatic-type malignant cells are associated with a 30% and <10% survival rate, respectively.[1]

REFERENCES

1. Moreira AL, Chan JKC, Looijenga LHJ, et al. Germ cell tumours of the mediastinum. In: Travis WD, et al., eds. *WHO Classification of Tumours of the Lung, Pleura, Thymus, and Heart*. Lyon, France: ARC Press; 2015:244–259.
2. Billmire D, Vinocur C, Rescorla F, et al. Malignant mediastinal germ cell tumors: an intergroup study. *J Pediatr Surg*. 2001;36:18–24.
3. Schneider DT, Calaminus G, Reinhard H, et al. Primary mediastinal germ cell tumors in children and adolescents: results of the German cooperative protocols MAKEI 83/86, 89, and 96. *J Clin Oncol*. 2000;18:832–839.
4. Yalcin B, Demir HA, Tanyel FC, et al. Mediastinal germ cell tumors in childhood. *Pediatr Hematol Oncol*. 2012;29:633–642.
5. Schneider DT, Schuster AE, Fritsch MK, et al. Genetic analysis of mediastinal nonseminomatous germ cell tumors in children and adolescents. *Genes Chromosomes Cancer*. 2002;34:115–125.
6. Beresford L, Fernandez CV, Cummings E, et al. Mediastinal polyembryoma associated with Klinefelter syndrome. *J Pediatr Hematol Oncol*. 2003;25:321–323.
7. Kesler KA, Rieger KM, Hammoud ZT, et al. A 25-year single institution experience with surgery for primary mediastinal nonseminomatous germ cell tumors. *Ann Thorac Surg*. 2008;85:371–378.
8. Moran CA, Suster S, Koss MN. Primary germ cell tumors of the mediastinum: III. Yolk sac tumor, embryonal carcinoma, choriocarcinoma, and combined nonteratomatous germ cell tumors of the mediastinum--a clinicopathologic and immunohistochemical study of 64 cases. *Cancer*. 1997;80:699–707.
9. Rivera C, Arame A, Jougon J, et al. Prognostic factors in patients with primary mediastinal germ cell tumors, a surgical multicenter retrospective study. *Interact Cardiovasc Thorac Surg*. 2010;11:585–589.
10. Rodney AJ, Tannir NM, Siefker-Radtke AO, et al. Survival outcomes for men with mediastinal germ-cell tumors: the University of Texas M. D. Anderson Cancer Center experience. *Urol Oncol*. 2012;30:879–885.
11. Sarkaria IS, Bains MS, Sood S, et al. Resection of primary mediastinal non-seminomatous germ cell tumors: a 28-year experience at memorial sloan-kettering cancer center. *J Thorac Oncol*. 2011;6:1236–1241.
12. Takeda S, Miyoshi S, Ohta M, et al. Primary germ cell tumors in the mediastinum: a 50-year experience at a single Japanese institution. *Cancer*. 2003;97:367–376.
13. Kiffer JD, Sandeman TF. Primary malignant mediastinal germ cell tumors: a study of eleven cases and a review of the literature. *Int J Radiat Oncol Biol Phys*. 1989;17:835–841.
14. Wood DE. Mediastinal germ cell tumors. *Semin Thorac Cardiovasc Surg*. 2000;12:278–289.
15. Moran CA, Suster S. Primary germ cell tumors of the mediastinum: I. Analysis of 322 cases with special emphasis on teratomatous lesions and a proposal for histopathologic classification and clinical staging. *Cancer*. 1997;80:681–690.
16. Andre F, Fizazi K, Culine S, et al. The growing teratoma syndrome: results of therapy and long-term follow-up of 33 patients. *Eur J Cancer*. 2000;36:1389–1394.
17. Sung MT, Maclennan GT, Lopez-Beltran A, et al. Primary mediastinal seminoma: a comprehensive assessment integrated with histology, immunohistochemistry, and fluorescence in situ hybridization for chromosome 12p abnormalities in 23 cases. *Am J Surg Pathol*. 2008;32:146–155.
18. Harms D, Zahn S, Gobel U, et al. Pathology and molecular biology of teratomas in childhood and adolescence. *Klin Padiatr*. 2006;218:296–302.
19. Dominguez Malagon H, Perez Montiel D. Mediastinal germ cell tumors. *Semin Diagn Pathol*. 2005;22:230–240.
20. Bokemeyer C, Nichols CR, Droz JP, et al. Extragonadal germ cell tumors of the mediastinum and retroperitoneum: results from an international analysis. *J Clin Oncol*. 2002;20:1864–1873.
21. Reuter VE. The pre and post chemotherapy pathologic spectrum of germ cell tumors. *Chest Surg Clin N Am*. 2002;12:673–694.

126 Mediastinal Germ Cell Tumor with Somatic-Type and Hematologic Malignancy

Borislav A. Alexiev, M.D., and Allen P. Burke, M.D.

Terminology

Germ cell tumor with somatic-type malignancy (GCT-STM) denotes a GCT containing a malignant somatic component of a type typically encountered in other organs or tissues, for example, carcinoma, sarcoma, and lymphoma/leukemia. A minimum size of one low-power field has been suggested as the threshold for the diagnosis of STM in GCTs. However, this size criterion is arbitrary. More important is the independent growth pattern demonstrated by the somatic-type malignancy.[1]

A unique type of somatic malignancy associated with mediastinal GCTs is that of hematologic malignancy, which, although not always within the mediastinal mass itself, is considered a manifestation of the GCT (Table 126.1).

Pathogenesis

The pathogenesis of GCT-STM is unknown. Divergent differentiation of a pluri- or totipotent primordial germ cell toward a GCT and the somatic-type malignancy has been suggested. This hypothesis is favored by the finding that "pure" mature mediastinal teratomas show no chromosome 12 abnormalities while a shared isochromosome 12p abnormality is characteristic of teratomas with somatic-type malignancies, including leukemias.[2]

Incidence and Clinical

GCT-STM has been classified into two clinical and pathologic types: GCT-STM induced by chemotherapy or irradiation[3-6] and naturally occurring GCT-STM.[7,8] The former type tends to occur in young patients (between 20 and 40 years of age) with an initial presentation of a mixed GCT.[8-11] Naturally occurring teratoma–somatic-type malignancy is more frequently seen in older patients, with a peak incidence in the fifth and sixth decades of life.[9]

GCT-STM account for up to 29% of all mediastinal GCTs of adults but are almost nonexistent in children.[2,6,8,11-20] The tumors occur predominantly in males.[10] The somatic-type malignancy may arise in the primary mediastinal tumor or only in the metastases.[1] The tumors show the same local symptoms as do other mediastinal GCTs, but they are more frequently symptomatic (~90%) than pure GCTs.[1] Tumor markers (α-fetoprotein, β-human chorionic gonadotropin, carcinoembryonic antigen) may be elevated according to the malignant components that are present.

Gross Pathology

GCT-STM usually exhibits a partially cystic and often variegated cut surface with focally necrotic areas. The carcinoma or sarcoma areas are firm and gray or hemorrhagic and often adherent to adjacent mediastinal structures.

TABLE 126.1 Characteristics of Somatic and Hematologic Malignancies Associated with Mediastinal GCTs

Primary Tumor	Somatic Malignancies	Hematologic Malignancies
Immature and mature teratoma, often mixed with yolk sac tumor and embryonal carcinoma	Rhabdomyosarcoma	Megakaryocytic leukemia
Pure seminoma (rare)	Angiosarcoma	Malignant histiocytosis
Embryonal carcinoma with or without yolk sac tumor (rare)	Leiomyosarcoma	Granulocytic sarcoma
	Undifferentiated sarcoma	
	Myxoid liposarcoma	
	Malignant peripheral nerve sheath tumor	
	Malignant "triton" tumor	
	Epithelioid hemangioendothelioma	
	Primitive neuroectodermal tumor	
	Nephroblastoma	
	Adenocarcinoma	
	Squamous cell carcinoma	
	High-grade neuroendocrine carcinoma	
	Melanoma	
	Pancreatic neuroendocrine tumor	
	Liposarcoma	
	Osteosarcoma	
	Glioma	
	Glioblastoma	

Microscopic Pathology

In the largest pathologic series of mediastinal GCT-STM (23 patients), there were 15 mature teratomas, 3 immature teratomas (with or without mature areas), 2 mature teratomas with other components (one seminoma and one choriocarcinoma), 1 immature teratoma with seminoma, and 1 each of pure yolk sac tumor and seminoma.[7] Associated somatic malignancies were, in this series, all sarcomas (13 rhabdomyosarcomas, 1 with glioblastoma; 4 angiosarcomas; 2 leiomyosarcomas; and 1 each of epithelioid hemangioendothelioma, undifferentiated

sarcoma, malignant peripheral nerve sheath tumor, and malignant "triton" tumor).[7]

A variety of other somatic malignancies, including carcinomas, have been reported in mediastinal GCTs, often as case reports[6,8,9,21-24] (see Table 126.1).

Embryonal rhabdomyosarcoma is the single most frequent somatic-type malignancy[11] (Figs. 126.1 and 126.2). The somatic malignancy can be intimately intermingled with the GCT component or forms an expansile nodular proliferation of atypical cells, often with increased mitotic rate and necrosis.[1] Neuroblastoma, which is relatively common as somatic malignancy in testicular GCTs, is rare in mediastinal GCTs.

Hematologic Malignancies in GCTs of the Mediastinum

Mediastinal GCTs are unique for two reasons: their frequent refractoriness to current treatment modality gives them the worst prognosis among GCTs of all sites, and they tend to give rise to secondary hematologic neoplasia. The hematologic malignancies are unusual and often morphologically resemble acute megakaryoblastic leukemia or malignant histiocytosis. The hematologic neoplasia is typically diagnosed on bone marrow biopsy but may occur within the GCT itself as granulocytic sarcoma.[21] The GCT is nonseminomatous and frequently shows immature teratoma and yolk sac tumor. The hematologic malignancy generally occurs at the time of or soon after the diagnosis of mediastinal GCT, indicating that it is not secondary to chemotherapy. Furthermore, the cytogenic marker i(12p), which is an isochromosome of the short arm of chromosome 12, typical of GCTs, has been identified in the leukemic infiltrates. The outcome is grave for patients with GCT-associated hematologic malignancies.[25-30]

Differential Diagnosis

Immature teratoma may be difficult to distinguish from teratoma with somatic-type malignancy. Frank atypia and infiltrative growth favor the latter interpretation. Likewise, chemotherapy-induced atypia is usually diffusely distributed throughout the tumor, while somatic-type malignancy is a focal process often forming a recognizable mass and invading adjacent structures.

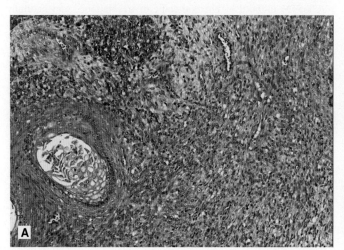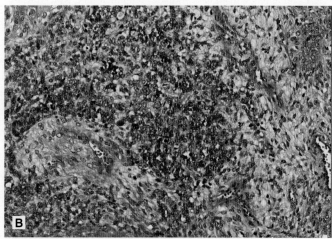

FIGURE 126.1 ▲ Mixed GCT with rhabdomyosarcoma. **A.** There is mature and immature teratoma with cellular stroma. **B.** A higher magnification of stroma shows increased cellularity with undifferentiated-appearing small round blue cells.

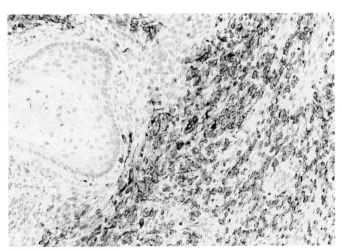

FIGURE 126.2 ▲ Mixed GCT with rhabdomyosarcoma. An immunohistochemical stain for desmin demonstrates myogenic differentiation.

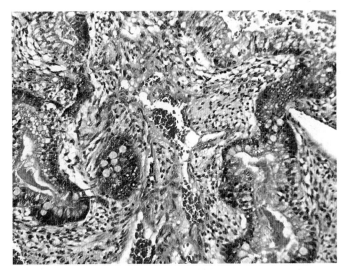

FIGURE 126.4 ▲ Mixed GCT with angiosarcoma. In this field there is teratoma with an atypical vascular proliferation. This photomicrograph is of the same tumor shown in Figure 126.3.

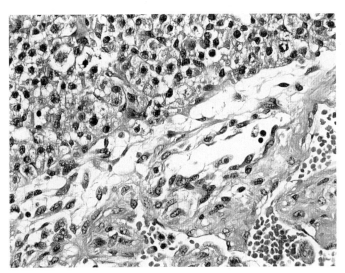

FIGURE 126.3 ▲ Mixed GCT with angiosarcoma. Above, there is seminoma, and below atypical vascular proliferation. The patient was a 12-year-old girl with anterior mediastinal mass.

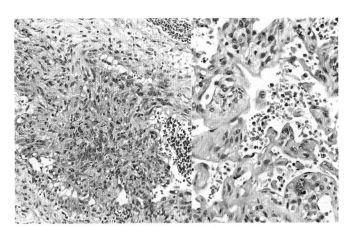

FIGURE 126.5 ▲ Mixed GCT with angiosarcoma. This photomicrograph is of the same tumor shown in the Figures 126.3 and 126.4.

Immature neural elements may be selected by chemotherapy and may resemble neuroblastoma, but a low mitotic and proliferative rate favors a GCT element over somatic-type malignancy[31] (Figs. 126.3 to 126.5).

Glandular yolk sac tumor may be difficult to distinguish from adenocarcinoma, which is less more likely to be glypican negative and EMA and cytokeratin-7 positive.[32] The spindled areas of yolk sac tumor can mimic sarcoma but tend to be SALL4 positive.[32]

Rhabdomyoblasts can rarely occur in thymic carcinomas. However, thymic carcinomas are morphologically different from GCTs and commonly express CD5, while the rhabdomyoblasts are devoid of atypia and proliferative activity.[1]

Treatment and Prognosis

The GCT-STM has been reported to be generally advanced at diagnosis, highly metastatic, resistant to standard chemotherapy, and associated with poorer prognosis than GCT without somatic-type malignancy.[6,17,18] In one series, nearly 90% of patients were dead of disease within 3 years.[7] Angiosarcoma in mediastinal GCTs is especially aggressive.[33] Metastatic sites include liver, bone, retroperitoneum, heart, lung, and lymph nodes.[3,6,7]

Results of the recently developed protocol using intensive therapy with cisplatin-containing agents and surgery are promising.[6]

REFERENCES

1. Moreira AL, Chan JKC, Looijenga LHJ, et al. Germ cell tumours of the mediastinum. In: Travis WD, et al., eds. *WHO Classification of Tumours of the Lung, Pleura, Thymus, and Heart.* Lyon, France: IARC Press; 2015:244–259.
2. Schneider DT, Schuster AE, Fritsch MK, et al. Genetic analysis of mediastinal nonseminomatous germ cell tumors in children and adolescents. *Genes Chromosomes Cancer.* 2002;34:115–125.
3. Aliotta PJ, Castillo J, Englander LS, et al. Primary mediastinal germ cell tumors. Histologic patterns of treatment failures at autopsy. *Cancer.* 1988;62: 982–984.
4. Kesler KA, Rieger KM, Hammoud ZT, et al. A 25-year single institution experience with surgery for primary mediastinal nonseminomatous germ cell tumors. *Ann Thorac Surg.* 2008;85:371–378.
5. Sarkaria IS, Bains MS, Sood S, et al. Resection of primary mediastinal non-seminomatous germ cell tumors: a 28-year experience at memorial sloan-kettering cancer center. *J Thorac Oncol.* 2011;6:1236–1241.
6. Asakura K, Izumi Y, Ikeda T, et al. Mediastinal germ cell tumor with somatic-type malignancy: report of 5 stage I/II cases. *Ann Thorac Surg.* 2010;90:1014–1016.

7. Dominguez-Malagon H, Perez Montiel D. Mediastinal germ cell tumors. *Semin Diagn Pathol.* 2005;22:230–240.

8. Moran CA, Suster S. Primary germ cell tumors of the mediastinum: I. Analysis of 322 cases with special emphasis on teratomatous lesions and a proposal for histopathologic classification and clinical staging. *Cancer.* 1997;80:681–690.

9. Kim JY, Lee CH, Park WY, et al. Adenocarcinoma with sarcomatous dedifferentiation arising from mature cystic teratoma of the anterior mediastinum. *Pathol Res Pract.* 2012;208:741–745.

10. Knapp RH, Hurt RD, Payne WS, et al. Malignant germ cell tumors of the mediastinum. *J Thorac Cardiovasc Surg.* 1985;89:82–89.

11. Manivel C, Wick MR, Abenoza P, et al. The occurrence of sarcomatous components in primary mediastinal germ cell tumors. *Am J Surg Pathol.* 1986;10:711–717.

12. Caballero C, Gomez S, Matias-Guiu X, et al. Rhabdomyosarcomas developing in association with mediastinal germ cell tumours. *Virchows Arch A Pathol Anat Histopathol.* 1992;420:539–543.

13. Kolodziejski L, Duda K, Niezabitowski A, et al. Occurrence of malignant non-germ cell components in primary mediastinal germ cell tumours. *Eur J Surg Oncol.* 1999;25:54–60.

14. Malagon HD, Valdez AM, Moran CA, et al. Germ cell tumors with sarcomatous components: a clinicopathologic and immunohistochemical study of 46 cases. *Am J Surg Pathol.* 2007;31:1356–1362.

15. Ulbright TM, Loehrer PJ, Roth LM, et al. The development of non-germ cell malignancies within germ cell tumors. A clinicopathologic study of 11 cases. *Cancer.* 1984;54:1824–1833.

16. Donadio AC, Motzer RJ, Bajorin DF, et al. Chemotherapy for teratoma with malignant transformation. *J Clin Oncol.* 2003;21:4285–4291.

17. Gonzalez-Vela JL, Savage PD, Manivel JC, et al. Poor prognosis of mediastinal germ cell cancers containing sarcomatous components. *Cancer.* 1990;66:1114–1116.

18. Wright CD, Kesler KA, Nichols CR, et al. Primary mediastinal nonseminomatous germ cell tumors. Results of a multimodality approach. *J Thorac Cardiovasc Surg.* 1990;99:210–217.

19. Bokemeyer C, Nichols CR, Droz JP, et al. Extragonadal germ cell tumors of the mediastinum and retroperitoneum: results from an international analysis. *J Clin Oncol.* 2002;20:1864–1873.

20. Takeda S, Miyoshi S, Ohta M, et al. Primary germ cell tumors in the mediastinum: a 50-year experience at a single Japanese institution. *Cancer.* 2003;97:367–376.

21. Saito A, Watanabe K, Kusakabe T, et al. Mediastinal mature teratoma with coexistence of angiosarcoma, granulocytic sarcoma and a hematopoietic region in the tumor: a rare case of association between hematological malignancy and mediastinal germ cell tumor. *Pathol Int.* 1998;48:749–753.

22. Schaefer IM, Zardo P, Freermann S, et al. Neuroendocrine carcinoma in a mediastinal teratoma as a rare variant of somatic-type malignancy. *Virchows Arch.* 2013;463:731–735.

23. Takanashi Y, Tajima S, Takahashi T, et al. Mediastinal mature teratoma with complete gastrointestinal and bronchial walls. *Respirol Case Rep.* 2015;3:89–91.

24. Chang YL, Wu CT, Lee YC. Mediastinal and retroperitoneal teratoma with focal gastrointestinal adenocarcinoma. *J Thorac Oncol.* 2006;1:729–731.

25. Hirai Y, Yoshimasu T, Oura S, et al. Mediastinal germ cell tumor with acute myeloid leukemia and growing teratoma syndrome. *Interact Cardiovasc Thorac Surg.* 2011;12:96–97.

26. Ikdahl T, Josefsen D, Jakobsen E, et al. Concurrent mediastinal germ-cell tumour and haematological malignancy: case report and short review of literature. *Acta Oncol.* 2008;47:466–469.

27. Nichols CR, Hoffman R, Einhorn LH, et al. Hematologic malignancies associated with primary mediastinal germ-cell tumors. *Ann Intern Med.* 1985;102:603–609.

28. Nichols CR, Roth BJ, Heerema N, et al. Hematologic neoplasia associated with primary mediastinal germ-cell tumors. *N Engl J Med.* 1990;322:1425–1429.

29. Nichols CR, Saxman S, Williams SD, et al. Primary mediastinal nonseminomatous germ cell tumors. A modern single institution experience. *Cancer.* 1990;65:1641–1646.

30. Zhao GQ, Dowell JE. Hematologic malignancies associated with germ cell tumors. *Expert Rev Hematol.* 2012;5:427–437.

31. Pelosi G, Sonzogni A, Solli P, et al. Differentiating neuroblastoma arising in mediastinal germ cell tumour. *Histopathology.* 2008;53:350–352.

32. Magers MJ, Kao CS, Cole CD, et al. "Somatic-type" malignancies arising from testicular germ cell tumors: a clinicopathologic study of 124 cases with emphasis on glandular tumors supporting frequent yolk sac tumor origin. *Am J Surg Pathol.* 2014;38:1396–1409.

33. Contreras AL, Punar M, Tamboli P, et al. Mediastinal germ cell tumors with an angiosarcomatous component: a report of 12 cases. *Hum Pathol.* 2010;41:832–837.

127 Primary Mediastinal Large B-Cell Lymphoma

Borislav A. Alexiev, M.D., and Rima Koka, M.D., Ph.D.

Terminology

Primary lymphomas of the mediastinum are believed to arise from mediastinal lymph nodes or, when in the anterior mediastinum, the thymus gland (Table 127.1). Primary mediastinal large B-cell lymphoma (PMLBL) is a subtype of diffuse large B-cell lymphoma arising in the mediastinum of putative thymic medullary B-cell origin with distinctive clinical, immunophenotypic, genotypic, and molecular features.[1]

Incidence and Clinical

PMLBL accounts for ~2% to 5% of patients with non-Hodgkin lymphoma.[2,3] The tumor typically affects young women, presenting in their third to fourth decade of life with rapidly growing mediastinal masses, often with respiratory symptoms and evidence of intrathoracic extension on imaging.[1,2,4,5] Up to 50% can have signs and symptoms of superior vena cava syndrome at presentation, with facial edema, neck vein distention, and, occasionally, upper extremity swelling and/or deep vein thrombosis.

Despite local invasiveness, distant spread, including bone marrow infiltration, is infrequent at initial presentation. At relapse, however, unusual extranodal sites, such as the liver, kidneys, and central nervous system, are not uncommon.[1,2,4,5]

Staging is performed according to the Ann Arbor scheme for lymphoma. Staging is established using both standard radiologic procedures and positron emission tomography (PET), which is helpful in assessing response to treatment.

Gross Pathology

PMLBL presents as a solid mass lesion, tan to light brown, sometimes with necrosis and hemorrhage.

Microscopic Pathology

PMLBL shows a wide morphologic spectrum from case to case.[1,2,4,5] The growth pattern is diffuse and the large cells usually form clusters or sheets (Fig. 127.1).[1,2,4,5] A frequent but not consistent feature is a distinctive fibrosis made up of irregular collagen bands compartmentalizing cellular areas of varying size.[1,2,4,5] The cells range from medium-sized to large (2 to 5 times the size of a small lymphocyte) and have abundant, frequently clear cytoplasm and irregularly round or ovoid nuclei, usually with small nucleoli. Some cases may contain cells with

TABLE 127.1 Mediastinal and Thymic Lymphomas

	Overall Proportion of Lymphomas (Any Site)	Mediastinal Involvement	Demographic Characteristics	Distinguishing Characteristics
Primary mediastinal B-cell lymphoma (PMBL)	2%–5%	100%, often with infiltration of surrounding structures	Young women predominantly	Frequent SVC syndrome; delicate "alveolar-like" sclerosis; high cure rate with current chemotherapy
Extranodal marginal zone lymphoma (mucosa associated)	7%–8% of B-cell lymphomas (all extranodal MZL)	<1%	Associated with autoimmune disorders, especially SS	Lymphoepithelial lesions
Precursor T-cell lymphoblastic lymphoma/leukemia (ALL)	15% childhood ALL; 25% of adulthood ALL	Frequent, usually with leukemic involvement	Late childhood to yearly adulthood	Pleural and pericardial effusions common; overlapping nuclei with dispersed chromatin and scant cytoplasm
Hodgkin lymphoma (classical; CHL)	30%	60% (usually with cervical lymph node involvement) (thymic or mediastinal lymph nodes)	Adolescents and young adults; no gender predilection	Contiguous spread typical; necrosis, fibrosis, and granulomatous reaction may obscure diagnosis in small specimens
Gray zone lymphoma	Uncommon, incidence unknown	Nearly 100%	Male predominance; adolescents and young adults	Histologic and immunohistochemical features intermediate between PMBL and CHL
Anaplastic large cell lymphoma	3% (adult) 15%–20% (children)	Common, usually with advanced disease, rare as primary site	Children (typically ALK positive) and adults	"Hallmark" cells with kidney-bean–shaped nuclei, may mimic carcinoma or melanoma
Follicular dendritic cell sarcoma	Rare	12%	Adults, mean age 50	Spindled appearance mimics myofibroblastic tumor; may occur with Castleman disease

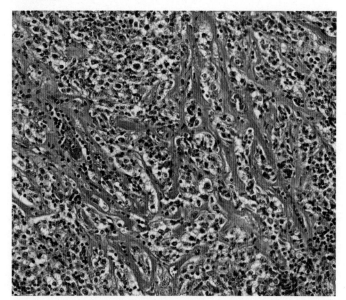

FIGURE 127.1 ▲ Primary mediastinal large B-cell lymphoma. Note diffuse growth pattern and fibrosis.

pleomorphic and/or multilobated nuclei and abundant amphophilic cytoplasm, which may resemble Reed-Sternberg cells and raise suspicion of Hodgkin lymphoma or nonlymphoid tumor. At the periphery of the mass, a variable number of reactive cells such as lymphocytes, macrophages, and granulocytes may be present. In case of regional lymph node involvement, the invasion pattern is carcinoma-like, starting from marginal sinuses, continuously infiltrating and replacing the normal lymphoid tissue.

Special Studies

PMLBL expresses B-cell lineage antigens such as CD19, CD20, CD22, and CD79a but characteristically lacks immunoglobulin expression.[1,2,4,5] There is functional immunoglobulin gene rearrangement and expression of the transcription factors PAX5, BOB.1, OCT-2, and PU.1.[6]

CD30 is present in more than 80% of cases (Fig. 127.2) but, in contrast to classical Hodgkin lymphoma, is usually weak and heterogeneous and often without membranous staining.[7] CD15 is occasionally present. Tumor cells are frequently positive for IRF4/MUM1 (75%)

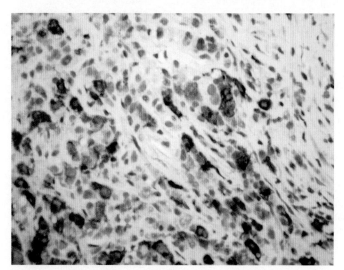

FIGURE 127.2 ▲ Primary mediastinal large B-cell lymphoma. Note positive staining for CD30.

and CD23 (70%) and have variable expression of BCL2 and BCL6.[8,9] CD10 expression is uncommon.[9] Expression of TNFAIP2 was recently identified to be aberrantly expressed in PMLBL as a feature in common with classical Hodgkin lymphoma but rarely found in diffuse large B-cell lymphoma.[10]

Recent microarray studies revealed a unique molecular signature of PMLBL, distinguishing it from diffuse large B-cell lymphoma, with striking overlap with the nodular sclerosis subtype of classical Hodgkin lymphoma.[4,11] The genomic profile typically contains gains including amplified regions in chromosome 9p24.1 including the JAK2/PDL2 locus (up to 75%) and 2p16.1 including the REL/BCL11A locus (51%), but also in chromosomes Xp11.4-21 (33%) and Xq24-26 (33%).[4,11,12]

Differential Diagnosis

The diagnosis of PMLBL requires a combination of pathologic and clinical information. Diffuse large B-cell lymphoma involving the mediastinum often shows involvement of mediastinal lymph nodes rather than the thymic area and more abundant extramediastinal involvement than PMLBL. Classical Hodgkin lymphoma can be ruled out by detection of surface B-cell antigens like CD79a and CD20 as well as CD45 in PMBL. However, lymphomas sharing histopathologic features of classical Hodgkin lymphoma and PMLBL have been described and are categorized as B-cell lymphoma, unclassifiable, with features intermediate between diffuse large B-cell lymphoma and classical Hodgkin lymphoma (sometimes referred to as "mediastinal gray zone lymphoma").[13,14]

Treatment and Prognosis

Gene expression profiling identified PMLBL as a subgroup of diffuse large B-cell lymphoma with a relatively favorable survival rate after therapy: the 5-year survival rate of PMLBL was 64% compared with 59% and 30% for the germinal center B-cell–like diffuse large B-cell lymphoma and activated B-cell–like diffuse large B-cell lymphoma subgroups, respectively.[15] Extension into adjacent thoracic viscera, pleura, or pericardial effusion and poor performance status are associated with inferior outcome.[15]

The optimal therapy for PMLBL remains undefined. The superiority of intensive chemotherapy regimens (methotrexate, doxorubicin, cyclophosphamide, vincristine, prednisone, bleomycin [MACOP-B]/etoposide, doxorubicin, cyclophosphamide, vincristine, prednisone, bleomycin [VACOP-B]) over cyclophosphamide, doxorubicin, vincristine, prednisone (CHOP)-like chemotherapy is upheld by some authors.[15]

REFERENCES

1. Gaulard P, Harris NL, Pileri SA, et al. Primary mediastinal B-cell lymphoma. In: Swerdlow SH, et al., eds. *WHO Classification of Tumours of Haematopoietic and Lymphoid Tissue.* Lyon, France: IARC Press; 2008.
2. Boleti E, Johnson PW. Primary mediastinal B-cell lymphoma. *Hematol Oncol.* 2007;25:157–163.
3. Gerrard M, Waxman IM, Sposto R, et al. Outcome and pathologic classification of children and adolescents with mediastinal large B-cell lymphoma treated with FAB/LMB96 mature B-NHL therapy. *Blood.* 2013;121:278–285.
4. Savage KJ, Monti S, Kutok JL, et al. The molecular signature of mediastinal large B-cell lymphoma differs from that of other diffuse large B-cell lymphomas and shares features with classical Hodgkin lymphoma. *Blood.* 2003;102:3871–3879.
5. Travis W, Brambilla E, Burke AP, et al. *WHO Classification of Tumours of the Lung, Pleura, Mediastinum, and Heart.* 5th ed. Lyon, France: IARC Press; 2015.
6. Pileri SA, Gaidano G, Zinzani PL, et al. Primary mediastinal B-cell lymphoma: high frequency of BCL-6 mutations and consistent expression of the transcription factors OCT-2, BOB.1, and PU.1 in the absence of immunoglobulins. *Am J Pathol.* 2003;162:243–253.

7. Higgins JP, Warnke RA. CD30 expression is common in mediastinal large B-cell lymphoma. *Am J Clin Pathol.* 1999;112:241–247.

8. Calaminici M, Piper K, Lee AM, et al. CD23 expression in mediastinal large B-cell lymphomas. *Histopathology.* 2004;45:619–624.

9. de Leval L, Ferry JA, Falini B, et al. Expression of bcl-6 and CD10 in primary mediastinal large B-cell lymphoma: evidence for derivation from germinal center B cells? *Am J Surg Pathol.* 2001;25:1277–1282.

10. Kondratiev S, Duraisamy S, Unitt CL, et al. Aberrant expression of the dendritic cell marker TNFAIP2 by the malignant cells of Hodgkin lymphoma and primary mediastinal large B-cell lymphoma distinguishes these tumor types from morphologically and phenotypically similar lymphomas. *Am J Surg Pathol.* 2011;35:1531–1539.

11. Feuerhake F, Kutok JL, Monti S, et al. NFkappaB activity, function, and target-gene signatures in primary mediastinal large B-cell lymphoma and diffuse large B-cell lymphoma subtypes. *Blood.* 2005;106:1392–1399.

12. Calvo KR, Traverse-Glehen A, Pittaluga S, et al. Molecular profiling provides evidence of primary mediastinal large B-cell lymphoma as a distinct entity related to classic Hodgkin lymphoma: implications for mediastinal gray zone lymphomas as an intermediate form of B-cell lymphoma. *Adv Anat Pathol.* 2004;11:227–238.

13. Eberle FC, Salaverria I, Steidl C, et al. Gray zone lymphoma: chromosomal aberrations with immunophenotypic and clinical correlations. *Mod Pathol.* 2011;24:1586–1597.

14. Traverse-Glehen A, Pittaluga S, Gaulard P, et al. Mediastinal gray zone lymphoma: the missing link between classic Hodgkin's lymphoma and mediastinal large B-cell lymphoma. *Am J Surg Pathol.* 2005;29:1411–1421.

15. Mazzarotto R, Boso C, Vianello F, et al. Primary mediastinal large B-cell lymphoma: results of intensive chemotherapy regimens (MACOP-B/VACOP-B) plus involved field radiotherapy on 53 patients. A single institution experience. *Int J Radiat Oncol Biol Phys.* 2007;68:823–829.

128 Thymic Extranodal Marginal Zone B-Cell Lymphoma of Mucosa-Associated Lymphoid Tissue

Borislav A. Alexiev, M.D., and Rima Koka, M.D., Ph.D.

Terminology

Primary thymic extranodal marginal zone B-cell lymphoma (MZBL) of mucosa-associated lymphoid tissue (MALT) is a lymphoma consisting predominantly of small B cells with a centrocyte-like or monocytoid appearance, which surround reactive follicles and infiltrate the thymic epithelium to produce lymphoepithelial lesions. This lymphoma is derived from post–germinal center marginal zone B cells.[1]

Incidence and Clinical

Extranodal MZBL of MALT arising in the thymus is a rare disorder with an apparent predilection for Asians and a strong association with autoimmune diseases, among which the strongest link appears to be with Sjögren syndrome. Most patients are in the fifth and sixth decades. There is female predominance (M:F = 1:4). The prevalence of autoimmunity is much lower in males with thymic MALT lymphoma compared to females (33% vs. 87%).[2] It is characterized by the frequent presence of thymic cysts, consistent plasma cell differentiation, tumor cells expressing IgA, and a lack of API2-MALT1 gene fusion.[2–13] There is no association with Epstein-Barr virus.[4] The bulk of the disease is in the anterior mediastinum, but the regional lymph nodes and other extranodal sites (e.g., stomach, salivary gland, lung) may be involved concurrently.

Gross Pathology

Grossly, the tumor is often encapsulated and comprises solid grayish-white fleshy tissue commonly interspersed with multiple variable-sized cysts. Invasion into the adjacent pericardium and pleura is sometimes found.

Microscopic Pathology

Histologically, the lymphoid infiltrates consist of monotonous centrocyte-like cells with interspersed aggregates of monocytoid cells, small lymphocytes, and plasma cells. They show extensive invasion of the Hassall corpuscles or the thymic epithelium-lined cystic spaces, forming lymphoepithelial lesions (Fig. 128.1).[5,7,13,14] Scattered centroblast-like cells or immunoblasts are frequently found. Transformation to diffuse large B-cell lymphoma has only been rarely reported.[1]

Special Studies

Immunohistochemically, the tumor cells express B-cell–specific markers (CD20 and CD79a) and BCL2. They are negative for CD3, CD5, CD10, CD23, CD43, and cyclin D1.[1,2,5] More than 75% of the cases express IgA.[4]

Immunoglobulin genes are clonally rearranged.[1] Although API2-MALT1 fusion resulting from t(11;18) is present in up to 50% of extranodal MZBLs in general, this chromosomal translocation is not detected in thymic extranodal MZBLs.[2,4,7,9,12] Trisomy 3 and an A20 deletion might play a role in the pathogenesis of thymic MALT lymphoma.[2]

Differential Diagnosis

The main differential diagnosis is reactive lymphoid hyperplasia of the thymus. In reactive lymphoid hyperplasia, which is most frequently associated with myasthenia gravis, the thymic lobular architecture

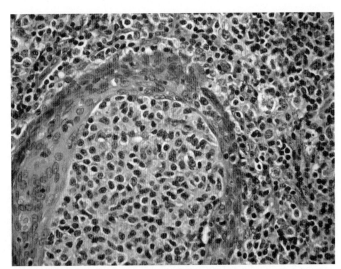

FIGURE 128.1 ▲ Thymic extranodal marginal zone B-cell lymphoma of mucosa-associated lymphoid tissue. Note small lymphocytes with a centrocyte-like or monocytoid appearance and lymphoepithelial lesion (H&E, ×400).

is preserved, and there is no band-like or sheet-like proliferation of centrocyte-like cells and monocytoid cells.[10] Appropriate sampling, cytokeratin staining, and molecular analyses may help to identify early MALT-type lymphoma developing in the setting of thymic lymphofollicular hyperplasia.[10]

Treatment and Prognosis

Thymic extranodal MZBL is associated with an excellent outcome. High tumor stage at presentation or concurrent involvement of other MALT sites is not necessarily associated with a poor prognosis. Surgical excision and chemoradiotherapy are usually effective, and when completely resected, long-term survival can be achieved. According to Inagaki et al., the overall survival rates at 3 years and 5 years were 89% and 83%, respectively.[4]

REFERENCES

1. Isaacson PG, Chott A, Nakamura S, et al. Extranodal marginal zone lymphoma of mucosa-associated lymphoid tissue (MALT lymphoma). In: Swerdlow SH, et al., eds. *WHO Classification of Tumours of Haematopoietic and Lymphoid Tissues.* Lyon, France: IARC Press; 2008.
2. Go H, Cho HJ, Paik JH, et al. Thymic extranodal marginal zone B-cell lymphoma of mucosa-associated lymphoid tissue: a clinicopathological and genetic analysis of six cases. *Leuk Lymphoma.* 2011;52:2276–2283.
3. Braham E, Capron J, Sene D, et al. Thymic marginal zone B-cell lymphoma of mucosa-associated lymphoid tissue-type in a patient with Sjogren's syndrome and cryoglobulinaemia. *Pathology.* 2009;41:701–703.
4. Inagaki H, Chan JK, Ng JW, et al. Primary thymic extranodal marginal-zone B-cell lymphoma of mucosa-associated lymphoid tissue type exhibits distinctive clinicopathological and molecular features. *Am J Pathol.* 2002;160:1435–1443.
5. Kim JM. Primary extranodal marginal zone B-cell lymphoma of mucosa-associated lymphoid tissue-type in the thymus of a patient with Sjogren's syndrome and rheumatoid arthritis. *J Korean Med Sci.* 2003; 18:897–900.
6. Kinoshita N, Ashizawa K, Abe K, et al. Mucosa-associated lymphoid tissue lymphoma of the thymus associated with Sjogren's syndrome: report of a case. *Surg Today.* 2008;38:436–439.
7. Kominato S, Nakayama T, Sato F, et al. Characterization of chromosomal aberrations in thymic MALT lymphoma. *Pathol Int.* 2012;62:93–98.
8. Kurabayashi A, Iguchi M, Matsumoto M, et al. Thymic mucosa-associated lymphoid tissue lymphoma with immunoglobulin-storing histiocytosis in Sjogren's syndrome. *Pathol Int.* 2010;60:125–130.
9. Ortonne N, Copie-Bergman C, Remy P, et al. Mucosa-associated lymphoid tissue lymphoma of the thymus: a case report with no evidence of MALT1 rearrangement. *Virchows Arch.* 2005;446:189–193.
10. Parrens M, Dubus P, Danjoux M, et al. Mucosa-associated lymphoid tissue of the thymus hyperplasia vs lymphoma. *Am J Clin Pathol.* 2002;117: 51–56.
11. Sakamoto T, Yamashita K, Mizumoto C, et al. MALT lymphoma of the thymus with Sjogren's syndrome: biphasic changes in serological abnormalities over a 4-year period following thymectomy. *Int J Hematol.* 2009;89: 709–713.
12. Sunohara M, Hara K, Osamura K, et al. Mucosa associated lymphoid tissue (MALT) lymphoma of the thymus with trisomy 18. *Intern Med.* 2009;48:2025–2032.
13. Yamasaki S, Matsushita H, Tanimura S, et al. B-cell lymphoma of mucosa-associated lymphoid tissue of the thymus: a report of two cases with a background of Sjogren's syndrome and monoclonal gammopathy. *Hum Pathol.* 1998;29:1021–1024.
14. Maeda A, Hayama M, Nakata M, et al. Mucosa-associated lymphoid tissue lymphoma in the thymus of a patient with systemic lupus erythematosus. *Gen Thorac Cardiovasc Surg.* 2008;56:288–291.

129 Precursor T-Cell Lymphoblastic Lymphoma/Leukemia

Borislav A. Alexiev, M.D., and Rima Koka, M.D., Ph.D.

Terminology

Precursor T-lymphoblastic lymphoma/leukemia is a neoplasm of lymphoblasts committed to the T-cell lineage, typically composed of small to medium-sized blasts with scant cytoplasm, moderately condensed to dispersed chromatin and indistinct nucleoli, variably involving bone marrow and blood (T-cell acute lymphoblastic leukemia), thymus, and/or lymph nodes (T-cell lymphoblastic lymphoma).[1]

Incidence and Clinical

Clinically, a case is defined as lymphoma if there is a mediastinal or other mass and <25% blasts in the bone marrow and as leukemia if there are >25% bone marrow blasts, with or without a mass.[1] However, the threshold of 25% blasts in the bone marrow is not firmly defined by the World Health Organization (WHO).[1]

Patients with ataxia telangiectasia are at increased risk for development of precursor T-cell lymphoblastic lymphoma, but the ATM gene has not been implicated in sporadic T-cell precursor neoplasia.[1]

Precursor T-cell lymphoblastic lymphoma is rare, accounting for 1% to 2% of all non-Hodgkin lymphomas.[1] The neoplasm occurs most frequently in late childhood, adolescence, and young adulthood, with a male predominance.[1] Patients usually present with a bulky anterior

mediastinal mass, associated with pleural or pericardial effusions, superior vena cava syndrome, and tracheal obstruction. The tumor typically involves the thymus and often mediastinal, cervical, supraclavicular, or axillary lymph nodes. The bone marrow and peripheral blood are involved in the majority of the cases.[1] Central nervous system (CNS) involvement is also common, but abdominal involvement (liver and spleen) is unusual.[1–3]

Gross Pathology

Grossly, the tumor often presents as a solid mass lesion with grayish-white fleshy cut surface involving the thymus or mediastinal lymph nodes. Invasion into the adjacent pericardium and pleura is sometimes found.

Microscopic Pathology

The thymus and mediastinal soft tissue as well as adjacent lymph nodes are typically involved. The neoplastic cells are of medium size with a high nuclear/cytoplasmic ratio (Fig. 129.1). There may be a considerable size range from small lymphoblasts with condensed chromatin and no evident nucleoli to larger blasts with finely dispersed chromatin and relatively prominent nucleoli. Nuclear contours range from round to

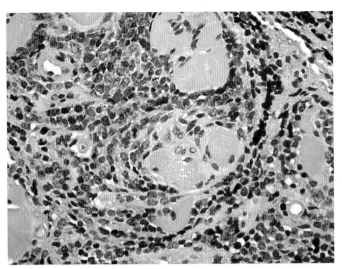

FIGURE 129.1 ▲ Mediastinal precursor T-cell lymphoblastic lymphoma. The neoplastic cells are of medium size with a high nuclear/cytoplasmic ratio.

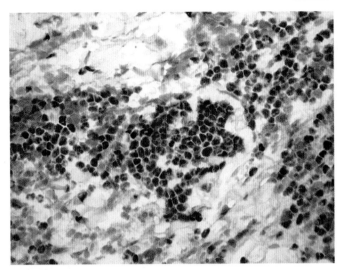

FIGURE 129.2 ▲ Mediastinal precursor T-cell lymphoblastic lymphoma. Note strong TdT expression (anti-TdT).

irregular to convoluted. Cytoplasmic vacuoles may be present. Mitotic figures are often numerous. A starry-sky pattern may be present but is usually less prominent than in Burkitt lymphoma. The thymic epithelial meshwork is destroyed, septa are effaced, and the tumor cells spread through the capsule into adjacent mediastinal tissue. The lymph nodes generally show capsular involvement and complete effacement of architecture. Recently, cases of mediastinal precursor T-cell lymphomas with significant infiltrate of eosinophils among the lymphoma cells and increased tissue and bone marrow eosinophils have been described.[1]

Special Studies

The lymphoblasts are usually TdT positive (Fig. 129.2) and variably express CD2, CD3, CD4, CD5, CD7, and CD8.[2] CD3 is considered lineage specific. In addition to TdT, the most specific markers to indicate the precursor nature of T lymphoblasts are CD99, CD34, and CD1a.[1,2] The presence of myeloid markers does not exclude the diagnosis of T-cell lymphoblastic lymphoma, nor does it indicate mixed phenotype T/myeloid leukemia.[1]

T-cell lymphoblastic lymphoma almost always shows clonal rearrangements of the T-cell receptor (TCR) genes, but there is simultaneous presence of immunoglobulin heavy chain gene rearrangements in ~20% of cases. An abnormal karyotype is found in 50% to 70% of T-cell lymphoblastic lymphoma cases. Translocations typically involve one of the TCR loci and a variety of partner genes; these include the transcription factors c-MYC (8q24), TAL1/SCL (1p32), RBTN1 (11p35), RBTN2 (11q13), and HOX11 (10q24) and the cytoplasmic tyrosine kinase LCK (1p34).[1]

Differential Diagnosis

The differential diagnosis may include thymoma with a prominent immature T-cell population (B1 or B2 thymoma). The immunophenotype of precursor T-cell lymphoblastic lymphoma and of the normal precursor T cells in thymoma can be identical. The infiltrative growth of the lymphoblasts with destruction of the epithelium, flow cytometric evidence of aberrant marker acquisition and/or demonstration of clonality by molecular genetic analysis can be helpful in confirming the diagnosis of lymphoma.

Treatment and Prognosis

Precursor T-cell lymphoblastic lymphoma is highly aggressive but frequently curable with current therapies.[2–4] The prognosis in all age groups has dramatically improved with the use of intensive chemotherapy regimens, with a disease-free survival of 73% to 90% in children and 45% to 72% in adults.[2–4] As CNS relapse is common, CNS prophylaxis with high-dose chemotherapy and intrathecal therapy is also standard.[5] The utility of consolidation radiation to the mediastinum remains uncertain.[5]

REFERENCES

1. Borowitz MJ, Chan JKC. T lymphoblastic leukemia/lymphoma. In: Swerdlow SH, et al., eds. *WHO Classification of Tumours of Haematopoietic and Lymphoid Tissues.* Lyon, France: IARC Press; 2008:176–178.
2. Ellin F, Jerkeman M, Hagberg H, et al. Treatment outcome in T-cell lymphoblastic lymphoma in adults—a population-based study from the Swedish Lymphoma Registry. *Acta Oncol.* 2014;53:927–934.
3. Jin X, Zhao HF, Yu Y, et al. Analysis of clinical characteristics and prognostic factors of primary mediastinal T-cell lymphoblastic lymphoma. *Zhongguo Shi Yan Xue Ye Xue Za Zhi.* 2013;21:377–382.
4. Bersvendsen H, Kolstad A, Blystad AK, et al. Multimodal treatment with ALL-like chemotherapy, auto-SCT and radiotherapy for lymphoblastic lymphoma. *Acta Oncol.* 2014;53:680–687.
5. Portell CA, Sweetenham JW. Adult lymphoblastic lymphoma. *Cancer J.* 2012;18:432–438.

130 Hodgkin Lymphoma

Borislav A. Alexiev, M.D., and Rima Koka, M.D., Ph.D.

Terminology

Hodgkin lymphoma (HL) is a monoclonal lymphoid neoplasm (in most instances derived from B cells) composed of mononuclear Hodgkin cells and multinucleated Reed-Sternberg (RS) cells residing in a reactive infiltrate containing a variable mixture of nonneoplastic small lymphocytes, eosinophils, neutrophils, histiocytes, plasma cells, fibroblasts, and collagen. There are two histologic types of HL: the nodular lymphocyte predominant HL (NLPHL) and the "classic" HL (CHL). Within CHL, four subtypes have been distinguished, based on the characteristics of the reactive infiltrate and to a certain extent on the morphology of the RS cells: nodular sclerosis CHL, lymphocyte-rich, CHL, mixed cellularity CHL, and lymphocyte-depleted CHL.[1] The most common type of HL to affect the mediastinum is nodular sclerosis CHL (NSCHL). NLPHL does not involve the mediastinum primarily, and fewer than 15% of cases have secondary mediastinal involvement.[2]

Pathogenesis

Epstein-Barr virus (EBV) is expressed in about 20% to 25% of NSCHL.[3,4] The incidence of EBV association in NSCHL is generally lower than in other subtypes and varies geographically.[3,5]

Incidence and Clinical

HL is an uncommon malignancy, with 7,000 to 7,500 new cases diagnosed annually in the United States.[6] NSCHL is the most frequent subtype, representing ~70% of all CHL.[7,8] The disease primarily affects young adults.[8,9] In contrast to other forms of CHL and NLPHL, NSCHL demonstrates a female predominance.[8]

Mediastinal Involvement

In 80% of patients with NSCHL, the mediastinum is involved, and 50% of patients present with bulky disease.[8] NSCHL of the anterior mediastinum often originates from the thymus or mediastinal lymph nodes, or both may be involved.[10,11] Some patients have simultaneous involvement of supraclavicular or lower cervical lymph nodes. Involvement of extralymphatic organs or bone marrow is not common. The patients often present with symptoms associated with the presence of a large anterior mediastinal mass, such as chest discomfort or dyspnea. Occasionally, asymptomatic patients may be diagnosed by finding an incidental mass lesion on imaging studies performed for other indications. B symptoms occur in ~40% of all patients.[6]

Mediastinal HL may be restricted to the mediastinum (single lymph node region or lymphoid structure) (stage I) or may involve two or more nodal groups on the same side of the diaphragm (stage II) or nodal groups on both sides of the diaphragm, and rarely the spleen (stage III) or extranodal site(s) such as the liver or bone marrow (designated E if there is, involvement of a single extranodal site, or contiguous or proximal to known nodal site of disease) (stage IV).

Gross Pathology

The thymus or mediastinal lymph nodes involved by NSCHL show multiple firm grayish-white nodules, with or without visible fibrous bands. The thymus commonly exhibits interspersed cystic spaces.[10]

Microscopic Pathology

Classical diagnostic RS cells are large with abundant, slightly basophilic cytoplasm and have at least two nuclear lobes or nuclei. The nuclei are large with prominent irregular nuclear membrane, pale chromatin, and usually one prominent eosinophilic nucleolus, with perinuclear clearing, resembling a viral inclusion. Diagnostic RS cells must have at least two nucleoli in two separate lobes. Mononuclear cells are termed Hodgkin cells. NSCHL differs from other subtypes in terms of the growth pattern and the characteristics of the neoplastic cells (Fig. 130.1). In NSCHL, the characteristic RS cell is termed a lacunar cell (Fig. 130.2), because the cytoplasmic membrane is often retracted in formalin-fixed tissues. Compared

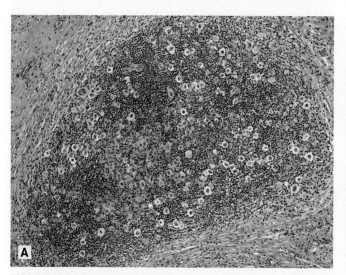 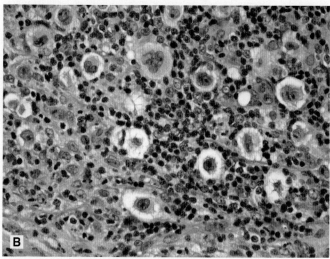

FIGURE 130.1 ▲ Nodular sclerosis classic Hodgkin lymphoma. **A.** Note nodular architecture, perinodular sclerosis, and Reed-Sternberg cells. **B.** Note numerous Reed-Sternberg (lacunar) cells with retraction artifact.

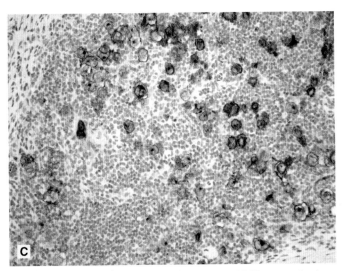

FIGURE 130.1 (*Continued*) ▲ **C.** Note strong CD30 expression in Reed-Sternberg (lacunar) cells (anti-CD30).

with classical RS cells, lacunar cells have smaller nuclei, less prominent nucleoli, and more abundant cytoplasm.[8] Classic RS cells usually are rare in NSCHL. Lacunar cells are found in cellular nodules, containing variable numbers of small lymphocytes. Neutrophils and eosinophils may be abundant, sometimes forming microabscesses within the nodules. The nodules are surrounded by dense collagen bands poor in fibroblasts. The fibrosis often begins in the lymph node capsule, with invagination into the lymph node along vascular septa.[8] The reactive background contains variable numbers of B and T lymphocytes, the latter forming inflammatory infiltrate occasional rosettes around individual tumor cells. Some morphologic variations of NSCHL exist. The "syncytial variant" of NSCHL is characterized by cohesive sheets of lacunar cells within the nodules.[12,13] In the "cellular phase" of NSCHL, a nodular growth pattern is present, but concentric fibrous bands are not formed.

Special Studies

In NSCHL, tumor cells strongly and consistently express CD30 (Fig. 130.3).[14] CD15 is detectable in more than 85% of the cases, although sometimes only focally.[8] Even though both tumor cell types

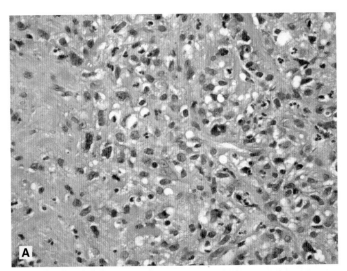

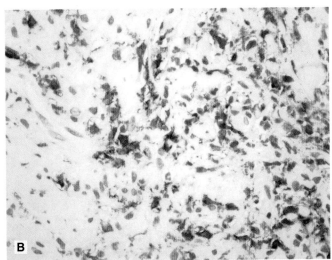

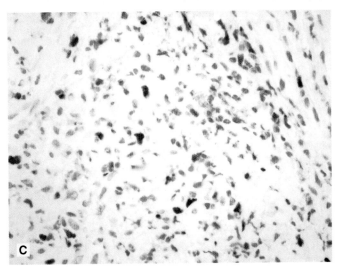

FIGURE 130.2 ▲ Classic Hodgkin lymphoma, mediastinal core biopsy. **A.** Mixed cellular infiltrate with eosinophils. There are scattered enlarged atypical cells (RS cells). **B.** CD30 staining is positive in RS cells. **C.** Pax-5 also highlights RS cells.

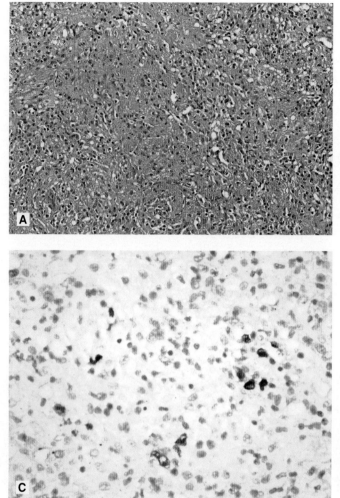

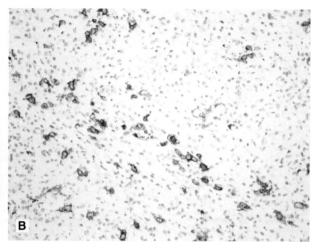

FIGURE 130.3 ▲ Classic Hodgkin lymphoma, mediastinal biopsy, with granulomatous reaction. **A.** Hematoxylin–eosin stain does not suggest lymphoma. **B.** CD30 stains RS cells that in this case were very inconspicuous on routine stains. **C.** EBER ISH is positive in this case, again highlighting RS cells.

(Hodgkin and RS cells) are genotypically of B-cell lineage, CD20 and CD79a are only expressed by a minority of CHL cases. The transcription regulating proteins, Oct-2 and BOB.1, that are involved in germinal center formation and immunoglobulin production are often negative in CHL.[8] EBV may be detected by immunohistochemistry for its latent membrane antigen or by EBER in situ hybridization probes.[3]

Array-based comparative genomic hybridization revealed gain of 2p, 7p, 9p, 11q, and Xq and loss of 4q and 11q.[6] Recent molecular studies applying gene expression profiling show that NSCHL and primary mediastinal large B-cell lymphoma (PMLBL) are closely related.[15–17] Like NSCHLs, PMLBLs also demonstrate high levels of expression of the interleukin-13 (IL-13) receptor and downstream effectors of IL-13 signaling (Janus kinase-2 [JAK2] and signal transducer and activator of transcription-1 [STAT1], tumor necrosis factor [TNF] family members, and TNF receptor–associated factor-1 [TRAF1]).[17] Despite these links between PMLBL and CHL, these two lymphoma types are clearly distinguishable by the expression of other genes.[18] A subset of PMBL signature genes and the mature B-cell genes (e.g., CD19, CD20, CD22, CD79a, and Oct-2) are not typically expressed in NSCHL.[15]

Differential Diagnosis

Because lymphoma of the mediastinum is treated primarily by chemotherapy, complete resection is not attempted, and diagnosis may depend on mediastinoscopic biopsies that are relatively small. The success rate in making a definitive biopsy with core needle biopsies

is <75%.[19] Although flow cytometry is important in the diagnosis of non-HL, it is of no use in HL, because of the relatively small number of neoplastic cells.

There should be a high index of suspicion for HL in biopsies of mediastinal masses in young adults.[19–21] Necrosis, fibrosis, and granulomatous reactions can obscure the diagnosis, which is established by identifying RS cells using a panel of markers, including CD20, CD15, CD30, EBER, and Pax5.

Lymphomas sharing histopathologic features of CHL and PMLBL have been described and are categorized as B-cell lymphoma, unclassifiable, with features intermediate between diffuse large B-cell lymphoma and CHL (sometimes referred to as "mediastinal gray zone lymphoma").

Treatment and Prognosis

Patients are usually treated with chemotherapy with or without radiotherapy, adapted to clinical stage. High-dose chemotherapy supported by autologous stem cell transplantation is considered the standard of care in patients with HL, which has relapsed after, or is refractory to conventional chemoradiotherapy.[6] Stage is the single most important prognostic factor.[1] NSCHL has a better prognosis overall than other subtypes (lymphocyte depletion, mixed cellularity) of CHL.[22] Massive mediastinal disease is an adverse prognostic factor.[1] The mortality due to HL has progressively reduced over the last 30 years. The most recent 5-year survival figure is 81%.[6]

Practical Points

▶ Lymphomas account for 15% of mediastinal masses.

▶ Fifty to seventy percent are nodular sclerosing classic HL.

▶ Most mediastinal CHL occurs between 15 and 34 years of age without gender predilection.

▶ Because treatment for all lymphomas is chemotherapy/radiation, diagnosis often rests on small biopsy samples.

▶ Flow cytometry is essential in the diagnosis of non-HL but not helpful in HL, which requires tissue diagnosis.

▶ Diagnosis can be difficult due to necrosis, fibrosis, and granulomatous reaction.

▶ A panel of antibodies is critical to detect RS cells including the following:

▷ CD30

▷ CD15

▷ EBER ISH

▷ PAX 5

▷ CD20

REFERENCES

1. Stein H, Delsol G, Pileri SA, et al. Classical Hodgkin lymphoma, introduction. In: Swerdlow SH, et al., eds. *WHO Classification of Tumours of Haematopoietic and Lymphoid Tissues.* Lyon, France: IARC Press; 2008:326–329.

2. Lee AI, LaCasce AS. Nodular lymphocyte predominant Hodgkin lymphoma. *Oncologist.* 2009;14:739–751.

3. Glaser SL, Lin RJ, Stewart SL, et al. Epstein-Barr virus-associated Hodgkin's disease: epidemiologic characteristics in international data. *Int J Cancer.* 1997;70:375–382.

4. Keegan TH, Glaser SL, Clarke CA, et al. Epstein-Barr virus as a marker of survival after Hodgkin's lymphoma: a population-based study. *J Clin Oncol.* 2005;23:7604–7613.

5. Harris NL. The many faces of Hodgkin's disease around the world: what have we learned from its pathology? *Ann Oncol.* 1998;9(Suppl 5):S45–S56.

6. Gobbi PG, Ferreri AJ, Ponzoni M, et al. Hodgkin lymphoma. *Crit Rev Oncol Hematol.* 2013;85:216–237.

7. Clavel J, Steliarova-Foucher E, Berger C, et al. Hodgkin's disease incidence and survival in European children and adolescents (1978–1997): report from the Automated Cancer Information System project. *Eur J Cancer.* 2006;42:2037–2049.

8. Eberle FC, Mani H, Jaffe ES. Histopathology of Hodgkin's lymphoma. *Cancer J.* 2009;15:129–137.

9. Engert A, Ballova V, Haverkamp H, et al. Hodgkin's lymphoma in elderly patients: a comprehensive retrospective analysis from the German Hodgkin's Study Group. *J Clin Oncol.* 2005;23:5052–5060.

10. Keller AR, Castleman B. Hodgkin's disease of the thymus gland. *Cancer.* 1974;33:1615–1623.

11. Krugmann J, Feichtinger H, Greil R, et al. Thymic Hodgkin's disease—a histological and immunohistochemical study of three cases. *Pathol Res Pract.* 1999;195:681–687.

12. Ben-Yehuda-Salz D, Ben-Yehuda A, Polliack A, et al. Syncytial variant of nodular sclerosing Hodgkin's disease. A new clinicopathologic entity. *Cancer.* 1990;65:1167–1172.

13. Strickler JG, Michie SA, Warnke RA, et al. The "syncytial variant" of nodular sclerosing Hodgkin's disease. *Am J Surg Pathol.* 1986;10:470–477.

14. Nakamura S, Jaffe ES, Harris NL, et al. Hodgkin lymphoma. In: Travis WD, et al., eds. *WHO Classification of Tumours of the Lung, Pleura, Mediastinum and Heart.* Lyon, France: IARC Press; 2015:277–279.

15. Calvo KR, Traverse-Glehen A, Pittaluga S, et al. Molecular profiling provides evidence of primary mediastinal large B-cell lymphoma as a distinct entity related to classic Hodgkin lymphoma: implications for mediastinal gray zone lymphomas as an intermediate form of B-cell lymphoma. *Adv Anat Pathol.* 2004;11:227–238.

16. Feuerhake F, Kutok JL, Monti S, et al. NFkappaB activity, function, and target-gene signatures in primary mediastinal large B-cell lymphoma and diffuse large B-cell lymphoma subtypes. *Blood.* 2005;106:1392–1399.

17. Savage KJ, Monti S, Kutok JL, et al. The molecular signature of mediastinal large B-cell lymphoma differs from that of other diffuse large B-cell lymphomas and shares features with classical Hodgkin lymphoma. *Blood.* 2003;102:3871–3879.

18. Rosenwald A, Wright G, Leroy K, et al. Molecular diagnosis of primary mediastinal B cell lymphoma identifies a clinically favorable subgroup of diffuse large B cell lymphoma related to Hodgkin lymphoma. *J Exp Med.* 2003;198:851–862.

19. Sklair-Levy M, Polliack A, Shaham D, et al. CT-guided core-needle biopsy in the diagnosis of mediastinal lymphoma. *Eur Radiol.* 2000;10:714–718.

20. Tantisattamo E, Bello EF, Acoba JD. Nodular sclerosing Hodgkin's lymphoma presenting with a pseudo-breast mass extending from a necrotizing granulomatous mediastinal tumor. *Hawaii J Med Public Health.* 2012;71:212–217.

21. Goknar N, Cakir E, Cakir FB, et al. A difficult case of hodgkin lymphoma with differential diagnosis of tuberculosis and sarcoidosis. *Hematol Rep.* 2015;7:5644.

22. Allemani C, Sant M, De Angelis R, et al. Hodgkin disease survival in Europe and the U.S.: prognostic significance of morphologic groups. *Cancer.* 2006;107:352–360.

131 Histiocytic and Dendritic Cell Neoplasms (Histiocytic Sarcoma, Tumors Derived from Langerhans Cells, Interdigitating Dendritic Cell Sarcoma, Follicular Dendritic Cell Sarcoma)

Borislav A. Alexiev, M.D., and Rima Koka, M.D., Ph.D.

Follicular Dendritic Cell Sarcoma

Terminology

Follicular dendritic cell sarcoma is a neoplastic proliferation of spindle to ovoid cells with a phenotype similar to that of follicular dendritic cells.

Incidence and Clinical

Malignant neoplasms showing follicular dendritic cell differentiation are uncommon. Most reported cases have involved lymph nodes of the neck, mediastinum, and axilla.[1–6] The patients are adults with a mean age of 46 years, and there is a slight female predominance.[1–6] The patients may be asymptomatic or present with cough, hemoptysis, or chest discomfort. A small proportion of cases have arisen against a background of Castleman disease of the hyaline-vascular type and others in association with Epstein-Barr virus infection.[7]

Microscopic Pathology

Follicular dendritic cell sarcomas are formed by oval to spindle cells with eosinophilic cytoplasm growing in sheets and fascicles, with a focal storiform pattern and whorls reminiscent of those seen in meningioma.[4-13] The nuclei are oval or elongated with thin nuclear membranes, inconspicuous or small eosinophilic nucleoli, and clear or dispersed chromatin. Nuclear pseudoinclusions are common. Typically, the tumor cells are intimately admixed with small lymphocytes, with a prominent perivascular cuffing. Occasional multinucleated tumor cells can be seen. Some cases can exhibit necrosis, marked cellular atypia, high mitotic rate, and/or abnormal mitoses.

A diagnosis of follicular dendritic cell sarcoma should be confirmed by immunohistochemical studies demonstrating expression of CD21, CD23, clusterin, and CD35 and by ultrastructural studies showing numerous long slender cytoplasmic processes and mature desmosomes.[13]

Treatment and Prognosis

The behavior of these tumors is more akin to that of a low-grade soft tissue sarcoma than a malignant lymphoma and is characterized by local recurrences in 36% of cases and metastases in 28%.[11] Complete surgical resection is the treatment of choice whenever feasible. Adjuvant radiotherapy or chemotherapy may be indicated in cases having adverse pathologic features and in recurrent or incompletely resected lesions.[5]

Interdigitating Dendritic Cell Sarcoma

Terminology

Interdigitating dendritic cell sarcoma is a neoplastic proliferation of spindle to ovoid cells with phenotypic features similar to those of interdigitating dendritic cells.[13-15]

Incidence and Clinical

Interdigitating dendritic cell sarcoma is very rare, and mediastinal involvement is even rarer. The few reported cases have involved the mediastinal lymph nodes as a component of disseminated disease. Patients may present with superior vena caval obstruction due to a mediastinal mass.[16]

Microscopic Pathology

Interdigitating dendritic cell sarcoma has a storiform architectural pattern with paracortical distribution in involved lymph nodes. Tumor cells form sheets or fascicles and whorls of spindled and ovoid cells with abundant, slightly eosinophilic cytoplasm and indistinct cell borders. The nuclei have small to large, distinct nucleoli and may show nuclear membrane indentations. The chromatin is often vesicular. Cytologic atypia is variable. Mitotic rate is usually low. Necrosis is not observed. There are numerous admixed nonneoplastic lymphocytes and, less commonly, plasma cells.[9,15] Immunohistochemical studies show that the tumor cells are positive for S100, fascin, and vimentin but uniformly negative for markers preferentially expressed in follicular dendritic cells (CD21, CD23). Myeloperoxidase, CD34, CD30, EMA, cytokeratins, and specific T-cell– and B-cell–associated antigens are not expressed.[9,15]

Tumors Derived from Langerhans Cells (Langerhans Cell Histiocytosis and Langerhans Cell Sarcoma)

Terminology

Langerhans cell histiocytosis is a clonal neoplastic proliferation of Langerhans-type cells that expresses CD1a, langerin, and S100 and demonstrates Birbeck granules by ultrastructural examination.[9,12]

Langerhans cell sarcoma differs from Langerhans cell histiocytosis in showing overtly malignant cytologic features.

Incidence and Clinical

Involvement of the thymus or mediastinal lymph nodes by Langerhans cell histiocytosis or sarcoma is rare.[17,18] It usually occurs in the setting of disseminated disease.[19,20] The peak incidence is during childhood, and there is a predilection for males. The disease is more common in whites of northern European descent.

Microscopic Pathology

The key histologic feature of Langerhans cell histiocytosis is a diffuse infiltrate of noncohesive Langerhans cells with grooved or markedly contoured nuclei, thin nuclear membranes, fine chromatin, and inconspicuous nucleoli.[19,20] Nuclear atypia is minimal. The cytoplasm is moderately abundant and eosinophilic. There are commonly admixed eosinophils, multinucleated giant cells, and variable numbers of histiocytes, neutrophils, and small lymphocytes in the background.

In contrast to Langerhans cell histiocytosis, Langerhans cell sarcoma demonstrates overtly malignant morphology. Thus far, only one case involving has been reported and this was secondary to direct extension from the lung.[21]

Histiocytic Sarcoma

Terminology

Histiocytic sarcoma, formerly designated as true histiocytic lymphoma, is a malignant proliferation of cells with the morphologic and immunophenotypic features of mature tissue histiocytes.[22]

Incidence and Clinical

Histiocytic sarcoma encompasses an exceedingly rare group of hematopoietic neoplasms, representing <1% of all non-Hodgkin lymphomas.[23] Among a recent case series of histiocytic sarcoma diagnosed using strict criteria (including over 50 cases), there is only a single case with predominant involvement of the mediastinum.[24] Most cases occur in the fifth decade of life (reported age range 20 to 73 years). Male and female patients are equally affected. Patients may present with a solitary mass, but systemic symptoms are relatively common.

Microscopic Pathology

Histiocytic sarcoma demonstrates a diffuse growth pattern composed of large polygonal cells, predominantly arranged in discohesive sheets.[24] There is expression of one or more histiocytic markers, including CD68, CD163, and lysozyme. In addition, CD45 and CD4 are usually positive. Weak and focal expression of S100 may also be noted. There is no positivity for specific B-cell (CD20), T-cell (CD3), Langerhans cell (CD1a, langerin), follicular dendritic cell (CD21, CD35), and myeloid cell (myeloperoxidase) markers.

REFERENCES

1. Ceresoli GL, Zucchinelli P, Ponzoni M, et al. Mediastinal follicular dendritic cell sarcoma. *Haematologica*. 2003;88:ECR04.
2. Chan JK, Fletcher CD, Nayler SJ, et al. Follicular dendritic cell sarcoma. Clinicopathologic analysis of 17 cases suggesting a malignant potential higher than currently recognized. *Cancer*. 1997;79:294–313.
3. Fassina A, Marino F, Poletti A, et al. Follicular dendritic cell tumor of the mediastinum. *Ann Diagn Pathol*. 2001;5:361–367.
4. Guettier C, Validire P, Emilie D, et al. Follicular dendritic cell tumor of the mediastinum: expression of fractalkine and SDF-1alpha as mast cell chemoattractants. *Virchows Arch*. 2006;448:218–222.
5. Jiang L, Admirand JH, Moran C, et al. Mediastinal follicular dendritic cell sarcoma involving bone marrow: a case report and review of the literature. *Ann Diagn Pathol*. 2006;10:357–362.

6. Leipsic JA, McAdams HP, Sporn TA. Follicular dendritic cell sarcoma of the mediastinum. *AJR Am J Roentgenol.* 2007;188:W554–W556.
7. Perez-Ordonez B, Erlandson RA, Rosai J. Follicular dendritic cell tumor: report of 13 additional cases of a distinctive entity. *Am J Surg Pathol.* 1996;20:944–955.
8. Grogg KL, Lae ME, Kurtin PJ, et al. Clusterin expression distinguishes follicular dendritic cell tumors from other dendritic cell neoplasms: report of a novel follicular dendritic cell marker and clinicopathologic data on 12 additional follicular dendritic cell tumors and 6 additional interdigitating dendritic cell tumors. *Am J Surg Pathol.* 2004;28:988–998.
9. Kanaan H, Al-Maghrabi J, Linjawi A, et al. Interdigitating dendritic cell sarcoma of the duodenum with rapidly fatal course: a case report and review of the literature. *Arch Pathol Lab Med.* 2006;130:205–208.
10. Krober SM, Marx A, Aebert H, et al. Sarcoma of follicular dendritic cells in the dorsal mediastinum. *Hum Pathol.* 2004;35:259–263.
11. Perez-Ordonez B, Rosai J. Follicular dendritic cell tumor: review of the entity. *Semin Diagn Pathol.* 1998;15:144–154.
12. Pileri SA, Grogan TM, Harris NL, et al. Tumours of histiocytes and accessory dendritic cells: an immunohistochemical approach to classification from the International Lymphoma Study Group based on 61 cases. *Histopathology.* 2002;41:1–29.
13. Saygin C, Uzunaslan D, Ozguroglu M, et al. Dendritic cell sarcoma: a pooled analysis including 462 cases with presentation of our case series. *Crit Rev Oncol Hematol.* 2013;88:253–271.
14. Fonseca R, Yamakawa M, Nakamura S, et al. Follicular dendritic cell sarcoma and interdigitating reticulum cell sarcoma: a review. *Am J Hematol.* 1998;59:161–167.
15. Kawachi K, Nakatani Y, Inayama Y, et al. Interdigitating dendritic cell sarcoma of the spleen: report of a case with a review of the literature. *Am J Surg Pathol.* 2002;26:530–537.
16. Feltkamp CA, van Heerde P, Feltkamp-Vroom TM, et al. A malignant tumor arising from interdigitating cells; light microscopical, ultrastructural, immuno- and enzyme-histochemical characteristics. *Virchows Arch A Pathol Anat Histol.* 1981;393:183–192.
17. Ben-Ezra J, Bailey A, Azumi N, et al. Malignant histiocytosis X. A distinct clinicopathologic entity. *Cancer.* 1991;68:1050–1060.
18. Lieberman PH, Jones CR, Steinman RM, et al. Langerhans cell (eosinophilic) granulomatosis. A clinicopathologic study encompassing 50 years. *Am J Surg Pathol.* 1996;20:519–552.
19. Bove KE, Hurtubise P, Wong KY. Thymus in untreated systemic histiocytosis X. *Pediatr Pathol.* 1985;4:99–115.
20. Junewick JJ, Fitzgerald NE. The thymus in Langerhans' cell histiocytosis. *Pediatr Radiol.* 1999;29:904–907.
21. Zwerdling T, Won E, Shane L, et al. Langerhans cell sarcoma: case report and review of world literature. *J Pediatr Hematol Oncol.* 2014;36:419–425.
22. Alexiev BA, Sailey CJ, McClure SA, et al. Primary histiocytic sarcoma arising in the head and neck with predominant spindle cell component. *Diagn Pathol.* 2007;2:7.
23. Vos JA, Abbondanzo SL, Barekman CL, et al. Histiocytic sarcoma: a study of five cases including the histiocyte marker CD163. *Mod Pathol.* 2005;18:693–704.
24. Kamel OW, Gocke CD, Kell DL, et al. True histiocytic lymphoma: a study of 12 cases based on current definition. *Leuk Lymphoma.* 1995;18:81–86.

132 Anaplastic Large Cell Lymphoma (ALK-Positive and ALK-Negative)

Borislav A. Alexiev, M.D., and Rima Koka, M.D., Ph.D.

Background

ALK-positive anaplastic large cell lymphoma (ALCL) is a T-cell lymphoma that is characterized by a pleomorphic cell population in which a variable proportion of cells have distinctive eccentric, horseshoe- or kidney-shaped nuclei, often with an eosinophilic region near the nucleus (hallmark cells).[1-6] In addition, the tumor cells express CD30 and exhibit genetic alterations involving the ALK gene on 2p23.[7-14]

ALK-negative ALCL is a CD30-positive T-cell non-Hodgkin lymphoma that morphologically resembles ALK-positive ALCL but lacks chromosomal rearrangements of the ALK gene.[3,15-19] Criteria to distinguish ALK-negative ALCL from other CD30-positive peripheral T-cell lymphomas remain imprecise, making this entity a diagnostic challenge; this difficulty is further compounded by a lack of specific genetic biomarkers for ALK-negative ALCL.[17]

Incidence and Clinical Findings

ALCL is a well-recognized clinicopathologic entity accounting for 2% of all adult non-Hodgkin's lymphomas (NHL) and about 13% of pediatric NHL.[1] ALCL frequently involves both lymph nodes and extranodal sites.[11] Mediastinal disease is less frequent than in classic Hodgkin lymphoma, occurring in 35% to 59% of patients.[4,20] The mediastinum is uncommonly the sole site of disease.[21,22]

ALK-positive ALCL occurs most commonly in children and young adults, although cases can occur at any age; there is also a male predominance (male-to-female ratio, 3.0).[4,8,21]

In contrast to ALK-positive ALCL, ALK-negative cases tend to occur in older individuals and show a lower male-to-female ratio (0.9) as well as lower incidence of stage III to IV disease and extranodal involvement at presentation.[8]

An association with hemophagocytosis has been reported with mediastinal ALCL.[23]

Gross Pathology

The tumor is firm in consistency with a gray-tan cut surface. Focal hemorrhages and necrosis may be present.

Microscopic Pathology

In most cases, the tissue architecture is effaced by solid, cohesive sheets of neoplastic cells.[6] ALCLs contain a variable proportion of large cells with eccentric, horseshoe- or kidney-shaped nuclei, often with an eosinophilic region near the nucleus (Fig. 132.1).[5,10,11,13] These cells have been referred to as hallmark cells because they are present in all ALK-positive and ALK-negative cases, including lymphohistiocytic, small cell, and Hodgkin-like variants.[6] Spindle and/or signet ring cells may be prominent in some cases and simulate sarcoma and carcinoma, respectively.[24-26]

Immunohistochemical Studies

The tumor cells are positive for CD30 (Fig. 132.2) and epithelial membrane antigen (EMA). The great majority of ALCLs express one or more T-cell antigens, cytotoxic-associated markers (TIA1, granzyme B, and/or perforin), and are variably positive for CD45 and/or CD25.[27,28]

ALCLs are consistently negative for EBV, even when occurring in transplant patients.[29] Generation of immunohistochemical monoclonal antibodies to the aberrantly expressed ALCL kinase (ALK, Fig. 132.3) protein has helped define the clinical and prognostic implications of this entity.[10]

Differential Diagnosis

ALK-positive ALCL must be distinguished from primary cutaneous ALCL and other subtypes of T-cell or B-cell lymphoma with anaplastic features and/or CD30 expression.[30]

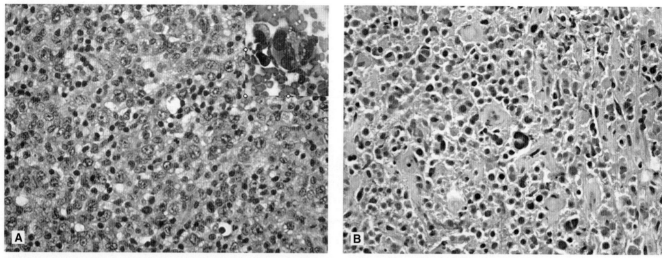

FIGURE 132.1 ▲ ALK-positive anaplastic large cell lymphoma. **A.** Note hallmark cell **(inset)**. **B.** Hallmark cell has a horseshoe shape.

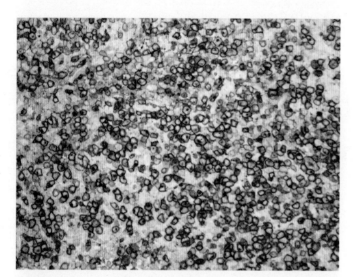

FIGURE 132.2 ▲ ALK-positive anaplastic large cell lymphoma. Note CD30 expression.

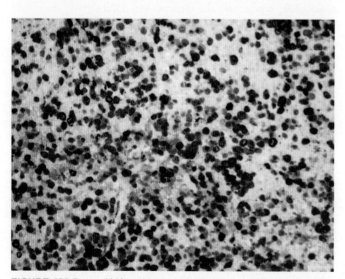

FIGURE 132.3 ▲ ALK-positive anaplastic large cell lymphoma. Note ALK1 expression.

Diffuse large B-cell lymphomas with immunoblastic/plasmablastic features expressing the ALK protein may resemble ALK-positive ALCL. These lymphomas express EMA, as do ALCLs, but lack CD30. Some nonhematopoietic neoplasms such as rhabdomyosarcoma and inflammatory myofibroblastic tumor may express ALK but are morphologically distinguishable from ALCL and are negative for both CD30 and EMA. The principal differential diagnoses of ALK-negative ALCL are classic Hodgkin lymphoma and peripheral T-cell lymphoma.[6]

Treatment and Prognosis

The prognosis of ALK-positive ALCL is remarkably better than that of other T-cell lymphomas.[31] Standard first-line treatment for ALK-positive ALCL consists of doxorubicin-containing polychemotherapy, which is associated with an overall response rate of 90%, a 5-year relapse-free survival of 60%, and a 5-year overall survival of 70%.[2]

The prognosis for ALK-negative ALCL is poor, with a 5-year overall survival of 30% to 49%, which is significantly worse when compared to overall survival reported in patients with ALK-positive ALCL.[17,32] ALK-negative ALCL is generally responsive to doxorubicin-containing chemotherapy, but relapses are frequent.[32]

REFERENCES

1. Drexler HG, Gignac SM, von Wasielewski R, et al. Pathobiology of NPM-ALK and variant fusion genes in anaplastic large cell lymphoma and other lymphomas. *Leukemia.* 2000;14:1533–1559.
2. Ferreri AJ, Govi S, Pileri SA, et al. Anaplastic large cell lymphoma, ALK-positive. *Crit Rev Oncol Hematol.* 2012;83:293–302.
3. Ferreri AJ, Govi S, Pileri SA, et al. Anaplastic large cell lymphoma, ALK-negative. *Crit Rev Oncol Hematol.* 2013;85:206–215.
4. Pileri S, Bocchia M, Baroni CD, et al. Anaplastic large cell lymphoma (CD30 +/Ki-1+): results of a prospective clinico-pathological study of 69 cases. *Br J Haematol.* 1994;86:513–523.
5. Stein H, Foss HD, Durkop H, et al. CD30(+) anaplastic large cell lymphoma: a review of its histopathologic, genetic, and clinical features. *Blood.* 2000;96:3681–3695.
6. Pletneva MA, Smith LB. Anaplastic large cell lymphoma: features presenting diagnostic challenges. *Arch Pathol Lab Med.* 2014;138:1290–1294.
7. Benharroch D, Meguerian-Bedoyan Z, Lamant L, et al. ALK-positive lymphoma: a single disease with a broad spectrum of morphology. *Blood.* 1998;91:2076–2084.
8. Falini B, Pileri S, Zinzani PL, et al. ALK+ lymphoma: clinico-pathological findings and outcome. *Blood.* 1999;93:2697–2706.

9. Gascoyne RD, Aoun P, Wu D, et al. Prognostic significance of anaplastic lymphoma kinase (ALK) protein expression in adults with anaplastic large cell lymphoma. *Blood.* 1999;93:3913–3921.
10. Jaffe ES. Anaplastic large cell lymphoma: the shifting sands of diagnostic hematopathology. *Mod Pathol.* 2001;14:219–228.
11. Kinney MC, Kadin ME. The pathologic and clinical spectrum of anaplastic large cell lymphoma and correlation with ALK gene dysregulation. *Am J Clin Pathol.* 1999;111:S56–S67.
12. Sherman CG, Zielenska M, Lorenzana AN, et al. Morphological and phenotypic features in pediatric large cell lymphoma and their correlation with ALK expression and the t(2;5)(p23;q35) translocation. *Pediatr Dev Pathol.* 2001;4:129–137.
13. Shiota M, Mori S. The clinicopathological features of anaplastic large cell lymphomas expressing p80NPM/ALK. *Leuk Lymphoma.* 1996;23:25–32.
14. Wellmann A, Otsuki T, Vogelbruch M, et al. Analysis of the t(2;5)(p23;q35) translocation by reverse transcription-polymerase chain reaction in CD30+ anaplastic large-cell lymphomas, in other non-Hodgkin's lymphomas of T-cell phenotype, and in Hodgkin's disease. *Blood.* 1995;86:2321–2328.
15. Agnelli L, Mereu E, Pellegrino E, et al. Identification of a 3-gene model as a powerful diagnostic tool for the recognition of ALK-negative anaplastic large-cell lymphoma. *Blood.* 2012;120:1274–1281.
16. Feldman AL, Dogan A, Smith DI, et al. Discovery of recurrent t(6;7)(p25.3;q32.3) translocations in ALK-negative anaplastic large cell lymphomas by massively parallel genomic sequencing. *Blood.* 2011;117:915–919.
17. Savage KJ, Harris NL, Vose JM, et al. ALK– anaplastic large-cell lymphoma is clinically and immunophenotypically different from both ALK+ ALCL and peripheral T-cell lymphoma, not otherwise specified: report from the International Peripheral T-Cell Lymphoma Project. *Blood.* 2008;111:5496–5504.
18. ten Berge RL, de Bruin PC, Oudejans JJ, et al. ALK-negative anaplastic large-cell lymphoma demonstrates similar poor prognosis to peripheral T-cell lymphoma, unspecified. *Histopathology.* 2003;43:462–469.
19. ten Berge RL, Oudejans JJ, Ossenkoppele GJ, et al. ALK-negative systemic anaplastic large cell lymphoma: differential diagnostic and prognostic aspects—a review. *J Pathol.* 2003;200:4–15.
20. Lowe EJ, Sposto R, Perkins SL, et al. Intensive chemotherapy for systemic anaplastic large cell lymphoma in children and adolescents: final results of Children's Cancer Group Study 5941. *Pediatr Blood Cancer.* 2009;52:335–339.
21. Kayao J, Tamaru J, Wakita H, et al. Anaplastic large cell lymphoma of the mediastinum diagnosed by transbronchial scratch cytology. A case report. *Acta Cytol.* 2002;46:405–411.
22. Taki M, Inada S, Ariyasu R, et al. Anaplastic large cell lymphoma mimicking fibrosing mediastinitis. *Intern Med.* 2013;52:2645–2651.
23. Sevilla DW, Choi JK, Gong JZ. Mediastinal adenopathy, lung infiltrates, and hemophagocytosis: unusual manifestation of pediatric anaplastic large cell lymphoma: report of two cases. *Am J Clin Pathol.* 2007;127:458–464.
24. Yu L, Yan LL, Yang SJ. Sarcomatoid variant of ALK– anaplastic large cell lymphoma involving multiple lymph nodes and both lungs with production of proinflammatory cytokines: report of a case and review of literature. *Int J Clin Exp Pathol.* 2014;7:4806–4816.
25. Chan JK, Buchanan R, Fletcher CD. Sarcomatoid variant of anaplastic large-cell Ki-1 lymphoma. *Am J Surg Pathol.* 1990;14:983–988.
26. Massone C, El-Shabrawi-Caelen L, Kerl H, et al. The morphologic spectrum of primary cutaneous anaplastic large T-cell lymphoma: a histopathologic study on 66 biopsy specimens from 47 patients with report of rare variants. *J Cutan Pathol.* 2008;35:46–53.
27. Takahashi E, Kajimoto K, Fukatsu T, et al. Intravascular large T-cell lymphoma: a case report of CD30-positive and ALK-negative anaplastic type with cytotoxic molecule expression. *Virchows Arch.* 2005;447:1000–1006.
28. Foss HD, Demel G, Anagnostopoulos I, et al. Uniform expression of cytotoxic molecules in anaplastic large cell lymphoma of null/T cell phenotype and in cell lines derived from anaplastic large cell lymphoma. *Pathobiology.* 1997;65:83–90.
29. Magro CM, Weinerman DJ, Porcu PL, et al. Post-transplant EBV-negative anaplastic large-cell lymphoma with dual rearrangement: a propos of two cases and review of the literature. *J Cutan Pathol.* 2007;34(suppl 1):1–8.
30. Querfeld C, Khan I, Mahon B, et al. Primary cutaneous and systemic anaplastic large cell lymphoma: clinicopathologic aspects and therapeutic options. *Oncology (Williston Park).* 2010;24:574–587.
31. Han JY, Suh JK, Lee SW, et al. Clinical characteristics and treatment outcomes of children with anaplastic large cell lymphoma: a single center experience. *Blood Res.* 2014;49:246–252.
32. Sibon D, Fournier M, Briere J, et al. Long-term outcome of adults with systemic anaplastic large-cell lymphoma treated within the Groupe d'Etude des Lymphomes de l'Adulte trials. *J Clin Oncol.* 2012;30:3939–3946.

133 Mediastinal Gray Zone Lymphoma (B-Cell Lymphoma, Unclassifiable, with Features Intermediate Between Diffuse Large B-Cell Lymphoma and Classical Hodgkin Lymphoma)

Borislav A. Alexiev, M.D., and Rima Koka, M.D., Ph.D.

Terminology

Mediastinal gray zone lymphoma (MGZL) has transitional morphologic and immunophenotypic features between the nodular sclerosis subtype of Hodgkin lymphoma and primary mediastinal large B-cell lymphoma.[1–4] Diagnostic criteria for MGZL are still being defined, and the optimal therapy is as yet undetermined.[5,6]

Incidence and Clinical

Clinical features of MGZL include young age, male predominance, and localized mediastinal presentation.[2,5,6] MGZL commonly presents as a bulky lesion in the anterior–superior mediastinum with symptoms related to local invasion or compression. Most reported cases have been in adults. MGZL is very rare in children.[3]

Gross Pathology

The lymph nodes are markedly enlarged. The cut surface is yellow-tan with hemorrhages and necrosis.

Microscopic Pathology

The lymphoma demonstrates a sheet-like growth pattern of pleomorphic neoplastic cells, sometimes in a fibrotic stroma. The neoplastic cells are large and pleomorphic, resembling lacunar Reed-Sternberg cells and Hodgkin cells (Figs. 133.1 and 133.2). A characteristic feature is the broad spectrum of cytologic appearances within different areas of the tumor. Some areas may more closely resemble classical Hodgkin lymphoma, while others appear more typical of diffuse large B-cell

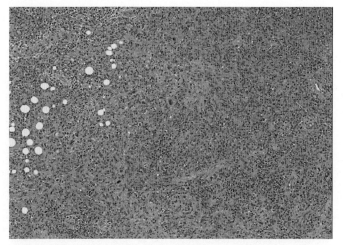

FIGURE 133.1 ▲ Gray zone lymphoma of the mediastinum. The tumor forms sheets, with occasional large pleomorphic cells.

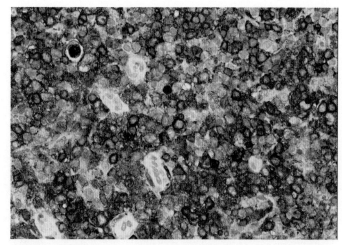

FIGURE 133.3 ▲ Gray zone lymphoma, mediastinum. CD30 is diffusely positive.

lymphoma. Necrosis is frequent. A sparse inflammatory infiltrate may be seen, including small lymphocytes, plasma cells, histiocytes, and eosinophils.[4]

Special Studies

Immunophenotypically, tumors share features of diffuse large B-cell lymphoma and classical Hodgkin lymphoma, with expression of CD30, CD15, and a full B-cell profile including CD45, CD20, and CD79a[7] (Figs. 133.3 and 133.4). The transcription factors OCT2 and BOB.1 are usually expressed. BCL6 is variably positive, but CD10 and ALK are negative. MAL, a marker associated with primary mediastinal large B-cell lymphoma, is expressed in at least a subset of the cases.[8,9] The background lymphocytes are predominantly CD3 positive and CD4 positive, as seen in classic Hodgkin lymphoma.

MGZL has a distinct epigenetic profile intermediate between classical Hodgkin lymphoma and primary mediastinal large B-cell lymphoma but remarkably different from that of diffuse large B-cell lymphoma.[5,6,10,11] Gains including amplifications in 2p16.1 (REL/BCL11A locus) were observed in 33% of all patients, whereas alterations affecting the JAK2/PDL2 locus in 9p24.1 were present in 55%.[5]

Differential Diagnosis

The rarity of these cases poses a tremendous challenge to both pathologists and oncologists because its differential diagnosis has direct implications for management strategies.[1] Diagnostic criteria for MGZL are not yet established. Although most experts agree that the deviation of a single marker or criterion, for example, CD20 expression in otherwise typical classical Hodgkin lymphoma, is not sufficient to put a case in the unclassifiable (gray zone) category, the expression of CD15 in an otherwise typical primary mediastinal large B-cell lymphoma would be.[2] From a practical point of view, strong and uniform expression of CD20 in classical Hodgkin lymphoma should be regarded as abnormal and prompt the pathologist to determine the complete phenotype.[2] MGZL should express at least two markers associated with B-cell lineage.[1]

Treatment and Prognosis

There is a paucity of prospective experience treating MGZL, given its rarity and relatively recent recognition.[12] Recent studies suggest that MGZLs have an aggressive clinical course and poorer outcome than does either classical Hodgkin lymphoma or primary mediastinal large B-cell lymphoma, which emphasizes the importance of accurate classification.[2]

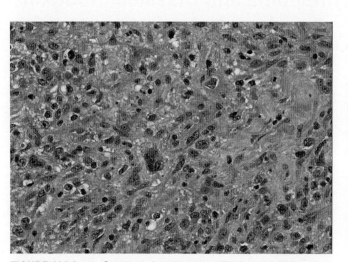

FIGURE 133.2 ▲ Gray zone lymphoma, mediastinum. A higher magnification shows a large multilobated pleomorphic tumor cells.

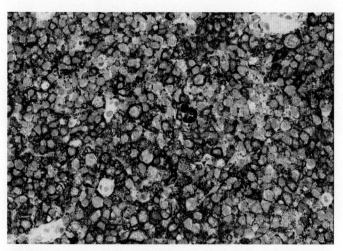

FIGURE 133.4 ▲ Gray zone lymphoma, mediastinum. CD20 is diffusely positive.

REFERENCES

1. Gualco G, Natkunam Y, Bacchi CE. The spectrum of B-cell lymphoma, unclassifiable, with features intermediate between diffuse large B-cell lymphoma and classical Hodgkin lymphoma: a description of 10 cases. *Mod Pathol.* 2012;25(5):661–674.
2. Quintanilla-Martinez L, Fend F. Mediastinal gray zone lymphoma. *Haematologica.* 2011;96(4):496–499.
3. Oschlies I, Burkhardt B, Salaverria I, et al. Clinical, pathological and genetic features of primary mediastinal large B-cell lymphomas and mediastinal gray zone lymphomas in children. *Haematologica.* 2011;96(2):492–498.
4. Dogan A. Gray zone lymphomas. *Hematology.* 2005;10(suppl 1):190–192.
5. Eberle FC, Salaverria I, Steidl C, et al. Gray zone lymphoma: chromosomal aberrations with immunophenotypic and clinical correlations. *Mod Pathol.* 2011;24(12):1586–1597.
6. Eberle FC, Rodriguez-Canales J, Wei L,et al. Methylation profiling of mediastinal gray zone lymphoma reveals a distinctive signature with elements shared by classical Hodgkin's lymphoma and primary mediastinal large B-cell lymphoma. *Haematologica.* 2011;96(4):558–566.
7. García JF, Mollejo M, Fraga M, et al. Large B-cell lymphoma with Hodgkin's features. *Histopathology.* 2005;47(1):101–110.
8. Traverse-Glehen A, Pittaluga S, Gaulard P, et al. Mediastinal gray zone lymphoma: the missing link between classic Hodgkin's lymphoma and mediastinal large B-cell lymphoma. *Am J Surg Pathol.* 2005;29(11):1411–1421.
9. Copie-Bergman C, Boulland ML, Dehoulle C, et al. Interleukin 4-induced gene 1 is activated in primary mediastinal large B-cell lymphoma. *Blood* 2003;101(7):2756–2761.
10. Savage KJ, Monti S, Kutok JL, et al. The molecular signature of mediastinal large B-cell lymphoma differs from that of other diffuse large B-cell lymphomas and shares features with classical Hodgkin lymphoma. *Blood.* 2003;102(12):3871–3879.
11. Rosenwald A, Wright G, Leroy K, et al. Molecular diagnosis of primary mediastinal B cell lymphoma identifies a clinically favorable subgroup of diffuse large B cell lymphoma related to Hodgkin lymphoma. *J Exp Med.* 2003;198(6):851–862.
12. Dunleavy K, Grant C, Eberle FC, et al. Gray zone lymphoma: better treated like Hodgkin lymphoma or mediastinal large B-cell lymphoma? *Curr Hematol Malig Rep.* 2012;7(3):241–247.

134 Mediastinal Nerve Sheath Tumors (Schwannoma, Neurofibroma, Malignant Peripheral Nerve Sheath Tumor)

Borislav A. Alexiev, M.D., and Jennifer M. Boland, M.D.

General

Peripheral nerve sheath tumors encompass a spectrum of well-defined clinicopathologic entities, ranging from benign tumors, including schwannoma, neurofibroma, and perineurioma, to high-grade malignant neoplasms termed malignant peripheral nerve sheath tumors (MPNSTs).[1] Perineuriomas, which express epithelial membrane antigen and possess wavy nuclei and slender, bipolar cytoplasmic processes, have rarely if ever been described in the mediastinum and will not be discussed further.[2]

Neural tumors constitute about 15% of mediastinal tumors in adults and are usually in the posterior mediastinum. Two-thirds are schwannomas, and the majority of the remainder are ganglioneuromas.[3] Ganglioneuromas and tumors with neuroblastic differentiation are discussed in Chapter 135.

Most benign peripheral nerves sheath tumors are sporadic, although multiple neurofibromas suggest neurofibromatosis type 1 (NF1 or von Recklinghausen disease) and multiple schwannomas suggest neurofibromatosis type 2 (NF2) or schwannomatosis. MPNSTs are rare; ~50% are NF1 associated, 10% are associated with prior therapeutic irradiation, and the remainder are sporadic.[4]

Schwannoma

Terminology

Schwannoma, also termed neurilemmoma, is a benign nerve sheath tumor arising from Schwann cells.

Incidence and Clinical Findings

Schwannoma is the most common neurogenic tumor of the mediastinum and may involve any thoracic nerve.[5–12] The vast majority originate in the posterior mediastinum, while anterior and middle mediastinal schwannomas are rare.[4,10] Approximately 10% of mediastinal schwannomas originate from the vagus nerve, and are almost twice as likely to be located on the left as on the right.[11]

Mediastinal schwannomas occur at all ages and may show a female predilection.[4] Almost two-thirds are incidental findings on imaging studies performed for other reasons. Presenting symptoms in the other third include shoulder, flank, back, or chest pain; symptoms of Horner syndrome; dysphagia; cough; and palpitations. Most patients do not have a clinical syndrome such as NF2, although there may be a history of sporadic schwannomatosis or familial adenomatous polyposis.[4] Mediastinal schwannomas may mimic pericardial or bronchogenic cysts, if cystic degeneration is extensive.[4,13]

Plexiform and melanotic schwannomas are two distinctive subtypes that are variably associated with schwannoma predisposition syndromes, including NF2 and schwannomatosis, or Carney complex, respectively.[14] Multiple schwannomas in a patient without café au lait spots, characteristic of NF1, are often seen in NF2.[15] Plexiform

schwannomas have rarely been reported in the mediastinum as an extension of a neck tumor,[16] and melanotic schwannomas have also rarely been reported in the mediastinum.[17]

Schwannomas very rarely undergo malignant change, most often in the form of epithelioid MPNST.[18]

Gross Pathology

The gross appearance of schwannomas is an encapsulated, round-to-ovoid, firm mass with cystic change. Lesions affecting spinal nerve roots are often dumbbell shaped. Sectioned tumors reveal firm or rubbery, light tan (conventional schwannoma) to gray-black (melanocytic schwannoma) glistening tissue, with patchy hemorrhage.

Microscopic Pathology

Conventional schwannomas are encapsulated biphasic tumors composed of compact hypercellular Antoni A areas and myxoid hypocellular Antoni B areas that resemble neurofibroma. Antoni B areas may be absent in small tumors or cellular schwannomas. The cells are narrow, elongate, and wavy with tapered ends interspersed with collagen fibers. Tumor cells have ill-defined cytoplasm and dense chromatin. Nuclear palisading around fibrillary process (Verocay bodies) is often seen in Antoni A areas (Fig. 134.1A). Schwannomas have characteristic irregularly spaced gaping tortuous vessels with thickened hyalinized walls (Fig. 134.1B). The tumors often display degenerative nuclear atypia (ancient change). Mitoses are rarely observed. Rare findings in schwannomas include large cellular palisades resembling neuroblastic rosettes (i.e., "neuroblastoma-like" schwannoma), pseudoglandular structures, benign epithelioid change, and lipoblastic differentiation.[1]

Cellular schwannoma, although relatively uncommon, is an important variant of schwannoma to recognize, because its high cellularity, fascicular growth pattern, increased mitotic activity, and occasional locally destructive behavior (including bone erosion) often prompt consideration of malignancy. Cellular schwannoma is defined as a schwannoma composed almost entirely of a compact, fascicular proliferation of well-differentiated, cytologically bland cells lacking Verocay bodies and showing no more than very focal Antoni B pattern growth. Important clues to this diagnosis include the presence of foamy histiocyte aggregates, the typical hyalinized vascular pattern of schwannoma, and a well-formed capsule containing lymphoid aggregates.

Plexiform schwannoma is a distinctive subtype of schwannoma that rarely occurs in the mediastinum and is defined by a plexiform (intraneural-nodular) pattern of growth.[1,19] Characteristic histologic features included hypercellularity, composed of spindled cells with elongate hyperchromatic nuclei, and indistinct cellular outlines. The nuclei vary minimally in size and shape but are at least three times the size of typical neurofibroma nuclei. Mitoses are frequently seen. Plexiform tumors differ from conventional schwannomas and nonplexiform cellular schwannomas by their lack of both well-formed capsules and degenerative changes.

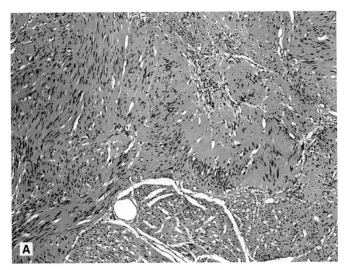

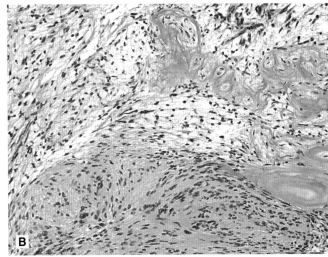

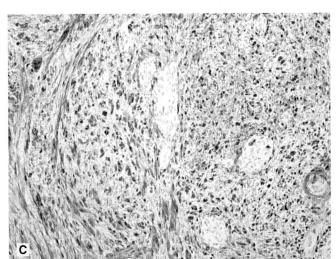

FIGURE 134.1 ▲ Schwannoma. **A**. Note nuclear palisading. **B**. Note alternating cellularity, and hyalinized vessels. **C**. Schwannomas characteristically show strong and diffuse S100 expression (**C**, Anti-S100, protein).

Melanotic schwannoma is a rare, distinctive, potentially malignant neoplasm characterized by spindled or epithelioid cells with variably sized nuclei, small distinct nucleoli, marked accumulation of melanin in neoplastic cells, and associated melanophages.[14,20] One of 13 in one series was present in the mediastinum.[17] In some areas, the nucleoli may be large and prominent. The presence of psammoma bodies in these tumors (i.e., psammomatous melanotic schwannoma) is associated in approximately half the cases with Carney complex.[1]

Special Studies

By immunohistochemistry, schwannomas characteristically show diffuse, strong expression of S100 protein (Fig. 134.1C) and abundant pericellular laminin and collagen type IV, consistent with the presence of a continuous pericellular basal lamina. Glial fibrillary acid protein (GFAP) is expressed in a subset of schwannomas. Recently described markers frequently positive in schwannomas include SOX10, which is a nuclear marker that can be diagnostically useful in evaluation of schwannian and melanocytic tumors, as well as more nonspecific markers podoplanin and calretinin.[1]

In melanocytic schwannomas, the pigment is positive for Fontana-Masson and negative for Prussian blue and PAS. Melanocytic schwannomas strongly express various schwannian, melanocytic, and basement membrane markers, including but not limited to S100, HMB-45, Melan-A, vimentin, laminin, and collagen IV.[14,20] Ultrastructurally, numerous elongated tumor-cell processes, duplicated basement membrane, and melanosomes are observed in all developmental stages.[1] Gene expression profiling shows significant differences between melanotic schwannoma, melanoma, and conventional schwannoma. Loss of *PRKAR1A* expression suggests a link to Carney complex in patients with melanotic schwannoma, even when this history is absent.[14,20]

Differential Diagnosis

The differential diagnosis of schwannoma depends on the morphology of the tumor, and may include other benign and malignant peripheral nerve sheath tumors, as well as other S100-positive neoplasms, specifically melanoma. It may be difficult to distinguish schwannoma from neurofibroma on small biopsies, since the Antoni B areas of schwannoma can be indistinguishable from neurofibroma histologically. Since this is typically not a critical distinction on a small biopsy, a diagnosis of benign peripheral nerve sheath tumor is usually adequate, and definitive subtyping can be performed if the tumor should be excised. Concern for malignancy may arise in cellular schwannomas. Diffuse S100 protein expression is exceedingly uncommon in spindled MPNST, and this finding should always raise the possibility of cellular schwannoma. Combined use of laminin and collagen IV is often helpful in distinguishing melanotic schwannoma from malignant melanoma.[1]

Treatment and Prognosis

Conventional schwannomas are benign lesions with indolent course.[4] A large study showed no recurrences after excision of mediastinal tumors.[4] Cellular schwannomas, despite their occasional alarming cellularity, lack malignant potential for practical purposes and never metastasize. Local recurrence is variable (5% to 40%) and may be higher than in conventional schwannomas. Plexiform schwannomas are also generally benign tumors, although some may show rapid growth, hypercellularity, and increased mitotic activity, along with occasional locally aggressive behavior and difficulty obtaining complete surgical resection, which are unsettling to pathologist and clinician alike. These features may lead to a misdiagnosis of malignancy, which could result in harmful overtreatment. The treatment of choice for mediastinal schwannomas is a complete resection using either thoracoscopic surgery or thoracotomy.[5,11]

The observed clinical course of disease in melanotic schwannomas, which only rarely occur in the mediastinum, differs somewhat in various studies, but they are generally considered to have unpredictable behavior based on well-documented examples of metastatic disease in a minority of cases. Clinical follow-up of melanotic schwannomas in a recent study showed an alarming rate of local recurrences in 35% and metastases in 44% of patients.[14] Of the reported patients with melanotic schwannoma, ~15% died of tumor.[17] Some authors have therefore proposed that melanotic schwannomas are distinctive malignant neoplasms and should be reclassified as "malignant melanotic schwannian tumors".[14] Wide local resection seems to be the current treatment of choice, and additional radiotherapy could be considered. Distinguishing between melanotic schwannomas and malignant melanoma is of paramount importance in planning of management; thus, correlation with staging studies and clinical–radiographic correlation is essential.

Neurofibroma

Terminology

Neurofibroma is a benign peripheral nerve sheath tumor consisting of a heterogeneous mix of cells, including differentiated Schwann cells, perineurial-like cells, fibroblasts, mast cells, and residual interspersed myelinated and unmyelinated axons embedded in extracellular matrix.

Incidence and Clinical

The mediastinum is an uncommon location for neurofibroma. In one series of 75 thoracic nerve sheath tumors, all 46 mediastinal lesions were schwannomas. Neurofibromas of the thorax in this series were found only in the lung and pleura.[4] Rare mediastinal neurofibromas generally are reported in association with the vagus nerve in the upper mediastinum.[21,22]

The majority of neurofibromas occur sporadically as solitary lesions. Less often, neurofibromas occur as multiple tumors in individuals with NF1. All races and ages and both sexes are affected. Neurofibromas are usually asymptomatic and most commonly present as a mass. Plexiform, diffuse, and solitary intraneural neurofibromas may be precursor lesions of MPNST, especially in patients with NF1.[23]

Gross Pathology

Intraneural neurofibromas present as solitary segmental fusiform enlargements of sizeable nerves. Plexiform neurofibromas may cause tortuous enlargement (worm-like growths) of involved nerves. The cut surfaces of neurofibromas are tan or gray-tan, firm, glistening, and more gelatinous than schwannomas.

Microscopic Pathology

In contrast to schwannomas, neurofibromas are not encapsulated and the cells are loosely arranged with diffuse infiltration of the involved nerve. Verocay bodies, nuclear palisading, or hyalinized thickening of vessel walls are not seen. Neurofibromas are composed in large part of Schwann cells, which are considerably smaller than those of schwannomas, with spindle-shaped, round, ovoid, and comma-shaped nuclei and scant amount of cytoplasm. There are also fibroblasts present within the tumor, separated by eosinophilic wiry collagen fibers, and in some cases myxoid matrix (Fig. 134.2). The stroma often contains scattered mast cells. In plexiform neurofibromas, the nerve fascicles are expanded by dispersed tumor cells enmeshed in abundant myxoid matrix and encompassed by a prominent perineurium. Onion-bulb-like proliferations of Schwann cells can also be seen. Mitotic figures are rare. Rarely, neurofibromas contain melanin pigment or have epithelioid morphology.[1]

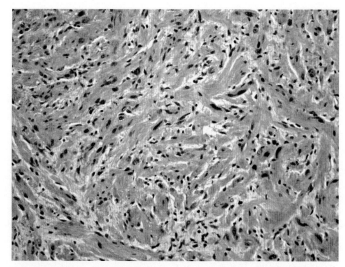

FIGURE 134.2 ▲ Neurofibroma. Note small bland spindle cells with elongate, wavy nuclei, and intervening wiry stromal collagen.

Differential Diagnosis

The differential diagnosis includes solitary fibrous tumor, schwannoma, and MPNST. Solitary fibrous tumor can usually easily be excluded by immunohistochemistry, since they are S100 negative and strongly positive for CD34 and STAT6. Differentiation from schwannoma may be difficult on small biopsies due to the aforementioned overlap between morphology of neurofibroma and Antoni B areas of schwannoma, but this distinction is usually not critical at the time of biopsy, and can be made using morphologic features if the lesion is surgically excised. MPNST is often a concern in patients with NF1, since these can arise from a preexisting neurofibroma. Most MPNSTs will show overt features of malignancy that are not observed in neurofibromas, including hypercellularity, nuclear atypia, necrosis, and mitotic activity. Some MPNSTs arising from neurofibroma may show low-grade features, and the distinction between "atypical neurofibroma" and low-grade MPNST may not be possible on small biopsies and in fact is often very challenging even when the entire lesion is removed.

Malignant Peripheral Nerve Sheath Tumor

Terminology

MPNSTs are malignant tumors arising from a peripheral nerve, from a preexisting benign nerve sheath tumor (usually neurofibroma) or in a patient with NF1. Outside of these settings, the diagnosis is based on the constellation of histologic, immunohistochemical, and ultrastructural features suggesting Schwann cell differentiation.[1,4]

Incidence

Mediastinal MPNSTs are rare, constituting 1% to 2% of thoracic neural tumors.[4,24] The mean age is 50 years at onset. There does not appear to be the same predisposition for location in the posterior mediastinum as benign neural tumors, as anterior,[24,25] middle, and posterior locations were equally prevalent in one series.[26]

Clinical Findings

MPNSTs may occur sporadically (approximately two-thirds), in association with NF1 (about one-third) and after prior radiation therapy.[26–28] They are generally tumors of adulthood, although they can also arise in children, especially those with NF1. The mediastinum is a rare primary site for MPNSTs, and the presenting symptoms are those of an enlarging mass with compression and/or invasion of adjacent structures.[4] The main recognizable benign precursor to MPNST is neurofibroma, particularly the plexiform type, in the setting of NF1. Malignant transformation of schwannoma into MPNST is an extremely rare phenomenon.[29]

Gross Pathology

MPNSTs usually present as a large fusiform mass involving a major nerve. Masses typically are elongated along the direction of nerve, with mean size of 11 cm.[26] The tumor has a tan-white, fleshy cut surface with areas of hemorrhage and necrosis.

Microscopic Pathology

Typical cases of MPNST are composed of relatively monomorphic spindle cells showing fascicular growth and a branching hemangiopericytoma-like vascular pattern, as well as alternating hypercellular and hypocellular areas (Fig. 134.3A). Frequent histologic findings, although not entirely specific, include palisading or rosette-like arrangements, perineural/intraneural spread when associated with nerve, subendothelial accentuation of tumor cellularity, and large areas of geographic necrosis. Heterologous differentiation in the form of cartilage and bone, or, less commonly, skeletal muscle (so-called malignant Triton tumor), smooth muscle, angiosarcoma, and even well-formed glands occur on occasion, particularly in patients with NF1.[1,4,31] Rare MPNSTs demonstrate perineurial differentiation.[32]

A distinctive subtype of MPNST is characterized by a predominance of large epithelioid cells, that is, epithelioid MPNST.[18] These tumors, in contrast to conventional MPNSTs, express S100 protein strongly and diffusely. For unknown reasons, the majority of MPNSTs arising within preexisting schwannoma (a very rare event) are of epithelioid type.

Standardized, reproducible grading systems for MPNST are generally lacking at the present time. A practical approach is to divide MPNST into low-grade and high-grade categories.[1] Most MPNSTs fall into a high-grade category, based on cytologic atypia, brisk mitotic activity (>5 per 10 high-power fields), and hypercellularity with or without necrosis (Fig. 134.3B). The term "low-grade MPNST" is applied to less

anaplastic tumors arising in transition from a neurofibroma precursor. The diagnosis of low-grade MPNST is generally quite difficult to make.

Special Studies

Immunohistochemically, MPNSTs are positive for S100 in <50% of cases. The staining is usually focal (Fig. 134.3C). Diffuse S100 staining should raise the possibility of other tumors, including cellular schwannoma or malignant melanoma, as well as more rare entities such as clear cell sarcoma and dendritic cell neoplasms. In contrast to the focal staining typical of classical MPNST, epithelioid MPNSTs are usually strongly positive for S100 but lack staining for other melanoma markers, and show loss of nuclear expression of SMARCB1 (INI1) in around 50% of cases.[8,14] GFAP is positive in 20% to 30% of MPNSTs.[14,17] Heterologous components such as skeletal muscle differentiation and angiosarcomatous components stain for appropriate markers.

Biallelic mutations of *NF1* are found in a significant portion of MPNSTs.[1] Most tumors exhibit complex karyotypes with numerous structural and numerical changes including gains from chromosome arms 7p, 8q, and 17q and losses from 9p and 17p. No consistent differences between NF1 and non-NF1-associated MPNSTs have been reported.[1]

Differential Diagnosis

The differential diagnosis of MPNST is wide and includes a variety of sarcomas, primarily the other monomorphic spindle cell sarcomas, which include adult-type fibrosarcoma and monophasic synovial sarcoma. Depending on morphology of a particular case, other entities such as rhabdomyosarcoma, leiomyosarcoma, dedifferentiated liposarcoma, and clear cell sarcoma could be considered. One of the most useful distinctions from benign Schwann cell tumors is the partial or even complete loss of S100 expression in MPNST. Conversely, isolated

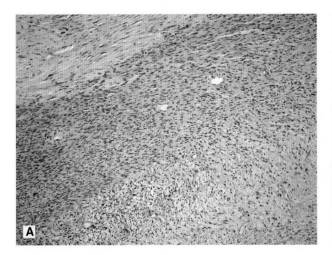
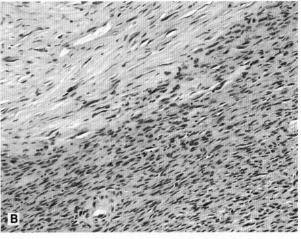
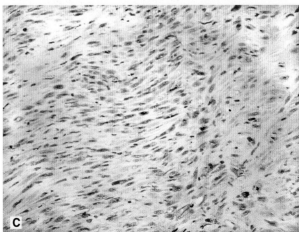

FIGURE 134.3 ▲ Malignant peripheral nerve sheath tumor. Note alternating areas of cellularity (**A**, H&E, ×100) and cytologic atypia (**B**, H&E, ×200). MPNSTs characteristically show only focal S100 expression (**C**, Anti-S100, ×200).

expression of S100 should not be considered definite evidence of MPNST, since S100 expression may be seen in synovial sarcomas, leiomyosarcomas, and rhabdomyosarcomas, among others. The tumor that perhaps most closely resembles MPNST is synovial sarcoma, in particular its monophasic variant. By immunohistochemistry, both synovial sarcoma and MPNST may express low molecular weight cytokeratins and EMA, although expression of high molecular weight cytokeratins is seen only in synovial sarcoma. S100 expression may be seen in both tumors, but CD34 expression is typically not seen in synovial sarcoma.[32] A history of NF1 and/or a coexisting neurofibroma precursor lesion would strongly suggest the diagnosis of MPNST. Demonstration of *SS18-SSX1* or *SS18-SSX2* gene fusions by RT-PCR or FISH, resulting from the characteristic X;18 translocation, may be required for a definitive diagnosis of synovial sarcoma in other scenarios.[33]

The differential diagnosis of epithelioid MPNST includes malignant melanoma, clear cell sarcoma, epithelioid sarcoma, and carcinoma. Lack of expression of melanocytic markers (e.g., Melan-A, HMB45, MITF) is very helpful in the distinction of epithelioid MPNST from malignant melanoma and clear cell sarcoma, and absence of cytokeratin expression distinguishes them from carcinoma and epithelioid sarcoma. Both epithelioid MPNST and epithelioid sarcoma may show loss of nuclear SMARCB1/INI1/BAF47 protein expression, a potential diagnostic pitfall in the differential diagnosis with malignant rhabdoid tumor.[1]

Treatment and Prognosis

Most MPNSTs are aggressive tumors with a poor outcome, and those occurring in the mediastinum are no different.[4] Data from all primary sites show a median survival of 43 months.[28] Radiologic and pathologic identification of invasion of adjacent structures is generally an indication for neoadjuvant or adjuvant chemoradiation.[26]

There is conflicting evidence regarding the impact of neurofibromatosis on prognosis, with one study showing none[28] and another showing decreased survival among NF1 patients.[35] Both NF1-associated and sporadic MPNSTs are associated with improved disease-specific survival compared with radiation-induced tumors, which share a dismal prognosis with those showing skeletal muscle differentiation (malignant Triton tumors).[27,28,35]

Margin status and size remain the most important predictors of disease-specific survival in patients with MPNST. In general, surgery is the treatment of choice whenever possible.[24,26,35]

Practical Points

▶ Benign peripheral nerve sheath tumors of the mediastinum constitute about 10% of mediastinal tumors, are almost always in the posterior mediastinum, and are usually schwannomas.

▶ Benign peripheral nerve sheath tumors arising in the vagus nerve or nerves of the pulmonary artery may occur in the anterior or middle mediastinum.

▶ Most mediastinal schwannomas are sporadic, although multiple tumors suggest the possibility of neurofibromatosis type 2 or schwannomatosis.

▶ Mediastinal neurofibromas are uncommon and may be associated with neurofibromatosis type 1, especially when multiple.

▶ Malignant peripheral nerve sheath tumors may occur anywhere in the mediastinum.

▶ Malignant peripheral nerve sheath tumors may be associated with neurofibromatosis or prior irradiation. Irradiation-induced sarcomas and those with heterologous elements such as rhabdomyosarcoma (Triton tumor) have an especially poor prognosis.

REFERENCES

1. Rodriguez FJ, Folpe AL, Giannini C, et al. Pathology of peripheral nerve sheath tumors: diagnostic overview and update on selected diagnostic problems. *Acta Neuropathol.* 2012;123:295–319.
2. Park JY, Park NJ, Kim SP, et al. A soft tissue perineurioma and a hybrid tumor of perineurioma and schwannoma. *Korean J Pathol.* 2012;46:75–78.
3. Shrivastava CP, Devgarha S, Ahlawat V. Mediastinal tumors: a clinicopathological analysis. *Asian Cardiovasc Thorac Ann.* 2006;14:102–104.
4. Boland JM, Colby TV, Folpe AL. Intrathoracic peripheral nerve sheath tumors—a clinicopathological study of 75 cases. *Hum Pathol.* 2015;46:419–425.
5. Eguchi T, Yoshida K, Kobayashi N, et al. Multiple schwannomas of the bilateral mediastinal vagus nerves. *Ann Thorac Surg.* 2011;91:1280–1281.
6. Huang TW, Yang MH, Cheng YL, et al. Vagus nerve schwannoma in the middle mediastinum. *Thorac Cardiovasc Surg.* 2010;58:312–314.
7. Mallios DI, Krassas A, Kakaris S, et al. Compression of the trachea by intrathoracic vagus nerve schwannoma. *Asian Cardiovasc Thorac Ann.* 2012;20:86.
8. Plotkin SR, Blakeley JO, Evans DG, et al. Update from the 2011 International Schwannomatosis Workshop: from genetics to diagnostic criteria. *Am J Med Genet A* 2013;161A:405–416.
9. Rammos KS, Rammos SK, Foroulis CN, et al. Schwannoma of the vagus nerve, a rare middle mediastinal neurogenic tumor: case report. *J Cardiothorac Surg.* 2009;4:68.
10. Vaish AK, Verma SK, Shakya S, et al. Schwannoma in anterior mediastinum with massive pericardial effusion. *BMJ Case Rep.* 2012. doi:10.1136/bcr-2012-007867.
11. Wu Z, Shi M, Wan H, et al. Thoracoscopic resection of a vagal schwannoma in the superior mediastinum: a case report. *Oncol Lett.* 2014;8:461–463.
12. Yamaguchi M, Yoshino I, Fukuyama S, et al. Surgical treatment of neurogenic tumors of the chest. *Ann Thorac Cardiovasc Surg.* 2004;10:148–151.
13. Taguchi S, Mori A, Suzuki R, et al. Mediastinal schwannoma diagnosed preoperatively as a cyst. *Tex Heart Inst J.* 2014;41:76–79.
14. Torres-Mora J, Dry S, Li X, et al. Malignant melanotic schwannian tumor: a clinicopathologic, immunohistochemical, and gene expression profiling study of 40 cases, with a proposal for the reclassification of "melanotic schwannoma". *Am J Surg Pathol.* 2014;38:94–105.
15. Evans DG, Huson SM, Donnai D, et al. A clinical study of type 2 neurofibromatosis. *Q J Med.* 1992;84:603–618.
16. Tomita K, Mori K, Miyajima Y, et al. Plexiform schwannoma of the neck extending deeply to the mediastinum. *Acta Otolaryngol Suppl.* 1998;539:106–109.
17. Zhang HY, Yang GH, Chen HJ, et al. Clinicopathological, immunohistochemical, and ultrastructural study of 13 cases of melanotic schwannoma. *Chin Med J (Engl).* 2005;118:1451–1461.
18. McMenamin ME, Fletcher CD. Expanding the spectrum of malignant change in schwannomas: epithelioid malignant change, epithelioid malignant peripheral nerve sheath tumor, and epithelioid angiosarcoma: a study of 17 cases. *Am J Surg Pathol.* 2001;25:13–25.
19. Woodruff JM, Scheithauer BW, Kurtkaya-Yapicier O, et al. Congenital and childhood plexiform (multinodular) cellular schwannoma: a troublesome mimic of malignant peripheral nerve sheath tumor. *Am J Surg Pathol.* 2003;27:1321–1329.
20. Vallat-Decouvelaere AV, Wassef M, Lot G, et al. Spinal melanotic schwannoma: a tumour with poor prognosis. *Histopathology.* 1999;35:558–566.
21. Kanzaki R, Inoue M, Minami M, et al. Bilateral mediastinal neurofibroma of the vagus nerves in a patient with neurofibromatosis type 1. *Ann Thorac Cardiovasc Surg.* 2013;19:293–296.
22. Okamoto J, Kubokura H, Ishii H, et al. Mediastinal neurofibroma originating from the pulmonary branch of the right vagus nerve in a patient without von Recklinghausen disease. *Thorac Cardiovasc Surg Rep.* 2013;2:29–31.
23. Tucker T, Wolkenstein P, Revuz J, et al. Association between benign and malignant peripheral nerve sheath tumors in NF1. *Neurology.* 2005;65:205–211.
24. Kalra B, Kingsley PA, Bedi HS, et al. Malignant peripheral nerve sheath tumor of the anterior mediastinum: a rare presentation. *Rare Tumors.* 2014;6:5528.
25. Koezuka S, Hata Y, Sato F, et al. Malignant peripheral nerve sheath tumor in the anterior mediastinum: a case report. *Mol Clin Oncol.* 2014;2:987–990.
26. Kamran SC, Shinagare AB, Howard SA, et al. Intrathoracic malignant peripheral nerve sheath tumors: imaging features and implications for management. *Radiol Oncol.* 2013;47:230–238.
27. LaFemina J, Qin LX, Moraco NH, et al. Oncologic outcomes of sporadic, neurofibromatosis-associated, and radiation-induced malignant peripheral nerve sheath tumors. *Ann Surg Oncol.* 2013;20:66–72.

28. Kamran SC, Howard SA, Shinagare AB, et al. Malignant peripheral nerve sheath tumors: prognostic impact of rhabdomyoblastic differentiation (malignant triton tumors), neurofibromatosis 1 status and location. *Eur J Surg Oncol.* 2013;39:46–52.

29. Nielsen GP, Stemmer-Rachamimov AO, Ino Y, et al. Malignant transformation of neurofibromas in neurofibromatosis 1 is associated with CDKN2A/p16 inactivation. *Am J Pathol.* 1999;155:1879–1884.

30. Woodruff JM, Selig AM, Crowley K, et al. Schwannoma (neurilemoma) with malignant transformation. A rare, distinctive peripheral nerve tumor. *Am J Surg Pathol.* 1994;18:882–895.

31. Rodriguez FJ, Scheithauer BW, Abell-Aleff PC, et al. Low grade malignant peripheral nerve sheath tumor with smooth muscle differentiation. *Acta Neuropathol.* 2007;113:705–709.

32. Hirose T, Tani T, Shimada T, et al. Immunohistochemical demonstration of EMA/Glut1-positive perineurial cells and CD34-positive fibroblastic cells in peripheral nerve sheath tumors. *Mod Pathol.* 2003;16:293–298.

33. Cote JF, de Saint-Maur PP, Coindre JM, et al. Unusual strong CD34 positivity in a thoracic monophasic fibrous synovial sarcoma. *Histopathology.* 2004;45:539–540.

34. Zhou H, Coffin CM, Perkins SL, et al. Malignant peripheral nerve sheath tumor: a comparison of grade, immunophenotype, and cell cycle/growth activation marker expression in sporadic and neurofibromatosis 1-related lesions. *Am J Surg Pathol.* 2003;27:1337–1345.

35. Lamm W, Schur S, Kostler WJ, et al. Clinical signs of neurofibromatosis impact on the outcome of malignant peripheral nerve sheath tumors. *Oncology.* 2014;86:122–126.

135 Neuroblastoma, Ganglioneuroblastoma, and Ganglioneuroma of the Mediastinum

Borislav A. Alexiev, M.D., Jennifer M. Boland, M.D., and Allen P. Burke, M.D.

Introduction

Neural tumors constitute 15% of mediastinal tumors in adults, and around one-third in children. They are almost always in the posterior mediastinum.[1,2] In children, 80% of mediastinal neural tumors are neuroblastomas or ganglioneuroblastomas, whereas in adults, most are benign peripheral nerve sheath tumors (see Chapter 134) and ganglioneuromas.[1,2]

Neuroblastoma and Ganglioneuroblastoma

Classification

The neuroblastic and schwannian stromal cells in neuroblastoma are derived from genetically identical neoplastic cells and support the classical paradigm that neuroblastoma arises from tumoral cells capable of development along multiple lineages.[3]

The neuroblastic tumors are a family of neoplasms composed of various degrees of immature and maturing neural elements. The International Neuroblastoma Pathology Committee has adopted a prognostic system for neuroblastic tumors modeled on the classification proposed by Shimada et al.[4] It is an age-linked risk stratification system dependent on the degree of differentiation observed in the neuroblasts (if present), the cellular turnover index in the neuroblastic component (mitosis- karyorrhexis index), and the presence or absence of schwannian stromal development.[4–6]

Based on morphologic criteria, neuroblastic tumors are classified into four categories: (1) neuroblastoma (schwannian stroma–poor); (2) ganglioneuroblastoma, intermixed (schwannian stroma–rich); (3) ganglioneuroblastoma, nodular; and (4) ganglioneuroma (schwannian stroma–dominant).

Neuroblastomas are defined as neuroblastic, schwannian stroma–poor tumors, although scattered Schwann cells can be detected in the fibrovascular septa demarcating more- or less-defined lobules of neuroblastic cells.[5,6] By definition, the proportion of tumor tissue with schwannian stroma–rich histology should not exceed 50%.[4]

Ganglioneuroblastomas have identifiable nests or nodules of neuroblasts and have schwannian stroma that constitutes >50% of the tumor. Ganglioneuroblastomas can be further subcategorized into *intermixed type* (randomly distributed nests of neuroblastic cells in varying stages of development in a background of schwannian stroma) or *nodular type* (one or more clonal nodules of neuroblasts in a background of ganglioneuroma-like or intermixed ganglioneuroblastoma-like tumor).

The neuroblastic component of neuroblastoma and nodular ganglioneuroblastoma should be further subclassified based on degree of differentiation. The undifferentiated subtype has no neuropil and no recognizable differentiation based on morphology (entirely small round blue cells). The poorly differentiated subtype has neuropil in the background of the tumor, with <5% of cells composed of differentiating neuroblasts (resembling ganglion-like cells, vesicular chromatin with prominent nucleoli and more ample cytoplasm). The differentiating subtype is composed of >5% differentiating neuroblasts, sometimes accompanied by mature ganglion cells.

Incidence and Clinical

Neurogenic tumors can arise from neural cells in any location; however, they commonly are found in the mediastinum (15.3%).[7] The posterior mediastinum is the second most common primary site for neuroblastoma and ganglioneuroblastoma (after the adrenals/abdominal paravertebral sympathetic chain).[8]

Neuroblastoma commonly occurs in children but is rare in adults.[9] Approximately one in six pediatric neuroblastomas occur in the mediastinum, the majority of the remainder occurring in the abdomen.[10]

The median age at presentation is 0.9 years, with 42% of patients presenting at <1 year of age.[11] There is a slight female predominance.[12] A posterior mediastinal mass is diagnosed on incidental chest roentgenograms performed for non–tumor-related symptoms in 49% of the cases. The patients may present with neurologic symptoms, acute respiratory distress, and elevated urinary catecholamines. Less common presentations include Horner syndrome and opsoclonus–myoclonus.[13]

Gross Pathology

Neuroblastoma is typically tan-grey with invasive margins. Tumors often show hemorrhagic and necrotic regions with calcifications.

Microscopic Pathology

Neuroblastomas are histologically separated from ganglioneuroblastomas by the proportion of neuroblasts and schwannian stroma: neuroblastomas have >50% neuroblasts (<50% schwannian stroma), while ganglioneuroblastomas have <50% neuroblasts (>50% schwannian stroma). Neuroblastomas and ganglioneuroblastomas should be subtyped into one of the following categories based on histologic characteristics[4]:

1. **Neuroblastoma, undifferentiated subtype** is composed of undifferentiated small to medium-size cells with round or elongated nuclei and "salt-and-pepper" chromatin, distinct nucleoli, and scant cytoplasm. Identifiable background neuropil is absent.

2. **Neuroblastoma, poorly differentiated subtype** is a tumor with background of neuropil (Fig. 135.1). Most tumor cells appear undifferentiated; only 5% or less of the tumor cell population has morphologic features of differentiation towards ganglion cells.

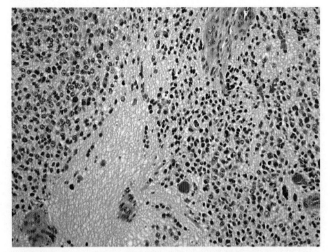

FIGURE 135.1 ▲ Neuroblastoma, poorly differentiated subtype. Note background of neuropil and absence of ganglion cells.

3. **Neuroblastoma, differentiating subtype** has abundant neuropil, with 5% or more of the tumor cells showing differentiation towards ganglion cells.
4. **Ganglioneuroblastoma, intermixed (schwannian stroma–rich)** shows a transitional appearance, often seeming to be on its way toward full differentiation/maturation; however, the process is not complete, as evidenced by scattered microscopic foci of neuroblastic cells, which occur in small nests, admixed with the schwannian stroma. The proportion of ganglioneuromatous component to neuroblastic foci should exceed 50% of the tumor volume.
5. **Ganglioneuroblastoma, nodular (composite schwannian stroma–rich/stroma-dominant and stroma-poor)** is composed of macroscopic, usually hemorrhagic neuroblastic nodule(s) (stroma-poor) coexisting with ganglioneuroblastoma, intermixed (schwannian stroma–rich) or ganglioneuroma (schwannian stroma–dominant) components. The term composite implies that the tumor is composed of biologically different clones.

Neuroblastomas are composed of neuroblasts exhibiting variable degrees of differentiation up to ganglion cells. Neuroblasts have small round nuclei with stippled ("salt and pepper") chromatin, distinct nucleoli, scant eosinophilic cytoplasm, and indistinct cell borders. Scattered large cells with nuclei 1.5 to 2 times larger than those of typical neuroblasts are usually seen in the undifferentiated and poorly differentiated subtypes of neuroblastoma.[14] Ganglion cells have large round nuclei with prominent nucleoli and abundant eosinophilic cytoplasm with Nissl substance (basophilic granules/bodies composed of endoplasmic reticulum). The tumoral background stroma also shows different levels of differentiation, and may consist of neuropil (pink, fibrillary extracellular material) and/or spindle cell schwannian stroma. Calcifications and dense lymphoid infiltrates are occasionally present. One characteristic feature of neuroblastoma is the formation of Homer-Wright rosettes, which are circular or ovoid collections of tumor cells arranged around a central core of neuropil. Homer-Wright rosettes are typical of neuroblastoma, but they are not always present.

The mitosis–karyorrhexis index (MKI) (number of mitoses and karyorrhectic nuclei per 5,000 neuroblastic cells) is a useful prognostic indicator and should be determined as an average of all tumor sections available.[5,6] According to the International Neuroblastoma Pathology Classification, morphologic features (grade of neuroblastic differentiation and MKI) along with patient's age at the time of diagnosis are taken into account for the prognostic distinction of neuroblastoma into favorable histology or unfavorable histology groups.[5,6]

The International Neuroblastoma Staging System is accepted as universally applicable and should always be recorded for new patients.[6,15] It should be noted that tumor maturation may occur in the setting of systemic chemotherapy, so classification is optimally performed on the initial pretreatment biopsy/resection material, if available. The core of

staging is the resectability of the primary tumor, lymph node status (ipsilateral or contralateral), growth across midline, and the presence of distant metastases.[6] Stage 4 disease denotes dissemination to distant lymph nodes, bone, bone narrow, liver, skin, and other organs. Stage 4S denotes localized primary tumor (stage 1, 2A, or 2B), with dissemination limited to skin, liver, and/or bone marrow, in infants <1 year of age.

Special Studies

The most commonly used immunohistochemical antibodies for supporting the diagnosis of neuroblastoma are synaptophysin, chromogranin, CD56, and NSE.[16] Schwannian stromal cells may be identified by S100 immunostaining. MYCN oncogene amplification is an important prognostic factor in neuroblastoma and is associated with poor prognosis/high-risk tumors. MYCN amplification may be assessed by FISH, which should routinely be performed in cases of neuroblastoma.

Differential Diagnosis

The histologic and immunohistochemical differentiation of neuroblastoma from other pediatric small round blue cell tumors may be difficult in undifferentiated tumors or on small biopsies: Ewing sarcoma/primitive neuroectodermal tumor (PNET), lymphoma/leukemia, desmoplastic small round cell tumor, rhabdomyosarcoma, and extrarenal nephroblastoma have to be excluded. Differential diagnosis is generally only a problem with the undifferentiated subtype, since the presence of neuropil and/or differentiating neuroblasts/ganglion cells strongly suggests the diagnosis of neuroblastoma. In difficult cases, immunohistochemistry and molecular studies may be required, and targeted testing using these means usually easily distinguishes neuroblastoma from other entities in the differential diagnosis. Correlation with clinical and radiographic findings is often very helpful, as neuroblastomas often have a typical posterior mediastinal/paraspinal location and often are associated with elevated catecholamine metabolites.

Treatment and Histologic Treatment Effect

Surgery is usually performed for stages I and II. Stage III nonresectable tumors are treated first with chemotherapy and then with salvage resection.[1,2] Most tumors respond to chemotherapy.

Those patients with residual tumor may be biopsied for evaluation of treatment effect, which generally shows decrease in cellularity with necrosis in about half, and tumor maturation with schwannian or ganglioneuroma formation in the other half. Calcification and hemosiderin are common. The pathologist should evaluate presence of stroma, differentiation, MKI, degree of necrosis (none, minimal, <20% or >20%), calcification (none/minimal, moderate, extensive), hemosiderin (none, minimal, moderate, extensive), and fibrosis (none, minimal, moderate, extensive), optimally comparing to pretreatment tumor histology.[10]

Prognosis

Neuroblastoma of all sites remains a relatively common pediatric malignancy with a 5-year survival of nearly 90%.[17] The prognosis of mediastinal neuroblastoma has been reported to be better than that of neuroblastomas at other sites with a 5-year survival rate of 78% compared to 59% for neuroblastomas at other primary sites.[18] A series of mediastinal neuroblastomas and ganglioneuroblastomas showed a 95% 3.5-year survival with the only deaths occurring in the neuroblastoma group.[2]

Early diagnosis and surgical therapy continue to provide the best chance for cure. More effective therapies for patients presenting over 1 year of age or those with advanced disease are still needed. Unfavorable indicators include undifferentiated neuroblastoma, especially in older patients, and high MKI.[4-6] MYCN amplification correlates with advanced-stage tumors. Patients with opsoclonus–myoclonus syndrome usually have an excellent prognosis.[19]

Ganglioneuroma

Terminology

Ganglioneuromas arise from the autonomic nervous system, most commonly the peripheral sympathetic system.[20,21] Ganglioneuroma is not considered a separate entity, but rather a tumor in the final stage of maturation along the spectrum of neuroblastic tumors. It is thought that all ganglioneuromas were once neuroblastomas at an earlier time in their development.[4]

Incidence and Clinical

The tumor is often seen in children and adolescents up through young adulthood, with a slight female predominance.[22] The most common location is the posterior mediastinum.[23] Ganglioneuromas constitute <5% of mediastinal tumors in adolescents and adults and are three times less common than benign peripheral nerve sheath tumors in the same location.[2]

Ganglioneuroma most often manifests as an asymptomatic mass discovered on a routine radiographic study, such as a chest radiograph. Large tumors can cause symptoms due to compression of adjacent structures, and may present with hypertension and flushing if they produce catecholamines.[24] Paravertebral ganglioneuromas may cause progressive scoliosis, and a careful examination for patients with progressive scoliosis is mandatory.[25]

Gross Pathology

The tumor is usually well circumscribed and firm (Fig. 135.2). The cut surface is yellowish to gray-tan, whorled or trabeculated, without evidence of hemorrhage or necrosis.

Microscopic Pathology

Ganglioneuromas can be subtyped based on the following histologic features[4]:

1. **Ganglioneuroma, maturing subtype,** is composed of bundles of longitudinal or transversely oriented Schwann cells and ganglion cells (Fig. 135.3). Scattered throughout the ganglioneuromatous stroma are evenly or unevenly distributed differentiating neuroblasts, but the number and distribution of these cells may be quite variable. The neuroblastomatous foci do not form distinct microscopic nests and blend into the ganglioneuromatous stroma. In general, the ganglion cells are not fully mature and lack satellite cells and Nissl bodies.
2. **Ganglioneuroma, mature subtype** is composed of ganglion cells and schwannian stroma (Fig. 135.4). A fascicular profile of neuritic processes, accompanied by Schwann cells and perineural cells, is characteristic of these tumors. Fully mature ganglion cells are usually surrounded by satellite cells. Complete maturation requires the absence of a neuroblastomatous component.

In some ganglioneuromas, there may be conspicuous finely granular brown pigment resembling lipofuscin or neuromelanin within the

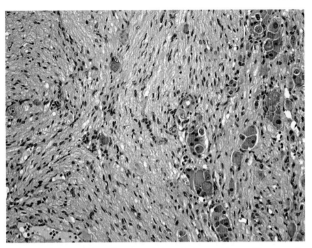

FIGURE 135.3 ▲ Ganglioneuroma, maturing subtype. The ganglion cells are not fully mature and lack satellite cells.

ganglion cells. Multifocal calcifications are frequently observed. Rarely, fat is present in the stroma.[26]

Special Studies

The cells of ganglioneuroma show expressions of S100, neurofilament protein, and calretinin. In addition, many spindle cells are positive for perineural cell markers EMA, claudin-1, and GLUT1. These cells are often arranged in an organoid fashion around the schwannian bundles. The findings indicate that the cells of ganglioneuroma can mature simultaneously towards both Schwann cell and perineural cell phenotypes.[27]

Differential Diagnosis

Individual tumors may have transitional or overlapping features between intermixed ganglioneuroblastoma and maturing ganglioneuroma. The distinctive feature of maturing ganglioneuroma is that neuroblastomatous cells do not form distinct microscopic nests, as in the intermixed subtype of ganglioneuroblastoma; rather, individual neuroblastic cells merge or blend into the predominant ganglioneuromatous stroma.

Treatment and Prognosis

Mediastinal ganglioneuromas, although benign, can grow aggressively and invade mediastinal structures and the spine. According to Hayat et al[24], patients with ganglioneuromas have an excellent prognosis with no tumor-related deaths. Surgical resection is the method of choice to achieve a complete cure and definitive classification.[21,24]

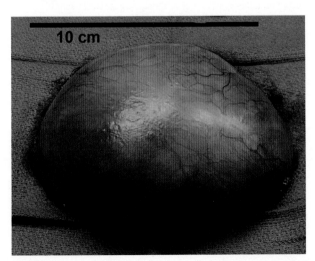

FIGURE 135.2 ▲ Ganglioneuroma, gross appearance. The anterior surface shown is smooth and covered with serosa. The posterior surface (not shown) was ragged and inked for margin evaluation. (Figure courtesy Dr. Joseph Friedberg.)

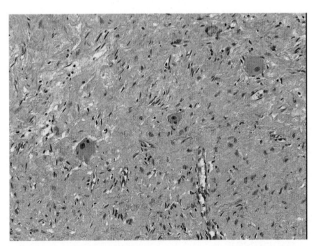

FIGURE 135.4 ▲ Ganglioneuroma, mature subtype. Most of the tumor resembled peripheral nerve sheath tumor. There were scattered ganglion cells confirming a diagnosis of ganglioneuroma. Same tumor as that shown in Fig. 135.2.

Teaching Points

▶ Neurogenic tumors constitute one-third of pediatric and 15% of adult mediastinal tumors.

▶ Almost all mediastinal neurogenic tumors are located in the posterior mediastinum.

▶ In children, most mediastinal neural tumors are neuroblastomas and ganglioneuroblastomas, followed by ganglioneuromas.

▶ In adults, most are benign peripheral nerve sheath tumors, followed by ganglioneuromas.

▶ About one in six pediatric neuroblastomas occur in the mediastinum adjacent to the thoracic spine.

▶ In neuroblastoma and ganglioneuroblastoma, the tumor should be reported similar to that of abdominal tumors in children using the International Neuroblastoma Staging System.[15]

▷ Histologic type

▷ Degree of differentiation

▷ Mitotic–karyorrhectic index

▷ Favorable versus unfavorable histopathology

▷ International neuroblastoma stage

▷ For *MYCN* and other molecular testing, air-dried touch preps for FISH, tumor cultures for cytogenetics and drug sensitivity, and snap frozen tissue should be procured[15]

REFERENCES

1. Fraga JC, Aydogdu B, Aufieri R, et al. Surgical treatment for pediatric mediastinal neurogenic tumors. *Ann Thorac Surg.* 2010;90:413–418.
2. Shrivastava CP, Devgarha S, Ahlawat V. Mediastinal tumors: a clinicopathological analysis. *Asian Cardiovasc Thorac Ann.* 2006;14:102–104.
3. Mora J, Cheung NK, Juan G, et al. Neuroblastic and Schwannian stromal cells of neuroblastoma are derived from a tumoral progenitor cell. *Cancer Res.* 2001;61:6892–6898.
4. Shimada H, Ambros IM, Dehner LP, et al. Terminology and morphologic criteria of neuroblastic tumors: recommendations by the International Neuroblastoma Pathology Committee. *Cancer.* 1999;86:349–363.
5. Peuchmaur M, d'Amore ES, Joshi VV, et al. Revision of the International Neuroblastoma Pathology Classification: confirmation of favorable and unfavorable prognostic subsets in ganglioneuroblastoma, nodular. *Cancer.* 2003;98:2274–2281.
6. Qualman SJ, Bowen J, Fitzgibbons PL, et al. Protocol for the examination of specimens from patients with neuroblastoma and related neuroblastic tumors. *Arch Pathol Lab Med.* 2005;129:874–883.
7. Reeder LB. Neurogenic tumors of the mediastinum. *Semin Thorac Cardiovasc Surg.* 2000;12:261–267.
8. Demir HA, Yalcin B, Buyukpamukcu N, et al. Thoracic neuroblastic tumors in childhood. *Pediatr Blood Cancer.* 2010;54:885–889.
9. Ohtaki Y, Ishii G, Hasegawa T, et al. Adult neuroblastoma arising in the superior mediastinum. *Interact Cardiovasc Thorac Surg.* 2011;13:220–222.
10. Marachelian A, Shimada H, Sano H, et al. The significance of serial histopathology in a residual mass for outcome of intermediate risk stage 3 neuroblastoma. *Pediatr Blood Cancer.* 2012;58:675–681.
11. Gutierrez JC, Fischer AC, Sola JE, et al. Markedly improving survival of neuroblastoma: a 30-year analysis of 1,646 patients. *Pediatr Surg Int.* 2007;23:637–646.
12. Takeda S, Miyoshi S, Minami M, et al. Intrathoracic neurogenic tumors—50 years' experience in a Japanese institution. *Eur J Cardiothorac Surg.* 2004;26:807–812.
13. Cooper R, Khakoo Y, Matthay KK, et al. Opsoclonus-myoclonus-ataxia syndrome in neuroblastoma: histopathologic features—a report from the Children's Cancer Group. *Med Pediatr Oncol.* 2001;36:623–629.
14. Tornoczky T, Kalman E, Kajtar PG, et al. Large cell neuroblastoma: a distinct phenotype of neuroblastoma with aggressive clinical behavior. *Cancer.* 2004;100:390–397.
15. Jarzemboski JA, Bowen J, Hill DA, et al. *Protocol for the Examination of Specimens from Patients with Neuroblastoma.* College of American Pathologists Cancer Protocols; 2012 [cited June 2012]. Available from: http://www.cap.org/apps/docs/committees/cancer/cancer_protocols/2012/Neuroblastoma_12.pdf
16. Park SJ, Park CJ, Kim S, et al. Detection of bone marrow metastases of neuroblastoma with immunohistochemical staining of CD56, chromogranin A, and synaptophysin. *Appl Immunohistochem Mol Morphol.* 2010;18:348–352.
17. Zhou Y, Li K, Zheng S, et al. Retrospective study of neuroblastoma in Chinese neonates from 1994 to 2011: an evaluation of diagnosis, treatments, and prognosis: a 10-year restrospective study of neonatal neuroblastoma. *J Cancer Res Clin Oncol.* 2014;140:83–87.
18. Suita S, Tajiri T, Sera Y, et al. The characteristics of mediastinal neuroblastoma. *Eur J Pediatr Surg.* 2000;10:353–359.
19. Rudnick E, Khakoo Y, Antunes NL, et al. Opsoclonus-myoclonus-ataxia syndrome in neuroblastoma: clinical outcome and antineuronal antibodies—a report from the Children's Cancer Group Study. *Med Pediatr Oncol.* 2001;36:612–622.
20. Geoerger B, Hero B, Harms D, et al. Metabolic activity and clinical features of primary ganglioneuromas. *Cancer.* 2001;91:1905–1913.
21. Guan YB, Zhang WD, Zeng QS, et al. CT and MRI findings of thoracic ganglioneuroma. *Br J Radiol.* 2012;85:e365–e672.
22. Dai X, Zhang R, Li Y, et al. Multiple ganglioneuromas: a report of a case and review of the ganglioneuromas. *Clin Neuropathol.* 2009;28:193–196.
23. Forsythe A, Volpe J, Muller R. Posterior mediastinal ganglioneuroma. *Radiographics.* 2004;24:594–597.
24. Hayat J, Ahmed R, Alizai S, et al. Giant ganglioneuroma of the posterior mediastinum. *Interact Cardiovasc Thorac Surg.* 2011;13:344–345.
25. Kara T, Oztunali C. Radiologic findings of thoracic scoliosis due to giant ganglioneuroma. *Clin Imaging.* 2013;37:767–768.
26. Ko SM, Keum DY, Kang YN. Posterior mediastinal dumbbell ganglioneuroma with fatty replacement. *Br J Radiol.* 2007;80:e238–e240.
27. Chlumska A, Ondrias F. Mediastinal ganglioneuroma with perineural cell differentiation. Report of a case. *Cesk Patol.* 2012;48:94–96.

136 Synovial Sarcoma

Borislav A. Alexiev, M.D., Jennifer M. Boland, M.D., and Allen P. Burke, M.D.

Terminology

Synovial sarcoma is a malignant mesenchymal tumor that displays a variable degree of epithelial differentiation, which may include gland formation, and has a specific chromosomal translocation t(X;18) (p11;q11). Synovial sarcomas of the thorax are rare, but most frequently occur in the mediastinum, followed by the pleura, lung parenchyma, pericardium, and myocardium. Synovial sarcomas of the pleura are discussed in Chapter 96, Part 1.

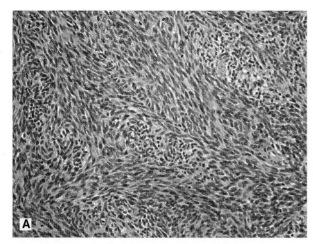
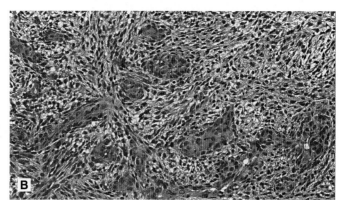

FIGURE 136.1 ▲ Synovial sarcoma, mediastinum. **A.** Monophasic subtype. The tumor is composed of uniform spindle cells arranged in fascicles. **B.** Biphasic type. There are nests of epithelioid cells. These stained for both epithelial membrane antigen and cytokeratins (not shown).

Incidence and Clinical

Synovial sarcoma accounts for up to 8% to 10% of all histologic types of soft tissue sarcoma, and can occur in almost any part of the body (i.e., it is unrelated to the synovium). It has been reported in children and adults, with a male-to-female ratio of 2:1, and most often affects the deep soft tissues of the extremities.

Primary synovial sarcoma of the mediastinum is rare, with ~50 reported cases.[1] The anterior mediastinum is the most common compartment involved, although it can also occur in the posterior mediastinum/paraspinal region and often presents with nonspecific regional symptoms including chest pain (69%), shortness of breath (63%), pericardial or pleural effusion (22%), and cough (16%).[1,2]

Gross Pathology

Synovial sarcoma is usually grossly circumscribed, although this may be deceptive as it may microscopically invade adjacent mediastinal structures. The cut surface is soft or firm, pink-tan to yellow-grey, and can be multinodular and cystic. Hemorrhage, necrosis, and calcifications may be present.

Microscopic Pathology

Histologically, synovial sarcoma may be monophasic fibrous (spindle cells only), biphasic (spindle cells and gland formation), or poorly differentiated, which have been divided into small, large and spindle cell variants, the latter with abundant necrosis and prominent hemangiopericytoma-like vascular pattern.[3]

It seems that monophasic examples outnumber biphasic tumors in the mediastinal location. The monophasic subtype is composed of uniform spindle cells, which are arranged in sheets, fascicles or herringbone patterns (Fig. 136.1). The tumor characteristically has a "staghorn" or "hemangiopericytoma-like" vascular pattern. The monomorphic spindle cells have sparse cytoplasm with ovoid, hyperchromatic nuclei, and inconspicuous nucleoli. The nuclear-to-cytoplasmic ratio is high, and nuclear overlapping is commonly observed. In biphasic synovial sarcoma, spindle cell and epithelial components are present in varying proportions. The spindle cells in biphasic synovial sarcoma are identical to the spindle cells in the monophasic subtype. The epithelial cells may be arranged in solid nests, cords, or glands. Some glandular lumina may contain mucin. The amount of stromal collagen is variable, but usually scant. Myxoid change, calcifications, and ossification may be present. Mast cells can be abundant. Poorly differentiated areas may be present in synovial sarcoma, usually admixed with more classic-appearing areas of monophasic or biphasic synovial sarcoma, but some examples may be entirely poorly differentiated. Poorly differentiated areas may show a small round blue cell, fascicular spindle cell, or epithelioid morphology (Fig. 136.2). Poorly differentiated areas typically have nuclear crowding, nuclear membrane irregularity, irregularly clumped chromatin,

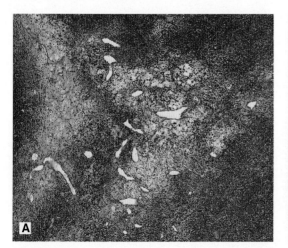
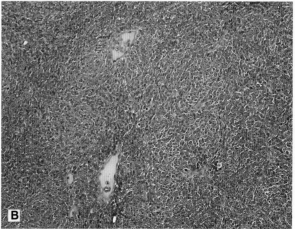

FIGURE 136.2 ▲ Synovial sarcoma, poorly differentiated. **A.** A low magnification showing hemangiopericytoma-like vascular pattern. **B.** Note the prominent nucleoli and plump ovoid shape of the tumor cells. The tumor still retains nuclear monotony and hemangiopericytoma-like vessels, which are clues to the diagnosis.

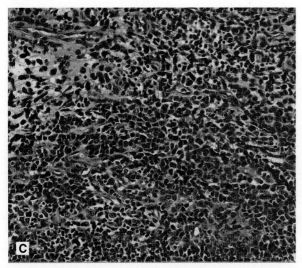

FIGURE 136.2 (*Continued*) ▲ **C.** This example showed a small cell pattern, and the clinical suspicion was mediastinal small cell carcinoma extending from the lung.

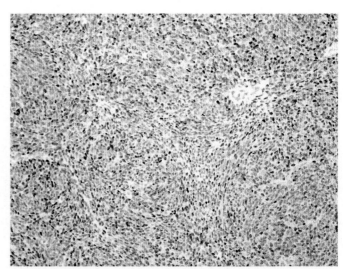

FIGURE 136.3 ▲ Synovial sarcoma. Synovial sarcoma often expresses nuclear TLE1, which is a sensitive marker but is not specific for this tumor type.

prominent nucleoli, and high mitotic activity (>15 mitoses/10 HPFs), but usually retain some degree of nuclear monotony that is typical of translocation-associated sarcomas.

Immunohistochemical Findings

Synovial sarcomas characteristically express epithelial markers (EMA and cytokeratins), usually in a focal manner. EMA is expressed more often and more widely than are cytokeratins, especially in the monophasic and poorly differentiated subtypes.[2–5] It should be noted that the absence of discernable EMA and cytokeratin expression does not exclude the diagnosis of synovial sarcoma if the morphology is typical, especially on small biopsies where sampling is an issue. Because of the variability in immunohistochemical and histologic findings, molecular testing is invaluable to confirm the diagnosis.

The nuclear marker TLE1 can be helpful in the evaluation of synovial sarcoma (Fig. 136.3), where it is a sensitive but nonspecific marker.[6]

CD99 expression is common in synovial sarcoma (Fig. 136.4A), which may lead to confusion with Ewing sarcoma/PNET in poorly differentiated examples.[2,3,5,7] Similarly, CD56 is usually diffusely positive (Fig. 136.4B),[2,7,8] but synaptophysin, another neuroendocrine marker, is generally negative.[8] A large majority of synovial sarcomas are positive for vimentin and bcl2, but these markers are very nonspecific and therefore usually not useful in the diagnostic workup.[3,9] Focal expression of S100 may be detectable in up 40% of cases, which can lead to confusion with malignant peripheral nerve sheath tumor (MPNST).[2,3] CD34 and desmin are generally negative, although there are occasional exceptions to this rule.[3]

Electron Microscopy

Ultrastructural examination of synovial sarcoma shows epithelial differentiation (abundant cytoplasmic intermediate filaments, and immature desmosome-type cell junctions).[5]

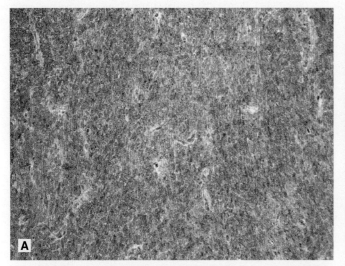

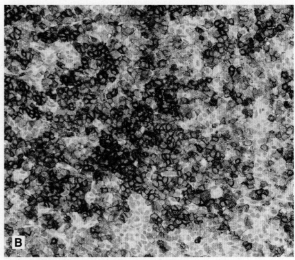

FIGURE 136.4 ▲ Synovial sarcoma. **A.** Note positive staining for CD99, which can be a potential diagnostic pitfall. **B.** Similarly, staining for CD56 is common and, in conjunction with epithelial marker staining, can be confusing with small cell carcinoma in the mediastinum.

Cytogenetics

Synovial sarcoma is characterized by the t(X;18)(p11;q11) translocation, leading to fusion of the *SS18* gene (also known as *SYT* or *SSXT*) on chromosome 18 with one of the *SSX* genes (*SSX1*, *SSX2* or *SSX4*) on the X chromosome. Testing for these characteristic fusion genes can be performed by RT-PCR, or using break-apart FISH for the *SS18(SYT)* gene. The characteristic translocation t(X;18)(p11;q11) has been noted in more than 95% of cases,[10] and thus testing for this characteristic genetic abnormality can be very helpful to confirm or refute the diagnosis of synovial sarcoma.

Differential Diagnosis

Monophasic synovial sarcoma is a monomorphic spindle cell sarcoma, and thus has overlapping morphologic features with MPNST, which can be further confounded by the occasional expression of S100 by synovial sarcoma and the anomalous keratin expression that is sometimes seen in MPNST. A history of neurofibromatosis type 1 would strongly support a diagnosis of MPNST, while many other cases require careful histologic examination and possible molecular testing for synovial sarcoma to make this distinction. The cytologic monotony and staghorn vascular pattern may lead to consideration of solitary fibrous tumor (SFT) or type A thymoma, but these entities are readily excluded using immunohistochemistry for CD34 and STAT6 (SFT) or cytokeratin and TdT (thymoma, which would show diffuse keratin and scattered TdT positive T cells). Biphasic examples may bring malignant mesothelioma to mind, but expression of specific mesothelial markers often makes this diagnosis straightforward. Sarcomatoid carcinomas generally show more pleomorphism than does synovial sarcoma, but molecular testing could be considered in difficult cases. Finally, poorly differentiated examples of synovial sarcoma may strongly resemble Ewing sarcoma/PNET and may express CD99; thus, testing for the translocations that characterize these tumors may be necessary.

Treatment and Prognosis

Mediastinal synovial sarcomas are aggressive high-grade tumors with poor prognosis, as tumors tend to be very large at presentation and are often advanced stage.[1] Completeness of resection is the only identified factor that influences survival and can result in outcomes similar to those observed in synovial sarcomas arising primarily in the extremities, but tumors often invade critical mediastinal structures at presentation and thus complete resection is often not possible.[1]

Practical Points

▶ Because the mediastinum is an unusual location for synovial sarcoma, the diagnosis may be initially overlooked.

▶ Undifferentiated synovial sarcoma can mimic primitive neuroectodermal tumor/Ewing's, and frequently expresses CD99.

▶ Undifferentiated synovial sarcoma can mimic small cell carcinoma, and frequently expresses CD56.

▶ Molecular testing for the t(x;18) translocation is the gold standard for diagnosis and should be performed in any tumor in which the histologic features are suggestive of the diagnosis.

REFERENCES

1. Salah S, Salem A. Primary synovial sarcomas of the mediastinum: a systematic review and pooled analysis of the published literature. *ISRN Oncol.* 2014;2014:412527.
2. Hartel PH, Fanburg-Smith JC, Frazier AA, et al. Primary pulmonary and mediastinal synovial sarcoma: a clinicopathologic study of 60 cases and comparison with five prior series. *Mod Pathol.* 2007;20:760–769.
3. Pelmus M, Guillou L, Hostein I, et al. Monophasic fibrous and poorly differentiated synovial sarcoma: immunohistochemical reassessment of 60 t(X;18)(SYT-SSX)-positive cases. *Am J Surg Pathol.* 2002;26:1434–1440.
4. Miettinen M, Limon J, Niezabitowski A, et al. Patterns of keratin polypeptides in 110 biphasic, monophasic, and poorly differentiated synovial sarcomas. *Virchows Arch.* 2000;437:275–283.
5. Suster S, Moran CA. Primary synovial sarcomas of the mediastinum: a clinicopathologic, immunohistochemical, and ultrastructural study of 15 cases. *Am J Surg Pathol.* 2005;29:569–578.
6. Foo WC, Cruise MW, Wick MR, et al. Immunohistochemical staining for TLE1 distinguishes synovial sarcoma from histologic mimics. *Am J Clin Pathol.* 2011;135:839–844.
7. Olsen SH, Thomas DG, Lucas DR. Cluster analysis of immunohistochemical profiles in synovial sarcoma, malignant peripheral nerve sheath tumor, and Ewing sarcoma. *Mod Pathol.* 2006;19:659–668.
8. Huang CC, Michael CW, Pang JC. Fine needle aspiration of primary mediastinal synovial sarcoma: cytomorphologic, immunohistochemical, and molecular study. *Diagn Cytopathol.* 2014;42:170–176.
9. Hirakawa N, Naka T, Yamamoto I, et al. Overexpression of bcl-2 protein in synovial sarcoma: a comparative study of other soft tissue spindle cell sarcomas and an additional analysis by fluorescence in situ hybridization. *Hum Pathol.* 1996;27:1060–1065.
10. Ferrari A, Gronchi A, Casanova M, et al. Synovial sarcoma: a retrospective analysis of 271 patients of all ages treated at a single institution. *Cancer.* 2004;101:627–634.

137 Miscellaneous Mediastinal Tumors (Paraganglioma, Vascular and Lipomatous Tumors, Other Sarcomas)

Borislav A. Alexiev, M.D., and Jennifer M. Boland, M.D.

Paraganglioma

Terminology

Paragangliomas are neuroendocrine tumors that arise in the extraadrenal sympathetic and parasympathetic paraganglia.

Incidence and Clinical

Paraganglioma in the mediastinum is extremely rare, accounting for 0.3% of all mediastinal tumors. The posterior mediastinum is the commonest site for mediastinal paraganglioma while anterior mediastinal localization is unusual.[1] Paragangliomas are tumors of adults, with a female predominance, and a peak incidence occurring during the third and fourth decade.[1] Most paragangliomas are asymptomatic and present as painless masses.[2,3] Clinical manifestations of mediastinal paraganglioma refer to a space-occupying mass and include hoarseness, dysphagia, chest pain, cough and, occasionally, superior vena cava syndrome. Patients may have symptoms related to excess secretion of catecholamines.[4] Multiple paragangliomas occur in 22% of patients.[4] Paragangliomas may occur sporadically or in association with several hereditary tumor syndromes, including neurofibromatosis type 1, von Hippel-Lindau disease, Carney triad, multiple endocrine neoplasia type 2, and pheochromocytoma–paraganglioma syndrome.[5-7] Therefore, genetic testing should be considered in all patients with paraganglioma. Aggressive growth and metastases are observed in ~20% of mediastinal paragangliomas.

Gross Pathology

Paragangliomas are solid tumors and are partially or completely encapsulated in a thin capsule. They frequently have a soft, heterogeneous, red-brown/mahogany cut surface.

Microscopic Pathology

Histologically, the organoid–nested pattern ("zellballen") of the normal paraganglion is seen in these tumors (Fig. 137.1). However, a wide range of variant morphology may be observed, including trabecular, spindled, or angioma-like patterns. Paragangliomas are composed of two cell types: (a) chief cells, which have abundant slightly granular cytoplasm with round or oval nuclei; and (b) sustentacular cells, which are inconspicuous spindled cells usually arranged around the periphery of the cell nests. There is a prominent delicate capillary vascular network. Mitotic figures are rare.

Special Studies

Immunohistochemically, neuroendocrine markers such as chromogranin A, synaptophysin, and CD56 are usually positive in chief cells (Fig. 137.2).[1,4] S100 and GFAP immunostaining is present in sustentacular cells. Electron microscopy demonstrates neurosecretory granules in tumor cells.

Differential Diagnosis

Tumors that should be differentiated from mediastinal paragangliomas include well-differentiated neuroendocrine tumor (carcinoid), metastatic medullary thyroid carcinoma, and glomangioma. Carcinoid

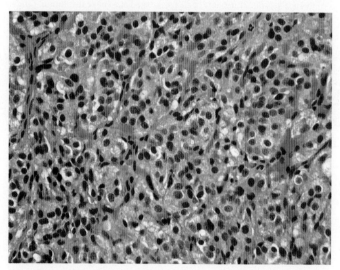

FIGURE 137.1 ▲ Paraganglioma. Note organoid pattern and prominent vascular network (H&E, ×200).

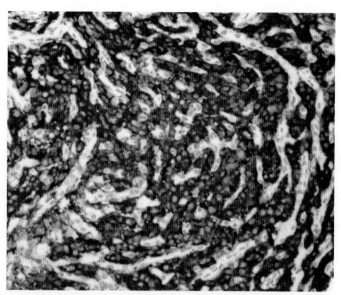

FIGURE 137.2 ▲ Paraganglioma. Note positive staining for synaptophysin (Antisynaptophysin, ×200).

tumors typically express keratin, in contrast to paragangliomas, and lack sustentacular cells. Medullary thyroid carcinoma usually expresses calcitonin, and may have recognizable amyloid deposits. Glomangiomas lack expression of neuroendocrine markers and usually express smooth muscle actin.

Treatment and Prognosis

It is generally accepted that a paraganglioma is determined to be malignant only when metastases are demonstrated, as histologic criteria do not reliably predict malignancy. The treatment of choice for paraganglioma is surgical resection; most tumors are benign and can be excised totally.[8,9] The surgery of anterior and middle mediastinal paragangliomas is challenging because of their close proximity to the central airways, heart, and great vessels, making complete resection difficult. Preoperative embolization is an established technique to reduce operative blood loss.[2] In these cases, the pathology may see evidence of intra-arterial microspheres with a foreign body reaction adjacent to the tumor.

Lymphangioma

Terminology

Lymphangioma is a benign cavernous/cystic vascular lesion composed of dilated lymphatic channels. Early or congenital age of onset favors a developmental malformation.

Incidence and Clinical

Mediastinal lymphangioma is rare, accounting for 0.7% to 4.5% of all mediastinal tumors.[10-16] The lesions may remain asymptomatic for years. Most are found incidentally in adulthood, or become apparent with manifestations related to compression of intrathoracic structures, including respiratory symptoms or dysphagia.[15] Preoperative diagnosis is difficult and most of them are diagnosed intra- or postoperatively. Computed tomographic scans generally show a homogeneous, low-attenuation mass that often involves vascular or airway structures.

Gross Pathology

Lymphangiomas may be well capsulated, smoothly marginated, unilocular, or multicystic, with cavities containing watery/milky fluid. They may involve adjacent structures and viscera, or infiltrate soft tissue.

Microscopic Pathology

Lymphangiomas are characterized by thin-walled, dilated lymphatic vessels, lined by flattened endothelium, and frequently surrounded by lymphocytic aggregates. Stromal fibrosis with chronic inflammation, mast cells, and hemosiderin deposits are common.

Special Studies

The endothelium in lymphangiomas expresses D2-40, PROX1, CD31, and CD34.

Differential Diagnosis

The differential diagnosis includes hemangioma and various subtypes of hemangioendothelioma. D2-40 expression in the endothelial cells is helpful to support a lymphatic phenotype, and Prox1 is generally absent in capillary and cavernous hemangiomas. The lymphocyte aggregates commonly seen in lymphangioma are also not commonly seen in other vascular lesions.

Treatment and Prognosis

The standard treatment has been surgical excision, but frequent involvement of adjacent vital structures often makes total excision virtually impossible.[15] Malignant transformation does not occur. However, recurrences occur in up to 20% of cases and are minimized by complete resection of the tumor.[15] Deaths due to mediastinal lymphangioma are rare, and overall survival matches that of the general population.[15]

Hemangioma

Terminology

Hemangiomas have been traditionally classified according to the vessel size, into capillary and cavernous types, although most are mixed. Hemangiomas can be composed almost exclusively of veins of variable size, often having thick muscular walls (venous hemangioma).

Incidence and Clinical

Hemangiomas are rare benign vascular lesions estimated to constitute about 0.5% of all mediastinal tumors.[17] Most mediastinal hemangiomas are located in the anterior mediastinum,[18,19] and a few have been reported in the posterior mediastinum.[17,19–21] A small number are of proven thymic origin.[18,22] Seventy-five percent of the lesions appear before the age of 35 years, though they have been found between 2 months to 76 years of age.[19,20,23,24] There is no gender preponderance. Nearly half of all patients are symptomatic. The main symptoms include cough, chest pain, dyspnea, hoarseness, and dysphagia. Rarely, patients with mediastinal hemangioma present with bloody pleural effusion.[21]

Gross Pathology

Grossly, the lesions are hemorrhagic, and may be cystic. Most are well circumscribed,[18,21,23,25] but they may infiltrate surrounding structures, including veins, resulting in aneurysms.[22]

Microscopic Pathology

Histologically, the tumors can be divided into capillary and cavernous types based on vessel size, although these types are often intermixed and do not have clinical relevance. Capillary hemangiomas are characterized by a lobular and solid growth pattern featuring anastomosing and dilated small vascular channels lined by flattened endothelial cells without atypia. Cavernous hemangioma (Fig. 137.3) is characterized by large dilated vascular spaces filled with blood, often with areas showing interstitial inflammatory changes, fibrosis, and smooth muscle proliferation. Prominent regressive changes, including stromal hyalinization, dystrophic ossification, cystic and perivascular myxoid changes, and extensive fatty overgrowth, may be observed.[19,24] In some cases, it may be difficult to determine whether the lesion represents

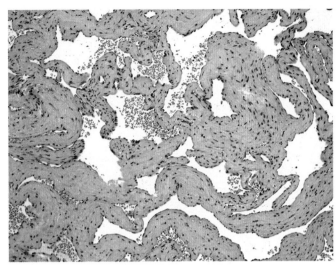

FIGURE 137.3 ▲ Cavernous hemangioma. Note large dilated vascular spaces (H&E, ×200).

a cavernous hemangioma or an arterial–venous malformation. The endothelial cells lining the vascular spaces are bland without atypia. Venous hemangiomas typically consist of large thick-walled muscular vessels, which are variably dilated and commonly display thrombosis.[25] Widely dilated vessels can show attenuation of their walls, mimicking a cavernous hemangioma.

Special Studies

Elastic stains reveal the absence of an internal elastic lamina. Immunohistochemical examination of the lining cells shows positivity for CD31, FLI1, FVIII, and CD34, consistent with a lesion of endothelial origin.

Differential Diagnosis

The differential diagnosis includes lymphangioma, arteriovenous malformation, and various subtypes of hemangioendothelioma. Absence of an internal elastic lamina aids in the distinction from an arteriovenous malformation, and this distinction is often clear on radiographic grounds, so correlation with radiographic and clinical features is often helpful. D2-40 and Prox1 expression is present in lymphangioma and is generally absent in capillary and cavernous hemangiomas. Hemangioendotheliomas are vascular tumors of intermediate malignancy. The subtype most commonly encountered in the mediastinum is epithelioid hemangioendothelioma (EHE), which generally does not form extracellular vascular structures, and therefore is readily distinguished from hemangioma based on morphologic features (see Chapter 93).

Treatment and Prognosis

The treatment of choice for mediastinal hemangioma is surgical resection. In general, tumors are excised without significant complication, although rarely bony invasion necessitates complex surgery.[26] Recurrences have not been reported for mediastinal hemangiomas.

Angiosarcoma

Terminology

Angiosarcoma is a malignant tumor that recapitulates the morphologic and functional features of endothelium to a variable degree.

Incidence and Clinical

Angiosarcoma is a rare neoplasm, accounting for only 1% to 2% of all sarcomas. It occurs most frequently in the skin and soft tissue and

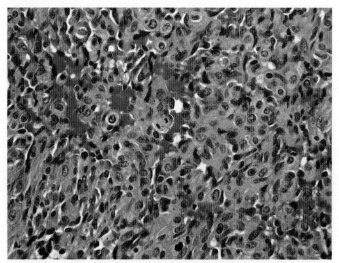

FIGURE 137.4 ▲ Angiosarcoma. Note high-grade epithelioid and spindled cells without clear vasoformation (H&E, ×200).

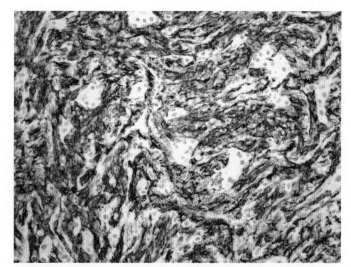

FIGURE 137.5 ▲ Angiosarcoma. Note positive staining for CD31 (anti-CD31, ×200).

rarely in the in the thoracic region. Those in the mediastinum occur most frequently in the pericardium, right side of the heart, and aorta.[27] Rarely, they involve the anterior mediastinum without involvement of the pericardial space.[28–31]

Angiosarcomas affect patients of all ages (mean 40.7 years). There is a slight male predominance. The main presenting symptoms of mediastinal angiosarcomas include chest pain, dyspnea, and cough.

The occurrence of an angiosarcomatous component in mediastinal germ cell tumors is an uncommon phenomenon.[30]

Gross Pathology

Macroscopically, the lesions are multinodular hemorrhagic masses with ill-defined margins.

Microscopic Pathology

Angiosarcomas display a wide range of morphologic appearances, ranging from areas of well-formed, anastomosing vessels to solid sheets of high-grade epithelioid, hobnailed or spindled cells without clear vasoformation (Fig. 137.4).[28–31] Multiple patterns may be present in the same tumor. Tumor cells have irregular, hyperchromatic, or vesicular nuclei and prominent nucleoli. Cytoplasm is eosinophilic with ill-defined borders. Hyaline globules may be seen. The tumor has infiltrative margins. Extensive hemorrhage is a characteristic feature.

Immunohistochemical Findings

Immunohistochemical studies show immunoreactivity for vascular markers including CD31, ERG, FLI-1, and CD34 (Fig. 137.5).[32] These stains often accentuate vessel lumen formation. Coexpression of epithelial antigens (low molecular weight cytokeratins) is not uncommon in epithelioid angiosarcoma (present in up to 20%), a fact that should be considered in distinguishing them from carcinoma.[32]

Differential Diagnosis

Angiosarcomas are often obviously high-grade malignant neoplasms, but some cases may show overlapping features with EHE. Morphologic features that favor a diagnosis of angiosarcoma include vasoformation of extracellular capillary-like spaces, blood lakes, papilla formation, prominent nucleoli, marked nuclear atypia, and high mitotic rate.[32] Conversely, histologic features including intracytoplasmic lumens, intranuclear vacuoles, and prominent matrix favor the diagnosis of EHE.[32] In particularly challenging cases, molecular testing for the *WWTR1-CAMTA1* fusion could be considered, as this is present in most EHEs, but not in angiosarcoma.[32]

In addition to other vascular lesions, the differential diagnosis includes malignant tumors that display cystic areas of hemorrhage, including carcinomas. Expression of endothelial markers is quite uncommon in epithelial malignancies. Epithelioid sarcoma with hemorrhagic foci (angiomatoid variant) may mimic angiosarcoma both morphologically and immunophenotypically: both tumors can express epithelial markers and CD34. Positive expression of other endothelial markers such as CD31, ERG, and FLI-1 are useful in excluding epithelioid sarcoma,[33] and nuclear loss of INI-1 (SMARCB1) expression would favor epithelioid sarcoma. Germ cell tumors with angiosarcomatous foci should also be considered in the differential diagnosis in the mediastinum, a diagnosis that would require identification of other germ cell elements.

Treatment and Prognosis

Management of primary mediastinal angiosarcoma needs a multidisciplinary approach, and is based mainly on radical resection. Despite their histologic similarity to angiosarcomas at other sites, primary angiosarcomas of the mediastinum appear to follow a more protracted clinical course than do their counterparts in other organ system including the heart, with pleural involvement a bad prognostic sign.[29,32]

The presence of an angiosarcomatous component in mediastinal germ cell tumor, even in a small amount, is associated with a poor clinical outcome.[30]

Lipoma

Terminology

Lipoma is a benign tumor composed of mature white adipocytes.[34]

Incidence and Clinical

Lipomas are common benign tumors that occur mostly in subcutaneous tissue but are rarely seen in the mediastinum.[35–39] Mediastinal lesions are classified as deep-seated lipomas. They typically arise within the anterior mediastinum, and are reported to represent 1.6% to 2.3% of all primary mediastinal tumors.[35–39] Although most mediastinal lipomas are asymptomatic and incidentally discovered, symptoms depend on their site and size. Mediastinal lipomas may occasionally lead to manifestations including coughing, dyspnea, heart disorder, or even death. Clinically, most tumors become apparent in patients at 40 to 60 years of age.[35–37,39–42]

Gross Pathology

Mediastinal lipomas are soft and usually well circumscribed.[42] The cut sections of the mass show multiple pale yellow lobules of different sizes separated from each other by fine septa of connective tissue.

Microscopic Pathology

Conventional lipoma is composed of lobules of mature adipocytes without any stromal atypia. Although in general benign lipomas can occasionally demonstrate fibrous tissue or thin-walled vessels, it is prudent to consider a diagnosis of well-differentiated liposarcoma (WDL) in all deep-seated fatty tumors and perform molecular studies when at all possible and thorough tumor sampling.

Special Studies

Immunohistochemistry is generally not helpful in the diagnosis of lipomas. Given the deep location in the mediastinum, the diagnosis of WDL must be carefully considered before the diagnosis of lipoma is rendered. Since some WDLs can appear very "lipoma-like," liberal use of FISH studies for *MDM2* or other genes in the amplified area of chromosome 12 should be considered before diagnosing lipoma at this site. Amplification of this area of chromosome 12 is typical of WDL but is not observed in lipoma; thus, this test can be very helpful in making this distinction.

Differential Diagnosis

Given the mediastinum is a deep location that shares many features with the retroperitoneum, mediastinal lipomas need to be carefully differentiated from WDLs, which are not uncommon at this site.[43] Careful morphologic examination should be performed for the atypical stromal cells, which characterize WDL. Methods to detect amplification of *MDM2* or nearby genes are very helpful to distinguish WDL from lipomas. Thymolipoma is also in the differential diagnosis, since the distribution of thymic tissue in those lesions can be patchy, so adequate sampling is important for correct classification.

Treatment and Prognosis

The outcome after resection of mediastinal lipomas is usually good.[44,45] However, they may recur locally, and the rate of recurrence after an excision has been reported to be <5%.[41]

Thymolipoma

Terminology

Thymolipoma is a benign tumor that contains an admixture of thymic parenchyma and mature adipose tissue.

Incidence and Clinical

Thymolipoma is a rare benign anterior mediastinal neoplasm of thymic origin. The pathogenesis remains controversial. The tumor accounts for 2% to 10% of all thymic neoplasms. Thymolipomas may occur at any age, but are most commonly encountered in young adults and are rarely described in children.[37,46,47] There is no sex predilection. Most patients are asymptomatic, with the lesion detected incidentally. Symptoms such as cough, dyspnea, arrhythmias, and chest pain may occur secondary to the displacement of mediastinal structures.[33,37,46–49] Similar to thymoma, thymolipoma has been reported to simultaneously occur with autoimmune diseases, such as myasthenia gravis, aplastic anemia, hypogammaglobulinemia and Graves disease.[33,50] Thymomas and thymic carcinoma arising within a thymolipoma are extremely rare.

Gross Pathology

The tumors are yellow, soft, and fairly well circumscribed. The cut sections of the mass show multiple pale yellow lobules of different sizes separated from each other by fine septa of connective tissue and focal solid areas.

Microscopic Pathology

Thymolipomas consist of abundant mature adipose tissue admixed with areas containing remnants of thymic tissue (Fig. 137.6). The

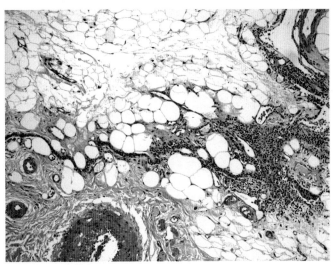

FIGURE 137.6 ▲ Thymolipoma. Note strands of atrophic thymic epithelium (H&E, ×200).

thymic tissue component may vary from strands of atrophic thymic epithelium to large areas containing inconspicuous thymic parenchyma with Hassall bodies.

Special Studies

Positive expression of cytokeratin markers such as CK5/6 and CK903 are useful in demonstrating the presence of atrophic thymic epithelium.

Differential Diagnosis

The main differential diagnoses include lipoma of the thymus (no epithelial component) and WDL (characteristic atypical stromal cells). Therefore, adequate sampling is important to make this distinction, and FISH studies for *MDM2* amplification could be considered if needed.

Treatment and Prognosis

Local excision is curative. There have been no reports of recurrences or tumor-related deaths.

Liposarcoma

Terminology

Liposarcomas of the mediastinum include most types reported in soft tissue. The most common is WDL, followed by dedifferentiated liposarcoma, pleomorphic liposarcoma, and myxoid liposarcomas.[43,51]

Incidence and Clinical

Primary liposarcomas of the mediastinum constitute <1% of all mediastinal tumors.[34,38,43,51–54] The tumors can attain massive sizes and can arise in all mediastinal compartments, most commonly in the anterior and posterior. The tumor affects patients of all ages, with a mean in the 50's, and a range from childhood (3 years) to 73 years.[43,51] There is no gender preponderance. Clinical manifestations of mediastinal liposarcomas refer to a space-occupying mass and may include hoarseness, dysphagia, chest pain, cough and, occasionally, superior vena cava syndrome.

Gross Pathology

Liposarcomas present as well-circumscribed, multinodular masses, showing yellow to white, firm and/or gelatinous cut surface, depending on the proportion of adipocytic, fibrous and/or myxoid areas. Areas of necrosis are common.

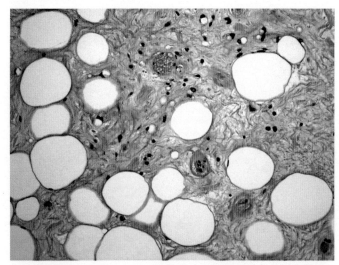

FIGURE 137.7 ▲ Well-differentiated liposarcoma. Note bizarre stromal cells with hyperchromatic nuclei (H&E, ×200).

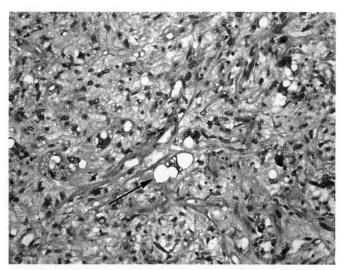

FIGURE 137.9 ▲ Pleomorphic liposarcoma. Note atypical pleomorphic cells with occasional lipoblasts with enlarged pleomorphic and hyperchromatic nuclei (*arrow*).

Microscopic Pathology

Almost 40% of reported mediastinal liposarcomas are of the well-differentiated type.[43,51] The morphologic hallmark of WDL is the hyperchromatic atypical stromal cells, which have dark, enlarged, angulated nuclei. These atypical cells are often concentrated in fibrous bands and around vascular structures (where they may be present in the wall of thick-walled vessels) but may be quite subtle when present in the lobules of mature adipocytes (Fig. 137.7). Careful examination and adequate sampling should be performed to look for areas of dedifferentiation, as this confers metastatic potential.

Dedifferentiated liposarcoma (almost 30% of mediastinal liposarcoma) is characterized by morphologic progression from WDL to a nonlipogenic sarcoma (Fig. 137.8). This transition is usually abrupt, and the nonlipogenic areas are usually high grade, although low-grade dedifferentiation can also occur. Classification of dedifferentiated liposarcoma into low and high grade is recommended, as this may have prognostic significance. Well-differentiated and dedifferentiated liposarcoma share the same genetic abnormality, characterized by giant marker and ring chromosomes composed of amplified material from chromosome 12q13-15, including the genes *MDM2*, *CDK4*, and *CPM*, among others.

Pleomorphic liposarcomas (almost 25% of mediastinal sarcomas)[43,51] are high-grade sarcomas with either a pleomorphic spindled or epithelioid pattern, showing variable numbers of pleomorphic lipoblasts. Pleomorphic lipoblasts are cells with enlarged pleomorphic and hyperchromatic nuclei, containing multiple lipid vacuoles in the cytoplasm, which characteristically indent the pleomorphic nucleus (Fig. 137.9). Identification of pleomorphic lipoblasts is the key morphologic feature of pleomorphic liposarcoma, since they are not typically seen in other types of liposarcoma. Very rare examples of dedifferentiated liposarcoma can show pleomorphic lipoblasts, so careful examination for a well differentiated component should be performed. Pleomorphic liposarcomas are generally not associated with a well-differentiated precursor. Rare tumors with well-differentiated and pleomorphic components have been shown to have amplification of chromosome 12q13-15, which supports classification as dedifferentiated liposarcoma.[44] Pleomorphic liposarcomas do not have a recurrent genetic abnormality identified to date, and instead show a complex karyotype typical of many high-grade sarcomas.

Myxoid liposarcoma constitutes <10% of mediastinal liposarcoma and is typically composed of a hypocellular proliferation of small

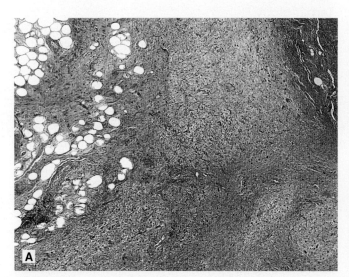

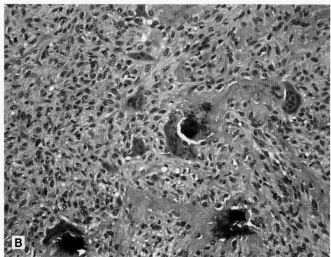

FIGURE 137.8 ▲ Dedifferentiated liposarcoma. **A.** Note areas of well-differentiated liposarcoma adjacent to differentiated areas. **B.** Higher magnification of dedifferentiated area. There are foci of bone formation.

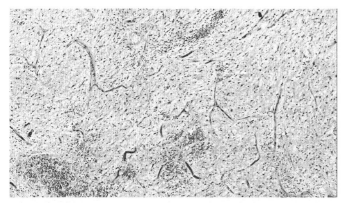

FIGURE 137.10 ▲ Myxoid liposarcoma. A key to diagnosis is the vascular pattern of thin-walled arborizing vessels in a paucicellular myxoid stroma.

primitive mesenchymal cells set in a myxoid background, and associated with a varying number of monovacuolated ("signet ring cell") lipoblasts (Fig. 137.10). A very helpful morphologic clue is the presence of a thin-walled capillary network organized in a plexiform pattern. Hypercellular areas that exhibit an undifferentiated round-cell morphology represent tumor progression to high-grade myxoid liposarcoma ("round cell liposarcoma"). Myxoid liposarcoma is characterized genetically by a recurrent t(12;16)(q13;p11), which leads to the *FUS-DDIT3* fusion gene.

Unusual histologic features that have been described in mediastinal liposarcomas include lipoleiomyosarcoma, dedifferentiated liposarcoma with "meningothelial"-like dedifferentiation, pleomorphic liposarcoma with epithelioid and myxoid change, and pleomorphic liposarcoma resembling myxofibrosarcoma with atypical hyperchromatic spindle cells.[43,51]

Differential Diagnosis

The differential diagnosis of WDL includes benign lipoma; the differential diagnosis of pleomorphic and dedifferentiated liposarcoma includes other subtypes of sarcoma; and the differentiated diagnosis of myxoid liposarcoma includes benign myxoid lesions that rarely if ever occur in the mediastinum (myxoma, myxoid dermatofibrosarcoma, myxoid chondrosarcoma) and myxoid undifferentiated pleomorphic sarcoma. Targeted genetic studies (as needed) and complete sampling of tumor are key in establishing the correct diagnosis.

Treatment and Prognosis

The histologic type and the success of surgical resection are the factors that influence the behavior and prognosis of mediastinal liposarcoma. Local recurrence occurs in 25% of patients. Death from disease is uncommon in WDL, but metastasis and progressive disease are not uncommon in dedifferentiated, pleomorphic, and myxoid liposarcoma.[43,51]

Rhabdomyosarcoma

The mediastinum is a rare site of rhabdomyosarcoma, which involves the thymus or the anterior mediastinum and most commonly occurs as a complication of a germ cell tumor.[30,55-57] The tumors can occur in adults and children, and follow a very aggressive clinical course with frequent recurrences and rapid dissemination.[30,55-57]

Other Rare Neoplasms

Other rare thymic/mediastinal soft tissue tumors include Ewing sarcoma/PNET,[45,58] leiomyosarcoma,[59] chondrosarcoma,[60] osteosarcoma,[61] pleomorphic sarcoma/malignant fibrous histiocytoma, inflammatory myofibroblastic tumor,[62] meningioma,[63,64] chordoma,[65] myelolipoma,[40] and extramedullary hematopoietic tumors.[66] Malignant melanoma may occur in the mediastinum without apparent extrathoracic primary.[67]

Metastatic Neoplasms

Most metastases to the mediastinum involve lymph node spread from lung cancers (see chapter 73). Other carcinomas may metastasize to mediastinal lymph nodes, including renal cell carcinomas, breast, and colon cancers.[68-70] Sarcomas metastatic to the mediastinum may rarely cause confusion with primary mediastinal tumors.[71,72] Melanomas not infrequently metastasize to mediastinal lymph nodes, occasionally mimicking a primary tumor.[73,74]

REFERENCES

1. Moran CA, Suster S, Fishback N, et al. Mediastinal paragangliomas. A clinicopathologic and immunohistochemical study of 16 cases. *Cancer.* 1993;72:2358–2364.
2. Shakir M, Blossom G, Lippert J. Anterior mediastinal paraganglioma: a case for preoperative embolization. *World J Surg Oncol.* 2012;10:134.
3. Suzawa K, Yamamoto H, Ichimura K, et al. Asymptomatic but functional paraganglioma of the posterior mediastinum. *Ann Thorac Surg.* 2014;97:1077–1080.
4. Gallivan MV, Chun B, Rowden G, et al. Intrathoracic paravertebral malignant paraganglioma. *Arch Pathol Lab Med.* 1980;104:46–51.
5. Takahashi T, Nogimura H, Kuriki K, et al. Superior mediastinal paraganglioma associated with von Hippel-Lindau syndrome: report of a case. *World J Surg Oncol.* 2014;12:74.
6. van Nederveen FH, Gaal J, Favier J, et al. An immunohistochemical procedure to detect patients with paraganglioma and phaeochromocytoma with germline SDHB, SDHC, or SDHD gene mutations: a retrospective and prospective analysis. *Lancet Oncol.* 2009;10:764–771.
7. Wichmann CL, Helmchen B, Weber A, et al. An unusual case of mediastinal mass and bilateral nodules. *Asian Cardiovasc Thorac Ann.* 2013;22:623–626.
8. Brown SM, Myssiorek D. Lateral thyrotomy for excision of laryngeal paragangliomas. *Laryngoscope.* 2006;116:157–159.
9. Lamy AL, Fradet GJ, Luoma A, et al. Anterior and middle mediastinum paraganglioma: complete resection is the treatment of choice. *Ann Thorac Surg.* 1994;57:249–252.
10. Charruau L, Parrens M, Jougon J, et al. Mediastinal lymphangioma in adults: CT and MR imaging features. *Eur Radiol.* 2000;10:1310–1314.
11. Choi SH, Kim L, Lee KH, et al. Mediastinal lymphangioma treated using endobronchial ultrasound-guided transbronchial needle aspiration. *Respiration.* 2012;84:518–521.
12. Fokkema JP, Paul MA, Vrouenraets BC. Mediastinal lymphangioma in an adult. *Ann R Coll Surg Engl.* 2014;96:e24–e25.
13. Handa R, Kale R, Upadhyay KK. Isolated mediastinal lymphangioma herniating through the intercostal space. *Asian J Surg.* 2004;27:241–242.
14. Oshikiri T, Morikawa T, Jinushi E, et al. Five cases of the lymphangioma of the mediastinum in adult. *Ann Thorac Cardiovasc Surg.* 2001;7:103–105.
15. Park JG, Aubry MC, Godfrey JA, et al. Mediastinal lymphangioma: Mayo Clinic experience of 25 cases. *Mayo Clin Proc.* 2006;81:1197–1203.
16. Shaffer K, Rosado-de-Christenson ML, Patz EF, Jr., et al. Thoracic lymphangioma in adults: CT and MR imaging features. *AJR Am J Roentgenol.* 1994;162:283–289.
17. Hammoumi MM, Sinaa M, Arsalane A, et al. Mediastinal cystic haemangiomas: a two cases report and review of the literature. *Heart Lung Circ.* 2014;23:e118–e121.
18. Yamazaki A, Miyamoto H, Saito Y, et al. Cavernous hemangioma of the anterior mediastinum: case report and 50-year review of Japanese cases. *Jpn J Thorac Cardiovasc Surg.* 2006;54:221–224.
19. Moran CA, Suster S. Mediastinal hemangiomas: a study of 18 cases with emphasis on the spectrum of morphological features. *Hum Pathol.* 1995;26:416–421.
20. Das A, Das SK, Basuthakur S, et al. Hemangioma in the posterior mediastinum. *Lung India.* 2014;31:186–188.
21. Kubokura H, Okamoto J, Hoshina H, et al. Mediastinal cystic hemangioma presenting as bilateral bloody pleural effusion: a case report. *J Nippon Med Sch.* 2012;79:381–384.
22. Akiba T, Morikawa T, Hirayama S, et al. Thymic haemangioma presenting with a left innominate vein aneurysm: insight into the aetiology. *Interact Cardiovasc Thorac Surg.* 2012;15:925–927.

23. McAdams HP, Rosado-de-Christenson ML, Moran CA. Mediastinal hemangioma: radiographic and CT features in 14 patients. *Radiology.* 1994;193:399–402.

24. Cohen AJ, Sbaschnig RJ, Hochholzer L, et al. Mediastinal hemangiomas. *Ann Thorac Surg.* 1987;43:656–659.

25. Odaka M, Nakada T, Asano H, et al. Thoracoscopic resection of a mediastinal venous hemangioma: report of a case. *Surg Today.* 2011;41:1455–1457.

26. Yun T, Suzuki H, Tagawa T, et al. Cavernous hemangioma of the posterior mediastinum with bony invasion. *Gen Thorac Cardiovasc Surg.* 2014.

27. Fatima J, Duncan AA, Maleszewski JJ, et al. Primary angiosarcoma of the aorta, great vessels, and the heart. *J Vasc Surg.* 2013;57:756–764.

28. Tane S, Tanaka Y, Tauchi S, et al. Radically resected epithelioid angiosarcoma that originated in the mediastinum. *Gen Thorac Cardiovasc Surg.* 2011;59:503–506.

29. Weissferdt A, Kalhor N, Suster S, et al. Primary angiosarcomas of the anterior mediastinum: a clinicopathologic and immunohistochemical study of 9 cases. *Hum Pathol.* 2010;41:1711–1717.

30. Contreras AL, Punar M, Tamboli P, et al. Mediastinal germ cell tumors with an angiosarcomatous component: a report of 12 cases. *Hum Pathol.* 2010;41:832–837.

31. Deyrup AT, Miettinen M, North PE, et al. Angiosarcomas arising in the viscera and soft tissue of children and young adults: a clinicopathologic study of 15 cases. *Am J Surg Pathol.* 2009;33:264–269.

32. Anderson T, Zhang L, Hameed M, et al. Thoracic epithelioid malignant vascular tumors: a clinicopathologic study of 52 cases with emphasis on pathologic grading and molecular studies of WWTR1-CAMTA1 fusions. *Am J Surg Pathol.* 2015;39:132–139.

33. Tsukioka T, Inoue K, Iwata T, et al. Thymolipoma associated with myasthenia gravis. *Gen Thorac Cardiovasc Surg.* 2007;55:26–28.

34. Marulli G, Rea F, Feltracco P, et al. Successful resection of a giant primary liposarcoma of the posterior mediastinum. *J Thorac Oncol.* 2007;2:453–455.

35. La Mantia E, Franco R, Rocco R, et al. Spindle cell lipoma: a rare tumor of the mediastinum. *J Thorac Dis.* 2013;5:E152–E154.

36. Marreez YM, Roy W, Roque R, et al. The rare mediastinal lipoma: a postmortem case report. *Int J Clin Exp Pathol.* 2012;5:991–995.

37. Gaerte SC, Meyer CA, Winer-Muram HT, et al. Fat-containing lesions of the chest. *Radiographics.* 2002;22 Spec No:S61–S78.

38. Klimstra DS, Moran CA, Perino G, et al. Liposarcoma of the anterior mediastinum and thymus. A clinicopathologic study of 28 cases. *Am J Surg Pathol.* 1995;19:782–791.

39. Williams WT, Parsons WH. Intrathoracic lipomas. *J Thorac Surg.* 1957;33:785–790.

40. Vaziri M, Sadeghipour A, Pazooki A, et al. Primary mediastinal myelolipoma. *Ann Thorac Surg.* 2008;85:1805–1806.

41. Sakurai H, Kaji M, Yamazaki K, et al. Intrathoracic lipomas: their clinicopathological behaviors are not as straightforward as expected. *Ann Thorac Surg.* 2008;86:261–165.

42. Vougiouklakis T, Mitselou A, Agnantis NJ. Giant lipoma: an unusual cause of intrathoracic mass. *Pathol Res Pract.* 2006;202:47–49.

43. Hahn HP, Fletcher CD. Primary mediastinal liposarcoma: clinicopathologic analysis of 24 cases. *Am J Surg Pathol.* 2007;31:1868–1874.

44. Boland JM, Weiss SW, Oliveira AM, et al. Liposarcomas with mixed well-differentiated and pleomorphic features: a clinicopathologic study of 12 cases. *Am J Surg Pathol.* 2010;34:837–843.

45. Schweigert M, Meyer C, Wolf F, et al. Peripheral primitive neuroectodermal tumor of the thymus. *Interact Cardiovasc Thorac Surg.* 2011;12:303–305.

46. Parakh A, Singh V, Subramaniam R, et al. Giant thymolipoma in an infant. *Paediatr Int Child Health.* 2014;34:230–232.

47. Moran CA, Rosado-de-Christenson M, Suster S. Thymolipoma: clinicopathologic review of 33 cases. *Mod Pathol.* 1995;8:741–744.

48. Ajaz B, Tran TA, Truong T, et al. Thymolipoma with sebaceous differentiation: a hitherto unreported variant of thymolipoma. *Int J Surg Pathol.* 2013;21:526–530.

49. Haddad H, Joudeh A, El-Taani H, et al. Thymoma and thymic carcinoma arising in a thymolipoma: report of a unique case. *Int J Surg Pathol.* 2009;17:55–59.

50. Huang CS, Li WY, Lee PC, et al. Analysis of outcomes following surgical treatment of thymolipomatous myasthenia gravis: comparison with thymomatous and non-thymomatous myasthenia gravis. *Interact Cardiovasc Thorac Surg.* 2014;18:475–481.

51. Boland JM, Colby TV, Folpe AL. Liposarcomas of the mediastinum and thorax: a clinicopathologic and molecular cytogenetic study of 24 cases, emphasizing unusual and diverse histologic features. *Am J Surg Pathol.* 2012;36:1395–1403.

52. Weissferdt A, Moran CA. Lipomatous tumors of the anterior mediastinum with muscle differentiation: a clinicopathological and immunohistochemical study of three cases. *Virchows Arch.* 2014;464:489–493.

53. Chen M, Yang J, Zhu L, et al. Primary intrathoracic liposarcoma: a clinicopathologic study and prognostic analysis of 23 cases. *J Cardiothorac Surg.* 2014;9:119.

54. Barbetakis N, Asteriou C, Kleontas A, et al. Primary pleomorphic liposarcoma: a rare mediastinal tumor. *Interact Cardiovasc Thorac Surg.* 2010;11:327.

55. Chu WP. Anterior mediastinal alveolar rhabdomyosarcoma in an infant: rare site for a common paediatric tumour. *Hong Kong Med J.* 2013;19:458–459.

56. Panasuk DB, Bauer TL, Davies AL, et al. Common malignancies with uncommon sites of presentation: case 1. Anterior mediastinal rhabdomyosarcoma. *J Clin Oncol.* 2003;21:4455–4456.

57. Suster S, Moran CA, Koss MN. Rhabdomyosarcomas of the anterior mediastinum: report of four cases unassociated with germ cell, teratomatous, or thymic carcinomatous components. *Hum Pathol.* 1994;25:349–356.

58. Manduch M, Dexter DF, Ellis PM, et al. Extraskeletal Ewing's sarcoma/primitive neuroectodermal tumor of the posterior mediastinum with t(11;22)(q24;q12). *Tumori.* 2008;94:888–891.

59. Moran CA, Suster S, Perino G, et al. Malignant smooth muscle tumors presenting as mediastinal soft tissue masses. A clinicopathologic study of 10 cases. *Cancer.* 1994;74:2251–2260.

60. Suster S, Moran CA. Malignant cartilaginous tumors of the mediastinum: clinicopathological study of six cases presenting as extraskeletal soft tissue masses. *Hum Pathol.* 1997;28:588–594.

61. Hishida T, Yoshida J, Nishimura M, et al. Extraskeletal osteosarcoma arising in anterior mediastinum: brief report with a review of the literature. *J Thorac Oncol.* 2009;4:927–929.

62. Meng X, Wang R. Inflammatory myofibroblastic tumor occurs in the mediastinum. *J Cancer Res Ther.* 2013;9:721–723.

63. Mogi A, Hirato J, Kosaka T, et al. Primary mediastinal atypical meningioma: report of a case and literature review. *World J Surg Oncol.* 2012;10:17.

64. Falleni M, Roz E, Dessy E, et al. Primary intrathoracic meningioma: histopathological, immunohistochemical and ultrastructural study of two cases. *Virchows Arch.* 2001;439:196–200.

65. Suster S and Moran CA. Chordomas of the mediastinum: clinicopathologic, immunohistochemical, and ultrastructural study of six cases presenting as posterior mediastinal masses. *Hum Pathol.* 1995;26:1354–1362.

66. Ramasamy K, Lim Z, Pagliuca A, et al. Acute myeloid leukaemia presenting with mediastinal myeloid sarcoma: report of three cases and review of literature. *Leuk Lymphoma.* 2007;48:290–294.

67. Bavi P, Shet T, Gujral S. Malignant melanoma of mediastinum misdiagnosed as a spindle cell thymoma in a fine needle aspirate: a case report. *Acta Cytol.* 2005;49:424–426

68. Carbonari A, Camunha M, Binato M, et al. A rare case of mediastinal metastasis of ovarian carcinoma diagnosed by endobronchial ultrasound-guided transbronchial needle aspiration (EBUS-TBNA). *J Thorac Dis.* 2015;7:E505–E508

69. Dhillon SS, Harris K, Pokharel S, et al. Calcified Mediastinal Metastasis of Ovarian Cancer Mimicking Broncholithiasis. *J Bronchology Interv Pulmonol.* 2016

70. Kuba H, Sato N, Uchiyama A, et al. Mediastinal lymph node metastasis of colon cancer: report of a case. *Surg Today.* 1999;29:375–377

71. Grover SB, Pathak A, Agarwal A, et al. An unusual mediastinal mass due to metastasis. *Indian J Chest Dis Allied Sci.* 1999;41:163–168

72. Hambleton C, Noureldine S, Gill F, et al. Myxofibrosarcoma with metastasis to the lungs, pleura, and mediastinum: a case report and review of literature. *Int J Clin Exp Med.* 2012;5:92–95

73. Kiparakis M, Lazopoulos G, Koutsopoulos A, et al. Metastatic Ocular Melanoma Presenting as a Heart-Compressing Mediastinal Mass. *Ann Thorac Surg.* 2015;100:1448–1450

74. Webb WR. Hilar and mediastinal lymph node metastases in malignant melanoma. *AJR Am J Roentgenol.* 1979;133:805–810

SECTION ONE
GENERAL TOPICS

138 Examination of Cardiovascular Specimens

Joseph J. Maleszewski, M.D., and Allen P. Burke, M.D.

Overview

Cardiac specimens may be procured for examination either at autopsy or surgery. Autopsy-derived specimens are in the context of a forensic (legal) investigation or a medical procedure (so-called hospital autopsy). Surgical specimens are removed in the course of biopsy, excision, repair, or replacement of diseased cardiovascular tissue and may be in the form of biopsies, valve resections or repairs, myectomies, repairs of congenital heart disease, explants, and other procedures.

Regardless of the setting in which cardiac tissue is to be examined, there are common principles that should be kept in mind prior to handling and/or processing. First and foremost, a thorough understanding of the clinical situation in which the tissue was procured is essential. The documentation, dissection, tissue processing, and reporting will all be contingent upon the clinical scenario. In this chapter and those that follow, emphasis is placed on how to handle and evaluate specimens in the context of different circumstances. Second, documentation of the examination and handling is necessary throughout the process and ideally includes both thorough written description as well as liberal photography. Finally, a uniform approach to documentation is strongly encouraged for consistency and efficiency.

Cardiac Examination at Autopsy

General Considerations

Autopsy-derived cardiovascular specimens may be evaluated in the context of either a forensic or medical autopsy. In the case of forensic evaluation, the objective is primarily to determine cause and manner of death. In establishing a natural manner of death, it is important to exclude noncardiac causes as the heart may be grossly and microscopically normal in cases of sudden arrhythmic death (see Chapter 141). Conversely, it is also important to keep in mind that arrhythmic substrates may exist in individuals who die of noncardiac causes.

Medical (nonforensic) autopsies may be performed for a number of reasons. Like their forensic counterparts, they also may be performed to more definitively establish a cause of death (though the manner is almost invariably natural). They also may be performed to document pathology and interventions (including potential complications thereof) (Table 138.1).

In either forensic or medical autopsy, it may be important to preserve tissue for molecular study, especially in the setting of sudden death (see Chapter 141). Such can typically be best accomplished by reserving whole blood in an EDTA (lavender top) tube until the autopsy is completed. Increasingly, paraffin samples can be utilized to answer many questions with newer-generation nucleic acid sequencing techniques.

Whether dealing with a forensic or medical autopsy, appropriate evaluation of the patient history and medical record is paramount. Information contained in the history will help to guide the examination, documentation, and handling. Important facts to know prior to autopsy include changes in circulatory status (abrupt or gradual), cardiac rhythms, and cardiac interventions. An example of a handout to be completed prior to autopsy is illustrated in Table 138.2.

Finally, the method of dissection and evaluation described below is a general dissection method. Although nearly all varieties of congenital and acquired heart disease can be evaluated and documented using

---

TABLE 138.1 Goals of Cardiac Evaluation at Autopsy

Forensic autopsy
- Establish the manner of death (natural, accident, homicide, suicide)
- Identify a natural cardiac cause if extracardiac and unnatural causes have been excluded
- Identify the cause as unexplained arrhythmia in the absence of significant cardiac and extracardiac findings (see Chapter 141)

Medical autopsy (and to a lesser extent forensic autopsies)
- Document cardiac pathology, including iatrogenic
- Correlate cardiac findings with history and interventions
- Determine a cardiac or noncardiac cause of death
- Determine possible contributing cardiac causes of death
- Preserve the specimen after proper dissection and diagnosis, if allowed in the autopsy permit, for a reasonable period of time for potential subsequent investigations
- Perform postmortem radiographs in cases of stents or prosthesis, when indicated
- Photograph the specimen as necessary

TABLE 138.2 Worksheet for Preautopsy Preparation

Date of admission _____

Date of admission at outside facility (if transferred) _____

Major problem at admission _____

Date of death and time interval between admission and death: _____

Recent medical history (cause for admission):_____

Important prior medical and surgical history[a]:_____

_____

Hospital course, surgical interventions, and dates, including complications:
_____
_____
_____

Hospital course, medical complications, and dates: _____
_____
_____
_____
_____

Circumstances of death[b]:_____

Presumed cause of death (clinical): _____

Questions to be answered: _____
_____
_____

[a]Prior cardiac operative notes are very helpful. If not immediately available, they can be accessed after autopsy and before cardiac dissection, which generally occurs after proper fixation.
[b]For example, hypotensive shock, hemorrhage, septic shock, cardiogenic shock, shock of unclear etiology; sudden death (witness or not), cardiac arrest, respiratory arrest, cardiorespiratory arrest or arrest of uncertain etiology; brain death with removal of life support.

this method, other dissection techniques (such as dissecting along tomographic planes or base-of-the heart dissections) can be of utility in certain circumstances.

Removal of the Heart at Autopsy

The examination of the adult heart begins after the anterior chest plate has been removed. The pericardium is inspected for effusions (abnormal amounts of fluid; normal <50 mL of straw-colored fluid) or blood, and the amount of pericardial fluid is measured. The surface of the visceral as well as parietal pericardium is also examined for exudates, adhesions, tumor nodules, or other lesions. The heart can then be removed from the thorax, or the heart and lungs can be removed en bloc. The latter approach is described as it allows the removal of the abdominal viscera to proceed while the thoracic block is being evaluated. The superior and inferior venae cavae should be cut leaving ~1 cm of each on the thoracic block. The aortic arch vessels should likewise be cut ~1 cm from their origins. Transection of the esophagus and trachea can proceed at the level of the thoracic inlet. At this point, reflection of the block from superior to inferior can proceed, using scissors to separate the periaortic tissue from the vertebral bodies. The esophagus may be tied off at the diaphragmatic crux and then transected distally as well.

Once the thoracic block is removed, a posterior approach is recommended to begin separation of the pulmonary venous connections. First, the esophagus is reflected upward and removed. In fetal autopsies, careful evaluation for a tracheoesophageal fistula is warranted (usually by first opening the esophagus posteriorly and visually inspecting the anterior luminal surface). Next, the posterior parietal pericardium is incised from the inferior edge up to the carina, effectively dividing it into left and right portions. Reflecting these respective portions will reveal the pulmonary venous drainage that typically includes a right-sided upper and lower pulmonary vein as well as a left-sided upper and lower pulmonary vein. Blunt dissection of the pericardium around these veins will enable the prosector to leave 1 cm of each vein attached to the left atrium.

After the pulmonary veins have been separated, the block may be turned over and approached from the anterior aspect. Excess anterior parietal pericardium may be removed at this time. The pulmonary artery should be transected ~1 cm above the infundibulum, and the aorta should be transected just beyond the sinotubular junction. It is important to keep in mind that the ascending aorta and main pulmonary artery are nearly perpendicular to one another, with the former directed toward the right shoulder and the latter directed toward the left shoulder. Thus, the cuts should be made at nearly 90 degrees with respect to one another to achieve perfect cross sections. The superior vena cava can then be reflected anteriorly and inferiorly.

At this point, the only connection the heart will have to the thoracic block is through a fold of fibroadipose tissue situated just inferior to right and left pulmonary arteries. Hence, careful separation just beneath the pulmonary bifurcation will effectively separate the heart from the rest of the thoracic block. The main pulmonary artery and branches can then be dissected with the lungs, including evaluation for pulmonary embolism.

Depending on the clinical/forensic questions to be addressed, it may be useful to fix the heart (by perfusion or otherwise) at this point for a specific dissection and/or consultation. Such perfusion may be achieved by placing the heart several feet below a formalin source. The aorta, one of the vena cava, and one of the pulmonary veins can be cannulated with clamps, tubes, and/or glass cannulas. All remaining vascular connections can be tied off. Simple perfusion for 20 minutes, followed by formalin submersion, will often allow adequate fixation. If such perfusion is not possible, a short-axis cut at the midventricular level, parallel to the cardiac base (dividing the heart into apical and basal halves), will usually allow for adequate fixation of the external and internal structures.

External Examination and Weighing the Heart

Following separation of the heart from the thoracic block (and fixation, if performed) (Fig. 138.1A), the remaining great arteries may be trimmed from the heart (~1 cm above the semilunar valves) (Fig. 138.1B, C).

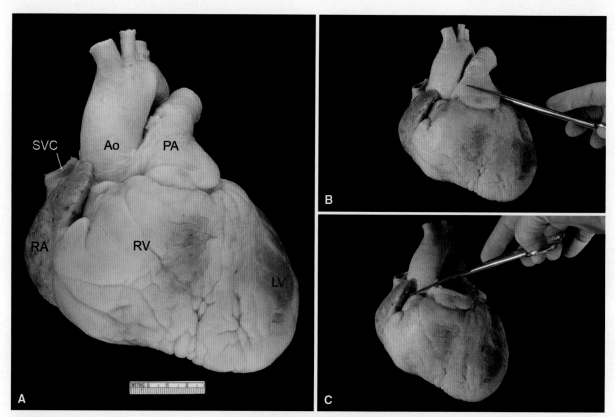

FIGURE 138.1 ▲ **A.** External, anterior, view of the heart procured at the time of autopsy. From this perspective, the following structures can be readily identified: right atrium (RA), right ventricle (RV), left ventricle (LV), superior vena cava (SVC), ascending aorta (Ao), and the main pulmonary artery (PA). **B.** Transection of the pulmonary artery, ~1 cm above the pulmonary valve commissures. **C.** Transection of the ascending aorta, ~1 cm above the aortic valve.

The great arteries are positioned ~60 to 90 degrees relative to one another, necessitating cuts in different planes. After removal of the great arteries, the heart should be weighed. The heart should be free of postmortem clot, and gentle manual removal through the venae cavae or pulmonary veins is usually adequate. The presence of a large or firm clot within the heart may necessitate reweighing the heart after dissection.

Heart weight should be compared to standard nomograms, given the individuals body size.[1,2] In general, body weight is a better correlate with heart weight than height, unless the decedent is morbidly obese or cachectic. As a rule of thumb, male heart weight is ~0.45% of body weight and female heart weight is ~0.4% of body weight.[3,4]

Heart weight is the single best indicator of cardiac hypertrophy. After weighing, the external surfaces of the heart should be inspected and described. The epicardial surface should be smooth and glistening.

Examination of the Coronary Arteries

In general, the epicardial coronary arteries are best evaluated after removal from the heart and decalcification (depending on the firmness of the vessels themselves). Radiographic evaluation of the heart specimen can help in the determination of the extent of coronary calcification, as well as calcification in other areas of the heart (Fig. 138.2). Such radiographic evaluation can also be useful in the identification and localization of intravascular stents or other intracardiac hardware.

The epicardial course should be described along with the dominance pattern (Fig. 138.3). Approximately 70% of hearts will exhibit right dominance, in which the posterior descending coronary artery is derived from the right coronary artery. About 20% of the time, the posterior descending coronary artery is derived from the left circumflex coronary artery, with the balance consisting of those that exhibit shared (derived from a combination of right coronary and left circumflex coronary arteries) dominance. The coronary arteries are best handled after removal from the heart (Fig. 138.4).

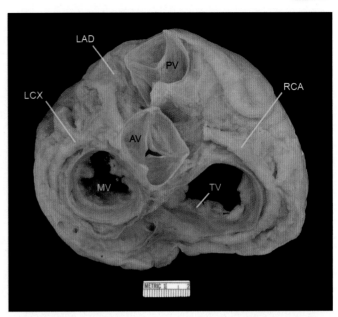

FIGURE 138.3 ▲ Base of the heart view, from an autopsy specimen (atria removed). This view is a particularly good perspective to evaluate the position of the four major cardiac valves with respect to one another. The aortic valve (AV) is centrally placed, with the pulmonary valve (PV) located anterior and slightly leftward. The mitral valve (MV) is situated leftward and posteroinferior to the AV, and the tricuspid valve (TV) is rightward and posteroinferior. The course of the epicardial coronary arteries, including the left anterior descending (LAD), left circumflex (LCX), and right coronary artery (RCA), can also be seen from this vantage.

Following decalcification (if necessary) the coronary arteries should be transversely sectioned at 2- to 3-mm intervals. Careful inspection of each cross section should commence with documentation of the areas of maximal narrowing. Areas of maximal narrowing should also typically be evaluated by microscopy.

If stents are present in the coronary tree, techniques for dissolving such have been previously described and can allow for subsequent histopathologic assessment of the stented arterial segment.[5,6]

Sectioning and Dissection of the Heart

After removal of the coronary arteries, the heart can be serially sectioned, beginning at the apex. Such sections should be made along the short axis, parallel to the cardiac base (or atrioventricular plane). Eight- to twelve-millimeter sections can be made serially to the midventricular level (Fig. 138.5). Typically, the last section should be just below the tips of the papillary muscles. The serially sectioned short-axis slices can then be laid out and the myocardium examined for uniformity and thickness (Fig. 138.5C).

Measurements of wall thickness should be documented to include the left ventricular free wall, ventricular septum, and right ventricle (Fig. 138.6). Such measurements should *not* include the trabeculations or papillary muscles. Mention of whether or not the thickness was uniform should be made. If disproportionate thickening is identified, indicating the measurement and the level (apical, midventricular, or basal) of said thickening should be documented. In general, the adult left ventricular free wall is 8 to 12 mm in thickness. The septum is usually between 10 and 15 mm in thickness. The normal septum to free wall ratio (VS:LVFW) is <1.3. VS:LVFW >1.2 is considered disproportionate and raises concern for the presence of disease (e.g., hypertrophic cardiomyopathy, amyloidosis).

The chamber dimensions should also be documented, to allow for assessment of dilatation. Because the left ventricle is circular in the short axis, two measurements perpendicular to one another can be taken and averaged. As above, these measurements should also

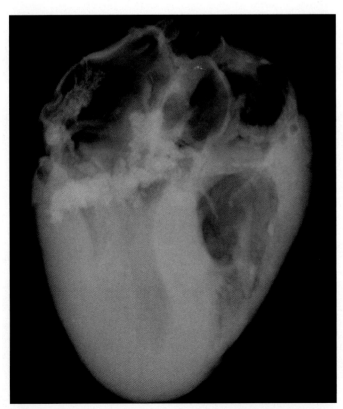

FIGURE 138.2 ▲ Postmortem radiograph of the heart. Radiographic study can reveal the location and extent of calcifications in the epicardial coronary vessels, myocardium, and cardiac valves. In this instance, the mitral valve annulus exhibits extensive calcification.

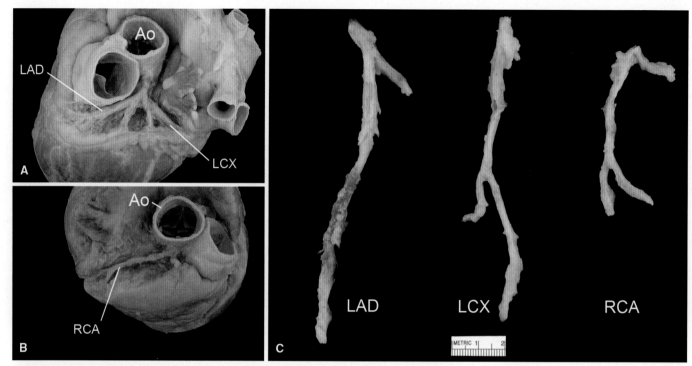

FIGURE 138.4 ▲ Dissection and removal of the coronary arteries. **A.** The left main is identified, arising from the left aortic sinus of the aortic root (Ao) and will bifurcate into the left anterior descending (LAD) and left circumflex (LCX) coronary arteries. The LAD will travel in the anterior interventricular sulcus, while the LCX travels in the left atrioventricular sulcus to give rise to the posterior descending coronary artery in this instance (as it does ~15% to 20% of the time. **B.** The right coronary artery (RCA) arises from the right aortic sinus and travels in the right atrioventricular sulcus. **C.** After dissection from the heart, the coronary arteries may be appropriately decalcified, sectioned, and processed.

not include the trabeculations or papillary muscles. The normal left ventricular chamber is <2.5 cm, though agonal/decompositional dilatation can occur depending on the postmortem interval. The right ventricle is crescent shaped in the short axis, and therefore, both anterior–posterior and left–right dimensions should be described. In general, the adult right ventricular chamber is ~5.0 × 2.5 cm. Measurements of wall thickness and chamber dimensions should all be taken at the midventricular level so long as there is relatively uniformity.

Attention can then be turned to the cardiac base (Fig. 138.7). Starting at the right atrium, a small incision is made just anterior to the inferior vena cava. This cut is extended upward, with scissors, to the tip of the right atrial appendage. A second cut is then made ~5 mm lateral to the atrial septum extending inferior to the right ventricle (through the posterior tricuspid valve leaflet). A third cut is then made into the right ventricular myocardium, immediately adjacent to the ventricular septum. Extending this cut up through the pulmonary artery will result in incision of the commissure between the anterior and left pulmonary valve cusps. Moving back around to the posterior aspect of the heart, a small incision is made in the left atrial dome between the pulmonary veins (Fig. 138.8). This cut (the fourth cut) is extended inferiorly to the level of the mitral valve and then laterally to the tip of the left atrial appendage. A blade can then be used to cut (fifth cut) through the mitral valve by placing the blade through the mitral orifice and cutting directly opposite the anterior mitral valve leaflet (at the midway point of the posterior leaflet). The final (sixth) cut is made by separating the pulmonary artery and aorta slightly and then cutting downward from the ascending aorta, through the commissure between the left and right aortic valve cusps into the left ventricular base. The sixth cut can then be extended just lateral to the septum, to open the left ventricular outflow tract.

Evaluation for a patent foramen ovale can be done after the heart is opened by gently probing the region of the valve of the fossa ovalis for probe patency. A patent foramen ovale may be seen in up to a third of individuals after birth with a decreasing incidence over the human life span.[7] Careful evaluation for mural thrombi should also be performed, paying particular attention to the atrial appendages.[8]

Examination of the Major Cardiac Valves

After opening the heart along the lines of flow (as described above), the major cardiac valves can be examined. As a point of nomenclature, typically the term *cusp* is used to describe the semilunar valves (aortic and pulmonic) and the term *leaflet* is used to describe the atrioventricular valves (mitral and tricuspid). Valvular abnormalities such as congenital anomalies (such as a bicuspid aortic valve), thickening, calcification, and/or vegetation should be documented at this time. In general, both atrioventricular valve leaflets and semilunar valve cusps should be translucent normally.

The valve annuli should also be measured and help to corroborate any ventricular dilatation that may have been suspected based on the cavity dimensions that were measured. Although the semilunar valve annuli are technically shaped like triradiate crowns, a simple linear measurement along the tips of the commissures is appropriate.

The atrioventricular valve apparatus consists of the valve annulus, leaflets (mitral anterior and posterior; tricuspid anterior, posterior, and septal), and tendinous cords (Fig. 138.8F). The tendinous cords insert down onto papillary muscles that are located beneath each valve commissure (the point where to leaflets or cusps meet). This strategic location allows for the papillary muscle to pull the leaflets into apposition during ventricular systole. The atrial aspects of the atrioventricular

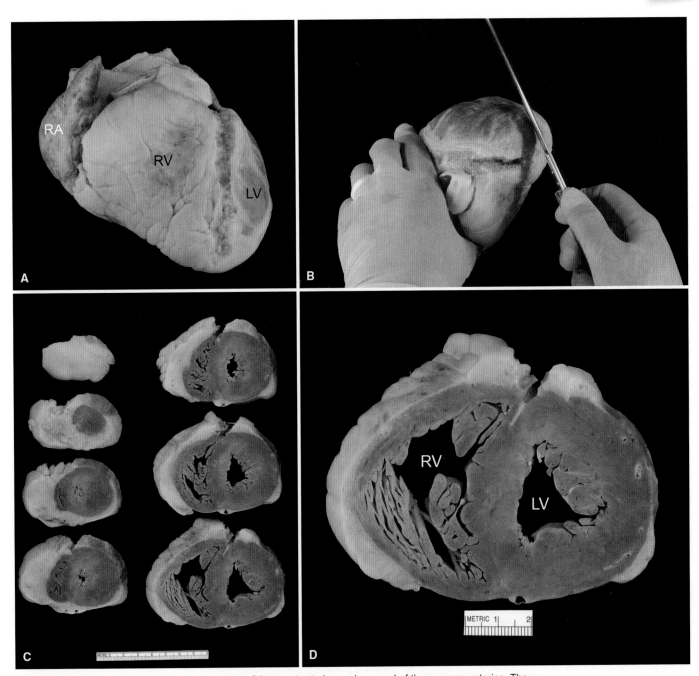

FIGURE 138.5 ▲ **A.** The heart after transection of the great arteries and removal of the coronary arteries. The right ventricle (RV) is again shown as the anterior-most chamber, with the right atrium (RA) in the right lateral position and the left ventricle (LV) in the left inferior/posterior position. **B.** Serial sectioning of the myocardium along the short axis (parallel to the atrioventricular plane), from apex to base, provides an excellent means of assessing the ventricular myocardium. **C.** Cuts should be made at ~8-mm intervals to at least the midventricular level (the level at which there are two distinct papillary muscles). **D.** The midventricular short-axis section reveals the circular left ventricle (LV) and the crescent-shaped right ventricle (RV)

valves, especially mitral valve, should be viewed for evidence of prolapse and atria for evidence of dilatation or focal endocardial fibrosis indicative of regurgitation (jet lesions) (Fig. 138.9).

The semilunar valves contain a valve annulus and cusps, but without a tensor apparatus. Instead of a tensor apparatus, the valve relies on pressure and flow dynamics to appropriately open and close throughout the cardiac cycle. The semilunar valve cusps contain a nodular area of thickening in the middle (nodule of Arantius), away from which extends a biscalloped ridge (the line of closure) that terminates at the commissure (Fig. 138.10). This line serves as the surfaces of apposition between adjacent cusps. It is not uncommon to identify age-related

fenestrations distal to the line of closure that do not typically have functional consequence given their distal location.

Examination of the Conduction System

In certain circumstances, evaluation of the cardiac conduction system can be of utility. Cases of sudden cardiac death, certain arrhythmic states (bundle-branch block), and documentation of ablations are just a few instances in which such evaluation may be necessary. Because evaluation of the conduction system is somewhat more resource intensive, a stepwise approach, whereby the nodal/perinodal conducting

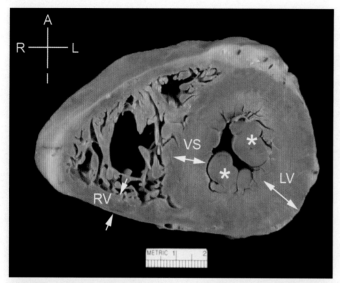

FIGURE 138.6 ▲ Short-axis section of the midventricular myocardium. The circular nature of the left ventricle (LV) can be compared with the crescent-shaped right ventricle (RV). Measurements of the free walls and ventricular septum (VS) should be taken and documented, excluding the papillary muscles and trabeculations. The two prominent papillary muscles (*asterisk*) seen in the LV cavity are an indicator that this is a midventricular section.

tissue is excised and reserved, is appropriate so that it can be evaluated at a later time.

Both the sinoatrial (SA) and atrioventricular (AV) conducting tissues are approached from the right atrium (Fig. 138.11). The SA node is located on the lateral aspect of the junction of the superior vena cava and the right atrial appendage. A rectangular section of atrial free wall, which includes the crista terminalis, at this location will allow for sampling of this epicardial structure. Histologically, the node consists of small specialized cardiomyocytes within fibrous and elastic tissue. The artery feeding the node is often identified in the vicinity.

The atrioventricular node is located within the triangle of Koch immediately posterior to the central fibrous body. The AV node is again approached from the right atrium, identifying the coronary sinus inferiorly, annulus of the tricuspid valve anteriorly, and membranous septum superiorly (Fig. 138.11A). The superior limit is formed by the tendon of Todaro, a microscopic bundle of fibrous tissue that is not seen grossly but extends from the commissure between the valve of the coronary sinus and the valve of the inferior vena cava to the commissure between the anterior and septal tricuspid valve leaflets. Sections are taken from posterior to superior, with evaluation of the atrioventricular node and branching bundles in more superior sections. Histologically, the atrioventricular node should be identified, with a note about increased vascularity or fat, abnormal conduction pathways between the node and the ventricular septum, and the continuation of the right and left bundle branches.

Cardiac Explant

General Considerations

In centers that perform heart transplants, the surgical pathologist evaluates the explant (recipient) heart. The gross description should be similar to that of an autopsy heart, but there are some important differences. Typically, only a small portion of the atria remains with the specimen, because the atria and vascular connections stay in the recipient to serve as the anastomotic site for the graft. Also, it is increasingly common to also receive attached left ventricular assist devices that served as the bridge to transplant for the patient.

A wide spectrum of pathologies can be encountered at explant, including both congenital and acquired forms of cardiovascular disease. Common indications for transplantation include ischemic heart disease (severe coronary atherosclerosis with healed infarction(s)), cardiomyopathy (dilated, hypertrophic, arrhythmogenic, and restrictive), amyloidosis, and congenital heart disease. Several important aspects to address with some of these more common entities are discussed below.

Ischemic Heart Disease

Ischemic heart disease refers to end-organ (heart) damage as a consequence of coronary artery disease (usually atherosclerotic). Infarcts should be documented by site (left or right ventricular), location (anterior, lateral, inferior/posterior, septal), level (apical, midventricular, basal), and extent (subendocardial or transmural).

Oftentimes, the heart has been previously intervened on and may contain coronary artery stents and/or bypass grafts. In the examination of a heart containing bypass grafts, the grafts should be removed with the native epicardial coronary arteries and appropriately decalcified. Sectioning and sampling of, at a minimum, the graft, anastomotic site, and distal native coronary artery should be performed. The distal native coronary arteries can be presumed to contain severe disease (prompting the original need for bypass). Stents can be identified, as described above, using radiography. Stent dissolution may be performed electrolytically so that the stented segments can also be processed for histology.

Cardiomyopathy

Cardiomyopathy refers to primary myocardial disease and can be classified in a number of different ways (see Chapter 156). In general, evaluation for disproportionate septal thickening, subaortic endocardial fibrosis, and abnormal papillary muscles will be helpful appropriate classification of hypertrophic cardiomyopathy. Excluding ischemic etiologies for dilated cardiomyopathy by careful evaluation of the short-axis slices will be useful. Special stains to evaluate for the presence of amyloidosis can be of particularly high yield in cases of suspected hypertrophic (owing to the phenotypic overlap) and restrictive cardiomyopathies.

Congenital Heart Disease

Appropriate classification of congenital heart disease rests on being able to accurately identify the venoatrial, atrioventricular, and ventriculoarterial connections. Documentation of any congenital obstructions or shunts is also necessary. Given that neither the atria nor the venoatrial connections are usually present in explant specimens, the evaluation will be somewhat limited.

Cardiac Biopsy

Transplant Biopsies

The minimum number of myocardium-containing specimens recommended for grading of rejection is three (see Chapter 31).[9] Importantly, dividing a sample into smaller portions at the time of grossing to meet the adequacy requirement is not permissible. Immunohistochemistry or immunofluorescence for complement (C4d and C3d) is recommended for the diagnosis of antibody-mediated rejection (see Chapter 32).[10] If paraffin-based tests are employed, all biopsy fragments can be processed routinely; if immunofluorescence is used, one fragment should be maintained fresh and frozen.

Nontransplant Biopsies

Today, one of the most common indications for native heart biopsy is to exclude infiltrative processes, especially in patients with restrictive hemodynamics or unexplained cardiac hypertrophy. The specific entities in the differential diagnosis include amyloidosis, eosinophilic endomyocardial disease, and storage disease (e.g., glycogen storage disease or Fabry disease) (see Chapter 23). In general, three hematoxylin

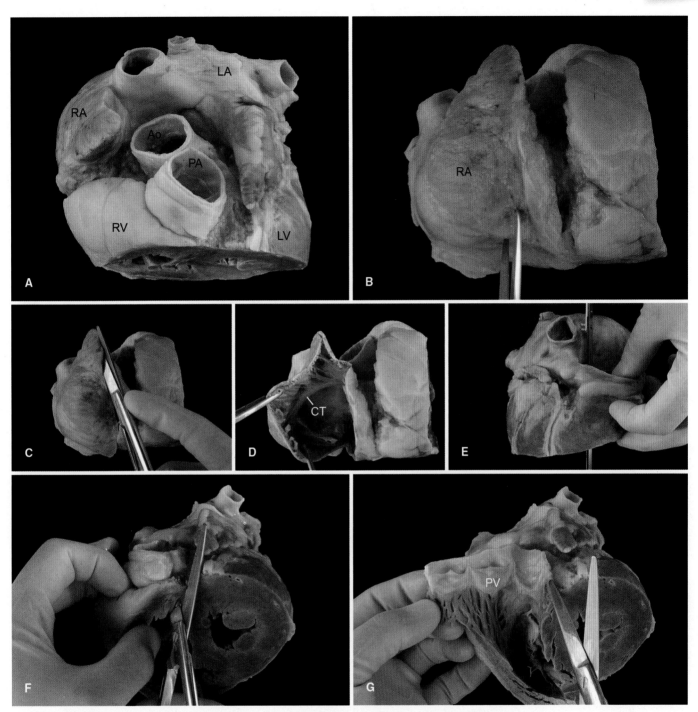

FIGURE 138.7 ▲ **A.** The cardiac base after short-axis sections have been taken. The right atrium (RA), right ventricle (RV), left atrium (LA), and left ventricle (LV) are in clear view, as are the pulmonary artery (PA) and the ascending aorta (Ao). **B.** The first cut is made just anterior to the inferior vena cava and **(C)** extended up to the tip of the right atrial appendage. **D.** The right atrial free wall is reflected to reveal the right atrium, including the pectinate muscles, crista terminalis (CT), and the atrial septum. **E.** The RV inflow is examined by cutting the posterior tricuspid valve, ~1 cm lateral to the ventricular septum. **F and G.** The RV outflow is examined by cutting along the ventricular septum, through the pulmonary valve (PV) at the commissure between the anterior and left cusps.

and eosin (H&E)-stained slides are recommended, in addition to ancillary studies appropriate for the clinical question.[11]

For cases in which an infiltrative disease is included in the differential diagnosis, a Congo red or sulfated Alcian blue stain may be ordered up-front, in addition to H&E-stained sections. If a storage disease or drug toxicity is included in the differential diagnosis, a single 1-mm portion of myocardium should be reserved for ultrastructural study.

Examination of three tissue fragments has excellent sensitivity for the evaluation for amyloidosis.

Another indication for native heart biopsy is acute-onset heart failure. In these cases, the exclusion of inflammatory processes, such as myocarditis (and especially giant cell myocarditis, which has urgent clinical implications), is vital. If the clinician specifically requests to exclude myocarditis, then all fragments should be processed routinely,

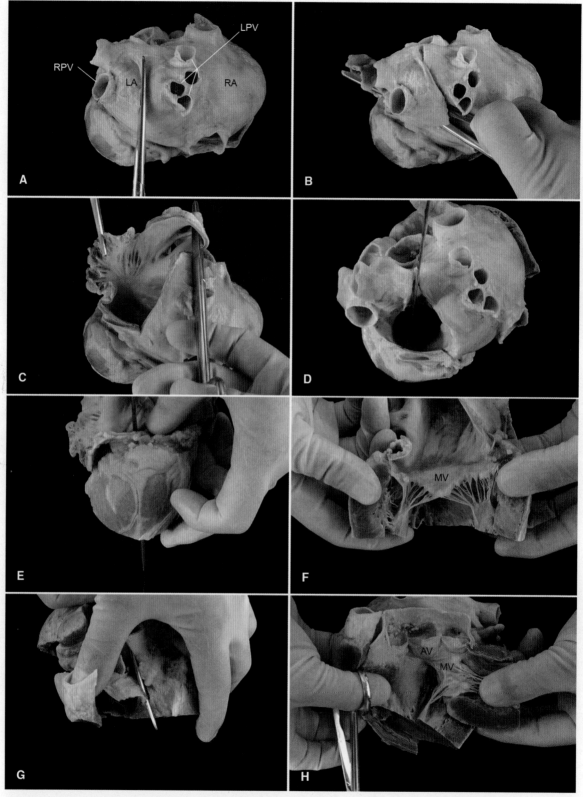

FIGURE 138.8 ▲ **A.** The left atrium (LA) is then incised between the left pulmonary veins (LPV) and right pulmonary veins (RPV), and the cut is extended both to the superior atrial dome and downward to the mitral orifice. **B.** The cut is extending around the mitral orifice to the tip of the left atrial appendage. **C and D.** The left atrial wall is reflected to inspect the left atrial cavity and internal structures. **E and F.** The left ventricular inflow tract is opened by passing a blade at the midway portion of the posterior mitral valve. **G.** The left ventricular outflow is assessed by cutting between the left and right aortic valve cusps and then down through the anteroseptal left ventricle. **H.** The continuity of the aortic valve (AV) and mitral valve (MV) can be appreciated after this cut.

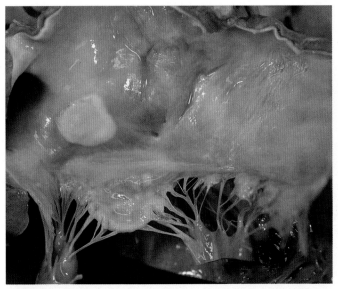

FIGURE 138.9 ▲ Left atrial dilatation in the setting of mitral regurgitation. Opening of the heart revealed a dilated left atrium and a mild rolling/thickening of the free edge of the anterior mitral valve leaflet. These changes, along with the discrete endocardial thickening in the left atrium ("jet lesion"), are indicators of the presence of mitral valve regurgitation.

in order to minimize sampling error. At least 10 H&E levels are recommended to evaluate for myocarditis.

Other Surgical Specimens

Apical Core Resections

Ventricular assist devices (left, right, or biventricular) are increasingly used as either a bridge to eventual cardiac allotransplantation or as destination therapy in cases of severe medically intractable heart failure. During the implantation, a full-thickness plug of myocardium is removed from the apical ventricle, through which a cannula is placed that will lead to the rotor pump.

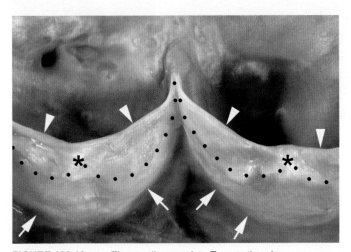

FIGURE 138.10 ▲ The semilunar valve. Two aortic valve cusps are shown in this gross photograph (the right aortic cusp on the left and the posterior aortic valve cusp on the right). The *asterisk* mark the nodule of Arantius, and the *dotted lines* indicate the biscalloped line of closure along the cusps. The *arrows* indicate the triradiate crown–shaped annulus of the semilunar valves. The free edge of the cusps (*white arrowheads*) can also be readily seen.

This apical core specimen generated should be evaluated histologically, in the context of the clinical history. Typical findings include those of ischemic heart disease such as myocyte hypertrophy and interstitial (both pericellular-type and replacement-type) fibrosis, cardiomyopathy such as hypertrophy and interstitial (usually pericellular-type) fibrosis, or any number of other conditions that culminated in heart failure (e.g., amyloidosis, sarcoidosis, myocarditis).

Septal Myectomy

In patients with dynamic left ventricular outflow tract obstruction, such as that seen in hypertrophic cardiomyopathy or chronic aortic stenosis, a portion of subaortic ventricular septal myocardium may be excised to open the outflow tract. In doing so, multiple endomyocardial samples are often generated.

Histologically, these specimens should be evaluated for the degree of myocyte hypertrophy, endocardial fibrosis, interstitial fibrosis, and myocyte disarray. Indicating that these findings are compatible with the clinical diagnosis of hypertrophic cardiomyopathy or chronic aortic stenosis is appropriate. Careful examination for amyloidosis is warranted, particularly when specimens are from individuals ≥65 years.

Atrial Appendage Resections

Atrial appendages are commonly removed in the setting of atrial fibrillation (as part of the Cox-maze procedure) or sometimes during the course of general cardiac surgery for prophylaxis of thromboembolism. Typical findings, in the setting of atrial fibrillation, include myocyte hypertrophy and interstitial fibrosis. When moderate or marked in nature, these features have been shown to have some correlation with the recurrence of atrial fibrillation in some patients.

Cardiac Valves

In general, cardiac valves should be photographed, measured, and described. A more comprehensive approach to cardiac valves in specific disease states is presented in Chapter 34.

Pericardial Tissue

Pericardial tissue is usually removed as a primary indication or incidentally during the course of surgery. Primary indications include recurrent pericarditis, recurrent pericardial effusion (pericardial window), or pericardial constriction.

The spectrum of pericardial pathology is wise and does not necessarily correlate with the clinical extent of disease. Areas of plate-like calcification are not uncommonly encountered in the setting of constriction, but pericardium may also be of normal thickness in ~10% of individuals with hemodynamic constriction. Sampling of the pericardium and histologic evaluation are important to document the presence of pericarditis and to exclude rare malignant processes such as lymphoma or mesothelioma.

Ascending Aortic Specimens

Portions of ascending aorta are usually removed in the setting of aneurysm. The specimen will typically come either as an obvious segmental resection (ring of tissue) or as a flat portion of tissue that may represent either a partial resection or a segmental resection that was opened by the surgical team. Either way, between four and six full-thickness portions of aorta should be examined histologically. Histologic evaluation of all vascular specimens should include an elastic stain in addition to H&E staining.[12]

Documentation of the presence of medial degeneration, dissection (acute or healed), aortitis (healed or active), laminar medial necrosis, and intimal atherosclerosis is recommended. In general, the presence of aneurysm in an individual <50 years should raise concerns for an underlying connection tissue disease, particularly in the absence of systemic hypertension.

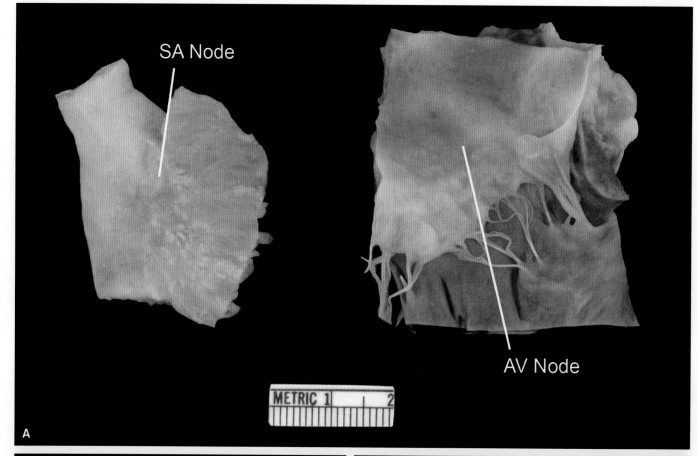

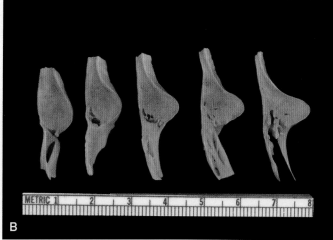

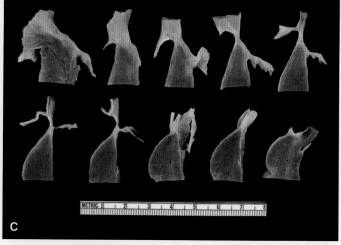

FIGURE 138.11 ▲ **A.** The nodal conduction tissue, including sinoatrial (SA) node and atrioventricular (AV) node, is removed by dissecting from the heart the lateral superior portion of the right atrium (where the superior vena cava connects to the right atrium) as well as the triangle of Koch. Serial sections of each tissue block, **(B)** the SA node and **(C)** the AV node, are then made and processed for histologic examination.

REFERENCES

1. Scholz DG, Kitzman DW, Hagen PT, et al. Age-related changes in normal human hearts during the first 10 decades of life. Part I (Growth): a quantitative anatomic study of 200 specimens from subjects from birth to 19 years old. *Mayo Clin Proc.* 1988;63:126–136.
2. Kitzman DW, Scholz DG, Hagen PT, et al. Age-related changes in normal human hearts during the first 10 decades of life. Part II (Maturity): a quantitative anatomic study of 765 specimens from subjects 20 to 99 years old. *Mayo Clin Proc.* 1988;63:137–146.
3. Hangartner JR, Marley NJ, Whitehead A, et al. The assessment of cardiac hypertrophy at autopsy. *Histopathology.* 1985;9:1295–1306.
4. Schulz DM, Giordano DA. Hearts of infants and children. Weights and measurements. *Arch Pathol.* 1962;74:464–471.
5. Bradshaw SH, Kennedy L, Dexter DF, et al. A practical method to rapidly dissolve metallic stents. *Cardiovasc Pathol.* 2009;18:127–133.
6. Mont E, Cresswell N, Burke A. Pathologic findings of coronary stents: a comparison of sudden coronary death versus non-cardiac death. *J Forensic Sci.* 2013;58:1542–1548.
7. Sweeney LJ, Rosenquist GC. The normal anatomy of the atrial septum in the human heart. *Am Heart J.* 1979;98:194–199.
8. Di Biase L, Santangeli P, Anselmino M, et al. Does the left atrial appendage morphology correlate with the risk of stroke in patients with atrial fibrillation? Results from a multicenter study. *J Am Coll Cardiol.* 2012;60:531–538.

9. Stewart S, Winters GL, Fishbein MC, et al. Revision of the 1990 working formulation for the standardization of nomenclature in the diagnosis of heart rejection. *J Heart Lung Transplant.* 2005;24:1710–1720.
10. Berry GJ, Burke MM, Andersen C, et al. The 2013 International Society for Heart and Lung Transplantation Working Formulation for the standardization of nomenclature in the pathologic diagnosis of antibody-mediated rejection in heart transplantation. *J Heart Lung Transplant.* 2013;32:1147–1162.
11. Leone O, Veinot JP, Angelini A, et al. 2011 consensus statement on endomyocardial biopsy from the Association for European Cardiovascular Pathology and the Society for Cardiovascular Pathology. *Cardiovasc Pathol.* 2012;21:245–274.
12. Stone JR, Basso C, Baandrup UT, et al. Recommendations for processing cardiovascular surgical pathology specimens: a consensus statement from the Standards and Definitions Committee of the Society for Cardiovascular Pathology and the Association for European Cardiovascular Pathology. *Cardiovasc Pathol.* 2012;21:2–16.

139 Myocardial Response to Injury

Allen P. Burke, M.D., and Fabio R. Tavora, M.D., Ph.D.

General

Myocyte injury results from a variety of insults, including ischemia, inflammation, toxic insults, and physical forces such as trauma or increased wall tension. The specific diseases or entities and their pathologic manifestations are covered in detail in other chapters. There are relatively few "final common pathways" that are seen from diverse causes and that are, in many cases, nonspecific for a particular disease. A list of terms describing myocardial injury is provided in Table 139.1.

Evaluation of Myocardial Injury

Clinically, cardiac injury is equated to myocyte necrosis and is assessed by measuring the release of cardiomyocyte constituents such as cardiac troponins and creatine kinase into the serum or plasma. Chronic injury causes abnormalities in cardiac function and wall motion, assessed by cardiac imaging. Experimentally, ischemic myocytes can be histologically detected by the in vivo injection of antimyosin antibody prior to animal sacrifice, allowing immunohistochemical visualization of irreversibly damaged myocytes with sarcolemmal disruption that have allowed intracytoplasmic passage of the antibody. A clinical correlate in human patients is the use of antimyosin nuclear medicine scanning to visualize areas of myocardial ischemia.

Histologically, light microscopic alterations in myocyte cytoplasm, nucleus, and cell size and shape allow assessment of myocyte injury from a practical standpoint. Because histologic manifestations of ischemia occur hours after onset, however, special techniques are necessary to diagnose recent myocardial infarction. Tetrazolium salts stain viable myocardium in gross heart specimens, but not ischemic regions, as tetrazolium compounds are cleaved into visible formazan dyes on exposure to dehydrogenase enzymes, which are exquisitely sensitive to ischemia.

Immunohistochemical staining for substances that enter the cell with sarcolemmal disruption, such as complement, troponin, fibronexin, and connexin-43, has been used to detect early ischemic cell death in forensic autopsies.[1,2] Ultrastructural evaluation of myocytes is helpful in determining changes in cell size, nuclear shape, cytoplasmic organelles, and other constituents, which reflect cardiac injury. However, other than in the evaluation of anthracycline toxicity and exclusion of specific cardiomyopathies, electron microscopy has limited practical diagnostic use, because many ultrastructural changes are nonspecific, and application for autopsy is hindered by postmortem changes that mimic ischemia.

TABLE 139.1 Terms Used in Describing Myocardial Injury

Designation	Context	Notes
Hypereosinophilia	Early ischemic necrosis	Loss of membrane integrity demonstrated by identifying leaked proteins into cytosol (oncosis)
Pyknosis and karyorrhexis	Myocardial infarction	Degeneration of cellular nuclei (including neutrophils and endothelial cells), predominantly apoptotic
Autophagy	Heart failure / Reperfusion injury	Lysosomal mediated process that eliminates damaged proteins and organelles
Coagulative necrosis	Myocardial infarction	Zones of necrotic myocytes with distinguishable borders and dissolving internal structure
Contraction bands	Acute catecholamine injury / Fixation artifact	May be seen in resuscitation or biopsy artifact (cold fixatives in biopsies)
Contraction band necrosis	Chronic catecholamine injury / Reperfusion injury	"Brain death" lesions / "Single cell necrosis"
Ischemia–reperfusion injury	Reperfusion infarction	Hemorrhagic infarct with contraction bands and diffuse sparse neutrophilic inflammation
Myocytolysis	Chronic ischemia / Contraction band necrosis (obsolete)	Vacuolization caused by intracellular edema and myofibrillar loss
Replacement fibrosis	Healed infarct, cardiomyopathy	Localized reparative fibrosis after infarction or large areas of necrosis of other cause
Interstitial fibrosis	Hypertensive hypertrophy, heart failure	Diffuse increased epimysial and perimysial collagen
Lipofuscin	Senescence	Autofluorescent, finely granular yellow-brown pigment containing lysosomal residues
Basophilic degeneration	Senescence, cardiomyopathy	Intracytoplasmic PAS-positive glycoprotein, resembles amyloid
Sarcoplasmic and T-tubular dilatation	Drug toxicity, cardiomyopathy	Enlargement and dilatation of sarcotubules and T tubules, leading to myocyte vacuolization if diffuse

Myocyte Cell Death

Ischemic Cell Death (Oncosis)

The initial phase in ischemic coagulative necrosis is marked by loss of cell membrane integrity, resulting in mitochondrial swelling and swelling of the nucleus and cytoplasm. The free passage of intracellular and extracellular materials results in "oncosis" (cell swelling) and can be histologically manifested by hypereosinophilia and eventual loss of cytoplasmic detail (Fig. 139.1). The demonstration of intracytoplasmic antigens not normally present, such as complement, may be useful in demonstrating small foci of ischemic cell death, such as seen in autopsy hearts in ischemic cardiomyopathy or heart biopsies soon after transplant. Individual myocytes with sarcolemmal damage, as evidenced by complement labeling, are present in biopsies of patients with heart failure in <0.1% of myocytes.[3]

In contrast to apoptosis, necrosis is considered to be an unregulated form of cell death. However, there has been described an intermediate form of necrotic cell death, seen especially in myocarditis, termed "necroptosis" or "programmed necrosis" that is initiated by tumor necrosis factor and characterized by mitochondrial fission resulting in cell death.[4]

Apoptosis (Programmed Cell Death)

Neutrophil apoptosis may be seen in the karyorrhectic inflammatory cells surrounding an evolving myocardial infarction. Apoptosis is uncommonly visualized in the cardiac myocytes, as cardiomyocytes undergo programmed cell death at a very low rate in failing hearts. Techniques such as in situ end labeling of DNA fragments, electron microscopy, or immunohistochemical staining for caspases are required to detect myocyte apoptosis. In heart failure of all causes, far fewer than 1% of cardiomyocytes are shown to have features of apoptosis by nick end labeling or immunohistochemistry, with a wide range reported, from <0.01% to <1% of cells.[3,5] Apoptotic myocytes are removed by macrophages through phagocytosis without triggering inflammation. Immunoelectron microscopy shows cytochrome c release from the mitochondria into the cytoplasm and annexin V translocation in the outer plasma cell layer.[6]

Pyknosis and Karyorrhexis

Pyknosis is the irreversible condensation of chromatin, and karyorrhexis is the subsequent fragmentation of cell nuclei undergoing apoptotic or other types of cell death. Pyknosis and karyorrhexis are features of cell death that are readily appreciated by light microscopy,

and involve myocytes, endothelial cells, and inflammatory cells in areas of myocardial infarction. These nuclear changes have been used in the evaluation of reperfusion injury in experimental models[7] and as a marker of early transplant rejection.[8] The terms "pyknosis" and "karyorrhexis" are most commonly used in reference to acute myocardial infarction, as indicators of breakdown of neutrophils at the margins of nonreperfused infarcts that occurs at about 3 days and thereafter.

Autophagy

Autophagy mediates the degradation of damaged cytoplasmic proteins and organelles that accumulate with cellular stress or hypoxia and is associated with myocardial necrosis and impairment of lysosomal degradation.[6] It may be present not only in heart failure but also in myocarditis and reperfusion injury. Prolonged activation of autophagy can lead to cell death.[9] Autophagy sequesters altered cytoplasmic proteins in lysosomes (autophagosomes) that can be visualized only by ultrastructural methods (Fig. 139.2). Morphologically, autophagic vacuoles contain mitochondria, glycogen granules, and myelin-like figures; by immunolabeling, proteins including ubiquitin, cathepsin D, and Rab7 can be identified within them.[10] Heart biopsies with idiopathic dilated cardiomyopathy may show evidence of autophagic vacuoles in over 10% of biopsies, and ultrastructural morphologic features of apoptosis, oncosis, and autophagocytosis often coexist.[6,11] *Danon cardiomyopathy* is characterized by a dramatic accumulation of autophagic vacuoles because of deficiency in LAMP-2 protein that inhibits uptake of proteins into lysosomes for degeneration. An early form of autophagy has been termed "mitophagy," a cardioprotective response that removes damaged

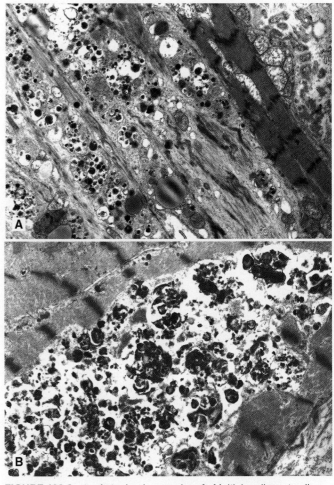

FIGURE 139.2 ▲ Autophagic vacuoles. **A.** Multiple adjacent cells are affected with myofibrillar loss and autophagic vacuoles. **B.** A portion of a myocyte is replaced by autophagic debris.

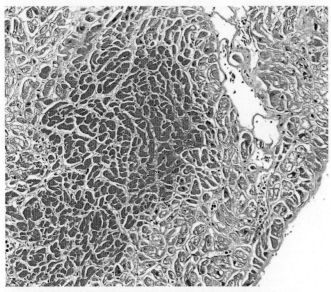

FIGURE 139.1 ▲ Myocyte necrosis (oncosis). There is a zone of hypereosinophilia in a case of acute subendocardial infarction.

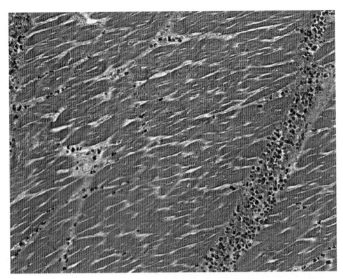

FIGURE 139.3 ▲ Coagulative necrosis. The infarct myocytes show patchy loss of cross-striations, nuclear loss, and hypereosinophilia, with visible cell borders.

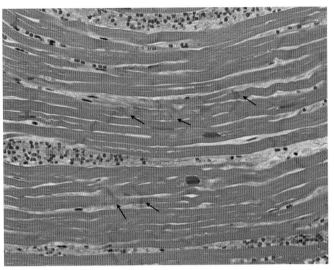

FIGURE 139.4 ▲ Contraction bands. There are thickened transverse bands corresponding to overlapping myofibrils (*arrows*). There is no evidence of necrosis.

mitochondria and that is inactivated by increased oxidative stress and apoptotic proteases, allowing for the programmed cell death to occur.

Myocyte Necrosis

Coagulative Necrosis

In general, coagulative necrosis indicates dead tissue that softens as in a gel but maintains its architecture and is seen in the heart and other organs typically in response to an infarct. Histologically, infarcted myocardium demonstrates necrotic myocytes with intact nuclei and cell borders (in early stages), hypereosinophilic cytoplasm indicative of denatured proteins, and an absence of identifiable cross-striations (Fig. 139.3). Later, a polymorphonuclear leukocytic infiltration is followed by macrophage digestion. The histologic evolution of myocardial ischemia is discussed in detail in Chapter 151.

Contraction Band Necrosis

Contraction bands are seen in both striated muscle and smooth muscle and represent a hypercontracted state of the cell in which

transverse bands of condensed myofilaments are visible at the light microscopic level. Although sometimes used interchangeably, "contraction bands" are not the same as "contraction band necrosis," in which there are also features of cell necrosis (hypereosinophilia and loss of normal striations). Contraction bands are a common finding at autopsy in patients who have been resuscitated with exogenous pressor agents (Fig. 139.4). Contraction band necrosis, on the other hand, can be extensive, especially in areas of reperfusion infarction, and is characterized by fragmentation of hypercontracted myocytes, irregular cross-bands of coagulated sarcomeres, and a macrophage reaction (Fig. 139.5).[12] Single or small clusters of necrotic cells with contraction bands and a mononuclear cell infiltrate are referred to as "single cell necrosis" and are an indicator of systemic increase in catecholamines. For this reason, the term "brain death lesions" has been used to describe focal contraction band necrosis because of their common occurrence in patients with cerebral hypoxia maintained on life support.[13] Contraction band necrosis may undergo calcification in patients on chronic pressor support for shock who have hypercalcemia and renal failure (Fig. 139.5B).

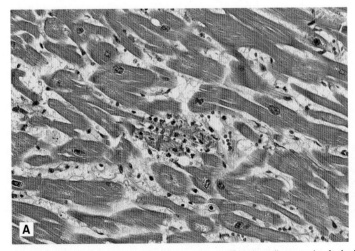
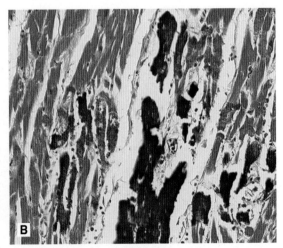

FIGURE 139.5 ▲ Contraction band necrosis. Single cell necrosis. **A.** A shrunken myocyte contains degenerated cytoplasm with contraction bands and degenerative inflammatory cells. **B.** Contraction band necrosis with calcification. An autopsy specimen with patchy calcified myocytes. Although the cytoplasm is not discernable, the pattern is characteristic of contraction band necrosis with calcification in the setting of shock, chronic pressor therapy, and hypercalcemia of chronic renal failure.

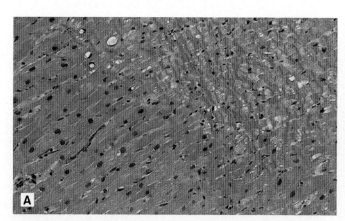
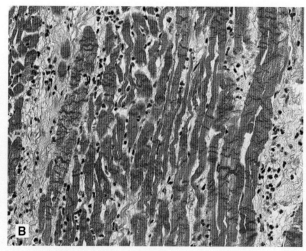

FIGURE 139.6 ▲ Reperfusion infarct. **A.** There is diffuse contraction band necrosis with myocyte degeneration in the upper right of a papillary muscle that ruptured (rupture site not shown). **B.** A slightly later reperfusion infarct shows diffuse contraction band necrosis, myocyte degeneration, and a sparse inflammatory infiltrate.

Necrosis in Myocarditis

Although myocyte necrosis is a hallmark of myocarditis, the histologic evidence may be relatively sparse, compared to the degree of inflammation, especially in lymphocytic myocarditis. The necrotic cells in myocarditis may be isolated, but in contrast to single cell (contraction band) necrosis, there is an abundance of inflammation far exceeding the degree of necrosis. Experimentally, T-cell–mediated myocyte injury in viral myocarditis is a form of programmed cell death involving TNF receptor ligand activation.[14] Histologically, myocyte necrosis in myocarditis is characterized by mixed infiltrate of macrophages and T lymphocytes that engulf single or small clusters of myocytes, which lose their cell integrity and identifiable cell borders.[15]

Ischemia Reperfusion Injury

Prolonged myocardial ischemia with subsequent reperfusion leads to "ischemia–reperfusion injury" characterized by the development of contractile dysfunction, arrhythmias, and reperfusion infarction. The lack of oxygen during the ischemic period causes a condition susceptible to oxidative stress upon restoration of circulation. Increased capillary permeability, production of reactive oxygen species by activated endothelial cells, and the influx of inflammatory cells producing free radicals culminate in tissue injury despite the restoration of oxygen. Mitochondria are also involved in the release of reactive oxygen species via the mitochondrial ATP-sensitive potassium channel, which is related to mitochondrial connexin-43. Autophagy and apoptotic cell death are pathways of cardiomyocyte death induced by acute ischemia–reperfusion injury.[16]

Light microscopic changes are seen only when there is end-stage reperfusion injury manifested by reperfusion infarction. In contrast to nonreperfused infarcts, reperfusion infarcts are characterized by interstitial hemorrhage, edema, and inflammatory infiltrates and diffuse contraction band necrosis (Fig. 139.6).

Myocytolysis

The term "myocytolysis" has been used to define internal myocyte disruption following acute myocardial ischemia or toxic myocyte injury in experimental animals[17,18] and has been occasionally applied to contraction band necrosis.[19] "Myocytolysis" is also used as a clinical designation for leakage of cardiac proteins into the serum indicative of myocyte death.[20] Possibly, the most accepted pathologic meaning of "colliquative myocytolysis" (corresponding to the German "Fibrillolyse") is chronic vacuolization with myofibrillar loss associated with chronic ischemia (Fig. 139.7).[21] Extensive subendocardial vacuolization indicative of chronic ischemia is present in ischemic cardiomyopathy, dilated cardio-

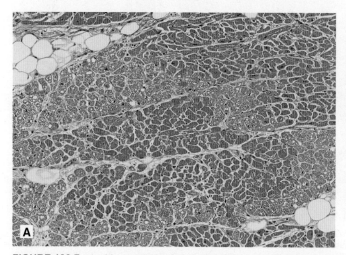
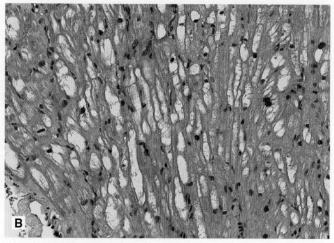

FIGURE 139.7 ▲ Myocytolysis and acute ischemia. **A.** There is an irregular zone of lighter staining myocytes with diffuse cytoplasmic vacuolization. Myocytolysis is generally considered a manifestation of chronic ischemia. In this example, the nonvacuolated myocytes show diffuse hypereosinophilia characteristic of early ischemic necrosis. **B.** A higher magnification of myocytolysis shows diffuse myocyte clearing indicative of chronic ischemia.

myopathy, and transplant vascular disease.[12] In contrast to contraction band necrosis, which is common in states with excess circulating catecholamines, myocytolysis is absent in patients dying with cocaine abuse, head trauma, or electrocution.[12] Because myocytolysis is evidence of chronic ischemia, it may be tempting to equate its presence with "hibernating myocardium," a functional designation of hypo- or akinetic left ventricular wall that regains function after revascularization. However, the presence of "cytoplasmic clearing" in left ventricles biopsied during bypass grafting showed no correlation with functional reserve or subsequent improvement in wall motion. These cells were more extensive in biopsies with extensive fibrosis, which had a strong negative correlation with a rebound in function.[21] Pathologic features of hibernating myocardium, usually assessed ultrastructurally, include decreased myofilaments, disorganization of desmin, reduction of connexin-43, chromatin clumping, glycogen accumulation, apoptosis, and interstitial fibrosis.[22]

Myocardial Fibrosis

Myocardial fibrosis has been classified clinically into "reparative" fibrosis, in which scar forms after ischemic necrosis, or "reactive" fibrosis, which is generally diffuse.[23] There terms roughly correspond, respectively, to pathologic "replacement" and "interstitial" fibrosis.

Clinically, diffuse *interstitial fibrosis* is known to increase ventricular stiffness and is considered a form of cardiac remodeling that impairs left ventricular diastolic dysfunction. Collagen that is deposited in heart failure or cardiac hypertrophy manifests as microscopic collagen in the epimysium (around individual myocytes) or perimysium (around cardiomyocyte bundles and along arterioles and small venules).[24]

By light microscopy, morphometric studies have shown that interstitial collagen constitutes 2% to 6% of myocardial area in normal individuals, depending on methodology.[23] In contrast, the proportion of myocardium comprised by collagen ranges from 15% to over 30% in hypertensive cardiomyopathy[23] and from 10% to 20% in left ventricular myocardial samples taken at insertion of assist devices for end-stage heart failure.[25] Histologically, the interstitium contains fibrillar collagen as well as fibroblasts (Fig. 139.8). Ultrastructurally, there is an excess of pericellular collagen weave fibers (endomysial matrix) and markedly thickened perimysial collagen fibrils.[23] Patients with chronic kidney disease and hypertension are especially prone to develop myocardial fibrosis and disturbances in diastolic function.[26] Microscopic fibrosis has also been described in stimulant abuse, possibly secondary to inflammation,[27] as well as in cases of hypertrophy in an athlete.[28]

Replacement fibrosis denotes areas of scar that have replaced previously viable myocytes, in healed infarcts, areas of scar after myocarditis, or nonspecific scars in nonischemic cardiomyopathy.

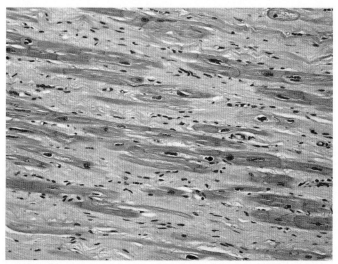

FIGURE 139.8 ▲ Interstitial fibrosis. The interstitium contains fibroblasts and collagen fibers. The underlying condition is idiopathic dilated cardiomyopathy.

Myofiber Disarray

Myofiber disarray may result secondarily as a reaction to scarring, for example, adjacent to prior biopsy sites, or after mitral valve surgery.[29] Myofiber disarray may also be seen at an ultrastructural level, typically in idiopathic cardiomyopathy.[30] Myofiber disarray with marked cellular hypertrophy and interstitial fibrosis is a hallmark of hypertrophic cardiomyopathy.

Heart Failure and Myocyte Changes

Heart failure of any cause results in nonspecific changes in cardiac myocytes and the interstitium. Secondary myocyte changes seen in heart failure include myocyte hypertrophy, variability in myofiber and nuclear size, increased lipofuscin, and myocyte vacuolization (myocytolysis, especially subendocardially in chronic ischemia). Interstitial fibrosis (increase in both fibroblasts and collagen) as well as patchy replacement fibrosis occur to variable degrees in failing hearts.[24]

Electron microscopic evaluation of heart biopsies in patients with unexplained heart failure is generally performed to exclude a specific etiology. There are a variety of changes that are nonspecific and are seen in heart failure of any cause in various degrees. A common finding in heart biopsies performed for heart failure is the increase in mitochondria, or mitochondriosis. In over 10% of biopsies, mitochondria have abnormal morphology, including enlarged organelles, abnormal cristae, calcification, and inclusion bodies. These findings have been associated with heteroplasmic mitochondrial mutations.[31] A variety of changes that are seen in heart failure and other forms of myocyte injury include T-tubular dilatation and aggregates, sarcotubular dilatation (similar to that seen in anthracycline toxicity), Z-disk abnormalities (rod bodies, streaming), and increased glycogen.[6,11,31]

Senescence

General

There is no direct correlation between the aging process and a decrease in systolic ventricular function. In addition, there are no observable changes in the myocardium of people of advanced age with normal ejection fractions, although there may be an increase in lipofuscin and basophilic degeneration. Recently, it has been shown that cardiac myocytes have the potential for replication,[32] suggesting that a potential consequence of aging could be an imbalance between myocyte growth and cell death resulting in an excess of senescent myocytes. A quantitative study of heart biopsies in the elderly showed that those from patients with a decreased ejection fraction differed from younger patients with idiopathic dilated cardiomyopathy. The study showed that both populations showed increased cell death, but apoptotic myocytes in the elderly, unlike those in younger patients, expressed the kinase inhibitor p16INK4a and showed telomeric shortening. Mitotic figures and telomerase were increased in the elderly patients with heart failure, but not enough to compensate for cell death and telomeric shortening.[33]

Lipofuscin

Senescent cells may be no longer in need of mitochondria, whose turnover is mediated by the autophagic–lysosomal pathway and the ubiquitin proteasome system. A decline in functioning autophagy results in an excess of lipofuscin in the normal (senescent) cell; in addition, autophagy may reflect increased cardiac damage, including necrosis or apoptosis. However, there is evidence that lipofuscin can form in the absence of autophagy.[9] Usually perinuclear, lipofuscin is an autofluorescent, finely granular yellow-brown pigment composed of lipid-containing residues of lysosomal digestion (Fig. 139.9). It is considered a natural manifestation of senescence and is composed of highly oxidized and covalently cross-linked proteins, unsaturated fatty acids, glycoproteins, and metals including mercury, aluminum, iron, copper, and zinc. The finding of increased lipofuscin in heart samples does not correlate with disease or decreased ventricular function.

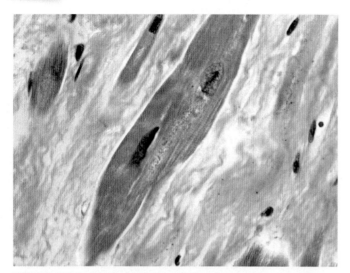

FIGURE 139.9 ▲ Lipofuscin. Lipofuscin is a golden-brown perinu-clear granular pigment composed of lysosomal breakdown products.

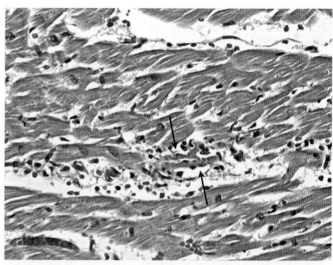

FIGURE 139.11 ▲ 5-Fluorouracil toxicity. Autopsy heart tissue from a patient dying while on second round of chemotherapy for colorectal carcinoma. There is acute inflammation with interstitial neutrophils, and contraction band necrosis is evident with necrotic myocyte (*arrows*).

Basophilic Degeneration

A less-understood form of cardiac myocyte degenerative is seen in basophilic degeneration, in which there are isolated PAS-positive amyloid-like intracytoplasmic inclusions within otherwise unremarkable myocytes (Fig. 139.10). Basophilic degeneration is caused by the accumulation of a glycoprotein with similar chemical composition as that seen in Lafora bodies of Lafora progressive myoclonic epilepsy. It is present in a small number of normal myocytes in virtually all individuals over age 60 years, and is seen more extensively in hearts from patients with cardiomyopathy and thyroid disease.[34]

Drug Toxicity

General

Cardiotoxicity may result from a variety of drug therapies, especially those used in oncology. Acute effects generally manifest as arrhythmias and chronic effects as decreased ventricular function and ejection fraction. The drug most often associated with cardiotoxicity is doxorubicin (Adriamycin), which causes cardiac complications in a dose-dependent manner in 4% to 36% of patients (usually after a cumulative dose of

500 mg/m^2 body surface area). The mechanism of cardiotoxicity and morphologic manifestations has been most thoroughly researched in the case of anthracycline drugs, especially doxorubicin, which bind to topoisomerase-2β. Other antineoplastic drugs that have adverse effects on cardiac function include 5-fluorouracil (with a fatality rate of 2% to 13% after high-dose treatment), trastuzumab, paclitaxel, sunitinib, and sorafenib. Treatment with beta-blockers and angiotensin-converting enzyme inhibitors can lessen the likelihood of side effects of many of these agents.[35]

The histologic changes of drug toxicity are nonspecific and not well described. In acute stage, there may be acute inflammation, contraction band necrosis, and vascular inflammation (Fig. 139.11).

Chronic opiate use is associated with myocardial changes of increased interstitial T lymphocytes and macrophages as well as interstitial fibrosis.[27]

Anthracycline Toxicity

Endomyocardial biopsies performed in human hearts after administration of doxorubicin reveal an increase in sarcoplasmic reticulum and

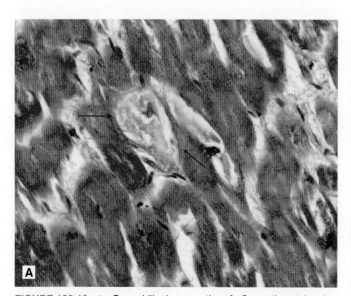

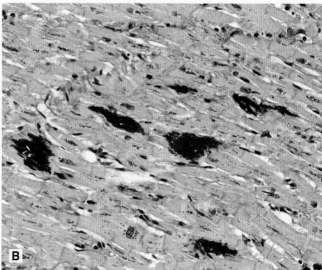

FIGURE 139.10 ▲ Basophilic degeneration. **A.** On routine stains, basophilic degeneration is intracytoplasmic, pale material (*arrows*). **B.** Basophilic degeneration is PAS positive and diastase resistant.

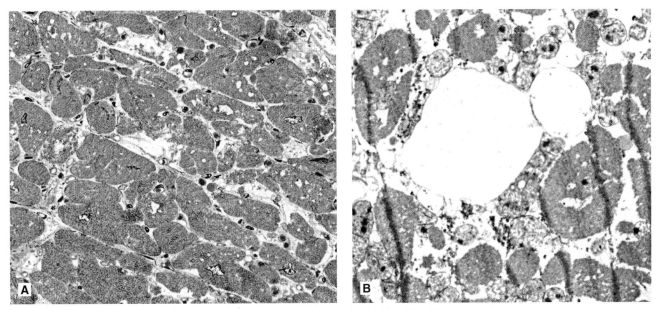

FIGURE 139.12 ▲ Anthracycline toxicity. **A.** On thick sections stained with *toluidine blue,* there are scattered myocardial vacuoles. **B.** On thin sections, myocyte shows membrane-lined vacuoles indicative of sarcotubular dilatation.

T-tubule size, which leads to sarcotubular and T-tubular dilatation, manifest on light microscopic, toluidine blue-stained thick sections as myocyte vacuolization (Fig. 139.12). Other ultrastructural findings include marked myofibrillar loss, characterized by absence of myofilaments with peripheral Z-band remnants, mitochondrial degeneration, and nuclear changes including clumping of chromatin and nucleolar shrinkage.[36,37] The degree of changes may be scored based on the proportion of cells showing abnormal features, primarily cytoplasmic vacuolization and marked myofibrillar loss.[36]

In vitro studies of myoblast cultures have demonstrated doxorubicin-induced disruption of the nuclear lamina, sarcomeric cardiac myosin, and mitochondrial membranes, which lead at higher concentrations to nuclear and mitochondrial swelling and extensive cytoplasmic vacuolization.[38]

REFERENCES

1. Kawamoto O, Michiue T, Ishikawa T, et al. Immunohistochemistry of connexin43 and zonula occludens-1 in the myocardium as markers of early ischemia in autopsy material. *Histol Histopathol.* 2014;29:767–775.
2. Jasra SK, Badian C, Macri I, et al. Recognition of early myocardial infarction by immunohistochemical staining with cardiac troponin-I and complement C9. *J Forensic Sci.* 2012;57:1595–1600.
3. Kostin S, Pool L, Elsasser A, et al. Myocytes die by multiple mechanisms in failing human hearts. *Circ Res.* 2003;92:715–724.
4. Kaczmarek A, Vandenabeele P, Krysko DV. Necroptosis: the release of damage-associated molecular patterns and its physiological relevance. *Immunity.* 2013;38:209–223.
5. Kuethe F, Sigusch HH, Bornstein SR, et al. Apoptosis in patients with dilated cardiomyopathy and diabetes: a feature of diabetic cardiomyopathy? *Horm Metab Res.* 2007;39:672–676.
6. Arbustini E, Brega A, Narula J. Ultrastructural definition of apoptosis in heart failure. *Heart Fail Rev.* 2008;13:121–135.
7. Tochinai R, Ando M, Suzuki T, et al. Histopathological studies of microtubule disassembling agent-induced myocardial lesions in rats. *Exp Toxicol Pathol.* 2013;65:737–743.
8. Herskowitz A, Soule LM, Mellits ED, et al. Histologic predictors of acute cardiac rejection in human endomyocardial biopsies: a multivariate analysis. *J Am Coll Cardiol.* 1987;9:802–810.
9. Hohn A, Sittig A, Jung T, et al. Lipofuscin is formed independently of macroautophagy and lysosomal activity in stress-induced prematurely senescent human fibroblasts. *Free Radic Biol Med.* 2012;53:1760–1769.
10. Miyata S, Takemura G, Kawase Y, et al. Autophagic cardiomyocyte death in cardiomyopathic hamsters and its prevention by granulocyte colony-stimulating factor. *Am J Pathol.* 2006;168:386–397.
11. Arbustini E, Gavazzi A, Dal Bello B, et al. Ten-year experience with endomyocardial biopsy in myocarditis presenting with congestive heart failure: frequency, pathologic characteristics, treatment and follow-up. *G Ital Cardiol.* 1997;27:209–223.
12. Turillazzi E, Baroldi G, Silver MD, et al. A systematic study of a myocardial lesion: colliquative myocytolysis. *Int J Cardiol.* 2005;104:152–157.
13. Perez Lopez S, Otero Hernandez J, Vazquez Moreno N, et al. Brain death effects on catecholamine levels and subsequent cardiac damage assessed in organ donors. *J Heart Lung Transplant.* 2009;28:815–820.
14. Seko Y, Takahashi N, Oshima H, et al. Expression of tumour necrosis factor (TNF) receptor/ligand superfamily co-stimulatory molecules CD40, CD30L, CD27L, and OX40L in murine hearts with chronic ongoing myocarditis caused by coxsackie virus B3. *J Pathol.* 1999;188:423–430.
15. Lieberman EB, Hutchins GM, Herskowitz A, et al. Clinicopathologic description of myocarditis. *J Am Coll Cardiol.* 1991;18:1617–1626.
16. Senturk T, Cavun S, Avci B, et al. Effective inhibition of cardiomyocyte apoptosis through the combination of trimetazidine and N-acetylcysteine in a rat model of myocardial ischemia and reperfusion injury. *Atherosclerosis.* 2014;237:760–766.
17. Chow LH, Yee SP, Pawson T, et al. Progressive cardiac fibrosis and myocyte injury in v-fps transgenic mice. A model for primary disorders of connective tissue in the heart? *Lab Invest.* 1991;64:457–462.
18. Tan LB, Jalil JE, Pick R, et al. Cardiac myocyte necrosis induced by angiotensin II. *Circ Res.* 1991;69:1185–1195.
19. Brander L, Weinberger D, Henzen C. Heart and brain: a case of focal myocytolysis in severe pneumococcal meningoencephalitis with review of the contemporary literature. *Anaesth Intensive Care.* 2003;31:202–207.
20. Manna A, Cadenotti L, Motto A, et al. Reversible cardiac dysfunction without myocytolysis related to all-trans retinoic acid administration during induction therapy of acute promyelocytic leukemia. *Ann Hematol.* 2009;88:91–92.
21. Hennessy T, Diamond P, Holligan B, et al. Correlation of myocardial histologic changes in hibernating myocardium with dobutamine stress echocardiographic findings. *Am Heart J.* 1998;135:952–959.
22. Wilson JM. Reversible congestive heart failure caused by myocardial hibernation. *Tex Heart Inst J.* 1999;26:19–27.
23. Abdullah OM, Drakos SG, Diakos NA, et al. Characterization of diffuse fibrosis in the failing human heart via diffusion tensor imaging and quantitative histological validation. *NMR Biomed.* 2014;27:1378–1386.
24. Drakos SG, Kfoury AG, Hammond EH, et al. Impact of mechanical unloading on microvasculature and associated central remodeling features of the failing human heart. *J Am Coll Cardiol.* 2010;56:382–391.

25. Saito S, Matsumiya G, Sakaguchi T, et al. Cardiac fibrosis and cellular hypertrophy decrease the degree of reverse remodeling and improvement in cardiac function during left ventricular assist. *J Heart Lung Transplant*. 2010;29:672–679.

26. Lopez B, Gonzalez A, Hermida N, et al. Myocardial fibrosis in chronic kidney disease: potential benefits of torasemide. *Kidney Int Suppl*. 2008: S19–S23.

27. Dettmeyer R, Friedrich K, Schmidt P, et al. Heroin-associated myocardial damages—conventional and immunohistochemical investigations. *Forensic Sci Int*. 2009;187:42–46.

28. Whyte G, Sheppard M, George K, et al. Post-mortem evidence of idiopathic left ventricular hypertrophy and idiopathic interstitial myocardial fibrosis: is exercise the cause? *Br J Sports Med*. 2008;42:304–305.

29. Pirolo JS, Hutchins GM, Moore GW, et al. Myocyte disarray develops in papillary muscles released from normal tension after mitral valve replacement. *Circulation*. 1982;66:841–846.

30. Gambarin FI, Tagliani M, Arbustini E. Pure restrictive cardiomyopathy associated with cardiac troponin I gene mutation: mismatch between the lack of hypertrophy and the presence of disarray. *Heart*. 2008;94:1257.

31. Arbustini E, Diegoli M, Fasani R, et al. Mitochondrial DNA mutations and mitochondrial abnormalities in dilated cardiomyopathy. *Am J Pathol*. 1998;153:1501–1510.

32. Beltrami AP, Urbanek K, Kajstura J, et al. Evidence that human cardiac myocytes divide after myocardial infarction. *N Engl J Med*. 2001;346: 5–15.

33. Chimenti C, Kajstura J, Torella D, et al. Senescence and death of primitive cells and myocytes lead to premature cardiac aging and heart failure. *Circ Res*. 2003;93:604–613.

34. Tamura S, Takahashi M, Kawamura S, et al. Basophilic degeneration of the myocardium: histological, immunohistochemical and immuno-electron microscopic studies. *Histopathology*. 1995;26:501–508.

35. Schlitt A, Jordan K, Vordermark D, et al. Cardiotoxicity and oncological treatments. *Dtsch Arztebl Int*. 2014;111:161–168.

36. Torti FM, Bristow MM, Lum BL, et al. Cardiotoxicity of epirubicin and doxorubicin: assessment by endomyocardial biopsy. *Cancer Res*. 1986;46: 3722–3727.

37. Unverferth DV, Magorien RD, Unverferth BP, et al. Human myocardial morphologic and functional changes in the first 24 hours after doxorubicin administration. *Cancer Treat Rep*. 1981;65:1093–1097.

38. Sardao VA, Oliveira PJ, Holy J, et al. Morphological alterations induced by doxorubicin on H9c2 myoblasts: nuclear, mitochondrial, and cytoskeletal targets. *Cell Biol Toxicol*. 2009;25:227–243.

140 Congenital Heart Disease

Allen P. Burke, M.D., and Joseph J. Maleszewski, M.D.

General

Epidemiology

Congenital abnormalities of the heart and aortic arch (excluding the congenitally bicuspid aortic valve) occur in slightly less than 1% of the population[1] and range from severe defects that result in life-threatening symptoms to incidental abnormalities. Congenital anomalies can affect multiple chambers or valves, resulting from a significant developmental defect (complex congenital heart disease). Isolated congenital disease of the valves or isolated atrial septal defects (ASDs) may remain asymptomatic for prolonged periods, and small ventricular septal defects may heal spontaneously. The approximate frequencies of various forms of congenital heart disease are presented in Table 140.1.

Genetics

There are several congenital syndromes associated with specific heart defects, the most common being Down syndrome and 22q11.2 deletion syndrome (see Table 140.2). In infants with heart defects, ~20% have a defined syndrome, about half of which have gross chromosomal defects and half with defects at the gene level. Overall, up to 45% of patients with congenital heart disease have extracardiac anomalies.

Trisomy 21 (Down syndrome) is associated with heart defects in about 40% of patients and, because of its high prevalence, accounts for the largest single group of chromosome-related heart disease. The most characteristic defect is the atrioventricular (AV) septal defect (AV canal defect), but other anomalies, including ventricular septal defect, ASD, and patent ductus arteriosus (PDA), also occur with increased frequency in Down syndrome.

The 22q11.2 deletion syndrome, which includes velocardiofacial and DiGeorge syndromes, is the most frequent known chromosomal microdeletion syndrome, with an incidence of 1 in 4,000 to 5,000 live births. It is characterized by a 3-Mb deletion on chromosome 22q11.2, T-cell deficits, cleft palate facial anomalies, and hypocalcemia. Mutations in *TBX1*, *LHX2*, and *TCF21* are associated with the 22q11.2 syndrome.[4,6] Approximately 80% of patients have heart defects

that include conotruncal anomalies, including truncus arteriosus, and anomalies of the aortic arch, including interruption of the aortic arch.[4]

A family history of congenital heart disease, from relatively simple to complex forms, increases the recurrence in siblings (Table 140.3). Therefore, genetics and epigenetics are likely to play a more significant role than we can directly account for at this time.

TABLE 140.1 Approximate Frequencies of Congenital Heart Diseases, as Proportion of Total

Ventricular septal defect	41%
Atrial septal defect	10%
Pulmonary valve stenosis	8%
Patent ductus arteriosus	8%
Tetralogy of Fallot	5%
Coarctation of the aorta	5%
Atrioventricular septal defect	4%
Transposition of the great arteries	4%
Aortic valve stenosis[a]	3%
Hypoplastic left heart	3%
Double outlet right ventricle	2%
Pulmonary atresia with VSD	1%
Pulmonary atresia with intact VS[b]	1%
Ebstein anomaly	1%
Double inlet left ventricle	1%
TAPVC	1%
Tricuspid atresia	1%
Other	1%

[a]Congenitally dysplastic stenotic valve.
[b]Hypoplastic right heart syndrome.
VS, ventricular septum; VSD, ventricular septal defect; TAPVC, total anomalous pulmonary venous connection.
From van der Bom T, et al. The prevalence of adult congenital heart disease, results from a systematic review and evidence based calculation. *Am Heart J*. 2012;164(4):568–575, Ref. [2]; Hoffman JI, Kaplan S. The incidence of congenital heart disease. *J Am Coll Cardiol*. 2002;39(12):1890–1900, Ref. [3].

TABLE 140.2   Syndromes and Congenital Heart Disease[a]

Syndrome	Heart Defect	Percentage with Heart Involvement
Chromosomal abnormalities		
Trisomy 21 (Down)	VSD, AVSD	40
Trisomy 18 (Edwards)	VSD, AVSD, PVD	95
Trisomy 13 (Patau)	DORV, ToF, VSD, ASD, PDA, PVD, Anomalous pulmonary veins	75
Monosomy X (Turner)	Coarctation, aortic stenosis	30
47,XXY (Klinefelter)	ASD, PDA, MVP	50
Partial chromosomal abnormalities (deletions and tetrasomies)		
22q11.2 syndrome[b] (Del 22q11.2)	DiGeorge (*TBX1, LHX2, TCF21*): TA, ToF, PA-VSD, AAA	75–80
	Velocardiofacial: ToF, TA, AAA	
Williams syndrome (Del 7q11.23)	Supravalvar aortic stenosis	65
Cat eye (tetrasomy 22p)	Anomalous pulmonary veins	50
Genetic abnormalities		
Noonan syndrome (*PTPN11, KRAS, SOS1*, and others)	Hypertrophic cardiomy-opathy, PS, PVD	85
Heterotaxy (*ZIC3, LEFTY2, CFC1, NODAL, ACVR2B*)	Anomalous pulmonary venous connection, AVSD, VI, TGA, DORV, PS	95
Alagille (*NOTCH2, JAG1*)	ToF, PS, PPAS, ASD	90
Holt-Oram (*TBX5*)	ASD, VSD, AVSD, ToF	80
CHARGE (*CHD7, SEMA3E*)	ASD, PDA, MVP	65
Ellis-van Creveld (*EVC, EVC2*)	AVSD, ASD	65
Smith-Lemli-Opitz (*DHCR7*)	AVSD, partial anomalous pulmonary veins	45

[a]Adapted from Blue GM, et al. Congenital heart disease: current knowledge about causes and inheritance. *Med J Aust.* 2012;197(3):155–159, Ref. [4]; Goldmuntz E, Crenshaw ML, Lin AE. Genetic aspects of congenital heart defects. In: Allen HD, et al., eds. *Moss and Adams' Heart Disease in Infants, Children, and Adolescents Including the Fetus and Young Adult.* Philadelphia, PA: Lippincott Williams & Wilkins; 2013:617–643, Ref. [5]. Implicated genes are in italics.
[b]Includes DiGeorge syndrome, velocardiofacial syndrome, Shprintzen syndrome, conotruncal anomaly face syndrome, Strong syndrome, congenital thymic aplasia.
Abbreviations: ToF, tetralogy of Fallot; AAA, aortic arch anomalies; AS, aortic stenosis; ASD, atrial septal defect; AVSD, atrioventricular septal defect (primum and complete types); DORV, double outlet right ventricle; TGA, transposition of the great arteries; PA-VSD, pulmonary atresia with ventricular septal defect; PS, pulmonary stenosis; PDA, patent ductus arteriosus; PPAS, peripheral pulmonary artery stenosis; PVD, polyvalvular dysplasia; TA, truncus arteriosus; VI, ventricular inversion.

Intrauterine Risk Factors

Intrauterine rubella infection is associated with congenital heart defects in up to 45% of fetuses and neonates, including PDA, ventricular septal defect, pulmonary stenosis, and peripheral pulmonary artery stenosis.

TABLE 140.3   Recurrence Risk Siblings, Percent, After Diagnosis of Infant or Fetus with Congenital Heart Disease, by Type

• VSD	4–6
• PDA	2.5–3
• Cushion	2–3
• Coarctation	2–7
• Tetralogy	2–3
• TGA	2
• HLHS	1–4

VSD, ventricular septal defect; PDA, patent ductus arteriosus; TGA, transposition of the great arteries; HLHS, hypoplastic left heart syndrome.

Intrauterine exposure to thalidomide results in a 30% risk of congenital heart defects, including atrial and ventricular septal defects and conotruncal anomalies. Retinoic acid has similar affects, with a 25% rate of defects including ventricular septal defect and tetralogy of Fallot.

Approach to Autopsy

Congenital heart disease is generally diagnosed clinically and known at the time of autopsy. Most patients with complex congenital heart disease have undergone surgical intervention. Familiarity with the surgical procedures and clinical complications, as well as knowledge of the clinicians' concerns, is important. Review of computed tomography angiography reports and other imaging studies and correlation of such with autopsy are critical. Often, the surgical team involved in any intervention will request attendance at the postmortem and can provide invaluable clinical information.

The pathologist may encounter untreated congenital heart disease in babies with inoperable congenital defects, often with extracardiac anomalies. Knowledge of fetal ultrasound findings is very helpful before dissection of the heart, but the pathologist should be guided by the observed anatomy and should not rely solely on imaging or intraoperative impressions.

The dissection of congenital heart specimens should accommodate answering specific questions of the clinicians, expose any abnormalities or complications, and maintain the specimen for photography and potential second opinion recognizing that few centers have the expertise to evaluate the full spectrum of congenital heart disease. Care should be taken to keep the great vessels attached. To these ends, keeping the lungs with the heart will help to document pulmonary venous connections. Thereafter, the lungs, pulmonary veins, ascending aorta, and pulmonary trunk, with the intervening ductus, can be kept as a separate block by transecting the aorta and pulmonary artery near the valves.

There are many facets to the autopsy of a child (or adult) with congenital heart disease, in addition to documenting the underlying malformation. It is important to diagnose extracardiac anomalies (which can help to establish a syndrome) and secondary changes, especially hypertensive changes in pulmonary arteries and chronic congestive changes in pulmonary and hepatic veins. Cardiac hypertrophy secondary to stenosis and shunting can be marked, and right ventricular hypertrophy is frequent in patients with pulmonary hypertension. Myocardial ischemia may occur postoperatively and should be described similar to that seen in native coronary disease. Dilatation of the ventricles and atria should be described.

Interventions (aided by review of the operative notes and imaging studies), including anastomoses, prior takedowns (especially systemic–pulmonary arterial shunts), anastomotic strictures, thrombosis, or narrowing of shunts, are all to be evaluated and documented. It is helpful to review the operative notes prior to autopsy and familiarize oneself with the specific procedure performed.

General Approach and Segmental Analysis

Specimens to be evaluated for congenital heart disease should be approached in a uniform and consistent fashion. Such evaluation begins with a description of the location and position of the heart within the chest, then a thorough description of all the connections (venoatrial, atrioventricular, and ventriculoarterial), and then documentation of any abnormal shunts.

Cardiac Position and Sidedness (Situs)

The normal location (or position) of the heart in the left hemithorax is termed "levoposition." Dextroposition (displacement into the right hemithorax) or mesoposition (midline displacement) often result from extracardiac causes, for example, pulmonary hypoplasia or scoliosis. The direction of the apex is usually described separately as leftward (normal), rightward, or midline.[7]

There are three asymmetric organs: the heart, lungs, and gut. The spleen is a unilateral organ that is left sided from inception. The situs of the three organs indicates the status of normally manifest sidedness: normal (situs solitus), mirror image (situs inversus), right isomerism (both sides have typical right-sided features), and left isomerism (both sides have typical left-sided features). The spleen, being left sided, is absent in right-sided isomerism, on the right in situs inversus, and multiple in left-sided isomerism.

The sidedness (situs) of the heart is determined solely by atrial morphology and can be described as normal (solitus), inverted (inversus), or duplicated (ambiguous). Right atrial features include the presence of the following: crista terminalis, coronary sinus ostium, limbus of the oval fossa, pyramidal atrial appendage, and a suprahepatic portion of the inferior vena cava. Left atrial morphology is defined by a lack of conspicuous pectinate muscles and a narrow-based atrial appendage with variable morphology.

Like atrial morphology, ventricular morphology is side specific. As a rule, the atrioventricular valves always ride with their corresponding ventricle. The inflow, apical trabeculated, and outflow portions of the ventricle each have unique features. The inflow of the morphologic right ventricle (RV) has an atrioventricular (tricuspid) valve with direct septal chordal insertions. The apical trabeculations of a morphologic RV are more coarse than those observed in a morphologic left ventricle (LV), and the outflow portion of the right ventricle is muscular. All tendinous cords on the left are attached to papillary muscles (without direct septal chordal insertions). The apex has finer trabeculations than those seen in a morphologic RV, and the outflow tract is musculomembranous owing to the continuity between the atrioventricular and semilunar valves.

The sidedness of the heart, lungs, and abdominal viscera is not always the same. In complete situs inversus, all three organs are inverted. However, in some cases of heterotaxy syndromes, the heart and possibly lungs may be the only organs involved. Pulmonary sidedness is defined by the relationship of the pulmonary arteries to the upper lobe bronchus. The right side pulmonary artery is normally anterior to the upper lobe bronchus and the left side superior to the upper lobe bronchus. Number of lobes (three on the right, two on the left) is not a reliable indicator of sidedness.

Venoatrial Connections

The inferior vena cava normally enters the right atrium. It may enter the left side of a common atrium or left-sided atrium in heterotaxy syndromes. It may also end in the liver, with azygous connection to the atria. The interrupted inferior vena cava syndrome is associated with heart defects in 85% of cases, especially polysplenia.[8]

The normal left-sided venoatrial connections consist of pulmonary veins (usually two left and two right) emptying into the chamber. Variability in number is not uncommon, but all connections should be documented.

Atrioventricular Connections

Atrioventricular connections can be described as concordant (morphologic atrium to respective morphologic ventricle) or discordant. Ventricular inversion (atrioventricular discordance) may be encountered and is the hallmark of congenitally corrected transposition of the great arteries (L-TGA). Univentricular connections may be the result of a single connection (e.g., tricuspid atresia, where there is absent right-sided and normal left-sided connection); double inlet ventricle (usually left), where two mirror-image mitral-like valves enter the ventricle, with a rudimentary right ventricle; or common inlet atrioventricular valve into a single ventricle (usually right), with a rudimentary left ventricle. The latter condition is highly associated with asplenia.

Ventriculoarterial Connections

Ventriculoarterial discordance is more common than atrioventricular discordance and is seen in all cases of transposition of the great arteries (both D and L types). In this condition, the morphologic right ventricle gives rise to the aorta and the morphologic left ventricle the pulmonary artery. The semilunar valve always accompanies the artery; therefore, the aortic valve is present in the artery that gives rise to the coronary and arch vessels and the pulmonary valve the artery that supplies the lungs.[7]

Other abnormal connections include double outlet ventricles (rare and more common on the right), single outlet (pulmonary atresia or hypoplastic left heart syndrome), and common outlet ventricles (truncus arteriosus).

Valvular Atresia, Stenosis, and Absence

The term "atresia" indicates lack of connection across two chambers normally connected through a valvular orifice. Stenosis indicates decreased flow with a gradient. Absent valve indicates no valve leaflets, but a widely patent outflow (seen exclusively in the pulmonary position in variants of tetralogy of Fallot, where there is marked dilatation of the annulus).

Shunts

A shunt is defined as an abnormal connection between two noncontiguous cardiac structures resulting in abnormal blood flow. The most common type of shunt is a left-to-right shunt (e.g., ASD, ventricular septal defect, patent ductal artery), which results in blood traveling from the systemic circulation into the pulmonary circulation. Clinically, untreated septal defects result in progressive heart failure and acyanotic heart disease, until there is reversal of flow and cyanosis ensues.

Aortic Arch Anomalies

Embryology and Interruption of the Aortic Arch

The dorsal aortas are initially connected to the aortic sac by three sets of arteries that originate from the pharyngeal arches III, IV, and VI. Those from arch III become the carotid and subclavian arteries, IV the aortic arch and innominate artery, and VI the pulmonary arteries and ductus. The ascending aorta and the C segment of the aorta (from the innominate to the left common carotid) are derived from the aortic sac, the B segment from the IV arch (left common carotid to left subclavian), and the A segment (isthmus) from the dorsal aorta. The numbers A, B, and C refer not only to the segments of the aorta but also to the sites of interruption in congenitally interrupted aortic arch. Type B, for example, is the most common seen in DiGeorge syndrome (Fig. 140.1).

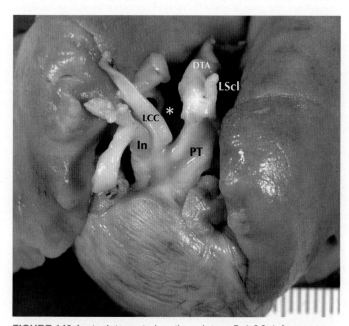

FIGURE 140.1 ▲ Interrupted aortic arch type B. LCC, left common carotid; PT, pulmonary trunk; LScl, left subclavian; DTA, descending thoracic aorta. *Asterisk* is the location of normal arch, which is absent. Interruption between left subclavian and left common carotid is in the B aortic segment, between the left common carotid and left subclavian.

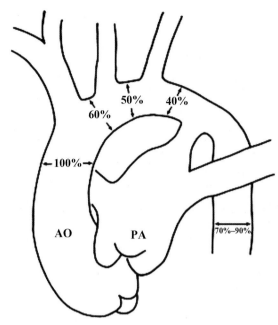

FIGURE 140.2 ▲ Normal diameters of the aortic arch in utero. Note that the isthmus is normally 40% that of the ascending aorta; narrowing of the isthmus should not be overcalled as coarctation. Reproduce with permission, Siewers RD, Ettedgui J, Pahl E, et al. Coarctation and hypoplasia of the aortic arch: will the arch grow? *Ann Thorac Surg.* 1991;52:608–614.

Coarctation of the Aorta

Aortic coarctation usually occurs at the level of the left subclavian artery (distal arch) (Figs. 140.2 to 140.4). In severe infantile coarctation, aortic flow is dependent on ductal flow ("preductal coarctation"). Less severe forms present as hypertension in children and adolescents and are often "postductal."

Most cases of congenital coarctation of the aorta are associated with other cardiac defects, usually congenital left-sided obstruction such as the bicuspid aortic valve, which is seen in approximately half of cases of aortic coarctation. The association of coarctation with supravalvar mitral ring, parachute mitral valve, and subaortic stenosis is termed "Shone complex."[9] There is also an association with cerebral aneurysms and Marfan syndrome.

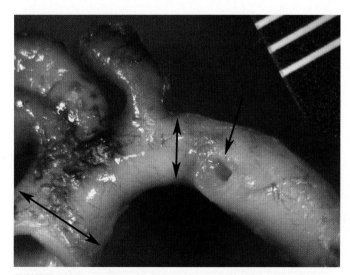

FIGURE 140.3 ▲ Normal infant aortic arch. *Double arrows* show ascending aorta (left) and isthmus (right). *Single arrow* shows the orifice of the ductus arteriosus.

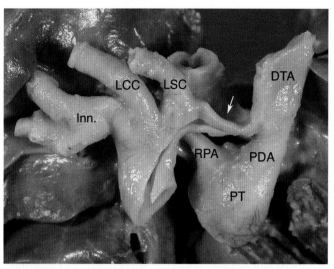

FIGURE 140.4 ▲ Aortic coarctation, preductal. The *arrow* points to the coarctation at the isthmus. Inn, innominate; LCC, left common carotid; LSC, left subclavian; RPA, right pulmonary artery; PT, pulmonary trunk; PDA, patent ductus arteriosus; DTA, descending thoracic aorta.

Surgical corrections of coarctation include balloon angioplasty and resection with placement of an interposition graft. Complications of balloon angioplasty include restenosis, postdilatation aneurysms for native coarctation, aortic dissection, and aortic perforation. Surgical repair of coarctation includes the subclavian flap, which sacrifices the subclavian artery. For this reason, it is recommended only for patients under 1 year of age, so that collateral may form. End-to-end anastomotic repair may be performed in older patients. Complications include recurrent stenosis, persistent left ventricular hypertrophy, and aneurysms at site of repair, especially with patch aortoplasty. Patch repair may be complicated by rupture and endocarditis.

Double Aortic Arch

In double aortic arch, there is duplication of the arch around the trachea and esophagus, forming a ring. The right arch is usually larger, with a left-sided ductus arteriosus (Fig. 140.5). It is commonly isolated but can be associated with transposition of the great arteries, ventricular septal defect, persistent truncus arteriosus, and tetralogy. Double arches are typically symptomatic, with findings of stridor, dysphagia, cough, and pneumonia. Imaging studies demonstrate esophageal and tracheal compression. Diagnosis is confirmed by magnetic resonance angiography.

Aberrant (Retroesophageal) Right Subclavian Artery

Aberrant right subclavian artery is a benign isolated condition affecting 0.5% of the population. The artery arises distal to left subclavian and travels posterior to the esophagus. Oftentimes, a saccular outpouching (diverticulum of Kommerell) may be seen at the takeoff of the right subclavian from the aorta. It rarely causes symptoms, usually in the form of dysphagia ("dysphagia lusoria"). When associated with coarctation, it can cause the subclavian steal syndrome.

Right Aortic Arch

Laterality of the aortic arch is determined by the bronchus over which it travels (left bronchus, left aortic arch; right bronchus, right aortic arch) (Fig. 140.6). Typically, the branching pattern of vessels will be mirror image, such that the innominate arises first giving rise to the left subclavian and common carotid, followed by the right common carotid and right subclavian in turn. Between 20% and 30% of patients with

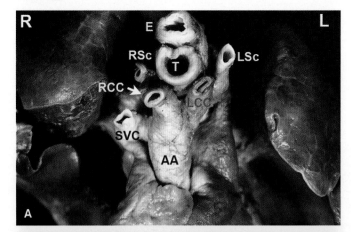

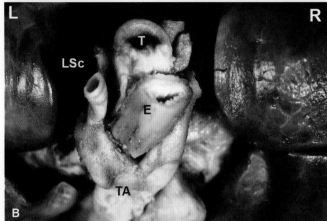

FIGURE 140.5 ▲ Double aortic arch, anterior/cranial view. **A.** The ascending aorta bifurcates into an anterior left branch, supplying the left common carotid artery and the left subclavian artery, and a posterior right branch, supplying the right common carotid and right subclavian arteries. **B.** Double aortic arch, posterior/cranial view. The continuation of the aorta viewed from behind demonstrates the anterior left branch wrapping around the trachea and esophagus as well as the right posterior branch emerging from under the esophagus. The distal aorta continues as a centrally located structure. Abbreviations: RCC, right common carotid artery; LCC, left common carotid artery; RSc, right subclavian artery; LSc, left subclavian artery; E, esophagus; T, trachea; AA, ascending aorta; TA, descending aorta; SVC, superior vena cava.

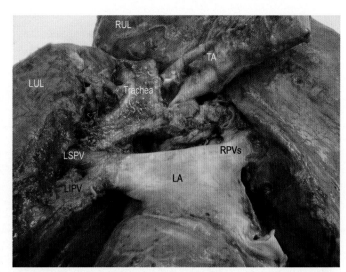

FIGURE 140.6 ▲ Right aortic arch, posterior view. The descending thoracic aorta (TA) is to the right of the trachea. RUL, right upper lobe; LUL, left upper lobe; LSPV, left superior pulmonary vein; RPV, right pulmonary vein; LA, left atrium.

tetralogy, persistent truncus arteriosus, and pulmonary atresia and ventricular septal defect have right-sided arches with mirror-image branching (see below), in addition to lower rates for double outlet right ventricle, tricuspid atresia, and transposition.

Abnormal Shunts

Patent Foramen Ovale

Patent foramen ovale (PFO) refers to failed fusion between the valve and limbus of the fossa ovalis, resulting in a *potential* interatrial communication (Figs. 140.7 and 140.8). It is evaluated for during life via echocardiography (with a bubble study) or at autopsy by the ability to pass a probe from the right atria to the left across the valve of the fossa ovalis. Its incidence is indirectly related with age, seen in approximately one in three individuals <30 years, one in four individuals between the ages of 30 and 80, and one in five individuals >80 years.

Most cases of PFO do not come to clinical attention and are incidental findings on imaging or autopsy. A small proportion, however, present with cerebrovascular symptoms of paradoxical small emboli

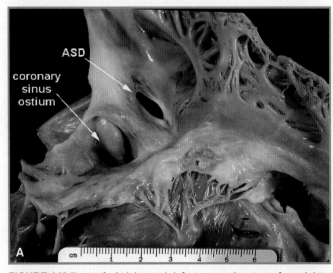

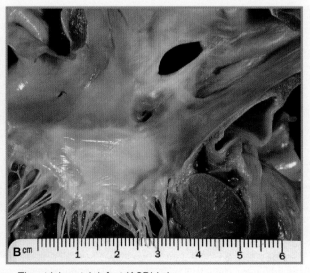

FIGURE 140.7 ▲ **A.** Atrial septal defect, secundum type, from right atrium. The atrial septal defect (ASD) is in the area of the oval fossa. The coronary sinus ostium appears dilated. **B.** Atrial septal defect, secundum type, from left atrium. This defect is the same as that illustrated in figure 8, from the left side. The anterior leaflet of the mitral valve is below.

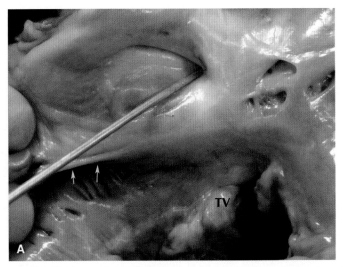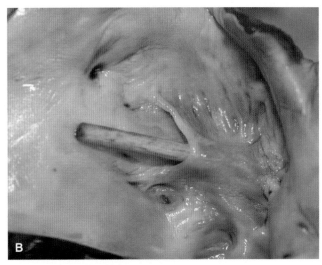

FIGURE 140.8 ▲ Patent foramen ovale, adult. **A.** The probe is present within the right side of the oval fossa. The eustachian valve is present at the bottom above the orifice of the coronary sinus. The septal leaflet of the tricuspid valve (TV) is present below. **B.** Viewed from the left, this patency was a tunnel within the foramen ovale. The characteristic "backward C" is present where the probe emerges.

that may range from sporadic migraine to transient ischemic attacks or stroke. Transthoracic echocardiography with contrast or transesophageal echocardiography is usually required to detect small PFO.

In cases of atrial dilatation, stretching of the atrial wall may cause the limbus and valve portions of a PFO to pull away from one another, resulting in what looks like an ASD (so-called acquired atrial septal defect). Therefore, in cases of atrial dilatation, care should be taken to not overcall the presence of an ASD.

Patent Ductus Arteriosus

Normally, the ductal artery functionally closes within 24 hours of birth and anatomically seals within the first few months of life. PDA refers to persistent communication between the pulmonary artery and aorta through the ductal artery, allowing for a left-to-right shunt early on, which may eventually reverse and become right to left.

In utero and at birth, the duct diameter is approximate to that of the pulmonary trunk and descending thoracic aorta; if significantly narrowed in stillborns, the diagnosis of premature closure of the duct should be considered. In adulthood, calcification and aneurysms may form of the patent duct as well as endocarditis (rarely).[10]

If isolated, it is usually repaired without sequelae. Surgical corrections of the ductus arteriosus include open ligation, vascular clipping, transection with oversewing, and pericardial patching if there are residual defects in the aorta of pulmonary artery or ductal calcification in older patients. Percutaneous closure with device is the current procedure of choice in many centers.[11]

Atrial Septal Defects

ASD refers to an abnormal communication between the atria owing to a deficiency in the atrial septum. They can be categorized into one of four varieties: secundum, coronary sinus, sinus venosus, and primum. The latter, primum type, is usually considered an atrioventricular septal defect and is therefore discussed under that heading.

The most common ASD is the secundum type, representing 70% of cases. The defect is present in the region of the fossa ovalis and is thought to be secondary to incomplete formation of septum secundum or too large of an ostium secundum (Figs. 140.9 and 140.10). The flap valve may be completely absent, or partly absent with fenestrations.

Sinus venosus ASDs are rare and usually associated with partial anomalous pulmonary venous return, because of the location near the superior vena cava and the right pulmonary veins (Fig. 140.11). The location is posterior to the fossa ovalis, on the superior surface of the septum. Sinus venosus defects are often seen in association with

anomalous drainage of right pulmonary veins into the right atrium (partial anomalous venous return).

The least common type of ASD is the coronary sinus type (so-called unroofed coronary sinus). Absence of the anterior portion of the coronary sinus as it enters the right atrium can result in connection to the adjacent left atrium and led to shunting of blood from the left atrium into the coronary sinus and subsequently into the right atrium. This type is often associated with a persistent left-sided superior vena cava.[12]

ASDs are more common in women than men with a 2 to 3:1 ratio. They are occasionally inherited.[13] Symptoms of ASDs result from left-to-right shunting with resultant increased pulmonary blood flow relative to systemic flow. Patients may present with dyspnea, fatigue, and palpitations. Sizeable defects may develop into severe hemodynamic consequences that warrant surgical treatment.

Uncommonly, ASDs may be specific causes of death that are related to atrial fibrillation, right heart failure, and pulmonary hypertension. Echocardiography reliably identifies most cases of ASDs. Cardiac catheterization is used in a few cases, when assessment of hemodynamics is required.[14] Surgery early in life dramatically increases life survival, especially if undertaken before the third decade of life.[15] Open surgical treatment is gradually being replaced by percutaneous closure by clamshell and other types of devices.[16]

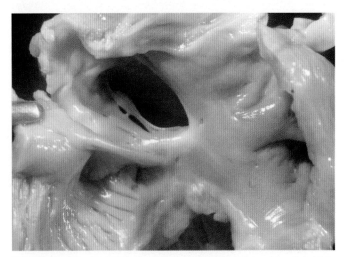

FIGURE 140.9 ▲ Atrial septal defect, secundum type, from the right. There is no septal tissue present in the oval fossa area, save a thin cord. The coronary sinus is present just below (posteriorly).

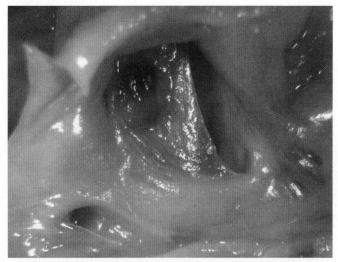

FIGURE 140.10 ▲ Patent foramen ovale, viewed from the right atrium. In this premature neonate, this is a normal finding. The oval fossa nearly covered by a thin, translucent membrane. It is easy to disrupt the ostium primum in fetal and neonatal hearts, and one should be careful not to overcall atrial septal defect.

Atrioventricular Septal Defect

Atrioventricular septal defects (AVSDs) (also called atrioventricular cushion defects) result from a defect in the region of the atrioventricular septum. By virtue of the deficient AV septum, the mitral valve is apically displaced to reside in the same plane as that of the tricuspid valve. AVSDs can be further categorized into complete and partial forms.

A partial AVSD indicates atrial septal involvement (so-called primum-type ASD) with separate mitral and tricuspid valve orifices. The mitral valve usually exhibits a cleft anterior leaflet (Fig. 140.12). There is no direct interventricular or atrioventricular communication. A complete AVSD results in a common atrioventricular valve, with five

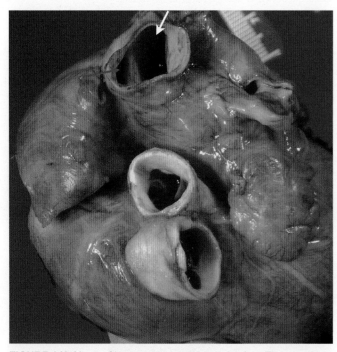

FIGURE 140.11 ▲ Sinus venosus atrial septal defect. The superior vena cava (above) is transected, revealing the superior rim of the atrial septal defect, exposing the right atrium (*blue arrow*) and left atrium (*white arrow*).

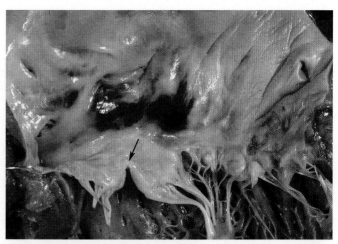

FIGURE 140.12 ▲ Partial atrioventricular canal defect. Note cleft of the anterior mitral valve leaflet (*arrow*).

distinct leaflets, and direct interventricular and atrioventricular communication (Figs. 140.13 to 140.16).

Associated anomalies include Down syndrome (75%), tetralogy of Fallot (almost 100% association with Down syndrome), single papillary muscle in the left ventricle (important to identify prior to surgery), double outlet right ventricle, transposition of great arteries, and hypoplastic left ventricle (unbalanced AVSD).

Surgical correction involves one or two synthetic patches to cover the defect, with suspension of mitral component to the patch and valve reconstruction/replacement. The cleft in the mitral valve (present in partial AV canal) is repaired if large. Postoperative complications include mitral valve stenosis (especially if single papillary muscle or double orifice mitral valve), mitral insufficiency, residual shunts, and arrhythmias in 25% of patients, a minority of whom require pacemakers. Progressive pulmonary hypertension is especially common if there is high pulmonary resistance preoperatively, which occurs most commonly in Down syndrome.

Ventricular Septal Defect

There are several classifications for ventricular septal defects (VSDs). The simplest includes perimembranous (adjacent to the membranous septum), muscular (generally trabeculated portion of the inlet ventricle), outflow or subpulmonic, and inlet/septal (atrioventricular canal defects).[12]

Perimembranous ventricular septal defects account for about 35% of clinically detected VSDs (Figs. 140.17 and 140.18). Synonyms include paramembranous, infracristal, and conoventricular defects. The posterior border is the membranous septum, with the aortic and tricuspid valves in direct continuity. In some hearts, there is a muscular band that separates the defect from membranous septum. The perimembranous defects have been subclassified by the direction to which they extend, including inlet, trabecular, and infundibular.

Small perimembranous ventricular septal defects can spontaneously close by adherence of the septal tricuspid leaflet to the defect. Occasionally, a windsock-type "aneurysm" of the tricuspid valve may form, which may form a nidus for infectious endocarditis (Fig. 140.19).

Muscular ventricular septal defects are the most common type of VSD, but because of their high propensity to spontaneously close, they are the second most common type identified clinically. They can be in the apical, inlet, or outlet portions of the ventricle, when defined as muscle surrounding the entire defect. The most common are apical ones, which can be easily missed at autopsy. Muscular defects close spontaneously by endocardial fibrotic covering over the defect (Fig. 140.20). Spontaneous closure usually occurs in small defects, by age 2 years. A large defect can be defined as the size of the aortic outflow, also called nonrestrictive, which cannot close spontaneously.

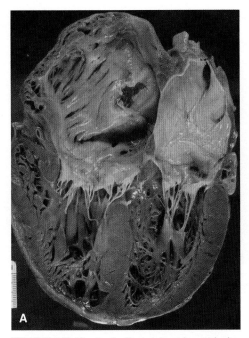
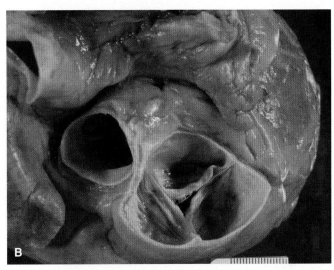

FIGURE 140.13 ▲ **A.** Complete atrioventricular canal defect. The posterior portion of the four-chamber view shows the right ventricle on the left and a defect at the crest of the ventricular septum. There is marked biatrial dilatation, especially on the right. **B.** Complete atrioventricular canal defect. The outflow of the great arteries shows a dilated pulmonary trunk, indicating increased pulmonary to systemic flow.

Outlet or subpulmonic ventricular septal defects are also called juxta-arterial, doubly committed, infundibular, subarterial, supracristal, and conal defects. By definition, there is continuity with pulmonary aortic valves, with a defect seen on the left side between the left and right coronary ostia (Fig. 140.21). The incidence of aortic prolapse/incompetence is higher than in other types of outlet defects (muscular or perimembranous).

Large ventricular septal defects are closed by patch repair, either autologous pericardium or synthetic patch repair. Postoperative complications include right bundle branch block, residual shunts with or without endocarditis, and aortic regurgitation. If the defect is closed before age 3, pulmonary hypertension tends to regress. Pulmonary banding procedures may be formed as a palliative procedure to avert pulmonary hypertension if a definition patch repair cannot be performed early. Untreated ventricular septal defects result in congestive heart failure, recurrent pneumonia, and pulmonary hypertension (usually over 10 years of age). Sudden death can occur secondary to pulmonary hypertension or ventricular arrhythmias.

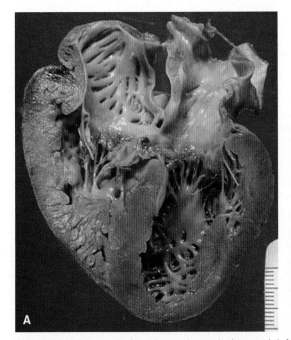
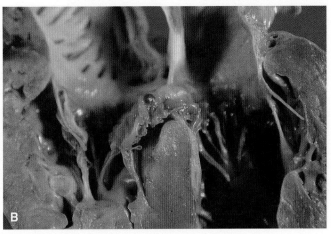

FIGURE 140.14 ▲ **A.** Complete atrioventricular canal defect. A posterior four-chamber view demonstrates focal chordal attachments of the posterior bridging leaflet on the crest of the ventricular septum. **B.** A higher magnification shows focal chordal attachments onto the crest of the posterior ventricular septum.

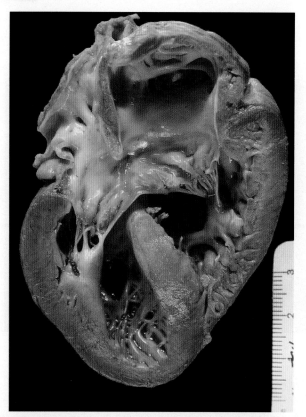

FIGURE 140.15 ▲ Complete atrioventricular canal defect. The anterior portion of this heart shows the anterior bridging leaflet, without chordal attachment onto the crest of the ventricular septum.

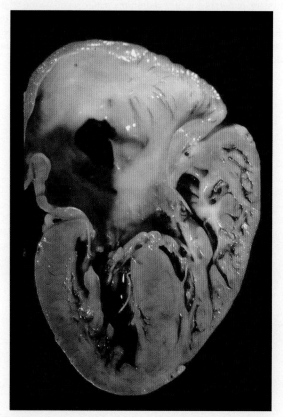

FIGURE 140.16 ▲ Complete atrioventricular canal defect. A four-chamber view from behind, showing the left ventricle at the left. There is massive atrial dilatation. Note that there is valve tissue on the crest of the ventricular septum.

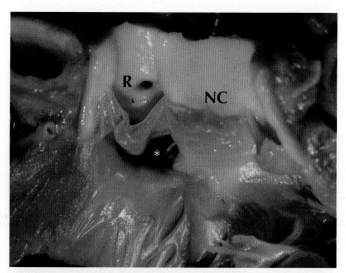

FIGURE 140.17 ▲ Perimembranous septal defect, viewed from left. The *asterisk* shows a large (nonrestrictive) ventricular septal defect in the region of the membranous septum between the right (R) and noncoronary (NC) sinuses of Valsalva.

Congenital Valve Disease

Pulmonary Valve Disease

Congenital pulmonary valve disease most often presents as isolated congenital stenosis, but may also occur in association with tetralogy of Fallot, Noonan syndrome, and chromosomal defects such as trisomies 13 and 18. As a general rule, pulmonary valve stenosis is not typically symptomatic at birth, and survival into adulthood is common. There are a variety of morphologic types, divided into abnormalities of cusp number, narrowing of the annulus, and valve thickening (increased myxomatous tissue resulting in dysplasia). The most common is the acommissural dome-shaped valve, followed by bicuspid valves, quadricuspid valves, tricuspid dysplastic valves with stenosis, hypoplastic valves, and unicuspid valves (with or without raphes) (Figs. 140.21 to 140.24).[17]

The incidence of bicuspid pulmonary valve in the adult population is not known, but is considerably less frequent than bicuspid aortic valve. Analogous to aortic bicuspid aortic valve, there is a risk of endocarditis as well as pulmonary aneurysm with cystic medial necrosis of the pulmonary artery.[18–20] Patients can be asymptomatic for their entire lives, in which case the finding is incidental at autopsy, often with no consequences other than mild pulmonary trunk dilatation. The gross appearance is that of a bicuspid valve similar to that seen in the aortic position (Fig. 140.25). Bicuspid pulmonary valve is the most common type in tetralogy but is uncommon in isolated pulmonary stenosis.

Quadricuspid pulmonary valve is a rare congenital anomaly, which is usually clinically quiescent (Fig. 140.26). Pathologists encounter it occasionally during autopsy. While rare, it is almost five times more common than quadricuspid aortic valve.[21] Autopsy series have estimated quadricuspid pulmonary valve from 0.0014% to 0033% frequency.[22] The majority of cases present as three equal cusps and one smaller rudimentary cusp, about 15% with two large and two smaller cusps, and 10% showing four cusps of equal size.[23] Most cases are clinically silent, but valvular insufficiency has been reported infrequently.[24]

Dysplastic pulmonary valves that result in stenosis may show concomitant dysplasia of the coronary arteries and ascending aorta as well as left ventricular hypertrophy.[25] Pulmonary valve dysplasia, either isolated or as part of polyvalvular dysplasia,[26] is associated with Noonan syndrome.[27,28]

The primary treatment for congenital pulmonary valve stenosis is percutaneous balloon valvuloplasty, which is especially effective

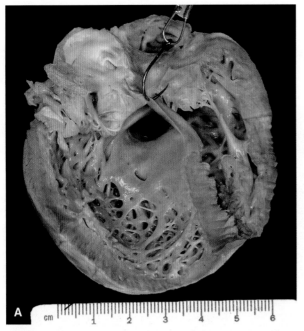

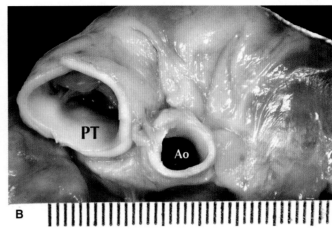

FIGURE 140.18 ▲ **A.** Ventricular septal defect, perimembranous, from left. The defect is large (nonrestrictive). The anterior portion of the heart is shown, with the left ventricle at the left. **B.** Ventricular septal defect, perimembranous, origin of great arteries. The heart demonstrated in Figure 8 shows dilatation of the pulmonary trunk (PT) and normal-sized aorta (Ao). The ventricular septal defect resulted in increased pulmonary blood flow.

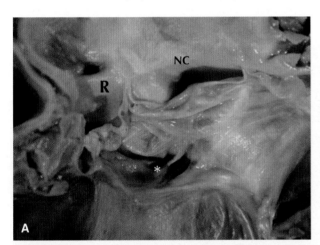

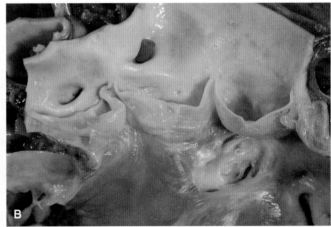

FIGURE 140.19 ▲ Perimembranous ventricular septal defect. **A.** The *asterisk* highlights the membranous septum as seen from the left. R, right coronary sinus, NC, noncoronary sinus. **B.** The membranous septum is enlarged, with a central defect exposing the tricuspid valve, which has partly covered the opening.

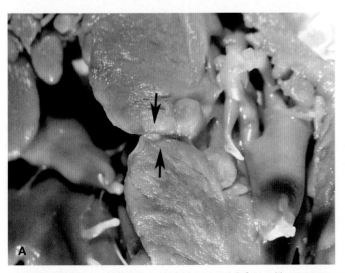

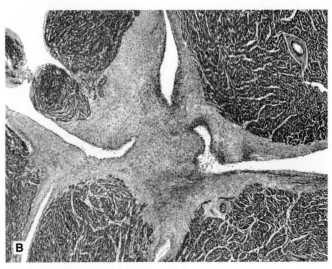

FIGURE 140.20 ▲ Muscular ventricular septal defect, with spontaneous closure. **A.** The *arrows* show an area in the ventricular septum of a defect with central fibrosis. **B.** A trichrome stained shows fibrosis with overgrowth of the defect by collagenous tissue.

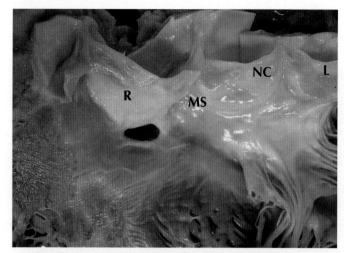

FIGURE 140.21 ▲ Subpulmonary ventricular septal defect, as seen from the left. R, right coronary sinus; MS, membranous septum; NC, noncoronary cusp; L, left sinus.

in the dome-shaped and bicuspid valves. Pulmonary insufficiency is a relatively common complication but is generally mild. However, it may increase with time and is more frequent in younger patients and patients with dysplastic valves.[29]

Tricuspid Valve Disease (Including Ebstein Anomaly)

Ebstein anomaly is a congenital malformation characterized by any degree of apical displacement of the functional tricuspid valve annulus, resulting in the basal ventricle becoming "atrialized" (Figs. 140.27 and 140.28). Formation of the tricuspid valve occurs, in part, due to delamination of the right ventricular endocardium. Failure of this process, so-called nondelamination, results in the Ebstein anomaly.

It represents <1% of all congenital heart diseases with a prevalence of 5.2 per 100,000 live births.[30] Among live births, 40% have other cardiac defects and 20% noncardiac anomalies. In a series surgically resected, 74% of patients had interatrial communication, 13% mitral valve prolapse, and 5% bicuspid aortic valve.[31] The majority of cases are sporadic, with a few familial cases reported; involvement of

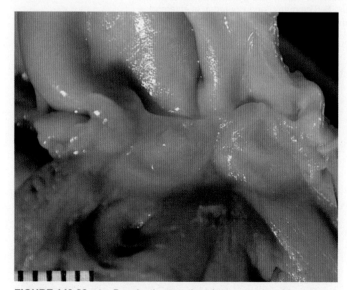

FIGURE 140.22 ▲ Dysplastic stenotic pulmonary valve, 33-week gestational age fetus. The valve leaflets are redundant, thickened, and opaque. The wall of the pulmonary artery was thickened as well.

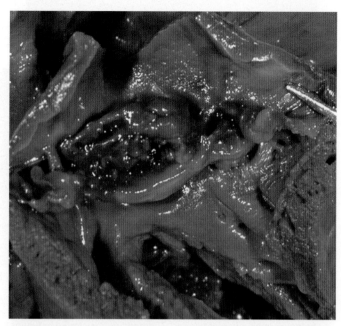

FIGURE 140.23 ▲ Dysplastic stenotic pulmonary valve, 28-week gestation fetus, trisomy 18. The pulmonary valve was markedly dysplastic, without distinct leaflets. The three other heart valves were similarly affected (polyvalvular dysplasia or congenital polyvalvular disease).

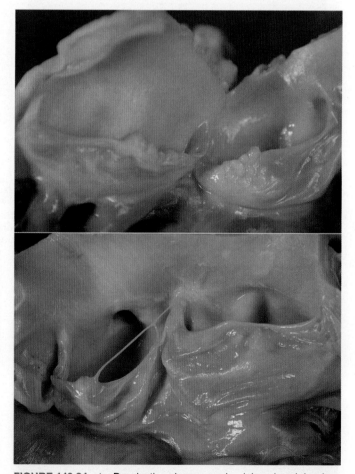

FIGURE 140.24 ▲ Dysplastic pulmonary valve (above) and dysplastic aortic valve (below), 40-year-old man with Noonan syndrome and hypertrophic cardiomyopathy. Note the nodular tissue at the free edge of the pulmonary valve. The third leaflet is out of the field. The aortic valve shows irregularities and a large fenestration. The mitral valve was also dysplastic (polyvalvular dysplasia).

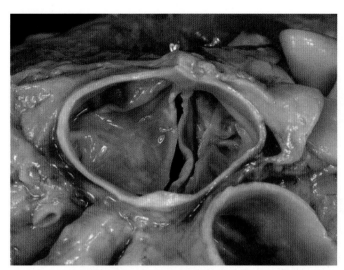

FIGURE 140.25 ▲ Bicuspid pulmonary valve, incidental finding, without dysplasia.

a nonidentical twin raises the risk eightfold over the general population and any family history of congenital heart disease sixfold.[30] Ebstein anomaly is relatively uncommon in African Americans.[30]

Grossly, the right ventricle is typically dilated and thinned; indeed, in a child, this is nearly pathognomonic for Ebstein anomaly. There is typically marked annular dilatation, of up to 20 cm.[32] Usually, the posterior and septal leaflets are adherent to the atrialized ventricle, while the anterior is larger and redundant. The right ventricle can be atrialized and yet show a normal anterior leaflet size and shape, but it can be stenotic in selected cases. A severe form is characterized by atrialization of the entire right ventricle, except for a small infundibular component.

This variable severity correlates with clinical severity, wherein some cases present with intractable heart failure, while others remain asymptomatic throughout life. Surgical resection is the rule with those that are symptomatic. The anterior tricuspid leaflet is resected or, in some instances, reconstructed.

Congenital dysplasia of the tricuspid valve without fusion of the leaflet to the endocardium occurs about one-half as often as Ebstein anomaly.[33] There are wide anatomic variations that lead to congenital tricuspid regurgitation in children without Ebstein malformation, including congenital absence of chordae and myxoid change with elongation and hooding of leaflets (Fig. 140.29). Tricuspid valve dysplasia often accompanies other cardiac defects, especially pulmonary atresia and intact ventricular septum.[34]

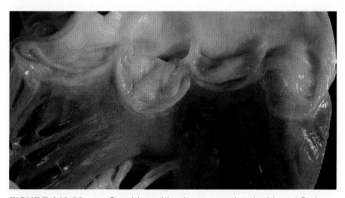

FIGURE 140.26 ▲ Quadricuspid pulmonary valve, incidental finding. Note four leaflets of approximately equal size, which is somewhat unusual; in most cases of quadricuspid valves, one leaflet is rudimentary.

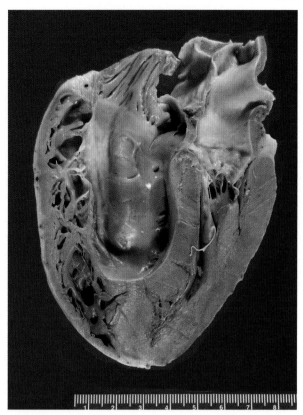

FIGURE 140.27 ▲ Ebstein anomaly, 12-year-old boy with a history of Ebstein anomaly and preexcitation syndrome (Wolff-Parkinson-White). Four-chamber view demonstrating dilated right side, with atrialized ventricle involving posterior free wall and septum.

Subvalvular Aortic Stenosis

The incidence of subvalvular aortic stenosis is about 0.1 per 1,000 live births.[35] There is a male predominance (2:1) and an association with ventricular septal defect, PDAs aortic coarctation, and interruption in about a third of patients.[36] About one-third of cases of isolated subvalvular aortic stenosis are associated with bicuspid aortic valve.[37] In addition to gradients below the valve, there is frequently insufficiency at the valve level itself, due to hemodynamic changes and in some cases dysplastic leaflets.[38] Patients generally become symptomatic before age 20, with a mean age at surgery between 7 and 10 years of age.[35] Patients may present with a heart murmur, or signs and symptoms related to associated cardiac conditions or aortic stenosis.

Subvalvular aortic stenosis is caused by a fibrous membrane in the majority of cases (Figs. 140.30 to 140.32) and a tunnel-like narrowing of the left ventricular outflow tract in the remainder.

Subvalvular membranes usually extend to the aortic valve and the anterior leaflet of the mitral valve.[37] The subvalvular membrane creates abnormal flow, which gives rise to jet lesions underneath the aortic leaflets. Surgical procedures for subvalvar aortic stenosis include fibrous or fibromuscular subaortic resection, apical aortic conduit insertion, aortic valve replacement with mechanical valve, Ross procedure (aortic valve replacement with pulmonary autograft), or Ross-Konno procedure (concomitant subaortic muscular resection).[39] Recurrence of subvalvar obstruction occurs more commonly with the tunnel type. The development of valvular regurgitation is more common if the membrane is <6 mm from the valve.[40-42]

When resected, there are fragments of muscle with attached thickened endocardium. Histologic evaluation shows a bland fibrous membrane, often with cardiac muscle underlying, depending on the type of surgical procedure.

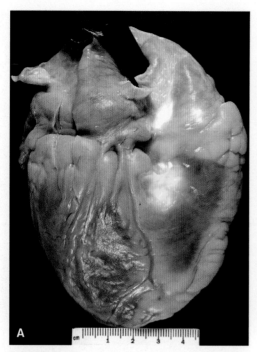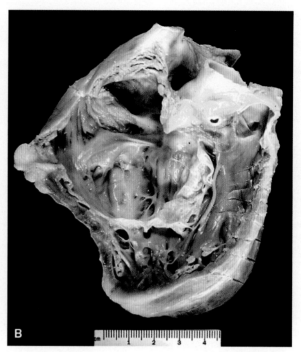

FIGURE 140.28 ▲ Ebstein anomaly. **A.** The heart is viewed from the inferior aspect. There is a light in the right ventricle demonstrating transillumination. **B.** The right ventricular inflow portion is thinned with the valve adhered to the posterior wall. The outflow is to the right.

Aortic Valve Disease

Supravalvar aortic stenosis is one of the least common causes of left ventricular outflow tract obstruction. It typically presents in childhood. It is in most cases associated with a localized aortic narrowing, but can also involve the aortic root diffusely.[43] Clinically, patients present with symptoms related to aortic stenosis and are at risk for sudden death and anesthetic complications. Symptoms include dyspnea, syncope, and angina.

Supravalvular aortic stenosis most typically demonstrates an external hourglass deformity with luminal narrowing of the aorta at a level just distal to the coronary artery ostia (Fig. 140.33A). In one in four patients, a fibrous diaphragm is present just distal to the coronary artery ostia. Least commonly, there is diffuse narrowing along a variable length of ascending aorta. The arch vessels may be involved (Fig. 140.33B).

The aortic valve is often thickened and dysplastic with concomitant thickening of the sinotubular junction. Aortic valve abnormalities occur in half of the patients, most commonly bicuspid aortic valve.[43]

There is a high rate of coronary lesions. There may be narrowing limited to the ostium, due to dysplasia or fusion of the aortic cusp to the supravalvar ridge, or diffuse narrowing of the coronary arteries. Histologic features include reduction and disorganization of

FIGURE 140.29 ▲ Tricuspid valve dysplasia with marked right atrial dilatation, fetal heart. Note the marked enlargement with elongation of the leaflets, but Ebsteinization was not present.

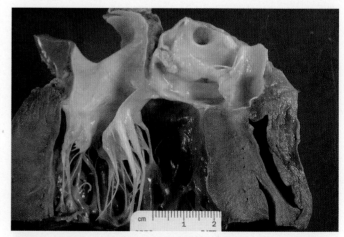

FIGURE 140.30 ▲ Subvalvar aortic stenosis. There is a discrete membrane underneath the valve. The left coronary ostium is visible. There are fenestrations on the left cusp of the aortic valve, which is often regurgitant in patients with subvalvar aortic stenosis.

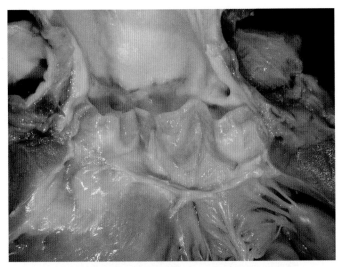

FIGURE 140.31 ▲ Subvalvar aortic stenosis, recurrence of membrane. In this case, there is evidence of prior surgery (see sutures in proximal ascending aorta). The valve itself is dysplastic. The membrane is quite close to the valve, which is a bad prognostic sign.

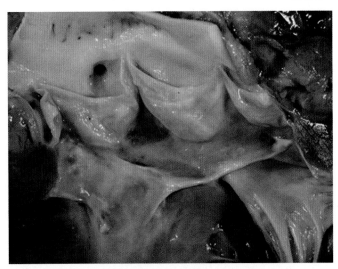

FIGURE 140.32 ▲ Subvalvar aortic stenosis, recurrence of membrane. In this example, there is again evidence of prior surgery in the proximal aorta. The free edges of the aortic valve show rolling and mild redundancy indicative of insufficiency. The membrane has recurred.

elastic fibers with the media, imparting the appearance of dysplasia (Fig. 140.34). Similar findings occur in the aortic wall.[44] There is also increased collagen deposition and smooth muscle hypertrophy.

Conotruncal Anomalies

Tetralogy of Fallot

The primary defect in tetralogy of Fallot is anterior displacement of the infundibular "septum" resulting in a large malalignment ventricular septal defect (Fig. 140.35). The ventriculoinfundibular fold (parietal band) inserts anterior to trabecula septomarginalis (septal band) instead of between limbs of septal band. There is overriding of the aorta over the right ventricle, with narrowing of the right ventricular outflow. The right ventricle is secondarily hypertrophied. The ventricular septal defect is typically perimembranous, large, and nonrestrictive.

The degree of pulmonary stenosis determines the pulmonary flow and the overall clinical severity. If there is critical stenosis, the pulmonary circulation depends on the ductal artery, which may be right or left sided. The pulmonary valve is either stenotic or dysplastic (75%), bicuspid (65%), and absent (3%).

The surgical correction is often in stages. The first is to increase pulmonary flow with a systemic–pulmonary shunt, such as the Blalock-Taussig shunt (ipsilateral subclavian to pulmonary artery, typically with an interposition graft). Next, there is a right ventricular reconstruction with patch enlargement of the outflow, with or without a transannular patch or pulmonary valve replacement. At this stage, there is generally the repair of the ventricular septal defect and takedown of the shunt. Surgical complications include right bundle branch block, left anterior hemiblock, residual right ventricular obstruction, aortic regurgitation, and late aortic dilatation.

Overall, postsurgically, actuarial 10-, 20-, and 30-year survival rates are 97%, 94%, and 89% respectively,[45] and sudden cardiac death occurs at the rate of 1%, 2%, and 5% at 10, 20, and 30 years, respectively.[46] Findings at autopsy in patients who die suddenly are nonspecific and demonstrate ventricular scarring consistent with prior surgery and various degrees of right ventricular dilatation.

Late complications included recurrent pulmonary valve disease, typically insufficiency, especially after transannular patch repair. The pathologist may receive pulmonary valve leaflets in adults treated with valve replacement decades after initial correction for tetralogy of Fallot.[47]

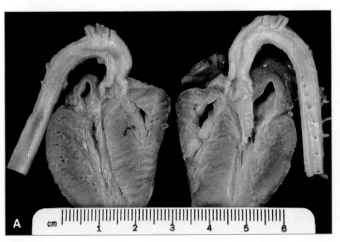

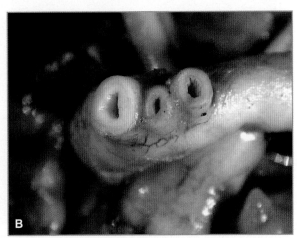

FIGURE 140.33 ▲ Supravalvar aortic stenosis. **A.** Note the narrowing of the aorta at the sinotubular junction. This patient suffered from Williams syndrome. **B.** Supravalvar aortic stenosis, involvement of arch vessels. This condition is associated with thickening and dysplasia of the coronary arteries, aorta, and proximal arch vessels.

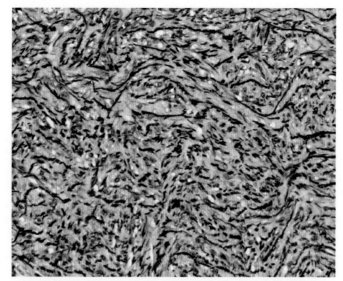

FIGURE 140.34 ▲ Supravalvar aortic stenosis, medial dysplasia. The pulmonary arteries demonstrate disorganization of the media (Movat elastic stain). Similar findings were seen in the coronary arteries and aortic wall (not illustrated).

Pulmonary Atresia with Ventricular Septal Defect (PA-VSD)

PA-VSD denotes the absence of a connection between the right ventricle, which is usually normally situated, and the pulmonary arteries. It is sometimes clinically considered the extreme form of tetralogy of Fallot,[48] but the lesions are anatomically different.[12,49,50] The atretic segment is cord-like in 70%, and there is no identifiable segment in the majority of the remainder. In <5% of cases, the atresia is isolated to the valve; these are the easiest to correct surgically. A clinical classification adopted by imaging specialists identifies four types: pulmonary trunk present but atretic (type I), both pulmonary arteries present (pulmonary artery confluence) without trunk (II), single artery present (III), and absent intrapericardial pulmonary arteries (IV); types II to IV have also been termed A to C, respectively.[50]

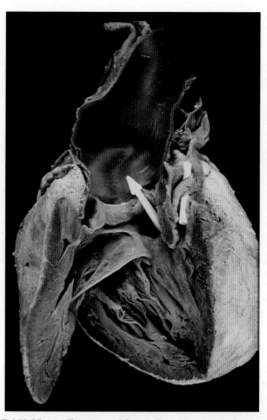

FIGURE 140.35 ▲ Tetralogy of Fallot. The right ventricular is opened to expose the ventricular septal defect and overriding aorta (*white plastic arrow*). The right ventricle is hypertrophied due to marked outflow obstruction (white plastic tube). Figure courtesy Dr. William Edwards.

A right-sided arch is present in about 25% of cases (Fig. 140.36A). Practically, pulmonary atresia with VSD can be separated into those with a significant portion of pulmonary blood flow from the pulmonary artery (via the ductus) and those with most arising from major

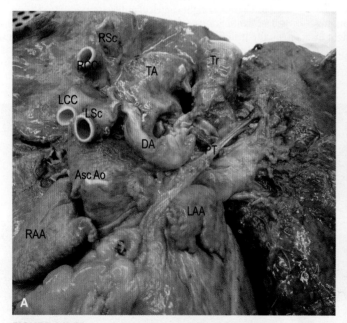

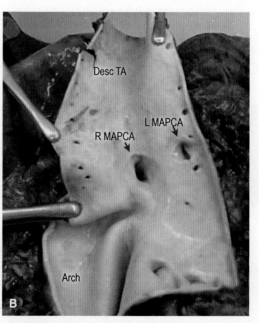

FIGURE 140.36 ▲ Pulmonary atresia with ventricular septal defect and major aortopulmonary collateral arteries. **A.** The pulmonary trunk (PT) is a thin cord. The ductus arteriosus (DA) supplies the right lung. TA, thoracic aorta; Asc ao, ascending aorta; LCC, left common carotid; LSc, left subclavian; RSc, right subclavian; Tr, trachea; RAA, right atrial appendage. The right is right sided, with mirror-image branching. **B.** The descending thoracic aorta is opened, revealing MAPCA (major aortopulmonary collateral artery) orifices. Desc, descending.

aortopulmonary collateral arteries (MAPCAs), which largely are derived from bronchial arteries (Fig. 140.36B). The surgical anatomy is defined by the presence or absence of pulmonary artery confluence.

If the ductus is patent, there is 80% chance of pulmonary artery confluence. If the duct supplies one lung, it is usually the *only* supply to this lung. In addition to MAPCAs, pulmonary flow may arise from subclavian arteries, abdominal aorta, coronary artery, bronchial plexuses, and pleural arteries.

The ventricular septal defect is usually the malalignment type (with override of the aorta), either membranous or infundibular, and is similar to that of truncus arteriosus. The arch is right sided in up to 30% of cases, similar in incidence to tetralogy of Fallot and truncus arteriosus. The ascending aorta is typically dilated. One-half of patients have a secundum-type ASD.

With confluent arteries, a complete repair with a valved graft is possible, with concomitant patch repair of the ventricular septal defect. Even with confluent arteries, if fewer than 14 of the 20 lung segments are not supplied, the treatment is the same as for nonconfluence.

With nonconfluent arteries ("pulmonary atresia with VSD and MAPCAs"), the pulmonary blood flow is supplied primarily by arteries that may have limited potential for growth. Often, a staged repair is performed to enlarge initially the central pulmonary arteries with a central aortopulmonary artery shunt, or if there is a hypoplastic pulmonary artery confluence, with a right ventricle–pulmonary artery conduit. One-stage procedure entails surgically combining collateral arteries (unifocalization) and anastomosing them to a reconstructed pulmonary artery confluence, which is connected to the right ventricle with a variety of conduits including cryopreserved homografts and various heterografts.[51,52] Generally, a VSD repair is performed and MAPCAs that are not used for unifocalization are embolized with coils or ligated or left alone.

Pulmonary Atresia with Intact Ventricular Septum (Hypoplastic Right Heart)

This variant of pulmonary atresia is less common than pulmonary atresia with ventricular septal defect and has a different clinical and surgical approach. The heart findings are somewhat analogous to hypoplastic left heart syndrome, but on the right side. The right ventricle is usually markedly hypoplastic, but may still be evident due to coronary cameral fistulae (ventriculocoronary shunts) allowing for intracavitary flow. The right ventricle, in <10% of cases, is dilated and thin walled; this configuration has a high mortality. The tricuspid valve is usually abnormal with regurgitation, and in some cases, coexistent Ebstein anomaly. The pulmonary outflow is atretic at the valve with or without infundibular atresia. The pulmonary trunk is unusually near normal in size with pulmonary flow from ductus arteriosus.[53]

Right ventricular fistulae are common, providing flow to the coronary arteries from the right ventricle. Therefore, the coronary ostia may be small and one or both completely atretic (absent ostium) (Fig. 140.37). In these cases, surgical repair with right ventricular decompression by right ventricular, oversewing of tricuspid valve may result in cardiac ischemia and postoperative death.

Surgical treatment is variable and an option only if right ventricular decompression is not contraindicated by fistulae with coronary ostial stenosis. If there is a hypoplastic right ventricle with infundibular atresia, atrial patency by balloon septostomy is necessary, with subsequent oversewing of the tricuspid valve and eventual Fontan procedure. The Fontan procedure establishes a communication between the right atrium and pulmonary artery, either with a conduit or without (direct anastomosis), and utilized the right atrium as a pumping chamber. An alternative procedure is anastomosis of the superior vena cava to the pulmonary artery (Glenn anastomosis).[54] Homograft valves are often chosen for the valved conduits, which may be composed entirely of tissue as opposed to synthetic grafts, because of improved longevity. Long-term complications of the Fontan procedure include the formation of arteriovenous malformations in the lung and cardiac cirrhosis.[55,56]

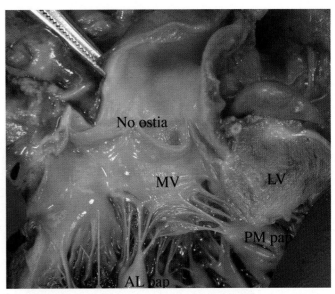

FIGURE 140.37 ▲ Pulmonary atresia with intact ventricular septum. There are no coronary ostia. These have regressed due to coronary cameral fistulae that were supplying blood flow to the ventricle before surgery, at which time the right-sided pressures were decreased. LV, left ventricle; MV, mitral valve; PM pap, posteromedial papillary muscle; AL pap, anterolateral papillary muscle.

Transposition of the Great Arteries

Transposition of the great arteries is characterized by ventriculoarterial discordance. The diagnosis can be recognized by inspection of the great arteries; instead of their normal perpendicular arrangement, the arteries arise in parallel with a right anterior aorta (Fig. 140.38A). In 21%, the aorta is directly anterior, and in 12%, the aorta is to the right of the pulmonary artery (side by side) (Fig. 140.38B).

Grossly, the coronary ostia and arch vessels branch from the aorta, which arises from the right ventricle. In 60% to 80%, there is an intact ventricular septum; 6% to 9% of these have subpulmonic (left ventricular outflow) obstruction. Obstruction is caused by a narrow annulus or subvalvar muscle. When there is a VSD, 25% to 30% of patients have subpulmonic obstruction, either by malalignment of the VSD or straddling of valves. Eight percent of patients have extracardiac anomalies, and fewer than 1% have chromosomal syndromes. Juxtaposition of the atrial appendages, usually with both appendages situation to the left of the great arteries, may be seen in transposition of the great arteries as well as tricuspid atresia (Fig. 140.38C).

Because the circulations are parallel, not serial, oxygenation depends on some type of shunt. If not coexistent, these shunts can be created medically (administration of prostaglandins to maintain ductal artery patency) or surgically (atrial septostomy). In many cases, children undergo definitive surgery within a few days of life without the need for palliative procedures.

Coronary artery patterns from the anteriorly located aorta are important in determining outcome of arterial switch.[57] In 75%, the right coronary artery arises from the posterior sinus and the left main from the anterior sinus (Fig. 140.38B). In 15%, the right coronary artery and left circumflex arise from the posterior sinus and the left anterior descending from the anterior sinus. In 5%, there is a single ostium posteriorly. Intramural coronary arteries are especially difficult to reimplant surgically.[58]

The arterial switch operation is the procedure of choice and is best performed within 2 weeks of birth.[59] The surgeon transects the aorta and pulmonary trunk and implants the coronary ostia into the pulmonary trunk, often with pericardial reconstruction (Fig. 140.39). Negative prognostic factors include age older than 1 month, preceding pulmonary artery banding, and adverse coronary artery patterns. Anatomic complications that can be evaluated at autopsy include stenosis of the arterial anastomoses, neoaortic valve regurgitation, and acute myocardial infarction.

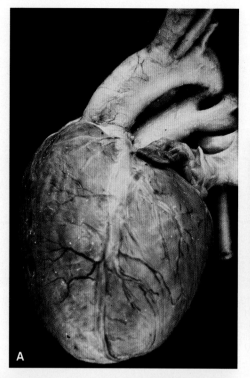

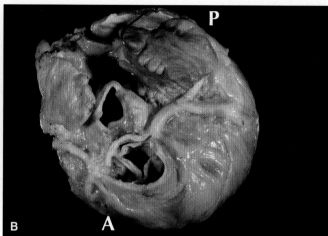

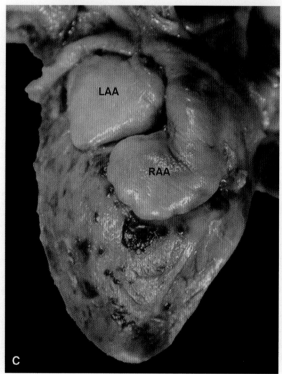

FIGURE 140.38 ▲ Transposition of the great arteries. **A.** The anterior aspect of the heart shows right ventricular prominence and the aorta anterior arising from this chamber. The pulmonary valve is posterior. (Figure courtesy William Edwards, M.D.) **B.** There is juxtaposition of the right atrial appendage to the left of the ascending aorta. Left-sided juxtaposition is usually associated with transposition of the great arteries or tricuspid atresia. LAA, left atrial appendage; RAA, right atrial appendage. **C.** As shown from above, the aorta (A) is anterior and to the left, instead of posterior (P) and to the right. The left anterior descending arises from the posterior leaflet and the right from the anterior leaflet.

Ventriculoarterial discordance may accompany a variety of congenital heart disease, including congenitally corrected transposition (by definition), tricuspid atresia, atrioventricular septal defects, arch anomalies, and double inlet ventricles (Fig. 140.40).

Truncus Arteriosus

Truncus arteriosus (TA) is failure of the common truncal artery to divide into the aorta and pulmonary artery. It accounts for <1% of complex congenital heart disease. Up to 40% of patients have the 22q11.2 deletion syndrome.[60] TA is frequently misdiagnosed by

autopsy pathologists in cases of pulmonary atresia or hypoplastic left heart syndrome, in which there is a single trunk consisting of the aorta and pulmonary trunk, respectively.

In TA, a common trunk gives rise to the coronary ostia, pulmonary arteries, and arch vessels. The valve for this trunk is the only outflow of ventricles; the truncal valve is often abnormal. There are three types of persistent truncus arteriosus:

- Type I: a main pulmonary artery arising from truncus, then bifurcating
- Type II: separate pulmonary arteries near each other from truncus

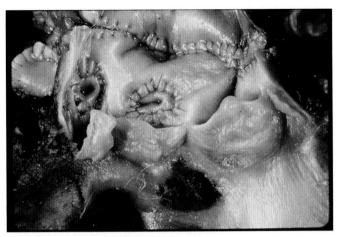

FIGURE 140.39 ▲ Transposition of the great arteries, status postre-pair. Sutures show implantation sites of the coronary arteries and the anastomosis between the native pulmonary trunk and distal aorta. Figure courtesy William D. Edwards, M.D.

- Type III: separate pulmonary arteries at opposite sides of the truncus
- (Type IV): pulmonary arteries arise from descending aorta; most of these represent pulmonary atresia with large collaterals

In 65% of cases, the truncal valve is tricuspid; it is bi- or quadricus-pid in the remainder. There is always a large ventricular septal defect, which is large and nonrestrictive. Associated conditions include right-sided arch (30%), interrupted arch (15%), and absence of the ductus arteriosus (50%).

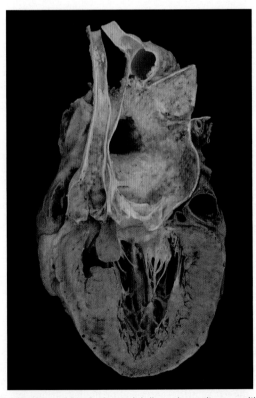

FIGURE 140.40 ▲ Ventriculoarterial discordance (transposition), with interrupted aortic and double inlet left ventricle. The right ven-tricle is rudimentary consisting of only an outflow portion and gives rise to the aorta, which is interrupted after the innominate artery. The pulmonary trunk is massively dilated and arises from the dominant left ventricle. The pulmonary trunk continues as the thoracic aorta, giving rise to distal arch vessels. Figure courtesy William Edwards, M.D.

Surgical correction includes construction of a valved conduit, often with a homograft valve, from the right ventricle to the pulmonary arteries, together with repair of the ventricular septal defect, such that the truncal valve (neoaortic valve) communicates with the left ventri-cle. The presence of the 22q11.2 deletion is a negative prognostic factor for length of hospital stay and adverse events.[60]

Double Outlet Right Ventricle

Double outlet right ventricle, in which both great arteries arise from the morphologic right ventricle, accounts for <1% of complex congeni-tal heart disease. Because the artery is assigned to whichever ventricle it is most over, there may be some overlap with cases of tetralogy of Fallot, where the overriding aorta may be assigned to the morphologic right ventricle by some observers.

Classification of double outlet right ventricle, with two semilunar valves arising from the right ventricular, without fibrous continuity with the atrioventricular valves, usually depends on the location of the septal defect:

- DORV with subaortic VSD (60% to 70%)
- DORV with subpulmonary VSD (Taussig-Bing heart) (20%)
- DORV with doubly committed VSD (5%)
- DORV with uncommitted VSD (10% to 15%)

Associated anomalies include aortic coarctation, if there is a sub-pulmonary ventricular septal defect and small aorta, and straddling atrioventricular valve, especially the tricuspid.

Surgical correction includes intraventricular tunnel repair, involv-ing baffling of the VSD to connect the left ventricle to the aorta, with right ventricular outflow reconstruction necessary in about one-half of cases. In cases other than subaortic VSD, tunnel repair to the pulmo-nary trunk, and arterial switch or similar procedure may be necessary. If there is severe outflow obstruction, then a LeCompte or Rastelli pro-cedure may be necessary (see Table 140.4). Concurrent valvuloplasties or enlargement of the VSD is needed in 12% of patients.[62]

CC-TGA (Congenitally Corrected Transposition of the Great Arteries)

Congenitally corrected transposition of the great arteries (CC-TGA, L-TGA) is characterized by the presence of both discordant atrioven-tricular and ventriculoarterial connections. It accounts for <1% of congenital heart disease and is several times less frequent than trans-position with normally related ventricles (D-TGA). Although the combination of atrioventricular and ventricular discordance results in normally connected circulation, associated anomalies result in severe cardiac dysfunction in the vast majority of patients. Even those without associated anomalies will ultimately exhibit symptoms of heart failure as the morphologic right ventricle is not capable of serving as a long-term systemic chamber.

Those with associated anomalies often exhibit significant pulmo-nary stenosis and ventricular septal defect; occasionally, the systemic atrioventricular valve ("tricuspid") shows Ebstein-like deformity. Straddling of one atrioventricular valve is common. One chamber may be relatively hypoplastic, forming a spectrum with univentricular heart (double inlet left or right ventricle). Partial or complete heart block is common. Complete atrioventricular canal can be present in asplenia cases associated with the asplenia syndrome; these commonly have common atria, pulmonary venous return abnormalities, and pulmo-nary stenosis. Treatment includes double atrial and arterial switch, with Senning often preferred.[63,64]

Functionally Univentricular Hearts

From an embryologic standpoint, there is no such thing as a uni-ventricular heart in mammals, because the normal looping results in two ventricles very early in cardiac development. However, function-ally univentricular hearts represent a significant proportion of com-plex congenital heart disease. There is almost always a rudimentary

TABLE 140.4 Selected Surgical Procedures for Congenital Heart Disease

Procedure	Examples of Underlying Condition	Description
Pulmonary artery banding	VSDs, large, multiple, complex Balanced atrioventricular canal defects CC-TGA TGA Double outlet right ventricle[61]	Synthetic band around pulmonary trunk (open procedure) Intraluminal pulmonary artery banding
Atrial septectomy	TGA (currently less common with early complete correction) HLHS/univentricular hearts Tricuspid atresia	Excision of atrial septum Balloon septostomy (more historical)
Blalock-Taussig shunt	Initial palliation hypoplastic left heart syndrome (during Norwood)	PTFE shunt between innominate right pulmonary artery (or ipsilateral pulmonary artery)
Central aortopulmonary shunt, with PTFE graft	PA-VSD, palliation	PTFE shunt between the ascending aorta and pulmonary artery
RV–PA conduit	Initial palliation, hypoplastic left heart	Alternative to BT shunt
Unifocalization of MAPCAs	PA-VSD with MAPCAs	Merging collaterals with the native pulmonary arteries or with each other by side-by-side anastomoses; patch augmenting the neoconstructed pulmonary arterial confluence
RVOT reconstruction	ToF PA-VSD, pulmonary confluence PA intact VS	Augmentation of outflow tract with synthetic patch, autologous patch, with or without valve replacement and conduit or pulmonary arteries
Arterial switch	TGA	Transection of ascending aorta and pulmonary trunk, with reanastomosis to native pulmonary trunk and aorta, respectively, and reimplantation of coronary arteries
Atrial switch	TGA, usually CC-TGA with arterial switch/Rastelli	Rerouting pulmonary veins to right ventricle with venae cavae to the left atrium, with (Mustard) or without (Senning) pericardial patch conduit
Rastelli	TGA or CC-TGA with subpulmonary obstruction DORV with outflow obstruction	Conduit between RVOT and pulmonary artery, with conduit (valved homograft conduit, bovine vein, PTFE, porcine aortic root, etc.)
LeCompte procedure (REV[a])	TGA with subpulmonary obstruction PA-VSD (with pulmonary confluence without MAPCAs) DORV and other anomalies with pulmonary stenosis	Resection of the conal septum with RVOT reconstruction, with arterial switch (for TGA) Augmentation of PA with segment of aorta (modification)
Norwood	Hypoplastic left heart "Univentricular" hearts	Aortic arch reconstruction with or without autologous or homograft pericardial patch; coarctation excision, with or without anastomosis of descending aorta to aortic arch; ascending aorta division with reimplantation to the right anterior neoaorta
Glenn bidirectional (bidirectional cavopulmonary anastomosis)	Hypoplastic left heart syndrome Pulmonary atresia with intact VS Double inlet left ventricle	Direct anastomosis of superior vena cava to pulmonary artery confluence, allowing bilateral pulmonary (nonpulsatile) flow, detaching SVC from right atrium
Fontan (original)	Pulmonary atresia with intact VS or VSD with intact PA confluence	Communication between right atrium and pulmonary arteries with or without conduit
Total cavopulmonary connection, intracardiac (modified Fontan)	Hypoplastic left heart syndrome Tricuspid atresia Univentricular hearts	After bidirectional Glenn, fenestrated baffle (PTFE) in the right atrium excludes blood flow through the tricuspid valve and connects right atrium to superior vena cava
Extracardiac TCPC (modified Fontan)		Extracardiac PTFE conduit from inferior vena cava (or hepatic vein if necessary in heterotaxy cases) and SVC-PA Glenn anastomosis
Damus-Kaye-Stansel	TGA with tricuspid atresia or hypoplastic right heart syndrome; double inlet left ventricle TGA (historical)	Anastomosis of the proximal end of the transected pulmonary artery to the side of the ascending aorta, RA–PA conduit or modified Fontan procedure
Ross procedure	Congenital aortic stenosis	Aortic valve replacement by pulmonary autograft
Ross-Konno procedure	Congenital aortic stenosis	Ross procedure with subaortic muscle resection (myectomy)
Sano shunt	Conduit between right ventricle and pulmonary artery confluence	First stage Norwood for hypoplastic left heart syndrome

[a]Réparation a l'étage ventriculaire.
[b]Left ventricle in normally related ventricles; right ventricle in inverted ventricle; dominant ventricle in hearts with univentricular dominance.

hypoplastic ventricle identifiable either grossly as a slit-like cavity or microscopically as an endocardial-lined space (Fig. 140.40). The "univentricular" hearts are embryologically diverse and are grouped together only because of some similarities in operative approach. The major types are:

• Hypoplastic left heart syndrome (aortic/mitral atresia)
• Absent right atrioventricular connection (tricuspid atresia)
• Other forms of single atrioventricular connection associated with ventricular inversion and heterotaxy (double inlet left ventricle and common inlet right ventricle)

Hypoplastic Left Heart Syndrome

Hypoplastic left heart syndrome is characterized by normal atrial situs, normally formed right ventricle, and absent or hypoplastic connection between the left ventricle–aorta and/or the left atrium–left ventricle. The left-sided valves are either absent (consisting of an imperforate membrane) or hypoplastic (Fig. 140.41). The mitral valve is atretic in 65% of cases and markedly stenotic in the balance. Coronary circulation is provided by ostia in the aortic root, which is intact, with flow provided retrograde down a narrow ascending aorta via the ductus arteriosus. Pulmonary venous return is accomplished across the oval fossa.

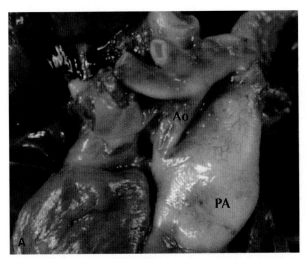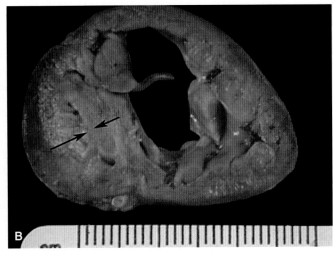

FIGURE 140.41 ▲ Hypoplastic heart syndrome, from anterior portion of heart. **A.** The aorta (Ao) is narrow, compared to the pulmonary artery (PA). The hypoplastic tubular ascending aorta supplies blood to the coronary arteries by retrograde flow. **B.** The left ventricular cavity is narrowed to a small slit (*arrows*).

The left ventricle may be small or rudimentary in other conditions, such as complete atrioventricular canal defect, and cases of transposition, in which cases the term "unbalanced ventricles" is sometimes used.

The right atrium is dilated, with a large right atrial appendage, and the tricuspid valve has a dilated annulus and may be redundant. The coronary sinus is usually large. The pulmonary valve is usually normal with large pulmonary arteries. The pulmonary veins are dilated due to obstruction. The left atrium is congenitally small, with mild endocardial thickening, and may eventually dilate somewhat.

The atrial septum often demonstrates a septal defect, across which the pulmonary venous blood returns to the right atrium. In 10% of cases, the atrial septum is intact, in which blood returns via pulmonary lymphangiectasia, anomalous pulmonary venous connections, or levoatriocardinal vein. The left ventricle is by definition small and may have thick fibroelastosis and spongy myocardium with thick sinusoids.

Because the diagnosis is readily made by fetal ultrasound, pregnancies are often terminated, as the condition is invariably lethal without surgery, which is often staged and complex. There is no adverse effect of hypoplastic left heart syndrome on fetal life; infants are born typically healthy with normal Apgar scores. After birth, the aortic flow depends on a large PDA; death occurs soon after functional closure without maintenance of ductal patency.

Treatment initially is prostaglandins for the ductus arteriosus and establishment of intra-atrial connection, for example, by balloon septostomy. Surgical repair is by several stages (Norwood procedure) (Table 140.4). Initially, the atrial septum is excised, the ductus arteriosus is divided, and the large pulmonary trunk and small ascending aorta are made into a single outflow, with reimplantation of the pulmonary arteries. The second stage includes a connection between the right atrium and pulmonary arteries (Fontan) and an intra-atrial baffle to direct systemic return to pulmonary arteries, in order to establish a single systemic ventricle and the right atrium as the right ventricular chamber. Because mortality is ~50% by age 4, and normal life expectancy is not possible, pediatric cardiac transplantation is a recommended treatment.

Tricuspid Atresia

Tricuspid atresia is best considered as an absent right-sided atrioventricular connection, as there is no valve tissue in most cases. Typically, there are normal ventriculoarterial connections (over 75%). There is usually a small right ventricle with a small ventricular septal defect and narrow pulmonary outflow. Less commonly, there is a large ventricular septal defect, more normal-sized right ventricle, and no pulmonary stenosis. Rarely, the ventricular septum is intact, with pulmonary atresia.

In less than one in four cases, there is ventriculoarterial discordance (D-transposition), in which case the aorta arises from the right ventricle, whose size depends on the size of the ventricular septal defect, as in cases with ventriculoarterial concordance.

The right atrium demonstrates a muscular or fibrous dimple without any valve tissue in most cases (Fig. 140.42). An ASD is necessary for systemic return to pass into the left atrium and mix with pulmonary venous return, resulting in right atrial dilatation. The atrial communication is usually a stretched patent foramen or true ASD. The right ventricle is usually small (depends on the size of the ventricular septal defect) and composed of trabecular and outlet components. There is subpulmonary stenosis in 75% of hearts, especially when there is a small ventricular septal defect and long narrow infundibular tract. Obstruction at the level of the valve is uncommon. The ventricular septal defect may become smaller with endocardial fibrosis and cause significant pulmonary stenosis. When there is transposition (ventriculoarterial discordance), the aorta arises from small anterior right ventricle, with a high rate of aortic coarctation.

The definitive correction involves the Fontan procedure, which is establishing direct connections between the right atrium and the right

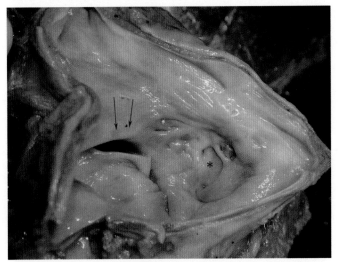

FIGURE 140.42 ▲ Tricuspid atresia, right atrium. The *arrows* show the patent foramen ovale, which has been stretched from blood forced through the left atrium. The *asterisk* shows the dimple in the right atrium where the tricuspid valve would normally be.

pulmonary artery, and the Glenn shunt (vena cava to pulmonary artery). A "modified" Fontan includes a pericardial or Dacron patch to augment the atrial–arterial connection, which is typically done. A "fenestrated" Fontan allows for stepwise closure of the ASD. This is important in patients with elevated pulmonary resistance, to limit right atrial pressures and to prevent sudden drop in cardiac output by maintaining a right-to-left atrial shunt. Complications of utilizing the right atrium as the right-sided pumping chamber include ascites, edema, chylothorax, impaired liver function, protein-losing enteropathy, and mural thrombi right atrium with pulmonary emboli. Other pathologic complications of the Fontan include thrombosis; calcification, or neointimal obstruction of conduit if present; patch dehiscence; complete heart block; and left ventricular dysfunction.

Patients who survive initial surgery showed, in one follow-up study, a 91% 1-month, 87% 6-month, and 83% 1-year survival with no subsequent deaths for subsequent 13 years.[65] One reported patient survived over 63 years with only Blalock-Taussig shunting.[66]

Anomalous Pulmonary Venous Connections

There are normally four pulmonary veins that connect to the left atrium: two on the left (superior, inferior) and two on the right. A common vein on one side (joining of the superior and inferior) is present in 24% of normal individuals. A third vein on one side is present in 2% of the population, and a common vein is rare. All are asymptomatic. Stenotic pulmonary veins are more common with anomalous connections.

Partial Anomalous Pulmonary Venous Connection

Partial anomalous pulmonary venous connection is characterized by two veins connecting normally into the left atrium and two connecting to the right atrium. Symptoms are similar to those of an ASD. The autopsy incidence is 0.6% to 0.7%. An ASD (sinus venosus type) may be present. Anomalous left pulmonary veins connect to derivatives of left cardinal veins (coronary sinus, left innominate vein), and right pulmonary veins connect to derivatives of right cardinal veins (venae cavae and venous portion of the right atrium).

The most common forms of partial anomalous veins are
- Right pulmonary veins to superior vena cava
- Right pulmonary veins right atrium
- Right pulmonary veins to supradiaphragmatic inferior vena cava (scimitar syndrome with intact atrial septum)
- Left pulmonary veins to innominate vein

Total Anomalous Pulmonary Venous Connection

Total anomalous pulmonary venous connection means that all four pulmonary veins connect anomalously. Heterotaxy syndrome is a frequent association, occurring in about one in three cases. There is always an ASD. Total anomalous veins can be classified as infradiaphragmatic versus supradiaphragmatic and have associated obstruction of the anomalous vessels.

Sites of connection, in approximate order of frequency, are
- Left innominate vein (left common cardinal system)
- Coronary sinus (left common cardinal system)
- Right atrium
- (Right) superior vena cava (right common cardinal system)
- Portal system (umbilicovitelline system)

Sites of possible obstruction in total anomalous veins are:
- Interatrial septum: size of ASD related to untreated survival
- Intrinsic obstruction due to scarring
- Extrinsic obstruction (50% of supradiaphragmatic, most cases of infradiaphragmatic connections)
- Vertical vein to innominate between left main pulmonary artery and left mainstem bronchus
- Anomalous vein to superior vena cava between right pulmonary artery and trachea
- Portal vein "obstructed" by hepatic sinusoids

Without pulmonary venous obstruction, patients are asymptomatic at birth, but most are symptomatic by 1 year, with 75% mortality. Presenting symptoms include cyanosis and congestive failure. With pulmonary venous obstruction, there may be immediate cyanosis (12 hours after birth) with rapid progression to heart failure.

Heterotaxy Syndromes

The heterotaxy syndromes are characterized by abnormal morphology of the asymmetric organs, in the sense that the features typical of one side are present on the other, or on both sides. The most straightforward is complete situs inversus, caused by ciliary abnormalities, and results in a normal heart that shows mirror-image inversion and absence of cardiac anomalies. The asplenia syndrome is also fairly distinct, with bilateral right-sidedness in the heart and often lungs and gut, with a typical constellation of abnormalities in the heart, including ventricular inversion, common atrioventricular valves, and anomalous venous return. Polysplenia syndrome is the most diverse, with a variety of cardiac findings and variable atrial morphologies.

Asplenia

With asplenia, there is typically right atrial isomerism, with a midline liver midline, mirror-image right hepatic lobes, a patent biliary tree, and single gallbladder. The bowel is typically rotated. There is a 1.7:1 male to female predominance. The presenting symptom is typically cyanosis because of anomalous pulmonary veins and single functional ventricle. About 80% of infants die before 1 year versus 50% for polysplenia. Heterotaxy of the gut is present in 70% versus 50% for polysplenia. Genitourinary abnormalities (horseshoe kidney or adrenal, hydroureter, and others) are seen in 15% of patients.

The cardiac finding include dextroposition of the heart (40%), right-sided aortic arch (38%), common atrium and atrioventricular valve (75%), single atrioventricular connection connected to dominant ventricle with right morphology (50% to 75%), anomalous pulmonary veins (90% to 100%), and left-sided superior vena cava (33%).

Polysplenia

In the polysplenia syndrome, left atrial isomerism is typical, but there is often ambiguous, inverted, or even normal atria. There are multiple spleens, and some are a significant size, unlike accessory spleens. There is usually azygous continuation between the inferior vena cava and superior vena cava. There is frequently a right-sided aortic arch. The superior vena cava is normal in one-third, bilateral in one-third, and right-sided in one-third of patients. Pulmonary veins are most often normal, but may be either side of the atrium in about 25% of patients. The coronary sinus is often absent. A common atrium is less common than in asplenia, seen in less than one-third. A common atrioventricular valve is seen in 10% to 50% of cases. The ventricular situs is either normal or inverted, and the left ventricle may be hypoplastic. Univentricular hearts with double inlet ventricle are uncommon. Pulmonary stenosis or atresia is present in 40% of patients.

REFERENCES

1. Dolk H, et al. Congenital heart defects in Europe: prevalence and perinatal mortality, 2000 to 2005. *Circulation.* 2011;123(8):841–849.
2. van der Bom T, et al. The prevalence of adult congenital heart disease, results from a systematic review and evidence based calculation. *Am Heart J.* 2012;164(4):568–575.
3. Hoffman JI, Kaplan S. The incidence of congenital heart disease. *J Am Coll Cardiol.* 2002;39(12):1890–1900.
4. Blue GM, et al. Congenital heart disease: current knowledge about causes and inheritance. *Med J Aust.* 2012;197(3):155–159.
5. Goldmuntz E, Crenshaw ML, Lin AE. Genetic aspects of congenital heart defects. In: Allen HD, et al., eds. *Moss and Adams' Heart Disease in Infants, Children, and Adolescents Including the Fetus and Young Adult*, Philadelphia, PA: Lippincott Williams & Wilkins; 2013:617–643.
6. Yagi H, et al. Role of TBX1 in human del22q11.2 syndrome. *Lancet.* 2003;362(9393):1366–1373.
7. Edwards WD, Maleszewsk JJ. Cardiac anatomy and examination of cardiac specimens. In: Allen HD, et al., eds. *Moss and Adams' Heart Disease in Infants, Children, and Adolescents Including the Fetus and Young Adult.* Philadelphia, PA: Lippincott Williams & Wilkins:1–31.

8. Mehta AJ, et al. Interrupted inferior vena cava syndrome. *J Assoc Physicians India.* 2012;60:48–50.

9. Narvencar KP, Jaques e Costa AK, Patil VR. Shone's complex. *J Assoc Physicians India.* 2009;57:415–416.

10. Wimpfheimer O, Haramati LB, Haramati N. Calcification of the ligamentum arteriosum in adults: CT features. *J Comput Assist Tomogr.* 1996;20(1):34–37.

11. Saliba Z, et al. The amplatzer duct occluder II: a new device for percutaneous ductus arteriosus closure. *J Interv Cardiol.* 2009;22(6):496–502.

12. Edwards WD, Maleszewsk JJ. Classification and terminology of cardiovascular anomalies. In: Allen HD, et al., eds. *Moss and Adams' Heart Disease in Infants, Children, and Adolescents Including the Fetus and Young Adult.* Philadelphia, PA: Lippincott Williams & Wilkins; 2013:32–51.

13. Bjornstad PG, Leren TP. Familial atrial septal defect in the oval fossa with progressive prolongation of the atrioventricular conduction caused by mutations in the NKX2.5 gene. *Cardiol Young.* 2009;19(1):40–44.

14. Wahl A, Windecker S, Meier B. Evaluation and treatment of abnormalities of the interatrial septum. *Catheter Cardiovasc Interv.* 2004;63(1):94–103.

15. Konstantinides S, et al. A comparison of surgical and medical therapy for atrial septal defect in adults. *N Engl J Med.* 1995;333(8):469–473.

16. Berger F, et al. Comparison of acute effects on right ventricular haemodynamics of surgical versus interventional closure of atrial septal defects. *Cardiol Young.* 1999;9(5):484–487.

17. Behjati-Ardakani M, et al. Immediate, short, intermediate and long-term results of balloon valvuloplasty in congenital pulmonary valve stenosis. *Acta Med Iran.* 2013;51(5):324–328.

18. Amonkar GP, Deshpande JR. Infective endocarditis of bicuspid pulmonary valve. *Cardiovasc Pathol.* 2006;15(2):119–120.

19. Jodocy D, et al. Left main compression syndrome by idiopathic pulmonary artery aneurysm caused by medial necrosis Erdheim-Gsell combined with bicuspid pulmonary valve. *J Thorac Cardiovasc Surg.* 2009;138(1):234–236.

20. Vedanthan R, Sanz J, Halperin J. Bicuspid pulmonic valve. *J Am Coll Cardiol.* 2009;54(8):e5.

21. Davia JE, et al. Quadricuspid semilunar valves. *Chest.* 1977;72(2):186–189.

22. Edwards WD. Acquired bicuspid aortic valves. *Am J Cardiol.* 1990;65(11):827.

23. Hedayat KM, et al. A quadricuspid pulmonic valve diagnosed in a live newborn by two-dimensional echocardiography. *Pediatr Cardiol.* 2000;21(3):279–281.

24. Fernandez-Armenta J, et al. Quadricuspid pulmonary valve identified by transthoracic echocardiography. *Echocardiography.* 2009;26(3):288–290.

25. Schieken RM, Friedman S, Pierce WS. Severe congenital pulmonary stenosis with pulmonary valvular dysplasia syndrome. Diagnostic and surgical experience in 3 children. *Ann Thorac Surg.* 1973;15(6):570–577.

26. Bendon R, Asamoah A. Perinatal autopsy findings in three cases of jugular lymphatic obstruction sequence and cardiac polyvalvular dysplasia. *Pediatr Dev Pathol.* 2008;11(2):133–137.

27. Becu L, Somerville J, Gallo A. 'Isolated' pulmonary valve stenosis as part of more widespread cardiovascular disease. *Br Heart J.* 1976;38(5):472–482.

28. Harinck E, et al. The left ventricle in congenital isolated pulmonary valve stenosis. A morphological study. *Br Heart J.* 1977;39(4):429–435.

29. Poon LK, Menahem S. Pulmonary regurgitation after percutaneous balloon valvoplasty for isolated pulmonary valvar stenosis in childhood. *Cardiol Young.* 2003;13(5):444–450.

30. Correa-Villasenor A, et al. Ebstein's malformation of the tricuspid valve: Genetic and environmental factors. *Tetralogy.* 1994;50:137–147.

31. Barbara DW, et al. Surgical pathology of 104 tricuspid valves (2000–2005) with classic right-sided Ebstein's malformation. *Cardiovasc Pathol.* 2008;17(3):166–171.

32. Waller BF, Howard J, Fess S. Pathology of tricuspid valve stenosis and pure tricuspid regurgitation—Part III. *Clin Cardiol.* 1995;18(4):225–230.

33. Barre E, et al. Ebstein's anomaly and tricuspid valve dysplasia: prognosis after diagnosis in utero. *Pediatr Cardiol.* 2012;33(8):1391–1396.

34. Said SM, Burkhart HM, Dearani JA. Surgical management of congenital (non-Ebstein) tricuspid valve regurgitation. *Semin Thorac Cardiovasc Surg Pediatr Card Surg Annu.* 2012;15(1):46–60.

35. Grech V. Incidence and management of subaortic stenosis in Malta. *Pediatr Cardiol.* 2001;22(5):431.

36. Newfeld EA, et al. Discrete subvalvular aortic stenosis in childhood. Study of 51 patients. *Am J Cardiol.* 1976;38(1):53–61.

37. Marasini M, et al. Discrete subaortic stenosis: incidence, morphology and surgical impact of associated subaortic anomalies. *Ann Thorac Surg.* 2003;75(6):1763–1768.

38. Frommelt MA, et al. Echocardiographic assessment of subvalvular aortic stenosis before and after operation [see comments]. *J Am Coll Cardiol.* 1992;19(5):1018–1023.

39. Mavroudis C, Mavroudis CD, Jacobs JP. The Ross, Konno, and Ross–Konno operations for congenital left ventricular outflow tract abnormalities. *Cardiol Young.* 2014;24(6):1121–1133.

40. Dodge-Khatami A, et al. Risk factors for reoperation after relief of congenital subaortic stenosis. *Eur J Cardiothorac Surg.* 2008;33(5):885–889.

41. Geva A, et al. Risk factors for reoperation after repair of discrete subaortic stenosis in children. *J Am Coll Cardiol.* 2007;50(15):1498–1504.

42. Ruzmetov M, et al. Long-term results of surgical repair in patients with congenital subaortic stenosis. *Interact Cardiovasc Thorac Surg.* 2006;5(3):227–233.

43. McElhinney DB, et al. Issues and outcomes in the management of supravalvar aortic stenosis. *Ann Thorac Surg.* 2000;69(2):562–567.

44. Perou ML. Congenital supravalvular aortic stenosis. A morphological study with attempt at classification. *Arch Pathol.* 1961;71:453–466.

45. Cuypers JA, et al. Unnatural history of tetralogy of Fallot: prospective follow-up of 40 years after surgical correction. *Circulation.* 2014;130(22):1944–1953.

46. Nollert GD, et al. Risk factors for sudden death after repair of tetralogy of Fallot. *Ann Thorac Surg.* 2003;76(6):1901–1905.

47. Mainwaring RD, et al. Late repair of the native pulmonary valve in patients with pulmonary insufficiency after surgery for tetralogy of Fallot. *Ann Thorac Surg.* 2012;93(2):677–679.

48. Lin MT, et al. Detection of pulmonary arterial morphology in tetralogy of Fallot with pulmonary atresia by computed tomography: 12 years of experience. *Eur J Pediatr.* 2012;171(3):579–586.

49. Jacobs JP, et al. Congenital Heart Surgery Nomenclature and Database Project: ventricular septal defect. *Ann Thorac Surg.* 2000;69(4 suppl):S25–S35.

50. Tchervenkov CI, Roy N. Congenital Heart Surgery Nomenclature and Database Project: pulmonary atresia–ventricular septal defect. *Ann Thorac Surg.* 2000;69(4 suppl):S97–S105.

51. Carotti A, et al. Determinants of outcome after surgical treatment of pulmonary atresia with ventricular septal defect and major aortopulmonary collateral arteries. *J Thorac Cardiovasc Surg.* 2010;140(5):1092–1103.

52. Davies B, et al. Unifocalization of major aortopulmonary collateral arteries in pulmonary atresia with ventricular septal defect is essential to achieve excellent outcomes irrespective of native pulmonary artery morphology. *J Thorac Cardiovasc Surg.* 2009;138(6):1269–1275 e1.

53. Choi YH, et al. Morphology of tricuspid valve in pulmonary atresia with intact ventricular septum. *Pediatr Cardiol.* 1998;19(5):381–389.

54. Chen Q, et al. Does the persistence of pulsatile antegrade pulmonary blood flow following bidirectional Glenn procedure affect long term outcome? *Eur J Cardiothorac Surg.* 2015;47(1):154–158; discussion 158.

55. Carlo WF, Nelson DP. Inhaled nitric oxide improves oxygen saturation in children with pulmonary arteriovenous malformations after the Fontan procedure. *Pediatr Crit Care Med.* 2011;12(3):e152–e154.

56. Kendall TJ, et al. Hepatic fibrosis and cirrhosis in the Fontan circulation: a detailed morphological study. *J Clin Pathol.* 2008;61(4):504–508.

57. Honjo O, et al. Anatomical factors determining surgical decision-making in patients with transposition of the great arteries with left ventricular outflow tract obstruction. *Eur J Cardiothorac Surg.* 2013;44(6):1085–1094; discussion 1094.

58. Cetrano E, Carotti A. Surgical treatment of transposition of the great arteries with bilateral intramural coronary arteries. *Ann Thorac Surg.* 2012;93(3):986–987.

59. Gorler H, et al. Long-term morbidity and quality of life after surgical repair of transposition of the great arteries: atrial versus arterial switch operation. *Interact Cardiovasc Thorac Surg.* 2011;12(4):569–574.

60. O'Byrne ML, et al. 22q11.2 Deletion syndrome is associated with increased perioperative events and more complicated postoperative course in infants undergoing infant operative correction of truncus arteriosus communis or interrupted aortic arch. *J Thorac Cardiovasc Surg.* 2014;148(4):1597–1605.

61. Dehaki MG, et al. Pulmonary artery banding in the current era: Is it still useful? *Ann Pediatr Cardiol.* 2012;5(1):36–39.

62. Li S, et al. Surgical outcomes of 380 patients with double outlet right ventricle who underwent biventricular repair. *J Thorac Cardiovasc Surg.* 2014;148(3):817–824.

63. Barron DJ, Jones TJ, Brawn WJ. The Senning procedure as part of the double-switch operations for congenitally corrected transposition of the great arteries. *Semin Thorac Cardiovasc Surg Pediatr Card Surg Annu.* 2011;14(1):109–115.

64. Hiramatsu T, et al. Long-term prognosis of double-switch operation for congenitally corrected transposition of the great arteries. *Eur J Cardiothorac Surg.* 2012;42(6):1004–1008.

65. Wald RM, et al. Outcome after prenatal diagnosis of tricuspid atresia: a multicenter experience. *Am Heart J.* 2007;153(5):772–778.

66. Scholtz W, et al. 63-year survival after Blalock–Taussig shunt operation in a patient with single ventricle, tricuspid atresia, and pulmonary stenosis. *Congenit Heart Dis.* 2011;6(2):179–182.

141 Sudden Cardiac Death

Allen P. Burke, M.D., and Joseph J. Maleszewski, M.D.

Definition

Sudden cardiac death (SCD) is an unexpected death due to cardiac causes occurring in a short time period (generally within 1 hour of symptom onset) in a person with or without known cardiac disease. In situations where the sudden death is not witnessed, careful investigation of the circumstances is necessary to conclude that it was due to a sudden cardiac event.

Epidemiology

SCD accounts for ~350,000 deaths annually in the United States, which represents an incidence of about 0.1% to 0.2% per year in the adult population or 1 to 2 deaths per 1,000 person-years.[1] The inci-

dence of sudden death in adolescents and young adults is far lower, about 0.003% per year, about 25% of which are unexplained, even with autopsy (sudden arrhythmic death syndrome [SADS]).[2] SCD can also occur in young, otherwise healthy-appearing athletes, where the incidence ranges from 1:3,000 person-years to 1:9,17,000 person-years, with the highest incidence seen in African American male basketball players.[3] Men, in general, have been reported to have at least a two- to fourfold increased risk when compared with women, depending somewhat on the population being considered.

Causes and mechanisms of SCD, discussed in detail below, differ by age group (Tables 141.1 to 141.4). In individuals more than 40 years of age, most causes are acquired, with coronary atherosclerosis and its

TABLE 141.1   Causes and Substrates Underlying Sudden Cardiac Arrhythmic Death

Cause	Mechanism	Arrhythmia	Comments
Acute narrowing of coronary artery • Coronary thrombosis • Coronary artery dissection • Coronary embolism	Acute ischemia, focal	Ventricular fibrillation Bradycardia Pulseless electrical activity	The focus of ischemia is not usually found because it is too early. May be signs of remote ischemia from prior events
Chronic narrowing of coronary artery or arteries • Coronary atherosclerosis without thrombosis • Anomalous coronary artery origin	Acute ischemia, unclear mechanism	Ventricular fibrillation Bradyarrhythmias Pulseless electrical activity (uncommon)	By convention, 75% luminal area narrowing required for atherosclerotic sudden death Other substrates common (hypertrophy, scars) Often with exertion (anomalous artery)
Heart failure • Dilated cardiomyopathy (primary or secondary) • Ischemic heart disease • Aortic/mitral insufficiency	Ventricular hypertrophy, microscopic scarring, ischemia	Ventricular fibrillation Bradyarrhythmias (uncommon)	Heart failure may be subclinical or not diagnosed and may be corroborated by ventricular dilatation and pulmonary and hepatic congestion.
Myocardial inflammation • Myocarditis • Sarcoidosis	Myocyte necrosis, inflammation	Ventricular fibrillation Bradyarrhythmias (uncommon)	Degree of inflammation/necrosis needed as a cause of death unclear
Myocardial scars • Healed ischemia • Cardiomyopathy • Healed myocarditis (sarcoid, lymphocytic)	Ventricular hypertrophy, microscopic scarring, ischemia	Ventricular fibrillation	The degree of scarring necessary to result in lethal arrhythmia unknown. Other causes of death need to be excluded, and there are often contributing heart findings.
Myocardial hypertrophy • Primary cardiomyopathy • Hypertensive and secondary cardiomyopathy	Cardiomyocyte hypertrophy, microscopic scarring	Ventricular fibrillation Bradyarrhythmias (uncommon)	Methods of determining hypertrophy are approximate. Other causes of death need to be excluded, and there are often contributing heart findings.
Aortic stenosis	Ventricular hypertrophy, ischemia	Ventricular fibrillation Bradyarrhythmias	Degree of stenosis typically severe, often with marked left ventricular hypertrophy
Mitral valve prolapse	Unclear, may include ischemia, hypertrophy, and autonomic dysfunction	Ventricular fibrillation	Conduction system study may be considered to rule out myxoid vascular and neural changes
Long QT syndrome	Congenital (mutations) Acquired (drugs)	Ventricular fibrillation (torsades de pointes)	Congenital syndromes result from mutations in ion channel genes. Diagnosis rests on premortem ECG or molecular autopsy.
Familial polymorphous ventricular tachycardia	Ryanodine receptor (RyR) mutations	Ventricular tachycardia, polymorphous	Diagnosis rests on genetic testing or clinical history.
Hypoxia resulting from pulmonary insufficiency • Severe pulmonary stenosis • Pulmonary hypertension	Global myocardial or generalized hypoxia	Baroreflex stimulation with bradyarrhythmias Ventricular tachyarrhythmias Bradyarrhythmias	Right ventricular hypertrophy usually contributing factor

AV, atrioventricular.

TABLE 141.2   Causes of SCDs in Adults

Cause of Death	Approximate Percentage[a]
Atherosclerosis with acute thrombosis[b]	30%–60%
Atherosclerosis with stable plaque (>75% area narrowing) and cardiomegaly[c]	20%–40%
Cardiomegaly[c] in the absence of atherosclerosis (<75% area narrowing)	10%–20%
Atherosclerosis with stable plaque (<75% area narrowing) without cardiomegaly	<10
No morphologic substrate	10%–30%[d]
Hypertrophic cardiomyopathy[e]	4%
Myocarditis[f]	3%
Sarcoidosis	2%
Aortic valve stenosis	2%
Aortic dissection	2%
Arrhythmogenic cardiomyopathy[e]	2%
Endocarditis	1%
Mitral valve prolapse	1%
Myocardial bridging, rheumatic mitral stenosis, anomalous coronary artery, coronary artery dissection, and acute myocardial infarction in the absence of significant coronary disease	<1%

[a]Depends on the population studied.
[b]Additional arrhythmogenic substrates (remote infarcts, cardiomegaly) present in >50% of cases; includes cases of ruptured acute myocardial infarction.
[c]When associated with hypertension and hypertensive LVH/cardiomyopathy.
[d]Rate has inverse correlation with age.
[e]Higher in exertional deaths in younger patients.
[f]Higher in adolescent and young adults, especially recruits.

consequences responsible for the death in more than 7 of every 10 cases (Table 141.3). Hypertensive heart disease is the second most common cause and has appreciable overlap with atherosclerotic heart disease, given the common risk factors.

In those <40 years of age, congenital disease is the most common cause of SCD, including anomalous coronary artery origin and genetic cardiomyopathies (Tables 141.3 and 141.4).[5] Myocarditis is also much more common among the young.

General Mechanisms of SCD

Electrical Arrest

Sudden arrhythmic events, electrical arrest, constitute the most common underlying mechanism in cases of SCD. Arrhythmogenic foci can

TABLE 141.3   Major Causes of SCD in the Young Adult < 30 Years of Age[a]

Cause of Death	Percentage
Atherosclerosis	28%
No morphologic substrate	21%
Idiopathic left ventricular hypertrophy	12%
Hypertrophic cardiomyopathy	7%
Myocarditis	6%
Anomalous coronary artery	4%
Dilated cardiomyopathy	3%
Rheumatic mitral stenosis	3%
Complex congenital heart disease	2%
Hypertensive LV hypertrophy	2%
Endocarditis	2%
Sarcoidosis, aortic stenosis, mitral valve prolapse, arrhythmogenic cardiomyopathy	1%
Coronary aneurysm, amyloid	<1%

[a]Adapted from Burke AP, Farb A, Virmani R, et al. Sports-related and non- sports-related sudden death in young adults. *Am Heart J.* 1991;121:568–575, Ref.[4]

TABLE 141.4   Major Causes of SCD in Children

Cause of Death	Percentage
Myocarditis	28%
Coronary artery anomalies	24%
No morphologic substrate	20%
Other findings[a]	16%
Hypertrophic cardiomyopathy	12%

[a]Nonspecific cardiomyopathy, supra- or subvalvar aortic stenosis, coronary artery dysplasia, histiocytoid cardiomyopathy (infants), complex congenital heart disease, cardiac tumors.

result from myocardial ischemia, scarring, or inflammation. The precise location of the arrhythmogenic focus in the ventricular myocardium is usually not definitively established by pathologic examination; rather, structural abnormalities in a broad sense are assumed to be culpable for such. In fact, there are often multiple coexisting potential substrates for arrhythmia identified in a given heart, including coronary artery disease (leading to presumed myocardial ischemia), myocyte hypertrophy (which increases the heart's oxygen demand), and scarring.

Mechanical Arrest

Some cases of SCD are caused by sudden catastrophic changes in hemodynamics, so-called mechanical arrest. These changes can involve the heart itself or the great arteries (Table 141.2). These may be relatively common (e.g., cardiac tamponade as a result of ischemic myocardial rupture or ruptured aortic aneurysm, pulmonary embolism) or rare (e.g., tumor obstructing normal blood flow).

Approach to the Heart in SCD

It is especially important to rule out noncardiac natural and unnatural causes of death before determining the manner and cause of sudden deaths. In the case of hospital-based or private autopsies, the manner is determined to be natural prior to autopsy and documented by the death certificate. Any case of suspicious or undetermined manner of death is referred to a medical examiner or coroner's office for clearance.

The standard approach to the heart is appropriate for the vast majority of cases of SCD. Given that most arrhythmogenic substrates for sudden death are within the myocardium (not the specialized conduction system), the heart should be cut serially along the short axis to maximize the area visualized and allow for accurate and complete description of the identified lesion(s).

The ventricular cavities should be measured (excluding trabeculations and papillary muscles). Additionally, the ventricular wall thicknesses including those of the free walls and septum (again, excluding trabeculations and papillary muscles) should be measured. Because recent ischemic foci (<12 hours) are usually not evident grossly, a careful evaluation of the coronary vessels, including their course, is necessary, which often necessitates removal of the coronary arteries from the heart and subsequent decalcification. Tetrazolium salts may be useful in evaluating for early ischemic changes (see Chapter 14). The coronary ostia should be carefully inspected for anomalous origins and patency.

Because many causes of SCD are underlying chronic conditions, there is no way to prove causation in an individual case, other than by exclusion. Exceptions to this rule are cardiac tamponade caused by aortic rupture or myocardial infarct, or saddle pulmonary embolism (technically not sudden *cardiac* death), which are never incidental findings. Acute occlusive coronary thrombosis and spontaneous coronary artery dissection are virtually never incidental, because of their acute nature. Acute myocardial infarctions are also seldom incidental, although uncommonly seen, because death generally occurs before histologic manifestations become manifest.

Routine evaluation of the cardiac conduction system study has fallen out of favor because arrhythmias in the face of negative autopsy are generally caused by channelopathies that have no gross or histopathologic correlate. Nevertheless, evaluation of the cardiac conduction system can occasionally yield relevant findings. In cases with an antemortem history of heart block, abnormalities of the region of the atrioventricular node (AVN) (including involvement by sarcoidosis) can be seen. Additionally, in cases of myxomatous mitral valve disease, abnormalities of the atrioventricular conduction system have been described.[6,7]

Dissection of the Sinoatrial and Atrioventricular Nodes

The sinoatrial node is located on the lateral aspect of the junction of the superior vena cava and the trabecular portion of the right atrium, in the superior aspect of the sulcus terminalis (which corresponds

internally to the crista terminalis). Dissection involves identification of junction between the muscular and venous portion of the right atrium, with cross sections to identify the sinoatrial nodal artery around which the nodal tissue resides. Histologically, the node consists of small specialized cardiomyocytes within fibrous and elastic tissue.

The AVN is located within the triangle of Koch immediately posterior to the central fibrous body (CFB) (Fig. 141.1). The dissection is generally approached from the right atrium, identifying the coronary sinus posteriorly, annulus of the tricuspid valve anteriorly, and membranous septum superiorly. The posterosuperior limit is formed by the tendon of Todaro, a microscopic bundle of fibrous tissue that is not seen grossly extending from the junction of the valves of the inferior vena cava and coronary sinus toward the commissure between the septal and anterior tricuspid valve leaflets. Sections are taken from inferior

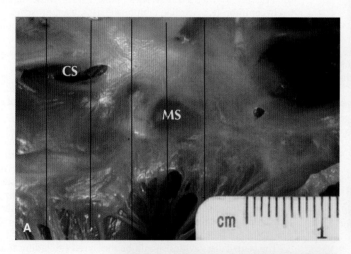

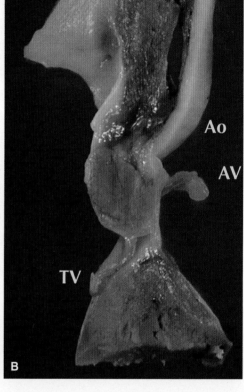

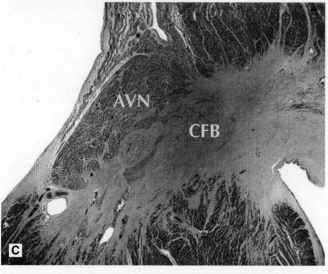

FIGURE 141.1 ▲ Conduction system study, right atrium. **A.** Bars indicate knife cuts to be made. CS, coronary sinus; MS, membranous septum. **B.** Gross cross section. The tricuspid valve (TV) annulus is inferior to the mitral and aortic valve (AV). The mitral valve is seen in more posterior portions of the conduction system sections. Ao, aorta. **C.** Histologic section of atrioventricular node (AVN). The central fibrous body (CFB) is the fibrous portion of the base of the heart adjacent to the atrioventricular and aortic valve insertions. The crest of the ventricular septum is below, and the atrial myocardium above.

to superior, with consecutive sampling of the compact AVN, penetrating bundle of His, and proximal left bundle branch (LBB) and right bundle branch (RBB).

Histologically, the nodal tissues should be identified, with attention to inflammation, tumor, and increased collagen. Other abnormal findings include dysplastic changes of the atrioventricular nodal artery, which have been associated with sudden death, and infiltrative processes such as amyloidosis. Rarely, necrosis of myocardium in the crest of the ventricular septum can be seen in association with isolated small vessel disease at the base of the heart, as well as small vessel disease associated with mitral valve prolapse.[7,8] In patients with heart block, either acquired or congenital, there may be scarring in the area of the node and the branching bundle.

Postmortem Genetic Testing

In selected autopsy cases of SCD where no pathologic substrate could be identified, including unexplained drowning deaths, sequencing candidate genes may be of some utility.[9] Testing in these individuals is important because it can serve as proband identification in families and allow for efficient screening of at-risk individuals. Such testing should be performed in a clinical laboratory. In the case of underlying channelopathies, identification of a causal mutation will be the only way of recognizing the disease. In a series of SCD cases in which an underlying channelopathy was identified, fewer than one-third of patients had a history of cardiac events.[9]

Postmortem genetic testing in those with cardiomyopathy has only uncovered a causal mutation in ~10% of cases. This relatively low number may be, in part, explained by wide diversity of mutations that can cause these diseases (often kindred specific) and our somewhat rudimentary variant classification techniques. Patients dying with hypertrophic cardiomyopathy (HCM), dilated cardiomyopathy, and arrhythmogenic cardiomyopathy showed mutations in *MYBPC3*, *MYH7*, *LMNA*, *PKP2*, or *TMEM43* genes, distributed across all three groups.[10]

Specific Causes of SCD

The cause of SCD is typically attributed to one or more *morphologic substrates* that increase the risk of electrical instability that can lead to a fatal dysrhythmia. Because of uncertainty in the relationship between the cause of death and the individual substrate in many cases, causes of SCD have been classified as certain, highly probable, and uncertain, with the majority falling in the highly probable group.[11]

Chronic occlusions of the epicardial coronary arteries impart an increased risk for sudden death, likely due to the increased potential for transient ischemic events during periods of increased myocardial oxygen demand. When secondary myocardial changes, such as remote infarctions (replacement-type fibrosis) and/or hypertrophy, are present, the designation of ischemic heart disease can be applied.

By convention, at least 75% cross-sectional narrowing (grade 4 stenosis) of an epicardial coronary artery needs to be found in order for the coronary lesion to be considered a likely cause of death. In cases of anomalous origin, especially of the left main coronary artery, the explanation for sudden death is also not clear in most cases, as the lesion is chronic and present from birth. There is often a history of exertion during or prior to death resulting in increased oxygen demand and histologic change of prior ischemic episodes. Aside from the origin of the coronary arteries, the ultimate course is important as well.

Coronary thrombosis, resulting in sudden occlusion of an epicardial artery, can arise in the setting of atherosclerosis (Fig. 141.2). This can cause focal ischemia or infarction and an ensuing arrhythmia. Because ischemic myocardium cannot be identified at autopsy until histologic changes are manifest (at least several hours), the ultimate cause (myocardial ischemia) will often not be identified but rather inferred by identification of the said thrombus. Uncommon causes of sudden narrowing of an epicardial artery include spontaneous coronary artery

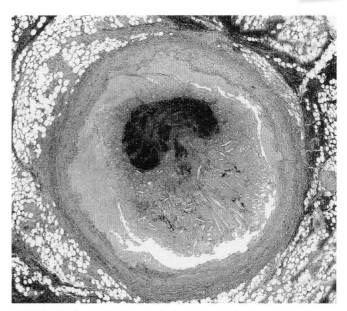

FIGURE 141.2 ▲ Sudden death due to acute plaque rupture with occlusive thrombus. In ~50% of sudden deaths with severe coronary artery disease, an acute thrombus will be identified. Most commonly, the etiology is plaque rupture.

dissection and embolic phenomenon, the latter of which can derive from thrombus or tumor.

Heart failure is known to increase the risk for ventricular arrhythmias and may serve as an intermediary mechanism behind SCD. Importantly, however, it is not technically a "cause" of death. Rather, it represents a constellation of symptoms resulting from the inability of the heart muscle to effectively pump blood to meet the metabolic demands of the body. This results from an underlying pathology, such as ischemic heart disease, hypertensive heart disease, valvular heart disease, or a cardiomyopathic state. In most cases, there is a history of heart disease, and the patient is taking cardiac medications.

Myocardial inflammation can be the only finding to explain SCD. The most common pattern is diffuse lymphocytic myocarditis with associated myocyte necrosis, usually seen in younger patients and caused by viruses and autoimmune disease. Predominantly, interstitial infiltrates with relatively little necrosis are characteristic of hypersensitivity (or drug-related) myocarditis, consisting of a mix of histiocytes, eosinophils, and occasional neutrophils. The role of focal myocarditis as a cause of sudden death is debated, and often ascribed as a contributing or possible cause.

Myocardial scarring is frequent in SCD and usually seen as a consequence of cardiomyopathy, coronary artery disease, myocarditis, or sarcoidosis. The pattern and size of scars are important to note, as well as the pattern of replacement or interstitial fibrosis. Small amounts of subendocardial fibrosis are common in dilated or hypertrophied hearts, and interstitial collagen is a normal finding in some areas of the myocardium, including near the CFB and near insertions of the atrioventricular valves.

Cardiomegaly, typically diagnosed when heart weight is more than 50% above the expected mean, can result from many of the abovementioned conditions (e.g., hypertension, chronic valvular disease, cardiomyopathy, and ischemic heart disease). The presence of cardiomegaly is associated with an increased risk of SCD.

Most (up to 80%) children dying suddenly (of apparent SCD) do not have an anatomic substrate identified by traditional gross and microscopic evaluation.[12] The proportion of so-called autopsy-negative SCD (SADS) is ~30% when young adults are considered[2,12] and is about 12% for all adults.[11] Cases of autopsy-negative SCD are likely to decrease with broader availability of advanced genomic and proteomic ancillary studies.

Coronary Atherosclerosis

SCD is often the first manifestation of coronary atherosclerosis, occurring in more than one-third of patients with coronary atherosclerosis. This occurs despite the fact that prior symptoms were reported to be present in more than half of these individuals.[13] Risk factors for sudden death in patients with ischemic heart disease include presence of heart failure, especially with an ejection fraction of <30%. The risk of SCD extends beyond the initial infarction with a high rate of ventricular arrhythmias persisting throughout the patient's life. Patients who have survived a prior cardiac arrest are also likely to have recurrent arrest.[14–16] The incidence of coronary disease increases with age in all populations, but the proportion of deaths that are sudden from coronary disease actually decreases with age.[14–16]

The arrhythmogenic foci in cases of coronary atherosclerosis are almost always in the left ventricular myocardium, but in sudden cases, this is usually not found because ischemic myocardium is not histologically manifest before 12 to 24 hours. This necessitates careful evaluation of the coronary arteries, where a culprit lesion may be found in about 30% to 80% of cases, depending on the population. Lesions should be graded based on extent of stenosis (0% to 25%, grade 1; 26% to 50%, grade 2; 51% to 75%, grade 3; 76% to 100%, grade 4). In case of atherosclerotic disease, plaque rupture, plaque erosion, or intraplaque hemorrhage should be noted (Figs. 141.2 and 141.3).

In most cases of coronary atherosclerosis without thrombi, there are other morphologic findings that increase the risk of ventricular arrhythmias, especially healed infarcts and ventricular hypertrophy.[17–19] Occasionally, only stable plaque (usually causing grade 3 to 4 stenosis) is found, in the setting of normal heart weight and no prior infarcts (Fig. 141.4). In these cases, which constitute about 15% of SCDs attributed to coronary disease, the real mechanism of death remains obscure.[20]

The estimation of the exact degree of coronary artery narrowing may become important in sudden coronary death autopsies, especially if there are no thrombi and if there are medicolegal concerns. There are many factors that render precise morphometric measurements somewhat meaningless in arteries that are not perfusion fixed at physiologic pressures. These include processing shrinkage and collapse of the artery, which can cause gross overestimations. Furthermore, assessment of narrowing angiographically during life is determined based

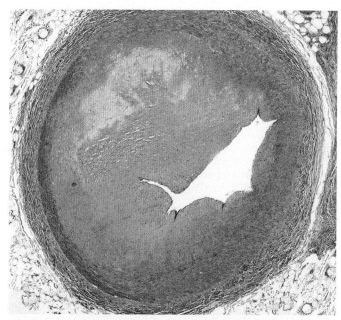

FIGURE 141.4 ▲ Sudden death with severe narrowing due to stable plaque. In this example, there is pathologic intimal thickening with significant luminal stenosis. There are no features of plaque instability (intraplaque hemorrhage or surface thrombus). The mechanism of death in such patients is unclear if there are no additional arrhythmogenic substrates.

on a proximal reference segment. At autopsy, the percent stenosis is estimated as an area within the internal elastic lamina at the same segment, which does not take into account positive arterial remodeling, resulting in further overestimation of luminal narrowing.

Acute myocardial infarcts are present in about 20% of SCD cases, healed infarcts in about 50%, and cardiomegaly in about 40% to 50%, most often due to multifactorial diseases that include hypertension and chronic ischemic changes.[21]

Coronary lesions are also present incidentally in noncardiac deaths, emphasizing the need to exclude noncardiac causes in all cases. Single-vessel coronary disease (≥1 epicardial artery with ≥75% area narrowing) is present in 10% to 40% of noncardiac deaths, depending on the population age and underlying disease. Plaque fissure may also be present incidentally, in about 10% to 15% of trauma and other hospital deaths, but an occlusive thrombus and one associated with acute plaque rupture is almost never incidental.[17,22,23]

Cardiomegaly

The term cardiomegaly refers to a heart that is larger than normal. In most circumstances, this increased size is reflected in increased weight (>50% above the expected mean). A heart can also be considered cardiomegalic if there is massive biatrial dilatation (which may not be reflected with significant increase in heart weight) or if there is massive acute ventricular dilatation, such as can be seen in certain inflammatory states (myocarditis, and allograft rejection). Cardiomegaly can result from either congenital or acquired forms of heart disease and, in some cases, may be multifactorial. The presence of cardiomegaly is itself a risk factor for sudden death and should warrant investigation for an underlying etiology.[21]

Multiple Arrhythmogenic Substrates in Adult Sudden Death

In many cases of SCD, there are multiple anatomic substrates found at autopsy, each of which contribute to the electrical instability of the heart. In patients with coronary artery disease, there are frequently changes of ventricular remodeling, such as cardiomegaly, ventricular

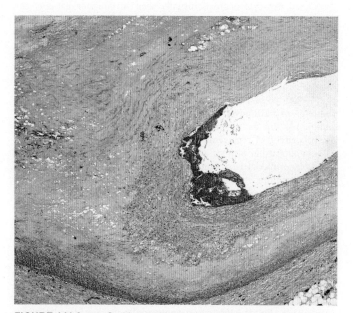

FIGURE 141.3 ▲ Sudden death due to acute plaque erosion and subocclusive thrombus. The mechanism of sudden death with nonocclusive thrombus is not entirely clear, but they are a reasonably certain cause of death in the absence of other causes.

dilatation, and scars from previous infarcts.[17] It is the role of the autopsy pathologist to enumerate the potential arrhythmogenic substrates, with the most likely first. Combining terms (e.g., hypertensive and atherosclerotic cardiovascular disease) is entirely appropriate when one entity is not favored over another.

Some individual diseases have multiple underlying mechanisms that can lead to SCD. In the case of hypertrophic obstructive cardiomyopathy, the hypertrophied and sometimes scarred myocardium may serve as arrhythmogenic substrate but the outflow tract obstruction that is present may result in poor coronary perfusion and subsequent ischemia. Similarly, aortic valve regurgitation, in addition to resulting in left ventricular hypertrophy (so-called volume hypertrophy), also impedes coronary filling during diastole.

Sudden Death due to Familial (Inherited) Cardiomyopathy

Mutations in genes encoding cardiac proteins may cause arrhythmias in the absence of gross or microscopic abnormalities or may underlie cardiomyopathies with gross and histologic findings that are usually nonspecific and sometimes subtle. Specific types of cardiomyopathies that cause sudden death in the young include HCM, arrhythmogenic (right ventricular) cardiomyopathy, histiocytoid cardiomyopathy, left ventricular noncompaction, and dilated cardiomyopathy. Some genetic storage disease (Danon disease) has also been associated with SCD.

Hypertrophic Cardiomyopathy

HCM is believed to be the underlying cause of death in 4% to 10% of SCDs (Tables 141.2 to 141.4; Fig. 141.5). HCM is a relatively common disease, with an estimated incidence of ~1/500. It is autosomal dominant with variable penetrance. The incidence of SCD in the setting of HCM is quite variable and, in large part, dependent on the disease severity and the number of defined risk factors present. Risk factors associated with SCD include young age at diagnosis, presence of symptoms, presence of hemodynamic obstruction, history of arrhythmia, and family history of SCD. Patients with no risk factors can have a relatively low risk of SCD (0.83% per year), while those with multiple risk factors can have a 5% risk per year (10,666,426, 11,127,463). An autopsy study showed that age at death was significantly younger in exertional (27+/−13 years) versus nonexertional sudden deaths (40+/−16 years) and that exertional deaths were more likely in women. The average heart weight was less in exertional sudden deaths as compared to stationary deaths.[24]

Grossly, hearts with HCM are typically enlarged and usually show thickening of the ventricular walls. This thickening may be either symmetric or asymmetric. In the latter instance, it is the ventricular septum that is usually disproportionately hypertrophied resulting in a ventricular septal-to-free wall ratio (VS:LVFW) >1.2.

Arrhythmogenic Cardiomyopathy

Arrhythmogenic cardiomyopathy (arrhythmogenic right ventricular dysplasia/cardiomyopathy) accounts for <3% of cases of SCD but is a relatively more common cause if exertional deaths are considered. Similar to HCM, arrhythmogenic cardiomyopathy is familial in up to 50% of cases, in which case the mode of inheritance is autosomal dominant with variable penetrance. Most patients are <40 years old at the time of death, and some deaths occur in children. Grossly at autopsy, biventricular scars situated under the epicardium are seen in the majority of hearts from patients dying suddenly. Heart weight is increased in slightly over 50%. Histologically, there are areas of fibrofatty change with vacuolated myocytes (Fig. 141.6).[25]

Familial Dilated Cardiomyopathy

SCD occurs in 2.4% of children with dilated cardiomyopathy over 5 years, which is at least 100 times that of the normal population.[26] These hearts exhibit hypertrophy (usually biventricular) and variable degrees of dilatation. A wide spectrum of mutations have been associated with dilated cardiomyopathy, including genes encoding for cardiac troponin T myosin heavy chain, myosin-binding protein, and titin.[27,28] Mutations in lamin A/C (*LMNA*)[29-31] are frequently observed in patients with aggressive clinical course.

Inherited Arrhythmia Syndromes

There is some overlap between congenital cardiomyopathy and inherited arrhythmia syndromes, because some genetic variants predisposing to sudden death are seen in various phenotypes, including specific cardiomyopathy and sudden death with an anatomically normal heart.

In up to 80% of forensic autopsies in young children dying with SCD,[32] and up to one-third of young adults, there are no gross or microscopic findings to explain the fatal arrhythmia. Unfortunately, postmortem genetic testing establishes a diagnosis in only a minority of cases (Table 141.5).

Channelopathies (ion channel disorders) are characterized by repolarization abnormalities, which are manifest on electrocardiogram as long QT syndrome and cause a ventricular tachyarrhythmia termed *torsade de pointes*. Gap junctions are agglomerates of multiple intercellular channels, which connect the cytoplasm of adjacent cardiomyocytes. Each gap junction channel is composed of 12 connexin molecules, assembled from two hexameric hemichannels (connexons). Mutations resulting in inactivation of the cardiac potassium channel subunits (*KCNQ1*, *KCNH2*, *KCNE1*, and *KCNE2*) cause electrocardiographic prolongation of the QT interval, ventricular tachyarrhythmias, syncope, and sudden death. HERG and MiRP1 are alpha and beta

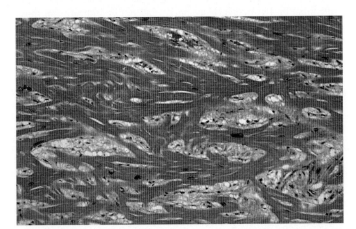

FIGURE 141.5 ▲ Sudden death due to hypertrophic cardiomyopathy. A histologic section shows typical myofiber disarray.

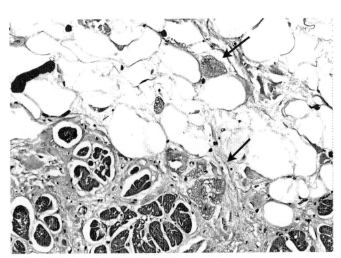

FIGURE 141.6 ▲ Arrhythmogenic right ventricular cardiomyopathy. There are typical vacuolated myocytes (*arrows*).

TABLE 141.5   Postmortem Identification of Ion Channel Mutations Causing Sudden Death in the Negative Autopsy[a]

Mutation Found	Incidence
None	65%
RYR2	14%
KCNQ1	10%
KCNH2	6%
SCN5A	4%

[a]Adapted from Tester DJ, Ackerman MJ. The role of molecular autopsy in unexplained sudden cardiac death. *Curr Opin Cardiol.* 2006;21:166–172, Ref. [33]; Tester DJ, Spoon DB, Valdivia HH, et al. Targeted mutational analysis of the RyR2-encoded cardiac ryanodine receptor in sudden unexplained death: a molecular autopsy of 49 medical examiner/coroner's cases. *Mayo Clin Proc.* 2004;79:1380–1384, Ref. [34]. Mutational analysis with gene sequencing was performed for ion channel genes, including long QT and ryanodine receptor, 49% cases.

subunits of the same channel protein, and likewise for KCNQ1 and minK, respectively. Mutations in *KCNQ1* or *LQT1* (long QT-1) have been identified as the cause of Romano-Ward syndrome, an autosomal dominant condition characterized by familial premature sudden death. The genes are on different chromosomes (with the exception of *KCNE1* and *KCNE2*, which share sequence identity) and are composed of multiple exons. Homozygous mutations in *KCNQ1* are the cause of the Jervell and Lange-Nielsen syndrome, an autosomal recessive disorder characterized by marked prolongation of the QT interval, sensorineural deafness, and sudden death. Mutations resulting in activation (as opposed to inactivation) of the cardiac sodium channel gene (*SCN5A* or *LQT3*) also cause long QT syndrome, *torsade de pointes*, and SCD. There are some differences in typical clinical presentation according to type of long QT syndrome.

The *Brugada syndrome* is characterized by electrocardiographic findings of RBB block with ST segment elevation in leads V1–V3, ventricular arrhythmias, syncope, and sudden death. The syndrome is related to sudden unexpected nocturnal death syndrome in Southeast Asia and Japan, which has many synonyms, including bangungut, lai tia, and pokkuri. Most cases are autosomal dominant. A relationship between Brugada syndrome and arrhythmogenic cardiomyopathy was previously proposed.

The most common mutation found in molecular autopsy of patients dying suddenly without apparent anatomic substrate involves the *cardiac ryanodine receptor* gene (*RyR2*), which resides in the sarcoplasmic reticulum and modulates the calcium channel, which is key to electric propagation in the heart. Mutations in this gene result in *familial polymorphic ventricular tachycardia*, an autosomal dominant syndrome characterized by ventricular arrhythmias, prolongation of the QT interval prior to the onset of tachycardia, and sudden death. Cardiac events, including sudden death, are often precipitated by exertion or adrenergic stimuli.

Desmosomal protein disorders have been associated with sudden death in a variety of settings, including sudden death with negative autopsy and sudden death due to arrhythmogenic cardiomyopathy,[35] dilated cardiomyopathy, and familial premature coronary artery disease.[35] The majority of research has centered on mutations in arrhythmogenic cardiomyopathy. The cardiac desmosomal proteins include the cadherins desmoglein-2 (*DSG2*) and desmocollin-2 (*DSC2*), which form the intercellular adhesive interface, and armadillo and plakin family desmoplakin (*DSP*), plakophilin-2 (*PKP2*), and plakoglobin (*JUP*). The cytoplasmic tails of the cadherins interact with plakoglobin, which binds to desmoplakin, in turn anchored to the desmin intermediate filaments.

Wolff-Parkinson-White Syndrome

The Wolff-Parkinson-White syndrome, a preexcitation syndrome diagnosed by electrocardiographic findings, has a prevalence of 1.5 to 3.1 per 1,000 persons, making it one of the more common arrhythmic

syndromes. Sudden death occurs due to ventricular fibrillation mediated by fast conduction over the accessory pathway (atrioventricular reciprocating tachycardia) during atrial fibrillation.[36] Sudden death in Wolff-Parkinson-White syndrome occurs with an incidence ≤1:1,000 per year[37]; however, <1% of sudden deaths that are aborted with successful resuscitation are shown due to Wolff-Parkinson-White syndrome with follow-up cardiac testing.[38]

Atrial Fibrillation

Atrial fibrillation is known to greatly increase the risk of sudden death.[39] While some of the risk appears to be mediated through other concomitant factors, such as presence of heart failure, adjusting for such variables still seems to show a fourfold increase in SCD in patients with AF. Patients who are treated with radiofrequency ablation of the AVN and pacing have a high rate of sudden death (nearly 2% annual rate), although this risk also appears largely related to the underlying organic heart disease and not from the scarring secondary to the procedure.[40]

Commotio Cordis

"Commotio cordis" is a fatal mechanoelectric arrhythmogenic syndrome caused by a blunt impact to the chest, without the occurrence of a rupture of a vessel or hemopericardium. Autopsy criteria for diagnosis include no cardiac or other organic fatal lesions with negative toxicologic screening. Most cases are accidental deaths in young men during sporting activities, but it may also be a form of homicide in instances of intentional striking with intent to harm.[41]

Lymphocytic Myocarditis

Inflammatory myocardial disease as a cause of death is most frequently seen in infants and children as lymphocytic myocarditis but occurs in adults as well. Usually associated with viral infection, lymphocytic myocarditis is the cause of SCD in 15% to 20% of children and young adolescents and less frequently in young adults. At autopsy, a pericardial effusion is often found. Histologically, there is myocyte necrosis with an accompanying lymphocytic infiltrate. The degree of infiltration may be especially marked in infants and young children, and there may be scattered neutrophils and histiocytes, in addition to lymphocytes. Areas of scarring are not uncommon and are indicative of chronicity and healing. Large areas of granulation tissue may be present in cases of extensive myocarditis. Those who survive the initial insult may go on to develop a postmyocarditic dilated cardiomyopathy phenotype. Some have hypothesized that in utero myocarditis may account for some cases of congenital dilated cardiomyopathy.

There is debate regarding the extent of inflammation and necrosis required to report a forensic diagnosis of myocarditis.[42] Sensitive techniques such as reverse transcriptase polymerase chain reaction to detect viral nucleic acid may aid in diagnosis where there is little inflammation but may lack specificity and not be indicative of infection. Histologic extent of inflammation has been classified as marked (mean >5 foci per slide), moderate (2 to 5 foci per slide), and mild (<2 per slide) myocarditis.[42] Focal myocardial inflammation (<5 microscopic foci) with or without necrosis has been reported as an incidental finding and appears more likely in deceased who were taking oral medications, especially antibiotics.[42]

Hypersensitivity Myocarditis

Interstitial cardiac infiltrates with a predominance of macrophages and scattered eosinophils and neutrophils are typically an incidental finding. However, there are cases of necrotizing eosinophilic myocarditis related to drug ingestion (see Chapter 27) that represent a cause of death. When there are only sparse infiltrates with minimal myocyte necrosis, hypersensitivity myocarditis could be considered a possible or contributory factor in cases of SCD. Coronary vasoconstriction secondary to mast cell degranulation may play a role in some cases.[43]

Aortic Stenosis

In children, sub- or supravalvular aortic stenosis may cause sudden death, whereas in adults, both congenitally bicuspid or degenerative tricuspid valves are the cause (see Chapters 3 and 35).[44-47] These conditions account for ~2% of sudden deaths in adults.

Mitral Valve Prolapse

Mitral valve prolapse is an uncommon cause of sudden death (see Chapter 39). The rate of sudden death in patients with mitral valve prolapse is greater in the setting of a flail leaflet or if mitral regurgitation is present. The lifetime risk of SCD in patients with mitral valve prolapse is around 1% to 3%.[48] The pathophysiology of SCD in mitral valve prolapse and competent valves is not completely understood but appears to be related to the increased propensity for an arrhythmic state. Vectorcardiograms suggest that the majority of ventricular arrhythmias in patients with mitral valve prolapse arise in the posterior basilar septum of the left ventricle. Autopsy studies have provided several theories for sudden death, including endocardial friction lesions resulting in ventricular arrhythmias, traction of an abnormally inserted valve on the conduction system, deposition of proteoglycans within the autonomic nerve supply to the heart, and small-vessel dysplasia at the base of the heart.[7]

Infectious Endocarditis

Infectious endocarditis is 300 times more likely a finding in sudden death in intravenous drug addicts as compared to nonaddicts. Healed lesions of the tricuspid valve are common, in addition to acute vegetations.[49] In sudden death due to endocarditis, 85% occur in previously normal valves and 70% are left sided. Sudden death may occur in patients with prosthetic heart valves; when the valve is the culprit, valve thrombosis with occlusion, embolization of vegetation material into coronary arteries, anticoagulation-related hemorrhage, and perivascular fistula are the most common etiologies. Strut fractures in mechanical valves are of historic interest and are no longer a complication with improvement in valve design.[50]

SCD due to Congenital Coronary Disease

Of SCDs occurring in individuals <20 years of age, a coronary etiology is found in only about 10%, usually in the form of anomalous origin of the coronary arteries[51] (Fig. 141.7). The estimated incidence of anomalous

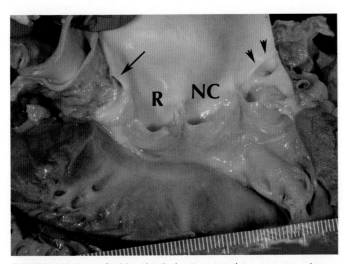

FIGURE 141.7 ▲ Sudden death due to anomalous coronary artery. An anomaly that is easily overlooked by forensic pathologists is the anomalous origin of a coronary artery. The *arrow* shows the slit-like orifice of the right coronary artery, and the *arrowheads* the normally located ostium of the left main in the left sinus of Valsalva. R, right sinus; NC, noncoronary sinus.

coronary artery from large series of angiographic studies is ~1% in the general population,[52] and autopsy studies report a rate of about 0.3%.[53]

Anomalous Left Coronary Artery from Pulmonary Artery (ALCAPA)

Ectopic origin of coronary arteries is the most common cause of sudden coronary death in children. The most common anomaly affecting infants and young children is the *anomalous left coronary artery from pulmonary artery* (ALCAPA or Bland-White-Garland syndrome) occurring in 1/50,000 to 1/300,000 autopsies, representing 0.25% to 0.5% of congenital heart disease.[52] Most cases are identified in the first year of life, and sudden death occurs in ~40% of cases. When unrecognized, mortality resulting from this lesion is high (80% to 90% in the first year of life). Sudden death usually occurs at rest but may occur after strenuous activity in older children. Pathologically, the aberrant artery arises in the left pulmonary sinus in 95% of cases.[54] Typically, the artery appears thin walled and vein-like, and the right coronary artery, while normal in location, is tortuous. The heart is typically enlarged, with extensive scarring and thinning of the anterolateral left ventricular wall and anterolateral papillary muscle. Dilatation of the left ventricle with endocardial fibroelastosis is common, and the gross appearance of the heart may mimic dilated cardiomyopathy.[5]

Anomalous Origin of the Left Main Coronary Artery from the Right Aortic Sinus

Anomalous left main coronary artery from the right aortic sinus is lethal in up to 75% of affected individuals and generally presents in adolescence or young adulthood. There is striking male predilection for the anomaly (M:F = 4 to 9:1). There are often premonitory symptoms of syncope or chest pain, but stress electrocardiograms and stress echocardiograms are often negative. Almost three-fourths of individuals die during or immediately after exertion.[55,56]

Pathologically, there are several variants to this anomaly. The common feature is the presence of the left main ostium within the right aortic sinus. This ostium is typically near the commissure and, in some cases, actually lies above the commissure between the right and left sinuses. Often, the ostium is somewhat malformed and slit-like, and an ostial ridge is present. The proximal artery lies within the aortic media and traverses between the aorta and pulmonary trunk.[52,55] In a minority of cases, the left main travels anterior to the pulmonary trunk, posterior to the aorta, or posterior to the right ventricular outflow tract within the ventricular septum. Because of the relatively high frequency of the conus coronary artery arising directly from the right aortic sinus, it is not uncommon to see two ostia within the said sinus. Therefore, two or three ostia may be seen in the setting of this anomaly.

The pathophysiology of sudden death in patients with aberrant left main coronary artery may be related to compression of the left main by the pulmonary trunk and aorta, diastolic compression of the vessel lying within the aortic media, and poor filling during diastole because of ostial ridges or slit-like ostia.

Anomalous Origin of the Right Coronary Artery from the Left Aortic Sinus

Anomalous origin of the right coronary artery from the left aortic sinus is lethal in about 1/3 of individuals. In contrast to anomalous left main coronary artery, anomalous right coronary artery from the left aortic sinus was thought to be an incidental finding, although cases of SCD have been attributed to this variant as well. Almost 50% of these deaths are exercise related, and most deaths occur in individuals <35 years of age.

Grossly, there are two ostia located in the left aortic sinus. The ostium supplying the right coronary artery may have similar features as anomalous left ostia located in the right sinus. Namely, there may be upward displacement, location near the commissure, and slit-like ostium with ostial ridges. The proximal anomalous right coronary generally also courses between the aorta and pulmonary trunk. The pathophysiology of sudden death is similar to that of anomalous left coronary artery, and evidence of acute or remote ischemia in the ventricular myocardium is not often found.[54,56–58] The actual focus of ischemia in the myocardium is not often identified by autopsy, but up to 50% of hearts will show areas of scarring.

Spontaneous Coronary Artery Dissection

Spontaneous coronary artery dissection should be suspected in SCDs in women of childbearing age. The dissection can usually be identified grossly. The specific etiology of the condition is unknown, but some authors consider a form of arterial dysplasia. In fact, there is emerging evidence that indeed there is a heritable component to this condition.[59] Histologically, there is medial dissection, usually accompanied by a reactive eosinophilic infiltrate surrounding the dissection tract (see Chapter 18).

Coronary Artery Spasm

Clinically, coronary artery spasm has been shown to result in life-threatening ventricular arrhythmias and sudden death.[60–64] At autopsy, the diagnosis can only be surmised based on clinical history and absence of significant coronary disease. If there are areas of acute and chronic ischemia in the myocardium of sudden death victims, with normal coronary arteries, then a presumptive diagnosis of coronary artery spasm can be made.[62]

Nonatherosclerotic Thrombosis

Epicardial coronary artery thrombosis in the absence of underlying atherosclerosis is rare and may be a complication of cocaine abuse and acquired coagulopathies. Late in-stent thrombosis may occur in segments that have undergone percutaneous coronary intervention and results from delayed intimal healing, other intimal injury, or hypersensitivity with eosinophilic arteritis. Thrombosis of arterioles and capillaries is a feature of thrombotic microangiopathies, such as thrombotic thrombocytopenic purpura. Cardiac arrhythmias may result from occlusion of small vessels and result in relatively rapid death. Histologically, there may be subepicardial interstitial hemorrhages and focal myocyte necrosis. *Antiphospholipid syndrome* may also result in small myocardial vessel occlusion, pulmonary embolism, and autonomic dysfunction, in addition to epicardial arterial thrombosis.[65]

Miscellaneous Nonatherosclerotic Coronary Disease

Rarely, intimal disease in coronary arteries may cause sudden coronary death in children. Fibromuscular dysplasia of an epicardial coronary artery is an extremely rare finding.[62] The cause is uncertain but is likely congenital. Coronary fibromuscular dysplasia can be associated with other vascular regions including renal, intracranial, and abdominal aortic branches and is also seen in cases of anomalous origins of coronaries.[66]

Coronary vasculitis may rarely cause sudden death, either as ostial extension from aortitis or as primarily necrotizing coronary arteritis (see Chapter 11). Rarely, acute myocardial infarction may occur in the absence of coronary artery disease, especially in women. In these cases, coronary artery spasm is presumed the etiology of the infarct, which is often of the reperfusion type.

Complex Congenital Heart Disease

Ventricular tachyarrhythmias and sudden death are known complications of surgical repairs of complex congenital heart disease and may occur years after surgery in adulthood. The mechanisms include longstanding hypertrophy and fibrosis caused by chronic hemodynamic overload and surgical scarring. These arrhythmias include re-entrant atrial and ventricular tachycardias, heart block, and sinus node dysfunction. Specifically, sudden death has been recognized as a late complication of surgical correction of tetralogy of Fallot, especially with transannular patch repair. The incidence of such an event appears to be between 1.5 and 4.5 deaths per 1,000 patient-years, most commonly occurring 4 years or more after repair.[67]

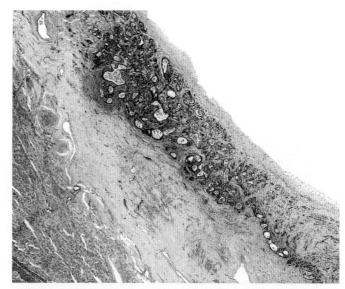

FIGURE 141.8 ▲ Atrioventricular nodal tumor. These lesions typically result in heart block and occasionally sudden death.

Cystic Tumor of the Atrioventricular Node

A developmental rest originally believed to be of ultimobranchial origin, cystic tumor of the AVN is a collection of endoderm-derived glands in the region of the AVN (Fig. 141.8). The condition is congenital and results in heart block from birth in most patients. Sudden death may occur at any age, from young childhood to late adulthood. In most patients, there is no clinical history, but when present, it is generally heart block.

Congenital Heart Block

Congenital heart block is often the result of maternal lupus autoantibodies, which cause in utero inflammation and scarring, often with calcification. Acquired inflammation and scarring may occur in children and adults, without known predisposing cause (Fig. 141.9). The risk of sudden death in patients with congenital or acquired heart block is small.[68]

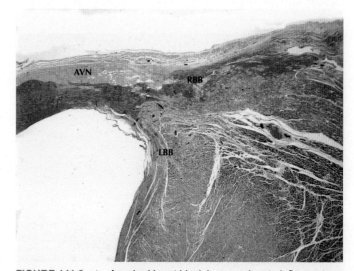

FIGURE 141.9 ▲ Acquired heart block is secondary to inflammatory conditions involving the atrioventricular nodal area such as ankylosing spondylitis, may be idiopathic or related to ischemic heart disease, and often involves the bundle branches only (incomplete heart block). In this example, there is fibrosis of the right bundle branch (RBB) and left bundle branch (LBB). The atrioventricular node (AVN) is seen at the left. Masson trichrome stain.

Miscellaneous Causes of SCD

Virtually any process that involves the myocardium can result in an increased risk of arrhythmias and sudden death. These include tumors and cysts, and prior surgeries.[69,70]

REFERENCES

1. Kucharska-Newton AM, Harald K, Rosamond WD, et al. Socioeconomic indicators and the risk of acute coronary heart disease events: comparison of population-based data from the United States and Finland. *Ann Epidemiol.* 2011;21:572–579.

2. Margey R, Roy A, Tobin S, et al. Sudden cardiac death in 14- to 35-year olds in Ireland from 2005 to 2007: a retrospective registry. *Europace.* 2011;13: 1411–1418.

3. Harmon KG, Asif IM, Maleszewski JJ, et al. Incidence, cause, and comparative frequency of sudden cardiac death in National Collegiate Athletic Association Athletes: a decade in review. *Circulation.* 2015;132:10–19.

4. Burke AP, Farb A, Virmani R, et al. Sports-related and non- sports-related sudden death in young adults. *Am Heart J.* 1991;121:568–575.

5. Tavora F, Li L, Burke A. Sudden coronary death in children. *Cardiovasc Pathol.* 2010;19:336–339.

6. Morales AR, Romanelli R, Boucek RJ, et al. Myxoid heart disease: an assessment of extravalvular cardiac pathology in severe mitral valve prolapse. *Hum Pathol.* 1992;23:129–137.

7. Burke AP, Farb A, Tang A, et al. Fibromuscular dysplasia of small coronary arteries and fibrosis in the basilar ventricular septum in mitral valve prolapse. *Am Heart J.* 1997;134:282–291.

8. Burke AP, Subramanian R, Smialek J, et al. Nonatherosclerotic narrowing of the atrioventricular node artery and sudden death. *J Am Coll Cardiol.* 1993;21:117–122.

9. Tester DJ, Medeiros-Domingo A, Will ML, et al. Cardiac channel molecular autopsy: insights from 173 consecutive cases of autopsy-negative sudden unexplained death referred for postmortem genetic testing. *Mayo Clin Proc.* 2012;87:524–539.

10. Larsen MK, Nissen PH, Berge KE, et al. Molecular autopsy in young sudden cardiac death victims with suspected cardiomyopathy. *Forensic Sci Int.* 2012;219:33–38.

11. Wang H, Yao Q, Zhu S, et al. The autopsy study of 553 cases of sudden cardiac death in Chinese adults. *Heart Vessels.* 2014;29:486–495.

12. Risgaard B, Winkel BG, Jabbari R, et al. Burden of sudden cardiac death in persons aged 1 to 49 years: nationwide study in Denmark. *Circ Arrhythm Electrophysiol.* 2014;7:205–211.

13. Jabbari R, Risgaard B, Holst AG, et al. Cardiac symptoms before sudden cardiac death caused by coronary artery disease: a nationwide study among young Danish people. *Heart.* 2013;99:938–943.

14. Kuller LH. Sudden death—definition and epidemiologic considerations. *Prog Cardiovasc Dis.* 1980;23:1–12.

15. Kannel WB, Cupples LA, D'Agostino RB. Sudden death risk in overt coronary heart disease: the Framingham study. *Am Heart J.* 1987;113:799–804.

16. Chugh SS, Reinier K, Teodorescu C, et al. Epidemiology of sudden cardiac death: clinical and research implications. *Prog Cardiovasc Dis.* 2008;51: 213–228.

17. Davies MJ. Anatomic features in victims of sudden coronary death. Coronary artery pathology. *Circulation.* 1992;85:I19–I124.

18. Burke AP, Farb A, Liang Y-H, et al. The effect of hypertension and cardiac hypertrophy on coronary artery morphology in sudden cardiac death. *Circulation.* 1996;94:3138–3145.

19. Mehta D, Curwin J, Gomes JA, et al. Sudden death in coronary artery disease: acute ischemia versus myocardial substrate. *Circulation.* 1997;96: 3215–3223.

20. Tavora F, Cresswell N, Li L, et al. Sudden coronary death caused by pathologic intimal thickening without atheromatous plaque formation. *Cardiovasc Pathol.* 2011;20:51–57.

21. Tavora F, Zhang Y, Zhang M, et al. Cardiomegaly is a common arrhythmogenic substrate in adult sudden cardiac deaths, and is associated with obesity. *Pathology.* 2012;44:187–191.

22. Arbustini E, Grasso M, Diegoli M, et al. Coronary thrombosis in non-cardiac death. *Coron Artery Dis.* 1993;4:751–759.

23. Warnes CA, Roberts WC. Sudden coronary death: comparison of patients with to those without coronary thrombus at necropsy. *Am J Cardiol.* 1984;54: 1206–1211.

24. Tavora F, Cresswell N, Li L, et al. Morphologic features of exertional versus nonexertional sudden death in patients with hypertrophic cardiomyopathy. *Am J Cardiol.* 2010;105:532–537.

25. Tavora F, Zhang M, Franco M, et al. Distribution of biventricular disease in arrhythmogenic cardiomyopathy: an autopsy study. *Hum Pathol.* 2012;43:592–596.

26. Pahl E, Sleeper LA, Canter CE, et al. Incidence of and risk factors for sudden cardiac death in children with dilated cardiomyopathy: a report from the Pediatric Cardiomyopathy Registry. *J Am Coll Cardiol.* 2012;59:607–615.

27. Hanson EL, Jakobs PM, Keegan H, et al. Cardiac troponin T lysine 210 deletion in a family with dilated cardiomyopathy. *J Card Fail.* 2002;8:28–32.

28. Merlo M, Sinagra G, Carniel E, et al. Poor prognosis of rare sarcomeric gene variants in patients with dilated cardiomyopathy. *Clin Transl Sci.* 2013;6:424–428.

29. Botto N, Vittorini S, Colombo MG, et al. A novel LMNA mutation (R189W) in familial dilated cardiomyopathy: evidence for a 'hot spot' region at exon 3: a case report. *Cardiovasc Ultrasound.* 2010;8:9.

30. Chen W, Huo J, Ma A, et al. A novel mutation of the LMNA gene in a family with dilated cardiomyopathy, conduction system disease, and sudden cardiac death of young females. *Mol Cell Biochem.* 2013;382:307–311.

31. Geiger SK, Bar H, Ehlermann P, et al. Incomplete nonsense-mediated decay of mutant lamin A/C mRNA provokes dilated cardiomyopathy and ventricular tachycardia. *J Mol Med (Berl).* 2008;86:281–289.

32. Pilmer CM, Kirsh JA, Hildebrandt D, et al. Sudden cardiac death in children and adolescents between 1 and 19 years of age. *Heart Rhythm.* 2014;11:239–245.

33. Tester DJ, Ackerman MJ. The role of molecular autopsy in unexplained sudden cardiac death. *Curr Opin Cardiol.* 2006;21:166–172.

34. Tester DJ, Spoon DB, Valdivia HH, et al. Targeted mutational analysis of the RyR2-encoded cardiac ryanodine receptor in sudden unexplained death: a molecular autopsy of 49 medical examiner/coroner's cases. *Mayo Clin Proc.* 2004;79:1380–1384.

35. Zhang M, Tavora F, Oliveira JB, et al. PKP2 mutations in sudden death from arrhythmogenic right ventricular cardiomyopathy (ARVC) and sudden unexpected death with negative autopsy (SUDNA). *Circ J.* 2012;76: 189–194.

36. Antz M, Weiss C, Volkmer M, et al. Risk of sudden death after successful accessory atrioventricular pathway ablation in resuscitated patients with Wolff-Parkinson-White syndrome. *J Cardiovasc Electrophysiol.* 2002;13:231–236.

37. Garcia-Cosio Mir F. [Sudden death in the Wolff-Parkinson-White syndrome]. *Rev Esp Cardiol.* 1989;42:234–239.

38. Rosman HS, Goldstein S, Landis JR, et al. Clinical characteristics and survival experience of out-of-hospital cardiac arrest victims without coronary heart disease. *Eur Heart J.* 1988;9:17–23.

39. Reinier K, Marijon E, Uy-Evanado A, et al. The association between atrial fibrillation and sudden cardiac death: the relevance of heart failure. *JACC Heart Fail.* 2014;2:221–227.

40. Darpo B, Walfridsson H, Aunes M, et al. Incidence of sudden death after radiofrequency ablation of the atrioventricular junction for atrial fibrillation. *Am J Cardiol.* 1997;80:1174–1177.

41. Zheng N, Liang M, Liu Y, et al. Commotio cordis—a report of two similar cases. *J Forensic Sci.* 2013;58:245–247.

42. De Salvia A, De Leo D, Carturan E, et al. Sudden cardiac death, borderline myocarditis and molecular diagnosis: evidence or assumption? *Med Sci Law.* 2011;51(suppl 1):S27–S29.

43. Kounis NG. Coronary hypersensitivity disorder: the Kounis syndrome. *Clin Ther.* 2013;35:563–571.

44. Gohlke-Barwolf C, Peters K, Petersen J, et al. Influence of aortic valve replacement on sudden death in patients with pure aortic stenosis. *Eur Heart J.* 1988;9(suppl E):139–141.

45. Suarez-Mier MP, Morentin B. Supravalvular aortic stenosis, Williams syndrome and sudden death. A case report. *Forensic Sci Int.* 1999;106:45–53.

46. Sun CC, Jacot J, Brenner JI. Sudden death in supravalvular aortic stenosis: fusion of a coronary leaflet to the sinus ridge, dysplasia and stenosis of aortic and pulmonic valves. *Pediatr Pathol.* 1992;12:751–759.

47. Turan AA, Guven T, Karayel F, et al. Subvalvular aortic stenosis as a cause of sudden death: two case reports. *Am J Forensic Med Pathol.* 2006;27: 90–92.

48. Franchitto N, Bounes V, Telmon N, et al. Mitral valve prolapse and out-of-hospital sudden death: a case report and literature review. *Med Sci Law.* 2010;50:164–167.

49. Burke AP, Kalra P, Li L, et al. Infectious endocarditis and sudden unexpected death: Incidence and morphology of lesions in intravenous addicts and non drug abusers. *J Heart Valve Dis.* 1997;6:198–203.

50. Burke AP, Farb A, Sessums L, et al. Causes of sudden cardiac death in patients with replacement valves: an autopsy study. *J Heart Valve Dis.* 1994;3:10–16.

51. Drezner JA, Courson RW, Roberts WO, et al. Inter-association task force recommendations on emergency preparedness and management of sudden cardiac arrest in high school and college athletic programs: a consensus statement. *Heart Rhythm.* 2007;4:549–665.

52. Angelini P, Velasco JA, Flamm S. Coronary anomalies: incidence, pathophysiology, and clinical relevance. *Circulation.* 2002;105:2449–2454.

53. Alexander RW, Griffith GC. Anomalies of the coronary arteries and their clinical significance. *Circulation.* 1956;14:800–805.

54. Roberts WC. Major anomalies of coronary arterial origin seen in adulthood. *Am Heart J.* 1986;111:941–963.

55. Eckart RE, Jones SO IV, Shry EA, et al. Sudden death associated with anomalous coronary origin and obstructive coronary disease in the young. *Cardiol Rev.* 2006;14:161–163.

56. Iino M, Kimura T, Abiru H, et al. Unexpected sudden death resulting from anomalous origin of the right coronary artery from the left sinus of Valsalva: a case report involving identical twins. *Leg Med (Tokyo).* 2007;9:25–29.

57. Kahali B, Roy DG, Batabyal S, et al. Study of sudden cardiac deaths in young athletes. *J Indian Med Assoc.* 2002;100:708–709.

58. Khan A, Stewart J, Smith W. Sudden cardiac death in the young: don't forget abnormal coronary arteries! *N Z Med J.* 2007;120:U2710.

59. Goel K, Tweet M, Olson TM, et al. Familial spontaneous coronary artery dissection: evidence for genetic susceptibility. *JAMA Intern Med.* 2015;175:821–826.

60. Chevalier P, Kirkorian G, Touboul P. Arrhythmic sudden cardiac death due to coronary artery spasm. *Card Electrophysiol Rev.* 2002;6:104–106.

61. Fiocca L, Di Biasi M, Bruno N, et al. Coronary vasospasm and aborted sudden death treated with an implantable defibrillator and stenting. *Ital Heart J.* 2002;3:270–273.

62. Hill SF, Sheppard MN. Non-atherosclerotic coronary artery disease associated with sudden cardiac death. *Heart.* 2010;96:1119–1125.

63. Letsas KP, Filippatos GS, Efremidis M, et al. Secondary prevention of sudden cardiac death in coronary artery spasm: is implantable cardioverter defibrillator always efficient? *Int J Cardiol.* 2007;117:141–143.

64. Mitchell LB. Use of the implantable cardioverter-defibrillator in patients with coronary artery spasm as the apparent cause of spontaneous life-threatening ventricular tachycardia or ventricular fibrillation: crossing the spasm sudden death chasm. *J Am Coll Cardiol.* 2012;60:914–916.

65. Nicklin A, Byard RW. Lethal manifestations of systemic lupus erythematosus in a forensic context. *J Forensic Sci.* 2011;56:423–428.

66. Maresi E, Becchina G, Ottoveggio G, et al. Arrhythmic sudden cardiac death in a 3-year-old child with intimal fibroplasia of coronary arteries, aorta, and its branches. *Cardiovasc Pathol.* 2001;10:43–48.

67. Steeds RP, Oakley D. Predicting late sudden death from ventricular arrhythmia in adults following surgical repair of tetralogy of Fallot. *QJM.* 2004;97:7–13.

68. Kumar AU, Sripriya R, Parthasarathy S, et al. Congenital complete heart block and spinal anaesthesia for caesarean section. *Indian J Anaesth.* 2012;56:72–74.

69. Cina SJ, Smialek JE, Burke AP, et al. Primary cardiac tumors causing sudden death: a review of the literature. *Am J Forensic Med Pathol.* 1996;17:271–281.

70. Hejna P, Janik M. Lipomatous hypertrophy of the interatrial septum: a possibly neglected cause of sudden cardiac death. *Forensic Sci Med Pathol.* 2014;10:119–121.

142   Pathology of Cardiac Devices and Interventions

Joseph J. Maleszewski, M.D., and Allen P. Burke, M.D.

Introduction

Open and percutaneous interventions performed on the heart and thoracic aorta are relatively commonplace. They are typically done in order to restore normal blood flow. Procedures can involve the valves (Chapter 41), coronary arteries (Chapters 16 and 17), thoracic aorta and branches (Chapter 53), as well as the myocardium itself (such as in congenital heart disease or cardiomyopathies) (Chapters 3, 19, 20, and 25).

This chapter addresses (1) interventions used in the treatment of arrhythmias, including placement of indwelling leads for pacing or defibrillation, and direct ablation of arrhythmogenic foci within the myocardium; (2) common interventions used in the treatment of heart failure; and (3) unexpected thoracic complications of percutaneous interventions.

At autopsy, the pathologist should describe the intervention, pathology in and around the intervened site, and any sequelae. Some interventions result in unexpected consequences that may be incidentally noted, for example, embolization of catheter-based hydrophilic polymers.

Pathologic reactions to treatments and devices have a common pathway of wound healing, which progresses through phases of acute and chronic inflammation, granulation tissue, and fibrosis, often with a tissue reaction to foreign material. In the case of intravascular interventions, there is a progression of acute thrombosis (composed of fibrin and platelets) to early organization with endothelialization and persistent fibrin and to mature organization often with recanalization. There may or may not be foreign body/inflammatory reactions complicating the healing process.

Pacemakers and AICDs

There are myriad devices implanted in the heart for treatment of arrhythmias, including pacemakers and automatic implantable cardiac defibrillators. Indications for cardiac pacing include acquired atrioventricular block such as seen after atrioventricular nodal ablation, myocardial infarction, or a number of syndromic states.

Pacemakers are generally either single chamber (lead in either right atrium or right ventricle) or dual chamber (leads in both right atrium and right ventricle). Each lead communicates with the pacemaker and provides pacing and/or monitoring capabilities. Pacemakers may be used in conjunction with defibrillators, which are similar in appearance. In patients with heart failure, a third pacing wire in the left ventricle, inserted through the coronary sinus and anterior cardiac vein, results in better contractility via synchronous biventricular contraction (cardiac resynchronization therapy).[1]

At autopsy, leads are identified in the heart, entering through the superior vena cava (Fig. 142.1). They can be separated from the device itself by cutting the wires within the superior vena cava. The device is usually positioned subcutaneously in the upper chest. The lead may be adherent to the tricuspid valve, which in some instances may tether the valve and cause significant hemodynamic regurgitation. Occasionally, tricuspid valve replacement is necessary in order to surgically extract an indwelling right ventricular lead or if the lead becomes infected.[2,3] A hollow, cylindrical, lead tract may be present extending from the tricuspid valve to the insertion in the ventricular wall (Fig. 142.2). This tract consists of endocardium that has grown around the foreign object.[2,3]

Care should be taken to avoid electric shocks to the prosecting pathologist or assistant. The status of the leads and their tips should be

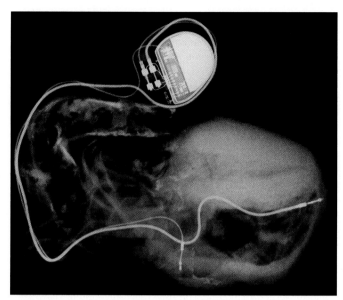

FIGURE 142.1 ▲ Pacemaker device seen at autopsy, postmortem radiography. The pacer is dual chamber, with one lead in the right atrium and the other in the right ventricle. The indication in this patient was acquired third-degree heart block.

TABLE 142.1   Sites of Ablation, by Common Types of Arrhythmia

	Common Sites of Ablation
Atrial fibrillation Paroxysmal Chronic	Pulmonary vein sleeve Linear posterior left atrial ablations (maze)
Atrial fibrillation, control of ventricular response	Atrioventricular junction ablation (insertion of pacemaker)
Atrial flutter	Isthmus between coronary sinus and inferior vena cava
Supraventricular atrial re-entrant tachycardia	Coronary sinus
WPW preexcitation syndrome	Atrioventricular groove, especially left atrial free wall > right atrial free wall
Supraventricular nodal re-entrant tachycardia	Atrioventricular node
Monomorphic ventricular tachycardia, monomorphic premature ventricular contractions	Left ventricular outflow near aortic valve and near any of the 4 valves (especially dilated cardiomyopathy) including outflow tracts Epicardial sites Areas of scar (ischemic cardiomyopathy)

ascertained, including their position and associated pathology (if any). Interrogation of the device can provide important clues as to the functioning of the device at the time of death and/or the terminal rhythm. Such interrogation can usually be performed by electrophysiology personnel or the device manufacturer and can be done without the leads being attached.[4]

Cardiac Ablations

General

Endocardial cardiac ablations are performed for a variety of indications. These include ablation of bypass tracts, re-entrant pathways, and arrhythmogenic foci determined by electrophysiologic mapping (Table 142.1). Arrhythmias that are treated include atrial and ventricular tachycardias and atrial fibrillation.

Ablation is most frequently accomplished by radiofrequency waves, but lasers, microwaves, and cryoablation have also been used. Radiofrequency causes thermal injury using alternating current and is usually delivered percutaneously via catheter. Cryoablation produces myocardial injury with tissue freezing and thawing. Cryoablation, which is more frequently done by open procedure, produces less endothelial or endocardial injury possibly with less endocardial thrombus.

An electrophysiologic study records electrical activity and determines where catheter ablation may eliminate cardiac arrhythmias. The success of catheter ablation is high for atrioventricular nodal reentry, accessory pathways, atrial flutter, and idiopathic ventricular tachycardia. The success rate is lower in patients with atrial fibrillation or structural heart disease.[5]

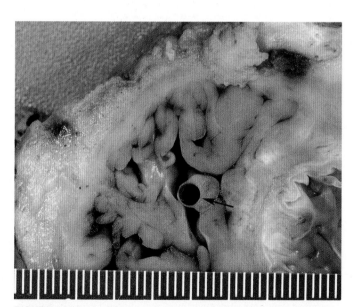

FIGURE 142.2 ▲ Right ventricular scar at site of indwelling lead. Right ventricular catheter site, manifest as hole from catheter, incidental finding. The *arrow* indicates the site where the catheter tip was pulled at explant. There is a fibrous capsule around the catheter lead, which had been removed from its entanglement in the tricuspid valve.

Atrioventricular Nodal Ablation

Atrioventricular nodal ablation is performed in patients who have atrial fibrillation with a rapid ventricular response who do not respond to medical treatment. Complete atrioventricular node ablation requires implantation of a permanent pacemaker. At autopsy, there will be scarring in the region of the membranous septum (Fig. 142.3).

Wolff-Parkinson-White Syndrome

Wolff-Parkinson-White (WPW) syndrome is a preexcitation syndrome caused by atrioventricular bypass tracts that are most common in the left free wall, followed by the right free wall and the posteroseptal region (see Chapter 4). Most patients are asymptomatic and do not require treatment. Catheter ablation is performed in patients who are refractory to drugs and are symptomatic with atrioventricular re-entrant tachycardia or paroxysmal atrial fibrillation. In the past, open surgical procedures were performed to interrupt the pathway, and currently, catheter-based radiofrequency ablation is used, with a success rate of near 100%.[6]

Of note, patients with certain types of congenital heart disease (e.g., Ebstein anomaly) (Chapter 34) have a high incidence of WPW and may have ablations in addition to their underlying structural heart disease.

Atrial Arrhythmias

Supraventricular arrhythmias are frequently treated with ablation and are often caused by reentry, especially near the coronary sinus. Of atrial arrhythmias in children, supraventricular re-entrant tachycardia

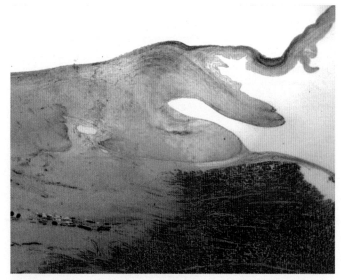

FIGURE 142.3 ▲ Ablation scarring, atrioventricular nodal area. Scarring under tricuspid valve after remote atrioventricular nodal ablation. This section is more anterior or distal, in the area of right bundle branch, which is completely scarred.

accounts for over 60%, the remainder including atrioventricular nodal re-entrant tachycardia, atrial tachycardia, and atrial flutter.[7–9] Supraventricular tachycardias also occur in adults, and ablation sites can be anywhere in the atria but most frequently in the area of the atrioventricular node and posteriorly at the coronary sinus. In junctional reciprocating tachycardia, the accessory pathway is often the posteroseptal area.[10] Occasionally, they may be associated with coronary sinus aneurysms (Fig. 142.4).

Atrial flutter is classified as counterclockwise or clockwise and is a re-entrant arrhythmia, which often involves the isthmus between the tricuspid valve and the inferior vena cava; this area is used for

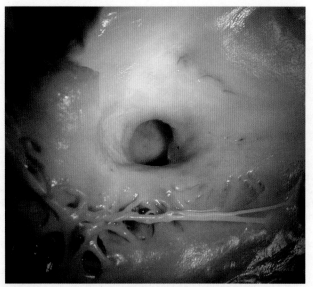

FIGURE 142.4 ▲ Coronary sinus seen from right atrium. There is marked endocardial fibrosis from remote endocardial ablation, performed in the coronary sinus area. This region is a common site of ablations for atrial tachycardias and atrial flutter (the latter typically at the isthmus between the coronary sinus and inferior vena cava).

treatment of atrial flutter, and ablation sites may be present in this area at autopsy from patients with prior treatment.

Atrial fibrillation is the most common arrhythmia treated by intervention. It may be chronic or paroxysmal and is frequently associated with organic heart disease, such as cardiomyopathy or ischemia. Chronic atrial fibrillation has been classified as persistent (>7 days) or permanent. Occasionally, there are no predisposing diseases (lone atrial fibrillation). Noncardiac conditions that increase the risk of atrial fibrillation include hypertension, lung disease, and hyperthyroidism. The most common cardiac conditions are mitral valve disease, especially stenosis, ischemic heart disease, and cardiomyopathy.

Patients with atrial fibrillation are treated with anticoagulation, because there is a sevenfold increase in the risk of stroke from embolized mural thrombosis. Other complications include heart failure and palpitations; the ventricular response is treated with beta-blockers and calcium channel blockers. Occasionally, ablation of the atrioventricular node is necessary, with dual-chamber pacing.

There are no specific pathologic findings in atrial fibrillation, but nonspecific features are commonly encountered such as gross atrial dilatation (which may be primary or secondary to the arrhythmic state) and histologic hypertrophy and fibrosis. These latter findings have been shown to have some correlation with recurrence of atrial fibrillation following the Cox maze procedure.[11] Mural thrombi are common findings in markedly dilated atria.

The arrhythmia is believed to propagate in the area of the pulmonary valve sleeves, or regions of smooth muscle that extend from the pulmonary vein media into the left atrial body. The sleeve length ranges from 2 to 25 mm and is longest in the upper veins. The concept of interruption of left atrial tracts has led to a variety of surgical approaches, which are generally termed "maze" procedure, after the irregular incisions made above the posterior leaflet of the mitral valve. Patients with atrial fibrillation due to mitral valve disease often undergo mitral valve replacement or repair. Approximately 40% of these patients have surgical ablation either by incisions or by other methods of ablation, typically cryotherapy (cryomaze). The latter procedure has been associated with over 75% freedom from recurrent atrial fibrillation at 1 year.[12] In general, the success of the maze procedure is correlated to the degree of atrial dilatation and is most successful if the atrium is <50 mm in diameter.

Ventricular Tachycardia in the Absence of Structural Heart Disease

Monomorphic ventricular tachycardias and premature ventricular impulses occur anywhere in the ventricles but most frequently in the left ventricular outflow tract beneath the aortic valve cusps,[13] right ventricular outflow tract,[14] and tricuspid annulus.[15] Ablation has a good success rate of ameliorating symptoms with prevention of recurrent arrhythmias. In patients with a history of ventricular ablation, these are sites that are likely to have been treated with prior ablations, which appear as white endocardial scars.

Ventricular Tachycardia in Structural and Ischemic Heart Disease

Cardiomyopathies, including hypertrophic and dilated cardiomyopathy, are prone to the development of monomorphic ventricular tachycardias that are amenable to ablation.[16] In dilated cardiomyopathy, they may be endocardial based, especially near a valve annulus, or deep and subepicardial.[17] The latter may be approached percutaneously by introducing the catheter to the epicardium through the pericardium. Ventricular tachycardia associated with healed myocardial infarction is also associated with areas of low-voltage scar. Histologic sections of these areas at autopsy show transmural scars in most cases.[18] Common ablation sites for monomorphic ventricular tachycardias in ischemic cardiomyopathy are the posterior papillary muscle and ventricular septum.[19]

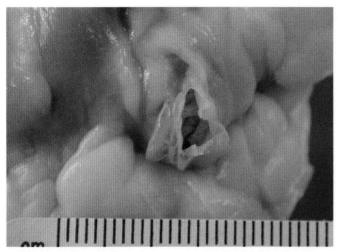

FIGURE 142.5 ▲ Complication of right ventricular outflow ablation. Months after a right ventricular outflow ablation for ventricular tachycardia, there was rupture of a pseudoaneurysm resulting in hemopericardium and sudden death. Perforation and sudden death rarely occurs and may happen years after procedure (from a published case report).[20]

Pathologic Findings

Radiofrequency ablation results in endocardial injury generally 5 to 6 mm diameter and up to 3 mm deep, sometimes associated with mural thrombus. Grossly, lesions are acutely pale and progress to fibrosis, which may disappear on gross inspection. Acutely, there is coagulative necrosis surrounded by neutrophils and then macrophages and granulation tissue, as in any wound healing response. In areas of healed injury, there may be transmural coagulation necrosis of mesh-like fibrotic tissue, with interspersed islands of myocardial cells, up to a maximum depth of 7 mm.[18] Chronically, there is fibrosis, which is nonspecific as to etiology.

Complications

Complications include perforation (Fig. 142.5) with possible tamponade,[20] pneumothorax, hemothorax, and mural thrombus (with or without embolization). Rare complications include aortic and coronary arterial injury, air embolism, valve injury, and atrioesophageal fistula after pulmonary vein ablation for atrial fibrillation.

Complications of Percutaneous Interventions

Cardiac Perforation

Complications of catheter-based interventions include vascular or cardiac perforation and may result from injury by the catheter/lead or the introducer sheath. For example, retroperitoneal hemorrhage is a known complication of femoral catheterizations.[21] The sheath that is used to guide the catheter into the artery, and which is relatively stiff, may be long enough to extend from the femoral site through the pelvis into the retroperitoneum and erode through the vessel if left in place for extended periods.[22]

Right ventricular perforation may occur from pacemaker or defibrillator leads and can occur days after the procedure[23,24] (Fig. 142.6). There is a very low risk of right ventricular perforation with tamponade after endomyocardial biopsy, even with mesothelium identified on the biopsy sample, and significant accumulation of blood in the pericardium is rare.[25–28] Extremely rare complications of biopsy include deployment of the bioptome in the wrong area (e.g., coronary sinus) due to errors in fluoroscopic guidance.

Coronary Artery Perforation

Currently, most coronary interventions include angioplasty as well as stent deployment. Those procedures that include removal of plaque have a higher incidence of complications such as perforation. These atheroablative procedures include direction atherectomy (rarely performed currently in the coronary artery), excimer laser, rotablator, and transluminal extraction catheters. Rotablators are used specifically for treatment of calcified plaques. The use of anticoagulation in the form of IIb/IIIa inhibitors, as well as oversized stents, also increases the risk of hemorrhage (Figs. 142.7 and 142.8).

The angiographic classifications of coronary perforations are type I (crater extending outside the lumen without angiographic evidence of dissection), type II (pericardial or myocardial blush without an exit hole or one <1 mm), and type III (frank streaming of contrast through an exit hole larger than 1 mm, with or without spilling into the coronary sinus or right ventricle).[29] Hemopericardium may cause tamponade and death or cause more isolated left atrial compression.[30] The traumatic injury may be caused by guidewire itself or the stent or atherectomy device. The risk of guidewire injury is greater in attempted ballooning of chronic total occlusions.[31] Calcified lesions treated with rotablator or other cutting balloons are at higher risk for medial perforation. Excimer laser coronary angioplasty with ballooning (usually

FIGURE 142.6 ▲ Right ventricular laceration from pacer lead. In this case, the tear (*arrow*) was incidental and secondary to pericardiocentesis during cardiac arrest caused by other causes. **A.** External surface shows barely discernable area of hemorrhage. **B.** Cross-section demonstrates clear perforation. There was hemopericardium at autopsy secondary to the defect (not shown).

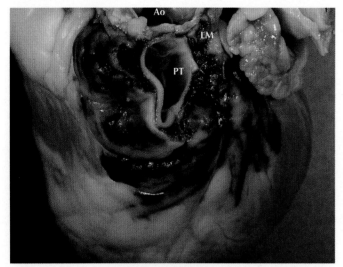

FIGURE 142.7 ▲ Epicardial hemorrhage, surrounding proximal arteries, secondary to perforation of artery during rotablator. The tear was diagnosed by angiography during the intervention and successfully treated with stenting. The patient died later from hemopericardium from right ventricular puncture. Ao, ; LM, ; PT, .

without the need of stents) has been used as treatment of an obstructive coronary artery lesions in native coronary atherosclerosis[32] as well as graft vasculopathy transplant patients.[33] Treatment of coronary perforations is generally by restenting and sometimes by open procedures involving vascular wrapping with Gore-Tex–coated Teflon.[34]

Hydrophilic Polymer Embolization

Although far more common in the pulmonary arterial circulation (see Chapter 61), hydrophilic gels that coat catheters and catheter sheaths may embolize and lodge into the coronary or cerebral vasculature after left-sided interventions (Fig. 142.9). Systemic embolization may also occur in the setting of venous instrumentation when a patent foramen ovale is present along with elevated right atrial pressures. Typically, hydrophilic embolization is an incidental finding but may cause a granulomatous reaction with giant cells, causing symptomatic abscess formation.[35]

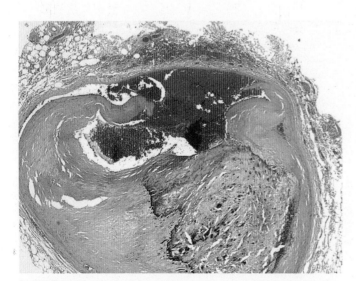

FIGURE 142.8 ▲ Perforation of artery during rotablator. Note defect in the media at the top of the figure. Cutting catheters are used for heavily calcified plaques, which are difficult to balloon and stent.

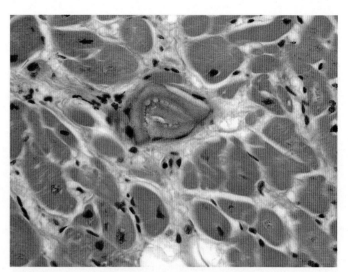

FIGURE 142.9 ▲ Hydrophilic polymer embolization, incidental, myocardium. Catheter sheaths are often coated with gels to decrease friction during passage of the catheter itself.

Complications of Stented Endografts

Stents are also used for treatment of aortic disease, especially thoracic and, to a lesser extent, abdominal aneurysms (Fig. 142.10). The latter are surgically repaired with minimal complications, but the significant complications of thoracic aneurysm repair may necessitate less invasive percutaneous procedures. The most common complication of aortic endovascular stenting is that of leakage of blood from the lumen to the space between the graft and the aneurysm wall. These leaks, which are called endoleaks, have been classified as type I (between arterial wall and endoprosthesis), type II (retrograde flow from lumbar arteries/internal mammary arteries (most common)), type III (endoprosthetic defects), and type IV (porosity/microleaks).

Greenfield Vena Cava Filter Complications

Metallic devices implanted in the inferior vena cava for the prevention of pulmonary embolism may be encountered by pathologists. The

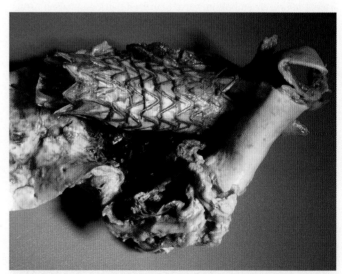

FIGURE 142.10 ▲ Aortic endograft, treatment for pseudoaneurysm. The patient had an atherosclerotic aneurysm with leakage and pseudoaneurysm formation. He was not a surgical candidate, due to stage IV colon cancer, and the procedure was largely palliative. The patient died of rupture of the pseudoaneurysm, which has not been adequately sealed due to a large type I endoleak.

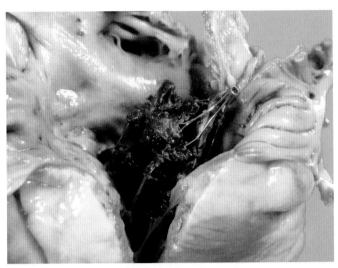

FIGURE 142.11 ▲ There is a thrombosed vena cava filter that dislodged and obstructed the tricuspid valve, resulting in sudden unexpected death.

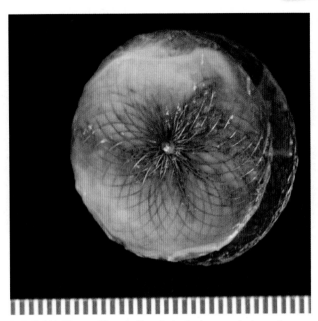

FIGURE 142.13 ▲ Clamshell occlude device, surgical specimen. The device was removed for persistent shunt.

devices have stood the test of time for safety and success in preventing pulmonary embolism, with a recurrence rate of 4% at 20 years and a thrombosis rate of 4% at 20 years.[36,37] Rare complications include rupture of the vena cava, rupture of the aorta,[38,39] detachment and embolization to the right atrium, migration to the pulmonary artery, perforation of the duodenum, and perforation of the right ventricle[40–45] (Fig. 142.11).

Septal and Ductal Closure Devices

Closure devices that are deployed via catheter, and have expandable discs seal over both sides of a central axle ("clamshell" shape), have been used for over 10 years for repair of atrial septal defects (Figs. 142.12 and 142.13) and patent ductus arteriosus, and less commonly patent foramen ovale, aortic pseudoaneurysms, and ventricular septal defects. The device is composed of nitinol (nickel titanium alloy) wire and Dacron fabric. Incomplete endothelialization can predispose to endocarditis. Initial complications include atrial fibrillation (<5%), hemopericardium with or without tamponade (<1%), and device embolization (<1%).

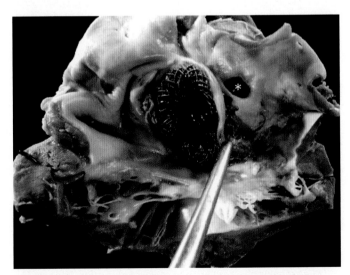

FIGURE 142.12 ▲ Clamshell occluder device, inserted in ductus arteriosus for closure. Clamshell occluder device, atrial septum, as seen from the left atrium. There is a persistent shunt (*asterisk*).

In cases of device failure or embolization,[46] excised occluders (mostly commonly the "Amplatzer" device) demonstrate endothelialization with fibrosis on the right and left atrial sides and organized thrombus between the metal wires. There is a reactive infiltrate of macrophages, multinucleate giant cells, and lymphocytes.[47–52]

A smaller version of the device (Amplatzer duct occluder) is utilized specifically for treatment of patent ductus arteriosus.[53]

A similar clamshell device (Amplatzer Vascular Plug device) is used for perivalvular leaks adjacent to prosthetic valves.[54]

Percutaneous Valve Interventions

Prosthetic valves are usually placed by open surgical procedures, although stented bioprosthetic valves can be deployed percutaneously in selected indications. Prosthetic valves are discussed in Chapter 41.

Transcatheter aortic valve implantation (TAVI) is an alternate to open valve replacement for high-risk and inoperable patients with severe aortic stenosis. Procedural complications include stroke, vascular complications related to deployment, paravalvular leak, and conduction disturbances.[55] Significant postprocedure aortic regurgitation may require open procedures or closed repair with Amplatzer Vascular Plug, which is between the valve skirt and the aortic annulus.[54] A rare complication is postprocedural acquired ventricular septal defect.[56] TAVI may be performed using balloon-expandable devices or those that are self-expanding.[55,57]

Mitral valve endovascular clip repair is an alternative for open mitral valve repair. In this procedure, clips are deployed by catheterization to close adjacent edges of the posterior leaflet of the mitral valve, in order to decrease regurgitation. Complications include need for subsequent open procedures because of persistent mitral insufficiency.[58]

Heart Failure Interventions

Ventricular Aneurysm

There are a variety of interventions for heart failure. In ischemic heart disease with postinfarction aneurysm, closure of aneurysm wall with partial aneurysmectomy and patch repair may be performed. The pathologist will get a portion of the left ventricle, which generally demonstrates transmural replacement-type interstitial fibrosis. The patch itself may be a synthetic material or homograft or xenograft pericardium.[59]

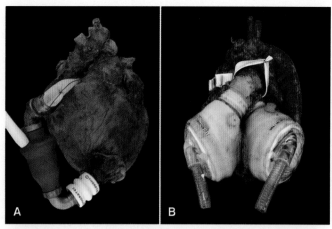

FIGURE 142.14 ▲ A. Left ventricular assist device (LVAD) with inflow cannula implanted in left ventricle and outflow cannula within the ascending aorta. **B.** TAH wherein both ventricles have been removed and replaced by the device.

Ventricular Assist Devices

Assist devices for heart failure are either implanted temporarily (bridge therapy) or for the life of the patient (destination therapy). They may be left, right, or biventricular (Fig. 142.14A). In addition, there are total artificial hearts (TAHs) that physically and functionally replace the ventricular chambers (Fig. 142.14B). There is an inflow cannula of the ventricular assist device at the left (or right or both) ventricular apex. The outflow cannula (away from the device back into the patient) is generally placed in the corresponding great artery. The conduits may contain either bioprosthetic valves or valves made of synthetic materials.

Currently, the most widely implanted assist devices are relatively small and provide nonpulsatile flow with a rotor or impeller encased in a metal housing. The HeartMate (Novacor) consists of an extraventricular rotor that is within the thorax near the cardiac apex and connected between the ventricle and the ascending aorta via a synthetic conduit. There is a driveline that provides power, which courses outside the body to an external battery. In other devices, the rotor may be within the left ventricular apex itself (e.g., Jarvik-2000).[60,61] The impeller or rotor draws blood from the ventricular cavity through the device out into the outflow cannula, such as a Dacron conduit anastomosed into the ascending aorta, with a porcine or other type of valve.

During surgical implant, a portion of the left ventricle will be removed, representing a core of the apex. Histologically, the cores will generally demonstrate nonspecific findings of cardiomyopathy, such as myocyte hypertrophy and interstitial fibrosis. In cases of ischemic heart disease, subendocardial myocyte vacuolization or healed myocardial infarctions may be present. Occasionally, a specific type of cardiomyopathy can be suggested. Incidental findings such as hypersensitivity myocarditis may be seen in ~5% to 10% of patients (Fig. 142.15).

Pump thrombosis is one of the main causes for device malfunction in ~6% of patients with nonpulsatile assist devices, with some cases being fatal.[62,63] Chronic complications include degenerative and calcific changes of the valves within the conduit.[64]

A serious complication of ventricular assist devices is infection, which may arise at the site of the driveline exiting the skin and result in cutaneous infections and mediastinitis. With the use of older devices, over 40% of patients developed sepsis in 1 year and over one-half at 2 years.[65] To lessen life-threatening thoracic infections, the driveline is often placed in remote locations, such as the peritoneum, tunneled to the extracorporeal controller unit. However, mediastinitis is still a potentially lethal complication of current assist devices. The most common organisms are staphylococci, *Pseudomonas*, enterococci, and *Candida*.

Other complications include hemorrhage, due to the need for anticoagulation,[61] and cerebrovascular accidents, either embolic or hemorrhagic. These occur in up to 25% of patients.

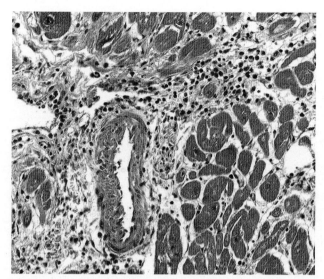

FIGURE 142.15 ▲ Left ventricular core excision at LVAD placement. In <10% of cases, incidental findings such as hypersensitivity myocarditis may be found (see Chapter 27).

An autopsy study of patients dying with ventricular assist devices demonstrated that the cause of death was related to device malfunction, cerebrovascular accidents, pulmonary hypertension, and other conditions; contributing findings included liver necrosis, acquired aortic valve disease, bowel infarction, abdominal aortic aneurysm, and intra-conduit porcine aortic valve degeneration.[66] In comparison to myocardium sampled at the time of insertion, the assist devices significantly reduced the amount of contraction band necrosis and myocytolysis (endocardial vacuolization related to ischemia) in the left ventricle.[66]

Intra-Aortic Balloon Pumps

Intra-aortic counterpulsation is an acute treatment for heart failure and consists of a cylindrical balloon that sits in the aorta and actively deflates in systole, increasing forward blood flow by reducing afterload, and actively inflates in diastole increasing blood flow to the coronary arteries. It is commonly used for patients with cardiogenic shock or perioperative cardiac failure. Complications occur in 6% to 15% of patients[67] and increase with prolonged duration.[68] Complications include compartment syndrome from femoral insertion, thromboembolism,[67] and rupture of the balloon, necessitating surgical extraction of the retained device.[69] The use for balloon pump placement for high-risk cardiac surgery is debated, some studies showing benefit[70] and others showing a higher risk of urinary tract infection, renal failure, and prolonged ventilatory support.[71]

Practical Points

▶ In evaluation of surgical specimens, it is necessary to have a clinical history of previous intervention in order to properly evaluate the specimen.

▶ Most cases of interventional pathology will be seen at autopsy.

▶ A careful clinical history is of vital importance to piece together the sequence of events linking the intervention to morbidity or mortality.

▶ Radiographs of the specimen are essential in cases of metallic device embolization.

▶ Knowledge of specific timing of procedures is important in assessing the significance of vascular perforations or other untoward sequelae of vascular interventions.

REFERENCES

1. Shandling A, Donohue D, Tobias S, et al. Use of an active-fixation coronary sinus lead to implant a biventricular pacemaker via the femoral vein. *Tex Heart Inst J.* 2010;37:92–94.

2. Lee JH, Kim TH, Kim WS. Permanent pacemaker lead induced severe tricuspid regurgitation in patient undergoing multiple valve surgery. *Korean J Thorac Cardiovasc Surg.* 2015;48:129–133.

3. Kaul P, Adluri K, Javangula K, et al. Successful management of multiple permanent pacemaker complications—infection, 13 year old silent lead perforation and exteriorisation following failed percutaneous extraction, superior vena cava obstruction, tricuspid valve endocarditis, pulmonary embolism and prosthetic tricuspid valve thrombosis. *J Cardiothorac Surg.* 2009;4:12.

4. Nazmul MN, Cha YM, Lin G, et al. Percutaneous pacemaker or implantable cardioverter-defibrillator lead removal in an attempt to improve symptomatic tricuspid regurgitation. *Europace.* 2013;15:409–413.

5. Veinot JP, Lemery R. Innovations in cardiovascular pathology: anatomic and electrophysiologic determinants associated with ablation of atrial arrhythmias. *Cardiovasc Pathol.* 2005;14:204–213.

6. Iesaka Y, Takahashi A, Chun YH, et al. Radiofrequency catheter ablation of atrioventricular accessory pathways in Wolff-Parkinson-White syndrome with drug-refractory and symptomatic supraventricular tachycardia—its high effectiveness irrespective of accessory pathway location and properties. *Jpn Circ J.* 1994;58:767–777.

7. Vida VL, Calvimontes GS, Macs MO, et al. Radiofrequency catheter ablation of supraventricular tachycardia in children and adolescents: feasibility and cost-effectiveness in a low-income country. *Pediatr Cardiol.* 2006;27:434–439.

8. Lee PC, Hwang B, Chen SA, et al. The results of radiofrequency catheter ablation of supraventricular tachycardia in children. *Pacing Clin Electrophysiol.* 2007;30:655–661.

9. Aiyagari R, Saarel EV, Etheridge SP, et al. Radiofrequency ablation for supraventricular tachycardia in children < or =15 kg is safe and effective. *Pediatr Cardiol.* 2005;26:622–626.

10. Meiltz A, Weber R, Halimi F, et al. Permanent form of junctional reciprocating tachycardia in adults: peculiar features and results of radiofrequency catheter ablation. *Europace.* 2006;8:21–28.

11. Castonguay MC, Wang Y, Gerhart JL, et al. Surgical pathology of atrial appendages removed during the cox-maze procedure: a review of 86 cases (2004 to 2005) with implications for prognosis. *Am J Surg Pathol.* 2013;37:890–897.

12. Watkins AC, Young CA, Ghoreishi M, et al. Prospective assessment of the CryoMaze procedure with continuous outpatient telemetry in 136 patients. *Ann Thorac Surg.* 2014;97:1191–1198; discussion 1198.

13. Yamada T, McElderry HT, Doppalapudi H, et al. Idiopathic ventricular arrhythmias originating from the aortic root prevalence, electrocardiographic and electrophysiologic characteristics, and results of radiofrequency catheter ablation. *J Am Coll Cardiol.* 2008;52:139–147.

14. Yamada T, Murakami Y, Yoshida N, et al. Efficacy of electroanatomic mapping in the catheter ablation of premature ventricular contractions originating from the right ventricular outflow tract. *J Interv Card Electrophysiol.* 2007;19:187–194.

15. Tada H, Tadokoro K, Ito S, et al. Idiopathic ventricular arrhythmias originating from the tricuspid annulus: prevalence, electrocardiographic characteristics, and results of radiofrequency catheter ablation. *Heart Rhythm.* 2007;4:7–16.

16. Lim KK, Maron BJ, Knight BP. Successful catheter ablation of hemodynamically unstable monomorphic ventricular tachycardia in a patient with hypertrophic cardiomyopathy and apical aneurysm. *J Cardiovasc Electrophysiol.* 2009;20:445–447.

17. Soejima K, Stevenson WG, Sapp JL, et al. Endocardial and epicardial radiofrequency ablation of ventricular tachycardia associated with dilated cardiomyopathy: the importance of low-voltage scars. *J Am Coll Cardiol.* 2004;43:1834–1842.

18. Deneke T, Muller KM, Lemke B, et al. Human histopathology of electroanatomic mapping after cooled-tip radiofrequency ablation to treat ventricular tachycardia in remote myocardial infarction. *J Cardiovasc Electrophysiol.* 2005;16:1246–1251.

19. Nogami A, Kubota S, Adachi M, et al. Electrophysiologic and histopathologic findings of the ablation sites for ventricular fibrillation in a patient with ischemic cardiomyopathy. *J Interv Card Electrophysiol.* 2009;24:133–137.

20. Wolf DA, Burke AP, Patterson KV, et al. Sudden death following rupture of a right ventricular aneurysm 9 months after ablation therapy of the right ventricular outflow tract. *Pacing Clin Electrophysiol.* 2002;25:1135–1137.

21. Sreeram S, Lumsden AB, Miller JS, et al. Retroperitoneal hematoma following femoral arterial catheterization: a serious and often fatal complication. *Am Surg.* 1993;59:94–98.

22. Ellis SG, Bhatt D, Kapadia S, et al. Correlates and outcomes of retroperitoneal hemorrhage complicating percutaneous coronary intervention. *Catheter Cardiovasc Interv.* 2006;67:541–545.

23. Foo NP, Lin HJ. Delayed perforation of right ventricle with cardiac tamponade: a complication of pacemaker implantation. *Eur J Emerg Med.* 2005;12:89–91.

24. Sassone B, Gabrieli L, Boggian G, et al. Management of traumatic implantable cardioverter defibrillator lead perforation of the right ventricle after car accident: a case report. *Europace.* 2009;11:961–962.

25. Rodrigues AC, de Vylder A, Wellens F, et al. Right ventricular pseudoaneurysm as a complication of endomyocardial biopsy after heart transplantation. *Chest.* 1995;107:566–567.

26. Shevland JE. Right ventricular perforation: a rare complication of percutaneous lung biopsy. *J Thorac Imaging.* 1991;6:85–86.

27. Patane F, Sansone F, Centofanti P, et al. Left ventricular pseudoaneurysm after pericardiocentesis. *Interact Cardiovasc Thorac Surg.* 2008;7:1112–1113.

28. Preis LK, Taylor GJ, Martin RP. Traumatic pericardiocentesis: two-dimensional echocardiographic visualization of an unfortunate event. *Arch Intern Med.* 1982;142:2327–2329.

29. Hatanaka K, Takase I, Kobayashi M, et al. A case of delayed shock due to dissection of the hyperplastic coronary artery after balloon angioplasty and stenting. *J Clin Forensic Med.* 2002;9:78–81.

30. Barbeau GR, Senechal M, Voisine P. Delayed abrupt tamponade by isolated left atrial compression following coronary artery perforation during coronary angioplasty. *Catheter Cardiovasc Interv.* 2005;66:562–565.

31. Mathew OP, Dugal JS, Jetley V, et al. Angioplasty for chronic total coronary occlusions: safety and efficacy. *J Assoc Physicians India.* 2002;50:1251–1254.

32. Topaz O, Ebersole D, Das T, et al. Excimer laser angioplasty in acute myocardial infarction (the CARMEL multicenter trial). *Am J Cardiol.* 2004;93:694–701.

33. Topaz O, Janin Y, Bernardo N, et al. Coronary revascularization in heart transplant recipients by excimer laser angioplasty. *Lasers Surg Med.* 2000;26:425–431.

34. Inoue Y, Ueda T, Taguchi S, et al. Teflon felt wrapping repair for coronary perforation after failed angioplasty. *Ann Thorac Surg.* 2006;82:2312–2314.

35. Kozak M, Adams DR, Ioffreda MD, et al. Sterile inflammation associated with transradial catheterization and hydrophilic sheaths. *Catheter Cardiovasc Interv.* 2003;59:207–213.

36. Greenfield LJ, Proctor MC. Twenty-year clinical experience with the Greenfield filter. *Cardiovasc Surg.* 1995;3:199–205.

37. Johnson SP, Raiken DP, Grebe PJ, et al. Single institution prospective evaluation of the over-the-wire Greenfield vena caval filter. *J Vasc Interv Radiol.* 1998;9:766–773.

38. Dabbagh A, Chakfe N, Kretz JG, et al. Late complication of a Greenfield filter associating caudal migration and perforation of the abdominal aorta by a ruptured strut. *J Vasc Surg.* 1995;22:182–187.

39. Mastrobattista JM, Caputo TA, Bush HS. Perforation of the inferior vena cava by a recently inserted Greenfield filter. *Gynecol Oncol.* 1995;56:399–401.

40. Bianchini AU, Mehta SN, Mulder DS, et al. Duodenal perforation by a Greenfield filter: endoscopic diagnosis. *Am J Gastroenterol.* 1997;92:686–687.

41. De Waele JJ, De Pauw M, Van Belleghem Y, et al. Diagnosis of myocardial perforation by a Greenfield filter made by transesophageal echocardiography. *J Am Soc Echocardiogr.* 2002;15:374–375.

42. Duperier T, Mosenthal A, Swan KG, et al. Acute complications associated with greenfield filter insertion in high-risk trauma patients. *J Trauma.* 2003;54:545–549.

43. Mitchell WB, Bonn J. Percutaneous retrieval of a Greenfield filter after migration to the left pulmonary artery. *J Vasc Interv Radiol.* 2005;16:1013–1017.

44. Mohan G, Kasmani R, Okoli K, et al. Right atrial foreign body: transvenous migration of Greenfield filter. *Interact Cardiovasc Thorac Surg.* 2009;8:245–246.

45. Promisloff RA. Pulmonary embolism after insertion of a Greenfield filter. *J Am Osteopath Assoc.* 2002;102:558–560.

46. Chan KT, Cheng BC. Retrieval of an embolized amplatzer septal occluder. *Catheter Cardiovasc Interv.* 2010;75(3):465–468.

47. Ahn E, Luk A, Mezody M, et al. Early morphological changes of an amplatzer septal occluder explanted at heart transplant. *Cardiovasc Pathol.* 2009;18:57–60.

48. Bialkowski J, Zabal C, Szkutnik M, et al. Percutaneous interventional closure of large pulmonary arteriovenous fistulas with the amplatzer duct occluder. *Am J Cardiol*. 2005;96:127–129.

49. Giombolini C, Notaristefano S, Santucci S, et al. Transcatheter closure of postinfarction ventricular septal defect using the amplatzer atrial septal defect occluder. *J Cardiovasc Med (Hagerstown)*. 2008;9:941–945.

50. Holzer R, Balzer D, Cao QL, et al. Device closure of muscular ventricular septal defects using the amplatzer muscular ventricular septal defect occluder: immediate and mid-term results of a U.S. registry. *J Am Coll Cardiol*. 2004;43:1257–1263.

51. Lin MC, Fu YC, Jan SL, et al. Transcatheter closure of secundum atrial septal defect using the amplatzer septal occluder: initial results of a single medical center in Taiwan. *Acta Paediatr Taiwan*. 2005;46:17–23.

52. Slesnick TC, Nugent AW, Fraser CD Jr, et al. Images in cardiovascular medicine. Incomplete endothelialization and late development of acute bacterial endocarditis after implantation of an amplatzer septal occluder device. *Circulation*. 2008;117:e326–e327.

53. Dua J, Chessa M, Piazza L, et al. Initial experience with the new amplatzer duct occluder II. *J Invasive Cardiol*. 2009;21:401–405.

54. Arri SS, Poliacikova P, Hildick-Smith D. Percutaneous paravalvular leak closure for symptomatic aortic regurgitation after core valve transcatheter aortic valve implantation. *Catheter Cardiovasc Interv*. 2015;85:657–664.

55. Ohno Y, Tamburino C, Barbanti M. Transcatheter aortic valve implantation experience with SAPIEN 3. *Minerva Cardioangiol*. 2015;63(3):205–216. Epub 2015 Apr 22.

56. Mauri L, Aldebert P, Cuisset T, et al. Percutaneous closure of a poorly tolerated post-transcatheter aortic valve implantation ventricular septal defect. *Ann Thorac Surg*. 2014;98:1823–1826.

57. Moretti C, D'Ascenzo F, Mennuni M, et al. Meta-analysis of comparison between self-expandable and balloon-expandable valves for patients having transcatheter aortic valve implantation. *Am J Cardiol*. 2015;115(12):1720–1725.

58. Attizzani GF, Ohno Y, Capodanno D, et al. Extended use of percutaneous edge-to-edge mitral valve repair beyond EVEREST (Endovascular Valve Edge-to-Edge Repair) criteria: 30-day and 12-month clinical and echocardiographic outcomes from the GRASP (Getting Reduction of Mitral Insufficiency by Percutaneous Clip Implantation) registry. *JACC Cardiovasc Interv*. 2015;8:74–82.

59. Henry MJ, Preventza O, Cooley DA, et al. Left ventricular aneurysm repair with use of a bovine pericardial patch. *Tex Heart Inst J*. 2014;41:407–410.

60. Zucchetta F, Tarzia V, Bottio T, et al. The Jarvik-2000 ventricular assist device implantation: how we do it. *Ann Cardiothorac Surg*. 2014;3:525–531.

61. Haj-Yahia S, Birks EJ, Rogers P, et al. Midterm experience with the Jarvik 2000 axial flow left ventricular assist device. *J Thorac Cardiovasc Surg*. 2007;134:199–203.

62. Chiu WC, Slepian MJ, Bluestein D. Thrombus formation patterns in the HeartMate II ventricular assist device: clinical observations can be predicted by numerical simulations. *ASAIO J*. 2014;60:237–240.

63. Kounis NG, Soufras GD, Davlouros P, et al. Thrombus formation patterns in HeartMate II continuous-flow left ventricular assist devices: a multifactorial phenomenon involving Kounis syndrome? *ASAIO J*. 2014;60:369–371.

64. Khan NA, Butany J, Zhou T, et al. Pathological findings in explanted prosthetic heart valves from ventricular assist devices. *Pathology*. 2008;40:377–384.

65. Rose EA, Gelijns AC, Moskowitz AJ, et al. Long-term mechanical left ventricular assistance for end-stage heart failure. *N Engl J Med*. 2001;345:1435–1443.

66. Rose AG, Park SJ. Pathology in patients with ventricular assist devices: a study of 21 autopsies, 24 ventricular apical core biopsies and 24 explanted hearts. *Cardiovasc Pathol*. 2005;14:19–23.

67. Kloppenburg GT, Sonker U, Schepens MA. Intra-aortic balloon pump related thrombus in the proximal descending thoracic aorta with peripheral emboli. *J Invasive Cardiol*. 2009;21:e110–e112.

68. Cook L, Pillar B, McCord G, et al. Intra-aortic balloon pump complications: a five-year retrospective study of 283 patients. *Heart Lung*. 1999;28:195–202.

69. Kirksey L, Woody DJ, Plazk L. Ruptured intra-aortic balloon pump. A case report. *J Cardiovasc Surg (Torino)*. 2002;43:461–464.

70. Elahi MM, Chetty GK, Kirke R, et al. Complications related to intra-aortic balloon pump in cardiac surgery: a decade later. *Eur J Vasc Endovasc Surg*. 2005;29:591–594.

71. Davoodi S, Karimi A, Ahmadi SH, et al. Coronary artery bypass grafting in patients with low ejection fraction: the effect of intra-aortic balloon pump insertion on early outcome. *Indian J Med Sci*. 2008;62:314–322.

143   Left Ventricular Hypertrophy and Failure

Allen P. Burke, M.D., and Joseph J. Maleszewski, M.D.

Left Ventricular Hypertrophy

Physiology and Causes

Cardiac hypertrophy is an adaptive response to an increased load (pressure or volume) on the ventricle (Table 143.1). It is integral to processes that govern both normal physiology (e.g., athletic hypertrophy) and abnormal pathology (e.g., heart failure). Ventricular hypertrophy is often secondary to conditions that result in increased *afterload* or tension experienced by the ventricular wall during systole. Left ventricular wall thickness inversely correlates with afterload, which is directly proportional to chamber diameter and chamber pressure (Laplace law). Left ventricular hypertrophy also causes decreased *preload,* or diastolic stretching that allows filling of the ventricle. Optimal ventricular filling increases stroke volume by the Frank-Starling law, allowing for compensated left ventricular function at early stages in conditions with increased preload.

A chronic volume load and high cardiac output result in compensatory left ventricular hypertrophy, similar to conditions causing increased afterload. Aortic and mitral insufficiency and left-to-right shunts cause increased ventricular volume and subsequent cardiac enlargement. Increased volumes associated with pregnancy will transiently cause an increase in ventricular size and mass that normalizes in the months after delivery.[1]

A chronic increase in afterload, such as systemic hypertension and aortic stenosis, results in *concentric left ventricular hypertrophy* (with an increase in ratio between wall thickness and internal radius), which is the result of increased numbers of sarcomeres with normal length, arrayed in parallel. Initially, the left ventricular chamber cavity is small. With persistent increases in afterload, compensatory ventricular hypertrophy can no longer occur, and progression to ventricular dilatation and heart failure ensues.

Nonconcentric (eccentric) left ventricular hypertrophy is a clinical and radiologic term indicating increased left ventricular mass with a normal ratio between relative wall thickness and internal cavity dimension (Fig. 143.1). Nonconcentric hypertrophy is theoretically the result of increased sarcomeres arranged in series, pathologically resembles a dilated ventricle with a thick wall, and is associated with conditions associated with volume overload and decompensated concentric left ventricular hypertrophy. It is important to note that the clinical term "concentric left ventricular hypertrophy" corresponds to the pathologic term, whereas "eccentric left ventricular hypertrophy" is not typically used in a pathologic context and should not be confused with "asymmetric hypertrophy" caused by predominant thickening of the septum. Moreover, the term *eccentric* is somewhat of a misnomer in that the hypertrophy is not "off-center" as the term would imply. "Eccentric left

TABLE 143.1 Causes of Left Ventricular Hypertrophy

	Phenotype	Associations
Increased afterload	Wall thickening (early stages)	Systemic hypertension
	Chamber dilatation (late stages)	Aortic stenosis
Volume overload	Chamber dilatation	Aortic insufficiency
		Mitral insufficiency
		Right-to-left shunts
		Atrial septal defect
		Ventricular septal defect
		Patent ductus arteriosus
		Arteriovenous malformations and shunts
Myocardial diseases	Wall thickening (may be asymmetric) or chamber dilatation	Amyloidosis
		Fabry disease
		Danon disease
		Hemochromatosis
		Sarcoidosis
		Hypertrophic cardiomyopathy
	Chamber dilatation	Dilated cardiomyopathy
Multifactorial	Wall thickening and/or chamber dilatation	Chronic renal disease
		Obesity

ventricular hypertrophy" is typically described as "cardiac hypertrophy with dilatation" in autopsy specimens, although the radiologic definition depends not on chamber diameter by itself but ratio of wall thickness to cavity dimensions.

In addition to increased ventricular load, there are a variety of conditions that result in hypertrophy. These include infiltrative diseases such as amyloidosis and cardiomyopathies. Cardiac hypertrophy of obesity and end-stage renal disease is often multifactorial and may involve hypertension and myocardial fibrosis. Ischemic heart disease has often been associated with left ventricular hypertrophy, also likely due to ischemic fibrosis, often with concomitant hypertension.[2]

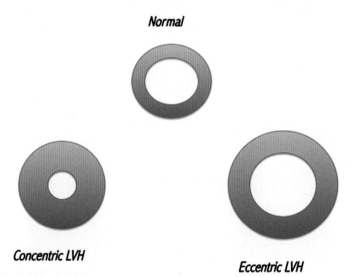

Normal

Concentric LVH

Eccentric LVH

FIGURE 143.1 ▲ Concentric and eccentric left ventricular hypertrophy. By imaging, there is increased free wall thickness to cavity diameter ratio in concentric but not eccentric left ventricular hypertrophy, because of chamber diameter increase in the latter.

"Asymmetric left ventricular hypertrophy" denotes increased left ventricular mass predominantly caused by septal hypertrophy. It is typical of hypertrophic obstructive cardiomyopathy and is seen in a minority of patients with hypertensive cardiomyopathy, aortic stenosis, and cardiac amyloidosis.

The concept of "idiopathic left ventricular hypertrophy" has been applied to patients with echocardiographic concentric left ventricular hypertrophy in the absence of other conditions that could explain it (ischemic, valvular, and hypertensive forms of heart disease).[3] Often used in series of sudden death, the term is linked often with athlete's heart.[4] For autopsy diagnosis, in which case a history of hypertension is not always available or there is not other end organ damage (e.g., hypertensive nephropathy), the term "idiopathic left ventricular hypertrophy" can be used as a cause of death or descriptive term, when there are no anatomic or histologic abnormalities reflecting underlying cardiac disease.

In order to get an idea about the factors governing left ventricular hypertrophy in an autopsy specimen, it is critical to evaluate ventricular thickness and left chamber diameter excluding trabeculae and papillary muscles, at the level of the papillary muscles (see Chapter 1). The ventricular septal thickness needs to be measured separately, for evaluation of asymmetry (normally, the VS:FW < 1.3).

Epidemiology

In a series of elderly American men with high cardiovascular risk, 83% of whom had systemic hypertension, 66% had left ventricular hypertrophy by transthoracic echocardiography, 22% severe.[5] In a relatively younger Han Chinese population, the prevalence of left ventricular hypertrophy was 43%, about evenly split between concentric and eccentric types.[6] In autopsy series of sudden cardiac death, left ventricular hypertrophy is a very common finding, present in over 80% of hearts.[7] Black race may be a risk factor for cardiomegaly in hypertension.[7,8]

Radiologic Findings

Echocardiographic assessment of left ventricular hypertrophy is more sensitive than electrocardiography, when corrected for body weight[9,10]. Currently, the radiologic gold standard for assessing left ventricular hypertrophy is magnetic resonance imaging, which can evaluate fibrosis.[11] Cardiac magnetic resonance imaging has been used to define subsets of hypertrophy, with dilated and nondilated forms of both eccentric and concentric hypertrophy.[12]

Gross Findings

In the absence of significant right ventricular hypertrophy, heart weight, as adjusted to body weight or body size, is the ultimate gold standard of the degree of hypertrophy. Heart weight must be evaluated in context of sex and body size, and there are several resources available for this adjustment.[13,14] Although it has been proposed that 383 g is the upper limit of normal for a man's heart,[15] this assessment was based on young men with a mean age of 23 and is therefore not useful for older individuals, as it is established that heart weight increases with age.[16] An estimation of cardiomegaly based on a ratio to body weight or body surface area (heart weight index) is often used in animal studies (using body weight) and occasionally in human autopsy studies (using body surface area as estimated by the square root of the height). By the latter formula, a normal heart weight index is 200 mg/m².[17] However, a more practical approach is by defining cardiomegaly as a heart that weighs >50% above the expected mean (based on the individual's size or weight).

Performing parallel short-axis sections from midventricle to the apex allows for good visual assessment of left ventricular hypertrophy. Traditionally, left ventricular wall thickness ≥15 mm is indicative of hypertrophy, but one must be aware that cardiac rigor (increased thickness) and decomposition (decreased thickness, so-called agonal dilatation) may affect the measurements. Care should be taken to avoid measuring recesses formed by trabeculations or papillary

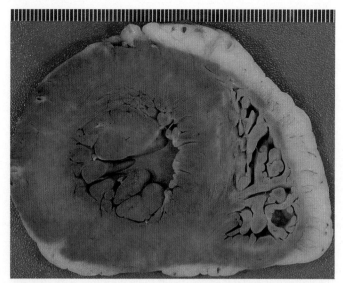

FIGURE 143.2 ▲ Concentric left ventricular hypertrophy. There is concentric thickening of the left ventricular wall, with a normal cavity diameter. The patient had hypertension and a 550-gram heart.

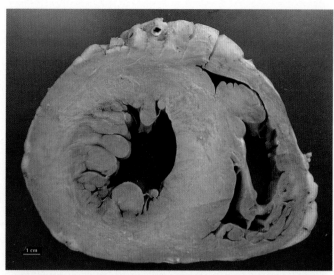

FIGURE 143.4 ▲ Concentric left ventricular hypertrophy with mild dilatation. The patient died suddenly and had marked concentric left ventricular hypertrophy (700 g) with mild chamber dilatation (4.5 cm). The patient had no history of hypertension, but renal vascular changes were highly suggestive of hypertensive renal disease.

muscles. In patients with hypertension, there is frequent coexistent right ventricular hypertrophy.[8] The degree of chamber dilatation is important to record, primarily for determination of the presence of pressure (Figs. 143.2 and 143.3) or volume hypertrophy (Figs. 143.4 to 143.6).

Microscopic Findings

Left ventricular hypertrophy, in the pathologic sense, is a form of cardiac remodeling that consists of myocyte hypertrophy and perivascular- and pericellular-type interstitial fibrosis (Figs 143.7 to 143.9). There may be medial thickening of intramyocardial coronary arteries.[18] Morphometric measurements of left ventricular samples taken from failing hearts demonstrate increased myocyte and nuclear size, increased interstitial collagen, and decreased microvascular density and microvascular lumen area.[19,20] The number of binucleated myocytes does not appear to increase significantly.[21]

Endomyocardial Biopsy in Left Ventricular Hypertrophy

Native heart biopsy is generally performed in patients with unexplained heart failure, or to exclude cardiac amyloidosis. In patients with a clinical and imaging diagnosis of concentric left ventricular hypertrophy, the histologic changes are generally nonspecific, with amyloidosis confirmed in a small proportion. In about 5% of patients, lysosome-associated membrane protein 2 mutations have been found, indicating a diagnosis of Danon cardiomyopathy.[22] In about 1% of patients, Fabry disease will be confirmed based on alpha-galactosidase A activity and mutation analysis of the GLA gene.[23]

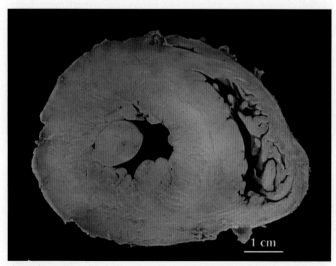

FIGURE 143.3 ▲ Concentric left ventricular hypertrophy. The appearance is similar to that shown in Figure 143.2. The patient had a severely stenotic (tricuspid) aortic valve with calcification (not shown).

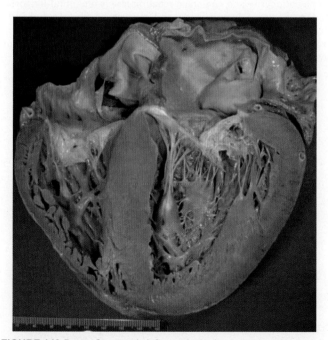

FIGURE 143.5 ▲ Concentric left ventricular hypertrophy with moderate dilatation. The heart weighed 600 g, and there was concentric thickening of the left ventricular wall (16 mm) with mild dilatation of the ventricular cavity (42 mm). The patient had long-standing hypertension and end-stage renal disease.

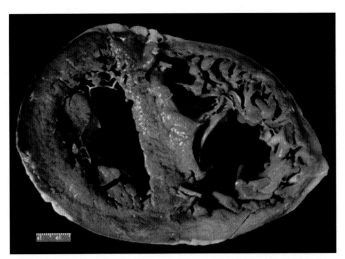

FIGURE 143.6 ▲ Cardiomegaly with biventricular dilatation. The heart weighed 750 g, in a morbidly obese patient who died suddenly after minor surgery.

Prognosis and Outcome

Left ventricular hypertrophy leads to an increased risk of ventricular arrhythmias and sudden death, especially if there is concomitant heart failure. The risk factor–adjusted hazard ratio for sudden death ranged from 1.5 to 2.2 in echocardiography-documented left ventricular hypertrophy, which was highly significant.[24] As assessed by two-dimensional echocardiography, increased left ventricular mass demonstrated a significant risk for cardiovascular death at 2 years, ranging from two to four times that of patients with normal-sized ventricles, depending on the severity of hypertrophy.[25] The persistence and development of left ventricular hypertrophy as assessed by electrocardiography are associated with an increased risk of atrial fibrillation, the mechanism of which may be mediated by left atrial enlargement.[26] Concentric left ventricular hypertrophy is an independent risk factor for both cardiovascular and all-cause mortality after heart transplant.[27]

Heart Failure

Epidemiology

Heart failure is defined as left ventricular dysfunction resulting in ineffective cardiac output and affects 1% of the adults in the United

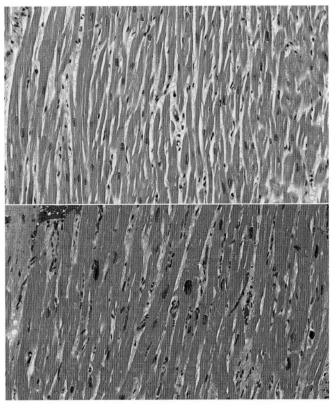

FIGURE 143.7 ▲ Cardiomyocyte hypertrophy. The top illustrates normal myocardium, and below a figure from a patient with hypertensive heart disease. Both are at the same level of magnification.

States over age 65. It is more frequent in men than in women under that age, after which there is an equal frequency between sexes. African Americans have the highest prevalence of heart failure at 4.6 per 1,000 per year, followed by Hispanic, Caucasian, and Asian Americans at 3.5, 2.4, and 1.0 per 1,000 per year, respectively. Heart failure is associated with a 50% 5-year mortality rate and is responsible for over one-third of all deaths in the United States from cardiovascular causes.[28]

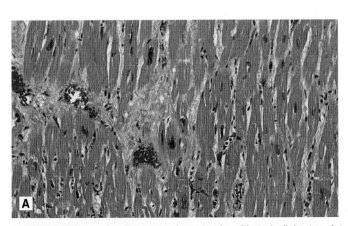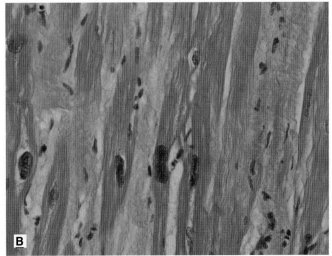

FIGURE 143.8 ▲ Cardiomyocyte hypertrophy with pericellular-type interstitial fibrosis. **A.** The nuclei are enlarged and there is interstitial fibrosis around a vessel. **B.** A higher magnification demonstrates interstitial fibroblasts and collagen and enlarged, "boxcar" nuclei.

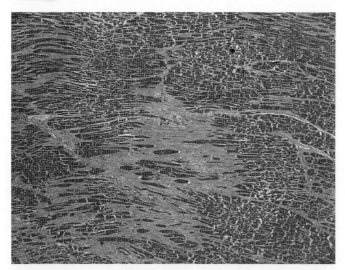

FIGURE 143.9 ▲ Cardiomyocyte hypertrophy with replacement-type interstitial fibrosis. Hypertensive hypertrophy as well as hypertrophy from other causes can result in patchy and small areas of replacement-type interstitial fibrosis. Typically, these areas are smaller than that seen in ischemic heart disease. The myocyte-surrounding scars are often enlarged to a greater degree than those away from the fibrosis.

Pathophysiology

Heart failure involves abnormalities or maladaptation of mechanical, neurohormonal, and cardiorenal factors relating to ventricular function. It is a complex clinical syndrome and not a specific pathologic entity. The definition involves the inability of the left ventricle to effect cardiac output that is adequate to meet metabolic requirements and accommodate venous return.[29]

Cardiac output is the product of heart rate and stroke volume and is typically 4 to 8 L/min. As noted above, stroke volume depends on preload (amount of end-diastolic myocardial fiber stretch), afterload (resistance that the ventricle must overcome to eject blood), and contractility (inotropic state of the ventricle).

Left ventricular dysfunction resulting in failure can be divided into *systolic dysfunction* (impaired ventricular contraction) and *diastolic dysfunction* (impaired relaxation and ventricular filling). The predominant cause of heart failure is systolic dysfunction in 70%, compared to 30% for diastolic dysfunction, although there is significant overlap. If the ejection fraction is lower than 40%, it is defined as systolic dysfunction, and if it is ≥40%, it is diastolic dysfunction.

The initial compensation for decreased contractility is ventricular dilatation, which causes increased end-diastolic tension and increased stroke volume by the Frank-Starling law. With irreversible myocyte change, this compensation is decreased, as increasing amounts of preload result in relatively little increase in cardiac output as the Starling curve flattens.

An integral component of mean arterial pressure is peripheral resistance, which, as a product with cardiac output, forms mean arterial pressure. Neurohormonal activation increases peripheral resistance by promoting sodium and water retention, which maximizes stroke volume and augments cardiac output via the Frank-Starling mechanism. The renal response to decreased blood flow increases circulating angiotensin II, which directly increases vasoconstriction and promotes the release of aldosterone. The up-regulation of local renin angiotensin system may contribute to myocardial changes, including interstitial fibrosis.

Heart failure involves the increase in circulating natriuretic peptides including atrial natriuretic peptide, brain natriuretic peptide, and C-type natriuretic peptide, which counteracts the vasoconstriction caused by the renal angiotensin system. These serum markers are useful diagnosis and in following response to treatment of heart failure.

Gross Findings

The gross findings observed in failing hearts consist of a combination of those responsible for the heart failure and changes that are considered secondary. The most common cause of heart failure in adults is ischemic heart disease, usually resulting in areas of transmural myocardial scarring, in combination with areas of subendocardial replacement fibrosis and areas of chronic ischemia (see Chapter 15). The second most common cause is dilated cardiomyopathy, including idiopathic dilated cardiomyopathy (see Chapter 19), end-stage hypertensive heart disease, and heart failure related to obesity, renal failure, and diabetes (see below and also Chapter 9). The causes often overlap, and overall, three-quarters of all heart failure patients have preexisting hypertension, the single most important risk factor for the disease.[29]

Increased cardiac size, assessed by a combination of weight and chamber dimensions, is the most common finding in patients with clinical heart failure. Weight >50% above the expected mean and/or left ventricular short-axis chamber diameter >4 cm is suggestive of the possibility that there was clinically significant cardiac dysfunction. As mentioned before, chamber size in isolation is rather limited owing to the possibility of agonal dilatation and postmortem autolysis, which may artifactually increase the chamber size (making weight a more reliable indicator in most settings).

In addition to ventricular dilatation, heart failure is also associated with left atrial dilatation. Left atrial enlargement is most marked with atrial fibrillation (there will also be right atrial or biatrial dilatation) and mitral valve disease, especially stenosis. In the absence of these conditions, left atrial dilatation is a barometer of left ventricular filling pressure, which is uniformly found in the presence of symptomatic congestive heart failure. Although difficult to precisely measure at autopsy, any dimension significantly >4 cm in the left atrium is suggestive of enlargement, correlating with clinical measurements using ultrasound. Slight enlargement of the left atrium, as assessed by echocardiography and indexed for body mass index, may predict the development of heart failure in asymptomatic patients at high risk.[30,31]

Histologic Findings

Histologically, interstitial fibrosis and myocyte hypertrophy are known to contribute to the pathogenesis of heart failure, with an adverse impact on mechanical and electric properties of the myocardium.[32] Interstitial fibrosis can be broadly dichotomized into two basic types: pericellular-type fibrosis and replacement-type fibrosis. While the former is very nonspecific and can be seen in valvular, hypertensive, and ischemic forms of heart disease as well as cardiomyopathic states, the latter is most usually seen in the setting of ischemic heart disease. Replacement-type interstitial fibrosis may also be seen in the setting of healed or ongoing myocarditis and surgical site changes.

Secondary Changes of Congestive Heart Failure in the Lung

Many of the acute findings of increased pulmonary venous pressures may occur terminally, with sudden decrease in cardiac output and fluid resuscitation during life. These include edema, which occurs in the interlobular septa and within the alveolar spaces, and small hemorrhages. Chronically, increased central venous pressure is transmitted to the pulmonary veins and capillaries, resulting in pulmonary congestion and edema as well as pleural effusion. Histologically, there are perivascular and interstitial transudates (amorphous pink proteinaceous deposits, alveolar septal edema, and accumulation of edema fluid in the alveolar spaces). Chronically, as red cells extravasate from the leaky capillaries into alveolar spaces, they are phagocytosed by macrophages, resulting in hemosiderin-laden alveolar macrophages—so-called *heart failure cells*. These are nonspecific reflections of prior hemorrhage and are generally scattered and few in number if caused by heart failure, and accompanied by interlobular septal edema, fibrosis, lymphangiectasia, and venous thickening.

Specific Causes of Left Ventricular Hypertrophy and Dilatation

Hypertensive Heart Disease

Among hypertensive patients, echocardiograms will demonstrate hypertrophy in the majority, half of which will demonstrate a degree of dilatation.[33] The degree of hypertension increases the likelihood of hypertrophy.[34] Left ventricular dilatation or concentric hypertrophy imparts a two- to fourfold risk of cardiovascular death in hypertensive patients.[33]

Although untreated hypertensive heart disease can lead to heart failure and dilated cardiomyopathy, treatment of hypertension can significantly decrease this risk and can result in normalization of left ventricular mass. However, diastolic dysfunction related to interstitial fibrosis is less frequently reversible and contributes significantly to overall heart failure morbidity.[18]

Angiotensin receptor blockade prevents progression of left ventricular hypertrophy in nearly 95% of patients at 3 to 4 years and allows for regression in 25% to 50%.[26,33] In general, inhibition of the renin–angiotensin–aldosterone system and sympathetic neuroendocrine pathways (valsartan and moxonidine) provides the greatest degree of regression.[35]

Histologically, hypertensive heart disease is characterized by myocyte hypertrophy and interstitial fibrosis. In autopsy specimens, Rossi found an increased myocyte diameter of 24 to 38 μm compared to a normal of 13.7 μm.[36] Interstitial fibrosis contains both collagen as well as fibroblasts. The proportion of myocardium constituted by collagen ranges from 15% to over 30% in hypertensive cardiomyopathy, compared to 2% to 5% in normal hearts.[19,36] Ultrastructurally, there is an excess of pericellular collagen weave fibers (endomysial matrix) and markedly thickened perimysial collagen fibrils.[36]

Heart Disease in the Setting of Renal Disease (So-Called Cardiorenal Syndrome)

Increasingly, it has been recognized that significant dysfunction in either the heart or the kidneys can lead to dysfunction in the other. This concept has been termed the cardiorenal syndrome. There is an increased prevalence of left ventricular hypertrophy in patients with chronic renal disease.[37] Mortality due to cardiovascular events is high with chronic kidney disease and is associated with left ventricular hypertrophy.[38] By imaging, left ventricular hypertrophy is associated with valve calcification in hypertensive patients with chronic renal failure.[39,40] Interstitial and perivascular fibrosis are constant findings in heart biopsies and autopsy studies in patients with chronic kidney disease and left ventricular hypertrophy, especially those with hypertension.[41,42]

Valvular Heart Disease

Aortic stenosis results in increased afterload with compensatory increases in wall thickness of the left ventricle. Although 88% of patients with aortic stenosis have increased left ventricular mass or thickened left ventricular walls by magnetic resonance imaging, there is no significant relation with the aortic valve area or degree of aortic stenosis; only the presence of hypertension increases the risk of ventricular remodeling.[12] The types of ventricular remodeling found by imaging have been described as concentric hypertrophy (37%); asymmetric hypertrophy (15%); concentric remodeling, or thickened ventricle without increased mass (12%); asymmetric remodeling, or increased septal thickness without increased mass (12%); and hypertrophy with dilated ventricle, or eccentric hypertrophy (11%).[12]

There are few autopsy studies of myocardial changes in aortic stenosis. Increase in heart weight and left ventricular thickness is universally found in patients requiring valve replacement, and gross patchy scars in a nonischemic distribution are present in 90% of cases.[17] Biopsy studies have shown that there is an increase in myocyte diameter (mean 31 to 33 μm) and interstitial fibrosis (16% to 18%) histologically.[43,44]

Left ventricular hypertrophy, as assessed by imaging, regresses after surgery in the majority of patients, generally within 3 months, with a decrease in end-diastolic left ventricular diameter.[45] Risk factors for persistent left ventricular hypertrophy include hypertension and undersized prosthetic valves.[46] An autopsy study showed that length of time between operation and death was inversely correlated with heart weight.[17] Histologic studies of regression after valve replacement show an early decrease in muscle hypertrophy with a later decrease in collagen constant.[43,44]

Aortic insufficiency increases left ventricular mass by a mechanism of chronic volume overload, which is especially harmful because of an increase in end-diastolic in addition to end-systolic stress in the compensated phase of chronic regurgitation. Aortic insufficiency is a high-impedance leak and therefore more harmful to the left ventricle than mitral regurgitation, which is low impedance. Therefore, for a given regurgitant volume, aortic insufficiency causes greater left ventricular enlargement and hypertrophy than does mitral insufficiency.[47,48] By cardiac imaging, patients with aortic insufficiency have more dilated ventricles and an increase in end-diastolic and end-systolic volumes, as compared to aortic stenosis, but the overall ventricular mass is less.[45,49] There is a strong positive correlation between aortic regurgitant volume and ventricular dilatation.[47]

Similar to aortic stenosis, myocyte diameter is increased in hearts with aortic insufficiency (mean 31 μm), with a similar increase in interstitial fibrosis (24%).[43]

By imaging, regression of ventricular remodeling occurs at a slower rate in aortic insufficiency than in aortic stenosis,[50] and the left ventricular diameter decreases more rapidly than does ventricular mass.[51] Histologic regression of myocyte hypertrophy up to 5 years postoperatively was similar to aortic stenosis, with a lesser decrease in interstitial and total collagen content.[43]

The Athletic Heart

Left ventricular hypertrophy is a well-known adaptation to endurance training and is manifest echocardiographically by increases in left ventricular chamber size, wall thickness, and mass. Two different morphologic forms of athlete's heart have been described: a strength-trained heart and an endurance-trained heart. The high cardiac output of endurance training results in eccentric left ventricular hypertrophy, characterized by an unchanged relationship between left ventricular wall thickness and left ventricular radius. In contrast, isometric exercise such as weight lifting causes pressure overload by intermittent increases in arterial pressure, with increased left ventricular wall thickness and unchanged left ventricular chamber size.[52,53]

"Athlete's heart" is a clinical and radiologic term applied to enlarged, sometimes dilated hearts in an athlete that may predispose to arrhythmias.[4] It is generally a benign adaptation that can be difficult to discern clinically from pathologic disease. About 15% of highly trained athletes have striking enlargement of the left ventricular cavity similar to dilated cardiomyopathy, and 20% of retired, deconditioned elite athletes show residual dilatation of cardiac chambers.[54,55] These findings suggest a potential deleterious effect of extreme conditioning on a susceptible minority of athletes.

Pathologic information on "athlete's heart" is largely restricted to autopsy studies of individuals who die suddenly of presumed heart disease. In this group, about 10% of deaths are attributed to "idiopathic left ventricular hypertrophy," with cardiac enlargement (weights of 400 to 499 g) and mild ventricular wall thickening (15 to 19 mm), without septal asymmetry or myofiber disarray of hypertrophic cardiomyopathy.[56,57] It is difficult to know if these patients have underlying cardiomyopathy or if the adaptation to training resulted in a pathologic condition. An autopsy study comparing hearts from fatal cycling accidents to motor vehicle accidents in nonathletes found a nonsignificant increase in heart weight, with a decrease in coronary artery disease. This study did not therefore support an entity of "athlete's heart" but suggested a protective antiatherosclerotic effect of exercise.[58] A case report of an endurance athlete dying suddenly during a marathon showed interstitial fibrosis of unclear cause.[59]

Obesity-Related Hypertrophy and Heart Disease

Cardiac abnormalities that are associated with obesity are often seen in other conditions associated with obesity, including hypertension, obstructive sleep apnea, and renal disease. The most important mechanisms in the development of so-called obesity cardiomyopathy are insulin resistance and related metabolic disturbances, activation of the renin–angiotensin–aldosterone and sympathetic nervous systems, myocardial hypertrophy, and small-vessel disease.[60] Left ventricular hypertrophy as assessed by echocardiography is associated with increased body mass index.[61]

Cardiomegaly is seen in virtually all hearts of obese subjects at autopsy,[62] although it is proportional to body weight.[63] There is an increase in myocyte size and nuclear area in hypertrophied hearts of obese patients similar to hypertensive left ventricular hypertrophy, but increases in interstitial fibrosis were not observed in one study.[63] Causes of sudden death in morbid obesity are most frequently dilated cardiomyopathy, presumably related to decompensated left ventricular hypertrophy, followed by coronary atherosclerosis and concentric left ventricular hypertrophy without dilatation.

REFERENCES

1. Ducas RA, Elliott JE, Melnyk SF, et al. Cardiovascular magnetic resonance in pregnancy: insights from the cardiac hemodynamic imaging and remodeling in pregnancy (CHIRP) study. *J Cardiovasc Magn Reson*. 2014;16:1.
2. Zhang M, Shields J, Zhang Y, et al. Correlation between coronary plaque burden and heart weight. *Pathol Res Pract*. 2012;208:610–614.
3. Morganroth J, Henry WL, Maron RJ, et al. Idiopathic left ventricular hypertrophy. *N Engl J Med*. 1974;290:1047–1050.
4. Maron BJ. Sudden death in young athletes. *N Engl J Med*. 2003;349:1064–1075.
5. Tsioufis C, Kokkinos P, Macmanus C, et al. Left ventricular hypertrophy as a determinant of renal outcome in patients with high cardiovascular risk. *J Hypertens*. 2010;28:2299–2308.
6. Wang SX, Xue H, Zou YB, et al. Prevalence and risk factors for left ventricular hypertrophy and left ventricular geometric abnormality in the patients with hypertension among Han Chinese. *Chin Med J (Engl)*. 2012;125:21–26.
7. Tavora F, Zhang Y, Zhang M, et al. Cardiomegaly is a common arrhythmogenic substrate in adult sudden cardiac deaths, and is associated with obesity. *Pathology*. 2012;44:187–191.
8. Sant'Anna MP, Mello RJ, Montenegro LT, et al. [Left and right ventricular hypertrophy at autopsy of hypertensive individuals]. *Rev Assoc Med Bras*. 2012;58:41–47.
9. Kahn JP, Gorman JM, King DL, et al. Cardiac left ventricular hypertrophy and chamber dilatation in panic disorder patients: implications for idiopathic dilated cardiomyopathy. *Psychiatry Res*. 1990;32:55–61.
10. Kiatchoosakun S, Mahanonda N, Phankingthongkum R, et al. Left ventricular hypertrophy: relationship of echocardiographic and electrocardiographic findings in idiopathic dilated cardiomyopathy. *J Med Assoc Thai*. 1996;79:103–107.
11. Brumback LC, Kronmal R, Heckbert SR, et al. Body size adjustments for left ventricular mass by cardiovascular magnetic resonance and their impact on left ventricular hypertrophy classification. *Int J Cardiovasc Imaging*. 2010;26:459–468.
12. Dweck MR, Joshi S, Murigu T, et al. Left ventricular remodeling and hypertrophy in patients with aortic stenosis: insights from cardiovascular magnetic resonance. *J Cardiovasc Magn Reson*. 2012;14:50.
13. de la Grandmaison GL, Clairand I, Durigon M. Organ weight in 684 adult autopsies: new tables for a Caucasoid population. *Forensic Sci Int*. 2001;119:149–154.
14. Kitzman DW, Scholz DG, Hagen PT, et al. Age-related changes in normal human hearts during the first 10 decades of life. Part II (Maturity): a quantitative anatomic study of 765 specimens from subjects 20 to 99 years old. *Mayo Clin Proc*. 1988;63:137–146.
15. Molina DK, DiMaio VJ. Normal organ weights in men: part I-the heart. *Am J Forensic Med Pathol*. 2012;33:362–367.
16. Sheikhazadi A, Sadr SS, Ghadyani MH, et al. Study of the normal internal organ weights in Tehran's population. *J Forensic Leg Med*. 2010;17:78–83.
17. Lund O, Larsen KE. Cardiac pathology after isolated valve replacement for aortic stenosis in relation to preoperative patient status. Early and late autopsy findings. *Scand J Thorac Cardiovasc Surg*. 1989;23:263–270.
18. Gradman AH, Alfayoumi F. From left ventricular hypertrophy to congestive heart failure: management of hypertensive heart disease. *Prog Cardiovasc Dis*. 2006;48:326–341.
19. Drakos SG, Kfoury AG, Hammond EH, et al. Impact of mechanical unloading on microvasculature and associated central remodeling features of the failing human heart. *J Am Coll Cardiol*. 2010;56:382–391.
20. Saito S, Matsumiya G, Sakaguchi T, et al. Cardiac fibrosis and cellular hypertrophy decrease the degree of reverse remodeling and improvement in cardiac function during left ventricular assist. *J Heart Lung Transplant*. 2010;29:672–679.
21. Olivetti G, Cigola E, Maestri R, et al. Aging, cardiac hypertrophy and ischemic cardiomyopathy do not affect the proportion of mononucleated and multinucleated myocytes in the human heart. *J Mol Cell Cardiol*. 1996;28:1463–1477.
22. Cheng Z, Cui Q, Tian Z, et al. Danon disease as a cause of concentric left ventricular hypertrophy in patients who underwent endomyocardial biopsy. *Eur Heart J*. 2012;33:649–656.
23. Terryn W, Deschoenmakere G, De Keyser J, et al. Prevalence of Fabry disease in a predominantly hypertensive population with left ventricular hypertrophy. *Int J Cardiol*. 2013;167:2555–2560.
24. Haider AW, Larson MG, Benjamin EJ, et al. Increased left ventricular mass and hypertrophy are associated with increased risk for sudden death. *J Am Coll Cardiol*. 1998;32:1454–1459.
25. Barbieri A, Bursi F, Mantovani F, et al. Left ventricular hypertrophy reclassification and death: application of the Recommendation of the American Society of Echocardiography/European Association of Echocardiography. *Eur Heart J Cardiovasc Imaging*. 2012;13:109–117.
26. Okin PM, Gerdts E, Wachtell K, et al. Relationship of left atrial enlargement to persistence or development of ECG left ventricular hypertrophy in hypertensive patients: implications for the development of new atrial fibrillation. *J Hypertens*. 2010;28:1534–1540.
27. Patel PC, Reimold SC, Araj FG, et al. Concentric left ventricular hypertrophy as assessed by cardiac magnetic resonance imaging and risk of death in cardiac transplant recipients. *J Heart Lung Transplant*. 2010;29:1369–1379.
28. Roger VL, Go AS, Lloyd-Jones DM, et al. Heart disease and stroke statistics—2012 update: a report from the American Heart Association. *Circulation*. 2012;125:e2–e220.
29. Kemp CD, Conte JV. The pathophysiology of heart failure. *Cardiovasc Pathol*. 2012;21:365–371.
30. Abhayaratna WP, Seward JB, Appleton CP, et al. Left atrial size: physiologic determinants and clinical applications. *J Am Coll Cardiol*. 2006;47:2357–2363.
31. Armstrong AC, Liu K, Lewis CE, et al. Left atrial dimension and traditional cardiovascular risk factors predict 20-year clinical cardiovascular events in young healthy adults: the CARDIA study. *Eur Heart J Cardiovasc Imaging*. 2014;15:893–899.
32. Abdullah OM, Drakos SG, Diakos NA, et al. Characterization of diffuse fibrosis in the failing human heart via diffusion tensor imaging and quantitative histological validation. *NMR Biomed*. 2014;27:1378–1386.
33. Bang CN, Gerdts E, Aurigemma GP, et al. Four-group classification of left ventricular hypertrophy based on ventricular concentricity and dilatation identifies a low-risk subset of eccentric hypertrophy in hypertensive patients. *Circ Cardiovasc Imaging*. 2014;7:422–429.
34. Matsui Y, Eguchi K, Shibasaki S, et al. Morning hypertension assessed by home monitoring is a strong predictor of concentric left ventricular hypertrophy in patients with untreated hypertension. *J Clin Hypertens (Greenwich)*. 2010;12:776–783.
35. Burns J, Ball SG, Worthy G, et al. Hypertensive left ventricular hypertrophy: a mechanistic approach to optimizing regression assessed by cardiovascular magnetic resonance. *J Hypertens*. 2012;30:2039–2046.
36. Rossi MA. Pathologic fibrosis and connective tissue matrix in left ventricular hypertrophy due to chronic arterial hypertension in humans. *J Hypertens*. 1998;16:1031–1041.
37. Bircan Z, Duzova A, Cakar N, et al. Predictors of left ventricular hypertrophy in children on chronic peritoneal dialysis. *Pediatr Nephrol*. 2010;25:1311–1318.
38. Simpson JM, Savis A, Rawlins D, et al. Incidence of left ventricular hypertrophy in children with kidney disease: impact of method of indexation of left ventricular mass. *Eur J Echocardiogr*. 2010;11:271–277.
39. Turkmen F, Emre A, Ozdemir A, et al. Relationship between aortic valve sclerosis and left ventricular hypertrophy in chronic haemodialysis patients. *Int Urol Nephrol*. 2008;40:497–502.

40. Yilmaz M, Unsal A, Oztekin E, et al. The prevalence of hypertension, valve calcification and left ventricular hypertrophy and geometry in peritoneal dialysis patients. *Kidney Blood Press Res.* 2012;35:431–437.

41. Lopez B, Gonzalez A, Hermida N, et al. Myocardial fibrosis in chronic kidney disease: potential benefits of torasemide. *Kidney Int Suppl.* 2008;111:S19–S23.

42. Gross ML, Ritz E. Hypertrophy and fibrosis in the cardiomyopathy of uremia—beyond coronary heart disease. *Semin Dial.* 2008;21:308–318.

43. Krayenbuehl HP, Hess OM, Monrad ES, et al. Left ventricular myocardial structure in aortic valve disease before, intermediate, and late after aortic valve replacement. *Circulation.* 1989;79:744–755.

44. Villari B, Vassalli G, Monrad ES, et al. Normalization of diastolic dysfunction in aortic stenosis late after valve replacement. *Circulation.* 1995;91:2353–2358.

45. Breitenbach I, Harringer W, Tsui S, et al. Magnetic resonance imaging versus echocardiography to ascertain the regression of left ventricular hypertrophy after bioprosthetic aortic valve replacement: results of the REST study. *J Thorac Cardiovasc Surg.* 2012;144:640.e1–645.e1.

46. Villa E, Troise G, Cirillo M, et al. Factors affecting left ventricular remodeling after valve replacement for aortic stenosis. An overview. *Cardiovasc Ultrasound.* 2006;4:25.

47. Uretsky S, Supariwala A, Nidadovolu P, et al. Quantification of left ventricular remodeling in response to isolated aortic or mitral regurgitation. *J Cardiovasc Magn Reson.* 2010;12:32.

48. Villari B, Sossalla S, Ciampi Q, et al. Persistent diastolic dysfunction late after valve replacement in severe aortic regurgitation. *Circulation.* 2009;120:2386–2392.

49. Ribeiro HB, Le Ven F, Larose E, et al. Cardiac magnetic resonance versus transthoracic echocardiography for the assessment and quantification of aortic regurgitation in patients undergoing transcatheter aortic valve implantation. *Heart.* 2014;100:1924–1932.

50. Bolcal C, Doganci S, Baysan O, et al. Evaluation of left ventricular functions after aortic valve replacement in a specific young male patient population with pure aortic insufficiency or aortic stenosis: 5-years follow-up. *Heart Surg Forum.* 2007;10:E57–E63.

51. Lamb HJ, Beyerbacht HP, de Roos A, et al. Left ventricular remodeling early after aortic valve replacement: differential effects on diastolic function in aortic valve stenosis and aortic regurgitation. *J Am Coll Cardiol.* 2002;40:2182–2188.

52. Pluim BM, Zwinderman AH, van der Laarse A, et al. The athlete's heart. A meta-analysis of cardiac structure and function. *Circulation.* 2000;101:336–344.

53. D'Andrea A, Caso P, Bossone E, et al. Right ventricular myocardial involvement in either physiological or pathological left ventricular hypertrophy: an ultrasound speckle-tracking two-dimensional strain analysis. *Eur J Echocardiogr.* 2010;11:492–500.

54. Pelliccia A, Culasso F, Di Paolo FM, et al. Physiologic left ventricular cavity dilatation in elite athletes. *Ann Intern Med.* 1999;130:23–31.

55. Pelliccia A, Maron BJ, De Luca R, et al. Remodeling of left ventricular hypertrophy in elite athletes after long-term deconditioning. *Circulation.* 2002;105:944–949.

56. Burke AP, Farb A, Virmani R, et al. Sports-related and non-sports-related sudden cardiac death in young adults. *Am Heart J.* 1991;121:568–575.

57. Maron BJ, Shirani J, Poliac LC, et al. Sudden death in young competitive athletes. Clinical, demographic, and pathological profiles. *JAMA.* 1996;276:199–204.

58. Kennedy A. Exercise and heart disease: cardiac findings in fatal cycle accidents. *Br J Sports Med.* 1997;31:328–331.

59. Whyte G, Sheppard M, George K, et al. Post-mortem evidence of idiopathic left ventricular hypertrophy and idiopathic interstitial myocardial fibrosis: is exercise the cause? *Br J Sports Med.* 2008;42:304–305.

60. Wong C, Marwick TH. Obesity cardiomyopathy: pathogenesis and pathophysiology. *Nat Clin Pract Cardiovasc Med.* 2007;4:436–443.

61. Rodrigues SL, Baldo MP, Sa Cunha R, et al. Anthropometric measures of increased central and overall adiposity in association with echocardiographic left ventricular hypertrophy. *Hypertens Res.* 2010;33:83–87.

62. Haque AK, Gadre S, Taylor J, et al. Pulmonary and cardiovascular complications of obesity: an autopsy study of 76 obese subjects. *Arch Pathol Lab Med.* 2008;132:1397–1404.

63. Duflou J, Virmani R, Rabin I, et al. Sudden death as a result of heart disease in morbid obesity. *Am Heart J.* 1995;130:306–313.

144 Cor Pulmonale

Allen P. Burke, M.D., and Adina Paulk, M.D.

Definition

Cor pulmonale, or pulmonary heart disease, is right ventricular enlargement with or without right heart failure resulting from pulmonary hypertension caused by structural or functional abnormalities of the pulmonary circulation.[1] "Cor pulmonale" may be used for right heart enlargement from all causes of pulmonary hypertension except left-sided heart disease.[2,3] Despite a lack of a clear consensus definition and a recent trend to abandon the use of the term altogether, Roberts et al. recently proposed a unifying definition. In a clinical and pathologic review, they define cor pulmonale as "dilatation of the right ventricular cavity without hypertrophy of its wall (acute and subacute cor pulmonale) or both dilatation of the right ventricular cavity and hypertrophy of its wall (chronic cor pulmonale), secondary to pulmonary hypertension not caused by a condition involving the left side of the heart.[2]

Pathophysiology

The pathophysiology of cor pulmonale is analogous to left-sided hypertrophy and failure brought on by increased afterload caused by systemic hypertension (see Chapter 143). The main responses to circulatory and pressure overload are right ventricular dilatation and

hypertrophy, respectively. When the onset of pulmonary hypertension is sudden, dilatation occurs. When it is gradual, there is right ventricular hypertrophy and dilatation, which progress concomitantly, with eventual right-sided failure.[1] A phase of right ventricular hypertrophy without dilatation, as is seen in the left ventricle, is not generally described.

Right ventricular hypertrophy is caused by chronic increased pulmonary vascular resistance, due to any of the causes of pulmonary hypertension (Table 144.1).

The general causes of cor pulmonale fall into three groups. Those characterized by a limitation to airflow (COPD and other causes of chronic bronchial obstruction) account for 80% of cases. Those characterized by a restriction of pulmonary volumes (restrictive lung diseases) account for the majority of the remainder and include idiopathic pulmonary fibrosis and pulmonary sarcoidosis. Idiopathic pulmonary arterial hypertension and associated pulmonary arterial hypertension are additional causes of cor pulmonale. Finally, there are those conditions where mechanical properties of the lungs and chest wall are preserved, but poor ventilatory drive causes gas exchange abnormalities, as in, for example, obesity–hypoventilation syndrome (formerly "pickwickian syndrome"), and obstructive sleep apnea.

Alveolar hypoxia is an important cause of pulmonary hypertension, chronic obstructive lung disease, kyphoscoliosis, and hypoventilation.

TABLE 144.1 Causes of Cor Pulmonale

Acute cor pulmonale
   Pulmonary embolism
   Acute respiratory distress syndrome
Chronic cor pulmonale
   Chronic lung disease, especially chronic obstructive lung disease
   Interstitial lung disease (idiopathic pulmonary fibrosis, sarcoidosis,
      pneumoconiosis)
   Loss of lung tissue following trauma or surgery
   Primary pulmonary hypertension
   Chronic thrombotic pulmonary hypertension, including sickle cell
      disease
Mechanical impedance to ventilation
   T1-4 Vertebral subluxation
   Severe thoracic kyphosis
Central causes of decreased ventilation
   Obstructive sleep apnea
   Obesity-hypoventilation syndrome
   Bronchopulmonary dysplasia (in infants)

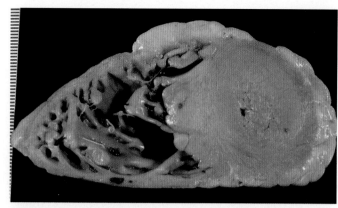

FIGURE 144.1 ▲ Right ventricular dilatation, subacute cor pulmonale. The apical most cross section demonstrates marked right ventricular dilatation. At this level, the right ventricular cavity should be inconspicuous or absent. There is associated concentric left ventricular hypertrophy.

In diffuse interstitial lung disease, destruction of vessels with intimal remodeling is a contributory factor.

Acute and Subacute Cor Pulmonale

In the clinical setting, acute cor pulmonale is mainly observed as a complication of massive pulmonary embolism or acute respiratory distress syndrome.

The diagnosis is generally made by echocardiography. When evaluated along the long axis, the area of the right ventricle is enlarged compared to the left at a ratio of 0.6 and 1 (moderate cor pulmonale) or >1 (severe cor pulmonale).[4] Pulmonary arterial wedge pressures are generally normal, indicating a lack of left ventricular dilatation.

In acute respiratory distress syndrome, the rate of cor pulmonale ranges from 14% to 50%.[5] The main cause of pulmonary artery vasoconstriction in mechanically ventilated ARDS patients is hypercapnia, with mechanical ventilation contributing by way of an alveolar distension compressing the capillary bed in undamaged areas of the lung.[4] There are various clinical strategies involving ventilator settings that have been developed to lessen the incidence of acute cor pulmonale in acute respiratory distress syndrome ("what is good for the lung is good for the right ventricle").[5]

In approximately 60% of patients with massive pulmonary embolism, acute cor pulmonale is seen. Hyperacute cor pulmonale caused by massive pulmonary emboli results in cardiac dilatation without hypertrophy. Similarly, subacute cor pulmonale, often caused by embolic malignancy,[2,6-9] also causes right ventricular dilatation without hypertrophy[2] (Fig. 144.2).

Cor Pulmonale in Chronic Obstructive Lung Disease

Chronic pulmonary hypertension is diagnosed by a mean pulmonary artery pressure of >20 mm Hg. The impact of cor pulmonale on morbidity and mortality in chronic obstructive lung disease is difficult to assess, because cor pulmonale is a complication among many others and is impossible to separate from respiratory failure.[1] The incidence depends on criteria for diagnosis and ranges from 20% to 91% of patients with chronic obstructive lung disease.[3]

Pulmonary hypertension in chronic obstructive lung disease is generally mild to moderate, and progresses at a slow rate. A minority of patients exhibit severe or "disproportionate" pulmonary hypertension, which can be defined by a resting pulmonary arterial pressure of >35 to 40 mm Hg. Mechanisms and appropriate treatment for this disease have yet to be fully elucidated.[10]

Gross Pathologic Findings

Grossly, dilatation caused by acute cor pulmonale results in enlargement without wall thickening, and is best assessed by evaluating an apical short axis section, where normally there is little or no right ventricular cavity present (Fig. 144.1). If present, there is evidence of dilatation, which is more subjectively evident towards the base of the heart and in the outflow region.

In chronic cor pulmonale, there is a thickened right ventricular wall with variable dilatation (Figs. 144.2 and 144.3). Right ventricular hypertrophy can be extreme, especially if congenital, in infants with persistent pulmonary hypertension of the newborn (Figs. 144.4 to 144.6). Ventricular dilatation is invariably associated with right atrial dilatation, and elongated, rolled, leaflets of the pulmonic and tricuspid valve. The right atrium is not generally dilated in acute or subacute cor pulmonale.[2] An increase in the tricuspid annulus (over 11 cm) is typical, and there may also be aneurysmal dilatation of the oval fossa reflective of increased atrial pressures (see below).

In general, the posterior right ventricle and muscular wall of the outflow tract is no >4 mm in thickness. Care must be taken to avoid measuring the fat in the epicardium, which is normally minimal in these locations.

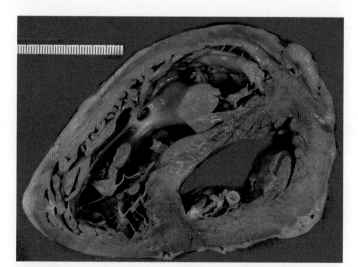

FIGURE 144.2 ▲ Right ventricular hypertrophy with marked ventricular dilatation (chronic cor pulmonale). The patient had pulmonary hypertension secondary to mitral stenosis. Note marked thickening of the right ventricle.

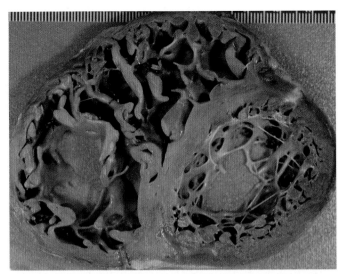

FIGURE 144.3 ▲ Right ventricular dilatation and hypertrophy, massive. This patient had congenital pulmonary atresia that was treated with right ventricular outflow tract reconstruction, with persistent pulmonary valve regurgitation. The right ventricle is massively dilated with prominent trabeculations. The left ventricle is also dilated. In both these examples the appearance is similar to cor pulmonale, but the term is not appropriate as cardiac disease was the underlying cause of right ventricular dilatation.

Histologic Findings

The histologic features of chronic cor pulmonale include myocyte hypertrophy, interstitial fibrosis, and occasional areas of replacement fibrosis. In acute cor pulmonale, there may be a right ventricular inflammatory infiltrate comprised predominantly of macrophages, T lymphocytes and neutrophils, with small foci of myocyte necrosis[11] (Fig. 144.7).

In the liver, chronic pulmonary hypertension results in progressive hepatic fibrosis, the degree of which correlates with right atrial pressures during life. Initially there is acute passive congestion, with sinusoidal dilatation in the centrilobular zone. Later, there is centrilobular necrosis (Fig. 144.8) that progresses to fibrosis that can be associated with hepatocyte atrophy.[12]

Oval Fossa Aneurysm

Aneurysm of the fossa ovalis is a septal structure that bulges into either atrium and can be detected incidentally at autopsy, or cause significant

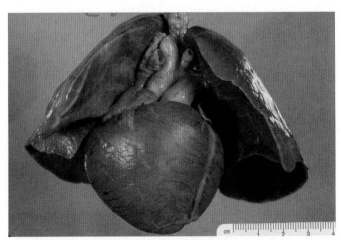

FIGURE 144.4 ▲ Cor pulmonale, infant with persistent pulmonary hypertension of the newborn. Anterior aspect of the heart shows marked right ventricular predominance.

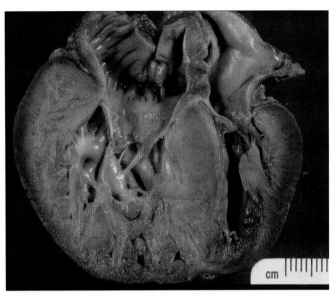

FIGURE 144.5 ▲ Cor pulmonale, infant with persistent pulmonary hypertension of the newborn. A four-chamber cut shows massive right ventricular hypertrophy.

clinical symptoms.[13] It is an uncommon anomaly, present in about 2% of the adult population, with an association with pulmonary hypertension and cor pulmonale.[14]

Patients can present with symptoms related to atrial inflow obstruction, in some instances similarly to an atrial tumor. Age of presentation is extremely varied, with reported cases from newborns to elderly. The majority of reported cases are aneurysms protruding into the right atrium, but they can occur on either side. In few cases, the side of protrusion changes from systole to diastole.[13]

Aneurysms range from a few millimeters to about 30 to 40 mm in maximum diameter. The surface of the aneurysm is usually an intact septum, but there may be associated patent foramen ovale (Fig. 144.9). In a significant proportion of cases, an extrinsic mechanism of increased atrial pressure can be elicited, and those include in addition to elevated pulmonary artery pressure, left-sided outflow obstruction, mitral regurgitation, and left ventricular hypertrophy.[13] The remainder of the cases can be attributed to a reduced size of the interatrial ostium.

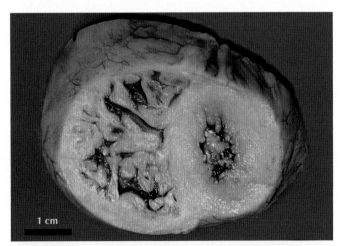

FIGURE 144.6 ▲ Chronic cor pulmonale, with right ventricular dilatation. In this case, the patient was a 6-month-old baby with the diagnosis of bronchopulmonary dysplasia and consequent right ventricular hypertrophy.

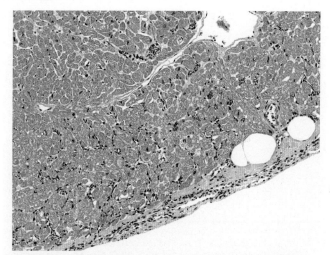

FIGURE 144.7 ▲ Reactive inflammation, right ventricular endo-cardium. The patient died of massive pulmonary embolism with right ventricular dilatation. There is a sparse chronic infiltrate in the endocardium and adjacent myocardium.

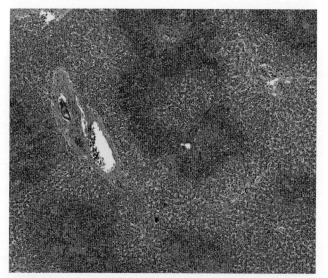

FIGURE 144.8 ▲ Centrilobular hepatic necrosis. There is severe acute centrilobular congestion with necrosis secondary to right heart failure.

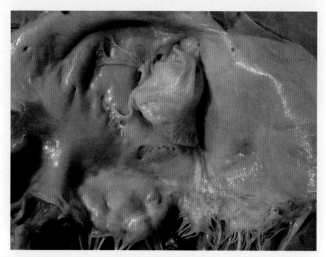

FIGURE 144.9 ▲ Oval fossa aneurysm. There is a bulging of the oval fossa, which may be closed or probe patent, into the left atrial cavity. It is frequently but not always a complication of elevated right-sided pressures.

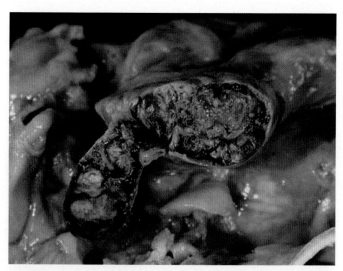

FIGURE 144.10 ▲ Isolated right atrial infarct. The thinned wall of the atrium showed acute infarction histologically (not shown) and there is extensive occlusive thrombus.

Isolated Atrial Infarction

Infarctions of the atria are usually related to ventricular infarcts (see Chapter 7). Occasionally, they can be isolated (Fig. 144.10). Autopsy studies have shown a 15% incidence of atrial infarct, 3% of which were isolated to the atria. Pulmonary hypertension has been suggested to play a role in some cases due to strain on the atrial wall. Embolic occlusion, iatrogenic vascular damage during surgery, vasculitis and atherosclerosis may be etiologic factors. Atrial infarcts may cause arrhythmias, thromboembolic events, and atrial rupture, although clinical pathologic correlative studies are few.[15]

REFERENCES

1. Weitzenblum E, Chaouat A. Cor pulmonale. *Chron Respir Dis.* 2009;6:177–185.
2. Roberts WC, Shafii AE, Grayburn PA, et al. Clinical and morphologic features of acute, subacute and chronic cor pulmonale (pulmonary heart disease). *Am J Cardiol.* 2015;115:697–703.
3. Shujaat A, Minkin R, and Eden E. Pulmonary hypertension and chronic cor pulmonale in COPD. *Int J Chron Obstruct Pulmon Dis.* 2007;2:273–282.
4. Jardin F and Vieillard-Baron A. Acute cor pulmonale. *Curr Opin Crit Care.* 2009;15:67–70.
5. Repesse X, Charron C, Vieillard-Baron A. Acute cor pulmonale in ARDS: rationale for protecting the right ventricle. *Chest.* 2015;147:259–265.
6. Schriner RW, Ryu JH, Edwards WD. Microscopic pulmonary tumor embolism causing subacute cor pulmonale: a difficult antemortem diagnosis. *Mayo Clin Proc.* 1991;66:143–148.
7. Lambert-Jensen P, Mertz H, Nyvad O, et al. Subacute cor pulmonale due to microscopic pulmonary tumour cell embolization. *J Intern Med.* 1994;236:597–598.
8. Kinuya K, Yamanouchi K, Terahata S. Diagnosis: pulmonary tumor thrombotic microangiopathy developing cor pulmonale. *Ann Nucl Med.* 2002;16:frontpage, 220.
9. Corradi D, Mormandi F, Tanzi G, et al. Fatal cor pulmonale caused by pulmonary tumor microembolism in a patient with occult gastric cancer. *Cardiovasc Pathol.* 2006;15:157–160.
10. Seeger W, Adir Y, Barbera JA, et al. Pulmonary hypertension in chronic lung diseases. *J Am Coll Cardiol.* 2013;62:D109–D116.
11. Orde MM, Puranik R, Morrow PL, et al. Myocardial pathology in pulmonary thromboembolism. *Heart.* 2011;97:1695–1699.
12. Dai DF, Swanson PE, Krieger EV, et al. Congestive hepatic fibrosis score: a novel histologic assessment of clinical severity. *Mod Pathol.* 2014;27:1552–1558.
13. Topaz O, Edwards JE, Bojack-Mackey S, et al. Aneurysm of fossa ovalis in adults: a pathologic study. *Cardiovasc Pathol.* 2003;12:219–225.
14. Khouzam RN, D'Cruz IA, Minderman DP. Pulmonary sarcoidosis with pulmonary hypertension, fossa ovalis aneurysm and interatrial shunt. *Clin Cardiol.* 2008;31:284–285.
15. Cunningham KS, Chan KL, Veinot JP. Pathology of isolated atrial infarction: case report and review of the literature. *Cardiovasc Pathol.* 2008;17:183–185.

145 Cardiac Disease in Hematologic Disorders

Allen P. Burke, M.D., and Adina Paulk, M.D.

Sickle Cell Disease

Sickle cell disease is a chronic hemolytic anemia caused by abnormal hemoglobin that polymerizes and deforms red blood cells into the characteristic sickle shape. There is a single nucleotide mutation in the gene coding of the β-hemoglobin chain that is inherited in an autosomal recessive fashion. Sickle cell crises cause episodes of microvascular occlusion and premature red blood cell destruction, which lead to chronic severe hemolytic anemia and microscopic infarcts in the brain, lung, bone, kidney, liver, spleen, and retina.

The most common cardiac manifestation of sickle cell disease is high-output heart failure secondary to chronic anemia. Left ventricular mass is increased secondary to compensatory hypertrophy, which occurs in response to ventricular dilatation.[1]

Primary cardiac damage in sickle cell disease is theoretically possible through two mechanisms: direct iron toxicity due to myocyte iron overload and ischemic change secondary to microscopic thrombosis. Despite the frequent assertion that there is increased iron within the myocytes of patients with sickle cell disease,[2] there is little if any evidence to support this view pathologically.

Clinically, iron overload in the heart, liver, and pancreas is assessed by magnetic resonance imaging. Myocardial iron overload as assessed by magnetic resonance imaging (T2) has been shown to occur in only a small percentage of chronically transfused sickle cell disease patients.[1] One study of 23 patients showed no myocardial iron accumulation.[3] Those patients at risk have exceptionally poor chelation control of total body iron stores and very high levels of hemoglobin S, reticulocytes, and serum transferrin.[4] There have been no reports of invasive procedures (i.e., endomyocardial biopsy) documenting the presence of myocardial iron related to iron overload in sickle cell disease.

Approximately 10% of patients with sickle cell crisis have evidence of enzyme leak with elevated troponins, and chest pain may occur.[5] Myocardial perfusion defects have been described by single photon emission computed tomography.[6] By cardiac magnetic resonance imaging using late gadolinium enhancement, only 13% of sickle cell patients had evidence of myocardial fibrosis.[1]

There is a paucity of autopsy studies documenting the pathologic features of ischemic lesions in sickle cell disease (Figs. 145.1 and 145.2).[8] Microvascular occlusions resulting in ischemic scars, sometimes termed "sludge infarcts,"[9] have been related to sickle cell "vasculopathy."[10] One autopsy study demonstrated acute infarcts in 3 and healed infarcts in 4 of 72 patients with sickle cell disease and documented intramural coronary thrombi.[11] A different autopsy study of over 50 patients did not demonstrate evidence of intramural coronary occlusion or infarcts, but showed secondary changes related to atherosclerosis, pulmonary hypertension, and systemic hypertension. The term "cardiomyopathy of sickle cell disease" was therefore not recommended.[12]

Sickle cell disease often causes right ventricular hypertrophy and dilatation secondary to pulmonary vascular occlusive disease and pulmonary hypertension.

Pathophysiology of Cardiac Iron Overload

As serum transferrin becomes saturated, iron that is not bound to transferrin is released into the circulation, which can enter hepatic, pancreatic, and other organ tissue including the myocardium. Ferrous iron enters

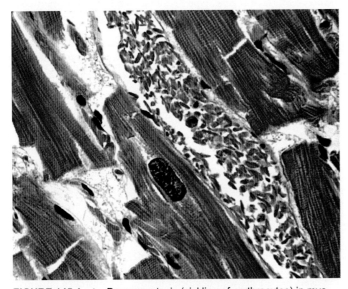

FIGURE 145.1 ▲ Drepanocytosis (sickling of erythrocytes) in myocardial vessel. This is a constant finding in patients dying with sickle cell disease but is also seen in 95% of patients dying with sickle cell trait. See reference.[7]

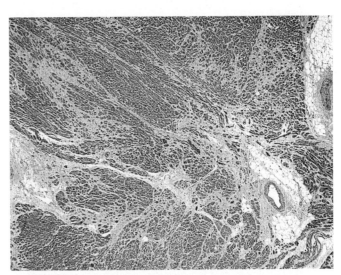

FIGURE 145.2 ▲ Sickle cell disease, patchy scarring. Sickle cell disease may cause patchy scarring in the myocardium, presumably caused by areas of healed ischemia from microvascular disease.

TABLE 145.1 Conditions Associated with Tissue Iron Overload, and Cardiac Involvement

Cause	Symptomatic Heart Involvement	Type of Cardiomyopathy	Cause of Cardiomyopathy	Iron in Myocardial Tissue
Primary (genetic)				
Hemochromatosis	15% of patients	Restrictive, arrhythmias	Iron overload	Yes
Secondary iron overload				
Thalassemia	7% of patients	Dilated	Iron overload, high-output failure, others	Yes
Sickle cell disease	Frequent, depending on degree of anemia	Dilated	High-output failure	No
Myelodysplastic syndromes	Infrequent	Dilated	High-output failure and iron overload[14]	No
Myelofibrosis	Rare	—	—	—
Aplastic anemia	Rare	Dilated	High-output failure and iron overload[15]	No
Intravenous iron supplementation	Rare	—	Iron overload	Rare[16]
Friedreich ataxia	Common	Dilated	Multifactorial, including iron overload	Yes
Increased dietary intake	Not reported	—	—	—
Cirrhosis	Infrequent	Right ventricular and biventricular failure	High-output failure, right ventricular hypertrophy (pulmonary hypertension)	Infrequent[17]

cardiac myocytes through L-type calcium channels where it is bound to ferritin. As the capacity of ferritin to store iron is exceeded, it is released in the form of hemosiderin and free iron into the cytoplasm. Cardiac damage is the result of oxidation and formation of free radical hydroxyl ions that cause lipid peroxidation and increased membrane permeability.[13]

Cardiac iron overload is caused by a variety of conditions including genetic (hemochromatosis) and acquired (see Table 145.1). Friedreich ataxia is considered in more detail in Chapter 160.

Transfusions are a major contributor to cardiac iron overload in cases of hemolytic anemias and hemoglobinopathies, with a minor contribution by hemolysis. Supplemental iron infusions may rarely result in iron overload involving the heart.[16,18] Cardiac iron overload is characteristic of hemochromatosis and thalassemia and plays a minor role in other hemoglobinopathies, such as sickle cell disease. Iron overload may interact with other processes that contribute to heart failure, such as anthracycline toxicity or, more commonly, high-output failure related to anemia.[13]

Histologically, iron deposited in cardiac tissues is within the cytoplasm (sarcoplasmic) and not the interstitium. Tissue iron quantity correlates well with the level of myocardial dysfunction and is the basis for scoring methods, similar to those employed in the liver, that have primarily been used in animal studies.[19]

Thalassemia

β-Thalassemia is the result of reduced synthesis of β-globin chains, caused by mutations in *HBB* (hemoglobin subunit B). There is ineffective erythropoiesis resulting in chronic hemolytic anemia. Increased patient survival due to routine blood transfusions has increased the risk for iron overload and the need for iron chelation therapy with parenteral deferoxamine. Cardiomyopathy accounts for almost 75% of deaths in thalassemia patients, with a prevalence at age 35 of around 7%.[20]

Cardiomyopathy in thalassemia is multifactorial and due in part to high-output heart failure in addition to iron overload. The correlation with myocardial iron overload and the development of heart failure is poor.[20] Nevertheless, in the era of systematic transfusion therapy, myocardial iron overload is traditionally thought to be the main cause of thalassemia cardiomyopathy. The actual cause of increased tissue iron is primarily transfusion related, but also due to ineffective erythropoiesis, peripheral hemolysis, and increased intestinal iron absorption.

Cardiomyopathy of thalassemia has both dilated and restrictive components that have not been shown to relate closely to high-output failure and iron overload, respectively. An increased incidence of allele e4 of apolipoprotein E, which is associated with impairment of antioxidant properties, was found in thalassemia patients with heart failure.[21] Myocarditis has also been associated with the development of heart failure in thalassemia major patients.[22]

Clinically, myocardial iron overload is determined by magnetic resonance imaging,[19] which has been correlated with myocardial iron in mouse studies.[23] Pathologically, the myocardium demonstrates fibrosis, iron deposits, and myocyte loss and hypertrophy. Reactive inflammation with myocarditis is not infrequent. In myocardial biopsies, stainable iron in more than 50% of the cardiomyocytes is graded as severe iron deposition and correlates with iron detected by magnetic resonance imaging.[24]

Myocardial disease is not common in sickle/β-thalassemia, and iron deposition is not seen in this hemoglobinopathy.[25]

Hemochromatosis

Primary hemochromatosis is caused by a genetic defect that occurs in 10% of Americans, most of whom are unaffected heterozygotes. The most common defect is a well-conserved homozygous missense mutation (C282Y) within the high iron gene *HFE*. Homozygotes represent 5 in 1,000 white Americans, who have hemochromatosis type 1, an autosomal recessive disease. Rare variants of hereditary hemochromatosis include type 2, or juvenile hemochromatosis, caused by mutations in hemojuvelin (HFE2) gene; type 3, caused by mutations in transferrin receptor 2 (TfR2) gene; and type 4, caused by mutations in ferroportin-1 (*FPN1*) gene.

The clinical diagnosis of iron overload is established by elevated serum transferrin saturation (>55%) and elevated serum ferritin (>300 ng/mL). Genetic testing for mutations in the *HFE* (high iron) gene and others are then indicated.

The cardiomyopathy of hemochromatosis is initially characterized by diastolic dysfunction and arrhythmias and in later stages by dilated cardiomyopathy. Cardiac magnetic resonance imaging with measurement of T2* relaxation times can help quantify myocardial iron overload.

Endomyocardial biopsy may be performed if the primary clinical manifestations are cardiac. Any stainable iron by Prussian blue (Perls) iron stain is abnormal. The amount of iron is greater in subepicardial compared with endocardial regions, accounting for decreased sensitivity of biopsies in the early phases of disease. Although histologically detectable myocardial iron is usually present in biopsies of patients with cardiac dysfunction from hemochromatosis, biopsies may be falsely negative.[26]

The most common cause of death is from cardiac failure and arrhythmias, followed by cirrhosis and hepatocellular carcinoma.[27] At autopsy, the heart in patients with hemochromatosis demonstrates intramyocyte iron, as demonstrated by Prussian blue stains, myocyte hypertrophy, and interstitial fibrosis (Figs. 145.3 and 145.4). Involvement of the atrioventricular node is associated with bradyarrhythmias and the need for cardiac pacing.[13]

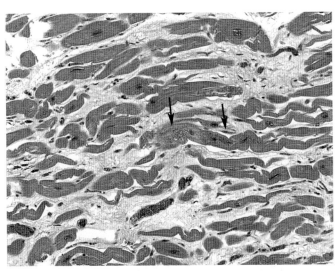

FIGURE 145.3 ▲ Hemochromatosis. Iron in the form of hemosiderin can be seen on routine stains (*arrows*).

Thrombotic Thrombocytopenic Purpura

Thrombotic thrombocytopenic purpura is a thrombotic microangiopathy characterized by thrombocytopenia, erythrocyte fragmentation, and organ failure of variable severity. Cardiac involvement is common and associated with a relatively high rate of mortality. Systemic platelet aggregation caused by the accumulation of unfolded high molecular weight von Willebrand factor multimers is caused by a deficiency in a disintegrin and metalloproteinase with thrombospondin motifs 1, member 13 (ADAMTS13). Biallelic mutations of the encoding gene cause a hereditary form of the disease (5% of patients). More commonly, thrombotic thrombocytopenic purpura is an acquired autoimmune process associated with polyclonal autoantibodies against ADAMTS13.[28,29]

Predisposing conditions include pregnancy, systemic disease, malignant hypertension, HIV infection, cancer, systemic lupus erythematosus, sickle cell disease, and treatment with anticancer drugs.[30–32]

Peripheral blood smears show anemia, red cell schistocytes, and thrombocytopenia. Characteristic cardiac findings include subepicardial hemorrhages, often seen grossly (Fig. 145.5). Microscopically, there are platelet thrombi within intramyocardial arterioles. Immunohistochemical stains for platelet glycoproteins (CD61 or CD31) and fibrin are helpful in the differential diagnosis (Figs. 145.6 and 145.7).[32]

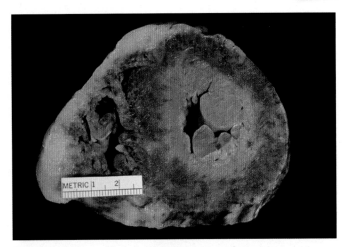

FIGURE 145.5 ▲ Thrombotic thrombocytopenic purpura. Subepicardial hemorrhage is pathognomonic for the disease. However, not all cases of rapid death due to thrombotic thrombocytopenic purpura result in gross hemorrhage. (Reproduced with permission from Burke AP, Mont E, Kolodgie F, et al. Thrombotic thrombocytopenic purpura causing rapid unexpected death: value of CD61 immunohistochemical staining in diagnosis. *Cardiovasc Pathol.* 2005;14:150–155.)

With current treatment, approximately 10% of patients die of the acute episode. Risk factors for death include hypertension, ischemic heart disease, seizures, renal failure, and advanced age.[28,29]

Antiphospholipid Syndrome

The antiphospholipid syndrome (APS) is a hypercoagulable state associated with vascular thrombosis and pregnancy loss. The primary form is isolated, and the secondary form is associated with other autoimmune disorders, especially systemic lupus erythematosus. Thrombosis occurs in both veins and arteries, including coronary vessels, as well as on valve surfaces.

The diagnosis is based on finding one or more autoantibodies in the serum, including antibodies against cardiolipin and the plasma protein β2-glycoprotein I, and on the presence of the lupus anticoagulant. The association with thrombosis is strong when all three autoantibodies are present and weak when a single test is positive.

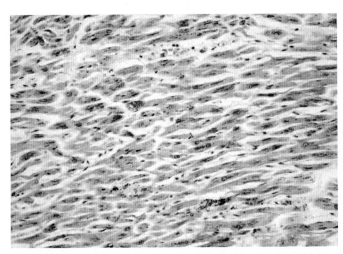

FIGURE 145.4 ▲ Hemochromatosis. Prussian blue stain highlights intramyocyte iron. Any amount of iron in the myocyte is abnormal.

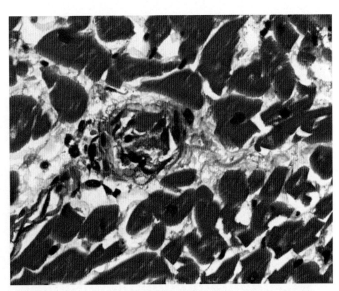

FIGURE 145.6 ▲ Thrombotic thrombocytopenic purpura. The histologic characteristic is that of microthrombi of fibrin, with endothelial swelling.

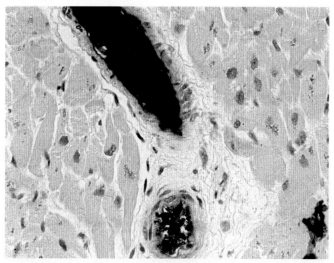

FIGURE 145.7 ▲ Thrombotic thrombocytopenic purpura. The thrombi also contain platelets (anti-CD31 immunohistochemistry). Anti-CD31 stains of hearts from patients dying of other causes do not show diffuse platelet plugs.

The mechanisms by which the antibodies cause the cardiac injury are unclear but are likely related to inflammation as well as thrombosis.

Among the varied cardiac manifestations of APS (Table 145.2), the most common is valve disease. Almost one-third of the patients with primary APS present with valve abnormalities, which are detected by echocardiography. Physiologically, they may be related to exposure of negative phospholipids on the surface of valve leaflets. Grossly, the findings are those of marantic endocarditis, with variable sized thrombi on the inflow or outflow portion of the valve, the mitral and aortic most commonly affected (Fig. 145.8). Histologically, there are

TABLE 145.2 Cardiac Manifestations of Antiphospholipid Syndrome

Arterial thrombosis
Aorta
Axillary
Carotid
Hepatic
Iliofemoral
Mesenteric
Pancreatic
Popliteal
Splenic
Subclavian arteries
Pulmonary (in situ)

Valve disease
Mitral insufficiency
Mitral stenosis (rare)
Leaflet thickening
Vegetations (nonbacterial thrombotic endocarditis)

Myocardial ischemia
Ventricular hypertrophy
Diastolic and systolic dysfunction
Myocarditis
Heart failure
Coronary artery disease
Embolization or atherosclerosis
Angina
Myocardial infarction
Microvascular damage

Venous thromboembolism
Venous thrombosis
Pulmonary emboli
Chronic thromboembolic pulmonary hypertension (CTPH).

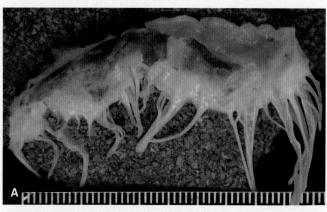
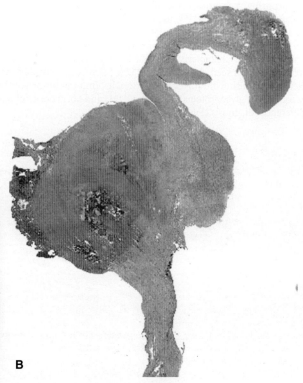

FIGURE 145.8 ▲ Antiphospholipid syndrome, mitral valve. **A.** Gross photograph of excised valve shows small nondestructive vegetations on the atrial surface. **B.** Histologic section shows thrombus on both valve surfaces.

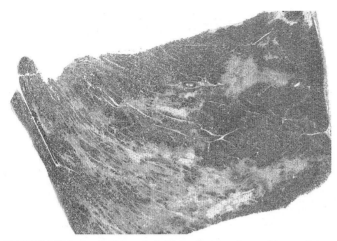

FIGURE 145.9 ▲ Antiphospholipid syndrome, primary. Myocardial ischemia. There is an epicardial artery with organizing thrombus, without significant atherosclerosis.

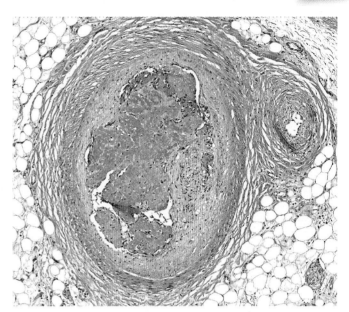

FIGURE 145.10 ▲ Antiphospholipid syndrome. A section of the kidney shows recanalized thrombi in muscular arteries.

fibrin-rich surface thrombi, with vascular proliferation, intravalvular fibrin, capillary thrombosis, and calcifications.[33] Although the term "Libman-Sacks" vegetations are often used for the valve lesions in primary APS, this term suggests an underlying autoimmune valvulitis with secondary thrombosis in patients with lupus erythematosus[34] (see Chapter 10).

Myocardial infarction is increased in frequency in patients with primary and secondary APS. The mechanisms include coronary thromboembolism (e.g., from mitral vegetations or from in situ thrombosis). Coronary thrombi in APS typically involve smaller intramural arteries but may involve epicardial arteries as well (Figs. 145.9 and 145.10). Atherosclerosis of epicardial arteries occurs at an accelerated rate in patients with APS, providing another mechanism for ischemic myocardial lesions.[34]

REFERENCES

1. Junqueira FP, Fernandes JL, Cunha GM, et al. Right and left ventricular function and myocardial scarring in adult patients with sickle cell disease: a comprehensive magnetic resonance assessment of hepatic and myocardial iron overload. *J Cardiovasc Magn Reson.* 2013;15:83.
2. Voskaridou E, Christoulas D, Terpos E. Sickle-cell disease and the heart: review of the current literature. *Br J Haematol.* 2012;157:664–673.
3. Inati A, Musallam KM, Wood JC, et al. Absence of cardiac siderosis by MRI T2* despite transfusion burden, hepatic and serum iron overload in Lebanese patients with sickle cell disease. *Eur J Haematol.* 2009;83:565–571.
4. Meloni A, Puliyel M, Pepe A, et al. Cardiac iron overload in sickle-cell disease. *Am J Hematol.* 2014;89:678–683.
5. Aslam AK, Rodriguez C, Aslam AF, et al. Cardiac troponin I in sickle cell crisis. *Int J Cardiol.* 2009;133:138–139.
6. de Montalembert M, Maunoury C, Acar P, et al. Myocardial ischaemia in children with sickle cell disease. *Arch Dis Child.* 2004;89:359–362.
7. Thogmartin JR, Wilson CI, Palma NA, et al. Histological diagnosis of sickle cell trait: a blinded analysis. *Am J Forensic Med Pathol.* 2009;30:36–39.
8. Mansi IA, Rosner F. Myocardial infarction in sickle cell disease. *J Natl Med Assoc.* 2002;94:448–452.
9. Westwood MA, Shah F, Anderson LJ, et al. Myocardial tissue characterization and the role of chronic anemia in sickle cell cardiomyopathy. *J Magn Reson Imaging.* 2007;26:564–568.
10. Kato GJ, Hebbel RP, Steinberg MH, et al. Vasculopathy in sickle cell disease: biology, pathophysiology, genetics, translational medicine, and new research directions. *Am J Hematol.* 2009;84:618–625.
11. Martin CR, Johnson CS, Cobb C, et al. Myocardial infarction in sickle cell disease. *J Natl Med Assoc.* 1996;88:428–432.
12. Gerry JL, Bulkley BH, Hutchins GM. Clinicopathologic analysis of cardiac dysfunction in 52 patients with sickle cell anemia. *Am J Cardiol.* 1978;42:211–216.
13. Gulati V, Harikrishnan P, Palaniswamy C, et al. Cardiac involvement in hemochromatosis. *Cardiol Rev.* 2014;22:56–68.
14. Oliva EN, Schey C, Hutchings AS. A review of anemia as a cardiovascular risk factor in patients with myelodysplastic syndromes. *Am J Blood Res.* 2011;1:160–166.
15. Nishio M, Endo T, Nakao S, et al. Reversible cardiomyopathy due to secondary hemochromatosis with multitransfusions for severe aplastic anemia after successful non-myeloablative stem cell transplantation. *Int J Cardiol.* 2008;127:400–401.
16. Kobayashi T, Tadokoro H, Matsumoto K. An autopsy case of secondary iron-overload cardiomyopathy. *Intern Med.* 2013;52:1369–1373.
17. Abu Rajab M, Guerin L, Lee P, et al. Iron overload secondary to cirrhosis: a mimic of hereditary haemochromatosis? *Histopathology.* 2014;65:561–569.
18. Ishizaka N, Yuki M, Kanzaki Y. An autopsy case of secondary iron-overload cardiomyopathy. *Intern Med.* 2014;53:351.
19. Wood JC. Use of magnetic resonance imaging to monitor iron overload. *Hematol Oncol Clin North Am.* 2014;28:747–764, vii.
20. Kremastinos DT, Farmakis D, Aessopos A, et al. Beta-thalassemia cardiomyopathy: history, present considerations, and future perspectives. *Circ Heart Fail.* 2010;3:451–458.
21. Aessopos A, Farmakis D, Andreopoulos A, et al. Assessment and treatment of cardiac iron overload in thalassemia. *Hemoglobin.* 2009;33(Suppl 1):S87–S92.
22. Kremastinos DT, Tiniakos G, Theodorakis GN, et al. Myocarditis in beta-thalassemia major. A cause of heart failure. *Circulation.* 1995;91:66–71.
23. Liu P, Henkelman M, Joshi J, et al. Quantification of cardiac and tissue iron by nuclear magnetic resonance relaxometry in a novel murine thalassemia-cardiac iron overload model. *Can J Cardiol.* 1996;12:155–164.
24. Mavrogeni SI, Markussis V, Kaklamanis L, et al. A comparison of magnetic resonance imaging and cardiac biopsy in the evaluation of heart iron overload in patients with beta-thalassemia major. *Eur J Haematol.* 2005;75:241–247.
25. Ghoti H, Goitein O, Koren A, et al. No evidence for myocardial iron overload and free iron species in multitransfused patients with sickle/beta-thalassaemia. *Eur J Haematol.* 2010;84:59–63.
26. Furth PA, Futterweit W, Gorlin R. Refractory biventricular heart failure in secondary hemochromatosis. *Am J Med Sci.* 1985;290:209–213.
27. Witte DL, Crosby WH, Edwards CQ, et al. Practice guideline development task force of the College of American Pathologists. Hereditary hemochromatosis. *Clin Chim Acta.* 1996;245:139–200.

28. Benhamou Y, Assie C, Boelle PY, et al. Development and validation of a predictive model for death in acquired severe ADAMTS13 deficiency-associated idiopathic thrombotic thrombocytopenic purpura: the French TMA Reference Center experience. *Haematologica.* 2012;97:1181–1186.

29. Benhamou Y, Boelle PY, Baudin B, et al. Cardiac troponin-I on diagnosis predicts early death and refractoriness in acquired thrombotic thrombocytopenic purpura. Experience of the French Thrombotic Microangiopathies Reference Center. *J Thromb Haemost.* 2015;13:293–302.

30. Hawkins BM, Abu-Fadel M, Vesely SK, et al. Clinical cardiac involvement in thrombotic thrombocytopenic purpura: a systematic review. *Transfusion.* 2008;48:382–392.

31. Perez L, Ramappa P, Guzman JA. Myocardial injury in thrombotic thrombocytopenic purpura: a frequent, perplexing complication. *Int J Cardiol.* 2008;128:257–260.

32. Burke AP, Mont E, Kolodgie F, et al. Thrombotic thrombocytopenic purpura causing rapid unexpected death: value of CD61 immunohistochemical staining in diagnosis. *Cardiovasc Pathol.* 2005;14:150–155.

33. Lev S, Shoenfeld Y. Cardiac valvulopathy in the antiphospholipid syndrome. *Clin Rev Allergy Immunol.* 2002;23:341–348.

34. Denas G, Jose SP, Bracco A, et al. Antiphospholipid syndrome and the heart: a case series and literature review. *Autoimmun Rev.* 2015;14:214–222.

146 Cardiac Disease in Endocrine Disorders

Allen P. Burke, M.D., and Adina Paulk, M.D.

Introduction

The effect of metabolism and endocrine disorders on the heart is multifaceted, and there are no specific cardiac features or findings to point to a specific systemic disease. Endocrine disorders such as thyroid disease and diabetes are known to profoundly affect cardiac function in ways that are not clearly understood.

Diabetes Mellitus

Maternal diabetes, especially insulin-dependent diabetes, results in transient and nonfamilial cardiomyopathy that is part of generalized organomegaly. The incidence is as high as 38%, as determined by echocardiography.[1] Pathologically, there is thickening of the septum, but typical histologic findings of myofiber disarray are absent.[2] The condition regresses with age and is considered transitory to the altered intrauterine environment of increased glucose exposure.

Diabetes' effects on the heart are mediated by alterations in serum lipids, direct effects of hyperglycemia and hyperinsulinemia, effects on the autonomic system, and changes in the cardiac microcirculation. The term "diabetic cardiomyopathy" is frequently used in the clinical literature to describe systolic and diastolic dysfunction in diabetic patients that appears to be independent of epicardial coronary disease and the effects of hypertension.[3,4]

There are several mechanisms by which diabetes affects cardiac contractility (Table 146.1). Diabetes is associated with dyslipidemia

TABLE 146.1 Diabetic Cardiomyopathy: Pathophysiology

Mechanisms
Dyslipidemia and oxidative stress
Advanced glycation end products

Experimental findings
Myocyte autophagy
Necrosis and apoptosis of myocytes, endothelial cells, fibroblasts
Up-regulation of cardiac sarcomeric genes

Clinical findings
Diastolic dysfunction
Systolic dysfunction
Cardiac hypertrophy

Histologic findings
Myocyte hypertrophy
Thickened small vessels
Interstitial and perivascular fibrosis

("metabolic syndrome") that accelerates atherosclerosis and may increase oxidative stress within the myocardium.[5] Increases in advanced glycation end products may lead to endothelial and myocyte damage[6] and have been demonstrated by immunolocalization techniques in the atherosclerotic plaques within the coronary arteries.[7] Glycation of apolipoprotein B may be associated with an increased risk of coronary events, and advanced glycation end products may result in the up-regulation of vascular adhesion molecules. An increased level of myocyte autophagy has been reported in experimental forms of diabetic cardiomyopathy.[8]

Epidemiologic data show a 2.5- to 5-fold increased risk of heart failure in diabetics, independent of hypertension and coronary disease.[9–11] Approximately 60% of adults with well-controlled type II diabetes have some evidence of cardiomyopathy based on echocardiographic findings of diastolic dysfunction and cardiac hypertrophy. Although clinical studies suggest the existence of "diabetic cardiomyopathy," causality has been questioned.[12,13] Echocardiographic studies in long-term diabetics have not supported a link between left ventricular dysfunction and type I diabetes.[14]

In addition to cardiomyopathy, the clinical manifestations of cardiac disease among diabetics include acute myocardial infarction and cardiac autonomic dysfunction. Pathologic studies of coronary artery disease in patients dying suddenly show diabetics are more likely to have extensive and distal disease, organized thrombi, and healed myocardial infarcts and are less likely to have acute thrombi than are normoglycemics.[15]

As mentioned above, pathologic findings in diabetic cardiomyopathy are nonspecific; many have been described in experimental models. Findings in the extracellular matrix include distortion of myocardial capillaries, thickening of capillary walls, and disorganization of contractile fibers within cardiac myocytes. A human study showed basement membrane thickening in the capillaries, small arterioles and venules, arteriolar hyalinization, and perivascular fibrosis.[14] Other findings include increased interstitial collagen and myocyte hypertrophy, which may be related to up-regulation of β-myosin heavy chain gene.[13] Increases in necrosis and apoptosis of myocytes, fibroblasts, and endothelial cells appear related to oxidative stress and are augmented by hypertension.[16]

Hypothyroidism

Hypothyroidism results from decreased levels of T4 and T3, with increases in serum thyroid-stimulating hormone. The cardiovascular manifestations of hypothyroidism include diastolic hypertension, sinus bradycardia due to sinus node dysfunction, and failure of the sinus node to accelerate normally under conditions of stress. Other cardiac manifestations may include heart block, pericarditis, and pericardial effusion. Approximately 4% of patients with hypothyroidism develop

TABLE 146.2 Cardiac Manifestations of Thyroid Disease

Hypothyroidism
Hypertension (especially diastolic)
Sinus bradycardia
Heart block
Pericarditis (especially "cholesterol" pericarditis)
Pericardial effusion
Cardiac tamponade
Dilated cardiomyopathy (low output)

Hyperthyroidism
High-output heart failure
Systolic hypertension
Left ventricular hypertrophy
Atrial fibrillation and flutter
Sinus tachycardia
Reversible dilated cardiomyopathy

pericarditis. Less commonly, there is cardiomyopathy, endocardial fibrosis, and myxomatous valvular changes[17] (Table 146.2).

Hypothyroidism, if long standing and untreated, may result in a constellation of cardiac effects historically termed "myxedema heart".[18-20] These include cardiac dilatation, low cardiac output, low electrical voltages on electrocardiogram, and flattened or inverted T waves: all findings that reverse with treatment. Massive pericardial effusions may also be the initial presentation of untreated hypothyroidism.[21] Physiologic effects of hypothyroidism on the circulation include decreased cardiac output, decreased stroke volume, and increased circulation time. There appears to be an increased risk of hypertension, due to a persistent low-renin state and increased peripheral vascular resistance. Even subclinical hypothyroidism is associated with decreased cardiac preload, increased afterload, and reductions in stroke volume and cardiac output.[22]

Biopsies of patients with heart failure secondary to myxedema are nonspecific and may show vacuolated myocytes indicative of chronic ischemia.[19] There is typically extensive basophilic degeneration of myocytes, although the finding is not specific for thyroid disease (Fig. 146.1).

The cause of pericardial effusion in hypothyroidism is not certain, but likely due to volume retention. The fluid may be golden in color due to cholesterol crystals (so-called cholesterol pericarditis, see Chapter 167).

Hyperthyroidism

Hyperthyroidism is characterized by a low serum thyroid stimulating hormone TSH level and elevated serum T4, T3, or both. Cardiovascular manifestations of hyperthyroidism include systolic hypertension, increased left ventricular mass, angina pectoris, and systolic murmurs due to high cardiac output. A minority of patients develop atrial fibrillation with its risk of stroke, atrial flutter, and high-output heart failure (Table 146.2). The most common rhythm is sinus tachycardia. In a series of patients with untreated hyperthyroidism, 15% had atrial fibrillation, the highest risk of stroke being in the elderly.[23]

The clinical differential diagnosis of heart failure associated with hyperthyroidism includes high-output failure (congestive state), tachycardia-induced cardiomyopathy (see Chapter 19), atrial fibrillation, and underlying organic heart disease. Types of structural heart disease that are increased in frequency in hyperthyroidism include coronary atherosclerosis, hypertensive heart disease, mitral valve prolapse, left ventricular dilatation leading to mitral regurgitation, and cardiac tamponade.

Pathologically, left ventricular hypertrophy is more prevalent in elderly patients who are hyperthyroid than in those who are euthyroid.[24] There is typically left or biventricular dilatation (Fig. 146.2). Histologically, the cardiac findings of hyperthyroidism are nonspecific and include myocyte necrosis, fibrosis, and rare lymphohistiocytic infiltrate.

Thyrotoxicosis has been associated with reversible dilated cardiomyopathy and takotsubo-like cardiomyopathy (stress-related cardiomyopathy, see Chapter 24).[25,26]

Hyperparathyroidism

Symptomatic primary hyperparathyroidism is associated with increased mortality due in large part to cardiovascular complications.[27,28] Up to 80% of patients with primary hyperparathyroidism have left ventricular hypertrophy, often complicated by systemic

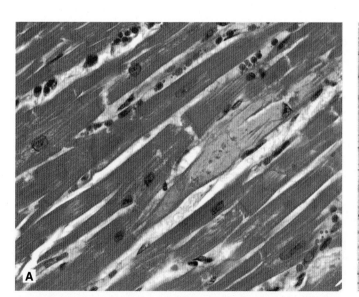
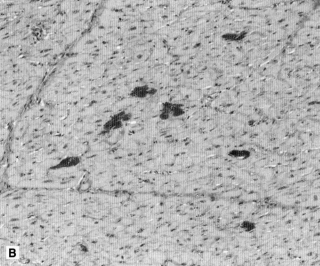

FIGURE 146.1 ▲ Basophilic degeneration in hypothyroidism. **A.** There is an inclusion in the myocyte cytoplasm. Although seen in hypothyroidism, basophilic degeneration is a nonspecific age-related change. **B.** Basophilic degeneration, PAS stain. The inclusions are strongly PAS positive. The deposits of basophilic degeneration are similar ultrastructurally and histochemically to the deposits of glycogenosis type IV, the glycogen deposits in Lafora type epilepsy, and corpora amylacea.

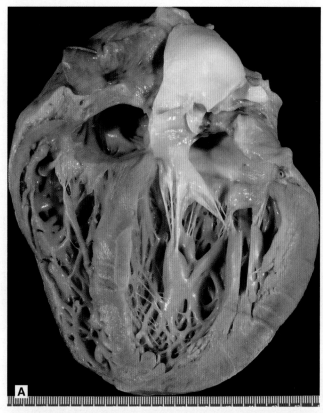

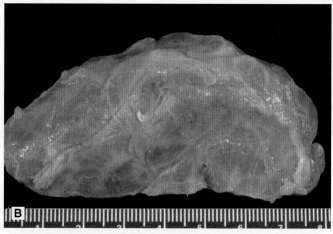

FIGURE 146.2 ▲ Dilated cardiomyopathy of thyrotoxicosis. The patient presented with signs of congestive heart failure and hyperthyroidism; the serum TSH was not measurable. **A.** Four-chamber view showing dilatation and left ventricular hypertrophy. **B.** The thyroid gland demonstrated diffuse enlargement; the histologic features (not shown) were typical of Graves disease.

arterial hypertension. By imaging, calcification of valves, especially aortic and mitral, is often present, in addition to myocardial calcifications[29] (Table 146.3). Marked calcification of the heart valves and myocytes in hyperparathyroidism has been designated "Stony heart."[30]

A direct effect of parathyroid hormone on cardiomyocytes has been shown only in vitro. Histologically, there can be myocyte hypertrophy and microscopic calcification (Fig. 146.3).

It is unclear if the cardiac hypertrophy seen in end-stage renal failure is mediated in part by secondary hyperparathyroidism or is due to other factors such as hypertension and anemia (see Chapter 6).

In patients with long-standing sepsis and multiorgan failure, calcification of contraction band necrosis can result in diffuse mineralization of the myocardium that can be seen by radiography and computed tomography.[31,32] The process is poorly understood but may be related to hyperparathyroidism secondary to renal failure resulting in dystrophic calcification of necrotic myocytes. In adults, myocardial calcification of infarcts is uncommon, although the accelerated metabolism in children leads to rapid calcification of ischemic myocytes (Figs. 146.4 and 146.5).

TABLE 146.3   Cardiac Manifestations of Hyperparathyroidism

- Left ventricular hypertrophy
- Diastolic dysfunction
- Mitral annular calcification
- Aortic valve calcification
- Myocardial calcification
- Sudden cardiac death

Adrenal Disease

Cushing syndrome results from increased levels of cortisol and may occur from oversecretion of ACTH by the pituitary (sometimes referred to as Cushing disease), primary tumors of the adrenal cortex, ectopic production of cortisol by nonadrenal tumors, or iatrogenic causes.

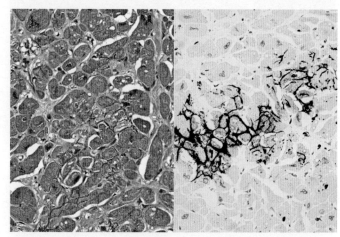

FIGURE 146.3 ▲ Cardiomyopathy of chronic renal failure with hyperparathyroidism. There is myocyte hypertrophy with prominent interstitial fibrosis and microscopic calcification (not evident on routine stains, **left**). von Kossa calcium stain (**right**) demonstrates interstitial calcifications. More commonly, there is calcification of the mitral annulus, aortic valve, and atherosclerotic plaques (not shown).

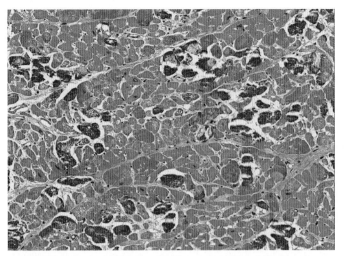

FIGURE 146.4 ▲ Contraction band necrosis with calcification. In patients with hyperparathyroidism secondary to chronic renal failure, areas of contraction band necrosis may calcify if there is sepsis and multiorgan failure. This process is in contrast to interstitial calcification. There are scattered individual calcified myocytes.

Cardiac complications of Cushing syndrome include accelerated atherosclerosis and concentric left ventricular hypertrophy. One in four patients with Cushing syndrome have left ventricular hypertrophy by echocardiogram.[33] The mechanism by which cortisol results in myocyte hypertrophy has not been elucidated. Reversible dilated cardiomyopathy has also been described in patients with Cushing syndrome, as a presenting symptom,[34,35] and has also been described in adrenal insufficiency (Addison syndrome).[36]

Cushing syndrome is associated with visceral obesity, systemic arterial hypertension, and the metabolic syndrome, which increase the risk of coronary artery disease, congestive heart failure, and cardiac stroke.[37]

Increased catecholamine levels due to *pheochromocytoma* or exogenous pressors may result in chronic myocardial damage and congestive heart failure. Patients with pheochromocytoma may present with a dilated cardiomyopathy reversed by normalization of circulating catecholamines by medical or surgical means.[38] Other causes of increased catecholamine release, such as brain death, or even severe emotional distress, may result in decreased left ventricular function (see Chapters 2 and 24). Histologically, the major features of cardiomyopathy related to catecholamines are isolated cells or groups of myocytes showing contraction band necrosis, with an associated inflammatory reaction composed of neutrophils and mononuclear cells. Catecholamine-mediated

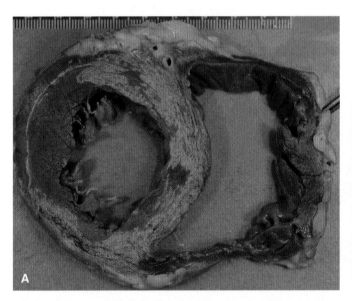

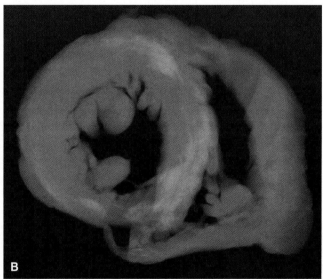

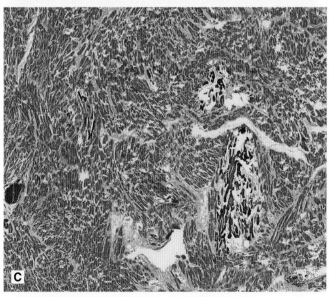

FIGURE 146.5 ▲ Sepsis-related calcification. Rarely, extensive myocyte necrosis can calcify in the setting of septic shock, treatment with pressors, and multiorgan failure, including renal failure with hyperparathyroidism. **A.** Grossly, the greenish areas of discoloration had a gritty texture on sectioning. **B.** The calcification can be extensive enough to be seen radiographically. **C.** Histologically, there are large areas of myocardial calcification.

toxicity is believed to be the result of beta-adrenoceptor–mediated cyclic adenosine monophosphate–dependent calcium overload of the cardiac myocyte.[39]

Acromegaly

The clinical manifestations of acromegalic cardiomyopathy include arrhythmias, valvular regurgitation, concentric left ventricular hypertrophy, and left ventricular diastolic dysfunction. Cardiovascular complications are the most common causes of morbidity and mortality in acromegaly with 50% to 60% of acromegalic patients dying from heart disease. Conduction defects are present in about 40% of patients. There are numerous supraventricular and ventricular arrhythmias that occur and are secondary to the underlying ventricular hypertrophy.

Eventually, systolic dysfunction with heart failure occurs. Heart failure from acromegalic cardiomyopathy is one of the most common causes of death in acromegaly.[40] In one large series of acromegalic patients, 4% had overt congestive heart failure, characterized by biventricular dysfunction and global hypokinesis. Aortic root diameters are also increased in patients with acromegaly compared with healthy controls.[41] Coexistent diseases that frequently affect cardiac function in acromegalic patients include diabetes mellitus, hypertension, and coronary artery disease.

Treatment of acromegalic heart disease includes octreotide therapy and resection of pituitary tumors.[42]

Autopsy findings are nonspecific and include concentric left ventricular hypertrophy, left ventricular dilatation, and myocyte hypertrophy with interstitial fibrosis.[42] Acromegalic cardiomyopathy is characterized by massive cardiac enlargement with myocyte hypertrophy and interstitial fibrosis. Sudden cardiac death has been reported, with autopsy findings of concentric left ventricular hypertrophy.[43]

REFERENCES

1. Abu-Sulaiman RM, Subaih B. Congenital heart disease in infants of diabetic mothers: echocardiographic study. *Pediatr Cardiol.* 2004;25:137–140.
2. Russell NE, Holloway P, Quinn S, et al. Cardiomyopathy and cardiomegaly in stillborn infants of diabetic mothers. *Pediatr Dev Pathol.* 2008;11:10–14.
3. Westermeier F, Navarro-Marquez M, Lopez-Crisosto C, et al. Defective insulin signaling and mitochondrial dynamics in diabetic cardiomyopathy. *Biochim Biophys Acta.* 2015;1853:1113–1118.
4. Seferovic PM, Paulus WJ. Clinical diabetic cardiomyopathy: a two-faced disease with restrictive and dilated phenotypes. *Eur Heart J.* 2015.
5. Liu Q, Wang S, Cai L. Diabetic cardiomyopathy and its mechanisms: role of oxidative stress and damage. *J Diabetes Investig.* 2014;5:623–634.
6. Bodiga VL, Eda SR, Bodiga S. Advanced glycation end products: role in pathology of diabetic cardiomyopathy. *Heart Fail Rev.* 2014;19:49–63.
7. Burke AP, Kolodgie FD, Zieske A, et al. Morphologic findings of coronary atherosclerotic plaques in diabetics: a postmortem study. *Arterioscler Thromb Vasc Biol.* 2004;24:1266–1271.
8. Kobayashi S, Liang Q. Autophagy and mitophagy in diabetic cardiomyopathy. *Biochim Biophys Acta.* 2015;1852:252–261.
9. Bertoni AG, Tsai A, Kasper EK, et al. Diabetes and idiopathic cardiomyopathy: a nationwide case–control study. *Diabetes Care.* 2003;26:2791–2795.
10. From AM, Leibson CL, Bursi F, et al. Diabetes in heart failure: prevalence and impact on outcome in the population. *Am J Med.* 2006;119:591–599.
11. Nichols GA, Hillier TA, Erbey JR, et al. Congestive heart failure in type 2 diabetes: prevalence, incidence, and risk factors. *Diabetes Care.* 2001;24:1614–1619.
12. Guha A, Harmancey R, Taegtmeyer H. Nonischemic heart failure in diabetes mellitus. *Curr Opin Cardiol.* 2008;23:241–248.
13. Letonja M, Petrovic D. Is diabetic cardiomyopathy a specific entity? *World J Cardiol.* 2014;6:8–13.
14. Konduracka E, Gackowski A, Rostoff P, et al. Diabetes-specific cardiomyopathy in type 1 diabetes mellitus: no evidence for its occurrence in the era of intensive insulin therapy. *Eur Heart J.* 2007;28:2465–2471.
15. Virmani R, Burke AP, Kolodgie F. Morphological characteristics of coronary atherosclerosis in diabetes mellitus. *Can J Cardiol.* 2006;22(Suppl B):81B–84B.
16. Frustaci A, Kajstura J, Chimenti C, et al. Myocardial cell death in human diabetes. *Circ Res.* 2000;87:1123–1132.
17. Grais IM, Sowers JR. Thyroid and the heart. *Am J Med.* 2014;127:691–698.
18. Dainauskas JR, Susmano A, Bogdonoff ML. Clinical-pathologic conference. Myxedema, and heart enlargement. *Am Heart J.* 1974;88:229–239.
19. Fujimoto K, Tagata M, Nagao M, et al. [A case of myxedema heart with serial endomyocardial biopsy]. *Kokyu To Junkan.* 1992;40:1019–1023.
20. Chaudhari D, Gangadharan V, Forrest T. Heart failure presenting as myxedema coma: case report and review article. *Tenn Med.* 2014;107:39–41.
21. Chiang WF, Wu KA, Liu KY, et al. Hypovolemia-induced cardiac Tamponade in a patient with hypothyroidism. *J Emerg Med.* 2012;43:e409–e412.
22. Ripoli A, Pingitore A, Favilli B, et al. Does subclinical hypothyroidism affect cardiac pump performance? Evidence from a magnetic resonance imaging study. *J Am Coll Cardiol.* 2005;45:439–445.
23. Petersen P, Hansen JM. Stroke in thyrotoxicosis with atrial fibrillation. *Stroke.* 1988;19:15–18.
24. de Carvalho Filho ET, Dias VL, Fernandes MC, et al. [Cardiac manifestations of hyperthyroidism in the elderly]. *Arq Bras Cardiol.* 1991;56:31–37.
25. Cakir M. Takotsubo cardiomyopathy in thyrotoxicosis. *Int J Cardiol.* 2010;145:499–500.
26. Rossor AM, Pearce SH, Adams PC. Left ventricular apical ballooning (takotsubo cardiomyopathy) in thyrotoxicosis. *Thyroid.* 2007;17:181–182.
27. Hedback G, Oden A. Increased risk of death from primary hyperparathyroidism—an update. *Eur J Clin Invest.* 1998;28:271–276.
28. Goswami S, Ghosh S. Hyperparathyroidism: cancer and mortality. *Indian J Endocrinol Metab.* 2012;16:S217–S220.
29. Andersson P, Rydberg E, Willenheimer R. Primary hyperparathyroidism and heart disease—a review. *Eur Heart J.* 2004;25:1776–1787.
30. Toniato A, Boschin IM. Stony heart and severe hyperparathyroidism. *ANZ J Surg.* 2007;77:802–803.
31. Rossi MA, Santos CS. Sepsis-related microvascular myocardial damage with giant cell inflammation and calcification. *Virchows Arch.* 2003;443:87–92.
32. Simonson S, Miller WT Jr, Perl A, et al. Diffuse left ventricular myocardial calcification in the setting of sepsis on CT imaging. *J Thorac Imaging.* 2007;22:343–345.
33. Muiesan ML, Lupia M, Salvetti M, et al. Left ventricular structural and functional characteristics in Cushing's syndrome. *J Am Coll Cardiol.* 2003;41:2275–2279.
34. Peppa M, Ikonomidis I, Hadjidakis D, et al. Dilated cardiomyopathy as the predominant feature of Cushing's syndrome. *Am J Med Sci.* 2009;338:252–253.
35. Marazuela M, Aguilar-Torres R, Benedicto A, et al. Dilated cardiomyopathy as a presenting feature of Cushing's syndrome. *Int J Cardiol.* 2003;88:331–333.
36. Derish M, Eckert K, Chin C. Reversible cardiomyopathy in a child with Addison's disease. *Intensive Care Med.* 1996;22:460–463.
37. De Leo M, Pivonello R, Auriemma RS, et al. Cardiovascular disease in Cushing's syndrome: heart versus vasculature. *Neuroendocrinology.* 2010;92(suppl 1):50–54.
38. Nanda AS, Feldman A, Liang CS. Acute reversal of pheochromocytoma-induced catecholamine cardiomyopathy. *Clin Cardiol.* 1995;18:421–423.
39. Baroldi G, Di Pasquale G, Silver MD, et al. Type and extent of myocardial injury related to brain damage and its significance in heart transplantation: a morphometric study. *J Heart Lung Transplant.* 1997;16:994–1000.
40. Schwarz ER, Jammula P, Gupta R, et al. A case and review of acromegaly-induced cardiomyopathy and the relationship between growth hormone and heart failure: cause or cure or neither or both? *J Cardiovasc Pharmacol Ther.* 2006;11:232–244.
41. van der Klaauw AA, Bax JJ, Smit JW, et al. Increased aortic root diameters in patients with acromegaly. *Eur J Endocrinol.* 2008;159:97–103.
42. Dutta P, Das S, Bhansali A, et al. Congestive heart failure in acromegaly: a review of 6 cases. *Indian J Endocrinol Metab.* 2012;16:987–990.
43. Comunello A, Dassie F, Martini C, et al. Heart rate variability is reduced in acromegaly patients and improved by treatment with somatostatin analogues. *Pituitary.* 2014;epub 27 Sept.

147 Cardiac Involvement in Rheumatologic Diseases

Allen P. Burke, M.D., and Fabio R. Tavora, M.D., Ph.D.

Acute Rheumatic Carditis

Incidence and Epidemiology

Acute rheumatic carditis is a common sequela of acute rheumatic fever. When it progresses to chronic rheumatic heart disease, it is a leading cause of heart failure in children and young adults, a common cause of cardiovascular mortality, and a predominant indication for cardiac surgery in poor countries.[1-4]

Acute rheumatic fever affects millions of people worldwide, and there are probably millions more that are not diagnosed.[5] The incidence in the United States is somewhat less than 1 in 100,000, compared to 19 per 100,000 worldwide, and over 50 per 100,000 in high-risk regions such as Northern India.[6]

The incidence of carditis in children with rheumatic fever is as high as 50% to 60%,[7] but the overall incidence is reported as 35% to 40%.[5,6] The most common manifestations are mitral insufficiency and pericarditis. Although myocardial inflammation with interstitial Aschoff nodules is frequent, true myocarditis with myocyte necrosis is rare.[8] Progression to chronic mitral and aortic valve disease occurs by adulthood in up to 60% of patients, almost half of whom do not recall a specific history of acute rheumatic fever.[6]

Risk factors for acute rheumatic fever include poverty, overcrowding, malnutrition, and maternal educational level and employment, but there are no identifiable risks for the development of acute pancarditis associated with the disease.[9,10]

Clinical Findings

The first episode of acute rheumatic fever usually occurs in children and young adolescents aged 5 to 14 years old. Presentation in those younger than 2 years or older than 35 years of age is rare.[6]

The clinical diagnosis of acute rheumatic fever is based on modified Jones criteria. Cardiac involvement is determined by significant apical systolic and/or basal diastolic murmurs, presence of pericarditis or unexplained congestive heart failure, and echocardiography or magnetic resonance imaging findings.[11-13] Carditis may be isolated, or associated with chorea or arthritis, or both.[7] Pericarditis and congestive heart failure almost never occur in the absence of valvular involvement, suggesting that primary myocarditis is uncommon.[13]

Rheumatic carditis is either *primary* or *recurrent*; recurrences are rare if the initial bout of rheumatic fever did not involve the heart. Recurrences are clinically defined as acute pericarditis or abrupt change in cardiac findings and are often difficult to diagnose if there is significant valvular disease. The use of Jones criteria in the evaluation of recurrent rheumatic fever is debated.[1] Despite antibiotic prophylaxis for secondary prevention, carditis frequently recurs especially when there is poor compliance. These recurrent episodes tend to mimic the initial attack and generally occur within the first 5 years.[6]

Clinically, acute rheumatic carditis results in sinus tachycardia, an extended PR interval on electrocardiogram and a pansystolic murmur. The most common functional lesion is mitral regurgitation due to acute valvulitis. Pericarditis may cause chest pain and pericardial friction in cases with effusion, but cardiac tamponade is rare.[14,15] Fulminant valvulitis causing death is also rare.[16] Subclinical valvulitis as seen on echocardiographic studies is not uncommon.[11,12,17] The risk of developing chronic rheumatic heart disease has been shown to directly correlate with the severity of carditis during the initial attack (Table 147.1).[6]

Pathogenesis

Acute rheumatic fever occurs as a sequel to upper respiratory tract infection by group A β-hemolytic streptococcal infections. The time interval between infection and systemic symptoms is commonly 2 to 5 weeks. The true pathogenesis of the carditis in rheumatic fever is unknown, and likely involves an altered immune response consisting of antibody-mediated and cellular components against cardiac proteins that show cross-reaction with epitopes from the bacteria. The adherence proteins M, T, and R of the microorganism probably share antigenic and molecular mimicry with several cardiac proteins such as cardiac myosin, tropomyosin, keratin, laminin, and vimentin. Different patterns of T-cell antigen cross-recognition have been identified in the process.[18] Another theory relates to the damage caused to the endothelial collagen matrix type IV collagen, which may explain the more systemic nature of the process in some individuals.[19] Cross-reactive antibodies bind to the endothelium with associated inflammatory infiltrates that mediate the up-regulation of VCAM-1.[20,21]

Pathologic Findings

The cardiac involvement by acute rheumatic fever usually involves endocardium, myocardium, and pericardium to various degrees, with at least half the patients presenting with cardiac inflammation involving the valvular endocardium (Table 147.2).[17,22]

Historically, Aschoff nodules have been described as the hallmark of rheumatic fever. Several studies have shown a high percentage of this finding in surgical specimens and endomyocardial biopsies in the older literature. The incidence of Aschoff bodies in the left atrial appendage ranges from 20% to 80% when these specimens were routinely removed during mitral commissurotomy for stenosis.[23,24] The presence of Aschoff nodules was also highly detected in autopsy studies from patients dying from acute rheumatic fever and can also be seen years after the initial illness, with no correlation with activity or severity of disease.[23-25] In endomyocardial biopsies, the frequency of finding Aschoff nodules is lower than in open surgical specimens, probably due to sampling, but one study found them in 22% of cases with suspected carditis clinically.[26] A more recent study observed Aschoff nodules in 21% of the myocardium of acute rheumatic fever patients undergoing valve replacement or repair procedures.[27]

Histologically, Aschoff nodules are characterized by a histiocytic-rich lesion that resembles a granuloma and that is round or oval, usually in the endocardium or in the perivascular regions of the myocardium (Figs. 147.1 and 147.2). There is a central area of fibrinoid necrosis surrounded by histiocytes that show a basophilic cytoplasm and a vesicular nucleus. These histiocytes have been denominated by Anitschkow cells or Aschoff cells (Fig. 147.3).

Established myocardial necrosis is only seldom present in endomyocardial biopsies from patients with confirmed rheumatic fever,[19,26] confirming clinical studies that only rarely show evidence of myocardial troponin elevations in the serum.[8,13]

In acute rheumatic fever, pericarditis is present in about one-fifth of the cases with confirmed histology, generally associated with underlying chronic inflammation. Pericarditis is usually fibrinous, with some cases showing the typical "bread and butter" appearance.[28] There is an overlying fibrin layer and associated inflammatory infiltrates in the stroma with edema and the presence of Aschoff nodules, especially in

TABLE 147.1   Evolution of Rheumatic Heart Disease

	Streptococcal Infection	Acute Rheumatic Fever (ARF)	Acute Rheumatic Carditis	Chronic Rheumatic Heart Disease
Incidence/ frequency	Ubiquitous	<1–50/100,000 incidence; 0.3% of streptococcal pharyngitis	30%–45% of ARF	60% over lifetime[a]
Age	All ages	5–14 years, common 2–5, 14–35 years, uncommon Other ages rare	Primary: same as ARF Recurrences: usually within 5 years	20–50 years of age typical
Time interval	—	2–5 weeks after acute infection	Usually occurs at same time as ARF; first manifestation at recurrent ARF is rare	For symptomatic disease, usually years
Characteristics	Groups A (*Streptococcus pyogenes*) pharyngitis Poststreptococcal glomerulonephritis Impetigo Necrotizing fasciitis	**Carditis**[b] **Polyarthritis** **Sydenham chorea** **Erythema marginatum** **Arthralgias** **Fever** Elevated inflammatory markers* Prolonged PR interval Preceding streptococcal infection Positive throat culture ASO titers	Pancarditis (see Table 147.2)	Mitral stenosis Mitral insufficiency Aortic stenosis and insufficiency
Risk factors	—	"Rheumatogenic" strains of *S. pyogenes* Ethnic subgroups[c] Overcrowding Low socioeconomic status Limited health care	Unknown; aggressive treatment of carditis with anti-inflammatory agents does not significantly decrease risk	Initially severe carditis; recurrences

[a]Many adults with typical findings of postinflammatory mitral/aortic valve disease (40%–50%) have no documented history of acute rheumatic fever as a child; therefore, true incidence is unknown.
[b]Major Jones criteria are in bold.
[c]Maori, aboriginal, Sub-Saharan Africans, Pacific Islanders.

TABLE 147.2   Most Common Gross and Histologic Findings in Specimens of Acute Rheumatic Carditis.

Site of Lesions	Gross Findings	Microscopic Findings
Endocardium	• Small friable vegetations on atrial surface of atrioventricular valves and ventricular surface of semilunar valves • Edema and granulation tissue • Valvular fibrosis and chordal fusion in chronic lesions	• Edema and inflammatory infiltrates in the various layers • Underlying chronic inflammation with lymphocytes and plasma cells • Aschoff bodies
Myocardium	• Most commonly no gross abnormalities • Globular enlargement if fatal cases	• Edema and nonspecific inflammation • Debatable if there are true foci of myocardial necrosis • Aschoff bodies, if present, are usually in the perivascular regions of the interventricular septum and posterior wall of LV
Pericardium	• Fibrinous pericarditis in about 1/5 of cases • Fibrous plaques may be present • Rarely the lesions persist with fibrous adhesions	• Fibrin layer with underlying acute and chronic inflammatory infiltrates • Aschoff bodies more common in younger patients

a perivascular distribution. Chronic fibrinous pericarditis is a rare phenomenon after resolution of the acute disease.[29]

Acute rheumatic fever may cause significant endocardial and consequently valvar inflammatory lesions, generally characterized by small 1- to 2-mm fibrinous vegetations seen on the atrial surface at sites of valve closure (Fig. 147.4). Histologically, they are associated with underlying chronic inflammatory infiltrates involving the valve leaflet, unlike marantic endocarditis. Aschoff bodies have been reported in the valvar tissue with variable prevalence.[23,28] Examination of valves reveals

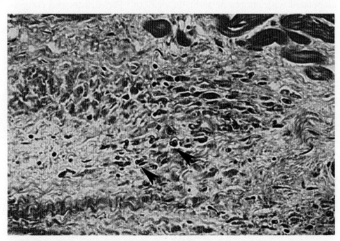

FIGURE 147.1 ▲ Aschoff nodule. There is an interstitial aggregate of macrophages and degenerating collagen. There are scattered Anitschkow cells (*arrows*).

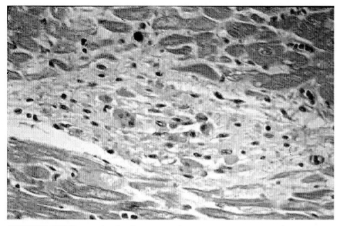

FIGURE 147.2 ▲ Aschoff nodule. There is vaguely granulomatous aggregate in the interstitium, with macrophages and lymphocytes.

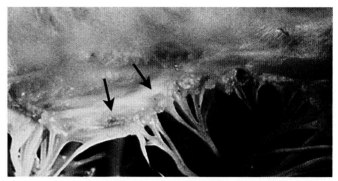

FIGURE 147.4 ▲ Verrucous vegetations, acute rheumatic fever. There are small uniform vegetations at the line of closure of the mitral valve (arrows).

that the mitral valve is most commonly affected, followed by the aortic, tricuspid, and, uncommonly, pulmonic valve. Valvular fibrosis occurs over time, when the disease progress to chronic rheumatic disease with regurgitation and/or stenosis clinically.

Treatment and Prognosis

The treatment of acute rheumatic fever aims first and foremost to eradicate the streptococci to avoid repetitive exposure to the bacterial antigens. However, antimicrobial therapy does not affect the frequency or severity of rheumatic carditis, and there is little consensus about therapy to prevent cardiac sequelae.[30] Treatment of the acute illness includes intravenous immunoglobulin, salicylates, and steroids.[6,10] The surgical treatment of valvular lesions is only rarely used in the acute setting and reserved for chronic rheumatic valvular disease.

Most patients recover from an episode of acute rheumatic carditis without sequelae, but the outcome worsens if the episodes recur.[4] Therefore, overall prognosis is mostly dependent on severity of carditis and recurrent episodes of rheumatic fever.[22] In all, it is estimated that 60% of patients will at one time in their lives develop chronic heart valve disease.[5,6]

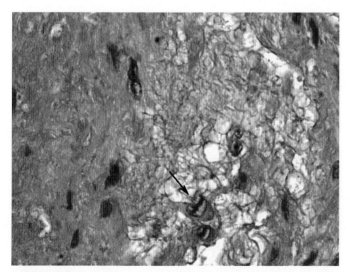

FIGURE 147.3 ▲ Anitschkow cell. This cell is present within Aschoff nodules but is nonspecific. The nucleus has a "caterpillar" appearance with a central linear groove (arrow).

Systemic Lupus Erythematosus

Incidence

Cardiac involvement in systemic lupus erythematosus is common and involves the pericardium, myocardium, and valves. By sensitive imaging techniques, up to 55% of patients have cardiovascular involvement, most frequently of the pericardium.[31] Symptomatic involvement of the heart with damage to valves or myocardium occurs in fewer than 5% of patients, however.[32] The risk for deep venous thrombosis and pulmonary embolism is 13 and 20 times the general population, respectively, with even higher risks in younger adults.[33] The risk is also increased in patients with antiphospholipid syndrome without overt lupus.[34]

Cardiovascular manifestations of lupus when they occur at the initial presentation of the disease include pericarditis with pericardial effusion (63%), followed by mitral regurgitation (63%), impairment of left ventricular systolic function (25%), and tricuspid regurgitation secondary to pulmonary hypertension (13%) (Table 147.3).[35]

A substantial proportion (6% to 40%) of deaths in patients with lupus is due to cardiovascular involvement, especially in late-onset systemic lupus erythematosus.[36,37]

Clinical

Pericarditis in patients with systemic lupus erythematosus is diagnosed primarily by echocardiography and is treated with steroids, intravenous immunoglobulin, and immunosuppressive drugs if necessary. Pericarditis is manifest by pericardial thickening with effusions. Progression to constrictive pericarditis or tamponade is uncommon.[38,39]

Valvular involvement in lupus involves the mitral and aortic valves and generally results in insufficiency. By echocardiography, there is thickening of the valve leaflets, often with characteristic verrucous vegetations (Libman-Sacks endocarditis). Mitral valve disease is typically asymptomatic and is detected in 40% to 60% of patients, higher rates seen with transesophageal echocardiography, a more sensitive modality.[31] Symptomatic patients may be treated with steroids, and if there is permanent valve damage, mitral valve replacement or repair is indicated.[39,40]

Myocardial involvement in lupus may be secondary to ischemia, drug toxicity (especially cyclophosphamide or chloroquine), or myocarditis. The incidence of myocarditis clinically is estimated as high as 10% and may be associated with anti-Ro/SSA autoantibodies.[31] The diagnosis is made by elevated serum troponins, antimyosin scintigraphy, and magnetic resonance imaging.[41,42] Treatment includes steroids, intravenous immunoglobulin, cyclophosphamide, and azathioprine.[39]

The risk of myocardial infarction is elevated four- to eightfold over that of the general population and is usually due to an increased

TABLE 147.3 Cardiac Involvement in Systemic Rheumatologic Disorders

	Incidence	Pericarditis	Myocardial Disease	Valve Disease	Coronary Arteritis
Systemic lupus erythematosus	55% (all) 5% (symptomatic)	60%	25% (myocarditis)	60% (Libman-Sacks mitral endocarditis and nonspecific insufficiency)	Rare
Idiopathic inflammatory myositis	25%	<10%	25% (myocarditis)	Rare	Rare
Systemic sclerosis	60%	50%	10%–30% (myocardial fibrosis)	Rare	Rare
Rheumatoid arthritis	33%	13%	33%	50%	10%
Wegener granulomatosis	10%–82%	20%	20%	10%	10%
Churg-Strauss	10%–70%	Uncommon	10% (eosinophilic myocarditis)	Uncommon	10%–20% (eosinophilic)
Polyarteritis nodosa*	20%	Uncommon	Uncommon	Uncommon	20%

prevalence of atherosclerosis in lupus patients. Other causes of myocardial infarction, especially in younger patients, include vasculitis and intramyocardial thrombosis.[31]

Pulmonary hypertension in patients with lupus occurs in up to 8% of patients and is multifactorial, including recurrent thromboembolism, left heart disease, and unknown causes.[43]

Pathologic Findings

The dominant cardiac findings in lupus include immune complex–mediated inflammation (myocarditis, valvulitis, and pericarditis), accelerated atherosclerosis, and intramural coronary thrombosis.[44] In classic autopsy series, pericarditis was found in 62%, myocarditis was found in 40%, and Libman-Sacks lesions were found in 43%.[45]

Pericarditis in lupus is indistinguishable from idiopathic pericarditis and is fibrinous in early stages, that can progress to a more fibrinous pericarditis with a serous effusion. Complement deposition can be documented by immunofluorescence in small vessels.[46]

The mitral valve most frequently shows nonspecific thickening and retraction resulting in insufficiency, presumably secondary to healed lesions. Libman-Sacks active lesions consist of fibrin on the surface of the valve, with focal necrosis and mononuclear cell infiltrates. Healed lesions show vascularized fibrous tissue sometimes associated with calcifications, which are indistinguishable from postinflammatory (rheumatic) valve disease (Fig. 147.5).[45]

Lupus myocarditis may be indistinguishable from viral myocarditis. However, the infiltrates are typically less diffuse, and there are small foci of fibrinoid necrosis of interstitial collagen, infiltrates of plasma cells and lymphocytes, and small patches of myocardial fibrosis (Fig. 147.6).[45–47]

Antiphospholipid Syndrome

The antiphospholipid syndrome has a high rate of cardiovascular complications and may be primary or associated with other autoimmune disorders, especially lupus erythematosus. The disorder is discussed in detail in Chapter 145.

Idiopathic Inflammatory Myositis (Polymyositis–Dermatomyositis)

Incidence

The true incidence of heart involvement with skeletal myositis is difficult to determine, because of lack of tissue sampling. Cardiac involvement as a cause of death in polymyositis has been reported as 10% to 20%.[48] A study 30 years ago showed a four-times increased overall mortality and a 16-times risk from myocardial infarction compared to the normal population.[49] The range in estimates of congestive heart failure observed in patients with idiopathic

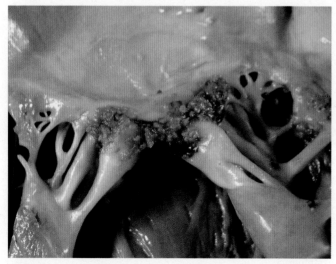

FIGURE 147.5 ▲ Libman-Sacks vegetations, lupus erythematosus. There is a small cluster of vegetations. The underlying valve shows chordal shortening and thickening.

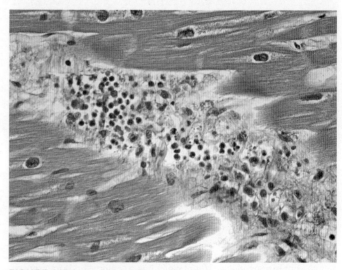

FIGURE 147.6 ▲ Lupus myocarditis. There is a sparse mixed inflammatory infiltrate with little necrosis.

inflammatory myositis is high, ranging between 3% and 45%.[48] Pericarditis is unusual in the inflammatory myopathies, occurring in fewer than 10% of patients.[48]

Clinical

The cardiac manifestations of idiopathic inflammatory myopathy include symptomatic heart failure and acute myocardial infarction, and subclinical conduction system disturbances and ventricular dysfunction. A small study showed that 25% of patients had heart failure.[50] Coronary heart disease with angina pectoris and myocardial infarction have been described, although the frequency is uncertain. Vasospastic angina that accompanied small vessel disease of the heart was reported in one case with dermatomyositis and Raynaud phenomenon.[51]

Subclinical left ventricular diastolic dysfunction has been reported in 12% to 42% of myositis patients.[48] Subclinical electrocardiographic changes are seen in 32.5% to 72% and include atrial and ventricular arrhythmias, bundle-branch block, atrioventricular blocks, prolongation of PR intervals, ventricular premature beats, abnormal Q waves, as well as nonspecific ST- and T-wave changes.[48]

Pathologic Findings

Although it could be predicted that myocardial involvement in idiopathic inflammatory myopathies would manifest as myocarditis, there are few histologic data to confirm this. Autopsy studies prior to the year 2000 have shown mononuclear inflammatory cell infiltrates localized to the endomysium and to the perivascular areas of the myocardium with necrosis of cardiac myocytes and cells of the conducting system.[52-54] A case report in a child with polymyositis demonstrated capillary necrosis and secondary thrombosis, associated with extensive hemorrhagic myocardial necrosis.[55] An endomyocardial biopsy performed in a woman with polymyositis/mixed connective tissue disease demonstrated myocarditis (Table 147.3).[56]

Systemic Sclerosis

Incidence

The most dominant cardiovascular manifestations of systemic sclerosis are peripheral vascular disease and pulmonary arterial hypertension. As with other autoimmune disorders, pericardial involvement is common, with 50% of patients showing at least subclinical pericardial inflammation and 16% to 30% of patients manifesting clinical pericarditis during the course of the disease.[57]

Clinically, 21% of patients demonstrate myocardial dysfunction, about half of which may be due to intrinsic cardiac involvement.[58] Autopsy and imaging studies suggest that one-third to one-half of patients have some degree of myocardial fibrosis intrinsic to the disease.[59,60]

Whether accelerated atherosclerosis arises in patients with systemic sclerosis remains controversial.[9] Valvular disease and fibrosis of the conduction system have been reported in systemic sclerosis.[61]

Clinical

Cardiac involvement in systemic sclerosis is recognized as a poor prognostic factor when clinically evident.[62] In patients without overt cardiac manifestations, magnetic resonance imaging using myocardial T1 mapping with extracellular volume quantification showed focal fibrosis in 53% of patients with areas of myocardial edema in one-third.[60] Right ventricular dysfunction is common and usually related to pulmonary hypertension but may also be due to intrinsic myocardial disease.[9] The use of serum troponin screening to identify phases of acute muscle injury has been proposed.[63] Overt left heart failure, conduction system abnormalities, and sudden cardiac death occur uncommonly, in <2% of patients, often in patients with coexistent skeletal myopathy.[58]

Pathologic Findings

Nonspecific interstitial fibrosis is seen in 33% of autopsy hearts with systemic sclerosis, when controlled for fibrosis in control hearts.[59] It has been proposed that recurrent vasospasm, together with irreversible structural lesions, leads to repeated focal ischemia and eventual myocardial fibrosis.[64] An anecdotal report of severe myocyte damage with contraction band necrosis, but without fibrosis or inflammation, in a scleroderma patient dying from heart failure, supports this concept.[58]

Rheumatoid Arthritis

Incidence

Rheumatoid arthritis is associated with an increased risk of coronary artery disease, myocardial infarction, and valve disease.[65] Rheumatoid arthritis increases the risk of sudden cardiac death, ischemic heart disease, and heart failure by 1.5- to twofold over the general population.[66] In a 10-year follow-up study, 2% to 3% of patients with rheumatoid arthritis developed pericarditis, with a similar proportion developing visceral, including coronary, arteritis.[67] Cross-sectional studies show that pericarditis is present in 13% of patients, with an increased rate of mitral insufficiency (80%) and left ventricular systolic dysfunction (37%).[68] Patients with rheumatoid arthritis are three to five times as likely to have echocardiographic evidence of mitral or aortic valve thickening or calcification.[65]

Clinical

Cardiac symptoms in rheumatoid arthritis are associated with abnormal cardiac enzymes in 25%, abnormal wall motion in 10%, and cardiac magnetic resonance imaging findings suggestive of myocarditis in the majority. Patients with presumed myocarditis have a predisposition for relapse and the development of heart failure.[69]

Pathologic Findings

Heart biopsies in rheumatoid arthritis patients and clinical evidence of myocarditis have shown nonspecific inflammation consistent with myocarditis.[69]

Autopsy studies have shown coronary arteritis in 10% with infarcts in a subset of these. Rheumatoid nodules may be present in the myocardium, valve leaflets, and epicardium.[70]

Atherosclerotic plaques in patients dying with rheumatoid arthritis show an increase in inflammation and vulnerable plaques compared to those in patients without rheumatoid arthritis.[71]

Systemic Vasculitic Syndromes

Granulomatosis with Polyangiitis

Cardiac involvement in granulomatosis with polyangiitis (Wegener granulomatosis) is often thought of as rare, although some studies show a rate of up to 44%. Pericarditis, coronary arteritis, myocarditis, valvulitis, and arrhythmias are the most common manifestations of cardiac involvement.[72]

In a series of patients with extensive disease refractory to treatment, cardiac involvement was present in 82%, manifest as regional wall motion abnormalities and necrotic inflammatory lesions seen on cardiac magnetic resonance imaging. Pericardial effusion was observed infrequently.[73] Valve disease, especially of the aortic valve, may manifest as sterile endocarditis and aortic insufficiency, necessitating valve replacement.[74]

Pathologically, valve lesions resemble infectious endocarditis,[75] but lesions are sterile, and no organisms are identified on tissue sections. Myocardial and pericardial involvement is generally manifest as vasculitis (Fig. 147.7A, B) that may focally involve epicardial arteries (Fig. 147.7C).

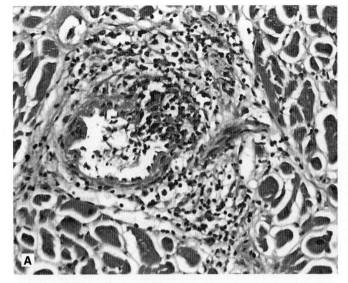

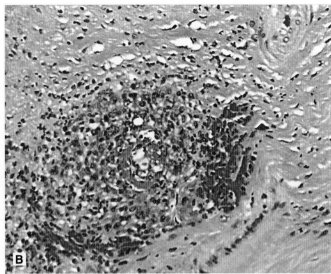

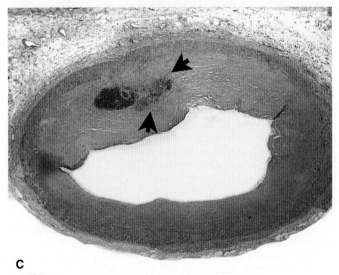

FIGURE 147.7 ▲ Granulomatosis with polyangiitis, heart. **A.** Myocardial involvement with segmental mixed inflammation of a small muscular artery. **B.** Pericardial involvement showing necrotizing vasculitis with fibrinoid necrosis. **C.** Area of necrosis in the intimal of an epicardial coronary artery (*arrows*).

Eosinophilic Granulomatosis with Polyangiitis

Heart involvement is the leading cause of death in patients with eosinophilic granulomatosis with polyangiitis (Churg-Strauss syndrome) and is more frequent in antineutrophil cytoplasmic antibody–negative patients. Overall, more than 50% of patients have cardiac involvement, which is the major cause of morbidity and mortality.[76] However, a prospective series demonstrated that only 2 of 19 patients with eosinophilic granulomatosis with polyangiitis developed cardiac involvement.[77] Cross-sectional studies have shown that two-thirds of patients show subclinical evidence of heart involvement, especially in ANCA-negative and younger patients.[78]

Autopsy studies have shown necrotizing, granulomatous arteritis of medium-sized arteries, extravascular granulomas and fibrosis in the interstitium of the heart, and tissue infiltration by eosinophils with myocyte necrosis (Fig. 147.8).[79] In some cases, the predominant finding is eosinophilic myocarditis.[80] An explant study of antineutrophil antibody–negative patients with end-stage cardiomyopathy secondary to eosinophilic granulomatosis with polyangiitis showed that heart failure was a presenting symptom in half and occurred between 1 and 24 years of onset of symptoms in the remainder. Endomyocardial biopsies performed prior to transplant showed eosinophilic infiltrates in 5/7, two of which had arteritis. One-third of explants showed arteritis with fibrinoid necrosis, nearly one-half showed eosinophilic myocarditis, one with giant cells, and the remainder with nonspecific findings, including interstitial fibrosis.[81]

Polyarteritis Nodosa

The incidence of coronary involvement in polyarteritis nodosa is unknown. One study showed that over one-fifth of patients have coronary involvement, which is a major factor increasing the risk for death. Cardiomyopathy is less common but also associated with overall mortality.[82]

Polyarteritis nodosa may also involve the pericardium and be diagnosed on pathologic evaluation of pericardiectomy specimens.[83]

Coronary involvement by polyarteritis nodosa typically results in aneurysms, which are typically concomitant with renal or mesenteric aneurysms.[84] Myocardial infarction may be the result of thrombosed aneurysms.[85] Coronary aneurysms caused by polyarteritis nodosa may be detected by magnetic resonance imaging or angiography.[86,87]

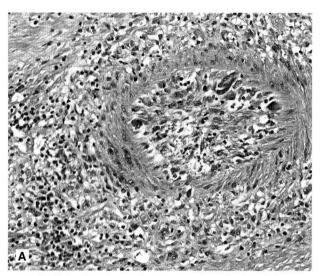
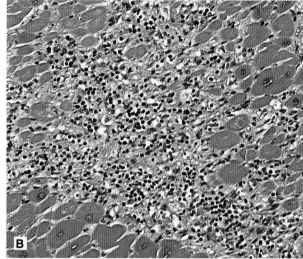

FIGURE 147.8 ▲ Eosinophilic granulomatosis with polyangiitis, heart. **A.** There is vasculitis obliterating a small muscular artery, with mixed inflammation including eosinophils. **B.** Myocarditis is manifest as mixed inflammation including abundant eosinophils.

REFERENCES

1. Narula J, Chandrasekhar Y, Rahimtoola S. Diagnosis of active rheumatic carditis. The echoes of change. *Circulation.* 1999;100:1576–1581.
2. Krishnaswami S, Joseph G, Richard J. Demands on tertiary care for cardiovascular diseases in India: analysis of data for 1960–89. *Bull World Health Organ.* 1991;69:325–330.
3. Ralph AP, Carapetis JR. Group a streptococcal diseases and their global burden. *Curr Top Microbiol Immunol.* 2013;368:1–27.
4. Carapetis JR, Steer AC, Mulholland EK, et al. The global burden of group A streptococcal diseases. *Lancet Infect Dis.* 2005;5:685–694.
5. Marijon E, Ou P, Celermajer DS, et al. Prevalence of rheumatic heart disease detected by echocardiographic screening. *N Engl J Med.* 2007;357:470–476.
6. Lee JL, Naguwa SM, Cheema GS, et al. Acute rheumatic fever and its consequences: a persistent threat to developing nations in the 21st century. *Autoimmun Rev.* 2009;9:117–123.
7. Tani LY, Veasy LG, Minich LL, et al. Rheumatic fever in children younger than 5 years: is the presentation different? *Pediatrics.* 2003;112:1065–1068.
8. Kamblock J. Does rheumatic myocarditis really exists? Systematic study with echocardiography and cardiac troponin I blood levels. *Eur Heart J.* 2003;24:855–862.
9. Goldblatt F, O'Neill SG. Clinical aspects of autoimmune rheumatic diseases. *Lancet.* 2013;382:797–808.
10. Marijon E, Mirabel M, Celermajer DS, et al. Rheumatic heart disease. *Lancet.* 2012;379:953–964.
11. Hilario MO, Andrade JL, Gasparian AB, et al. The value of echocardiography in the diagnosis and followup of rheumatic carditis in children and adolescents: a 2 year prospective study. *J Rheumatol.* 2000;27:1082–1086.
12. Shivaram P, Ahmed MI, Kariyanna PT, et al. Doppler echocardiography imaging in detecting multi-valvular lesions: a clinical evaluation in children with acute rheumatic fever. *PLoS One.* 2013;8:e74114.
13. Xavier JL, Jr, Matos Soeiro A, Lopes AS, et al. Clinically manifested myocarditis in acute rheumatic fever. *Arq Bras Cardiol.* 2014;102:e17–e20.
14. Special Writing Group of the Committee on Rheumatic Fever E, and Kawasaki Disease of the Council on Cardiovascular Disease in the Young of the American Heart Association. Guidelines for the diagnosis of rheumatic fever. Jones Criteria, 1992 update. Special Writing Group of the Committee on Rheumatic Fever, Endocarditis, and Kawasaki Disease of the Council on Cardiovascular Disease in the Young of the American Heart Association. *JAMA.* 1992;268:2069–2073.
15. Chockalingam A, Gnanavelu G, Elangovan S, et al. Current profile of acute rheumatic fever and valvulitis in southern India. *J Heart Valve Dis.* 2003;12:573–576.
16. Crain FE, Pham N, Wagoner SF, et al. Fulminant valvulitis from acute rheumatic fever: successful use of extracorporeal support. *Pediatr Crit Care Med.* 2011;12:e155–e158.
17. Caldas AM, Terreri MT, Moises VA, et al. What is the true frequency of carditis in acute rheumatic fever? A prospective clinical and Doppler blind study of 56 children with up to 60 months of follow-up evaluation. *Pediatr Cardiol.* 2008;29:1048–1053.
18. Cunningham MW. Pathogenesis of group A streptococcal infections. *Clin Microbiol Rev.* 2000;13:470–511.
19. Tandon R, Sharma M, Chandrashekhar Y, et al. Revisiting the pathogenesis of rheumatic fever and carditis. *Nat Rev Cardiol.* 2013;10:171–177.
20. Galvin JE, Hemric ME, Ward K, et al. Cytotoxic mAb from rheumatic carditis recognizes heart valves and laminin. *J Clin Invest.* 2000;106: 217–224.
21. Roberts S, Kosanke S, Terrence Dunn S, et al. Pathogenic mechanisms in rheumatic carditis: focus on valvular endothelium. *J Infect Dis.* 2001;183:507–511.
22. Meira ZM, Goulart EM, Colosimo EA, et al. Long term follow up of rheumatic fever and predictors of severe rheumatic valvar disease in Brazilian children and adolescents. *Heart.* 2005;91:1019–1022.
23. Thomas WA, Averill JH, Castleman B, et al. The significance of Aschoff bodies in the left atrial appendage; a comparison of 40 biopsies removed during mitral commissurotomy with autopsy material from 40 patients dying with fulminating rheumatic fever. *N Engl J Med.* 1953;249:761–765.
24. Virmani R and Roberts WC. Aschoff bodies in operatively excised atrial appendages and in papillary muscles. Frequency and clinical significance. *Circulation.* 1977;55:559–563.
25. Gross L, Ehrlich JC. Studies on the myocardial Aschoff body: II. Life cycle, sites of predilection and relation to clinical course of rheumatic fever. *Am J Pathol.* 1934;10:489–504.1.
26. Narula J, Chopra P, Talwar KK, et al. Does endomyocardial biopsy aid in the diagnosis of active rheumatic carditis? *Circulation.* 1993;88:2198–2205.
27. Sampaio RO, Fae KC, Demarchi LM, et al. Rheumatic heart disease: 15 years of clinical and immunological follow-up. *Vasc Health Risk Manag.* 2007;3:1007–1017.
28. Virmani R, Farb A, Burke AP, et al. In: Virmani R, Reddy KS, Tandon R, eds. *Rheumatic Fever.* Washington, DC: American Registry of Pathology; 1999:217–234.
29. Okada R. [Clinicopathological analysis of rheumatic heart disease]. *J Cardiol.* 1996;27(suppl 2):3–11; discussion 12–13.
30. Cilliers A, Manyemba J, Adler AJ, et al. Anti-inflammatory treatment for carditis in acute rheumatic fever. *Cochrane Database Syst Rev.* 2012;(6):CD003176.
31. Doria A, Iaccarino L, Sarzi-Puttini P, et al. Cardiac involvement in systemic lupus erythematosus. *Lupus.* 2005;14:683–686.
32. Cervera R, Doria A, Amoura Z, et al. Patterns of systemic lupus erythematosus expression in Europe. *Autoimmun Rev.* 2014;13:621–629.
33. Chung WS, Lin CL, Chang SN, et al. Systemic lupus erythematosus increases the risks of deep vein thrombosis and pulmonary embolism: a nationwide cohort study. *J Thromb Haemost.* 2014;12:452–458.

34. Reynaud Q, Lega JC, Mismetti P, et al. Risk of venous and arterial thrombosis according to type of antiphospholipid antibodies in adults without systemic lupus erythematosus: a systematic review and meta-analysis. *Autoimmun Rev.* 2014;13:595–608.
35. Chen PY, Chang CH, Hsu CC, et al. Systemic lupus erythematosus presenting with cardiac symptoms. *Am J Emerg Med.* 2014;32:1117–1119.
36. Cartella S, Cavazzana I, Ceribelli A, et al. Evaluation of mortality, disease activity, treatment, clinical and immunological features of adult and late onset systemic Lupus erythematosus. *Autoimmunity.* 2013;46:363–368.
37. Jakes RW, Bae SC, Louthrenoo W, et al. Systematic review of the epidemiology of systemic lupus erythematosus in the Asia-Pacific region: prevalence, incidence, clinical features, and mortality. *Arthritis Care Res (Hoboken).* 2012;64:159–168.
38. Kruzliak P, Novak M, Piler P, et al. Pericardial involvement in systemic lupus erythematosus: current diagnosis and therapy. *Acta Cardiol.* 2013;68:629–633.
39. Tincani A, Rebaioli CB, Taglietti M, et al. Heart involvement in systemic lupus erythematosus, anti-phospholipid syndrome and neonatal lupus. *Rheumatology (Oxford).* 2006;45(suppl 4):iv8–iv13.
40. Foroughi M, Hekmat M, Ghorbani M, et al. Mitral valve surgery in patients with systemic lupus erythematosus. *Scientific World Journal.* 2014;2014:216291.
41. Singh JA, Woodard PK, Davila-Roman VG, et al. Cardiac magnetic resonance imaging abnormalities in systemic lupus erythematosus: a preliminary report. *Lupus.* 2005;14:137–144.
42. Manautou L, Jerjes-Sanchez C, Meraz M, et al. Myopericarditis with predominantly right ventricular involvement with normal B-type natriuretic peptide and cardiac tamponade as the initial manifestation of systemic lupus erythematosus. *Lupus.* 2014;23:935–938.
43. Akdogan A, Kilic L, Dogan I, et al. Pulmonary hypertension in systemic lupus erythematosus: pulmonary thromboembolism is the leading cause. *J Clin Rheumatol.* 2013;19:421–425.
44. Ashrafi R, Garg P, McKay E, et al. Aggressive cardiac involvement in systemic lupus erythematosus: a case report and a comprehensive literature review. *Cardiol Res Pract.* 2011;2011:578390.
45. Doherty NE, Siegel RJ. Cardiovascular manifestations of systemic lupus erythematosus. *Am Heart J.* 1985;110:1257–1265.
46. Bidani AK, Roberts JL, Schwartz MM, et al. Immunopathology of cardiac lesions in fatal systemic lupus erythematosus. *Am J Med.* 1980;69:849–858.
47. Bulkley BH, Roberts WC. The heart in systemic lupus erythematosus and the changes induced in it by corticosteroid therapy. A study of 36 necropsy patients. *Am J Med.* 1975;58:243–264.
48. Lundberg IE. The heart in dermatomyositis and polymyositis. *Rheumatology (Oxford).* 2006;45(suppl 4):iv18–iv21.
49. DeVere R, Bradley WG. Polymyositis: its presentation, morbidity and mortality. *Brain.* 1975;98:637–666.
50. Oka M, Raasakka T. Cardiac involvement in polymyositis. *Scand J Rheumatol.* 1978;7:203–208.
51. Riemekasten G, Opitz C, Audring H, et al. Beware of the heart: the multiple picture of cardiac involvement in myositis. *Rheumatology (Oxford).* 1999;38:1153–1157.
52. Denbow CE, Lie JT, Tancredi RG, et al. Cardiac involvement in polymyositis: a clinicopathologic study of 20 autopsied patients. *Arthritis Rheum.* 1979;22:1088–1092.
53. Haupt HM, Hutchins GM. The heart and cardiac conduction system in polymyositis-dermatomyositis: a clinicopathologic study of 16 autopsied patients. *Am J Cardiol.* 1982;50:998–1006.
54. Lightfoot PR, Bharati S, Lev M. Chronic dermatomyositis with intermittent trifascicular block. An electrophysiologic-conduction system correlation. *Chest.* 1977;71:413–416.
55. Jimenez C, Rowe PC, Keene D. Cardiac and central nervous system vasculitis in a child with dermatomyositis. *J Child Neurol.* 1994;9:297–300.
56. Pardo J, Meruane J, Staeding J, et al. [Cardiac involvement in polymyositis–dermatomyositis associated with Sjogren's syndrome]. *Rev Med Chil.* 1995;122:550–555.
57. Gowda RM, Khan IA, Sacchi TJ, et al. Scleroderma pericardial disease presented with a large pericardial effusion—a case report. *Angiology.* 2001;52:59–62.
58. Follansbee WP, Zerbe TR, Medsger TA Jr. Cardiac and skeletal muscle disease in systemic sclerosis (scleroderma): a high risk association. *Am Heart J.* 1993;125:194–203.
59. Follansbee WP, Miller TR, Curtiss EI, et al. A controlled clinicopathologic study of myocardial fibrosis in systemic sclerosis (scleroderma). *J Rheumatol.* 1990;17:656–662.
60. Ntusi NA, Piechnik SK, Francis JM, et al. Subclinical myocardial inflammation and diffuse fibrosis are common in systemic sclerosis—a clinical study using myocardial T1-mapping and extracellular volume quantification. *J Cardiovasc Magn Reson.* 2014;16:21.
61. Lambova S. Cardiac manifestations in systemic sclerosis. *World J Cardiol* 2014;6:993–1005.
62. Allanore Y, Meune C. Primary myocardial involvement in systemic sclerosis: evidence for a microvascular origin. *Clin Exp Rheumatol.* 2010;28:S48–S53.
63. Hughes M, Lilleker JB, Herrick AL, et al. Cardiac troponin testing in idiopathic inflammatory myopathies and systemic sclerosis-spectrum disorders: biomarkers to distinguish between primary cardiac involvement and low-grade skeletal muscle disease activity. *Ann Rheum Dis.* 2015;74(5):795–798.
64. Ngian GS, Sahhar J, Wicks IP, et al. Cardiovascular disease in systemic sclerosis—an emerging association? *Arthritis Res Ther.* 2011;13:237.
65. Corrao S, Messina S, Pistone G, et al. Heart involvement in rheumatoid arthritis: systematic review and meta-analysis. *Int J Cardiol.* 2013;167:2031–2038.
66. Lazzerini PE, Capecchi PL, Acampa M, et al. Arrhythmic risk in rheumatoid arthritis: the driving role of systemic inflammation. *Autoimmun Rev.* 2014;13:936–944.
67. Turesson C, O'Fallon WM, Crowson CS, et al. Occurrence of extraarticular disease manifestations is associated with excess mortality in a community based cohort of patients with rheumatoid arthritis. *J Rheumatol.* 2002;29:62–67.
68. Guedes C, Bianchi-Fior P, Cormier B, et al. Cardiac manifestations of rheumatoid arthritis: a case–control transesophageal echocardiography study in 30 patients. *Arthritis Rheum.* 2001;45:129–135.
69. Mavrogeni S, Bratis K, Sfendouraki E, et al. Myopericarditis, as the first sign of rheumatoid arthritis relapse, evaluated by cardiac magnetic resonance. *Inflamm Allergy Drug Targets.* 2013;12:206–211.
70. Bely M, Apathy A, Beke-Martos E. Cardiac changes in rheumatoid arthritis. *Acta Morphol Hung.* 1992;40:149–186.
71. Aubry MC, Maradit-Kremers H, Reinalda MS, et al. Differences in atherosclerotic coronary heart disease between subjects with and without rheumatoid arthritis. *J Rheumatol.* 2007;34:937–942.
72. Goodfield NE, Bhandari S, Plant WD, et al. Cardiac involvement in Wegener's granulomatosis. *Br Heart J.* 1995;73:110–115.
73. Miszalski-Jamka T, Szczeklik W, Sokolowska B, et al. Cardiac involvement in Wegener's granulomatosis resistant to induction therapy. *Eur Radiol.* 2011;21:2297–2304.
74. Morelli S, Gurgo Di Castelmenardo AM, Conti F, et al. Cardiac involvement in patients with Wegener's granulomatosis. *Rheumatol Int.* 2000;19:209–212.
75. Mishell JM. Cases from the Osler Medical Service at Johns Hopkins University: cardiac valvular lesions in Wegener's granulamatosis. *Am J Med.* 2002;113:607–609.
76. Nadeau PL, Kumar A, O'Connor K, et al. Usefulness of cardiac resonance imaging in Churg-Strauss syndrome. *J Cardiovasc Med (Hagerstown).* 2014.
77. Whyte AF, Smith WB, Sinkar SN, et al. Clinical and laboratory characteristics of 19 patients with Churg-Strauss syndrome from a single South Australian centre. *Intern Med J.* 2013;43:784–790.
78. Vinit J, Bielefeld P, Muller G, et al. Heart involvement in Churg-Strauss syndrome: retrospective study in French Burgundy population in past 10 years. *Eur J Intern Med.* 2010;21:341–346.
79. Sasaki A, Hasegawa M, Nakazato Y, et al. Allergic granulomatosis and angiitis (Churg-Strauss syndrome). Report of an autopsy case in a nonasthmatic patient. *Acta Pathol Jpn.* 1988;38:761–768.
80. Setoguchi M, Okishige K, Sugiyama K, et al. Sudden cardiac death associated with Churg-Strauss syndrome. *Circ J.* 2009;73:2355–2359.
81. Groh M, Masciocco G, Kirchner E, et al. Heart transplantation in patients with eosinophilic granulomatosis with polyangiitis (Churg-Strauss syndrome). *J Heart Lung Transplant.* 2014;33:842–850.
82. Bourgarit A, Le Toumelin P, Pagnoux C, et al. Deaths occurring during the first year after treatment onset for polyarteritis nodosa, microscopic polyangiitis, and Churg-Strauss syndrome: a retrospective analysis of causes and factors predictive of mortality based on 595 patients. *Medicine (Baltimore).* 2005;84:323–330.
83. Hu PJ, Shih IM, Hutchins GM, et al. Polyarteritis nodosa of the pericardium: antemortem diagnosis in a pericardiectomy specimen. *J Rheumatol.* 1997;24:2042–2044.
84. Hwang J, Yang JH, Kim DK, et al. Polyarteritis nodosa involving renal and coronary arteries. *J Am Coll Cardiol.* 2012;59:e13.
85. Kastner D, Gaffney M, Tak T. Polyarteritis nodosa and myocardial infarction. *Can J Cardiol.* 2000;16:515–518.
86. Kobayashi H, Yokoe I, Hattan N, et al. Cardiac magnetic resonance imaging in polyarteritis nodosa. *J Rheumatol.* 2010;37:2427–2429.
87. Maillard-Lefebvre H, Launay D, Mouquet F, et al. Polyarteritis nodosa-related coronary aneurysms. *J Rheumatol.* 2008;35:933–934.

148 Cardiac Amyloidosis

Joseph J. Maleszewski, M.D., and Allen P. Burke, M.D.

Introduction

General

Amyloidosis is the deposition of misfolded protein with an antiparallel β-pleated sheet configuration in a variety of organs including the heart.[1] Amyloidosis is generally systemic, although localized forms involving particular types of amyloid have been described, including in both the heart and lung (Chapter 27). Although the histologic appearance and histochemical staining characteristics are identical regardless of the protein precursor, amyloid typing has become essential, as treatment is directed at the underlying disease process or, in some instances, the protein itself.

Classification

The classification of the amyloidoses is evolving, but currently is driven primarily by the type of misfolded protein present in tissue (Table 148.1). Cardiac amyloidosis can be broadly divided into acquired and hereditary forms, the latter characterized by the deposition of mutant proteins. While light chain (AL)-type amyloidosis is responsible for most (~80%) cases of cardiac amyloidosis overall, the majority (approximately two-thirds) of cases seen at cardiac biopsy for symptomatic amyloidosis are of the transthyretin (ATTR) variety, owing to selection biopsy of those that undergo endomyocardial sampling.

All amyloidoses are named by designating the abbreviated name of the protein with the letter "A" (meaning *amyloid*).[2] Therefore, transthyretin-type amyloidosis is abbreviated ATTR, (A [amyloid] +TTR [the abbreviated name of the protein]). ATTR-type amyloidosis includes both mutant (hereditary) and acquired (wild-type) forms. The latter instance is sometimes referred to as *senile systemic amyloidosis*; however, the term *wild-type ATTR amyloidosis* is now strongly preferred. Alternatively, wild-type and mutant ATTR have been designated ATTRwt and ATTRm, respectively. Variants such as the V122I polymorphism can also be designated by indicating the variation after the amyloid type (e.g., ATTR V122I).[3]

Light chain amyloid is designated AL-type amyloidosis and is the result of an underlying plasma cell dyscrasia. Although amyloid derived from serum amyloid A protein (AA) is a relatively common form of systemic amyloidosis, it rarely if ever causes cardiac symptoms.

By far the most frequent hereditary amyloidosis to involve the heart is mutant or hereditary ATTR.

So-called isolated atrial amyloidosis, caused by deposition of atrial natriuretic factor (AANF), is characterized by relatively sparse amyloid depositions within the atrial walls. Such deposits usually occur in older individuals, though its relationship with disease has not yet been established.

Methods of Typing Amyloid

It has been shown that the presence of a monoclonal gammopathy is not adequate for typing of amyloid, because 15% of patients with AL-type amyloidosis have no evidence of such in their serum or urine

TABLE 148.1 Cardiac Amyloidosis, Clinical Findings by Protein Precursor

Type	Amyloid Subunit	Age (mean)	Cardiac Involvement	Frequency of Patients Diagnosed with Cardiac Amyloid by Biopsy	Extracardiac Involvement
ATTR (senile systemic amyloidosis)	Trans-thyretin, wild type[a]	70–83	Invariable, usually mild but may be severe	30% (overall 26%–57%)	Predominantly in vessels, especially lung
ATTR (hereditary)	Trans-thyretin, mutant	57	Usual, especially severe with Leu55Pro, Val30Met, Val122Ile, Tyr78Phe mutations	12%–25%	Nerves, endocrine tissues, various viscera with sparing of liver and relative sparing of kidney
AL	Immunoglobulin light chains	56–60	Frequent	44% (λ) 43% all (M) 9% (κ) Range 45–82	Multiorgan involvement, frequent involvement of liver, spleen, and kidney
Apo A1	Mutant apolipoprotein A1	Few cases	May be severe	<1	Skin Kidney Stomach Larynx Bowel Liver Gynecologic tract Lymph nodes
AANF	Atrial natriuretic peptide	80+	Invariable (atria)	0	None
AA	Amyloid protein A		Frequent, rarely symptomatic	0	Typical
Aβ₂M	β₂-Microglobulin	Variable	Usually asymptomatic	0	Blood vessels in various organs

[a]Including V112I ATTR, which increases the risk for amyloid. It is prevalent in >1% of African Americans and therefore considered a polymorphism as opposed to mutation (defined as <1%).

("nonsecretors"). Furthermore, up to 25% of patients with ATTR-type amyloidosis have monoclonal immunoglobulins in their serum or urine.[4,5] Because treatment is driven by the amyloid protein present, it is necessary to type amyloid when it is identified in cardiac biopsy samples.

Immunohistochemical techniques are generally performed as panels for kappa land lambda light chains, transthyretin, AA protein, and amyloid P protein. Although some centers have demonstrated very accurate results in the majority (95%) of their samples,[1] the reliability of immunohistochemistry, especially for AL, has been questioned.[6] In one series, transthyretin staining was 100% sensitive and specific, but light chain staining was only 38% sensitive.[4] Immunofluorescence staining on frozen tissue shows a high specificity and sensitivity for subtyping of amyloid deposits but requires frozen sections and equipped laboratories.[6]

There are a number of problems inherent to immunohistochemical or immunofluorescent techniques. First and foremost, while ~98% of cardiac amyloidosis is either of the AL or ATTR variety, rare forms do exist and would necessitate relatively large and broad panels. Second, codeposition of multiple types has been described and is difficult to sort out with antigen-based methods alone. Finally, formalin fixation and tissue processing may result in high background staining, rendering accurate interpretation difficult.[7]

Another direct form of interrogation of the amyloid protein, laser-capture tandem mass spectrometry-based proteomics has recently been employed as a means of very effective amyloid typing on paraffin-embedded tissues. It has the added benefit of also having excellent sensitivity for detecting mutant forms of the protein as well.[8] However, such mutant forms still must be confirmed by gene sequencing.

Clinical Findings

Patients with cardiac amyloidosis often present with restrictive hemodynamics, arrhythmias, conduction disturbances, and/or congestive heart failure. Amyloidosis has been attributed to ~10% of all nonischemic cardiomyopathies, although there is debate about whether the disease itself is considered a cardiomyopathy.[1]

The average age of patients presenting with cardiac amyloidosis is ~60 years for AL type and 70 years for ATTR type.[1,5] Males are disproportionately affected by nonhereditary ATTR-type amyloidosis (>25:1 in most series), while AL-type cardiac amyloidosis shows no such sex predilection.[3] Syncope is often a manifestation of late stages of disease and may herald sudden death.[9] Cardiac involvement is the most serious complication of systemic amyloidosis and has been attributed to the cause of death in more than half of patients.[1]

Electrocardiogram shows low voltage with a mean of <0.5 mV in all limb leads. Serum N-terminal pro B-type natriuretic peptide is frequently elevated (>332 ng/L).

Echocardiographic study generally reveals a mean left ventricular wall thickness >12 mm, which is likely a result of the accumulation of the abnormal protein and concomitant myocyte hypertrophy.[10] Speckling of the myocardial interstitium, seen on echocardiography, can also be a clue to the diagnosis. This is particularly true in cases of ATTR-type cardiac amyloidosis, which often exhibits the most striking hypertrophy. In 10% to 20% of patients, the echocardiographic features are suggestive of dilated cardiomyopathy or hypertrophic cardiomyopathy.

Magnetic resonance imaging may differentiate amyloid deposits from idiopathic cardiomyopathy by high-resolution evaluation of the myocardial wall.[11] Diffuse, late enhancement with gadolinium is typical, and focal enhancement, especially in the inferior basal segment, may occur before there is significant ventricular hypertrophy.[12]

Gross Pathologic Findings

Grossly, the heart at autopsy is generally enlarged (Fig. 148.1) and of firm consistency, and with advanced amyloid shows a waxy beaded endocardial surface of the atria and of the atrioventricular valves, which have propensity for the deposits. The mean heart weight at autopsy is about 550 g.[13] In autopsies of cases of AL-type amyloidosis, there is typically gross enlargement of the spleen (Fig. 148.2). The gross

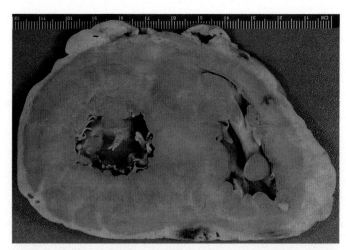

FIGURE 148.1 ▲ Cardiac amyloidosis. A short-axis section demonstrates ventricular hypertrophy with septal asymmetry. The heart was an explant from a patient with cardiomyopathy; a diagnosis of amyloid was made first at pathologic examination of the explanted heart.

consistency of the myocardium is often described as firm, rubbery or waxy. Atrial dilatation is a constant feature (owing to the underlying restrictive hemodynamics), but ventricular dilatation is uncommon. In cases of AL-type cardiac amyloidosis, either primary or secondary to multiple myeloma, gross involvement of viscera, especially liver and spleen, may occur. The hypertrophy resulting from amyloid may occasionally result in septal asymmetry, mimicking hypertrophic cardiomyopathy both by cardiac imaging as well as pathologically[14] (Fig. 148.1).

Microscopic Findings

The histologic appearance of cardiac amyloid is identical to that of amyloidosis of other organs (Figs. 148.3 to 148.11). Namely, the proteinaceous deposits show reactivity with Congo red stain and exhibit birefringence when placed in cross-polarized light (Fig. 148.12). In native heart biopsies, amyloid is the most common specific diagnosis rendered, and there should always be a high index of suspicion, especially if there is a clinical suggestion. On low magnification, there is patchy, haphazard deposition of eosinophilic to amphophilic

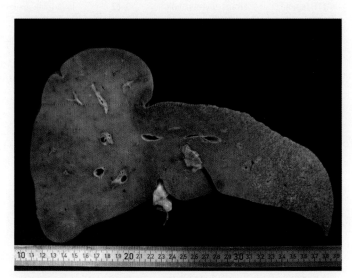

FIGURE 148.2 ▲ Systemic amyloidosis. The liver from a patient with amyloidosis shows firm waxy involvement with amyloid. Visceral involvement, including the spleen and liver, is more common in AL amyloid than other types.

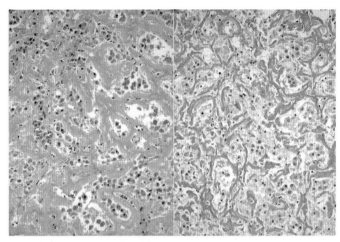

FIGURE 148.3 ▲ Systemic amyloidosis, spleen. The hematoxylin eosin stain is at the left and Congo red stain at the right.

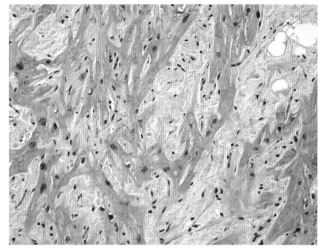

FIGURE 148.6 ▲ Cardiac amyloidosis. In this example, there is myofiber disarray as a reaction to the amyloid, as can be seen adjacent to scarring or in hypertrophic cardiomyopathy.

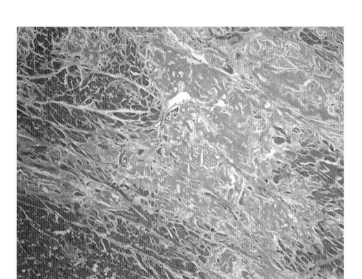

FIGURE 148.4 ▲ Cardiac amyloidosis. The majority of the field is replaced by amyloid. In some instances, the amount of amyloid may be estimated based on multiple cardiac samples.[15] In some medicolegal cases, the approximate amyloid burden by percent myocardial involvement may have bearing on estimating patient survival.

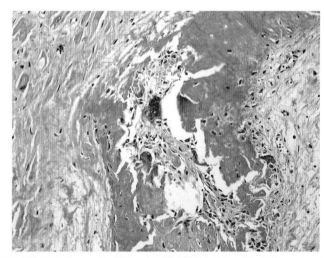

FIGURE 148.7 ▲ Cardiac amyloidosis. There may be an occasional macrophage giant cell reaction to nodular amyloid deposits.

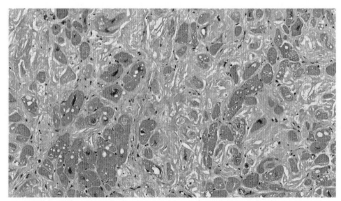

FIGURE 148.5 ▲ Cardiac amyloidosis. There is diffuse interstitial amyloid around individual myocytes. The differential diagnosis includes interstitial fibrosis; the diagnosis of amyloid is made based on the homogenous, nonfibrillar appearance of the deposits and confirmed by Congo red or trichrome stains.

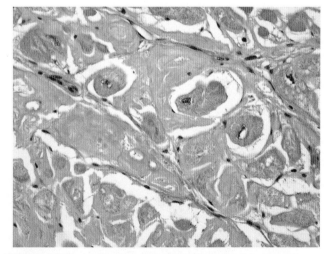

FIGURE 148.8 ▲ Cardiac amyloidosis. There is encircling of the myocytes by the amyloid deposits, which are slate-gray, homogenous, nonfibrillar, with the typical cracking artifact. In addition, a retraction artifact between the myocytes and amyloid may be present.

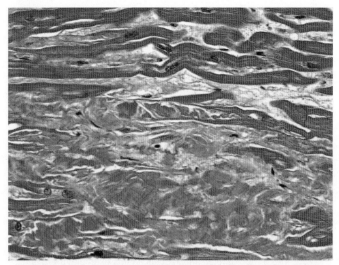

FIGURE 148.9 ▲ Cardiac amyloidosis, nodular pattern. There are unaffected myocytes oriented longitudinally above and a mass of extracellular amyloid below, which is amorphous, nonfibrillar, and typical of amyloid. In the myocardium, there is essentially nothing that could cause this histologic appearance other than amyloid.

homogenous material (Fig. 148.4) that may exhibit a cracked appearance. In some examples, there may be only interstitial amyloid that may be focal, necessitating careful review of all biopsies (Fig. 148.5). There may be associated myofiber disarray, interstitial fibrosis, and/or hypertrophy (Fig. 148.6). Occasionally, as in other organs, a foreign body–type giant cell reaction is present (Fig. 148.7). The differential diagnosis is fibrosis, which is generally not as randomly distributed, and shows a more fibrillar appearance.

In most cases, cardiac amyloid is readily diagnosed on the basis of routine stains. Confirmatory stains such as sulfated Alcian blue, metachromatic stains (crystal or methyl violet), Congo red stain, Sirius red, and thioflavin T stains highlight the amyloid deposits.[15] Congo red staining is probably the most commonly employed of these and yields excellent results. Although apple-green birefringence is required for the specific diagnosis, technical limitations related to optics of a specific microscope and subjectivity of interpretation should be considered, and a diagnosis should not be excluded based solely on this aspect of diagnosis, as long as the typical orange-red staining (so-called congophilia) is seen with bright field microscopy.

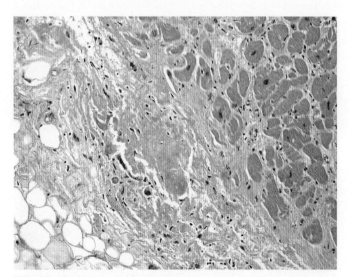

FIGURE 148.10 ▲ Cardiac amyloidosis. There may be extension into the epicardium as seen here.

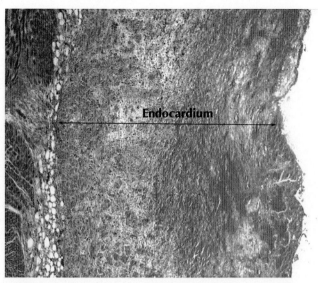

FIGURE 148.11 ▲ Cardiac amyloidosis, endocardial involvement. There is marked expansion of the atrial endocardium.

There are three patterns of cardiac amyloidosis that may be seen on biopsy, which usually overlap: interstitial (either pericellular [surrounding myocytes] or [Fig. 148.8] nodular [Fig. 148.9], endocardial [Fig. 148.10], epicardial [Fig. 148.11], and vascular [Fig. 148.12]). The interstitial pattern may have a fine pseudofibrillar pattern, sometimes referred to as reticular (Fig. 148.13). On Masson trichrome stain, amyloid has a slate gray appearance in contrast to bright blue collagen. Congo red stains show characteristic birefringence (usually applegreen) when viewed in cross-polarized light (Fig. 148.12). AL-type amyloidosis is associated with extensive infiltrates that are both interstitial and vascular amyloid. In contrast, ATTR-type amyloid is often associated with less extensive infiltrates, which correlate with overall fewer cardiac symptoms, and a higher incidence of nodular deposits.[1,16,17]

Immunohistochemical staining for amyloid P protein is highly specific and, although not routinely required, may confirm the diagnosis of amyloid, regardless of the subtype. Because of the need for typing in all cases, confirmation of the diagnosis will occur with special testing generally performed at a reference laboratory (see above). Immunohistochemical stains for free kappa light chains, lambda light chains, and transthyretin will show specific results in some cases.

The epicardial coronary arteries and valves may show amyloid deposits, but rarely if ever result in obstruction or functional abnormalities.[17]

In SSA-type, there is typically arterial amyloid involvement in the lungs, liver, and kidneys.[18] AL-type amyloidosis virtually always affects viscera with extensive deposits that are extravascular, and there is a high frequency of splenic involvement. The distribution of amyloidosis in hereditary ATTR-type amyloidosis is more extensive than in the wild-type ATTR (senile systemic amyloidosis) variety, with subcutaneous fat and rectal biopsy positivity in 75% of cases.[19]

Light Chain (AL) Amyloidosis

The heart is affected in ~50% of AL amyloidosis patients. Monoclonal gammopathies are not detected in 14%; therefore, their absence does not exclude light chain derivation of the abnormal protein.[4] Over 20% of patients with primary amyloidosis present with cardiac symptoms, most with congestive heart failure. A rare complication is that of atrial hemorrhage.[20]

In contrast to plasma cell neoplasms, in which κ light chain restriction is more common than λ light chain restriction, λ is more common than κ in patients with AL amyloid by a 3–4:1 margin. In addition to being more amyloidogenic than κ light chains, amyloidogenic λ light chains appear to have greater tropism for the heart and kidneys than do amyloidogenic κ light chains.[6]

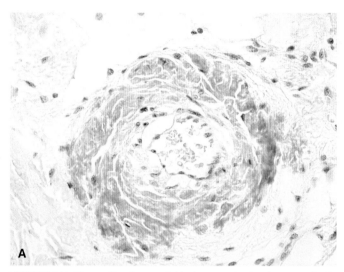
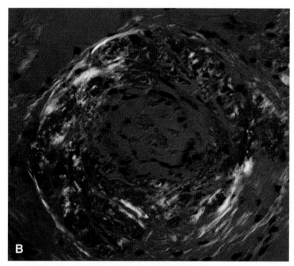

FIGURE 148.12 ▲ Cardiac amyloidosis, vascular involvement. **A.** The vascular pattern can be seen in amyloid of various types and is not specific. **B.** When viewed by polarized light, there is apple-green birefringence.

Transthyretin (ATTR) Amyloidosis

Wild Type ("Senile Systemic Amyloidosis")

Wild-type ATTR amyloidosis is almost exclusively a disease of elderly men. The echocardiographic appearance is indistinguishable from other forms of amyloidosis. Because of the indolent course, management is conservative, including treatment of heart failure and atrial fibrillation, and occasionally ventricular pacing if there is high-degree AV block. Severe left ventricular dysfunction may rarely occur. Wild-type ATTR was the cause of cardiac amyloid in 8% of patients undergoing transplant for end-stage amyloid heart disease.[21]

Isoleucine-122 (V122I) ATTR Amyloidosis

One form of ATTR is caused by a polymorphism in the *TTR* gene and is intermediate in clinical course. The isoleucine-122 (V122I) variant in *TTR*, present in ~3% to 4% of Blacks, but rarely in Caucasians, is responsible for about 20% of senile systemic amyloidosis in Blacks, with no significant impact on Caucasian statistics. The majority of

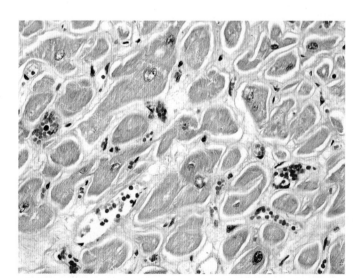

FIGURE 148.13 ▲ Cardiac amyloidosis, interstitial deposits. In some instances, the amyloid can appear as fine strands (so-called reticular pattern).

Blacks possessing this variant harbor microscopic quantities of amyloid in their cardiac ventricles.[22]

Although there is no overall significant difference in mortality between carriers, the TTR variant may increase the risk for heart failure in African Americans, presumably because of amyloid deposits.[23] Elderly African Americans with a diagnosis of amyloidosis due to V122I ATTR are more likely to die or require hospitalization, compared to patients with wild-type ATTR amyloidosis, at a follow-up averaging 15 months.[3]

Mutated TTR Amyloidosis

More than 100 different mutations in *TTR* can cause hereditary amyloidosis, many of which involve the heart. The Val30Met is the commonest mutation of transthyretin seen clinically with heart involvement. This mutation represents 85% of *TTR* mutations reported to the Familial Amyloid Polyneuropathy World Transplant Registry.[10]

Up to one-fourth of patients with hereditary amyloidosis have monoclonal serum or urine gammopathies,[4,5] underscoring the need for direct typing of the amyloid protein.

Hereditary amyloidosis is characterized by nerve involvement and is manifest by polyneuropathy and autonomic dysfunction. The median age at presentation is in the 6th to 7th decade, and cardiac involvement is present in 25% of patients, with heart disease the most common cause of death. Over three-fourths of patients have peripheral neuropathy and one-third have autonomic neuropathy.[19] Renal disease is uncommon, and liver involvement is rare. The sensitivity of subcutaneous fat aspirates or rectal biopsy specimens is similar to that seen in AL-type amyloidosis and is about 75%; bone marrow biopsy is positive in less than half of patients.[19] Autopsy studies show multiple organ involvement with large deposits in the endocrine and nervous system, with sparing of the liver parenchyma and bone marrow.[24,25]

Cardiac Involvement in Other Hereditary Forms of Amyloidosis

Apolipoprotein A1–derived amyloidosis (AApoA1) is due to germ-line mutations in the APOA1 gene; currently 13 are known to be associated with amyloidosis. Various organs may be involved, including the skin, larynx, small intestine, large intestine, heart, liver, kidney, uterus, ovary, and lymph nodes.[26] The diagnosis is generally made by immunohistochemical confirmation of the protein subtype with DNA sequencing. In a series of heart transplants for cardiac amyloid, AApoA1 was present in 8% of patients.[21] In a series of organ transplants for AApoA1, only one of ten was a cardiac transplant, and most of the remainder were renal transplants.[27]

Cardiac conduction disturbances have been described in Gelsolin amyloidosis (AGel), a polyneuropathy caused by G654A or G654T mutation in the gelsolin gene at 9q32-34.[28]

Isolated Atrial Amyloid

Isolated atrial amyloid is localized amyloid deposition within the atria of the aging heart. The main amyloid constituents are atrial natriuretic factor (ANF) and the N-terminal part of its precursor form (NT-proANF). Isolated atrial amyloidosis is seen as an incidental autopsy finding in about 80% of patients over 80 years of age, but deposits are inconspicuous on routine staining and electron microcopy or immunohistochemistry is necessary for their detection. Atrial amyloid has not been clearly linked to cardiac dysfunction or cardiomyopathy, although there appears to be a likely association with atrial fibrillation and prominent atrial deposition.[29,30] Deposits are more pronounced in women and in the left atrium, especially the posterior wall.[29] There is a suggestion that it is more prominent in patients with heart failure.[31]

Dialysis-Related Amyloid

β2-Microglobulinemia–related amyloid is found in patient on chronic hemodialysis and is deposited primarily in joints and synovium, causing carpal tunnel syndrome. Most patients have undergone hemodialysis for 10 years or more. Histologically, there is exclusive involvement of cardiac microvasculature.[32] Cardiac involvement is mild and usually does not result in symptoms. Rarely, there can be massive cardiac infiltration by amyloid and heart failure.[33]

Amyloid A

Systemic AA amyloidosis rarely causes symptomatic heart disease.[34] Amyloid deposits are frequently present upon endomyocardial biopsy but are of no clinical consequence in over 95% of patients.[35]

Nonspecific Components of Amyloid

In addition to the protein that is responsible for the pathogenic β-pleated sheet configuration that is the basis for classification, other proteins and glycoproteins are consistently found in the amyloid deposits. Serum amyloid P is a 25-kDa protein that forms doughnut-shaped pentamers that are stacked at right angles to the fibril. It is useful in the immunohistochemical detection of amyloid (regardless of the type) in tissues as well as scintigraphic localization of amyloid within patients. Heparan sulfate, perlecan, laminin, collagen IV, fibronectin, and entactin are also deposited in many or all forms of amyloid.

Treatment

Treatment of AL amyloidosis includes chemotherapy, especially oral melphalan and dexamethasone, and stem cell transplant.[10] Cardiac transplantation does not affect the production of the amyloid protein precursor, resulting in recurrence of amyloid in the graft. Cardiac transplantation followed by autologous stem cell transplant has been used, with conditioning chemotherapy consisting of high- or low-dose melphalan.[36]

Treatment of hereditary ATTR-type amyloidosis includes orthotopic liver transplantation, which eliminates more than 95% of variant transthyretin from the circulation.[21] Concomitant or subsequent heart transplantation is often required.[37] Recently, newer generation pharmacotherapeutics have shown a great deal of promise in ATTR-type amyloidosis. Drugs such as Diflunisal act by stabilizing the tetrameric form of the protein and may slow, or even cause regression of, the abnormal protein deposition.

The 1- and 3-year survival rates of AL-type cardiac amyloid are 68% and 63%, respectively, and are affected by degree of cardiac involvement by clinical evaluation. Cardiac involvement in ATTR-type amyloidosis shows better survival, with 1- and 3-year survival rates of 91% and 83%, respectively.[38]

Practical Points

▶ Endomyocardial biopsies should be carefully evaluated for amyloid, even if the history indicates dilated as opposed to restrictive cardiomyopathy.

▶ Carefully screen for amyloid at autopsy in individuals >65 years old. Irregular or unusual areas of fibrosis-like change in a nonischemic pattern can be a helpful clue.

▶ If Masson trichrome stain is not typical of collagen (slate gray), and Congo red stain shows typical orange staining, the diagnosis of amyloid is highly likely, even in apple-green birefringence is not demonstrated due to technical or other reasons.

▶ Direct typing of the amyloid protein should be performed on all amyloid heart biopsies, with mass spectroscopy or immunofluorescence showing the highest accuracy.

▶ Tandem mass spectrometry–based proteomics provides information on the amyloid type as well as serves as an effective screen for mutations

▶ Immunohistochemistry usually shows good results for amyloid P protein and transthyretin, but for subtyping kappa and lambda light chains, there is often extensive background staining.

REFERENCES

1. Kieninger B, Eriksson M, Kandolf R, et al. Amyloid in endomyocardial biopsies. *Virchows Arch.* 2010;456:523–532.
2. Sipe JD, Benson MD, Buxbaum JN, et al. Nomenclature 2014: amyloid fibril proteins and clinical classification of the amyloidosis. *Amyloid.* 2014;21:221–224.
3. Ruberg FL, Maurer MS, Judge DP, et al. Prospective evaluation of the morbidity and mortality of wild–type and V122I mutant transthyretin amyloid cardiomyopathy: the Transthyretin Amyloidosis Cardiac Study (TRACS). *Am Heart J.* 2012;164:222–228 e1.
4. Lachmann HJ, Booth DR, Booth SE, et al. Misdiagnosis of hereditary amyloidosis as AL (primary) amyloidosis. *N Engl J Med.* 2002;346:1786–1791.
5. Maleszewski JJ, Murray DL, Dispenzieri A, et al. Relationship between monoclonal gammopathy and cardiac amyloid type. *Cardiovasc Pathol.* 2013;22:189–194.
6. Collins AB, Smith RN, Stone JR. Classification of amyloid deposits in diagnostic cardiac specimens by immunofluorescence. *Cardiovasc Pathol.* 2009;18:205–216.
7. Picken MM, Herrera GA. The burden of "sticky" amyloid: typing challenges. *Arch Pathol Lab Med.* 2007;131:850–851.
8. Vrana JA, Gamez JD, Madden BJ, et al. Classification of amyloidosis by laser microdissection and mass spectrometry-based proteomic analysis in clinical biopsy specimens. *Blood.* 2009;114:4957–4959.
9. Chamarthi B, Dubrey SW, Cha K, et al. Features and prognosis of exertional syncope in light-chain associated AL cardiac amyloidosis. *Am J Cardiol.* 1997;80:1242–1245.
10. Dubrey SW, Comenzo RL. Amyloid diseases of the heart: current and future therapies. *QJM.* 2012;105:617–631.
11. Suri A, Moon JC, Dhamrait SS, et al. Cardiac amyloid by cardiovascular magnetic resonance. *Heart.* 2007;93:1496.
12. Deux JF, Damy T, Rahmouni A, et al. Noninvasive detection of cardiac involvement in patients with hereditary transthyretin associated amyloidosis using cardiac magnetic resonance imaging: a prospective study. *Amyloid.* 2014;21:246–255.
13. Roberts WC, Waller BF. Cardiac amyloidosis causing cardiac dysfunction: analysis of 54 necropsy patients. *Am J Cardiol.* 1983;52:137–146.
14. Morner S, Hellman U, Suhr OB, et al. Amyloid heart disease mimicking hypertrophic cardiomyopathy. *J Intern Med.* 2005;258:225–230.

15. Kosma VM, Collan Y, Kulju T, et al. Quantitation of staining for amyloid in histological sections: sources of variation, correlation analysis, and interstain reproducibility. *Appl Pathol.* 1986;4:74–82.
16. Sharma PP, Payvar S, Litovsky SH. Histomorphometric analysis of intramyocardial vessels in primary and senile amyloidosis: epicardium versus endocardium. *Cardiovasc Pathol.* 2008;17:65–71.
17. Wittich CM, Neben-Wittich MA, Mueller PS, et al. Deposition of amyloid proteins in the epicardial coronary arteries of 58 patients with primary systemic amyloidosis. *Cardiovasc Pathol.* 2007;16:75–78.
18. Pitkanen P, Westermark P, Cornwell GG III. Senile systemic amyloidosis. *Am J Pathol.* 1984;117:391–399.
19. Gertz MA, Kyle RA, Thibodeau SN. Familial amyloidosis: a study of 52 North American-born patients examined during a 30-year period. *Mayo Clin Proc.* 1992;67:428–440.
20. Edibam C, Playford D, Texler M, et al. Isolated left atrial amyloidosis: acute premitral stenosis secondary to spontaneous intramural left atrial hemorrhagic dissection. *J Am Soc Echocardiogr.* 2006;19:938 e1–e4.
21. Dubrey SW, Burke MM, Hawkins PN, et al. Cardiac transplantation for amyloid heart disease: the United Kingdom experience. *J Heart Lung Transplant.* 2004;23:1142–1153.
22. Jacobson DR, Pastore RD, Yaghoubian R, et al. Variant-sequence transthyretin (isoleucine 122) in late-onset cardiac amyloidosis in black Americans. *N Engl J Med.* 1997;336:466–473.
23. Quarta CC, Buxbaum JN, Shah AM, et al. The amyloidogenic V122I transthyretin variant in elderly black Americans. *N Engl J Med.* 2015;372:21–29.
24. Tanimura A, Cho T, Shinohara Y, et al. Familial amyloidosis. A histopathological study. *Acta Pathol Jpn.* 1984;34:335–344.
25. Hofer PA, Anderson R. Postmortem findings in primary familial amyloidosis with polyneuropathy. *Acta Pathol Microbiol Scand A.* 1975;83:309–322.
26. Eriksson M, Schonland S, Yumlu S, et al. Hereditary apolipoprotein AI-associated amyloidosis in surgical pathology specimens: identification of three novel mutations in the APOA1 gene. *J Mol Diagn.* 2009;11:257–262.
27. Gillmore JD, Stangou AJ, Lachmann HJ, et al. Organ transplantation in hereditary apolipoprotein AI amyloidosis. *Am J Transplant.* 2006;6:2342–2347.
28. Pihlamaa T, Suominen S, Kiuru-Enari S. Familial amyloidotic polyneuropathy type IV—gelsolin amyloidosis. *Amyloid.* 2012;19(suppl 1):30–33.
29. Steiner I, Hajkova P. Patterns of isolated atrial amyloid: a study of 100 hearts on autopsy. *Cardiovasc Pathol.* 2006;15:287–290.
30. Podduturi V, Armstrong DR, Hitchcock MA, et al. Isolated atrial amyloidosis and the importance of molecular classification. *Proc (Bayl Univ Med Cent).* 2013;26:387–389.
31. Millucci L, Ghezzi L, Bernardini G, et al. Prevalence of isolated atrial amyloidosis in young patients affected by congestive heart failure. *Scientific World Journal.* 2012;2012:293863.
32. Saito A, Gejyo F. Current clinical aspects of dialysis-related amyloidosis in chronic dialysis patients. *Ther Apher Dial.* 2006;10:316–320.
33. Kawano M, Muramoto H, Yamada M, et al. Fatal cardiac beta2-microglobulin amyloidosis in patients on long-term hemodialysis. *Am J Kidney Dis.* 1998;31:E4.
34. Helder MR, Schaff HV, Nishimura RA, et al. Impact of incidental amyloidosis on the prognosis of patients with hypertrophic cardiomyopathy undergoing septal myectomy for left ventricular outflow tract obstruction. *Am J Cardiol.* 2014;114:1396–1399.
35. Lachmann HJ, Goodman HJ, Gilbertson JA, et al. Natural history and outcome in systemic AA amyloidosis. *N Engl J Med.* 2007;356:2361–2371.
36. Lacy MQ, Dispenzieri A, Hayman SR, et al. Autologous stem cell transplant after heart transplant for light chain (Al) amyloid cardiomyopathy. *J Heart Lung Transplant.* 2008;27:823–829.
37. Singer R, Mehrabi A, Schemmer P, et al. Indications for liver transplantation in patients with amyloidosis: a single-center experience with 11 cases. *Transplantation.* 2005;80:S156–S159.
38. Kristen AV, Dengler TJ, Katus HA. Suspected cardiac amyloidosis: endomyocardial biopsy remains the diagnostic gold-standard. *Am J Hematol.* 2007;82:328.

149 Cardiac Sarcoidosis

Fabio R. Tavora, M.D., Ph.D. and Allen P. Burke, M.D.

Epidemiology

The prevalence of sarcoidosis is difficult to ascertain, because many patients are asymptomatic, and the clinical symptoms and histologic findings are nonspecific. In the United States, the overall prevalence of sarcoidosis is estimated at 10 to 40/100,000 persons with an annual incidence of 40/100,000 in blacks compared to 5 to 11/100,000 in whites.[1–3] Outside the United States, the highest rate of occurrence is reported in Scandinavia, especially Finland and Sweden (yearly incidence of 5 to 40/100,000 people, prevalence of 64/100,000 population).[1,2] There is a female predominance, especially among African Americans, among whom there is a 2:1 female-to-male ratio.

Cardiac involvement in sarcoidosis occurs in 20% to 30% of patients in autopsy studies, although only 5% of patients with sarcoidosis have clinical manifestations of cardiac disease.[3]

Etiology

The etiology of sarcoidosis is unknown. It is presumed to be an immunologic disorder involving acquired cellular immunity directed against an unknown antigen or antigens and possibly environmental factors in predisposed individuals. A number of infectious organisms, including *Mycobacteria*, *Propionibacteria*, *Borrelia*, *Rickettsia*, and herpes virus have been implicated.[1–3] Although nucleotide sequences specific for several organisms have been identified in sarcoid granulomas, the only cultured bacterium has been *Propionibacterium acnes*, at a higher frequency and concentration than in nonsarcoid lymph nodes.[4,5] A subset of patients demonstrates T- and B-cell responses to mycobacterial antigens.[6] Environmental factors such as pollen, pica, fireplaces, and mold are epidemiologically associated with systemic sarcoidosis.[7–9]

Clinical Findings

Cardiac involvement by sarcoid granulomas was reported as early as 1929,[10] and there have been several subsequent autopsy series.[11–16] Although cardiac involvement is generally around 30% in autopsy series,[11] it occurs at a higher rate in Asians, especially Japanese, in whom cardiac manifestations account for as many as 85% of deaths.[13,14,17]

There are various clinical manifestations of cardiac sarcoid, including chest pain, palpitations, dyspnea, syncope, conduction abnormalities, ventricular or supraventricular arrhythmias, and heart failure. Conduction abnormalities vary from isolated bundle branch block to complete heart block, which can be detected in 23% to 30% of patients with cardiac sarcoid. There is a poor correlation between cardiac symptoms and extent of cardiac involvement, underscoring the need for better imaging techniques for diagnosing cardiac disease.[11]

In up to two-thirds of patients with biopsy-confirmed cardiac sarcoidosis, clinical symptoms are limited to the heart.[18]

Sudden Death

The incidence of sudden cardiac death from sarcoid-induced arrhythmia ranges from 12% to 65% and is associated with extensive myocardial involvement at autopsy.[11,19] Most sudden deaths occur in patients without previously identified cardiac involvement.[11,15,19-22] Predictors of sudden death in patients with a clinical diagnosis are similar to other clinical presentations of heart failure and include ventricular arrhythmias, increased left ventricular diastolic diameter, and New York Heart Association functional class.[1-3]

Cardiac Imaging

Echocardiography is not sensitive in detecting heart involvement.[23] Cardiac magnetic resonance imaging has a better sensitivity and is relatively specific, depending on the stage of disease.[24] Myocardial thickening and regional wall motion abnormalities characterize the inflammatory phase, corresponding to active granulomas with little fibrosis. The use of sequences to evaluate late gadolinium enhancement demonstrates transmural, subepicardial, or midmyocardial lesions in a nonischemic pattern.[24]

Nuclear medicine imaging may demonstrate uptake in the lung parenchyma, mediastinal lymph nodes, as well as the myocardium, where it is patchy and focal.[24] The presence of positron emission tomographic avidity was associated with increased rates of ventricular tachycardia or sudden death especially if there was right ventricular involvement.[25]

Association with Lung Involvement

Although chest radiograph is a sensitive screening tool for diagnosing pulmonary and mediastinal sarcoid, myocardial involvement requires other imaging modalities. Although one study found an inverse correlation between cardiac and pulmonary involvement,[20] this has not been found subsequently.[11,16,23] In a series of cardiac sarcoidosis from a single medical examiner (unpublished observations), 80% of cases had pulmonary parenchymal involvement.

Gross Findings

All layers of the heart can be involved by sarcoidosis, but the myocardium is most frequently involved, followed by the epicardium and endocardium. The heart weight is increased due to presence of granulomas and scar, and cardiac remodeling due to valve disease or heart failure. Grossly, lesions are typically zonal and well demarcated (Fig. 149.1) but can occasionally be diffuse and difficult to identify or result in wall thinning mimicking old myocardial infarction (Fig. 149.2). In cases of pulmonary sarcoid, the heart will show cor pulmonale, with or without sarcoid lesions microscopically (Fig. 149.3). Because there is typically an extensive fibrous reaction to the granulomas, the lesions appear as scars and are generally firmer than lymphomatous deposits, which they can resemble. In descending order of cardiac involvement, sarcoid lesions involve the interventricular septum (basal aspect most often), left ventricular free wall, right ventricular free wall, atria, pericardium, and endocardium. In the left ventricle, the lateral wall is least often involved.[19]

In unusual cases, the lesions may be limited to the atria, subepicardium, or right ventricle. Scarring can lead to the formation of ventricular aneurysms, which have been reported in 8% to 10% of patients with cardiac sarcoidosis, which may grossly resemble infarcts (Fig. 149.2)[26] and which may rarely rupture.[27] Valvular infiltration by sarcoidosis is uncommon, although mitral insufficiency is not uncommon with left ventricular dilatation.[28]

In rare instances of diffuse granulomatous involvement of early phase granulomas, the gross findings may be subtle.[19,29] In incidental sarcoid, in which there are few granulomas that are seen only microscopically, the gross appearance is normal.

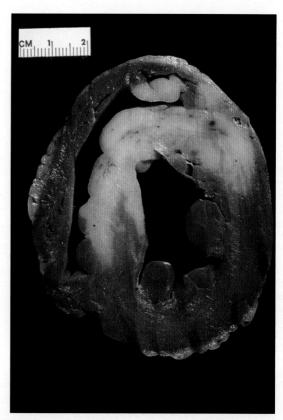

FIGURE 149.1 ▲ Cardiac sarcoidosis. There is a homogeneous white scar. Because the lesion is not in an ischemic distribution, the appearance is nearly pathognomonic for sarcoidosis.

Histologic Findings

The characteristic lesion of sarcoidosis is a discrete, compact, noncaseating epithelioid cell granuloma, similar to extracardiac sarcoid. The diagnosis is established by the presence of epithelioid granulomas with or without giant cells, in the absence of necrosis, organisms as seen on special stains, or myocyte necrosis.

Early lesions contain numerous lymphocytes (Fig. 149.4); typical lesions are primarily granulomatous (Figs. 149.5 and 149.6) and late or

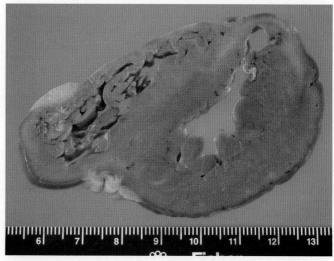

FIGURE 149.2 ▲ Cardiac sarcoidosis. In this explant, there is a transmural scar mimicking a healed infarct.

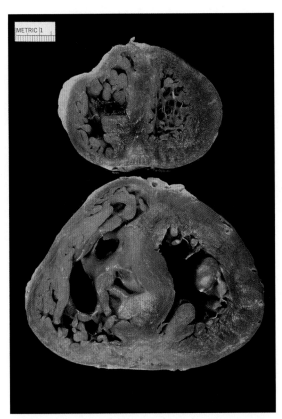

FIGURE 149.3 ▲ Cor pulmonale, pulmonary sarcoidosis. There is no cardiac involvement by sarcoid, but pulmonary involvement led to severe pulmonary hypertension and marked right ventricular hypertrophy.

"healed" lesions are largely collagen with few granulomas and chronic inflammation. Although there is tremendous overlap, the intermediate phase is predominant in autopsied hearts from patients dying suddenly.[19]

The need for special stains is debatable, as infectious myocarditis with nonnecrotizing granulomas is exceedingly rare. In early lesions, lymphocytes are plentiful; sampling of edges of these lesions may lead to diagnosis of lymphocytic myocarditis. In later lesions, scar tissue predominates, granulomas are sparse or restricted to scattered giant cells, and the differential diagnosis includes scarring from ischemia or

cardiomyopathy. The granulomas are composed of activated T lymphocytes with increased CD8/CD4 ratios and activated monocytes and macrophages.[30]

Differential Diagnosis

Grossly and microscopically, autopsy or explant hearts with sarcoid may demonstrate areas resembling ischemia, myocarditis, and arrhythmogenic cardiomyopathy, underscoring the need for thorough histologic evaluation.[29,31] Clinically, the diagnosis may be ischemic cardiomyopathy due to left ventricular transmural scars.[31]

The most difficult differential diagnosis is that of giant cell myocarditis, which can also have areas of fibrosis (see Chapter 28). In general, necrosis is seen to a great degree in giant cell myocarditis and does not occur in sarcoid. Eosinophils are more common in giant cell myocarditis, but epicardial involvement does not occur. Well-formed granulomas and extracardiac involvement are typical of sarcoid and do not occur in giant cell myocarditis.

Role of Endomyocardial Biopsy

Although heart biopsy is highly specific for cardiac sarcoid, it is an insensitive diagnostic test (only 20% to 50% cardiac sarcoid cases are positive) because myocardial involvement often spares the right ventricular apex.[32] Despite its low sensitivity, a common indication for endomyocardial biopsy of native hearts is the exclusion of so-called infiltrative processes, including sarcoid, amyloid, and Fabry disease. A positive biopsy for sarcoidosis has been associated with a shorter median survival, presumably reflecting extensive myocardial involvement.[32]

Histologic findings are those of granulomas with or without giant cells (Fig. 149.7). Because of limited sampling, histologic findings on biopsy may not be classic and contain only lymphocytes with or without occasional giant cells, instead of well-formed granulomas, so a descriptive diagnosis may be necessary including myocarditis or giant cell myocarditis in the differential diagnosis.

Treatment and Prognosis

Cardiac sarcoidosis has 60% to 75% 5-year overall survival.[18] In a study of biopsy-confirmed cases, most patients received immunosuppressive therapy including steroids, over one-half required an intracardiac defibrillator, and 10% required cardiac transplantation. The Kaplan-Meier estimates for 1-, 5-, and 10-year transplantation-free cardiac survival were 97%, 90%, and 83%, respectively, with heart failure at presentation the strongest predictor for poor outcome.[18]

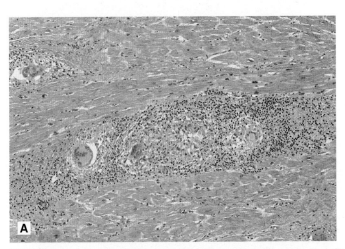

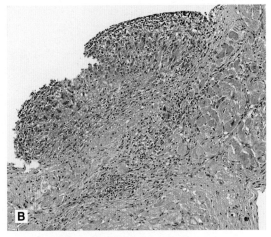

FIGURE 149.4 ▲ Sarcoid granulomas with prominent lymphocytic infiltrate. **A.** The granuloma is midmyocardial and surrounded by lymphocytes. **B.** The granuloma is endocardial and demonstrates an area of inflammation resembling myocarditis deep to it.

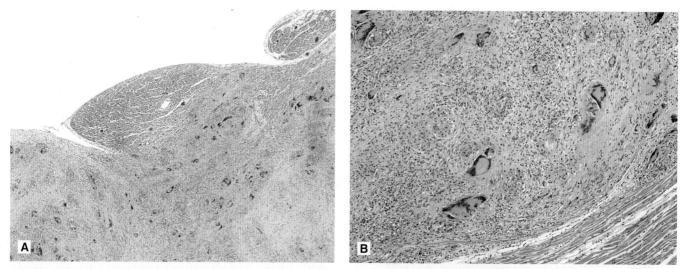

FIGURE 149.5 ▲ Cardiac sarcoidosis. **A.** All layers of the myocardium may be involved. However, endocardial involvement is usually an extension of transmural sarcoidosis. **B.** Cardiac sarcoidosis. Some lesions are quite cellular, but there is a fairly circumscribed border.

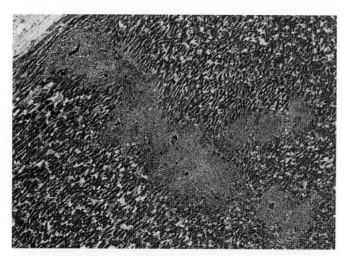

FIGURE 149.6 ▲ Cardiac sarcoidosis, sudden death. There are irregularly shaped granulomas in the myocardium extending toward the epicardial surface.

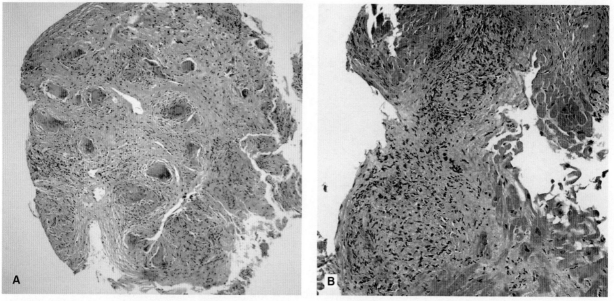

FIGURE 149.7 ▲ Cardiac sarcoidosis, endomyocardial biopsy. **A.** The sarcoid lesion practically replaces the entire biopsy sample. **B.** A different example showing abundant chronic inflammation.

REFERENCES

1. Dubrey S, Shah S, Hardman T, et al. Sarcoidosis: the links between epidemiology and aetiology. *Postgrad Med J.* 2014;90:582–589.
2. Lazarus A. Sarcoidosis: epidemiology, etiology, pathogenesis, and genetics. *Dis Mon.* 2009;55:649–660.
3. Sekhri V, Sanal S, Delorenzo LJ, et al. Cardiac sarcoidosis: a comprehensive review. *Arch Med Sci.* 2011;7:546–554.
4. Homma JY, Abe C, Chosa H, et al. Bacteriological investigation on biopsy specimens from patients with sarcoidosis. *Jpn J Exp Med.* 1978;48:251–255.
5. Abe C, Iwai K, Mikami R, et al. Frequent isolation of *Propionibacterium acnes* from sarcoidosis lymph nodes. *Zentralbl Bakteriol Mikrobiol Hyg A.* 1984;256:541–547.
6. Hance AJ. The role of mycobacteria in the pathogenesis of sarcoidosis. *Semin Respir Infect.* 1998;13:197–205.
7. Kreider ME, Christie JD, Thompson B, et al. Relationship of environmental exposures to the clinical phenotype of sarcoidosis. *Chest.* 2005;128:207–215.
8. Dunner E, Williams JH Jr. Epidemiology of sarcoidosis in the United States. *Am Rev Respir Dis.* 1961;84(5 pt 2):163–168.
9. Nikoskelainen J, Hannuksela M, Palva T. Antibodies to Epstein-Barr virus and some other herpesviruses in patients with sarcoidosis, pulmonary tuberculosis and erythema nodosum. *Scand J Infect Dis.* 1974;6:209–216.
10. Berstein M, Konzelmann FW, Sidlick DM. Boeck's sarcoid. *Arch Intern Med.* 1929;44:721–734.
11. Silverman KJ, Hutchins GM, Bulkley BH. Cardiac sarcoid: a clinicopathologic study of 84 unselected patients with systemic sarcoidosis. *Circulation.* 1978;58:1204–1211.
12. Longcope WT, Freiman DG. A study of sarcoidosis; based on a combined investigation of 160 cases including 30 autopsies from The Johns Hopkins Hospital and Massachusetts General Hospital. *Medicine (Baltimore).* 1952;31:1–132.
13. Iwai K, Tachibana T, Takemura T, et al. Pathological studies on sarcoidosis autopsy. I. Epidemiological features of 320 cases in Japan. *Acta Pathol Jpn.* 1993;43:372–376.
14. Iwai K, Sekiguti M, Hosoda Y, et al. Racial difference in cardiac sarcoidosis incidence observed at autopsy. *Sarcoidosis.* 1994;11:26–31.
15. Virmani R, Bures JC, Roberts WC. Cardiac sarcoidosis; a major cause of sudden death in young individuals. *Chest.* 1980;77:423–428.
16. Perry A, Vuitch F. Causes of death in patients with sarcoidosis. A morphologic study of 38 autopsies with clinicopathologic correlations. *Arch Pathol Lab Med.* 1995;119:167–172.
17. Iwai K, Takemura T, Kitaichi M, et al. Pathological studies on sarcoidosis autopsy. II. Early change, mode of progression and death pattern. *Acta Pathol Jpn.* 1993;43:377–385.
18. Kandolin R, Lehtonen J, Airaksinen J, et al. Cardiac sarcoidosis: epidemiology, characteristics, and outcome over 25 years in a nationwide study. *Circulation.* 2015;131:624–632.
19. Tavora F, Cresswell N, Li L, et al. Comparison of necropsy findings in patients with sarcoidosis dying suddenly from cardiac sarcoidosis versus dying suddenly from other causes. *Am J Cardiol.* 2009;104:571–577.
20. Roberts WC, McAllister HA Jr, Ferrans VJ. Sarcoidosis of the heart. A clinicopathologic study of 35 necropsy patients (group 1) and review of 78 previously described necropsy patients (group 11). *Am J Med.* 1977;63:86–108.
21. Thomsen TK, Eriksson T. Myocardial sarcoidosis in forensic medicine. *Am J Forensic Med Pathol.* 1999;20:52–56.
22. Lubitz SA, Goldbarg SH, Mehta D. Sudden cardiac death in infiltrative cardiomyopathies: sarcoidosis, scleroderma, amyloidosis, hemachromatosis. *Prog Cardiovasc Dis.* 2008;51:58–73.
23. Kim JS, Judson MA, Donnino R, et al. Cardiac sarcoidosis. *Am Heart J.* 2008;157:9–21.
24. Jeudy J, Burke AP, White CS, et al. Cardiac sarcoidosis: the challenge of radiologic-pathologic correlation: from the radiologic pathology archives. *Radiographics.* 2015;35:657–679.
25. Blankstein R, Osborne M, Naya M, et al. Cardiac positron emission tomography enhances prognostic assessments of patients with suspected cardiac sarcoidosis. *J Am Coll Cardiol.* 2014;63:329–336.
26. Lynch JP III, Sharma OP, Baughman RP. Extrapulmonary sarcoidosis. *Semin Respir Infect.* 1998;13:229–254.
27. Halushka MK, Yuh DD, Russell SD. Right ventricle-dominant cardiac sarcoidosis with sparing of the left ventricle. *J Heart Lung Transplant.* 2006;25:479–482.
28. Barton JH, Tavora F, Farb A, et al. Unusual cardiovascular manifestations of sarcoidosis, a report of three cases: coronary artery aneurysm with myocardial infarction, symptomatic mitral valvular disease, and sudden death from ruptured splenic artery. *Cardiovasc Pathol.* 2010;19(4):e119–e123.
29. Bagwan IN, Hooper LV, Sheppard MN. Cardiac sarcoidosis and sudden death. The heart may look normal or mimic other cardiomyopathies. *Virchows Arch.* 2011;458:671–678.
30. Litovsky SH, Burke AP, Virmani R. Giant cell myocarditis: an entity distinct from sarcoidosis characterized by multiphasic myocyte destruction by cytotoxic T cells and histiocytic giant cells. *Mod Pathol.* 1996;9:1126–1134.
31. Zhang M, Tavora F, Huebner T, et al. Allograft pathology in patients transplanted for idiopathic dilated cardiomyopathy. *Am J Surg Pathol.* 2012;36:389–395.
32. Ardehali H, Howard DL, Hariri A, et al. A positive endomyocardial biopsy result for sarcoid is associated with poor prognosis in patients with initially unexplained cardiomyopathy. *Am Heart J.* 2005;150:459–463.

150 Coronary Atherosclerosis

Allen P. Burke, M.D., and Fabio R. Tavora, M.D., Ph.D.

Methods of Sampling

The practicing pathologist will encounter coronary atherosclerosis primarily at autopsy. Because of the high prevalence of the disease in adults, the majority of autopsies will demonstrate some degree of coronary artery disease, whether incidental or relevant.

There are two major methods of in vivo sampling of coronary atherosclerosis as a surgical specimen: percutaneous via catheters, and open procedures. Coronary atherectomy was at one time a standard treatment for coronary stenosis, with catheter-based removal of the plaque or thrombus. Studies of directional coronary atherectomy showed an increase in hemorrhage into plaque, thrombosis, and lipid-rich plaque in patients with unstable coronary syndromes compared to those with stable angina.[1] "Plain old balloon angioplasty" (POBA) is still occasionally performed, however, which is a procedure that includes balloon dilatation of the lesion without stenting.[2]

Coronary thrombosuction, or thrombus aspiration, is occasionally performed in conjunction with balloon angioplasty studies, yielding pathologic information about the type and duration of the thrombus, including the presence of organizing thrombus, which is associated with a poor prognosis, and plaque components such as cholesterol crystals and calcification.[3,4]

Coronary endarterectomy (surgical removal of intimal disease, usually with concomitant bypass grafting) is not commonly performed because of relatively high rates of restenosis. However, in patients with severe diffuse disease not amenable to bypass, the surgeon may excise lengths of coronary plaques, which will be sent for pathologic examination.[5] Multiple arteries may undergo endarterectomy, with patch plasty of the left internal mammary artery. Minimally invasive surgery with off-pump techniques has been employed.[5–7]

Examination of the Coronary Arteries at Autopsy

Ideally, coronary arteries should be sampled at 3- to 5-mm intervals to exclude coronary atherosclerotic lesions and thrombi (see Chapter 138). Postmortem radiographs for assessment of the degree of calcification and time necessary for decalcification may be indicated for coronary deaths (Fig. 150.1). When arteries are significantly calcified, they should be removed from the heart prior to sectioning for decalcification.

If accurate measurements of cross-sectional luminal narrowing are to be undertaken, perfusion fixation is necessary, as there is collapse of arterial walls rendering overestimation of percent stenosis, especially in eccentric lesions (Fig. 150.2). The coronaries are perfusion fixed with 10% buffered formaldehyde retrograde from the ascending aorta at 100 mm Hg pressure for at least 5 minutes. A synthetic or rubber plug or stopper with central tubing is inserted into the aorta, taking care that the plug does not touch the aortic valve. The plug is attached to the tubing that is connected to the perfusion chamber that is placed 135 cm above the specimen, approximately equivalent to 100 mm Hg.

If a perfusion apparatus is not available, one can connect a polyethylene tube to a formalin spigot at one end and place the other end of the tube in the ascending or descending thoracic aorta, with the heart in a container on the floor. The spigot is opened, and leakage of formalin from the aorta is prevented with clamps.

The coronary arteries are then fixed in a distended state that approximate the dimensions observed in living patients. The method requires patency of the aortic valve to allow pressure filling of the coronaries.

FIGURE 150.1 ▲ Postmortem radiograph of coronary arteries. If heavily calcified, the epicardial arteries should be removed if there is a suspicion of coronary cause of death. LAD, left anterior descending; LCx, left circumflex; RCA, right coronary artery.

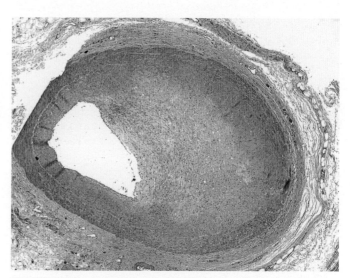

FIGURE 150.2 ▲ Pathologic intimal thickening. There is significant narrowing without necrotic core formation.

Assessing Degree of Stenosis of Coronary Atherosclerosis at Autopsy

The accepted level of critical stenosis at autopsy that could result in ischemia or sudden death is 75% cross-sectional area narrowing of the lumen. By angiography, percent stenosis is determined as diameter narrowing of the column of contrast, compared to a proximal reference segment. However, at autopsy, cross sections of the arteries are taken, and percent narrowing is defined by cross-sectional area luminal narrowing. If plaques are concentric, a critical 75% area reduction (as seen on the glass slide) is comparable to a 50% narrowing as seen by angiography.

For correlation with premortem angiography, and for medicolegal civil matters, accurate percent stenosis is often important to determine. There are three factors limiting accuracy in this regard: lack of perfusion fixation, subsequent tissue shrinkage during fixation and processing, and use of reference segment to determine percent narrowing.

Firstly, if the arteries are not perfusion fixed, then medial collapse of an uninvolved quadrant of the vessel can greatly overestimate percent stenosis, as the lumen is artifactually compromised. This artifact is greatest in eccentric plaques and those with mild to moderate stenosis; indeed, a 25% lesion could be seen as >90% if the vessel is collapsed.

The second source of error is tissue shrinkage. In reality, because of differential shrinkage of intimal tissues versus smooth muscle wall, the affect on percent stenosis is minimal. For segments with about 50% stenosis before processing, there is an increase to about 65% after processing. However, for 80% stenosis, there is actually a decrease in percent stenosis after processing to almost 70%.[8]

Thirdly, angiographic assessment of coronary narrowing is performed comparing the culprit segment with a proximal, presumably normal, segment. At autopsy, the assessment of coronary narrowing is performed comparing the intimal area to the area within the internal elastic lamina at the same segment. Therefore, affects of positive remodeling are not taken into account; therefore, the degree of stenosis is further exaggerated compared to angiographic methods.

Pathologic Staging of Atherosclerosis

Atherosclerotic plaques enlarge over time, resulting in progressive luminal narrowing. In reality, the decrease in lumen is not linear, because of episodic thrombi that suddenly enlarge the plaque. Also, the narrowing is not directly depending on plaque area, because compensatory remodeling expands the wall and counteracts the decrease in luminal area.

The American Heart Association has adopted a scheme of plaque stages denoted by Roman numerals (Table 150.1).[9] Some of the terms

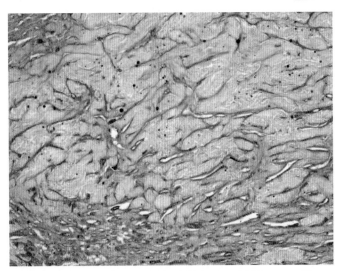

FIGURE 150.3 ▲ Pathologic intimal thickening. A higher magnification of the artery shown in Figure 150.2 shows extracellular lipid pools, apoptotic smooth muscle cells with prominent basement membranes, and microcalcifications.

have been adopted from aortic lesions that were traditionally staged by gross inspection and after staining with lipophilic substances such as oil red O. A type I plaque is a fibromuscular intimal lesion without significant lipids. A type II plaque has intimal foam cells (predominantly macrophages), and a type III plaque has extracellular lipid, primarily esterified, with little free cholesterol (Fig. 150.3). The type III plaques are sometimes referred to as preatheroma. Type II and III lesions are not distinct and occur simultaneously as plaques progress[10] (Figs. 150.3 and 150.4). The lipids are of two types, cholesterol and triglycerides, reflecting the low-density lipoprotein particles, which enter preferentially if oxidized. Stage IV plaques have a necrotic core, which is richer in free cholesterol and fatty acids, reflecting apoptotic breakdown of smooth muscle cells and macrophages (Fig. 150.5). Stage V plaques have a thick cap, which is frequently calcified, and stage VI plaques show hemorrhage, surface disruption, or thrombus (Fig. 150.6).

The traditional numerical classification does not identify the so-called thin-cap fibroatheroma, an important form of "vulnerable" plaque, or one prone to thrombosis.[11] Also, plaques with multiple

TABLE 150.1   Stages of Coronary Atherosclerotic Plaque (Lipid Rich)[a]

AHA Type	Descriptive Designation	Histologic Features
I	Adaptive intimal thickening	Mild intimal thickening with smooth muscle cells
II	Fatty streak/intimal xanthoma	Collection of intimal foamy macrophages
III	Pathologic intimal thickening	Pools of extracellular lipids, little or no free cholesterol (crystals)
IV	Fibroatheroma	Fibrous cap, poorly formed
V	Fibroatheroma with thick cap and calcification	Thick fibrous cap, often with calcification
		Healed plaque rupture with multiple cores
-	Thin-cap fibroatheroma	Fibrous cap < 65 μm overlying lipid-rich core
VI	Disrupted plaque	Acute plaque rupture/fissure Acute plaque erosion

[a]There are often coexisting multiple types in a single arterial segment. Plaques can also progress in the absence of significant lipid accumulation (pathologic intimal thickening with plaque erosion).
AHA, American Heart Association.

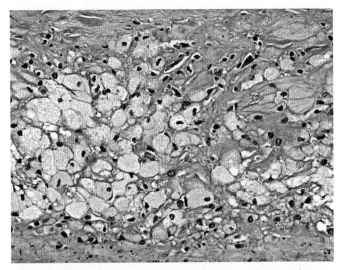

FIGURE 150.4 ▲ Foam cell–rich lesion (intimal xanthoma or fatty streak). There is a collection of foamy macrophages, which are filled in part with lipid derived from low density lipoprotein (LDL) particles that enter the intimal through receptors on endothelial cells.

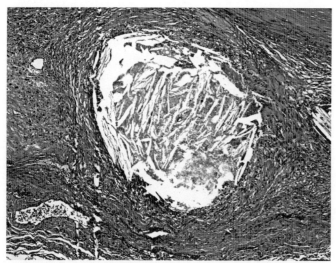

FIGURE 150.5 ▲ Fibroatheroma. High magnification of a small necrotic core shows free cholesterol crystals, which are dissolved in processing.

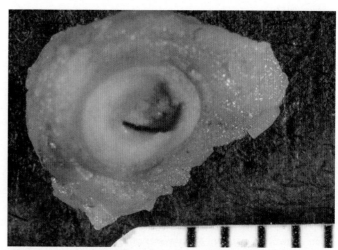

FIGURE 150.7 ▲ Acute plaque rupture with occlusive thrombus. The disrupted fibrous cap is seen in the center of the lumen filled with thrombus. There is an eccentric bright yellow necrotic core at the left.

necrotic cores are frequently the result of healed plaque ruptures, so the numerical classification does not accurately reflect chronology of plaque progression.

Morphologic Features of Coronary Atherothrombosis

In patients dying after *acute myocardial infarct*, thrombi are found in 98% of autopsies[1] (Fig. 150.7). In the autopsy evaluation of hearts with acute myocardial infarction, histologic evaluation of the entire coronary tree, comparing sites of acute myocardial necrosis with thrombosed arteries supplying the infarcted region, is important for clinicopathologic correlation.

The frequency of acute thrombosis in *unstable angina* is less than that seen in acute myocardial infarction and ranges from <50% to nearly 80%.[1]

Patients dying suddenly due to an arrhythmic event, with severe coronary atherosclerosis as the presumed cause of death, often have

an absence of thrombi and may show only relatively early (though obstructive) coronary lesions.[12] The types of atherosclerotic lesions seen in *sudden coronary death* include stable plaque with severe narrowing, hemorrhage into a necrotic core, and occlusive or nonocclusive thrombi (see Chapter 4).

The degree of luminal narrowing by stable plaque underlying coronary thrombosis may be important from a medicolegal standpoint and is relevant in formulating prevention strategies against coronary thrombosis. Pathologic studies have shown that a majority of underlying lesions is narrowed >50% (by area).[13–16] The only study comparing ruptures and erosions showed a mean area luminal narrowing of 78% in the former and 70% in the latter.[17] Sequential angiographic studies have shown that at least 50% of patients with acute coronary thrombosis had preexisting severe stenosis (>50% lumen diameter narrowing by angiography).[18]

Plaque ruptures are characterized by a luminal thrombus overlying a lipid-rich fibroatheroma, often with areas of hemorrhage, usually with a visibly interrupted cap (Figs. 150.8 and 150.9). Serial sections may be necessary to demonstrate the actual rupture site. Plaque ruptures account for the majority of coronary thrombi in sudden unexpected

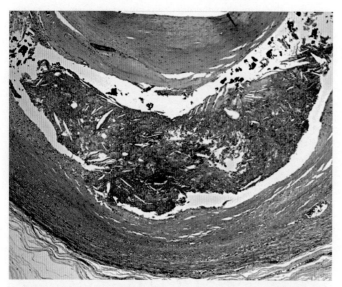

FIGURE 150.6 ▲ Fibroatheroma, with hemorrhage into plaque. One mechanism of plaque enlargement is the accumulation of blood within the necrotic cores, which generally occurs by rupture of small intimal neovessels (vasa vasorum). The leaked blood then becomes resorbed, and the cholesterol in the red blood cell membranes combines with that of apoptotic macrophages and smooth muscle cells to enlarge the necrotic core.

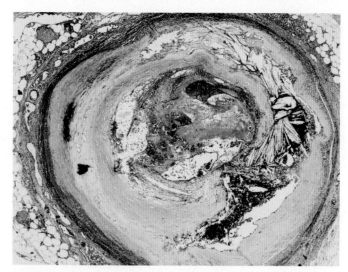

FIGURE 150.8 ▲ Acute plaque rupture with occlusive thrombus. The necrotic core with hemorrhage into plaque is at the bottom right adjacent to the rupture site. The contact between the tissue factor–rich core and the flowing blood resulted in occlusive luminal thrombus by activation of the extrinsic pathway. Movat pentachrome.

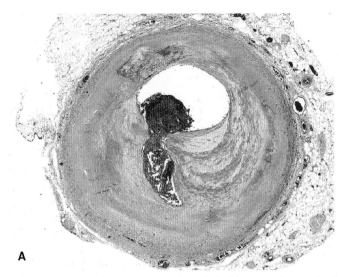
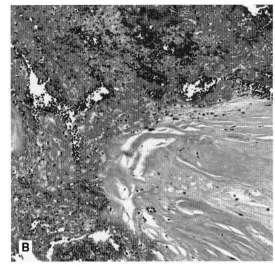

FIGURE 150.9 ▲ Acute plaque rupture. **A.** In this unusual example, the rupture site (at least at this level) appears fairly thick; in over 90% of cases, the cap is thin (<65 μm). **B.** A higher magnification shows the rupture site and adjacent fibrin–platelet thrombus.

death and myocardial infarction. The thinned, inflamed fibrous cap demonstrates an area of discontinuity, allowing the underlying lipid-rich core to contact the luminal blood, resulting in fibrin–platelet luminal thrombus. The overlying thrombus may be small and nonocclusive or occlusive, completely filling the lumen.

The thrombus may propagate antegrade or retrograde to the area of cap disruption and often shows some degree of organization, even in cases of sudden unexpected death. Distal embolization of the thrombus and necrotic core may occur; therefore, histologic evaluation of perfused myocardial beds should entail not only the assessment of myocyte necrosis but also *microembolization* of thrombotic material and plaque gruel.[19] Microembolization in the myocardial small vessels is more common with plaque erosion than plaque rupture.[19]

Acute thrombi that result in sudden death or acute myocardial infarct are generally visible to the naked eye, allowing the pathologist to adequately sample and histologically prepare the specimen, provided that proper coronary sectioning after decalcification has been achieved.

Plaque fissure is an early form of plaque rupture, in which there has break in the fibrous cap without significant luminal thrombus, or little exposure of lipid core to the lumen, resulting in intraplaque fibrin deposits without luminal thrombus.[20] The distinction between plaque fissure and rupture may be difficult and sometimes arbitrary. *Plaque ulceration* is a form of plaque rupture in which the contents of the lipid core have been extruded into the lumen and then embolized, resulting in a scooped-out lesion covered by organizing thrombus.

Most acute plaque ruptures do not result in sudden death or acute coronary syndromes. *Healed plaque ruptures* represent a mechanism of plaque enlargement[21] (Fig. 150.10). Old plaque ruptures are identified morphologically by the presence of a break in the fibrous cap, surrounded by granulation tissue with overlying organized thrombus. Although healed plaque ruptures are a form of stable plaque and do not result in acute coronary syndromes, they are associated with similar risk factors as are acute ruptures and are important for the autopsy pathologist to identify. Multiple old ruptures may be identified in a single site representing successive events increasing plaque size.

Plaque erosion is an often-overlooked cause of sudden death in young men and women accounting for about 35% of fatal coronary thrombi[17,22] (Fig. 150.11). Plaque erosion is uncommon after age 60 and is defined by the lack of surface disruption of the fibrous cap. Typically, there is not a prominent necrotic core, in contrast to plaque rupture.[12]

Plaque erosion is characterized by lesser degrees of calcification and overall plaque burden. Histologically, plaque erosion shows a denuded endothelial surface with luminal thrombus. The plaque underlying the thrombus is rich in proteoglycans and smooth muscle cells; there is often a small lipid core near the internal elastic lamina, but prominent cholesterol crystals and hemorrhage into plaque are absent.

Dating of acute coronary thrombi at autopsy is not precisely possible, although a dating system has been proposed.[4] It has been shown, both in autopsy studies and by thrombosuction from patients with acute coronary syndromes, that days or even weeks have passed between onset of thrombosis and acute coronary syndrome. In general, a thrombus is considered acute or subacute as long as fibrin is still present. Fresh thrombus occurs from 0 to 1 day and is composed of layers of platelets and fibrin, and few neutrophils without signs of lysis. Lytic thrombus occurs from 1 to 3 days and shows nuclear inflammatory cell

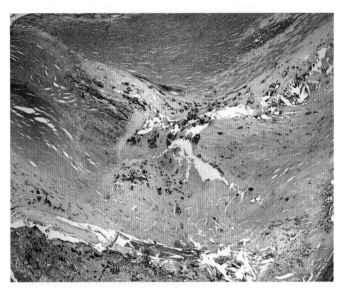

FIGURE 150.10 ▲ Healed plaque rupture. The prior rupture has healed over with granulation tissue and the healed thrombus above (*green*). Plaque rupture provides a mechanism for plaque enlargement and progression if nonocclusive. Movat pentachrome.

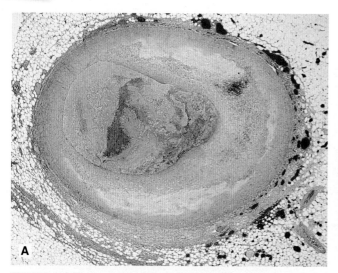
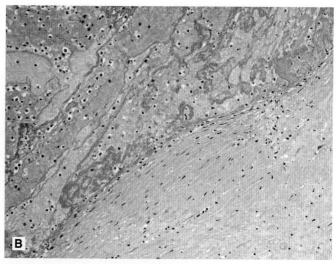

FIGURE 150.11 ▲ Acute plaque erosion with occlusive thrombus. **A.** In this case, there are early fibroatheromatous cores, but no thin-cap or surface disruption. **B.** The surface of the cap shows endothelial denudation, which is barely discernable, with an overlying fibrin–platelet thrombus.

degradation but no organization. Healing thrombus occurs from 4 to 7 days and has basal ingrowth of smooth muscle cells and endothelial cells without deposition of proteoglycans. Partially organized thrombus, >7 days, is composed of layers of smooth muscle cells or the presence of microvessels and proteoglycan deposition.

Thin-Cap Fibroatheroma

The concept of "vulnerable plaque" was first proposed by Muller more than 15 years ago.[23] The identification of precursor lesions for an acute thrombosis in the coronary arteries was the first step in eventual stabilization and prevention of not only thrombosis but also plaque progression. The first histologic description was described later and defined as a fibroatheroma with a fibrous cap 65 μm or thinner[24] (Fig. 150.12). Thin-cap fibroatheromas are characterized by a necrotic core and overlying fibrous cap that is infiltrated by macrophages. Markers of plaque growth and instability have focused on macrophage markers, matrix metalloproteinases, apoptosis, angiogenesis within necrotic cores, physicochemical properties of the plaque, cholesterol

crystals, calcification, and proteolytic enzymes such as myeloperoxidase.[25] The concept of vulnerable plaque has been expanded to that of a "vulnerable patient," because of the known increased risks of acute coronary syndromes in patients with increased levels of inflammatory markers such as C-reactive protein.

The distribution of thin-cap fibroatheroma favors the proximal arteries, especially the left anterior descending (LAD), and mirrors the distribution of acute and healed plaque ruptures.

Calcification and Coronary Atherosclerosis

Calcification is a reliable marker of coronary plaque burden, especially over the age of 40 years for men and 50 years for women. It is not sensitive for lipid-poor plaques in patients dying with plaque erosion, who tend to be young. Calcium can be detected by computed tomography (multislice CT) and scored by a number of quantitative measures.

The calcification process occurs in several cell types, including smooth muscle cells in pathologic intimal thickening, which undergo apoptosis

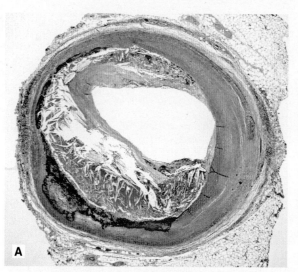
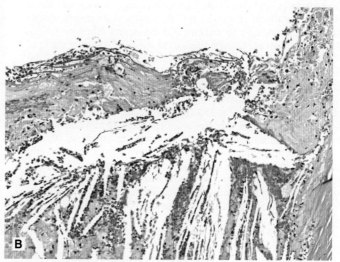

FIGURE 150.12 ▲ Thin-cap fibroatheroma. **A.** The necrotic core shows an overlying cap with focal thinning < 65 μm. **B.** Thin-cap fibroatheroma. A higher magnification shows prominent cholesterol crystals at the narrowed site, with marked narrowing of the fibrous cap, rendering the lesion prone to rupture and thrombosis.

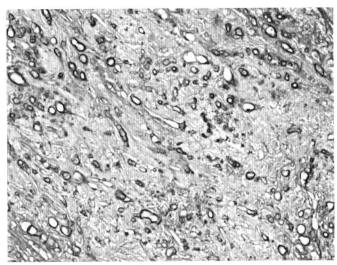

FIGURE 150.13 ▲ Calcification in an atherosclerotic plaque. Pathologic intimal thickening with diffuse calcification shows extracellular lipid pools with diffuse calcification.

and calcification (Fig. 150.13). The calcification in intimal smooth muscle cells has been likened to an active process, similar to that of membrane calcification in osteoblasts. Less studied is the calcification process in macrophages within atherosclerotic plaques that undergo apoptosis. Macroscopic calcification is not a reliable marker of plaque instability. Histologic studies have shown that calcification is frequent in "stable" plaques such as fibrocalcific plaques, and not particularly frequent in thin-cap fibroatheroma.

Microscopic calcifications are theoretically detrimental to plaque stability, however. The calcification in acute plaque ruptures tends to be fragmented and "speckled," as opposed to dense "pipestem" calcification of stable plaques with large lumens. Bioengineering studies using finite element analysis have attributed cap rupture to microcalcifications in the fibrous cap proper.[26]

A distinct form of calcification has been termed "nodular calcification" and may rarely rupture causing acute thrombosis.[27] Nodular calcification is typically present on sclerotic aortic valves and common in the aorta and carotid arteries. In the coronary circulation, it may be seen especially in proximal arteries (Fig. 150.14).

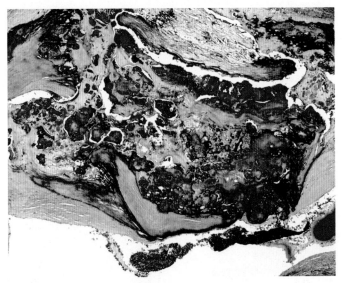

FIGURE 150.14 ▲ Nodular calcification, left anterior descending coronary artery. There are irregular blocks of calcified plaque surrounded by hemorrhage and fibrin.

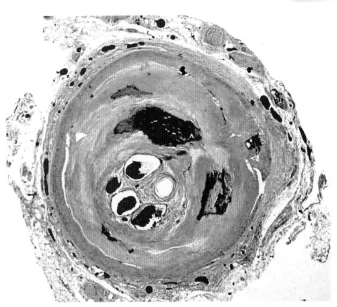

FIGURE 150.15 ▲ Chronic total occlusion with recanalized thrombus. There are multiple channels of recanalization and focal calcification.

Pathology of Chronic Total Occlusion

Chronic total occlusions indicate the presence of complete obstructions of the arterial lumen and are typically caused by organized thrombi (Fig. 150.15). Approximately one-third of patients undergoing angiography for coronary artery disease demonstrate total occlusions, and less than half are amenable to percutaneous revascularization. The most common artery involved is the right coronary and the least common the circumflex. Morphologically, chronic total occlusions are organized thrombi without calcification in two-thirds and fibrous or fibrocalcific plaques in one-third. The mean length of organized thrombi is longer if there is no calcification (mean 2 cm) as compared to 0.5 to 1 cm for total occlusion due to fibrous or fibrocalcific plaques.[28]

Coronary Remodeling and Adventitial Inflammation

Initially described by Glagov,[29] the phenomenon of positive remodeling results in compensatory enlargement of the artery with plaque growth, decreasing the narrowing effect of atherosclerosis. Coronary artery remodeling is associated with inflammation and is greatest in arteries with healed ruptures and large necrotic cores.[30] The mechanism may be the elaboration of proteases and elastases (matrix metalloproteinases) by macrophages. Negative remodeling denotes narrowing of the vessel in relation to a proximal reference segment and occurs in plaque erosion. Inflammation in atherosclerotic plaques of the coronary arteries does not only occur within the plaques themselves, but is also common in the adventitia, especially in plaques with large necrotic cores and in the segments adjacent to the necrotic core.[12]

The enlargement of the area within the internal elastic artery can be segmental and extreme, resulting in atherosclerotic aneurysms. Most aneurysms detected angiographically are associated with coronary atherosclerosis, and few are idiopathic or congenital (see Chapter 11). Atherosclerotic aneurysms are often distal to stenoses, suggesting a poststenotic dilatation. Coronary aneurysms have been defined as a diameter 1.5 times greater than the length of the dilated area.[31]

Practical Points

▶ Assessment of luminal narrowing is difficult in nonperfusion fixed autopsy hearts. In general, 75% area narrowing is considered a significant stenosis, corresponding to 50% diameter narrowing as seen angiographically.

▶ Decalcification is critical before sectioning arteries, in order to establish the presence or absence of thrombus. In general, a disrupted plaque with thrombus is rarely if ever an incidental finding.

▶ The epicardial arteries should be carefully sectioned to exclude thrombi and other lesions. Arteries typically overlooked include the left main artery and the proximal circumflex, which courses closely under the left atrial appendage.

▶ Assessment of luminal narrowing without considering luminal thrombus may be important for clinicopathologic correlation, especially if angiography had been performed during life.

REFERENCES

1. Burke AP, Farb A, Virmani R. Coronary thrombosis: What's new? *Pathol Case Rev.* 2001;6:244–252.
2. Tada T, Kadota K, Hosogi S, et al. Association between tissue characteristics evaluated with optical coherence tomography and mid-term results after paclitaxel-coated balloon dilatation for in-stent restenosis lesions: a comparison with plain old balloon angioplasty. *Eur Heart J Cardiovasc Imaging.* 2014;15:307–315.
3. Noguchi M, Yamada Y, Sakakura K, et al. Coronary thrombus aspiration revealed tumorous embolism of myxofibrosarcoma from the left atrium. *Cardiovasc Interv Ther.* 2016;31(1):75–78.
4. Rittersma SZ, van der Wal AC, Koch KT, et al. Plaque instability frequently occurs days or weeks before occlusive coronary thrombosis: a pathological thrombectomy study in primary percutaneous coronary intervention. *Circulation.* 2005;111:1160–1165.
5. Nemati MH, Astaneh B, Khosropanah S. Outcome and graft patency in coronary artery bypass grafting with coronary endarterectomy. *Korean J Thorac Cardiovasc Surg.* 2015;48:13–24.
6. Dawood MY, Lehr EJ, de Biasi A, et al. Robotically assisted coronary endarterectomy. *Innovations (Phila).* 2011;6:391–394.
7. Schmitto JD, Kolat P, Ortmann P, et al. Early results of coronary artery bypass grafting with coronary endarterectomy for severe coronary artery disease. *J Cardiothorac Surg.* 2009;4:52.
8. Siegel RJ, Swan K, Edwalds G, et al. Limitations of postmortem assessment of human coronary artery size and luminal narrowing: differential effects of tissue fixation and processing on vessels with different degrees of atherosclerosis. *J Am Coll Cardiol.* 1985;5:342–346.
9. Li T, Li X, Zhao X, et al. Classification of human coronary atherosclerotic plaques using ex vivo high-resolution multicontrast-weighted MRI compared with histopathology. *AJR Am J Roentgenol.* 2012;198:1069–1075.
10. Nakashima Y, Fujii H, Sumiyoshi S, et al. Early human atherosclerosis. Lipid and proteoglycans in intimal thickenings followed by macrophage infiltration. *Arterioscler Thromb Vasc Biol.* 2007;27:1159–1165.
11. Virmani R, Kolodgie FD, Burke AP, et al. Lessons from sudden coronary death: a comprehensive morphological classification scheme for atherosclerotic lesions. *Arterioscler Thromb Vasc Biol.* 2000;20:1262–1275.
12. Tavora F, Cresswell N, Li L, et al. Sudden coronary death caused by pathologic intimal thickening without atheromatous plaque formation. *Cardiovasc Pathol.* 2011;20:51–57.
13. Horie T, Sekiguchi M, Hirosawa K. Coronary thrombosis in pathogenesis of acute myocardial infarction. Histopathological study of coronary arteries in 108 necropsied cases using serial section. *Br Heart J.* 1978;40:153–161.
14. Falk E. Plaque rupture with severe pre-existing stenosis precipitating coronary thrombosis. Characteristics of coronary atherosclerotic plaques underlying fatal occlusive thrombi. *Br Heart J.* 1983;50:127–134.
15. Qiao JH, Fishbein MC. The severity of coronary atherosclerosis at sites of plaque rupture with occlusive thrombosis. *J Am Coll Cardiol.* 1991;17:1138–1142.
16. Davies MJ. Anatomic features in victims of sudden coronary death. Coronary artery pathology. *Circulation.* 1992;85:I19–I24.
17. Farb A, Burke AP, Tang AL, et al. Coronary plaque erosion without rupture into a lipid core. A frequent cause of coronary thrombosis in sudden coronary death. *Circulation.* 1996;93:1354–1363.
18. Mancini GB, Hartigan PM, Bates ER, et al. Angiographic disease progression and residual risk of cardiovascular events while on optimal medical therapy: observations from the COURAGE Trial. *Circ Cardiovasc Interv.* 2011;4:545–552.
19. Schwartz RS, Burke A, Farb A, et al. Microemboli and microvascular obstruction in acute coronary thrombosis and sudden coronary death relation to epicardial plaque histopathology. *J Am Coll Cardiol.* 2009;54:2167–2173.
20. Davies MJ, Thomas AC. Plaque fissuring—the cause of acute myocardial infarction, sudden ischaemic death, and crescendo angina. *Br Heart J.* 1985;53:363–373.
21. Burke AP, Kolodgie FD, Farb A, et al. Healed plaque ruptures and sudden coronary death: evidence that subclinical rupture has a role in plaque progression. *Circulation.* 2001;103:934–940.
22. Virmani R, Burke AP, Farb A. Plaque rupture and plaque erosion. *Thromb Haemost.* 1999;82(suppl 1):1–3.
23. Muller JE, Abela GS, Nesto RW, et al. Triggers, acute risk factors and vulnerable plaques: the lexicon of a new frontier. *J Am Coll Cardiol.* 1994;23:809–813.
24. Burke AP, Farb A, Malcom GT, et al. Coronary risk factors and plaque morphology in men with coronary disease who died suddenly. *N Engl J Med.* 1997;336:1276–1282.
25. Virmani R, Burke AP, Farb A, et al. Pathology of the vulnerable plaque. *J Am Coll Cardiol.* 2006;47:C13–C18.
26. Kelly-Arnold A, Maldonado N, Laudier D, et al. Revised microcalcification hypothesis for fibrous cap rupture in human coronary arteries. *Proc Natl Acad Sci USA.* 2013;110:10741–10746.
27. Rodriguez-Olivares R, Garcia-Touchard A, Diletti R, et al. First observation of acute coronary syndrome triggered by calcified nodules. Angiographic and optical coherence assessment. *Int J Cardiol.* 2014;173:e70–e71.
28. Srivatsa SS, Edwards WD, Boos CM, et al. Histologic correlates of angiographic chronic total coronary artery occlusions: influence of occlusion duration on neovascular channel patterns and intimal plaque composition. *J Am Coll Cardiol.* 1997;29:955–963.
29. Glagov S, Bassiouny HS, Sakaguchi Y, et al. Mechanical determinants of plaque modeling, remodeling and disruption. *Atherosclerosis.* 1997;131(suppl):S13–S14.
30. Burke AP, Kolodgie FD, Farb A, et al. Morphological predictors of arterial remodeling in coronary atherosclerosis. *Circulation.* 2002;105:297–303.
31. Harikrishnan S, Sunder KR, Tharakan JM, et al. Saccular coronary aneurysms: angiographic and clinical profile and follow-up of 22 cases. *Indian Heart J.* 2000;52:178–182.

151 Myocardial Infarction

Allen P. Burke, M.D., and Fabio R. Tavora, M.D., Ph.D.

Types of Acute Infarcts

Acute myocardial infarction indicates irreversible myocardial injury resulting in coagulative necrosis of the myocardium. Ischemia resulting in clinical or electrocardiographic manifestations is generally >1 cm.

"Acute" indicates infarction <5 days old, when the inflammatory infiltrate is primarily neutrophilic. Acute myocardial infarction may be either of the nonreperfusion type, in which case the obstruction to blood flow is permanent, or of the reperfusion type, in which the obstruction or lack of blood flow is long enough in duration (generally hours) but reversed or restored after there is myocardial cell death. "Subacute" of "healing" generally implies the onset of healing, as in granulation tissue with ingrowth of capillaries and fibrosis that begins at about 1 week. A "healed" infarct denotes the presence of dense scar, which begins at around 1 month, and is generally complete at 3 months.

Grossly, infarcts are classified by extent into subendocardial infarcts (less than one-third to one-half of the myocardial thickness) and transmural infarcts. Ischemic lesions caused by epicardial occlusions are endocardial based.

Clinically, acute coronary syndromes are classified as unstable angina/non-ST elevation myocardial infarction (NSTEMI) and ST elevation myocardial infarction (STEMI). Troponin "leak" in the proper clinical setting is indicative of myocardial damage and is the basis for the distinction between unstable angina and NSTEMI.

Incidence

Acute myocardial infarctions are common and result in hospitalizations of approximately four men and two women per 1,000 people in the United States yearly.[1]

It has been estimated that an acute myocardial infarction occurs every 44 seconds in the United States.[2] There is an annual incidence of 620,000 acute coronary events resulting in hospitalization or death and there are more than twice that rate of silent myocardial infarcts.[2]

Although the incidence has held steady in the United States, there has been a trend to a decrease in hospital mortality.[1,2]

Sudden Death and Heart Failure After Acute Infarction

Of all patients with STEMI, 25% to 35% will die of sudden cardiac death before receiving medical attention, most often from ventricular fibrillation.[3] Ventricular fibrillation complicates 5% to 6% of acute myocardial infarctions and imparts an increased risk of in-hospital mortality, but no increased long-term risk of sudden death.[4]

After hospital discharge for patients surviving acute myocardial infarction, there is a 1% to 2% risk of sudden death yearly for up to 5 years.[5,6] The rate of sudden death is increased in patients with heart failure. For this reason, patients are often treated with implantation of a cardioverter defibrillator when malignant ventricular arrhythmias occur more than 48 hours after the infarction and when the ejection fraction is decreased.[3]

Up to one-third of patients have recurrent ischemia in a 5-year period, with half that rate developing heart failure. Heart failure is the most significant risk factor for sudden death.[5]

Etiology

Autopsies of hospital inpatients dying with acute myocardial infarction will reveal an acute thrombus overlying atherosclerotic plaque in over 95% of cases, with careful inspection of the coronary arteries.[7,8]

Most fatal infarcts are transmural STEMIs that are presumed caused by occlusive thrombi.[9]

In autopsy studies of sudden deaths, there is a range of data regarding the frequency of occlusive versus nonocclusive lesions. Occlusive lesions have been described at a rate of 30% to 40%.[10,11]

The thrombi in NSTEMIs have often been presumed to be primarily nonocclusive, although because they rarely result in deaths, confirmatory autopsy studies are lacking. More recent studies using intravascular ultrasound have shown a significant increase in plaque volume and thrombus size comparing unstable angina and acute myocardial infarction, but no difference between NSTEMI and STEMI other than the size of the arc of the ruptured plaque.[12]

In the remaining hearts in patients with acute myocardial infarction, which represents <5%, there will be severe coronary diseases without thrombus.[13] Rare causes of acute myocardial infarction include no apparent cause (usually attributed to coronary spasm), coronary embolism (various causes, including valve vegetations and tumors), and thrombosis in nonatherosclerotic normal coronary arteries (hypercoagulable states) (see Chapter 155).

Reperfusion Infarction

Most myocardial infarcts in the preintervention era were nonreperfused, which indicates that the occlusion of a coronary artery is fixed, and not lysed by natural or iatrogenic means. Typically, a nonreperfused infarct is caused by an acute occlusive thrombus, which eventually organizes into a recanalized thrombus that may eventually allow some blood flow to occur.

When infarcts are diagnosed within hours of onset of symptoms, the thrombus is lysed pharmacologically or relieved by percutaneous intervention, preferably before irreversible injury occurs. If the infarct has resulted in irreversible injury prior to intervention (generally more than 6 to 8 hours after onset of chest pain), a reperfusion-type infarct occurs. In cases of reperfusion, the *area at risk*, or myocardium supplied by the thrombosed artery, is prone to irreversible ischemia from the occlusion itself as well as *reperfusion injury*. Components of reperfusion-induced myocardial damage include oxidative stress, Ca^{++} overload, rapid restoration of physiologic pH, and release of neutrophil granules, which open mitochondrial membranes and induce cardiomyocyte death.[14] Histologically, revascularization of the necrotic myocardium results in hemorrhage and edema, and endothelial swelling brought by the diffuse influx of neutrophils.[8]

Distribution of Ischemia

Whether an infarct is of the nonreperfused or perfused type, a proximal occlusion at the level of an epicardial artery results in a typical distribution starting at the subendocardium and progressing toward the epicardium (so-called wavefront phenomenon).[15] Therefore, an area of necrosis or scarring is considered to have an "ischemic pattern" if it is largest at the endocardium, with a wedge-shaped extending up to the epicardial surface. Ischemic injury may, however, be located in the midmyocardium or even subepicardium, if the level of the coronary occlusion is distal within the myocardium.[8]

The area of infarct occurs in the distribution of the occluded vessel (Table 151.1). Left main occlusion generally results in a large anterolateral infarct, whereas occlusion of the left anterior descending causes necrosis limited to the anterior wall. There is often extension to the anterior portion of the ventricular septum with proximal left coronary occlusions. In hearts with a right coronary dominance (right supplying

TABLE 151.1   Expected Distribution of Infarct, by Occluded Epicardial Vessel

Location of Infarct in Left Ventricle	Expected Occlusion Site(s)	Alternate Occlusion Site(s)
Anteroseptal	LAD	LM
Anterior	LAD	LD
Anterolateral	PLCx	LM, LOM
Lateral	LOM	LCx
Posterior	RCA	LCx (left dominant)
		LAD (wraparound LAD)
		LOM (LOM supplying PDA)

the posterior descending branch), a right coronary occlusion causes a posterior (inferior) infarct. With a left coronary dominance (about 15% of the population), a proximal circumflex occlusion will infarct the posterior wall; in the right dominant pattern, a proximal obtuse marginal thrombus will cause a lateral wall infarct only, and the circumflex distal is a small vessel. The anatomic variation due to microscopic collateral circulation, which is not evident at autopsy, plays a large factor in the size of necrosis and distribution. Unusual patterns of supply to the posterior wall, such as wraparound left anterior descending or posterior descending supplied by the obtuse marginal, may also result in unexpected areas of infarct in relation to the occluded proximal segment.

Gross Pathologic Findings

The earliest change that can be grossly discerned in the evolution of acute myocardial infarction is pallor of the myocardium, which is evident 12 hours or later after the onset of irreversible ischemia. The gross detection of infarction can be enhanced by the use of tetrazolium salt solutions, which form a colored precipitate on gross section of fresh heart tissue in the presence of dehydrogenase-mediated activity. Myocardial necrosis can be detected as early as 2 to 3 hours by this method.

In nonreperfused infarction, the area of the infarct is well defined at 2 to 3 days with a central area of yellow discoloration that is surrounded by a thin rim of highly vascularized hyperemia. In a reperfused infarct, the infarcted region will appear red from trapping of the red cells and hemorrhage from the rupture of the necrotic capillaries.

At 5 to 7 days, the regions are much more distinct, with a central soft area and a depressed hyperemic border. At 1 to 2 weeks, the infarct begins to be depressed, especially at the margins where organization takes place, and the borders are white; a clear gray color may be seen at the granulation tissue border. Healing may be complete as early as 4 to 6 weeks in small infarcts, or may take as long as 2 to 3 months when the area of infarction is large.

Healed infarcts are white from the scarring, and the ventricular wall may be thinned (aneurysmal), especially in transmural infarction.

The size of the infarct, whether acute, healing, or healed, should be estimated my assessing the largest dimension in any slice and giving an extent of the infarct from apex to the base of the heart. For example, an infarct could be described as 4 cm in greatest dimension, extending from 1 cm from the apex to midmyocardium, involving three contiguous 1-cm slides.

Figures 151.1 to 151.3 show examples of gross findings in different stages of acute myocardial infarction.

Histopathology of Nonreperfused Infarcts

The border zone between necrotic myocardium and viable myocardium is the focus of dating, which depends on the reaction of viable myocardium to the area of infarct (Table 151.2).

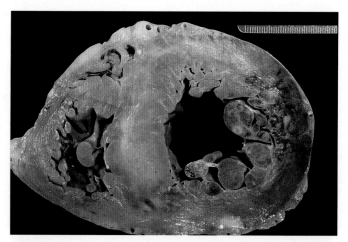

FIGURE 151.1 ▲ Acute myocardial infarction, lateral left ventricle. There is irregular mottling that is transmural in the lateral wall of the left ventricle, consistent with a thrombotic occlusion of the left circumflex artery.

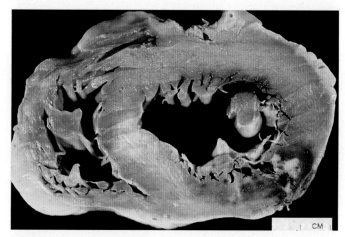

FIGURE 151.2 ▲ Acute myocardial infarction, posterolateral left ventricle. There is a yellow necrotic area surrounded by a hyperemic border, typical of a 2- to 4-day-old infarct. There was an occlusive thrombus in the mid-distal right coronary artery.

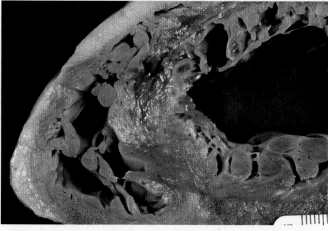

FIGURE 151.3 ▲ Healing myocardial infarction, anterior ventricular septum. The gelatinous appearance is that of granulation tissue with early scarring and edema. There was an organizing thrombus in the proximal first diagonal artery.

TABLE 151.2   Histologic Evolution of Nonreperfused Myocardial Infarction[a]

Injury Response	Initiation	Peak
Hypereosinophilia, myocytes	12–24 h	24–48 h[b]
Neutrophilic infiltrate at periphery	24 h	2–4 d
Neutrophil karyorrhexis	1.5 d	3–5 d
Macrophages with hemosiderin	4–5 d	5–10 d
Endothelial cell sprouts/granulation tissue	7 d	10 d–2 wk
Fibroblasts	7–14 d	2–4 wk
Collagen strands	2–3 wk	4 wk
Dense collagen	4 wk	>2–3 mo

[a]All times are approximate. Injury response should be evaluated at the border zone between the infarct and viable myocardium. In the first 30 to 40 minutes of ischemia, the changes are only appreciable by ultrastructure. After 3 to 4 hours, acute ischemia may be identified by triphenyl tetrazolium chloride, which detects dehydrogenase enzymes in viable myocardium applied to gross unfixed heart sections, staining it brick red.
[b]Dead, "mummified" myocytes devoid of cross-striations may persist within the center of nonreperfused infarcts for months.

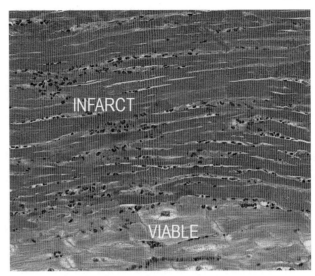

FIGURE 151.4 ▲ Acute myocardial infarction. **A.** The earliest change of acute myocardial ischemia is hypereosinophilic of myocytes, seen above (*infarct*). The non-infarcted myocardium is below (*viable*).

The earliest morphologic characteristic of myocardial infarction occurs between 12 and 24 hours after onset of chest pain.[8] Hypereosinophilia of the cytoplasm is characteristic of myocardial ischemia (Figs. 151.4 and 151.5). Neutrophil infiltration is present by 24 hours at the border. As the infarct progresses between 24 and 48 hours, coagulation necrosis is established with various degrees of nuclear pyknosis, early karyorrhexis, and karyolysis. The myocyte striations are preserved and the sarcomeres elongate. The border areas show prominent neutrophil infiltration by 48 hours (Fig. 151.6). At 3 to 5 days, the central portion of the infarct shows loss of myocyte nuclei and striations; in smaller infarcts, neutrophils invade within the infarct and fragment, resulting in more severe karyorrhexis (nuclear dust) (Fig. 151.7). Markers of ischemia include hypoxia inducible factor 1, complement leaking into myocytes, and cyclooxygenase-2, which can be demonstrated immunohistochemically. Macrophages and fibroblasts begin to appear in the border areas by 5 to 7 days. By 1 week, neutrophils are inconspicuous and granulation tissue is established. Eosinophils may be seen within the inflammatory infiltrate but are only present in one in four infarcts. There is phagocytic removal of the necrotic myocytes by macrophages, and pigment is seen within macrophages at about 1 week (Figs. 151.8 and 151.9).

By the second week, there is continued removal of the necrotic myocytes as the fibroblasts are actively producing collagen and angiogenesis occurs in the area of healing (Figs. 151.8 and 151.9). The healing continues, and depending on the extent of necrosis, the healing may be complete as early as 4 weeks, or require 8 weeks or longer to complete. The central area of infarction may remain unhealed showing mummified myocytes for extended periods, despite the fact that the infarct borders are completely healed. As mentioned above, infarcts caused by emboli from proximal ruptured plaques may have a random or subepicardial distribution.

Pathology of Reperfused Acute Myocardial Infarction

Reperfusion infarcts are usually hemorrhagic. If there is reperfusion of an epicardial occlusion, the distribution of the infarct is identical to nonreperfused infarcts (Fig. 151.10). If reperfusion occurs as a result of resuscitation after global myocardial ischemia, then there is diffuse subendocardial hemorrhage (Fig. 151.11).

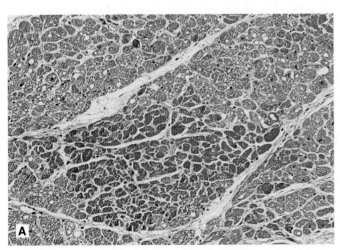

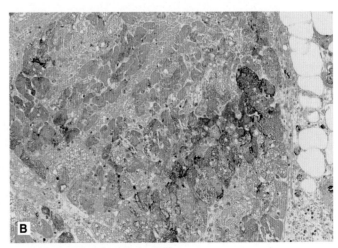

FIGURE 151.5 ▲ Acute myocardial infarct. **A.** There is patchy hypereosinophilia in an acutely ischemic area within chronic ischemic vacuolated myocytes (see Figure 139.7). **B.** Immunohistochemical staining for complement shows intracytoplasmic uptake in the ischemic areas.

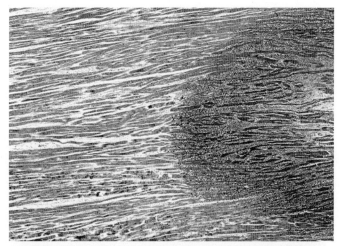

FIGURE 151.6 ▲ Acute infarct, 2 to 3 days. The infarct is at the left; there is an influx of neutrophils at the right, coming from viable myocardium.

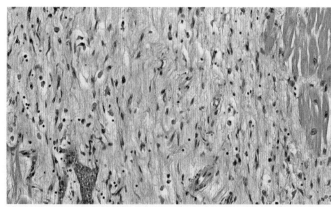

FIGURE 151.9 ▲ Healing infarct, 2 weeks. There is granulation tissue composed of fibroblasts, chronic inflammation, and neocapillaries. There are loose fibrosis and scattered hemosiderin macrophages.

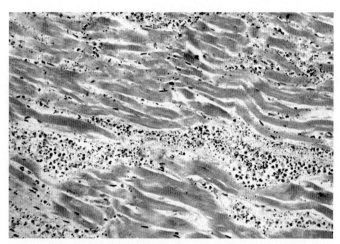

FIGURE 151.7 ▲ Neutrophil karyorrhexis. By 4 to 5 days, there is apoptosis of neutrophils, which are then taken up by macrophages.

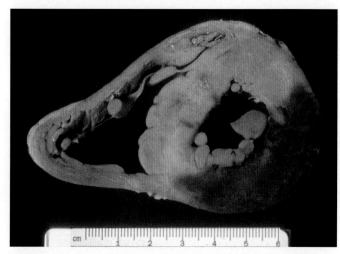

FIGURE 151.10 ▲ Acute reperfusion infarct, posterolateral left ventricle. Reperfusion infarcts may be caused by delayed thrombolytic therapy given after irreversible myocyte damage. (Reproduced from Burke AP, Virmani R. Pathophysiology of acute myocardial infarction. *Med Clin North Am.* 2007;91:553, with permission.)

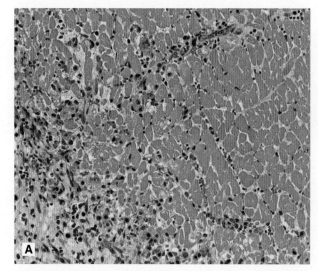

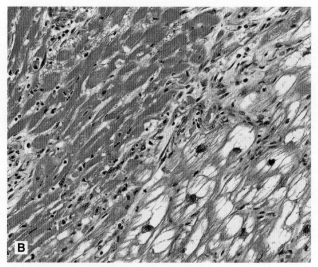

FIGURE 151.8 ▲ Subacute infarct. Acute infarct, 5 days. **A.** The myocytes are hypereosinophilic with loss of cross-striations and nuclei. The adjacent inflammatory reaction is that of chronic inflammation and macrophages. **B.** In this example, there are chronic ischemic changes with myocyte vacuolization and myofibrillar loss (**bottom right**) with an acute infarct at the top left.

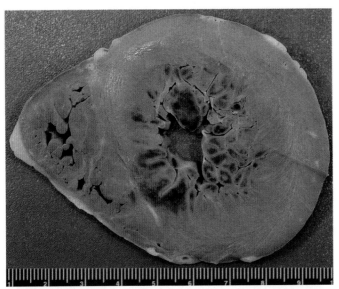

FIGURE 151.11 ▲ Acute reperfusion infarct, concentric, subendo-cardial, secondary to resuscitation. This heart shows subendocardial hemorrhage in the papillary muscles of the left ventricle, which resulted from a cardiac arrest with delayed resuscitation 1.5 days prior to death. The cause of death was somewhat unclear, but likely related to cardio-myopathy related to ventricular noncompaction, with contributing factor of coronary disease.

Histologically, there is a confluent area of hemorrhage within the infarcted myocardium, with extensive contraction band necrosis (Fig. 151.12). Within a few hours of reperfusion, sparse neutrophils are evident within the area of necrosis, but they are usually sparse. Macrophages begin to appear by day 2 to 3; by day 3 to 5, fibroblasts appear, with an accelerated rate of healing as compared to nonreper-fused infarcts. As early as 2 to 3 weeks, subendocardial infarcts may be fully healed. Larger infarcts, and those reperfused after 6 hours, take longer to heal. Infarcts reperfused after 6 hours show larger areas of hemorrhage as compared to occlusions with more immediate reperfusion.

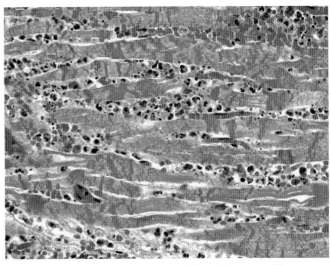

FIGURE 151.12 ▲ Acute reperfusion infarct. There are diffuse con-traction bands, hemorrhage, and neutrophilic apoptosis.

Pathologic Consequences of Acute Infarction

Rupture of the Left Ventricular Free Wall

When the pathologist encounters hemopericardium in cases of sud-den unexpected death, two entities should be immediately consid-ered: rupture of the ascending aorta and rupture of the myocardium. The ventricular defect in rupture infarcts may be obvious, or rela-tively subtle when viewed from the epicardial surface. Bread loafing the myocardium will demonstrate transmural acute infarction, with or without a grossly identified rupture track. Associated aneurysm formation with rupture is also a common complication (Figs. 151.13 to 151.15).[17]

Factors associated with cardiac rupture include female gender, age over 60 years, hypertension, and first MI. Additional risk factors include multivessel atherosclerotic disease, absence of ventricular hypertrophy, poor collateral flow, transmural infarct involving at least

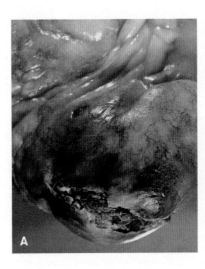

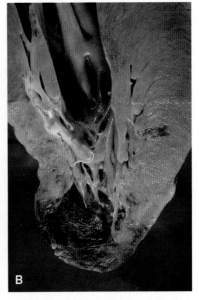

FIGURE 151.13 ▲ Acute infarction, with aneurysm and rupture. **A.** The infarct resulted in an apical aneurysm, which ruptured causing hemopericardium and sudden death. **B.** Acute infarction, with aneurysm and rupture. A high magnification shows the transmural infarct with acute thinning of the ventricle. (Part A is reproduced from Burke AP, Virmani R. Pathophysiology of acute myocardial infarc-tion. *Med Clin North Am.* 2007;91:553, with permission.)

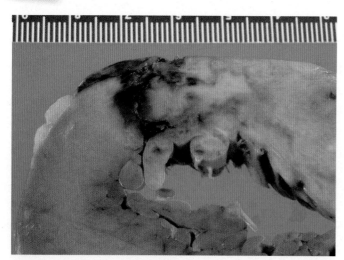

FIGURE 151.14 ▲ Acute infarction with rupture, anterolateral left ventricle. There is a mottled area at the junction of the anterior septum and free wall. The rupture track is hemorrhagic. There was hemopericardium at autopsy.

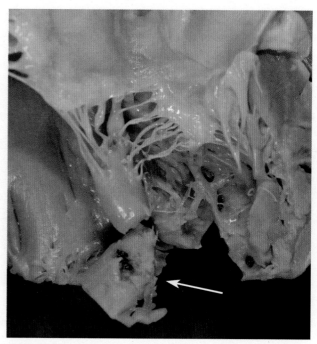

FIGURE 151.16 ▲ Acute rupture, papillary muscle. The *arrow* shows the hemorrhagic area that ruptured; the patient had acute respiratory failure and a holosystolic murmur of mitral regurgitation. He had complained of severe chest pain 10 days prior, but was discharged home without cardiac evaluation.

20% of the wall, and location of the infarct in the midanterior or lateral wall of the left ventricle.

An autopsy study from 2015 showed that risk factors for cardiac rupture after myocardial infarction included advanced age, excessive fat in the epicardium, absence of healed infarcts, absence of diabetes, and a higher rate of thrombolytic therapy.[19] Intense interstitial neutrophil infiltration may increase the risk of the myocardial rupture after infarction.[20]

Cardiac rupture usually occurs in the first few days (1 to 4 days) following the infarct when coagulation necrosis and neutrophilic infiltration are at their peak and have weakened the left ventricular wall. A recent study reported a median of 3 days (mean 5 days) after infarct.[19]

Rupture of the Posteromedial Papillary Muscle

Myocardial rupture may involve the papillary muscle only or the papillary muscle and the posterolateral ventricular wall (Figs. 151.16

and 151.17). Most involve the posteromedial papillary muscle with occlusion of the right circulation and are associated with a posterior free wall infarct. A thrombus in the left anterior descending thrombus may rarely cause a rupture of the posterior papillary muscle.[21]

Rupture of the Ventricular Septum

Ruptures of the ventricular septum result in an *acquired ventricular septal defect* and are often accompanied by a free wall rupture.[19] Simple ventricular septal ruptures have a discrete defect and have a

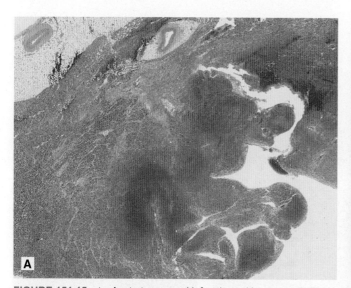
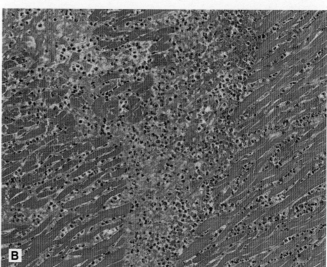

FIGURE 151.15 ▲ Acute transmural infarction, with rupture. **A.** The ventricle wall shows a predominantly subendocardial infarction with extension to the epicardial surface. **B.** A higher magnification shows a dense neutrophilic infiltrate at the rupture site. Metalloproteinases elaborated by neutrophils may play a role in destruction of the myocardium in myocardial rupture.

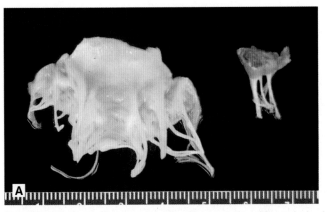
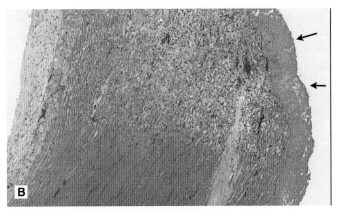

FIGURE 151.17 ▲ Acute rupture, papillary muscle, with surgical valve replacement. **A.** A gross photograph shows the mitral valve and the detached papillary muscle that was severed by the infarct. **B.** Histologically, there are necrotic myocytes (below), granulation tissue in the center (indicating some evidence of healing), and the rupture track at the right lined by platelets (*arrows*).

direct through-and-through communication across the septum, are usually associated with anterior myocardial infarction, and are located in the apex. Complex ruptures are characterized by extensive hemorrhage with irregular serpiginous borders of the necrotic muscle, usually occur in inferior infarcts, and involve the basal inferoposterior septum.

Intramural Thromboembolism and Focal Ischemic Lesions

It is not uncommon to find focal microscopic ischemic-like lesion in the hearts of patients dying of cardiac and noncardiac causes. These so-called anginal lesions are often attributed to small embolic events in intramyocardial small coronaries. Often, no evidence of embolism is present (Fig. 151.18).

Postinfarction Pericardial Effusion and Pericarditis

Pericardial effusion is reported in 25% of patients with acute myocardial infarcts and is more common in patients with anterior

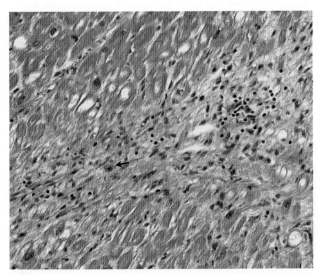

FIGURE 151.18 ▲ Focal ischemic lesion, myocardium. In this example, the hemosiderin macrophages are evident (*arrow*). These are more commonly seen in ischemic lesions than postmyocarditis foci.

myocardial infarction, large infarcts, and congestive heart failure. Pericarditis occurs less often than pericardial effusion and is seen only in transmural acute myocardial infarction. Postinfarction syndrome (Dressler syndrome), previously reported to occur in 3% to 4% of all myocardial infarction, has been greatly reduced in incidence because of the extensive use of thrombolysis and treatments that dramatically decreased the size of myocardial necrosis and modulated the immune system.[18]

Postinfarction Mural Thrombus and Embolization

Mural thrombus forming on the endocardial surface over the area of the acute infarction occurs in 20% of all patients, 40% for anterior infarcts, and 60% for apical infarcts.[22] The risk of embolization is greatest in the first few weeks of acute myocardial infarction. The usual sites of symptomatic embolization are the brain, eyes, kidney, spleen, bowel, legs, and coronary arteries.

Acute Respiratory Failure

In ~5% of patients who die of unexplained acute respiratory failure, autopsy will demonstrate an undiagnosed acute myocardial infarction. The histologic findings in the lungs are usually those of acute respiratory distress syndrome (diffuse alveolar damage).[23]

Prognosis

The 5-year survival rate for patients hospitalized for acute myocardial infarction is ~75%.[4] The mortality from ST elevation myocardial infarcts depends largely on infarct size. Other factors associated with poor prognosis include advanced age, renal failure, diabetes, heart failure, three-vessel coronary disease, and delayed treatment of reperfusion.[14]

Right Ventricular and Atrial Infarction

Right ventricular infarcts typically involve the posterior wall as extensions of posterior left ventricular infarcts, occurring in up to one-third of patients.[25] Right ventricular extension of inferior infarcts is associated with a poorer prognosis[26] especially if there is concomitant high-degree atrioventricular block. Inferior infarcts with right ventricular involvement may be clinically silent.[27] Atrial involvement occurs in up to 10% of ventricular infarcts. Isolated right ventricular infarcts are generally associated with pulmonary hypertension and right ventricular hypertrophy, and rarely rupture.[28–30]

Practical Points

► Hemopericardium resulting in sudden death is caused by one of two processes: ascending aortic rupture and myocardial rupture. The latter can be subtle from inspection of the epicardial surface of the heart; as the rupture site can be relatively small, blood may accumulate from a relatively slow leak. Hemopericardium is only rarely caused by perforation by chest compressions, in which case there is rib fracture.

► Acute myocardial infarction is not seen in surgical pathology, unless there is mitral valve replacement due to rupture of the posteromedial papillary muscle (see Chapter 33).

► Dating of myocardial infarction may be important, especially in medicolegal situations. Dating is essentially based on temporal progression of reactions to wound repair, which overlap temporally and are especially imprecise after 2 weeks. It is important to remember that the findings must be applied to the junction of the viable myocardium to the infarcted area and that dating of small lesions (1 to 2 mm or smaller) is impossible.

REFERENCES

1. Rosamond WD, Chambless LE, Folsom AR, et al. Trends in the incidence of myocardial infarction and in mortality due to coronary heart disease, 1987 to 1994. *N Engl J Med.* 1998;339:861–867.
2. Mozaffarian D, Benjamin EJ, Go AS, et al. Heart disease and stroke statistics—2015 update: a report from the American Heart Association. *Circulation.* 2015;131:e29–e322.
3. Manolis AS. The clinical challenge of preventing sudden cardiac death immediately after acute ST-elevation myocardial infarction. *Expert Rev Cardiovasc Ther.* 2014;12:1427–1437.
4. Bougouin W, Marijon E, Puymirat E, et al. Incidence of sudden cardiac death after ventricular fibrillation complicating acute myocardial infarction: a 5-year cause-of-death analysis of the FAST-MI 2005 registry. *Eur Heart J.* 2014;35:116–122.
5. Adabag AS, Therneau TM, Gersh BJ, et al. Sudden death after myocardial infarction. *JAMA.* 2008;300:2022–2029.
6. Yu H, Pi-Hua F, Yuan W, et al. Prediction of sudden cardiac death in patients after acute myocardial infarction using T-wave alternans: a prospective study. *J Electrocardiol.* 2012;45:60–65.
7. Arbustini E, Dal Bello B, Morbini P, et al. Plaque erosion is a major substrate for coronary thrombosis in acute myocardial infarction. *Heart.* 1999;82:269–272.
8. Burke AP, Virmani R. Pathophysiology of acute myocardial infarction. *Med Clin North Am.* 2007;91:553–572, ix.
9. Davies MJ, Woolf N, Robertson WB. Pathology of acute myocardial infarction with particular reference to occlusive coronary thrombi. *Br Heart J.* 1976;38:659–664.
10. Davies MJ. Anatomic features in victims of sudden coronary death. Coronary artery pathology. *Circulation.* 1992;85:I19–I24.
11. Farb A, Burke AP, Tang AL, et al. Coronary plaque erosion without rupture into a lipid core. A frequent cause of coronary thrombosis in sudden coronary death. *Circulation.* 1996;93:1354–1363.
12. Lee CW, Hwang I, Park CS, et al. Comparison of intravascular ultrasound and histological findings in culprit coronary plaques between ST-segment elevation and non-ST-segment elevation myocardial infarction. *Am J Cardiol.* 2013;112:68–72.
13. Reynolds HR. Myocardial infarction without obstructive coronary artery disease. *Curr Opin Cardiol.* 2012;27:655–660.
14. McAlindon E, Bucciarelli-Ducci C, Suleiman MS, et al. Infarct size reduction in acute myocardial infarction. *Heart.* 2015;101:155–160.
15. Reimer KA, Jennings RB. The "wavefront phenomenon" of myocardial ischemic cell death. II. Transmural progression of necrosis within the framework of ischemic bed size (myocardium at risk) and collateral flow. *Lab Invest.* 1979;40:633–644.
16. Lambert JM, Lopez EF, Lindsey ML. Macrophage roles following myocardial infarction. *Int J Cardiol.* 2008;130:147–158.
17. Batts KP, Ackermann DM, Edwards WD. Postinfarction rupture of the left ventricular free wall: clinicopathologic correlates in 100 consecutive autopsy cases. *Hum Pathol.* 1990;21:530–535.
18. Hayashi T, Miyataka M, Kimura A, et al. Recent decline in hospital mortality among patients with acute myocardial infarction. *Circ J.* 2005;69:420–426.
19. Roberts WC, Burks KH, Ko JM, et al. Commonalities of cardiac rupture (left ventricular free wall or ventricular septum or papillary muscle) during acute myocardial infarction secondary to atherosclerotic coronary artery disease. *Am J Cardiol.* 2015;115:125–140.
20. Zidar N, Jera J, Maja J, et al. Caspases in myocardial infarction. *Adv Clin Chem.* 2007;44:1–33.
21. Cherian PS, Clarke AJ, Burstow DJ. Unusual case of acute posteromedial papillary muscle rupture after acute anterior myocardial infarction. *Heart Lung Circ.* 2014;23:e16–e19.
22. Keeley EC, Hillis LD. Left ventricular mural thrombus after acute myocardial infarction. *Clin Cardiol.* 1996;19:83–86.
23. Soeiro Ade M, Ruppert AD, Canzian M, et al. Postmortem diagnosis of acute myocardial infarction in patients with acute respiratory failure: demographics, etiologic and pulmonary histologic analysis. *Clinics (Sao Paulo).* 2012;67:213–217.
24. Botker HE, Kharbanda R, Schmidt MR, et al. Remote ischaemic conditioning before hospital admission, as a complement to angioplasty, and effect on myocardial salvage in patients with acute myocardial infarction: a randomised trial. *Lancet.* 2010;375:727–734.
25. Pirzada AM, Zaman KS, Mahmood K, et al. High degree atrioventricular block in patients with acute inferior myocardial infarction with and without right ventricular involvement. *J Coll Physicians Surg Pak.* 2009;19:269–274.
26. Khan S, Kundi A, Sharieff S. Prevalence of right ventricular myocardial infarction in patients with acute inferior wall myocardial infarction. *Int J Clin Pract.* 2004;58:354–357.
27. Manka R, Fleck E, Paetsch I. Silent inferior myocardial infarction with extensive right ventricular scarring. *Int J Cardiol.* 2008;127:e186–e187.
28. Hurley RW, Subramanian R, Rahko PS, et al. Isolated right atrial infarction with rupture. *N Engl J Med.* 1990;322:1611.
29. Stanescu DC, Teculescu DB. Isolated atrial infarction. *Dis Chest.* 1967;51:643–644.
30. Ventura T, Colantonio D, Leocata P, et al. Isolated atrial myocardial infarction: pathological and clinical features in 10 cases. *Cardiologia.* 1991;36:345–350.

152   Chronic Ischemic Heart Disease

Allen P. Burke, M.D., and Joseph J. Maleszewski, M.D.

Background and Terminology

"Ischemic cardiomyopathy" denotes the presence of obstructive epicardial coronary atherosclerosis with decreased left ventricular systolic dysfunction. An obsolete use of the term "ischemic cardiomyopathy" was "a dilated cardiomyopathy with impaired contractile performance not explained by the extent of coronary artery disease or ischemic damage."[1] Although the commonly used term *ischemic cardiomyopathy* is not supported by the American Heart Association[2] or by the European Society of Cardiology,[3] it is still in widespread use to distinguish clinically dilated cardiomyopathy from ischemic heart disease with heart failure.[4–14]

Clinically, ischemic cardiomyopathy is defined as left ventricular ejection fraction <35% to 40%, increased left end-diastolic diameter (6.5 cm), and evidence of coronary occlusive disease. The latter is generally defined as >70% stenosis (diameter narrowing) in ≥1 epicardial coronary vessel on angiography, history of myocardial infarction or revascularization, or demonstrable ischemia.[8,12] "Demonstrable ischemia" generally indicates evidence of segmental wall motion abnormalities or documented myocardial infarction.

Epidemiology

Chronic ischemic heart disease affects an estimated 3 million people in the United States and is the most common cause of heart failure worldwide.[15,16] Overall, there are more than 5 million Americans with heart failure, most caused by the sequelae of coronary ischemia, with over 80,000 new cases annually.[16]

Pathophysiology

After a myocardial infarction heals, the scarred area remodels, with compensatory left ventricular dilatation in the surrounding myocardium. The normal left ventricular elliptical shape changes as the ventricular volume increases, leading to ventricular dyssynchrony and nonuniform contraction. As the normal elliptical shape transforms to a spherical shape, the ejection fraction declines significant, and the prognosis becomes poor.[9]

Clinical Findings in Chronic Ischemic Heart Disease

Although coronary artery frequently disease presents as stable angina or acute coronary syndromes (ST elevation and non–ST elevation infarcts and sudden death), a substantial proportion of patients present with signs and symptoms of heart failure. The clinical findings are similar to those in heart failure of any cause, but angiography will demonstrate coronary artery stenoses, with irreversible wall motion abnormalities in areas of occlusion. In many cases of "ischemic cardiomyopathy," the clinical course is initially that of acute infarction, treated by percutaneous interventions or open surgery, and then progresses to end-stage heart failure.

Between 75% and 90% of patients with ischemic cardiomyopathy are men, with a mean age of about 60 at the time of surgery.[8,12] Risk factors are frequently present, including hypertension (50% to 70%) and diabetes mellitus (30% to 45% of patients). Hyperlipidemia and smoking are also common, with a minority of patients with concomitant cerebrovascular or peripheral vascular disease. Between 20% and 50% of patients have no prior history of acute coronary syndrome.[8,12]

Arrhythmias in Ischemic Heart Disease

Patients with ischemic cardiomyopathy are at increased risk for ventricular tachycardia, ventricular fibrillation, and sudden cardiac death.[17] Up to one-third of patients require implantable defibrillators.[8,17] Various findings on electrocardiograms are associated with increased risk for ventricular fibrillation, including voltage criteria for left ventricular hypertrophy.[17]

The size of the infarct, as characterized by late gadolinium enhancement cardiac magnetic resonance, correlates with the risk of sustained monomorphic ventricular tachycardia, which may progress to ventricular fibrillation.[5] Because monomorphic tachycardias may be mapped to specific sites by electrophysiologic studies, hearts from patients with ischemic cardiomyopathy frequently show patches of endocardial scarring indicative of prior ablation sites.

At explant or autopsy, approximately one-third of hearts will demonstrate implantable cardioverter defibrillators. These may be either single lead (tip of right ventricular apex) or dual (atrioventricular), with a second lead in the right atrium. Atrioventricular defibrillators are indicated in those at risk for bradycardia from intrinsic sinus node dysfunction or conduction system disease, or use of medications with negative chronotropic properties.

Cardiac Resynchronization Therapy

In heart failure of any cause, including that caused by ischemic heart disease, intraventricular dyssynchrony may necessitate biventricular pacing. In order to access the left ventricle, a lead is placed in the coronary sinus coursing to an anterior cardiac vein, in addition to the right atrial and ventricular pacemaker leads. These three pacing wires are often found at autopsy in patients with chronic ischemic heart disease and will have been removed in explanted hearts. Indications for resynchronization therapy include a QRS duration of ≥120 ms with moderate or severe heart failure and a QRS duration of ≥150 ms for patients with mild symptoms.[11]

Revascularization in Ischemic Heart Disease

There are several surgical approaches to the treatment of chronic ischemic heart disease: coronary bypass grafting, mitral valve repair or replacement, and, in the case of aneurysm, surgical ventricular reconstruction.

The rationale behind coronary bypass surgery in patients with stable, healed infarcts is based on the presence of myocardial tissue that is not irreversibly damaged by ischemia, but is not contracting. The pathologic features of these areas have not been characterized, although the extent of transmural extent of scar has been negatively correlated with functional recovery after revascularization. Survival after coronary artery bypass surgery is better in patients with lower scar burden and lesser degrees of cardiac dilatation (as assessed by end-systolic volume).[8]

There is some evidence that bypass surgery may be superior to medical treatment in selected patients.[13] Patients who are candidates for surgery include those with <50% stenosis of the left main coronary artery by angiography, no recent myocardial infarction (7 days or earlier), and no evidence of unstable angina.[13]

Postoperative complications include arrhythmias (33%), renal failure, infection, multiorgan failure, stroke, and respiratory failure (all <5%).[12]

Mitral Insufficiency in Ischemic Heart Disease

In ischemic heart disease (and also idiopathic dilated cardiomyopathy), left ventricular systolic dysfunction is frequently complicated by functional mitral regurgitation, which is a relatively common cause of mitral valve repair and replacement. Mitral insufficiency is the result of posteromedial papillary muscle scarring or, more commonly, remodeling of the ventricle without necessarily dilatation of the annulus. Morbidity and mortality are directly related to the severity of mitral regurgitation, leading to mitral valve surgery in about 25% of patients with chronic ischemic heart disease.[7]

The surgical options include mitral annuloplasty using an undersized ring as well as valve replacement, which are frequently performed concomitantly with coronary artery bypass surgery. In contrast to mitral valve prolapse, a portion of the valve is typically not removed during the repair. If the valve is replaced, the valve appears essentially unremarkable. Long-term complications of annuloplasty rings include recurrent regurgitation, which eventually results in reoperation with removal of the ring and valve replacement. In such cases, the pathologist will receive as a surgical specimen both the explanted ring and the valve itself, which may show nonspecific fibrosis.

Hospital mortality is as high as 2.3% for mitral repair and 12.5% for mitral replacement in the setting of ischemic cardiomyopathy with concomitant bypass grafting.[4] Medium-term survival at 2.5 years was reported as 92% for mitral repair and 73% for valve replacement in the same study.[4]

Atrial and Ventricular Thrombi

With idiopathic dilated cardiomyopathy, there is an increased risk of thrombi developing in the left side of the heart, especially in areas of healed infarct. Left ventricular thrombi are detected in up to 20% of patients and left atrial thrombin up to 40%.[18]

Because of the increased risk of thrombosis, it is not uncommon to receive as pathologic specimens left atrial appendages in patients undergoing coronary artery bypass graft procedures for coronary artery disease and concomitant heart failure.

Pathologic Findings in Chronic Ischemic Heart Disease

In surgical pathology, evaluation of chronically ischemic myocardium is limited to incidental examinations of tissues removed for left ventricular assist device placement (apical plugs), aneurysmectomies, and explanted hearts. In such specimens, the presence of replacement fibrosis, transmural infarcts, calcification, and adipose metaplasia in the scars should be noted. In addition, myocyte vacuolization indicative of chronic ischemic heart disease should be described.

At autopsy and at explant, the extent and degree of epicardial coronary atherosclerosis, degree of chamber dilatation, presence of scars, and aneurysms should be noted (Table 152.1). Old infarcts should be described as subendocardial or transmural, and their location radially (anterior, lateral, posterior, and septal) and longitudinally (base, apex, midventricle) should be stated. Approximate size of old infarcts should be noted as well. The mitral valve annulus should be measured, and any scars in the papillary muscle described (especially the posteromedial, which is the most sensitive to ischemia). Any degree of thinning at sites of old infarcts should be noted, with term aneurysm used if there is a bulge and transmural scar (Figs. 152.1 to 152.6). Acute necrosis or infarct should be carefully excluded. Often at autopsy, and invariably in explants, there will evidence of prior revascularization, in the form of coronary stents or bypass grafts.

Histologically, there is invariably irreversible ischemia in the form of replacement fibrosis (healed infarct), either subendocardial or transmural. In addition, there is increased interstitial fibrosis, as well as myocyte hypertrophy. The findings in the noninfarcted zones are nonspecific and similar to those of heart failure from idiopathic nonischemic cardiomyopathy.

In subendocardial regions, there is chronic ischemic change, as evidenced by myocyte vacuolization reflecting loss of sarcomeres (Figs. 152.7 and 152.8). These areas of "hibernating myocardium" are

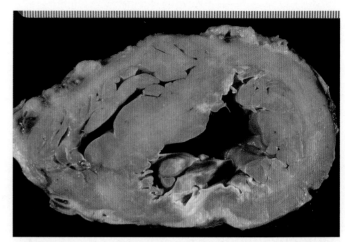

FIGURE 152.1 ▲ Ischemic heart disease with end-stage cardiomyopathy. The section is from an explanted heart from a patient with an ejection fraction of 10%. The left ventricular cavity diameter was ~5 cm, and there is a healed transmural infarct in the posterior left ventricle.

thought to be amenable to repopulation of sarcomeres with restoration of contractile function upon revascularization.

There is typically variability in the histologic findings in chronic ischemic heart disease. Grossly, the heart shows hypertrophy and left ventricular dilatation and typically two- or three-vessel disease with multifocal obstruction. Histologically, there may be multiple foci of subendocardial necrosis, patchy replacement fibrosis of varying age and size, and subendocardial vacuolization indicative of chronic ischemia. Congestion with dilatation of subendocardial vessels is common.[19]

Left Ventricular Aneurysms

One feature that contributes to the development of heart failure after myocardial infarction is the formation of ventricular aneurysms and pseudoaneurysms (Table 152.2). A large acute transmural myocardial infarct that has undergone expansion is the most likely infarct that will result in a true aneurysm.[20] The pulsatile force from the blood in the

---

TABLE 152.1   Pertinent Autopsy Findings in Chronic Ischemic Heart Disease

Coronary arteries
- Sites and degree of stenoses
- 1–3 vessel disease (number of epicardial arteries with >75% stenosis)
- Presence of acute coronary thrombi

Myocardium
- Degree of left ventricular cavity dilatation
- Site of healed infarcts (anterior, lateral, posterior, septal, and combinations)
- Extent of infarcts and dimensions in cm (transmural, subendocardial, apical, basal, midventricular)
- Presence of aneurysms
- Right ventricular and atrial dilatation (indication of pulmonary hypertension)

Endocardium
- Mural thrombi
- Endocardial fibrosis

Previous interventions
- Coronary stents (see Chapter 9)
- Coronary bypass grafts (see Chapter 10)

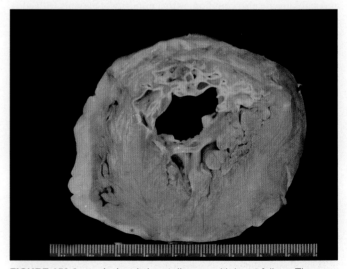

FIGURE 152.2 ▲ Ischemic heart disease with heart failure. The cross section, which is toward the apex, shows a healed transmural infarct in the anterior wall. The trabeculations are more prominent in this region with organized mural thrombus within and among the trabeculae.

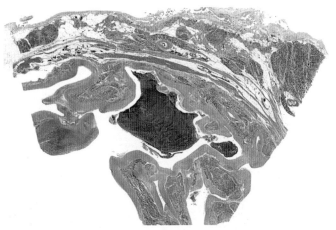

FIGURE 152.3 ▲ Masson trichrome stain. There is a mural thrombus and transmural fibrosis. There is, in addition, scattered fatty metaplasia within the scar.

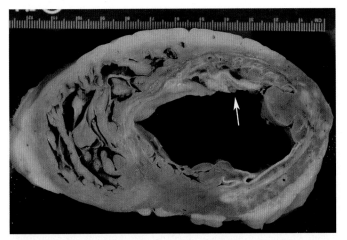

FIGURE 152.4 ▲ Chronic ischemic heart disease with healed infarction ("ischemic cardiomyopathy"). There are a healed posterolateral healed infarct, a healed transmural anteroseptal infarct, and a mural thrombus (arrow).

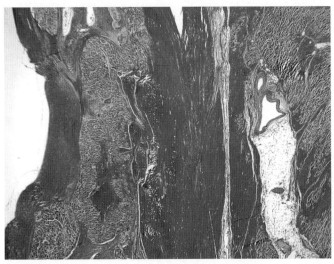

FIGURE 152.5 ▲ Healed transmural infarct. A histologic section shows a healed infarct with dense scar. Masson trichrome stain. There is focal fatty metaplasia at the right. There are islands of viable myocardium. The endocardium is at the left.

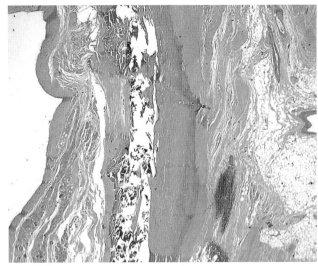

FIGURE 152.6 ▲ Healed transmural infarct, with calcification. In healed infarcts with aneurysms, the pericardium may calcify, of the fibrous tissue within the scar itself. In this case, there is fragmented calcification (center) within the scar of the infarct.

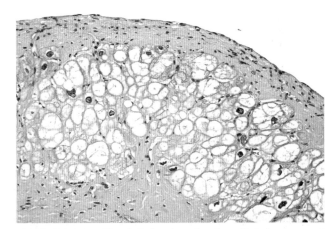

FIGURE 152.7 ▲ Chronic ischemia, subendocardium, in an area of subendocardial fibrosis. There is a cluster of chronically ischemic vacuolated myocytes within an area of scarring.

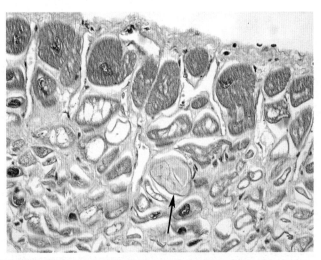

FIGURE 152.8 ▲ Chronic ischemia, subendocardium, with viable endocardial single cell layer. Frequently, there may be one layer of viable myocytes along the endocardial layer, which obtain oxygen from the ventricular cavity. Incidentally, there was a focus of basophilic degeneration (arrow), which is a nonspecific finding.

TABLE 152.2   Left Ventricular True Versus False Aneurysm (Aneurysm Versus Pseudoaneurysm)

	Aneurysm	Pseudoaneurysm
Clinical signs	Nonspecific	Nonspecific
Origin	Thinned infarct wall	Acute rupture of infarct, with localized containment of hematoma within pericardium instead of diffuse hemopericardium
Composition of wall	Begins acutely as infarcted myocardium, develops into healed infarct with dense collage, possible calcification	Granulation tissue developing fibrous capsule contained by pericardium
Base of cavity	Broad bulge	Narrow base with wider pseudoaneurysm cavity
Usual site	Apex	Base
Treatment	Medical or surgical (patch repair)	Surgical excision (primary repair or patch repair)

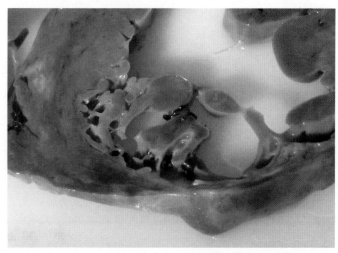

FIGURE 152.10 ▲ Healed infarct with wall thinning. A higher magnification of an area toward the apex (same heart as shown in Figure 19) shows an area of scarring with marked thinning with early bulging.

cavity stretches and thins the necrotic muscle, which heals forming the wall of a true aneurysm. The incidence of postinfarction aneurysm varies greatly from series to series and depends on definitions used. The autopsy definition of transmural scar or ventricular wall thinning with the presence of a bulge may be overly inclusive.[21] Surgical definitions include the presence of a bulge, myocardial thinning or scar, loss or trabecular pattern on the endocardium, and akinesis or dyskinesis. A proposed definition was "anatomically distinct area of the left ventricle that collapsed when the ventricle was vented." Echocardiographic studies emphasize systolic deformity over diastolic abnormalities. An aneurysm is defined pathologically by a transmural scar with a distinct bulge (Figs. 152.9 and 152.10).[21]

Morphologically, the wall of a true aneurysm consists of fibrous tissue with interspersed myocytes. There is often fat in the aneurysm wall, as with healed infarcts, and there may be calcification of fibrous tissue.

The incidence of true aneurysm following a myocardial infarction is 5% to 10% and is more frequent in transmural infarction than subendocardial infarction. Aneurysms are usually associated with two or more vessel coronary disease with poorly developed collaterals.[22] Over

three-fourths of left ventricular aneurysms involve the anteroapical wall. The pericardium is usually adherent to the aneurysm and may calcify. True aneurysm rarely ruptures, whereas rupture is more common of a false aneurysm. The cavity of the aneurysm usually contains an organizing thrombus and the patient may present with embolic complications (see below). The mortality is six times higher in patients with aneurysm than without, although the decrease in survival is not independent of ejection fraction, bifascicular block, number of diseased vessels, and postinfarct angina.[23]

Treatment of left ventricular aneurysm includes surgical repair and medical therapy for heart failure.[24]

Surgical Ventricular Restoration

Repair of true fibrous aneurysms that are nonviable by functional nuclear studies results in improved survival compared to repair of aneurysms with residual viable myocardium.[25] Surgical repair may be accompanied by coronary revascularization or bypass procedures. Surgical repair includes suturing the autologous pericardium or other patch at the interface between scarred and normal tissue. If there is extensive septal involvement, a portion of the septum is excised and repaired as well.[26] Pathologically, the excised specimen demonstrates full-thickness myocardium, the endocardial fibrosis, transmural scarring, and in some cases calcification.

Candidates for surgical ventricular restoration include dilated ventricle, a healed left anterior descending artery territory infarct, akinetic or dyskinetic anterior wall segment, and reasonable preserved basal and lateral wall motion. Often, coronary artery bypass graft surgery is performed concomitantly. A tailored Dacron patch may be secured to the opening.[9]

The typical hospital mortality of aneurysm repair is nearly 10%.[14] The mean increase in ejection fraction after the surgery, compared to preoperative status, is between 10% and 15%.[27] At a mean follow-up of 3 years, there was an 80% survival in a recent study.[14]

Left Ventricular Pseudoaneurysms

A postmyocardial infarction left ventricular pseudoaneurysm occurs when a rupture of the ventricular free wall is contained by the pericardium. Pericardial adhesions that have formed either prior to the infarct or prior to rupture (if late after an infarction) contain the hematoma.

Clinically, the most common presentations are heart failure and angina. Pseudoaneurysms are rarely suspected at clinical presentation. Echocardiography is 97% sensitive for the diagnosis.[28]

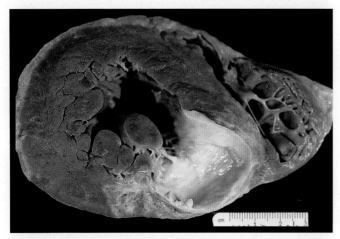

FIGURE 152.9 ▲ Ventricular aneurysm, chronic. There is a healed infarct with aneurysm, posteroseptal left ventricle. There is dense white scar, indicative of an old infarct, with thinning of the fibrous wall and aneurysm formation.

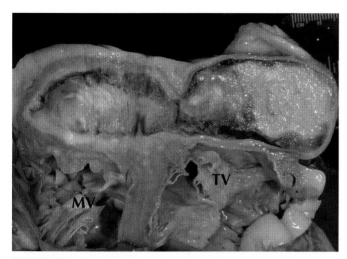

FIGURE 152.11 ▲ Ventricular pseudoaneurysm, remote. There is a large elongated cavity along the posterior aspect of the heart contained by a fibrous capsule. The cavity is filled with partly calcified organized thrombus. The ventricular septum is in the center, with mitral valve (MV) on the left, and the tricuspid valve (TV) on the right. The appearance is that of a hematoma with organization; the site of the blood was an old rupture infarct.

The cavity of the false aneurysm is usually filled with large blood clots, both old and new. The neck of the pseudoaneurysm is narrow, corresponding to the prior rupture site, compared to broad-based true aneurysms (Figs. 152.11 and 152.12). The wall of a pseudoaneurysm

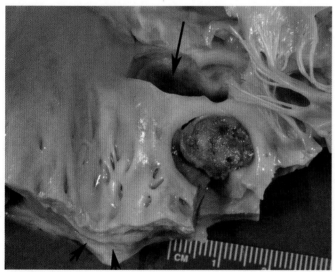

FIGURE 152.12 ▲ The posterior left ventricle of the heart in the previous figure has a cavity with a mural thrombus; the neck of the pseudoaneurysm was ~11 mm in diameter. A portion of the posterior left ventricular free wall has been cut away exposing the cavity shown in Figure 22 (*arrow*). The mitral valve posterior leaflet has been pushed aside. The endocardial surface is that of the posterior left ventricle, the ventricular septum is toward the left. A healed transmural infarct (which had ruptured months or years ago) can barely be seen on cut surface (*arrowheads*) in the posterior left ventricular wall. In most cases of rupture infarction, death occurs rapidly because of hemopericardium; if there are prior fibrous adhesions in the posterior left ventricle near the base, there may be localized pericardial containment of the extravasated blood without tamponade.

is granulation tissue progressing to scar, lacking cardiac muscle. Once recognized clinically, the usual treatment for it is urgent surgical repair. However, the imaging characteristics of pseudoaneurysm and aneurysm, for which treatment is more conservative, are quite similar.[29]

Left ventricular pseudoaneurysm may be surgically treated by excision and primary repair or more commonly by patch closure. Concurrent coronary revascularization or mitral valve repair is common. Hospital mortality is 20%, and late survival is ~60% at 5 years. Poor long-term survival is associated with poor preoperative left ventricular function.[28]

Treatment and Prognosis

The treatment of chronic ischemic heart disease includes heart failure therapy (medical treatment), coronary artery bypass graft surgery, mitral valve surgery, implantable defibrillators with or without cardiac resynchronization therapy, stem cell therapy, left ventricular assist devices, and heart transplantation.

Stem cell therapy may improve the left ventricular ejection fraction, with intramyocardial injection possibly being superior to intracoronary infusion.[6]

The prognosis of ischemic cardiomyopathy is poor, varies by study, and depends on the degree of heart failure, degree of cardiac hypertrophy, and comorbid conditions. Overall, there is a 5-year survival rate of 65% to 89%. Overall, actual survival was 96% at 1 year, 89% at 3 years, 83% at 5 years, and 75% at 10 years.[12] Another series showed that over one-third of patients died within 6 years after bypass surgery, with advanced age, body mass index, hypertension, diabetes, and hyperlipidemia being poor prognostic factors. Severe mitral regurgitation and large infarcts are also poor prognostic factors.[8]

Cerebrovascular disease and preoperative arrhythmias independently predict poor long-term survival.[12] Patients with implanted defibrillators for chronic ischemic heart disease have a 20% mortality at 3 years.[17]

Left ventricular assist devices and heart transplantation have become the standard of care for patients with ischemic cardiomyopathy when medical treatment has failed. Left ventricular assist devices are used as either bridge to transplant or destination devices (destination therapy). From a study at the Mayo Clinic, there was a 3% hospital mortality rate and 15% mortality rate at 1 year, numbers that were better than those for coronary artery bypass graft surgery with mitral valve replacement.[10]

Practical Points

▶ Ischemic heart disease is often treated with percutaneous interventions or surgery. At autopsy, the pathologist should be familiar with the evaluation of stents and bypass grafts in patients with chronic heart failure secondary to atherosclerosis (see Chapters 9 and 10).

▶ A clinical history with types of intervention, if any, and dates of prior infarctions is helpful in clinicopathologic correlation at autopsy.

▶ Occasionally, ischemic heart disease will be an incidental or unexpected finding in patients with sudden death or those dying of noncardiac causes; in these cases, the extent of epicardial disease and myocardial scarring is less than in previously symptomatic patients.

REFERENCES

1. Richardson P, McKenna W, Bristow M, et al. Report of the 1995 World Health Organization/International Society and Federation of Cardiology Task Force on the Definition and Classification of cardiomyopathies. *Circulation.* 1996;93:841–842.
2. Maron BJ, Towbin JA, Thiene G, et al. Contemporary definitions and classification of the cardiomyopathies: an American Heart Association Scientific Statement from the Council on Clinical Cardiology, Heart Failure and Transplantation Committee; Quality of Care and Outcomes Research and Functional Genomics and Translational Biology Interdisciplinary Working Groups; and Council on Epidemiology and Prevention. *Circulation.* 2006;113:1807–1816.
3. Elliott P, Andersson B, Arbustini E, et al. Classification of the cardiomyopathies: a position statement from the European Society of Cardiology Working Group on Myocardial and Pericardial Diseases. *Eur Heart J.* 2008;29:270–276.
4. De Bonis M, Ferrara D, Taramasso M, et al. Mitral replacement or repair for functional mitral regurgitation in dilated and ischemic cardiomyopathy: is it really the same? *Ann Thorac Surg.* 2012;94:44–51.
5. Gouda S, Abdelwahab A, Salem M, et al. Scar characteristics for prediction of ventricular arrhythmia in ischemic cardiomyopathy. *Pacing Clin Electrophysiol.* 2015;38:311–318.
6. Kandala J, Upadhyay GA, Pokushalov E, et al. Meta-analysis of stem cell therapy in chronic ischemic cardiomyopathy. *Am J Cardiol.* 2013;112:217–225.
7. Kische S, Nienaber C, Ince H. Use of four MitraClip devices in a patient with ischemic cardiomyopathy and mitral regurgitation: "zipping by clipping". *Catheter Cardiovasc Interv.* 2012;80:1007–1013.
8. Kwon DH, Hachamovitch R, Popovic ZB, et al. Survival in patients with severe ischemic cardiomyopathy undergoing revascularization versus medical therapy: association with end-systolic volume and viability. *Circulation.* 2012;126:S3–S8.
9. Liu J, Liu Z, Zhao Q, et al. Role of surgical ventricular restoration in the treatment of ischemic cardiomyopathy. *Ann Thorac Surg.* 2013;95:1315–1321.
10. Maltais S, Tchantchaleishvili V, Schaff HV, et al. Management of severe ischemic cardiomyopathy: left ventricular assist device as destination therapy versus conventional bypass and mitral valve surgery. *J Thorac Cardiovasc Surg.* 2014;147:1246–1250.
11. Muto C, Solimene F, Gallo P, et al. A randomized study of cardiac resynchronization therapy defibrillator versus dual-chamber implantable cardioverter-defibrillator in ischemic cardiomyopathy with narrow QRS: the NARROW-CRT study. *Circ Arrhythm Electrophysiol.* 2013;6:538–545.
12. Pinto N, Haluska B, Mundy J, et al. Ischemic cardiomyopathy: midterm survival and its predictors. *Asian Cardiovasc Thorac Ann.* 2012;20:669–674.
13. Velazquez EJ, Williams JB, Yow E, et al. Long-term survival of patients with ischemic cardiomyopathy treated by coronary artery bypass grafting versus medical therapy. *Ann Thorac Surg.* 2012;93:523–530.
14. Wakasa S, Matsui Y, Isomura T, et al. Risk scores for predicting mortality after surgical ventricular reconstruction for ischemic cardiomyopathy: results of a Japanese multicenter study. *J Thorac Cardiovasc Surg.* 2014;147:1868–1874, 1874 e1–2.
15. Ailawadi G, Kron IL. New strategies for surgical management of ischemic cardiomyopathy. *Expert Rev Cardiovasc Ther.* 2008;6:521–530.
16. Mozaffarian D, Benjamin EJ, Go AS, et al. Heart disease and stroke statistics—2015 update: a report from the American Heart Association. *Circulation.* 2015;131:e29–e322.
17. Bender SR, Friedman DJ, Markowitz SM, et al. Electrocardiographic left ventricular hypertrophy predicts arrhythmia and mortality in patients with ischemic cardiomyopathy. *J Interv Card Electrophysiol.* 2012;34:237–245.
18. Bakalli A, Georgievska-Ismail L, Kocinaj D, et al. Left ventricular and left atrial thrombi in sinus rhythm patients with dilated ischemic cardiomyopathy. *Med Arch.* 2012;66:155–158.
19. Taube JM, Hutchins GM. Multifocal ischemic necroses of varying age (MINOVA): a distinctive form of atherosclerotic heart disease. *Pathol Res Pract.* 2008;204:113–120.
20. Erlebacher JA, Weiss JL, Weisfeldt ML, et al. Early dilation of the infarcted segment in acute transmural myocardial infarction: role of infarct expansion in acute left ventricular enlargement. *J Am Coll Cardiol.* 1984;4:201–208.
21. Hamer DH, Lindsay J, Jr. Redefining true ventricular aneurysm. *Am J Cardiol.* 1989;64:1192–1194.
22. Forman MB, Collins HW, Kopelman HA, et al. Determinants of left ventricular aneurysm formation after anterior myocardial infarction: a clinical and angiographic study. *J Am Coll Cardiol.* 1986;8:1256–1262.
23. Heras M, Sanz G, Betriu A, et al. Does left ventricular aneurysm influence survival after acute myocardial infarction? *Eur Heart J.* 1990;11:441–446.
24. Daneshmand MA, Milano CA. Surgical treatments for advanced heart failure. *Surg Clin North Am.* 2009;89:967–999, x.
25. Zhang X, Liu XJ, Hu S, et al. Long-term survival of patients with viable and nonviable aneurysms assessed by 99mTc-MIBI SPECT and 18F-FDG PET: a comparative study of medical and surgical treatment. *J Nucl Med.* 2008;49:1288–1298.
26. Erbasan O, Turkay C, Mete A, et al. Surgical treatment of left ventricular aneurysms: a comparison of long-term follow-up of left ventricular function for classic aneurysmectomy and endoaneurysmorrhaphy techniques. *Heart Surg Forum.* 2009;12:E272–E278.
27. Dor V. Left ventricular reconstruction for ischemic cardiomyopathy. *J Card Surg.* 2002;17:180–187.
28. Atik FA, Navia JL, Vega PR, et al. Surgical treatment of postinfarction left ventricular pseudoaneurysm. *Ann Thorac Surg.* 2007;83:526–531.
29. Brown SL, Gropler RJ, Harris KM. Distinguishing left ventricular aneurysm from pseudoaneurysm. A review of the literature. *Chest.* 1997;111:1403–1409.

153   Coronary Stents

Allen P. Burke, M.D., and Joseph J. Maleszewski, M.D.

Introduction

Percutaneous balloon angioplasty with stenting has become standard treatment for obstructive coronary artery disease, including patients who present with myocardial infarction. Coronary stenting shows similar efficacy for the treatment of coronary artery disease as open surgical procedures.[1-4] In general, bypass is recommended for multivessel or left main disease, and coronary stenting is feasible for either single or multivessel disease. Stents are currently approved for deployment in stenotic segments. Overlapping stents, bifurcating stents, deployment in ostial or left main disease, and use in acute coronary syndromes are considered investigational ("off-label"). Various acronyms have been used for percutaneous interventions (Table 153.1).

Types of Stents

Stents vary by design, composition, and presence of drug. The composition is generally either stainless steel or cobalt chromium; self-expanding nitinol (nickel titanium alloy) stents are generally used for peripheral vascular disease.

There are three main types of stents currently seen by pathologists: bare metal stents, first-generation drug-eluting stents, and second-generation drug-eluting stents. Drug-eluting stents are coated with an antiproliferative drug embedded in a polymer, which elutes from the stent for several months after implantation and decreases the rate of restenosis. First-generation drug-eluting stents included sirolimus-eluting and paclitaxel-eluting stents that are composed of stainless steel

TABLE 153.1 Acronyms Associated with Percutaneous Interventions

Acronym	Meaning
PCI	Percutaneous intervention
PTCA	Percutaneous transluminal coronary angioplasty
POBA	Plain old balloon angioplasty (without stent)
BMS	Bare metal stent
DES	Drug-eluting stent
RX	Rapid exchange
OTW	Over the wire

struts measuring 130 to 140 μm thick and are similar in design to their bare metal counterparts. Second-generation drug-eluting stents were developed in part to decrease the risk for late stent thrombosis. In the case of first-generation drug-eluting stents, the rate of late stent thrombosis significantly exceeds that of bare metal stents and necessitates long-term antiplatelet therapy.[5] Second-generation stents are made of cobalt–chromium, which allows for thinner struts (80 to 90 μm), more rapid endothelialization, and decreased likelihood of thrombosis.[6] There are several available second-generation stents: everolimus-eluting cobalt–chromium stent (Xience V and Promus) and a zotarolimus-eluting cobalt–chromium stent (Endeavor and Resolute). Randomized clinical trials have shown a reduction in stent thrombosis, myocardial infarction, and rate of repeat intervention (target lesion revascularization) using these new stents compared to first-generation stents.[7]

Technical Considerations at Autopsy

At autopsy, the stented artery is radiographed to determine the location of the stent and degree of intimal calcification and dissected free of the epicardial fat (Fig. 153.1).[8] There are three methods of histologic evaluation: removal of stents with diamond scissors, with paraffin embedding; electrolytic dissolution of the stent with paraffin embedding[9]; and processing in methylmethacrylate and sectioning using special microtomes.[10]

Paraffin-based methods are preferred for immunohistochemical techniques. Scanning electron microscopy is used in research to examine the extent of endothelialization, although a surrogate for extent of endothelialization is the ratio of uncovered to covered stent struts seen on routine stains.[11]

In practice, evaluation of the contents of the stent only rarely contributes to the determination of the cause of death.[12] However, a registry of stented coronary arteries has led to important discoveries regarding the nature of human restenosis and late stent thrombosis and is available as a resource for pathologists.[10]

Incidence and Time Course of Restenosis (Neoatherosclerosis)

Autopsy studies that examine stents with various durations of implantation have elucidated the evolution of intimal healing, which, if exaggerated, results in in-stent restenosis, generally caused by neoatherosclerosis or thrombosis.[11,13–19] At autopsy, the rate of restenosis is between 5% and 10%, excluding late stent thrombosis that likely resulted in death.[20] No difference was found between the degree of intimal thickening and frequency of neoatherosclerosis between first- and second-generation drug-eluting stents in a different autopsy study.[10]

Angiographically, restenosis is defined as 50% diameter luminal narrowing (binary angiographic restenosis). Clinical endpoints for restenosis include late lumen loss, as measured angiographically by mm diameter narrowing, and the need for target lesion revascularization. Using the latter parameter, restenosis occurs at a rate of ~3% to 6% for currently employed drug-eluting stents.[10]

The time course of neoatherosclerosis varies by type of stent. Bare metal stents develop maximal restenosis with 6 to 12 months after implantation, after which there may be regression. In contrast, drug-eluting stents are characterized by delayed healing that results in continued growth of neoatherosclerotic lesions even after 1 year.[21] In addition, neoatherosclerosis develops more frequently within first-generation DES compared with bare metal stents.[22]

Histologic Findings of Neoatherosclerosis

Phases of intimal changes after stent deployment are, sequentially, thrombosis, inflammation, endothelialization, and finally smooth muscle cell migration with matrix deposition.[12,23] The typical finding is that of concentric intima thickening, which is generally fibrotic in bare metal stents (Fig. 153.2) and more inflamed with drug-eluting stents (Fig. 153.3).

Initially, there is deposition of platelets, hemorrhage, and foam cells around struts, more accentuated in drug-eluting stents (Fig. 153.4).[19]

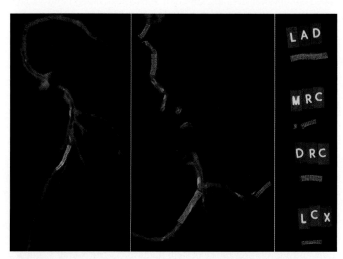

FIGURE 153.1 ▲ Postmortem radiographs of intracoronary stents. **Left**, a single stent in the left anterior descending artery. **Middle**, multiple stents in the left coronary circulation **(bottom)** as well as right **(top)**. **Right**, stents from the middle panel, excised separately after decalcification. LAD, ; MRC, ; DRC, ; LCX, .

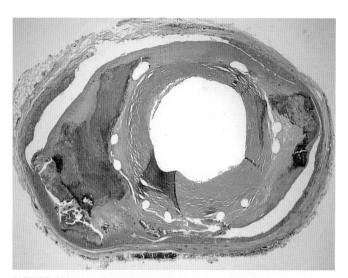

FIGURE 153.2 ▲ Neoatherosclerosis, bare metal stent. There is relatively mild intimal thickening, <75% cross-sectional narrowing. Restenosis is defined as narrowing >75%, as in this example. The lesion is relatively acellular. The stent struts are seen as gaps around the periphery of the arterial lumen.

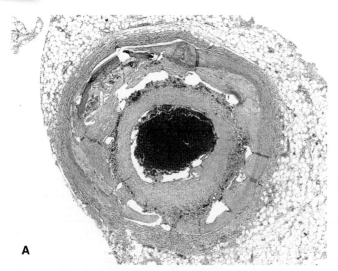

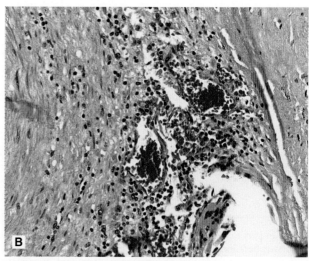

FIGURE 153.3 ▲ Neoatherosclerosis, drug-eluting stent. **A.** Low magnification shows stent struts with luminal concentric thickening. There is a calcified fibroatheroma peripheral to the stent. **B.** A higher magnification shows an increased amount of inflammation around the struts, a characteristic of drug-eluting stents. The example was an everolimus-coated first-generation stent.

Fibrin-rich thrombus around stent struts is always present within 11 days poststenting and is infrequent after 30 days. Thrombus in the first month is associated with acute and chronic inflammation, and giant cells may be seen at later time points. Persistent chronic inflammation beyond 90 days is associated with increased neointimal thickness and restenosis.[24]

Neointimal smooth muscle cells are only observed beyond 11 days and are a constant finding beyond 30 days. Immunophenotyping has shown that the early cells are dedifferentiated myofibroblasts, which over time mature into α-actin–positive smooth muscle cells.[13]

In-stent neoatherosclerosis is histologically characterized by an accumulation of lipid-laden foamy macrophages. There is no communication between the lesion within the neointima and the underlying native atherosclerosis, however. Hemorrhage into neoatherosclerosis may occur via fissure or rupture or from leaky vasa vasorum originating in the adventitia.[21]

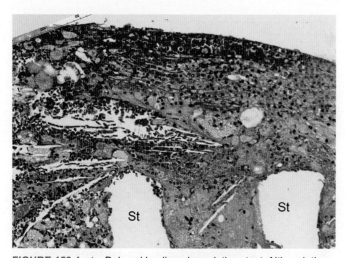

FIGURE 153.4 ▲ Delayed healing, drug-eluting stent. Although the stent had been in place for several months, there were areas where there was no endothelialization or healing over the struts. St, .

Risk Factors for Neoatherosclerosis and In-Stent Thrombosis

Both stent-related and patient-related factors play a role in the development of neoatherosclerosis and in-stent thrombosis (Table 153.2). Stent-related factors (in addition to the stent type) that increase the risk of restenosis include off-label use, longer stents, overlapping stents, strut fracture during deployment, and malapposition. Types of malapposition include medial perforation (Fig. 153.5) and lack of contact with the intima (uncovered struts). Medial perforation is associated with an inflammatory and angiogenic reaction that may contribute to restenosis (Fig. 153.6).

Patient-related risk factors include genetic factors,[25,26] diabetes and other risk factors for atherosclerosis, a history of acute coronary syndromes, small-vessel caliber, and long lesion length.

Late Stent Thrombosis

Stent thrombosis is considered as acute when occurring between 0 and 24 hours after stent implantation, subacute between 1 and 30 days, late between 30 days and 1 year, and very late after 1 year. Thirty days separates the general categories of early and late stent thrombosis.[27]

There is an increased risk for late stent thrombosis in early-generation drug-eluting stents, which seems to be reduced with second-generation stents. Delayed healing characterized by poor strut coverage has been the pathologic explanation for this phenomenon. Late stent thrombosis may cause sudden death or result in recurrent acute coronary syndromes without death, requiring target lesion revascularization therapy. Histologically, remote in-stent thrombosis undergoes recanalization (Fig. 153.7).

Other factors related to late stent thrombosis include hypersensitivity reactions, especially to sirolimus-eluting stents.[21] Pathologically, there will be abundant eosinophils in and around the stent thrombus, as well as in the arterial adventitia (Fig. 153.8). Mast cells have also been implicated in late stent thrombosis.[28,29]

An autopsy study has shown that second-generation cobalt–chromium everolimus-eluting stents have a substantially lower prevalence of late (and very late) stent thrombosis with decreased incidence of malapposition (uncovered struts), less inflammation and fibrin deposition, and a lower prevalence of stent fracture.[10,30] The overall frequency of very late stent thrombosis was shown in an autopsy study as 3.0% in bare metal stents, 19% in first-generation drug-eluting stents, and 0% in second-generation drug-eluting stents.[20]

TABLE 153.2   Risk Factors for Late Stent Thrombosis

Type of Factor	Risks
Procedural	Incomplete apposition
	Excessive stent length
	Overlapping stents
Device related	Hypersensitivity to polymer
	Uneven distribution of drug
	Incomplete apposition due to poor flexibility
	Use of first-generation drug-eluting stent
Factors related to under-lying lesion	Penetration of necrotic core or preexisting thrombus in acute coronary syndromes
	Bifurcation or ostial stenting
	Late malapposition due to inflammation
Systemic factors	Diabetes
	Renal failure
	Low ejection fraction
	Contraindications to long-term antiplatelet therapy
	Premature discontinuation of long-term antiplatelet therapy

Adapted from Burke AP, Ladich E, Virmani R, eds. Pathology of angioplasty and stenting. In: McManus B, ed. *Atlas of Cardiovascular Pathology for the Clinician.* 2nd ed. Philadelphia, PA: Current Medicine; 2008:93–100.

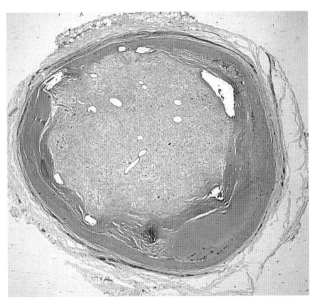

FIGURE 153.7 ▲ Late stent thrombosis, chronic. In this case, the thrombus is healed, occlusive, and partly recanalized.

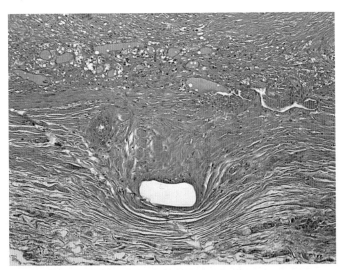

FIGURE 153.5 ▲ Malapposition with medial perforation. The stent strut is outside the adventitia, with a collagenous reaction surrounding it.

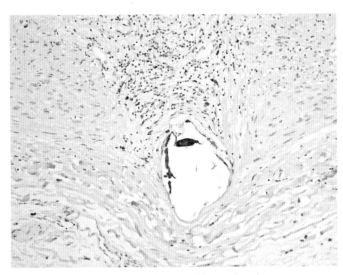

FIGURE 153.6 ▲ Medial perforation with reactive changes. Immunohistochemical stain, CD68 shows macrophages, with a foreign body giant cell around the hole where the stent strut had been.

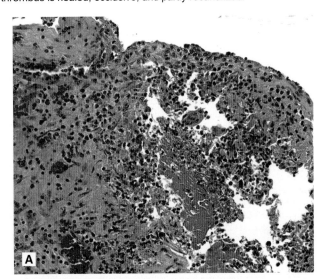

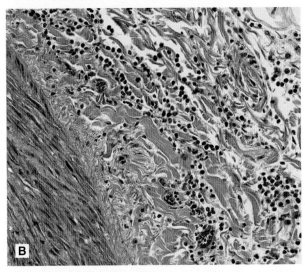

FIGURE 153.8 ▲ Late stent thrombosis, acute. **A.** The thrombus contained abundant eosinophils. **B.** There was an eosinophilic reaction that spreads along the adventitia of nonstented coronary arteries. Allergic reactions to first-generation everolimus-eluting stents have been well documented. The patient in this example died suddenly 16 months after stenting (very late stent thrombosis).

REFERENCES

1. Booth J, Clayton T, Pepper J, et al. Randomized, controlled trial of coronary artery bypass surgery versus percutaneous coronary intervention in patients with multivessel coronary artery disease: six-year follow-up from the stent or surgery trial (SoS). *Circulation.* 2008;118:381–388.
2. Gao G, Wu Y, Grunkemeier GL, et al. Long-term survival of patients after coronary artery bypass graft surgery: comparison of the pre-stent and post-stent eras. *Ann Thorac Surg.* 2006;82:806–810.
3. Kimura T, Morimoto T, Furukawa Y, et al. Long-term outcomes of coronary-artery bypass graft surgery versus percutaneous coronary intervention for multivessel coronary artery disease in the bare-metal stent era. *Circulation.* 2008;118:S199–S209.
4. Yang JH, Gwon HC, Cho SJ, et al. Comparison of coronary artery bypass grafting with drug-eluting stent implantation for the treatment of multivessel coronary artery disease. *Ann Thorac Surg.* 2008;85:65–70.
5. Kaiser C, Galatius S, Jeger R, et al. Long-term efficacy and safety of biodegradable-polymer biolimus-eluting stents: main results of the Basel Stent Kosten-Effektivitats Trial-PROspective Validation Examination II (BASKET-PROVE II), a randomized, controlled noninferiority 2-year outcome trial. *Circulation.* 2015;131:74–81.
6. Chitkara K, Pujara K. Drug-eluting stents in acute coronary syndrome: is there a risk of stent thrombosis with second-generation stents? *Eur J Cardiovasc Med.* 2010;1:20–24.
7. Stone GW, Rizvi A, Sudhir K, et al. Randomized comparison of everolimus- and paclitaxel-eluting stents. 2-year follow-up from the SPIRIT (clinical evaluation of the XIENCE V everolimus eluting coronary stent system) IV trial. *J Am Coll Cardiol.* 2011;58:19–25.
8. Burke AP, Ladich E, Virmani R, eds. Pathology of angioplasty and stenting. In: McManus B, ed. *Atlas of Cardiovascular Pathology for the Clinician.* 2nd ed. Philadelphia, PA: Current Medicine; 2008:93–100.
9. Bradshaw SH, Kennedy L, Dexter DF, et al. A practical method to rapidly dissolve metallic stents. *Cardiovasc Pathol.* 2009;18:127–133.
10. Otsuka F, Vorpahl M, Nakano M, et al. Pathology of second-generation everolimus-eluting stents versus first-generation sirolimus- and paclitaxel-eluting stents in humans. *Circulation.* 2014;129:211–223.
11. Joner M, Finn AV, Farb A, et al. Pathology of drug-eluting stents in humans: delayed healing and late thrombotic risk. *J Am Coll Cardiol.* 2006;48:193–202.
12. Mont E, Cresswell N, Burke A. Pathologic findings of coronary stents: a comparison of sudden coronary death versus non-cardiac death. *J Forensic Sci.* 2013;58:1542–1548.
13. Farb A, Kolodgie FD, Hwang JY, et al. Extracellular matrix changes in stented human coronary arteries. *Circulation.* 2004;110:940–947.
14. Guagliumi G, Virmani R, Musumeci G, et al. Drug-eluting versus bare metal coronary stents: long-term human pathology. Findings from different coronary arteries in the same patient. *Ital Heart J.* 2003;4:713–720.
15. Farb A, Burke AP, Kolodgie FD, et al. Pathological mechanisms of fatal late coronary stent thrombosis in humans. *Circulation.* 2003;108:1701–1706.
16. Virmani R, Liistro F, Stankovic G, et al. Mechanism of late in-stent restenosis after implantation of a paclitaxel derivate-eluting polymer stent system in humans. *Circulation.* 2002;106:2649–2651.
17. Farb A, Weber DK, Kolodgie FD, et al. Morphological predictors of restenosis after coronary stenting in humans. *Circulation.* 2002;105:2974–2980.
18. Virmani R, Farb A. Pathology of in-stent restenosis. *Curr Opin Lipidol.* 1999;10:499–506.
19. Farb A, Sangiorgi G, Carter AJ, et al. Pathology of acute and chronic coronary stenting in humans. *Circulation.* 1999;99:44–52.
20. Nakazawa G, Finn AV, Vorpahl M, et al. Coronary responses and differential mechanisms of late stent thrombosis attributed to first-generation sirolimus- and paclitaxel-eluting stents. *J Am Coll Cardiol.* 2011;57:390–398.
21. Otsuka F, Byrne RA, Yahagi K, et al. Neoatherosclerosis: overview of histopathologic findings and implications for intravascular imaging assessment. *Eur Heart J.* 2015.
22. Nakazawa G, Finn AV, Vorpahl M, et al. Incidence and predictors of drug-eluting stent fracture in human coronary artery a pathologic analysis. *J Am Coll Cardiol.* 2009;54:1924–1931.
23. Zhang M, Cresswell N, Tavora F, et al. In-stent restenosis is associated with neointimal angiogenesis and macrophage infiltrates. *Pathol Res Pract.* 2014;210:1026–1030.
24. Anderson PG, Bajaj RK, Baxley WA, et al. Vascular pathology of balloon-expandable flexible coil stents in humans. *J Am Coll Cardiol.* 1992;19:372–381.
25. Nozari Y, Vosooghi S, Boroumand M, et al. The impact of cytochrome P450 2C19 polymorphism on the occurrence of one-year in-stent restenosis in patients who underwent percutaneous coronary intervention: a case-match study. *Anatol J Cardiol.* 2015;15:348–353.
26. Fragoso JM, Zuniga-Ramos J, Arellano-Gonzalez M, et al. The T29C (rs1800470) polymorphism of the transforming growth factor-beta1 (TGF-beta1) gene is associated with restenosis after coronary stenting in Mexican patients. *Exp Mol Pathol.* 2015;98:13–17.
27. Lemesle G, Delhaye C, Bonello L, et al. Stent thrombosis in 2008: definition, predictors, prognosis and treatment. *Arch Cardiovasc Dis.* 2008;101:769–777.
28. Kounis NG, Almpanis GC, Tsigkas GG, et al. Kounis syndrome is the likely culprit in devastating stent thrombosis. *J Invasive Cardiol.* 2011;23:3 p preceding 88.
29. Kounis NG. Kounis syndrome should be considered the culprit cause of the most feared stent thrombosis. *J Am Coll Cardiol.* 2011;58:885; author reply 886-7.
30. Montone RA, Sabato V, Sgueglia GA, et al. Inflammatory mechanisms of adverse reactions to drug-eluting stents. *Curr Vasc Pharmacol.* 2013;11:392–398.

154 Coronary Artery Bypass Grafts

Allen P. Burke, M.D., and Fabio R. Tavora, M.D., Ph.D.

Clinical

Incidence and Indications

Coronary artery bypass graft surgery is performed 350,000 times annually in the United States.[1] The general indications are multivessel or left main coronary disease.[2,3] Recently, there has been a shift toward percutaneous revascularization for multivessel disease as well as single-vessel stenoses, suggesting that the rate of coronary artery bypass graft surgery may decrease.

However, the pendulum has not made a full swing away from bypass graft surgery. Isolated severe stenosis of the left anterior descending, as well as multifocal stenoses, is currently being treated with minimally invasive direct coronary artery bypass surgery with results comparable to stenting.[4]

Types of Bypass Grafts

The most common types of grafts are aortocoronary saphenous vein grafts and left internal mammary grafts, followed by right internal mammary grafts, radial artery grafts, and gastroepiploic artery grafts.

Mammary grafts are generally anastomosed directly to the left anterior descending artery. Vein grafts and radial artery grafts are often sequential, meaning that there are "touchdown" or side-to-side anastomoses along the course of the graft before the terminal anastomosis. Furthermore, vein and radial artery grafts may be inserted proximally into other vein grafts ("Y" conduits), minimizing proximal aortic anastomotic sites.

Graft Failure Rates

Vein grafts show poor long-term patency and limit the long-term success of coronary artery bypass grafting; ~60% to 70% will be narrowed or closed down within a decade. In contrast, 90% of internal mammary artery grafts remain patent at 10 years.[5] A recent 1-year angiographic study showed 100% patency rate for mammary artery grafts compared to only 70% for vein grafts.[6]

Because of the known increased longevity of mammary grafts over saphenous vein grafts, some centers perform bilateral mammary grafting; however, there has been no demonstrable difference in survival to single left internal mammary grafting.[7] Similarly, patients who received multiple grafts to each major diseased artery territory had early outcomes similar to those who received single grafts per territory, and constructing multiple grafts to each major diseased artery territory increases operative time and does not improve long-term survival.[8] Radial artery grafts have an intermediate failure rate between saphenous veins and internal mammary arteries, about 30% in 5 years.[9]

Survival

Long-term survival after coronary artery bypass surgery is generally excellent. Meta-analyses have shown 96% and 85% survival at 1 and 5 years, respectively,[10] and 86%, 48%, 19%, and 7% at 5, 15, 25, and 35 years after surgery, respectively.[11]

There are many factors that affect survival adversely, including multivessel disease, diabetes, prior bypass grafting, preoperative low ejection fraction or myocardial infarct, older age, emergency surgery, mitral incompetence, smoking, respiratory disease, and hypertension.[12-14]

In regard to mortality, coronary artery bypass grafting is superior to medical therapy. Most recent meta-analyses have shown general equal or superior outcome as compared to stenting with first-general drug-eluting stents, including patients with diabetes.[4,15-17]

Surgical Techniques

There are several techniques used for cardiac immobilization in order to perform bypass surgery. The classic procedure is cold cardioplegia with extracorporeal bypass. "Off-pump" denotes lack of bypass, with the heart stabilizers (such as the Octopus) used for suturing. In general, completeness of revascularization is more important for survival than technique employed.[18] Minimally invasive bypass often uses a robotic system (e.g., the Da Vinci robotic system used for cancer surgeries), with a keyhole opening. Minimally invasive procedures are generally limited to left anterior descending disease with internal mammary grafts, however. Completely robotic surgery via endoscopy is also possible using special bypass procedures. Such procedures are termed total endoscopic coronary artery bypass (TECAB) or endoscopic atraumatic coronary artery bypass (endoACAB).

Currently, the term "minimal invasive direct coronary artery bypass" (MIDCAB) is used to designate coronary bypass procedures that do not require sternotomy, cardiopulmonary bypass, or even blood transfusions.[19,20] These procedures employ minimal invasive extracorporeal circulation techniques (off-pump) that have replaced the heart–lung machine and reduced the need for transfusion.[19,20]

Pathologic Evaluation

Postmortem Radiography

Radiographic assessment is of great benefit in identifying sites of anastomosis, mammary grafts (with multiple surgical clips), and presence of stents, in either native vessels or grafts. In addition, postmortem radiography identifies the degree of coronary and graft calcification and will additionally demonstrate calcification of the aortic valve and mitral annulus (Fig. 154.1).

Postmortem Angiography

Used generally as a research tool, angiography can be performed on fresh autopsy hearts after injection of barium–formalin mixtures. Injection can be done after perfusion fixation at ~100 mm Hg or into fresh specimens with controlled pressures.[21]

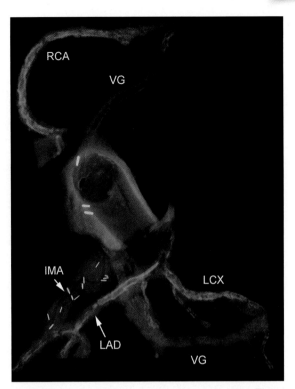

FIGURE 154.1 ▲ Postmortem radiograph, bypass heart. The radiograph is helpful in demonstrating calcification in native vessels and bypasses, as well as detecting stents (none in this example). The internal mammary artery graft typically demonstrates numerous clips for ligation of branch vessels (IMA). LAD, left anterior descending; LCX, left circumflex; VG, vein graft; RCA, right coronary artery.

Dissection Techniques

Gross dissection of bypass grafts is made difficult by pericardial adhesions, which are invariably present. The proximal aorta and pulmonary artery need to be freed of adhesions, such that the proximal trunks can be transected for exposure of the semilunar valves (Figs. 154.2 and 154.3).

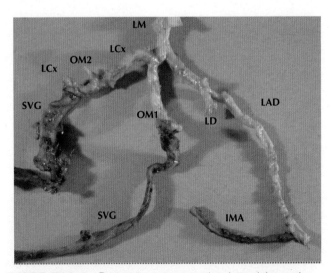

FIGURE 154.2 ▲ Postmortem coronary artery tree, status post coronary artery bypass surgery. The arteries were removed from the heart prior to decalcification. LM, left main; LAD, left anterior descending; LD, left diagonal; IMA, internal mammary artery; OM1, first obtuse marginal; SVG, saphenous vein graft; LCX, left circumflex; OM2, second obtuse marginal. The patient died of postoperative pulmonary complications and terminal sepsis after difficulties with reinflation of the left lung after total endoscopic coronary artery bypass.

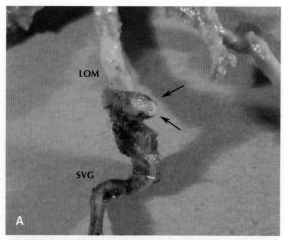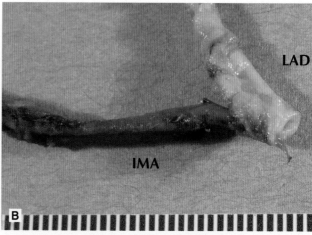

FIGURE 154.3 ▲ **A.** The obtuse marginal distal to the anastomosis shown in the prior figure demonstrated atherosclerotic narrowing (*arrows*). LOM, left obtuse marginal; SVG, saphenous vein graft. **B.** The distal runoff of the left anterior descending (LAD) was patent. IMA, internal mammary artery.

The proximal right and left ostia are then identified, and the arteries are removed for decalcification and further radiography, if desired. Sections of grafts themselves, if taken, can be identified by arterial target (e.g., saphenous vein graft to left obtuse marginal, SVG LOM). Sections of anastomotic sites can be identified by graft, vessel, and anastomosis (e.g., IMA LAD ANA). To obtain histologic sections of anastomotic sites, the native artery should be sectioned at cross sections as usual, with three sections: one just proximal to, one at, and one just distal to the anastomosis (Figs. 154.4 and 154.8). Sections of native arteries are especially important for evaluation of early deaths. Runoff vessels should be examined for luminal diameter and degree of atherosclerotic narrowing. Side-to-side anastomoses are harder to document histologically, but an attempt should be made to evaluate degree of stenosis before and after the "touchdown" site (Table 154.1).

Types of Conduits

The internal mammary artery is an elastic artery and is as such easily identified histologically with its multiple elastic laminae. Radial arteries are also elastic arteries and differ from mammary conduits in that they are sutured proximally to the aorta or a saphenous graft (Y graft). Saphenous vein grafts demonstrate histologic features of veins, namely, absence of discrete internal and external elastic lamina and abundant relatively disorganized elastic tissue in the outer media surrounding bundles of smooth muscle.

Proximal Disease

It is especially important to document atherosclerotic disease in native vessels proximal to the anastomotic sites in early deaths, in order to compare to preoperative angiography. The types of plaque, degree of luminal narrowing, and presence of thrombus should be ascertained.

Anastomotic Sites and Complications, Such as Dissections and Thrombosis

Histologic evaluation of anastomotic sites should document underlying atherosclerotic disease in the native vessel, presence of neointima as a reaction to the sutures, presence of acute or organized thrombus, and evidence of dissection (Figs. 154.4 to 154.8; Table 154.1).

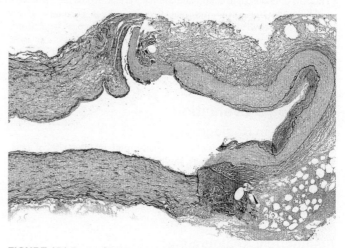

FIGURE 154.4 ▲ Saphenous vein anastomosis to native coronary. Above is proximal to the anastomosis, mid is at the anastomosis, and below is just distal, demonstrating the runoff vessel. The anastomosis is intact without significant preexisting coronary disease.

FIGURE 154.5 ▲ Saphenous vein anastomosis, acute postoperative death. There is no preexisting coronary disease, and the anastomosis is widely patent. At the right is the native artery, and at the left the vein graft.

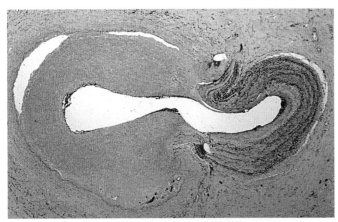

FIGURE 154.6 ▲ Radial artery anastomosis. The elastic artery is seen at the right, and there is moderate neointima **(left)** in the native vessel.

Runoff Vessels

It is important to document that the bypassed artery was adequate in size for revascularization. In non–perfusion-fixed specimens, there is collapse of the vessel, and the true luminal diameter is underestimated.

Evaluation of Early Deaths (<30 Days After Bypass)

Incidence

The rate of early deaths is currently between 2% and 3%.[11] Operative mortality with combined coronary artery bypass grafting and aortic valve replacement is similar, unless only right or left circumflex arteries are bypass, in which case it is over 5%.[22]

Cardiac Findings

The majority of early deaths are related to cardiogenic shock. The rate of intraoperative infarct is often difficult to establish clinically, because the cardiac damage induced by the surgery obscures ischemic necrosis. Clinical criteria that suggest intraoperative infarction include new Q

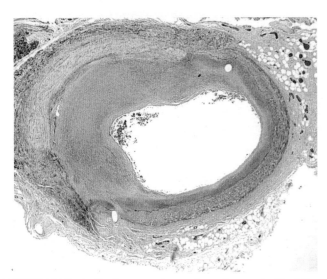

FIGURE 154.7 ▲ Saphenous vein anastomosis, remote. The left shows the vein graft, with mild neointimal proliferation. At the right is the native artery, with minimal intimal disease. The suture defects are seen at ~2 and 7 o'clock.

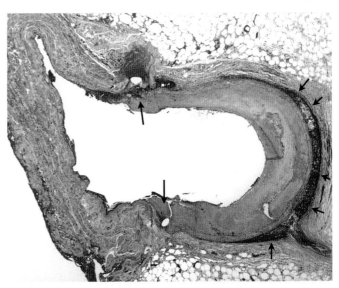

FIGURE 154.8 ▲ Acute dissection, anastomotic site. At the right is a dissection plane with hemorrhage between the media and adventitia (*short arrows*). Small degrees of dissection are not uncommon at anastomosis, although in this case it is more extensive than usual. The suture holes are seen (*long arrows*).

wave (found in about 4% of patients), new intraventricular conduction disturbance (7%), cardiogenic shock (4%), and excessively elevated cardiac enzymes (4%).[23] In an autopsy study of 32 patients who died postoperatively, there was no myocyte necrosis in those patients who could not be separated from bypass, presumably because the histologic changes did not have time to manifest; acute infarcts were found in 4 of 14 patients who lived up to 24 days.[24] Of patients who die postoperatively with autopsy, acute graft occlusion or other complication is found in over 50% of cases,[21] suggesting that they play an important role in the heart failure. Complications include twisting of grafts, thrombosis at the anastomosis, dissection at the anastomosis, and anastomoses into calcified atherosclerotic plaques. The degree of narrowing of native coronary lesions is generally found to be greater than estimated on angiography.[24] It is important at autopsy to describe the narrowing in the proximal and runoff vessels, as well as the anastomotic sites.

Extracardiac Causes of Early Death

Extracardiac complications of coronary artery bypass graft surgery include stroke, which occurs in 1% to 2% or patients and rarely

TABLE 154.1 Anatomic Findings of Importance in Autopsy Evaluation of Bypass Grafts

Proximal native vessels	Degree of narrowing
	Unstable lesions
Aortic anastomosis	Probe patency
Course of grafts	Fibrointimal thickening
	Atherosclerosis
	Aneurysm
	Cord-like graft
Coronary anastomotic site	Patency
	Underlying plaque
	Acute or organized thrombus
	Presence of dissection
Runoff vessel	Approximate luminal diameter
	Atherosclerotic narrowing

spinal artery infarct.[1] The incidence of stroke is no different between conventional and off-pump bypass surgery.[10] Infections and sepsis, sometimes complicating deep sternal infections, occur more frequently in patients with diabetes.[25] In general, the postoperative infection rate is 2% to 5% and involves the surgical site, septic shock, and multiorgan failure. The most common pathogens are gram-positive cocci, especially staphylococcal species and methicillin-resistant *Staphylococcus aureus*.[26] Perioperative mortality is nearly 10% in patients with sternal wound infections.[27] Acute mesenteric ischemia occurs in 0.5% of patients undergoing coronary artery bypass graft surgery and has a high mortality; risk factors include peripheral vascular disease, postoperative cardiogenic shock, and smoking.[28] Often, no anatomic occlusion is found in the mesenteric vessels at autopsy.[29] When fatal pulmonary embolism occurs after cardiopulmonary bypass for cardiac surgery, it usually occurs in the 2nd postoperative week.[30]

Evaluation of Late Deaths (>30 Days After Bypass)

Types of Deaths and Approach to Dissection

The autopsy pathologist will frequently encounter hearts from patients with a remote history of bypass surgery. In these cases, the cardiac findings may be incidental, a contributing factor, or the cause of sudden unexpected death. The approach to dissection depends somewhat on which of these three groups the patient falls into. For incidental cases in patients with a clear-cut noncardiac cause of death, detailed dissection may be done primarily for academic purposes. Similarly, in sudden natural deaths with no extracardiac cause, documentation of arrhythmogenic substrates (cardiomegaly, ventricular hypertrophy, cardiac scarring, severe native disease, and cardiac scarring) is adequate to establish a cardiac cause of death. For patients who fall in the category of uncertain or multifactorial causes of death, a detailed dissection including description of proximal anastomosis (saphenous vein or radial grafts), graft patency, distal anastomoses, and runoff vessels, in addition to cardiac findings, is indicated.

Chronic Graft Disease

There are several types of chronic graft disease. The most frequent, and occurring in virtually all vein grafts to some extent, is

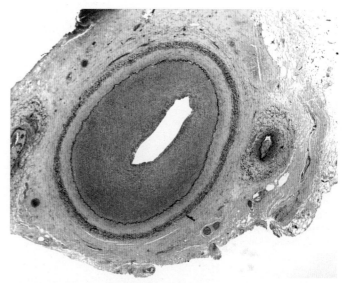

FIGURE 154.9 ▲ Diffuse intimal thickening, radial artery graft. There is a proteoglycan-rich neointima with severe luminal narrowing. Movat pentachrome.

fibrointimal proliferation (Fig. 154.9). Typically concentric, it is composed of smooth muscle cells in a background of proteoglycan matrix and progresses to significant stenosis only after many years. Secondly, lipid-rich atherosclerosis frequently occurs in vein grafts and is associated with typical risk factors associated with native coronary atherosclerosis[31,32] (Fig. 154.10). The pathologic features of saphenous vein atherosclerosis are similar to those of native arteries, but there tends to be abundant necrotic core and calcification (Fig. 154.11). These features cause difficulties for vein graft stenting, because of embolization of necrotic material and risk for perforation. Typical atherosclerosis with atheroma formation is uncommon in mammary grafts. Thirdly, there can be a cord-like saphenous graft without patency (Fig. 154.12). When thrombosis occurs early, the graft never sees blood flow and undergoes diffuse thrombosis and fibrosis, with occlusion along the length of the graft resulting in a cord-like appearance.

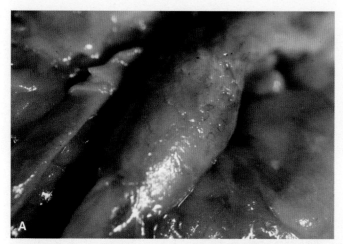
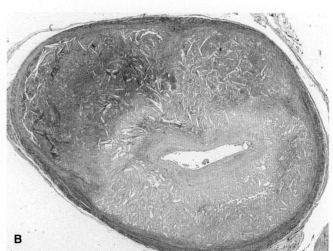

FIGURE 154.10 ▲ Saphenous vein graft with dilatation. **A.** In cases of fibroatheroma formation, there is extensive inflammation and lipid, resulting in atherosclerotic aneurysm. The gross appearance shows a dilated vessel. **B.** Microscopically, there is a lipid-rich plaque with extensive hemorrhage. Fibroatheromas occurring in vein grafts are typically rich in cholesterol clefts and necrotic gruel. Movat pentachrome.

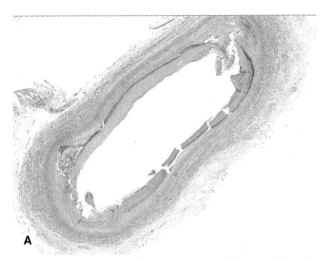
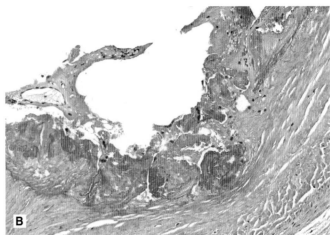

FIGURE 154.11 ▲ Calcification in patent saphenous vein graft removed at surgery for revascularization procedure. **A.** At low magnification, there is diffuse subintimal calcification. **B.** A different area shows fragmentation of the calcification with a calcified nodule.

Unusual complications of saphenous vein grafts include the formation of giant atherosclerotic aneurysms (Figs. 154.13 and 154.14), which may rupture; these occur in the setting of atheromatous change in the vein graft.[33] Infectious aneurysms involving bypass grafts are rare.[34]

Myocardial Evaluation

In most cases, there will be changes of ischemic cardiomyopathy, namely, healed infarcts, left ventricular diameter dilatation, and evidence of chronic congestion in the lungs and liver. Areas of acute infarction will be demonstrated in ~25% of patients dying in cardiogenic shock.

Surgical Pathologic Evaluation of Bypass Grafts

Rarely, the surgeon may remove bypass grafts during a second (redo) operation or at transplant for chronic ischemic heart disease. In such instances, grafts are often heavily calcified, necessitating decalcification procedures. Pathologic findings may include atherosclerosis, fibrointimal thickening, or aneurysm formation (Fig. 154.11).

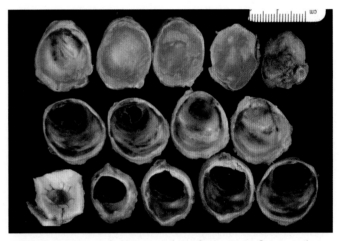

FIGURE 154.13 ▲ Saphenous vein graft aneurysm. Cross sections demonstrate layered thrombus. The ostium is at the lower left.

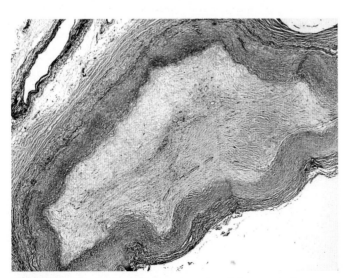

FIGURE 154.12 ▲ Cord-like thrombosed graft. In some instances, there is occlusion of a saphenous vein graft early postoperative. In these instances, there is diffuse organized thrombus with retraction and a cord-like graft.

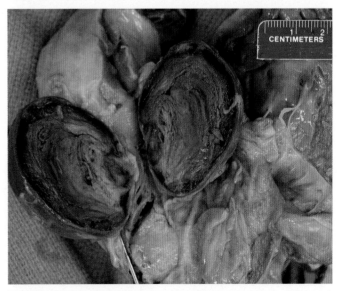

FIGURE 154.14 ▲ Saphenous vein graft aneurysm. There is layered thrombus within the lumen. In this example, the graft ruptured resulting in thoracic hemorrhage and death.

Practical Points

▶ To sample bypass grafts, the native artery should be cross-sectioned proximal to distal across the anastomotic site.

▶ Anastomoses are either terminal (end to side) or sequential ("touchdown") that are side to side and continue to the terminal anastomosis.

▶ Mammary grafts are generally single and to the left anterior descending, and tend to demonstrate multiple clips along the length that are evident radiographically.

▶ When labeling cassettes at autopsy, it is helpful to notate sections such as "SVG," "SVG LOM anastomosis," LOM runoff, "IMA LAD anastomosis," etc.

REFERENCES

1. Rossi D, Goodwin D, Cruzzavala J. Spinal cord infarction following coronary artery bypass grafting surgery. *W V Med J.* 2008;104:24–25.

2. Aupart M, Neville P, Tahir A, et al. Indications of coronary artery bypass graft in 2003. *J Cardiovasc Surg (Torino).* 2003;44:313–318.

3. Dean LS. Class I indications for coronary artery bypass graft surgery: what is the appropriate therapy for patients with multivessel coronary disease? *JACC Cardiovasc Interv.* 2009;2:622–623.

4. Blazek S, Rossbach C, Borger MA, et al. Comparison of sirolimus-eluting stenting with minimally invasive bypass surgery for stenosis of the left anterior descending coronary artery: 7-year follow-up of a randomized trial. *JACC Cardiovasc Interv.* 2015;8:30–38.

5. Nordgaard H, Vitale N, Haaverstad R. Transit-time blood flow measurements in sequential saphenous coronary artery bypass grafts. *Ann Thorac Surg.* 2009;87:1409–1415.

6. Taggart DP, Ben Gal Y, Lees B, et al. A randomized trial of external stenting for saphenous vein grafts in coronary artery bypass grafting. *Ann Thorac Surg.* 2015;99(6):2039–2045.

7. Bakaeen FG, Chu D, Dhaliwal AS, et al. Does the use of bilateral internal mammary artery grafts impact survival of veterans undergoing coronary artery bypass surgery? *Am J Surg.* 2008;196:726–731.

8. Chu D, Bakaeen FG, Wang XL, et al. The impact of placing multiple grafts to each myocardial territory on long-term survival after coronary artery bypass grafting. *J Thorac Cardiovasc Surg.* 2009;137:60–64.

9. Schwann TA, Zacharias A, Riordan CJ, et al. Sequential radial artery grafts for multivessel coronary artery bypass graft surgery: 10-year survival and angiography results. *Ann Thorac Surg.* 2009;88:31–39.

10. Filsoufi F, Rahmanian PB, Castillo JG, et al. Incidence, topography, predictors and long-term survival after stroke in patients undergoing coronary artery bypass grafting. *Ann Thorac Surg.* 2008;85:862–870.

11. Gao G, Wu Y, Grunkemeier GL, et al. Long-term survival of patients after coronary artery bypass graft surgery: comparison of the pre-stent and post-stent eras. *Ann Thorac Surg.* 2006;82:806–810.

12. Kofidis T, Gerd Paeschke H, Lichtenberg A, et al. Factors affecting post minimally invasive direct coronary artery bypass grafting incidence of myocardial infarction, percutaneous transluminal coronary angioplasty, coronary artery bypass grafting and mortality of cardiac origin. *Interact Cardiovasc Thorac Surg.* 2009;8:49–53.

13. Ahmed WA, Tully PJ, Baker RA, et al. Survival after isolated coronary artery bypass grafting in patients with severe left ventricular dysfunction. *Ann Thorac Surg.* 2009;87:1106–1112.

14. Toumpoulis IK, Chamogeorgakis TP, Angouras DC, et al. The impact of left ventricular hypertrophy on early and long-term survival after coronary artery bypass grafting. *Int J Cardiol.* 2009;135:36–42.

15. Wan YD, Sun TW, Kan QC, et al. Long-term outcomes of percutaneous coronary intervention with stenting and coronary artery bypass graft surgery—a meta-analysis. *Int J Cardiol.* 2013;168:e161–e164.

16. Li X, Kong M, Jiang D, et al. Comparing coronary artery bypass grafting with drug-eluting stenting in patients with diabetes mellitus and multivessel coronary artery disease: a meta-analysis. *Interact Cardiovasc Thorac Surg.* 2014;18:347–354.

17. Sipahi I, Akay MH, Dagdelen S, et al. Coronary artery bypass grafting vs percutaneous coronary intervention and long-term mortality and morbidity in multivessel disease: meta-analysis of randomized clinical trials of the arterial grafting and stenting era. *JAMA Intern Med.* 2014;174:223–230.

18. Lattouf OM, Thourani VH, Kilgo PD, et al. Influence of on-pump versus off-pump techniques and completeness of revascularization on long-term survival after coronary artery bypass. *Ann Thorac Surg.* 2008;86:797–805.

19. Rufa M, Schubel J, Ulrich C, et al. A retrospective comparative study of minimally invasive extracorporeal circulation versus conventional extracorporeal circulation in emergency coronary artery bypass surgery patients: a single surgeon analysis dagger. *Interact Cardiovasc Thorac Surg.* 2015;21(1):102–107.

20. Nakagawa H, Nabuchi A, Terada H, et al. Minimally invasive direct coronary artery bypass surgery with right gastroepiploic artery for redo patients. *Ann Thorac Cardiovasc Surg.* 2015;21(4):378–381.

21. Weman SM, Salminen US, Penttila A, et al. Post-mortem cast angiography in the diagnostics of graft complications in patients with fatal outcome following coronary artery bypass grafting (CABG). *Int J Legal Med.* 1999;112:107–114.

22. Jones JM, Lovell D, Cran GW, et al. Impact of coronary artery bypass grafting on survival after aortic valve replacement. *Interact Cardiovasc Thorac Surg.* 2006;5:327–330.

23. Olthof H, Middelhof C, Meijne NG, et al. The definition of myocardial infarction during aortocoronary bypass surgery. *Am Heart J.* 1983;106:631–637.

24. Waller BF, Roberts WC. Amount of narrowing by atherosclerotic plaque in 44 nonbypassed and 52 bypassed major epicardial coronary arteries in 32 necropsy patients who died within 1 month of aortocoronary bypass grafting. *Am J Cardiol.* 1980;46:956–962.

25. Marcheix B, Vanden Eynden F, Demers P, et al. Influence of diabetes mellitus on long-term survival in systematic off-pump coronary artery bypass surgery. *Ann Thorac Surg.* 2008;86:1181–1188.

26. Mastoraki E, Michalopoulos A, Kriaras I, et al. Incidence of postoperative infections in patients undergoing coronary artery bypass grafting surgery receiving antimicrobial prophylaxis with original and generic cefuroxime. *J Infect.* 2008;56:35–39.

27. Salehi Omran A, Karimi A, Ahmadi SH, et al. Superficial and deep sternal wound infection after more than 9000 coronary artery bypass graft (CABG): incidence, risk factors and mortality. *BMC Infect Dis.* 2007;7:112.

28. Venkateswaran RV, Charman SC, Goddard M, et al. Lethal mesenteric ischaemia after cardiopulmonary bypass: a common complication? *Eur J Cardiothorac Surg.* 2002;22:534–538.

29. Omoto T, Kamiya K, Akita S, et al. Nonocclusive mesenteric ischemia after cardiopulmonary bypass. *J Artif Organs.* 2004;7:161–163.

30. Masiello P, Mastrogiovanni G, Iesu S, et al. Massive pulmonary embolism 3 hours after cardiopulmonary bypass. An exceeding rare case. *Tex Heart Inst J.* 1994;21:314–316.

31. Domanski MJ, Borkowf CB, Campeau L, et al. Prognostic factors for atherosclerosis progression in saphenous vein grafts: the postcoronary artery bypass graft (Post-CABG) trial. Post-CABG Trial Investigators. *J Am Coll Cardiol.* 2000;36:1877–1883.

32. Korpilahti K, Engblom E, Syvanne M, et al. Angiographic changes in saphenous vein grafts and atherosclerosis risk factors. A 5-year study with serial measurements of serum lipids and lipoproteins. *Scand Cardiovasc J.* 1998;32:343–351.

33. Tavora FR, Jeudy J, Burke AP. Multiple aneurysms of aortocoronary saphenous vein grafts with fatal rupture. *Arq Bras Cardiol.* 2007;88:e107–e110.

34. Geneidy AA, Weise WJ. Coronary artery bypass graft mycotic aneurysms in a dialysis patient. *Am J Kidney Dis.* 2005;46:962–966.

155 Nonatherosclerotic Coronary Artery Disease

Allen P. Burke, M.D., and Fabio R. Tavora, M.D., Ph.D.

Congenital Anomalies of Coronary Circulation

Overview

Congenital anomalies of the origin and course of coronary arteries are relatively uncommon with a reported incidence of 0.2% to 1.2%.[1] They are generally divided into anomalies of origin, course, and termination (Table 155.1).

Symptoms shared by most anomalous coronary patterns include syncope and chest pain and frequently occur immediately before death or during exercise. Unfortunately, screening tests, including stress electrocardiography and echocardiography, are often negative, underscoring the need for more sensitive noninvasive imaging studies. Clinically, arteriography remains the gold standard method for evaluation of anomalous coronaries and evaluation of ischemic episodes in young patients with a suspected anomalous artery. The application of multislice computed tomography and cardiac magnetic resonance for cardiac imaging is increasing and becoming, along with other techniques, recognized methods of examination of the coronary arteries.[2]

Anomalous Origin of Coronary Circulation from Pulmonary Artery

Coronaries arising in the pulmonary circulation represent a rare cause of sudden death and heart failure in infants and children and are generally fatal if not surgically corrected. Most cases are identified within the first year of life, but some patients live well into the second and even third decade without a diagnosis.[3,4] Approximately 75% of patients will die before age 1 year, and the remainder dies or comes to clinical attention between 1 and 20 years of age. Symptoms occur in the majority of patients, although sudden unexpected death in the absence of prior symptoms has been reported. Anomalous origin of one coronary artery from the pulmonary trunk occurs in ~1 in 300,000 live births and accounts for 40% of pediatric coronary anomalies.[5]

The most common form of this anomaly, sometimes referred to as Bland-White-Garland syndrome,[6] is the *anomalous left coronary artery from the pulmonary artery (ALCAPA)*. The origin of the left main coronary artery from the pulmonary trunk should always be considered in cases of infantile and pediatric sudden death, as well as in infantile and childhood cases of dilated cardiomyopathy or endocardial fibroelastosis. The incidence of this anomaly ranges from 1/50,000 to 1/300,000 per live births. There is female-to-male ratio in incidence of 2 to 1. In adolescents surviving with the disease, sudden death may be exertional, which is typical for adults dying suddenly with anomalous origin of the left from the aorta. As infants, the clinical course in the adolescent can mimic dilated cardiomyopathy. Pathologically, the left main coronary artery arises from the pulmonary trunk, generally the left pulmonary sinus, or rarely from the anterior pulmonary sinus (Fig. 155.1). The left main coronary artery is thin walled and appears like a vein.

The treatment of ALCAPA is surgical reimplantation of the left coronary artery onto the ascending aorta, which may be complicated by restenosis necessitating revascularization including stenting.[7]

TABLE 155.1 Types of Congenitally Anomalous Coronary Arteries

Conditions involving ostia
Anomalous origin
  Anomalous origin of coronary circulation from pulmonary artery
  Anomalous origin of left main coronary artery from right sinus of Valsalva
  Anomalous origin of right coronary artery from the left sinus of Valsalva
  High–take-off origin
Ostial stenosis
Takayasu disease

Conditions involving epicardial arteries
Tunnel coronary artery/myocardial bridge
Inflammatory coronary diseases
  Kawasaki disease
  Vasculitis as part of systemic syndrome
    Takayasu disease
    Polyarteritis nodosa
    Giant cell arteritis
  Isolated coronary arteritis
Coronary artery dissection, spontaneous
Radiation-induced coronary disease
Epicardial coronary artery dysplasia
Congenital coronary artery aneurysms
Idiopathic calcification of infancy
Epicardial endocardial dysfunction
  Coronary artery spasm/Prinzmetal angina
  Diffuse endocardial dysfunction
Nonatherosclerotic coronary thrombosis
Coronary artery embolism

Conditions involving epicardial arteries and small vessels
Transplant arteriopathy (cardiac allograft vasculopathy)

Conditions involving intramural arteries
Small-vessel dysplasia/disease, area of AV node
  Isolated; associated with mitral valve prolapse
Small-vessel dysplasia, ventricular septum
  Isolated; associated with hypertrophic cardiomyopathy

Conditions involving arterioles and capillaries
Microvascular angina/cardiac syndrome X
Thrombotic thrombocytopenic purpura
Coronary artery fistulae

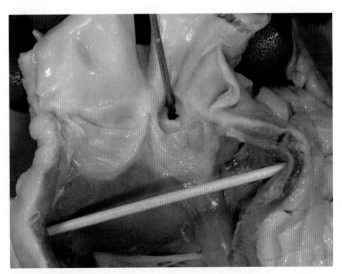

FIGURE 155.1 ▲ Anomalous origin, pulmonary trunk. The probe is inserted into the left main ostium, which arose in the anterior sinus of the pulmonary valve.

Rare variants of coronary arteries arising from the pulmonary circulation include origin of the right coronary arising from the pulmonary trunk,[8] origin of both left and right coronary arteries from the main pulmonary artery,[8,9] and origin of the coronary circulation from a branch of the pulmonary artery.[10]

Anomalous Origin of Left Main Coronary Artery from Right Sinus of Valsalva

The two most common congenital coronary anomalies resulting in sudden death are anomalous origination of a coronary artery from the opposite sinus (ACAOS), either the left or the right.[11] This anomaly is one of the most common causes of sudden death, especially exertional sudden death, in young men and women.[12] The rate of *left coronary artery originating from the right sinus* to the *right coronary artery originating from the left sinus* is about 5:1.5.[11]

More than half of the patients with this anomaly die suddenly, and the great majority of the ones dying suddenly die during exertion.[11] Most individuals who die suddenly from an anomalous left coronary artery are <30 years of age, and virtually all are younger than 40.[13] The course of the left main arising at the right sinus of Valsalva is generally between the aorta and pulmonary trunk, and often, the proximal artery is of small caliber compared to the normally positioned right coronary artery (Figs. 155.2 to 155.4). The ostium is often higher than that of the right coronary and near the commissure. Fibrosis of the myocardium in the region of the artery is common, and signs of myocardial infarct can be seen in as high as 80% of the sudden death cases.

The mechanism of death is related to myocardial ischemia and can be explained by several mechanisms. The anomalous coronary usually shows an acute-angle takeoff and the ostium is slit-like, distinct from the normally round orifice of a normal coronary.[13] The course of the anomalous artery in close relationship with the aortic media is also a possible explanation, since the aortic wall layers are very thin in the intramural segment and susceptible to luminal compression during systole.[11]

Anomalous Origin of Right Coronary Artery from the Left Sinus of Valsalva

The right coronary artery arising from the left sinus of Valsalva is less common and less lethal than the anomalous left coronary. While sudden death in the anomalous left is reported in the majority of cases, anomalous right is associated with sudden death in 20% to 45%

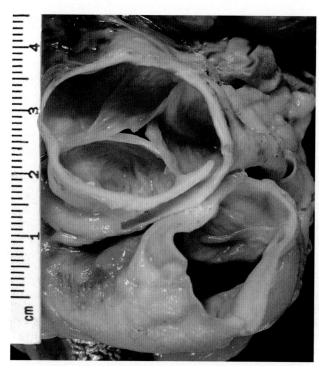

FIGURE 155.3 ▲ Anomalous origin, right coronary from the left sinus of Valsalva. Viewed from above, note the right artery arising from the left sinus of Valsalva. The pulmonary trunk is below and to the right. There is a long course between great vessels, which may become compressed during diastole when the artery normally fills.

of cases.[11] In this abnormality, both ostia arise from the left sinus of Valsalva. The proximal vessel, as the anomalous left described above, courses between the aorta and the pulmonary artery (Fig. 155.5). When present, acute or chronic ischemic changes are present in the inferior left ventricle, in the distribution of the right circulation. Evidence of ischemia essentially proves that the anomaly is potentially lethal and is corroborating evidence for causation of death. As with other potential causes of sudden death, other causes of death must be excluded carefully, especially if the death is nonexertional or occurs in someone over the age of 35 years.

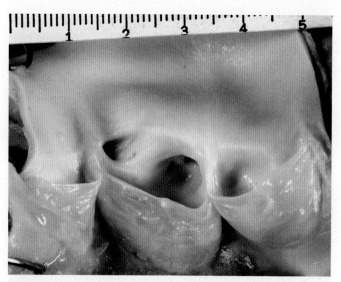

FIGURE 155.2 ▲ Anomalous origin, left main from right sinus of Valsalva. Note the left main ostium just to the right of the commissure, in the same sinus as the right (right sinus of Valsalva).

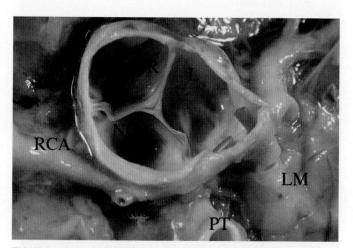

FIGURE 155.4 ▲ Anomalous origin, right coronary from the left sinus of Valsalva. There are red plastic tubes present within the ostia. The left main (LM) is normal, whereas the right coronary artery (RCA) arises from the left sinus to the left of the pulmonary trunk (PT). R, right sinus of Valsalva; L, left sinus of Valsalva; NC, noncoronary sinus.

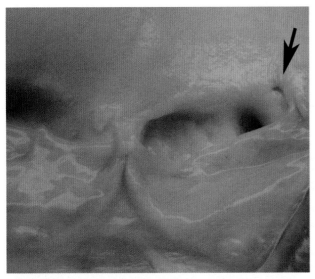

FIGURE 155.5 ▲ Anomalous origin, right coronary from the left sinus of Valsalva. In the left sinus of Valsalva, there are two ostia, one compressed (*arrow*) (anomalous right).

Miscellaneous Coronary Artery Anomalies that May Result in Ischemia and Sudden Death

Tunnel Left Anterior Descending Artery (Myocardial Bridge)

Tunneled coronary artery, or myocardial bridge, is defined as a segment of epicardial artery that goes intramurally beneath a muscle bridge and then becomes epicardial distal to the tunnel (Fig. 155.6). Virtually all tunnels involve the left anterior descending artery, although myocardial bridges involving the right coronary and left circumflex arteries have been reported.[15]

Most tunnels of the left anterior descending artery are incidental, occurring in 30% of autopsy heart specimens, and frequently occur in the presence of other cardiac findings.[16] However, bridging of coronary arteries into the myocardium can precipitate myocardial ischemia and sudden death, especially in the setting of strenuous exercise, arrhythmias, acute coronary syndromes, and coronary spasm.[17] Angiographically, systolic compression of the involved segment with "milking" of contrast is evidence of clinically significant disease.[18] There is an association between myocardial bridges and hypertrophic cardiomyopathy, especially in children.[19]

The degree of coronary obstruction by the myocardial bridge depends on location, thickness, length of the muscle bridge, and degree of cardiac contractility.[17] A tunneled artery of more than 3 mm in depth within the myocardium is considered a potential cause for ischemia or sudden death. Because most deaths due to coronary artery anomalies

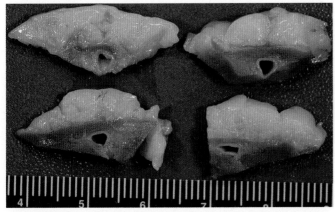

FIGURE 155.6 ▲ Tunnel coronary artery. The left anterior descending artery is separated from the epicardial fat by a rim of cardiac muscle.

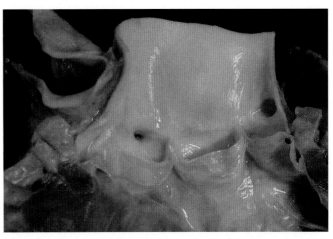

FIGURE 155.7 ▲ High takeoff, left coronary ostium. The ostium is normally within the sinus under (proximal to) the sinotubular junction; in this example, it is above (distal to) the sinotubular junction, which is the area along the aortic annulus.

are exertional, the finding of a deep tunnel in an exercise-related death is more likely significant than in a death that occurred at rest.[20]

High–Take-Off Coronary Ostia

The coronary artery ostia are normally present within the sinus of Valsalva beneath the sinotubular junction (Fig. 155.7). High takeoffs are considered a form of ostial anomaly that may be a causative factor for sudden death. In adults, a distance of 3 to 5 mm from the sinotubular junction is considered abnormal and may occur as high as 17 mm above it.[21] The diagnosis is made during life at angiography or CT angiograms.[22]

Ostial Stenosis and Atresia

Hearts with otherwise normal coronary artery may demonstrate stenosis of the coronary ostium attributable to a valve-like ridge with a fold in the elastic tunica media of the aorta. Ostial stenosis may be isolated, or a component of a more diffuse process, such as coronary and aortic dysplasia characteristic of supravalvar aortic stenosis. Coronary ostia may regress in utero, if there are significant coronary–cameral fistulae, as is characteristic of pulmonary atresia with intact ventricular septum (Fig. 155.8). Isolated ostial stenosis can be a cause of sudden death especially in infants and children.[23] Histologic

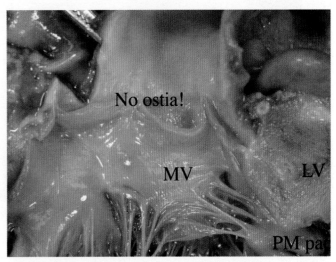

FIGURE 155.8 ▲ Absence of coronary ostia. In this infant's heart, there was atresia of the ostia, secondary to complex congenital heart disease (pulmonary atresia with intact ventricular septum). MV, mitral valve; LV, left ventricular outflow; PM pap, posteromedial papillary muscle.

evaluation is indicated, in order to distinguish congenital ostial stenosis to that caused by vasculitis, especially Takayasu disease, or coronary atherosclerosis.

Incidental Coronary Artery Anomalies and Variations

Conus Origin from Right Sinus

The origin of the conus branch from the right sinus of Valsalva is a common and incidental variation that does not cause any hemodynamic compromise. Angiographic studies estimate that this variation is present in as high as 30% of the population. At autopsy, there will be two ostia in the right sinus of Valsalva; always note the normal presence of the left anterior descending in the left sinus. Furthermore, the conus ostium is small and invariably immediately adjacent to the origin of the right, well below the sinotubular junction, unlike the anomalous left main.

Anomalous Left Circumflex from Right Sinus of Valsalva

The left circumflex artery can originate from the right aortic sinus or from the very proximal right coronary artery (Fig. 155.9). This anomaly is also common and usually incidentally found at autopsy or angiographic studies. Hemodynamic compromise is rare. The anomalous vessel usually arises with an acute angle and follows a course behind the aorta toward the left atrioventricular groove. This anomaly should be suspected if no circumflex is seen taking off from the left main coronary artery.

Single Coronary Ostium

When both main coronaries arise from a single sinus of Valsalva, as described above with anomalous right and left coronaries, one possible variation is only a single ostium, giving rise to each main artery, after a course of variable length. This anomaly is usually not associated with the problematic ostial ridges and acute takeoffs of single anomalous right or left coronaries. Therefore, association of single ostium with sudden death is uncommon. Single coronary artery is more liable to atherosclerotic changes because of decreased possibility of collateralization.

Coronary Arteritis

Kawasaki Disease

Kawasaki disease is an acute febrile syndrome, first described in 1967,[24] affecting the skin, mucosa, and lymph nodes. Subsequent reports related the acute syndrome, referred to as mucocutaneous lymph node syndrome, with coronary artery aneurysms. The incidence of Kawasaki disease ranges from 20 to 100/100,000 in Japan in children <5 years and to 4 to 15/100,000 in the United States. It is the cause of 1.3% of sudden cardiovascular deaths in persons younger than 35 years.[25] There is a male-to-female ratio of 1.5:1. More than 80% of cases occur between 6 months and 4 years of age. In Japan, a small proportion of cases have a positive family history, with a higher incidence in siblings overall.[26]

Angiographic studies have shown coronary aneurysms develop in about 5% of treated patients and 20% of untreated ones. Once established, the behavior is varied and the lesion may regress spontaneously, stay stable, progress to obstructive lesions, expand, and, in rare cases, rupture, which is the most feared complication. Infants <6 months may present a more severe form of disease and develop coronary aneurysms without any other signs and symptoms of Kawasaki disease. In adults, there are no specific gross findings and the diagnosis of Kawasaki is either assumed or established based on history (Fig. 155.10).

Pathologically, small-vessel vasculitis is believed to be the initial event in the pathogenesis in the heart and then followed by panvasculitis of the epicardial coronary arteries, aneurysms of the proximal portions, and later scarring with aneurysm of the coronary arteries. The initial phase of small-vessel vasculitis can be associated in some cases with pericarditis, myocarditis, inflammation of the atrioventricular node, and endocarditis with valvulitis. Calcification and aneurysms develop at a later stage and are detectable by imaging studies.

The histologic findings of the acutely affected artery show chronic inflammation of the media, without changes of fibrinoid necrosis as seen in polyarteritis nodosa (Fig. 155.11). The arteritis progresses through phases of healing with eventual chronic aneurysm formation, which may be recanalized and cause infarcts months and years after the initial diagnosis.[27] Death is rare in the acute stage and may be caused by myocarditis, arteritis, or noncardiac causes.

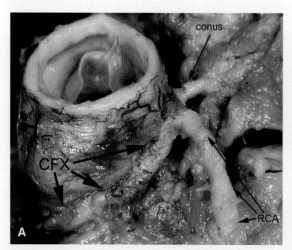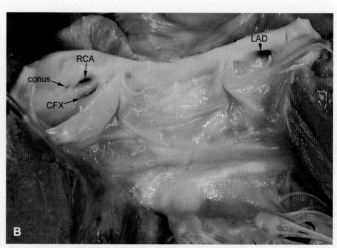

FIGURE 155.9 ▲ Anomalous origin of the left circumflex artery. **A.** This benign condition occurs when the left circumflex artery (CFX) arises from the right sinus near the ostium of the right coronary artery (RCA). In this case, there was a separate ostium for the conus artery, the first branch of the right coronary, also a benign condition. **B.** The valve is opened, demonstrating the ostia of the left circumflex (CFX), right coronary artery (RCA), and conus artery, all within the right sinus. The left main (LM) ostium is in the left sinus. LAD, left anterior descending.

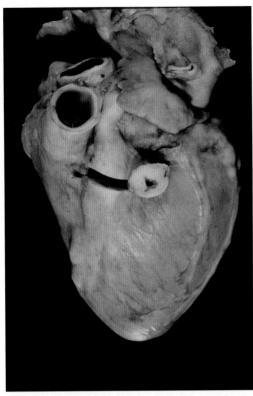

FIGURE 155.10 ▲ Kawasaki disease, adult aneurysm. There is an aneurysm of the proximal left anterior coronary artery with intimal thickening. The circumflex artery is also prominent. (Figure courtesy William Edwards, M.D.)

Thrombosis of coronary aneurysms may lead to ischemic damage to the myocardium. Aneurysms are characterized angiographically or by intravascular ultrasound (IVUS) by the presence of calcification and their size, which is classified as small (<1.5× normal), moderate (1.5 to 4× normal), and "giant" (>4× normal or larger than 8 mm).

Over 80% of small or moderate-sized aneurysms regress within 5 years, whereas giant aneurysms show a much slower rate of regression. Sudden death is a known late complication of thrombosed aneurysms in Kawasaki disease.[28-30]

Histologically, the aneurysms show organized mural thrombi, medial thinning with focal destruction of the elastic laminae, frequent calcification, and variable numbers of residual chronic inflammatory cells in the adventitia. Vessels other than the coronary arteries may be involved with vasculitis and aneurysm formation. Any artery may be involved, including in approximate order of incidence, the axillary artery, common iliac artery, renal artery, subclavian artery, internal iliac artery, superior mesenteric artery, internal thoracic artery, and femoral artery. Patients with extracoronary aneurysms almost invariably have giant coronary aneurysms.

Takayasu Aortitis with Coronary Ostial Involvement

Takayasu arteritis is an idiopathic large-vessel vasculitis that involves the aorta and its major branches (Chapter 189). In 10% to 30% of confirmed cases of Takayasu disease, coronary involvement, usually restricted to the ostia, is present and may result in acute coronary syndromes.[31-33] The pathology of coronary involvement in Takayasu arteritis involves stenotic lesions of the ostium or proximal lumen of major coronary arteries: multiple lesions with uninvolved intervening areas (skip lesions) (Fig. 155.12). Coronary thrombosis may also occur (Fig. 155.13).

Coronary Arteritis in Rheumatologic Diseases

Patients with lupus have an increased risk of premature coronary artery disease and unstable coronary syndromes (see Chapter 10). Coronary disease in lupus may include arteritis, thrombosis related to antiphospholipid syndrome, or typical atherosclerosis (the most frequent finding).

Autopsy series from the late 1900s showed coronary arteritis in 4 of 188 patients dying from complications of rheumatoid arthritis and vasculitis at a large tertiary center[34] and 10% of 179 patients with lupus in Hungary.[35] The involvement of coronary arteries in patients with rheumatoid arthritis tends to occur in patients with long-standing disease and high titers of rheumatoid factor.[36] Histologically, rheumatoid arteritis can reveal nonspecific features such as chronic inflammation

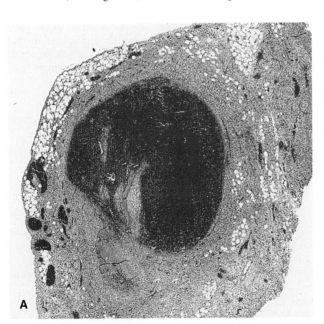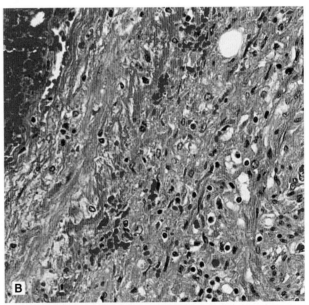

FIGURE 155.11 ▲ Kawasaki disease, acute-phase aneurysm. The patient, a 3-year-old child, died from complications of mucocutaneous lymph node syndrome and hemophagocytic lymphohistiocytosis, an uncommon association. **A.** At low magnification, there is ectasia of the artery with occlusive thrombus. **B.** The media shows chronic inflammation and thinning. There is no fibrinoid necrosis, as would be present in necrotizing arteritis such as polyarteritis nodosa.

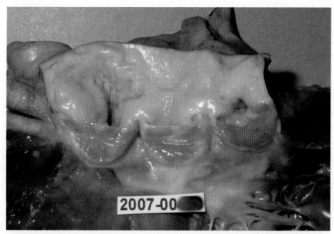

FIGURE 155.12 ▲ Takayasu disease, involving coronary ostia. The right coronary ostium is narrowed, with characteristic aortic wrinkling of the intima surrounding it.

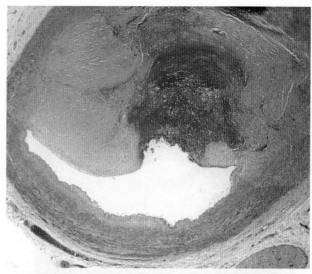

FIGURE 155.13 ▲ Takayasu disease, coronary artery. The right coronary ostium demonstrates eccentric intimal thickening with coronary thrombosis. There was extensive inflammation and destruction of the elastic laminae.

and disruption of the elastic lamina; rheumatoid nodules, while pathognomonic, are uncommon.

Coronary Arteritis in Systemic Vasculitis Syndromes

Coronary arteritis may be a manifestation of systemic vasculitis, such as polyarteritis nodosa, granulomatosis with polyangiitis, and eosinophilic granulomatosis with polyangiitis (Chapter 10). Giant cell arteritis uncommonly affects the coronary arteries and usually does so when there is aortic disease (Chapter 52). Although there is no statistically significant increase in the incidence of symptomatic coronary artery disease in patients with giant cell arteritis of the temporal artery, acute coronary syndromes and sudden death may occur secondary to giant cell arteritis of the coronary arteries with findings indistinguishable from the temporal artery lesions (Fig. 155.14).[37–40]

Isolated Coronary Arteritis

Isolated coronary arteritis is rare and denotes vasculitis of the epicardial arteries in the absence of extracardiac disease. The histologic features include inflammatory destruction of the media and elastic laminae, often with fibrinoid necrosis typical of polyarteritis nodosa. A predominance of eosinophils has been reported in isolated coronary arteritis.[41,42] Recently, an IgG4-mediated periarteritis has been described involving the coronary arteries as well as the aorta.[43]

Coronary Artery Dissection, Spontaneous

The incidence of *spontaneous coronary artery dissection (SCAD)* resulting in sudden death is ~ 2 per 1,000,000 young and middle-aged women annually, and there is an association with pregnancy. Up to 25% of pregnant patients with acute myocardial infarction have SCAD as the underlying cause.[44] The incidence of coronary artery dissection at angiography for chest pain is between 0.28% and 1.1%.[45]

The etiology of SCAD has long been considered unknown. It is currently thought to be a form of fibromuscular dysplasia, an entity which itself is largely idiopathic. A majority of patients with SCAD have abnormalities of extracardiac arteries, similar to those seen in fibromuscular dysplasia.[46] The classic "string-of-beads" appearance of dysplastic peripheral arteries is not present in presumed cases of coronary artery dysplasia and SCAD.[47]

SCAD is diagnosed by angiography in patients with chest pain, often in patients without cardiac risk factors. In clinical series, the mean age at presentation is 42 years, with a strong female predominance. Pregnant and peripartum patients with SCAD are younger (mean age 32 years).

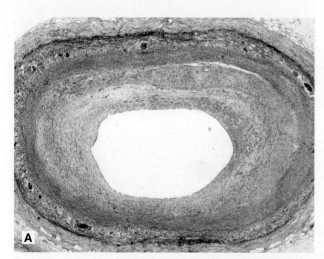

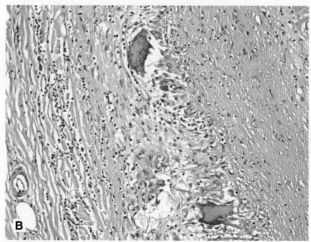

FIGURE 155.14 ▲ Giant cell arteries, coronary artery. **A.** A Movat pentachrome stain shows diffuse intimal thickening. **B.** A routine hematoxylin–eosin stain showing the granulomatous inflammation of the arterial media.

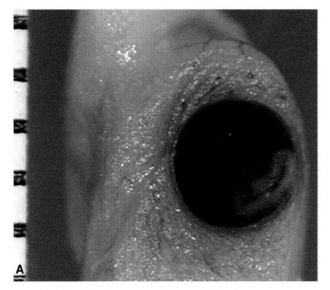

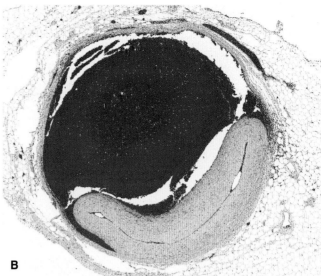

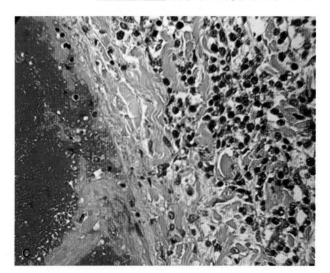

FIGURE 155.15 ▲ Spontaneous coronary artery dissection. **A.** A cross section of the epicardium shows the left anterior descending artery with a hematoma surrounding and compressing the artery. **B.** A histologic cross section showing the eccentric hematoma between the media and the adventitia. **C.** There is an infiltrate of reactive eosinophils in the adventitia.

In autopsy series, over 80% patients are women aged 20 to 50.[50] Over 75% of dissections involve the left anterior descending artery. Multiple dissections are not uncommon in autopsy series.[51] Although most patients are women in childbearing years, only a minority of deaths in autopsy studies occur in the peripartum period.[50] Traditional risk factors for coronary disease are generally absent, although hypertension has been proposed as a risk factor.[52]

The histologic findings in the majority of dissections seen at autopsy include relatively normal media, with an intramural hematoma in the space between the adventitia and media (Fig. 155.15). There is often an adventitial reaction that progresses from acute inflammation (hours) to eosinophils (days) and then fibroblasts. Abnormal media described as cystic medial necrosis was found in one of eight autopsy cases[52] as well as angiomatosis of the adventitia.[52] Acute myocardial infarction is found in 50% of patients, and healed infarction in 10%. Chronic dissections are characterized by a double-lumen chamber, one of which is lined by elastica and the other by organizing fibrointimal cells.

In patients diagnosed during life, patients are treated with intervention or bypass in over one-half of cases. Percutaneous intervention is associated with a high rate of failure.[44,48]

Syndrome X and Coronary Vasospasm

Anginal chest pain in the absence of fixed lesions on coronary angiography has been termed "angina pectoris with a normal angiogram"[54] and includes endothelial dysfunction resulting in coronary spasm and microcirculatory

disease (microvascular angina).[55] Epicardial spasm has been termed "Prinzmetal angina," after the first patients described by Prinzmetal et al.[56] The diagnosis is generally made by demonstrating complete angiographic response to coronary occlusions by the infusion of nitroglycerin.[57] Acetylcholine may also provoke spasm in patients with Prinzmetal angina.[58]

"Cardiac syndrome X" was initially defined as exertional angina in the case of normal coronary angiography. Current terms include microvascular angina and microvascular coronary dysfunction.[59] There is a strong association with female gender, as up to 50% of women with chest pain will have nonobstructive coronary artery disease (<50% narrowing by angiography). An association with left coronary artery dominance has also been described.

There are few pathologic correlates to function epicardial disease and microvascular disease (coronary spasm and syndrome X, respectively). In some cases at autopsy, concentric lipid-poor lesions are found that were not detected clinically (false-negative angiogram). Myocardial hypertrophy and sclerosis of small arteries and arterioles with perivascular fibrosis have been described in endomyocardial biopsies (Fig. 155.16).[61]

Acute myocardial infarction may occur rarely in the absence of coronary artery disease.[62–64] In autopsies of such patients, a premortem diagnosis of coronary artery spasm is often not available, and the etiology of the infarct is not apparent. From a practical standpoint, autopsied cases of syndrome X should include a thorough examination of the coronary arteries to detect obstructive coronary lesions that may have been overlooked by imaging and document the dominance (left vs. right) of the coronary circulation.

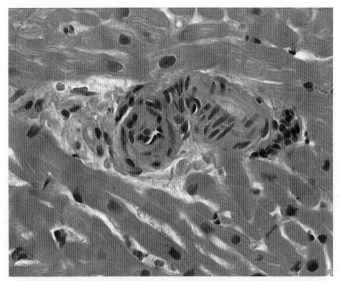

FIGURE 155.16 ▲ Syndrome X (microvascular angina), endomyocardial biopsy. There is thickening of the arterioles, a nonspecific finding but one that has been associated with microvascular angina, which this patient had by clinical criteria.

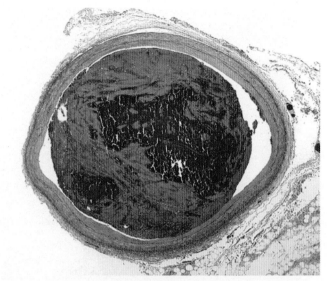

FIGURE 155.17 ▲ Nonatherosclerotic thrombosis, coronary artery. There is no underlying intimal disease. There is layering of the thrombus (lines of Zahn) that indicates that it was premortem. The patient had antiphospholipid syndrome.

Nonatherosclerotic Coronary Thrombosis

Cocaine

Cocaine abuse is known to predispose to coronary thrombosis, often in association with arterial spasm, as well as thrombosis in peripheral arteries.[65,66] In autopsy reports of cocaine-induced coronary thrombosis, over one-half of patients had underlying atherosclerosis, generally over eroded plaques.[67]

There are several potential mechanisms of cocaine-induced myocardial ischemia, in addition to vasospasm. Cocaine-induced enhancement of sympathetic activity may increase oxygen demand and decrease myocardial reserve by producing coronary constriction. One autopsy study showed increased numbers of mast cells in the adventitia of cocaine abusers, indicating a possible link to vasospasm.[67]

Thrombotic Disorders and Epicardial Thrombosis

Although rarely reported, protein C and S deficiency may result in an increased risk of coronary thrombosis in the absence of coronary atherosclerosis.[68-70] Protein C and S deficiency are also associated with intracardiac thrombi.[71,72] The antiphospholipid syndrome has also been associated with premature coronary thrombosis, in-stent thrombosis, and thrombosis of saphenous vein bypass grafts (Fig. 155.17).[73-75]

Coronary Artery Embolism

Causes

The etiology of coronary embolism includes thrombotic, infectious, and neoplastic conditions. The most common cause is embolism from valve vegetations, tumors such as myxoma or papillary fibroelastoma, and cardiac mural thrombi, especially after myocardial infarction. Rarer causes include postoperative air embolism, embolism of calcified valve fragments after surgery, and bone marrow embolism. Paradoxical embolism, or traversal of a probe-patent foramen ovale, is a requirement for embolic material originating from the peripheral circulation. Prior to the 1960s and the routine anticoagulation, the incidence of coronary embolism was as high as 5% after acute myocardial infarction.[77]

Septic Embolism

Myocardial infarction secondary to infectious endocarditis occurs via coronary embolization of fragmented septic vegetations. Staphylococcal

aortic valve endocarditis is a common underlying cause, but other organisms have also been reported in coronary embolism from endocarditis.[78] Treatment includes embolectomy via percutaneous catheterization.[79] If valve replacement is necessary, intraoperative transesophageal echocardiography may be helpful in identifying valve morphology and patency of coronaries.[80] Complications include myocardial abscess, infarction and ventricular aneurysm,[81] and near sudden death.[82]

Thrombotic Embolism

Thromboembolism is a common complication in patients with nonbacterial thrombotic endocarditis or patients with mural thrombi due to ischemic heart disease or cardiomyopathy. Cardiac sources include atrial thrombi associated with atrial fibrillation, thrombi on prosthetic heart valves and postrheumatic mitral stenosis, and atrial or ventricular thrombi in patients after myocardial infarction and with cardiomyopathy.[83] The coronary circulation is not a common site of embolization, however. Patients with myocardial infarction secondary to embolized marantic vegetations typically have underlying malignancy and concomitant central nervous system embolism, which is more common than cardiac embolism.[84]

Small-Vessel Coronary Dysplasia (Intramyocardial Small-Vessel Disease)

Isolated

Intramyocardial small-vessel abnormalities are not commonly recognized.[85] Isolated fibromuscular dysplasia of the sinoatrial or atrioventricular nodal arteries has been associated with sudden death (Fig. 155.18).[86] In contrast to syndrome X, the involved vessels are larger muscular arteries. The mechanism is uncertain but may be related to ischemia and fibrosis at the crest of the ventricular septum.[87] Isolated small-vessel disease throughout the ventricular septum without myofiber disarray or other features of hypertrophic cardiomyopathy has also been described in sudden death.[88]

Association with Myxoid Valve Disease and Cardiomyopathy

Small-vessel disease with myxoid change has been proposed as cause of sudden death in mitral valve prolapse.[89] Small-vessel disease is a recognized finding in patients with hypertrophic cardiomyopathy and is seen with myofiber disarray and scarring (Chapter 14).

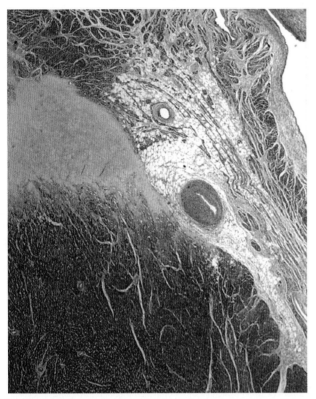

FIGURE 155.18 ▲ Coronary artery dysplasia, small vessel. There is a branch of the atrioventricular nodal artery near the node itself, which is thickened. Movat pentachrome stain demonstrates the central fibrous body to the left of the artery.

Miscellaneous Nonatherosclerotic Coronary Disease

Idiopathic Arterial Calcification of Infancy

Also known as idiopathic infantile coronary calcification, this rare condition presents in utero or at birth in up to 50% of cases as hydrops fetalis, maternal hydramnios, heart failure, or respiratory distress. Children present at a median age of 3 months, with sudden onset of fever, vomiting, irritability, or respiratory distress in a previously healthy infant. The disease can occur in patients up to 11 years old.[90] Histologically, there is diffuse calcification of coronary arteries, involving the intima and media.

Idiopathic Aneurysms

Coronary aneurysms are typically atherosclerotic, and in children caused by Kawasaki disease. In rare instances, they may be congenital or idiopathic.[91] Unlike Kawasaki aneurysms, they are more often single. Histologically, there is less inflammation and medial destruction than in postvasculitis aneurysms, although secondary changes may make the distinction difficult. Mycotic aneurysms are rare in the coronary circulation and demonstrate pseudoaneurysm histologically with a granulation tissue wall and areas of acute inflammation.

Coronary Artery Fistula

Abnormal connections may occur between the epicardial coronary arteries and the veins, cardiac chambers (ventricles or atria), or great arteries and may be congenital or the result of postinflammatory or iatrogenic injury. Coronary aneurysms, especially inflammatory, may erode into an adjacent structure with fistula formation. Congenital coronary fistulae occur in ~ 0.002% of the population[92] and constitute 13% of coronary anomalies diagnosed by angiography.[93] Diagnosis is made by imaging (Doppler echocardiography, magnetic resonance imaging)

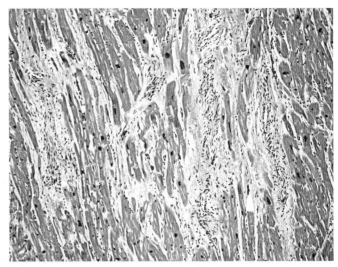

FIGURE 155.19 ▲ Coronary artery fistula. At autopsy, the exact fistulous connection can be difficult to pinpoint. In this case, there was diffuse proliferation of arterioles and capillaries in the right ventricle in a patient with a coronary–cameral fistula.

and confirmed by angiography.[94] The most common form of acquired coronary fistula is the left anterior descending artery to the pulmonary artery.[95]

Pathologically, histologic evaluation of excised tissue during open procedures may demonstrate an inflammatory etiology, although findings of noninflammatory of congenital fistulae are nonspecific. At autopsy, documentation of a congenital fistula may be difficult but is suggested by enlarged, tortuous feeder artery and dilated vessels in the myocardium, in the case of coronary–cameral or coronary venous fistula (Fig. 155.19).

Radiation-Induced Coronary Disease

Radiation coronary disease is characterized by fibrous lesions developing in the absence of lipid and foam cell accumulation (Fig. 155.20).[96,97] Patients typically have a remote history of mediastinal radiation, often for Hodgkin lymphoma. The most common artery involved is the left main. There may be concomitant radiation-induced valve disease.[98,99]

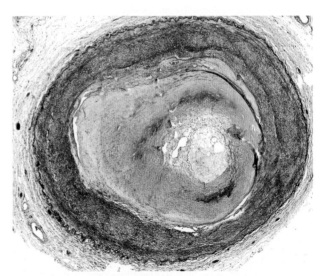

FIGURE 155.20 ▲ Radiation-induced coronary stenosis. There is total occlusion of the vessel with a bland, noninflamed fibrointimal stenosis. Verhoeff elastic stain.

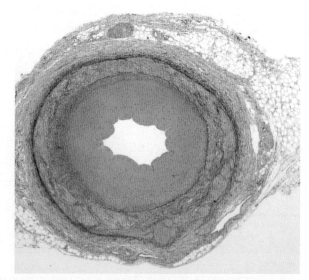

FIGURE 155.21 ▲ Epicardial coronary artery dysplasia. In most cases of epicardial fibromuscular dysplasia, the pattern is the intimal type showing prominent concentric intimal thickening. Often, there is less prominent medial involvement seen in this case as irregular deposits of proteoglycan with disorganized smooth muscle.

Coronary Artery Dysplasia (Epicardial Arteries)

Fibromuscular dysplasia of epicardial arteries is rare and is uncommonly diagnosed antemortem, often in association with SCAD.[47,100] It may be associated with renal artery fibromuscular dysplasia.[101] Epicardial coronary dysplasia typically involves the proximal arteries, especially the left anterior descending coronary artery, with diffuse intimal thickening, corresponding most closely to the intimal type in the peripheral arteries[102,103] (Fig. 155.21). Pathologically, the differential diagnosis includes concentric lipid-poor atherosclerotic disease as seen in young patients, especially women, with healed erosions. The presence of any area of pathologic intimal thickening favors atherosclerotic disease or dysplasia; in children, a healed arteritis should be considered. However, classic medial dysplasia does not result in interruption or destruction of the elastic laminae.

REFERENCES

1. Frescura C, Basso C, Thiene G, et al. Anomalous origin of coronary arteries and risk of sudden death: a study based on an autopsy population of congenital heart disease. *Hum Pathol.* 1998;29:689–695.
2. Clemente A, Del Borrello M, Greco P, et al. Anomalous origin of the coronary arteries in children: diagnostic role of three-dimensional coronary MR angiography. *Clin Imaging.* 2010;34:337–343.
3. Donataccio MP, Li W, Ramasamy M, et al. Anomalous origin of left coronary artery from the pulmonary artery (ALCAPA): a rare presentation in late adulthood. *Int J Cardiol.* 2015;182:179–180.
4. Toumpourleka M, Belitsis G, Alonso R, et al. Late presentation and surgical repair of ALCAPA. *Int J Cardiol.* 2015;186:207–209.
5. Ochoa-Ramirez E, Valdez-Garza HE, Reyes-Gonzalez R, et al. Double anomalous coronary origin from the pulmonary artery: successful surgical correction in an infant. *Tex Heart Inst J.* 2005;32:348–350.
6. Hsu HT, Wu MT. Bland-White-Garland syndrome. *QJM.* 2015;108:71–72.
7. Hallbergson A, Rome JJ. Percutaneous left main coronary artery stent for acute myocardial ischemia after repaired ALCAPA. *Catheter Cardiovasc Interv.* 2015;85:1017–1020.
8. Virmani R, Rogan K, Cheitlin MD. Congenital coronary artery anomalies: pathologic aspects. In: *Nonatherosclerotic Ischemic Heart Disease.* New York, NY: Raven Press; 1989:153–183.
9. Lipsett J, Cohle SD, Berry PJ, et al. Anomalous coronary arteries: a multi-center pediatric autopsy study. *Pediatr Pathol.* 1994;14:287–300.
10. Tavora F, Burke A, Kutys R, et al. Total anomalous origin of the coronary circulation from the right pulmonary artery. *Cardiovasc Pathol.* 2008;17:246–249.
11. Angelini P, Velasco JA, Flamm S. Coronary anomalies: incidence, pathophysiology, and clinical relevance. *Circulation.* 2002;105:2449–2454.
12. Burke AP, Farb A, Virmani R, et al. Sports-related and non-sports-related sudden cardiac death in young adults. *Am Heart J.* 1991;121:568–575.
13. Taylor AJ, Byers JP, Cheitlin MD, et al. Anomalous right or left coronary artery from the contralateral coronary sinus: "high-risk" abnormalities in the initial coronary artery course and heterogeneous clinical outcomes. *Am Heart J.* 1997;133:428–435.
14. Pascual DA, Soria F, Valdes M. Unusual congenital coronary anomaly and myocardial ischaemia. *Heart.* 1999;82:e7.
15. Tuncer C, Sokmen G, Acar G, et al. A case of myocardial bridging of the left circumflex coronary artery. *Turk Kardiyol Dern Ars.* 2008;36:562–563.
16. Quaranta F, Guerra E, Sperandii F, et al. Myocarditis in athlete and myocardial bridge: an innocent bystander? *World J Cardiol.* 2015;7:293–298.
17. Alegria JR, Herrmann J, Holmes DR, Jr., et al. Myocardial bridging. *Eur Heart J.* 2005;26:1159–1168.
18. Schwarz ER, Klues HG, vom Dahl J, et al. Functional, angiographic and intracoronary Doppler flow characteristics in symptomatic patients with myocardial bridging: effect of short-term intravenous beta-blocker medication. *J Am Coll Cardiol.* 1996;27:1637–1645.
19. Sunbul M, Kepez A, Tigen K, et al. Successful treatment of myocardial bridge with alcohol septal ablation in hypertrophic obstructive cardiomyopathy. *Int J Angiol.* 2014;23:69–70.
20. Corrado D, Thiene G, Cocco P, et al. Non-atherosclerotic coronary artery disease and sudden death in the young. *Br Heart J.* 1992;68:601–607.
21. Eren B, Turkmen N, Gundogmus UN. Sudden death due to high take-off right coronary artery. *Soud Lek.* 2013;58:45–46.
22. Kadakia J, Gupta M, Budoff MJ. Anomalous "High Take-Off" of the right coronary artery evaluated by coronary CT angiography. *Catheter Cardiovasc Interv.* 2013;82:E765–E768.
23. Kuremoto K, Matsuda S, Kanoh T. Isolated coronary ostial stenosis. *Nippon Rinsho.* 2007;(suppl 5, pt 2):114–116.
24. Kawasaki T. Acute febrile mucocutaneous syndrome with lymphoid involvement with specific desquamation of the fingers and toes in children. *Arerugi.* 1967;16:178–222.
25. Shimizu C, Sood A, Lau HD, et al. Cardiovascular pathology in 2 young adults with sudden, unexpected death due to coronary aneurysms from Kawasaki disease in childhood. *Cardiovasc Pathol.* 2015;24.
26. Nakamura Y, Yashiro M, Uehara R, et al. Epidemiologic features of Kawasaki disease in Japan: results from the nationwide survey in 2005–2006. *J Epidemiol.* 2008;18:167–172.
27. Takahashi K, Oharaseki T, Yokouchi Y, et al. Kawasaki disease arteritis and polyarteritis nodosa. *Pathol Case Rev.* 2007;12:193–199.
28. Ponniah U. Coronary artery thrombus resulting in sudden cardiac death in an infant with Kawasaki disease and giant coronary artery aneurysms. *Ann Pediatr Cardiol.* 2013;6:197–199.
29. Hartopo AB, Setianto BY. Coronary artery sequel of Kawasaki disease in adulthood, a concern for internists and cardiologists. *Acta Med Indones.* 2013;45:69–75.
30. Okura N, Okuda T, Shiotani S, et al. Sudden death as a late sequel of Kawasaki disease: postmortem CT demonstration of coronary artery aneurysm. *Forensic Sci Int.* 2013;225:85–88.
31. Camuglia AC, Randhawa VK, Lavi S. Takayasu arteritis involving the left main coronary artery treated with a bioresorbable vascular scaffold. *Int J Cardiol.* 2015;190:1–3.
32. Spagnolo EV, Cannavo G, Mondello C, et al. Unexpected death for Takayasu aortitis associated with coronary ostial stenosis: case report. *Am J Forensic Med Pathol.* 2015;36:88–90.
33. Yang M, Bai X, Xu J, et al. Two young women with severe coronary arterial ostial narrowing: a potential subtype of Takayasu arteritis. *Int J Cardiol.* 2015;189:94–95.
34. Gravallese EM, Corson JM, Coblyn JS, et al. Rheumatoid aortitis: a rarely recognized but clinically significant entity. *Medicine (Baltimore).* 1989;68:95–106.
35. Bely M, Apathy A, Beke-Martos E. Cardiac changes in rheumatoid arthritis. *Acta Morphol Hung.* 1992;40:149–186.
36. Morris PB, Imber MJ, Heinsimer JA, et al. Rheumatoid arthritis and coronary arteritis. *Am J Cardiol.* 1986;57:689–690.

37. Ungprasert P, Koster MJ, Warrington KJ. Coronary artery disease in giant cell arteritis: a systematic review and meta-analysis. *Semin Arthritis Rheum.* 2015;44:586–591.

38. Gonzalez-Gay MA, Garcia-Porrua C, Gonzalez-Juanatey C, et al. Biopsy-proven giant cell arteritis patients with coronary artery disease have increased risk of aortic aneurysmal disease and arterial thrombosis. *Clin Exp Rheumatol.* 2013;31:S94.

39. Godoy P, Araujo Sde A, Paulino E, Jr., et al. Coronary giant cell arteritis and acute myocardial infarction. *Arq Bras Cardiol.* 2007;88:e84–e87.

40. Karger B, Fechner G. Sudden death due to giant cell coronary arteritis. *Int J Legal Med.* 2006;120:377–379.

41. Omalu B, Hammers J, DiAngelo C, et al. Autopsy features of sudden death due to isolated eosinophilic coronary arteritis: report of two cases. *J Forensic Nurs.* 2011;7:153–156.

42. Arena V, Valerio L, Arena E, et al. Isolated eosinophilic coronary arteritis. *J Clin Pathol.* 2010;63:469–471.

43. Patel NR, Anzalone ML, Buja LM, et al. Sudden cardiac death due to coronary artery involvement by IgG4-related disease: a rare, serious complication of a rare disease. *Arch Pathol Lab Med.* 2014;138:833–836.

44. Higgins GL, 3rd, Borofsky JS, Irish CB, et al. Spontaneous peripartum coronary artery dissection presentation and outcome. *J Am Board Fam Med.* 2013;26:82–89.

45. Kamran M, Guptan A, Bogal M. Spontaneous coronary artery dissection: case series and review. *J Invasive Cardiol.* 2008;20:553–559.

46. Liang JJ, Prasad M, Tweet MS, et al. A novel application of CT angiography to detect extracoronary vascular abnormalities in patients with spontaneous coronary artery dissection. *J Cardiovasc Comput Tomogr.* 2014;8:189–197.

47. Michelis KC, Olin JW, Kadian-Dodov D, et al. Coronary artery manifestations of fibromuscular dysplasia. *J Am Coll Cardiol.* 2014;64:1033–1046.

48. Tweet MS, Hayes SN, Pitta SR, et al. Clinical features, management, and prognosis of spontaneous coronary artery dissection. *Circulation.* 2012;126:579–588.

49. Jaffe BD, Broderick TM, Leier CV. Cocaine-induced coronary-artery dissection. *N Engl J Med.* 1994;330:510–511.

50. Virmani R, Forman MB. Coronary artery dissections. In: Virmani R, Forman MB, eds. *Nonatherosclerotic Ischemic Heart Disease.* New York, NY: Raven Press; 1989:325–354.

51. Azzarelli S, Fiscella D, Amico F, et al. Multivessel spontaneous coronary artery dissection in a postpartum woman treated with multiple drug-eluting stents. *J Cardiovasc Med (Hagerstown).* 2009;10:340–343.

52. Basso C, Morgagni GL, Thiene G. Spontaneous coronary artery dissection: a neglected cause of acute myocardial ischaemia and sudden death. *Heart.* 1996;75:451–454.

53. Angelini P. Spontaneous coronary artery dissection: where is the tear? *Nat Clin Pract Cardiovasc Med.* 2007;4:636–637.

54. Yang EH, Lerman A. Angina pectoris with a normal coronary angiogram. *Herz.* 2005;30:17–25.

55. Petersen JW, Mehta PK, Kenkre TS, et al. Comparison of low and high dose intracoronary adenosine and acetylcholine in women undergoing coronary reactivity testing: results from the NHLBI-sponsored Women's Ischemia Syndrome Evaluation (WISE). *Int J Cardiol.* 2014;172:e114–e115.

56. Prinzmetal M, Ekmekci A, Toyoshima H, et al. Angina pectoris. III. Demonstration of a chemical origin of ST deviation in classic angina pectoris, its variant form, early myocardial infarction, and some noncardiac conditions. *Am J Cardiol.* 1959;3:276–293.

57. Ghadri JR, Ruschitzka F, Luscher TF, et al. Prinzmetal angina. *QJM.* 2014;107:375–377.

58. Michels HR, Baars HF. Multifocal spasm with acetylcholine in Prinzmetal angina. *Neth Heart J.* 2008;16:134–136.

59. Agrawal S, Mehta PK, Bairey Merz CN. Cardiac syndrome X: update 2014. *Cardiol Clin.* 2014;32:463–478.

60. Makarovic Z, Makarovic S, Bilic-Curcic I. Sex-dependent association between coronary vessel dominance and cardiac syndrome X: a case-control study. *BMC Cardiovasc Disord.* 2014;14:142.

61. Suzuki H, Takeyama Y, Koba S, et al. Small vessel pathology and coronary hemodynamics in patients with microvascular angina. *Int J Cardiol.* 1994;43:139–150.

62. Aldrovandi A, Cademartiri F, Menozzi A, et al. Evaluation of coronary atherosclerosis by multislice computed tomography in patients with acute myocardial infarction and without significant coronary artery stenosis: a comparative study with quantitative coronary angiography. *Circ Cardiovasc Imaging.* 2008;1:205–211.

63. Cortell A, Sanchis J, Bodi V, et al. Non-ST-elevation acute myocardial infarction with normal coronary arteries: predictors and prognosis. *Rev Esp Cardiol.* 2009;62:1260–1266.

64. Middlemost S, Mabin T. Takotsubo cardiomyopathy: an acute and reversible cardiomyopathy mimicking acute myocardial infarction. *Cardiovasc J Afr.* 2008;19:33–38.

65. Edgecombe A, Milroy C. Sudden death from superior mesenteric artery thrombosis in a cocaine user. *Forensic Sci Med Pathol.* 2012;8:48–51.

66. Apostolakis E, Tsigkas G, Baikoussis NG, et al. Acute left main coronary artery thrombosis due to cocaine use. *J Cardiothorac Surg.* 2010;5:65.

67. Kolodgie FD, Farb A, Virmani R. Pathobiological determinants of cocaine-associated cardiovascular syndromes. *Hum Pathol.* 1995;26:583–586.

68. Eshtehardi P, Ghassemi-Kakroodi P, Garachemani A, et al. Coronary thrombosis and myocardial infarction as the initial manifestation of protein C deficiency in a 20-year-old man. *Heart Lung.* 2011;40:e112–e114.

69. Goel PK, Batra A. Protein C and/or protein S deficiency and occurrence of stent thrombosis: a hitherto unrecognized association. *J Interv Cardiol.* 2010;23:560–564.

70. Sayin MR. Left main coronary artery thrombus resulting from combined protein C and S deficiency. *Intern Med.* 2013;52:697.

71. Sabzi F, Faraji R. Right atrial thrombosis associated with sagittal sinus thrombosis caused by protein C–S deficiency. *JNMA J Nepal Med Assoc.* 2013;52:378–383.

72. Sabzi F, Faraji R. Cardiac left ventricular thrombus in protein C deficiency. *Niger Med J.* 2014;55:354–355.

73. Denas G, Jose SP, Bracco A, et al. Antiphospholipid syndrome and the heart: a case series and literature review. *Autoimmun Rev.* 2015;14:214–222.

74. Lee YH, Yang HM, Tahk SJ, et al. Recurrent stent thrombosis in a patient with antiphospholipid syndrome and dual anti-platelet therapy non-responsiveness. *Korean Circ J.* 2015;45:71–76.

75. Smukowska-Gorynia A, Mularek-Kubzdela T, Araszkiewicz A. Recurrent acute myocardial infarction as an initial manifestation of antiphospholipid syndrome: treatment and management. *Blood Coagul Fibrinolysis.* 2015;26:91–94.

76. Singer RL, Mannion JD, Bauer TL, et al. Complications from heparin-induced thrombocytopenia in patients undergoing cardiopulmonary bypass. *Chest.* 1993;104:1436–1440.

77. Atkinson JB, Forman MB, Virmani R. Emboli and thrombi in coronary arteries. In: Virmani R, Forman MB, eds. *Nonatherosclerotic Ischemic Heart Disease.* New York, NY: Raven Press; 1989:355–385.

78. Acar G, Ozok A, Donmez C, et al. Myocardial infarction due to septic coronary artery embolism in the course of Brucella endocarditis. *Herz.* 2015;40:335–337.

79. Taniike M, Nishino M, Egami Y, et al. Acute myocardial infarction caused by a septic coronary embolism diagnosed and treated with a thrombectomy catheter. *Heart.* 2005;91:e34.

80. Eltzschig HK, Lekowski RW, Jr., Shernan SK, et al. Intraoperative transesophageal echocardiography to assess septic coronary embolism. *Anesthesiology.* 2002;97:1627–1629.

81. Adachi I, Kobayashi J, Nakajima H, et al. Coronary embolism and subsequent myocardial abscess complicating ventricular aneurysm and tachycardia. *Ann Thorac Surg.* 2005;80:2366–2368.

82. Yavari A, Paul G, Jackson G. Aborted sudden cardiac death—a rare presentation of septic coronary embolism. *Eur J Intern Med.* 2008;19:559.

83. Ricci S. Embolism from the heart in the young patient: a short review. *Neurol Sci.* 2003;24(suppl 1):S13–S14.

84. Dutta T, Karas MG, Segal AZ, et al. Yield of transesophageal echocardiography for nonbacterial thrombotic endocarditis and other cardiac sources of embolism in cancer patients with cerebral ischemia. *Am J Cardiol.* 2006;97:894–898.

85. Veinot JP, Johnston B, Acharya V, et al. The spectrum of intramyocardial small vessel disease associated with sudden death. *J Forensic Sci.* 2002;47:384–388.

86. James TN, Posada-de la Paz M, Abaitua-Borda I, et al. Histologic abnormalities of large and small coronary arteries, neural structures, and the conduction system of the heart found in postmortem studies of individuals dying from the toxic oil syndrome. *Am Heart J.* 1991;121:803–815.

87. Burke AP, Subramanian R, Smialek J, et al. Nonatherosclerotic narrowing of the atrioventricular node artery and sudden death. *J Am Coll Cardiol.* 1993;21:117–122.

88. Burke AP, Virmani R. Intramural coronary artery dysplasia of the ventricular septum and sudden death. *Hum Pathol.* 1998;29:1124–1127.

89. Burke AP, Farb A, Tang A, et al. Fibromuscular dysplasia of small coronary arteries and fibrosis in the basilar ventricular septum in mitral valve prolapse. *Am Heart J.* 1997;134:282–291.

90. Hault K, Sebire NJ, Ho SY, et al. The difficulty in diagnosing idiopathic arterial calcification of infancy, its variation in presentation, and the importance of autopsy. *Cardiol Young.* 2008;18:624–627.

91. Alioglu E, Turk UO, Engin C, et al. Left main coronary artery aneurysm in young patient with acute myocardial infarction. *J Cardiovasc Med (Hagerstown).* 2009;10:494–496.

92. Maleszka A, Kleikamp G, Minami K, et al. Giant coronary arteriovenous fistula. A case report and review of the literature. *Z Kardiol.* 2005;94:38–43.

93. Yamanaka O, Hobbs RE. Coronary artery anomalies in 126,595 patients undergoing coronary arteriography. *Cathet Cardiovasc Diagn.* 1990;21:28–40.

94. Rathi VK, Mikolich B, Patel M, et al. Coronary artery fistula; non-invasive diagnosis by cardiovascular magnetic resonance imaging. *J Cardiovasc Magn Reson.* 2005;7:723–725.

95. Abdelmoneim SS, Mookadam F, Moustafa S, et al. Coronary artery fistula: single-center experience spanning 17 years. *J Interv Cardiol.* 2007;20:265–274.

96. Mert M, Arat-Ozkan A, Ozkara A, et al. Radiation-induced coronary artery disease. *Z Kardiol.* 2003;92:682–685.

97. Notaristefano S, Giombolini C, Santucci S, et al. Radiation-induced ostial stenosis of the coronary artery as a cause of acute coronary syndromes: a novel mechanism of thrombus formation? *Ital Heart J.* 2003;4:341–344.

98. Akboga MK, Akyel A, Sahinarslan A, et al. Radiotherapy-induced concomitant coronary artery stenosis and mitral valve disease. *Wien Klin Wochenschr.* 2014;126:243–245.

99. Alsara O, Alsarah A, Kalavakunta JK, et al. Isolated left main coronary artery stenosis after thoracic radiation therapy: to operate or not to operate. *Case Rep Med.* 2013;2013:834164.

100. Makino Y, Inokuchi G, Yokota H, et al. Sudden death due to coronary artery dissection associated with fibromuscular dysplasia revealed by postmortem selective computed tomography coronary angiography: a case report. *Forensic Sci Int.* 2015;253:e10–e15.

101. Pate GE, Lowe R, Buller CE. Fibromuscular dysplasia of the coronary and renal arteries? *Catheter Cardiovasc Interv.* 2005;64:138–145.

102. Mogler C, Springer W, Gorenflo M. Fibromuscular dysplasia of the coronary arteries: a rare cause of death in infants and young children. *Cardiol Young.* 2015:1–4.

103. Garcia RA, deRoux SJ, Axiotis CA. Isolated fibromuscular dysplasia of the coronary ostium: a rare cause of sudden death. Case report and review of the literature. *Cardiovasc Pathol.* 2015;24:327–331.

104. Camuglia A, Manins V, Taylor A, et al. Case report and review: epicardial coronary artery fibromuscular dysplasia. *Heart Lung Circ.* 2009;18:151–154.

156 Dilated Cardiomyopathy

Allen P. Burke, M.D., and Joseph J. Maleszewski, M.D.

Classification

Primary Versus Secondary Dilated Cardiomyopathy

Dilated cardiomyopathy (DCM) is heart disease usually characterized by four-chamber dilatation in the absence of significant valvular, ischemic, or hypertensive disease. In the past, some have referred to ischemic heart disease as a form of DCM; hence, the generic division between "ischemic" and "nonischemic" cardiomyopathy is frequently made clinically.[1] However, it is important to note that while ischemic heart disease may cause ventricular dilatation, it should not be considered a cardiomyopathy. Moreover, despite the frequent use of the term "nonischemic dilated cardiomyopathy," it is considered both nonspecific and redundant and is therefore not accepted among pathologists.[2,3]

In the past, DCM was divided into "idiopathic," familial, and secondary types. Currently, it is understood that genetics plays a role in the majority of cases of DCM, even though a family history is elicited in only one-third.[4] There is no clear distinction between a cause and an association, blurring the lines between primary and secondary cardiomyopathy. For example, alcoholism may be a risk factor but not necessarily a cause for cardiomyopathy, and myocarditis may play a role in the development of heart disease in patients with cardiomyopathic mutations. For these reasons, there is a trend away from the designation "idiopathic dilated cardiomyopathy" as the line between genetic and environmental blurs.

In general, the term DCM should be employed by pathologists when no secondary factor is identified to explain the pathology.[5] However, if a nongenetic condition (e.g., myocarditis, hemochromatosis, etc.) is identified, the condition is best characterized as heart disease secondary to such (e.g., myocarditis-associated heart disease, cardiac hemochromatosis, etc.). Tables 156.1 and 156.2 present two currently accepted classifications of cardiomyopathy, and Table 156.3 a functional pathologic classification.

Phenotype–Genotype Correlation

Sampling limitations of endomyocardial biopsy, biases of autopsy studies, and lack of specificity of histologic findings have hampered the development of a pathologic classification of cardiomyopathy, especially DCM. It was hoped in the early years of this century that molecular studies would reveal a good correlation between classes of mutated proteins and type of cardiomyopathy as defined by imaging, hemodynamics, and electrocardiographic findings. However, molecular investigations of patients with cardiomyopathy have resulted in a large number of mutations that lack specificity for a specific clinical type and have thus far shown little correlation between phenotype and genotype. The American Heart Association classification, which relied heavily on genetics, was criticized by the European Society of Cardiology, who continued to rely primarily on morphology[6,8] (Table 156.2).

The major genes implicated in the pathogenesis of DCM include those encoding for proteins in the sarcomere (e.g., myosin heavy chain and titin), cytoskeleton (e.g., sarcoglycans and dystrophin), and nuclear membrane (e.g., lamin A) (Table 156.4; Fig. 156.1). Mutations in sarcomeric genes were originally discovered in familial hypertrophic cardiomyopathy (HCM) but are also found in DCM.

Currently, there is a movement to use a more descriptive classification system for clinicians, which relies on five criteria. The "MOGES" system uses morphofunctional phenotype (M), organ involvement (O), genetic or familial inheritance pattern (G), etiologic description (E) of genetic defect or nongenetic underlying cause, and the functional status (S) to characterize patients with cardiomyopathy of all types, including DCM.[11]

From the standpoint of the pathologist, it is important at a gross level to identify the phenotype of cardiomyopathy. There are currently five (Table 156.3): DCM, HCM, arrhythmogenic cardiomyopathy (AC), restrictive cardiomyopathy (RCM), and left ventricular noncompaction (LVNC). As will be addressed in Chapter 25, of these designations, there is the greatest pathologic variation in RCM, which is a phenotypic manifestation of diverse unrelated conditions.

The current chapter is devoted to DCM in adults, focusing on both the genetic varieties as well as those cases associated with drugs, pregnancy, viruses, and nutritional deficiency. Cardiomyopathy of childhood and those with extracardiac manifestations are discussed in Chapter 23. DCM occurring as a consequence of systemic diseases is discussed in detail in Section 3.

Autopsy Evaluation of Dilated Cardiomyopathy

The autopsy evaluation of cardiomyopathy should begin with review of clinical data. Some cases may have limited or no information (particularly in relatively young individuals who experience sudden death) and others may have extensive clinical and even molecular genetic data

TABLE 156.1   Classification of Primary Cardiomyopathy, AHA 2006[6]

Genetic	Mixed	Acquired
Hypertrophic cardiomyopathy	DCM	Inflammatory (myocarditis)
AC	Restrictive (nonhypertrophied and nondilated)	Takotsubo
LVNC		Peripartum
Conduction defects (Lenegre, sick sinus syndrome, WPW)		Tachycardia induced
		Infants of diabetic mothers
Mitochondrial myopathies		
Ion channel disorders (LQTS, Brugada, SQTS, SVPT, Asian SUNDS)[a]		

[a]The ion channel disorders are not usually classified under cardiomyopathy; see Chapter 4.

TABLE 156.2   Classification of Cardiomyopathies, ESC 2008[7]

	HCM	DCM	AC	RCM	Unclassified
Familial	Unknown gene Sarcomeric mutations Glycogen storage (Pompe, PRKAG2, Forbes, Danon) Lysosomal storage (Fabry, Hurler) Disorders of fatty acid metabolism Carnitine deficiency Phosphorylase B kinase deficiency Mitochondrial myopathies Syndromic[a]	Unknown gene Sarcomeric mutations Z-band mutations Cytoskeletal mutations Nuclear membrane Mildly dilated CM Desmosomal mutations Mitochondrial myopathy	Unknown gene Intercalated disc protein mutation Ryanodine receptor (Ryr2) TGFβ-3	Unknown gene Sarcomeric protein mutations Familial amyloidosis Desminopathy Pseudoxanthoma elasticum Hemochromatosis Fabry disease Glycogen storage disease	Left ventricular noncompaction (Barth syndrome, lamin A/C, ZASP, α-dystro-brevin mutations)
Nonfamilial	Obesity Infants of diabetic mothers Athletic training Amyloid	Postinflammatory[b] Drugs Peripartum Endocrine Nutritional[c] Alcohol Tachycardio-myopathy	Postmyocarditis ()	Amyloid Scleroderma Endomyocardial fibrosis Hypereosinophilic syndrome Drugs (serotonin, methysergide, ergotamine, mercurial agents, busulfan) Carcinoid heart disease Metastatic cancers Radiation drugs (anthracyclines)	Takotsubo (stress) cardiomyopathy

[a]Noonan, LEOPARD, Friedreich ataxia, Beckwith-Wiedemann, Swyer.
[b]Infectious, toxic immune myocarditis; Kawasaki; eosinophilic; viral persistence.
[c]Thiamine, carnitine, selenium, hypophosphatemia, hypocalcemia.

available. In the former scenario, the main purpose of the autopsy is to establish cause of death, (see Chapter 141), including cardiac arrhythmia, thromboembolism, and extracardiac or nonnatural causes, and to try and identify potential risk factors (hypertension, chronic renal disease, obesity, etc.). In the cases of a medical autopsy with abundant clinical data, the purpose of autopsy generally revolves around aspects of therapy, for example, ventricular assist devices or defibrillators, and the evaluation of extracardiac causes of death, such as infections and thromboembolism.

The first gross heart parameters to establish are the presence of cardiomegaly (preferably using tables based on body weight and height)[12] and the absence of other causes of myocardial disease, such as ischemic, valvular, and hypertensive diseases. In general, a heart weight >50% above the expected mean is in keeping with cardiomegaly. It should be noted that there may be coexistence of true cardiomyopathy with moderate coronary or moderate valve disease, in which case the extent of disease should be estimated.

In the end, it is a judgment call as to whether or not the extent of the underlying diseases is sufficient to explain the observed cardiac phenotype. Evaluation of clinical records, if available, can be helpful in determining the severity of comorbid states such as hypertension and valvular disease. However, evaluating for extracardiac manifestations of the disease can also be helpful. For example, if no hypertensive changes are observed in the kidney, it is unlikely that the hypertension alone could explain cardiomegaly.

TABLE 156.3   Morphofunctional (Clinicopathologic) Types/Patterns of Cardiomyopathy[a]

	Gross Pathologic Features	Microscopic Features	Causes/Associations
Dilated	Left ventricular dilatation (>4 cm) Normal or mildly increased wall thickness Dilated atria Gross scars possible	Nonspecific	Sarcomeric, cytoskeletal, and other myocyte protein mutations Inflammatory, nutritional, toxic, others
Hypertrophic	Left ventricular hypertrophy, especially septal Areas of scar common	Myofiber disarray[b]	Sarcomeric mutations (classic HCM)
Restrictive	Normal-appearing ventricles, dilated atria	Various, depending on cause	Amyloid Endocardial fibrosis Eosinophilic endomyocarditis (Loeffler) Various cardiomyocyte proteins (e.g., desminopathy)
Left ventricular noncompaction	Hypertrabeculated myocardium Sinusoidal recesses Poorly formed papillary muscles	Sinusoidal recesses	Barth syndrome Various mutations (LMNA, ZASP, α-dystrobrevin)
Arrhythmogenic	Biventricular subepicardial scars Ventricular wall thinning (usually right ventricular)	Fibrofatty change	Desmosomal mutations, sarcomeric mutations Postmyocarditis

[a]There is overlap among the groups; the most common features are presented. See Chapters 20 to 25 for a discussion of types of cardiomyopathy that are not typically of the dilated phenotype.
[b]Myofiber disarray is typical of classic hypertrophic cardiomyopathy (see Chapter 20). There may be distinct findings in some forms of cardiomyopathy that frequently present as a hypertrophic phenotype, for example, lamellated inclusions, (Fabry) and membrane-bound autophagosomes (Danon) by ultrastructure.

TABLE 156.4 Most Frequent Genes Implicated in the Pathogenesis of Dilated Cardiomyopathy

Gene Designation	Gene Name	Other Cardiomyopathy Phenotype Associations
LMNA[a]	Lamin A	LVNC
PKP2[b]	Plakophilin-2	AC
TTN[c]	Titin	HCM, AC
ANKRD1	Ankyrin repeat domain 1 (cardiac muscle)	HCM
DSP	Desmoplakin	AC
DSC2	Desmocollin 2	AC
LDB3	LIM domain binding 3	LVNC
MYH7	Myosin, heavy chain 7, cardiac muscle	HCM, LVNC
MYBPC3	Myosin binding protein C, cardiac	HCM, LVNC
RBM20	RNA binding motif protein 20	—
RYR2	Ryanodine receptor 2 (cardiac)	CPVT
SCN5A	Sodium channel, voltage-gated, type V, subunit	Long QT syndrome
TNNT2	Troponin T type 2 (cardiac)	HCM and LVNC
TPMI	Tropomyosin 1 (α)	DCM

CPVT, catecholaminergic polymorphous ventricular tachycardia; HCM, hypertrophic cardiomyopathy; LVNC, left ventricular noncompaction; RCM, restrictive cardiomyopathy.
[a]Historically considered the most common mutation, characteristic of DCM.
[b]Most common using next-generation sequencing.[9]
[c]Most frequent with multigene sequencing.[10]

Occasionally, the pathologist will be asked to perform molecular testing in cases that have been undertaken during life. Such molecular genetic testing affords the ability to formally characterize a process that cannot otherwise be explained. More importantly, it allows for more complete characterization of a disease that often has heritable implications. Confirming a genotype (or even absence of an identifiable mutation) can be immensely valuable when screening the kindred and assessing risk of surviving family members.

Explant

The diagnosis of cardiomyopathy at cardiac explant is generally straightforward, as the patient has been extensively evaluated prior to transplant and the diagnosis is not in doubt. In some cases, an unexpected diagnosis may be found, if a biopsy has not been performed. For example, a pattern of subepicardial replacement-type fibrosis may be indicative of prior myocarditis. Small foci of active myocarditis ("smoldering myocarditis") can also be identified. Sarcoidosis and hemochromatosis may also manifest as ventricular dilatation and failure. Although unusual, ischemic heart disease may occasionally be missed clinically, so it is important to carefully evaluate for such.[13] Similarly, there may be areas of extensive fibrofatty replacement of the ventricle, suggestive of a diagnosis of AC (Chapter 21).

Endomyocardial Biopsy

Because of limited sampling and lack of specific histologic features, endomyocardial biopsy is useful in excluding a specific pathologic entity, most commonly sarcoidosis or myocarditis. Ultrastructural evaluation is of limited use in most cases, although a search for membrane-bound autophagic vacuoles (Danon cardiomyopathy) or lamellar inclusions (Fabry disease) should be performed if indicated, as these conditions may occasionally present as a dilated phenotype (the former more so than the latter, which usually manifests as a hypertrophic phenotype).

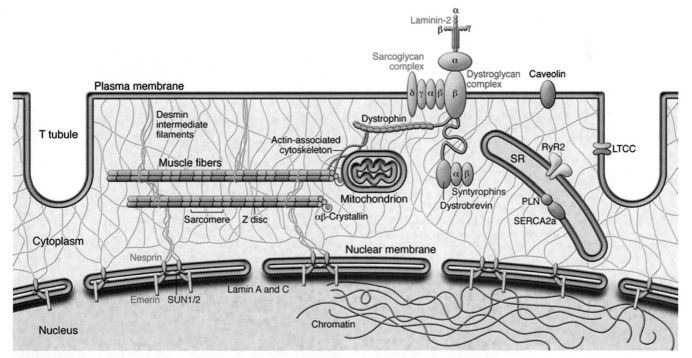

FIGURE 156.1 ▲ Schematic representation of cardiomyocyte proteins. The cytoplasm of the cardiomyocyte contains sarcomeres, which contain thin and thick filaments. Mutations in sarcomeric genes can be associated with either hypertrophic or dilated cardiomyopathy; these are most commonly titin, myosin (thick), actin (thin filaments), and associated proteins. Plasma membrane–associated proteins (dystrophin, dystrophin-associated proteins, and sarcoglycans) are associated with cardiac and skeletal muscle disease. Mutations of genes encoding nuclear membrane proteins (lamin A/C, emerin) lead to dilated cardiomyopathy typically without skeletal muscle disease. Nuclear membrane genes may also induce cardiac conduction system disease. (Reproduced with permission, McNally EM, Golbus JR, Puckelwartz MJ. Genetic mutations and mechanisms in dilated cardiomyopathy. J Clin Invest. 2013;123:19–26.)

Dilated Cardiomyopathy (Genetic or Likely Genetic)

Definition

DCM is defined clinically by global left ventricular systolic dysfunction and increased left ventricular cavity diameter in the absence of significant hypertension, valvular disease, or ischemia.[6,7] Because of this absence of a specific nongenetic etiology, it is sometimes referred to as "idiopathic" DCM—even when a genetic underpinning is identified. DCM produces a prominent increase in chamber volumes as well as ventricular wall thickening.[14] Wall thickening may not be apparent as dilatation becomes more pronounced. It is an irreversible form of primary heart muscle disease usually with a genetic (or likely genetic) etiology.[4]

Epidemiology

DCM accounts for 30% to 40% of all heart failure cases in large clinical trials and is a leading cause of heart transplantation.[9] The estimated prevalence of DCM is 1:2,700 with an incidence of 7/100,000/year. It is the most common cardiomyopathy. Of 845 patients with recent-onset heart failure referred to a tertiary center, 529 were idiopathic.[15] In most centers, it is the most frequent cause of heart transplantation. Incidence of the disease discovered at autopsy is estimated at 4.5/100,000/year while clinical incidence is 2.45/100,000/year.[16]

Etiology

DCM is considered a "mixed" form of cardiomyopathy (caused by acquired and genetic factors) by the AHA classification.[6] Mutations in cardiac genes involve both cytoskeletal and sarcomeric proteins. Among the most common are mutations of the following genes: *LMNA*, *MYH7*, *TNNT2*, *SCN5A*, *DES*, *MYBPC3*, *TNNI3*, *TPMI*, *ACTC*, *PLN*, *LDB3*, and *TAZ*.[4]

There are at least 60 genes encoding myocyte proteins that have been implicated in human cardiomyopathies, as of 2015, more than half of which have been associated with DCM; many of these are also associated with hypertrophic or arrhythmogenic cardiomyopathy.[17,18] Using current-generation sequencing techniques, 37% to 46% of patients (both with and without a family history) are found to have mutations that are likely pathogenic and more than a third will carry multiple mutations.[9,10] When inherited, the vast majority is transmitted in an autosomal dominant fashion, with X-linked and autosomal recessive forms being much less common.

A study screening a panel of genetic mutations found that titin (*TTN*) was the most frequently mutated gene, followed by lamin A (*LMNA*), myosin heavy chain 7 (*MYH7*), and desmoplakin (*DSP*).[10] A more recent study using next-generation sequencing found that genes typically associated with arrhythmogenic right ventricular cardiomyopathy (plakophilin-2, and desmoplakin) and HCM (myosin-binding protein C-3) are among the most common found in DCM.[9] These studies underscore the lack of specificity between genetic mutations and phenotype and the variability that depends on population studied and genetic testing methods.

Some genes are relatively specific to given populations. For example, nonsense mutations in *BAG3* have been found in 15% of familial cardiomyopathy in French Canadians.[19] *BAG3* is associated with chaperone-assisted selective autophagy. The ultrastructural findings in cardiomyopathy caused by *BAG3* mutations have not been investigated, and if there are autophagic vacuoles as seen in Danon cardiomyopathy.[20]

Sarcomeric protein mutations occur in up to 25% of patients with DCM.[9,10] It is important to note that many of these may reflect HCM that has "burnt out" and resolved into a dilated phenotype. Once again, this nonspecificity of phenotype for given genotype reflects a great need for further study into the variable and defining characteristics of cardiomyopathies and likely will ultimately result in a much different approach to diagnostic categorization.

Clinical Features

DCM is usually characterized by progressive heart failure frequently complicated by ventricular and supraventricular arrhythmias, conduction system abnormalities, thromboembolism, and often death (sudden or related to heart failure).[6] The mean age at presentation is 53 years, with familial cases typically symptomatic at an earlier age.[3] There is a male predisposition from 66% to 77%.[3,9] It is generally stated that a family history is present in 30% of cases, although if careful family screening is performed, this proportion increases to 37% to 49%.[9,10]

The course is that of steady decline in most patients, although there may be improvement or leveling off of symptoms with treatment in up to one-third of patients.[21] Echocardiography shows global hypokinesis with decreased ejection fraction and increased end-diastolic volume and diameter.

Arrhythmias and syncope are frequent, necessitating insertion of a defibrillator in about one-third of patients at some time in the course of disease.[3,9] Arrhythmias are typically prominent only after the onset of significant heart failure. However, familial disease, especially those associated with lamin A/C mutations, may present early with ventricular tachyarrhythmias.[22]

Mitral annular dilatation and ventricular dysfunction may result in severe mitral insufficiency that may be treated by annuloplasty or valve replacement, similar to functional mitral insufficiency in ischemic cardiomyopathy (see Chapter 15).[23] Tricuspid valve regurgitation is a frequent result of pulmonary hypertension and is treated by annuloplasty in select patients. In a pathologic series of explants, 6% of hearts had prosthetic mitral valves.[13] Surgical ventricular restoration involving partial resection of akinetic left ventricular segments, particular of the posterior wall, may be performed in conjunction with mitral annuloplasty.[24,25]

Gross Findings

The gross findings of DCM range from mild dilatation and cardiac enlargement (corresponding to minimal DCM, clinically) to a markedly enlarged, dilated heart with a "globoid" appearance (Figs. 156.2 to 156.4). The hallmark gross finding at autopsy four chamber dilatation, most prominently involving the left ventricle, which is >4 cm in

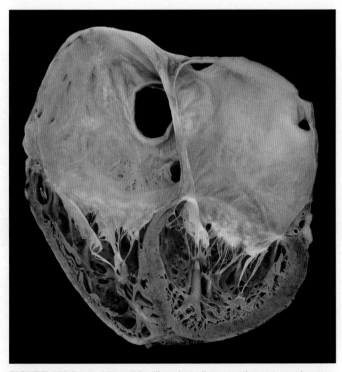

FIGURE 156.2 ▲ Idiopathic dilated cardiomyopathy, autopsy heart. There is marked four-chamber dilatation, shown in this four-chamber dissection.

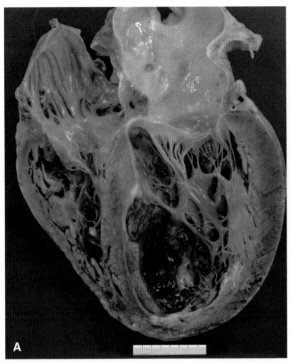
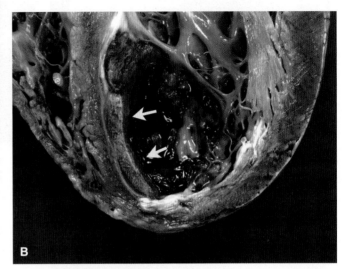

FIGURE 156.3 ▲ Idiopathic dilated cardiomyopathy, autopsy, four-chamber cut. **A.** The heart is viewed from the front (anterior). The right ventricle is at the left. The bar shows 4 cm. The left ventricular cavity, excluding the papillary muscles, is about 5.5 cm in diameter. **B.** A higher magnification shows mural thrombus (*arrows*) and endocardial fibrosis (*white areas*).

diameter (Fig. 156.2). Atrial dilatation may not be apparent in explant specimens, owing to the fact that the atria are left in the recipient for graft anastomosis.

Chamber dimensions should be measured along the short-axis, at the mid-ventricular level (see Chapter 1). The left ventricular wall may be normal (up to 14 to 15 mm) or thickened.[26] Either chamber dimensions or wall thickness alone is relatively meaningless, owing to artifactual dilatation after death or removal of the heart from the body, usually associated with wall thinning. Likewise, in the early postmortem period,

the heart may be in rigor and the wall thicknesses may be artifactually thickened. Therefore, weight is the best indicator of cardiomegaly.

Cardiomegaly is generally considered a requisite for the diagnosis of DCM.[27] Some cases (thought to be <5%) may be subtle and do not meet general criteria for cardiomegaly may be seen, particularly in children and young adults. For these instances, histology and molecular genetic testing may be of utility.[28]

The mean heart weight in a large series of DCM was 615 g (range 360 to 940 g).[29] Hearts weighing more than 700 g can be seen.[26,30] In addition to left ventricular dilatation, right ventricular dilatation results in the typical globular appearance of the heart.

Gross scarring is present in about 25% of cases (Fig. 156.5). The presence of scars has been associated with an increased risk of arrhythmias and sudden death (see below). Prior assist device placement results in decompression of the ventricle, and typical dilated features of cardiomyopathy are masked (Fig. 156.6). Frequently, there is an implanted cardioverter–defibrillator, and if there was cardiac resynchronization therapy, an addition lead will be present in the coronary sinus with the tip in the anterior cardiac vein. If the patient received prior ablations, there may be evidence of radiotherapy-induced scars (Fig. 156.7).

The mitral valve annulus has been described as relatively normal in circumference. Mitral insufficiency may result from displacement of the papillary muscles from their subcommissural location by ventricular remodeling.[27] In contrast, tricuspid regurgitation usually results from frank annular dilatation, owing to the incomplete nature of the right-sided fibrous annulus.[29] In ~5% of patients, there will be evidence of prior valve replacement in the mitral position, mechanical or bioprosthetic (see Chapter 36) (Fig. 156.8). A tricuspid valve ring may be present.

Right-sided mural thrombi are present in approximately one-third of hearts, and left-sided thrombi in nearly one-half (Fig. 156.3). Endocardial fibrous plaques in the ventricles are less common, occurring in about 10% of cases.[26,27] Endocardial plaques are believed to be the result of organized thrombi, unless there is a history of prior ablation. Mild diffuse or patchy endocardial fibrosis, especially toward the ventricular outflow tracts, is frequent and is likely a result of stasis and abnormal hemodynamics in the poorly functioning chamber.

FIGURE 156.4 ▲ Dilated cardiomyopathy, explant. Biventricular dilatation (*left > right*) is seen in the short-axis. The myocardium is uniformly red-brown without obvious scars in this instance.

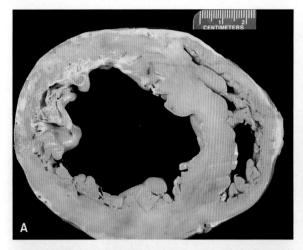

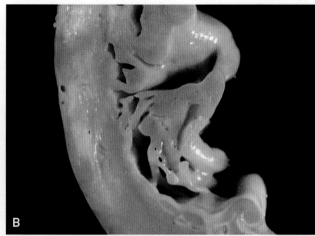

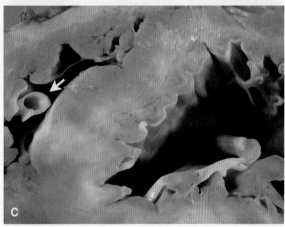

FIGURE 156.5 ▲ Dilated cardiomyopathy, explant, with gross scarring. **A.** A short-axis cut shows marked ventricular dilatation (left ventricular cavity diameter 7 cm), with normal ventricular wall thickness. There is subendocardial scarring in the posterior wall and patchy scarring in the lateral wall. **B.** A higher magnification demonstrates patchy fibrosis in the free wall of the ventricle. **C.** There is patchy fibrosis in the ventricular septum in this example, and note ring of fibrosis at prior pacing lead site (*arrow*). Fibrosis in the septum is more characteristic of hypertrophic cardiomyopathy.

Histologic Findings

The histologic features of DCM are nonspecific. In biopsies, the findings range from minimal variation in myocyte size to typical features of myofiber loss, interstitial fibrosis (usually pericellular type), and marked variation in myofiber size (Figs. 156.9 to 156.11). The important features are negative findings, such as the lack of inflammation/granulomas, iron deposition, or features suggestive of a storage disease. In fact, the role of endomyocardial biopsy in the diagnosis of DCM is primarily to exclude secondary causes.

A series of patients with unexplained heart failure has shown that endomyocardial biopsy may establish a specific diagnosis in ~25% of patients; these were primarily patients with amyloidosis, hemochromatosis, and adriamycin toxicity.[15,31] In addition, Fabry disease, Duchenne cardiomyopathy (dystrophinopathy), and Danon cardiomyopathy may occasionally manifest as a dilated phenotype clinical and have specific ultrastructural features (see Chapter).

Diffuse interstitial replacement-type fibrosis is characteristic of some familiar forms of DCM[32] and is also typical of DCM secondary to end-stage renal disease. Quantitation of collagen has shown up to four times the normal collagen concentration, with a decrease in mature cross-linked collagen, correlating with an increase in neutrophil-type collagenase activity.[33] Increased interstitial collagen is seen in many forms of heart failure (see Chapters 2 and 6).

DCM is characterized by abnormalities of desmin expression by immunohistochemical stains, in almost three-fourths of biopsies. Normally, desmin is visualized only in the intercalated disks and Z-lines. There is increased staining in these areas, often with abnormal aggregates, in about half of biopsies of patients with idiopathic DCM. Abnormal accumulations have been associated with decreased survival.[34]

Ultrastructurally, there are hypertrophied as well as atrophied myocytes, the volume density of myofibrils is reduced, and mitochondrial

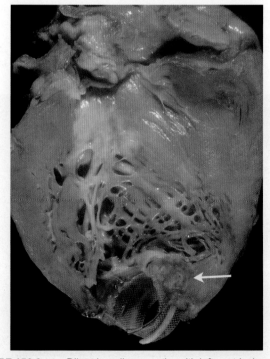

FIGURE 156.6 ▲ Dilated cardiomyopathy with left ventricular assist device, explanted heart. There is hypertrabeculation of the left ventricle toward the apex and mild endocardial fibrosis toward the left ventricular outflow tract. The conduit is present at the apex. There was an area of calcification near the LVAD conduit (*arrow*).

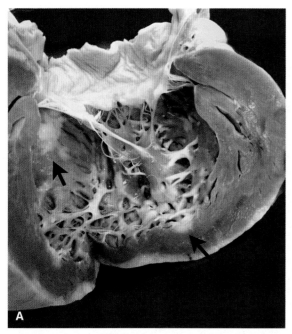
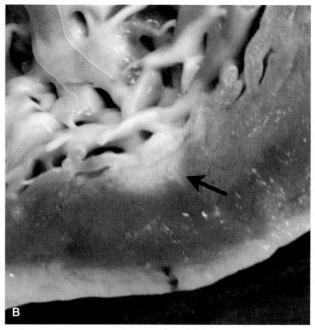

FIGURE 156.7 ▲ Idiopathic dilated cardiomyopathy, explant, with prior evidence of radiofrequency ablation for ventricular tachyarrhythmia. **A.** There is patchy endocardial fibrosis in the left ventricle. One area shows myocardial scar (*arrow*). **B.** A higher magnification demonstrates the site of an ablation. The cardiac electrophysiologist corroborated at explant that the site corresponded to the prior intervention.

density is normal, but the mitochondria are more numerous and small.[35]

In explants, up to 10% of cases of DCM show areas of fibrofatty change, sometimes with associated subepicardial scars typical of arrhythmogenic right ventricular cardiomyopathy.[13] There also may be patchy replacement fibrosis with chronic inflammation suggestive of prior myocarditis[13] (Fig. 156.12).

Treatment and Prognosis

The medical treatment of DCM includes angiotensin-converting enzyme inhibitors, angiotensin receptor blockers, and beta-blockers for heart failure. Cardioverter–defibrillators are implanted in 10% to 20% of patients.[36]

The prognosis for DCM has improved in the past decades, with more aggressive treatments for heart failure and arrhythmias. In the past, there was <50% survival at 10 years. With better supportive care, survival as high as 87% (transplant-free) at 8 years has been reported,[36] although 75% 5-year survival is more typical.[2]

The risk for sudden death is increased when there is a markedly depressed ejection fraction and is lower if there is an implanted defibrillator. There are no good risk stratifiers for predicting sudden death in DCM, however.[3] There is recent evidence that myocardial scarring, when identified by late gadolinium enhancement seen on magnetic resonance imaging, increases the risk for arrhythmias and sudden death.[2,5]

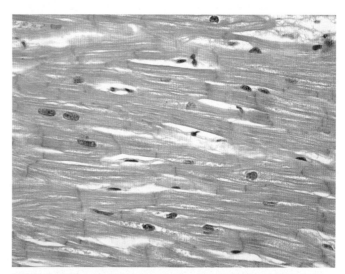

FIGURE 156.8 ▲ St. Jude bileaflet mechanical valve. The left atrium shows a mechanical valve that had been placed for severe mitral insufficiency secondary to heart failure. There is a pacing lead in the coronary sinus (*arrow*).

FIGURE 156.9 ▲ Dilated cardiomyopathy, minimal histologic findings. In this case, there was minimal myocyte enlargement or nuclear changes, and no evidence of interstitial fibrosis. The patient was transplanted for an ejection fraction of <10%. The intercalated discs are well seen in this photograph.

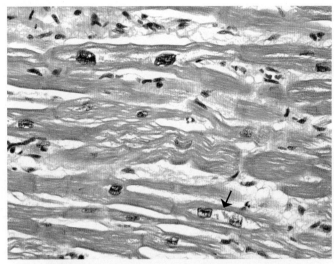

FIGURE 156.10 ▲ Dilated cardiomyopathy, nuclear myocyte variation. There is severalfold variation in length and diameter of myocyte nuclei. There is focal lipofuscin deposition (*arrow*). At the top of the field is an interstitial focus of cellular fibrosis. The findings are nonspecific.

Cardiotoxicity

While heart disease owing to exposure to toxic (either endogenous or exogenous) substances is occasionally referred to as "toxic cardiomyopathy," the authors prefer the term cardiotoxicity to help underscore the etiology in the diagnosis. Etiologic modifiers in the "MOGES" system of cardiomyopathy classification include pheochromocytoma-related cardiomyopathy, alcoholic cardiotoxicity, and drug-induced cardiomyopathy (e.g., chloroquine induced).[37]

Drugs of Abuse

Cardiotoxicity, often reversible, has been associated with drugs in the sympathomimetic amine class. The mechanism of myocyte injury may be related to catecholamine toxicity. Drug-induced cardiomyopathy has been reported with abuse of "ecstasy" (3,4-methylenedioxy-*N*-methylamphetamine), crystal methamphetamine, solvents, ipecac for weight loss, and cocaine. Cocaine abuse is reported in as high as 2% of patients with DCM.[38] There are no specific histologic alterations

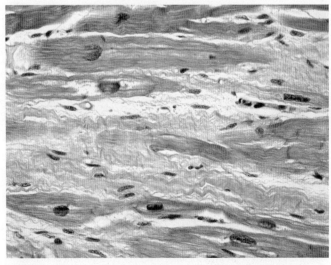

FIGURE 156.11 ▲ Dilated cardiomyopathy, interstitial fibrosis. In addition to myocyte hypertrophy and variation in myofiber size, there is interstitial fibrosis, seen as wavy collagen bundles.

associated with cocaine-related cardiomyopathy, although a small proportion of autopsies show patchy myocarditis.[39] Acute cocaine intoxication can result in multifocal contraction band necrosis.

Ethanol

Prolonged ingestion of large quantities of alcohol increases the risk of cardiotoxicity. Ethanol intake of >80 g/day (eight drinks) over a period of at least 5 years is an accepted criterion for ethanol-associated cardiotoxicity. Using this criterion, 10% to 40% of cases of DCM occur in alcoholics.[40] Ethanol-associated ("alcoholic") cardiomyopathy is not a specific pathologic term, as the distinction is entirely clinical and based on accuracy of patient history.

Ethanol-associated cardiotoxicity has been reported to have a prognosis than idiopathic DCM, with a higher rate of recovery or disease stabilization. There did not appear to be a difference in survival among patients who abstained versus those who decreased alcohol intake after diagnosis, however.[40]

The pathologic findings are nonspecific and indistinguishable from idiopathic DCM.[41] As in other forms of heart failure, mitochondrial DNA mutations have been identified. It is likely that certain genetic variations act synergistically with environmental factors (such as ethanol) to result in cardiotoxicity.

Anthracyclines and Chemotherapeutic Drugs (see Chapter 3)

Anthracyclines

Cardiac damage, usually in the form of a dilated or restrictive cardiomyopathy, occurs as a dose-related effect in patients receiving anthracycline drugs doxorubicin and daunorubicin. It represents ~1% of patients with DCM referred for tertiary care.[42] A lifetime limited cumulative dose of 450 to 550 mg/m² for conventional doxorubicin has been recommended, as cardiotoxicity is frequent above this level. Endomyocardial biopsy is considered to be the most sensitive and specific test for anthracycline cardiotoxicity. The entire specimen should be submitted for plastic embedding, and 10 blocks reviewed for ultrastructural study. The most obvious changes of anthracycline toxicity include distended sarcotubular reticulum in the form of vacuoles and myofibrillar loss. A three-point grading system has been devised by Billingham, which guides the clinician regarding the safety of further therapy.[41]

Mitoxantrone

Mitoxantrone is an anthracenedione drug that is structurally related to anthracyclines. It is used as a solid tumor chemotherapeutic agent as well as a treatment for multiple sclerosis. Endomyocardial biopsies have shown dilatation of the sarcoplasmic reticulum with vacuole formation, similar to the early changes of anthracycline cardiomyopathy. Clinical trials show that cardiotoxicity occurs in 2% of patients.[43]

Chloroquine

Chloroquine is a drug used to treat malaria and connective tissue diseases, particularly (e.g., systemic lupus erythematosus). It and related drugs induce a lysosomal dysfunction with an accumulation of inclusions in the cytoplasm by ultrastructural evaluation. Cardiac side effects are rarely reported and include third-degree atrioventricular block, which may require a permanent pacemaker, and cardiomyopathy that may have a dilated, restrictive, or hypertrophic phenotype.[44,45] Light microscopic findings are nonspecific and show vacuolar degeneration of myocytes that appears similar to changes of Fabry disease. Curvilinear bodies on electron microscopy are suggestive of chloroquine cardiotoxicity.[46]

Cobalt Cardiomyopathy

Cobalt cardiomyopathy was reported primarily in the last century when cobalt was used to stabilize the head on beer. It rarely occurs with exposure to cobalt from metal-on-metal joint prostheses, and presents as

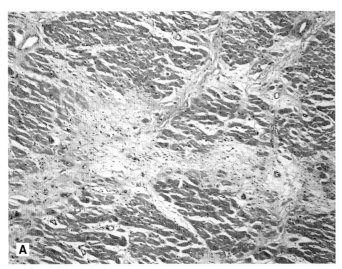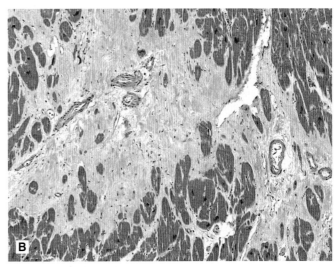

FIGURE 156.12 ▲ Dilated cardiomyopathy, pattern of healed myocarditis. **A.** This explant demonstrates patchy replacement fibrosis with chronic inflammation. **B.** A different area demonstrates a large area of replacement fibrosis.

congestive heart failure.[47] The diagnosis is suggested by history and increased serum levels of cobalt, as the histologic and ultrastructural changes are nonspecific.[48] Myofibrillar loss and myocyte atrophy without fibrosis have been described[49] as well as significant myocardial fibrosis.[47] Inflammation has not been reported.

Myocarditis-Associated Cardiomyopathy

About 15% of cases of dilated are considered to be postmyocarditis, based on identification of viral genome, as well as histopathologic patterns of myocardial injury (Fig. 156.12). Nonviral inflammation caused by sarcoidosis or autoimmune diseases, especially lupus and scleroderma, may also underlie DCM. Familial studies have shown that DCM attributed to prior myocarditis may also be associated with familial and genetic abnormalities.[4]

In the "MOGES" clinical classification system of cardiomyopathy, a notation of "m" for "myocarditis" is placed in the etiology ("E") descriptor.[4] Clinically, a prior episode of myocarditis, which can predate the onset of heart failure by months or years, is based on serologic, electrocardiographic, and imaging criteria. Myocarditis that presents as heart failure (fulminant myocarditis) may progress to cardiomyopathy (see Chapter 26).

There are no standardized criteria for the histologic diagnosis of healed myocarditis, as areas of fibrosis are relatively common in DCM without a clinical history of myocarditis. Importantly, the quality of fibrosis in myocarditis is slightly different than in other forms of DCM, manifesting as subepicardial replacement-type scarring rather than the diffuse pericellular-type fibrosis seen in the latter (Fig. 156.12). In a study of explants with DCM, 3 of 55 (5%) showed features of healed myocarditis.[13]

Human Immunodeficiency Virus–Associated Cardiomyopathy

Left ventricular dysfunction is found in 27% of patients with acquired immunodeficiency syndrome (AIDS), and <3% of human immunodeficiency virus (HIV)-infected individuals with normal T-cell counts.[50] An 8% overall rate of DCM was reported in an early series of HIV-infected individuals, prior to highly active antiretroviral therapy (HAART), with a higher rate in immunocompromised patients.[51] Myocardial involvement in HIV infection is multifactorial and has been variously attributed to viral, drug-related, nutritional, and autoimmune causes.[52] The histologic findings are nonspecific, but inflammatory infiltrates (myocarditis on endomyocardial biopsy) are seen

in 21% to 60% of cases, suggesting an inflammatory etiology in most cases of HIV cardiomyopathy.[51,53] HAART therapy has dramatically decreased the incidence of cardiomyopathy in HIV disease, especially in children.[54]

Miscellaneous Secondary Cardiomyopathies That May Have Dilated Phenotype

Tachycardia-Induced and Premature Ventricular Contraction–Induced Cardiomyopathy

An underrecognized and at least partially reversible form of secondary DCM with decreased left ventricular function occurs secondary to prolonged periods of tachycardia, including junctional tachycardia, atrial tachycardia, ventricular tachycardia, and atrial fibrillation with rapid ventricular response. The diagnosis is usually made retrospectively after marked improvement in systolic function is noted following control of the heart rate. Radiofrequency ablation is frequently useful in decreasing episodes of tachycardia and normalizing ventricular function.[55] There are no specific pathologic findings, which include interstitial fibrosis and myocyte hypertrophy.[56]

Premature ventricular contraction–associated cardiomyopathy, originally considered a form of tachycardia-induced cardiomyopathy, is characterized by numerous premature ventricular contractions, decreased left ventricular ejection fraction, increased left ventricular systolic and diastolic dimensions, and global wall motion abnormalities.[57] The link between the PVCs, which are common in the general population, and DCM is based on observations that radiofrequency catheter ablation of the right ventricular outflow tract improves left ventricular dilatation by suppressing arrhythmias.[58] There are no specific histologic findings in premature ventricular contraction–induced cardiomyopathy.

Peripartum Cardiomyopathy

Peripartum cardiomyopathy presents as left ventricular dysfunction and heart failure in the third trimester of pregnancy or the first 5 months postpartum. By definition, there is no underlying structural heart disease; in other words, there is not concomitant valvular, hypertensive, or ischemic forms of heart disease present.[59]

Peripartum cardiomyopathy occurs in 0.3% to 1% of pregnancies in developing countries, compared to rates one-tenth that in developed countries such as the United States.[59] In California, the pregnancy-related mortality rate from cardiomyopathy is 0.015%.[60] Risk factors include obesity, multiparity, preeclampsia, black race, twin gestation, and age over 30 years.[60]

There is an overlap between peripartum and familial cardiomyopathy. Mutations in cardiac troponin C (TNNC1), titin, *BAG3*, myosin heavy chain, SCN5A, and other cardiac myocyte genes have been identified in families with idiopathic and peripartum cardiomyopathy.[61] Approximately 5% of heart transplants in patients with idiopathic cardiomyopathy have their onset during pregnancy. There is debate about the role of myocarditis in the pathogenesis of peripartum cardiomyopathy. There are few autopsy studies of fatal cases, which have shown nonspecific findings consistent with DCM.[62] The rate of inflammation in endomyocardial biopsies is variable in reported studies.[59]

There are no specific pathologic findings in peripartum cardiomyopathy; indeed, autopsy findings may be relatively minimal or show nonspecific features of DCM. A low rate of borderline myocarditis has been described on endomyocardial biopsy as well as viral genomic material.[63]

About one-half of patients have complete or nearly complete recovery within 6 months. However, the remainder have a clinical course similar to idiopathic DCM characterized by progressive clinical deterioration, only one-quarter have complete normalization of the ejection fraction, and subsequent pregnancies carry a very high risk of mortality. A follow-up study reported a 7-year fatality rate of 16.5% with Black non-Hispanic women experiencing an almost fourfold increased fatality compared to Caucasian women.[64]

Cardiomyopathy Related to Deficiencies

The cardiac manifestations of severe malnutrition include autonomic dysfunction, long QT interval, valvular dysfunction, congestive heart failure, and sudden death. Reduced left ventricular mass may impair myocardial performance and result in congestive heart failure.[65] Echocardiographic studies of women with anorexia have shown abnormalities of mitral valve motion, ventricular function, and ventricular size. Pathologically, heart weight may be decreased, myocytes are diminished in diameter with increased lipofuscin, and the epicardial fat undergoes brown fat change.

More recently, there has been an association between Takotsubo cardiomyopathy (stress cardiomyopathy) and anorexia, as severe malnutrition may result in elevated serum catecholamines (Chapter 24).[66,67] Patients with eating disorder may suffer from *magnesium deficiency* and secondary cardiomyopathy after repeated ingestion of ipecac.[68]

Severe malnutrition states such as beriberi (thiamine deficiency), pellagra (niacin deficiency), scurvy, and kwashiorkor are associated decreased ventricular function and cardiomyopathy.[69] A peculiar form of cardiomyopathy with some features of DCM is termed *Keshan disease*. It results from selenium deficiency and is endemic in some regions of China and Africa. It is currently considered a form of secondary mitochondrial cardiomyopathy, characterized by enlarged and swollen mitochondria with distended crista membranes, resulting from oxidative stress.[70] The histopathologic feature is that of *multifocal myocardial necrosis* with fibrosis, which is present in the mid left ventricle and, to a lesser extent, the right ventricle and the atria. These necrotic lesions are not accompanied by an inflammatory reaction.[71]

Radiation-Induced Cardiomyopathy

Radiation to the mediastinum can cause myriad forms of cardiovascular disease. The most common effect pericardial disease, although accelerated coronary artery disease is an important late effect, especially in patients treated with radiation before the age of 21 years. Cardiomyopathy is rare and is characterized by patchy fibrosis.[72]

REFERENCES

1. Kadish AH, Rubenstein JC. Connecting the dots: the relevance of scar in nonischemic cardiomyopathy. *J Am Coll Cardiol.* 2009;53:1146–1147.
2. Gulati A, Jabbour A, Ismail TF, et al. Association of fibrosis with mortality and sudden cardiac death in patients with nonischemic dilated cardiomyopathy. *JAMA.* 2013;309:896–908.
3. Goldberger JJ, Subacius H, Patel T, et al. Sudden cardiac death risk stratification in patients with nonischemic dilated cardiomyopathy. *J Am Coll Cardiol.* 2014;63:1879–1889.
4. Arbustini E, Narula N, Tavazzi L, et al. The MOGE(S) classification of cardiomyopathy for clinicians. *J Am Coll Cardiol.* 2014;64:304–318.
5. Perazzolo Marra M, De Lazzari M, Zorzi A, et al. Impact of the presence and amount of myocardial fibrosis by cardiac magnetic resonance on arrhythmic outcome and sudden cardiac death in nonischemic dilated cardiomyopathy. *Heart Rhythm.* 2014;11:856–863.
6. Maron BJ, Towbin JA, Thiene G, et al. Contemporary definitions and classification of the cardiomyopathies: an American Heart Association Scientific Statement from the Council on Clinical Cardiology, Heart Failure and Transplantation Committee; Quality of Care and Outcomes Research and Functional Genomics and Translational Biology Interdisciplinary Working Groups; and Council on Epidemiology and Prevention. *Circulation.* 2006;113:1807–1816.
7. Elliott P, Andersson B, Arbustini E, et al. Classification of the cardiomyopathies: a position statement from the European Society Of Cardiology Working Group on Myocardial and Pericardial Diseases. *Eur Heart J.* 2008;29:270–276.
8. Kaski JP, Elliott P. The classification concept of the ESC Working Group on myocardial and pericardial diseases for dilated cardiomyopathy. *Herz.* 2007;32:446–451.
9. Haas J, Frese KS, Peil B, et al. Atlas of the clinical genetics of human dilated cardiomyopathy. *Eur Heart J.* 2015;36:1123–1135.
10. Pugh TJ, Kelly MA, Gowrisankar S, et al. The landscape of genetic variation in dilated cardiomyopathy as surveyed by clinical DNA sequencing. *Genet Med.* 2014;16:601–608.
11. Hazebroek MR, Moors S, Dennert R, et al. Prognostic relevance of gene-environment interactions in patients with dilated cardiomyopathy: applying the MOGE(S) classification. *J Am Coll Cardiol.* 2015;66:1313–1323.
12. Kitzman DW, Scholz DG, Hagen PT, et al. Age-related changes in normal human hearts during the first 10 decades of life. Part II (Maturity): A quantitative anatomic study of 765 specimens from subjects 20 to 99 years old. *Mayo Clin Proc.* 1988;63:137–146.
13. Zhang M, Tavora F, Huebner T, et al. Allograft pathology in patients transplanted for idiopathic dilated cardiomyopathy. *Am J Surg Pathol.* 2012;36:389–395.
14. Morimoto S. Sarcomeric proteins and inherited cardiomyopathies. *Cardiovasc Res.* 2008;77:659–666.
15. Ardehali H, Qasim A, Cappola T, et al. Endomyocardial biopsy plays a role in diagnosing patients with unexplained cardiomyopathy. *Am Heart J.* 2004;147:919–923.
16. Rakar S, Sinagra G, Di Lenarda A, et al. Epidemiology of dilated cardiomyopathy. A prospective post-mortem study of 5252 necropsies. The Heart Muscle Disease Study Group. *Eur Heart J.* 1997;18:117–123.
17. McNally EM, Golbus JR, Puckelwartz MJ. Genetic mutations and mechanisms in dilated cardiomyopathy. *J Clin Invest.* 2013;123:19–26.
18. Kimura A. Molecular genetics and pathogenesis of cardiomyopathy. *J Hum Genet.*
19. Chami N, Tadros R, Lemarbre F, et al. Nonsense mutations in BAG3 are associated with early-onset dilated cardiomyopathy in French Canadians. *Can J Cardiol.* 2014;30:1655–1661.
20. Cheng Z, Cui Q, Tian Z, et al. Danon disease as a cause of concentric left ventricular hypertrophy in patients who underwent endomyocardial biopsy. *Eur Heart J.* 2012;33:649–656.
21. Park JS, Kim JW, Seo KW, et al. Recurrence of left ventricular dysfunction in patients with restored idiopathic dilated cardiomyopathy. *Clin Cardiol.* 2014;37:222–226.
22. Nguyen TP, Wang DW, Rhodes TH, et al. Divergent biophysical defects caused by mutant sodium channels in dilated cardiomyopathy with arrhythmia. *Circ Res.* 2008;102:364–371.
23. De Bonis M, Ferrara D, Taramasso M, et al. Mitral replacement or repair for functional mitral regurgitation in dilated and ischemic cardiomyopathy: is it really the same? *Ann Thorac Surg.* 2012;94:44–51.

24. Isomura T, Hirota M, Notomi Y, et al. Posterior restoration procedures and the long-term results in indicated patients with dilated cardiomyopathy dagger. *Interact Cardiovasc Thorac Surg.* 2015;20:725–731.

25. Shudo Y, Taniguchi K, Takeda K, et al. Restrictive mitral annuloplasty with or without surgical ventricular restoration in ischemic dilated cardiomyopathy with severe mitral regurgitation. *Circulation.* 2011;124:S107–S114.

26. Edwards WD. Cardiomyopathies. *Hum Pathol.* 1987;18:625–635.

27. Roberts WC, Ferrans VJ. Pathologic anatomy of the cardiomyopathies. Idiopathic dilated and hypertrophic types, infiltrative types, and endomyocardial disease with and without eosinophilia. *Hum Pathol.* 1975;6:287–342.

28. Keren A, Billingham ME, Weintraub D, et al. Mildly dilated congestive cardiomyopathy. *Circulation.* 1985;72:302–309.

29. Roberts WC, Siegel RJ, McManus BM. Idiopathic dilated cardiomyopathy: analysis of 152 necropsy patients. *Am J Cardiol.* 1987;60:1340–1355.

30. Rose AG, Beck W. Dilated (congestive) cardiomyopathy: a syndrome of severe cardiac dysfunction with remarkably few morphological features of myocardial damage. *Histopathology.* 1985;9:367–379.

31. Felker GM, Thompson RE, Hare JM, et al. Underlying causes and long-term survival in patients with initially unexplained cardiomyopathy. *N Engl J Med.* 2000;342:1077–1084.

32. Ellinor PT, Sasse-Klaassen S, Probst S, et al. A novel locus for dilated cardiomyopathy, diffuse myocardial fibrosis, and sudden death on chromosome 10q25-26. *J Am Coll Cardiol.* 2006;48:106–111.

33. Gunja-Smith Z, Morales AR, Romanelli R, et al. Remodeling of human myocardial collagen in idiopathic dilated cardiomyopathy. Role of metalloproteinases and pyridinoline cross-links. *Am J Pathol.* 1996;148:1639–1648.

34. Pawlak A, Gil RJ, Grajkowska W, et al. Significance of low desmin expression in cardiomyocytes in patients with idiopathic dilated cardiomyopathy. *Am J Cardiol.* 2013;111:393–399.

35. Kostin S, Hein S, Arnon E, et al. The cytoskeleton and related proteins in the human failing heart. *Heart Fail Rev.* 2000;5:271–280.

36. Merlo M, Pivetta A, Pinamonti B, et al. Long-term prognostic impact of therapeutic strategies in patients with idiopathic dilated cardiomyopathy: changing mortality over the last 30 years. *Eur J Heart Fail.* 2014;16:317–324.

37. Arbustini E, Narula N, Dec GW, et al. The MOGE(S) classification for a phenotype-genotype nomenclature of cardiomyopathy: endorsed by the World Heart Federation. *J Am Coll Cardiol.* 2013;62:2046–2072.

38. Frustaci A, Russo MA, Morgante E, et al. Oxidative myocardial damage in human cocaine-related cardiomyopathy. *Eur J Heart Fail.* 2015;17:283–290.

39. Virmani R, Robinowitz M, Smialek JE, et al. Cardiovascular effects of cocaine: an autopsy study of 40 patients. *Am Heart J.* 1988;115:1068–1076.

40. Guzzo-Merello G, Segovia J, Dominguez F, et al. Natural history and prognostic factors in alcoholic cardiomyopathy. *JACC Heart Fail.* 2015;3:78–86.

41. Piano MR. Alcoholic cardiomyopathy: incidence, clinical characteristics, and pathophysiology. *Chest.* 2002;121:1638–1650.

42. Felker GM, Hu W, Hare JM, et al. The spectrum of dilated cardiomyopathy. The Johns Hopkins experience with 1,278 patients. *Medicine (Baltimore).* 1999;78:270–283.

43. Mulroy E, Joyce E, Scott J, et al. Long-term risk of leukaemia or cardiomyopathy after mitoxantrone therapy for multiple sclerosis. *Eur Neurol.* 2012;67:45–47.

44. Tonnesmann E, Kandolf R, Lewalter T. Chloroquine cardiomyopathy—a review of the literature. *Immunopharmacol Immunotoxicol.* 2013;35:434–442.

45. Tonnesmann E, Stroehmann I, Kandolf R, et al. Cardiomyopathy caused by longterm treatment with chloroquine: a rare disease, or a rare diagnosis? *J Rheumatol.* 2012;39:1099–1103.

46. Lopez-Ruiz N, Uribe CE. Chloroquine cardiomyopathy: beyond ocular adverse effects. *BMJ Case Rep.* 2014;2014.

47. Khan AH, Verma R, Bajpai A, et al. Unusual case of congestive heart failure: cardiac magnetic resonance imaging and histopathologic findings in cobalt cardiomyopathy. *Circ Cardiovasc Imaging.* 2015;8.

48. Allen LA, Ambardekar AV, Devaraj KM, et al. Clinical problem-solving. Missing elements of the history. *N Engl J Med.* 2014;370:559–566.

49. Centeno JA, Pestaner JP, Mullick FG, et al. An analytical comparison of cobalt cardiomyopathy and idiopathic dilated cardiomyopathy. *Biol Trace Elem Res.* 1996;55:21–30.

50. El Hattaoui M, Charei N, Boumzebra D, et al. [Prevalence of cardiomyopathy in HIV infection: prospective study on 158 HIV patients]. *Med Mal Infect.* 2008;38:387–391.

51. Barbaro G, Di Lorenzo G, Grisorio B, et al. Incidence of dilated cardiomyopathy and detection of HIV in myocardial cells of HIV-positive patients. Gruppo Italiano per lo Studio Cardiologico dei Pazienti Affetti da AIDS. *N Engl J Med.* 1998;339:1093–1099.

52. Frustaci A, Petrosillo N, Francone M, et al. Biopsy-proven autoimmune myocarditis in HIV-associated dilated cardiomyopathy. *BMC Infect Dis.* 2014;14:3855.

53. Shaboodien G, Maske C, Wainwright H, et al. Prevalence of myocarditis and cardiotropic virus infection in Africans with HIV-associated cardiomyopathy, idiopathic dilated cardiomyopathy and heart transplant recipients: a pilot study: cardiovascular topic. *Cardiovasc J Afr.* 2013;24:218–223.

54. Patel K, Van Dyke RB, Mittleman MA, et al. The impact of HAART on cardiomyopathy among children and adolescents perinatally infected with HIV-1. *AIDS.* 2012;26:2027–2037.

55. Aykan HH, Karagoz T, Akin A, et al. Results of radiofrequency ablation in children with tachycardia-induced cardiomyopathy. *Anadolu Kardiyol Derg.* 2014;14:625–630.

56. Gerloni R, Abate E, Pinamonti B, et al. A life-threatening manifestation of tachycardia-induced cardiomyopathy. *J Cardiovasc Med (Hagerstown).* 2014;15:164–166.

57. Lee GK, Klarich KW, Grogan M, et al. Premature ventricular contraction-induced cardiomyopathy: a treatable condition. *Circ Arrhythm Electrophysiol.* 2012;5:229–236.

58. Taieb JM, Maury P, Shah D, et al. Reversal of dilated cardiomyopathy by the elimination of frequent left or right premature ventricular contractions. *J Interv Card Electrophysiol.* 2007;20:9–13.

59. Bhattacharyya A, Basra SS, Sen P, et al. Peripartum cardiomyopathy: a review. *Tex Heart Inst J.* 2012;39:8–16.

60. Hameed AB, Lawton ES, McCain CL, et al. Pregnancy-related cardiovascular deaths in California: beyond peripartum cardiomyopathy. *Am J Obstet Gynecol.* 2015.

61. van Spaendonck-Zwarts KY, Posafalvi A, van den Berg MP, et al. Titin gene mutations are common in families with both peripartum cardiomyopathy and dilated cardiomyopathy. *Eur Heart J.* 2014;35:2165–2173.

62. Aroney C, Khafagi F, Boyle C, et al. Peripartum cardiomyopathy: echocardiographic features in five cases. *Am J Obstet Gynecol.* 1986;155:103–106.

63. Lamparter S, Pankuweit S, Maisch B. Clinical and immunologic characteristics in peripartum cardiomyopathy. *Int J Cardiol.* 2007;118:14–20.

64. Harper MA, Meyer RE, Berg CJ. Peripartum cardiomyopathy: population-based birth prevalence and 7-year mortality. *Obstet Gynecol.* 2012;120:1013–1019.

65. Birmingham CL, Gritzner S. Heart failure in anorexia nervosa: case report and review of the literature. *Eat Weight Disord.* 2007;12:e7–e10.

66. Volman MN, Ten Kate RW, Tukkie R. Tako Tsubo cardiomyopathy, presenting with cardiogenic shock in a 24-year-old patient with anorexia nervosa. *Neth J Med.* 2011;69:129–131.

67. Kim KH, Youn HJ, Lee WH, et al. A case of anorexia nervosa complicated with strongly suspected stress-induced cardiomyopathy and mural thrombus. *Korean Circ J.* 2011;41:615–617.

68. Kurnik BR, Marshall J, Katz SM. Hypomagnesemia-induced cardiomyopathy. *Magnesium.* 1988;7:49–53.

69. Tejedor A, Sole M, Prieto-Gonzalez S, et al. Acute dilated cardiomyopathy in a patient with beriberi and cryoglobulinaemic vasculitis: an unusual potential complication of two rare disorders. *Clin Exp Rheumatol.* 2014;32:S66–S69.

70. Pei J, Fu W, Yang L, et al. Oxidative stress is involved in the pathogenesis of Keshan disease (an endemic dilated cardiomyopathy) in China. *Oxid Med Cell Longev.* 2013;2013:474203.

71. Li GS, Wang F, Kang D, et al. Keshan disease: an endemic cardiomyopathy in China. *Hum Pathol.* 1985;16:602–609.

72. Wyman RA, Rahko PS. Patchy myocardial fibrosis 20 years after radiation therapy. *Echocardiography.* 2007;24:68–70.

Hypertrophic Cardiomyopathy

Allen P. Burke, M.D., Fabio R. Tavora, M.D., Ph.D., and Joseph J. Maleszewski, M.D.

General Considerations

Hypertrophic cardiomyopathy (HCM) is a heart muscle disease that results in cardiac hypertrophy and oftentimes left ventricular outflow tract (LVOT) obstruction. Both the structural and hemodynamic alterations impart risk of arrhythmia, heart failure, and sudden death in those affected. In >50% of patients, causative mutations in genes that encode proteins related to the structure and function of the sarcomere are found.

HCM is characterized by ventricular hypertrophy in the absence of ventricular dilatation in initial stages. The hypertrophy often shows a predilection for the ventricular septum at the base of the heart, resulting in asymmetric (nonconcentric) thickening, though midventricular, apical, and diffuse (neutral) forms can also be seen. Concentric hypertrophy can also occur.[1]

The septal hypertrophy results in LVOT obstruction, previously called "idiopathic hypertrophic subaortic stenosis" and currently designated "hypertrophic obstructive cardiomyopathy" (HOCM). Obstruction to LVOT is caused, in part, by bulging of the thickened septum. This altered LVOT geometry causes abnormal drag forces to be applied to the anterior mitral leaflet (posterior portion of the LVOT) and causes it to move anteriorly, which can further obstruct blood from ejection into the aorta. The designation HCM should be used for all morphologic variants, however, as the pathogenesis and genetics are similar.

HCM is most often inherited in an autosomal dominant fashion with variable and commonly incomplete penetrance. Symptoms and presentation vary substantially between cohorts and can range from in utero presentation to late adulthood.[2,3] Because patients often present initially as sudden death, typically during exertion, HCM is one of the best known cardiomyopathies.

Epidemiology

Defined by echocardiographic measurements, HCM affects about 1:500 of the general population.[4] With molecular genetic screening, some believe the rate may be higher, although most data show a similar rate to that seen with imaging.[5,6] Relatives of probands have some morphologic evidence of the disease in up to 25% of cases. HCM most commonly presents in the second or third decade of life but may present at any age. It is the most common identified substrate for sudden unexpected death among young athletes, although it is significantly more common to find nothing at all by conventional autopsy.[7] The incidence is low, however, in screening studies of competitive athletes.[8]

Clinical Features and Diagnosis

HCM is diagnosed in three groups of patients. First are patients who present with symptoms that are nonspecific and include dyspnea, especially during exercise; chest pain; palpitations; dizziness; and syncope. This first group is commonly young in the 2nd to 4th decades of life, and the diagnosis is confirmed by echocardiography and other imaging techniques.[9,10] The second and largest group is composed of either relatives of patients with the disease or patients who are found to have HCM incidentally. These patients are either asymptomatic or minimally symptomatic. The third group consists primarily of those who die suddenly without a prior history. In this group, the pathologist has a key role in establishing the diagnosis and establishing a basis for genetic counseling for family members.

Echocardiography

HCM is diagnosed by unexplained left ventricular hypertrophy, small left ventricular cavity size, and increased or normal left ventricular systolic function. Left ventricular hypertrophy may be either nonconcentric or concentric, with the former being more specific for the diagnosis than the latter. On echocardiography, a left ventricular thickness of more than 15 mm is suspicious for the disease. Tissue Doppler imaging has been recently applied to obtain an early diagnosis of HCM, making echocardiography, including Doppler evaluation, the most commonly used diagnostic technique.[11]

There are several conditions that may mimic the imaging features, especially amyloidosis and Fabry disease. Over 5% of patients over 40 years referred for the treatment of HCM are found to actually suffer from Fabry disease after serum levels of serum alpha-galactosidase are measured.[12,13] Additionally, the preferential deposition of amyloid in the basal ventricular septum can mimic the asymmetric hypertrophy seen in HCM.

Cardiac Magnetic Resonance Imaging

Cardiac magnetic resonance imaging is useful both diagnostically and prognostically in the assessment of patients with suspected HCM.[14] The presence of myocardial scar detected by late gadolinium enhancement (LGE) on cardiac magnetic resonance (CMR) imaging has been described as a good independent predictor of mortality and the risk of sustained ventricular tachycardia in patients with HCM.[15,16]

Arrhythmias in HCM

The prognosis of HCM is based primarily on the propensity for ventricular tachyarrhythmias and secondarily based on the development of late heart failure. A history of syncope is associated with a higher incidence of sudden death, and patients with a significant LVOT obstruction are more susceptible to clinical deterioration.[17,18] Risk stratification to evaluate the need for implantable defibrillation is based on clinical and electrocardiographic features.[19] The degree of ventricular hypertrophy or outflow obstruction is not particularly helpful, as certain genotypes (e.g., troponin mutations) are associated with arrhythmias in the absence of marked cardiomegaly.

Atrial fibrillation occurs in up to 20% of patients with HCM and is associated with older age, symptomatic disease, and decreased overall survival, but not sudden death. Radiofrequency ablation for atrial fibrillation may be effective in some patients.[20,21]

Genetics

More than half of patients with HCM have a family history of the disease, and the pattern of inheritance is usually autosomal dominant. In 1990, a seminal work led to the identification of a causal gene and mutation for HCM, a missense mutation in the cardiac β-myosin heavy chain gene (*MYH7*).[22]

Since then, multiple genes have been identified in HCM patients. Dominant pathogenic variants in HCM genes include sarcomeric genes that involve thick filaments (myosin-binding protein C [*MYBPC3*], β-myosin heavy chain [*MYH7*], and myosin light chains 2 and 3 [*MYL2* and *MYL3*]) and thin filaments (actinin1 [*ACTC1*], cardiac troponin I type 3 [*TNNI3*], cardiac troponin T type 2 [*TNNT2*], and tropomyosin-1 [*TPM1*]) (Table 157.1; Fig. 157.1). Additional genes, including *ACTN2*,

TABLE 157.1 Prevalence of Mutations in Hypertrophic Cardiomyopathy and Their Respective Clinical Characteristics

Gene	Characteristics	Frequency
Myosin-binding protein C (*MYBPC3*)	Incomplete and late penetrance, relatively benign course	~45%
β-Myosin heavy chain (*MYH7*) [α-myosin heavy chain (*MYH6*)][a]	High penetrance and severe hypertrophy	~30%
Troponin I type 3 (cardiac) (*TNNI3*)	Heterogeneous phenotypes, associated with apical hypertrophy	3%–5%
Troponin T type 2 (cardiac) (*TNNT2*)	Low penetrance and mild hypertrophy, but association with early sudden death (20% of families)[35] Normal echos and ECGs in most children	3%–5%
α-Actin cardiac muscle 1 (*ACTC1*)	Less hypertrophy, slight increased risk of arrhythmias (similar to other thin filament mutations)	<5%
α2-Actinin (*ACTN2*)	AV block, AFib, restrictive parameters[49]; heterogeneous[50]	<5%
Myosin, light chain 2, regulatory (*MYL2*)	Variable[51]	<5%
Myosin, light chain 3, alkali (*MYL3*)	Variable[51]	<5%
Tropomyosin-1 (α) (*TPM1*)	Variation in phenotypes, variable prognosis	<5%
Multiple genes (e.g., *MYBPC3* + *TNNI3*, compound *MYBPC3*)	Early age, adverse outcome[52]	5%

Additional genes, including *ACTN2, CSRP3, MYOZ2, NEXN, PLN, TNNC1,* and *TTN,* have been implicated but not definitively proven as causing disease. Pathogenic variants in other genes (*GLA*/Fabry disease, *LAMP2*/Danon cardiomyopathy, and *PRKAG2*/glycogenosis) also cause left ventricular hypertrophy but result in metabolic disorders distinct in their origin from HCM.[23]
[a]*MYH6* and *MYH7* are isoforms of the myosin heavy chain, the latter primarily expressed in the myocardium. There is a high degree of homology between them, so most studies do not test for MYH6 separately. Recently, a high rate of MYH6-specific mutations confirmed by sequencing was found in a series of HCM.[10]

CSRP3, MYOZ2, NEXN, PLN, TNNC1, and *TTN,* have been implicated but not definitively proven as causing HCM.

Other gene mutations in *GLA, LAMP2,* and *PRKAG2* cause left ventricular hypertrophy that may mimic HCM but are distinct disorders (Fabry disease, Danon cardiomyopathy, and *PRKAG2*-associated cardiomyopathy, respectively, the latter generally classified as a glycogenosis) (see Chapter 23).[23] Noonan syndrome, associated with mutations in a number of genes, *PTPN11, SOS1,* and *RAF1* being the most common, is also usually associated with cardiomegaly that mimics HCM. Importantly, these should NOT be considered HCM but rather heart disease associated with those conditions.

The detection rate of causative mutations in unselected probands with HCM varies, depending on the method used and definition of causation. The rate ranges from 32%[23] to 46%[24] and 64%.[10]

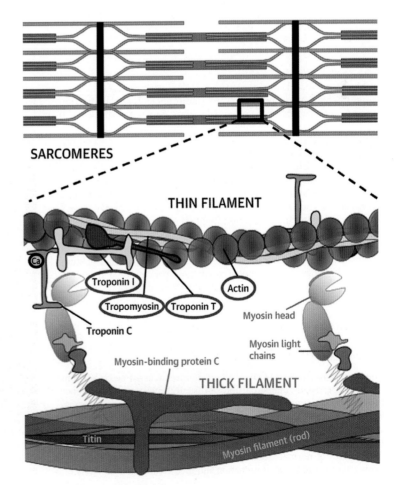

FIGURE 157.1 ▲ Genes associated with the pathogenesis of hypertrophic cardiomyopathy (HCM). Genes encoding proteins in the *thick filament* that cause hypertrophic cardiomyopathy include myosin-binding protein C and myosin heavy chain. Mutations in titin are associated primarily with dilated cardiomyopathy. Genes encoding proteins in the *thin filament* associated with HCM include troponins, tropomyosin, and actin (*circled*). Less commonly, HCM is caused by mutations in myosin light chains and actinin (not shown, involved in the attachment of actin filaments to the Z-line). (Reproduced with permission, Coppini R, Ho CY, Ashley E, et al. Clinical phenotype and outcome of hypertrophic cardiomyopathy associated with thin filament gene mutations. *J Am Coll Cardiol.* 2014;64:2589–2600.)

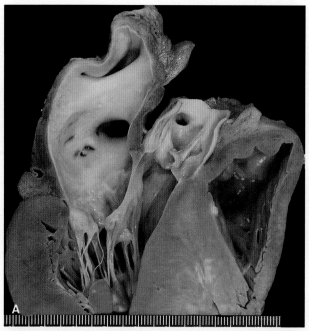
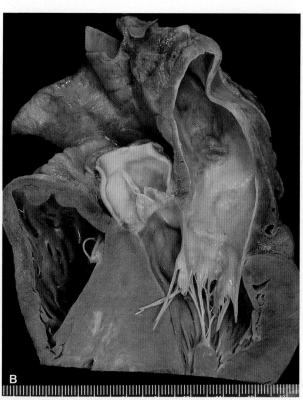

FIGURE 157.2 ▲ Hypertrophic cardiomyopathy. **A.** Long-axis section, base of heart, anterior left side of heart. There is thickening of the ventricular septum with focal gross scars. No outflow tract plaque is present in this case. **B.** Long-axis section. There is left atrial dilatation, typical of the disease, secondary to stiffening of the ventricle. There is no ventricular dilatation in early stages of disease. (Reprinted from Tavora F, Cresswell N, Li L, et al. Morphologic features of exertional versus nonexertional sudden death in patients with hypertrophic cardiomyopathy. *Am J Cardiol.* 2010;105:532–537, with permission.)

Mutations are classified as pathogenic, likely pathogenic, likely benign, benign, or of undetermined significance. This classification is based on frequency of the observed variant, functional studies, and computer-based prediction tools. These variants can be further categorized by the effect they have on the RNA transcript: missense, nonsense, insertions, deletions, or splice site.[23] The art and science of these genetic variant cells are ever improving and will likely have significant impact on the understanding of this disease over the next decade.

Multiple mutations are found in as many as 6% of patients, who tend to present at a younger age and have a more aggressive clinical course.[25] These include combined mutations in different genes and homozygous mutations in patients inheriting mutated alleles from both parents.[26]

Although specific mutations cannot predict the clinical course of patients with HCM, some trends can be inferred by a number of studies regarding phenotype–genotype correlations, penetrance, and severity of disease (Table 157.1). Mutations of thin filament genes (troponin I, troponin T, actin, and tropomyosin) are associated with less hypertrophy, but an equal or higher rate of arrhythmias compared to HCM associated with other genes.[27]

Gross Cardiac Findings

The main characteristics of HCM are cardiomegaly, asymmetric left ventricular hypertrophy, interstitial fibrosis (usually septal), and the presence of a mitral valve contact lesion in the outflow tract (evidence of abnormal systolic anterior mitral valve motion) (Figs. 157.2 to 157.5). The heart is usually enlarged and often more than twice the expected mean.[28] While heart weight and degree of hypertrophy may be predictors of sudden death, cases of normal-sized hearts have been reported, and the diagnosis relies on histologic examination and molecular genetic analysis.[29]

The hearts are usually enlarged due to left ventricular hypertrophy, which is commonly asymmetric with septal prominence. A ventricular septal-to-free wall ratio should be obtained routinely at the time of gross evaluation in all hearts. A ratio of ≥1.3 is considered abnormal and should warrant additional evaluation for HCM.[30]

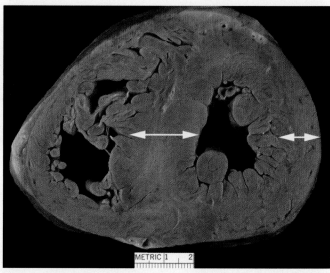

FIGURE 157.3 ▲ Hypertrophic cardiomyopathy, short-axis section. There is marked thickening of the ventricular septum compared with the left ventricular free wall (*arrows*).

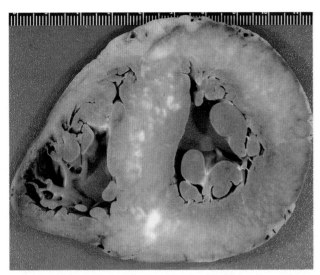

FIGURE 157.4 ▲ Hypertrophic cardiomyopathy, short-axis section from the heart illustrated in Figure 157.1. There is septal hypertrophy as well as gross scarring in the septum. In this case, the ventricular cavity is of normal diameter. (Reprinted from Tavora F, Cresswell N, Li L, et al. Morphologic features of exertional versus nonexertional sudden death in patients with hypertrophic cardiomyopathy. *Am J Cardiol.* 2010;105:532–537, with permission.)

The mitral valve is often thickened or may have been repaired or replaced. Associated with a thickened anterior leaflet is a discrete subaortic endocardial thickening, which is often the mirror image of the anterior mitral valve leaflet. A mitral valve contact lesion, while not specific for HCM, does warrant a careful examination for such (Fig. 157.6). Gross interstitial fibrosis is frequently seen, as patches of whitish scar, most prominent in the septum (Fig. 157.4). The presence of fibrosis seen grossly has been reported to occur in 40% to 50% of hearts of patients dying with HCM.[30]

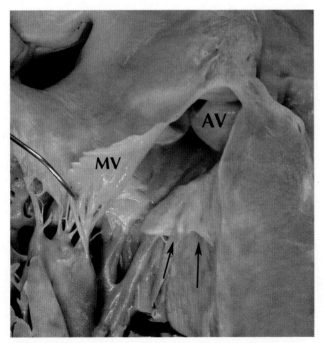

FIGURE 157.5 ▲ Hypertrophic cardiomyopathy, left ventricular outflow tract plaque. The *arrows* point to a discrete area of endocardial fibrosis that corresponds to a friction lesion adjacent to the anterior leaflet of the mitral valve (MV). The aortic valve (AV) is seen in the outflow.

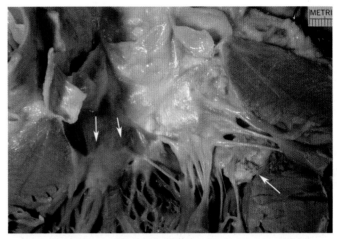

FIGURE 157.6 ▲ Left ventricular outflow tract plaque, secondary to mitral annular calcification. Other forms of valve disease can result in outflow tract plaques, such as in this case of mitral annular calcification. The plaque is on the left ventricular outflow endocardium (*arrows*). In addition to calcifications on the mitral and aortic valves, there is annular calcification forming a nodular mass (*arrow*).

Abnormalities in papillary muscle morphology and/or configuration have also been described in the setting of HCM in imaging series. The precise reason for such is not known.[31]

Microscopic Features

The main microscopic features of HCM are myocyte hypertrophy, myofiber disarray, and interstitial (pericellular-type) fibrosis. Myocyte hypertrophy is almost invariably seen, but while it is very sensitive, it is entirely nonspecific. Myocyte disarray, often touted as the pathologic hallmark, is also fairly nonspecific and can be seen in older patients and those with chronic hypertension. Nevertheless, the presence of these features, particularly in constellation, should cause consideration of HCM.

Myocyte hypertrophy can be assessed by both enlargement of the myocytes (usually <3 erythrocytes in diameter) and abnormal nuclear features (such as karyomegaly and multinucleation). Interstitial fibrosis is usually more prominent in the ventricular septum and is typically of the pericellular variety. However, it is not uncommon for individuals with HCM to have areas of infarction owing to supply–demand imbalance. The supply issues created by abnormally hypertrophied myofibers are often compounded by unusual ("dysplastic") intramural coronary arteries.

Histologic evaluation of myofiber disarray depends on taking cross sections of the ventricular septum, to avoid artifacts of tangential or longitudinal sections. Two main patterns of myofiber disarray have been described: the cartwheel or pinwheel pattern, characterized by hypertrophied myocytes misaligned perpendicular or oblique to each other, often with branching of myocytes, and the herringbone pattern, where fascicles of myocytes are aligned in groups perpendicular to each other but have a "swirled" appearance within the bundles[32] (Figs. 157.7 to 157.11).

Myofiber disarray should not be confused with physiologic disorganization of heart muscle cells at the junction of the septum and ventricles, particularly posterior, or near valve insertions. In contrast to pathologic disarray of HCM, the myocytes are not enlarged. It is sometimes useful to compare myocyte size in areas of disarray in the central septum to areas of the subendocardium on the same slide, where disarray does not occur, and note the marked difference in nuclear and cellular size in cases of HCM. Myofiber disarray may also occur adjacent to healed infarcts and as in areas of amyloidosis. The latter may be especially important to distinguish, as the gross features of amyloidosis may also mimic HCM.

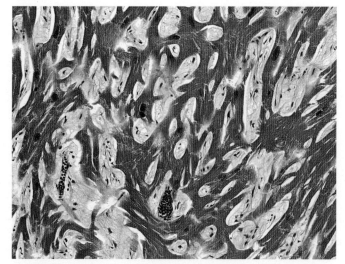

FIGURE 157.7 ▲ Myofiber disarray, hypertrophic cardiomyopathy. The typical appearance is that of branching, anastomosing myocytes with marked hypertrophy and nuclear enlargement.

Intramural coronary arteries are thickened in over 50% of hearts with HCM, depending on how extensive they are sampled (Fig. 157.12). Intramural coronary artery thickening is more common in hearts with fibrosis than those without significant fibrosis[33] and more frequent in sudden death compared to death with heart failure.[30]

Epicardial coronary arteries are usually normal in HCM. However, the presence of a myocardial bridge (which may be present in a third of patients) at the left anterior descending artery (tunnel) has been associated with an increased risk of sudden death, especially in the young. The obstructive effect of the tunnel can be surgically treated at the time of septal ablation.[34]

Treatment and Prognosis

Currently, most patients with a new diagnosis of HCM are either asymptomatic or minimally symptomatic. The disease is incidentally detected during workup for other conditions, during exam of

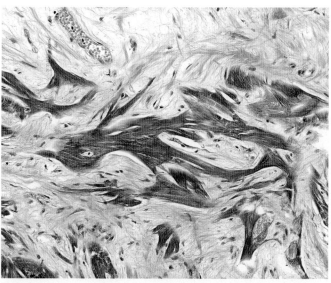

FIGURE 157.9 ▲ Myofiber disarray, hypertrophic cardiomyopathy. Fibrosis is often associated with areas of disarray, which suggest that it may be a part of the cardiomyopathic process and not always a sequela of ischemia.

relatives from index patients, or during screening in clinics and athletic facilities. For these patients, the aim is to prevent syncopal or sudden death episodes.

Treatment of arrhythmias in HCM involves pharmacotherapy (β-blockers, calcium channel blockers), antiarrhythmic interventions (ablations for atrial fibrillation and monomorphous ventricular tachycardia), and implanted cardioverter–defibrillators. Treatment for outflow obstruction includes both pharmacologic agents as well as surgical myectomy or ablation. Treatment for heart failure includes pharmacology, repair or replacement of the mitral valve, and cardiac transplant.

The prognosis of HCM is not well understood. The overall risk of nonsudden death, need for defibrillation, and need for transplant combined has been estimated at 1.6% yearly for patients with HCM with thin filament–related mutations. Added to this was an ~1% yearly

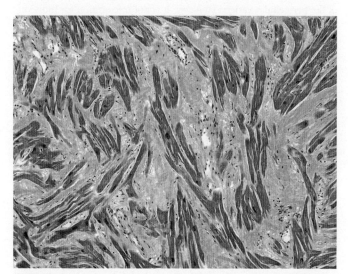

FIGURE 157.8 ▲ Myofiber disarray, hypertrophic cardiomyopathy. There is the typical cartwheel pattern, in this case with abundant background fibrosis. The cells are markedly enlarged, in contrast to so-called "physiologic" disarray seen at the junction of the posterior septum and right ventricle.

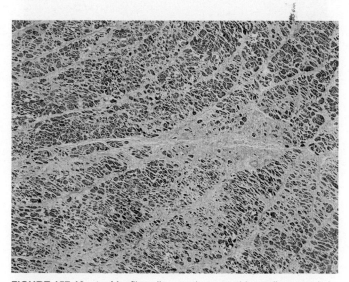

FIGURE 157.10 ▲ Myofiber disarray, hypertrophic cardiomyopathy. In some cases, there are ribbons of myocyte separated by collagen bands; the cells within these ribbons are often whorled and not oriented longitudinally. This type of disarray has been designated as type II disarray.

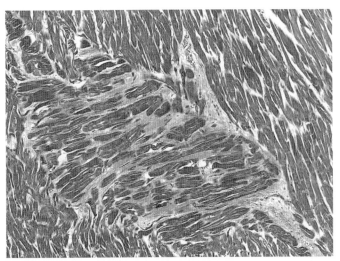

FIGURE 157.11 ▲ Myofiber disarray, hypertrophic cardiomyopathy. In this example, there are blocks of myocytes that are arrayed at right angles with other more normally oriented fibers.

risk for sudden unexpected death.[35] The overall 15-year survival in this study was about 75%.[35]

A study evaluating not only probands but also asymptomatic relatives, in a group with a genetic background that may be less arrhythmogenic, reported an annual rate of sudden cardiac death of only 0.1%.[36] The yearly mortality in high-risk groups, such as those with prior septal ablations, is 3%.[37]

Septal Interventions

The pathologist will often see hearts at autopsy or explant that have had prior interventions for the treatment of outflow tract obstruction. Procedures to remove the outflow obstruction include excision with a scalpel (myectomies) and ablations, which are typically done with alcohol. It is unclear whether the scarring brought about by the ablation increases the risk for arrhythmic death by forming a nidus for ventricular tachyarrhythmias.[37]

Alcohol ablations may be performed as an open procedure or transluminally via left heart catheterization.[38] Typically, they produced an area of scarring or myocardial mummification owing to the alcohol installed into the septal perforator artery.

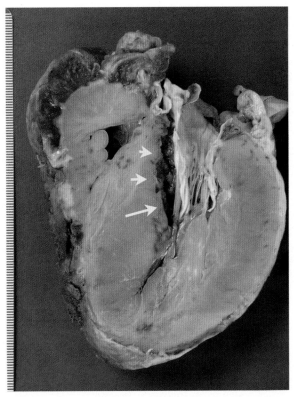

FIGURE 157.13 ▲ Hypertrophic cardiomyopathy, explanted heart, status post myectomy. The atria are not present. There is marked biventricular hypertrophy. *Arrows* demonstrate area of recent myectomy to relieve left ventricular outflow obstruction.

Open surgery, considered by some as the "gold standard" treatment, has an equal or higher success rate and a lower rate of subsequent pacemaker for atrioventricular block. The gross appearance may suggest relatively recent (Fig. 157.13) or remote surgery with dense scar (Fig. 157.14). The surgical pathologist may occasionally encounter myectomy specimens (Fig. 157.15) from those with either HCM or chronic aortic stenosis. Attention should be given to the changes in the tissue in order to correctly report the findings to the surgeon and to rule out mimics such as Fabry disease or amyloidosis.

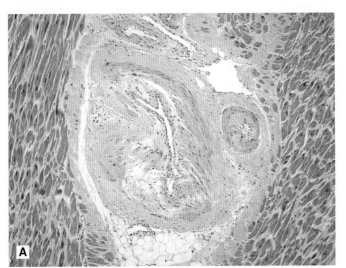

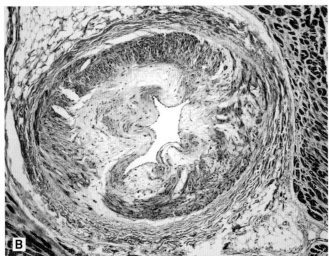

FIGURE 157.12 ▲ Intramural coronary artery thickening, hypertrophic cardiomyopathy. **A.** The arterial branch within the myocardium shows medial hypertrophy with disorganization and increased proteoglycans. **B.** Masson trichrome stain demonstrates the medial thickening with disorganized medial layer.

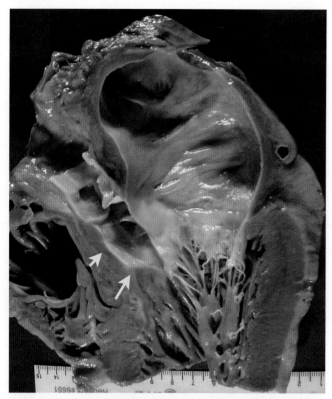

FIGURE 157.14 ▲ Hypertrophic cardiomyopathy, autopsy, status post remote myectomy. *Arrows* point to a scooped out area in the left ventricular outflow tract with endocardial scarring.

Catheter-Based Ablations for Arrhythmias

As with dilated cardiomyopathy, patients with HCM (especially the apical variant) have an increased risk for the development of monomorphic ventricular tachycardias that are amenable to treatment by ablation procedures. Arrhythmogenic foci may be endocardial or epicardial and occur in the ventricular apex or right ventricular outflow tract. Radiofrequency ablation after electrophysiologic mapping may result in effective control of arrhythmias. At explant or autopsy, areas of endocardial fibrosis may be seen consistent with prior ablative therapy.[39]

Because patients with HCM have a relatively high rate of atrial fibrillation, atrial ablation may be performed to restore normal sinus rhythm. The heart will show areas of endocardial fibrosis around the pulmonary veins, indicative of bilateral pulmonary vein isolation. Other sites that may be ablated include the left atrial roof, mitral isthmus, and tricuspid isthmus.[40]

Mitral Valve Replacement and Repair

The mitral valve often demonstrates abnormal movement in HCM and may become thickened and dysfunctional. Up to 20% of patients eventually require open repair or replacement of the mitral valve (Fig. 157.16).[41] The surgical pathologic findings of the mitral valves are nonspecific and include leaflet and cord thickening, with fibrosis histologically.

Apical and Midventricular HCM

Apical HCM was first described in the 1970s and this pattern of disease involvement has become increasingly recognized. The heart weight may be only mildly increased, and the apex of the ventricular septum demonstrates scarring and myofiber disarray. Apical forms of the disease seem to have a better prognosis than other types of HCM, but apical ischemia and/or infarction with aneurysm formation can occur.

The apical form of HCM occurs in ~25% of Asians diagnosed with HCM, but fewer than 10% of non-Asian HCM patients.[42] Among the non-Asian apical variants, patients are typically somewhat older than the typical asymmetric form of disease. Mutations are found in <25% of patients with apical HCM.[43]

Another variant is midventricular HCM (so-called "reverse curve" type),[44] characterized on echocardiogram by hypertrophied myocardium most prominent in the midventricular septum with markedly thickened papillary muscles (Fig. 157.17). In contrast to apical HCM, it is marked by progressive clinical deterioration.[45] Areas of hypertrophy and myofiber disarray may occur anywhere in the left ventricle and ventricular septum and occasionally be localized to the posterolateral left ventricular wall.[46]

Effect of Age on Phenotype of HCM

There are two age peaks at onset of HCM: adolescence and young adulthood and the 6th decades and above. An autopsy study comparing older and younger patients dying with HCM showed that asymmetric septal hypertrophy, subaortic mitral valve contact lesions, myocyte disarray, intramural coronary artery thickening, and sudden death were

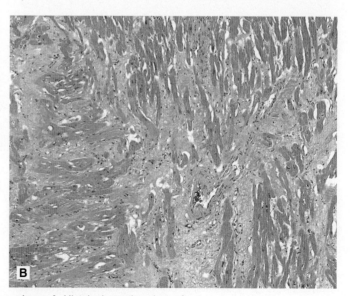

FIGURE 157.15 ▲ Hypertrophic cardiomyopathy, surgical myectomy specimen. **A.** Histologic section shows fragments of muscle and endocardial scarring. **B.** There were areas of myofiber disarray consistent with HCM.

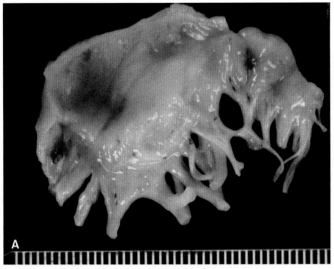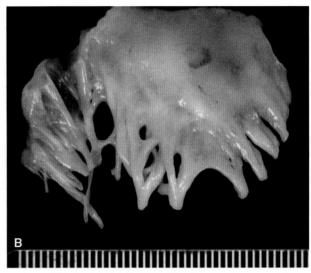

FIGURE 157.16 ▲ Hypertrophic cardiomyopathy, mitral valve replacement. The gross findings are those of fibrosis and chordal thickening. **A.** Atrial surface. **B.** Ventricular surface.

more prevalent in the young.[33] These findings suggest that HCM in the elderly may be a heterogeneous disorder, and the presence of known mutations in this age group may identify a pure subgroup of patients with the disease.

Postmortem Genetic Testing

Postmortem molecular testing is increasingly performed to provide more comprehensive evaluation of cases of sudden death and allow

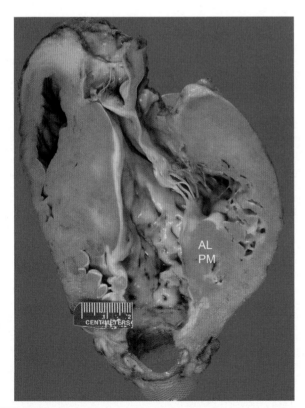

FIGURE 157.17 ▲ Hypertrophic cardiomyopathy with marked hypertrophy of papillary muscle. The anterolateral papillary muscle (AL PM) is markedly thickened. The septum is also thick, toward midventricle, with patchy fibrosis. There is an apical left ventricular assist conduit seen.

for more complete proband characterization. Ultimately, mutation-specific screening will likely allow for more cost-effective follow-up of kindreds and allow for more complete understanding of the correlation between phenotype and genotype.[47,48]

Practical Points

▶ Hypertrophic cardiomyopathy (HCM) should be considered in exertional sudden death cases at forensic autopsy, primarily if there is cardiomegaly.

▶ The major differential diagnosis is idiopathic left ventricular hypertrophy or hypertensive heart disease; histologic documentation of myofiber disarray with multiple sections of ventricular septum is recommended.

▶ Sections of ventricular septum must be taken transversely in order to identify correctly the extent and patterns of disarray.

▶ Pathologic disarray is distinguished from "physiologic" disarray in the posterior septum by the presence of marked enlargement of the myocytes in comparison to areas not involved near the endocardium.

▶ Less common mimickers of HCM include amyloidosis and Fabry disease; these are diagnosed by typical histologic findings.

▶ Myectomy specimens in patients with subaortic stenosis include two entities: HCM and congenital subaortic stenosis.

▶ Myectomy specimens show myofiber disarray in the majority, but not all cases; nonspecific findings of endocardial fibrosis and myocyte hypertrophy may not distinguish from congenital subaortic stenosis, which requires clinical correlation.

▶ Myectomy may also occasionally be performed in patients with aortic stenosis and asymmetric hypertrophy and subaortic obstruction, and the histologic findings are nonspecific without myofiber disarray.

REFERENCES

1. Roberts R, Sigwart U. New concepts in hypertrophic cardiomyopathies, part II. *Circulation.* 2001;104:2249–2252.

2. Pedra SR, Smallhorn JF, Ryan G, et al. Fetal cardiomyopathies: pathogenic mechanisms, hemodynamic findings, and clinical outcome. *Circulation.* 2002;106:585–591.

3. Lever HM, Karam RF, Currie PJ, et al. Hypertrophic cardiomyopathy in the elderly. Distinctions from the young based on cardiac shape. *Circulation.* 1989;79:580–589.

4. Klues HG, Schiffers A, Maron BJ. Phenotypic spectrum and patterns of left ventricular hypertrophy in hypertrophic cardiomyopathy: morphologic observations and significance as assessed by two-dimensional echocardiography in 600 patients. *J Am Coll Cardiol.* 1995;26:1699–1708.

5. Semsarian C, Ingles J, Maron MS, et al. New perspectives on the prevalence of hypertrophic cardiomyopathy. *J Am Coll Cardiol.* 2015;65:1249–1254.

6. Baudhuin LM, Kotzer KE, Kluge ML, et al. What is the true prevalence of hypertrophic cardiomyopathy? *J Am Coll Cardiol.* 2015;66:1845–1846.

7. Harmon KG, Asif IM, Maleszewski JJ, et al. Incidence, cause, and comparative frequency of sudden cardiac death in National Collegiate Athletic Association Athletes: a decade in review. *Circulation.* 2015;132:10–19.

8. Basavarajaiah S, Wilson M, Whyte G, et al. Prevalence of hypertrophic cardiomyopathy in highly trained athletes: relevance to pre-participation screening. *J Am Coll Cardiol.* 2008;51:1033–1039.

9. Landstrom AP, Adekola BA, Bos JM, et al. PLN-encoded phospholamban mutation in a large cohort of hypertrophic cardiomyopathy cases: summary of the literature and implications for genetic testing. *Am Heart J.* 2011;161:165–171.

10. Lopes LR, Zekavati A, Syrris P, et al. Genetic complexity in hypertrophic cardiomyopathy revealed by high-throughput sequencing. *J Med Genet.* 2013;50:228–239.

11. Marian AJ. Contemporary treatment of hypertrophic cardiomyopathy. *Tex Heart Inst J.* 2009;36:194–204.

12. Sachdev B, Takenaka T, Teraguchi H, et al. Prevalence of Anderson-Fabry disease in male patients with late onset hypertrophic cardiomyopathy. *Circulation.* 2002;105:1407–1411.

13. Geske JB, Jouni H, Aubry MC, et al. Fabry disease with resting outflow obstruction masquerading as hypertrophic cardiomyopathy. *J Am Coll Cardiol.* 2014;63:e43.

14. Noureldin RA, Liu S, Nacif MS, et al. The diagnosis of hypertrophic cardiomyopathy by cardiovascular magnetic resonance. *J Cardiovasc Magn Reson.* 2012;14:17.

15. Sakamoto N, Sato N, Oikawa K, et al. Late gadolinium enhancement of cardiac magnetic resonance imaging indicates abnormalities of time-domain T-wave alternans in hypertrophic cardiomyopathy with ventricular tachycardia. *Heart Rhythm.* 2015;12:1747–1755.

16. Prinz C, Schwarz M, Ilic I, et al. Myocardial fibrosis severity on cardiac magnetic resonance imaging predicts sustained arrhythmic events in hypertrophic cardiomyopathy. *Can J Cardiol.* 2013;29:358–363.

17. Kofflard MJ, Ten Cate FJ, van der Lee C, et al. Hypertrophic cardiomyopathy in a large community-based population: clinical outcome and identification of risk factors for sudden cardiac death and clinical deterioration. *J Am Coll Cardiol.* 2003;41:987–993.

18. Robinson K, Frenneaux MP, Stockins B, et al. Atrial fibrillation in hypertrophic cardiomyopathy: a longitudinal study. *J Am Coll Cardiol.* 1990;15:1279–1285.

19. Christiaans I, Wilde AA. The never ending story of risk stratification for sudden death in hypertrophic cardiomyopathy. *Am J Cardiol.* 2011;107:1871.

20. Contreras-Valdes FM, Buxton AE, Josephson ME, et al. Atrial fibrillation ablation in patients with hypertrophic cardiomyopathy: long-term outcomes and clinical predictors. *J Am Coll Cardiol.* 2015;65:1485–1487.

21. Siontis KC, Geske JB, Ong K, et al. Atrial fibrillation in hypertrophic cardiomyopathy: prevalence, clinical correlations, and mortality in a large high-risk population. *J Am Heart Assoc.* 2014;3:e001002.

22. Geisterfer-Lowrance AA, Kass S, Tanigawa G, et al. A molecular basis for familial hypertrophic cardiomyopathy: a beta cardiac myosin heavy chain gene missense mutation. *Cell.* 1990;62:999–1006.

23. Alfares AA, Kelly MA, McDermott G, et al. Results of clinical genetic testing of 2,912 probands with hypertrophic cardiomyopathy: expanded panels offer limited additional sensitivity. *Genet Med.* 2015;17:319.

24. Das KJ, Ingles J, Bagnall RD, et al. Determining pathogenicity of genetic variants in hypertrophic cardiomyopathy: importance of periodic reassessment. *Genet Med.* 2014;16:286–293.

25. Berge KE, Leren TP. Genetics of hypertrophic cardiomyopathy in Norway. *Clin Genet.* 2014;86:355–360.

26. Richard P, Charron P, Carrier L, et al. Hypertrophic cardiomyopathy: distribution of disease genes, spectrum of mutations, and implications for a molecular diagnosis strategy. *Circulation.* 2003;107:2227–2232.

27. Coppini R, Ho CY, Ashley E, et al. Clinical phenotype and outcome of hypertrophic cardiomyopathy associated with thin-filament gene mutations. *J Am Coll Cardiol.* 2014;64:2589–2600.

28. Kocovski L, Fernandes J. Sudden cardiac death: a modern pathology approach to hypertrophic cardiomyopathy. *Arch Pathol Lab Med.* 2015;139:413–416.

29. Maron BJ, Kragel AH, Roberts WC. Sudden death in hypertrophic cardiomyopathy with normal left ventricular mass. *Br Heart J.* 1990;63:308–310.

30. Tavora F, Cresswell N, Li L, et al. Morphologic features of exertional versus nonexertional sudden death in patients with hypertrophic cardiomyopathy. *Am J Cardiol.* 2010;105:532–537.

31. Maron MS. Clinical utility of cardiovascular magnetic resonance in hypertrophic cardiomyopathy. *J Cardiovasc Magn Reson.* 2012;14:13.

32. Maron BJ, Wolfson JK, Roberts WC. Relation between extent of cardiac muscle cell disorganization and left ventricular wall thickness in hypertrophic cardiomyopathy. *Am J Cardiol.* 1992;70:785–790.

33. Litovsky SH, Rose AG. Clinicopathologic heterogeneity in hypertrophic cardiomyopathy with regard to age, asymmetric septal hypertrophy, and concentric hypertrophy beyond the pediatric age group. *Arch Pathol Lab Med.* 1998;122:434–441.

34. Sunbul M, Kepez A, Tigen K, et al. Successful treatment of myocardial bridge with alcohol septal ablation in hypertrophic obstructive cardiomyopathy. *Int J Angiol.* 2014;23:69–70.

35. Pasquale F, Syrris P, Kaski JP, et al. Long-term outcomes in hypertrophic cardiomyopathy caused by mutations in the cardiac troponin T gene. *Circ Cardiovasc Genet.* 2012;5:10–17.

36. Christiaans I, Birnie E, van Langen IM, et al. The yield of risk stratification for sudden cardiac death in hypertrophic cardiomyopathy myosin-binding protein C gene mutation carriers: focus on predictive screening. *Eur Heart J.* 2010;31:842–848.

37. Veselka J, Zemanek D, Jahnlova D, et al. Risk and causes of death in patients after alcohol septal ablation for hypertrophic obstructive cardiomyopathy. *Can J Cardiol.* 2015;31:1245–1251.

38. Rigopoulos AG, Seggewiss H. Twenty years of alcohol septal ablation in hypertrophic obstructive cardiomyopathy. *Curr Cardiol Rev.* 2015.

39. Inada K, Seiler J, Roberts-Thomson KC, et al. Substrate characterization and catheter ablation for monomorphic ventricular tachycardia in patients with apical hypertrophic cardiomyopathy. *J Cardiovasc Electrophysiol.* 2011;22:41–48.

40. Wen SN, Liu N, Li SN, et al. QTc interval prolongation predicts arrhythmia recurrence after catheter ablation of atrial fibrillation in patients with hypertrophic cardiomyopathy. *Circ J.* 2015;79:1024–1030.

41. Vassileva CM, Boley T, Markwell S, et al. Mitral valve repair is underused in patients with hypertrophic obstructive cardiomyopathy. *Heart Surg Forum.* 2011;14:E376–E379.

42. Klarich KW, Attenhofer Jost CH, Binder J, et al. Risk of death in long-term follow-up of patients with apical hypertrophic cardiomyopathy. *Am J Cardiol.* 2013;111:1784–1791.

43. Towe EC, Bos JM, Ommen SR, et al. Genotype–phenotype correlations in apical variant hypertrophic cardiomyopathy. *Congenit Heart Dis.* 2015;10:E139–E145.

44. Said SM, Dearani JA, Ommen SR, et al. Surgical treatment of hypertrophic cardiomyopathy. *Expert Rev Cardiovasc Ther.* 2013;11:617–627.

45. Cai C, Duan FJ, Yang YJ, et al. Comparison of the prevalence, clinical features, and long-term outcomes of midventricular hypertrophy vs apical phenotype in patients with hypertrophic cardiomyopathy. *Can J Cardiol.* 2014;30:441–447.

46. Seki A, Perens G, Fishbein MC. Posterolateral hypertrophic cardiomyopathy: a rare, but clinically significant variant of hypertrophic cardiomyopathy. *Cardiovasc Pathol.* 2014;23:381–382.

47. Kane DA, Triedman J. Post-mortem genetic testing in a family with long-QT syndrome and hypertrophic cardiomyopathy. *Cardiovasc Pathol.* 2014;23:107–109.

48. Loporcaro CG, Tester DJ, Maleszewski JJ, et al. Confirmation of cause and manner of death via a comprehensive cardiac autopsy including whole exome next-generation sequencing. *Arch Pathol Lab Med.* 2014;138:1083–1089.

49. Girolami F, Iascone M, Tomberli B, et al. Novel alpha-actinin 2 variant associated with familial hypertrophic cardiomyopathy and juvenile atrial arrhythmias: a massively parallel sequencing study. *Circ Cardiovasc Genet.* 2014;7:741–750.

50. Chiu C, Bagnall RD, Ingles J, et al. Mutations in alpha-actinin-2 cause hypertrophic cardiomyopathy: a genome-wide analysis. *J Am Coll Cardiol.* 2010;55:1127–1135.

51. Kabaeva ZT, Perrot A, Wolter B, et al. Systematic analysis of the regulatory and essential myosin light chain genes: genetic variants and mutations in hypertrophic cardiomyopathy. *Eur J Hum Genet.* 2002;10:741–748.

52. Maron BJ, Maron MS, Semsarian C. Double or compound sarcomere mutations in hypertrophic cardiomyopathy: a potential link to sudden death in the absence of conventional risk factors. *Heart Rhythm.* 2012;9: 57–63.

158 Arrhythmogenic Cardiomyopathy

Allen P. Burke, M.D., and Fabio R. Tavora, M.D., Ph.D.

Background

The concept of arrhythmogenic cardiomyopathy (AC) has evolved over the last 25 years, resulting in a variety of synonyms for this disease. Over the years, the disease has been referred to as arrhythmogenic right ventricular dysplasia/cardiomyopathy, owing to its predilection for the right ventricle. However, is it become increasingly common to refer to it as arrhythmogenic cardiomyopathy (AC) in recognition of primarily left ventricular and biventricular forms of the disease. Gradually, the concept emerged that the right ventricle was infiltrated by fat and scar and that aneurysms were not uniformly present. Electrocardiographic and imaging studies expanded the phenotypic profile of the disease, which was consistently characterized by ventricular tachyarrhythmias and clinically resembled cardiomyopathy ("arrhythmogenic right ventricular dysplasia/cardiomyopathy (ARVD/C)" or "arrhythmogenic right ventricular cardiomyopathy (ARVC)"). The etiologic significance of the fat portion of the infiltrates was debated, and eventually it was agreed that the fibrotic portion of the pathologic process was indeed the *sine qua non* for diagnosis. Finally, as further autopsy studies have emerged, as well as more sensitive imaging, such as cardiac CT and MR, it has been recognized that left ventricular involvement is typical and possibly more common than the right ventricular changes.[1-3]

Definition

AC has been defined by electrocardiographic and imaging criteria (Table 158.1), by genetic criteria based on mutations in desmosomal genes, and pathologically. The pathologic diagnosis unfortunately can only be made at autopsy or explant, as the histologic findings in right ventricular biopsies are nonspecific. Because fat is normal in the right ventricle, fibrosis is considered a diagnostic feature of AC in biopsy (Table 158.1), even though fibrosis may be a component of any "morphofunctional phenotype," including hypertrophic, dilated, and restrictive cardiomyopathy.

Etiology

Between 30% and 50% of patients with AC have a family history of cardiomyopathy, and pathogenic mutations in genes encoding cardiac proteins are identified in 46% of patients.[4]

In addition to genetic causes, other possible etiologies for AC include a congenital malformation (dysplasia), now considered unlikely, and a healed myocarditis. The presence of inflammation in a large proportion of autopsy cases, as well as clinical documentation of myocarditis progressing to AC,[5,6] is in support of an inflammatory etiology for at least some cases and was once considered the likely cause.[7,8] It is likely that there is a "two-hit" phenomenon, namely, that myocarditis (viral or other types) progresses to AC if there is a predisposing genetic basis, such as those involving the desmosome or ryanodine receptor, affecting cardiomyocytes diffusely.

Genetics

Genetic studies based on animal models, rare families with coincidental skin lesions, and family studies of isolated cardiomyopathy have led to the discovery of mutations in genes related to the desmosome. These include plakophilin-2 (*PKP2*), desmoplakin (*DSP*), and desmoglein-2

TABLE 158.1 Major Criteria for the Clinicopathologic Diagnosis of Arrhythmogenic Right Ventricular Cardiomyopathy/Dysplasia, Simplified

Category of Finding	Specific
Imaging	Regional RV akinesia, dyskinesia, or aneurysm, by echocardiogram, MRI, or RV angiography
ECG	Inverted T waves in right precordial leads (V1, V2, and V3) or beyond in individuals >14 years of age (in the absence of complete right bundle-branch block QRS ≥120 ms)
	Epsilon wave (reproducible low-amplitude signals between end of QRS complex to onset of the T wave) in the right precordial leads (V1–V3)
ECG/arrhythmias	Nonsustained or sustained ventricular tachycardia of left bundle-branch morphology with superior axis (negative or indeterminate QRS in leads II, III, and aVF and positive in lead aVL)
Biopsy findings	>50% fibrous tissue on endomyocardial biopsy
Family history and genetics	• AC/D confirmed in a first-degree relative who meets current Task Force criteria
	• AC/D confirmed pathologically at autopsy or surgery in a first-degree relative
	• Identification of a pathogenic mutation categorized as associated or probably associated with AC/D in the patient under evaluation

Reprinted from Marcus FI, McKenna WJ, Sherrill D, et al. Diagnosis of arrhythmogenic cardiomyopathy/dysplasia: proposed modification of the Task Force Criteria. *Eur Heart J.* 2010;31:806–814.

(*DSG2*).[9,10] Many distinct mutations have been described for each, including over 25 for *PKP2* alone.[11] Up to 40% of all mutations are unique or "private," limited to a single proband or family.[4] Other desmosomal genes mutated in AC include plakoglobin (*JUP*) and desmocollin-2 (*DSC2*).[9]

Mutations unrelated to desmosomal proteins have also been identified in families of patients with AC as well as series of unrelated probands. These include the cardiac ryanodine receptor (*RYR2*),[12] transmembrane protein 43 encoding gene (*TMEM43*), phospholamban (*PLN*),[13–15] transforming growth factor beta-3 (*TGFβ3*), αT-catenin (*CTNNA3*), lamin A/C (*LMNA*), desmin (*DES*), and titin (*TTN*).[9]

Linkage analyses have identified loci not containing the above genes, and no causative genes have been identified in these regions yet. These loci (14q12-q22, 2q32.1-q32.3, 10p14-p12 and 10q22.3) and most of the identified genes listed above form the basis for a numbering system for AC from 1 to 12 (Online Mendelian Inheritance in Man, www.omim.org) (Table 158.1).[10]

The reported strong association between AC and mutations in desmosomal proteins may be somewhat biased. Firstly, series of unrelated patients only looked for mutations in desmosomal proteins, ignoring others,[4] leading to their inclusion as a major diagnostic criterion for the disease thereby boosting their frequency in AC (Table 158.2). Only recently have pathogenic nondesmosomal mutations been sought and found in a large proportion of unrelated patients with AC.[12] Secondly, desmosomal mutations were evaluated only recently in series of unrelated patients with other types of cardiomyopathy, which has led to the discovery of a high rate of desmosomal mutations in diseases other than AC, such as dilated cardiomyopathy.[20] Third and most importantly, pathologic confirmation of the diagnosis is only rarely accomplished by biopsy, and the clinical criteria are somewhat nonspecific, making genotypic/phenotypic correlation difficult. Autopsy series of AC with high throughput analysis of cardiomyopathic genes are not yet available, and cardiac imaging studies are not at this time sophisticated enough to make a reliable diagnosis of AC.

Incidence

The incidence of arrhythmogenic cardiomyopathy is unknown. It has been estimated, based on clinical criteria, to occur in 1:5,000 individuals, affecting men more frequently than women with a ratio of 3:1.[10]

It is a common cause of sudden exertional deaths in certain regions of Europe,[21,22] but accounts for a smaller proportion in the United States and Canada, about 2% of natural deaths in the young adult age.

Clinical Features

The primary symptoms are related to arrhythmias and conduction disturbances.[23] Arrhythmogenic cardiomyopathy with primary left ventricular involvement is distinguished from DCM by a propensity toward arrhythmia exceeding the degree of ventricular dysfunction.[24]

The pathologist is likely to encounter the disease at autopsy in cases of sudden death.[21] In autopsy series, there is a 6:1 male-to-female ratio, with a possible predilection for African Americans.[25] Approximately three-quarters of sudden deaths due to arrhythmogenic cardiomyopathy are exertional, with a higher rate in the predominantly right ventricular form.[25] Arrhythmogenic cardiomyopathy is generally limited to the young, especially males under the age of 40, although the disease has been described up to the ninth decade.[26] It is extremely uncommon under the age of 10 years.

Several clinical criteria for diagnosis have been proposed, including the Task Force of 2000[27] and a revision in 2002.[28] Symptoms and hemodynamic and ECG findings are relatively nonspecific, but advances in cardiac imaging, especially MR, have increased the reproducibility of clinical diagnosis. Cardiac magnetic resonance imaging is useful in detecting right ventricular tissue and motion abnormalities, as well as left ventricular involvement, manifest by late enhancement in a subepicardial and midwall distribution, corresponding to fibrofatty replacement and fibrosis on histopathology.[24]

Pathology

The gross evaluation of a heart for AC begins at external inspection. A suspicion of the diagnosis occurs if the right ventricle appears dilated, especially fatty (Fig. 158.1). Aneurysm-like dilatations occur in only 35% of patients when evaluated by imaging and gross examination, however. The heart is enlarged in only 50% of cases, more frequently when there is left ventricular involvement.[25]

On cut section, fibrofatty involvement of the right ventricle is typically patchy, but can also be diffuse (Figs. 158.2 to 158.4). Left ventricular scarring is generally subepicardial, but it has an otherwise

TABLE 158.2   Mutations in Patients with the Clinical Diagnosis of Arrhythmogenic Cardiomyopathy[a]

Mutation	Protein Function	Percent of Mutations	OMIM TYPE[8]
Plakophilin-2 *PKP2*	Present in desmosomes and nuclei, link cadherins to intermediate filaments in cytoskeleton	31%[4] 42%[5]	Type 9
Desmoplakin *DSP*[1]	Desmosomal protein, binds plakoglobin and plakophilin, anchor intermediate filaments	4.5%[4] 21.2%[5]	Type 8
Desmoglein-2 *DSG2*	Calcium-binding desmosome glycoprotein, type of cadherin	10%[4] 12.2%[5]	Type 10
Cardiac ryanodine receptor[3] *RYR2*	Calcium channel protein in sarcoplasmic reticulum	9%[6]	Type 2
(Junction) plakoglobin (gamma catenin) *JUP*	Component of desmosomes, binds desmoglein-1 (cadherin)	0%[4] 3.6%[5]	Type 12
Desmocollin-2 *DSC2*	Desmosomal glycoprotein, calcium-dependent cadherin	1.5%[4] 9.7%[5]	Type 11
Transmembrane protein 43 *TMEM43*	Maintains nuclear envelope structure	5%[7]	Type 5

[a]Most patients in reported families and series have no pathologic documentation. These are generally heterozygous variants that are considered pathogenic based on standard genetic criteria[4]: 1: Recessive (homozygous) mutations cause Carvajal syndrome, a form of dilated cardiomyopathy; 2: recessive mutations cause Naxos syndrome, a form of cardiomyopathy sometimes considered ARVC; 3: most often associated with polymorphous catecholaminergic polymorphic ventricular tachycardia, with normal gross heart at autopsy and most common mutation found in sudden death with normal autopsy 4[4]; 5[9]; 6[12]; 7[16]. Other pathogenic variants associated with ARVC involve genes *TGBβ3* (only rare reports[13] considered type 1 ARVC; αT-catenin (*CTNNA3*), usually resulting in a more dilated phenotype[17]; lamin A/C (*LMNA*), more frequently associated with dilated cardiomyopathy[15]; desmin (*DES*), rare, usually restrictive or dilated cardiomyopathy[18]; titin (*TTN*)[19]; phospholamban (*PLN*). 8. Some ARVC numbered types in OMIM have only chromosomal loci assigned (see text) and are not included in this table.

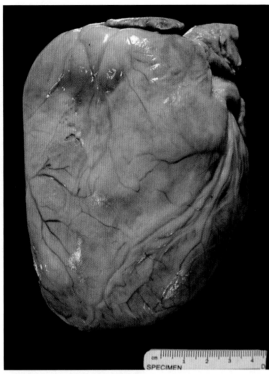

FIGURE 158.1 ▲ Arrhythmogenic cardiomyopathy. External anterior surface demonstrates right ventricular prominence.

random distribution (Figs. 158.5 to 158.6). On cross section, careful examination for fibrofatty infiltrates is necessary for adequate sampling that will lead to diagnosis. The changes can be subtle and the diagnosis made initially at histologic examination.[29]

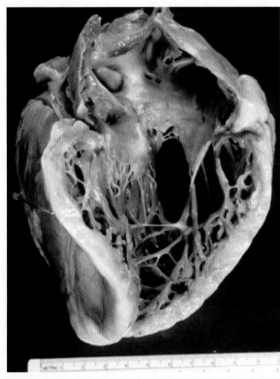

FIGURE 158.2 ▲ Arrhythmogenic cardiomyopathy. The right ventricle is opened, demonstrating diffuse fatty replacement of the right ventricle from base to apex.

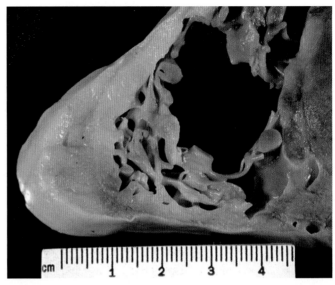

FIGURE 158.3 ▲ Arrhythmogenic cardiomyopathy. There is patchy replacement of the lateral and posterior right ventricle with fat.

In 50% of autopsy hearts, fibrofatty change is balanced nearly equally between the ventricles, followed by left predominant and right predominant pattern.[25]

Histologically, there is fibrosis and fat in random areas of the right ventricle and in subepicardium of the left ventricular free wall, with typical sparing of the septum. The adipose replacement can be prominent with various degrees of fibrosis (Figs. 158.7 to 158.9). The adipose tissue is believed to be metaplastic or secondary to an area of prior myocyte destruction. The left ventricular fibrosis is subepicardial, occasionally with a rim of uninvolved myocardium, or with rimming of the fatty metaplasia. The areas of fat are irregular, in contrast to the normal "marbling" appearance seen in the anterior right ventricle, in which there are relatively even linear fatty areas. In contrast to the right ventricle, the areas of involvement in the left ventricle are often less composed of fat and more of fibrous tissue. At higher magnification, altered myocytes with vacuoles can be seen in all areas of fibrofatty infiltration (Figs. 158.7 and 158.8).

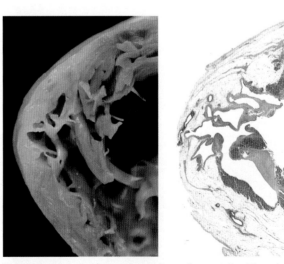

FIGURE 158.4 ▲ Arrhythmogenic cardiomyopathy. There is patchy fat replacement of the lateral right ventricle, which corresponds to fibrofatty replacement histologically.

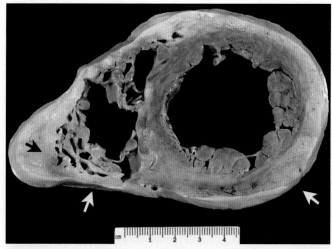

FIGURE 158.5 ▲ Arrhythmogenic cardiomyopathy. The right ventricle shows irregular fat replacement (*arrow*), with a prominent area in the posterior wall, which is typically devoid of fat (*arrow*).

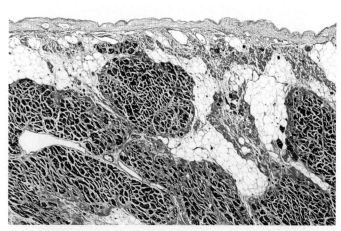

FIGURE 158.8 ▲ Arrhythmogenic cardiomyopathy, subepicardial fibrosis. In this example, a layer of fibrous tissue rims the fatty metaplasia in the subepicardium of the left ventricle. Masson trichrome.

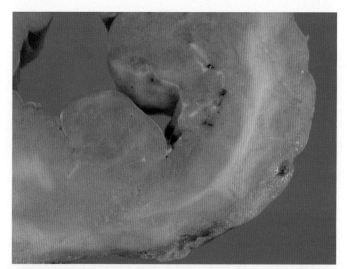

FIGURE 158.6 ▲ Arrhythmogenic cardiomyopathy, left ventricular involvement. Not fibrofatty change in the subepicardial layer of the posterolateral left ventricle.

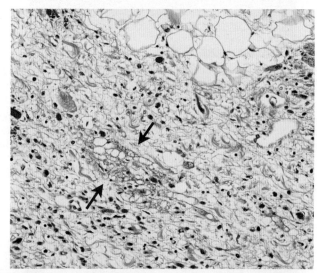

FIGURE 158.9 ▲ Healing myocarditis, progressing to arrhythmogenic cardiomyopathy. There are typical vacuolated, degenerating myocytes (*arrows*).

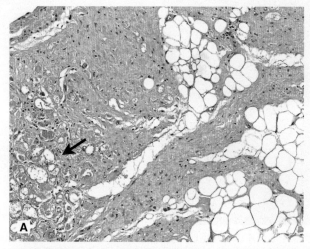

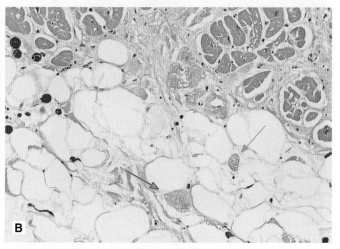

FIGURE 158.7 ▲ Arrhythmogenic cardiomyopathy. **A.** There is fibrofatty change with vacuolated, degenerated myocytes (*arrow*). This image corresponds to the gross figure in Figure 158.6. **B.** A high magnification shows degenerating vacuolated myocytes (*arrows*) within fat and strands of fibrous tissue.

Depending on the degree of sampling and definition of myocarditis, inflammation with myocyte necrosis is seen in over 25% of cases and over 80% of the predominantly right ventricular form[25] (Fig. 158.9).

Heart Biopsy

The utility of heart biopsy in the diagnosis of arrhythmogenic cardiomyopathy is limited, because changes are typically not present in the ventricular septum, and the right ventricular free wall may have spotty involvement. In addition, the presence of fat in the right ventricle is a normal finding; therefore, one must identify the characteristic features of fat and fibrous tissue, with morphologically altered myocytes. The current criteria state that 50% or 60% of the biopsy should be composed of fibrous tissue, in order to be a supporting finding for AC (Table 158.1). Endomyocardial biopsy may have an increased yield for the diagnosis of arrhythmogenic cardiomyopathy if guided by electrophysiologic voltage mapping.[30]

Differential Diagnosis at Autopsy

At autopsy, arrhythmogenic cardiomyopathy should be considered in the differential diagnosis in any unexpected death in a young adult, especially exertional.[22,29,31,32] Normal fat in the right ventricle is occasionally mistaken for arrhythmogenic cardiomyopathy[33]; the typical distribution of physiologic right ventricular adipose tissue is the anterior and lateral walls, sparing the outflow and posterior walls. The absence of fibrosis histologically excludes the diagnosis of arrhythmogenic cardiomyopathy.[33] Excessive fat without fibrosis, or massive fat infiltration of the right (and sometimes left) ventricle, is a rare finding in otherwise unexplained sudden death (Figs. 158.10 to 158.12).[34] Ongoing myocarditis with scarring may in fact be impossible to distinguish from arrhythmogenic cardiomyopathy, especially if there is subepicardial scarring in the left ventricle with fat infiltration.[8,35] Occasionally, there may be coexistent phenotypic features of multiple cardiomyopathies, for example, arrhythmogenic and hypertrophic, in the same heart.

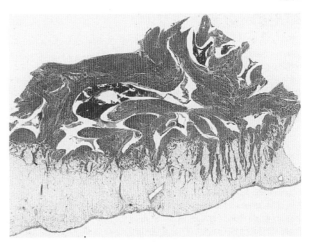

FIGURE 158.11 ▲ Normal right ventricular fat. The epicardial fat is at the bottom, and there is focal infiltration into the superficial myocardium. It has been shown that epicardial fat is related to increasing age, heart weight, and waist circumference. (Reprinted from Silaghi A, Piercecchi-Marti MD, Grino M, et al. Epicardial adipose tissue extent: relationship with age, body fat distribution, and coronaropathy. *Obesity (Silver Spring)*. 2008;16:2424–2430, with permission.)

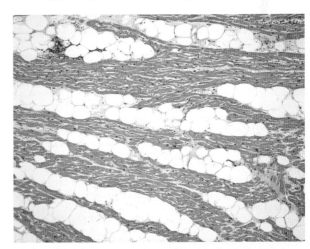

FIGURE 158.12 ▲ Normal right ventricular fat. Regular strands of adipose tissue, without fibrosis, are a normal finding in the right ventricle, especially in the anterior and lateral walls.

Practical Points

▶ Arrhythmogenic cardiomyopathy should be considered in cases of sudden death, with adequate sampling of the right ventricle.

▶ Intramyocardial fat can be considerable in the right ventricle and, in the absence of fibrosis, is a normal variant related to increased heart weight and body fat.

▶ Excessive fat in the right ventricle, without fibrosis, should not be diagnosed as arrhythmogenic cardiomyopathy.

▶ Subepicardial scars are seen in most cases of arrhythmogenic cardiomyopathy and can be a helpful diagnostic feature.

▶ The diagnostic features of arrhythmogenic cardiomyopathy are histologic fibrofatty change with vacuolated myocytes.

▶ Other features that initially constituted the diagnosis, such as right ventricular thinning or aneurysms, or grossly increased fat, are variably seen.

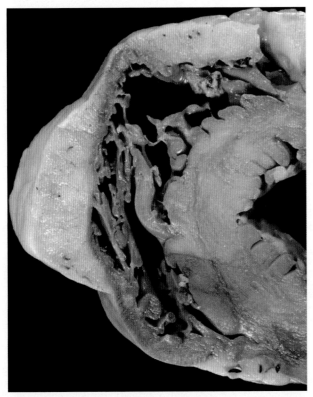

FIGURE 158.10 ▲ Increased right ventricular fat. The lateral and anterior wall show increased fat, but the posterior wall is spared; this is a normal variant.

REFERENCES

1. Lindstrom L, Nylander E, Larsson H, et al. Left ventricular involvement in arrhythmogenic right ventricular cardiomyopathy—a scintigraphic and echocardiographic study. *Clin Physiol Funct Imaging.* 2005;25:171–177.
2. Lobo FV, Silver MD, Butany J, et al. Left ventricular involvement in right ventricular dysplasia/cardiomyopathy. *Can J Cardiol.* 1999;15:1239–1247.
3. Michalodimitrakis M, Papadomanolakis A, Stiakakis J, et al. Left side right ventricular cardiomyopathy. *Med Sci Law.* 2002;42:313–317.
4. Fressart V, Duthoit G, Donal E, et al. Desmosomal gene analysis in arrhythmogenic right ventricular dysplasia/cardiomyopathy: spectrum of mutations and clinical impact in practice. *Europace.* 2010;12:861–868.
5. Tandri H, Asimaki A, Dalal D, et al. Gap junction remodeling in a case of arrhythmogenic right ventricular dysplasia due to plakophilin-2 mutation. *J Cardiovasc Electrophysiol.* 2008;19:1212–1214.
6. Zhang M, Tavora F, Huebner T, et al. Allograft pathology in patients transplanted for idiopathic dilated cardiomyopathy. *Am J Surg Pathol.* 2012;36:389–395.
7. Basso C, Thiene G, Corrado D, et al. Arrhythmogenic right ventricular cardiomyopathy. Dysplasia, dystrophy, or myocarditis? *Circulation.* 1996;94:983–991.
8. Thomas B, Tavares NJ. Is it myocarditis or arrhythmogenic right ventricular cardiomyopathy? *J Am Coll Cardiol.* 2009;54:663; author reply 665–666.
9. Lazzarini E, Jongbloed JD, Pilichou K, et al. The ARVD/C genetic variants database: 2014 update. *Hum Mutat.* 2015;36:403–410.
10. Romero J, Mejia-Lopez E, Manrique C, et al. Arrhythmogenic right ventricular cardiomyopathy (ARVC/D): a systematic literature review. *Clin Med Insights Cardiol.* 2013;7:97–114.
11. Gerull B, Heuser A, Wichter T, et al. Mutations in the desmosomal protein plakophilin-2 are common in arrhythmogenic right ventricular cardiomyopathy. *Nat Genet.* 2004;36:1162–1164.
12. Roux-Buisson N, Gandjbakhch E, Donal E, et al. Prevalence and significance of rare RYR2 variants in arrhythmogenic right ventricular cardiomyopathy/dysplasia: results of a systematic screening. *Heart Rhythm.* 2014;11:1999–2009.
13. Beffagna G, Occhi G, Nava A, et al. Regulatory mutations in transforming growth factor-beta3 gene cause arrhythmogenic right ventricular cardiomyopathy type 1. *Cardiovasc Res.* 2005;65:366–373.
14. Merner ND, Hodgkinson KA, Haywood AF, et al. Arrhythmogenic right ventricular cardiomyopathy type 5 is a fully penetrant, lethal arrhythmic disorder caused by a missense mutation in the TMEM43 gene. *Am J Hum Genet.* 2008;82:809–821.
15. Quarta G, Syrris P, Ashworth M, et al. Mutations in the Lamin A/C gene mimic arrhythmogenic right ventricular cardiomyopathy. *Eur Heart J.* 2012;33:1128–1136.
16. Milting H, Klauke B, Christensen AH, et al. The TMEM43 Newfoundland mutation p.S358L causing ARVC-5 was imported from Europe and increases the stiffness of the cell nucleus. *Eur Heart J.* 2015;36:872–881.
17. van Hengel J, Calore M, Bauce B, et al. Mutations in the area composita protein alphaT-catenin are associated with arrhythmogenic right ventricular cardiomyopathy. *Eur Heart J.* 2013;34:201–210.
18. van Tintelen JP, Van Gelder IC, Asimaki A, et al. Severe cardiac phenotype with right ventricular predominance in a large cohort of patients with a single missense mutation in the DES gene. *Heart Rhythm.* 2009;6:1574–1583.
19. Taylor M, Graw S, Sinagra G, et al. Genetic variation in titin in arrhythmogenic right ventricular cardiomyopathy-overlap syndromes. *Circulation.* 2011;124:876–885.
20. Haas J, Frese KS, Peil B, et al. Atlas of the clinical genetics of human dilated cardiomyopathy. *Eur Heart J.* 2015;36:1123–1135.
21. Thiene G, Corrado D, Basso C. Arrhythmogenic right ventricular cardiomyopathy/dysplasia. *Orphanet J Rare Dis.* 2007;2:45.
22. Thiene G, Nava A, Corrado D, et al. Right ventricular cardiomyopathy and sudden death in young people. *N Engl J Med.* 1988;318:129–133.
23. Richardson P, McKenna W, Bristow M, et al. Report of the 1995 World Health Organization/International Society and Federation of Cardiology Task Force on the Definition and Classification of cardiomyopathies. *Circulation.* 1996;93:841–842.
24. Sen-Chowdhry S, Syrris P, Ward D, et al. Clinical and genetic characterization of families with arrhythmogenic right ventricular dysplasia/cardiomyopathy provides novel insights into patterns of disease expression. *Circulation.* 2007;115:1710–1720.
25. Tavora F, Zhang M, Franco M, et al. Distribution of biventricular disease in arrhythmogenic cardiomyopathy: an autopsy study. *Hum Pathol.* 2012;43:592–596.
26. Ferreira AC, Garcia SA, Pasquale MA, et al. Arrhythmogenic right ventricular dysplasia in the elderly. *Heart Dis.* 2003;5:393–396.
27. Corrado D, Fontaine G, Marcus FI, et al. Arrhythmogenic right ventricular dysplasia/cardiomyopathy: need for an international registry. Study Group on Arrhythmogenic Right Ventricular Dysplasia/Cardiomyopathy of the Working Groups on Myocardial and Pericardial Disease and Arrhythmias of the European Society of Cardiology and of the Scientific Council on Cardiomyopathies of the World Heart Federation. *Circulation.* 2000;101:E101–E106.
28. Hamid MS, Norman M, Quraishi A, et al. Prospective evaluation of relatives for familial arrhythmogenic right ventricular cardiomyopathy/dysplasia reveals a need to broaden diagnostic criteria. *J Am Coll Cardiol.* 2002;40:1445–1450.
29. Burke AP, Robinson S, Radentz S, et al. Sudden death in right ventricular dysplasia with minimal gross abnormalities. *J Forensic Sci.* 1999;44:438–443.
30. Avella A, d'Amati G. Diagnosis of myocarditis mimicking arrhythmogenic right ventricular cardiomyopathy: the role of endomyocardial biopsy guided by electroanatomic voltage map. *J Am Coll Cardiol.* 2009;54:664–665; author reply 665–666.
31. Burke AP, Farb A, Tashko G, et al. Arrhythmogenic right ventricular cardiomyopathy and fatty replacement of the right ventricular myocardium: are they different diseases? *Circulation.* 1998;97:1571–1580.
32. Wingenfeld L, Freislederer A, Schulze-Bahr E, et al. Life-threatening hobbies in the youth? Two autoptic cases suggesting arrhythmogenic right ventricular cardiomyopathy. *Forensic Sci Int.* 2007;171:e1–e4.
33. Tansey DK, Aly Z, Sheppard MN. Fat in the right ventricle of the normal heart. *Histopathology.* 2005;46:98–104.
34. Voigt J, Agdal N. Lipomatous infiltration of the heart. An uncommon cause of sudden, unexpected death in a young man. *Arch Pathol Lab Med.* 1982;106:497–498.
35. Christensen AH, Svendsen JH. Myocarditis mimicking arrhythmogenic right ventricular cardiomyopathy. *J Am Coll Cardiol.* 2009;54:663–664; author reply 665–666.
36. Marcus FI, McKenna WJ, Sherrill D, et al. Diagnosis of arrhythmogenic right ventricular cardiomyopathy/dysplasia: proposed modification of the Task Force Criteria. *Eur Heart J.* 2010;31:806–814.
37. Silaghi A, Piercecchi-Marti MD, Grino M, et al. Epicardial adipose tissue extent: relationship with age, body fat distribution, and coronaropathy. *Obesity (Silver Spring).* 2008;16:2424–2430.

159 Left Ventricular Noncompaction

Allen P. Burke, M.D.

Definition

Left ventricular noncompaction is defined by prominent ventricular trabeculations, deep trabecular recesses, and a thin compacted layer, mostly involving the left ventricle, especially toward the apex.[1]

It is debated if it is a distinct cardiomyopathy or a secondary finding associated with other cardiomyopathies and congenital heart malformations.[1] It likely forms a spectrum, with secondary hypertrabeculation at one end and a primary cardiomyopathy at the other.

Incidence

Left ventricular noncompaction has been estimated to occur most often in infants (0.81 per 100,000 infants/year), followed by children (0.12 cases per 100,000 children/year) (21), and adults (prevalence 0.014%).[1]

The frequency of ventricular noncompaction among patients with established cardiomyopathy is 9.5% in children[2] and ranges from 3%[3] to 16%[4] in adults. In a clinical series of heart failure patients, ventricular noncompaction represented 3% of patients and 2% of all heart transplants.[5]

Clinical Findings

Left ventricular noncompaction may be an isolated finding or may be associated with other congenital heart anomalies (Table 159.1). When not associated with congenital heart disease, it can have dilated, hypertrophic, and restrictive phenotypes.[6] A substantial proportion of children improve clinically, but most of these have recurrent deterioration of their ejection fraction at a median interval of 6.3 years.[2]

In adults, the noncompaction form of nonischemic cardiomyopathy occurs at a somewhat younger age than does idiopathic dilated cardiomyopathy (mean age at diagnosis: 39 years). The prognosis is similar.[7]

Acquired, diagnosed by cardiac imaging, has been described in highly trained athletes, patients with sickle cell anemia, and pregnant patients and can be reversible.[1]

There have been rare reports with concomitant histiocytoid cardiomyopathy, suggesting a link with mitochondrial disease.[8,9]

Genetics

A proportion of cases of ventricular noncompaction are familial.[1,10] Mutations of several genes have been associated with LVNC. None is specific for the disease, and all have been reported in other phenotypes, most commonly dilated cardiomyopathy. Associated genes include *ACTC1* (actin, alpha, cardiac muscle); *DTNA* (dystrobrevin alpha); *LDB3* (domain-binding 3); *MIB1* (homolog of Drosophila mind bomb); *MYBPC3* (myosin-binding protein C, cardiac); *MYH7* (β-myosin heavy chain 7, cardiac muscle); *PRDM16* (PR domain-containing protein 16); *TAZ* (tafazzin); *TNNT2* (troponin T2); *TPM1* (tropomyosin 1); and *LMNA* (lamin A).[1,6,11] The association with tafazzin mutations suggests a pathogenetic link between noncompaction and Barth syndrome. Approximately one-half of patients with Barth syndrome demonstrate imaging features of ventricular noncompaction (see Chapter).

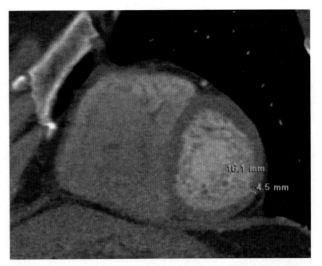

FIGURE 159.1 ▲ Left ventricular noncompaction. The diagnostic criterion by cardiac magnetic resonance is a noncompacted trabecular layer 2.4× thicker than the outer compact layer. (Figure courtesy Dr. Todd Villines.)

Imaging

The major finding in echocardiography and cardiac magnetic resonance is the presence of prominent trabeculations in the left ventricle, with involvement of apical and midsegments of the lateral and inferior walls. A noncompacted/compacted ratio >2.3 on cardiac magnetic resonance is considered the cutoff for the diagnosis of left ventricular noncompaction (Fig. 159.1).[1,6]

Gross Findings

Left ventricular noncompaction most frequently involves the apex and the adjacent parts of the lateral and inferior wall. It can be quite variable and focal.[1] Hypertrabeculations of the interventricular septum are rare.[10]

Three morphologic patterns have been described: polypoid trabeculations (Fig. 159.2), anastomosing trabeculae (Figs. 159.3 and 159.4),

TABLE 159.1   Conditions Associated with Ventricular Noncompaction (Selected)

- Coronary artery anomalies
- Conotruncal anomalies
  - Pulmonary atresia
  - Transposition of the great arteries
- Valve malformations
  - Absence of the pulmonary valve
  - Pulmonic stenosis
  - Tricuspid atresia
  - Ebstein anomaly
- Ventricular septal defect
- Atrial septal defect
- Hypoplastic heart syndrome
- Histiocytoid cardiomyopathy
- Barth syndrome
- DiGeorge syndrome (velocardiofacial/22q11.2 deletion syndrome)

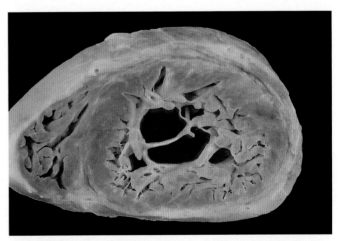

FIGURE 159.2 ▲ Left ventricular noncompaction. There is circumferential trabeculation of the left ventricle, without good formation of papillary muscles, even at the ventricular septum, which is said to be rare. Note the anomalous chord across the cavity, which is nonspecific but common in left ventricular noncompaction. (Figure courtesy Dr. Erik Mont.)

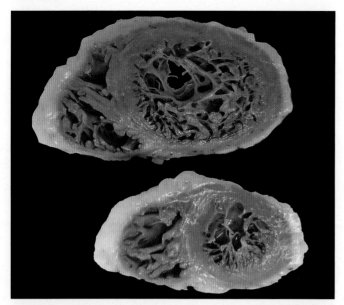

FIGURE 159.3 ▲ Left ventricular noncompaction, explant heart. The patient had end-stage ventricular function and clinical diagnosis of idiopathic dilated cardiomyopathy.

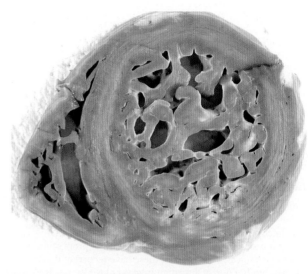

FIGURE 159.5 ▲ Left ventricular noncompaction. In this example, the ventricular cavity is replaced by anastomosing trabeculae of cardiac muscle, with areas of dense white endocardial fibrosis. (Reproduced with permission, Burke A, Mont E, Kutys R, et al. Left ventricular noncompaction: a pathological study of 14 cases. *Hum Pathol.* 2005;36:403–411, figure 1A.)

and spongy myocardium (Figs. 159.5 and 159.6).[9] A frequent additional finding is the presence of aberrant bands and false tendons in the left ventricular endocardium.

As has been appreciated by imaging, the diagnosis of left ventricular noncompaction requires an arbitrary cutoff between mildly hypertrabeculated myocardium and obvious disease. In normal hearts, more than three deep trabeculations were found in 4% of left ventricles, and more than five trabeculations were never found.[12]

Histologic Findings

Left ventricular noncompaction is diagnosed only at autopsy or explant and cannot be diagnosed by biopsy. The histologic findings are not specific and include endocardial fibrosis and a thickened trabecular layer, at least as thick as the compact layer (Fig. 159.7). The trabeculae are

often anastomosing, causing dilated endocardial-lined spaces, often with a staghorn configuration. There may be associated ischemic lesions in the thickened subendocardium.[9,13]

Prognosis

Complications of left ventricular noncompaction include heart failure, ventricular tachyarrhythmias, sudden cardiac death, and systemic embolic events. Atrial tachycardia and fibrillation are common.[1,6]

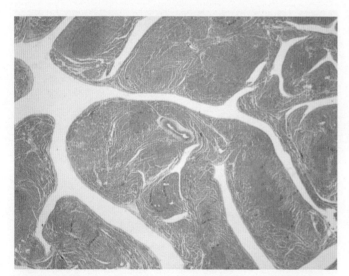

FIGURE 159.4 ▲ Left ventricular noncompaction. A histologic section hypertrabeculation, as well as patchy hypereosinophilia consistent with acute ischemia.

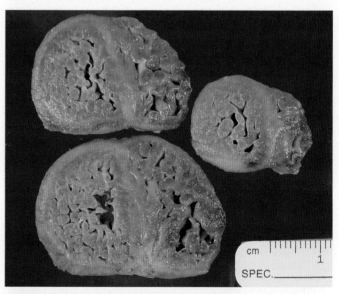

FIGURE 159.6 ▲ Left ventricular noncompaction, spongy myocardium. In infants, the appearance is that of a sponge. In these cases, there is a high incidence of associated anomalies. In this case, there was a coexistent ventricular septal defect (not shown).

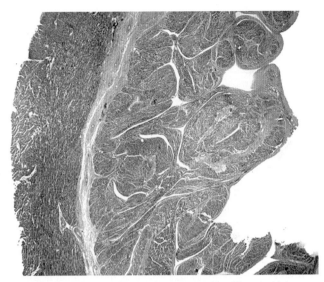

FIGURE 159.7 ▲ Left ventricular noncompaction, Masson trichrome stain. In some examples of noncompaction, the border zone between the compact myocardium (*left*) and the spongy myocardium (*right*) is well demarcated. Note the endocardial recesses among the trabeculae, with characteristic staghorn appearance. The noncompact region is much greater in thickness than the compact region at the left.

REFERENCES

1. Arbustini E, Weidemann F, Hall JL. Left ventricular noncompaction: a distinct cardiomyopathy or a trait shared by different cardiac diseases? *J Am Coll Cardiol.* 2014;64:1840–1850.

2. Pignatelli RH, McMahon CJ, Dreyer WJ, et al. Clinical characterization of left ventricular noncompaction in children: a relatively common form of cardiomyopathy. *Circulation.* 2003;108:2672–2678.
3. Sandhu R, Finkelhor RS, Gunawardena DR, et al. Prevalence and characteristics of left ventricular noncompaction in a community hospital cohort of patients with systolic dysfunction. *Echocardiography.* 2008;25:8–12.
4. Belanger AR, Miller MA, Donthireddi UR, et al. New classification scheme of left ventricular noncompaction and correlation with ventricular performance. *Am J Cardiol.* 2008;102:92–96.
5. Kovacevic-Preradovic T, Jenni R, Oechslin EN, et al. Isolated left ventricular noncompaction as a cause for heart failure and heart transplantation: a single center experience. *Cardiology.* 2009;112:158–164.
6. Parent JJ, Towbin JA, Jefferies JL. Left ventricular noncompaction in a family with lamin A/C gene mutation. *Tex Heart Inst J.* 2015;42:73–76.
7. Stanton C, Bruce C, Connolly H, et al. Isolated left ventricular noncompaction syndrome. *Am J Cardiol.* 2009;104:1135–1138.
8. Edston E, Perskvist N. Histiocytoid cardiomyopathy and ventricular noncompaction in a case of sudden death in a female infant. *Int J Legal Med.* 2009;123:47–53.
9. Burke A, Mont E, Kutys R, et al. Left ventricular noncompaction: a pathological study of 14 cases. *Hum Pathol.* 2005;36:403–411.
10. Stollberger C, Finsterer J, Blazek G. Left ventricular hypertrabeculation/noncompaction and association with additional cardiac abnormalities and neuromuscular disorders. *Am J Cardiol.* 2002;90:899–902.
11. Zuccarino F, Vollmer I, Sanchez G, et al. Left ventricular noncompaction: imaging findings and diagnostic criteria. *AJR Am J Roentgenol.* 2015;204:W519–W530.
12. Boyd MT, Seward JB, Tajik AJ, et al. Frequency and location of prominent left ventricular trabeculations at autopsy in 474 normal human hearts: implications for evaluation of mural thrombi by two-dimensional echocardiography. *J Am Coll Cardiol.* 1987;9:323–326.
13. Jenni R, Oechslin E, Schneider J, et al. Echocardiographic and pathoanatomical characteristics of isolated left ventricular non-compaction: a step towards classification as a distinct cardiomyopathy. *Heart.* 2001;86:666–671.

160 Miscellaneous Genetic Cardiomyopathies

Allen P. Burke, M.D., and Joseph J. Maleszewksi, M.D.

Infantile and Genetic Cardiomyopathy

A genetic basis underlies a majority of nonischemic cardiomyopathies (Chapters). In most cases of cardiomyopathy in adults, there are multiple genes and mutations that are associated with a particular phenotype (i.e., dilated, hypertrophic, arrhythmogenic, or noncompaction). In many examples, however, specific mutations or genes are associated with cardiomyopathy that typically presents at an early age and has extracardiac manifestations.

Although there is an overlap between familial cardiomyopathy and those associated with specific syndromes, the current chapter focuses on diseases that have a genetic basis, that often have extracardiac manifestations, that often occur in infants and children, and that are known by the specific mutation or by a specific eponym. The practice of renaming cardiomyopathy after a new mutational finding (e.g., desminopathy, laminopathy) has been discouraged.[1] Cardiomyopathies that are not defined by the mutational status or clinical syndrome but rather by cardiac clinicopathologic features are discussed in previous chapters.

Noonan Syndrome

Noonan syndrome is an autosomal dominant condition characterized by short stature, heart defects, pectus excavatum, webbed neck, learning problems, cryptorchidism, and facial dysmorphism.[2] It occurs in up to 1 in 1,000 live births.[3] Cardiovascular manifestations occur in 20% of patients and include cardiac hypertrophy (hypertrophic cardiomyopathy [HCM]-like phenotype), valvular dysplasias, atrial septal defect, ventricular septal defect, and patent ductus arteriosus (see Chapter 3).

Noonan syndrome and related conditions are caused by the dysregulation of the RAS–MAPK signaling pathway. Overall, mutations are found only in a subset of patients and include variants in *PTPN11* (about 50% of identified mutations), *SOS1* (13%), *RAF1* (5% to 15%), and *RIT1* (9%). Mutations of *KRAS, NRAS, SHOC2, BRAF, MEK1,* and *CBL* have also been reported.[2,3]

Pulmonary valve stenosis is the most common cardiovascular manifestation. The rate of HCM-like phenotype is as high as 70% in mutation-positive individuals and is frequently associated with pulmonary valve dysplasia with stenosis. There may be associated atrial and ventricular septal defects and mitral valve disease in up to one-third of these patients.[3]

The pathologic cardiac manifestations include generalized left ventricular hypertrophy and dome-shaped dysplastic pulmonic valves. Autopsy studies are few, and the pathologic features of the cardiomyopathy have not been studied.[4]

Myofiber disarray can occur in association with fibrosis (Fig. 160.1), but classic whorled appearance of sarcomeric HCM is not generally

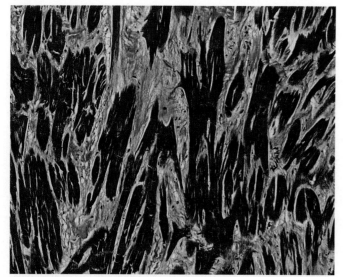

FIGURE 160.1 ▲ Noonan syndrome. There is myocyte hypertrophy and fibrosis, with mild disarray of myofibers. The histologic appearance is nonspecific. The diagnosis rests of constellation of clinical findings, including valve disorders, especially pulmonary stenosis (not shown) in addition to cardiomyopathy.

seen. Magnetic resonance imaging has demonstrated a subset of patients with myocardial bridges and left ventricular diverticula, crypts, and crevices.[5]

Friedreich Ataxia

Friedreich ataxia is the most common cause of inherited childhood-onset ataxia. It is an autosomal recessive disease caused by mutations in the human frataxin gene, *FXN*. Frataxin functions as a mitochondrial iron chaperone protein. Mutations result in abnormal accumulation of intramitochondrial iron, mitochondrial dysfunction, and oxidative damage.[6,7]

Cardiac manifestations of *Friedreich ataxia* occur at an older age than do the neurologic symptoms, generally in early adulthood. Up to 90% of patients will demonstrate cardiac abnormalities on echocardiography. Approximately 20% of patients will develop a hypokinetic dilated cardiomyopathy phenotype that may be fatal. Earlier phases of the cardiomyopathy are characterized by cardiac hypertrophy, which may be asymmetric or concentric.

The severity of left ventricular hypertrophy is related to the number of GAA repeats in the first intron of *FXN*. Pathologically, the heart is dilated and hypertrophied.[6] Histologically, there is diffuse interstitial fibrosis, patchy chronic inflammation, and endocardial fibrosis.[6] Small-vessel disease of intramural coronary arteries has also been described.[8]

Cardiomyopathy in patients with Friedreich ataxia may be exacerbated by diabetic ketoacidosis and Graves disease.[9] Sudden death has been reported as the initial manifestation of cardiac symptoms with diagnosis made by postmortem molecular testing.[6]

Myotonic Dystrophy

Myotonic dystrophy is an autosomal recessive disease involving facial, neck, and distal limb muscles. There are two types with differing genetic etiologies. Type 1 (Steinert disease) is caused by mutations in *DMPK*. Type 2 (proximal myotonic myopathy) is a milder form of the disease caused by mutations in *ZNF9*.

Cardiac involvement manifests most commonly as conduction defects, which may occur in the absence of severe skeletal disease and occur in the majority of patients. First-degree heart block is the most common abnormality, followed by ventricular tachycardia. Rarely, the

progression of the disease can lead to sudden, unpredictable death. Conduction electrophysiologic studies are generally performed to guide implantation of defibrillators.[10]

Histologic findings are nonspecific. There is typically fibrosis of the bundle of His and proximal bundle branches.[11] Myocytes show nonspecific hypertrophy with occasional vacuoles and disarray.[11] Electron microscopic findings include prominent I bands and myofibrillar degeneration.[12]

X-Lined Muscular Dystrophy

Duchenne and the milder *Becker* muscular dystrophies are caused by mutations in the dystrophin gene *DMD*, located at Xp21. *Dystrophin* is a cytoskeletal protein that provides structural support to the myocyte and links the sarcomeric contractile apparatus to the sarcolemma and extracellular matrix.

Duchenne muscular dystrophy (DMD) is most commonly caused by deletion of one or more exons, with duplications, single nucleotide variant, and splicing variants causing a lower percentage of total cases. In patients that survive past the age of 18, development of cardiomyopathy (dilated phenotype) is the rule. In fact, with improvements in treatment for respiratory and other complications, the cardiomyopathy is thought to account for most deaths in DMD (either heart failure or arrhythmia). Pathologically, there is myocardial fibrosis that is typically interstitial, although transmural scars may occur. The changes are most marked in the posterobasal region and adjacent lateral wall of the left ventricle.[13]

In ~6% of men with idiopathic dilated cardiomyopathy without skeletal myopathy, defects in the dystrophin gene may be identified.[14] Overall, X-linked inheritance accounts for between 2% and 5% of familial cases of dilated cardiomyopathy that manifests in young men with rapidly progressive heart failure.[15]

The presence of increased serum creatine phosphokinase (SCPK) is suggestive of the disease in men with a history of X-linked cardiomyopathy. Mutational analysis for pathogenic mutations in the dystrophic gene DMD is diagnostic, and immunohistochemical staining for dystrophin may also be helpful (Fig. 160.2).

Female carriers develop a milder form of cardiomyopathy, usually in their 50s. Immunohistochemical stains for dystrophin reveal a patchy loss of dystrophin, with scattered myocytes showing no staining in a mosaic pattern.[16] Cardiac findings are similar to those in males, with biventricular dilation and diffuse fibrous replacement.[16] The right ventricular free wall may become thin and replaced by fibrofatty tissue, mimicking arrhythmogenic right ventricular cardiomyopathy.[16]

Becker dystrophy is also the result of mutations in the *DMD* gene, but unlike DMD, some protein is produced. These individuals usually manifest a milder phenotype, but most (70%) will also develop cardiomyopathy, which, like DMD, is a common cause of mortality.[17]

Cardiac Involvement in Emery-Dreifuss and Myofibrillar Myopathies/Muscular Dystrophies

Emery-Dreifuss muscular dystrophy is a myopathy that causes cardiac dysrhythmias, late-onset heart failure, and progressive skeletal myopathy characterized by contractures of the neck, elbows, and ankles. It was generally considered an X-linked disease, although autosomal dominant forms have been more recently described. It is an example of a nuclear "envelopathy," or "laminopathy" caused by mutations of genes that encode proteins of the nuclear envelope. Mutations in the *EMD* gene, encoding emerin, cause the X-linked form, while *LMNA* gene mutations are responsible for autosomal forms, which manifest as a dilated phenotype (see Chapter 19).[18]

Mutations in *LMNA* also cause a related condition, limb girdle myotonic dystrophy type 1B.[19] Endomyocardial biopsy specimens show only nonspecific findings.[20]

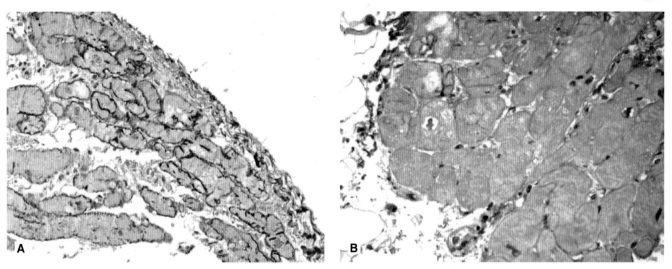

FIGURE 160.2 ▲ Duchenne cardiomyopathy. **A.** Immunohistochemical staining showing normal cytoplasmic dystrophin reactivity. **B.** Decreased expression is seen in male with sporadic cardiomyopathy in whom cardiac symptoms predated skeletal muscle disease. (Reproduced Arbustini E, Narula N, Dec GW, et al. The MOGE(S) classification for a phenotype-genotype nomenclature of cardiomyopathy: endorsed by the World Heart Federation. *J Am Coll Cardiol.* 2013;62:2046–2072, with permission.)

The "myofibrillar myopathies" (see Chapter 27) are characterized by myofibrillar disorganization of the Z-disk progressing to myofibrillar degradation in the adjacent sarcomere.[21] The pathologic diagnosis of myofibrillar myopathy is established by skeletal muscle biopsy in which hyaline deposits are present that may be congophilic. Cardiac involvement is most frequent in myofibrillar myopathies caused by mutations in desmin and zaspin (so-called desminopathy and zaspopathy, respectively).

Barth Syndrome

X-linked dilated cardiomyopathy in male infants is most frequently caused by Barth syndrome (dilated cardiomyopathy, skeletal myopathy, growth retardation, and neutropenia).[22] Male neonates or young infants present with congestive heart failure, neutropenia, and 3-methylglutaconic aciduria. Children die in infancy from progressive heart failure, sudden death, or sepsis. The pathologic findings are nonspecific, but imaging studies demonstrate that at least one-half of patients have left ventricular noncompaction.[23]

Barth syndrome is caused by mutations in the tafazzin gene (*TAZ*) on chromosome Xq28. Heart failure is common as patients survive childhood and is caused by cardiomyopathy with both a dilated and noncompaction phenotype, as well as endocardial fibroelastosis (EFE).[24]

Inborn Errors of Carbohydrate Metabolism (Tables 160.1 to 160.4)

Pompe Disease

Pompe disease is an autosomal recessive glycogen storage disease (infantile type IIa) caused by α-1,4 glycosidase (acid maltase) deficiency. Of the glycogen storage diseases, types II to IV may cause cardiac dysfunction in infants and young children. Type V glycogen storage disease (McArdle disease) rarely involves the heart.[35] Affected infants have profound cardiac dysfunction, with large accumulations of glycogen in cardiac myocytes. There is massive cardiomegaly and typically biventricular dilatation (Fig. 160.3). Diagnosis is made by accumulation of PAS-positive (diastase-labile) vacuoles diffusely throughout myocytes (Fig. 160.4) and, at autopsy, in other affected organs (skeletal muscles, liver, and nervous system).

Danon Cardiomyopathy

Defects in lysosome-associated membrane protein 2 (LAMP-2) cause the X-linked cardiomyopathy "Danon disease" (type IIb). Clinical manifestations are limited largely to the heart, usually with massive degrees of LV hypertrophy and ventricular preexcitation.[36] Skeletal myopathy occurs in about 20% of patients.[37]

TABLE 160.1   Cardiac Involvement in Glycogen Storage Diseases[a]

Inborn Error	Cardiac Involvement	Dominant Involvement	Diagnostic Tests
Type IIa (Pompe), lysosomal acid α-glucosidase (*GAA*)	Cardiomyopathy, infantile	Skeletal myopathy, hypotonia, macroglossia	Glycogen vacuoles in myocytes Decreased enzyme activity in skin fibroblasts/genetic testing
Type IIb (Danon) lysosomal membrane protein-2 (*LAMP2*)	Hypertrophic cardiomyopathy	Similar to Pompe, degree dependent on residual enzyme activity	Decreased enzyme activity in muscle/genetic testing Ultrastructural lysosomal vacuoles in heart muscle
Over 10 entities, including McArdle, Andersen, von Gierke, Hers (type VI), Forbes disease	None/minimal	Hypoglycemia, myopathy, various others	Decrease enzyme activity in liver (types I, III, VI, VIII/IX), muscle (III, VII, VIII/IX), skin fibroblasts (IV), RBCs (VII), lack of increased venous lactate with forearm ischemia (V, VII)
PRKAG2 mutation	Cardiomyopathy Conduction defect	Skeletal myopathy	Glycogen vacuoles in heart muscle Genetic testing

[a]There is no significant cardiac involvement in other carbohydrate metabolism disorders, such as galactosemia, fructose disorders, and pyruvate carboxylase/dehydrogenase deficiency.

TABLE 160.2   Cardiac Involvement in Inborn Errors of Metabolism: Fatty Acid Oxidation and Glycerol Metabolism Disorders

Inborn Error	Cardiac Involvement	Dominant Involvement	Diagnostic Tests
Fatty acid (β-oxidation cycle)			
Medium-chain acyl dehydrogenase	Minimal	Neonatal vomiting, lethargy, acidosis, SIDS like; episodic	Plasma/urine medium-chain fatty acid conjugates of carnitine; enzyme deficiency in cultured fibroblasts Genetic testing
Long-chain hydroxyacyl-CoA dehydrogenase	Cardiomyopathy	Myopathy with exertion; HELLP in mothers of affected fetuses	Plasma acylcarnitine and acylglycine profile; enzyme study in skin fibroblasts
Very long-chain hydroxyacyl-CoA dehydrogenase	Cardiomyopathy dominant	Myopathy	Acylcarnitine profile in serum or blood; enzyme activity in skin fibroblasts
Glycerol metabolism			
Glycerol kinase	Association with Duchenne muscular dystrophy	Acidosis, hypoglycemia	Elevated blood and urine glycerol

TABLE 160.3   Cardiac Involvement in Lysosomal Storage Disease

Inborn Error	Cardiac Involvement	Dominant Involvement	Diagnostic Tests
Mucopolysaccharidoses			
MPS I, Hurlers (α-L-iduronidase) MPS II, Hunter, (iduronate sulfate sulfatase) MPS IV, Morquio MPS VI, Maroteaux-Lamy	Mitral and aortic valve disease, infiltration of macrophages MPS I, II, IV, VI[25-28]	Coarse facies, CNS symptoms, joint and skeletal involvement, organomegaly, airway obstruction	Enzyme analysis of cultured fibroblasts (prenatal) or peripheral WBCs (postnatal)
Sphingolipidoses[a]			
Gaucher (glucocerebrosidase)	Cardiomyopathy with interstitial infiltrates of Gaucher cells[29]	Hepatosplenomegaly, skeletal disease, growth failure, delayed puberty, ecchymoses	Enzyme analysis of WBC
Niemann-Pick (sphingomyelinase)	Uncommon; coronary and valve disease[30]	Neonatal hepatosplenomegaly, rapidly progressive neurodegeneration	WBC enzyme assay; neonatal screening
Fabry (α-galactosidase A)	Cardiomyopathy	Angiokeratomas, acroparesthesias, corneal opacities, recurrent febrile episodes, renal failure	Enzyme assay on serum or WBCs Vacuolated cardiomyocytes, with lamellar bodies

[a]There is no significant cardiac involvement in Tay-Sachs disease or Wolman disease (liposomal acid lipase deficiency).

TABLE 160.4   Cardiac Involvement in Inborn Errors of Metabolism: Mitochondrial and Peroxisomal Disorders

Inborn Error	Cardiac Involvement	Dominant Involvement	Diagnostic Tests
Mitochondrial oxidative phosphorylation disorders[a]			
MELAS (Mutations in the mitochondrial *tRNA leu* gene)	Cardiomyopathy	Neurodegenerative, myopathy, periodic lactic acidosis	Lactic acidosis with increase in the lactate to pyruvate ratio Genetic testing for gene mutation
Kearns-Sayre Mitochondrial transfer RNA genes	Cardiomyopathy Atrioventricular block[31] Bradycardia-related polymorphic ventricular tachycardia	Ophthalmoplegia, ptosis, atypical retinitis pigmentosa, ragged red fiber myopathy, ataxia, deafness	Clinical, skeletal biopsy findings (ragged red fibers), genetic testing (mitochondrial DNA deletions); elevated lactic acid; cardiac ultrastructure (mitochondrial abnormalities)[32]
Leber hereditary optic neuropathy (mtDNA mutations m.11778G>A, m.3460G>A m.14484T>C)	Arrhythmias[33]	Blindness, children and young adults, maternal inheritance	Clinical; genetic testing
Leigh syndrome (heterogeneous; LRPPRC and mitochondrial DNA mutations)	Conduction disorders, Wolff-Parkinson-White syndrome[34] Hypertrophic cardiomyopathy	Encephalopathy, basal ganglia degeneration, lactic academia, ptosis, infantile apnea	CNS imaging with increased lactate in CSF; genetic testing
Peroxisomal disorders			
Refsum disease (phytanoyl-CoA hydroxylase)	Conduction defects Cardiomyopathy (uncommon)	Early adult peripheral neuropathy, retinitis pigmentosa, hearing deficit, anosmia, ichthyosis	Elevated VLCFA levels Elevated serum phytanic acid Decreased pristanic acid

[a]There is no significant cardiac involvement in myoclonic epilepsy with ragged red fibers (mitochondrial *tRNA lys* gene mutations).

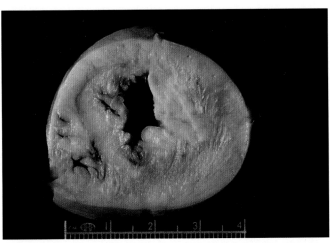

FIGURE 160.3 ▲ Pompe disease (acid maltase deficiency, infantile type II glycogen storage disease). The gross appearance is nonspecific and consists of biventricular hypertrophy.

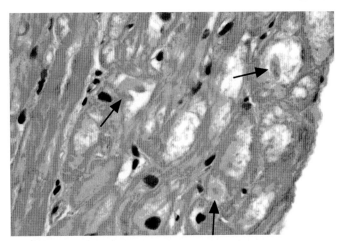

FIGURE 160.5 ▲ *PRKAG2*-associated cardiomyopathy. Endomyocardial biopsy shows nonspecific vacuolization. (Reproduced from Selcen D. Myofibrillar myopathies. *Curr Opin Neurol.* 2010;23:477–481, with permission.)

The diagnosis is confirmed by sequencing *LAMP2* gene from peripheral lymphocytes. It has been shown that 4% of children with HCM actually have *LAMP-2* mutations diagnostic of Danon cardiomyopathy.[38] The disease often progresses from a hypertrophic to dilated phenotype. The disease should be suspected in children with HCM, preexcitation of Wolff-Parkinson-White syndrome, and skeletal myopathy.

There are few pathologic studies of Danon cardiomyopathy. Grossly, the hearts are characterized by marked concentric hypertrophy.[37] Vacuolization may be minimal on endomyocardial biopsy and is often more pronounced in skeletal muscle. The vacuoles are the result of increased autophagic vacuoles seen ultrastructurally.[39] Women may develop disease in adulthood, unlike males that usually present in childhood.

PRKAG2-Associated Cardiomyopathy

A recently described autosomal dominant cardiac syndrome combines cardiac hypertrophy, ventricular preexcitation (Wolff-Parkinson-White syndrome), and progressive atrioventricular conduction block. *PRKAG2*-associated cardiomyopathy has been related to mutations in the gene encoding the G2 subunit of AMP-activated protein kinase (*PRKAG2*). Because decreased activity of the protein results in glycogen

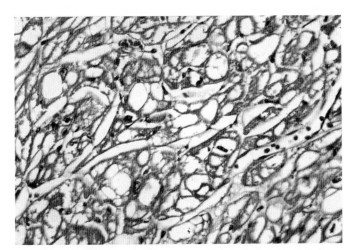

FIGURE 160.4 ▲ Pompe disease (acid maltase deficiency). There is diffuse vacuolization of myocytes. The material is PAS-positive (not shown) glycogen.

deposition in striated muscle cells, it has been considered a novel form of glycogen storage disease.[40]

The major effect of mutations in *PRKAG2* is to reduce activation of AMPK in response to stress. Affected patients present in late adolescence with paroxysmal supraventricular tachycardia, preexcitation, and progression to heart block. There is a frequent requirement for placement of a pacemaker device by fourth to fifth decades of life. Symptomatic skeletal myopathy occurs in fewer than half of patients.

The phenotype of the cardiomyopathy is hypertrophic. The clinical triad of cardiac hypertrophy, progressive conduction system disease, and ventricular preexcitation is also encountered in Pompe disease and Danon disease, two other glycogen storage diseases (see above).[41]

There are few pathologic studies of *PRKAG2*-associated cardiomyopathy. Cardiac findings include PAS-positive, diastase-labile, vacuoles containing polysaccharides diffusely throughout the myocardium[42] (Fig. 160.5). Skeletal muscle biopsies show PAS-positive, diastase-labile subsarcolemmal vacuoles, and ultrastructure shows nonlysosomal glycogen accumulation, with abundant granular nonmembrane-bound electron-dense material.[40]

Cardiac Involvement in Disorders of Fatty Acid Oxidation

Disorders of fatty acid oxidation include defects in medium-chain, long-chain, and very long-chain hydroxyacyl-CoA dehydrogenase (Table 160.2), with increasing incidence of cardiac involvement. Most infants present with skeletal myopathy and diffuse weakness. Presentation is typically in neonates, and often, there is a request for postmortem genetic testing for children who die in the hospital. Culture of skin fibroblasts may be requested to test for enzyme activities. Acylcarnitine and acylglycine blood profiles are also helpful in establishing a diagnosis.

Genetic tests for mutations underlying the disorders include probes for mutations in medium-chain acyl-CoA dehydrogenase (*MCAD*) gene, short-chain acyl-CoA dehydrogenase (*SCAD*) gene, long-chain 3-hydroxy acyl-CoA dehydrogenase (*LCHAD*) gene, and carnitine-palmitoyl-CoA transferase II (*CPTII*) gene.[43,44]

Lysosomal Storage Diseases

This group of diseases includes the mucopolysaccharidoses (MPS I to VI) and the sphingolipidoses. Cardiac involvement is not infrequent (Table 160.3). The pathologic manifestations generally include the accumulation of intracytoplasmic material, especially in macrophages, but also in the myocardium.

Mucopolysaccharidoses are characterized by defects in the ability of lysosomes to catabolize glycosaminoglycans and result often in short stature, progressive coarsening of facial features, skeletal abnormalities, corneal clouding, mental retardation, and cardiovascular effects. Valve disease is the most common cardiac manifestation. Enzyme deficiencies that prevent glycosaminoglycan breakdown cause accumulation of glycosaminoglycan fragments in lysosomes.

Sphingolipidoses characteristically result in the lysosomal accumulation of sphingolipids, which are normal lipid components of cell membranes, because of congenital enzyme deficiencies.

Hurler Syndrome

Hurler syndrome (type I) is the most common mucopolysaccharidoses and is caused by α-L-iduronate deficiency. Children develop progressive cardiac symptoms due to increased proteoglycans primarily in the heart valves. Other areas of cardiac involvement include the endocardium, myocardium, and coronary arteries. Large vacuolated fibroblasts, known as Hurler cells, are seen by light microscopy.

By ultrastructure, granular cells are observed in the coronary arteries, in the atrioventricular valves, and in the myocardial interstitium. Deposits of acid mucopolysaccharides can be seen in smooth muscle cells by routine microscopy but usually not in cardiomyocytes, where electron microscopy is necessary. Narrowing of the extramural coronary arteries, thickening of the cardiac valves (the left-sided more than the right-sided valves), and endocardial fibrosis can be appreciated grossly. Microscopically, "Hurler cells" in the valves are clear and immunophenotypically resemble activated myofibroblasts.[25,45] Other mucopolysaccharidoses may result in valve disease (Table 160.3).

Gaucher Disease

Gaucher disease is a sphingolipidosis caused by deficiency of glucocerebrosidase. It is the most common of the lysosomal storage disorders with an incidence of ~1:40,000. The main clinical features of adult Gaucher disease are hepato- and splenomegaly, bone marrow infiltration leading to cytopenias, and skeletal involvement leading to bone pain and pathologic fracture. Cardiac involvement is uncommon and may lead to cardiomyopathy, valve disease, and pericardial thickening due to infiltration of glucocerebroside within myocytes and stromal cells.[46] Valve involvement can lead to progressive calcification.[47-49]

Fabry Disease

Fabry disease (Anderson-Fabry disease; angiokeratoma corporis diffusum) is an X-linked genetic disorder caused by the deficiency of α-galactosidase A, resulting in the lysosomal accumulation of glycosphingolipids, including globotriaosylceramide. It affects ~1 in 40,000 to 60,000 men. Endothelial accumulation is thought to cause the progressive renal insufficiency and CNS pathology in Fabry patients, whereas the accumulation of lamellar bodies is seen with cardiac myocytes.

The diagnosis is made on the basis of low plasma α-galactosidase A activity and mutational analysis of the *GLA* gene. Dermal and extremities signs of the disease first appear in the childhood and include severe pain in the extremities, corneal and lenticular changes, and skin lesions (angiokeratomas). It has been suggested that ~3% of men with unexplained left ventricular hypertrophy suffer from a homozygous form of Fabry disease.[50] Cardiac disease also occurs in female heterozygotes, albeit at a later age than in males.

Up to 60% of affected men have cardiac abnormalities, including left ventricular hypertrophy, arrhythmias, valvular dysfunction, and conduction abnormalities. Disease onset is typically in the fourth decade for men and the fifth for women. Infiltration of the conduction system is responsible for heart block and tachy- and bradyarrhythmias. Accumulation of lipid causes fibrosis of the valves, especially the mitral and aortic leaflets.[51]

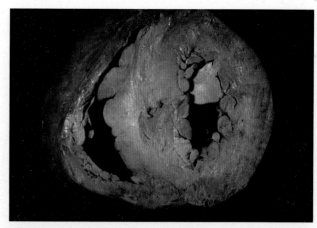

FIGURE 160.6 ▲ Fabry disease. The gross appearance is that of biventricular hypertrophy, often with septal asymmetry mimicking hypertrophic cardiomyopathy.

Isolated cardiac Fabry disease without extracardiac manifestations may represent 5% to 15% of men evaluated for left ventricular hypertrophy/HCM.[52]

Grossly, Fabry disease shows concentric hypertrophy, but a gross appearance indistinguishable from asymmetric hypertrophy seen in HCM can occur (Fig. 160.6). Histologically, there are vacuolated myocytes diffusely throughout the ventricles (Fig. 160.7). However, in women, mosaicism may lead to a more focal or patchy distribution of vacuolization. Areas of disarray may be present around scars. Electron microscopy shows characteristic myelin-like inclusions in hypertrophic vacuolated cells with electron-dense concentric lamellar bodies corresponding to glycosphingolipid, which is predominantly globotriaosylceramide.[53]

Histologically, vacuolated cells are present in valves as well as myocytes. The presence of atrioventricular block is correlated with glycosphingolipid accumulation in the atrioventricular node and bundle of His.[54]

Endomyocardial biopsy has been used to assess the response to treatment with recombinant alpha galactosidase. Specifically, treatment results in a decrease in capillary endothelial deposits of globotriaosylceramide as assessed by ultrastructure.[55]

Mitochondrial and Peroxisomal Disorders (Table 160.4)

Mitochondrial disease is the most common metabolic cause of dilated cardiomyopathy, accounting for 46% of cases.[56] After mitochondrial conditions, the most common metabolic disorders are Barth syndrome (24% of metabolic causes) and primary or systemic fatty acid oxidation deficiencies (11%).[57] These disorders include MELAS (mitochondrial encephalomyopathy, lactic acidosis, and stroke-like episodes), myoclonic epilepsy with ragged red fibers, Kearns-Sayre syndrome, Leber hereditary optic neuropathy, and Leigh syndrome (Table 160.4).

Electron microscopy may show altered mitochondrial morphology, including concentric cristae that form bizarre, haphazard, and often undulating shapes, sometimes associated with giant mitochondria measuring >4 to 5 times the normal (up to 10 μm). Electron-dense mitochondrial inclusions and calcifications may also be present. About one-fifth of cases with mitochondrial abnormalities demonstrate potentially pathogenetic heteroplasmic mutations of mitochondrial DNA.[58]

Kearns-Sayre Syndrome

Kearns-Sayre syndrome is a mitochondrial disorder caused by mutations in mitochondrial transfer RNA genes. Kearns and Sayre first described a constellation of features constituting progressive external ophthalmoplegia, pigmentary retinopathy, and cardiac conduction disorder in 1958.[59] The classic triad, which occurs before age 20, is progressive external ophthalmoplegia, pigmentary retinal degeneration,

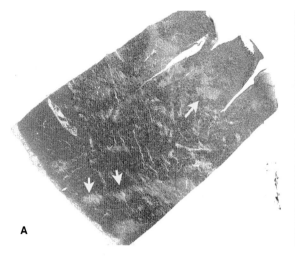

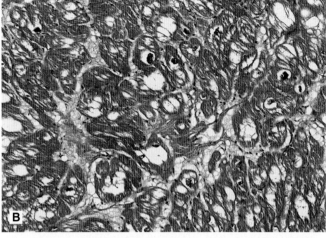

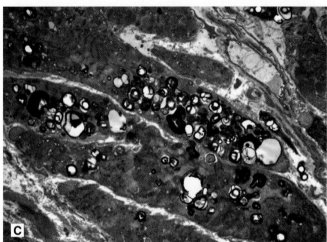

FIGURE 160.7 ▲ Fabry disease. **A.** A low magnification shows patchy areas of lighter staining (*arrows*). **B.** There areas correspond to generalized vacuolization of cardiomyocytes. The histologic appearance is not specific; the diagnosis rests on the finding of decreased α-galactosidase A levels and mutations in the *GLA* gene. **C.** Ultrastructure will demonstrate myelin figures. (Reproduced from Arbustini E, Narula N, Dec GW, et al. The MOGE(S) classification for a phenotype-genotype nomenclature of cardiomyopathy: endorsed by the World Heart Federation. *J Am Coll Cardiol.* 2013;62:2046–2072, with permission.)

and one of the following: complete heart block, cerebellar dysfunction, and cerebrospinal fluid protein above 100 mg/dL.[60] Other abnormalities include nystagmus, ataxia, vestibular dysfunction, corticospinal dysfunction, and widespread muscular dystrophy.

Kearns-Sayre syndrome typically affects the heart, causing cardiac conduction defects, progressing to complete heart block manifesting as congestive heart failure, syncope, or sudden death in up to 57% of patients.[60]

Peroxisomal Diseases

Peroxisomes are intracellular organelles that contain enzymes for β-oxidation. These enzymes overlap in function with those in mitochondria, although mitochondria lack enzymes to metabolize very long-chain fatty acids. Therefore, peroxisomal disorders generally manifest with elevated levels of very long-chain fatty acids.

Refsum disease is most often caused by mutations in *PHYH* (phytanoyl-CoA-2 hydroxylase), a peroxisomal protein, resulting in its

deficiency. Other genes, such as *PEX7*, have also been implicated.[61] Phytanic acid accumulates in tissue lipids and in plasma. Neurologic symptoms include retinitis pigmentosa, night blindness, and anosmia. Cardiac symptoms include conduction defects and arrhythmias.[62]

Diseases of Amino Acid Metabolism (Table 160.5)

Ochronosis

Ochronosis is a rare disorder of tyrosine metabolism due to a deficiency of the enzyme homogentisic acid oxidase. Also called alkaptonuria, it is characterized by homogentisic aciduria, bluish-black discoloration of connective tissues and arthropathy. Less common manifestations include cardiovascular abnormalities, renal, urethral, and prostatic calculi. The cardiovascular system is affected primarily on the valves. The aortic valve is the most commonly affected, with stenosis and black discoloration. Coronary disease can also occur in up to 50% of cases by

TABLE 160.5 Cardiac Involvement in Inborn Errors of Metabolism: Amino Acid Metabolism[a]

Inborn Error	Cardiac Involvement	Dominant Involvement	Diagnostic Tests
Alkaptonuria	Black pigment in valves, aorta	Joints	Elevated urine homogentisic acid
Methionine (homocystinuria) cystathionine-β-synthase, methionine synthase, MTHFR	Increased risk for thromboembolism and atherosclerosis	Ectopia lentis, intellectual impairment, ataxia, megaloblastic anemia	Elevated serum methionine, urine homocysteine; enzyme levels

[a]There is no significant cardiac involvement in phenylketonuria, tyrosinemia, branched-chain amino acid deficiencies or urea cycle disorders.

imaging and is characterized by discoloration and calcification. Other manifestations include pigmentation of the endocardium, mitral valve, pericardium, and aortic intima.[63,64] It is thought that the deposition of homogentisic acid within the valves may hasten calcific degeneration.

Homocystinuria

Homocystinuria is a disorder of methionine metabolism, resulting in abnormal accumulation of homocysteine and its metabolites (e.g., homocysteine, homocysteine–cysteine complex) in blood and urine. Patients with homocystinuria may first be recognized because of downward dislocation of the lens (ectopia lentis), Marfan-like appearance, mental retardation, and seizures. Abnormalities manifest themselves by age 3 to 4 years. Heterozygous have hyperhomocysteinemia—raised plasma homocysteine levels with no homocystinuria. Their risk of premature cardiovascular disease is increased and includes increased risk for thromboembolism, premature and accelerated coronary artery disease, and mitral valve prolapse.[65–67] Coronary artery lesions in patients with elevated homocysteine tend to be rich in fibrous tissue.[68]

Hyperoxaluria

Primary hyperoxaluria is a hereditary disease that comes in three forms: types I and II primary hyperoxaluria are alterations of metabolism resulting in the production of excess oxalate ions, while type III is caused by increased oxalate absorption by the gastrointestinal tract. All three types are characterized by chronic renal failure. The disease most commonly affects multiple organ systems, especially the kidney, myocardium, and thyroid, where deposits of oxalate crystals can be found.[69] In the heart, the deposits can cause a restrictive hemodynamics, heart blocks, and calcification of the coronary arteries.[69] Oxalate crystal deposits can be observed in vessels with polarized light. Cardiac manifestations have been reported to reverse with normalization of serum oxalate levels.

Primary Endocardial Fibroelastosis

Definition

EFE in children is considered by some to be a manifestation of otherwise dilated cardiomyopathy (owing to abnormal flow dynamics in poorly functioning ventricles) and by others to be a distinct entity.[70] It is defined pathologically as diffuse thickening of the left ventricular endocardium with elevation of the papillary muscles and thickening of the free edge of the mitral valve leaflets.

Incidence

Although the incidence of EFE is not known, it accounted for over 25% of pediatric heart transplants with dilated cardiomyopathy.[70]

Etiology

The etiology of EFE is unknown, although theories include viral myocarditis, metabolic disorders, genetic (*EFE1* and *EFE2*), abnormal immune responses, and congenital malformations.

Clinical

Patients are children with intractable heart failure. Most have a clinical diagnosis of idiopathic dilated cardiomyopathy. Mean age at transplant is 10 months; there may be a female predilection.[70]

Pathologic Findings

There is diffuse thickening of the endocardium, typically left ventricular, with a ceramic white appearance (Fig. 160.8). Unlike dilated cardiomyopathy, mural thrombi are not found, and there is little if any interstitial fibrosis. The endocardium is greatly thickened by fibrosis and elastic tissue, and the subendocardial layer typically shows myocytolysis.

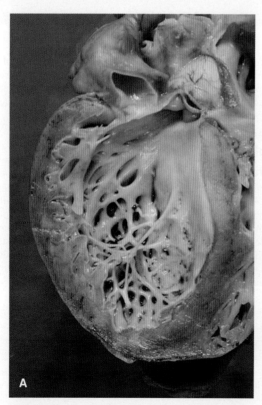
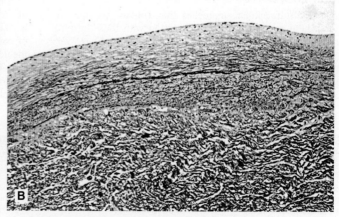

FIGURE 160.8 ▲ Idiopathic endocardial fibroelastosis. The patient was a 6½-month-old girl who was found dead. **A.** The left ventricular endocardium shows diffuse thickening, and the mitral valve is elevated. **B.** The thickened endocardium shows both fibrosis and elastosis.

REFERENCES

1. Arbustini E, Narula N, Dec GW, et al. The MOGE(S) classification for a phenotype-genotype nomenclature of cardiomyopathy: endorsed by the World Heart Federation. *J Am Coll Cardiol.* 2013;62:2046–2072.

2. Carapito R, Paul N, Untrau M, et al. A new mutation in the C-SH2 domain of PTPN11 causes Noonan syndrome with multiple giant cell lesions. *J Hum Genet.* 2014;59:57–59.

3. Aoki Y, Niihori T, Banjo T, et al. Gain-of-function mutations in RIT1 cause Noonan syndrome, a RAS/MAPK pathway syndrome. *Am J Hum Genet.* 2013;93:173–180.

4. Tanimura A, Hayashi I, Adachi K, et al. Noonan syndrome with hypertrophic obstructive cardiomyopathy. *Acta Pathol Jpn.* 1977;27:225–230.

5. Martinez-Quintana E, Rodriguez-Gonzalez F, Junquera-Rionda P. Noonan syndrome and different morphologic expressions of hypertrophic cardiomyopathy. *Pediatr Cardiol.* 2013;34:1871–1873.

6. Quercia N, Somers GR, Halliday W, et al. Friedreich ataxia presenting as sudden cardiac death in childhood: clinical, genetic and pathological correlation, with implications for genetic testing and counselling. *Neuromuscul Disord.* 2010;20:340–342.

7. Gulati V, Harikrishnan P, Palaniswamy C, et al. Cardiac involvement in hemochromatosis. *Cardiol Rev.* 2014;22:56–68.

8. Meyer C, Schmid G, Gorlitz S, et al. Cardiomyopathy in Friedreich's ataxia-assessment by cardiac MRI. *Mov Disord.* 2007;22:1615–1622.

9. Snyder M, Seyer L, Lynch DR, et al. Cardiac dysfunction exacerbated by endocrinopathies in Friedreich ataxia: a case series. *J Child Neurol.* 2012;27:1316–1319.

10. Khalighi K, Kodali A, Thapamagar SB, et al. Cardiac involvement in myotonic dystrophy. *J Community Hosp Intern Med.* 2015;5:25319.

11. Nguyen HH, Wolfe JT III, Holmes DR Jr, et al. Pathology of the cardiac conduction system in myotonic dystrophy: a study of 12 cases. *J Am Coll Cardiol.* 1988;11:662–671.

12. Motta J, Guilleminault C, Billingham M, et al. Cardiac abnormalities in myotonic dystrophy. Electrophysiologic and histopathologic studies. *Am J Med.* 1979;67:467–473.

13. van Westering TL, Betts CA, Wood MJ. Current understanding of molecular pathology and treatment of cardiomyopathy in Duchenne muscular dystrophy. *Molecules.* 2015;20:8823–8855.

14. Feng J, Yan J, Buzin CH, et al. Mutations in the dystrophin gene are associated with sporadic dilated cardiomyopathy. *Mol Genet Metab.* 2002;77:119–126.

15. Ferlini A, Sewry C, Melis MA, et al. X-linked dilated cardiomyopathy and the dystrophin gene. *Neuromuscul Disord.* 1999;9:339–346.

16. Melacini P, Fanin M, Angelini A, et al. Cardiac transplantation in a Duchenne muscular dystrophy carrier. *Neuromuscul Disord.* 1998;8:585–590.

17. Tsuda T, Fitzgerald K, Scavena M, et al. Early-progressive dilated cardiomyopathy in a family with Becker muscular dystrophy related to a novel frameshift mutation in the dystrophin gene exon 27. *J Hum Genet.* 2015;60:151–155.

18. Bonne G, Quijano-Roy S. Emery-Dreifuss muscular dystrophy, laminopathies, and other nuclear envelopathies. *Handb Clin Neurol.* 2013;113:1367–1376.

19. Hong JS, Ki CS, Kim JW, et al. Cardiac dysrhythmias, cardiomyopathy and muscular dystrophy in patients with Emery-Dreifuss muscular dystrophy and limb-girdle muscular dystrophy type 1B. *J Korean Med Sci.* 2005;20:283–290.

20. Kanada M, Demirtas M, Guzel R, et al. Cardiomyopathy and atrioventricular block in Emery-Dreifuss muscular dystrophy—a case report. *Angiology.* 2002;53:109–112.

21. Selcen D. Myofibrillar myopathies. *Curr Opin Neurol.* 2010;23:477–481.

22. Barth PG, Valianpour F, Bowen VM, et al. X-linked cardioskeletal myopathy and neutropenia (Barth syndrome): an update. *Am J Med Genet A.* 2004;126A:349–354.

23. Spencer CT, Bryant RM, Day J, et al. Cardiac and clinical phenotype in Barth syndrome. *Pediatrics.* 2006;118:e337–e346.

24. Jefferies JL. Barth syndrome. *Am J Med Genet C Semin Med Genet.* 2013;163C:198–205.

25. Schroeder L, Orchard P, Whitley CB, et al. Cardiac ultrasound findings in infants with severe (Hurler phenotype) untreated mucopolysaccharidosis (MPS) type I. *JIMD Rep.* 2013;10:87–94.

26. Madireddi J, Sarada P, Shetty RK, et al. Hunter syndrome with its typical heart: a close mimic to rheumatic heart. *BMJ Case Rep.* 2015;2015.

27. Nicolini F, Corradi D, Bosio S, et al. Aortic valve replacement in a patient with morquio syndrome. *Heart Surg Forum.* 2008;11:E96–E98.

28. Brands M, Roelants J, de Krijger R, et al. Macrophage involvement in mitral valve pathology in mucopolysaccharidosis type VI (Maroteaux-Lamy syndrome). *Am J Med Genet A.* 2013;161A:2550–2553.

29. Solanich X, Claver E, Carreras F, et al. Myocardial infiltration in Gaucher's disease detected by cardiac MRI. *Int J Cardiol.* 2012;155:e5–e6.

30. McGovern MM, Lippa N, Bagiella E, et al. Morbidity and mortality in type B Niemann-Pick disease. *Genet Med.* 2013;15:618–623.

31. Kabunga P, Lau AK, Phan K, et al. Systematic review of cardiac electrical disease in Kearns-Sayre syndrome and mitochondrial cytopathy. *Int J Cardiol.* 2015;181:303–310.

32. Schwartzkopff B, Frenzel H, Breithardt G, et al. Ultrastructural findings in endomyocardial biopsy of patients with Kearns-Sayre syndrome. *J Am Coll Cardiol.* 1988;12:1522–1528.

33. Sorajja P, Sweeney MG, Chalmers R, et al. Cardiac abnormalities in patients with Leber's hereditary optic neuropathy. *Heart.* 2003;89:791–792.

34. Monlleo-Neila L, Toro MD, Bornstein B, et al. Leigh syndrome and the mitochondrial M.13513G>A mutation: expanding the clinical spectrum. *J Child Neurol.* 2013;28:1531–1534.

35. Lepoivre T, Legendre E, Pinaud M. [Anesthesia for cesarean section in a patient with McArdle disease and hereditary dilated cardiomyopathy]. *Ann Fr Anesth Reanim.* 2002;21:517–520.

36. Dougu N, Joho S, Shan L, et al. Novel LAMP-2 mutation in a family with Danon disease presenting with hypertrophic cardiomyopathy. *Circ J.* 2009;73:376–380.

37. Cottinet SL, Bergemer-Fouquet AM, Toutain A, et al. Danon disease: intrafamilial phenotypic variability related to a novel LAMP-2 mutation. *J Inherit Metab Dis.* 2011;34:515–522.

38. Taylor MR, Ku L, Slavov D, et al. Danon disease presenting with dilated cardiomyopathy and a complex phenotype. *J Hum Genet.* 2007;52:830–835.

39. Cheng Z, Cui Q, Tian Z, et al. Danon disease as a cause of concentric left ventricular hypertrophy in patients who underwent endomyocardial biopsy. *Eur Heart J.* 2012;33:649–656.

40. Laforet P, Richard P, Said MA, et al. A new mutation in PRKAG2 gene causing hypertrophic cardiomyopathy with conduction system disease and muscular glycogenosis. *Neuromuscul Disord.* 2006;16:178–182.

41. Aggarwal V, Dobrolet N, Fishberger S, et al. PRKAG2 mutation: an easily missed cardiac specific non-lysosomal glycogenosis. *Ann Pediatr Cardiol.* 2015;8:153–156.

42. Arad M, Benson DW, Perez-Atayde AR, et al. Constitutively active AMP kinase mutations cause glycogen storage disease mimicking hypertrophic cardiomyopathy. *J Clin Invest.* 2002;109:357–362.

43. Gregersen N, Andresen BS, Bross P. Prevalent mutations in fatty acid oxidation disorders: diagnostic considerations. *Eur J Pediatr.* 2000;159(suppl 3):S213–S218.

44. Joost K, Ounap K, Zordania R, et al. Prevalence of long-chain 3-hydroxyacyl-CoA dehydrogenase deficiency in Estonia. *JIMD Rep.* 2012;2:79–85.

45. Braunlin E, Tolar J, Mackey-Bojack S, et al. Clear cells in the atrioventricular valves of infants with severe human mucopolysaccharidosis (Hurler syndrome) are activated valvular interstitial cells. *Cardiovasc Pathol.* 2011;20:315–321.

46. Edwards WD, Hurdey HP III, Partin JR. Cardiac involvement by Gaucher's disease documented by right ventricular endomyocardial biopsy. *Am J Cardiol.* 1983;52:654.

47. George R, McMahon J, Lytle B, et al. Severe valvular and aortic arch calcification in a patient with Gaucher's disease homozygous for the D409H mutation. *Clin Genet.* 2001;59:360–363.

48. Veinot JP, Elstein D, Hanania D, et al. Gaucher's disease with valve calcification: possible role of Gaucher cells, bone matrix proteins and integrins. *Can J Cardiol.* 1999;15:211–216.

49. Chabas A, Cormand B, Grinberg D, et al. Unusual expression of Gaucher's disease: cardiovascular calcifications in three sibs homozygous for the D409H mutation. *J Med Genet.* 1995;32:740–742.

50. Nakao S, Takenaka T, Maeda M, et al. An atypical variant of Fabry's disease in men with left ventricular hypertrophy. *N Engl J Med.* 1995;333:288–293.

51. Becker AE, Schoorl R, Balk AG, et al. Cardiac manifestations of Fabry's disease. Report of a case with mitral insufficiency and electrocardiographic evidence of myocardial infarction. *Am J Cardiol.* 1975;36:829–835.

52. Chimenti C, Pieroni M, Morgante E, et al. Prevalence of Fabry disease in female patients with late-onset hypertrophic cardiomyopathy. *Circulation.* 2004;110:1047–1053.

53. Sadick N, Thomas L. Cardiovascular manifestations in Fabry disease: a clinical and echocardiographic study. *Heart Lung Circ.* 2007;16:200–206.

54. Sheppard MN, Cane P, Florio R, et al. A detailed pathologic examination of heart tissue from three older patients with Anderson-Fabry disease on enzyme replacement therapy. *Cardiovasc Pathol.* 2010;19:293–301.

55. Thurberg BL, Fallon JT, Mitchell R, et al. Cardiac microvascular pathology in Fabry disease: evaluation of endomyocardial biopsies before and after enzyme replacement therapy. *Circulation.* 2009;119:2561–2567.

56. Towbin JA, Lowe AM, Colan SD, et al. Incidence, causes, and outcomes of dilated cardiomyopathy in children. *JAMA.* 2006;296:1867–1876.

57. Gilbert-Barness E. Review: metabolic cardiomyopathy and conduction system defects in children. *Ann Clin Lab Sci.* 2004;34:15–34.

58. Arbustini E, Diegoli M, Fasani R, et al. Mitochondrial DNA mutations and mitochondrial abnormalities in dilated cardiomyopathy. *Am J Pathol.* 1998;153:1501–1510.

59. Kearns TP, Sayre GP. Retinitis pigmentosa, external ophthalmophegia, and complete heart block: unusual syndrome with histologic study in one of two cases. *AMA Arch Ophthalmol.* 1958;60:280–289.

60. Chawla S, Coku J, Forbes T, et al. Kearns-Sayre syndrome presenting as complete heart block. *Pediatr Cardiol.* 2008;29:659–662.

61. Van Veldhoven PP. Biochemistry and genetics of inherited disorders of peroxisomal fatty acid metabolism. *J Lipid Res.* 2010;51:2863–2895.

62. Claridge KG, Gibberd FB, Sidey MC. Refsum disease: the presentation and ophthalmic aspects of Refsum disease in a series of 23 patients. *Eye (Lond).* 1992;6(pt 4):371–375.

63. Wauthy P, Seghers V, Mathonet P, et al. Cardiac ochronosis: not so benign. *Eur J Cardiothorac Surg.* 2009;35:732–733.

64. Erek E, Casselman FR, Vanermen H. Cardiac ochronosis: valvular heart disease with dark green discoloration of the leaflets. *Tex Heart Inst J.* 2004;31:445–447.

65. Ogawa S, Katayama T, Kaikita K, et al. Chronic thromboembolic pulmonary hypertension complicated with homocystinuria. *Intern Med.* 2014;53:2605–2608.

66. Profitlich LE, Kirmse B, Wasserstein MP, et al. High prevalence of structural heart disease in children with cblC-type methylmalonic aciduria and homocystinuria. *Mol Genet Metab.* 2009;98:344–348.

67. Evangelisti L, Lucarini L, Attanasio M, et al. Vascular and connective tissue features in 5 Italian patients with homocystinuria. *Int J Cardiol.* 2009;134:251–254.

68. Burke AP, Fonseca V, Kolodgie F, et al. Increased serum homocysteine and sudden death resulting from coronary atherosclerosis with fibrous plaques. *Arterioscler Thromb Vasc Biol.* 2002;22:1936–1941.

69. Fishbein GA, Micheletti RG, Currier JS, et al. Atherosclerotic oxalosis in coronary arteries. *Cardiovasc Pathol.* 2008;17:117–123.

70. Seki A, Patel S, Ashraf S, et al. Primary endocardial fibroelastosis: an underappreciated cause of cardiomyopathy in children. *Cardiovasc Pathol.* 2013;22:345–350.

161 Stress Cardiomyopathy

Allen P. Burke, M.D., and Joseph J. Maleszewski, M.D.

Terminology

Stress cardiomyopathy refers to catecholamine-induced myocardial injury that results in transient left ventricular systolic dysfunction. There are two recognized varieties of stress cardiomyopathy: (1) that caused by acute emotional or physical stress (Takotsubo cardiomyopathy or apical ballooning syndrome), and (2) that associated with catecholamine release secondary to central nervous system trauma (so-called neurogenic stress cardiomyopathy).

Takotsubo cardiomyopathy, originally described in the early 1990s, refers to a type of stress cardiomyopathy characterized by acute but rapidly reversible left ventricular systolic dysfunction in the absence of atherosclerotic coronary artery disease, triggered by profound psychological stress.[1] Neurogenic stress cardiomyopathy, described nearly a decade later, is also mediated by catecholamine-induced myocardial injury but is the result of CNS injury (such as head trauma or cerebral infarction.[2-5] Although some consider both stress cardiomyopathy and neurogenic cardiomyopathy part of the same disease,[5] there are characteristics that separate the two (Table 161.1).

Takotsubo Cardiomyopathy

Clinical Findings

Takotsubo cardiomyopathy is a form of ventricular stunning manifested by apical ballooning. It typically affects older women (82% to 100% of cases,) usually aged 62 to 75 years.[5] Although a trigger is not always found, there is typically a history of recent intense emotional or physical stress.[6]

Electrocardiographically, there is usually anterior lead ST-segment elevation. Serologically, markers of myocardial injury (CK-MB and troponins) will be elevated, and angiography shows an absence of significant coronary artery disease.

Imaging, including echocardiograms and cardiac magnetic resonance imaging, shows apical ballooning and hypokinesis, with a decreased ejection fraction.

Pathologic Findings

There are few histopathologic reports of findings in takotsubo cardiomyopathy. Biventricular dilatation with nonspecific features of nonischemic cardiomyopathy with occasional contraction bands has been reported in a fatal case at autopsy.[7] In the acute stage, there is diffuse catecholamine injury in the form of contraction band necrosis (Fig. 161.1). In chronic stage when the ventricular dysfunction does not reverse, there is apical aneurysm with transmural scarring (Fig. 161.2).

In autopsy cases of clinically diagnosed takotsubo cardiomyopathy, the pathologist should carefully evaluate the coronary arteries for evidence of disease that may have been missed on angiogram.

Prognosis

A 1% to 3% mortality rate has been estimated for takotsubo cardiomyopathy.[2]

Neurogenic Stress Cardiomyopathy

Although there is overlap with takotsubo cardiomyopathy,[8] *neurogenic stress cardiomyopathy* is generally reserved for patients with cardiac dysfunction related to head trauma or cerebral infarction.

Compared to takotsubo cardiomyopathy, there is less frequent apical involvement, more global hypokinesis, and basal patterns (so-called inverted takotsubo cardiomyopathy).

TABLE 161.1   Clinical Diagnostic Criteria for Takotsubo Syndrome/Stress Cardiomyopathy[a]

	Takotsubo Cardiomyopathy	Neurogenic Cardiomyopathy
Typical cause	Emotional stress "Classic" takotsubo excludes CNS disease or pheochromocytoma	Acute brain injury, brain death, subarachnoid hemorrhage Pheochromocytoma (rare) Scorpion sting (reported case) Amphetamines (reported case) Sepsis[b]
Incidence	2% of ACS, up to 6% in women	25%–45% of acute brain injury
ECG	Transient ST-segment elevations Diffuse T-wave inversion	50%; long QT, peaked T waves, T-wave abnormalities, ST-segment depression or elevation, prominent U waves
Serum troponin	Usually elevated	Usually low level
Ejection fraction	Decreased; can be exacerbated by dynamic LV outflow obstruction with systolic anterior motion of MV mimicking HOCM	Decreased ejection fraction (45% cutoff for transplantation)
Echocardiogram/imaging	Apical ballooning	Global hypokinesis Basal patterns ("inverted takotsubo" pattern)
Angiogram	No fixed coronary lesions or thrombi	Usually normal
Outcome	Reversible; 1%–2% mortality	Usually reversible, within hours to days

[a]Some authors consider them identical Madias JE. "Neurogenic stress cardiomyopathy in heart donors" is a form of Takotsubo syndrome. *Int J Cardiol.* 2015;184:612–613.
[b]Probably other factors in addition to hypercatecholamine state, including inflammatory response, TNF-α, anaphylatoxins, complement.

Neurogenic stress cardiomyopathy has been studied most extensively in context with heart donors. Between 23% and 45% of brain-dead patients from subarachnoid hemorrhage have left ventricular dysfunction.[2]

Histologically, there are areas of contraction band necrosis and "brain death lesions." Because there is a sparse inflammatory infiltrate, stress cardiomyopathy is sometimes considered a form of "toxic myocarditis" (see Chapter 27). The term "myocytolysis" is often used in the clinical literature for these lesions, although the term is also used for myofibrillar loss (see Chapter 2).[2,9,10]

In setting of brain injury, the clinical relevance of decreased left ventricular dysfunction and catecholamine-induced heart injury involves their impact on suitability for heart transplant. Generally, if the ejection fraction improves to >45% after transient left ventricular suppression, there is no impact on graft viability.[11]

Other Forms of Catecholamine-Related Cardiomyopathy

Transient left ventricular dysfunction has been reported after exposure to scorpion venom, with a clinical course similar to stress cardiomyopathy.[12] Because no histologic findings were reported, it is unclear whether a form of toxic myocarditis occurred. Because α toxins in scorpion venom cause massive autonomic stimulation and adrenergic storm, it was reasoned that the mechanism of cardiotoxicity was mediated through catecholamines. A similar argument has been used for transient left ventricular dysfunction with apical ballooning following amphetamine use.[13]

Sepsis causes left ventricular dysfunction, sometimes mimicking takotsubo cardiomyopathy.[14] Generally, however, there is more global left ventricular dysfunction, and the cardiac damage is multifactorial, including inflammation-mediated injury in addition to excess catecholamines.[14] Histologically, there is often calcification, because of renal failure association with multiorgan failure (Fig. 161.3) (see Chapter 9).

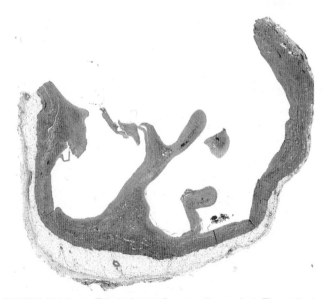

FIGURE 161.2 ▲ Takotsubo cardiomyopathy, explant. The patient was a middle-aged woman who experienced emotional trauma after unwanted separation from a partner. An apical transmural infarction was diagnosed. The patient survived 2 years until transplant. The coronary arteries were normal. The histologic sections show transmural fibrosis. The features are nonspecific and require exclusion of coronary obstruction and clinical information to assess the etiology of the infarct.

FIGURE 161.1 ▲ Takotsubo cardiomyopathy. The patient was a middle-aged woman who suffered from apical acute myocardial infarction after experiencing tremendous fear from a large falling object. Coronary arteries were normal at autopsy, and gross findings were unremarkable. There is diffuse contraction band necrosis.

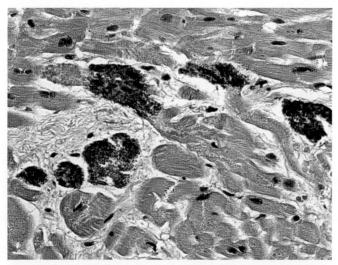

FIGURE 161.3 ▲ Sepsis-induced contraction necrosis. The patient had multiorgan and renal failure, diffuse myocardial calcification, and decreased left ventricular ejection fraction. The individual calcified myocytes indicate calcified necrotic myocytes (calcified contraction band necrosis).

REFERENCES

1. Pavin D, Le Breton H, Daubert C. Human stress cardiomyopathy mimicking acute myocardial syndrome. *Heart.* 1997;78:509–511.
2. Bybee KA, Prasad A. Stress-related cardiomyopathy syndromes. *Circulation.* 2008;118:397–409.
3. Prasad A, Lerman A, Rihal CS. Apical ballooning syndrome (Tako-Tsubo or stress cardiomyopathy): a mimic of acute myocardial infarction. *Am Heart J.* 2008;155:408–417.
4. Wittstein IS. Stress cardiomyopathy: a syndrome of catecholamine-mediated myocardial stunning? *Cell Mol Neurobiol.* 2012;32:847–857.
5. Madias JE. "Neurogenic stress cardiomyopathy in heart donors" is a form of Takotsubo syndrome. *Int J Cardiol.* 2015;184:612–613.
6. Hurst RT, Prasad A, Asker JW, et al. Takotsubo cardiomyopathy: a unique cardiomyopathy with variable ventricular morphology. *J Am Coll Cardiol Img.* 2010;3:641–649.
7. Tran K, Milne N, Duhig E, et al. Inverted Takotsubo cardiomyopathy—clinicopathologic correlation. *Am J Forensic Med Pathol.* 2013;34:217–221.
8. Pinnamaneni S, Dutta T, Melcer J, et al. Neurogenic stress cardiomyopathy associated with subarachnoid hemorrhage. *Future Cardiol.* 2015;11:77–87.
9. Berman M, Ali A, Ashley E, et al. Is stress cardiomyopathy the underlying cause of ventricular dysfunction associated with brain death? *J Heart Lung Transplant.* 2010;29:957–965.
10. Banki NM, Kopelnik A, Dae MW, et al. Acute neurocardiogenic injury after subarachnoid hemorrhage. *Circulation.* 2005;112:3314–3319.
11. Mohamedali B, Bhat G, Tatooles A, et al. Neurogenic stress cardiomyopathy in heart donors. *J Card Fail.* 2014;20:207–211.
12. Miranda CH, Braggion-Santos MF, Schmidt A, et al. The first description of cardiac magnetic resonance findings in a severe scorpion envenomation: is it a stress-induced (Takotsubo) cardiomyopathy like? *Am J Emerg Med.* 2015;33:862 e5–e7.
13. Movahed MR, Mostafizi K. Reverse or inverted left ventricular apical ballooning syndrome (reverse Takotsubo cardiomyopathy) in a young woman in the setting of amphetamine use. *Echocardiography.* 2008;25:429–432.
14. Madias JE. Pathophysiology of sepsis-triggered takotsubo syndrome. *Acute Card Care.* 2014;16:134.

162 Restrictive Cardiomyopathy, Endocardial Fibrosis, and Eosinophilic Endomyocarditis

Fabio R. Tavora, M.D., Ph.D., and Allen P. Burke, M.D.

Restrictive Heart Disease

Restrictive heart disease refers to hemodynamic cardiac alterations that result from increased stiffness of the ventricles (diastolic dysfunction) causing impaired ventricular filling with preserved systolic function. The decrease in ventricular compliance is secondary to infiltrative disease of the myocardium (most frequently amyloid), endocardial disease, or nonischemic cardiomyopathy.

"Idiopathic" restrictive cardiomyopathy generally denotes today a form of nonischemic cardiomyopathy that may overlap genetically and clinically with dilated cardiomyopathy (see Chapter 19) but is marked primarily by restrictive hemodynamics. Primary acquired endocardial disease in adults is generally classified as tropical (idiopathic endocardial fibrosis) or eosinophilic. Congenital endocardial fibrosis is considered a form of infantile dilated cardiomyopathy (see Chapter 23).

Hemodynamic Findings

Because of increased ventricular stiffness, there is reduced diastolic ventricular volume with normal or near-normal systolic function (ejection fraction) and wall thickness. Ventricular pressures rise markedly with small increases in volume, and left ventricular end-diastolic volume is <100 mL/m² with pressures >18 mm Hg. The atria are dilated with nonhypertrophied, nondilated ventricles. Pressure tracings show a characteristic diastolic dip and a plateau or a square root sign. Atrial fibrillation is noted in three-fourths of patients.[1]

Idiopathic Restrictive Cardiomyopathy

Genetic Findings

Patients with familial restrictive cardiomyopathy have familial phenotypes and genetic alterations that reflect hypertrophic, dilated, and noncompaction-type cardiomyopathy. One-third have sarcomere protein gene mutations involving cardiac troponin I gene (*TNNI3*), troponin T (*TNNT2*) desmin (*DES*), and alpha-cardiac actin (*ACTC*).[2,3] Recently, mutations in TNNI3 (cardiac troponin I type 3) have been described in children with restrictive cardiomyopathy.[4,5]

Restrictive cardiomyopathy may be a manifestation of the *myofibrillar myopathies*, which are characterized by disintegration of the Z-disk, accumulation of cytoplasmic myofibrillar osmiophilic bodies ultrastructurally, and sometimes congophilic material on skeletal muscle biopsies. Myofibrillar myopathies may also manifest as arrhythmogenic and dilated cardiomyopathy.[6] Mutations involved in myofibrillar myopathies include desmin, αB-crystallin, myotilin, ZASP, filamin C, and BAG3. Of these, desmin, αB-crystallin, and *BAG3* have been implicated in cardiomyopathy.[7]

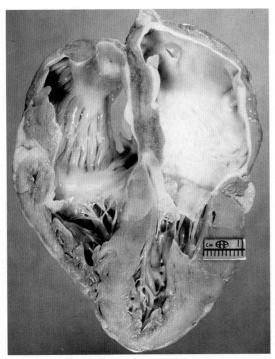

FIGURE 162.1 ▲ Restrictive cardiomyopathy. An autopsy heart from a child with idiopathic restrictive cardiomyopathy. Note relatively normal-appearing ventricles and marked dilatation of atria.

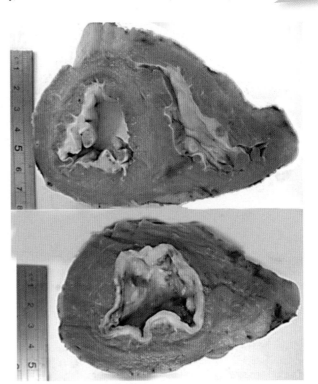

FIGURE 162.2 ▲ Endocardial fibrosis, adult (tropical) type. **A.** There is fibrosis in the left ventricle predominantly in the apex.

Gross Pathologic Findings

Grossly, the ventricles are relatively normal, but there is marked biatrial dilatation (Fig. 162.1).

Histologic Findings

The histologic features of idiopathic restrictive cardiomyopathy are nonspecific, including interstitial fibrosis and myocyte hypertrophy. Most cases with histologic evaluation have demonstrated myofiber disarray, but in the absence of significant hypertrophy.[8]

A subset of restrictive cardiomyopathy is associated with intramyocyte desmin deposition (desminopathy, a form of myofibrillar myopathy) involving the heart and skeletal muscle. Atrioventricular block is common. Electron microscopy is necessary to demonstrate filamentous desmin deposits[9,10].

Idiopathic Endomyocardial Fibrosis

Clinical Findings

Idiopathic endomyocardial fibrosis is a disorder of the tropical and subtropical regions that is clinically characterized by restrictive cardiomyopathy. The eponym term "Davies disease" has been used because of descriptions of the disease by Davies in the 1950s and 1960s in Africa.[11–14] It affects predominantly children and young adults.[15] The disease is endemic in India and South America, as well as Africa.[16] It is rare in the United States.

In contrast to eosinophilic endomyocarditis, most patients do not have peripheral eosinophilia. Ventriculograms demonstrate changes in ventricular morphology with restriction or obliteration in the inflow tract or apex, reduction in the diastolic ventricular dimension, endocardial irregularities, and, in severe cases, a tubular distortion of the ventricle due to obliteration of the inflow tract. Mitral and tricuspid regurgitation are typical. Magnetic resonance imaging findings include ventricular diastolic dysfunction, systolic dysfunction, and extensive subendocardial delayed contrast enhancement with atrial enlargement and organized ventricular thrombus.[17] Surgical treatment includes valve replacement or repair, and resection of the endocardial fibrotic tissue.[16]

In instances, surgical treatment is curative. Even though bilateral disease is typical, there may be isolated left or right ventricular involvement.[15]

Etiology

The specific etiology is unknown, but abnormalities in the recruitment of eosinophils inducing subendocardial inflammation have been found.[18] Endomyocardial fibrosis is believed to start as eosinophilic infiltration of the myocardium with myocyte necrosis and endocardium damage, despite the lack of peripheral eosinophilia at the time of symptom onset. One theory postulates that cerium excess stimulates collagen synthesis and endomyocardial fibrosis, following cardiac necrosis triggered by helminths and the associated hypereosinophilia. Later, the damaged endocardium predisposes to mural thrombi that may organize. There is no consensus regarding the role of viruses in the pathogenesis.[19]

Pathologic Findings

Scarring and fibrosis of the endocardium are the hallmarks of the disease, but only occur after about 1 year of the first initiation event. Patchy fibrosis of the endocardium leads to reduced compliance and subsequently to restrictive physiology as the disease becomes more diffuse (Fig. 162.2).

Histologic findings in resected surgical samples demonstrate bland fibrosis with superficial acellular hyaline collagen fibers type I more predominant than type III (Fig. 162.3). There may be associated chronic inflammation and a lymphatic-rich vascular pattern in the deep endocardium.

Eosinophilic Endomyocarditis (Hypereosinophilic Syndrome Involving the Heart)

Etiology and Classification

Degranulation of eosinophils within the eosinophil infiltrated myocardium causes myocardial necrosis from the release of toxic cationic proteins and mural thrombi, which can occur anywhere in the ventricles.

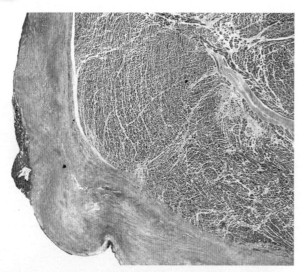

FIGURE 162.3 ▲ Endocardial fibroelastosis, adult (tropical) type. Masson trichrome stain demonstrates a dense band of collagenized tissue. There is a small surface thrombus.

Synonyms of cardiac manifestations of hypereosinophilic syndrome include Loeffler endocarditis, nontropical eosinophilic endomyocardial disease, eosinophilic endomyocarditis, and eosinophilic endomyocardial disease.

Loeffler eosinophilic endomyocarditis, similar to idiopathic hypereosinophilic syndrome, can be secondary, and idiopathic forms. Primary hypereosinophilic syndrome is a myeloproliferative disorder associated with the chromosomal rearrangement resulting in PDGFRA fusion kinase. Secondary hypereosinophilic syndrome is a polyclonal expansion of eosinophils in reaction to lymphoproliferative disease. Most cases are idiopathic, which include "overlap" forms, which are limited to a specific organ, such as the heart or gastrointestinal tract.[20]

Eosinophilic endomyocarditis is usually idiopathic but may be associated with primary hypereosinophilic syndrome, or eosinophilic granulomatosis with eosinophilia (see Chapter 10).[21,22]

Imaging

Eosinophilic endomyocarditis affects both ventricles, but rare cases of isolated left ventricular processes have been reported.[23] The mitral valve is most commonly involved, although tricuspid and pulmonic valves may also be affected by the mural thrombus.[24]

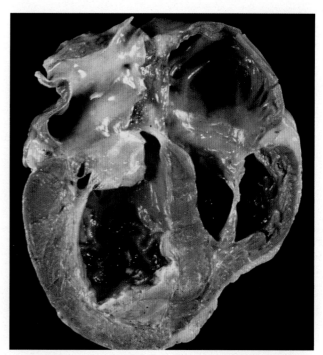

FIGURE 162.4 ▲ Hypereosinophilic syndrome (eosinophilic endomyocardial disease). There is a thrombus covering the surface of the left atrial endocardium.

Contrast-enhanced magnetic resonance imaging is helpful to demonstrate thrombus, endomyocardial fibrosis, and inflammation in eosinophilic endomyocardial disease.[23] Complications include embolic phenomena, atrial fibrillation, ventricular arrhythmias, and heart failure.

Pathologic Findings

Grossly, there is mural thrombus, often at the apex, resulting in entrapment of the atrioventricular valve (Fig. 162.4). The presence of eosinophils, intramural arterial thrombi, and mural thrombi confirms the diagnosis (Fig. 162.5); often, there is myocardial necrosis. Extracardiac autopsy findings include bone marrow hypereosinophilia, biventricular thrombi with eosinophilia, liver involvement of hypereosinophilic syndrome, and systemic and pulmonary emboli.[25]

On endomyocardial biopsy, presence of any eosinophils should be carefully noted, especially if there is a history of restrictive parameters.[26]

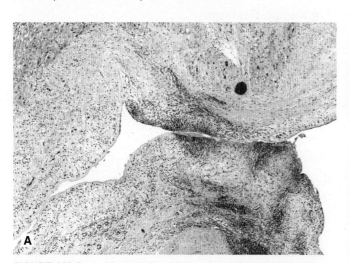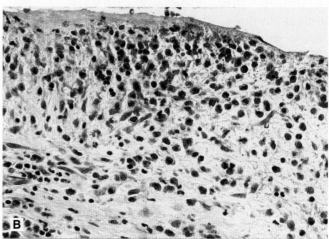

FIGURE 162.5 ▲ Hypereosinophilic syndrome (eosinophilic endomyocarditis), autopsy. **A.** At low magnification, there is endocardial thickening with inflammation. **B.** At higher magnification, there are numerous eosinophils.

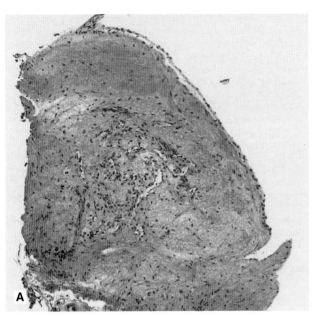
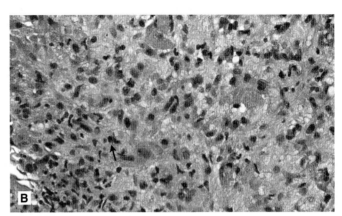

FIGURE 162.6 ▲ Eosinophilic endomyocarditis, endomyocardial biopsy. **A.** Low magnification shows inflammation, granulation tissue, and endocardial fibrosis. **B.** There is granulation tissue, with rare eosinophils (*arrow*).

Histologically, resection of thrombus may lead to diagnosis because of the presence of eosinophils in the clot[27] (Fig. 162.6). Any biopsy with eosinophils should warrant a comment including hypereosinophilic syndrome in the differential diagnosis.[28]

Because of endocardial involvement, the mitral valve may become damaged and require replacement.[29] Mitral valve repair has also been reported.[30] Similarly, right ventricular involvement may necessitate tricuspid valve replacement.[31] Aortic valve involvement is rare.[32]

Prognosis

The mortality rate is high due to cardiac complications. In addition to surgery, medical treatment of hypereosinophilic syndrome includes steroids and cytotoxic agents[25,33] as well as interferon.[34] Hypereosinophilic syndrome that manifests as restrictive cardiomyopathy may necessitate heart transplantation.[35,36]

Practical Points

▶ Endomyocardial biopsies of patients with restrictive cardiomyopathy are often performed to rule out, in addition to amyloid, eosinophilic endomyocarditis. The presence of eosinophils should carefully be evaluated in this setting.

▶ Endocardial fibrosis is common as a secondary finding in idiopathic dilated and hypertrophic cardiomyopathy, adjacent to abnormal valves, and in areas of prior ablation or other instrumentation. Idiopathic endocardial fibrosis is very rare in developed countries and is a diagnosis made only in conjunction with imaging and clinical findings or at autopsy or explant.

REFERENCES

1. Ammash NM, Seward JB, Bailey KR, et al. Clinical profile and outcome of idiopathic restrictive cardiomyopathy. *Circulation.* 2000;101:2490–2496.
2. Parvatiyar MS, Pinto JR, Dweck D, et al. Cardiac troponin mutations and restrictive cardiomyopathy. *J Biomed Biotechnol.* 2010;2010:350706.
3. Akhter S, Bueltmann K Jr, Huang X, et al. Restrictive cardiomyopathy mutations demonstrate functions of the C-terminal end-segment of troponin I. *Arch Biochem Biophys.* 2014;552–553:3–10.
4. Chen Y, Yang S, Li J, et al. Pediatric restrictive cardiomyopathy due to a heterozygous mutation of the TNNI3 gene. *J Biomed Res.* 2014;28:59–63.
5. Mouton JM, Pellizzon AS, Goosen A, et al. Diagnostic disparity and identification of two TNNI3 gene mutations, one novel and one arising de novo, in South African patients with restrictive cardiomyopathy and focal ventricular hypertrophy. *Cardiovasc J Afr.* 2015;26:63–69.
6. Selcen D. Myofibrillar myopathies. *Neuromuscul Disord.* 2011;21:161–171.
7. Sanbe A. Molecular mechanisms of alpha-crystallinopathy and its therapeutic strategy. *Biol Pharm Bull.* 2011;34:1653–1658.
8. Gambarin FI, Tagliani M, Arbustini E. Pure restrictive cardiomyopathy associated with cardiac troponin I gene mutation: mismatch between the lack of hypertrophy and the presence of disarray. *Heart.* 2008;94:1257.
9. Arbustini E, Morbini P, Grasso M, et al. Restrictive cardiomyopathy, atrioventricular block and mild to subclinical myopathy in patients with desmin-immunoreactive material deposits. *J Am Coll Cardiol.* 1998;31:645–653.
10. Arbustini E, Pasotti M, Pilotto A, et al. Desmin accumulation restrictive cardiomyopathy and atrioventricular block associated with desmin gene defects. *Eur J Heart Fail.* 2006;8:477–483.
11. Davies JN. Endomyocardial fibrosis in Uganda. *Cent Afr J Med.* 1956;2:323–328.
12. Davies JN. The reactions of the endocardium to disease. *East Afr Med J.* 1962;39:5–11.
13. Davies JN. Pathology and pathogenesis of endocardial disease. *Cardiologia.* 1963;42:161–175.
14. Davies JN, Ball JD. The pathology of endocardial fibrosis in Uganda. *Br Heart J.* 1955;17:337–359.
15. Mocumbi AO, Yacoub MH, Yokohama H, et al. Right ventricular endomyocardial fibrosis. *Cardiovasc Pathol.* 2009;18:64–65.
16. Mady C, Barretto AC, Oliveira SA, et al. Evolution of the endocardial fibrotic process in endomyocardial fibrosis. *Am J Cardiol.* 1991;68:402–403.
17. Paydar A, Ordovas KG, Reddy GP. Magnetic resonance imaging for endomyocardial fibrosis. *Pediatr Cardiol.* 2008;29:1004–1005.
18. Sezi CL. Endomyocardial fibrosis and eosinophilia. *Lancet.* 1993;342:1233–1234.
19. Iglezias SD, Benvenuti LA, Calabrese F, et al. Endomyocardial fibrosis: pathological and molecular findings of surgically resected ventricular endomyocardium. *Virchows Arch.* 2008;453:233–241.
20. Hsieh FH. Hypereosinophilic syndrome. *Ann Allergy Asthma Immunol.* 2014;112:484–488.

21. Arbustini E, Narula N, Tavazzi L, et al. The MOGE(S) classification of cardiomyopathy for clinicians. *J Am Coll Cardiol.* 2014;64:304–318.

22. Campbell RT, Jhund PS, Dalzell JR, et al. Diagnosis and resolution of Loeffler endocarditis secondary to eosinophilic granulomatosis with polyangiitis demonstrated by cardiac magnetic resonance-T2 mapping. *Circulation.* 2015;131:114–117.

23. Bonanad C, Monmeneu JV, Lopez-Lereu MP. Loeffler endocarditis of the left ventricle: cardiac magnetic resonance findings. *Heart Lung Circ.* 2013;22:1056–1057.

24. Garg A, Nanda NC, Sungur A, et al. Transthoracic echocardiographic detection of pulmonary valve involvement in Loeffler's endocarditis. *Echocardiography.* 2014;31:83–86.

25. Chao BH, Cline-Parhamovich K, Grizzard JD, et al. Fatal Loeffler's endocarditis due to hypereosinophilic syndrome. *Am J Hematol.* 2007;82:920–923.

26. Inoue T, Watanabe C, Ayukawa H, et al. Biopsy-proven Loeffler endocarditis successfully treated with steroids. *Circulation.* 2015;131:e353–e354.

27. Blauwet LA, Breen JF, Edwards WD, et al. Atypical presentation of eosinophilic endomyocardial disease. *Mayo Clin Proc.* 2005;80:1078–1084.

28. Kawagoshi H, Shimizu M, Suematsu T, et al. A case of eosinophilic heart disease diagnosed by endomyocardial biopsy findings. *Jpn Heart J.* 1990;31:259–264.

29. Boustany CW Jr, Murphy GW, Hicks GL Jr. Mitral valve replacement in idiopathic hypereosinophilic syndrome. *Ann Thorac Surg.* 1991;51:1007–1009.

30. Fuzellier JF, Chapoutot L, Torossian PF. Mitral valve repair in idiopathic hypereosinophilic syndrome. *J Heart Valve Dis.* 2004;13:529–531.

31. Carnero-Alcazar M, Reguillo-Lacruz F, O'Connor F, et al. Hypereosinophilic syndrome and myocardial fibrosis. *Interact Cardiovasc Thorac Surg.* 2008;7:928–930.

32. Gudmundsson GS, Ohr J, Leya F, et al. An unusual case of recurrent Loffler endomyocarditis of the aortic valve. *Arch Pathol Lab Med.* 2003;127:606–609.

33. Kim CH, Vlietstra RE, Edwards WD, et al. Steroid-responsive eosinophilic myocarditis: diagnosis by endomyocardial biopsy. *Am J Cardiol.* 1984;53:1472–1473.

34. Baratta L, Afeltra A, Delfino M, et al. Favorable response to high-dose interferon-alpha in idiopathic hypereosinophilic syndrome with restrictive cardiomyopathy—case report and literature review. *Angiology.* 2002;53:465–470.

35. Korczyk D, Taylor G, McAlistair H, et al. Heart transplantation in a patient with endomyocardial fibrosis due to hypereosinophilic syndrome. *Transplantation.* 2007;83:514–516.

36. Syed IS, Martinez MW, Feng DL, et al. Cardiac magnetic resonance imaging of eosinophilic endomyocardial disease. *Int J Cardiol.* 2008;126:e50–e52.

163 Lymphocytic Myocarditis

Fabio R. Tavora, M.D., Ph.D., and Allen P. Burke, M.D.

Pathogenesis

"Lymphocytic myocarditis" describes the histologic pattern of the most common form of myocarditis, which is associated with viruses and autoimmune responses. It is hypothesized that after viral entry, viral replication causes acute myocyte injury, myocyte necrosis, exposure of intracellular antigens, and activation of the immune system. After an acute phase of infiltration of natural killer cells, macrophages, and neutrophils, a second autoimmune phase is defined by activated virus-specific T lymphocytes, which may target the host's organs by molecular mimicry. It is in this phase, when virus has largely been cleared, that diagnosis is generally made by biopsy or at autopsy.[1]

A causative link between viruses and myocardial inflammation is difficult to prove, because viral cultures and serology are often unrewarding, with low yields.[2] A large number of studies that have utilized molecular techniques have investigated the presence of biopsies in tissue samples of patients with myocarditis and dilated cardiomyopathy. Because of the presence of transmembrane receptor CAR (coxsackievirus and adenovirus receptor) and the established murine model for coxsackievirus myocarditis, coxsackieviruses and adenoviruses were among the first viruses studied by polymerase chain reaction. Early studies based on tissue samples with acute myocarditis showed a high rate of positivity for viruses, especially adenoviruses, with confirmation by culture in a small subset of patients.[2,3] Subsequent studies using polymerase chain reaction, primarily on endomyocardial biopsies, showed a smaller and widely variable number of samples with enteroviruses or adenoviruses, ranging from 1% to 60% (reviewed in Ref. [4]).

Molecular techniques have greatly increased the scope of viruses detected in cardiac tissues, including cytomegalovirus, parvovirus, human herpes virus 6, and Epstein-Barr virus.[4] There is an especially high rate of detection of HHV6 and parvovirus 19, which have been localized to macrophages and endothelial cells in the heart, respectively, leading to a "shift" in the focus of viral etiology away from adeno- and enteroviruses. Whether these agents are causative or "innocent bystanders" has yet to be determined, however.

Because an autoimmune reaction is believed to play a role in viral myocarditis, it is not unexpected that the histologic features are similar with those of myocarditis associated with rheumatologic autoimmune diseases (see Chapter 10).

Clinical Findings

Myocarditis is generally a disease of infants, children, and young adults. The most commonly implicated etiologies—entero- and adenoviruses—are ubiquitous with widespread serologic immunity across the adult population. There is no known genetic predisposition to the development of myocarditis after viral infection; familial cases are rare,[5] although families with dilated cardiomyopathy have been found to harbor antimyocardial antibodies.[6]

The clinical diagnosis is made on the basis of electrocardiographic changes, myocardial damage evidenced by elevated troponin, evidence of systemic inflammation, lack of epicardial coronary artery disease, and generally mild and transient ventricular dysfunction. Relatively uncommonly, there is severe ventricular dysfunction ("fulminant myocarditis"), which responds to steroids and other immunosuppressive therapies.[7] Fulminant myocarditis is diagnosed on the basis of clinical features at presentation, including the presence of severe hemodynamic compromise, rapid onset of symptoms, and fever.

Most patients present with symptoms of concomitant pericardial inflammation, chest pain, and palpitations. Patients with the combination of myocarditis and pericarditis (myopericarditis) typically have chest pain, flu-like symptoms, and pericardial friction rubs, in addition to significant increases in serum troponins. Most patients respond to treatment with nonsteroidal anti-inflammatory drugs, and the prognosis appears to be better than that of pure myocarditis.[8]

Long-term follow-up studies in patients with acute myocarditis show that ~20% develop dilated cardiomyopathy in 3 years.[9]

Coxsackie B viral myocarditis may occasionally present at birth and present with signs and symptoms of heart failure. Virus is detected in the blood, cerebrospinal fluid, nasopharyngeal swab, or stool by PCR or culture. The mortality is nearly one-third, and the survivors typically develop left ventricular aneurysms.[10]

Magnetic Resonance Imaging

The magnetic resonance changes in myocardial tissue during the first phase of myocardial inflammation include edema on T2-weighted images, which is generally consistent with inflammation. Late gadolinium enhancement imaging generally reveals an intramural, rim-like pattern in the septal wall or patchy subepicardial distribution in the left ventricular lateral free wall.[1]

Diagnosis of Myocarditis at Autopsy

Myocarditis is present in 8% to 12% of cases of sudden death in young adults[11] and is one of the more common diagnoses in medicolegal autopsies of infants and children (see Chapter 4).

Gross Findings

Grossly, myocarditis reveals nonspecific findings ranging from normal to dilatation of all four chambers, depending on the specific agents and the duration of illness. Ventricular softening and pallor is typical but not always evident. Fibrinous pericarditis can be associated with cases of myocarditis and does not necessarily indicate bacterial etiology. Fibrosis is a component of healed myocarditis, and the distribution is random, as opposed to subendocardial-based scars of ischemia.[12] Scars that are subepicardial, as opposed to subendocardial or transmural, are rarely ischemic, unless secondary to embolization from coronary thrombosis. Subepicardial scars should raise the differential diagnosis of healed myocarditis or arrhythmogenic cardiomyopathy. Rare cases of diffuse calcification of the myocardium following myocarditis have been reported.[13] Figure 163.1 shows a series of axial cuts on a case of myocarditis with the typical myocardium pallor and healed fibrosis.

Microscopic Findings

In cases of sudden death due to myocarditis, the infiltrate is generally diffuse, in all sections examined, and there is no question as to

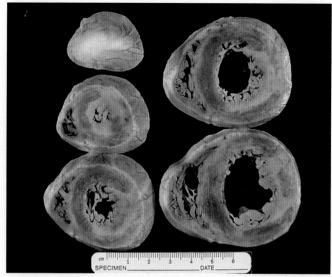

FIGURE 163.1 ▲ Myocarditis. A 4-year-old child died after complaining of weakness and shortness of breath; there was a history of recent diarrhea and vomiting. Short-axis sections of the heart show irregular mottling of the myocardium, corresponding to areas of hyperemia or lymphocytic infiltration. In most cases of fatal myocarditis, the heart appears grossly normal.

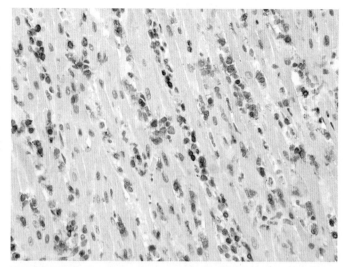

FIGURE 163.3 ▲ The lymphocytes in lymphocyte myocarditis are predominantly T cells (anti-CD3).

diagnosis or mechanism of death, which is attributed to ventricular arrhythmia (Fig. 163.2). There may be variability in the extent of inflammation from slide to slide, and endocardial as well as inflammation in the epicardial fat is not uncommon.

The inflammatory cells are most frequently mature T lymphocytes with a large population of accompanying macrophages, but small numbers of plasma cells and neutrophils can be seen in any given case (Fig. 163.3). The T cells are a mixture of CD4+ and CD8+ cells. Neutrophils are usually associated with bacterial infection, but may also be prominent in infants with acute viral myocarditis.

The infiltrate of lymphocytic myocarditis is generally centered around myocytes, although the interstitial may also be involved. Necrosis is invariably present, but is relatively mild in extent in relationship to the degree of inflammation (Fig. 163.2).

In ~25% of fatal cases, there are areas of healing fibrosis or scar, but these are typically small in comparison to the areas of inflammation (Fig. 163.4). It is presumed that the finding on healing with fibrosis is associated with the development of dilated cardiomyopathy.

Significance of Focal Myocardial Inflammation at Autopsy

Histologically, the degree of inflammation in cases of myocarditis can vary considerably. Most cases of fatal myocarditis show diffuse inflammation involving most of the regions of the ventricles, with less in the atria.[12,14,15]

A common scenario is the finding of focal infiltrates of uncertain significance, with or without myocyte necrosis (Fig. 163.5). If there is an established cause of death such as associated cardiomyopathy, or extracardiac cause, the finding is incidental or may be considered a factor contributing to death. In the absence of a cause of death, the significance of isolated infiltrates can be controversial. It has been demonstrated that lymphohistiocytic infiltrates are found in ~1 in 5 autopsies in noncardiac deaths,[16] an infiltrate defined as at least 10 cells. Focal myocarditis has been described as resulting in clinical symptoms and may be localized to one portion of the left ventricle or more commonly the right ventricle (Fig. 163.3).[17] An autopsy study of an established cause of death unrelated to myocarditis showed that up to one-third of hearts show focal inflammation as an incidental finding, but that focal inflammation with necrosis occurred in <5% and that the finding of focal infiltrates was associated with antibiotic use.[18]

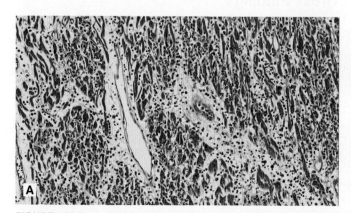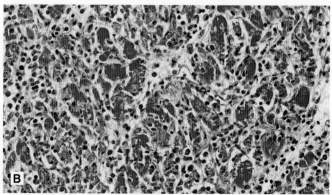

FIGURE 163.2 ▲ Myocarditis, autopsy, sudden death. **A.** There is a diffuse lymphocytic infiltrate surrounding individual cardiomyocytes. **B.** There is extensive myocyte necrosis in this field.

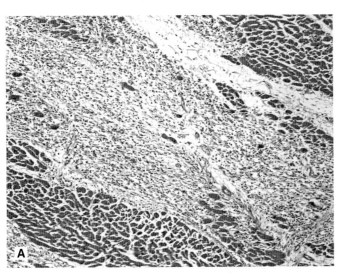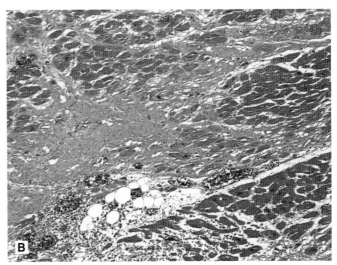

FIGURE 163.4 ▲ Lymphocytic myocarditis, with healing. In ~25% of sudden deaths with myocarditis, there are areas of healing. **A.** There is an area of granulation tissue with early fibroblast response. **B.** There is an area of remote scarring with active inflammation.

Differential Diagnosis

Catecholamine-induced injury and ischemic injury show a large extent of necrosis compared to the inflammation. Single cell necrosis shows clearly necrotic myocytes with only few surrounding lymphocytes. On occasion, the distinction between ischemia (especially reperfusion type) with adjacent neutrophilic response and acute myocarditis can be difficult, but zonal necrosis with abundant necrosis favors the former.

A significant number of B lymphocytes and plasma cells should raise the possibility of a bacterial infection as well as of a toxic etiology. Eosinophils can be found in most types of myocarditis, but are typically numerous in hypersensitivity myocarditis, eosinophilic endomyocardial disease, parasitic infections, and giant cell myocarditis. Giant cells

can be seen in mycobacterial and fungal infections, sarcoidosis, or giant cell myocarditis.

Diagnosis of Myocarditis on Endomyocardial Biopsy

One of the more common indications for endomyocardial biopsy in native hearts is to exclude the diagnosis of myocarditis (Fig. 163.6). The rate of myocarditis in biopsies for new-onset heart failure has been reported at 5%[19] to up to 15%,[20] partly dependent on histologic criteria. The proportion of patients with the clinical diagnosis of myocarditis as a cause of recent-onset heart failure may exceed those with positive biopsy, as the diagnosis of myocarditis is in part clinical, and sampling sensitivity is lower than 40%.[21] An autopsy study with simulated endomyocardial biopsies, predicted 60% positivity rate for endomyocardial biopsies of patients dying with myocarditis (Fig. 163.6).[22]

The classic criteria for the endomyocardial biopsy diagnosis of myocarditis were established in 1987 in Dallas, Texas.[23] In this system, myocyte necrosis is required for the diagnosis of myocarditis; necrosis is somewhat subjective, but is diagnosed by the presence of myocyte with degenerated cytoplasm, lack of cross striations, and intracytoplasmic lymphocytes. This diagnostic category, inflammation with myocyte necrosis, has been designated as "active myocarditis."[20] The borderline-positive category was used for a lymphocytic infiltrate without myocyte necrosis. The Dallas criteria, however, lack sensitivity, have a high level of interobserver variability, and, most importantly, did not predict those patients who respond to immunosuppressive treatment.[24] For these reasons, it has been recommended to abandon the Dallas criteria and make the diagnosis of myocarditis with any significant inflammation on biopsy.[25] Clinical criteria of fulminant disease and circulating myocardial antibodies may predict those patients who respond to steroids; histologic features, such as the presence of HLA antigens in T cells and endothelial cells of biopsies, have not been shown to consistently guide treatment.[19]

A tentative semiquantitative criteria for the diagnosis of myocarditis have been proposed and include the detection of more than 14 T cells per mm^2 (~4 high-power fields) in an endomyocardial biopsy specimen by immunohistochemistry[26] or the consistent finding of 5 lymphocytes per high-power field on routine microscopy.[27]

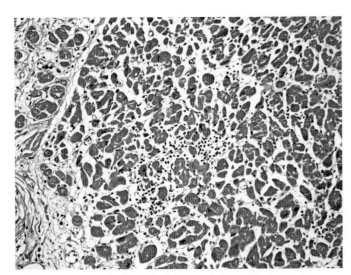

FIGURE 163.5 ▲ Focal myocarditis may occasionally be an incidental finding at autopsy. Uncommonly, nodules of lymphocytic infiltrates can be seen; this patient died of unrelated causes.

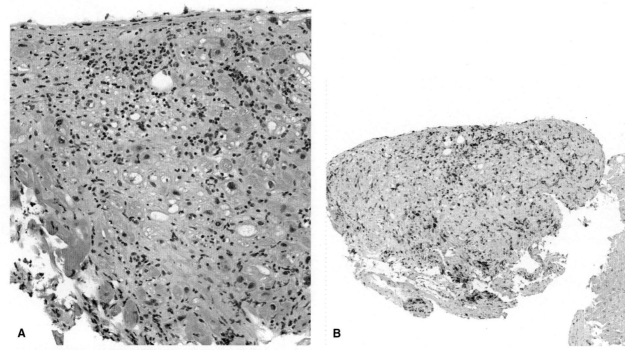

FIGURE 163.6 ▲ Myocarditis, endomyocardial biopsy. **A.** There is an area of necrosis and chronic inflammation. **B.** The inflammatory infiltrate shows an infiltrate rich in T lymphocytes (anti-CD3).

Autoimmune Myocarditis and Myocarditis Associated with Connective Tissue Disease

The myocarditis of acute rheumatic fever (rheumatic myocarditis) is classically described as a pancarditis characterized by interstitial Aschoff nodules composed of macrophages, lymphocytes, and a central necrotic zone of collagen (see Chapter 10).

In lupus, clinical fulminant myocarditis is uncommon, but subclinical involvement has been detected in autopsy studies in as high as 40% of the patients[28] (Fig. 163.7). Diagnosis is confirmed by endomyocardial biopsy, which shows inflammation with or without necrosis.[29]

Rheumatoid myocarditis is uncommon, but has been described to produce clinical symptoms.[30] Most reports are of individual cases.

Mixed connective tissue disease may also be complicated by lymphocytic myocarditis. Patients present with heart failure, with increased serum troponin.[31,32]

REFERENCES

1. Kindermann I, Barth C, Mahfoud F, et al. Update on myocarditis. *J Am Coll Cardiol.* 2012;59:779–792.
2. Martin AB, Webber S, Fricker FJ, et al. Acute myocarditis. Rapid diagnosis by PCR in children. *Circulation.* 1994;90:330–339.
3. Bowles NE, Ni J, Kearney DL, et al. Detection of viruses in myocardial tissues by polymerase chain reaction. evidence of adenovirus as a common cause of myocarditis in children and adults. *J Am Coll Cardiol.* 2003;42:466–472.
4. Pankuweit S, Klingel K. Viral myocarditis: from experimental models to molecular diagnosis in patients. *Heart Fail Rev.* 2013;18:683–702.
5. O'Connell JB, Fowles RE, Robinson JA, et al. Clinical and pathologic findings of myocarditis in two families with dilated cardiomyopathy. *Am Heart J.* 1984;107:127–135.
6. Caforio AL, Iliceto S. Genetically determined myocarditis: clinical presentation and immunological characteristics. *Curr Opin Cardiol.* 2008;23:219–226.
7. Gupta S, Markham DW, Drazner MH, et al. Fulminant myocarditis. *Nat Clin Pract Cardiovasc Med.* 2008;5:693–706.
8. Buiatti A, Merlo M, Pinamonti B, et al. Clinical presentation and long-term follow-up of perimyocarditis. *J Cardiovasc Med (Hagerstown).* 2013;14:235–241.
9. D'Ambrosio A, Patti G, Manzoli A, et al. The fate of acute myocarditis between spontaneous improvement and evolution to dilated cardiomyopathy: a review. *Heart.* 2001;85:499–504.
10. Freund MW, Kleinveld G, Krediet TG, et al. Prognosis for neonates with enterovirus myocarditis. *Arch Dis Child Fetal Neonatal Ed.* 2010;95:F206–F212.
11. Fabre A, Sheppard MN. Sudden adult death syndrome and other non-ischaemic causes of sudden cardiac death. *Heart.* 2006;92:316–320.
12. Guarner J, Bhatnagar J, Shieh WJ, et al. Histopathologic, immunohistochemical, and polymerase chain reaction assays in the study of cases with fatal sporadic myocarditis. *Hum Pathol.* 2007;38:1412–1419.
13. Oka K, Oohira K, Yatabe Y, et al. Fulminant myocarditis demonstrating uncommon morphology—a report of two autopsy cases. *Virchows Arch.* 2005;446:259–264.

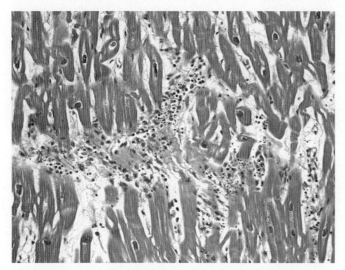

FIGURE 163.7 ▲ Lupus myocarditis. Inflammation tends to be interstitial, with necrosis of interstitial collagen and apoptotic debris.

14. Tavora F, Burke A, Li L, et al. Postmortem confirmation of Lyme carditis with polymerase chain reaction. *Cardiovasc Pathol.* 2008;17:103–107.

15. Tavora F, Gonzalez-Cuyar LF, Dalal JS, et al. Fatal parvoviral myocarditis: a case report and review of literature. *Diagn Pathol.* 2008;3:21.

16. Fineschi V, Wetli CV, Di Paolo M, et al. Myocardial necrosis and cocaine. A quantitative morphologic study in 26 cocaine-associated deaths. *Int J Legal Med.* 1997;110:193–198.

17. Di Bella G, de Gregorio C, Minutoli F, et al. Early diagnosis of focal myocarditis by cardiac magnetic resonance. *Int J Cardiol.* 2007;117:280–281.

18. Zhang M, Tavora F, Zhang Y, et al. The role of focal myocardial inflammation in sudden unexpected cardiac and noncardiac deaths—a clinicopathological study. *Int J Legal Med.* 2013;127:131–138.

19. Arbustini E, Gavazzi A, Dal Bello B, et al. Ten-year experience with endomyocardial biopsy in myocarditis presenting with congestive heart failure: frequency, pathologic characteristics, treatment and follow-up. *G Ital Cardiol.* 1997;27:209–223.

20. McCarthy RE III, Boehmer JP, Hruban RH, et al. Long-term outcome of fulminant myocarditis as compared with acute (nonfulminant) myocarditis. *N Engl J Med.* 2000;342:690–695.

21. Ardehali H, Qasim A, Cappola T, et al. Endomyocardial biopsy plays a role in diagnosing patients with unexplained cardiomyopathy. *Am Heart J.* 2004;147:919–923.

22. Hauck AJ, Kearney DL, Edwards WD. Evaluation of postmortem endomyocardial biopsy specimens from 38 patients with lymphocytic myocarditis: implications for role of sampling error. *Mayo Clin Proc.* 1989;64:1235–1245.

23. Aretz H, Billingham M, Edwards W, et al. Myocarditis: a histologic definition and classification. *Am J Cardiovasc Pathol.* 1987;1:3–14.

24. Mason JW. Myocarditis. *Adv Intern Med.* 1999;44:293–310.

25. Baughman KL. Diagnosis of myocarditis: death of Dallas criteria. *Circulation.* 2006;113:593–595.

26. Pankuweit S, Lottspeich F, Maisch B. Characterization of relevant membrane antigens by two-dimensional immunoblot and n-terminal sequence analysis in patients with myocarditis. *Eur Heart J.* 1995;16(suppl O):81–84.

27. Edwards WD, Holmes DR Jr, Reeder GS. Diagnosis of active lymphocytic myocarditis by endomyocardial biopsy: quantitative criteria for light microscopy. *Mayo Clin Proc.* 1982;57:419–425.

28. Doherty NE, Siegel RJ. Cardiovascular manifestations of systemic lupus erythematosus. *Am Heart J.* 1985;110:1257–1265.

29. Frustaci A, Gentiloni N, Caldarulo M. Acute myocarditis and left ventricular aneurysm as presentations of systemic lupus erythematosus. *Chest.* 1996;109:282–284.

30. Wu CH, Sung SH, Wu TC. Focal myocarditis mimicking myocardial infarction in a patient with rheumatoid arthritis. *Clin Rheumatol.* 2009;28:479–481.

31. Hammann C, Genton CY, Delabays A, et al. Myocarditis of mixed connective tissue disease: favourable outcome after intravenous pulsed cyclophosphamide. *Clin Rheumatol.* 1999;18:85–87.

32. Lash AD, Wittman AL, Quismorio FP Jr. Myocarditis in mixed connective tissue disease: clinical and pathologic study of three cases and review of the literature. *Semin Arthritis Rheum.* 1986;15:288–296.

164 Hypersensitivity, Eosinophilic, and Toxic Myocarditis

Allen P. Burke, M.D.

Definitions

"Hypersensitivity myocarditis" is an etiologic definition that denotes a reaction to an ingested substance, usually a drug, that usually, but not always, has an eosinophilic reaction. "Eosinophilic myocarditis" is applied to symptomatic myocarditis with documented tissue or peripheral eosinophilia and often also has an allergic or hypersensitivity etiology. Eosinophils are not specific for cause, however, as they may be present in infectious as well as giant cell myocarditis.

Toxic myocarditis is a heterogeneous group of disorders. As is the case with hypersensitivity, drugs commonly cause toxic insults to the heart. However, the mechanism is believed to be direct myocyte toxicity, as opposed to immune-mediated mechanisms. Catecholamine-induced myocardial injury is often considered a form of toxic myocarditis, but because inflammation is relatively minimal, it is usually considered a form of cardiomyopathy (see Chapters 2 and 24). Chemotherapy-induced myocyte injury often goes through an inflammatory phase, but is also considered a form of cardiomyopathy (see Chapters 2 and 19). Other toxic compounds, such as arsenic, have historically been linked to a form of myocarditis. For all intents and purposes, the term "toxic myocarditis" is of limited use currently and will be addressed only briefly in this chapter.

Hypersensitivity and Eosinophilic Myocarditis

Incidence

Symptomatic hypersensitivity myocarditis, especially when documented histologically, is rare and generally the subject of case reports. The incidence of incidental hypersensitivity myocarditis diagnosed initially at autopsy is high, about 2% to 5%, depending on the population and history of medication use. In patients awaiting transplant, who are often on multiple medications, the incidence is 2% to 7%, as diagnosed histologically in the explanted heart or left ventricular apex removed at time of assist device insertion.[1,2]

Pathogenesis

Hypersensitivity is due to a delayed hypersensitivity reaction, and not a toxic effect of the offending drug. It has been postulated that modified collagen may be a trigger for eosinophilic reaction and degranulation.[3]

Many drugs have been histologically associated with hypersensitivity myocarditis.[4] A smaller number have been implicated in symptomatic hypersensitivity myocarditis diagnosed histologically (generally by endomyocardial biopsy) (Table 164.1).

In incidentally found hypersensitivity myocarditis at autopsy and explants, a specific drug is rarely identified, because of multiple medication history.

Eosinophilic myocarditis may also be the result of mechanisms other than hypersensitivity. Churg-Strauss syndrome, parasitic infection, and chronic eosinophilic leukemia can result in eosinophilic infiltrates in the myocardium, often with myocyte necrosis. In some patients, an underlying cause or offending agent is never found.[26]

Clinical Findings

Clinical manifestations of hypersensitivity myocarditis fall into two groups of patients: those diagnosed during life, who have severe, often life-threatening symptoms (more often termed "eosinophilic myocarditis)," and those diagnosed at explant or autopsy, who often have no symptoms. The term "acute necrotizing eosinophilic myocarditis" has been used for the most severe form of hypersensitivity myocarditis that causes rapidly progressive congestive heart failure.[27,28]

TABLE 164.1   Drugs Associated with Hypersensitivity Myocarditis Diagnosed Pathologically

Medication	Symptom	Reference
Amoxicillin	Heart failure, chest pain, acute coronary syndrome	5
		6 (Giant cells)
		7 (No giant cells)
	Sudden death	
Ciprofloxacin	Cardiogenic shock	8
Cephalosporin (cefaclor)	Heart failure	9
Cephalosporins (2)	Heart failure and death	10
Dobutamine	Heart failure	11
		12
Clozapine	Sudden death[a]	13
	Heart failure, fever	14
Metoprolol	Heart failure	15
Azithromycin	Fever, rash, heart failure, DRESS syndrome	16
Mesalamine	Chest pain, heart failure	17
Ephedra	Heart failure	18
Sulfasalazine	Cardiogenic shock (Fatal)	19 (Had giant cells on biopsy)
		20 (No giant cells)
Isoniazid	Rash, myocarditis	21
Antituberculous drugs (multiple)	Myocarditis, heart failure	22
Herbal supplements	Heart failure, ventricular arrhythmias	23
Adalimumab	Fatal cardiogenic shock	24
No agent identified	Heart failure	25

[a]Diagnosed made at autopsy. Others in table were diagnosed by biopsy.

Patients with symptomatic hypersensitivity myocarditis often present with signs and symptoms of myocarditis, often with heart failure. The symptoms generally occur within weeks after exposure to agent and generally resolve after withdrawal of the drug. The cardiac symptoms may be accompanied by a skin rash. Other manifestations of systemic hypersensitivity, including peripheral eosinophilia, may accompany hypersensitivity myocarditis (drug-induced rash with eosinophilia and systemic symptoms).[5,21,29,30] Hypersensitivity myocarditis causing severe heart failure has been reported complicating Stevens-Johnson syndrome.[19]

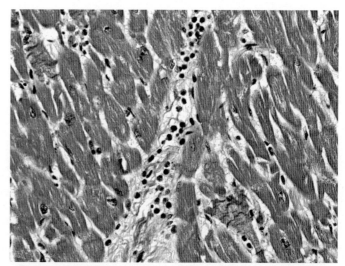

FIGURE 164.1 ▲ Hypersensitivity myocarditis. There is a sparse interstitial infiltrate, without any myocyte damage. Focal interstitial infiltrates are a common finding at autopsy, especially in patients on multiple medications.

Most patients respond to steroids and drug cessation.[22,23,25,31,32] Irreversible heart failure may lead to cardiogenic shock and death, or heart transplantation.[7,19,20]

Histologic Findings

There is a spectrum of histologic findings in hypersensitivity myocarditis. Incidental, asymptomatic disease is typically manifested by sparse interstitial infiltrates of macrophages and lymphocytes, with occasional plasma cells; eosinophils may be difficult to find. Symptomatic myocarditis is characterized by cellular infiltrates of eosinophils, macrophages, and lymphocytes, with myocyte destruction and abundant myocyte necrosis. The degree of necrosis in some cases is such that there is a macrophage giant cell reaction mimicking giant cell myocarditis.

Incidental hypersensitivity myocarditis shows interstitial and perivascular infiltrates that do not infiltrate among individual myocytes and that are often overlooked at low magnification (Figs. 164.1 and 164.2). The infiltrates are composed of macrophages, lymphocytes, and eosinophils, with a

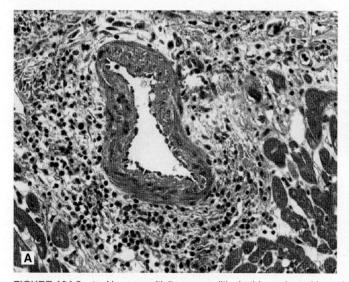

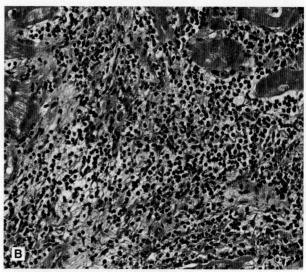

FIGURE 164.2 ▲ Hypersensitivity myocarditis. In this explanted heart in a transplant recipient, there are scattered interstitial infiltrates, without myocyte damage. **A.** There is interstitial inflammation with eosinophils and mononuclear cells. **B.** A higher magnification shows marked interstitial inflammation with prominent eosinophils.

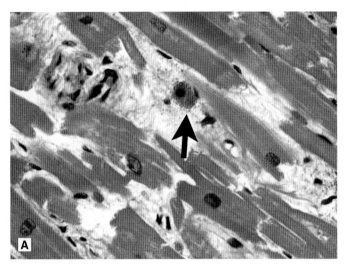
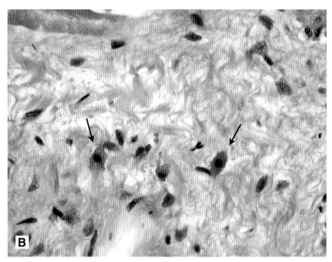

FIGURE 164.3 ▲ Hypersensitivity myocarditis, mast cells. **A.** Degranulating mast cells may be present near myocytes. **B.** Mast cells may also accompany the interstitial infiltrate.

subpopulation of plasma cells in some cases. Small, poorly formed granulomas may occur around vessels and in the interstitium. The incidence of myocyte necrosis depends on the extent of disease; in general, there is no myocyte damage and therefore no resulting fibrosis. However, in some autopsy series, necrosis has been found in up to half of cases, but are typically described as small or inconspicuous.[4] At autopsy, infiltrates in other organs such as the lung and liver are present in more than half of patients.[4]

Mast cells may contribute to symptoms by degranulating and causing vasoconstriction (Fig. 164.3). Symptomatic eosinophilic myocarditis shows a diffuse inflammatory infiltrate with predominant eosinophils with extensive myocyte necrosis (Fig. 164.4). Plasma cells may be prominent, and occasionally there is little necrosis, despite symptoms of heart failure.[33]

Incidental Hypersensitivity Myocarditis in Explanted Hearts

Hypersensitivity myocarditis is seen in 3% to 10% of cardiac explants[1,2] and may develop while the patient is on a ventricular assist device.[34]

There has been an association with increased risk for rejection, but not with decreased graft survival.[2]

Giant Cell Myocarditis as Manifestation of Hypersensitivity

The extent of necrosis in cases of hypersensitivity myocarditis may be so great that there is a macrophage giant cell reaction (Fig. 164.5).[6,19] Whether these cases should be considered a form of hypersensitivity with giant cell reaction, or giant cell myocarditis, is unclear. Giant cell myocarditis is generally considered an autoimmune disease that may have a minority component of eosinophils in the inflammatory reaction (Chapter 28).

Kounis Syndrome

A reversible acute coronary syndrome caused by hypersensitivity has been called "Kounis syndrome." It is diagnosed in patients who have systemic allergic or anaphylactic symptoms and signs and symptoms of acute myocardial infarction, which usually responds to

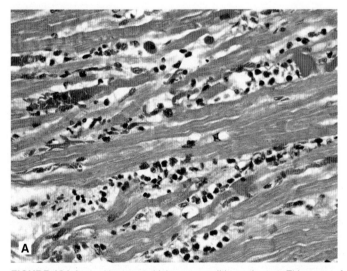
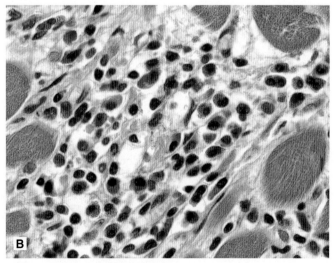

FIGURE 164.4 ▲ Hypersensitivity myocarditis, patient on Zithromax. **A.** Infiltrates related to hypersensitivity may be relatively expensive with borderline myocyte necrosis; this patient had focal severe coronary disease, but the myocarditis may have played a contributing role in the patient's death. **B.** In this patient, plasma cells were relatively numerous.

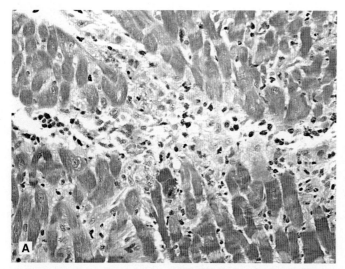
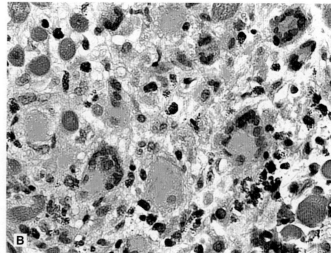

FIGURE 164.5 ▲ Eosinophilic myocarditis (necrotizing eosinophilic myocarditis), with giant cells, fatal. In rare instances, reactions to drugs may result in an intense inflammatory reaction with granulomas or giant cells. This patient had a severe reaction to ceftriaxone with cutaneous manifestations. **A.** Note interstitial inflammation with eosinophils. **B.** In other areas, there were giant cells and myocyte necrosis.

nitroglycerin and steroids. Allergic coronary spasm resulting from presumed mast cell degranulation may be associated with hypersensitivity myocarditis.[35,36]

Catecholamine-Induced Myocarditis

Catecholamines typically induce contractions band necrosis (see Chapters 2 and 24). Contraction band necrosis is a well-described entity that is related to catecholamine toxicity, mediated by calcium ion influx or microvascular spasm. Prolonged resuscitation in adults produces a recognizable pattern of myocardial injury characterized by contraction band necrosis, focal hemorrhage, and coagulation necrosis (Table 164.2). Studies of donor hearts awaiting explantation for transplant have shown that contraction band necrosis is especially prevalent in patients with intracranial hemorrhage, followed by patients with brain trauma who have survived several hours, followed by fewer than 5% of patients with instantaneous death following trauma.[37] These studies have lent the term "brain death lesions" to myocardial contraction band necrosis in patients with anoxic encephalopathy and absence of brain function, but did not demonstrate significant myocardial damage.

Contraction band necrosis, in its earliest stage, is the prominence of thick Z-bands in intact myocytes; this change is a common artifact of resuscitation and has minimal to absent inflammatory reaction (Fig. 164.6). Later stages, which presumably occur after hours of catecholamine damage, include single cell necrosis, with contraction bands variably discernable, with occasional

macrophages at the sarcolemmal membrane (Fig. 164.7). Later, there may be groups of necrotic cells, a sparse inflammatory infiltrates, and extracellular edema, which eventually progresses to interstitial hemorrhage and focal necrosis of small vessels. While the histologic finding of contraction band necrosis is usually easily seen at conventional histology, it can be highlighted by Masson trichrome stain (Fig. 164.8).

Toxic Myocarditis

The term toxic myocarditis has been used in a variety of settings. Toxic myocarditis connotes drug-induced injury that is dose related, not mediated by hypersensitivity, and that persists after cessation of the drug, similar to cardiotoxicity due to chemotherapeutic agents.[38,39] Rarely, a form of myocarditis may occur after venom

TABLE 164.2   Stages of Myocardial Catecholamine-Induced Injury

Necrosis	Inflammation	Interstitial Changes
Contraction bands with wide Z-bands	None	None
Coagulative single cell necrosis	Rare macrophages within sarcolemma	None
Groups of necrotic myocytes	Macrophages, neutrophils in interstitium	Edema
Diffuse injury	Mixed	Edema and hemorrhage

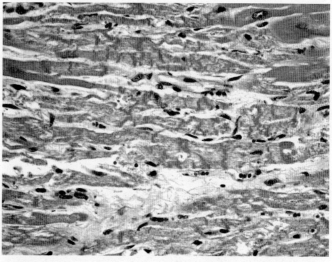

FIGURE 164.6 ▲ Hypersensitivity myocarditis with extensive necrosis and sudden death. Another area of the myocardium illustrated in Figure 164.5 demonstrates extensive myocyte necrosis, an atypical feature in hypersensitivity myocarditis.

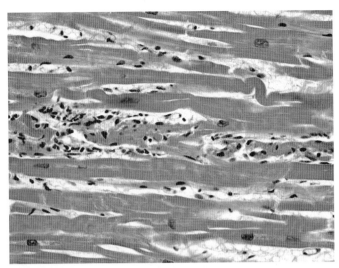

FIGURE 164.7 ▲ Contraction band necrosis. There is a zone of contraction bands with minimal inflammation. The patient died in hypotensive shock after a gastrointestinal bleed.

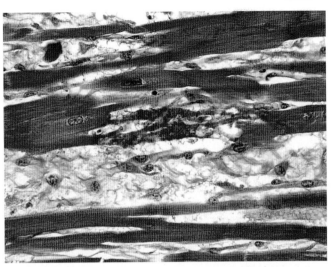

FIGURE 164.8 ▲ Focal contraction band necrosis. Such lesions at autopsy are sometimes referred to as "brain death lesions"; in this case of sudden unexpected death, the cause of contraction bands was related possibly to the patient's use of catecholaminergic drugs (Ephedra).

exposure, for example, to black widow spiders. In these cases, the diagnosis of myocarditis was made clinically without pathologic confirmation.[40,41]

Histologic features of toxic myocarditis have included contraction band necrosis, vasculitis, intracellular edema, and mixed inflammatory infiltrate. The inflammatory infiltrate of toxic myocarditis has been described, however, as variably mixed, with neutrophils, B lymphocytes, and macrophages, with areas of fibrosis in different stages of development, namely, with temporal heterogeneity. Many single reports of toxic myocarditis lack detailed histologic characterization and clear association with the offending agent.[42,43] Therefore, the diagnosis of "toxic myocarditis" has little meaning from a histopathologic standpoint currently.

Practical Points

▶ Hypersensitivity myocarditis is a subset of eosinophilic myocarditis that occurs days to weeks after exposure to allergen (usually medication).

▶ Unlike eosinophilic endomyocardial disease (hypereosinophilic syndrome), hypersensitivity myocarditis resolves upon cessation of the drug and is not associated with vascular or mural thrombosis.

▶ The histologic spectrum of hypersensitivity myocarditis ranges from sparse interstitial infiltrates without necrosis (asymptomatic without myocyte damage) to a fulminant reaction with aggressive infiltrates and myocyte necrosis (heart failure with elevated cardiac enzymes).

▶ Toxic myocarditis is not a specific histologic entity, but is an etiologic designation indicating dose-related inflammatory myocardial inflammation.

▶ The most common type of toxic myocardial injury is that of catecholamine-related myocyte damage from endogenous or exogenous catecholamines or related drugs of abuse.

REFERENCES

1. Gravanis MB, Hertzler GL, Franch RH, et al. Hypersensitivity myocarditis in heart transplant candidates. *J Heart Lung Transplant.* 1991;10:688–697.
2. Kanai-Yoshizawa S, Sugiyama Kato T, Mancini D, et al. Hypersensitivity myocarditis and outcome after heart transplantation. *J Heart Lung Transplant.* 2013;32:553–559.
3. Kendell KR, Day JD, Hruban RH, et al. Intimate association of eosinophils to collagen bundles in eosinophilic myocarditis and ranitidine-induced hypersensitivity myocarditis. *Arch Pathol Lab Med.* 1995;119:1154–1160.
4. Burke AP, Saenger J, Mullick F, et al. Hypersensitivity myocarditis. *Arch Pathol Lab Med.* 1991;115:764–769.
5. Park Y, Ahn SG, Ko A, et al. Hypersensitivity myocarditis confirmed by cardiac magnetic resonance imaging and endomyocardial biopsy. *Korean J Intern Med.* 2014;29:236–240.
6. Martinez S, Miranda E, Kim P, et al. Giant cell myocarditis associated with amoxicillin hypersensitivity reaction. *Forensic Sci Med Pathol.* 2013;9:403–406.
7. Huston B, Froloff V, Mills K, et al. Death due to eosinophilic necrotizing myocarditis despite steroid treatment. *Am J Forensic Med Pathol.* 2013;34:95–97.
8. Aggarwal A, Bergin P, Jessup P, et al. Hypersensitivity myocarditis presenting as cardiogenic shock. *J Heart Lung Transplant.* 2001;20:1241–1244.
9. Beghetti M, Wilson GJ, Bohn D, et al. Hypersensitivity myocarditis caused by an allergic reaction to cefaclor. *J Pediatr.* 1998;132:172–173.
10. Chikwava KR, Savell VH Jr, Boyd TK. Fatal cephalosporin-induced acute hypersensitivity myocarditis. *Pediatr Cardiol.* 2006;27:777–780.
11. Butany J, Nair V, Ahluwalia MS, et al. Hypersensitivity myocarditis complicating hypertrophic cardiomyopathy heart. *Can J Cardiol.* 2004;20:911–914.
12. Lee CC, Luthringer DJ, Czer LS. Dobutamine-induced fever and isolated eosinophilic myocarditis in a 66-year-old male awaiting heart transplantation: a case report. *Transplant Proc.* 2014;46:2464–2466.
13. Fineschi V, Neri M, Riezzo I, et al. Sudden cardiac death due to hypersensitivity myocarditis during clozapine treatment. *Int J Legal Med.* 2004;118:307–309.
14. Pieroni M, Cavallaro R, Chimenti C, et al. Clozapine-induced hypersensitivity myocarditis. *Chest.* 2004;126:1703–1705.
15. Frustaci A, Verardo R, Sale P, et al. Hypersensitivity myocarditis induced by beta-blockers: an unexpected cause of abrupt deterioration in hypertrophic cardiomyopathy. *Intensive Care Med.* 2007;33:1848–1849.
16. Pursnani A, Yee H, Slater W, et al. Hypersensitivity myocarditis associated with azithromycin exposure. *Ann Intern Med.* 2009;150:225–226.
17. Stelts S, Taylor MH, Nappi J, et al. Mesalamine-associated hypersensitivity myocarditis in ulcerative colitis. *Ann Pharmacother.* 2008;42:904–905.
18. Zaacks SM, Klein L, Tan CD, et al. Hypersensitivity myocarditis associated with ephedra use. *J Toxicol Clin Toxicol.* 1999;37:485–489.

19. Mitoff PR, Mesana TG, Mielniczuk LM, et al. Giant cell myocarditis in a patient with a spondyloarthropathy after a drug hypersensitivity reaction. *Can J Cardiol.* 2013;29:1138 e7-8.
20. Jeremic I, Vujasinovic-Stupar N, Terzic T, et al. Fatal sulfasalazine-induced eosinophilic myocarditis in a patient with periodic fever syndrome. *Med Princ Pract.* 2015;24:195–197.
21. Zhang SN, He QX, Yang NB, et al. Isoniazid-induced drug rash with eosinophilia and systemic symptoms (DRESS) syndrome presenting as acute eosinophilic myocarditis. *Intern Med.* 2015;54:1227–1230.
22. Li H, Dai Z, Wang B, et al. A case report of eosinophilic myocarditis and a review of the relevant literature. *BMC Cardiovasc Disord.* 2015;15:15.
23. Allen SF, Godley RW, Evron JM, et al. Acute necrotizing eosinophilic myocarditis in a patient taking Garcinia cambogia extract successfully treated with high-dose corticosteroids. *Can J Cardiol.* 2014;30:1732.e13-5.
24. Adamson R, Yazici Y, Katz ES, et al. Fatal acute necrotizing eosinophilic myocarditis temporally related to use of adalimumab in a patient with relapsing polychondritis. *J Clin Rheumatol.* 2013;19:386–389.
25. Aslan I, Fischer M, Laser KT, et al. Eosinophilic myocarditis in an adolescent: a case report and review of the literature. *Cardiol Young.* 2013;23:277–283.
26. Kawano S, Kato J, Kawano N, et al. Clinical features and outcomes of eosinophilic myocarditis patients treated with prednisolone at a single institution over a 27-year period. *Intern Med.* 2011;50:975–981.
27. Watanabe N, Nakagawa S, Fukunaga T, et al. Acute necrotizing eosinophilic myocarditis successfully treated by high dose methylprednisolone. *Jpn Circ J.* 2001;65:923–926.
28. Kontani M, Takashima S, Okura K, et al. Survival after acute necrotizing eosinophilic myocarditis complicating a massive left ventricular mural thrombus: a case report. *J Cardiol.* 2007;50:127–133.
29. Pereira CM, Vaz M, Kotha S, et al. Dapsone hypersensitivity syndrome with myocarditis. *J Assoc Physicians India.* 2014;62:728–731.
30. Kanno K, Sakai H, Yamada Y, et al. Drug-induced hypersensitivity syndrome due to minocycline complicated by severe myocarditis. *J Dermatol.* 2014;41:160–162.
31. Eppenberger M, Hack D, Ammann P, et al. Acute eosinophilic myocarditis with dramatic response to steroid therapy: the central role of echocardiography in diagnosis and follow-up. *Tex Heart Inst J.* 2013;40:326–330.
32. Komatsu T, Isoda K, Niida T, et al. A good outcome of a case with eosinophilic myocarditis. *Intern Med.* 2012;51:2483–2484.
33. Raje VP, Lewis NP, Katlaps GJ, et al. Dobutamine induced eosinophilic myocarditis and right heart failure requiring emergent biventricular assist device implantation. *ASAIO J.* 2015;61:213–215.
34. Pereira NL, Park SJ, Daly RC, et al. De novo development of eosinophilic myocarditis with left ventricular assist device support as bridge to transplant. *Ann Thorac Surg.* 2010;90:1345–1347.
35. Cardillo MT, Della Bona R, Basile E, et al. Hypersensitivity myocarditis or Kounis syndrome? *Intern Emerg Med.* 2014;9:247–248.
36. Almpanis GC, Mazarakis A, Dimopoulos DA, et al. The conundrum of hypersensitivity cardiac disease: hypersensitivity myocarditis, acute hypersensitivity coronary syndrome (Kounis syndrome) or both? *Int J Cardiol.* 2011;148:237–240.
37. Baroldi G, Mittleman RE, Parolini M, et al. Myocardial contraction bands. Definition, quantification and significance in forensic pathology. *Int J Legal Med.* 2001;115:142–151.
38. Ansari A, Maron BJ, Berntson DG. Drug-induced toxic myocarditis. *Tex Heart Inst J.* 2003;30:76–79.
39. Berry G. Pathology of myocarditis. In: Cooper LT, ed. *Myocarditis: From Bench to Bedside.* New York, NY: Humana Press, Springer; 2002:325–370.
40. Golcuk Y, Velibey Y, Gonullu H, et al. Acute toxic fulminant myocarditis after a black widow spider envenomation: case report and literature review. *Clin Toxicol (Phila).* 2013;51:191–192.
41. Sari I, Zengin S, Davutoglu V, et al. Myocarditis after black widow spider envenomation. *Am J Emerg Med.* 2008;26:630 e1-3.
42. Fagan E, Forbes A, Williams R. Toxic myocarditis in paracetamol poisoning. *Br Med J (Clin Res Ed).* 1988;296:63–64.
43. Gradinger R, Jung C, Reinhardt D, et al. Toxic myocarditis due to oral ingestion of hydrofluoric acid. *Heart Lung Circ.* 2008;17:248–250.

165 Giant Cell Myocarditis

Allen P. Burke, M.D.

Pathogenesis

Historically termed *"Fiedler myocarditis,"*[1] giant cell myocarditis is a rare disorder with unclear cause. An autoimmune cause is likely, because patients often have concomitant autoimmune disorders (up to 8% in one series).[2] Table 165.1 lists diseases that have been associated disease with giant cell myocarditis.

The etiology of the giant cells, which are present by definition, is unclear, but likely related to macrophage engulfment of necrotic myocytes. There is some overlap with necrotizing eosinophilic myocarditis, which may elicit a giant cell reaction due to extensive necrosis (see Chapter 27).[20] There are occasional reported cases that suggest an enteroviral trigger.[21]

Incidence

Giant cell myocarditis is rare, accounting for fewer than 1% of myocarditis cases.[22]

Clinical Findings

Giant cell myocarditis most often affects young to middle-aged adults, although several case reports in children as early as 10 days old have been documented.[23,24] There is a slight male predominance.

Most cases of giant cell myocarditis follow a rapidly deteriorating course (days to months) from congestive heart failure to cardiogenic shock that is often unresponsive to conventional treatments. During the course of the illness, ventricular tachycardia is noted in a high percentage of the patients.[25] The initial presenting symptoms may also be sudden death.[26]

In a subset of patients, early symptoms are those of lymphocytic myocarditis or myopericarditis with more gradually progressive heart failure.[27]

TABLE 165.1 Selected Reported Autoimmune Disorders Associated with Giant Cell Myocarditis

Associated Disease
Myasthenia gravis and or thymoma[3–6]
Inflammatory bowel disease[7,8]
Idiopathic generalized myositis[3,9]
Orbital myositis[10–12]
Systemic lupus erythematosus[13]
Common variable immunodeficiency syndrome[14]
Autoimmune hepatitis[13]
Sjogren syndrome[15,16]
Vitiligo[12,16]
Hashimoto thyroiditis[17]
Behçet disease[18]
Spondyloarthropathy, HLA B27 associated[19]

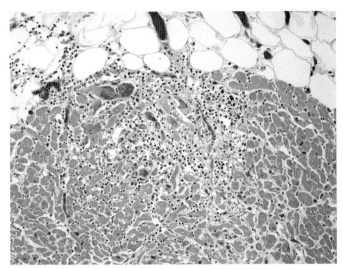

FIGURE 165.1 ▲ Giant cell myocarditis. There is an area of inflammation with giant cells at the epicardium. The epicardial fat is not involved in giant cell myocarditis, which is a process targeted at the myocyte. The focus was an incidental finding at autopsy.

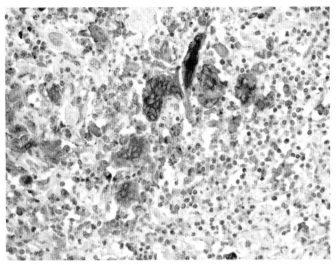

FIGURE 165.3 ▲ Giant cell myocarditis, CD68 immunohistochemical stain. The giant cells are predominantly macrophages.

Rarely, giant cell myocarditis can be an incidental finding, especially if isolated to the atria (see below)[28] (Fig. 165.1).

Imaging

The imaging findings of giant cell myocarditis are similar to those of lymphocytic myocarditis. On cardiac magnetic resonance, T2-weighted images show high-intensity signals in a patchy ventricular distribution. Late gadolinium enhancement, which is seen in fibrosis, necrosis, inflammation, and edema, is seen in multiple myocardial areas in different myocardial layers.[29]

Gross Pathology Findings

The gross findings at autopsy reflect those of inflammation and fibrosis and range from minimal findings to irregular areas of scarring and mottling. The presence of gross abnormalities is more common than in lymphocytic myocarditis, because of frequent progression to fibrosis. At autopsy, cardiomegaly is present in about one-half of cases.[30] Most

cases have involvement of the left ventricle with a diffuse yellow-brown discoloration and without sharp demarcation from the surrounding myocardium. In some cases, subendocardial necrosis may mimic acute myocardial infarction.[30] Unusual findings include mural thrombi and ventricular wall rupture.[22]

Microscopic Findings

Giant cell myocarditis is histologically characterized by diffuse infiltration of the myocardium by a heterogeneous infiltrate composed of abundant lymphocytes, some eosinophils and plasma cells, occasional neutrophils, and scattered prominent giant cells (Fig. 165.2). The giant cells are predominantly macrophages, although there may be occasional myocyte giant cells in areas of necrosis. Myocyte giant cells are not specific for giant cell myocarditis and are seen adjacent to infarcts. In giant cell myocarditis, T lymphocytes are more numerous than B cells with a predominance of CD8 T lymphocytes.[30] There are invariably myocyte degenerative changes and myocyte necrosis, especially in early stages of the disease. Most of the giant cells are macrophages of Langhans type (Fig. 165.3), measuring 40 to 50 μm in diameter and usually

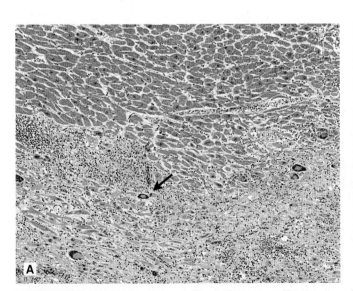

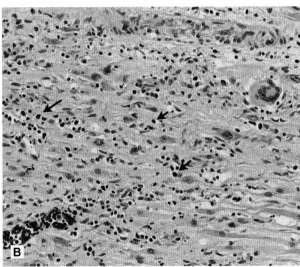

FIGURE 165.2 ▲ Giant cell myocarditis. **A.** At low magnification, there is an area of inflammation with extensive myocyte necrosis (below), with scattered giant cells (*arrow*). **B.** At higher magnification, the inflammatory infiltrate contains scattered eosinophils (*arrows*).

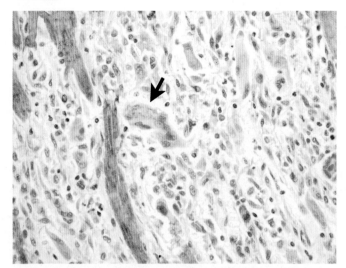

FIGURE 165.4 ▲ Giant cell myocarditis, muscle-specific actin. There are fragments of cardiomyocyte cytoplasm in the giant cells. Cardiomyocyte giant cells also occur at the edges of necrosis in giant cell myocarditis, as around the edge of infarcts.

found on the borders of active lesions, within normal myocardium. Myocyte cytoplasm may be detected within the macrophage giant cells (Fig. 165.4). The nuclei vary in number from 2 to 20 with small nucleoli.[30]

In association with the inflammation and tissue damage, evolving and healed lesions show a fewer number of giant cells and are characterized by large zones of fibrosis, collage deposition, and granulation tissue. In these chronic lesions, active myocyte necrosis is far less prominent. Even later in the stage of the disease, it is very difficult to find giant cells, and the tissue is replaced by scar with a very sparse lymphocytic infiltrate.

Eosinophils are frequently present at low numbers (Fig. 165.2B). Giant cell myocarditis associated with drug hypersensitivity, as defined by antibiotic or other drug exposure with an associated rash, has an especially high density of eosinophils in the infiltrate.[31]

Differential Diagnosis

In contrast to cardiac sarcoidosis, in giant cell myocarditis, the giant cells are not part of well-formed granulomas, and there is abundant

TABLE 165.2 Differential Features Between Giant Cell Myocarditis and Cardiac Sarcoidosis

	Giant Cell Myocarditis	Cardiac Sarcoidosis
Myocyte necrosis	+++	+/−
Well-formed granulomas	−	+/−
Fibrosis	+/−	++
Giant cells adjacent to myocyte necrosis	++	−
Epicardial involvement	−	+/−
Eosinophils	−	+/−

myocyte necrosis in active areas. Eosinophils can be present in most cases of giant cell myocarditis and rare in cardiac sarcoidosis (Table 165.2).[30]

A large number of eosinophils raise the possibility of necrotizing eosinophilic myocarditis (see Chapter 27), which is generally considered a hypersensitivity reaction and not an autoimmune disorder. Whether eosinophilic myocarditis with necrosis and macrophage giant cell reaction, and giant cell myocarditis form part of a spectrum or are distinct entities has yet to be clarified.

Biopsy Diagnosis

Giant cell myocarditis is usually diagnosed at autopsy, by endomyocardial biopsy (Fig. 165.5), or upon examination of left ventricular apical tissue removed to insertion of assist devices.[32] Endomyocardial biopsies, because of their small size, often show borderline results or changes indistinguishable from lymphocytic myocarditis.[19,33] There are no precise guidelines regarding rebiopsy in patients suspected of having giant cell myocarditis in whom biopsies show equivocal results.[34]

Atrial Giant Cell Myocarditis

Atrial giant cell myocarditis differs from typical giant cell myocarditis, in that the disease is generally benign. Atrial giant cell myocarditis can be an incidental finding in removal of atrial during surgery for atrial fibrillation.[28]

Patients with isolated atrial giant cell myocarditis often have atrial fibrillation and atrial thrombi. Histologically, there are giant cell and lymphocytic infiltrates, lymphocytic myocarditis-like foci,

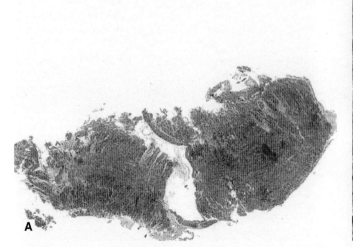

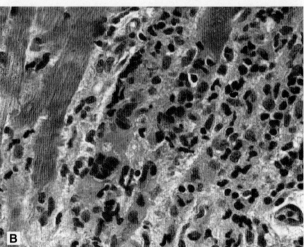

FIGURE 165.5 ▲ Giant cell myocarditis, endomyocardial biopsy. **A.** Low magnification shows a large area of inflammation and myocyte dropout. **B.** Higher magnification shows cardiomyocyte necrosis and a lymphocytic infiltrate with macrophage giant cells.

cardiomyocyte necrosis, and cardiomyocyte hypertrophy. As with ventricular disease, interstitial fibrosis and scattered eosinophils are common.[35]

Treatment

Treatment for giant cell myocarditis includes immunosuppression with combined corticosteroids and calcineurin inhibitors[27] and ventricular assist devices or cardiac transplantation in patients refractory to therapy.[36]

Patients with atrial giant cell myocarditis generally respond to conventional therapies and have an excellent prognosis.[35]

REFERENCES

1. Hertzog AJ, Hayford WD. Acute isolated myocarditis (Fiedler's myocarditis). *Minn Med.* 1947;30:54–56.
2. Cooper LT Jr, Berry GJ, Shabetai R. Idiopathic giant-cell myocarditis—natural history and treatment. Multicenter Giant Cell Myocarditis Study Group Investigators. *N Engl J Med.* 1997;336:1860–1866.
3. Burke JS, Medline NM, Katz A. Giant cell myocarditis and myositis. Associated with thymoma and myasthenia gravis. *Arch Pathol.* 1969;88:359–366.
4. Joudinaud TM, Fadel E, Thomas-de-Montpreville V, et al. Fatal giant cell myocarditis after thymoma resection in myasthenia gravis. *J Thorac Cardiovasc Surg.* 2006;131:494–495.
5. Kon T, Mori F, Tanji K, et al. Giant cell polymyositis and myocarditis associated with myasthenia gravis and thymoma. *Neuropathology.* 2013;33:281–287.
6. Koul D, Kanwar M, Jefic D, et al. Fulminant giant cell myocarditis and cardiogenic shock: an unusual presentation of malignant thymoma. *Cardiol Res Pract.* 2010;2010:185896.
7. Ariza A, Lopez MD, Mate JL, et al. Giant cell myocarditis: monocytic immunophenotype of giant cells in a case associated with ulcerative colitis. *Hum Pathol.* 1995;26:121–123.
8. Nash CL, Panaccione R, Sutherland LR, et al. Giant cell myocarditis, in a patient with Crohn's disease, treated with etanercept—a tumour necrosis factor-alpha antagonist. *Can J Gastroenterol.* 2001;15:607–611.
9. Tanahashi N, Sato H, Nogawa S, et al. A case report of giant cell myocarditis and myositis observed during the clinical course of invasive thymoma associated with myasthenia gravis. *Keio J Med.* 2004;53:30–42.
10. Leib ML, Odel JG, Cooney MJ. Orbital polymyositis and giant cell myocarditis. *Ophthalmology.* 1994;101:950–954.
11. Lind-Ayres MR, Abramowsky C, Mahle WT. Pediatric giant cell myocarditis and orbital myositis. *Pediatr Cardiol.* 2009;30(4):510–512.
12. Stevens AW, Grossman ME, Barr ML. Orbital myositis, vitiligo, and giant cell myocarditis. *J Am Acad Dermatol.* 1996;35:310–312.
13. Shariff S, Straatman L, Allard M, et al. Novel associations of giant cell myocarditis: two case reports and a review of the literature. *Can J Cardiol.* 2004;20:557–561.
14. Laufs H, Nigrovic PA, Schneider LC, et al. Giant cell myocarditis in a 12-year-old girl with common variable immunodeficiency. *Mayo Clin Proc.* 2002;77:92–96.
15. Lindvall K, Edhag O, Erhardt LR, et al. Complete heart block due to granulomatous giant cell myocarditis: report of 3 cases. *Eur J Cardiol.* 1978;8:349–358.
16. Schumann C, Faust M, Gerharz M, et al. Autoimmune polyglandular syndrome associated with idiopathic giant cell myocarditis. *Exp Clin Endocrinol Diabetes.* 2005;113:302–307.
17. Kanzato N, Nakasone I, Sunagawa O, et al. [Giant-cell myocarditis without a symptom of heart failure seen in a patient with myasthenia gravis and concurrent Hashimoto's disease]. *Rinsho Shinkeigaku.* 2001;41:813–817.
18. Maeda S, Tamura A, Zaizen H, et al. Behcet's disease complicated by giant-cell myocarditis. *Intern Med.* 2014;53:1721.
19. Mitoff PR, Mesana TG, Mielniczuk LM, et al. Giant cell myocarditis in a patient with a spondyloarthropathy after a drug hypersensitivity reaction. *Can J Cardiol.* 2013;29:1138.e7-8.
20. Micozzi S, Pinto C, Seoane M, et al. Giant cell myocarditis in hypersensitivity reactions: is an early diagnose possible? *Ann Allergy Asthma Immunol.* 2015;115(3):247–248.
21. Lee M, Kwon GY, Kim JS, et al. Giant cell myocarditis associated with Coxsackievirus infection. *J Am Coll Cardiol.* 2010;56:e19.
22. Vaideeswar P, Cooper LT. Giant cell myocarditis: clinical and pathological features in an Indian population. *Cardiovasc Pathol.* 2013;22:70–74.
23. Cooper LT. Giant cell myocarditis in children. *Prog Pediatr Cardiol.* 2007;24:47–49.
24. Pyun KS, Kim YH, Katzenstein RE, et al. Giant cell myocarditis. Light and electron microscopic study. *Arch Pathol.* 1970;90:181–188.
25. Cooper LT Jr, Berry GJ, Rizeq M, et al. Giant cell myocarditis. *J Heart Lung Transplant.* 1995;14:394–401.
26. Hazebroek MR, van Paassen P, Weerwind PW, et al. A passionate endurance cyclist ultimately survives sudden death in right ventricular giant cell myocarditis. *Int J Cardiol.* 2014;170:e74–e75.
27. Tompkins R, Cole WJ, Rosenzweig BP, et al. Giant cell myocarditis: not always a presentation of cardiogenic shock. *Case Rep Cardiol.* 2015;2015:173826.
28. Bose AK, Bhattacharjee M, Martin V, et al. Giant cell myocarditis of the left atrium. *Cardiovasc Pathol.* 2010;19:e37–e38.
29. Sujino Y, Kimura F, Tanno J, et al. Cardiac magnetic resonance imaging in giant cell myocarditis: intriguing associations with clinical and pathological features. *Circulation.* 2014;129:e467–e469.
30. Litovsky SH, Burke AP, Virmani R. Giant cell myocarditis: an entity distinct from sarcoidosis characterized by multiphasic myocyte destruction by cytotoxic T cells and histiocytic giant cells. *Mod Pathol.* 1996;9:1126–1134.
31. Martinez S, Miranda E, Kim P, et al. Giant cell myocarditis associated with amoxicillin hypersensitivity reaction. *Forensic Sci Med Pathol.* 2013;9:403–406.
32. Eid SM, Schamp D, Halushka MK, et al. Resolution of giant cell myocarditis after extended ventricular assistance. *Arch Pathol Lab Med.* 2009;133:138–141.
33. Anderson K, Carrier M, Romeo P, et al. An unusual case of giant cell myocarditis missed in a Heartmate-2 left ventricle apical-wedge section: a case report and review of the literature. *J Cardiothorac Surg.* 2013;8:12.
34. Kalra A, Kneeland R, Samara MA, et al. The changing role for endomyocardial biopsy in the diagnosis of giant-cell myocarditis. *Cardiol Ther.* 2014.
35. Larsen BT, Maleszewski JJ, Edwards WD, et al. Atrial giant cell myocarditis: a distinctive clinicopathologic entity. *Circulation.* 2013;127:39–47.
36. Bendayan I, Crespo-Leiro MG, Paniagua-Martin MJ, et al. Giant cell myocarditis and heart transplantation. *J Heart Lung Transplant.* 2008;27:698–699.

166 Infections of the Myocardium

Fabio R. Tavora, M.D., Ph.D., and Allen P. Burke, M.D.

Viral and Postviral Myocarditis

Coxsackievirus type B is a type of enterovirus that causes a flu-like systemic illness that frequently involves the heart. Coxsackievirus type B is associated with epidemic disease and is frequently symptomatic; it is relatively uncommon, however, in prospective series of acute myocarditis that include subclinical cases.[1,2] It usually occurs in infants and children, in whom systemic disease is frequent. The mean age at presentation in symptomatic patients requiring hospitalization is a little under 3 years. Extracardiac symptoms include herpangina in three-fourths of patients and meningitis in about one-fourth. Most children survive, and type CB3 is associated with a worse prognosis.[3] In adults, coxsackieviral myocarditis is rare, especially with associated systemic disease.[4,5]

Adenovirus is the most frequent viral etiology in subclinical myocarditis as well as tissue diagnosis based on polymerase chain reaction; both receptors for adeno- and enterovirus have been demonstrated in human myocytes.[6] A recent autopsy study, however, found no case of adenoviral DNA in cardiac tissue with myocarditis.[7] The difficulty in detecting viral organisms and establishing causation is in part because the virus is largely cleared before significant inflammation or symptoms develop. The use of the term "postviral" myocarditis reflects this phenomenon.[8]

Other viruses that have been associated with myocarditis include parvovirus, influenza, poliomyelitis, Epstein-Barr virus, HIV-1, viral hepatitis, mumps, rubeola, varicella, variola/vaccinia, arbovirus, respiratory syncytial virus, herpes simplex virus, yellow fever virus, parvovirus, and rabies.[9,10] In endemic areas, high rates of dengue fever myocarditis with sudden death cases have been reported.[11,12] A specific etiologic relationship has not always been proven, however. For example, in the case of parvovirus, which is implicated in dilated cardiomyopathy,[13] there is a high rate of detection of viral-specific DNA in control tissue.[7]

The histologic features of inflammation are not specific for any virus, and a lymphocytic myocarditis is typically described in reports of unusual viral etiologies, with some exceptions. See Chapter 21 for detailed histologic description of lymphocytic myocarditis.

Immunocompromised patients, especially transplant recipients, are susceptible to cytomegaloviral infections including myocarditis. In immunocompetent individuals, cytomegalovirus infection may cause an infectious mononucleosis-like syndrome that uncommonly involves the heart as myocarditis.[14,15]

Bacterial Myocarditis

Acute neutrophilic myocarditis is rare and may be seen as an early phase in viral infections or as a result of bacterial myocarditis, often complicating endocarditis, in which case microabscesses are common (Figs. 166.1 to 166.4).

In immunocompetent patients, bacterial myocarditis in the absence of valvular endocarditis is unusual but may occur concomitantly with extensive bacterial pneumonia, caused especially by mycoplasma[16–18] or chlamydia.[19] Diagnosis is only rarely confirmed by endomyocardial biopsy, which shows lymphocytic infiltrates with myocyte necrosis.[20] In addition to microbiologic studies, clinical and laboratory studies consistent with myocarditis (ECG, serology for troponins, elevations of acute phase reactants, exclusion of coronary and other cardiac disease), myocarditis can also be suggested by cardiac magnetic resonance imaging.[19]

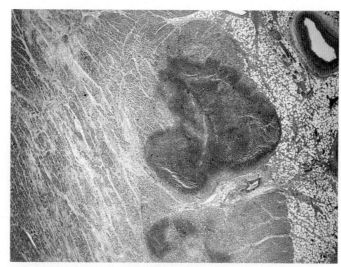

FIGURE 166.2 ▲ Bacterial myocarditis. Microabscesses are common, with necrosis and purulent exudate.

Disseminated leptospirosis, when fatal, involves the heart in over one-third of cases.[21] Histologic findings include hemorrhage and lymphocytic infiltrates. The organisms can be identified by immunohistochemical methods or silver stains and are most numerous in the kidneys.[21]

Other infections that may result in myocarditis include legionella, leptospirosis,[22] syphilis,[23] and tuberculosis. The latter presents typically as pericardial disease,[24] but nodular and miliary cardiac lesions can occur.[25] A variety of bacteria have been implicated in myocarditis in immunosuppressed patients. Histologically, the infection is similar to bacterial infections elsewhere and is characterized by neutrophilic infiltrates and microabscess formation. Focal tissue necrosis and myocyte loss are invariably seen. In sepsis, the myocardium can be secondarily involved and show intravascular inflammatory cells extending to the interstitium (Fig. 166.5).

Lyme disease (infection with *Borrelia burgdorferi*) results in cardiac symptoms in about 5% of patients, especially in the early stage of disseminated disease. Symptoms include conduction disturbances (especially heart block), pericarditis, and heart failure. There have been only a handful of reports with histologic confirmation of myocarditis, which shows intense interstitial inflammation with myocyte necrosis and mixed chronic inflammatory infiltrate (Figs. 166.6 and 166.7).[26] Cardiac magnetic resonance may demonstrate nonspecific changes of myocarditis.[27]

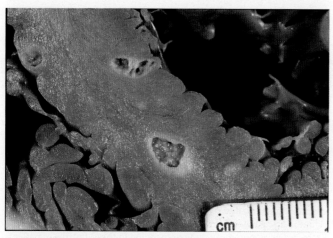

FIGURE 166.1 ▲ Bacterial myocarditis with abscesses. These are seen in the ventricular septum in this case.

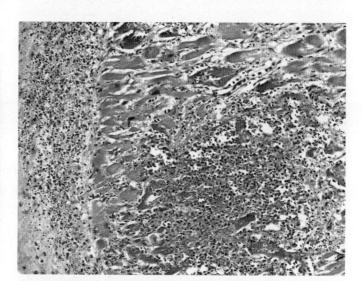

FIGURE 166.3 ▲ Bacterial myocarditis. There is extensive tissue destruction and neutrophilic exudate.

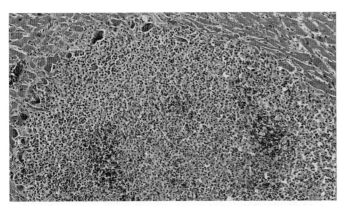

FIGURE 166.4 ▲ Bacterial myocarditis with microabscess. The neutrophils in this example infiltrate around myocytes with myocyte necrosis.

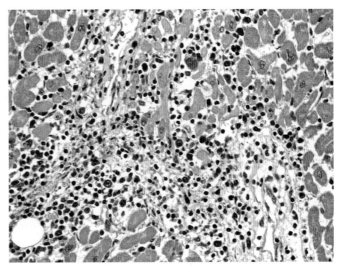

FIGURE 166.6 ▲ Lyme myocarditis. There is a mixed chronic inflammatory infiltrate with myocyte necrosis.

Whipple disease may occasionally involve the heart and valves,[28] resulting in heart failure in rare instances. Intracellular organisms are identified in macrophages by PAS staining and may be accompanied by neutrophils and chronic inflammation.[28]

Rickettsial myocarditis may be a manifestation of Rocky Mountain spotted fever[29] and rarely Q fever.[30] Generally, it is part of a systemic illness. Histologically, there is primarily interstitial inflammation, with rickettsial organisms occasionally identified by silver impregnation stains in a perivascular location (Fig. 166.8).

Fungal Myocarditis

Fungal myocarditis is rare and typically associated with immunosuppression in the setting of transplantation, chemotherapy, and HIV disease.[31] *Candida, Aspergillus, Cryptococcus,* and *Mucor* are the most common fungi involved, and patients usually have evidence of systemic disease (Figs. 166.9 to 166.11).[32]

Myocarditis Caused by Parasites

Parasitic myocarditis caused by toxoplasmosis occurs primarily in the immunocompromised setting.[33,34] Pathologic confirmation is usually only performed at autopsy, since endomyocardial biopsy has a very low sensitivity. On light microscopy, intracytoplasmic cysts can be seen (Fig. 166.12). There is generally minimal if any inflammatory reaction, because of immunosuppression.

Endemic Chagas disease has become established through Latin America, especially in the Amazon river basin, and it is estimated that 15 to 16 million people are infected with *Trypanosoma cruzi*. Initially, patients are most often asymptomatic, but an acute manifestation with fever, adenopathy, hepatosplenomegaly, and myocarditis can occur. Then the disease may evolve to the cardiac or digestive form. In cases with immunosuppression, the chronic infection may become acute again, with diffuse myocarditis.[35] Myocarditis is typically diagnosed clinically[36] and by cardiac magnetic resonance imaging.[37] Chronic Chagas disease happens most often in young adults, from 3 to 15 years after the initial infection. Histologically, acute forms are characterized by dense lymphocytic infiltrates that can be prominent in eosinophils with our without necrosis and parasitism of myofibers. Chronic Chagas disease reveals cardiomegaly, mostly on the right side, with dilatation more important than hypertrophy (Fig. 166.13). A peculiar thinning of the apex, especially on the left ventricle, with aneurysm formation is present in more than 50% of the cases.[38] May recur as myocarditis in transplanted hearts.[39]

Echinococcus may infest the heart as cysts, with little inflammatory reaction. They may be surgically excised if they lead to hemodynamic disturbances or ischemic symptoms.[40] Intraoperative sterilization is generally performed to prevent spread of scolices. Cysticercosis can

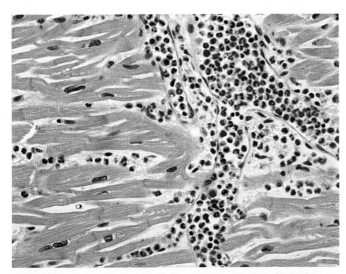

FIGURE 166.5 ▲ Myocarditis in bacterial sepsis. There is intravascular expansion of inflammatory cells, primarily neutrophils, which extend into tissue septa.

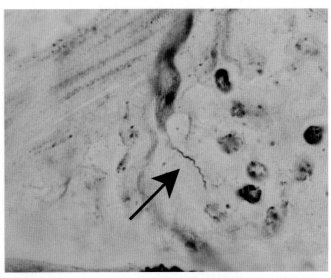

FIGURE 166.7 ▲ Lyme myocarditis (*Borrelia burgdorferi*). Silver impregnation stain demonstrates spirochetal organism.

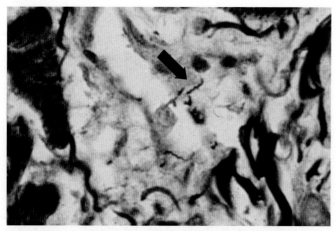

FIGURE 166.8 ▲ Relapsing fever with myocarditis. *Borrelia recurrentis* may also cause myocarditis (silver impregnation stain).

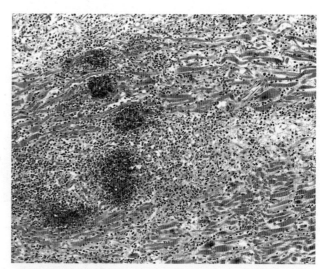

FIGURE 166.10 ▲ Fungal myocarditis. There is extensive inflammation with necrotizing inflammation.

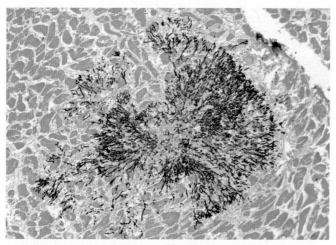

FIGURE 166.9 ▲ Aspergillus myocarditis. There is a centrifugal growth of branching hyphae. Gomori methenamine silver.

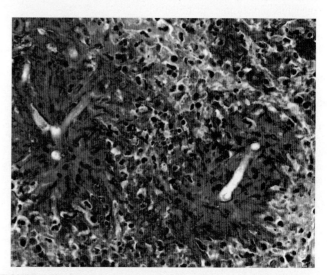

FIGURE 166.11 ▲ Fungal myocarditis. In this rare example of cardiac basidiobolomycosis, the fungal hyphae elicit a strong eosinophilic response with palisading granulomas. The hyphae are visible without special stains.

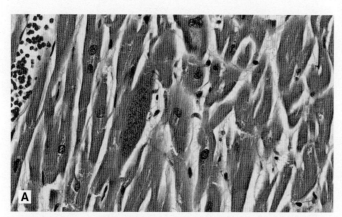

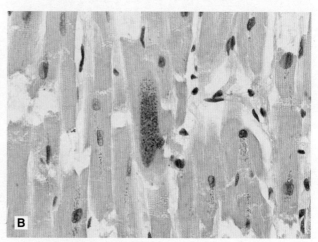

FIGURE 166.12 ▲ Cardiac toxoplasmosis. The patient was an immunocompromised child with disseminated toxoplasmosis. **A.** The intracytoplasmic cysts are seen on routine stains. **B.** Immunohistochemical stains confirm the diagnosis.

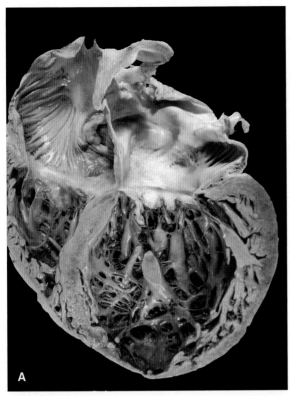
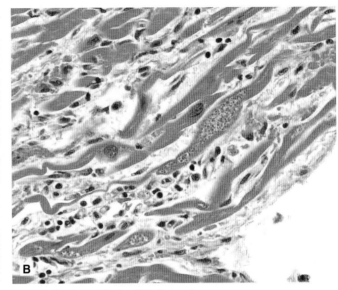

FIGURE 166.13 ▲ Chagas disease. **A.** The four-chamber photograph shows ventricular dilatation and aneurysm formation toward the apex. (Courtesy of Drs. Vera Aiello and Paulo Gutierrez, Sao Paulo, Brazil.) **B.** There are multiple intracytoplasmic cysts containing organisms.

also involve the heart and usually occurs in patients with disseminated disease. Heart involvement is commonly asymptomatic and detected at autopsy, but cysts and calcification can be detected by echocardiogram (Fig. 166.14).

Identification of Infectious Agents Causing Myocarditis

Special stains for organisms are rarely if ever useful in native biopsies, but may be helpful in autopsy diagnosis of bacterial myocarditis. Immunohistochemical staining is useful for toxoplasmosis, leptospirosis, and cytomegalovirus (*Toxoplasma gondii* and *T. cruzi*).[41] There are

reports of immunohistochemical identification of enteroviral capsid protein in cases of coxsackieviral myocarditis.[42]

The identification of viral DNA or RNA from biopsy or autopsy samples by molecular techniques is hampered by frequent absent findings, presumably due to the transient nature of viral infection with adeno- and coxsackieviruses, and the high frequency of detection of viral-specific nucleotide sequences in control tissues.[7] There is currently a large range (0% to 100%) of positive results for viral identification in human tissue samples with histologic myocarditis.[7,41,43-45] Immunohistochemical and in situ hybridization assays are available for bacteria and parasites (including *T. gondii* and *T. cruzi*).[41] In one large autopsy study of myocarditis samples, 43% yielded viral DNA, the largest group represented by cytomegalovirus.[46] In another, there were no cases of adenovirus or enterovirus, with a high rate of parvovirus in control tissues.[7]

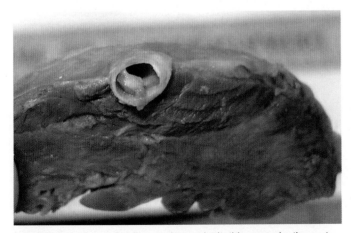

FIGURE 166.14 ▲ Cardiac cysticercosis. In this example, the cyst was on the epicardial surface. Virtually all areas of the heart can be affected. (Courtesy of Dr. Luciano Franco, Fortaleza, Brazil.)

Practical Points

▶ Infectious agents are rarely identified in cases of myocarditis.

▶ Most cases of lymphocytic myocarditis are thought secondary to an immune response following common viruses, such as coxsackieviruses and adenoviruses, that are cleared quickly from the immune system.

▶ There are a variety of organisms, both bacterial and fungal, that infect the heart in immunocompromised patients, usually in the form of microabscesses.

▶ The only endemic infection of the heart is caused by *T. cruzi*, which causes Chagas cardiomyopathy in South America.

REFERENCES

1. Karjalainen J, Heikkila J. Incidence of three presentations of acute myocarditis in young men in military service. A 20-year experience. *Eur Heart J.* 1999;20: 1120–1125.

2. Karjalainen J, Heikkila J, Nieminen MS, et al. Etiology of mild acute infectious myocarditis. Relation to clinical features. *Acta Med Scand.* 1983;213: 65–73.

3. Lee CJ, Huang YC, Yang S, et al. Clinical features of coxsackievirus A4, B3 and B4 infections in children. *PLoS One.* 2014;9: e87391.

4. Akuzawa N, Harada N, Hatori T, et al. Myocarditis, hepatitis, and pancreatitis in a patient with coxsackievirus A4 infection: a case report. *Virol J.* 2014;11:3.

5. Saikia UN, Mishra B, Sharma M, et al. Disseminated coxsackievirus B fulminant myocarditis in an immunocompetent adult: a case report: case of disseminated coxsackievirus myocarditis. *Diagn Microbiol Infect Dis.* 2014;78:98–100.

6. Ruppert V, Meyer T, Pankuweit S, et al. Activation of STAT1 transcription factor precedes up-regulation of coxsackievirus-adenovirus receptor during viral myocarditis. *Cardiovasc Pathol.* 2008;17:81–92.

7. Nielsen TS, Hansen J, Nielsen LP, et al. The presence of enterovirus, adenovirus, and parvovirus B19 in myocardial tissue samples from autopsies: an evaluation of their frequencies in deceased individuals with myocarditis and in non-inflamed control hearts. *Forensic Sci Med Pathol.* 2014;10: 344–350.

8. Berry G. Pathology of myocarditis. In: Cooper LT, ed. *Myocarditis: From Bench to Bedside.* New York, NY: Humana Press, Springer; 2002: 325–370.

9. Ludwig A, Lucero-Obusan C, Schirmer P, et al. Acute cardiac injury events ≤30 days after laboratory-confirmed influenza virus infection among U.S. veterans, 2010–2012. *BMC Cardiovasc Disord.* 2015;15:109.

10. Niu L, An XJ, Tian J, et al. 124 cases of clinical analysis of children with viral myocarditis. *Eur Rev Med Pharmacol Sci.* 2015;19:2856–2859.

11. Torres AF, Braga DN, Muniz F, et al. Lymphocytic myocarditis at autopsy in patients with dengue fever. *Braz J Infect Dis.* 2013;17:619–621.

12. Kirawittaya T, Yoon IK, Wichit S, et al. Evaluation of cardiac involvement in children with dengue by serial echocardiographic studies. *PLoS Negl Trop Dis.* 2015;9:e0003943.

13. Bock CT, Duchting A, Utta F, et al. Molecular phenotypes of human parvovirus B19 in patients with myocarditis. *World J Cardiol.* 2014;6: 183–195.

14. Vandamme YM, Ducancelle A, Biere L, et al. Myopericarditis complicated by pulmonary embolism in an immunocompetent patient with acute cytomegalovirus infection: a case report. *BMC Res Notes.* 2014;7:193.

15. Vanstechelman F, Vandekerckhove H. Cytomegalovirus myocarditis in an immunocompetent patient. *Acta Cardiol.* 2012;67:257–260.

16. Hartleif S, Wiegand G, Kumpf M, et al. Severe chest pain caused by Mycoplasma myocarditis in an adolescent patient. *Klin Padiatr.* 2013;225:423–425.

17. Takei T, Morozumi M, Ozaki H, et al. Clinical features of *Mycoplasma pneumoniae* infections in the 2010 epidemic season: report of two cases with unusual presentations. *Pediatr Neonatol.* 2013;54:402–405.

18. Zhou Y, Zhang Y, Sheng Y, et al. More complications occur in macrolide-resistant than in macrolide-sensitive *Mycoplasma pneumoniae* pneumonia. *Antimicrob Agents Chemother.* 2014;58:1034–1038.

19. Dellegrottaglie S, Russo G, Damiano M, et al. A case of acute myocarditis associated with *Chlamydia trachomatis* infection: role of cardiac MRI in the clinical management. *Infection.* 2014;42:937–940.

20. Hoefer D, Poelzl G, Kilo J, et al. Early detection and successful therapy of fulminant chlamydia pneumoniae myocarditis. *ASAIO J.* 2005;51: 480–481.

21. Salkade HP, Divate S, Deshpande JR, et al. A study of sutopsy findings in 62 cases of leptospirosis in a metropolitan city in India. *J Postgrad Med.* 2005;51:169–173.

22. Chakurkar G, Vaideeswar P, Pandit SP, et al. Cardiovascular lesions in leptospirosis: an autopsy study. *J Infect.* 2008;56:197–203.

23. Carrada-Bravo T. [Cardiovascular syphilis: diagnosis, treatment]. *Arch Cardiol Mex.* 2006;76(Suppl 4):S189–S196.

24. Dada MA, Lazarus NG, Kharsany AB, et al. Sudden death caused by myocardial tuberculosis: case report and review of the literature. *Am J Forensic Med Pathol.* 2000;21:385–388.

25. Rose AG. Cardiac tuberculosis. A study of 19 patients. *Arch Pathol Lab Med.* 1987;111:422–426.

26. Tavora F, Burke A, Li L, et al. Postmortem confirmation of Lyme carditis with polymerase chain reaction. *Cardiovasc Pathol.* 2008;17:103–107.

27. Maher B, Murday D, Harden SP. Cardiac MRI of Lyme disease myocarditis. *Heart.* 2012;98:264.

28. Gunia S, Behrens MH, Stosiek P. A rare course of Whipple's disease with atypical cardiac manifestation. *APMIS.* 2004;112:222–224.

29. Walker DH, Paletta CE, Cain BG. Pathogenesis of myocarditis in Rocky Mountain spotted fever. *Arch Pathol Lab Med.* 1980;104:171–174.

30. Vogiatzis I, Dimoglou G, Sachpekidis V. Q fever myocarditis. *Hippokratia.* 2008;12:46–49.

31. Kuttin ES. Fungal infections of the cardiovascular system—a review. *Mycoses.* 1997;40:3–24.

32. Basti A, Taylor S, Tschopp M, et al. Fatal fulminant myocarditis caused by disseminated mucormycosis. *Heart.* 2004;90:e60.

33. Schmidt B, Wieneke H, Fahrenkamp A, et al. Encephalitic and myocardial toxoplasmosis masquerading as cytomegalovirus infection in a renal allograft recipient. *Nephrol Dial Transplant.* 1995;10:284–286.

34. Dixit PG, Umap PS, Bardale RV. Toxoplasma myocarditis presenting as myocardial infarction. *Indian J Med Sci.* 2007;61:218–220.

35. Coura JR. Chagas disease: what is known and what is needed—a background article. *Mem Inst Oswaldo Cruz.* 2007;102(Suppl 1):113–122.

36. Marques J, Mendoza I, Noya B, et al. ECG manifestations of the biggest outbreak of Chagas disease due to oral infection in Latin-America. *Arq Bras Cardiol.* 2013;101:249–254.

37. Regueiro A, Garcia-Alvarez A, Sitges M, et al. Myocardial involvement in Chagas disease: insights from cardiac magnetic resonance. *Int J Cardiol.* 2013;165:107–112.

38. Rossi MA, Ramos SG, Bestetti RB. Chagas' heart disease: clinical-pathological correlation. *Front Biosci.* 2003;8:e94–e109.

39. Bern C. Chagas disease in the immunosuppressed host. *Curr Opin Infect Dis.* 2012;25:450–457.

40. Rezaian GR, Aslani A. Endocardial hydatid cyst: a rare presentation of echinococcal infection. *Eur J Echocardiogr.* 2008;9:342–343.

41. Guarner J, Bhatnagar J, Shieh WJ, et al. Histopathologic, immunohistochemical, and polymerase chain reaction assays in the study of cases with fatal sporadic myocarditis. *Hum Pathol.* 2007;38:1412–1419.

42. Gaaloul I, Riabi S, Harrath R, et al. Coxsackievirus B detection in cases of myocarditis, myopericarditis, pericarditis and dilated cardiomyopathy in hospitalized patients. *Mol Med Rep.* 2014;10:2811–2818.

43. Winters GL, Costanzo-Nordin MR. Pathological findings in 2300 consecutive endomyocardial biopsies. *Mod Pathol.* 1991;4:441–448.

44. Ueno H, Yokota Y, Shiotani H, et al. Significance of detection of enterovirus RNA in myocardial tissues by reverse transcription-polymerase chain reaction. *Int J Cardiol.* 1995;51:157–164.

45. Nagai N, Ogura R, Seki A, et al. Cardiac rescue of an infant with fulminant myocarditis using extracorporeal membrane oxygenation. *Jpn Circ J.* 1996;60:699–702.

46. Kyto V, Saukko P, Lignitz E, et al. Diagnosis and presentation of fatal myocarditis. *Hum Pathol.* 2005;36:1003–1007.

167 Pericarditis

Fabio R. Tavora, M.D., Ph.D., and Allen P. Burke, M.D.

Incidence and Clinical Findings

Pericardial inflammation can be the result of infections, autoimmune disease, renal failure, radiation, malignancy, or trauma (Tables 167.1 and 167.2). In most cases, no specific etiology is found. Pericarditis is frequently associated with pleuritis, as the pericardium and pleura are contiguous.

Acute pericarditis accounts for ~1 in 1,000 hospital admissions and causes chest pain and ST-segment elevation in 1% of patients admitted to the emergency room.[37] The clinical presentation is characterized by chest pain, dyspnea, and fever. In children, abdominal pain may be the presenting symptom. In addition, a pericardial friction rub tachypnea is present, and if the fluid accumulation causes cardiac tamponade, hypotension and jugular venous distention can occur. The diagnosis of pericardial effusion can be easily detected by echocardiogram, which is capable of detecting an excess of 50 mL of fluid, beyond the physiologic amount in the pericardial sac.[38]

Acute idiopathic pericarditis (with or without associated myocarditis) is usually treated with anti-inflammatory drugs unless there is significant fluid accumulation necessitating pericardiocentesis or progressive fibrosis requiring pericardial resection. Recurrent pericarditis may be caused by recurrent viral infection or may represent an isolated autoimmune condition. In cases of recurrence, exclusion of bacterial and viral infection by PCR of pericardial fluid has been recommended before initiating aggressive anti-inflammatory treatment, which includes steroids, colchicine, and other anti-inflammatory agents.[39]

Etiology

Idiopathic or nonspecific pericarditis is by far the most common cause of acute pericarditis, accounting for 199 of 213 patients admitted for acute pericarditis in one series.[40] Many idiopathic cases are believed to be viral/postviral analogous to myocarditis.[41] The most common suspected and proven viral agent is cytomegalovirus, especially in immunocompromised patients; in immunocompetent individuals, coxsackievirus A and B, echovirus, and adenovirus have been implicated (Table 167.1). Viral detection may be difficult and may depend on PCR of pericardiocentesis fluid.

The clinical differential diagnoses of pericarditis are pericardial neoplasms, myocardial infarction, radiation therapy, tuberculosis and other mycobacterial infection, bacterial and fungal pericarditis, viral infections, and connective tissue diseases.

Inflammatory noninfectious pericarditis can occur by involvement of systemic collagen diseases, most commonly lupus erythematous and rheumatoid arthritis. Pericarditis can present in the acute phases of the diseases or be subclinically detected as small effusions.

Bacterial pericarditis including the purulent form is uncommon. Risk factors include immunodeficiency, recent thoracic surgery, pneumonia, meningitis, chest trauma, or malignancy. Staphylococci, meningococci, pneumococci, and *Haemophilus influenzae* are the most common etiologic agents. Uncommonly, pericarditis can represent extension from endocarditis.

About 5% to 7% of patients with pericardial effusion will bear a neoplastic process involving the pericardial space.[42] Metastatic tumors are by far more common than primary pericardial tumors, and lung tumor, breast tumor, and lymphoma are the three prevalent tumors that have a predilection to the pericardium. In cases of primary pericardial mesothelioma or pleural mesotheliomas involving the pericardium, constrictive pericarditis can occur. Cytologic aspirate material and biopsy have a high specificity and moderate sensitivity in cases of effusions unexplained but other causes or in patients unresponsive to medical treatment with NSAIDs.

TABLE 167.1 Organisms Implicated in Infectious Pericarditis

Class of Organism	Specific Organism
Viral (postviral)	CMV[1,2]
	Coxsackievirus[3–5]
	Echovirus[4,5]
	Vaccinia[6]
	Epstein-Barr virus[7]
	Adenovirus[8]
	Varicella[9,10]
	Herpes simplex[11]
	Parvovirus B19[12]
Bacterial (including mycobacterial)	Tuberculosis
	Staphylococci
	Pneumococcus[13–16]
	Meningococcus[17–19]
	Haemophilus[20–23]
	C. burneti[24,25]
	M. pneumoniae[26]
	Bartonella, Legionella pneumophila[26]
	Brucella[27]
	Actinomycetes[28]
Fungal	Histoplasmosis[29,30]
	Aspergillosis[31,32]
	Candida[33,34]
Parasitic	*Echinococcus*[35]
	Toxoplasmosis[26]
	Entamoeba histolytica[36]

TABLE 167.2 Causes of Noninfectious Pericarditis

Idiopathic	
Autoimmune or immune-mediated pericarditis	Lupus erythematosus systemic
	Rheumatoid arthritis
	Sjögren syndrome
	Systemic sclerosis
Postinfarction pericarditis (Dressler syndrome)	
Neoplastic pericarditis	Metastatic or direct extension
	Breast, lung, mediastinum, lymphoma
	Primary tumors:
	Mesothelioma, teratoma
Traumatic pericarditis	
Uremic pericarditis	
Other	Sarcoid
	Pericarditis associated with pancreatitis
	Posttransplant pericarditis
	Pericarditis associated with hypereosinophilic syndrome
	Hypo- and hyperthyroidism

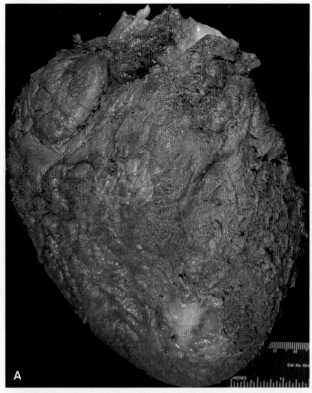

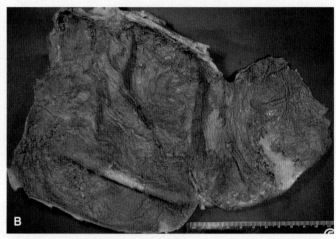

FIGURE 167.1 ▲ Chronic fibrinous pericarditis. **A.** The epicardial surface is shaggy, with a brown exudate. **B.** The pericardium shows the brown exudate on the visceral surface.

Pathologic Evaluation of Acute Pericarditis

Pathologic evaluation of pericarditis and pericardial disease includes analysis and cytology of pericardiocentesis fluid and routine histopathology of pericardial biopsies resulting from pericardiotomy with biopsy or percutaneous pericardial biopsy. Biopsy can be undertaken by direct visualization by video or pericardiotomy. Pericardial fluid is analyzed similar to pleural or peritoneal fluid including red blood cell count, white blood cell count with differential, pH, total protein, glucose, lactic acid dehydrogenase, culture for viruses, bacteria and fungi, Gram stain and stain for acid-fast bacilli, and cytologic examination.

The histologic findings of acute pericarditis include acute and chronic inflammation with loss or mesothelial lining and fibrin deposition. Biopsy greatly increases the sensitivity for specific causes such as malignancies and granulomatous processes (sarcoid and infection, especially tuberculosis). Cytologic findings in viral or autoimmune (lymphocytic fibrinous pericarditis) include a paucity of neutrophils, and abundant lymphocytes, macrophages, and reactive mesothelial cells. The differential diagnosis of acute pericarditis includes metastatic carcinoma and other malignancies, which typically result in a hemorrhagic effusion. An abundance of neutrophils or granulomas points to a bacterial or mycobacterial infection, respectively.

In patients with suspected infectious pericarditis, PCR tests for bacterial, mycobacterial, fungal, protozoal, and viral etiologies complement routine culture.[43–45] Serologic tests to exclude lupus erythematosus, rheumatoid arthritis, and acute rheumatic fever may be performed in selected patients based on history and clinical findings.

Chronic Fibrinous Pericarditis

Grossly, the classic "bread and butter" appearance is characteristic of chronic fibrinous pericarditis, regardless of cause (Fig. 167.1). Hemorrhage is not prominent, unless the patient is on anticoagulant treatment (Fig. 167.2). Fibrin deposition on the surface of pericardium persists in the subacute and early chronic phase (Figs. 167.3 to 167.5) and is accompanied by chronic inflammation, granulation tissue, and reactive mesothelial hyperplasia.

Chronic Fibrosing Pericarditis

Fibrotic thickening of the pericardium, the end result of fibrinous pericarditis, causes fibrosis of the pericardium and constrictive pericarditis (Fig. 167.6). The most frequent cause of pericardial fibrosis at autopsy

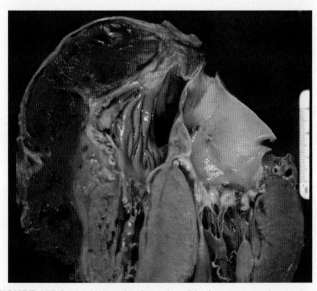

FIGURE 167.2 ▲ Hemorrhagic pericarditis. In postoperative pericarditis, anticoagulation can lead to localized areas of hemorrhage in the pericardial space.

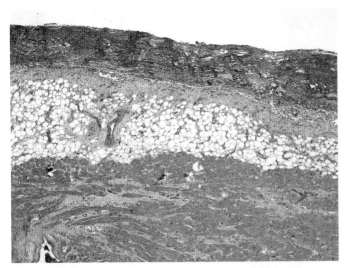

FIGURE 167.3 ▲ Acute fibrinous pericarditis. There is a fibrin layer outside the epicardial fat on the epicardial surface.

is prior cardiac surgery. Because of the clinical presentation of cardiac constriction, patients sometimes require surgery for decompression, and the pathologist will evaluate specimens characterized by fibrosis with variable ongoing chronic inflammation. Fibrin is usually absent in this late stage of the disease. In surgical series of pericardial resections for constriction, ~40% of patients will demonstrate pericardial calcification.[46]

Mesothelial cell hyperplasia is common in the fibrotic stage and is typically present in a linear distribution, unlike carcinoma, often forming tubular structures (Figs. 167.7 and 167.8). Reactive mesothelial cells may be difficult to distinguish from adenocarcinoma, which typically expresses markers such as ber-EP4 or TTF-1 (in the case of lung primaries), in contrast to mesothelial markers, such as calretinin (see Chapter 110, Section 1).

Hemorrhagic Pericarditis

Hemorrhagic pericarditis is a descriptive term that refers to blood mixed with a fibrinous or suppurative effusion. Most commonly, hemorrhagic pericarditis is caused by malignant effusions; historically, and in developing countries, hemorrhagic pericarditis is

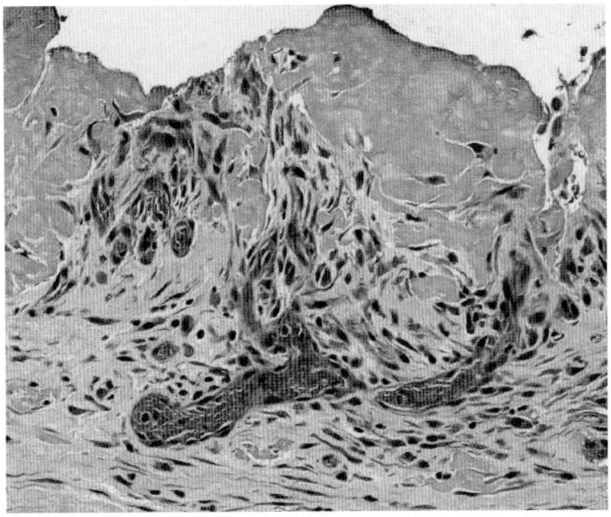

FIGURE 167.5 ▲ Radiation pericarditis. The visceral mesothelial cells show reactive hyperplasia with papillary formation.

attributed typically to tuberculosis. In cases of malignant pericarditis, metastatic disease is several times more prevalent than primary pericardial tumors. Hemorrhage can complicate acute and fibrinous pericarditis of any cause if there is a history of anticoagulation or coagulopathy.

Infectious Pericarditis

Bacterial/Purulent Pericarditis

Purulent pericarditis is defined as a collection of fluid that is either grossly or microscopically purulent.[33] The disease is usually caused by bacteria and less commonly fungi; it may be diffuse or form localized pericardial abscesses. Most cases of bacterial pericarditis are complications of pneumonia.[47,48] Other sources of infection include acute mediastinitis, especially from esophageal or postsurgical complications,[49] hematogenous spread in patients with sepsis,[50] infectious endocarditis,[51] and subdiaphragmatic abscesses.[52] Purulent pericarditis is rarely an iatrogenic complication following interventions for coronary disease or lung biopsy[53] and as a complication of dialysis.[54]

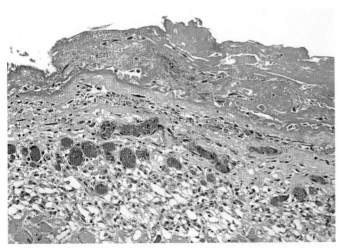

FIGURE 167.4 ▲ Acute fibrinous pericarditis. In this example, there are reactive fibroblasts among the layers, indicative of at least several days duration.

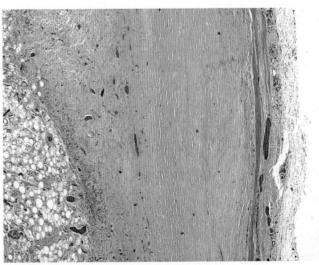

FIGURE 167.6 ▲ Chronic constrictive pericarditis. There is a thick band of collagen between the epicardial fat to the left and the epicardial surface on the right.

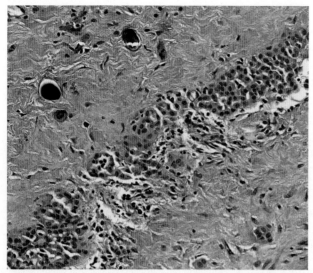

FIGURE 167.7 ▲ Chronic constrictive pericarditis with reactive mesothelial hyperplasia. Nests of mesothelial cells are present in the fibrosis, in a linear distribution.

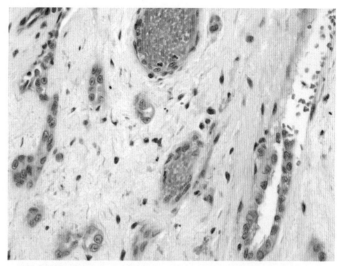

FIGURE 167.8 ▲ Chronic pericarditis with reactive mesothelial hyperplasia. Nests of mesothelial cells are present in the loose connective tissue.

The most common organisms are meningococcus,[17] pneumococcus,[55] *H. influenzae*,[20] and *Staphylococcus aureus*,[56] including methicillin-resistant strains.[57] Less common organisms that cause bacterial pericarditis include brucellosis, actinomycetes, nocardia, *Coxiella burnetii*, and *Haemophilus parainfluenzae*.[26–28,47,58]

Tuberculous Pericarditis

Tuberculosis involving the pleura is prone to serious complications and has a high mortality rate. While it has been increasingly rare in the United States and other developed countries, it is still prevalent in selected populations that include immunocompromised patients.

Approximately 50% of tuberculous pericarditis with pericardial effusions will have evidence of pericardial constriction.[59] Acute tamponade is relatively rare.[60] In developing countries, over 80% of HIV patients with pericardial effusions will demonstrate tuberculous pericarditis.[61]

The progression of the disease involves an acute fibrinous phase, with subsequent effusion rich in inflammatory cells and chronic fibrosis and constrictive pericarditis. Cystic loculated cavities may occur.[62]

Patients with suspected tuberculous pericarditis undergo diagnostic and therapeutic pericardiotomy, with drainage and biopsy. A definite diagnosis of tuberculous pericarditis is based on the demonstration of the bacilli in the fluid or biopsy specimen, by smear and culture. The presence of granulomas is variable on biopsy (Fig. 167.9), and AFB stains should be performed even if they are absent. The sensitivity of a pericardial biopsy for tuberculosis is low, with a low negative predictive value.[63] Molecular methods using PCR can be used in the tissue or aspirate to detect tuberculosis in the specimen.[64,65]

Postinfarction Pericarditis (Dressler Syndrome)

Pericarditis is the most common cause of chest pain following a myocardial infarction. Pericardial effusion can be detected in up to 25%

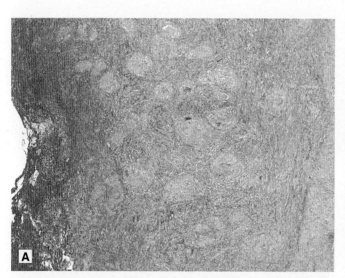
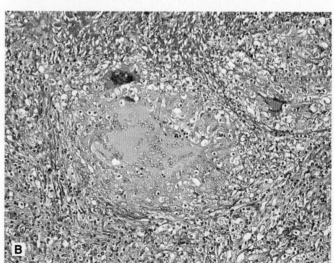

FIGURE 167.9 ▲ Tuberculous pericarditis. **A.** There is marked thickening of the pericardium with granulomas noted at this magnification. **B.** Higher magnification of necrotizing granuloma with giant cells.

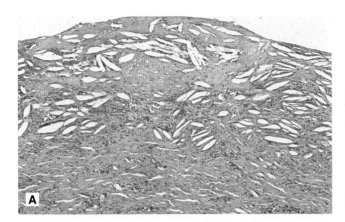

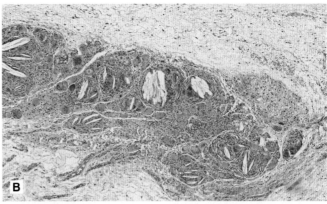

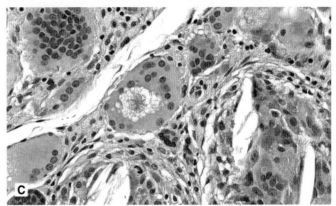

FIGURE 167.10 ▲ Cholesterol pericarditis. **A.** There are numerous cholesterol crystals in chronic inflammation. **B.** A different example shows chronic inflammation and cholesterol crystals. **C.** A higher magnification shows a macrophage with an *asteroid body*, a nonspecific finding in foreign body–type macrophage giant cells.

(10% to 40% in various series) of patients with acute myocardial infarcts and is more common in patients with anterior myocardial infarction, infarcts with large area of involvement, and congestive heart failure.[66,67]

Postinfarction syndrome (Dressler syndrome) denotes delayed (usually 2 to 3 weeks) occurrence of pericarditis after infarct associated with fever and chest pain. The incidence has been greatly diminished because of the extensive use of thrombolysis and treatments that dramatically decreased the size of myocardial necrosis and modulated the immune system.[68]

Miscellaneous Types of Pericarditis

Pancreatitis-Associated Pericarditis

Serous effusions are common in patients with acute pancreatitis. Pericarditis is rare, may be secondary to increased amylase levels in the pericardial fluid, and may cause tamponade. There may be an association with chronic periaortitis and IgG4-related disease in rare instances.[69]

Sarcoid

Pericardial involvement in sarcoid is uncommon, detected in <5% of patients by echocardiography. Up to 10% of patients with sarcoid have pericardial effusions, and pericardial involvement at autopsy is ~3%. Sarcoidosis should be considered in patients with constrictive pericarditis, accounting for 1% of cases.[70]

Cholesterol Pericarditis

Cholesterol pericarditis denotes the presence of cholesterol crystals within the inflammatory infiltrate, classically imparting a glittering gold

appearance. Although associated with myxedema, cholesterol crystals can be present also in tuberculous and rheumatoid pericarditis.[71,72] Diagnosis is made by the gross findings of yellow-gold, paint-like fluid and cytologic findings of lymphocytes and cholesterol crystals.[73] Histologically, there are abundant crystals in a background of chronic inflammation and variable fibrosis (Fig. 167.10).

Treatment includes stripping of the pericardium, especially in cases of constriction, and diagnosis is made on histologic finding.[71] Occasionally, there may be large accumulations of pericardial fluid with tamponade.[72]

Hypereosinophilic Syndrome

Endocardial and myocardial involvement in the hypereosinophilic syndrome results in a restrictive cardiomyopathy. Rarely, the pericardium may have the primary cardiovascular manifestation, resulting in effusions and pericardial constriction.[74]

Thyroid Disease

Hypothyroidism, and less often hyperthyroidism, may be associated with pericardial disease, generally effusions in the absence of significant inflammation. There may be concomitant viral pericarditis, however, as a first manifestation of pericarditis with effusion.[75]

Iatrogenic Pericarditis

Postoperative pericardial constriction has been described in patients after intraoperative instillation with povidone–iodine into the pericardial sac and as a consequence of a granulomatous reaction to talc, silicone, or asbestos.[76] The histologic findings in these cases are foreign body granulomas with the presence of crystalline deposits (Fig. 167.11).

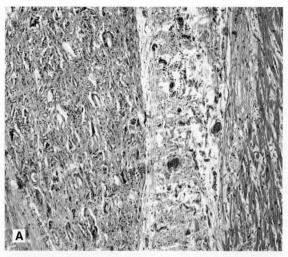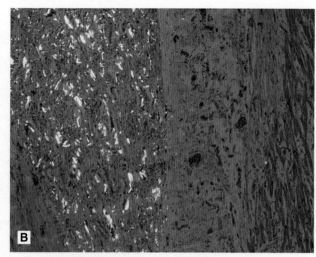

FIGURE 167.11 ▲ Talc pericarditis. **A.** The inflammation of the visceral pericardial layer is at the left and the myocardium at the right. **B.** Seen under polarized light. The talc crystals are seen at the left.

REFERENCES

1. Campbell PT, Li JS, Wall TC, et al. Cytomegalovirus pericarditis: a case series and review of the literature. *Am J Med Sci.* 1995;309:229–234.
2. Kwon CM, Jung YW, Yun DY, et al. A case of acute pericarditis with hemophagocytic syndrome, cytomegalovirus infection and systemic lupus erythematosus. *Rheumatol Int.* 2008;28:271–273.
3. Tilzey AJ, Signy M, Banatvala JE. Persistent coxsackie B virus specific IgM response in patients with recurrent pericarditis. *Lancet.* 1986;1:1491–1492.
4. Fairley CK, Ryan M, Wall PG, et al. The organisms reported to cause infective myocarditis and pericarditis in England and Wales. *J Infect.* 1996;32:223–225.
5. Ferreira Junior AG, Ferreira SM, Gomes ML, et al. Enteroviruses as a possible cause of myocarditis, pericarditis and dilated cardiomyopathy in Belem, Brazil. *Braz J Med Biol Res.* 1995;28:869–874.
6. de Meester A, Luwaert R, Chaudron JM. Symptomatic pericarditis after influenza vaccination: report of two cases. *Chest.* 2000;117:1803–1805.
7. Zafrir B, Aviv A, Reichman N, et al. Epstein-Barr virus-associated pericarditis and pericardial effusion: case report and diagnostic aspects. *Eur J Intern Med.* 2005;16:528–530.
8. Canas JA, Balsam D, Leggiadro RJ. Adenovirus pericarditis. *N Y State J Med.* 1986;86:269–270.
9. Cohen SN, Affleck AG, Littlewood SM. Varicella pericarditis mimicking myocardial infarction. *Br J Hosp Med (Lond).* 2007;68:680.
10. Winfield CR, Joseph SP. Herpes zoster pericarditis. *Br Heart J.* 1980;43:597–599.
11. Freedberg RS, Gindea AJ, Dieterich DT, et al. Herpes simplex pericarditis in AIDS. *N Y State J Med.* 1987;87:304–306.
12. Richards M, Johns J. Effusive-constrictive pericarditis associated with human parvovirus B19 infection. *Scand J Infect Dis.* 2005;37:609–611.
13. Tatli E, Buyuklu M, Altun A. An unusual complication of pneumococcal pneumonia: acute tamponade due to purulent pericarditis. *Int J Cardiol.* 2007;119:e1–e3.
14. Foo NH, Chen CT, Chow JC. Disseminated pneumococcal infection with pericarditis and cardiac tamponade: report of one case. *Acta Paediatr Taiwan.* 2005;46:301–304.
15. Kan B, Ries J, Normark BH, et al. Endocarditis and pericarditis complicating pneumococcal bacteraemia, with special reference to the adhesive abilities of pneumococci: results from a prospective study. *Clin Microbiol Infect.* 2006;12:338–344.
16. Blohm ME, Schroten H, Heusch A, et al. Acute purulent pericarditis in pneumococcal meningitis. *Intensive Care Med.* 2005;31:1142.
17. Zeidan A, Tariq S, Faltas B, et al. A case of primary meningococcal pericarditis caused by *Neisseria meningitidis* serotype Y with rapid evolution into cardiac tamponade. *J Gen Intern Med.* 2008;23:1532–1535.
18. de Souza AL, Seguro AC. Meningococcal pericarditis in the intensive care unit. *Crit Care Med.* 2008;36:651.
19. Falcao SN, Tsutsui JM, Ramires FJ, et al. The role of echocardiography in diagnosis and management of isolated meningococcal pericarditis. *Echocardiography.* 2007;24:263–266.
20. Elwood RL, DeBiasi RL. Purulent pericarditis caused by nontypeable *Haemophilus influenzae* in a pediatric patient. *Diagn Microbiol Infect Dis.* 2008;62:113–115.
21. Garg P, Gupta R, Szalados JE. Bacterial pericarditis and tamponade due to nonencapsulated *Haemophilus influenzae* complicating a case of adult community-acquired pneumonia. *MedGenMed.* 2006;8:48.
22. Taube JM, Hutchins GM, Carroll KC, et al. *Haemophilus influenzae* serotype f purulent pericarditis: a cause of death in a child with Down syndrome. *Diagn Microbiol Infect Dis.* 2006;56:87–89.
23. Yeh YH, Chu PH, Yeh CH, et al. *Haemophilus influenzae* pericarditis with tamponade as the initial presentation of systemic lupus erythematosus. *Int J Clin Pract.* 2004;58:1045–1047.
24. Levy PY, Gouriet F, Habib G, et al. Diagnosis of *Coxiella burnetii* pericarditis by using a systematic prescription kit in cases of pericardial effusion: an 8-year experience. *Clin Microbiol Infect.* 2009;15(suppl 2):173–175.
25. Levy PY, Carrieri P, Raoult D. *Coxiella burnetii* pericarditis: report of 15 cases and review. *Clin Infect Dis.* 1999;29:393–397.
26. Levy PY, Thuny F, Habib G, et al. Diagnosis of *Coxiella burnetii* pericarditis using a systematic prescription kit in case of pericardial effusion. *Ann N Y Acad Sci.* 2006;1078:248–251.
27. Kaya S, Eskazan AE, Elaldi N. Brucellar pericarditis: a report of four cases and review of the literature. *Int J Infect Dis.* 2013;17:e428–e432.
28. Mack R, Slicker K, Ghamande S, et al. *Actinomyces odontolyticus*: rare etiology for purulent pericarditis. *Case Rep Med.* 2014;2014:734925.
29. Wang JJ, Reimold SC. Chest pain resulting from histoplasmosis pericarditis: a brief report and review of the literature. *Cardiol Rev.* 2006;14:223–226.
30. Wheat LJ, Stein L, Corya BC. Pericarditis as a manifestation of histoplasmosis during two large urban outbreaks. *Medicine.* 1983;62:110–119.
31. Gokahmetoglu S, Koc AN, Patiroglu T. Case report. Fatal *Aspergillus flavus* pericarditis in a patient with acute myeloblastic leukaemia. *Mycoses.* 2000;43:65–66.
32. Salanitri GC, Huo E, Miller FH, et al. MRI of mycotic sinus of valsalva pseudoaneurysm secondary to *Aspergillus* pericarditis. *AJR Am J Roentgenol.* 2005;184:S25–S27.
33. Parikh SV, Memon N, Echols M, et al. Purulent pericarditis: report of 2 cases and review of the literature. *Medicine (Baltimore).* 2009;88:52–65.
34. Puius YA, Scully B. Treatment of *Candida albicans* pericarditis in a heart transplant patient. *Transpl Infect Dis.* 2007;9:229–232.
35. Shojaee S, Hutchins GM. Echinococcosis complicated by purulent pericarditis. *Chest.* 1978;73:512–514.
36. Costa Guimaraes A, Azevedo Vinhaes L, Santos Filho A, et al. Acute suppurative amebic pericarditis. *Am J Cardiol.* 1974;34:103–106.
37. Brady WJ, Perron AD, Martin ML, et al. Cause of ST segment abnormality in ED chest pain patients. *Am J Emerg Med.* 2001;19:25–28.

38. Galve E, Garcia-Del-Castillo H, Evangelista A, et al. Pericardial effusion in the course of myocardial infarction: incidence, natural history, and clinical relevance. *Circulation.* 1986;73:294–299.

39. Maisch B. Recurrent pericarditis: mysterious or not so mysterious? *Eur Heart J.* 2005;26:631–633.

40. Permanyer-Miralda G, Sagrista-Sauleda J, Soler-Soler J. Primary acute pericardial disease: a prospective series of 231 consecutive patients. *Am J Cardiol.* 1985;56:623–630.

41. Spodick DH. Risk prediction in pericarditis: who to keep in hospital? *Heart.* 2008;94:398–399.

42. Imazio M, Trinchero R, Shabetai R. Pathogenesis, management, and prevention of recurrent pericarditis. *J Cardiovasc Med (Hagerstown).* 2007;8:404–410.

43. Benson C, Gantt S, Zerr DM, et al. Use of 16S ribosomal DNA polymerase chain reaction to identify *Haemophilus influenzae* type b as the etiology of pericarditis in an infant. *Pediatr Infect Dis J.* 2005;24:287–288.

44. de Souza AL, Salgado MM, Alkmin MD, et al. Purulent pericarditis caused by *Neisseria meningitidis* serogroup C and confirmed through polymerase chain reaction. *Scand J Infect Dis.* 2006;38:143–145.

45. Meyburg J, Schmidt KG, Nutzenadel W, et al. Tuberculous pericarditis in an infant evolving during triple chemotherapy. *Eur J Pediatr.* 2002;161:138–141.

46. Anyanwu CH, Umeh BU. Pericarditis: a persisting surgical problem. *Cardiovasc Surg.* 1994;2:711–715.

47. Latyshev Y, Mathew A, Jacobson JM, et al. Purulent pericarditis caused by *Haemophilus parainfluenzae. Tex Heart Inst J.* 2013;40:608–611.

48. Lu S, Tsai JD, Tsao TF, et al. Necrotizing pneumonia and acute purulent pericarditis caused by *Streptococcus pneumoniae* serotype 19A in a healthy 4-year-old girl after one catch-up dose of 13-valent pneumococcal conjugate vaccine. *Paediatr Int Child Health.* 2015.

49. Takayama T, Okura Y, Funakoshi K, et al. Esophageal cancer with an esophagopericardial fistula and purulent pericarditis. *Intern Med.* 2013;52: 243–247.

50. Browatzki M, Borst MM, Katus HA, et al. Purulent pericarditis and pleural empyema due to *Staphylococcus aureus* septicemia. *Int J Cardiol.* 2006;107:117–118.

51. Natrajsetty HS, Vijayalakshmi IB, Narasimhan C, et al. Purulent pericarditis with quadruple valve endocarditis. *Am J Case Rep.* 2015;16:236–239.

52. Reddy G, Chatterjee A, Brott BC. Transdiaphragmatic rupture of hepatic abscess producing purulent pericarditis and pericardial tamponade. *Circulation.* 2015;131:e1–e2.

53. Tachjian A, Shafer KM, Denkinger C, et al. Purulent pericarditis after transbronchial biopsy. *Can J Cardiol.* 2014;30:1250 e19–e21.

54. Nwiloh JO, Egbe PA, Tagoe AT, et al. *Staphylococcus aureus* pericarditis masquerading as anterior mediastinal mass: mediastinal mass from pericarditis. *Chest.* 2000;118:1832–1833.

55. Flores-Gonzalez JC, Rubio-Quinones F, Hernandez-Gonzalez A, et al. Pneumonia and purulent pericarditis caused by *Streptococcus pneumoniae*: an uncommon association in the antibiotic era. *Pediatr Emerg Care.* 2014;30:552–554.

56. Bernadette NN, Kamgaing N, Monebenimp F, et al. Human immunodeficiency virus infection in a child revealed by a massive purulent pericarditis mistaken for a liver abscess due to *Staphylococcus aureus. Afr J Paediatr Surg.* 2015;12:71–73.

57. Lutmer JE, Yates AR, Bannerman TL, et al. Purulent pericarditis secondary to community-acquired, methicillin-resistant *Staphylococcus aureus*

58. Sirijatuphat R, Niltwat S, Tiangtam O, et al. Purulent pericarditis and cardiac tamponade caused by *Nocardia farcinica* in a nephrotic syndrome patient. *Intern Med.* 2013;52:2231–2235.

59. Ntsekhe M, Matthews K, Syed FF, et al. Prevalence, hemodynamics, and cytokine profile of effusive-constrictive pericarditis in patients with tuberculous pericardial effusion. *PLoS One.* 2013;8:e77532.

60. Couture T, Demondion P, Leprince P. Tuberculous pericarditis: an unusual cause of cardiac tamponade. *Ann Thorac Surg.* 2014;98:2234.

61. Ntsekhe M, Mayosi BM. Tuberculous pericarditis with and without HIV. *Heart Fail Rev.* 2013;18:367–373.

62. Lin TW, Tsai MD, Roan JN, et al. Cystic tuberculous pericarditis. *J Am Coll Cardiol.* 2013;62:1393.

63. Imazio M, Cecchi E, Ierna S, et al. Investigation on colchicine for acute pericarditis: a multicenter randomized placebo-controlled trial evaluating the clinical benefits of colchicine as adjunct to conventional therapy in the treatment and prevention of pericarditis; study design and rationale. *J Cardiovasc Med (Hagerstown).* 2007;8:613–617.

64. Pandie S, Peter JG, Kerbelker ZS, et al. Diagnostic accuracy of quantitative PCR (Xpert MTB/RIF) for tuberculous pericarditis compared to adenosine deaminase and unstimulated interferon-gamma in a high burden setting: a prospective study. *BMC Med.* 2014;12:101.

65. Mehta PK, Raj A, Singh N, et al. Diagnosis of extrapulmonary tuberculosis by PCR. *FEMS Immunol Med Microbiol.* 2012;66:20–36.

66. Widimsky P, Gregor P. Pericardial involvement during the course of myocardial infarction. A long-term clinical and echocardiographic study. *Chest.* 1995;108:89–93.

67. Aydinalp A, Wishniak A, van den Akker-Berman L, et al. Pericarditis and pericardial effusion in acute ST-elevation myocardial infarction in the thrombolytic era. *Isr Med Assoc J.* 2002;4:181–183.

68. Bendjelid K, Pugin J. Is Dressler syndrome dead? *Chest.* 2004;126: 1680–1682.

69. Rebelo M, Lima J, Ramos L, et al. The intriguing co-existence of a chronic periaortitis, a pericarditis and a pancreatitis: case report. *Acta Reumatol Port.* 2011;36:160–166.

70. Darda S, Zughaib ME, Alexander PB, et al. Cardiac sarcoidosis presenting as constrictive pericarditis. *Tex Heart Inst J.* 2014;41:319–323.

71. Adamson VW, Slim JN, Leclerc KM, et al. A rare case of effusive constrictive cholesterol pericarditis: a case report and review. *Case Rep Med.* 2013;2013:439505.

72. Setty NS, Sadananda KS, Nanjappa MC, et al. Massive pericardial effusion and cardiac tamponade due to cholesterol pericarditis in a case of subclinical hypothyroidism: a rare event. *J Am Coll Cardiol.* 2014;63:1451.

73. Barcin C, Yalcinkaya E, Kabul HK. Cholesterol pericarditis associated with rheumatoid arthritis: a rare cause of pericardial effusion. *Int J Cardiol.* 2013;166:e56–e58.

74. Ucar Elalmis O, Mansuroglu C, Cicekcioglu H, et al. An unusual case of idiopathic hypereosinophilic syndrome presenting with myopericarditis and a polypoid cardiac mass. *Turk Kardiyol Dern Ars.* 2014;42:281–284.

75. Gupta R, Munyak J, Haydock T, et al. Hypothyroidism presenting as acute cardiac tamponade with viral pericarditis. *Am J Emerg Med.* 1999;17:176–178.

76. Fraker TD Jr, Walsh TE, Morgan RJ, et al. Constrictive pericarditis late after the Beck operation. *Am J Cardiol.* 1984;54:931.

in previously healthy children. A sign of the times? *Ann Am Thorac Soc.* 2013;10:235–238.

SECTION SIX
TRANSPLANT PATHOLOGY

168 Acute Cellular Rejection

Allen P. Burke, M.D., and Fabio R. Tavora, M.D., Ph.D.

Introduction

Endomyocardial biopsy surveillance, with frequent biopsies in the early months and standardized treatments for particular clinical situations, is the gold standard procedure in follow-up and assessment of rejection.[1,2] Most biopsy samples are performed via the jugular or subclavian veins.[1] Access through the right femoral vein for access to the right ventricle is also feasible.

Cardiac Rejection: Overview

Cardiac rejection is classified by type of immune response, target tissue, and time of onset (Table 168.1). Acute or cellular rejection is an immune response aimed primarily at the cardiac myocyte[3]; it typically occurs within weeks to months of transplant, but can recur even years later if immunosuppressive treatment is insufficient. The histologic hallmarks are those of myocardial inflammation and myocyte necrosis. The second major type of rejection, antibody-mediated rejection (also known as humoral rejection), is manifest by immune complex deposition in small vessels, often in the absence of inflammation (Chapter 169). The immune target of chronic rejection, or graft vasculopathy, is also the endothelial cell, but primarily of arteries and, to a lesser extent, veins (Chapter 170).

One of the main challenges facing transplant biologists is clarifying the relationship of the three forms of rejection, especially in the context of identifying risk factors for and eventually preventing graft vascular disease, which is the main cause of graft failure after 1 year. A challenge in pathologic study of chronic rejection is the lack of sampling of larger vessels at biopsy and a paucity of autopsy studies.

Handling of Endomyocardial Biopsies

Biopsies of the right ventricular septum should comprise a few (at least 2) pieces of myocardium. Ideally, the evaluated tissue will be comprised of myocardium tissue and devoid of thrombus or scarred tissue. Since patients are usually biopsied multiple times throughout the lifetime of the allograft, it is common to identify a prior biopsy site (see below). For mechanical reasons, the bioptome in repeat biopsies tends to sample similar regions of the interventricular septum.

The tissue can be fixed in formalin and paraffin embedded, or a piece can be frozen and saved for immunofluorescence study with

the main purpose of performing C4d staining. Since this antibody is now available for paraffin immunohistochemistry, all the tissue can be fixed and processed routinely. Multiple sections should be taken for evaluation, and intervening unstained slides can be saved for further stains. Phenotyping of lymphocytes (CD3, CD4, CD8, CD20, CD68) is a way of confirming rejection, better evaluating the compartment of inflammation and differentiating rejection from Quilty effect or infection.[4,5] Masson trichrome can aid in the pathologic diagnosis. Immunohistochemical studies for CMV and silver stains for fungi can be performed in suspected cases.

Acute (Cellular) Rejection

Acute rejection occurs generally within weeks to months after transplant and results in clinical and electrocardiographic changes that do not reliably reflect the severity of myocardial damage. The gold standard for transplant rejection remains the endomyocardial biopsy, although antimyosin scintigraphy shows promise as a less invasive method to follow transplant rejection. Histologic diagnosis rests on the identification of one or more "infiltrates" of T lymphocytes and presence of myocyte damage; the definition of infiltrate has not been defined quantitatively, but includes an aggregate of cells that is in the interstitial or in a perivascular location. The cellular infiltrate in acute allograft rejection is primarily T lymphocytes, both CD4 and CD8 positive, as well as macrophages and occasional eosinophils.

In addition to establishing a diagnosis of cellular rejection, it is essential to grade the degree of inflammation. The grading of rejection is based on one primary feature: the presence or absence of myocyte necrosis. Because necrosis is rare in the absence of extensive inflammation, the degree of inflammation is also of importance in grading.

In 1990, the International Society of Heart Lung Transplantation (ISHLT) issued a grading system, which is based on the degree of inflammation and myocyte damage and presence of interstitial changes.[6] The ISHLT simplified the grading system in 2004 (Table 168.2).[7] The simplified system reflects a 3-tiered system of mild (inflammation without myocyte necrosis) (Figs. 168.1 and 168.2), moderate (inflammation with focal myocyte necrosis) (Figs. 168.3 to 168.5), and severe (extensive necrosis with other features such as edema, vasculitis, and

TABLE 168.1 Major Types of Cardiac Allograft Rejection

Type of Rejection	Onset Posttransplant	Clinical Criteria	Histologic Hallmarks
Acute (cellular)	Days–years	Graft dysfunction	T-cell infiltrates, with myocyte necrosis (when moderate to severe)
Antibody mediated (humoral)	Days–months	Graft dysfunction; alloantibodies[a]	Complement deposition in capillaries, especially C4d[b]
Chronic (graft vascular disease)	Months–years	Graft dysfunction, coronary narrowing by IVUS	Concentric intimal thickening, epicardial arteries, extending into smaller branches

[a]Panel-reactive antibodies and donor-specific antibodies, to both class I and II HLA antigens.
[b]The importance of a cellular reaction, in the form of capillary endothelial cell swelling, intraluminal macrophages, and intraluminal lymphocytes, is currently appreciated in symptomatic AMR.

TABLE 168.2 Grading of Acute (Cellular) Cardiac Rejection

Grade (ISHLT, 1990)	Histologic Features	Revised Nomenclature (ISHLT, 2004)
0	No infiltrates or necrosis	Grade 0 R
1A	Focal (perivascular or interstitial) infiltrate without necrosis	Grade 1 R, mild
1B	Diffuse, sparse infiltrate without necrosis	
2	One focus only with aggressive infiltration and/or focal myocyte damage	
3A	Multifocal aggressive infiltrates and/or myocyte damage	Grade 2 R, moderate
3B	Diffuse inflammatory process with necrosis	Grade 3 R, severe
4	Diffuse aggressive polymorphous infiltrate with edema, hemorrhage, vasculitis, and myocyte necrosis	

ISHLT, International Society for Heart and Lung Transplantation.
Adapted from Stewart S, Winters GL, Fishbein MC, et al. Revision of the 1990 working formulation for the standardization of nomenclature in the diagnosis of heart rejection. *J Heart Lung Transplant.* 2005;24:1710–1720, Ref. [7].

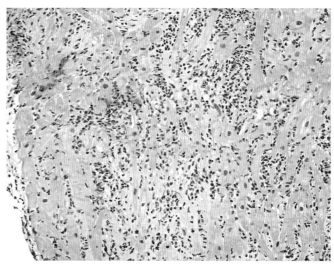

FIGURE 168.3 ▲ Moderate acute (cellular) rejection, grade 2R (3B). There is diffuse inflammation with myocyte necrosis.

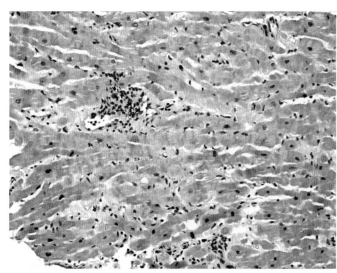

FIGURE 168.1 ▲ Mild acute (cellular) rejection, grade 1R (1A). R refers to revised grading system. There are two perivascular chronic inflammatory infiltrates.

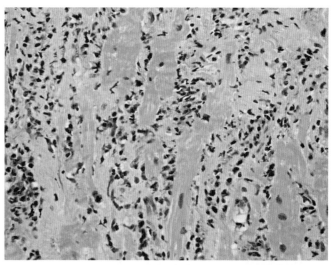

FIGURE 168.4 ▲ Moderate acute (cellular) rejection, grade 2R (3B). The myocyte necrosis is characterized by inflammation within myocytes, resulting in cytoplasmic fragmentation and lack of clear-cell borders.

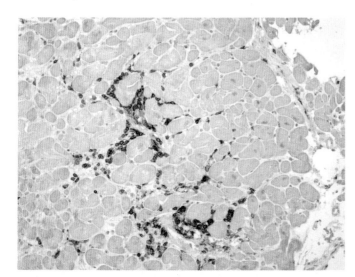

FIGURE 168.2 ▲ Mild acute (cellular) rejection, grade 1R (1R). CD3 immunohistochemical stain highlights the lymphocytes as T lymphocytes.

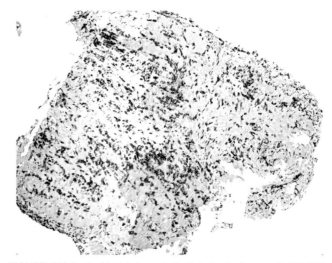

FIGURE 168.5 ▲ Moderate acute (cellular) rejection, grade 2R (3B). Low magnification stained with anti-CD8 demonstrates T lymphocytes diffusely infiltrating the biopsy specimen. The patient was noncompliant with medications and presented to the clinic in heart failure.

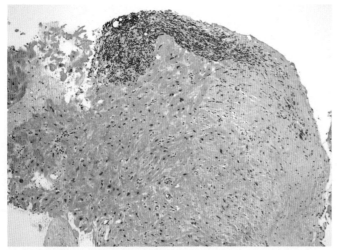

FIGURE 168.6 ▲ Quilty effect. There is a nodular infiltrate of lymphocytes in the endocardium.

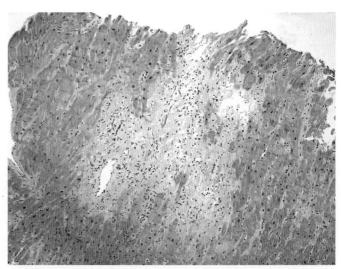

FIGURE 168.8 ▲ Myocardial ischemia. Areas of ischemic cell necrosis are generally zonal, with comparatively little inflammation, in contrast with necrosis secondary to rejection. In this example, the ischemia is associated with early fibrosis and is seen in a biopsy that is 3 weeks after transplant.

hemorrhage). The previous distinction between mild focal inflammation and mild diffuse inflammation (previous grades 1A and 1B, respectively) has been abandoned, as well as a single focus of "aggressive" inflammation (previous grade 2).

The interobserver variability in the grading of acute cellular rejection is significant, other than grade 0 (lack of rejection), underscoring the subjectivity of the criteria.[8]

Differential Diagnosis of Acute (Cellular) Rejection

Quilty Effect

Previously known as Quilty "lesion" and named after a patient, the Quilty effect is a subendocardial collection of lymphocytes that occurs at some point in up to 50% of transplant patients. The infiltrate is predominantly lymphocytic and, when large, contains a central B-cell follicle with small vascular channels and dendritic cells (Figs. 168.6 and 168.7). Quilty A signifies a well-defined endocardial lesion, whereas Quilty B infiltrates into the underlying myocardium; in the revised ISHLT

system, the A and B designations are dropped. Quilty lesions are weakly associated with cellular rejection, although they are not considered rejection *per se*, and are more frequent in women and younger patients. There has been no concrete evidence that they are associated with graft vascular disease.

To distinguish Quilty effect from rejection, it is necessary only to establish a subendocardial location. If tangential sectioning or biopsy artifact obscures the location of the inflammation, then immunohistochemical stains for B cells or dendritic cells (such as CD21) can help substantiate the diagnosis.

Acute Ischemic Changes

Perioperative ischemic myocardial injury is common in cardiac allografts, especially those with a history of increased cold ischemic time, and must be differentiated by the pathologist from acute rejection. Ischemia-related inflammation is characterized by a predominantly polymorphonuclear and histiocytic infiltrate with relative few T or B lymphocytes and relatively significant amounts of necrosis (Figs. 168.8 to 168.10). If immunohistochemical stains for complement

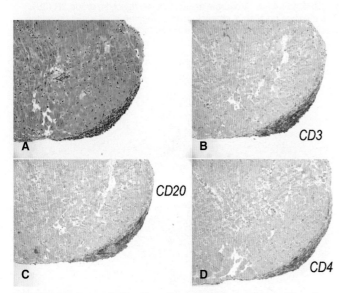

FIGURE 168.7 ▲ Quilty effect. The infiltrate is a mixture of lymphocytes and macrophages. Illustrated are routine hematoxylin–eosin **(A)**, pan T-cell marker **(B)**, B-lymphocyte marker **(C)**, and CD4 T-lymphocyte subset **(D)**.

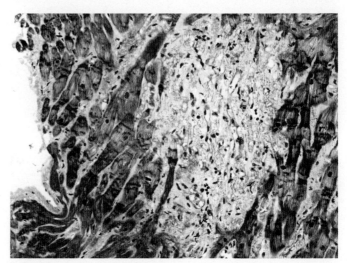

FIGURE 168.9 ▲ Myocardial ischemia. Masson trichrome stain demonstrates minimal fibrosis in the area.

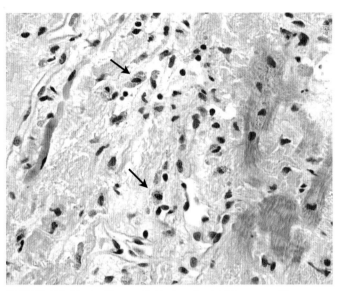

FIGURE 168.10 ▲ Myocardial ischemia. A higher magnification demonstrates hemosiderin-laden macrophages and scant lymphocytes.

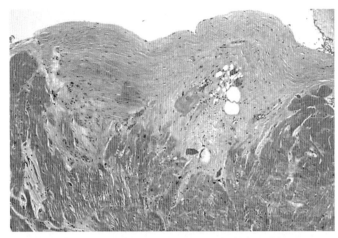

FIGURE 168.11 ▲ Biopsy site scar. A high proportion of biopsies shows previous scarring from prior biopsies, as the bioptome is directed to the apex of the right ventricle and patients are biopsied serially for surveillance. There is irregular endocardial scarring with irregular hypertrophy myocytes at the base of the scar.

are performed, in order to diagnose antibody-mediated rejection, "leaky" necrotic myocytes will strongly stain, establishing the diagnosis of ischemia.

Prior Biopsy Artifact

Because patients with allografts are often biopsied multiple times, it is common to direct the bioptome to sites of previous biopsy. Histologically, biopsy site is characterized by localized endocardial fibrosis, with underlying myocardial fiber disarray (Fig. 168.11). If the biopsy is recent, there may be abundant inflammatory cells; unlike rejection, however, these often include B cells. In cases of significant inflammation, there is generally evidence of organizing or organized thrombus, which should aid in the distinction between inflamed prior biopsy site and Quilty effect (Table 168.3).

Infections in the Allograft

If histologic findings are not typical of rejection or ischemic damage, an infection should be considered in the differential diagnosis. However, primary cardiac infections in allografts, diagnosed by endomyocardial biopsy, are rare. The overall incidence of infections in cardiac allograft continues to decrease due to advances in immunosuppression, the use of selective prophylaxis, and more effective treatment regimens.[2] In general, the presence of B cells and plasma cells in an infiltrate should raise the suspicion of infection. The diagnosis of cytomegalovirus may be made by identification of characteristic intranuclear and intracytoplasmic inclusion. Fungal infections are decreasing in prevalence, as well as *Pneumocystis jirovecii* and *Nocardia* infections. Rarely, tachyzoites and bradyzoites of *Toxoplasma gondii* may be observed in biopsy specimens of allografts and diagnosed by PCR. Even less common are cases of tuberculosis and other parasites such as *Giardia* that have been reported.[2]

TABLE 168.3 Differential Diagnosis of Acute (Cellular) Rejection

Diagnosis	Histologic Pointers	Immunohistochemistry	Incidence (in Biopsies)
Acute (cellular) rejection	Interstitial, perivascular infiltrates (at least 5–10 cells in contiguous focus); eosinophils only in moderate/severe with myocyte necrosis	T lymphocytes (CD4 and CD8), macrophages, B cells generally absent or small proportion	Common
Quilty (tangential)	Step sections may demonstrate endocardial location.	Central B-cell aggregate, often with CD21 dendritic cells	Common
Biopsy site inflammation	Adjacent disorganized myocytes, near the endocardium, may see organizing thrombus.	Prominent macrophages, also T cells and B cells	Common
Acute ischemia	Myocyte necrosis (hypereosinophilia)	Complement positivity within necrotic myocytes	Common in first 2 weeks of transplant
Infection	Viral inclusions, diffuse inflammation; plasma cells, eosinophils	B cells in addition to T cells, macrophages	Very rare
Posttransplant lymphoproliferative disease	Nodules of lymphocytes, without myocyte necrosis	B cells	Very rare

REFERENCES

1. Kilo J, Laufer G, Antretter H. Endomyocardial biopsy—jugular/subclavian vein approach. *Multimed Man Cardiothorac Surg.* 2006;2006:mmcts 2005 001149.
2. Haddad H, Isaac D, Legare JF, et al. Canadian Cardiovascular Society Consensus Conference update on cardiac transplantation 2008: executive summary. *Can J Cardiol.* 2009;25:197–205.
3. Wong BW, Rahmani M, Rezai N, et al. Progress in heart transplantation. *Cardiovasc Pathol.* 2005;14:176–180.
4. Frank R, Dean SA, Molina MR, et al. Correlations of lymphocyte subset infiltrates with donor-specific antibodies and acute antibody-mediated rejection in endomyocardial biopsies. *Cardiovasc Pathol.* 2015;24: 168–172.
5. Tavora F, Munivenkatappa R, Papadimitriou J, et al. Endotheliitis in cardiac allograft biopsy specimens: possible relationship to antibody-mediated rejection. *J Heart Lung Transplant.* 2011;30:435–444.
6. Berry GJ, Brunt EM, Chamberlain D, et al. A working formulation for the standardization of nomenclature in the diagnosis of heart and lung rejection: Lung Rejection Study Group. The International Society for Heart Transplantation. *J Heart Transplant.* 1990;9:593–601.
7. Stewart S, Winters GL, Fishbein MC, et al. Revision of the 1990 working formulation for the standardization of nomenclature in the diagnosis of heart rejection. *J Heart Lung Transplant.* 2005;24:1710–1720.
8. Angelini A, Andersen CB, Bartoloni G, et al. A web-based pilot study of inter-pathologist reproducibility using the ISHLT 2004 working formulation for biopsy diagnosis of cardiac allograft rejection: the European experience. *J Heart Lung Transplant.* 2011;30:1214–1220.

169 Antibody-Mediated Cardiac Allograft Rejection

Allen P. Burke, M.D.

Introduction

Antibody-mediated rejection is an immunologic response to the cardiac allograft distinct from cellular rejection by its biology and histologic findings. It is characterized by complement-mediated endothelial damage to the allograft and is classically considered to be devoid of a significant lymphocytic response. The main mechanism of injury in antibody-mediated rejection involves the activation of the classical pathway of the complement cascade. In contrast to acute cellular rejection (see Chapter 168), which has been extensively studied and well defined both clinically and pathologically, there is little consensus regarding the histopathologic diagnosis of antibody-mediated rejection.

The first recognition of antibody-mediated rejection described a small-vessel vasculitis associated with a poor graft outcome.[1] Later, immunofluorescence demonstrated immunoglobulin and complement deposition in the absence of a significant inflammatory reaction,[2] and the term "vascular rejection" was often used.[3] The concept that antibody-mediated rejection causes heart graft dysfunction in the absence of lymphocytic infiltrates has gradually been modified to include intravascular macrophages and possibly endotheliitis (or intimitis) as a component.[4,5]

The pathophysiology of antibody-mediated rejection involves a stepwise progression that begins with circulating immunoglobulins, followed by deposition of the endothelium of myocardial capillaries with complement activation, then involves tissue damage with or without inflammation, and finally culminates in graft dysfunction. The relationship between antibody-mediated rejection and the development of cardiac allograft vasculopathy in epicardial vessels remains unclear.

Clinical Features

Antibody-mediated rejection usually occurs within the first month after transplantation, but episodes of antibody-mediated rejection can happen many months or years after transplantation.[3] The alleged prevalence for cardiac antibody-mediated rejection is 7% to 18%, and antibody-mediated rejection associated with acute cellular rejection can be detected in as high as 23% of patients.[6] The clinical findings are generally those of graft dysfunction that mimic cellular rejection. Graft dysfunction ranges from decreased cardiac output with a rise in capillary wedge and pulmonary artery pressures to hypotension and shock.[6] Depending on the clinical and pathologic criteria for diagnosis, antibody-mediated rejection can be detected in asymptomatic patients.[5] The treatment of cardiac antibody-mediated rejection consists of increase in immunosuppression, plasmapheresis, intravenous immunoglobulin, and rituximab (anti-CD20). Associated cellular rejection is not uncommon, in both the adult and pediatric populations.[7]

Allosensitized patients are at increased risk of developing a rejection. The most common clinical settings are pregnancy, prior transplantation, and previous ventricular assist device use, and others include blood transfusions, cytomegalovirus seropositivity, elevated response to a panel of reactive antibodies, and sensitization by OKT3 induction therapy.[8]

Patients with a diagnosis of antibody-mediated rejection have worse graft survival, possibly an increased risk for cardiac allograft vasculopathy (see Chapter 29) and decreased overall survival.[5,6] It has been suggested that even asymptomatic antibody-mediated rejection may portend a higher risk of developing cardiac allograft vasculopathy.[5] This may suggest that attempts of early detection and treatment even for patients without symptoms may be advisable.

Pathologic Findings

The pathogenesis of antibody-mediated rejection involves endothelial cell activation with immune complex deposition in the absence of lymphocytic infiltration that characterizes cellular rejection.[3] The pathologic feature is that of "activated mononuclear cells," which result from interstitial capillary injury with swollen endothelial cells and intravascular macrophages.[9] The density of intracapillary macrophages has been shown to correlate with the presence of donor-specific and panel-reactive antibodies in patient's serum.[10]

The grading of antibody-mediated rejection is based on the extent of endothelial cell swelling, intravascular macrophages in and around capillaries, along with identification of immunoglobulin or complement by immunofluorescence or immunohistochemistry in myocardial capillaries (Table 169.1; Figs. 169.1 to 169.5). Other features that have been described, such as interstitial hemorrhage, edema, and acute inflammation, are rarely seen and are features of severe antibody-mediated rejection (Fig. 169.6). Although only intravascular macrophages are considered in the grading of antibody-mediated rejection, small-vessel inflammation (endotheliitis) also involves

TABLE 169.1   Classification of Antibody-Mediated Rejection by Recommendation of the International Society for Heart and Lung Transplantation

Grade	Definition	Substrates
pAMR 0	Negative for pathologic AMR	Histologic and immunopathologic studies are both negative.
pAMR 1 (H+)	Histopathologic AMR alone	Histologic findings are present and immunopathologic findings are negative.
pAMR 1 (I+)	Immunopathologic AMR alone	Histologic findings are negative and immunopathologic findings are positive.
pAMR 2	Pathologic AMR	CD68+ and/or C4d+. Histologic and immunopathologic findings are both present.
pAMR 3	Severe pathologic AMR	Interstitial hemorrhage, capillary fragmentation, mixed inflammatory infiltrates, endothelial cell pyknosis and/or karyorrhexis, and marked edema and immunopathologic findings are present. These cases may be associated with profound hemodynamic dysfunction and poor clinical outcomes.

AMR, antibody-mediated rejection.
From Berry GJ, Burke MM, Andersen C, et al. The 2013 International Society for Heart and Lung Transplantation Working Formulation for the standardization of nomenclature in the pathologic diagnosis of antibody-mediated rejection in heart transplantation. *J Heart Lung Transplant.* 2013;32:1147–1162.

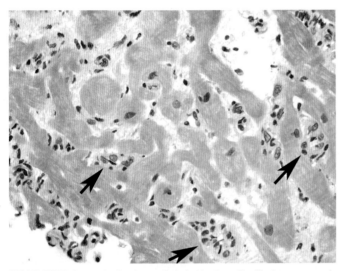

FIGURE 169.1 ▲ Antibody-mediated rejection. Capillaries are prominent with swollen endothelial cells (*arrows*).

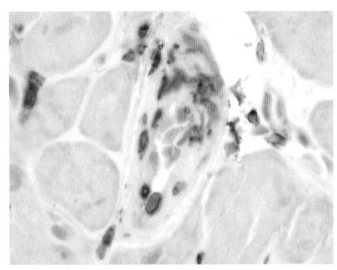

FIGURE 169.3 ▲ Anti-CD3 immunohistochemical staining. CD3-positive T lymphocytes are present in the capillary lumen and within the capillary wall.

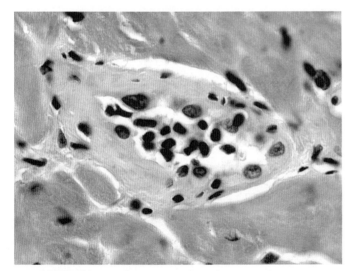

FIGURE 169.2 ▲ Antibody-mediated rejection. Intraluminal chronic inflammation with endothelial cell swelling.

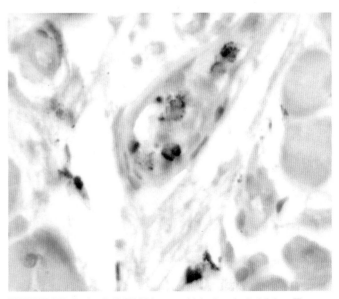

FIGURE 169.4 ▲ Anti-CD68 immunohistochemical staining. There are intraluminal macrophages, in association with swollen endothelial cell capillaries.

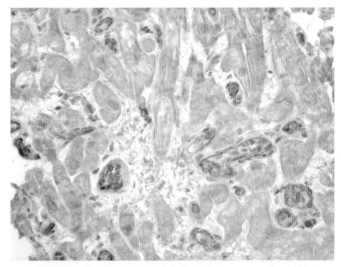

FIGURE 169.5 ▲ Anti-C4d immunohistochemical staining. Note diffuse endothelial capillary positivity.

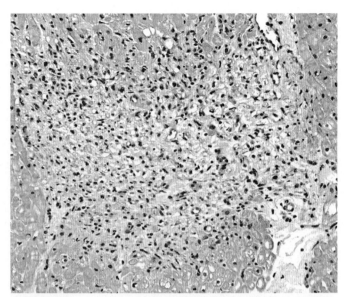

FIGURE 169.7 ▲ Ischemic injury. Endothelial changes can occur with ischemia, but there is generally an area of necrosis often with hemosiderin macrophages. Ischemic injury is rare after 3 months of transplant.

the recruitment of lymphocytes and neutrophils. Autopsy studies have described necrotizing vasculitis associated with intimal thickening and complement deposition, which has been associated with cytomegalovirus infection and the development of cardiac allograft vasculopathy.[11–13]

The relative diagnostic sensitivity and specificity of immunohistochemistry versus immunofluorescence and C4d versus C3d and other components of complements are under current study. The most commonly used marker for antibody-mediated rejection currently is C4d, and the easiness of use by immunohistochemistry has made this marker the most commonly used for aiding in the diagnosis of histologic antibody-mediated rejection.

Ischemic injury, which is also seen soon after transplant, also demonstrates prominent macrophages, but is in the setting of an area of healing necrosis (Fig. 169.7). Complement stains are frequently positive in capillaries and myocytes of ischemic lesions.

REFERENCES

1. Herskowitz A, Soule LM, Ueda K, et al. Arteriolar vasculitis on endomyocardial biopsy: a histologic predictor of poor outcome in cyclosporine-treated heart transplant recipients. *J Heart Transplant.* 1987;6:127–136.
2. Hammond EH, Yowell RL, Nunoda S, et al. Vascular (humoral) rejection in heart transplantation: pathologic observations and clinical implications. *J Heart Transplant.* 1989;8:430–443.
3. Olsen SL, Wagoner LE, Hammond EH, et al. Vascular rejection in heart transplantation: clinical correlation, treatment options, and future considerations. *J Heart Lung Transplant.* 1993;12:S135–S142.
4. Stewart S, Winters GL, Fishbein MC, et al. Revision of the 1990 working formulation for the standardization of nomenclature in the diagnosis of heart rejection. *J Heart Lung Transplant.* 2005;24:1710–1720.
5. Wu GW, Kobashigawa JA, Fishbein MC, et al. Asymptomatic antibody-mediated rejection after heart transplantation predicts poor outcomes. *J Heart Lung Transplant.* 2009;28:417–422.
6. Michaels PJ, Espejo ML, Kobashigawa J, et al. Humoral rejection in cardiac transplantation: risk factors, hemodynamic consequences and relationship to transplant coronary artery disease. *J Heart Lung Transplant.* 2003;22:58–69.
7. Zales VR, Crawford S, Backer CL, et al. Spectrum of humoral rejection after pediatric heart transplantation. *J Heart Lung Transplant.* 1993;12:563–571; discussion 572.
8. Tan CD, Baldwin WM III, Rodriguez ER. Update on cardiac transplantation pathology. *Arch Pathol Lab Med.* 2007;131:1169–1191.
9. Berry GJ, Burke MM, Andersen C, et al. The 2013 International Society for Heart and Lung Transplantation Working Formulation for the standardization of nomenclature in the pathologic diagnosis of antibody-mediated rejection in heart transplantation. *J Heart Lung Transplant.* 2013;32:1147–1162.
10. Xu L, Collins J, Drachenberg C, et al. Increased macrophage density of cardiac allograft biopsies is associated with antibody-mediated rejection and alloantibodies to HLA antigens. *Clin Transplant.* 2014;28:554–560.
11. Paavonen T, Mennander A, Lautenschlager I, et al. Endothelialitis in accelerated allograft arteriosclerosis in human cardiac transplant recipients. *Transplant Proc.* 1992;24:342–343.
12. Paavonen T, Mennander A, Lautenschlager I, et al. Endothelialitis and accelerated arteriosclerosis in human heart transplant coronaries. *J Heart Lung Transplant.* 1993;12:117–122.
13. Foerster A. Vascular rejection in cardiac transplantation. A morphological study of 25 human cardiac allografts. *APMIS.* 1992;100:367–376.

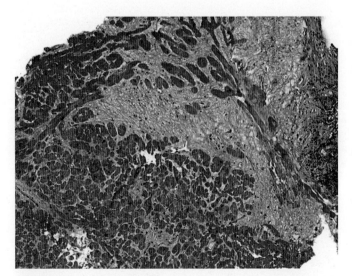

FIGURE 169.6 ▲ Intracellular edema. In contrast to artifactual separate between myocytes, intracellular myxoid material is clearly present.

170 Cardiac Allograft Vasculopathy

Joseph J. Maleszewski, M.D., and Allen P. Burke, M.D.

Overview

Cardiac allograft vasculopathy (CAV, or, loosely, chronic rejection) is a primarily intimal disease that is unique to allograft hearts.[1] It remains the main limitation of long-term success in heart transplantation.[2,3]

CAV involves the indirect allorecognition pathway of cell-mediated response, when antigens from the donor are processed by host dendritic cells and presented as peptides, which in turn trigger lymphocyte activation and vessel injury.[4,5] CAV predominantly affects arteries, but occasionally veins can exhibit similar changes.

Incidence and Risk Factors

Any degree of CAV is detectable in 7% of recipients within the first year, in 31.5% of recipients within 5 years, and in 52.7% of survivors within 10 years of transplant.[6] The cumulative incidence of obstructive CAV was 7% at 5 years and 23% by 10 years with an 11% cumulative probability of requiring a percutaneous intervention.[7]

Risk factors for the development of CAV include traditional ones (hypertension, dyslipidemia, diabetes, and metabolic syndrome) and those related to transplant and immunosuppression (cytomegalovirus infection, HLA mismatches, and rejection diagnosed by biopsy). A history of cellular or antibody-mediated rejection increases the risk of the development of CAV to 36% at 5 years.[6,8]

Clinical Diagnosis

CAV presents clinically as congestive heart failure, ventricular arrhythmias, or sudden death. Because CAV is concentric and diffuse, angiography, which is best in locating eccentric and focal lesions, is not the modality of choice. Furthermore, CAV frequently affects intramyocardial branches of the epicardial arteries that cannot be detected by imaging.

Modalities that have been used to measure CAV severity and intimal proliferation are dipyridamole myocardial perfusion scanning, dobutamine stress echocardiography, positron emission tomography (PET), cardiac magnetic imaging, computed tomography, and intravascular ultrasound, which is the diagnostic tool of choice.

Endomyocardial biopsy is of little use in the diagnosis of CAV, as chronic ischemic changes, while relatively specific, are insensitive diagnostic markers for the disease.[9]

Histopathology

In a series of 27 transplant autopsies with a mean of 3 years after surgery, 6 patients had CAV, compared to 13 with typical atherosclerosis and 8 without epicardial coronary disease, indicating that only a minority of transplant autopsies show features of CAV.[10] A series of hearts explanted for retransplantation showed that severe (>75%) cross-sectional area luminal narrowing was found in about 25% of hearts and involved the left anterior descending, circumflex, and right coronary arteries about equally.[11] Atheromas were described as frequent, even in pediatric hearts, suggesting that not all lipid-rich lesions are from the donor.[11]

The histologic findings are those of a mainly immune-mediated process characterized by intimal hyperplasia composed by smooth muscle cells with mild chronic inflammation. The internal elastic lamina is intact. Inflammation involves all layers of the vessel, including intima (intimitis or endotheliitis), media, and adventitia[12] (Figs. 170.1 to 170.3).

Small epicardial branch arteries and subepicardial intramyocardial arteries, as well as veins, may also be involved (Figs. 170.4 and 170.5). A typical feature is the presence of vasculitis, with thrombosis, which may be occlusive or nonocclusive (Fig. 170.6).[13,14]

Myocardial sections often show signs of chronic ischemia and patchy interstitial fibrosis. Intramyocardial vessels are affected first; thus, areas of large infarcts are uncommon unless the major arteries are affected[13,15] (Fig. 170.7).[9]

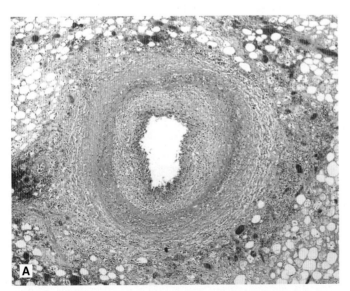
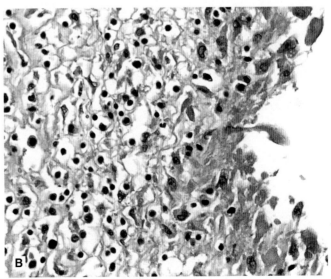

FIGURE 170.1 ▲ Cardiac allograft vasculopathy. **A.** Epicardial coronary artery shows concentric thickening; there are no lipid pools. **B.** A higher magnification shows inflammation on the luminal surface. Often, there is a band of inflammation at the lumen with a less cellular myxoid zone toward the internal elastic lamina.

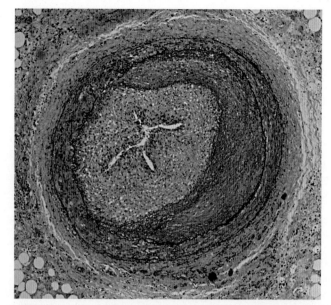

FIGURE 170.2 ▲ Cardiac allograft vasculopathy, Movat elastic stain. There is near total occlusion, with concentric narrowing and focal elastosis.

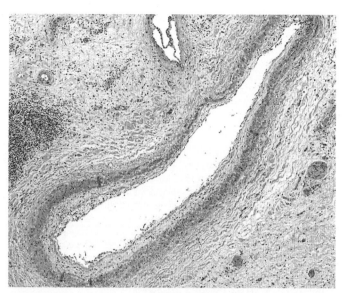

FIGURE 170.3 ▲ Cardiac allograft vasculopathy, involving epicardial vein. There is mild intimal thickening with inflammation.

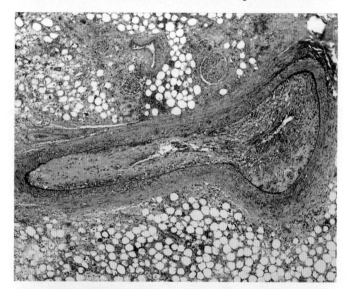

FIGURE 170.4 ▲ Cardiac allograft vasculopathy, branch point. In contrast to atherosclerosis, allograft vasculopathy typically involves intramural branches of the coronary arteries. Note that the internal elastic lamina is intact. Movat pentachrome stain.

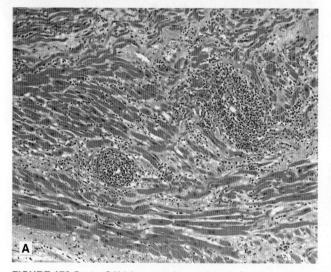

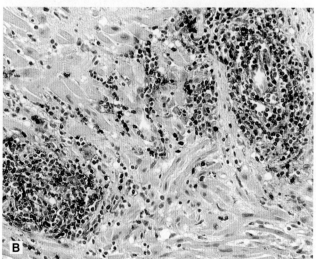

FIGURE 170.5 ▲ CAV, intramural vasculitis. **A.** Small muscular arteries and veins in the left ventricle are targeted by inflammation. **B.** CD4 immunohistochemical staining. A majority of the infiltrate is composed of CD4-positive T lymphocytes.

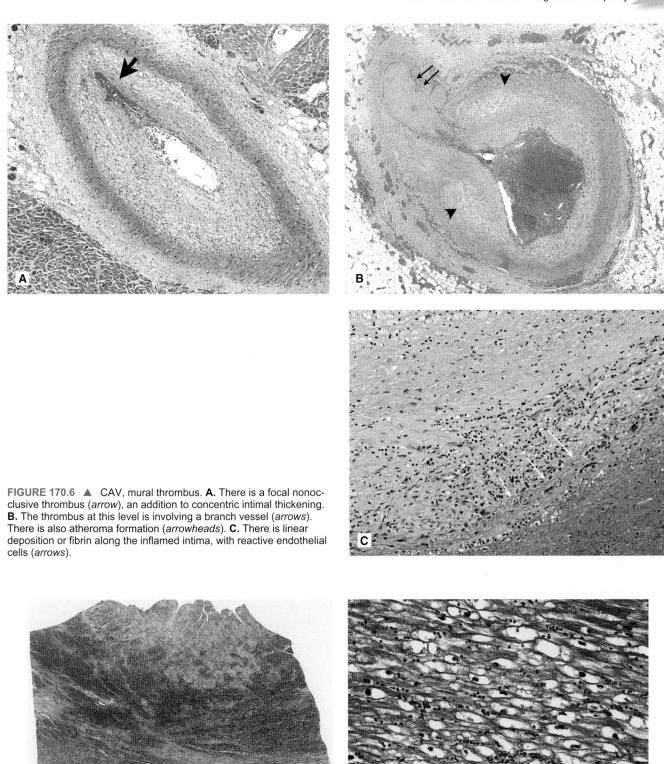

FIGURE 170.6 ▲ CAV, mural thrombus. **A.** There is a focal nonocclusive thrombus (*arrow*), an addition to concentric intimal thickening. **B.** The thrombus at this level is involving a branch vessel (*arrows*). There is also atheroma formation (*arrowheads*). **C.** There is linear deposition or fibrin along the inflamed intima, with reactive endothelial cells (*arrows*).

FIGURE 170.7 ▲ Chronic ischemia, heart explant, allograft. Graft failure necessitated repeat transplant, and the specimen is a surgical resection. **A.** There are patchy pale areas. **B.** Higher magnification demonstrates these to represent myocyte vacuolization typical of chronic ischemia. Because of small vessel involvement, the ischemic distribution may not be typical of epicardial occlusion as seen in atherosclerosis.

Prognosis

Although the overall survival from heart transplant has improved significantly over the last 3 decades, primarily due to improved immunosuppressive agents, CAV continues to be a significant cause of mortality after the first year of transplant. CAV, along with late graft failure, which may also represent unrecognized CAV, accounts for 32% of deaths after the fifth transplant year.[6]

REFERENCES

1. Mitchell RN. Graft vascular disease: immune response meets the vessel wall. *Annu Rev Pathol.* 2009;4:19–47.
2. Schmauss D, Weis M. Cardiac allograft vasculopathy: recent developments. *Circulation.* 2008;117:2131–2141.
3. Taylor DO, Edwards LB, Boucek MM, et al. Registry of the International Society for Heart and Lung Transplantation: twenty-third official adult heart transplantation report—2006. *J Heart Lung Transplant.* 2006;25: 869–879.
4. Lechler R, Ng WF, Steinman RM. Dendritic cells in transplantation—friend or foe? *Immunity.* 2001;14:357–368.
5. Rogers NJ, Lechler RI. Allorecognition. *Am J Transplant.* 2001;1:97–102.
6. Colvin-Adams M, Agnihotri A. Cardiac allograft vasculopathy: current knowledge and future direction. *Clin Transplant.* 2011;25:175–184.
7. Hamour IM, Khaghani A, Kanagala PK, et al. Current outcome of heart transplantation: a 10-year single centre perspective and review. *QJM.* 2011;104:335–343.
8. Skoric B, Cikes M, Ljubas Macek J, et al. Cardiac allograft vasculopathy: diagnosis, therapy, and prognosis. *Croat Med J.* 2014;55:562–576.
9. Winters GL, Schoen FJ. Graft arteriosclerosis-induced myocardial pathology in heart transplant recipients: predictive value of endomyocardial biopsy. *J Heart Lung Transplant.* 1997;16:985–993.
10. Alexander RT, Lathrop S, Vollmer R, et al. Graft vascular disease after cardiac transplantation and its relationship to mean acute rejection score. *Arch Pathol Lab Med.* 2005;129:1283–1287.
11. Lu WH, Palatnik K, Fishbein GA, et al. Diverse morphologic manifestations of cardiac allograft vasculopathy: a pathologic study of 64 allograft hearts. *J Heart Lung Transplant.* 2011;30:1044–1050.
12. Angelini A, Castellani C, Fedrigo M, et al. Coronary cardiac allograft vasculopathy versus native atherosclerosis: difficulties in classification. *Virchows Arch.* 2014;464:627–635.
13. Johnson DE, Gao SZ, Schroeder JS, et al. The spectrum of coronary artery pathologic findings in human cardiac allografts. *J Heart Transplant.* 1989;8:349–359.
14. Higuchi ML, Benvenuti LA, Demarchi LM, et al. Histological evidence of concomitant intramyocardial and epicardial vasculitis in necropsied heart allografts: a possible relationship with graft coronary arteriosclerosis. *Transplantation.* 1999;67:1569–1576.
15. Tan CD, Baldwin WM III, Rodriguez ER. Update on cardiac transplantation pathology. *Arch Pathol Lab Med.* 2007;131:1169–1191.

171 Evaluation of Excised Cardiac Valves

Allen P. Burke, M.D.

General Considerations

A gross photograph generally provides significantly more information than do histologic sections or long gross descriptions. However, histologic evaluation is essential in ruling out endocarditis, which may not always be grossly obvious.

The distinction between valve replacement and repair should be made. In general, aortic valves and stenotic mitral valves are replaced, and insufficient mitral valves are either repaired or replaced.

Aortic Valve

For replaced aortic valves, the number of tissue fragments and intact leaflets should be described, as well as intact (fused) commissures, raphes, and calcification. With any valve, roughened areas, vegetations, and perforations should be sectioned to exclude endocarditis (Table 171.1). The most common conditions encountered are degenerative calcific aortic stenosis (trileaflet somewhat more common than bileaflet), followed by insufficient valves (trileaflet or bileaflet) that look relatively normal, and postinflammatory (rheumatic) valve disease. Depending on the population, aortic valve endocarditis may be a relatively common diagnosis and is generally known prior to surgery (Table 171.2).

Mitral Valve

Mitral valves are frequently repaired, especially in cases of regurgitation, most frequently for prolapse. In such cases, only a fragment of the posterior leaflet may be encountered. For stenotic valves (usually a result of postinflammatory mitral valve disease and rarely calcific mitral valve disease), the valve is typically replaced. For the mitral valve, the chordae tendineae should be described, as they are important to distinguish prolapse (thin, elongated) from rheumatic disease (thickened, fused) (Table 171.3). Mitral valves that have been previously operated that have been previously infected may also show thickened chordae. Common conditions requiring mitral valve replacement are presented in Table 171.4.

Tricuspid and Pulmonary Valves

The tricuspid valve is often repaired for the treatment of insufficiency, generally in the setting of pulmonary hypertension. Usually, no tissue is excised, and a C-shaped annuloplasty device is placed.

In cases of infectious endocarditis involving the tricuspid valve, which generally occurs in intravenous drug addicts, the valve may be resected, if there is significant destruction of the leaflets (see Chapter 177).

The pulmonary valve is repaired or replaced, often with right ventricular outflow tract reconstruction, in children with tetralogy of Fallot. Adults may have revisions of right ventricular outflow procedures decades after the initial surgery, and portions of native valve, prosthetic valve, transannular patch, or conduit may be removed during surgery (see Chapter 140).

Vegetations

In some patients, only a vegetation from a valve is removed (vegetectomy). Most of these are infectious endocarditis, and histologic

---

TABLE 171.1 Gross Findings, Aortic Valve, Surgical Specimens[a]

Intact valve _____ Intact separate leaflets _____ Fragmented _____

Number of leaflets: Three _____ Two _____ One _____ Indeterminate _____

Fused commissures (0,1,2,3) _____

Bicuspid valves: presence of raphe _____ angle of conjoint cusp (if fused) _____

Fibrosis (absent, mild, marked) _____

Calcification (mild, nodular) _____

Free edge of valve (rolled edges, fibrotic, normal)

Vegetations _____ Perforations _____ Fenestrations _____

Examples of diagnoses:[b]
- Degenerative calcific sclerosis/stenosis, trileaflet valve
- Degenerative calcific sclerosis/stenosis, bicuspid valve
- Degenerative calcific sclerosis/stenosis, indeterminate number of leaflets
- Bicuspid valve, changes consistent with insufficiency (often with aneurysm repair)
- Trileaflet valve, changes consistent with insufficiency (sometimes with aneurysm repair)
- Postinflammatory (rheumatic) valve disease (primarily stenotic/insufficient)
- Infectious endocarditis
- Unicuspid/unicommissural valve (teardrop shape)
- Nonspecific fibrosis, indeterminate
- Focal calcification, indeterminate (may rarely cause insufficiency instead of stenosis)

[a]Gross photography is recommended and eliminates the need for long gross descriptions.
[b]Access to operative report and surgeon's description is very helpful.

TABLE 171.2   Aortic Valve Replacements: Pathologic Diagnoses, Gender, Age, and Frequency of Ascending Aortic Disease Requiring Repair[a]

Pathologic Designation	%	% Men	Age ± SD (years)	Ascending Aortic Disease
Degenerative calcific aortic stenosis, trileaflet	48%	59	76 ± 8	0.4% aneurysm 1% calcification requiring repair
Degenerative calcific aortic stenosis, bicuspid valve	27%	74	63 ± 10	25% aneurysm 75% normal by TEE
Aortic insufficiency trileaflet valve[b]	13%	80	62 ± 12	26% dissections 19% aneurysms 3% aortitis aneurysm 1% sinus of Valsalva aneurysm 51% normal by TEE
Aortic insufficiency, bicuspid valve[b]	6%	88	52 ± 13	41% dissections 16% aneurysms 3% aortitis aneurysm 40% normal by TEE
Postinflammatory valve disease[c]	3%	67	60 ± 12	7% aneurysm 93% normal by TEE
Nodular calcific aortic stenosis, unicommissural	1.5%	63	51 ± 8	25% aneurysm
Radiation injury[d]	<1% (n = 2)	0	57 ± 3	None
Degenerative calcific trileaflet disease with insufficiency	<1% (n = 2)	100	77 ± 8	None
Bicuspid valve with inflammatory stenosis	<1% (n = 1)	100	41	Aortitis
Quadricuspid aortic valve with stenosis	<1% (n = 1)	0	66	None
Congenitally dysplastic aortic valve	<1% (n = 1)	100	17	None

[a]Based on 530 consecutive aortic valve replacements, ages > 15 years, excluding for endocarditis or trauma, University of Maryland Medical Center.
[b]These appear relatively normal grossly, with variable myxoid change and thickened, rolled edges.
[c]10 of 15 were predominantly stenotic; the remainder insufficient.
[d]One insufficient, one stenotic.
Reproduced with permission from Burke AP. Cardiovascular pathology. In Silverberg SG, et al., eds. *Silverberg's Principles and Practice of Surgical Pathology and Cytopathology.* 5th ed. New York: Cambridge University Press; 2015, Ref. [1].

examination will show fibrin thrombus with entrapped neutrophils, and often bacteria. Occasionally, marantic (sterile) vegetations are removed, and histology shows bland fibrin thrombus. Another form of vegetation is represented by papillary fibroelastoma, which may be removed without incising the underlying valve leaflet (see Chapter 176).

Prosthetic Valve Replacement

Previously replaced valves can undergo degeneration or infection, primarily bioprosthetic valves. In such cases, the type of valve (porcine, pericardial, homograft) should be ascertained (see Chapter 173). In addition, perforations, calcifications, thrombosis, and exuberant fibrous

TABLE 171.3   Gross Findings, Mitral Valve, Surgical Specimens

Repair[a] _____ Fragments (number) _____
Replacement[a] _____ Intact valve _____ Number of fragments _____
Commissural fusion (if intact) _____
Leaflet color[b] _____
Leaflet thickness (fibrotic vs. thin and billowed) _____
Chordae (elongated, thin, thick, fused, ruptured) _____
Evidence of prior or intraoperative repair (e.g., clip or suture) _____
Papillary muscle: present _____ appearance _____
Vegetations, perforations _____
Calcification: none _____ leaflet _____ separate fragments _____

Diagnoses (examples):
• Changes consistent with mitral valve prolapse
• Postinflammatory (postrheumatic) mitral valve disease (stenosis, insufficiency)
• Normal-appearing valve (consistent with insufficiency, cardiomyopathy)
• Mitral annular calcification with/without leaflet calcification
• Acute infarction, papillary muscle, with acute mitral insufficiency
• Leaflet fibrosis, indeterminate, descriptive
• Infectious endocarditis

[a]Repair vs. replacement can sometimes be difficult, because the mitral valve is usually not completely removed when a prosthetic valve is replaced. If the valve is intact (e.g., rheumatic valve disease), it is obviously a case of replacement. In cases of insufficient valves secondary to prolapse or cardiomyopathy, it may be necessary to review the operative report to determine if the valve was replaced with a valve prosthesis or repaired with an annuloplasty ring.
[b]Mitral valve prolapse (floppy valves) are typically pearl white and glistening.

TABLE 171.4 Pathology of Mitral Valve Replacement[a]

Condition	%	Indication for Surgery	Procedure	Gross and Histologic Findings
Postinflammatory mitral valve disease	37%	Predominantly stenosis (49%) Insufficiency with or without stenosis (51%)	97% replacement 3% repair	Thickened, with chordal fusion
Mitral valve prolapse	36%	Insufficiency	86% repair 14% replacement	White mucoid valve, portion of posterior leaflet only (repairs)
Calcification (annular and leaflet)	13%	Insufficiency (57%) Stenosis (38%) Stroke (5%)	Replacement	
Functional regurgitation, ischemic heart disease	8%	Insufficiency	91% replacement 9% repair	
Functional regurgitation, cardiomyopathy	3%	Insufficiency	Replacement	
Congenital heart disease	1%	Insufficiency	Replacement	Variable
Radiation fibrosis	1%	Stenosis	Replacement	Nonspecific fibrosis

[a]or repairs with partial resection, excluding endocarditis. Based on 158 consecutive mitral valve replacements and repairs with partial resection and ring placement in patients > 15 years, University of Maryland Medical Center.
Reproduced with permission from Burke AP. Cardiovascular pathology. In Silverberg SG, et al., eds. *Silverberg's Principles and Practice of Surgical Pathology and Cytopathology.* 5th ed. New York: Cambridge University Press; 2015, Ref. 1.

tissue on the ring (pannus) should be described. Histologic sections to document infection are indicated.

Failed valve repairs (annuloplasty) may be treated with removal of the annuloplasty ring and valve replacement. In such cases, the ring can be described as a gross-only specimen; it is optional to submit attached soft tissue for histologic analysis. In cases of removal for annular abscess, histologic evaluation is indicated.

REFERENCE

1. Burke AP. Cardiovascular pathology. In Silverberg SG, et al., eds. *Silverberg's Principles and Practice of Surgical Pathology and Cytopathology.* 5th ed. New York: Cambridge University Press; 2015.

172 Degenerative Valve Disease—Calcific Aortic Stenosis and Mitral Annular Calcification

Allen P. Burke, M.D., and Joseph J. Maleszewski, M.D.

Introduction

Degenerative aortic valve disease extensively involves the cusps themselves and results in fibrotic thickening and nodular calcification. Inflammation and neovascularization are not dominant features, in distinction to rheumatic valve disease. Degenerative calcification has a propensity for congenitally bicuspid or unicuspid valves and usually causes stenosis with variable insufficiency.[1] Degenerative aortic stenosis is currently the most common indication for valve surgery, as the population ages and newer techniques, such as minimally invasive surgery and transcutaneous methods, become available (see Chapter 178).

Another common location for degenerative calcific changes in the heart is the mitral annulus, occasionally with involvement of the cusps themselves.[2,3]

Degenerative Aortic Stenosis (Tricuspid Valve)

Aortic sclerosis, which is clinically defined as valve thickening without obstruction to outflow, is present in about 25% of patients over 65 years of age, who have tricuspid valves. The incidence of symptomatic stenosis is ~5 in 10,000 and is generally a disease of the elderly. Risk factors overlap with those predisposing to atherosclerosis, and hypertension, smoking, diabetes, and obesity.[1,4,5] The role of hyperlipidemia

and statin treatment in the prevention of aortic stenosis is unclear, although hypercholesterolemia is an often-cited risk factor.[4,6]

Clinical Findings

Patients with calcific degenerative aortic stenosis present in the 6th to 9th decades and account for more than 70% of the patients undergoing valve replacement in the United States. Those patients with tricuspid valves are usually older than 65 to 70 years. Patients with chronic renal failure and secondary hyperparathyroidism have symptomatic disease at an earlier age, because of an increased risk for tissue calcification.[7]

There is a male predominance ranging from 1.6:1 to 4:1, depending on etiology. Clinically, most patients have stenosis or combined stenosis and insufficiency. The natural history of aortic stenosis is characterized by a prolonged period in which the disease is only incidentally detected. During the initial phases, the left ventricle adapts to the increased systolic pressure overload and develops hypertrophy with normal chamber volume. This is followed by concentric left ventricular hypertrophy, which may cause reduced coronary blood flow and subendocardial ischemia, even in the absence of epicardial coronary disease. Eventually, symptoms of angina, syncope, and heart failure develop. The development of symptoms usually signifies advanced disease with hemodynamic compromise.

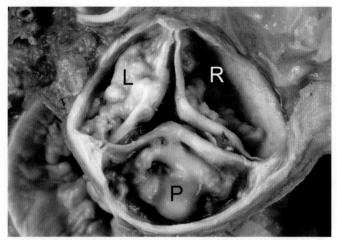

FIGURE 172.1 ▲ Degenerative (tricuspid) aortic valve disease, autopsy. There are nodular calcifications on the aortic surfaces of the cusps, filling the cusp pockets. (L, left aortic valve cusp; R, right aortic valve cusp; P, posterior aortic valve cusp.)

Gross Pathologic Findings

Degenerative calcific aortic valve disease is characterized by nodules of calcification on the aortic (nonflow) side of the cusps, usually near the base of the sinuses (Fig. 172.1). The degree of stenosis at autopsy is estimated by assessing the stiffness of the valves, as by palpation or passage of an instrument or finger through the opening the outflow tract, though only when concentric left ventricular hypertrophy is present should one presume stenosis was present.

The evaluation should also document degree and location of calcified deposits, presence of median raphe that would indicate a congenitally bicuspid valve (Fig. 172.2), commissural fusion, intimal calcification of the ascending aorta (Fig. 172.3), and evaluation of the aortic root for signs of dilatation. Occasionally, mild fusion of one or more commissures may be seen in the setting of degenerative sclerosis, but it is usually less than half way to the midpoint of the cusp free edge, distinguishing it from chronic rheumatic valve disease.

Heart weight and measurements of left ventricular free wall and left ventricular chamber diameter (excluding papillary muscles) are important to document the degree of cardiac hypertrophy and remodeling.

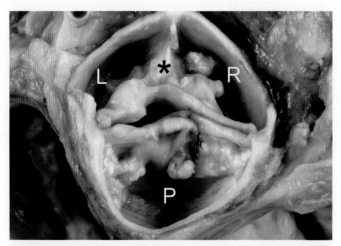

FIGURE 172.2 ▲ Degenerative (bicuspid) aortic valve disease, autopsy. Nodular calcifications fill the cusp pockets and can be seen on both the acquired and fused cusps. There is also calcification along the point of fusion (raphe) (*asterisk*). (L, remnant left aortic valve cusp; R, remnant right aortic valve cusp; P, posterior [nonconjoined] aortic valve cusp.)

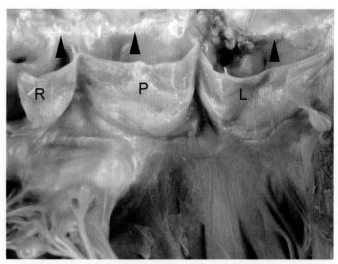

FIGURE 172.3 ▲ Calcification of the aortic sinotubular junction, autopsy. In some instances, nodular calcification (*arrowheads*) is primarily at the sinotubular junction and not involving sinuses of Valsalva. There was no valve stenosis. (L, left aortic valve cusp; R, right aortic valve cusp; P, posterior aortic valve cusp.)

In about 5% of patients, there is asymmetric hypertrophy with an increase in septal to free wall ratio. There is frequently coexistent atherosclerosis of the coronary arteries and calcification of the mitral annulus.

Normally, aortic valve cusps should be thin and translucent (Fig. 172.4A). As part of the degenerative process, aortic valve cusps become increasingly thickened until they are no longer translucent (Fig. 172.4B) and can be considered sclerotic. Surgically excised valves for nodular calcific aortic stenosis may be fragmented during surgical procedure due to heavy calcification, or the valve cusps may be relatively intact (Fig. 172.4C). The calcification begins in the base of the cusp and spares the free margins; thus, commissural fusion is rare but may occur (Fig. 172.5). Gross inspection and documentation of degree of calcification are sufficient for a diagnosis of degenerative calcific aortic disease. Endocarditis is an infrequent complication of calcific aortic stenosis but can be easily missed without histologic evaluation.

The presence of calcification is an important determinant of the degree of stenosis or gradient measured clinically.[8]

Microscopic Findings

The histologic findings include nodules of calcification at the base of the cusps on the aortic surface, which occur on pools of fibrin, similar to nodular calcified plaques seen in nodular calcific deposits in coronary and carotid atherosclerosis (Fig. 172.6). In addition to nodular calcification, there is mild chronic inflammation.[9,10] The sparse inflammation is composed of macrophages, plasma cells, and lymphocytes. If there are dense macrophage infiltrates or any neutrophilic inflammation, then superimposed endocarditis should be excluded by special stains or clinical correlation. Rarely, small foci of neutrophils may be identified adjacent to calcific deposits.

In the myocardium of patients with left ventricular hypertrophy secondary to aortic stenosis, the amount of myocardial fibrosis has been shown to affect long-term survival after aortic valve replacement.[11]

Treatment

The standard treatment for aortic stenosis is surgical replacement of the valve, with or without coronary artery bypass surgery for coronary atherosclerotic obstruction, which is commonly present. The operative mortality is 2% to 5%.[12]

Patients who are inoperable, due to functional status or ascending aortic calcification, may be treated by balloon valvuloplasty or transcatheter aortic valve replacement. The 5-year survival after

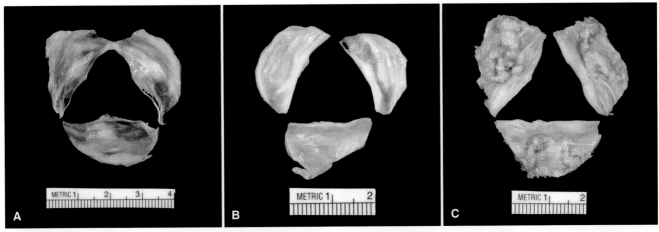

FIGURE 172.4 ▲ Aortic valve findings (tricuspid), surgery. **A.** Normal aortic valve cusps, thin and translucent. **B.** Sclerotic aortic valve cusps are no longer translucent but have little to no calcification. Hemodynamic stenosis may be present but is usually mild. **C.** Degenerative calcification of the aortic valve will show nodules of calcification involving one or more valve cusps.

either procedure is < 25%.[13] Transcatheter aortic valve implantation is performed with balloon-expandable or self-expandable valves (see Chapter 41).[14]

Degenerative Aortic Stenosis, Bicuspid Aortic Valve

Bicuspid Aortic Valve, General Aspects

Congenitally bicuspid aortic valve is present in about 1% to 2% of the population. There is male predominance of up to 4:1. Familial studies suggest that congenital bicuspid aortic valves follow autosomal dominant inheritance patterns with reduced penetrance. Congenitally bicuspid aortic valves are over 20 times more likely to become stenotic than normally formed aortic valves, and calcify at a younger age.

Although the rate of complications of bicuspid aortic valve is not well documented, it has been stated that the majority of patients will eventually require surgery before reaching old age.[15] Aortic stenosis is the most common complication of bicuspid aortic valve, as 80% of symptomatic patients have pure stenosis, 10% pure insufficiency, and 10% combined stenosis and insufficiency. About one in three patients with bicuspid valves eventually require valve replacement for stenosis, typically in the 6th to 8th decades. The pathologic features are identical to degenerative calcific disease occurring at an older age in patients with normal tricuspid valves. The risk factors are also shared and include smoking and hyperlipidemia.[16]

The rate of bicuspid aortic valve as a proportion of aortic valve replacement has been reported at 27%,[17] 32%,[18] 33%,[19] and 49%.[20] Stenotic bicuspid valves are 2 to 4 times as common as insufficient ones, which often require aortic aneurysm repair or resection. The pathologic features of aortic insufficiency with bicuspid aortic valve are discussed in the following chapter.

Gross Findings

Occasionally, a nondegenerative bicuspid valve will be encountered (Fig. 172.7A). The gross findings of degenerative calcified bicuspid aortic valves are similar to those seen in tricuspid valves, with the heaviest calcification seen at the point of congenital fusion (raphe), when one is present (Fig. 172.7B). Fewer than 25% of congenitally bicuspid aortic valves show equal-sized, symmetric cusps without raphes. A raphe, or abortive commissure in the midpoint of the fused

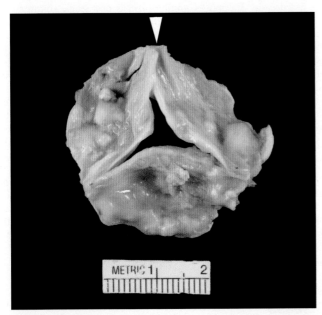

FIGURE 172.5 ▲ Degenerative calcific aortic stenosis, with fusion of one commissure (*arrowhead*). Commissural fusion may occasionally occur and signify the possibility of concurrent postinflammatory valve disease. In contrast to congenitally bicuspid valves, the angle formed by the conjoint cusp is acute.

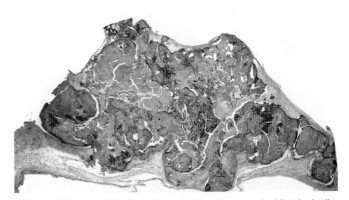

FIGURE 172.6 ▲ Degenerative calcific aortic stenosis. Histologically, there are plates of calcified acellular material intermixed with degenerative fibrin (red). In most cases, inflammation is minimal, as in this one.

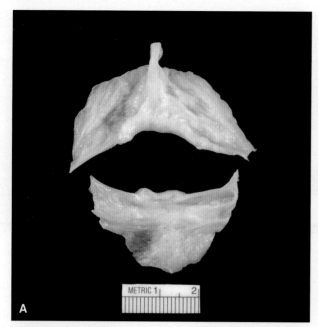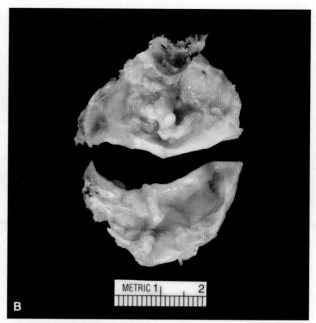

FIGURE 172.7 ▲ Aortic valve findings (bicuspid), surgery. **A.** Early sclerosis of the bicuspid aortic valve without significant calcification manifested, like with that of tricuspid aortic valve disease, with loss of translucency.
B. Degenerative calcification will typically begin around the point of fusion (raphe) and then fill the cusp pockets of both the conjoined and nonconjoined cusps.

cusp, is present in about 75% of bicuspid valves[21] and does not extend to the aortic wall at the level of the sinotubular junction but lower in the sinus. This feature helps the pathologist distinguish from acquired postinflammatory fusion. In those cases, the angle formed by the two cusps, with the vertex at the commissure, is generally <90%, whereas it is >90% in congenitally bicuspid valves (Fig. 172.8).

Fusion occurs of the right and left cusps in more than 80% of the cases, between the right and posterior in about 10% to 12% and the left and posterior in <5%.[22] In the most common form, both main coronaries arise from the sinus of the anterior conjoint cusp.

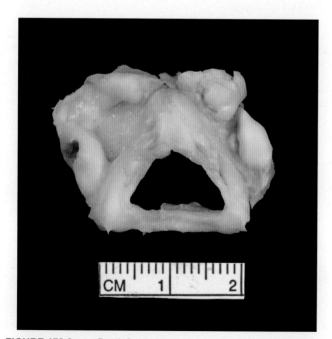

FIGURE 172.8 ▲ Postinflammatory aortic valve disease. With fusion of all three commissures and dense fibrosis. The valve has the appearance of having been dipped in wax.

Calcification is a constant finding in bicuspid aortic valve with clinical stenosis. It begins on the raphe and extends to the cusps, forming nodules on the aortic surface. Secondary left ventricular hypertrophy occurs similar to aortic stenosis from any cause.

Unicommissural (Unicuspid) and Quadricuspid Aortic Valve

Unicommissural aortic valves are heavily calcified with rigid cusps and have a classic "teardrop" shape (Fig. 172.9A). Symptomatic valve disease occurs earlier than with bicuspid valves and typically before the 5th decade. The most common form is of a single commissure, whereas underdeveloped conjoint three commissures with two raphes present and a central orifice can be seen in the minority of cases. Cusp dysplasia is common, and calcification variable. The incidence is low, estimated at 0.02% of patients referred for echocardiography.[23] In series of resected valves, they represent 3% to 5% of resected aortic valves.[18,20] Ascending aortic repair is often required for associated aneurysm.[18]

Clinically, the valves are usually both stenotic and insufficient, due to the lack of coaptation of the cusp. Most patients require repair by age 40 for severe insufficiency. Patients are at risk of developing infective endocarditis and aortic dissection. The risk for aortic dissection is greater than that of bicuspid aortic valves, ~14 times the general population.

Quadricuspid aortic valves are exceedingly rare, with an estimated incidence of <0.03%.[24] They are generally absent in series of resected valves or include one case.[17,19] This condition is not often associated with other congenital heart defects, as is bicuspid aortic valves. Aortic insufficiency is common, as usually there is abnormal cusp coaptation. Only in a very small proportion of cases do the cusps have similar sizes.[25] Grossly, there are four recognizable cusps (Fig. 172.9B).

Miscellaneous Acquired Aortic Valve Disease

Alkaptonuria (endogenous ochronosis) is a rare metabolic disorder caused by a deficiency of homogentisic acid oxidase, an enzyme responsible for the metabolic degradation of tyrosine. Patients with alkaptonuria present with arthritis and pigmentation of the ear

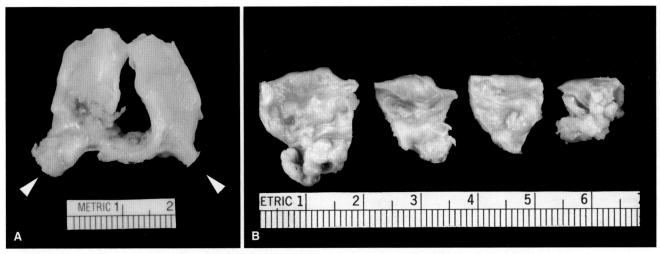

FIGURE 172.9 ▲ Aortic valves with unusual cusp numbers. **A.** Congenitally unicommissural aortic valve with two distinct raphes (*arrowheads*) showing moderate degenerative changes. The singe commissure can be seen at the top. **B.** Congenitally quadricuspid aortic valve with calcific degeneration of each of the four resected cusps.

cartilage and sclera. A small proportion of patients develop cardiac symptoms, primarily valve stenosis. Rarely, aortic valve stenosis is the first symptom.[26] The pathogenesis of cardiovascular ochronosis is unclear but is probably related to the extensive extracellular deposits of ochronotic pigment, homogentisic acid. Accumulation of this pigment can lead to an inflammatory reaction and to progressive valve dysfunction.[27]

Approximately 0.1% of patients with mediastinal radiation develop cardiac complications, usually decades later. Fibrosis with calcification of the aortic valve can lead to stenosis, often in association with coronary ostial stenosis[28] and rarely with diffuse aortic calcification ("porcelain aorta")[29] (Fig. 172.10). Echocardiographically, there is a unique and consistent pattern of thickening of the aortic and mitral valves involving the aortic–mitral curtain.[30] Most reported cases of aortic stenosis after radiation are case reports.[31]

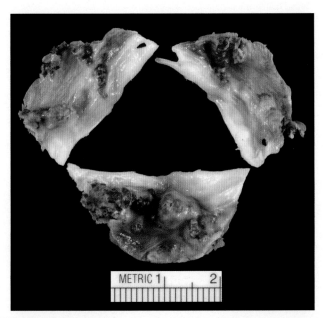

FIGURE 172.10 ▲ Aortic stenosis secondary to ochronosis, autopsy. Note the black pigment on the valve cusps.

Mitral Annular Calcification

Clinical Findings

Mitral annular calcification is seen most commonly in women over 65. It is also encountered in patients with mitral valve prolapse and patients with chronic renal failure and secondary hyperparathyroidism.[32] Its prevalence is 40% in renal transplant patients.[3] It is also not uncommon in elderly men, with an incidence of 37% in patients underlying coronary angiography for suspected coronary artery disease.[2]

Mitral annular calcification is generally asymptomatic, identified as an incidental finding on imaging or at autopsy. It is an uncommon cause of mitral insufficiency, in which case there is frequently mitral valve prolapse.[33] Mitral stenosis is a rare sequela and occurs when there is extension of the calcification onto the leaflets themselves, especially the anterior leaflet.[34,35] Mitral annular calcification has been identified as a risk factor for cardiovascular events and increased mortality in patients with coronary artery disease.[2,3]

Incidental mitral annular calcification is found in over 50% of patients undergoing isolated aortic valve replacements and is associated with end-stage renal disease and tricuspid aortic valves.[36]

Occasionally, mitral annular calcification can cause left atrial calcified masses that are clinically considered to be tumors or abscesses (see Chapter 42). Secondary bacterial infection in the form of endocarditis may also occur.

Gross Pathology Findings

Mitral annular calcification is encountered typically in patients with mitral insufficiency. The posterior "annulus" is involved, as the anterior leaflet does not rest along the atrioventricular groove and does not have an annulus *per se*. In a large surgical series of patients with mitral annular calcification involving at least one-third of the posterior mitral valve annulus and insufficiency necessitating valve replacement, the entire posterior annulus was involved in 10%, the entire anterior leaflet in 1.5%, the myocardium in 12%, leaflet tissue in 6%, and papillary muscle in 4.5%.[33]

At autopsy (or occasionally at surgical resection), there is a calcified mass at the annulus of the posterior leaflet. It may be difficult to identify without palpation, and radiography can be helpful in assessing the extent. Involvement of the anterior leaflet is rare. Mitral annular calcification is present at an increased rate in patients with mitral valve prolapse. Most often, mitral annular calcification is found incidentally at autopsy. In rare occasions, the calcified mass may become cystic or hemorrhagic and clinically mimic a tumor. Central softening of the calcium (so-called caseous degeneration of the mitral annulus) can be

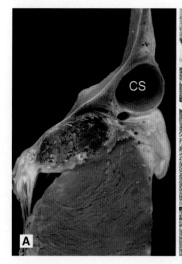
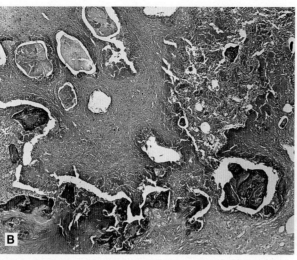

FIGURE 172.11 ▲ Mitral annular calcification. **A.** There is a calcified mass at the annulus, adjacent to the coronary sinus (CS). There is central softening of the annular calcium, which can radiologically mimic an abscess. **B.** Histologically, the material is calcified and may have a giant-cell reaction nearby.

mistaken for an abscess (Fig. 172.11). The calcified rind around such can also fissure, in which case the softened gruel-like substance may be expelled from the interior and embolize, thrombose, or incorporate into the subjacent endocardial surface. Infective endocarditis can complicate mitral annular calcification and can be grossly difficult to identify.[37]

After surgical excision of stenotic valves, in which case the calcification extends onto the leaflet, the annular debris is removed separately, with or without a recognizable valve.

Microscopic Pathologic Findings

Microscopically, there is a fibrocalcific capsule containing calcium that may be degenerated, with variable chronic inflammation.[32] There is diffuse calcification of the contents of the fibrous cavity.

Differential Diagnosis

Clinically, the differential diagnosis includes tumor and abscess; the clinician or surgeon is often skeptical of the pathologic diagnosis of mitral annular calcification. Microscopically, there is little in the differential diagnosis. Abscess is rare and is easily diagnosed by the presence of abundant neutrophils and the presence of microorganisms.

REFERENCES

1. Thaden JJ, Nkomo VT, Enriquez-Sarano M. The global burden of aortic stenosis. *Prog Cardiovasc Dis.* 2014;56:565–571.
2. Willens HJ, Chirinos JA, Schob A, et al. The relation between mitral annular calcification and mortality in patients undergoing diagnostic coronary angiography. *Echocardiography.* 2006;23:717–722.
3. Sharma R, Pellerin D, Gaze DC, et al. Mitral annular calcification predicts mortality and coronary artery disease in end stage renal disease. *Atherosclerosis.* 2007;191:348–354.
4. Tziomalos K, Athyros VG, Karagiannis A, et al. Established and emerging vascular risk factors and the development of aortic stenosis: an opportunity for prevention? *Expert Opin Ther Targets.* 2008;12:809–820.
5. Eveborn GW, Schirmer H, Lunde P, et al. Assessment of risk factors for developing incident aortic stenosis: the Tromso Study. *Eur J Epidemiol.* 2014;29:567–575.
6. Arsenault BJ, Boekholdt SM, Mora S, et al. Impact of high-dose atorvastatin therapy and clinical risk factors on incident aortic valve stenosis in patients with cardiovascular disease (from TNT, IDEAL, and SPARCL). *Am J Cardiol.* 2014;113:1378–1382.
7. Miura S, Arita T, Kumamaru H, et al. Causes of death and mortality and evaluation of prognostic factors in patients with severe aortic stenosis in an aging society. *J Cardiol.* 2015;65:353–359.
8. Chitsaz S, Gundiah N, Blackshear C, et al. Correlation of calcification on excised aortic valves by micro-computed tomography with severity of aortic stenosis. *J Heart Valve Dis.* 2012;21:320–327.
9. Mohler ER III, Gannon F, Reynolds C, et al. Bone formation and inflammation in cardiac valves. *Circulation.* 2001;103:1522–1528.
10. Veinot JP. Pathology of inflammatory native valvular heart disease. *Cardiovasc Pathol.* 2006;15:243–251.
11. Milano AD, Faggian G, Dodonov M, et al. Prognostic value of myocardial fibrosis in patients with severe aortic valve stenosis. *J Thorac Cardiovasc Surg.* 2012;144:830–837.
12. Kuwaki K, Inaba H, Yamamoto T, et al. Performance of the EuroSCORE II and the Society of Thoracic Surgeons Score in patients undergoing aortic valve replacement for aortic stenosis. *J Cardiovasc Surg (Torino).* 2015;56:455–462.
13. Kapadia SR, Leon MB, Makkar RR, et al. 5-year outcomes of transcatheter aortic valve replacement compared with standard treatment for patients with inoperable aortic stenosis (PARTNER 1): a randomised controlled trial. *Lancet.* 2015;385:2485–2491.
14. Covolo E, Saia F, Napodano M, et al. Comparison of balloon-expandable versus self-expandable valves for transcatheter aortic valve implantation in patients with low-gradient severe aortic stenosis and preserved left ventricular ejection fraction. *Am J Cardiol.* 2015;115:810–815.
15. Fedak PW, Verma S, David TE, et al. Clinical and pathophysiological implications of a bicuspid aortic valve. *Circulation.* 2002;106:900–904.
16. Chan KL, Ghani M, Woodend K, et al. Case-controlled study to assess risk factors for aortic stenosis in congenitally bicuspid aortic valve. *Am J Cardiol.* 2001;88:690–693.
17. Butany J, Collins MJ, Demellawy DE, et al. Morphological and clinical findings in 247 surgically excised native aortic valves. *Can J Cardiol.* 2005;21:747–755.
18. Collins MJ, Butany J, Borger MA, et al. Implications of a congenitally abnormal valve: a study of 1025 consecutively excised aortic valves. *J Clin Pathol.* 2008;61:530–536.
19. Burke AP. Cardiovascular pathology. In Silverberg SG, et al., eds. *Silverberg's Principles and Practice of Surgical Pathology and Cytopathology.* New York: Cambridge University Press; 2015.
20. Roberts WC, Ko JM. Frequency by decades of unicuspid, bicuspid, and tricuspid aortic valves in adults having isolated aortic valve replacement for aortic stenosis, with or without associated aortic regurgitation. *Circulation.* 2005;111:920–925.
21. Subramanian R, Olson LJ, Edwards WD. Surgical pathology of pure aortic stenosis: a study of 374 cases. *Mayo Clin Proc.* 1984;59:683–690.
22. Sabet HY, Edwards WD, Tazelaar HD, et al. Congenitally bicuspid aortic valves: a surgical pathology study of 542 cases (1991 through 1996) and a literature review of 2,715 additional cases. *Mayo Clin Proc.* 1999;74:14–26.
23. Novaro GM, Mishra M, Griffin BP. Incidence and echocardiographic features of congenital unicuspid aortic valve in an adult population. *J Heart Valve Dis.* 2003;12:674–678.
24. Feldman BJ, Khandheria BK, Warnes CA, et al. Incidence, description and functional assessment of isolated quadricuspid aortic valves. *Am J Cardiol.* 1990;65:937–938.
25. Hurwitz LE, Roberts WC. Quadricuspid semilunar valve. *Am J Cardiol.* 1973;31:623–626.
26. Folkes LV, Brull D, Krywawych S, et al. Aortic stenosis in cardiovascular ochronosis. *J Clin Pathol.* 2007;60:92–93.
27. Butany JW, Naseemuddin A, Moshkowitz Y, et al. Ochronosis and aortic valve stenosis. *J Card Surg.* 2006;21:182–184.

28. Chenu PC, Schroeder E, Buche M, et al. Bilateral coronary ostial stenosis and aortic valvular disease after radiotherapy. *Eur Heart J.* 1994;15:1150–1151.

29. Daitoku K, Fukui K, Ichinoseki I, et al. Radiotherapy-induced aortic valve disease associated with porcelain aorta. *Jpn J Thorac Cardiovasc Surg.* 2004;52:349–352.

30. Brand MD, Abadi CA, Aurigemma GP, et al. Radiation-associated valvular heart disease in Hodgkin's disease is associated with characteristic thickening and fibrosis of the aortic-mitral curtain. *J Heart Valve Dis.* 2001;10:681–685.

31. Adabag AS, Dykoski R, Ward H, et al. Critical stenosis of aortic and mitral valves after mediastinal irradiation. *Catheter Cardiovasc Interv.* 2004;63:247–250.

32. Kato M, Nakatani S, Okazaki H, et al. Unusual appearance of mitral annular calcification mimicking intracardiac tumor prompting early surgery. *Cardiology.* 2006;106:164–166.

33. Carpentier AF, Pellerin M, Fuzellier JF, et al. Extensive calcification of the mitral valve anulus: pathology and surgical management. *J Thorac Cardiovasc Surg.* 1996;111:718–729; discussion 729–730.

34. Muddassir SM, Pressman GS. Mitral annular calcification as a cause of mitral valve gradients. *Int J Cardiol.* 2007;123:58–62.

35. Akpinar I, Karabag T, Sayin MR, et al. Large caseous mitral annular calcification with mitral stenosis, dynamic left ventricular outflow obstruction, and syncope. *Tex Heart Inst J.* 2012;39:910–912.

36. Takami Y, Tajima K. Mitral annular calcification in patients undergoing aortic valve replacement for aortic valve stenosis. *Heart Vessels.* 2016;31(2):183–188.

37. Nishida J, Maeda T, Yuda S, et al. Massive cerebral embolism originated from ruptured infective mitral annular calcification in a chronic hemodialysis patient. *Echocardiography.* 2009;26:107–108.

173 Aortic Insufficiency

Allen P. Burke, M.D., and Fabio R. Tavora, M.D., Ph.D.

Etiology

In the previous century, aortic insufficiency was most commonly secondary to postinflammatory (rheumatic) valve disease. Postinflammatory fibrosis causes retracted and incompetent leaflets that are stiff and scarred, resulting in a component of stenosis. Pure aortic insufficiency is caused by infectious endocarditis with perforation of a leaflet (Chapter 177), dilated aortic root with lack of coaptation of the leaflets during diastole, and prolapse of one or more leaflets, often with myxoid or "floppy" change. Bicuspid valve can lead to isolated prolapse, is associated with aortic aneurysms, and is therefore overrepresented in not only aortic stenosis but also aortic insufficiency.

The 4 anatomic causes of aortic incompetence are therefore cusp retraction (chronic rheumatic disease), cusp perforation (endocarditis or trauma), cusp prolapse (myxomatous valve), and lack of coaptation or "diastasis" (dilated aortic root) (Table 173.1).

In a classic series of valve resections reported in 1984, the most common causes of aortic regurgitation were postinflammatory disease (46%), aortic root dilatation with or without bicuspid valve (21%), incomplete closure of a congenitally bicuspid aortic valve with normal aortic root (20%), infective endocarditis (9%), and other (4%).[1]

Since the 1980s, the prevalence of rheumatic valve disease has decreased, and the incidence of aortic aneurysm has increased. A more recent study of 107 purely insufficient resected valves the causes to be ascending aortic aneurysm with trileaflet valve (34%), aortic prolapse of trileaflet valve without aortic aneurysm (31%), aortic aneurysm with bicuspid valve (19%), bicuspid valve with prolapse and normal aortic root (12%), and postinflammatory aortic insufficiency (5%)[2] (see Chapter 35). The types of aneurysms were most commonly due to medial degeneration, followed by dissection, aortitis, and sinus of Valsalva aneurysm.

Gross Findings, Heart

Aortic insufficiency results in volume overload and cardiomegaly with left ventricular dilatation and concentric hypertrophy (see Chapter 143) (Fig. 173.1).

TABLE 173.1 Causes of Aortic Insufficiency

Mechanism	Most Common Etiology	Other Causes/Associations
Lack of coaptation	Noninflammatory aortic root dilatation	Bicuspid aortic valve Aortitis Sinus of Valsalva aneurysm
Cusp retraction due to fibrosis	Postinflammatory/rheumatic	Bicuspid aortic valve with degenerative changes but not severe to cause primary stenosis[a] Postendocarditis fibrosis Valvulitis (syphilitic, autoimmune) Degenerative calcification (rare as isolated insufficiency)
Prolapse	Myxomatous degeneration	Connective tissue disorders
Cusp perforation	Infective endocarditis	Trauma

[a]Often, there is associated aneurysm, an example of multifactorial cause for insufficiency.

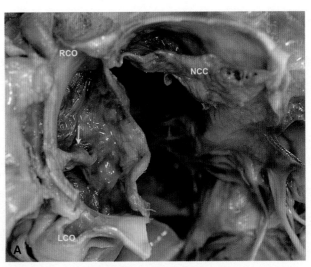

FIGURE 173.1 ▲ Aortic insufficiency with left ventricular dilatation, autopsy heart. **A.** The valve is opened with a cut at the commissure between the noncoronary and left side of the conjoint cusp and viewed from above. The arrow points to the raphe. RCO, right coronary ostium; NCC, noncoronary cusp; LCO, left coronary ostium. The deceased died suddenly and unexpectedly after refusing medical care for cough and shortness of breath.

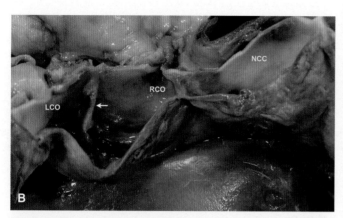

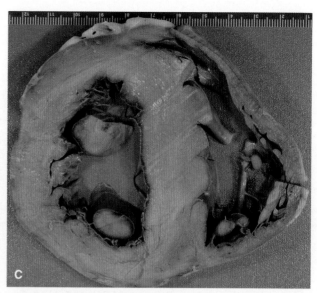

FIGURE 173.1 (*Continued*) ▲ **B.** Viewed from the side is the raphe. **C.** A short-axis section through the heart shows marked left ventricular dilatation.

Aortic Insufficiency with Bicuspid Aortic Valve

Patients with bicuspid aortic valves develop valvular insufficiency at lower rate than that of stenosis, by about a factor of five.[2,3] The mean age at valve surgery is in the early 50s for insufficiency, which is about 10 years younger than the typical age for severely symptomatic bicuspid aortic valve stenosis.[2,4] Men are affected 7 to 17 times frequently than women, a higher differential than bicuspid aortic stenosis.[2,3]

Aortic insufficiency in this group of patients is caused by cusp prolapse or restriction (retraction) or the aortic root dilatation. Retraction is caused by degenerative fibrosis, which leads more commonly to calcified (stenotic) valves, although there can be an overlap in pathologic findings. Approximately 43% of patients with insufficient bicuspid aortic valves have isolated valve disease, the remainder with ascending aneurysms.[5]

Treatment involves raphe repair, aortic annuloplasty, ascending aortic replacement with a tube graft, and aortic root and valve replacement.[5] In cases of valve replacements, the pathologist will receive a valve and perhaps ascending aorta. In valve-sparing operations, a specimen is sent to the surgical pathology laboratory only if there is ascending aneurysm repair. In some patients, aortic valve insufficiency will resolve with aneurysm repair, with or without repair of the aortic sinuses, and the valve is not removed.

Pathologically, the valves may be clear and translucent, especially if there is no aneurysm and there is isolated prolapse (Figs. 173.2 to 173.7). There may be variable fibrosis and mild calcification, which corresponds to an increased likelihood of mixed insufficiency and stenosis. There may or may not be a raphe. Histologic evaluation is not generally rewarding but should be done in all cases to exclude the

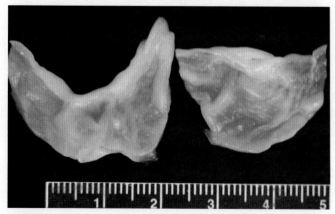

FIGURE 173.2 ▲ Bicuspid valve, resection for insufficiency. The conjoint leaflet **(left)** shows an area of thickening at the raphe. There is fibrosis of the conjoint cusp primarily at the raphe and the free edge. The pathogenesis of insufficiency with bicuspid valve can involve several mechanisms, including fibrous retraction, prolapse, and dilatation of the aortic root. In this case, the aorta was normal.

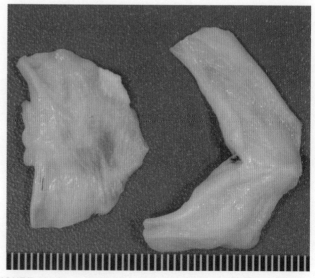

FIGURE 173.3 ▲ Bicuspid valve, resection for insufficiency. The conjoint cusp with a raphe is seen at the right. There is mild myxoid degeneration. The aorta was normal, and the insufficiency was the result of cuspal retraction at the site of the raphe and prolapse.

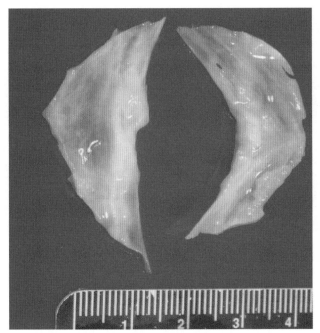

FIGURE 173.4 ▲ Bicuspid valve, resection for insufficiency. The valve is thin, and translucent, with a raphe indicating the cusp on the right is conjoint. The mechanism of insufficiency was aortic root dilatation, which necessitated aortic aneurysm repair. The leaflets tend to be wider with aortic root dilatation (compare Figs. 173.2 to 173.3).

possibility of superimposed endocarditis. Generally, the diagnosis of endocarditis is known clinically, although it is important after treatment to describe the absence of acute inflammation, in which case there will be only minimal chronic inflammation, fibroblast reaction, or surface fibrin (Chapter 40).

Aortic Insufficiency with Tricuspid/Trileaflet Aortic Valve

The most common cause of pure aortic insufficiency is ascending aortic aneurysms, especially when they involve the aortic root. In a series

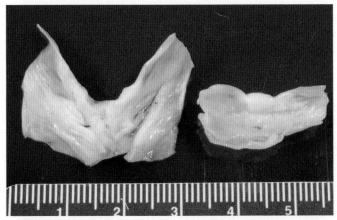

FIGURE 173.5 ▲ Bicuspid valve, resection for insufficiency. In this case, there is significant fibrosis resulting in retraction of the conjoint cusp on the left. In addition, there was marked aortic dilatation resulting in aneurysm repair and partial ascending aortic resection.

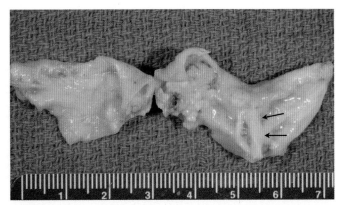

FIGURE 173.6 ▲ Bicuspid valve, resection for insufficiency. In this case, there are also features of degenerative calcific aortic valve disease. The valve was primarily insufficient, however, due to marked aortic root dilatation that resulted in aortic resection. *Arrows* indicate the raphe of the conjoint cusp.

from 1990s, 59% of pure aortic insufficiency was associated with a dilated aorta and trileaflet valves. The proportion of valve resections with nonaneurysmal aorta is higher in insufficient trileaflet than bicuspid valves, however.[6]

Although classically the aortic root is dilated in syphilis, Marfan syndrome, and bicuspid valve syndrome, aortic root dilatation is also not uncommon in isolated ascending aortic aneurysms. The treatment is similar to that of bicuspid aortic insufficiency and involves repair of the aneurysm with resection of a sleeve of aorta, with or without valve replacement and aortic root repair.

The gross findings are those of thin, translucent leaflets that may be elongated or show rolling of the free edges. An aortic specimen often accompanies the valve (Fig. 173.8).

Aortic Insufficiency Without Ascending Aortic Aneurysm (Myxomatous Aortic Valves)

Insufficient trileaflet aortic valves can occur with normal aortas in the absence of perforation or postrheumatic cusp retraction. The proportion of insufficient valves caused by "floppy" or "myxomatous" aortic valves varies widely by report. In one series, isolated myxomatous valves represented nearly 20% of cases of pure aortic regurgitation.[6]

Myxomatous change in aortic valves has been described as thinned, translucent cusps and thickened, gelatinous cusps, with thickening of the free edges.[7] Histologically, there is an increase in proteoglycans in the spongiosa with irregular collagen fibers.[7] Because these findings are similar to valves resected for insufficiency secondary to aortic root dilatation, the diagnosis of isolated aortic prolapse can only be done with knowledge of a normal ascending aorta (Fig. 173.9). If the intraoperative transesophageal echocardiogram or surgical note confirms an absence of aortic root disease, then an insufficient trileaflet valve is presumed to be myxomatous, unless there is postinflammatory valve retraction with scarring.

Myxomatous aortic valve has been associated with ventricular septal defect, Marfan syndrome, Ehlers-Danlos syndrome, and ventricular septal defect. The mean age at presentation is in the late 50s, and men are 2.5 times more likely to be affected.[7]

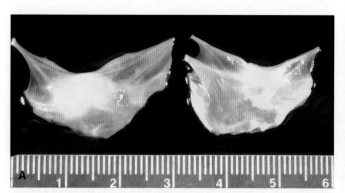

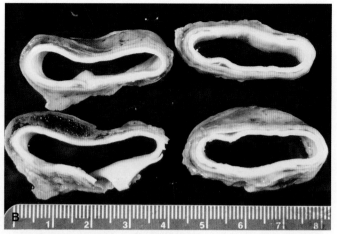

FIGURE 173.7 ▲ Bicuspid valve, resection during aortic dissection repair. The patient underwent operation for emergent repair of ascending dissection. **A.** The valve is bicuspid and translucent. **B.** Cross sections of aorta show hematoma between the media and adventitia. In some cases, the valve remains insufficient after repair of the aorta and replacement is necessary.

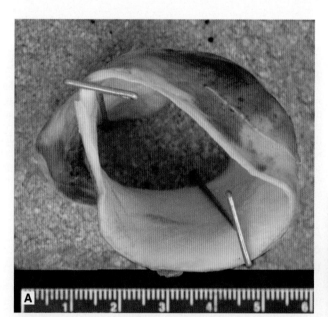

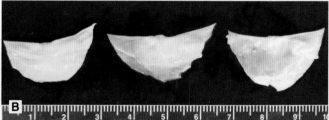

FIGURE 173.8 ▲ Trileaflet aortic insufficiency with ascending aortic aneurysm. **A.** The aneurysm was several centimeters in diameter. **B.** The valve shows mild fibrosis and the leaflet somewhat elongated.

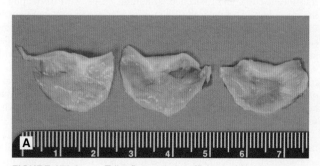

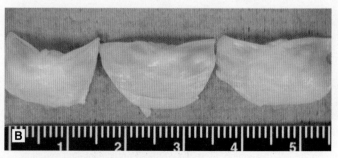

FIGURE 173.9 ▲ Trileaflet aortic insufficiency with normal ascending aorta diameter (myxomatous aortic valve disease). **A.** The valves are thin and translucent. **B.** In this case, there is mild thickening. Without knowledge of the imaging, it is impossible to distinguish isolated aortic prolapse from insufficiency secondary to dilated aortic root.

REFERENCES

1. Olson LJ, Subramanian R, Edwards WD. Surgical pathology of pure aortic insufficiency: a study of 225 cases. *Mayo Clin Proc.* 1984;59:8935–8941.
2. Burke AP. The cardiovascular system. In Silverberg, SG, et al., eds. *Silverberg's Principles and Practice of Surgical Pathology and Cytopathology.* Cambridge: Cambridge University Press; 2015.
3. Sabet HY, Edwards WD, Tazelaar HD, et al. Congenitally bicuspid aortic valves: a surgical pathology study of 542 cases (1991 through 1996) and a literature review of 2,715 additional cases. *Mayo Clin Proc.* 1999; 74:14–26.
4. Collins MJ, Butany J, Borger MA, et al. Implications of a congenitally abnormal valve: a study of 1025 consecutively excised aortic valves. *J Clin Pathol.* 2008;61:530–536.
5. Boodhwani M, de Kerchove L, Glineur D, et al. Repair of regurgitant bicuspid aortic valves: a systematic approach. *J Thorac Cardiovasc Surg.* 2010;140:276–284 e1.
6. Agozzino L, de Vivo F, Falco A, et al. Surgical pathology of the aortic valve: gross and histological findings in 1120 excised valves. *Cardiovasc Pathol.* 1994;3:155–161.
7. Tamura K, I-Ida T, Fujii T, et al. Floppy aortic valves without aortic root dilatation: clinical, histologic, and ultrastructural studies. *J Nippon Med Sch.* 2002;69:355–364.

174 Chronic Rheumatic and Autoimmune Valve Disease

Allen P. Burke, M.D.

Introduction

Postrheumatic or postinflammatory valve disease refers to scarring of the valve that occurs secondary to an autoimmune reaction following infection with group A streptococci. Acute valve disease occurs with the pancarditis of acute rheumatic fever and is associated with small sterile vegetations on the lines of closure of the mitral valve (see Chapter 147). The risks of the long-term development of chronic valve disease, which involves primarily the mitral and aortic valves, are discussed in Chapter 147.

Autoimmune valve disease also includes Libman-Sacks endocarditis with thrombotic vegetations associated with lupus erythematosus, as well as thrombotic endocarditis associated with antiphospholipid syndrome (Chapter 177). Chronic autoimmune valvulitis in autoimmune syndromes occurs most often in ankylosing spondylitis.

Chronic Rheumatic Mitral Valve Disease

Mitral Stenosis

There is a 20- to 40-year typical latent period between infection and initiation of symptoms, which are indolent for 10 years and then accelerate (see Chapter 147). The mean age at valve replacement has become later in developed countries. Most patients, who are more likely women than men, are over 60 at the time of valve repair or replacement.[1]

Medical treatment of postinflammatory mitral stenosis involves treatment of atrial fibrillation, endocarditis prophylaxis, and anticoagulation. Surgical treatment includes balloon valvuloplasty, if echocardiography demonstrates an absence of thrombus and significant regurgitation and shows favorable morphology. If there is marked distortion due to fibrosis and calcification, then open valve replacement is performed. The echocardiographic evaluation includes a score grading mobility, valve thickness, subvalvular thickening, and calcification; the score affects the decision between closed transcutaneous balloon procedure and open commissurotomy with possible valve replacement.

Mitral Insufficiency

Approximately one-fifth of patients with postinflammatory mitral valve disease have pure insufficiency; in all, 46% of patients have stenosis with insufficiency, and 34% pure stenosis.[1] Mitral insufficiency is more likely caused by floppy mitral valve, and ischemia and endocarditis are other important causes (see Chapter 176).[2]

Gross Pathologic Findings

At autopsy, findings involve the valve itself and secondary effects of mitral stenosis or insufficiency on the atria and ventricles. The valve is usually white and scarred, with fibrosis at the two commissures, leaflets, as well as chordae (Figs. 174.1 and 174.2). The chords are thickened and fused. The chordae are normal in a minority of patients, but generally showing fusion and thickening.[3] Lastly, the papillary muscles can also show scarring. Functionally, leaflet thickening and calcification, commissural fusion, chordal fusion, and the funnel-shaped orifice narrow the valve orifice. The valve ostium has a "fish-mouth" appearance when viewed from the atrial aspect, because of the thickened chordae and stenotic valve orifice (Fig. 174.2).

Secondary cardiac changes result in atrial dilatation, which may be massive and may be associated with mural thrombi. A characteristic, but nonspecific finding in the atrium is an area of endocardial fibrosis secondary to regurgitant jet stream called the "MacCallum plaque."[4] With long-standing disease, pulmonary hypertensive changes result in right ventricular hypertrophy and dilatation with tricuspid regurgitation[5] (Figs. 174.3 and 174.4).

The surgical specimen is typically a valve replacement showing an intact valve with two intact leaflets (Fig. 174.5). Valve replacements are the preferred procedure, as most patients are not candidates for percutaneous valvotomy or surgical commissurotomy. The entire valve is excised because marked scarring prevents valve repair. Up to 69% of mitral valve replacements for postinflammatory disease have a

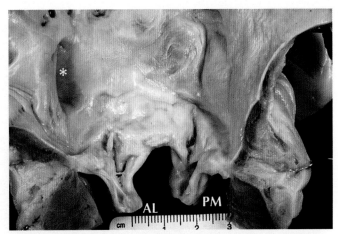

FIGURE 174.1 ▲ Postrheumatic mitral stenosis. There is marked chordal thickening and fusion. The endocardium of the left atrium is thickened and dense white from fibrosis. The orifice of the left atrial appendage is above left (*asterisk*). The anterolateral (AL) and posteromedial (PM) papillary muscles have thick, scarred chordae.

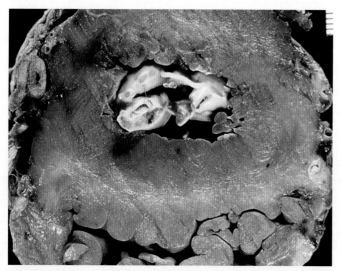

FIGURE 174.2 ▲ Postrheumatic mitral stenosis. A short-axis section demonstrates the papillary muscles are thickened and fibrotic near the chordal insertions and are white with scarring. The right ventricular trabeculae (shown partially at the bottom) are hypertrophic, due to pulmonary hypertension secondary to mitral stenosis. The term "fishmouth" applied to the mitral orifice derives from a catfish-like appearance when viewed from the apex.

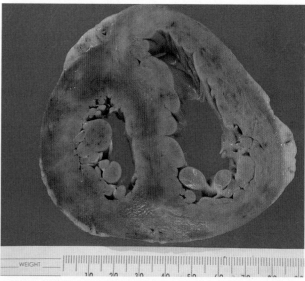

FIGURE 174.3 ▲ Postrheumatic mitral stenosis, with secondary right ventricular hypertrophy and dilatation. Long-standing mitral stenosis results in chronic pulmonary hypertension. As a result, the right ventricle is markedly thickened from pulmonary hypertensive changes. There was, in addition, right ventricular dilatation.

concomitant aortic valve replacement, a common association of valve disease in rheumatic fever.[1,6,7]

The gross appearance of the excised valve reveals thickened chordae and thickening of the valve leaflets (Fig. 174.5 and 174.6), in contrast to mitral valve prolapse. A fibrotic ridge is usually seen on the atrial surface at the line of closure.[5] Calcification is common, usually at the ventricular aspects of the leaflets, giving rise to a rigid conical structure. Fracture and calcified foci with secondary deposits can be observed in some cases.[7] Rheumatic valve disease predisposes to infectious endocarditis, which may be the cause for valve replacement (Fig. 174.7).

The morphology of postinflammatory mitral stenosis is distinct from postinflammatory regurgitation in the extent of calcification and fibrosis. In pure regurgitation, the leaflets are thickened, but commissural fusion is rarely seen. The fibrous thickening is less severe, and

calcification is not commonly found.[6] However, on gross examination, it is difficult to assess preoperative valve function, and it is helpful to refer to operative data and prior echocardiograms.

Complications

Elevated left atrial pressure caused by the stenotic mitral valve is transmitted to the pulmonary veins and pulmonary capillaries. To compensate, pulmonary vasoconstriction develops, causing pulmonary hypertension and right ventricular dilatation and hypertrophy. Increased pressure and distension of the pulmonary veins and capillaries also lead to pulmonary edema and congestion. Over time, chronic pulmonary arterial hypertension may develop and result in medial hypertrophy and intimal thickening of the pulmonary arteries (see Section 1, Chapter 67).

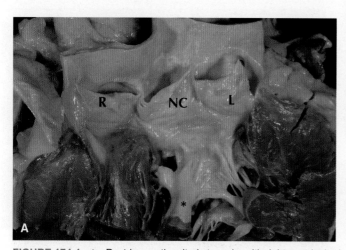

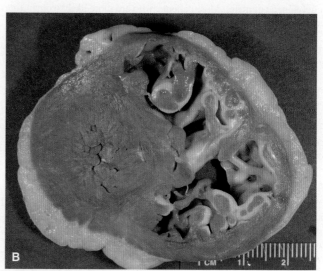

FIGURE 174.4 ▲ Postrheumatic mitral stenosis, with right ventricular hypertrophy. **A.** There is discrete endocardial fibrosis of the anterolateral papillary muscle (*asterisk*). The chords to the posteromedial papillary muscle are also thick. The aortic valve is relatively spared (L, left; NC noncoronary; R, right coronary cusps). There is a small fenestration of the noncoronary cusp. **B.** A short-axis section shows marked right ventricular dilatation and endocardial fibrosis. There is thickening of the right ventricular wall, up to 7 mm.

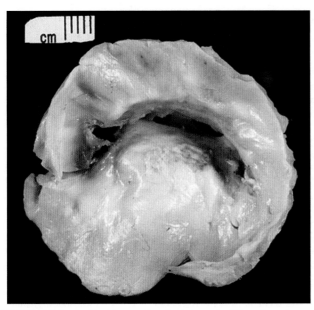

FIGURE 174.5 ▲ Postrheumatic mitral stenosis. When there is marked fibrosis and commissural fusion, the valve may be excised in total. The anterior leaflet is below.

Atrial fibrillation is a common late manifestation of mitral stenosis with atrial enlargement. Endocarditis, both sterile (marantic) and infectious, is increased in incidence in stenotic mitral valves (Fig. 174.8). The increased risk for endocarditis forms the basis for antibiotic prophylaxis during dental and other procedures for patients with rheumatic valve disease (see Chapter 177).

Microscopic Pathologic Findings

The histologic findings of postinflammatory mitral valve are nonspecific. In the majority of valves, there are fibrosis, neovascularization, and chronic inflammation, which is often mild. There is thickening of

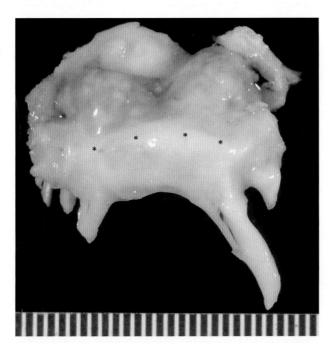

FIGURE 174.6 ▲ Postrheumatic mitral stenosis, surgical excision. There is marked fibrosis of the leaflet with thickening and thick chordae tendineae. There are nodules of calcification and a prominent ridge at the line of closure (*asterisks*).

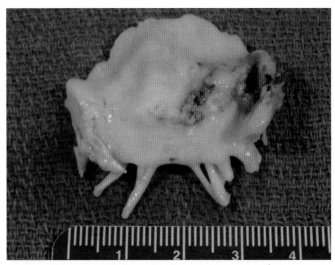

FIGURE 174.7 ▲ Postrheumatic mitral stenosis, superimposed endocarditis. There is an irregular surface with an irregular hemorrhagic surface and focal perforation (**right**).

overall leaflet tissue by collagen deposition, and there are foci of calcification and fibrosis. The layers are indistinct. In contrast, myxoid valve disease lacks inflammation and neovascularization.

Postinflammatory Aortic Valve Disease

Postinflammatory aortic valve disease is virtually always associated with mitral disease. The surgical pathologist usually encounters a mitral valve specimen in addition to the aortic valve, unless the mitral valve was repaired without excision.

There is a slight male predominance, with a mean age at surgery between 60 and 70 years.

About 40% of symptomatic postinflammatory aortic valves are both stenotic and insufficient; 35% are purely stenotic and 25% are purely insufficient.[5,8,9] Postinflammatory aortic stenosis may affect congenitally bicuspid valves as well as trileaflet valves.

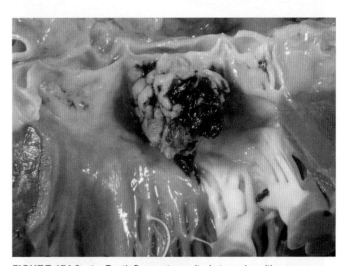

FIGURE 174.8 ▲ Postinflammatory mitral stenosis, with superimposed endocarditis. The chordae of the mitral valve are markedly thickened typical of rheumatic valve disease. The aortic valve has a large vegetation on the noncoronary cusp. The large size of the vegetation is indicative of an infection as opposed to thrombotic (marantic) endocarditis.

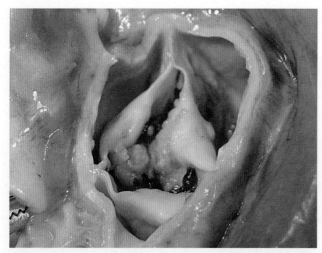

FIGURE 174.9 ▲ Postrheumatic aortic valve disease, autopsy heart. The valve leaflets are thickened and fibrotic, with commissural fusion. There are vegetations on the valve leaflets, which were seen when the valve was opened (previous figure).

Gross Pathology

There is diffuse fibrosis of the valve cusps, resulting in shortening that results almost invariably in a component of aortic insufficiency as well as stenosis, by preventing leaflet coaptation (Fig. 174.9). Calcification can be present, but nodules do not typically form at the base, as in degenerative calcification. When present, calcification may occur in the fused commissures and extend to the cusps (Fig. 174.10). Commissures are often fused, in contrast to nodular degenerative calcific aortic stenosis. If commissural fusion is present, the valve was likely mixed stenotic and insufficient. If only one commissure is fused, there may be confusion with congenital bicuspid aortic valve disease (see Chapter 172).

Histologic Findings

There is neovascularization, chronic inflammation rich in T cells, and fibrosis, similar to postinflammatory mitral stenosis.

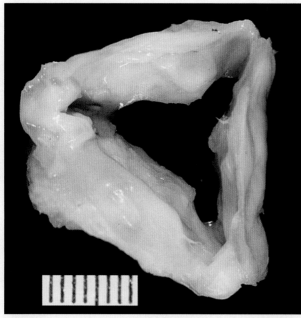

FIGURE 174.10 ▲ Aortic stenosis and insufficiency, secondary to postinflammatory (postrheumatic) valve disease. Note, in contrast to degenerative aortic stenosis, that there is thickening of the free edges and commissures, without nodules of calcium at the base.

Ankylosing Spondylitis and HLA-B27–Related Aortic Insufficiency

Background

Several seronegative spondyloarthropathies, such as Reiter syndrome and psoriatic arthritis, can affect the heart, but the most common is ankylosing spondylitis. Given the association of these entities with HLA-B27 antigens, HLA-B27–associated heart disease is also a generically used term.[10] The most common site affected by this disease is the ascending aorta, which can progress proximally and involve the aortic root and aortic cusps, causing clinically aortic insufficiency.[11] The incidence of aortic regurgitation in ankylosing spondylitis ranges from 10% to 50% of affected patients and increases with age, disease duration, and presence of peripheral arthritis.[11]

Pathologic Findings

With chronic involvement of the aortic valve by HLA-B27 disease, the valve cusps are thickened and markedly fibrotic, which cause regurgitation. In addition, there is inward rolling of valve cusp free edges that can be seen grossly. A subaortic fibrous ridge can be caused by extension of the inflammatory process downward. Aortic root dilatation can be severe in cases of Reiter disease and produce severe insufficiency. Histologic findings are nonspecific and include chronic inflammation and fibrosis.

Miscellaneous Autoimmune Valvulitis

The association between systemic lupus erythematosus and valvular disease goes beyond the presence of marantic (thrombotic) vegetations (Chapter 147). Although there are few histologic reports, the pathogenesis of valvular thickening is thought to be due to immune complex and complement deposition onto the valves and the infiltration of inflammatory cells around and into valve leaflets. Furthermore, there may also be acute infiltrates with hematoxylin bodies (neutrophils with intracytoplasmic inclusions).[12]

Lupus-associated valvulitis is usually asymptomatic, although in some cases, valve replacement is necessary.[13] In endocarditis related to antiphospholipid syndrome–related endocarditis, the lesions are typically on the atrial side of the mitral valve and do not show acute valve inflammation or hematoxylin bodies as classically described in Libman-Sacks endocarditis.[14]

Drug-induced lupus has been associated with valvulitis, although there are few reports of histologic descriptions, blurring the distinction between marantic thrombotic lesions and leaflet inflammation.[15]

Valvular disease is relatively common in rheumatoid arthritis but is rarely symptomatic (Chapter 147). Histologic features of rheumatoid valvulitis are nonspecific (Fig. 174.11).

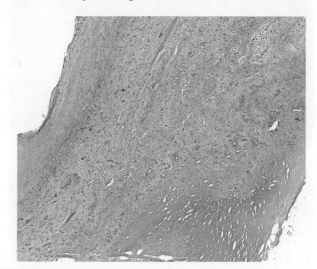

FIGURE 174.11 ▲ Autoimmune valvulitis. The aortic valve leaflet is diffusely scarred with chronic inflammation and neovascularity. The patient had aortic stenosis and mixed rheumatologic syndrome (lupus erythematosus and rheumatoid arthritis).

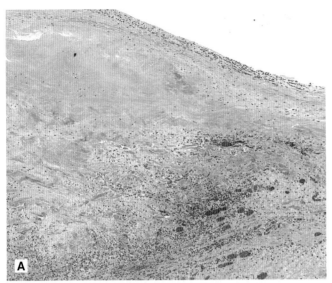
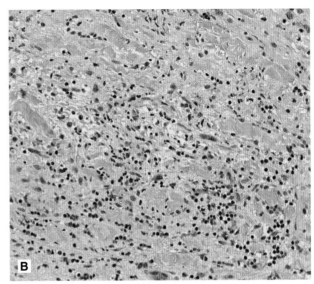

FIGURE 174.12 ▲ Autoimmune valvulitis. **A.** There is chronic inflammation of the valve leaflet. **B.** Higher magnification shows a mixed mononuclear cell infiltrate. The histologic features are nonspecific and overlap with healed infectious endocarditis. In this case, the patient had an ankylosing spondylitis associated with aortitis.

Autoimmune valvulitis resulting in sterile inflammatory vegetations has been described in granulomatosis with polyangiitis (Wegener granulomatosis).[16–18] Histologically, these valves, which may cause insufficiency and heart failure, demonstrate acute inflammation, and lymphohistiocytic infiltrates, sometimes with palisading. Complicating the distinction between infectious and autoimmune valvulitis is the fact that ANCA may be secondarily elevated in infections, including infectious endocarditis. However, reactive ANCA in patients with infected valves is typically of the cytoplasmic type, whereas the perinuclear type is associated with perinuclear myeloperoxidase ANCA.

Autoimmune valvulitis has been associated with isolated aortitis, especially with ankylosing spondylitis, Behçet disease, and Takayasu disease[19–22] (Fig. 174.12).

REFERENCES

1. Dare AJ, Harrity PJ, Tazelaar HD, et al. Evaluation of surgically excised mitral valves: revised recommendations based on changing operative procedures in the 1990s. *Hum Pathol.* 1993;24:1286–1293.
2. Olson LJ, Subramanian R, Ackermann DM, et al. Surgical pathology of the mitral valve: a study of 712 cases spanning 21 years. *Mayo Clin Proc.* 1987;62:22–34.
3. van der Bel-Kahn J, Becker AE. The surgical pathology of rheumatic and floppy mitral valves. Distinctive morphologic features upon gross examination. *Am J Surg Pathol.* 1986;10:282–292.
4. Lu TM, Yeh YC, Lu YW, et al. MacCallum plaque causes acute myocardial infarction in a young man. *Circulation.* 2015;131:1121–1122.
5. Veinot JP. Pathology of inflammatory native valvular heart disease. *Cardiovasc Pathol.* 2006;15:243–251.
6. Cheunsuchon P, Chuangsuwanich T, Samanthai N, et al. Surgical pathology and etiology of 278 surgically removed mitral valves with pure regurgitation in Thailand. *Cardiovasc Pathol.* 2007;16:104–110.
7. Hanson TP, Edwards BS, Edwards JE. Pathology of surgically excised mitral valves. One hundred consecutive cases. *Arch Pathol Lab Med.* 1985;109:823–828.
8. Subramanian R, Olson LJ, Edwards WD. Surgical pathology of pure aortic stenosis: a study of 374 cases. *Mayo Clin Proc.* 1984;59:683–690.
9. Subramanian R, Olson LJ, Edwards WD. Surgical pathology of combined aortic stenosis and insufficiency: a study of 213 cases. *Mayo Clin Proc.* 1985;60:247–254.
10. Bergfeldt L. HLA-B27-associated cardiac disease. *Ann Intern Med.* 1997;127: 621–629.
11. Klingberg E, Svealv BG, Tang MS, et al. Aortic regurgitation is common in ankylosing spondylitis: time for routine echocardiography evaluation? *Am J Med.* 2015;128(11):1244–1250.e1.
12. Godman GC, Deitch AD, Klemperer P. The composition of the LE and hematoxylin bodies of systemic lupus erythematosus. *Am J Pathol.* 1958;34: 1–23.
13. Einav E, Gitig A, Marinescu LM, et al. Valvulitis requiring triple valve surgery as an initial presentation of systemic lupus erythematosus. *J Am Soc Echocardiogr.* 2007;20:1315 e1–e3.
14. Eiken PW, Edwards WD, Tazelaar HD, et al. Surgical pathology of nonbacterial thrombotic endocarditis in 30 patients, 1985–2000. *Mayo Clin Proc.* 2001;76:1204–1212.
15. Chadha T, Hernandez JE. Infliximab-related lupus and associated valvulitis: a case report and review of the literature. *Arthritis Rheum.* 2006;55:163–166.
16. Anthony DD, Askari AD, Wolpaw T, et al. Wegener granulomatosis simulating bacterial endocarditis. *Arch Intern Med.* 1999;159:1807–1810.
17. Jimenez Caballero PE, Segura Martin T. Cardioembolic stroke secondary to non-bacterial endocarditis in Wegener disease. *Eur J Neurol.* 2007;14:683–685.
18. Oliveira GH, Seward JB, Tsang TS, et al. Echocardiographic findings in patients with Wegener granulomatosis. *Mayo Clin Proc.* 2005;80:1435–1440.
19. Xu L, Heath J, Burke A. Ascending aortitis: a clinicopathological study of 21 cases in a series of 300 aortic repairs. *Pathology.* 2014;46:296–305.
20. Looi JL, Pui K, Hart H, et al. Valvulitis and aortitis associated with ankylosing spondylitis: early detection and monitoring response to therapy using cardiac magnetic resonance imaging. *Int J Rheum Dis.* 2011;14:e56–e58.
21. Poppas A, Coady M. Echocardiographic findings and cardiac surgical implications of aortitis and valvulitis in Behçet's disease. *J Am Soc Echocardiogr.* 2009;22:1275–1278.
22. Rushing L, Schoen FJ, Hirsch A, et al. Granulomatous aortic valvulitis associated with aortic insufficiency in Takayasu aortitis. *Hum Pathol.* 1991;22:1050–1053.

175 Carcinoid Heart Disease

Allen P. Burke, M.D., and Fabio R. Tavora, M.D., Ph.D.

Pathogenesis

Carcinoid heart disease occurs when active secretory products of low-grade neuroendocrine tumors damage the endocardium of the heart. The most common setting involves jejunoileal carcinoids metastatic to the liver, allowing access to the right heart (Table 175.1). Because pulmonary endothelium, like the liver, also inactivates carcinoid secretory products, left-sided cardiac involvement is rare.

Carcinoid heart disease refers to valvular damage related to elevated serum tachykinins, serotonin (5-hydroxytryptophan), and 5-hydroxyindoleacetic acid, a metabolite of serotonin.[2-5] These circulating agents induce fibroblast proliferation, with possible thrombus formation and increased permeability of vascular endothelium on valve surfaces.[6] Cardiac involvement is almost always on the right side, with fibrous endocardial plaques formed on the leaflets of the tricuspid and pulmonary valves and subvalvular apparatus. Left-sided involvement implies a cardiac shunt or excess tumor burden that overcomes the capacity of lung endothelial cells to metabolize serotonin. The role of serotonin in the pathogenesis of the valvular disease has been reinforced by the fact that fenfluramine, a serotonin agonist used as appetite suppressant, induces a valvular disease similar to the one in carcinoid heart disease.[7] Drugs used to treat Parkinson disease, which are dopamine agonists, have been found to have similar effects.[8]

Incidence

Jejunoileal carcinoids have a 50% to 75% rate of liver metastasis. Among patients with liver metastases, about 20% show symptoms of carcinoid syndrome,[9] of whom ~40% develop carcinoid heart disease.[5] Therefore, overall, carcinoid syndrome occurs in fewer than 10% of patients with jejunoileal carcinoid tumors.

Clinical

The most frequent symptoms of carcinoid syndrome are cutaneous flushing, gastrointestinal hypermotility, and cardiac involvement.[2] Carcinoid heart disease is the initial presentation of the tumor in as many as 20% of patients. Most patients diagnosed with carcinoid heart disease have liver metastases. The vast majority of patients with carcinoid heart disease have signs of right heart failure, initially resulting in fatigue, peripheral edema, and dyspnea on exertion. Echocardiography is the principal imaging modality used in the assessment of carcinoid heart disease. Cardiac magnetic resonance imaging enables more accurate quantification of regurgitant volumes and right ventricular ejection fraction. Furthermore, carcinoid plaques can be directly visualized using delayed enhancement imaging with gadolinium.[10,11]

Ovarian carcinoid heart disease is rare, as only 0.3% of carcinoid tumors are ovarian in origin. Cardiac involvement may occur at the initial presentation or years after excision of the primary tumor.[12,13]

Gross Pathologic Features

Valves and chordae tendineae are thickened and shortened and have a pearly white appearance not dissimilar to postrheumatic heart disease (Figs. 175.1 to 175.3). The retraction and stiffening of the valves render results in retrograde valvular leakage (insufficiency) often combined with an antegrade outflow obstruction (stenosis).[11] In autopsy examples, the liver typically shows extensive involvement by metastatic carcinoid (Fig. 175.4).

The left heart is rarely affected because of pulmonary deactivation of hormonal substances. Patent foramen ovale appears to be more common in patients with carcinoid syndrome compared to the general population. Their prevalence has been reported to be as high as 41% in patients with carcinoid syndrome and up to 59% in those with carcinoid heart disease.[14]

In a series of patients with carcinoid heart disease, left-sided valvular involvement was present in five patients (7%), involving the mitral valve in all five and the aortic valve in two (Table 175.2). In one of these cases, carcinoid tumor involved the lung; in three patients, a patent foramen ovale was present; and one had neither pulmonary involvement nor a patent foramen ovale but had extensive disease with markedly increased 24-hour urinary 5-HIAA that was markedly increased.[1]

In a series of surgically resected valves, 53% were tricuspid valves, 40% pulmonary valves, 4% mitral valves, and 3% aortic valves.[15]

Microscopic

Histologically, the leaflet is intact with a superimposed plaque (Fig. 175.5). All plaques show a proliferation of myofibroblasts with collagen, along with myxoid ground substance, neovascularization, and mild chronic inflammation in more than 90%.[15] Elastic tissue is deposited in one-fifth of valves within the onlay lesion.[15]

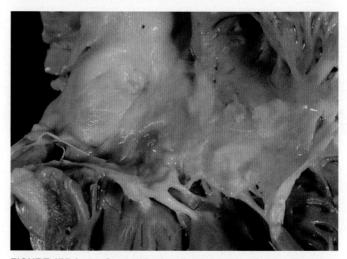

FIGURE 175.1 ▲ Carcinoid valve disease, tricuspid valve. There is thickening and shortening of the chordae. Note patchy endocardial fibrosis in the atrium, which may be secondary to regurgitant jet lesions or toxic effects of carcinoid tumor products. There are anomalous cords adjacent to the valve of the coronary sinus.

TABLE 175.1   Sites of Primary Tumor in Carcinoid Heart Disease

Small bowel	72%
Undetermined	18%
Lung	4%
Cecum/large bowel	4%
Pancreas	1%
Appendix	1%

Data from Pellikka PA, Tajik AJ, Khandheria BK, et al. Carcinoid heart disease. Clinical and echocardiographic spectrum in 74 patients. *Circulation*. 1993;87:1188–1196.

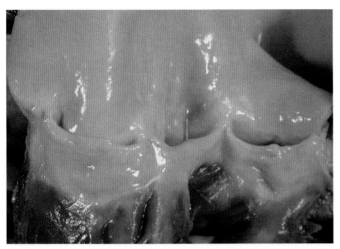

FIGURE 175.2 ▲ Carcinoid valve disease, pulmonary valve. Unlike the mitral and tricuspid valves, carcinoid disease of the pulmonary valve often results in stenosis. In this case, there is diffuse thickening with a glistening white appearance of the leaflets.

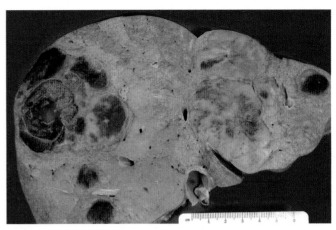

FIGURE 175.4 ▲ Liver with metastatic carcinoid tumor.

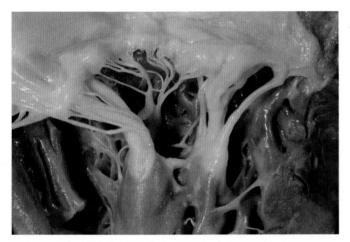

FIGURE 175.3 ▲ Carcinoid valve disease, mitral valve. The appearance is not dissimilar to that of postrheumatic heart disease, but the color is glistening white.

TABLE 175.2 Frequency of Valve Involvement (by Echocardiography) in Patients with Carcinoid Heart Disease

Valve	Frequency of Involvement	% Insufficient[a]	% Insufficient and Stenotic[a]	% Stenotic[a]
Tricuspid	97%–100%	80%	20%	0
Pulmonic	88%–92%	30%–46%	38%–52%	15%–18%
Mitral	7%–44%	97%	3%	0
Aortic	3%–32%	95%	5%	0

[a]of involved valves.
Data from Pellikka PA, Tajik AJ, Khandheria BK, et al. Carcinoid heart disease. Clinical and echocardiographic spectrum in 74 patients. *Circulation.* 1993;87:1188–1196.; Simula DV, Edwards WD, Tazelaar HD, et al. Surgical pathology of carcinoid heart disease: a study of 139 valves from 75 patients spanning 20 years. *Mayo Clin Proc.* 2002;77:139–147.

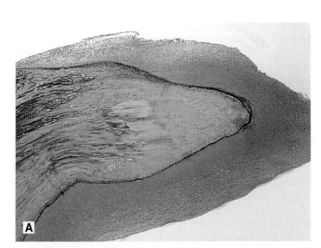
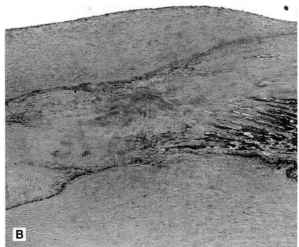

FIGURE 175.5 ▲ Carcinoid valve, disease, histologic findings, Movat pentachrome stain. **A.** The underlying valve is intact, but there is an onlay of proteoglycan-rich smooth muscle cell proliferation. **B.** A higher magnification demonstrates the smooth muscle cells within a myxoid matrix and sparse inflammation.

Treatment and Prognosis

A multidisciplinary approach is necessary in the management of patients with carcinoid heart disease. Digoxin may improve right ventricular contractility. Nonsurgical antitumor interventions such as somatostatin analogue treatment, hepatic artery embolization, and systemic chemotherapy do not alter progression of valvular disease. However, there are limited data suggesting that hepatic oligometastasectomy may increase survival. Valve surgery is the definitive treatment, with valve repair unfortunately not usually possible due to the degree of leaflet restriction, thereby necessitating valve replacement.[10] Less than one-half of patients with carcinoid heart disease eventually require valve repair or replacement.[15]

REFERENCES

1. Pellikka PA, Tajik AJ, Khandheria BK, et al. Carcinoid heart disease. Clinical and echocardiographic spectrum in 74 patients. *Circulation.* 1993;87:1188–1196.
2. Yao JC, Hassan M, Phan A, et al. One hundred years after "carcinoid": epidemiology of and prognostic factors for neuroendocrine tumors in 35,825 cases in the United States. *J Clin Oncol.* 2008;26:3063–3072.
3. Dobson R, Burgess MI, Valle JW, et al. Serial surveillance of carcinoid heart disease: factors associated with echocardiographic progression and mortality. *Br J Cancer.* 2014;111:1703–1709.
4. Moller JE, Connolly HM, Rubin J, et al. Factors associated with progression of carcinoid heart disease. *N Engl J Med.* 2003;348:1005–1015.
5. Castillo JG, Milla F, Adams DH. Surgical management of carcinoid heart valve disease. *Semin Thorac Cardiovasc Surg.* 2012;24:254–260.
6. Gustafsson BI, Hauso O, Drozdov I, et al. Carcinoid heart disease. *Int J Cardiol.* 2008;129:318–324.
7. Pena-Silva RA, Miller JD, Chu Y, et al. Serotonin produces monoamine oxidase-dependent oxidative stress in human heart valves. *Am J Physiol Heart Circ Physiol.* 2009;297:H1354–H1360.
8. Antonini A, Poewe W. Fibrotic heart-valve reactions to dopamine-agonist treatment in Parkinson's disease. *Lancet Neurol.* 2007;6:826–829.
9. Lundin L, Norheim I, Landelius J, et al. Carcinoid heart disease: relationship of circulating vasoactive substances to ultrasound-detectable cardiac abnormalities. *Circulation.* 1988;77:264–269.
10. Dobson R, Burgess MI, Pritchard DM, et al. The clinical presentation and management of carcinoid heart disease. *Int J Cardiol.* 2014;173:29–32.
11. Patel C, Mathur M, Escarcega RO, et al. Carcinoid heart disease: current understanding and future directions. *Am Heart J.* 2014;167:789–795.
12. Damen N. Ovarian carcinoid presenting with right heart failure. *BMJ Case Rep.* 2014;2014. doi: 10.1136/bcr-2014-204518.
13. Mordi IR, Bridges A. A rare case of ovarian carcinoid causing heart failure. *Scott Med J.* 2011;56:181.
14. Mansencal N, Mitry E, Pilliere R, et al. Prevalence of patent foramen ovale and usefulness of percutaneous closure device in carcinoid heart disease. *Am J Cardiol.* 2008;101:1035–1038.
15. Simula DV, Edwards WD, Tazelaar HD, et al. Surgical pathology of carcinoid heart disease: a study of 139 valves from 75 patients spanning 20 years. *Mayo Clin Proc.* 2002;77:139–147.

176 Mitral Insufficiency

Allen P. Burke, M.D.

Etiology

Similar to the aortic valve, regurgitation of the mitral valve may be caused by intrinsic mitral valve disease (myxoid degeneration resulting in prolapse), postinflammatory scarring with leaflet retraction, or factors not directly related to valve leaflets. In the last group are cardiomyopathies (ischemic or nonischemic) and ischemic damage (acute or chronic) involving the papillary muscles, most importantly the posteromedial papillary muscle.

Mitral Valve Prolapse

Background

Mitral valve prolapse is a disease of unclear etiology, genetics, and pathophysiology that has been recognized for more than a century.[1,2] In the 1960s, Barlow et al. described the association between mitral prolapse and mitral insufficiency using cineventriculography.[3] The eponymous term "Barlow mitral valve disease" is still used today for mitral valve prolapse.

Mitral valve prolapse is a spectrum of valve disease ranging from functional prolapse without insufficiency to a billowed, thickened valve with chordal disarray and mitral insufficiency. The pathologic terms "floppy mitral valve" or "myxomatous mitral valve" are sometimes used for prolapsed valves with thickened, elongated leaflets.[4]

Mitral valve prolapse is defined echocardiographically as the systolic movement of mitral valve leaflets into the left atrium that exceeds 2 mm. By this definition, mitral valve prolapse is common, ranging from 1% to 2.5% in the United States.[1] Pathologically, floppy mitral valve (or myxomatous mitral valve) is defined by valve elongation and chordal disarray, especially of the posterior leaflet, with accumulation of mucoid ground substance (myxoid change.)

The incidence floppy mitral valve is less than one-third that of functional mitral valve prolapse. Surgeons use the term "Barlow disease" specifically for prolapse with diffuse bileaflet thickening, ballooning of the leaflet and chordae, and annular dilatation. Mitral valve prolapse is frequently complicated by mitral regurgitation, but prolapse may occur in the absence of a regurgitant jet stream.[1]

Genetics of Mitral Valve Prolapse

Mitral valve prolapse is usually sporadic or nonsyndromic. Familial mitral valve prolapse occurs as an autosomal dominant trait with variable expressivity. Three loci for autosomal dominant, nonsyndromic mitral valve prolapse have been identified on chromosomes 16, 11, and 13.[1] Although there is an association between mitral valve prolapse and Marfan syndrome, no connection has been made between sporadic mitral valve prolapse and fibrillin-1 mutations.

Mitral valve prolapse is also associated with Marfan syndrome, Ehlers-Danlos syndrome, osteogenesis imperfecta, Loeys-Dietz syndrome, pseudoxanthoma elasticum, and aneurysms–osteoarthritis syndrome.[1] The incidence of mitral valve prolapse in Marfan syndrome is about 25%.[1]

Clinical Findings

Patients with mitral valve prolapse are usually asymptomatic. The diagnosis is most often made incidentally at auscultation or echocardiography. There is a female predominance for functional mitral valve prolapse, but symptomatic disease with thickened regurgitant valves has no gender predisposition. Symptoms include heart palpitations and syncope and shortness of breath, chest pain, and panic attacks. Patients with mitral valve prolapse tend to have a low body mass index.

By echocardiography, both leaflets are involved in 40% of patients; in 60%, the disease is limited to the posterior leaflet. If mitral regurgitation complicates mitral valve prolapse, a pansystolic murmur can be heard. Other findings of mitral regurgitation, such as left

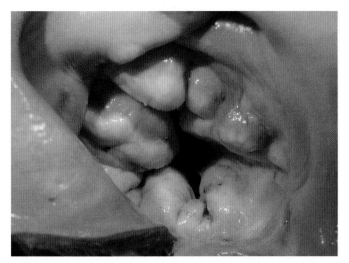

FIGURE 176.1 ▲ Mitral valve prolapse, autopsy. When inspected from above, it is immediately obvious that there is prolapse of the mitral valve. In this case, the prolapse involves all segments of both leaflets.

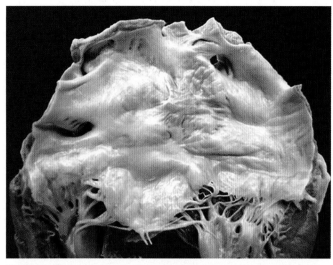

FIGURE 176.3 ▲ Mitral valve prolapse, autopsy. The specimen is opened to demonstrate the marked left atrial dilatation, with multifocal endocardial plaques, indicative of chronic mitral insufficiency.

ventricular enlargement and left atrial dilatation, can also occur in late stages of the disease. Association with other valvular disorders is common and includes prolapse of the other three heart valves, with up to 40% of patients demonstrating tricuspid valve prolapse.[1,5] The association between mitral valve prolapse and atrial septal defect is also recognized; in this case, the anterior, instead of the posterior, leaflet is generally involved, probably related to flow-induced valve billowing.

Complications are uncommon, but can lead to serious morbidity and mortality, including heart failure, progressive mitral regurgitation, bacterial endocarditis, thromboembolism, atrial fibrillation, and sudden death. These comorbidities affect <3% of subjects with mitral valve prolapse.[6] Sudden death from mitral valve prolapse is rare, and ventricular arrhythmias are the most likely cause (see Chapter 141). The mechanism of sudden death is poorly understood. Extravalvular cardiac pathology, in particular intramural artery dysplasia and fibrosis in the base of

the interventricular septum, has been reported in a high percentage of cases of mitral valve prolapse and may play a role in the formation of arrhythmias.[7]

Gross Pathologic Findings, Autopsy

The most common autopsy finding in patients with a clinical history of functional mitral valve prolapse without valve thickening echocardiographically is the absence of valvular abnormality.

In patients with thickened floppy mitral valve or myxomatous valve disease, mitral valve prolapse typically involves the posterior leaflet, often with the posterior portion of the anterior leaflet involved as well (Figs. 176.1 to 176.4). Involvement of both leaflets diffusely is unusual and may be an indication for valve replacement instead of the more typical valve repair. When viewed from the atrial surface, there is unmistakable billowing and elongation of the posterior

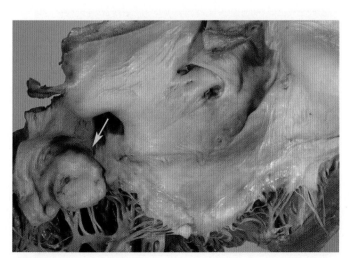

FIGURE 176.2 ▲ Mitral valve prolapse, autopsy. The lateral left ventricle was cut open, such that the posterior leaflet is seen in two parts, flanking the anterior leaflet in the center. There is a large billowed portion of the posterior leaflet under the left atrial appendage orifice (**left**, *arrow*). The anterior leaflet is relatively spared.

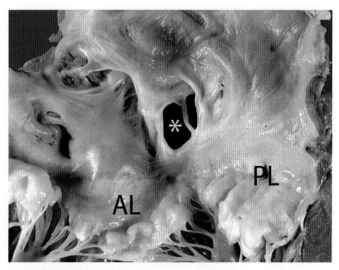

FIGURE 176.4 ▲ Mitral valve prolapse and atrial septal defect. The defect (*asterisk*) is above the posterior commissure of the valve, between the anterior and posterior leaflets (AL and PL, respectively). The prolapse involves both, but is more prominent in the posterior leaflet.

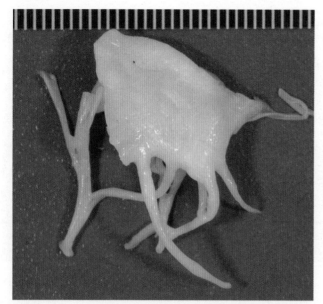

FIGURE 176.5 ▲ Mitral valve prolapse, surgical specimen from mitral valve repair, atrial aspect. The valve is glistening and white, with long, branched, irregular cords. Although nonspecific, the small fragment excised and gross findings are typical of mitral valve prolapse.

leaflet, often with demarcation of the three posterior scallops, which are difficult to identify in a normal valve. When opened, the posterior leaflet is seen to prolapse into the atrium, which may be dilated (Fig. 176.4). Prolapsed posterior leaflets show redundancy and increase of the surface area and ballooning of the scallops. There is frequently a "friction lesion" on the posterior left ventricular endocardium under the valve. The latter is characterized by subvalvular whitish slightly indurated plaque that, if extensive, can lead to fusion of the left mural endocardium to chordae and shortening of the latter, which can also serve as basis for mitral regurgitation. Rupture of chordae can be seen and may result in sudden mitral regurgitation due to a resulting "flail leaflet." Unlike postinflammatory (rheumatic)

mitral disease, fibrosis and leaflet calcification are uncommon and, if present, not extensive.

The chordae tendineae in mitral valve prolapse are disorganized, often arising from the "rough" zone of the ventricular surface of the valve, instead of the free edge. They frequently lack attachments to progressively larger chordae ("strut" or "stem" chordae) that attach directly to the papillary muscles.[8] In general, the length of the posterior leaflet is 17 mm or greater, although there is no specific length criterion.

If mitral valve prolapse is isolated, without regurgitation, there are no cardiac abnormalities other than those related to the valve itself. With regurgitation, there will be left atrial dilatation and, with long-standing regurgitation, generalized cardiomegaly with left atrial and ventricular dilatation. Pulmonary hypertension may cause right ventricular dilatation in addition to the other findings. Complications of atrial dilatation, specifically mural thrombi, and atrial endocardial fibrosis at the sites of regurgitant jet lesions should be assessed.

Secondary changes that may be present include vegetations and annular calcification. As with any structural valve disease, thrombotic and infectious endocarditis is seen at increased frequency. Additionally, the development of annular calcification is accelerated in mitral valve prolapse, especially if there are predisposing factors such as chronic renal insufficiency.

Surgical Pathology Diagnosis

Surgical approaches include leaflet resection, valvuloplasty, chordal transfer, neochordoplasty (use of prosthetic cords), commissuroplasty, and, when necessary, annular decalcification. The specimen generally received in the pathology laboratory is a portion of the posterior leaflet. The findings are nonspecific, but consistent of a glistening, white, soft valve fragment, without significant scarring or calcification, and with a mass of disorganized, thin chordae on the ventricular surface (Figs. 176.5 and 176.6). Microscopic assessment is generally unnecessary, unless there are vegetations. The gross diagnosis can generally be a short description with the designation "consistent with mitral valve prolapse."

In rare cases of bileaflet disease, a valve replacement may be performed, in which case a more extensive valve specimen including both leaflets is received. In some cases, valve repair is attempted and then aborted, with chordal repairs or insertion of prosthetic cords on the anterior leaflet of the surgical specimen.

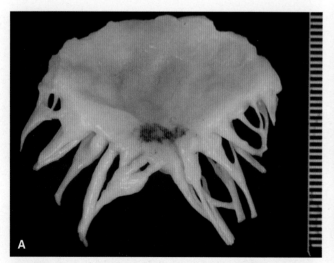
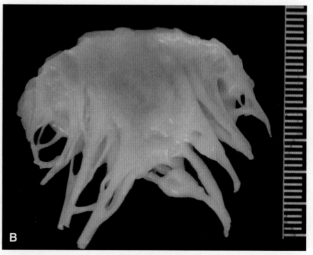

FIGURE 176.6 ▲ Mitral valve repair, mitral insufficiency secondary to rheumatic heart disease. There is thickening of the chordae and mild fibrotic changes, less than expected from a stenotic valve. In some cases, insufficient postrheumatic valves are difficult to diagnose on small specimens, and clinical history is necessary. **A.** Atrial aspect. **B.** Ventricular aspect.

Microscopic Findings

The histologic features of mitral valve prolapse are expansion of the spongiosa of the mitral valve posterior leaflets and mucopolysaccharide replacement of leaflet collagen, causing myxomatous leaflet thickening. The central part of the valve, the spongiosa layer, is the most common affected area of myxomatous degeneration, but the involvement of the fibrosa is believed to be the reason for weakening of the valve with prolapse. In contrast to postinflammatory mitral disease, there is little scarring and no neovascularization.

In cases of idiopathic sudden death complicating mitral valve prolapse, evaluation of the conduction system may demonstrate proteoglycan deposition not in the valve itself but involving the arteries at the base of the heart[7] and nerves and ganglia.[9] These changes are postulated to result in ischemia of the crest of the ventricular septum and alterations in neural conduction predisposing to autonomic imbalance and arrhythmias.

Postrheumatic Mitral Insufficiency

Approximately 1/5 of patients with postinflammatory mitral valve disease have pure insufficiency; in all, 46% of patients have stenosis with insufficiency and 34% pure stenosis.[10] Postinflammatory mitral valve disease is the second most common indication for repair or resection, after mitral valve prolapse. See Chapter 174 for a discussion of postrheumatic valve disease.

Functional Mitral Insufficiency

Mitral insufficiency is a frequent complication of cardiomyopathy, because of cardiac dilatation and remodeling (see Chapters 152 and 156). In ischemic cardiomyopathy, scarring of the posteromedial papillary muscle caused by inferior wall infarcts may also contribute to valvular insufficiency.[11] Mitral valve replacement or repair is a common procedure to slow the progression of heart failure in patients with end-stage cardiomyopathy.[12] Mitral valve replacement may successfully improve left ventricular function in end-stage ischemic cardiomyopathy, idiopathic cardiomyopathy, Chagas disease, postviral cardiomyopathy, and postpartum cardiomyopathy.[13]

Grossly, excised valve leaflets appear entirely normal, or have mild fibrotic or myxomatous degeneration (Fig. 176.7).

Acute Ischemic Mitral Insufficiency

Patients with an acute rupture of the papillary muscle undergo surgery on an emergency basis, with either valve repair or replacement, for acute mitral insufficiency. Posteromedial papillary muscle rupture

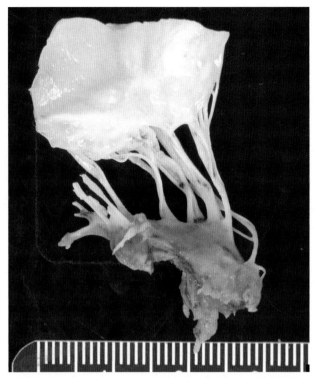

FIGURE 176.8 ▲ Acute mitral insufficiency secondary to infarction and rupture of the papillary muscle. The gross specimen shows the valve leaflet and attached papillary muscle with perforation.

occurs in the majority of cases, with 10% anterolateral papillary rupture. Bilateral papillary rupture is rare.[14]

Grossly, the specimen consists of a portion of the anterior leaflet, chordae, and attached papillary muscle with evident tear (Fig. 176.8). Histologically, acute infarct with fibrin-lined rupture site will be evident in the papillary muscle (Fig. 176.9).

Mitral Annular Calcification

Mitral annular calcification frequently complicates insufficient valves, especially prolapsed valves, and may be the primary cause of mitral insufficiency, and less often stenosis. See Chapter 172 for a further discussion of this entity.

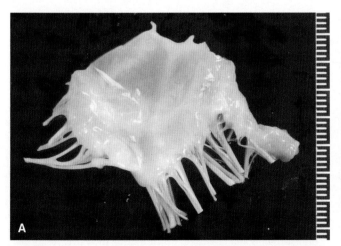
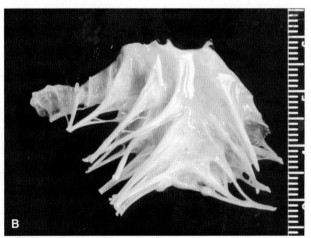

FIGURE 176.7 ▲ Mitral replacement for functional mitral insufficiency. Both the atrial (A) and ventricular (B) aspects of the valve appear normal. The patient has nonischemic (idiopathic dilated) cardiomyopathy.

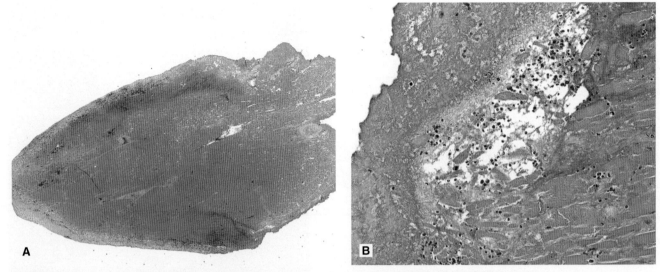

FIGURE 176.9 ▲ Acute mitral insufficiency secondary to infarction and rupture of the papillary muscle. **A.** Microscopic section shows the papillary muscle, which is largely infarcted. **B.** The rupture site is lined by platelets and fibrin.

REFERENCES

1. Delling FN, Vasan RS. Epidemiology and pathophysiology of mitral valve prolapse: new insights into disease progression, genetics, and molecular basis. *Circulation.* 2014;129:2158–2170.
2. Guy TS, Hill AC. Mitral valve prolapse. *Annu Rev Med.* 2012;63:277–292.
3. Barlow JB, Pocock WA. The significance of late systolic murmurs and mid-late systolic clicks. *Md State Med J.* 1963;12:76–77.
4. Shah PM. Current concepts in mitral valve prolapse—diagnosis and management. *J Cardiol.* 2010;56:125–133.
5. Devereux RB, Brown WT, Kramer-Fox R, et al. Inheritance of mitral valve prolapse: effect of age and sex on gene expression. *Ann Intern Med.* 1982;97:826–832.
6. Freed LA, Levy D, Levine RA, et al. Prevalence and clinical outcome of mitral-valve prolapse. *N Engl J Med.* 1999;341:1–7.
7. Burke AP, Farb A, Tang A, et al. Fibromuscular dysplasia of small coronary arteries and fibrosis in the basilar ventricular septum in mitral valve prolapse. *Am Heart J.* 1997;134:282–291.
8. Butany J, Privitera S, David TE. Mitral valve prolapse: an atypical variation of the anatomy. *Can J Cardiol.* 2003;19:1367–1373.
9. Morales AR, Romanelli R, Boucek RJ, et al. Myxoid heart disease: an assessment of extravalvular cardiac pathology in severe mitral valve prolapse. *Hum Pathol.* 1992;23:129–137.
10. Dare AJ, Harrity PJ, Tazelaar HD, et al. Evaluation of surgically excised mitral valves: revised recommendations based on changing operative procedures in the 1990s. *Hum Pathol.* 1993;24:1286–1293.
11. Kumanohoso T, Otsuji Y, Yoshifuku S, et al. Mechanism of higher incidence of ischemic mitral regurgitation in patients with inferior myocardial infarction: quantitative analysis of left ventricular and mitral valve geometry in 103 patients with prior myocardial infarction. *J Thorac Cardiovasc Surg.* 2003;125:135–143.
12. Geha AS, El-Zein C, and Massad MG. Mitral valve surgery in patients with ischemic and nonischemic dilated cardiomyopathy. *Cardiology.* 2004;101:15–20.
13. Buffolo E, Branco JN, Catani R, et al. End-stage cardiomyopathy and secondary mitral insufficiency surgical alternative with prosthesis implant and left ventricular restoration. *Eur J Cardiothorac Surg.* 2006;29(suppl 1):S266–S271.
14. Bouma W, Wijdh-den Hamer IJ, Koene BM, et al. Long-term survival after mitral valve surgery for post-myocardial infarction papillary muscle rupture. *J Cardiothorac Surg.* 2015;10:11.

177   Endocarditis

Joseph J. Maleszewski, M.D., Fabio R. Tavora, M.D., Ph.D., and Allen P. Burke, M.D.

Infectious Endocarditis

Terminology

Infectious (or infective) endocarditis denotes a bacterial or fungal infection of the endocardium. Although most cases involve the valve surfaces, endocarditis may occur on other areas of turbulent flow, for example, at ventricular or septal defects or at areas of instrumentation.[1] It may occur on native valves (native valve endocarditis [NVE]) or prosthetic valves (prosthetic valve endocarditis [PVE]).

There is a great variation in time course of endocarditis, depending in part on virulence factors of the offending organism. The term "subacute bacterial endocarditis" is often used for smoldering infections, for example, by low-virulence bacteria such as those belonging to the HACEK (*Haemophilus* species, *Actinobacillus actinomycetemcomitans*, *Cardiobacterium hominis*, *Eikenella corrodens*, and *Kingella* sp.) group.[2]

Risk Factors and Pathogenesis

NVE can occur on either structurally normal valves or structurally abnormal valves, which are prone to surface disruption. Patients with normal valves often have predisposing conditions such as intravenous drug use, intravenous lines, end-stage renal disease, poor oral hygiene, compromised immune systems, or malignancy (Table 177.1). In ~25% of patients, neither structural valve abnormalities nor predisposing conditions are evident.

The pathogenesis of infectious endocarditis begins presumably as sterile thrombi, which become secondarily infected, with the proliferation of organisms, enlargement of the thrombus, and recruitment of neutrophils and proteases, which destroy the valve. Abnormal flow around the valve, which increases the risk for infection, is caused by congenital valve abnormalities, especially bicuspid aortic valve and mitral valve prolapse (Table 177.1).

TABLE 177.1 Conditions Predisposing to Infectious Endocarditis

Structural Valve Lesions Predisposing to Infectious	Sources of Bacteremia Predisposing to Infectious Endocarditis[a]
Rheumatic valve disease 2%–6%	Hemodialysis 2%–27%
Mitral valve prolapse 4%–13%	Intravenous drug abuse 2%–27%
Bicuspid aortic valve 12%–18%	Intravascular procedures (peripheral and central lines, pacemakers, angiography)
Congenital heart disease 0%–4%	0%–2%
Hypertrophic cardiomyopathy 2%	Surgeries or procedures 2%–7%
Degenerative aortic stenosis (tricuspid) 0%–5%	Immunosuppression: 3%–7%
	Cutaneous infection 1%–2%
	Colon cancer 0%–1%

[a]Excluding chronic alcoholism and diabetes mellitus.
Data derived from Castonguay MC, et al. Surgical pathology of native valve endocarditis in 310 specimens from 287 patients (1985–2004). *Cardiovasc Pathol.* 2013;22(1):19–27; Collins JA, Zhang Y, Burke AP. Pathologic findings in native infective endocarditis. *Pathol Res Pract.* 2014;210(12):997–1004, Refs.[3,4]

Infectious Agents

Nosocomial infections are most often caused by staphylococci (47%), followed by alpha-hemolytic streptococci (14%), enterococci (5%), and other organisms (29%).[5] In two recent series of primarily community-acquired endocarditis, the relative frequency of staphylococcal infection approached that of streptococcal disease (Table 177.2).[3,4]

Some cases of culture-negative endocarditis are caused by fastidious Gram-negative organisms of the HACEK group,[6-8] which constitute ~1% to 3% of cases of community-acquired endocarditis on native and prosthetic valves, and may have a relatively good prognosis. Some organisms are especially virulent; for example, bacteremia with *Staphylococcus aureus* imparts a 13% risk,[9] whereas pneumococcus <2%.[10]

In children, more than 75% of endocarditis patients have preexisting congenital heart disease, often with prior surgery. Similar to adults, *Streptococcus viridans* and *S. aureus* are the predominant organisms.[11]

TABLE 177.2 Organisms Causing Infectious Endocarditis in Series of Surgically Excised Valves

Organism	Percent
Streptococci (total)	**39%–54%**
Viridans	*32%–28%*
Enterococcus/group D	*4%–13%*
Other	*7%–9%[a]*
***Staphylococcus* (total)**	**32%–37%**
Aureus	*20%–35%*
MRSA	*5%–20%*
Epidermidis	*2%–8%*
Other	**6%–7%[b]**
HACEK	**0%–3%**
Fungi	**1%–3%**
Culture negative	**2%–11%**

[a]Including one case of *Abiotrophia* spp.
[b]*Corynebacterium, Pseudomonas, Serratia.*
Data derived from Castonguay MC, et al. Surgical pathology of native valve endocarditis in 310 specimens from 287 patients (1985–2004). *Cardiovasc Pathol.* 2013;22(1):19–27; Collins JA, Zhang Y, Burke AP. Pathologic findings in native infective endocarditis. *Pathol Res Pract.* 2014;210(12):997–1004, Refs.[3,4] HACEK: Haemophilus, Aggregatibacter (previously Actinobacillus), Cardiobacterium, Eikenella, Kingella.

TABLE 177.3 Causes of Culture-Negative Endocarditis

Agent	Type of Organism	Method of Identification
Coxiella burnetii	Intracellular bacteria (previously rickettsia)	Serology, PCR, immunohistochemistry
Bartonella (henselae, quintana)	Intracellular bacteria (previously rickettsia)	Serology, silver impregnation stains, PCR, culture
Tropheryma whipplei	Bacteria	Histology using PAS, immunohistochemistry, silver impregnation stains, PCR
HACEK[a]	Bacteria, various Gram-negative rods	Culture
Mycoplasma hominis	Bacteria	Culture
Abiotrophia elegans	Bacteria, related to streptococci	Culture
Legionella pneumophila	Bacteria	Culture, serology, immunofluorescence

[a]HACEK organisms include *Haemophilus parainfluenzae, Actinobacillus actinomycetemcomitans, Cardiobacterium hominis, Eikenella corrodens, Kingella kingae.*

Clinical Findings

The clinical symptoms arise from valvular insufficiency in the majority of patients, with concomitant infectious symptoms. Uncommonly, large vegetations can obstruct the valve orifice and cause stenosis. Such large, obstructive, vegetations are indicative of fungal infection. The classic signs of Osler nodes and Janeway lesions are increasingly uncommon, but embolic phenomena such as splinter hemorrhages, Roth spots, and glomerulonephritis are frequently observed. The Duke criteria previously classified cases into possible and probable endocarditis, although current diagnosis rests largely on cardiac imaging, evidence of embolization, signs and symptoms of infection, and blood cultures. Clinical evidence of embolism, especially to the central nervous system, is common. Less symptomatic are emboli to the nail beds (splinter hemorrhages) and infarcts to the kidneys and spleen.

Culture-Negative Endocarditis

The rate of culture-negative endocarditis is about 10% and is higher in community-acquired infections, due to antibiotic treatment prior to diagnosis.[3,4] Extensive serologic testing, culture for esoteric organisms, and polymerase chain reaction testing reveal an etiology in over 75% of cases of endocarditis with initial negative culture. The most common organisms that are not detected routinely are *Coxiella burnetii* and *Bartonella* species.[12] The HACEK organisms and *Tropheryma whipplei* (Whipple disease) may also be frequent causes of culture-negative endocarditis (Table 177.3).[13] HACEK refers to the bacterial species Haemophilus, Aggregatibacter (previously Actinobacillus), Cardiobacterium, Eikenella, and Kingella.

Gross Pathologic Findings

Left-sided valves are most commonly infected, with approximately equal frequency between mitral and aortic valves. Left-sided valves are more frequent even in intravenous drug users than right-sided endocarditis, although infections of the tricuspid and pulmonary valves are highly suspicious of intravenous drug abuse. Tricuspid valve endocarditis may occur in community-acquired infection, usually in intravenous drug addicts, or hospital-acquired infections from implanted devices.

The gross hallmarks of infectious endocarditis are the presence of irregular vegetations and, in later stages, perforation or destruction of the valve apparatus (Figs. 177.1 to 177.3). The finding of a true perforation is nearly pathognomonic for endocarditis, as long as the distinction between perforation and fenestration is made (Chapter 138) (Fig. 177.4). Fenestrations, in contrast to perforations, are a normal finding in older patients and are present distal to the closing edge of semilunar valves.

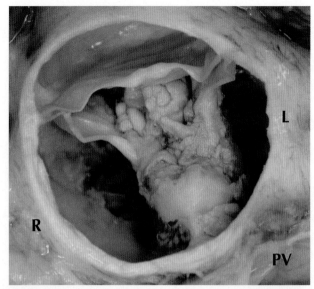

FIGURE 177.1 ▲ Infectious endocarditis, aortic valve. Note large vegetation in the orifice as well as the vegetation obscuring the commissure between the left (L) and right (R) aortic sinuses. The pulmonary valve is partially seen (PV). The underlying valve was normal; the patient was an intravenous drug addict.

At gross evaluation, documentation of the following is paramount: site(s) and size(s) of the vegetation(s), presence and size(s) of perforation(s), and underlying valve morphology should be documented. At autopsy or explant, any secondary effects of the regurgitant valve should be noted. These include jet lesions (evidence of valve regurgitation) and ventricular dilatation and hypertrophy (in cases of chronic regurgitation).

Fewer than one-third of patients with clinically diagnosed endocarditis have valvular destruction that requires surgery. In cases of valve replacement, any underlying malformation should be noted, such as congenital abnormality (e.g., bicuspid valve), mitral valve prolapse, or postinflammatory (rheumatic) valve disease.

The gross appearance of surgically resected valves varies by duration of infection and extent of leaflet destruction (Figs. 177.5 to 177.7). Occasionally, there can be aneurysmal thinning at the site of perforation. If there has been a history of prolonged antibiotic treatment, and the valve is excised for persistent regurgitation, then the only finding may be a perforation with little residual vegetation. If the valve was removed

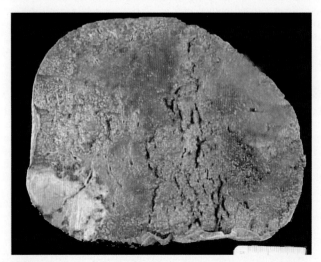

FIGURE 177.2 ▲ Splenic infarct. At autopsy, there were infarcts in various viscera including the spleen.

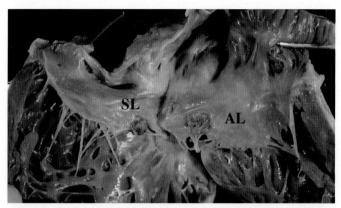

FIGURE 177.3 ▲ Tricuspid endocarditis, without leaflet destruction. There are two vegetations on both the anterior leaflet (AL) and septal leaflet (SL). When the valve apposed, these areas were touching ("kissing lesions"). Grossly, a marantic vegetation cannot be completely excluded, particularly in the absence of frank valve damage.

in the acute phase, because of irreversible destruction of the valve, then there may be bulky vegetations and barely discernable residual valve.

Tricuspid valve endocarditis may occur in community-acquired infection, usually in intravenous drug addicts, or hospital-acquired infections from implanted devices (Figs. 177.5 and 177.6).

Histologic Findings

Histologic changes, like gross alterations, depend on the length of treatment. In acute infectious endocarditis with bulky vegetations, there are large fibrin thrombi usually with abundant microorganisms and variable

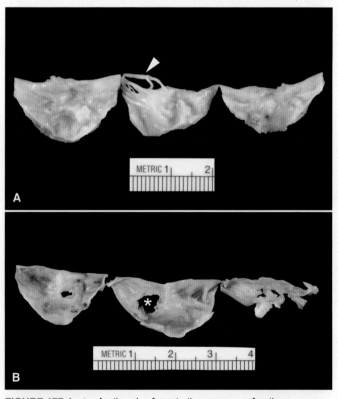

FIGURE 177.4 ▲ Aortic valve fenestration versus perforation. **A.** Fenestrations (*arrowhead*) are limited to the closing surface of the valve (distal to the line of closure) and are often associated with degenerative changes (nodular, calcific, aortic sclerosis). **B.** Perforations (*asterisk*) are not limited to the closing surface of the valve and, in the acute/subacute phase, are often associated with vegetations. When fully healed, perforations may exhibit a rolled appearance around their edges.

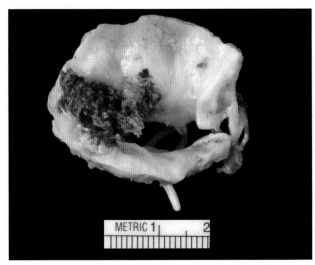

FIGURE 177.5 ▲ Infectious endocarditis, surgical resection, superimposed on postinflammatory (rheumatic) valve disease. Note the fibrotic thickening of the leaflet and cords. There is a destructive vegetation on the atrial side of the valve.

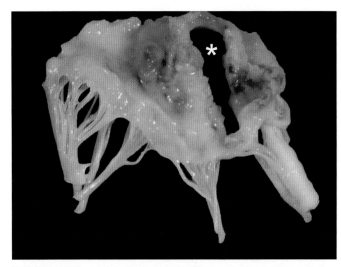

FIGURE 177.7 ▲ Infectious endocarditis, surgical resection, mitral valve, with large perforation (*asterisk*). In case of extensive valve destruction and secondary regurgitation, valve replacement is often necessary. The patient was on hemodialysis complicated by infection with methicillin-resistant *S. aureus*.

destruction of the underlying valve tissue. After long-standing antibiotic treatment, the histologic changes are subtle, with a fibroblastic reaction under the valve surface with chronic inflammation. In between these two time frames, granulation tissue is prominent. In the subacute phase, a macrophage reaction with palisading and giant cells may occur, more frequently in streptococcal than staphylococcal infections.[4] Special stains for microorganisms are generally positive in the acute phases when there is abundant acute inflammation (Figs. 177.8 to 177.11).

The inflammatory reaction in *C. burnetii* and *Bartonella* endocarditis has been described as primarily mononuclear inflammatory cells predominantly by foamy macrophages.[14] Foamy macrophages may also point to the possibility of Whipple endocarditis, which can be diagnosed by PAS, silver stains, and/or immunohistochemistry (Fig. 177.12).

Complications of Infectious Endocarditis

Embolic complications of endocarditis can result in cerebral infarction, transient ischemic attacks, renal infarction, splenic infarction (Fig. 177.2), and myocardial infarction. This dead tissue can then be seeded by microorganisms contained within the embolus and cause spread of infection. Infected emboli, for example, can lodge into the aortic intima resulting in infectious aneurysms.[15] In children with infectious endocarditis, septic emboli occur in nearly 50% of patients, causing permanent strokes in a significant number.[11]

Chronic valve regurgitation may result in heart failure, either primarily right or left sided, depending on the affected valve. Infection can spread from the valve to the valve annulus, resulting in paravalvular abscesses and fistulae. From the aortic valve, fistulae often connect to the right atrium[16]; from the mitral annulus, fistulae tend to connect the left atrium and left ventricle, causing a paravalvular leak. Infectious complications of the aortic valve can lead to severe cardiac failure and widespread contiguous lesions by the involvement of subaortic structures such as destruction of the aortic ring, aortic abscesses, true or false aneurysms, and acquired ventricular septal defects.[17,18]

Prosthetic Valve Endocarditis

Endocarditis occurs in 1% to 6% of prosthetic valves and results in nearly 50% high mortality. It occurs most frequently in the first few months after surgery. Immediate postoperative infections are currently rare, are thought to be due to organisms on the implanted valve, and occur generally in patients treated for NVE. This group of patients is at greatest risk for PVE, especially intravenous drug users.

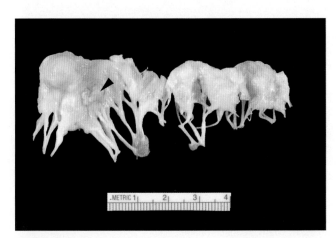

FIGURE 177.6 ▲ Infectious endocarditis, surgical resection, complicating mitral valve prolapse. There is a subtle vegetation on the rubbery and redundant anterior mitral valve leaflet.

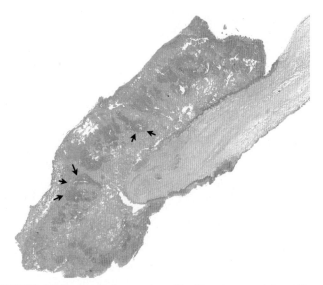

FIGURE 177.8 ▲ Infectious endocarditis. There is a vegetation at the free edge of the valve with barely discernable bacterial colonies (*arrows*).

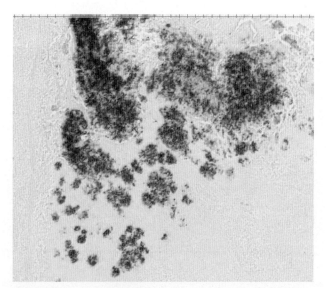

FIGURE 177.9 ▲ Infectious endocarditis, tissue Gram stain. There are clusters of Gram-positive cocci, morphologically consistent with staphylococci.

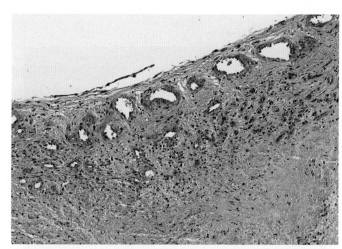

FIGURE 177.11 ▲ Infectious endocarditis, organizing phase. There is granulation tissue with prominent neovascularity at the surface of the valve.

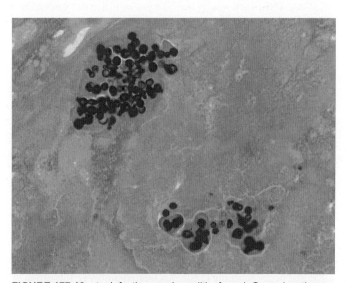

FIGURE 177.10 ▲ Infectious endocarditis, fungal. Gomori methenamine silver staining shows candida yeasts.

The rate is similar in patients with bioprosthetic and mechanical valves. In bioprosthetic valves, the valve leaflets themselves become infected, causing destruction of the leaflets, perforations, and valve insufficiency. Embolization of infected material may result in septic emboli and myocarditis, as with NVE. Mechanical valve infections result in ring abscesses and paravalvular leaks. Microorganisms are varied, but are most commonly Staphylococcal species. Infected tissue may involve the pannus surrounding the valve ring. Previously, skin contaminants, such as coagulase-negative staphylococci (epidermidis), represented a large proportion of PVE. Fungal endocarditis occurs at a higher rate than in NVE. Patients with prosthetic heart valves who develop nosocomial candidemia are at notable risk of either having or developing Candida endocarditis months or years later.[19]

Noninfectious Endocarditis (Nonbacterial Thrombotic Endocarditis)

Etiology

Nonbacterial thrombotic endocarditis (NBTE) (or marantic endocarditis) refers to the presence of sterile thrombi on heart valves occurring

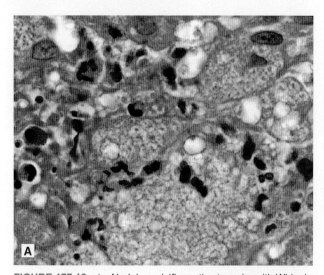

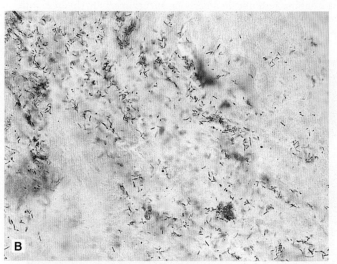

FIGURE 177.12 ▲ Nodular calcific aortic stenosis, with Whipple endocarditis. **A.** There are macrophages filled with intracellular organisms. In cases of suspected endocarditis, even if no vegetations are evident, histologic evaluation is mandatory. **B.** Diagnosis was confirmed by PAS, Warthin-Starry staining (shown), and molecular testing.

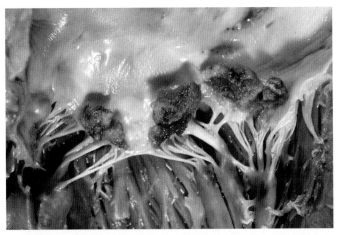

FIGURE 177.13 ▲ Nonbacterial thrombotic endocarditis, mitral valve. In contrast to infectious endocarditis, there is no underlying valve destruction, and the vegetations appear homogenous. However, an infectious endocarditis could not be completely excluded by gross examination.

because of abnormal flow causing stasis and endothelial damage. Predisposing factors include structural valve disease, as is the case with infectious endocarditis, autoimmune disorders, and hypercoagulable states, such as antiphospholipid syndrome, idiopathic thrombocytopenic purpura, and malignancy-related coagulopathy.

Clinical Findings

NBTE is often asymptomatic, but may cause cerebral embolism and other forms of thromboembolic disease. It has been estimated that 18% of strokes in cancer patients occur from embolism arising from NBTE.[20] Similar to infectious vegetations, valve-sparing procedures and vegetation removals are performed when possible in patients with symptoms.[21]

Pathologic Findings

In a series of valves excised for noninfectious (nonbacterial thrombotic) endocarditis, the mitral valve was the most common (2/3), with most of the remainder aortic valve resections.[21] In a large autopsy series, the aortic and mitral valves were affected equally, with one-fourth the rate in the tricuspid valve, and the pulmonic valve, as is the case with infectious endocarditis, only rarely affected.[22]

Grossly, noninfectious endocarditis results in thrombi on the surface of the valve, typically at the line of closure (atrial surface of the mitral valve and ventricular surface of the aortic valve). The vegetations grossly are similar to those of infectious endocarditis, although there

is no underlying valve destruction (Fig. 177.13). The thrombi may be firm and gritty or pink and soft.

The histologic findings of noninfectious vegetations include fibrin platelet thrombus, with intact interface with the underlying valve, often exhibiting a "stuck-on" appearance. The vegetation itself may demonstrate reactive fibroblasts and ingrowth of endothelial cells, with occasional iron deposition and uncommonly calcification. The underlying valve is typically devoid of acute inflammation and may demonstrate chronic fibrosis, if there is underlying postinflammatory valve disease.[21]

Autoimmune Valvulitis

"Autoimmune valvulitis" is a term generally used in animal models for autoimmune heart disease.[23] In humans, the term generally refers to vegetations occurring in patients with known autoimmune connective tissue diseases, especially lupus and rheumatoid arthritis. Valvulitis in patients with autoimmune connective tissue diseases overlaps with NBTE. In the largest series of vale resections for NBTE, 18 patients had evidence of autoimmunity (8 antiphospholipid syndrome, 6 rheumatic valve disease, 2 lupus erythematosus, and 2 rheumatoid arthritis).[21]

Lupus valvulitis was originally described in the 1920s by Libman and Sacks as a form of thrombi occurring on the valves and endocardium.[24] Almost 50% of patients with lupus have echocardiographic valve abnormalities, and 4% to 10% have verrucous valve vegetations, most commonly on the mitral valve.[25,26] Underlying valve thickening similar to rheumatic valve disease is not uncommon.[26]

Grossly, the vegetations are small and cluster along the line of closure and are typically on the ventricular surface of the mitral valve (Fig. 177.14A). Histologically, there may be acute infiltrates with hematoxylin bodies (neutrophils with intracytoplasmic inclusions), with acute and chronic inflammation (Fig. 177.14B).[27] More frequently, there is loose fibrosis with minimal inflammation at the interface between the thrombus and valve.[28] In most cases, especially if there is antiphospholipid syndrome, the histologic findings are indistinguishable from marantic endocarditis, with minimal inflammation or fibrosis.[21]

In addition to Libman-Sacks endocarditis, which by definition is a manifestation of lupus and antiphospholipid syndrome, autoimmune valvulitis resulting in sterile inflammatory vegetations has been described in other autoimmune syndromes, including Wegener granulomatosis[29] and rheumatoid arthritis.[21,30] Autoimmune aortic valvulitis has also been described in ankylosing spondylitis with aortitis and valve involvement, in which case vegetations may be absent[31,32] (Fig. 177.15).

The fact that ANCA may be secondarily elevated in infections, including infectious endocarditis, may complicate the distinction between infectious and noninfectious valvular vegetations in patients with autoimmune disorders. Furthermore, infectious endocarditis may occur in patients treated for autoimmune disorders such as rheumatoid arthritis.[33]

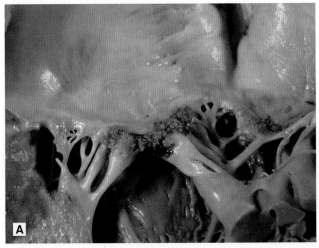

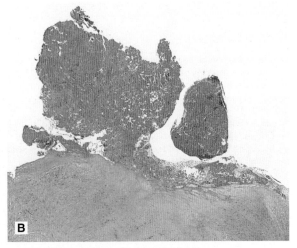

FIGURE 177.14 ▲ Libman-Sacks endocarditis. **A.** There are small vegetations at the lines of closure of the mitral valve. **B.** Histologically, the vegetations consist of bland aggregates of fibrin adherent to the endocardium of the valves without damage to the underlying valve.

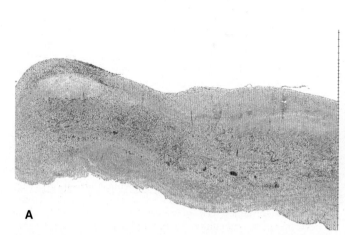
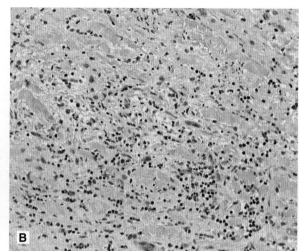

FIGURE 177.15 ▲ Autoimmune aortic valvulitis, ankylosing spondylitis. **A.** There is mild thickening and inflammation at low magnification. **B.** Higher magnification shows mixed chronic inflammatory infiltrate.

Practical Points

▶ The gross features of infectious endocarditis are two: vegetations and valve perforation. In early cases, the latter may not be present. Size, location of vegetations, and size of perforations should be noted.

▶ The differential diagnosis is nonbacterial thrombotic endocarditis (marantic endocarditis), which never results in valve perforation.

▶ Secondary hemodynamic effects in the heart at autopsy should be examined including evidence of valvular regurgitation and infection extending to the annulus (ring abscess) and rarely adjacent structures.

▶ Embolic complications should be looked for at autopsy, including septic emboli to the kidneys, mesenteric vessels, spleen, and brain.

▶ Surgical treatment of endocarditis is necessary if there is significant valvular regurgitation. In most cases, there has been treatment, and the amount of acute inflammation varies. Special stains for organisms are not necessary unless there is a history of culture-negative endocarditis.

REFERENCES

1. Krantz SB, Lawton JS. Subacute endocarditis of an atrial septal closure device in a patient with a patent foramen ovale. *Ann Thorac Surg.* 2014;98(5):1821–1823.
2. Wong D, Carson J, Johnson A. Subacute bacterial endocarditis caused by *Cardiobacterium hominis*: a case report. *Can J Infect Dis Med Microbiol.* 2015;26(1):41–43.
3. Castonguay MC, et al. Surgical pathology of native valve endocarditis in 310 specimens from 287 patients (1985–2004). *Cardiovasc Pathol.* 2013;22(1):19–27.
4. Collins JA, Zhang Y, Burke AP. Pathologic findings in native infective endocarditis. *Pathol Res Pract.* 2014;210(12):997–1004.
5. Chen SC, Dwyer DE, Sorrell TC. A comparison of hospital and community-acquired infective endocarditis. *Am J Cardiol.* 1992;70(18):1449–1452.
6. Das M, et al. Infective endocarditis caused by HACEK microorganisms. *Annu Rev Med.* 1997;48:25–33.
7. Tornos MP, et al. Prosthetic valve endocarditis caused by gram-negative bacilli of the HACEK group. *Am J Med.* 1990;88(1N):64N.
8. Meyer DJ, Gerding DN. Favorable prognosis of patients with prosthetic valve endocarditis caused by gram-negative bacilli of the HACEK group. *Am J Med.* 1988;85(1):104–107.
9. Chang FY, et al. A prospective multicenter study of *Staphylococcus aureus* bacteremia: incidence of endocarditis, risk factors for mortality, and clinical impact of methicillin resistance. *Medicine (Baltimore).* 2003;82(5):322–332.
10. Lindberg J, et al. Incidence of pneumococcal endocarditis: a regional health register-based study in Denmark 1981–1996. *Scand J Infect Dis.* 2005;37(6–7):417–421.
11. Hickey EJ, et al. Infective endocarditis in children: native valve preservation is frequently possible despite advanced clinical disease. *Eur J Cardiothorac Surg.* 2009;35(1):130–135.
12. Houpikian P, Raoult D. Blood culture-negative endocarditis in a reference center: etiologic diagnosis of 348 cases. *Medicine (Baltimore).* 2005;84(3):162–173.
13. Geissdorfer W, et al. High frequency of *Tropheryma whipplei* in culture-negative endocarditis. *J Clin Microbiol.* 2012;50(2):216–222.
14. Siciliano RF, et al. Infective endocarditis due to *Bartonella* spp. and *Coxiella burnetii*: experience at a cardiology hospital in Sao Paulo, Brazil. *Ann NY Acad Sci.* 2006;1078:215–222.
15. Araki T, Ogane K. Images in cardiovascular medicine. Rupture of infected splenic artery aneurysm secondary to infective endocarditis. *Circulation.* 2008;118(6):684–686.
16. Novak PG, et al. Transesophageal echocardiographic identification of an aortic root to right atrial fistula in a patient with acute streptococcal aortic valve bacterial endocarditis. *J Am Soc Echocardiogr.* 2003;16(5):497–498.
17. Lahdhili H, et al. Aortic endocarditis complicated with a large ventricular septal defect and septic pulmonary embolism. *Tunis Med.* 2007;85(7):600–603.
18. Ashmeik K, Pai RG. An unusual case of acquired ventricular septal defect as a complication of aortic valve endocarditis: echocardiographic delineation of multiple subvalvular complications in one patient. *J Am Soc Echocardiogr.* 2000;13(7):693–695.
19. Nasser RM, et al. Incidence and risk of developing fungal prosthetic valve endocarditis after nosocomial candidemia. *Am J Med.* 1997;103(1):25–32.
20. Dutta T, et al. Yield of transesophageal echocardiography for nonbacterial thrombotic endocarditis and other cardiac sources of embolism in cancer patients with cerebral ischemia. *Am J Cardiol.* 2006;97(6):894–898.
21. Eiken PW, et al. Surgical pathology of nonbacterial thrombotic endocarditis in 30 patients, 1985–2000. *Mayo Clin Proc.* 2001;76(12):1204–1212.
22. Biller J, et al. Nonbacterial thrombotic endocarditis. A neurologic perspective of clinicopathologic correlations of 99 patients. *Arch Neurol.* 1982;39(2):95–98.
23. Myers JM, et al. Autoimmune myocarditis, valvulitis, and cardiomyopathy. *Curr Protoc Immunol.* 2013;Chapter 15:Unit 15.14.1–51.
24. Libman E, Sacks B. A hitherto undescribed form of valvular and mural endocarditis. *Arch Intern Med.* 1924;33:701–737.
25. Cervera R, et al. Cardiac disease in systemic lupus erythematosus: prospective study of 70 patients. *Ann Rheum Dis.* 1992;51(2):156–159.
26. Galve E, et al. Prevalence, morphologic types, and evolution of cardiac valvular disease in systemic lupus erythematosus. *N Engl J Med.* 1988;319(13):817–823.

27. Rawsthorne L, et al. Lupus valvulitis necessitating double valve replacement. *Arthritis Rheum.* 1981;24(3):561–564.

28. Bouma W, et al. Mitral valve surgery for mitral regurgitation caused by Libman-Sacks endocarditis: a report of four cases and a systematic review of the literature. *J Cardiothorac Surg.* 2010;5:13.

29. Jimenez Caballero PE, Segura Martin T. Cardioembolic stroke secondary to non-bacterial endocarditis in Wegener disease. *Eur J Neurol.* 2007;14(6):683–685.

30. DeLong CE, Roldan CA. Noninfective endocarditis in rheumatoid arthritis. *Am J Med.* 2007;120(12):e1–e2.

31. Xu L, Heath J, Burke A. Ascending aortitis: a clinicopathological study of 21 cases in a series of 300 aortic repairs. *Pathology.* 2014;46(4):296–305.

32. Yuan SM. Cardiovascular involvement of ankylosing spondylitis: report of three cases. *Vascular.* 2009;17(6):342–354.

33. Letranchant L, et al. Fatal Histoplasma capsulatum mitral endocarditis in a French patient treated for rheumatoid arthritis. *Mycopathologia.* 2012;173(2–3):183–186.

178 Prosthetic Heart Valves

Allen P. Burke, M.D.

Background

Starr and Edwards described the first successful prosthetic valve replacement in 1961.[1] The ball-and-cage mechanical prosthesis was replaced by the (single) tilting disc valve in the 1970s and then, in the 1980s, by the St. Jude Medical bileaflet prosthesis. Although the durability of mechanical valves is superior, the risk of thromboembolic complications and bleeding related to anticoagulation has led to the widespread use of bioprosthetic valves, including porcine valves, homografts, and valves constructed from bovine pericardium.

Types of Prosthetic Valves

Just over half of implanted valves are mechanical, and of these, most are of the bileaflet tilting disc type.

Porcine aortic valve bioprostheses have been the most commonly implanted tissue valves, although bioprosthetic valves fabricated from xenograft pericardium, especially bovine, are becoming increasingly popular. Bioprosthetic valves are usually stented, but may lack a rigid structure and use, for example, porcine aorta as the valve ring.

Bioprosthetic valves are usually inserted during an open surgical procedure that may be minimally invasive or be inserted via a transcatheter approach, in the case of degenerative trileaflet aortic stenosis. Self- or balloon-expanding valves, in addition to transcatheter insertions, have been designed for surgical valve replacements, for ease of insertion with minimal if any suturing.

Tissue Valves

Tissue valves are either *xenografts* or *homografts* (Table 178.1).

Xenografts are made from preserved animal tissues that are usually mounted on a fabric-covered prosthetic frame or stent (Figs. 178.1 to 178.3). There are two common types, intact porcine aortic valves and valves constructed from bovine or porcine pericardium. The frame consists of posts (struts) and the intervening valve ring. Stentless xenografts are porcine aortic valves without a rigid stent and often have a portion of porcine aorta attached (full root valves) or lack porcine aorta (subcoronary valves).[2]

Pericardial xenograft bioprostheses are made of bovine parietal pericardium that is produced by computer-aided design to simulate valve leaflets (Figs. 178.4 to 178.6).

Homografts are human tissue grafts, generally cryopreserved allografts harvested from cadavers or from live donors. These are also

TABLE 178.1 Types of Prosthetic Valves

Bioprosthetic	
Xenograft	Animal valves, either intact aortic porcine valve or valves constructed from three separate semilunar fragments of bovine pericardium
Stented (sewing ring)	Valve or valve fragments attached to mechanical ring
Porcine valve	Intact porcine aortic valve, native, sewed onto metallic ring
Pericardial valve	Fashioned from three separate fragments of bovine pericardium, attached to sewing ring
Unstented	Portion of aorta and porcine aortic valve sewn into tubular cloth graft without sewing ring
Homograft	Human valves
Allograft	Donor's beating heart or cryopreserved human valves
Autograft	Patient's own tissue
Pulmonic valve	Transfer of patient's pulmonic valve to aortic position in congenital aortic valve disease
Transcatheter bioprosthetic	
Aortic	Tissue valve mounted on expandable stent
Pulmonary	Tissue valve mounted on expandable stent
Mechanical	
Ball cage	Obsolete
Tilting disc	Single disc
Bileaflet	Most common design in use today

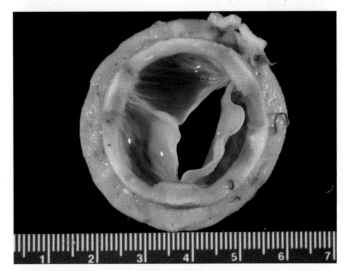

FIGURE 178.1 ▲ Bioprosthetic valve, porcine, removed surgically. The valve shows no evidence of degeneration. One leaflet is open.

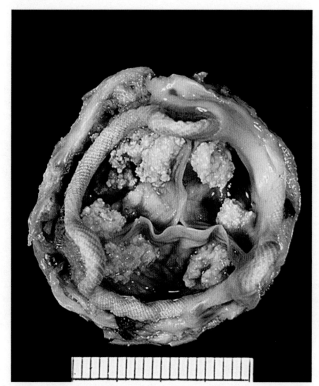

FIGURE 178.2 ▲ Calcific degenerative changes, bioprosthetic por-cine valve, necessitating valve replacement. In this case, the calcifica-tions are present as bulky nodules on the leaflet surfaces.

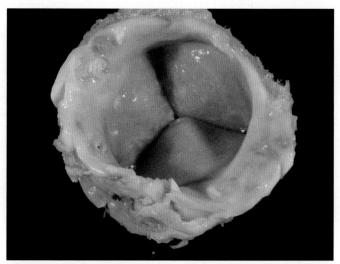

FIGURE 178.4 ▲ Pericardial valves. Replacement for excessive pannus overgrowth. In this valve, there is a fibrotic reaction encasing the sewing ring sutures. This response resulted in a degree of stenosis necessitating valve replacement.

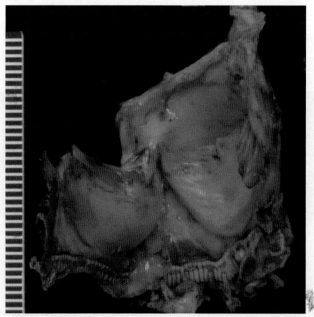

FIGURE 178.3 ▲ Unstented porcine valve, aortic position, removed surgically for degeneration. Two of the porcine leaflets are evident, as well as the cloth sewing ring (**bottom**), and a portion of the aortic root (**above**).

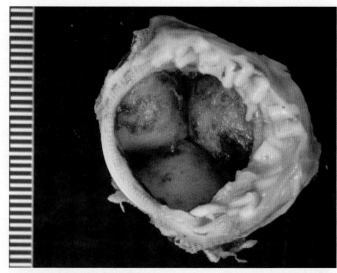

FIGURE 178.5 ▲ Pericardial valve, explant at autopsy. This example has a low profile (Sorin Mitroflow) without metal stent. The cause of death was not related to the valve. The flow surface and sewing ring are shown. There is a small amount of fibrin on the leaflets.

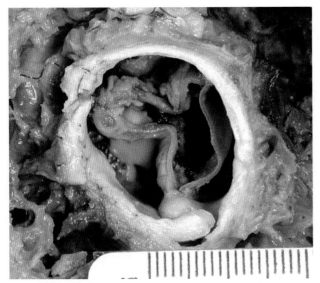

FIGURE 178.6 ▲ Infectious endocarditis, bovine pericardial valve. Two of the three synthetic leaflets demonstrate vegetations.

TABLE 178.2   Types of Bioprosthetic Valves, Selected

Class	Examples
Porcine stented	Supra-annular aortic porcine bioprosthesis, Carpentier-Edwards Duraflex mitral prosthesis, Carpentier-Edwards Hancock II, Mosaic, Medtronic St. Jude Medical Biocor Duraflex
Porcine stentless (full root includes part of pig aorta; subcoronary without root)(aortic position only)	Prima Plus (Carpentier-Edwards) Freestyle (Medtronic) SPV Stentless (St. Jude Medical Toronto)
Pericardial stented	Perimount Magna (Carpentier-Edwards) Theon, Mitral Ease (Carpentier-Edwards) St. Jude—Biocor Pericarbon More (Sorin Biomedica)
Pericardial stentless	Freedom Solo, Solo Smart (aortic), Mitroflow (Mitral)(Sorin Biomedica)
Pericardial self expanding (sutureless)	3f Enable (aortic position)(Medtronic)

stentless, or transplanted directly into the aortic root, without a supporting synthetic frame (Fig. 178.7). Autografts are homografts derived from the patient, usually the pulmonic valve translocated to the aortic position in cases of congenital aortic stenosis.

A list of the more common bioprosthetic valves and their characteristics are presented in Table 178.2.

Mechanical Valves

Bileaflet mechanical valves have largely replaced models of single tilting disc valves (Fig. 178.8). Because of symmetric flow, they offer excellent hemodynamic performance. Most use pyrolytic carbon as the structural component of the leaflets. The current types of bileaflet mechanical valves are presented in Table 178.3.

Single tilting disc valves were initially introduced as the Bjørk-Shiley valve, which, although largely successful with over 360,000 replacements, had complications of strut fracture with disc embolization[3] and were eventually withdrawn. More recent examples include the Medtronic Hall valves (Fig. 178.9) (see Table 178.3).

Transcatheter Valve Implantation

The most common percutaneous valve implant is the aortic valve (*transcatheter aortic valve implantation, TAVI*). Its use is for calcified stenotic or combined stenotic and regurgitant valves, with bicuspid valves a relative contraindication. TAVI was introduced in the early 2000s via a transfemoral vein approach requiring transatrial septal perforation and antegrade insertion through the mitral valve. Currently, TAVI uses a retrograde approach, first attempted in 2006, most commonly via the

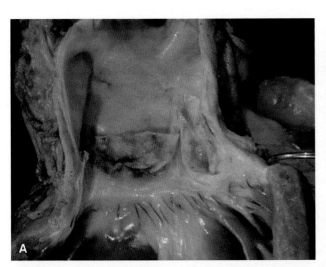
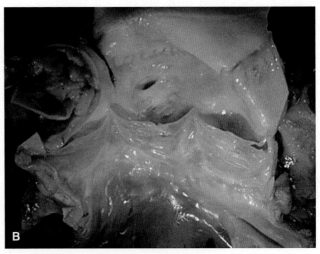

FIGURE 178.7 ▲ Homograft valve, allograft. Tissue valves may be harvested from human tissue, usually cryopreserved from autopsy. In this example, a human aortic valve was grafted into the pulmonary position in a child with aortic stenosis. **A.** The native pulmonary valve was normal and was used for an autograft. **B.** The native pulmonary valve that was removed in from the heart illustrated in Figure 178.9 was moved over into the aortic position, with reimplantation of the coronary ostia (note sutures).

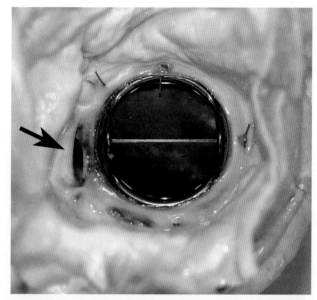

FIGURE 178.8 ▲ Bileaflet mechanical valve, paravalvular leak, mitral position. The *arrow* demonstrates an area of incomplete surgical closure. The leak was hemodynamically insignificant, and the patient died of noncardiac causes.

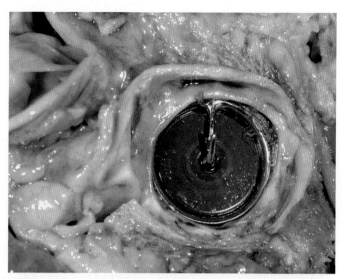

FIGURE 178.9 ▲ Medtronic Hall tiling disc mechanical valve. The valve was an incidental finding at autopsy. Note the central orifice and mild pannus overgrowth.

femoral artery. Alternative approaches utilize a transapical insertion through the left ventricle, or transaortic insertion through an incision in the ascending aorta. These techniques are usually accomplished via minimally invasive surgery (Table 178.4).

Transcatheter pulmonary valve implantation is used for pulmonary valve replacement and is done antegrade via a direct femoral vein approach.

Complications and Survival

The major complications of mechanical prosthetic valves are thromboembolism, thrombosis, and hemorrhage. The major drawback of bioprostheses is structural valve deterioration with the need for reoperation. Endocarditis can complicate both types of valves and involves the annulus or sewing ring area in cases of mechanical valves (Table 178.5).

In general, bioprosthetic valves are recommended for patients 65 years or older and for patients who cannot tolerate anticoagulation, such as women who may wish to become pregnant. A recent study showed virtually identical survival rates after aortic valve replacement between mechanical and bioprosthetic valves, with a 60% 15-year actuarial survival rate.[4] The risk of stroke was similar in both groups (cumulative incidence of 8% after 15 years), with a lower rate of major hemorrhage and higher rate of reoperation (12% at 15 years) for bioprosthetic valves.

In most patients, there is a gradual reduction in left ventricular mass after aortic valve surgery.[5] In general, patients with valve replacements for aortic insufficiency have a lower overall survival than do those with aortic stenosis.[6]

Bioprosthetic Valve Degeneration

Degenerative changes with calcification are an inevitable complication of bioprosthetic tissue valves (Figs. 178.2, 178.5, 178.10, and 178.11). Freedom from degenerative changes is nearly 100% at 5 years, 80% at 10 years, and 60% at 15 years. Durability is reduced in the mitral position because of greater closing pressure, and in younger patients who have higher calcium metabolism turnover.

Pathologic Complications

Pannus, or fibrous reactive to devices, occurs at the host–fabric or host–tissue interface and is generally mild (Fig. 178.4). Occasionally,

TABLE 178.3   Types of Mechanical Valves, Selected

Class	Manufacturer
Bileaflet	St Jude Medical
	Sorin CarboMedics
	Sorin Biomedica (Sorin Bicarbon Fitline)
	Medtronic Open Pivot
	ON-X mechanical prosthesis
Monoleaflet (tilting disk)	Medtronic Hall
	Sorin Biomedica All Carbon[a]
	Omnicarbon (CV Medical)[b]

[a]Discontinued, 2010.
[b]Discontinued, 2005.

TABLE 178.4   Types of Transcatheter Valve Implants

Aortic valve

Edwards Lifesciences Percutaneous Aortic Heart Valve (Sapien XT)	Bovine pericardium tricuspid valve mounted on a cobalt–chromium frame, balloon expandable	FDA approved for calcific trileaflet aortic stenosis with high operative risk
Medtronic CoreValve Percutaneous Pericardial Aortic Valve	Trileaflet porcine pericardial tissue valve in nitinol frame, self-expandable	FDA approved for calcific trileaflet aortic stenosis with high operative risk and for failure of surgical valve replacement

Pulmonary valve

Medtronic Melody Transcatheter Pulmonary Valve	Bovine jugular valve mounted within a platinum stent	Transfemoral venous approach, for native or prosthetic right ventricular outflow delivery

TABLE 178.5 Major Pathologic Complications of Prosthetic Valves

Mechanical or bioprosthetic
Paravalvular leak
Ring abscess
Coronary ostial occlusion
Excessive pannus formation

Mechanical valves
Thrombosis
Decreased leaflet movement (oversized valve, long sutures)

Bioprosthetic valves
Calcification
Leaflet endocarditis

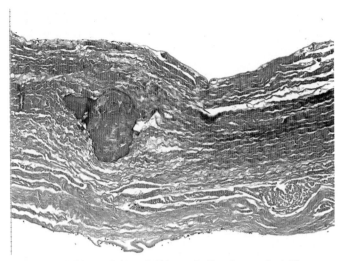

FIGURE 178.11 ▲ Pericardial bioprosthetic valve, explant. The histologic appearance is quite different from that of porcine valves and shows linear collagen bundles within the pericardium. There is focal calcification.

it can progress onto the sewing cuff and further into the biologic components, leading to their stiffening and progressive stenosis and dysfunction.[7,8]

Paravalvular leaks can occur from the time of surgery, if there is incomplete closure of the anastomotic site. Leaks are generally small and hemodynamically insignificant (Fig. 178.8). Acquired paravalvular leaks are almost always the result of infection of the sewing ring and are associated with ring abscesses and high morbidity and mortality.

Acute ischemia with myocardial infarction may occur in aortic valve replacements when the strut is positioned over the coronary ostium, especially the right coronary ostium in bioprosthetic porcine valves. This complication is more common in valve replacement for bicuspid aortic valve because of variation in anatomy.[9]

Thrombosis on valve surfaces is generally firmly stuck to the leaflets and difficult to remove, unlike soft, postmortem clots. The thrombi may occlude the valve opening resulting in restricted motion and may embolize causing coronary occlusion (Fig. 178.12) or stroke. The rate of thrombosis in patients on oral coagulation with mechanical valve prostheses is 1% to 4% per year and is higher in the elderly patients with atrial fibrillation or left ventricular dysfunction and patients with mitral prostheses.

Endocarditis is a complication of the valve surfaces in bioprosthetic valves (Figs. 178.13 and 178.14)[10] and does not occur after mechanical valve implantation, except for ring abscesses. Infective endocarditis is a common indication for excision of bioprosthetic valves, especially nonstented valves.[10]

Bioprosthetic Valve Inflammation and Endocarditis

Prosthetic valve endocarditis is generally highest in the first few months after surgery; however, it can occur for years after surgery.[11] Endocarditis rates are highest for patients who undergo valve replacement for infective endocarditis.[11] Pathologically, there are vegetations with or without perforation of the leaflets (Fig. 178.6).

Most common bacteria infecting bioprosthetic valves are staphylococci, followed by Gram-negative bacilli and fungi. Because the leaflets are avascular, host defenses and antibiotics are relatively ineffective. The rate of endocarditis is low, ~2% for the lifetime of the implant.[11]

Inflammation related to immunologic reactions in bioprosthetic valves is characterized by a macrophage infiltrate along the surface,

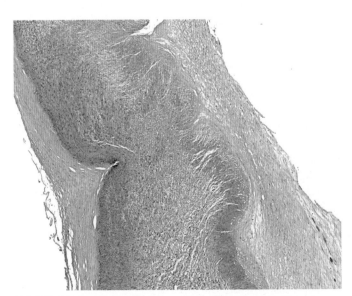

FIGURE 178.10 ▲ Porcine bioprosthetic valve, explant. There is fibrosis on both sides of the valve.

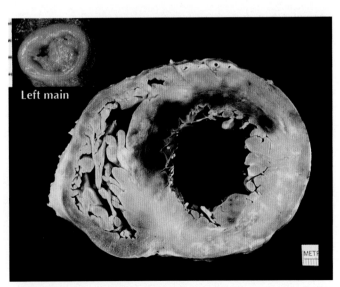

FIGURE 178.12 ▲ Thrombosis, mechanical valves, with embolization. There was a thromboembolus in the left main coronary artery (inset upper left), resulting in a hemorrhagic infarct involving the anterior septum and anterior wall.

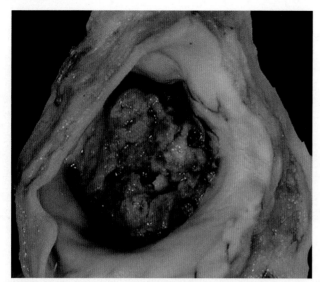

FIGURE 178.13 ▲ Infectious endocarditis, homograft valve
(allograft). The patient had a remote Ross procedure (autograft aortic
valve replacement with patient's native pulmonary valve and allograft
pulmonary valve replacement with cryopreserved aortic valve from
another patient). There was marked degeneration of the valve leaflets
with complete destruction by infected thrombus.

especially in pericardial valves. The macrophages typically demonstrate
a palisaded appearance at the valve edge. Infectious endocarditis of the
leaflet itself may result in valve perforation and vegetations.

Annuloplasty Rings

Valve repair in the tricuspid position is nearly always limited to annuloplasty with either a full ring or C-shaped flexible prosthesis. In the
mitral position, mitral repair with annuloplasty is typically associated with resection of a portion of the leaflet, typically the posterior. Annuloplasty rings may be resected surgically, if a repair valve
remains incompetent and needs to be replaced with a prosthetic valve
(Fig. 178.15).

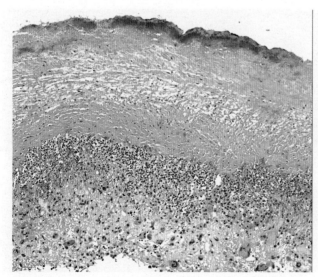

FIGURE 178.14 ▲ Infectious endocarditis, porcine bioprosthesis.
There is a rim of bacteria on the flow surface (**above**) and acute and
chronic inflammation with macrophage giant cells of the nonflow surface (**below**).

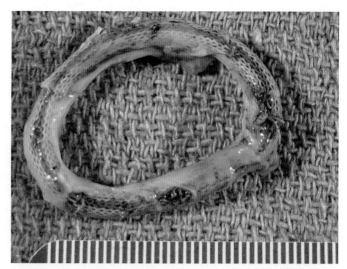

FIGURE 178.15 ▲ Annuloplasty ring, mitral valve. Annuloplasty
rings of either the mitral or tricuspid position may be removed if the
valve is persistently regurgitant and total valve replacement is necessary. Annuloplasty rings may be closed rings, as in this case, or open
C-shaped rings (not shown).

Teaching Points

▶ When encountering a prosthetic valve at **autopsy**, determine type and note any complications.

▶ Describe the type as tissue or mechanical; if mechanical,
note if tilting (single) disk or bileaflet.

▶ If tissue, attempt to distinguish porcine valve from
mechanical, if stented or not, or if an allograft (human)
valve (always unstented).

▶ Note complications of paravalvular leak, thrombosis, and
ring abscess in the case of mechanical valves, and note
normal excursion of disk or excessive pannus.

▶ Note complications of calcification, perforation, vegetations, perivascular leak, and ring abscess in the case of
bioprosthetic valves.

▶ Document any evidence of embolization in the case of
thrombosis.

▶ Document hemodynamic changes related to the underlying valve disease before valve replacement (e.g.,
left atrial and right-sided dilatation in the case of mitral
stenosis).

▶ Explanted prosthetic valves as a **surgical specimen** are
nearly always bioprosthetic.

▶ Attempt to determine the type of valve.

▶ Note calcification, perforation, vegetation, pannus, and
thrombosis.

REFERENCES

1. Starr A, Edwards ML. Mitral replacement: the shielded ball valve prosthesis.
J Thorac Cardiovasc Surg. 1961;42:673–682.
2. Greve HH, Farah I, Everlien M. Comparison of three different types of stentless valves: full root or subcoronary. *Ann Thorac Surg.* 2001;71:S293–S296.

3. Silver MA. Strut fracture and embolization of a Bjork-Shiley valve from the tricuspid valve position. *Am J Cardiol.* 1991;68:1253.

4. Chiang YP, Chikwe J, Moskowitz AJ, et al. Survival and long-term outcomes following bioprosthetic vs. mechanical aortic valve replacement in patients aged 50 to 69 years. *JAMA.* 2014;312:1323–1329.

5. Christ T, Grubitzsch H, Claus B, et al. Hemodynamic behavior of stentless aortic valves in long term follow-up. *J Cardiothorac Surg.* 2014;9:197.

6. Christ T, Grubitzsch H, Claus B, et al. Long-term follow-up after aortic valve replacement with Edwards Prima Plus stentless bioprostheses in patients younger than 60 years of age. *J Thorac Cardiovasc Surg.* 2014;147:264–269.

7. Butany J, Collins MJ. Analysis of prosthetic cardiac devices: a guide for the practising pathologist. *J Clin Pathol.* 2005;58:113–124.

8. Butany J, Leask RL, Desai ND, et al. Pathologic analysis of 19 heart valves with silver-coated sewing rings. *J Card Surg.* 2006;21:530–538.

9. Roberts WC, Patterson BA, Ko JM, et al. Massive acute infarction of the right ventricular wall without or only minimal infarction of the left ventricular wall after aortic valve replacement with or without simultaneous replacement of the ascending aorta. *Cardiovasc Pathol.* 2010;19(3):187–190.

10. Butany J, Zhou T, Leong SW, et al. Inflammation and infection in nine surgically explanted Medtronic Freestyle stentless aortic valves. *Cardiovasc Pathol.* 2007;16:258–267.

11. Jegatheeswaran A, Butany J. Pathology of infectious and inflammatory diseases in prosthetic heart valves. *Cardiovasc Pathol.* 2006;15:252–255.

179 Cardiac Thrombi and Pseudotumors

Joseph J. Maleszewski, M.D., and Allen P. Burke, M.D.

Mural Thrombi

Clinical Features and Pathogenesis

Thrombosis may occur in any cardiac chamber and evolve from acute masses formed primarily of fibrin, platelets, and entrapped blood to fibrotic, organized, masses. The majority of mural thrombi occur in association with underlying heart disease. Left atrial thrombi are frequently associated with mitral valvular disease, especially mitral stenosis,[1] and thrombi occur in either atrium in patients with atrial fibrillation and/or cardiac amyloidosis.[2] There is an increased risk for their development after cardiac surgery.[3]

Right atrial thrombi are frequently incidental findings at autopsy in patients with indwelling catheters or pacemakers and may occur in the setting of right heart failure, tricuspid regurgitation, or underlying coagulopathy. Rarely, they are the result of atrial infarctions, either isolated or with ventricular infarctions.[4] When occurring without underlying heart disease, atrial thrombi may be misdiagnosed as myxomas.[5]

In the majority of patients with mural thrombus and no structural heart disease, a coagulation defect is either suspected or documented.

Complications of mural thrombi include embolization, either pulmonary or systemic. Left-sided thrombi may be a source of transient ischemic attacks or stroke.

Pathologic Findings

Mural thrombi are occasionally removed surgically, if mistaken for a neoplastic process, or if there is no response to anticoagulation. In one surgical series of heart tumors, 13 of 84 resected tumors were thrombi that clinically mimicked neoplasms.[6]

Grossly, mural thrombi may be broad based and organized with little risk for embolization or polypoid and friable imparting higher risk for embolic phenomena. The former have been termed membranous thrombi and histologically are smooth muscle cell rich with variable proteoglycan matrix and fibroelastic tissue at the base. Polypoid thrombi are rich in fibrin and platelets, are more friable, and often superimposed on membranous type. The site of either type is usually within left atrial appendage, especially if there is atrial fibrillation[7] (Fig. 179.1).

Histologic findings in atrial thrombi are variable (Figs. 179.2 to 179.4). They are composed of fibrin, platelets, and entrapped blood cells, especially near the surface. Ingrowth of endothelium may result in a hemangioma-like appearance. Organization, often occurring at the base, usually has a fibroblastic appearance, which, in concert with a myxoid matrix, may mimic a myxoma. Importantly, vasocentric rings, and Gamna-Gandy bodies are not typically seen in organizing thrombus. Layering of thrombus (lines of Zahn) may be seen in early thrombi without organization. In later stages, the surface is endothelialized.

Aggregates of entrapped leukocytes (including neutrophils) may be encountered and should not be necessarily interpreted as infection. Septic thrombi are generally diagnosed clinically and will histologically demonstrate microabscesses and bacterial organisms.[8] The presence of leukocyte necrosis and debris often raises suspicion for underlying infection and helps to differentiate such from entrapped leukocytes in a noninfected thrombus.

Calcified Pseudotumors

Calcified Amorphous Tumor

Calcified amorphous tumor was initially described as pseudotumor, clinically mistaken for a neoplasm that occurred in adults in all four chambers.[9] Patients are usually symptomatic adults and suffer cardiorespiratory complaints or complications of embolism, such as stroke or digital gangrene.[10]

Grossly, resected specimens are often fragmented (Fig. 179.5) and usually have areas of dense calcification. Histologically, they consist of paucicellular eosinophilic material, with areas of dense calcification and admixed chronic inflammation and hemosiderin (Fig. 179.6), often with surface fibrin. Surgery is generally curative.[9]

Calcified amorphous tumors are generally considered a form of degenerating calcified thrombi.[6] They may be associated with chronic renal failure and antiphospholipid syndrome.[10] Those adjacent to the mitral annulus may be extensions of mitral annular calcification.[11-13]

Mitral Annular Calcification

Annular calcification refers to degenerative deposition of calcium and variable amounts of lipid, along the fibrous annulus of the mitral valve most often along the posterior leaflet (Chapter 172). It may occasionally protrude into the left atrial or ventricular cavity, producing a mass lesion, with features of calcified amorphous tumor. Occasionally, the lesion may undergo degenerative central softening ("caseous" degeneration of the mitral annulus).

In addition to obstructing leaflet excursion, mitral annular calcification may form a mass extending into the left atrium or left ventricular outflow tract.[13] This may occur by continued deposition of calcium and

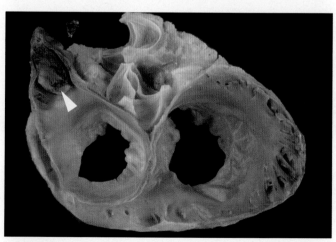

FIGURE 179.1 ▲ Left atrial appendage with mural thrombus. The appendage is a typical site for atrial thrombi. (Reproduced with permission from Burke AP, Tavora F, Maleszewski J, et al. *Atlas of Tumor Pathology, Tumors of the Heart and Great Vessels*. Washington, DC: American Registry of Pathology; 2014.)

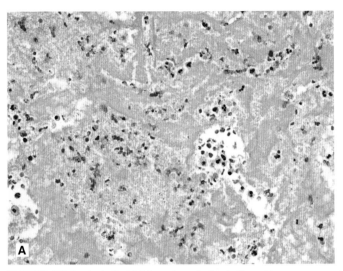
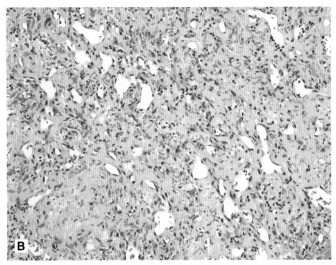

FIGURE 179.2 ▲ Left atrial thrombus. **A.** Acute thrombi are composed primarily of fibrin and platelets. **B.** A different area with organization mimicking a hemangioma.

growth of the mass or the fissuring of the calcified shell of centrally softened annular calcium. In the case of the latter, the gritty material may be extruded out onto the surface of the valve leaflet or onto a cardiac chamber wall (like toothpaste from a tube). Occasionally, giant cells can be identified in association with the tissue reaction to this partially calcified debris.

Histopathologically, discriminating between cardiac calcified amorphous tumor and extruded annular calcification can be difficult and is based primarily on location of the lesion. Grossly, mitral annular calcification often has soft and gummous areas, whereas calcified amorphous tumors are rock hard. Histologically, the presence of fresh thrombus and giant cells on the surface favors a diagnosis of annular calcification.

Mesothelial/Monocytic Incidental Cardiac Excrescence

Definition and Histogenesis

Mesothelial/monocytic incidental cardiac excrescences (MICEs) are collections of detached, avascular mesothelial cells, adipocytes, and macrophages that lack intervening stroma. They are generally found within the heart, aorta, or pericardium and have also been described in other mesothelial-lined surfaces. They are also called "lesions of aggregate monocytes and mesothelial cells (LAMM)"[14] and "nodular mesothelial hyperplasia."[15]

MICEs are considered artifacts of instrumentation (cardiac surgery or other interventional procedures) in most cases.[16,17] Most have been described as incidental fragments of tissue either found floating in the heart or attached to another process. In some cases, the location and history do not explain their formation via an iatrogenic route,[18-20] and the etiology remains obscure.

Pathologic Findings

Histologically, MICEs are compact clusters of histiocytes, fat, and mesothelial cells, without intervening stroma (Fig. 179.7). The mesothelial components of these lesions stain strongly with antibodies directed against calretinin and the monocytes with anti-CD68 or CD163. It is important to recognize the incidental nature of the lesions and not to mistake them for neoplasms.

Inflammatory Pseudotumor

Definition and Histogenesis

"Inflammatory pseudotumor" denotes a nonneoplastic mass composed primarily of inflammation, of unknown cause. "Inflammatory myofibroblastic tumor" is a distinct low-grade neoplasm of myofibroblastic cells and is considered separately (Chapter 180). The distinction

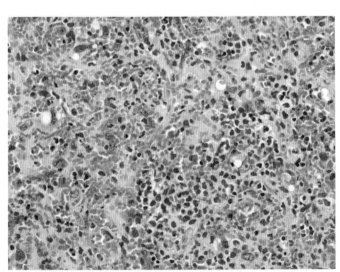

FIGURE 179.3 ▲ Left atrial thrombus. In some cases, there is abundant inflammation. Unless there are pockets of neutrophils with microabscesses, inflammation does not indicate septic thrombus.

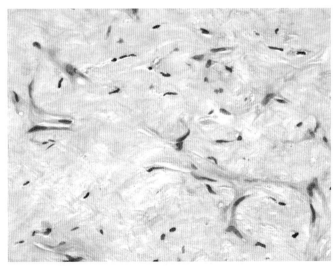

FIGURE 179.4 ▲ Right atrial thrombus, myxoid change. Myxoid areas may suggest the diagnosis of myxoma, but there are no myxoma cells or other features of myxoma.

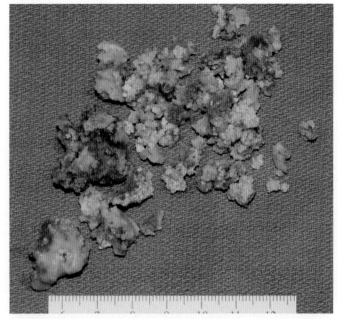

FIGURE 179.5 ▲ Calcified amorphous tumor. These are excised often in pieces, because of their rock-like nature.

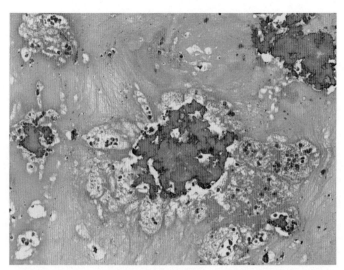

FIGURE 179.6 ▲ Calcified amorphous tumor. Histologically, there is abundant calcification with little cellularity.

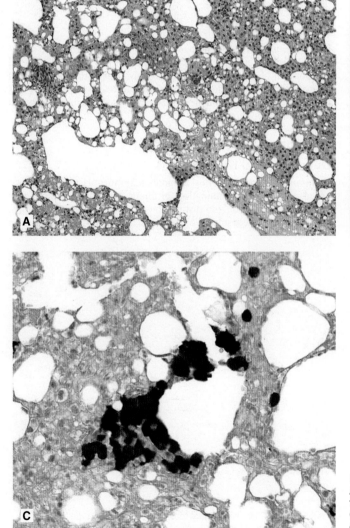

FIGURE 179.7 ▲ Incidental monocyte–mesothelial excrescence. A. Low magnification shows avascular collection of macrophages and fat cells. B. Higher magnification shows nests of mesothelial cells. C. Immunohistochemical staining for calretinin supports mesothelial origin. Macrophages do not stain.

in the heart has not always been consistently made[21] and is similar to that for inflammatory masses in the lung (see Chapter 68).

The etiology of inflammatory pseudotumors is unknown and likely heterogeneous. In the case of a defined condition (e.g., sarcoidosis or infection) that results in a mass, the term "pseudotumor" may be used descriptively. For example, an intracardiac abscess caused by *L. monocytogenes* has been described as a cardiac inflammatory pseudotumor.[22]

Clinical Features

Clinical manifestations related to inflammatory masses are due to either mechanical compressive effects or systemic signs and symptoms of inflammation.

Pathologic Findings

The histopathology of inflammatory masses is varied. IgG4-related disease has histologic features similar to sclerosing mediastinitis,[23] which may manifest as a paucicellular fibrous mass within a cardiac atrium.[24] Intracardiac masses composed of chronic inflammation and fibroblasts have been described in patients with Behçet disease.[25,26] Intracardiac lesions with abundant macrophages should be discerned from histiocytic proliferations that may also occur in the heart (see Chapter 180).[27]

REFERENCES

1. Bansal M, Kasliwal RR. Images in clinical medicine. Mobile large left atrial thrombus. *N Engl J Med*. 2015;372:e2.
2. D'Aloia A, Vizzardi E, Chiari E, et al. Cardiac arrest in a patient with a mobile right atrial thrombus in transit and amyloidosis. *Eur J Echocardiogr*. 2008;9: 141–142.
3. Arif S, Aktuerk D, Barron DJ. Giant, pedunculated right atrial thrombus formation after surgical atrial septal defect repair. *J Thorac Cardiovasc Surg*. 2015;149:e46–e48.
4. Lanjewar DN, Ramraje S, Lanjewar SD. Right atrial appendage thrombus with atrial infarct in a case of thyrotoxicosis: an autopsy report. *Indian J Pathol Microbiol*. 2010;53:532–534.
5. Kodali S, Yamrozik J, Biederman RW. Left atrial thrombus masquerading as a myxoma in a patient with mitral stenosis. *Echocardiography*. 2010;27:E98–E101.
6. Strecker T, Rosch J, Weyand M, et al. Primary and metastatic cardiac tumors: imaging characteristics, surgical treatment, and histopathological spectrum: a 10-year-experience at a German heart center. *Cardiovasc Pathol*. 2012;21: 436–443.
7. Saito T, Tamura K, Uchida D, et al. Histopathological evaluation of left atrial appendage thrombogenesis removed during surgery for atrial fibrillation. *Am Heart J*. 2007;153:704–711.
8. Dedeilias P, Roussakis A, Koletsis EN, et al. Left atrial giant thrombus infected by *Escherichia coli*. Case report. *J Cardiothorac Surg*. 2008;3:18.
9. Reynolds C, Tazelaar HD, Edwards WD. Calcified amorphous tumor of the heart (cardiac CAT). *Hum Pathol*. 1997;28:601–606.
10. Sabzi F, Karim H, Eizadi B, et al. Calcified amorphous tumor of the heart with purple digit. *J Cardiovasc Thorac Res*. 2014;6:261–264.
11. Yasui H, Takahama H, Kanzaki H, et al. Time-course changes of cardiac-specific inflammation in a patient with left ventricular calcified amorphous tumor. *Circ J*. 2015;79(9):2069–2071.
12. Seo H, Fujii H, Aoyama T, et al. Cardiac calcified amorphous tumor in a hemodialysis patient. *Asian Cardiovasc Thorac Ann*. 2015, doi: 10.1177/0218492315574795.
13. Mohamedali B, Tatooles A, Zelinger A. Calcified amorphous tumor of the left ventricular outflow tract. *Ann Thorac Surg*. 2014;97:1053–1055.
14. Erinanc H, Gunday M, Saba T, et al. Lesion of aggregated monocytes and mesothelial cells: mesothelial/monocytic incidental cardiac lesion. *Case Rep Pathol*. 2013;2013:836398.
15. Walley VM, Veinot JP, Tazelaar H, et al. Lesions described as nodular mesothelial hyperplasia. *Am J Surg Pathol*. 1999;23:994–995.
16. Walley VM, Peters HJ, Veinot JP, et al. The clinical and pathologic manifestations of iatrogenically produced mesothelium-rich fragments of operative debris. *Eur J Cardiothorac Surg*. 1997;11:328–332.
17. Courtice RW, Stinson WA, Walley VM. Tissue fragments recovered at cardiac surgery masquerading as tumoral proliferations. Evidence suggesting iatrogenic or artefactual origin and common occurrence. *Am J Surg Pathol*. 1994;18:167–174.
18. Argani P, Sternberg SS, Burt M, et al. Metastatic adenocarcinoma involving a mesothelial/monocytic incidental cardiac excrescence (cardiac MICE). *Am J Surg Pathol*. 1997;21:970–974.
19. Ng MT, Trendell-Smith NJ. A case of mesothelial/monocytic incidental cardiac excrescence (MICE) associated with squamous cell carcinoma of lung. *Pathology*. 2012;44:563–565.
20. Hu ZL, Lu H, Yin HL, et al. A case of mesothelial/monocytic incidental cardiac excrescence and literature review. *Diagn Pathol*. 2010;5:40.
21. Rao N, Gajjar T, Ghosal N, et al. Inflammatory pseudotumor arising from the right ventricular outflow tract causing pulmonary stenosis. *J Card Surg*. 2012;27:696–698.
22. Adler A, Fimbres A, Marcinak J, et al. Inflammatory pseudotumor of the heart caused by Listeria monocytogenes infection. *J Infect*. 2009;58:161–163.
23. Ishizaka N. Letter to the editors: IgG4-related inflammatory pseudotumor in the heart. *Methodist Debakey Cardiovasc J*. 2014;10:58.
24. Pereira-da-Silva T, Galrinho A, Ribeiro A, et al. Intracardiac mass due to fibrosing mediastinitis: the first reported case. *Can J Cardiol*. 2013;29:1015.e5-7.
25. Yao FJ, Liu D, Zhang Y, et al. Inflammatory pseudotumor of the right ventricle in a 35-year-old woman with Behçet's disease: a case report. *Echocardiography*. 2012;29:E134–E136.
26. Leitao B, Machado F, Soares F, et al. Myocardial inflammatory pseudotumor and multiple thromboses as a manifestation of Behcet disease. *J Clin Rheumatol*. 2009;15:252–253.
27. Obikane H, Ariizumi K, Yutani C, et al. Inflammatory pseudotumor (inflammatory myofibroblastic tumor) of the mitral valve of the heart. *Pathol Int*. 2010;60:533–537.

180 Pediatric and Congenital Tumors

Joseph J. Maleszewski, M.D., and Allen P. Burke, M.D.

General

Incidence

Pediatric heart tumors are rare and are the primary indication in <1% of heart surgeries in a children.[1]

Clinical

There is no obvious sex predilection for most of the cardiac tumors that arise in children. In surgically resected tumors, the mean age is ~4 years, with a range of 1 day to 18 years, or the definition of the upper limit of a pediatric age group.[2] Intrauterine detection of heart tumors has become common, especially for intrapericardial teratoma.[3]

Histopathologic Types

In general, there are five entities that are considered pediatric and/or congenital tumors of the heart. These include rhabdomyoma, fibroma, histiocytoid cardiomyopathy, and inflammatory myofibroblastic tumor (IMT). Cardiac hamartomas (discussed in Chapter 183) and cystic

TABLE 180.1   Cardiac Tumors in Children: Histologic Types and Frequency in 257 Tumors[a]

Tumor Type	
Rhabdomyoma	43%
Fibroma	13%
Teratoma	10%
Myxoma	20%
Hemangioma	3%
Sarcoma	5%
Inflammatory myofibroblastic tumor	1%
Papillary fibroelastoma	<1%
Metastases	3.5%
Leiomyoma	<1%
Schwannoma	<1%

From 3 series [1, 6, 2], 2 of which were resections only [1, 2]. Series including unoperated tumors have a much higher rate of rhabdomyoma, which are usually followed without excision.

tumor of the atrioventricular node are likely also present at birth and could be classified as pediatric/congenital tumors, but often do not present until adulthood.

The most common pediatric heart tumor in children < age 5 is rhabdomyoma, followed by cardiac fibroma (Tables 180.1 and 180.2). In neonates and fetuses, intrapericardial teratomas tend to be more common (see Chapter 186). In older children, myxomas are more common.

Myxomas are discussed in Chapter 181. In children, myxomas are rare under age 10 and are usually recognized during investigation of a murmur. As in adults, most are located in the left atrium. In children and young adults, there is a higher incidence of Carney complex than in adults with cardiac myxoma.[1]

Imaging

Echocardiography, ultrasound, and magnetic resonance imaging are used most commonly to image cardiac masses in children and fetuses. Echocardiography is noninvasive and radiation free, but has poor soft tissue characterization in larger children and suboptimal evaluation of extracardiac structures. Ultrasound is the modality of choice for evaluating fetal abnormalities and has excellent sensitivity for such.

Magnetic resonance imaging is the modality of choice for cardiac masses, especially in children. There is no use of ionizing radiation. With the use of intravenous contrast, it is excellent in differentiating neoplasms from thrombus as well as discriminating between benign and malignant cardiac masses. The extent of myocardial, pericardial,

valvular, and coronary arterial involvement can also be gauged well by this modality.

Computed tomography can provide additional anatomic information and tissue characterization such as calcification and offers assessment of patients with suspected metastatic disease, especially in conjunction with positron emission tomography.[4]

Treatment and Prognosis

The treatment of most heart tumors is surgical resection, with the exception of rhabdomyoma, which may spontaneously regress. The prognosis for excised benign tumors is excellent, with a 93% 5-year survival.[2] The highest intraoperative mortality is seen with cardiac fibroma, because of the frequent large size.[1] The prognosis for malignant tumors is poor, with a 40% 5-year survival.[2]

Rhabdomyoma
Clinical Findings

Children with rhabdomyomas typically present, before the age of 10 years, with murmurs, arrhythmias, or heart failure. There are extracardiac manifestations of tuberous sclerosis in >50% of patients.[1,2,5]

Only 23% of children with cardiac rhabdomyoma require heart surgery, because the tumors have a propensity to spontaneously regress. Those that require surgery generally have luminal obstructive lesions that usually require intervention prior to age 3 months.[6]

Gross Pathology

Cardiac rhabdomyomas usually involve the ventricles, with atrial involvement in fewer than 10% of cases. Most (>60%) occur in multiples, particularly those associated with tuberous sclerosis.

On gross examination, cardiac rhabdomyomas are lobulated, tan-white or yellow nodules with a distinct demarcation from the surrounding myocardium. They range from a few millimeters up to 10 cm. Rarely, they may occur as a miliary studding of the myocardium.[7]

Microscopic Pathology

Cardiac rhabdomyomas form well-demarcated unencapsulated lobules of vacuolated tumor cells identified easily on low magnification (Fig. 180.1). The lobules consist of round polygonal cells with cytoplasmic clearing and small nuclei (Fig. 180.2). Strands of eosinophilic cytoplasm often emanate from the center of the rhabdomyoma cell and extent radially to the sarcoplasmic membrane, giving the appearance of a spider (so-called *spider cells*).

Calcification is usually absent, in contrast to a large proportion of fibromas. On immunohistochemical studies, the tumor cells reflect

TABLE 180.2   Cardiac Tumors in Children, Associations, and Location

Tumor type	Associations, Comments	Location
Rhabdomyoma	Tuberous sclerosis (high frequency) Frequent regression	Ventricles
Fibroma	Gorlin syndrome (low frequency) Regression unusual May remain asymptomatic until late adult life	Ventricles
Histiocytoid cardiomyopathy	Congenital heart defects X-linked and mitochondrial mutations	Myocardium, endocardium, predilection for conduction system
Inflammatory myofibroblastic tumors	May be underreported as myxoma	Right ventricular endocardium, valves
Hemangioma	Associated with extracardiac hemangiomas May regress	Variable
Teratoma	Relatively common fetuses and neonates	Pericardium, rare in heart (see Chapter 49)
Myxoma	Rare in children <10 years High association with Carney complex in pediatric age group	Left atrium > right atrium
Cystic tumor of the AV node	Usually presents in adults, patients usually have congenital heart block. Occasional other midline defects	AV nodal area

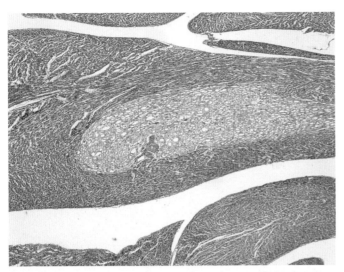

FIGURE 180.1 ▲ Cardiac rhabdomyoma. At low magnification, there are discrete areas of sarcoplasmic clearing.

their myogenous origin and show positivity for vimentin, actin, desmin, and myoglobin. Hamartin and tuberin, the protein products of the genes associated with TSC, namely, *TSC1* and *TSC2*, respectively, are also positive in rhabdomyomas, with some evidence pointing to a down-regulation status of these proteins in rhabdomyoma cells when compared to normal myocytes.[8]

Differential Diagnosis

The major differential diagnosis is histiocytoid cardiomyopathy. The vacuoles of rhabdomyoma are larger and contain PAS-positive (diastase-sensitive) glycogen, in contrast to histiocytoid cardiomyopathy.

Treatment and Prognosis

The prognosis for cardiac rhabdomyoma is excellent, as the tumor is benign and generally undergoes spontaneous regression. In those

children who require surgery for obstructive lesions, there is an operative mortality of around 7%.[1] More recently, drugs that inhibit the mTOR pathway have proven effective in hastening regression and may greatly reduce the number of surgical resections for this tumor.[9]

Cardiac Fibroma

Incidence and Clinical

Cardiac fibromas account for about 15% of excised heart tumors in children and are located mainly in the right ventricle, the ventricular septum, and the left ventricular free wall. There is a weak association with Gorlin syndrome, or nevoid basal cell carcinoma syndrome, which is associated with *PTCH* mutations.[10,11]

Although generally considered a congenital tumor, cardiac fibroma may remain undetected until adulthood.[11,12]

Gross Pathology

Cardiac fibromas are rounded masses, that, upon sectioning, exhibit a whilte and worled (often bulging) surface (Fig. 180.3) that resembles a uterine leiomyoma.

Microscopic Pathology

Cardiac fibroma is a homogeneous proliferation of monomorphic fibroblasts that demonstrate little or no atypia (Figs. 180.4 and 180.5). The degree of cellularity generally decreases with age of the patient, whereas the amount of collagen increases.[11] There can be a focally myxoid background, and calcification is common. Mitoses are generally present only in tumors of patients less than a few months of age.

Prognosis

There is a mortality of up to 20% with surgery in young children, because of the bulky and infiltrative nature of some tumors.[1] Otherwise, prognosis is excellent, as recurrences are exceptional. Malignant degeneration has not been reported.

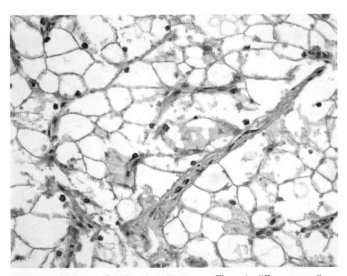

FIGURE 180.2 ▲ Cardiac rhabdomyoma. There is diffuse vacuolization of myocytes. The differential diagnosis is storage disease, which would not form discrete nodules or masses, and histiocytoid cardiomyopathy. The cells are much larger and have cytoplasmic clearing to a greater extent than histiocytoid cardiomyopathy. The vacuoles of rhabdomyoma are filled with glycogen; those of histiocytoid cardiomyopathy mitochondria (oncocytes).

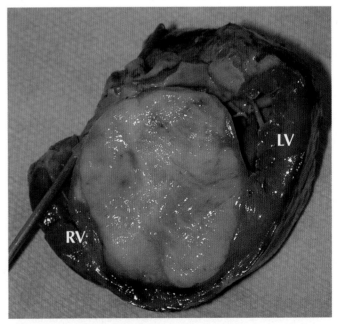

FIGURE 180.3 ▲ Cardiac fibroma. The appearance is that of a relatively circumscribed, whorled fibrous tumor. The tumor replaced the ventricular septum, a site of predilection for this tumor.

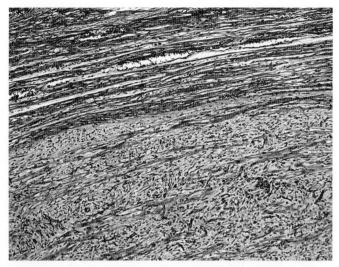

FIGURE 180.4 ▲ Cardiac fibroma. In infants, the tumors are relatively cellular. The differential diagnosis includes IMT, which has more inflammation and is endocardial in location.

Histiocytoid Cardiomyopathy

Clinical

Histiocytoid cardiomyopathy is an extremely rare condition characterized by incessant ventricular tachycardia in newborns and infants caused by multiple small cardiac tumors. Previously termed simply "hamartomas," these lesions were excised or treated by open ablation procedures and diagnosed by histopathologic examination.[13–15] Currently, transcatheter ablation is the primary treatment, and pathologic diagnosis is rarely made during life with many cases causing sudden death.[16] There is an association with other cardiac defects, including ventricular noncompaction and septal defects.

Gross Pathology

Histiocytoid cardiomyopathy is identified as pale, typically subendocardial, nodules that may occur anywhere in the heart, but with a predilection for areas near the specialized conduction system.

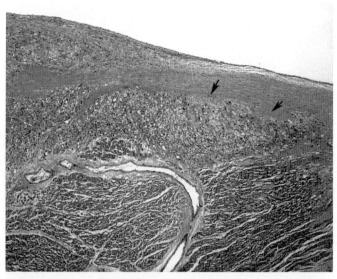

FIGURE 180.6 ▲ Histiocytoid cardiomyopathy. This illustration is from a heart of an expected SIDS death, with no gross abnormalities. Microscopically, there were nests of cleared cells (*arrows*) in the subendocardium. The lesions of histiocytoid cardiomyopathy may occur at all sites (endocardium, valvular, myocardium, and subepicardium) although there is a predilection for subendocardial regions.

Microscopic Pathology

Histiocytoid cardiomyopathies, as the name suggests, are nodules of small, macrophage-like cells with fine cytoplasmic vacuoles and small ovoid nuclei (Figs. 180.6 and 180.7). They are modified myocytes and express skeletal muscle antigens. Ultrastructurally, the vacuolization is the result of mitochondriosis.

Molecular Findings

Histiocytoid cardiomyopathy is associated with X-linked mutations, including those of *NDUFB11* and various mitochondrial genes.[17,18]

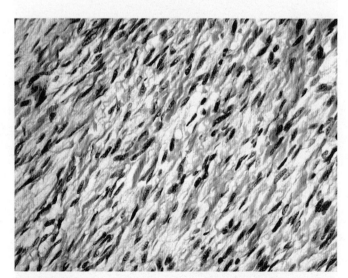

FIGURE 180.5 ▲ Cardiac fibroma. A higher magnification of the tumor illustrated in Figures 180.3 and 180.4 shows fibroblasts with intersperse bundles of dense collagen. The collagen deposition in IMT is less diffuse and may be absent.

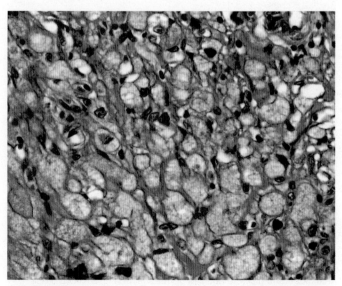

FIGURE 180.7 ▲ Histiocytoid cardiomyopathy. A higher magnification of the tumor illustrated in Figure 180.6 shows vacuolated cells. In contrast to rhabdomyoma, the cells are bubbly, not enlarged, and lack large vacuoles.

Differential Diagnosis

The differential diagnosis of histiocytoid cardiomyopathy includes artifactual pallor of endocardial myocytes caused by inadequate fixation and rhabdomyoma. The cells and vacuoles of cardiac rhabdomyoma are far larger than those of histiocytoid cardiomyopathy.

Inflammatory Myofibroblastic Tumor

Clinical

IMT of the heart is rare, with fewer than 50 reported cases. Several childhood cardiac IMTs have been reported as sarcomas and have had a benign course.[19-23]

The median age at presentation is 5.5 years, without a clear sex predilection. Cardiac symptoms related to IMT include heart failure, cyanosis, peripheral edema, dyspnea, and syncope. Systemic embolization to the brain or lower extremities is common.[24] Prolapse into the coronary arteries by lesions on the mitral or aortic valve can result in ischemia, myocardial infarction, and sudden death.[25] A few patients present with inflammatory symptoms and with fever, malaise, and elevated serum acute phase reactants.[26]

Gross Pathology

Cardiac IMTs are endocardial-based tumors that often have a stalk. Typically, they are multilobulated, often with a "grape-like" or clustered appearance (Fig. 180.8).[24] They may have a glistening, mucoid appearance that grossly mimics cardiac myxoma.[27]

The most frequent site is the right ventricular endocardium, followed by valves and the atria. Most tumors are single, although they may be multicentric.[28]

Microscopic Pathology

Cardiac IMTs are polypoid lesions, often with surface fibrin.[24,29] The spindle cells resemble myofibroblasts, with abundant cytoplasm and open, vesicular nuclei (Fig. 180.9). Mitotic figures are infrequent and are generally fewer than 2 per 10 high-power fields.[24] Atypical mitotic figures are absent. There is variable inflammation, but lymphoid aggregates or germinal centers are rare.

Immunohistochemically, tumor cells express smooth muscle actin and occasionally desmin.[26] Anaplastic lymphoma kinase (ALK-1) expression is absent or weak.[24] Tumors show a low proliferative index by immunohistochemical staining with Ki-67.[30]

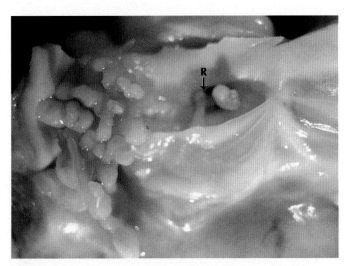

FIGURE 180.8 ▲ Inflammatory myofibroblastic tumor. There is an endocardial-based polypoid or filiform mass filling the left coronary ostium (not seen) and prolapsing into the right ostium (R). The patient, a young boy, died suddenly after experiencing episodes of chest pain for several days.

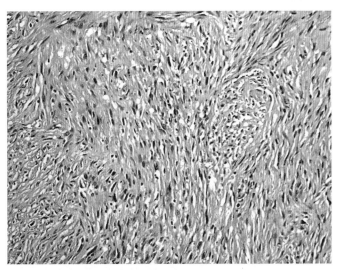

FIGURE 180.9 ▲ Inflammatory myofibroblastic tumor. A histologic section of the tumor illustrated in Figure 180.8 shows a proliferation of bland myofibroblastic cells, with little pleomorphism and, in this area, little inflammation.

Differential Diagnosis

The differential diagnosis of cardiac IMT is sarcoma and myxoma. Sarcomas are exceptionally rare in children and usually show a higher mitotic rate and a greater degree of pleomorphism and necrosis than IMT.

Those IMTs with a myxoid background can resemble cardiac myxoma, as both are endocardial-based lesions. Immunohistochemical staining for calretinin is negative in IMT.

Cystic Atrioventricular Nodal Tumor

Incidence and Clinical

There are fewer than 75 reports of atrioventricular nodal tumors, approximately twice the number of intrapericardial bronchogenic cysts. The true incidence may be higher than the literature suggests, because cases may be overlooked at autopsy. Atrioventricular nodal tumors have sometimes been referred to as "choristomas."[31] There is an association with other midline defects, suggesting that these lesions represent misplaced embryologic tissue.[32]

Atrioventricular nodal tumor is a rare cause of congenital heart block. Most atrioventricular nodal tumors are diagnosed at autopsy in patients dying suddenly (see Chapter 141). Death is usually unexpected, with a mean age at death in the fourth decade, although there is a wide range, from birth to the eighth decade.[33,34]

Gross Pathology

Grossly, atrioventricular tumors may appear in the region of the membranous septum as a cyst-like structure or as an area of thickening with small, fluid-filled cysts that are barely perceptible to the naked eye. They range in size from 2 to 20 mm. The gross examination of the heart is normal in 60%, with the tumor diagnosed microscopically after sections are taken of the atrioventricular node.[35]

Microscopic Pathology

Histologically, the tumor is located in the region of the AV node and proximal His bundles and respects the boundary of the central fibrous body without extending into the ventricular myocardium or into valvular tissues (Fig. 180.10). There are nests of cells that often form cysts of variable sizes and solid nests. The cells themselves are flattened or cuboidal and may contain transitional, sebaceous, and endocrine cells Immunohistochemically, most atrioventricular nodal

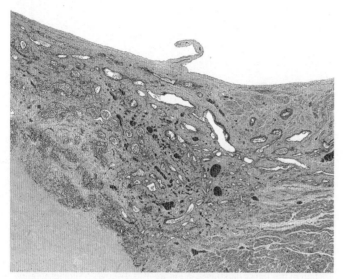

FIGURE 180.10 ▲ Cystic tumor of the atrioventricular node. There are small cysts and nests of epithelial cells in the area of the AV node. The patient had heart block diagnosed prenatally.

tumors are positive for carcinoembryonic antigen, B72.3 antigen, EMA, and CA19-9.[32]

Differential Diagnosis

Rarely, teratomas of the heart may be intramyocardial, within the ventricular septum. In contrast to atrioventricular nodal tumors, there are typically neuroectodermal and glandular structures present, and the tumors are larger. Intrapericardial germ cell tumors are discussed in Chapter 186.

REFERENCES

1. Bielefeld KJ, Moller JH. Cardiac tumors in infants and children: study of 120 operated patients. *Pediatr Cardiol.* 2013;34:125–128.
2. Padalino MA, Vida VL, Boccuzzo G, et al. Surgery for primary cardiac tumors in children: early and late results in a multicenter European Congenital Heart Surgeons Association study. *Circulation.* 2012;126:22–30.
3. Isaacs H Jr. Fetal and neonatal cardiac tumors. *Pediatr Cardiol.* 2004;25: 252–273.
4. Tao TY, Yahyavi-Firouz-Abadi N, Singh GK, et al. Pediatric cardiac tumors: clinical and imaging features. *Radiographics.* 2014;34:1031–1046.
5. Thomas-de-Montpreville V, Nottin R, Dulmet E, et al. Heart tumors in children and adults: clinicopathological study of 59 patients from a surgical center. *Cardiovasc Pathol.* 2007;16:22–28.
6. Linnemeier L, Benneyworth BD, Turrentine M, et al. Pediatric cardiac tumors: a 45-year, single-institution review. *World J Pediatr Congenit Heart Surg.* 2015;6:215–219.
7. Uzun O, McGawley G, Wharton GA. Multiple cardiac rhabdomyomas: tuberous sclerosis or not? *Heart.* 1997;77:388.
8. Kotulska K, Larysz-Brysz M, Grajkowska W, et al. Cardiac rhabdomyomas in tuberous sclerosis complex show apoptosis regulation and mTOR pathway abnormalities. *Pediatr Dev Pathol.* 2009;12:89–95.
9. Kocabas A, Ekici F, Cetin II, et al. Cardiac rhabdomyomas associated with tuberous sclerosis complex in 11 children: presentation to outcome. *Pediatr Hematol Oncol.* 2013;30:71–79.
10. Boutet N, Bignon YJ, Drouin-Garraud V, et al. Spectrum of PTCH1 mutations in French patients with Gorlin syndrome. *J Invest Dermatol.* 2003;121:478–481.
11. Burke AP, Rosado-de-Christenson M, Templeton PA, et al. Cardiac fibroma: clinicopathologic correlates and surgical treatment. *J Thorac Cardiovasc Surg.* 1994;108:862–870.
12. Strecker T, Rosch J, Weyand M, et al. Primary and metastatic cardiac tumors: imaging characteristics, surgical treatment, and histopathological spectrum: a 10-year-experience at a German heart center. *Cardiovasc Pathol.* 2012;21:436–443.
13. Garson A Jr, Smith RT Jr, Moak JP, et al. Incessant ventricular tachycardia in infants: myocardial hamartomas and surgical cure. *J Am Coll Cardiol.* 1987;10:619–626.
14. Kearney DL, Titus JL, Hawkins EP, et al. Pathologic features of myocardial hamartomas causing childhood tachyarrhythmias. *Circulation.* 1987;75:705–710.
15. Tazelaar HD, Locke TJ, McGregor CG. Pathology of surgically excised primary cardiac tumors. *Mayo Clin Proc.* 1992;67:957–965.
16. Gilbert-Barness E, Barness LA. Pathogenesis of cardiac conduction disorders in children genetic and histopathologic aspects. *Am J Med Genet A.* 2006;140:1993–2006.
17. Shehata BM, Cundiff CA, Lee K, et al. Exome sequencing of patients with histiocytoid cardiomyopathy reveals a de novo NDUFB11 mutation that plays a role in the pathogenesis of histiocytoid cardiomyopathy. *Am J Med Genet A.* 2015;167A(9):2114–2121.
18. Vallance HD, Jeven G, Wallace DC, et al. A case of sporadic infantile histiocytoid cardiomyopathy caused by the A8344G (MERRF) mitochondrial DNA mutation. *Pediatr Cardiol.* 2004;25:538–540.
19. Han P, Drachtman RA, Amenta P, et al. Successful treatment of a primary cardiac leiomyosarcoma with ifosfamide and etoposide. *J Pediatr Hematol Oncol.* 1996;18:314–317.
20. Itoh K, Matsumura T, Egawa Y, et al. Primary mitral valve sarcoma in infancy. *Pediatr Cardiol.* 1998;19:174–177.
21. Lee JR, Chang JM, Lee C, et al. Undifferentiated sarcoma of the mitral valve with unique clinicopathologic presentation. *J Cardiovasc Surg (Torino).* 2003;44:621–623.
22. McElhinney DB, Carpentieri DF, Bridges ND, et al. Sarcoma of the mitral valve causing coronary arterial occlusion in children. *Cardiol Young.* 2001;11: 539–542.
23. Takach TJ, Reul GJ, Ott DA, et al. Primary cardiac tumors in infants and children: immediate and long-term operative results. *Ann Thorac Surg.* 1996;62:559–564.
24. Burke A, Li L, Kling E, et al. Cardiac inflammatory myofibroblastic tumor: a "benign" neoplasm that may result in syncope, myocardial infarction, and sudden death. *Am J Surg Pathol.* 2007;31:1115–1122.
25. Li L, Burke A, He J, et al. Sudden unexpected death due to inflammatory myofibroblastic tumor of the heart: a case report and review of the literature. *Int J Legal Med.* 2011;125:81–85.
26. Elkiran O, Karakurt C, Erdil N, et al. An unexpected cause of respiratory distress and cyanosis: cardiac inflammatory myofibroblastic tumor. *Congenit Heart Dis.* 2013;8(6):E174–E177.
27. Li L, Cerilli LA, Wick MR. Inflammatory pseudotumor (myofibroblastic tumor) of the heart. *Ann Diagn Pathol.* 2002;6:116–121.
28. de Montpreville VT, Zemoura L, Vaksmann G, et al. Endocardial location of familial myofibromatosis revealed by cerebral embolization: cardiac counterpart of the frequent intravascular growth of the disease? *Virchows Arch.* 2004;444:300–303.
29. de Montpreville VT, Serraf A, Aznag H, et al. Fibroma and inflammatory myofibroblastic tumor of the heart. *Ann Diagn Pathol.* 2001;5:335–342.
30. Obikane H, Ariizumi K, Yutani C, et al. Inflammatory pseudotumor (inflammatory myofibroblastic tumor) of the mitral valve of the heart. *Pathol Int.* 2010;60:533–537.
31. Declich P, Sironi M, Isimbaldi G, et al. Atrio-ventricular nodal tumor associated with polyendocrine anomalies. *Pathol Res Pract.* 1996;192:54–59; discussion 60–61.
32. Burke AP, Anderson PG, Virmani R, et al. Tumor of the atrioventricular nodal region. A clinical and immunohistochemical study. *Arch Pathol Lab Med.* 1990;114:1057–1062.
33. Pan Y, Chen JL, Li ZJ, et al. Cystic tumour of the atrioventricular node: a case report and review of the literature. *Chin Med J (Engl).* 2012;125:4514–4516.
34. Oost E, Vermeulen T. Cystic tumour of the atrioventricular node: a case report. *Pathology.* 2012;44:487–489.
35. Sharma G, Linden MD, Schultz DS, et al. Cystic tumor of the atrioventricular node: an unexpected finding in an explanted heart. *Cardiovasc Pathol.* 2010;19:e75–e78.

181 Cardiac Myxoma

Joseph J. Maleszewski, M.D., and Allen P. Burke, M.D.

Definition and Histogenesis

Cardiac myxoma is a benign neoplasm characterized by stellate, ovoid, or plump spindle cells (so-called myxoma cells) embedded in a vascular myxoid stroma.[1] While myxoid tumors occur with some frequency in the heart, cardiac myxomas are distinct neoplasms with characteristic histopathologic findings.

While initially thought to represent a reactive phenomenon, heterotopic tissue rests, or organizing thrombi, cardiac myxomas are now considered a neoplastic process by virtue of their location, characteristic histopathology, protein expression, and genetics.[2–4] The precise etiology of the neoplastic cell, the "myxoma" (or *lepidic*) cell, is largely unknown. The diversity of cell types found in myxomas, such as endothelial cells, glandular elements, and apparently undifferentiated cells, has led many investigators to conclude that myxomas are of primitive multipotential mesenchymal origin.[5,6]

Epidemiology

Cardiac myxoma is the most common primary neoplasm of the heart. While other tumors (e.g., papillary fibroelastoma [PFE]) may occur at higher frequency, they do not appear to represent neoplastic processes.[7] They can occur at any age, but most present in the fourth to sixth decades of life. In individuals <65 years of age, there is a female predilection with a male to female ratio of ~1:2.[8] In older individuals, the ratio is much closer to 1:1.[9,10]

Clinical and Radiologic Features

Symptoms

Like all cardiac tumors, the symptoms of cardiac myxoma can be quite diverse and are generally related to tumor size, location, and consistency (Table 181.1). Cardiac myxoma may present with symptoms of hemodynamic obstruction, ranging in presentation from relatively mild (e.g., presyncope or dizziness), to more overt (e.g., syncope), to striking (e.g., frank heart failure or sudden death).[9,11] Symptoms resulting from thromboembolism (from either the tumor itself or adherent surface thrombus) may also occur. Finally (and somewhat curiously), constitutional symptoms have been described in the setting of cardiac myxoma. These include fever, weight loss, cachexia, fatigue, malaise, and arthralgias. These constitutional symptoms are thought to be the result of elaboration of cytokines (namely, IL-6) by the tumor.[12] Importantly, 10% to 20% of cardiac myxomas are found incidentally on routine workup for other conditions not directly related to the tumor.

The Carney Complex

Approximately 3% to 10% of cardiac myxomas occur in the setting of the Carney complex (CNC; also known as the myxoma syndrome).[4] This autosomal dominant condition is characterized by the constellation of myxomas (cardiac or otherwise), endocrinopathy (Cushing syndrome and/or acromegaly), and spotty skin pigmentation (particularly of the vermillion border of the lips). Diagnosis rests on recognition of major criteria or a combination of major and supplemental criteria in a given patient (Table 181.2).[13]

Aside from clinical criteria, inactivating mutations in the *PRKAR1A* gene have been found to be associated with CNC. Pathogenic *PRKAR1A* mutations have been found in more than 60% of individuals with CNC.[13] Genetic testing for such mutations is available clinically and can help to identify and screen CNC kindreds.

Cardiac myxomas arising in the setting of CNC are often multiple and found in atypical locations (outside of the left atrium). Additionally, they are more likely to occur in younger individuals (average age of 25 years) and recur throughout life.

Imaging

Chest radiography may show cardiomegaly and/or pleural effusions.[14] Calcification may be seen in up to 30% of cases and seems to be slightly more common in right atrial myxomas.[9,14] Echocardiography is a sensitive test of cardiac masses, including myxoma. Computed tomography (CT) and cardiac magnetic resonance imaging are often performed for preoperative characterization of tissue density and documentation of the relationship of the tumor to adjacent structures.[15] On CT, there is often a heterogeneous signal of the endocardium-based lesion.[16]

Prognosis

Despite the benign nature of the neoplasm, like other benign cardiac tumors, myxomas can rarely result in devastating consequences, depending on their size, location, and gross characteristics. Villous tumors and tumors containing >50% myxomatous stroma are more likely to embolize, and large tumors are more likely to obstruct. Either of these phenomena could result in sudden death.

Following recognition of the tumor, the prognosis of cardiac myxomas is largely driven by whether or not the tumor is arising in a

TABLE 181.1   Symptoms at Presentation

Symptom	Frequency at Presentation (%)
Valvular obstruction	20–70
Embolic phenomena	35–50
Fever, fatigue, malaise	5–35
Cardiac arrhythmia	10
Chest pain	5
Syncope	5
Sudden death	5
None	10–20

TABLE 181.2   Diagnostic Criteria for Carney Complex[a]

Major criteria
  Cardiac myxoma
  Other myxoma (e.g., cutaneous, mucosal, breast)
  Lentigines (particularly at the vermillion border)
  Cushing syndrome
  Acromegaly
  Large cell calcifying Sertoli cell tumor
  Psammomatous melanotic schwannoma
  Osteochondromyxoma
Supplemental criteria
  Affected first-degree relative
  Inactivating mutation of the *PRKAR1A* gene

[a]Diagnosis requires 2 major criteria or 1 major + 1 supplemental criterion.
Adapted from Stratakis CA, Kirschner LS, Carney JA. Clinical and molecular features of the Carney complex: diagnostic criteria and recommendations for patient evaluation. *J Clin Endocrinol Metab.* 2001;86:4041–4046.

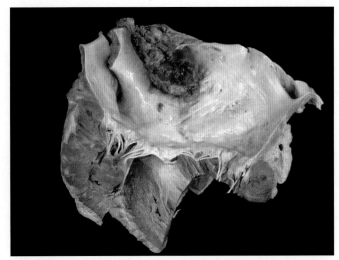

FIGURE 181.1 ▲ Left atrial cardiac myxoma arising from the septum. The sizeable tumor is protruding into the left atrial cavity and partially obstructed blood flow through the mitral valve.

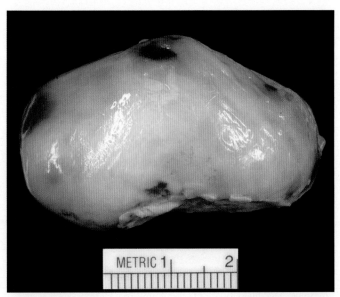

FIGURE 181.3 ▲ A smooth surface tumor with a relatively broad base (**bottom**).

syndromic context. Those tumors occurring in the setting of CNC have a relatively high rate of recurrence (10% to 20%), while those outside of CNC have a very low recurrence rate (<5%).[17,18] Most recurrences occurring in nonsyndromic tumors occur as a result of incomplete tumor resection, which is why it is recommended that the cardiac surgeon take a rim of normal tissue at the attachment site to ensure complete excision.

Pathologic Features

Location and Gross Pathology

Cardiac myxomas are endocardial lesions that protrude into the cardiac chamber from which they arise. Most (80% to 90%) arise in the left atrium, with attachment to the atrial septum in the region of the fossa ovalis (Fig. 181.1). As benign neoplasms, cardiac myxomas do not (by definition) invade, a point that serves to differentiate these lesions from malignant cardiac sarcomas or metastatic lesions. While

these tumors have been described in all cardiac chambers, the finding of a cardiac myxoma outside of the left atrium should raise concern for the possibility of a CNC-associated lesion. Valvular myxomas have been reported, but are distinctly unusual.

The tumors range in size from only a few millimeters to more than 15 cm. They may either arise from a stalk or be sessile and broad based (Fig. 181.2). Grossly, they can be either smooth surfaced or villous (Figs. 181.3 and 181.4). The latter appear to be more associated with

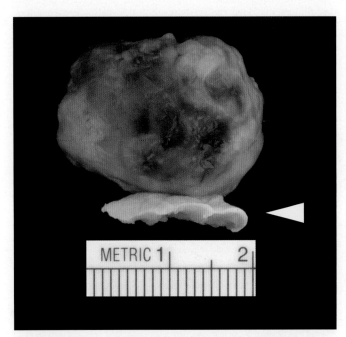

FIGURE 181.2 ▲ Cardiac myxoma with endocardial attachment (*arrowhead*). A rim of the myocardium is typically taken with the tumor at surgical resection to ensure completeness of excision.

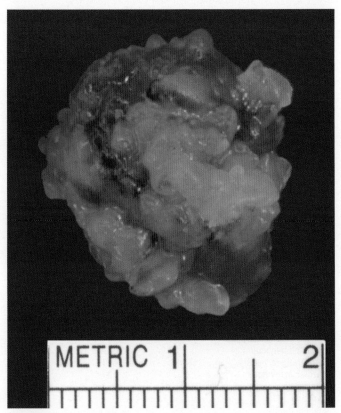

FIGURE 181.4 ▲ A villous and somewhat friable surface, which is more likely to have adherent surface thrombus and be associated with thromboembolic events.

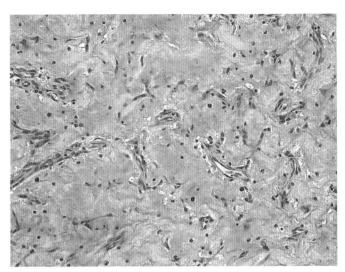

FIGURE 181.5 ▲ Cardiac myxoma exhibiting numerous spindle-shaped myxoma cells within a myxoid matrix. The cells form focal cords and small nests.

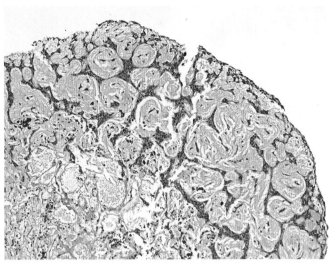

FIGURE 181.7 ▲ Myxoma cells forming cords throughout a myxoid matrix.

thromboembolic symptoms, either from adherent surface thrombus on the finger-like projections of tumor or from the friable tumor itself.[19]

Cardiac myxomas are typically soft but may have areas of dense calcification. The cut surface is usually mucoid or gelatinous, from which the tumor gets name "myxo" (Greek for slimy). Intratumoral hemorrhage is often present and gives the cut surface a variegated appearance. Cystic change is relatively uncommon.

Histopathology

Cardiac myxomas are characterized by the proliferation of myxoma cells in a basophilic or amphophilic, myxoid, stroma with variable degenerative changes that may include thrombosis, calcification, ossification, hemorrhage, and extramedullary hematopoiesis (Figs. 181.5 to 181.10). Mitotic figures may be present, but cellular atypia is uncommon.[1] Myxoma (or lepidic) cells are bland, spindle cells that are either ovoid or stellate in shape. The cells can occur singly or form clusters or rings, the latter of which typically occur around small capillaries (so-called vasocentric rings).

The stroma is usually myxoid, but those tumors with extensive (<50% of area) myxoid stroma have been found more prone to embolization.[9]

Conversely, those tumors with a fibrotic or calcified stroma are less likely to be associated with thromboembolic phenomena.

The background myxoid stroma may also be populated by variable numbers of inflammatory cells and blood vessels. Large thick-walled vessels are often seen in the stalk or attachment of the tumor to the subjacent cardiac wall. The large vessels can occasionally display rather striking thickening with disorganized media, probably owing to the motion of the tumor throughout the cardiac cycle and the to-and-fro traction on them. In addition to the reactive changes in larger vessels, the small vessels are prone to rupture with hemorrhage into the tumor. Accordingly, hemosiderin deposition is very common. In some instances, the iron from said hemorrhage will encrust on endogenous elastin fibers within the tumor, creating dark blue-to-black fibers known as Gamna-Gandy bodies (Fig. 181.11).

Less than 5% of cardiac myxomas show areas of heterologous differentiation. These areas include gland formation (Fig. 181.12) and metaplastic bone formation.[9,20] Glands are seen in 2% of myxoma, typically near the stalk, and may be confused with metastatic adenocarcinoma. Along with the ossification, extramedullary hematopoiesis may

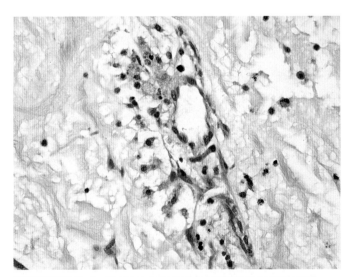

FIGURE 181.6 ▲ Myxoma cells tend to aggregate around small intratumor vessels (so-called vasocentric rings).

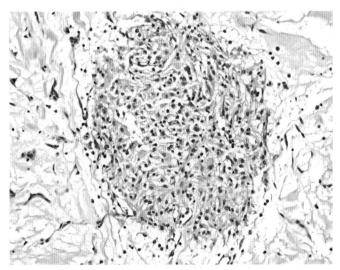

FIGURE 181.8 ▲ Myxoma cells occasionally can form solid aggregates within the tumor.

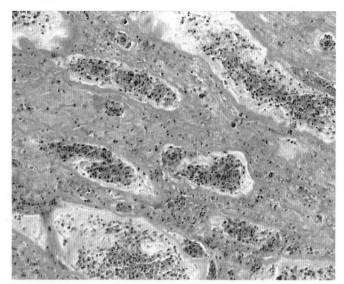

FIGURE 181.9 ▲ Artifactual halos often surround tumor nests and rings. Chronic inflammatory cells are frequently seen both in and out of these aggregates of lesional cells.

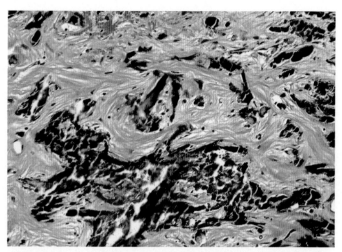

FIGURE 181.11 ▲ Gamna-Gandy bodies (*brown-black* crystals and fibers) are also commonly encountered and are the result of iron encrustation of the elastic fibers within the tumor.

be seen in these tumors as well.[21] Rare instances of chondroid differentiation and oncocytic change have also been reported.

The inflammatory cells that are usually seen in the background are usually polymorphous and may contain scattered giant cells. Rarely, a very exuberant or monotonous population of lymphoid cells may be encountered, raising concern for a lymphoproliferative process. Indeed, cases of diffuse large B-cell lymphoma associated with chronic inflammation have been described arising within cardiac myxomas.[22,23] They are associated with the presence of Epstein-Barr virus and generally have a good prognosis.

Immunohistochemistry

In most cases of cardiac myxoma, the diagnosis can be made on hematoxylin and eosin staining alone. In cases where only a small amount of material was procured or when considering another entity included in the relatively small differential diagnosis of these lesions, a limited panel of immunohistochemical studies may prove useful (Table 181.3). Calretinin reactivity is usually strong and diffuse in cardiac myxoma cells, helping to distinguish cardiac myxoma from hemangioma and organizing thrombus (Fig. 181.13).[24]

Areas of heterologous differentiation may exhibit antigenic features that are compatible with their morphology. Glandular elements, for example, usually react with cytokeratins and other epithelial markers.[20] They may even exhibit enteric differentiation, reacting with antibodies directed against CDX2.

Reactivity with endothelial antibodies (CD31, Fli-1, ERG, factor VIII, and ulex europaeus agglutinin) is predictably seen within the endothelium present in the many blood vessel populating these tumors.[25] Some have also reported variable reactivity of myxoma cells themselves with these antibodies.[19,26] CD34 is invariably expressed within tumor cells (Fig. 181.14).[27]

More recently, antibodies directed against PRKAR1A have shown some utility in the workup of cardiac myxomas.[4] Myxomas arising in the setting of CNC will typically not exhibit reactivity of myxoma cells with PRKAR1A antibodies (Fig. 181.15). Importantly, nonsyndromic tumors may also show this loss of reactivity; therefore, additional germline genetic testing is warranted in the setting of a PRKAR1A-negative tumor.

Genetics

The most compelling evidence for a genetic basis in cardiac myxomas has come from the study of those tumors that arise in the setting of

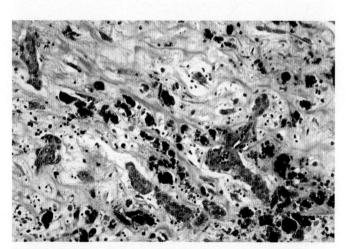

FIGURE 181.10 ▲ Hemosiderin deposition is a usual finding in cardiac myxomas owing to their vascular nature and their propensity to be traumatized throughout the cardiac cycle.

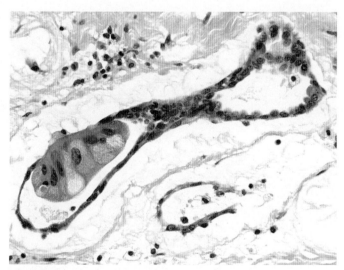

FIGURE 181.12 ▲ Glandular formation within cardiac myxomas is a rare finding that can be confused with a metastatic carcinoma.

TABLE 181.3 Immunohistochemical Profile of Cardiac Myxomas

Antibody	Myxoma Cells
Calretinin	+
CD34	+
Vimentin	+
Thrombomodulin	+
PRKAR1A	+/−[a]
CD31	+/−
Factor VIII	−[b]
S100	−[b]
Desmin	−[b]
SMA	−
NSE	−
EMA	−
Cytokeratins	−[c]

[a]Weak reactivity has been reported.
[b]Tumors arising in the setting of the Carney complex (CNC) are typically (−), while those arising in a nonsyndromic context may be +/−. A (−) result warrants further evaluation to exclude CNC.
[c]Positive in rare tumors (2%) in areas of glandular differentiation.

CNC. Linkage analysis has shown two independent loci to be implicated in CNC: 17q23-24 and 2p16.[13] Inactivating mutations in the *PRKAR1A* gene at the former locus have been described in about two-thirds of cases of CNC. There is also a growing body of evidence to suggest a role for *PRKAR1A* in the development of nonsyndromic myxomas as well.[4]

Cytogenetic studies have thus far not revealed recurrent cytogenetic anomalies in either syndromic or nonsyndromic tumors.[3,28] Nevertheless, advances in somatic nucleic acid sequencing technology are likely to shed more light on the nature of these lesions.

Differential Diagnosis

The differential diagnosis of cardiac myxoma includes organizing thrombus (as well as calcified amorphous tumors), hemangiomas, PFE, sarcomas, and metastatic carcinoma (Table 181.4). Identification of myxoma cells is necessary for a diagnosis of cardiac myxoma and is an important defining characteristic from histologically similar tumors like intracardiac thrombi and cardiac hemangiomas, both of which may have variably myxoid stroma but will lack said myxoma cells. Grossly, a PFE may mimic a cardiac myxoma.

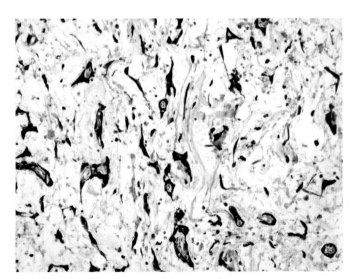

FIGURE 181.13 ▲ Strong reactivity of the myxoma cells with antibodies directed against calretinin.

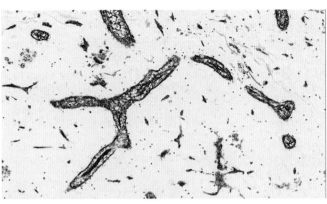

FIGURE 181.14 ▲ Strong reactivity of the myxoma cells with antibodies against CD34.

When not submerged in aqueous solution, the finger-like projections may condense down and impart a mucoid gross appearance on these tumors. Additionally, PFEs may also mimic a villous myxoma, but histologic examination will show PFEs to consist of avascular fibroelastic fronds.

Differentiating cardiac myxomas from metastatic carcinoma becomes important on the rare occasions that heterotopic glandular elements are encountered. In these instances, a thorough history to evaluate for prior malignancy as well as careful examination for myxoma cells will usually lead to the correct interpretation.

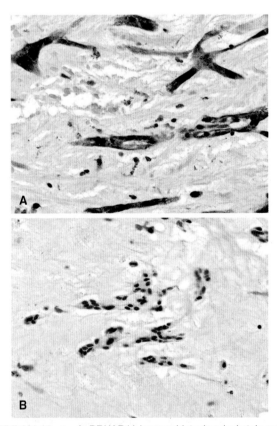

FIGURE 181.15 ▲ **A.** PRKAR1A immunohistochemical stain exhibiting strong reactivity with the myxoma cells in a case of a nonsyndromic myxoma. **B.** Loss of PRKAR1A reactivity is seen in cases of the Carney complex (CNC). While loss of PRKAR1A reactivity can also be seen in nonsyndromic tumors, this lack of staining may warrant additional genetic testing for CNC.

TABLE 181.4   Differential Diagnosis

Lesion	Location	Gross Features	Histologic Features	Immunohistochemistry
Cardiac myxoma	Left atrium (usually septum), endocardial	Mucoid, variegated with hemorrhage	Myxomas cells, myxoid stroma, hemorrhage	Calretinin (+)
Papillary fibroelastoma	Valvular, endocardial	Many fronds (when submerged)	Avascular fibroelastic fronds with endothelial lining	Calretinin (–)
Thrombus	Atrium (usually appendage), endocardial	Relatively homogenous or laminated	Fibrin- or red blood cell rich, +/– organization	Calretinin (–)
Hemangioma	Any chamber, usually mural	Dark red and solid	Blood vessels (often back to back)	Only vascular markers (+)
Sarcoma	Left atrium, usually mural	Solid or mucoid with infiltration of adjacent structures	Pleomorphism, brisk mitotic activity, necrosis	Calretinin (–) Desmin (+/–) Smooth muscle actin (+/–) Myogenin (+/–) MDM2 (+/–) Vascular markers (+/–)
Metastatic carcinoma	Right atrium or right ventricle, usually mural	Firm, well circumscribed	Infiltrating epithelial elements	Primary site dependent

Practical Points

▶ Cardiac myxoma is the most common primary cardiac *neoplasm*.

▶ They usually occur in the left atrium, in the region of the fossa ovalis.

▶ A diagnosis of cardiac myxoma should prompt consideration of the Carney complex, especially for tumors in young (<50 years) individuals and when tumors occur in multiple or in non–left atrial locations.

▶ Cardiac myxomas must be completely excised to reduce the risk of recurrence as much as possible. As such, inking the surface of resection and commenting on the margin status are important.

▶ Differentiation from organizing thrombus and PFE is important and can be achieved by careful gross and histologic evaluation, sometimes with the use of immunohistochemistry.

▶ Heterotopic elements such as glands and bone may be seen in cardiac myxomas and should not be mistaken for a metastatic lesion.

REFERENCES

1. Jain D, Maleszewski JJ. Cardiac myxoma. In: Travis WD, et al., eds. *WHO Classification of Tumours of the Lung, Pleura, Thymus and Heart.* Lyon, France: IARC Press; 2015.
2. Acebo E, Val-Bernal JF, Gomez-Roman JJ. Prichard's structures of the fossa ovalis are not histogenetically related to cardiac myxoma. *Histopathology.* 2001;39:529–535.
3. Dobin S, Speights VO Jr, Donner LR. Addition (1)(q32) as the sole clonal chromosomal abnormality in a case of cardiac myxoma. *Cancer Genet Cytogenet.* 1997;96:181–182.
4. Maleszewski JJ, Larsen BT, Kip NS, et al. PRKAR1A in the development of cardiac myxoma: a study of 110 cases including isolated and syndromic tumors. *Am J Surg Pathol.* 2014;38:1079–1087.
5. Amano J, Kono T, Wada Y, et al. Cardiac myxoma: its origin and tumor characteristics. *Ann Thorac Cardiovasc Surg.* 2003;9:215–221.
6. Vaideeswar P, Butany JW. Benign cardiac tumors of the pluripotent mesenchyme. *Semin Diagn Pathol.* 2008;25:20–28.
7. Tamin SS, Maleszewski JJ, Scott CG, et al. Prognostic and bioepidemiologic implications of papillary fibroelastomas. *J Am Coll Cardiol.* 2015;65:2420–2429.
8. Burke AP, Tavora F, Maleszewski JJ, et al. Cardiac myxoma. In: *Atlas of Tumor Pathology, Tumors of the Heart and Great Vessels.* Washington, DC: American Registry of Pathology; 2015.
9. Burke AP, Virmani R. Cardiac myxoma. A clinicopathologic study. *Am J Clin Pathol.* 1993;100:671–680.
10. Yoon DH, Roberts W. Sex distribution in cardiac myxomas. *Am J Cardiol.* 2002;90:563–565.
11. Scott N, Veinot JP, Chan KL. Symptoms in cardiac myxoma. *Chest.* 2003;124:2408.
12. Vaughan CJ, Gallagher M, Murphy MB. Left ventricular myxoma presenting with constitutional symptoms and raised serum interleukin-6 both suppressed by naproxen. *Eur Heart J.* 1997;18:703.
13. Stratakis CA, Kirschner LS, Carney JA. Clinical and molecular features of the Carney complex: diagnostic criteria and recommendations for patient evaluation. *J Clin Endocrinol Metab.* 2001;86:4041–4046.
14. Grebenc ML, Rosado-de-Christenson ML, Green CE, et al. Cardiac myxoma: imaging features in 83 patients. *Radiographics.* 2002;22:673–689.
15. Jain S, Maleszewski JJ, Stephenson CR, et al. Current diagnosis and management of cardiac myxomas. *Expert Rev Cardiovasc Ther.* 2015;13:369–375.
16. Tsuchiya F, Kohno A, Saitoh R, et al. CT findings of atrial myxoma. *Radiology.* 1984;151:139–143.
17. McCarthy PM, Piehler JM, Schaff HV, et al. The significance of multiple, recurrent, and "complex" cardiac myxomas. *J Thorac Cardiovasc Surg.* 1986;91:389–396.
18. Vidaillet HJ Jr, Seward JB, Fyke FE III, et al. "Syndrome myxoma": a subset of patients with cardiac myxoma associated with pigmented skin lesions and peripheral and endocrine neoplasms. *Br Heart J.* 1987;57:247–255.
19. Pinede L, Duhaut P, Loire R. Clinical presentation of left atrial cardiac myxoma. A series of 112 consecutive cases. *Medicine (Baltimore).* 2001;80:159–172.
20. Pucci A, Bartoloni G, Tessitore E, et al. Cytokeratin profile and neuroendocrine cells in the glandular component of cardiac myxoma. *Virchows Arch.* 2003;443:618–624.
21. Joukhadar R, De Las Casas LE, Lalude O, et al. Cardiac myxoma showing extramedullary hematopoiesis in a patient with beta thalassemia. *South Med J.* 2009;102:769–771.
22. Aguilar C, Beltran B, Quinones P, et al. Large B-cell lymphoma arising in cardiac myxoma or intracardiac fibrinous mass: a localized lymphoma usually associated with Epstein-Barr virus? *Cardiovasc Pathol.* 2015;24:60–64.
23. Svec A, Rangaiah M, Giles M, et al. EBV+ diffuse large B-cell lymphoma arising within atrial myxoma. An example of a distinct primary cardiac EBV+ DLBCL of immunocompetent patients. *Pathol Res Pract.* 2012;208:172–176.
24. Acebo E, Val-Bernal JF, Gomez-Roman JJ. Thrombomodulin, calretinin and c-kit (CD117) expression in cardiac myxoma. *Histol Histopathol.* 2001;16:1031–1036.
25. Silverman JS, Berrutti L. Cardiac myxoma immunohistochemistry: value of CD34, CD31, and factor XIIIa staining. *Diagn Cytopathol.* 1996;15:455–456.
26. Berrutti L, Silverman JS. Cardiac myxoma is rich in factor XIIIa positive dendrophages: immunohistochemical study of four cases. *Histopathology.* 1996;28:529–535.
27. Burke A, Tavora F, Maleszewski JJ, et al. Cardiac myxoma. In: *Tumors of the Heart and Great Vessels.* ARP Press; 2015.
28. Dijkhuizen T, de Jong B, Meuzelaar JJ, et al. No cytogenetic evidence for involvement of gene(s) at 2p16 in sporadic cardiac myxomas: cytogenetic changes in ten sporadic cardiac myxomas. *Cancer Genet Cytogenet.* 2001;126:162–165.

182 Papillary Fibroelastoma

Joseph J. Maleszewski, M.D., and Allen P. Burke, M.D.

Definition and Histogenesis

Papillary fibroelastomas are benign endocardial growths that consist of arborizing, avascular, fibroelastotic fronds enveloped by endothelium. Their nature is somewhat unclear, but there is increasing evidence that they represent reactive phenomena, often arising on traumatized or damaged endocardial surfaces.

Incidence

With the increased usage of cardiac imaging, along with the improved resolution of such studies, papillary fibroelastomas have been found to be more common than cardiac myxoma in the adults.[1,2] In a recent series of surgically resected heart tumors, 11 of 77 tumors were papillary fibroelastomas.[3]

Clinical

Papillary fibroelastoma is somewhat more common in women, with nearly all cases presenting in adults (mean age of ~60 years).[4-7] Most symptoms arise from left-sided lesions that embolize surface thrombus or the papillary fronds themselves into the cerebral circulation or prolapse into the coronary orifice.[8-10] The most common manifestations of embolism are transient neurologic defects and myocardial ischemia[11,12] and rarely sudden death.[13-15]

There is an association with valvular heart disease, such as rheumatic disease, likely owing to the endocardial injury that such imparts.[16] About 20% of papillary fibroelastomas develop as a result of iatrogenic factors,[15,17] including thoracic irradiation and open heart surgery (sub-aortic septal myectomy, valve repair, valve replacement, and repair of congenital defects).[15,18,19]

Imaging

Papillary fibroelastomas are often first visualized by two-dimensional echocardiography, and the tumor may be an incidental finding or be detected after cerebral ischemia.[20-27] They usually arise singly, but multiple lesions are found in between 10% and 30% of cases.[28] The added resolution of transesophageal echocardiography is helpful in cases of those papillary fibroelastomas that arise in unusual sites, such as nonvalvular surfaces.[29,30]

Location

Papillary fibroelastomas are invariably located on an endocardial surface, with 90% located on valves. The most common site, especially of symptomatic lesions, is the aortic or mitral valve; right-sided tumors, such as those located on the tricuspid valve, are often asymptomatic.[31] Unusual nonvalvular sites include the papillary muscles, the ostium of the right coronary artery, ventricular septum, left ventricular outflow tract, left atrium, right atrium, right ventricular outflow tract, pulmonary valve, and Chiari network.[32-34]

Gross Pathologic Findings

Grossly, papillary fibroelastomas are filiform papillary tumors that open up to a somewhat pom-pom-like mass when placed under water (Fig. 182.1). The appearance has been likened to that of a sea

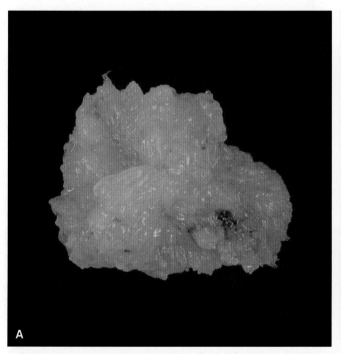
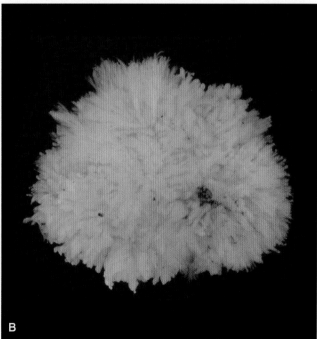

FIGURE 182.1 ▲ Papillary fibroelastoma, gross findings. **A.** Surgically resected papillary fibroelastoma outside of aqueous medium takes on an almost myxoid appearance as the papillary fronds collapse on themselves. **B.** When placed in solution, the tumor fronds unfurl and the tumor exhibits its resemblance to a sea anemone.

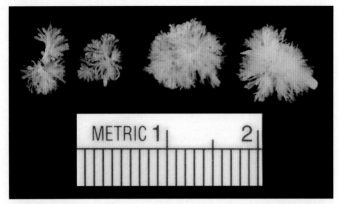

FIGURE 182.2 ▲ Papillary fibroelastomas, gross findings. Tumors can be multiple, as in this example of four different sized lesions.

anemone, although most of the sea animals have thicker tentacles than do the thin papillae of the cardiac tumor. When outside of aqueous solution, the fronds aggregate together, often imparting a myxoid quality to the lesion causing diagnostic confusion with the cardiac myxoma (Fig. 182.1). Papillary fibroelastomas range in size from 2 to 50 mm in greatest dimension and are usually attached to the endocardial surface by a short single stalk (Figs. 182.2 and 182.3). The lower end of the size spectrum is somewhat arbitrary, as the tumors overlap with Lambl excrescences with which they form a spectrum.

Microscopic Pathology

The papillary fronds of papillary fibroelastoma are usually narrow, elongated, and branching (Figs. 182.4 and 182.5). The papillae resemble tendinous cords but have a slightly different arrangement of elastic fibers when present. The matrix consists of mucopolysaccharides, elastic fibers, and rare spindle cells resembling smooth muscle cells or fibroblasts (Figs. 182.6 and 182.7). Elastic tissue is frequently absent or inconspicuous, despite the name of the tumor (Figs. 182.5 and 182.7).

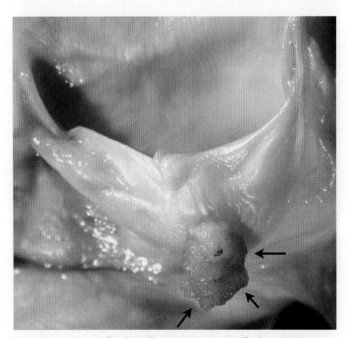

FIGURE 182.3 ▲ Papillary fibroelastoma, gross findings in situ. A 4- to 5-mm papillary fibroelastoma (*arrows*) is seen arising centrally on the posterior aortic valve cusp near the line of closure.

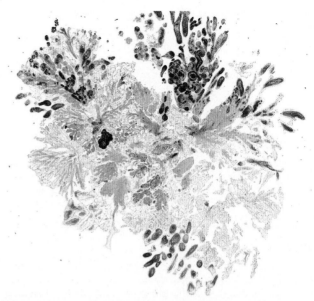

FIGURE 182.4 ▲ Papillary fibroelastoma, histologic findings. Numerous papillary fronds are evident on microscopic examination, analogous to the gross appearance (Verhoeff-van Gieson stain).

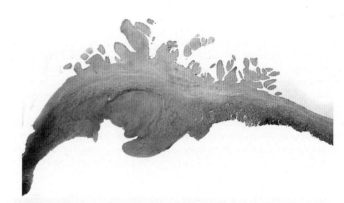

FIGURE 182.5 ▲ Papillary fibroelastoma, histologic findings. A more sessile lesion is seen arising on a valvular surface (Verhoeff-van Gieson stain).

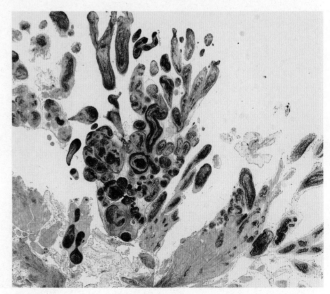

FIGURE 182.6 ▲ Papillary fibroelastoma, histologic findings. The elastic nature of the fronds is often evident when viewed with an elastic stain.

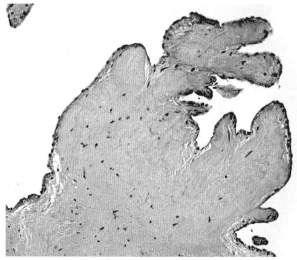

FIGURE 182.7 ▲ Papillary fibroelastoma, histologic findings. The avascular fronds can be devoid of elastic fibers, containing only rare, stromal, spindle cells, with the endothelial surface.

The papillary cores contain a proteoglycan-rich stroma, and layers of elastic fibers and collagen are prominent near the base of the lesion. There may be adherent surface fibrin (Fig. 182.8).

Treatment and Prognosis

The treatment of symptomatic papillary fibroelastoma is simple excision, which is curative.[35] Most often, the tumor can be removed without excision of significant areas of adjacent tissue, with minimal repair of the valve leaflet.[36,37] Valve-sparing excision produces good long-term results in most instances.[38] Valve replacement, as was performed in the past, is rarely necessary with current valve-sparing techniques.[39,40]

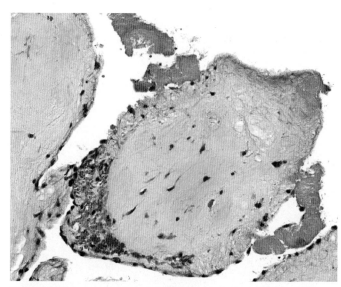

FIGURE 182.8 ▲ Papillary fibroelastoma, histologic findings. Occasionally, surface fibrin may be seen on the fronds. In addition to the tumor itself, the fibrin may embolize and be responsible for systemic symptoms in left-sided lesions.

REFERENCES

1. Tamin SS, Maleszewski JJ, Scott CG, et al. Prognostic and bioepidemiologic implications of papillary fibroelastomas. *J Am Coll Cardiol.* 2015;65:2420–2429.
2. Fleischmann KE, Schiller NB. Papillary fibroelastoma: move over myxoma. *J Am Coll Cardiol.* 2015;65:2430–2432.
3. Bossert T, Gummert JF, Battellini R, et al. Surgical experience with 77 primary cardiac tumors. *Interact Cardiovasc Thorac Surg.* 2005;4:311–315.
4. Amr SS, Abual Ragheb SY. Sudden unexpected death due to papillary fibroma of the aortic valve. Report of a case and review of the literature. *Am J Forensic Med Pathol.* 1991;12:143–148.
5. Edwards FH, Hale D, Cohen A, et al. Primary cardiac valve tumors. *Ann Thorac Surg.* 1991;52:1127–1131.
6. Fishbein MC, Ferrans VJ, Roberts WC. Endocardial papillary elastofibromas. Histologic, histochemical, and electron microscopical findings. *Arch Pathol.* 1975;99:335–341.
7. Heath D, Best PV, Davis BT. Papilliferous tumours of the heart valves. *Br Heart J.* 1961;23:20–24.
8. Anastacio MM, Moon MR, Damiano RJ Jr, et al. Surgical experience with cardiac papillary fibroelastoma over a 15-year period. *Ann Thorac Surg.* 2012;94:537–541.
9. Raju V, Srinivasan M, Padmanaban C, et al. Left main coronary artery embolus: unusual presentation of papillary fibroelastoma of the aortic valve. *Tex Heart Inst J.* 2010;37:365–367.
10. Itrat A, George P, Khawaja Z, et al. Pathological evidence of cardiac papillary fibroelastoma in a retrieved intracranial embolus. *Can J Neurol Sci.* 2015;42:66–68.
11. Bruno VD, Mariscalco G, De Vita S, et al. Aortic valve papillary fibroelastoma: a rare cause of angina. *Tex Heart Inst J.* 2011;38:456–457.
12. Vivacqua A, Shafii A, Kalahasti V, et al. Images in cardiology. Ventricular outflow tract papillary fibroelastoma presenting with non-ST-segment elevation myocardial infarction. *J Am Coll Cardiol.* 2010;55:2607.
13. Bottio T, Pittarello D, Bonato R, et al. Echocardiographic diagnosis of aortic valve papillary fibroelastoma. *Tex Heart Inst J.* 2004;31:322–323.
14. Boulmier D, Ecke JE, Verhoye JP. Recurrent myocardial infarction due to obstruction of the RCA ostium by an aortic papillary fibroelastoma. *J Invasive Cardiol.* 2002;14:686–688.
15. Kurup AN, Tazelaar HD, Edwards WD, et al. Iatrogenic cardiac papillary fibroelastoma: a study of 12 cases (1990 to 2000). *Hum Pathol.* 2002;33:1165–1169.
16. Kalman JM, Lubicz S, Brennan JB, et al. Multiple cardiac papillary fibroelastomas and rheumatic heart disease. *Aust N Z J Med.* 1991;21:744–746.
17. Kumar TK, Kuehl K, Reyes C, et al. Multiple papillary fibroelastomas of the heart. *Ann Thorac Surg.* 2009;88:e66–e67.
18. Kim RW, Jeffery ME, Smith MJ, et al. Minimally invasive resection of papillary fibroelastoma in a high-risk patient. *J Cardiovasc Med (Hagerstown).* 2007;8:639–641.
19. Zamora RL, Adelberg DA, Berger AS, et al. Branch retinal artery occlusion caused by a mitral valve papillary fibroelastoma—correction. *Am J Ophthalmol.* 1995;120:126.
20. Matsumoto N, Sato Y, Kusama J, et al. Multiple papillary fibroelastomas of the aortic valve: case report. *Int J Cardiol.* 2007;122:e1–e13.
21. Shub C, Tajik AJ, Seward JB, et al. Cardiac papillary fibroelastomas. Two-dimensional echocardiographic recognition. *Mayo Clin Proc.* 1981;56:629–633.
22. Frumin H, O'Donnell L, Kerin NZ, et al. Two-dimensional echocardiographic detection and diagnostic features of tricuspid papillary fibroelastoma. *J Am Coll Cardiol.* 1983;2:1016–1018.
23. Fowles RE, Miller DC, Egbert BM, et al. Systemic embolization from a mitral valve papillary endocardial fibroma detected by two-dimensional echocardiography. *Am Heart J.* 1981;102:128–130.
24. Mann J, Parker DJ. Papillary fibroelastoma of the mitral valve: a rare cause of transient neurological deficits. *Br Heart J.* 1994;71:6.
25. McFadden PM, Lacy JR. Intracardiac papillary fibroelastoma: an occult cause of embolic neurologic deficit. *Ann Thorac Surg.* 1987;43:667–669.
26. Richard J, Castello R, Dressler FA, et al. Diagnosis of papillary fibroelastoma of the mitral valve complicated by non-Q-wave infarction with apical thrombus: transesophageal and transthoracic echocardiographic study. *Am Heart J.* 1993;126:710–712.

27. Narang J, Neustein S, Israel D. The role of transesophageal echocardiography in the diagnosis and excision of a tumor of the aortic valve. *J Cardiothorac Vasc Anesth.* 1992;6:68–69.

28. Le Tourneau T, Pouwels S, Gal B, et al. Assessment of papillary fibro-elastomas with live three-dimensional transthoracic echocardiography. *Echocardiography.* 2008;25:489–495.

29. Baba Y, Tsuboi Y, Sakiyama K, et al. Cardiac papillary fibroelastoma as a cause of recurrent ischemic strokes: the diagnostic value of serial trans-esophageal echocardiography. *Cerebrovasc Dis.* 2002;14:256–259.

30. Vora TR. Unusual presentation of papillary fibroelastoma: utility of serial transesophageal echocardiograms. *Echocardiography.* 2004;21:69–71.

31. Massarenti L, Benassi F, Gallerano A, et al. Papillary fibroelastoma of the tricuspid anterior leaflet. *J Cardiovasc Med (Hagerstown).* 2009;10:933–935.

32. Valente M, Basso C, Thiene G, et al. Fibroelastic papilloma: a not so benign cardiac tumor. *Cardiovasc Pathol.* 1992;1:161–166.

33. Yagoub H, Abdullah AS, Ibrahim A, et al. Pulmonary valve papillary fibro-elastoma: a rare tumor and rare location. *Rev Cardiovasc Med.* 2015;16:90–93.

34. Taha A, Carr S, Beckwith LG, et al. Papillary fibroelastoma involving chor-dae of the mitral valve with two aortic valve excrescences. *J Heart Valve Dis.* 2015;24:270–271.

35. Topol EJ, Biern RO, Reitz BA. Cardiac papillary fibroelastoma and stroke. Echocardiographic diagnosis and guide to excision. *Am J Med.* 1986;80:129–132.

36. Di Marco L, Al-Basheer A, Glineur D, et al. Aortic valve repair for papillary fibroelastoma. *J Cardiovasc Med (Hagerstown).* 2006;7:362–364.

37. Chavanon O, Hlal M, Bakkali A, et al. Multiple microthrombi on a papillary fibroelastoma of the aortic valve. *Ann Thorac Surg.* 2012;93:304–306.

38. Gopaldas RR, Atluri PV, Blaustein AS, et al. Papillary fibroelastoma of the aortic valve: operative approaches upon incidental discovery. *Tex Heart Inst J.* 2009;36:160–163.

39. Marvasti MA, Obeid AI, Cohen PS, et al. Successful removal of papillary endocardial fibroma. *Thorac Cardiovasc Surg.* 1983;31:254–255.

40. Georghiou GP, Shapira Y, Stamler A, et al. Surgical excision of papillary fibroelastoma for known or potential embolization. *J Heart Valve Dis.* 2005;14:843–847.

183 Miscellaneous Benign and Low-Grade Tumors

Allen P. Burke, M.D., and Fabio R. Tavora, M.D., Ph.D.

Hemangioma

Clinical

Cardiac hemangiomas constitute fewer than 10% of benign cardiac tumors. Approximately 200 have been reported.[1] They occur in all ages with a mean in the 5th decade. Up to 25% of cardiac hemangiomas occur in infants and young children.[2]

Most cardiac hemangiomas are discovered incidentally. Cardiac hemangiomas may cause arrhythmias, pericardial effusions, conges-tive heart failure, outflow tract obstruction, and rarely sudden death.[2] Extracardiac hemangiomas can occur in association with cardiac lesions, especially in the gastrointestinal tract.[3]

Pathologic Findings

Grossly, cardiac hemangiomas are usually mural lesions but can also be found in the subendocardial space, as dark red well-circumscribed nodules that measure from <1 to 4 cm or larger in maximum diameter.

Those endocardial lesions are usually of the capillary type histologi-cally. In contrast, the less common intramural hemangiomas that arise with the ventricular wall resemble intramuscular hemangiomas of soft tissue.[3] Approximately half of these show at least focal thickened vessel walls that suggest arteriovenous malformations, and fat and fibrous tis-sue are not uncommon.

Endocardial-based hemangiomas of the heart are occasionally misdiagnosed as myxomas, because of their vascularity and myxoid stroma (Fig. 183.1). However, their vessels are mature and, in contrast to myxoma, are invested with actin-positive pericytes. In further dis-tinction from myxoma, hemangiomas are calretinin negative.

Endocardial-based hemangiomas may also be confused with organized thrombus. However, organized thrombi will in some areas demonstrate typical features of entrapped blood, fibrin, and hemosid-erin. Hemangiomas that infiltrate the trabeculae of the right atrium may be particularly difficult to distinguish from organized thrombus (Fig. 183.2).

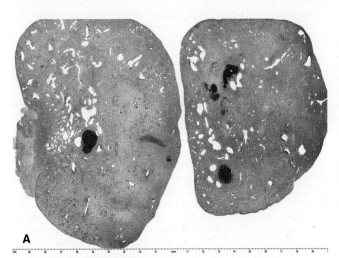
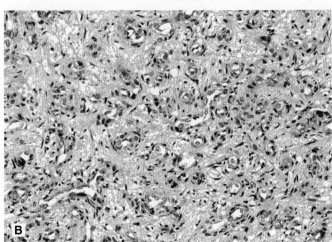

FIGURE 183.1 ▲ Cardiac hemangioma. **A.** Low magnification demonstrates a cellular tumor with scat-tered spaces (dilated vascular channels). **B.** Higher magnification of a cellular area shows features of capillary hemangioma.

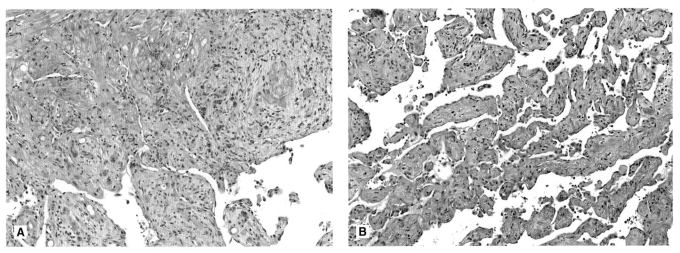

FIGURE 183.2 ▲ Cardiac hemangioma. **A.** The interface between the right atrial muscle (above) and tumor (below) is seen. The diagnosis is subtle in this area. **B.** Another area of the same tumor showing a papillary growth pattern that can occasionally cause diagnostic difficulties with angiosarcoma.

Benign Fatty Tumors

Lipomatous Hypertrophy of the Atrial Septum

Lipomatous hypertrophy of the atrial septum (LHAS) is a tumor-like condition characterized by excessive deposition of fat in the interatrial septum and a thickness of >2 cm[4,5] (Fig. 183.3A). It has been considered a form of hamartoma of immature brown fat. It has also been speculated to be part of a metabolic condition since there seems to be a strong correlation of LHAS with obesity.[5] LHAS, although anatomically located within the atrial septum, has a tendency to bulge into the right atrium. For this reason, the lesions are often interpreted by computed tomography or magnetic resonance as right atrial tumors.

Of the clinically apparent cases, the two most common signs are related to supraventricular arrhythmias and atrioventricular or right atrial inflow obstruction.[4] Computed tomography and magnetic resonance can also be useful investigations for diagnosis and in planning surgery. Surgical excision of the septal fat necessitates atrial reconstruction with pericardial or Dacron patches.

Macroscopically, LHAS cannot be distinguished from normal epicardial fat. There is usually no tumor capsule.[4]

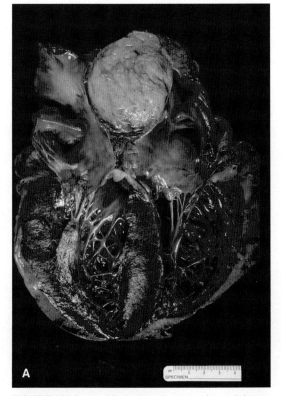

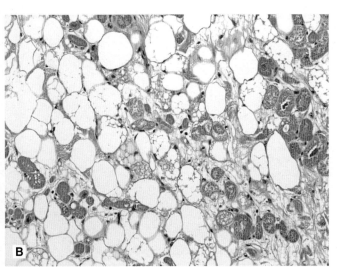

FIGURE 183.3 ▲ Lipomatous hypertrophy, atrial septum. **A.** Gross photograph demonstrates incidental atrial septal thickening by fat. The ventricles are dilated (dilated cardiomyopathy). **B.** Histologic section shows vacuolated brown fat cells and interspersed myocytes, which typically have enlarged hyperchromatic nuclei.

Histologically, there is a mixture of adipose tissue, fibrotic stroma, and hypertrophied myocytes. The adipocytes are vacuolated and resemble hibernoma-like brown fat (Fig. 183.3B). Enlarged hypertrophic myocytes are present in the areas of fibrosis with a haphazard arrangement, which sometimes leads to an erroneous impression of liposarcoma.

Cardiac Lipoma

Lipomas represent 1% to 3% of surgically excised tumors of the heart.[6] True cardiac lipomas are circumscribed lesions with a predilection to the epicardium. Lipomas of the cardiac valves, which usually occur on the mitral valve, have been referred to as fibrolipomas and lipomatous hamartomas.[7,8]

There is an association between tuberous sclerosis and multiple cardiac lipomas, which are seen primarily by magnetic resonance imaging. Histologic confirmation of lipoma has only rarely been reported.[9]

Cardiac lipomas are pathologically similar to lipomas elsewhere. Grossly, they are fatty-appearing tumors that can show a thin capsule. They are most frequent on the epicardial surface but may also occur within the cardiac walls and fill a cardiac chamber. Microscopically, mature adipocytes indistinguishable from normal fat form the tumor mass.

Paraganglioma

Terminology and Clinical Findings

Cardiac paragangliomas constitute a small proportion of extra-adrenal paragangliomas. The term "pheochromocytoma" is generally reserved for functional tumors. Over 75% of cardiac paragangliomas are functional and may cause episodic hypertension.[10]

Paraganglial cells are found normally in the atrial walls, and that is the location of the majority of these tumors when they occur in the heart. Tumors of the aorticopulmonary window, another site of paraganglial tissue, may protrude into the atrial and atrioventricular valves and also form tumors involving the heart.[11,12]

The age of presentation can range from children to the elderly, but most patients present between 20 and 60 years of age. Like paragangliomas elsewhere in the body, the majority of cardiac paragangliomas are benign and cured by complete excision. Invasion of cardiac structures may necessitate radical surgery or transplantation, however. In addition, there have been reports of malignant paragangliomas in the heart.[12,13]

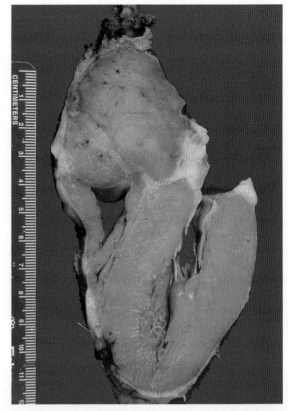

FIGURE 183.4 ▲ Cardiac paraganglioma, explant. The tumor has a copper bronze color. It is adherent to the aortic wall. The tumor could not be excised surgically. The tumor presumably arose from paraganglial cells of the aorticopulmonary window.

Pathologic Findings

The gross pathology of cardiac paragangliomas is characterized by a large poorly circumscribed mass that can measure up to 15 cm[14] (Fig. 183.4). Focal hemorrhage can be seen grossly, as these tumors are highly vascular. Paragangliomas of the heart are similar histologically and immunohistochemically to extracardiac paragangliomas (Fig. 183.5). Occasionally, cytoplasmic clearing is a prominent feature.

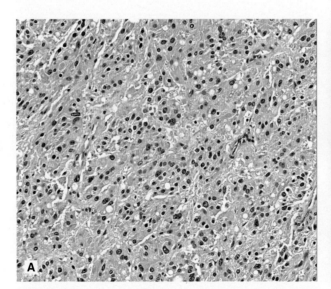

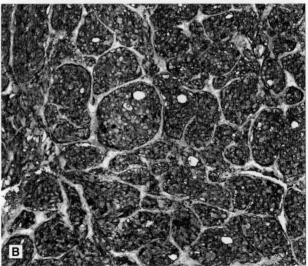

FIGURE 183.5 ▲ Cardiac paraganglioma. **A.** Hematoxylin–eosin stain shows abundant eosinophilic cytoplasm and variably sized nuclei. **B.** Immunohistochemical staining for synaptophysin highlights the compartmentalized "Zellballen" growth pattern.

The diagnosis is made on regular hematoxylin and eosin stains and can be confirmed by tumor expression of chromogranin or synaptophysin. S100 highlights sustentacular cells.[10]

Other Benign Heart Tumors

Adult cellular rhabdomyoma is an extremely rare cardiac neoplasm of striated muscle cells, pathologically similar to those occurring in the head and neck region. Because the latter are termed "extracardiac rhabdomyoma" in order to distinguish them from benign cardiac rhabdomyomas, which are hamartomas (see Chapter 180), those that occur in the heart have a separate designation.[15]

Hamartoma of mature cardiac myocytes is a poorly defined mass of large, disorganized cardiac muscle cells that may represent a very localized form of hypertrophic cardiomyopathy.[16,17] Histologically, the enlarged tumor cells merge imperceptibly with normal cardiac muscle and show evidence of disarray and interstitial fibrosis.[18]

Neurogenic tumors that occur in the heart include *schwannomas*[19] and *granular cell tumors*.[20]

REFERENCES

1. Li W, Teng P, Xu H, et al. Cardiac hemangioma: a comprehensive analysis of 200 cases. *Ann Thorac Surg.* 2015;99:2246–2252.
2. Thomas de Montpréville V, Maleszewski JJ. Haemangioma. In: Travis WD, et al., eds. *WHO Classification of Tumours of the Lung, Pleura, Thymus and Heart.* Lyon, France: IARC Press; 2015:318–320.
3. Burke A, Johns JP, Virmani R. Hemangiomas of the heart. A clinicopathologic study of ten cases. *Am J Cardiovasc Pathol.* 1990;3:283–290.
4. Burke A, Litovsky S, Virmani R. Lipomatous hypertrophy of the atrial septum presenting as a right atrial mass. *Am J Surg Pathol.* 1996;20:678–685.
5. Shirani J, Roberts W. Clinical, electrocardiographic and morphologic features of massive fatty deposits ("lipomatous hypertrophy") in the atrial septum. *J Am Coll Cardiol.* 1993;22:226–238.
6. Veinot JP. Lipoma. In: Travis WD, et al., eds. *WHO Classification of Tumours of the Lung, Pleura, Thymus and Heart.* Lyon, France: IARC Press; 2015:322–323.
7. Francisco A, Gouveia R, Anjos R. Mitral valve lipomatous hamartoma: a rare entity. *Cardiol Young.* 2014;24:923–925.
8. Bhat SP, Gowda SIG, Chikkatur R, et al. Lipomatous hamartoma of mitral valve. *Asian Cardiovasc Thorac Ann.* 2016;24(1):34–35.
9. Jabir S, Al-Hyassat S. Histological diagnosis of cardiac lipoma in an adult with tuberous sclerosis. *BMJ Case Rep.* 2013. doi: 10.1136/bcr-2012-007484.
10. Burke AP, Thomas de Montpréville V, Fletcher CDM, et al. Paraganglioma. In: Travis WD, et al., eds. *WHO Classification of Tumours of the Lung, Pleura, Thymus and Heart.* Lyon, France: IARC Press; 2015:326–327.
11. Abad C, Jimenez P, Santana C, et al. Primary cardiac paraganglioma. Case report and review of surgically treated cases. *J Cardiovasc Surg (Torino).* 1992;33:768–772.
12. Cruz PA, Mahidhara S, Ticzon A, et al. Malignant cardiac paraganglioma: follow-up of a case. *J Thorac Cardiovasc Surg.* 1984;87:942–944.
13. Jirari A, Charpentier A, Popescu S, et al. A malignant primary cardiac pheochromocytoma. *Ann Thorac Surg.* 1999;68:565–566.
14. Lupinski RW, Shankar S, Agasthian T, et al. Primary cardiac paraganglioma. *Ann Thorac Surg.* 2004;78:e43–e44.
15. Burke AP, Gatto-Weis C, Griego JE, et al. Adult cellular rhabdomyoma of the heart: a report of 3 cases. *Hum Pathol.* 2002;33:1092–1097.
16. Dell'Amore A, Lanzanova G, Silenzi A, et al. Hamartoma of mature cardiac myocytes: case report and review of the literature. *Heart Lung Circ.* 2011;20:336–340.
17. Raffa GM, Tarelli G, Balzarini L, et al. Hamartoma of mature cardiac myocytes: a cardiac tumour with preserved contractility. *Eur Heart J Cardiovasc Imaging.* 2013;14:1216.
18. Burke AP, Ribe JK, Bajaj AK, et al. Hamartoma of mature cardiac myocytes. *Hum Pathol.* 1998;29:904–909.
19. Burke AP, Thomas de Montpréville V, Fletcher CDM, et al. Schwannoma. In: Travis WD, et al., eds. *WHO Classification of Tumours of the Lung, Pleura, Thymus and Heart.* Lyon, France: IARC Press; 2015:325.
20. Burke AP, Thomas de Montpréville V, Fletcher CDM, et al. Granular cell tumour. In: Travis WD, et al., eds. *WHO Classification of Tumours of the Lung, Pleura, Thymus and Heart.* Lyon, France: IARC Press; 2015:324.

184 Sarcomas of the Heart and Great Vessels

Joseph J. Maleszewski, M.D., and Allen P. Burke, M.D.

Sarcomas of the Heart

General Features

Approximately 10% of primary cardiac tumors are malignant, and the vast majority of these are sarcomas. The current accepted classification is based on histologic appearance. The most frequent cardiac sarcoma that exhibits lineage-specific differentiation is angiosarcoma, but most cardiac sarcomas exhibit little (if any) differentiation.

Owing to their rarity, it is difficult to conduct large series to evaluate histologic grading and staging of cardiac sarcomas. Nevertheless, the current WHO classification has largely adapted the schemes used in noncardiac mesenchymal malignances to those seen in the heart. Such includes evaluation of cellular differentiation, necrosis, and mitotic activity. Grading systems such as the Fédération Nationale des Centres de Lutte Contre le Cancer, which are available in the College of American Pathologist Cancer Protocols as well as the American Joint Committee on Cancer, have also been employed.[1]

Regardless of the grading/staging system employed, most of these lesions carry a grave prognosis, with death often occurring within months of the diagnosis. Treatment is typically aimed at palliation and typically consists of surgical resection and/or adjuvant chemotherapy/radiotherapy.

Angiosarcoma

Definition

Cardiac angiosarcoma is a primary cardiac sarcoma exhibiting primarily endothelial differentiation.

Epidemiology

Angiosarcoma is the most common primary cardiac malignancy with differentiation, accounting for ~40% of cardiac sarcomas in the larger series reported.[2] Because they are often infiltrative and not amenable to surgical excision, they tend to represent a relatively small proportion of cardiac tumors in surgical series.

Clinical and Radiologic Features

Cardiac angiosarcomas occur over a wide age range (mean, 40 years), with no strong sex predilection. Nearly all lesions are sporadic in nature, but familial cases have been rarely reported.[3]

Cardiac angiosarcoma results in a variety of cardiac symptoms, including chest pain, shortness of breath, and pericarditis. When the pericardium is involved, hemopericardium and tamponade may occur and are more commonly seen in the setting of angiosarcoma (compared to other cardiac malignancies) owing to the vascular nature of the lesion. There may be a misdiagnosis of chronic pericarditis leading to delay in diagnosis. The first clinical manifestations may relate to metastatic disease, which is common.[4]

Echocardiographically, cardiac angiosarcomas are usually echogenic and lobulated. Pericardial effusion is also frequently seen. Computed tomography (CT) and cardiac magnetic resonance imaging (cMRI) usually reveal a heterogeneous, nodular mass. The vascular nature of the tumor is well demonstrated with contrast studies.[4] Multimodality imaging is useful in characterization of the tumor and in guiding biopsy of the lesion of interest.

Cardiac angiosarcoma is diagnosed by open biopsy, mediastinoscopy, echocardiogram-guided fine needle aspiration, and pericardial biopsy. Cytologic examination of pericardial effusion has not proven very sensitive. Transvenous endomyocardial biopsy guided by transesophageal echocardiography is relatively a noninvasive mode of diagnosis.[5]

Location and Gross Pathology

Most cardiac angiosarcomas arise in the right atrium, usually in the region of the atrioventricular sulcus. The tumor frequently replaces the right atrial free wall and protrudes into the chamber and/or pericardial space. The tumor often involves the pericardium as well. Left atrial angiosarcomas have also been described, but occur in <10% of cases (Table 184.1).

Grossly, cardiac angiosarcomas are red-brown (hemorrhagic), irregular masses that generally range from 2.0 to 10 cm in size. Occasionally, the tumors can appear more fleshy and yellow-white. The tumors usually exhibit extensive infiltration of the adjacent myocardial tissue and may significantly protrude into the atrial cavity or into the pericardial space.

Histopathology

Histologically, cardiac angiosarcomas have a rather variable appearance. Nearly two-thirds of tumors are relatively well differentiated, with the bulk of the tumor composed of malignant endothelial cells forming papillary structures and/or anastomosing, irregular, vascular spaces. The lining cells are atypical and usually pleomorphic. Mitotic activity is usually abundant (Fig. 184.1).

The remaining third consist of poorly differentiated, spindle cell, lesions. These lesions often contain abundant red blood cells, some of which appear to be contained within intracytoplasmic vacuoles (intracellular lumina).

As noted above, there is no established grading system for cardiac angiosarcomas. They are generally considered high grade regardless of histologic features. Nevertheless, the presence of necrosis and a high proliferative index may portend an incrementally more aggressive process.

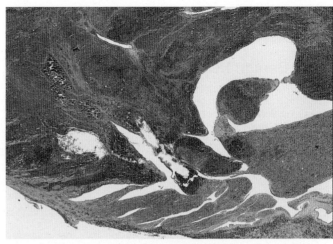

FIGURE 184.1 ▲ Cardiac angiosarcoma. A cellular hemorrhagic tumor infiltrates the right atrial wall. High magnification shows a cellular spindle cell neoplasm with interspersed erythrocytes.

Immunohistochemistry

Immunohistochemical staining for endothelial markers is useful. The most sensitive markers include CD31, ERG, and Fli-1. CD34 is not as specific for endothelial cells, but is usually reactive with the neoplastic cells.

Prognosis

The survival of patients with angiosarcoma of the heart is relatively poor in comparison with other cardiac sarcomas. A median survival of 13 months has been reported, with better survival among patients with localized disease.[6] A recent report showed a mean survival of 29 months.[7]

Cardiac angiosarcomas have an especially poor prognosis because they typically present with metastatic disease, often in multiple sites, including the lung and bone.

Differential Diagnosis

Well-differentiated cardiac angiosarcomas are uncommon, but may be confused with hemangiomas. The latter can be intramyocardial and appear infiltrative, but lack the pleomorphism and mitotic activity of angiosarcoma.

Papillary endothelial hyperplasia may occur within atrial thrombi and can mimic the anastomosing growth pattern of cardiac angiosarcoma; however, infiltrative growth and atypia are absent.

TABLE 184.1   Frequency of Histologic Subtypes of Cardiac Sarcomas

Type	Frequency (n, %)	Mean Age, Years ± S.D.	% Men
Pleomorphic spindle sarcoma (undifferentiated pleomorphic sarcoma)	50 (26%)	48 ± 21	46%
Angiosarcoma	47 (24%)	40 ± 17	79%
Undifferentiated sarcoma	20 (10%)	51 ± 20	45%
Osteosarcoma (matrix-forming sarcoma)	19 (10%)	40 ± 18	37%
Fibromyxosarcoma	18 (9%)	42 ± 19	56%
Leiomyosarcoma	14 (7%)	27 ± 16	57%
Synovial sarcoma	9 (5%)	46 ± 13	89%
Rhabdomyosarcoma	8 (4%)	20 ± 16	25%
MPNST	2 (<1%)	52 ± 5	100%
Liposarcoma	2 (<1%)	67 ± 4	50%
EHE, malignant SFT, malignant mesenchymoma	1 each (1.5% total)	71, 21, 46	0%
Total	192 (100%)	43 ± 20	56%

EHE, epithelioid hemangioendothelioma; MPNST, malignant peripheral nerve sheath tumor; SFT, solitary fibrous tumor.
From a database of 192 tumors seen by one coauthor in consultation.

Other cardiac sarcomas may also be confused with angiosarcoma, particularly in cases of spindle cell angiosarcomas. In these instances, immunohistochemistry is very useful to demonstrate endothelial antigenicity.

Undifferentiated Pleomorphic Sarcoma

Definition
Undifferentiated pleomorphic sarcomas are high-grade sarcomas showing no specific pattern of differentiation based on ancillary studies. In the past, these lesions have been referred to as undifferentiated sarcomas, intimal sarcomas, and malignant fibrous histiocytoma. The precise cell of origin is unknown.

Epidemiology
Undifferentiated pleomorphic sarcomas are as or slightly more common than cardiac angiosarcoma. They typically occur at an average age between 40 and 50 years with no obvious sex predilection.

Clinical and Radiologic Features
Undifferentiated pleomorphic sarcomas of the heart may present with symptoms related to direct effects of the primary tumor such obstruction (e.g., mitral stenosis, pulmonary vein stenosis, etc.) or symptoms related to metastases to other sites. The latter are particularly common with this aggressive entity.

As with other cardiac tumors, echocardiography can establish the presence of a mass lesion in most instances. CT and cMRI can provide additional information on the tissue characterization (presence of fat and/or calcification). They also provide more spatial resolution that can help to assess for invasion and improve surgical planning as well as posttreatment follow-up.

Location and Gross Pathology
Cardiac undifferentiated pleomorphic sarcomas usually arise in the left atrium and have prominent luminal growth, which occurs before extensive infiltration into the myocardium and pericardium.[5] The site of attachment is commonly the posterior wall or atrial septum. These lesions occur much less commonly in the ventricles and right atrium.[6]

Grossly, undifferentiated pleomorphic sarcomas may be sessile or pedunculated. Invasion into adjacent structures (such as the mitral apparatus) is not uncommon and serves as a good indicator of a malignant process. The tumors are usually tan-white or variegated, with hemorrhage and/or necrosis often present.

Histopathology
The histologic appearance of undifferentiated pleomorphic sarcomas is highly variable, but in general, there are areas of striking pleomorphism. The cells may be epithelioid, spindle shaped, or a combination thereof. The cells are often arranged in a storiform pattern within a variably collagenized stroma (Figs. 184.2 and 184.3).

Areas of myxoid change can occur, which is why there is somewhat of a spectrum between this lesion and so-called myxofibrosarcoma (see below). Mitotic activity and necrosis are usually readily identifiable.

As a point of nomenclature, some authors have applied the term *intimal sarcoma* to lesions that arise primarily within the heart. This term has been employed primarily because of the recognition that *MDM2* gene amplification may be seen in a subset of these lesions, a feature common to intimal sarcomas of the pulmonary artery.[8] Because *MDM2* amplification is not lineage specific, and "intima" is not anatomically correct in the atrium, this term is not currently recommended for sarcomas arising primarily within the heart.[9]

Immunohistochemistry
There is no specific antigenic pattern to undifferentiated pleomorphic sarcomas of the heart. Expression of cytokeratin, smooth muscle actin, and endothelial markers can be seen. In general, reactivity with these

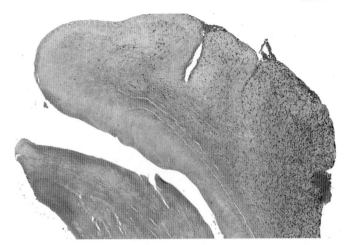

FIGURE 184.2 ▲ Cardiac myxofibrosarcoma. The tumor in this area is deceptively bland and covered by fibrin.

antibodies is usually focal and weak throughout the tumor owing to the overall undifferentiated nature of these lesions. In situ hybridization studies have shown *MDM2* amplification in a subset of these lesions.

Prognosis
As with other cardiac sarcomas, the prognosis for these tumors is poor, with most patients succumbing to disease within a few years of diagnosis. Treatment generally includes resection and some combination of chemotherapy and radiotherapy. Regardless, local recurrence or metastases are common. Isolated reports of increased survival associated with complete tumor resection do exist.[10]

Differential Diagnosis
The differential diagnosis includes other cardiac sarcomas, with the lack of a primary differentiation serving as the primary discriminating characteristic of undifferentiated sarcomas. The pleomorphism seen in undifferentiated pleomorphic sarcoma is helpful in differentiating this lesion from myxofibrosarcoma.

In differentiation of cardiac undifferentiated pleomorphic sarcoma from benign entities, such as myxoma, an invasive growth pattern is often most helpful. Additionally, reactivity of myxoma cells with antibodies directed against calretinin can help to distinguish the two as well.

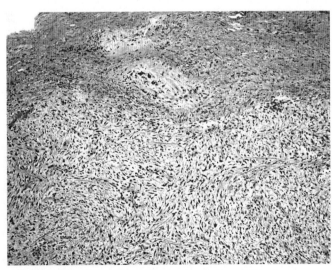

FIGURE 184.3 ▲ Cardiac undifferentiated pleomorphic sarcoma. A low magnification shows spindled cells with a vague storiform pattern.

Other Sarcomas

Myxofibrosarcoma

Myxofibrosarcoma was previously described as "myxoid malignant fibrous histiocytoma" and denotes a relatively more indolent tumor than that of an undifferentiated sarcoma (described above). Cardiac myxofibrosarcomas have been described in the left atrium most frequently, but occur in other sites in the heart as well.[11,12]

Histologically, fibromyxosarcomas demonstrate spindle cells within a fibrous matrix, without significant pleomorphism or a storiform pattern, or rounded cells in a myxoid matrix without marked atypia (Fig. 184.2). Although there is a continuum with undifferentiated sarcomas, there is no storiform pattern or marked pleomorphism.[12]

Leiomyosarcoma

Cardiac leiomyosarcoma represents ~6% of cardiac sarcomas. Most cardiac leiomyosarcomas are located in the left atrium (posterior wall) and usually involve pulmonary veins with or without involvement of the mitral apparatus. There is no sex predilection, and most occur in patients between 40 and 50 years of age. Dyspnea is the main clinical feature.[13]

Histologically, cardiac leiomyosarcomas are similar to those of soft tissue, express desmin intermediate filament, and have interdigitating fascicles of spindle cells with blunt-ended nuclei and frequent cytoplasmic vacuoles.

Osteosarcoma

Focal areas of osteosarcomatous or chondrosarcomatous differentiation occurs in ~15% of otherwise undifferentiated left atrial cardiac sarcomas. When the bulk of the lesion consists of osteosarcomatous features, the designation of cardiac osteosarcoma is appropriate. Men and women are equally affected. The mean is 40 years, with a range of 14 to 70; these tumors appear to occur in slightly younger patients than do pleomorphic sarcomas and have been reported in patients as young as 14 years.[14]

Dyspnea is the most common presenting symptom, often related to mitral valve obstruction secondary to their common cavitary location within the left atrium.

Histologically, cardiac osteosarcoma contains malignant osteoid-forming cells often with areas of chondrosarcomatous differentiation and sometimes with focal undifferentiated areas (Fig. 184.4). Chondrosarcomatous areas occur in about one-half of cases. There also may be myxoid areas in association with undifferentiated spindle cell regions, as well as areas containing numerous osteoclastic giant cells.[15]

The prognosis of cardiac osteosarcoma is poor. Cardiac osteosarcoma has an aggressive course with early metastases, to sites including

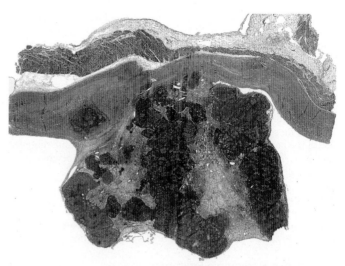

FIGURE 184.4 ▲ Cardiac osteosarcoma (chondrosarcoma predominant). The tumor is exophytic, projecting from the left atrial wall into the atrial cavity.

the lungs, skin, skeleton, and thyroid gland. Survival beyond one year is unusual.[15]

Rhabdomyosarcoma

Cardiac rhabdomyosarcoma is a rare tumor that occurs primarily in children.[16] The mean age at presentation is about 14 years. Clinical symptoms are diverse and depend on site of the tumor within the heart. In contrast to other cardiac sarcomas, most rhabdomyosarcomas arise in ventricular walls.[17]

Histologically, most cardiac rhabdomyosarcomas are of the embryonal type, although there are reports of alveolar botryoid and spindle cell growth patterns.[16]

Synovial Sarcoma

Synovial sarcoma represents about 3% to 5% of primary cardiac sarcomas. The mean age at presentation of cardiac synovial sarcoma is 41 years, and tumors have been described in children as young as 13 years.[18] The atria (left > right) are the most common location of cardiac synovial sarcoma. The presenting symptom is typically dyspnea, as with other heart tumors.

Synovial sarcomas may also arise in the pericardium and secondarily infiltrate the myocardium. Histologically, the tumor is usually biphasic (Fig. 184.5). The spindle component is generally dominant and may have a hemangiopericytoma-like vascular pattern.

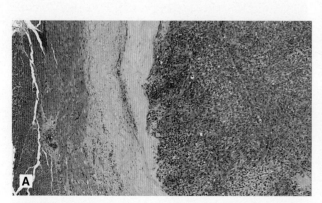

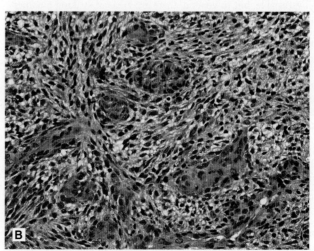

FIGURE 184.5 ▲ Cardiac synovial sarcoma. **A.** A cellular tumor is at the right, arising from the endocardium of the atrial wall (left). **B.** A higher magnification shows a biphasic growth pattern of synovial sarcoma.

Molecular studies confirm the diagnosis of synovial sarcoma of the heart, as in extracardiac locations. The *SYT-SSX* gene fusion product resulting from the t(X;18) translocation can be demonstrated by cytogenetics, RT-PCR and COBRA-FISH, the latter two methods on paraffin sections.

Sarcomas of the Great Arteries

General Features

Sarcomas of the great arteries typically arise in the intimal layer of the vessel and usually exhibit an intraluminal growth pattern. Because of this, the term *intimal sarcoma* is often employed. The intima is composed of endothelial and supporting cells (such as myofibroblasts). Because of this mixed population of cells, malignant tumors in this region may differentiate down a number of mesenchymal lineages. Nevertheless, the designation of intimal sarcoma is generally appropriate.

Aortic Intimal Sarcoma

Sarcomas of the aorta are rare and generally cause obstructive or embolic symptoms because of their luminal growth patterns, before invading into the adventitia. Of these rare tumors, ~30% occur in the thoracic aorta, almost always the descending portion. Most occur in the abdominal aorta.[19]

Grossly, aortic sarcomas are intraluminal, soft, gelatinous masses, which are easily separated from the wall of the aorta.

Histologically, intimal aortic sarcomas are of two general types. Undifferentiated intimal sarcomas are characterized by a layer of discohesive, epithelioid, pleomorphic cells that lie over a layer of fibrin and thrombus (Fig. 184.6). About one-half of these express endothelial markers, specifically CD31, and are therefore often designated as epithelioid angiosarcomas.[19] The other type of aortic intimal sarcoma resembles left atrial sarcomas, forming a spectrum between myxofibrosarcoma and undifferentiated pleomorphic sarcoma (Fig. 184.7).[19]

Regardless of the intraluminal appearance, tumors that invade into the adventitia adopt an appearance indistinguishable from that of undifferentiated pleomorphic sarcoma.[19]

Pulmonary Artery Sarcoma

Pulmonary artery sarcomas (or intimal sarcomas of pulmonary arteries) are rare and occur approximately at twice the rate of aortic intimal sarcomas. The most common presenting symptom is dyspnea, followed by chest or back pain, cough, hemoptysis, weight loss, malaise,

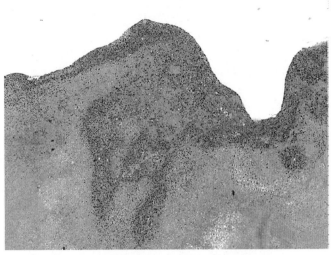

FIGURE 184.6 ▲ Aortic intimal sarcoma, undifferentiated type. Low magnification shows a cellular tumor overlying fibrin thrombus. In this case, endothelial markers were negative (not shown).

syncope, and fever. The clinical manifestations mimic acute or chronic thromboembolism and pulmonary hypertension, because of obstruction of the pulmonary circulation.[20]

Pulmonary artery sarcomas occur in the proximal elastic arteries, from the level of the pulmonary valve to the lobar branches. Most cases have bilateral involvement, although one side is usually dominant (Fig. 184.8).

Like their aortic counterparts, intimal sarcomas of the pulmonary arteries resemble mucoid or gelatinous clots filling vascular lumens. Distal extension may show smooth tapering of the mass.

The most common histologic type is differentiated pleomorphic sarcomas, followed by myxofibrosarcoma (Fig. 184.9). About one in six pulmonary artery intimal sarcomas show heterologous elements in the form of osteosarcoma or chondrosarcoma.[20]

MDM2 amplification has been observed in most pulmonary artery sarcomas, along with immunohistochemical overexpression of the protein product, often coexisting with amplification of *PDGFRA*.[21]

The prognosis of pulmonary artery sarcoma is generally poor, with a mean survival of 1 to 3 years. Rare intraluminal inflammatory myofibroblastic tumors have a relatively good prognosis.[20]

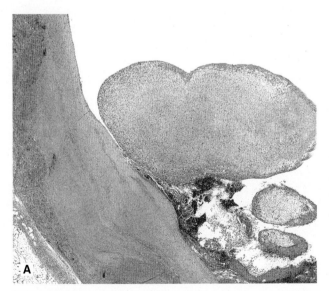

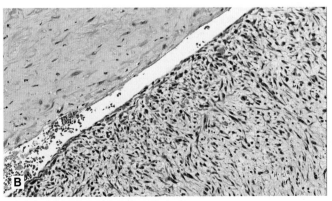

FIGURE 184.7 ▲ Aortic intimal sarcoma, myxofibrosarcoma type. **A.** A low magnification shows luminal tumor. **B.** A higher magnification shows a low-grade fibrous sarcoma with a myxoid matrix. The tumor was in the thoracic aorta and caused embolic symptoms in the lower extremities in a middle-aged woman.

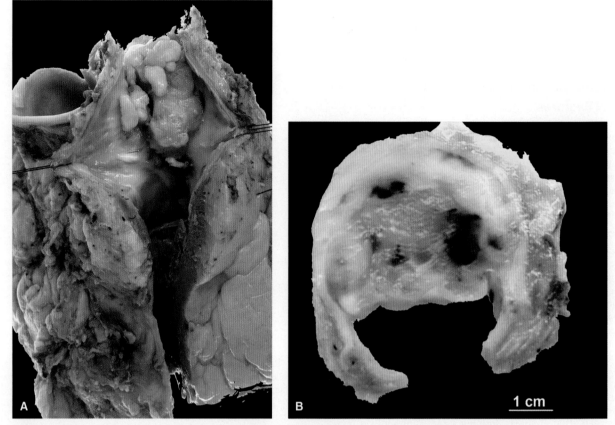

FIGURE 184.8 ▲ Pulmonary artery sarcoma, cardiac explant. **A.** The tumor is endoluminal and exophytic about 1cm above the pulmonary artery valve. **B.** Cross section of the pulmonary artery showing that the tumor fills about 70% of the pulmonary artery lumen. Invasion into the arterial wall is not seen.

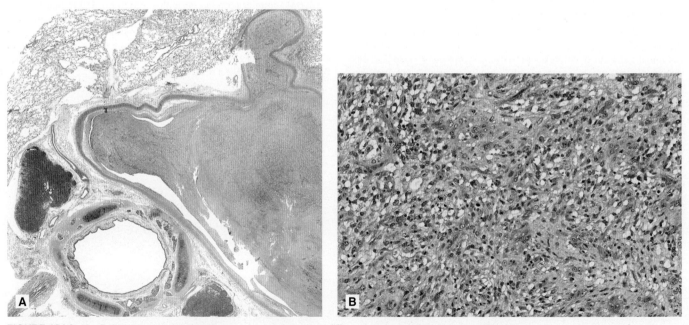

FIGURE 184.9 ▲ Pulmonary artery intimal sarcoma, pleomorphic undifferentiated type. **A.** A low magnification shows tumor filling the lumen of the pulmonary artery. **B.** Higher magnification shows undifferentiated pleomorphic sarcoma.

REFERENCES

1. Coindre JM. Grading of soft tissue sarcomas: review and update. *Arch Pathol Lab Med.* 2006;130:1448–1453.
2. Butany J, Bohle RM, Burke AP, et al. Angiosarcoma. In: Travis WD, et al., eds. *WHO Classification of Tumours of the Lung, Pleura, Thymus and Heart.* Lyon, France: IARC Press; 2015:329–330.
3. Keeling IM, Ploner F, Rigler B. Familial cardiac angiosarcoma. *Ann Thorac Surg.* 2006;82:1576.
4. Khanji M, Lee E, Ionescu A. Blushing primary cardiac angiosarcoma. *Heart.* 2014;100:266.
5. Savoia MT, Liguori C, Nahar T, et al. Transesophageal echocardiography-guided transvenous biopsy of a cardiac sarcoma. *J Am Soc Echocardiogr.* 1997;10:752–755.
6. Look Hong NJ, Pandalai PK, Hornick JL, et al. Cardiac angiosarcoma management and outcomes: 20-year single-institution experience. *Ann Surg Oncol.* 2012;19:2707–2715.
7. Pacini D, Careddu L, Pantaleo A, et al. Primary malignant tumors of the heart: outcomes of the surgical treatment. *Asian Cardiovasc Thorac Ann.* 2015;23:645–651.
8. Neuville A, Collin F, Bruneval P, et al. Intimal sarcoma is the most frequent primary cardiac sarcoma: clinicopathologic and molecular retrospective analysis of 100 primary cardiac sarcomas. *Am J Surg Pathol.* 2014;38:461–469.
9. Maleszewski JJ, Tavora F, Burke AP. Do "intimal" sarcomas of the heart exist? *Am J Surg Pathol.* 2014;38:1158–1159.
10. Furukawa N, Gummert J, Borgermann J. Complete resection of undifferentiated cardiac sarcoma and reconstruction of the atria and the superior vena cava: case report. *J Cardiothorac Surg.* 2012;7:96.
11. Lazaros GA, Matsakas EP, Madas JS, et al. Primary myxofibrosarcoma of the left atrium: case report and review of the literature. *Angiology.* 2008;59:632–635.
12. Butany J, Fletcher CDM. Myxofibrosarcoma. In: Travis WD, et al., eds. *WHO Classification of Tumours of the Lung, Pleura, Thymus and Heart.* Lyon, France: IARC Press; 2015:334–335.
13. Burke AP. Leiomyosarcoma. In: Travis WD, et al., eds. *WHO Classification of Tumours of the Lung, Pleura, Thymus and Heart.* Lyon, France: IARC Press; 2015:336.
14. Lurito KJ, Martin T, Cordes T. Right atrial primary cardiac osteosarcoma. *Pediatr Cardiol.* 2002;23:462–465.
15. Burke AP, Tavora F. Osteosarcoma. In: Travis WD, et al., eds. *WHO Classification of Tumours of the Lung, Pleura, Thymus and Heart.* Lyon, France: IARC Press; 2015:333.
16. Butany J, Fletcher CDM. Rhabdomyosarcoma. In: Travis WD, et al., eds. *WHO Classification of Tumours of the Lung, Pleura, Thymus and Heart.* Lyon, France: IARC Press; 2015:337.
17. Castorino F, Masiello P, Quattrocchi E, et al. Primary cardiac rhabdomyosarcoma of the left atrium: an unusual presentation. *Tex Heart Inst J.* 2000;27:206–208.
18. Tazelaar H, Fletcher CD. Synovial sarcoma. In: Travis WD, et al., eds. *WHO Classification of Tumours of the Lung, Pleura, Thymus and Heart.* Lyon, France: IARC Press; 2015:338.
19. Blondeau P. Primary cardiac tumors—French studies of 533 cases. *Thorac Cardiovasc Surg.* 1990;38(Suppl 2):192–195.
20. Burke AP, Yi ES. Pulmonary artery intimal sarcoma. In: Travis WD, et al., eds. *WHO Classification of Tumours of the Lung, Pleura, Thymus and Heart.* Lyon, France: IARC Press; 2015:128.
21. Bode-Lesniewska B, Zhao J, Speel EJ, et al. Gains of 12q13-14 and overexpression of MDM2 are frequent findings in intimal sarcomas of the pulmonary artery. *Virchows Arch.* 2001;438:57–65.

185 Cardiac Lymphomas, Histiocytic Proliferations, and Metastatic Tumors

Fabio R. Tavora, M.D., Ph.D., and Allen P. Burke, M.D.

Cardiac Lymphoma

Incidence

Primary cardiac lymphoma is rare, accounting for 1.3% of primary cardiac tumors and 0.5% of extranodal lymphomas.[1]

Clinical Presentation

Adults are typically affected with a mean age of ~60 years at presentation (range, 12 to 86 years).[2] The presenting symptoms are most commonly related to congestive heart failure, pleural effusions, or conduction system disturbances. Anginal pain may indicate infiltration of a coronary artery.[3]

There have been occasional reports of cardiac lymphoma, generally associated with extracardiac disease, in patients with AIDS or solid organ transplant.[2,4] Cardiac lymphoma after orthotopic heart transplant is rare.

Location in the Heart

The sites of the heart most often affected by lymphoma are the right atrium, followed by the right ventricle, left ventricle, left atrium, atrial septum, and ventricular septum[2,5] (Table 185.1). More than one cardiac chamber is involved in over 75% of cases.

Gross Findings

Primary cardiac lymphomas typically occur as multiple masses of firm, white, homogeneous nodules with the "fish flesh" consistency (Figs. 185.1 and 185.2). The heart is usually enlarged at autopsy or explant.[2,6] The gross appearance may suggest sarcoidosis. However, sarcoid granulomas do not usually form large nodules that extend onto epicardium/pericardium, as is typical for lymphoma, and are generally more firm and fibrous.

Microscopic Findings

The most common types of lymphomas involving the heart are diffuse large B-cell lymphoma, followed by Burkitt lymphoma, follicular lymphoma, effusion lymphoma, anaplastic large cell lymphoma, and peripheral T-cell lymphoma (Table 185.1)[2] (Figs. 185.3 to 185.6).

Prognosis

Survival is generally less than a month without treatment, but survival up to 5 years has been documented.[1] Patients treated with the CHOP (cyclophosphamide, hydroxydaunorubicin/adriamycin, oncovin, prednisone) survive up to 18 months; those treated with the BACOP (bleomycin, doxorubicin, cyclophosphamide, vincristine, and prednisone) survive up to 49 months; patients who are treated surgically survive more than 18 months; and those who undergo radiation therapy survive for up to 15 months.[6]

Histiocytosis Proliferations

Erdheim-Chester Disease

Considered a histiocytosis in the juvenile xanthogranuloma group, Erdheim-Chester histiocytosis typically involves the eyes, lungs, retroperitoneum, and pituitary glands, with characteristic radiologic abnormalities of the long bones (see Chapter 92). Clinical cardiovascular involvement occurs in 5% to 10% (although this estimate may be low[7]) and is manifest as aortic, myocardial, or pericardial disease.[8] The heart or aorta is rarely biopsied for diagnosis, which is generally made

TABLE 185.1   Cardiac Lymphomas

	Total (n = 21)	Primary (n = 14)	Secondary (n = 7)
Histologic type			
Diffuse large B-cell lymphoma	9	6	3
Burkitt lymphoma	4	4	0
Follicular B-cell lymphoma	2	1	1
Primary effusion lymphoma	2	2	0
Peripheral T-cell lymphoma	2	0	2
Anaplastic large cell lymphoma	2	1	1
Primary site in the heart			
Right atrium	7	5	2
Right ventricle	4	2	2
Pericardium	4	3	1
Left ventricle	3	2	1
Biatrial/atrial septum	2	1	1
Left atrium	1	1	0
Diagnostic procedure			
Open biopsy	8	7	1
Lymph node/liver biopsy	4	0	4
Endomyocardial biopsy	2	1	1
Pericardial cytology	2	2	0
Autopsy	2	1	1
Needle biopsy	1	1	0
Pleural cytology	1	1	0

From Jeudy J, Kirsch J, Tavora F, et al. From the radiologic pathology archives: cardiac lymphoma: radiologic-pathologic correlation. *Radiographics*. 2012;32:1369–1380, Ref.[2]

by computed tomography or magnetic resonance imaging.[9] By sensitive imaging study, 56% of patients with Erdheim-Chester disease have periaortic fibrosis, 44% pericardial involvement, and 31% myocardial involvement, often involving the right atrium.[7]

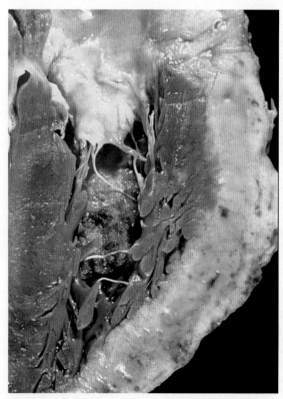

FIGURE 185.1 ▲ Cardiac lymphoma. The tumor is infiltrating the right ventricular muscle with marked thickening of the epicardium.

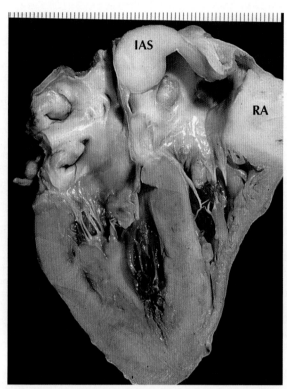

FIGURE 185.2 ▲ Cardiac lymphoma. There are tumor masses in the interatrial septum (IAS) and right atrium (RA), lateral wall.

Histologically, Erdheim-Chester disease is characterized by xanthogranulomatous lesions, which contain foamy and lipid-laden macrophages, multinucleated giant cells, monocytes, and lymphocytes in a mesh of fibrosis. There is typically infiltration of fibrous tissues and myocytes in the case of myocardial involvement. Immunohistochemically, Erdheim-Chester macrophages express CD14, CD68, factor XIIIa, and fascin and are negative for HLADr, CD1a, CD163, langerin, S100, and lysozyme (see Chapter 92).

Rosai-Dorfman Disease

Also known as sinus histiocytosis with massive lymphadenopathy, Rosai-Dorfman disease typically presents as a painless cervical

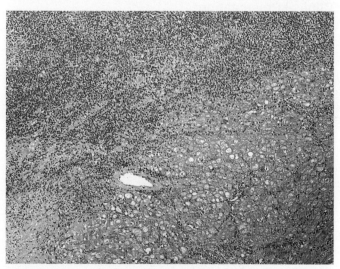

FIGURE 185.3 ▲ Cardiac lymphoma. There is infiltration of the cardiac muscle (top). The tumor was of follicular type.

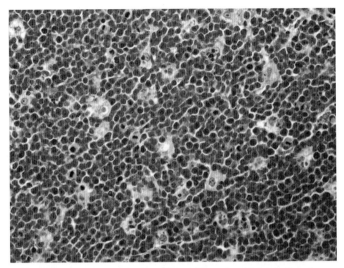

FIGURE 185.4 ▲ Cardiac lymphoma. There is a high mitotic rate, numerous macrophages, and small cell size, features of Burkitt lymphoma. Immunophenotyping was consistent with follicular center cell origin with nearly 100% Ki 67 positivity.

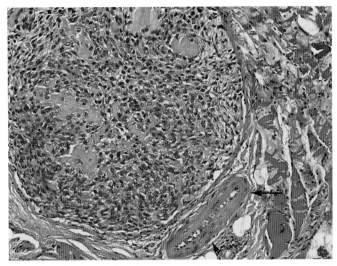

FIGURE 185.6 ▲ Metastatic osteosarcoma, heart. Sarcomas spread to the heart generally by hematogenous spread. There is a small artery (*arrows*) adjacent to a massively dilated vein filled with tumor.

adenopathy in young individuals. Lung involvement is relatively common (see Chapter 92). Involvement of the heart is rare.[10] Lesions may arise in any cardiac chamber from epicardium, myocardium, or endocardium.[10,11] Immunohistochemically, the histiocytes in Rosai-Dorfman disease express CD14, CD68, S100, lysozyme, CD163, HLADr, and fascin and are negative for CD1a, factor XIIIa, and langerin.

Langerhans Cell Histiocytosis

Cardiac involvement with Langerhans cell histiocytosis is rare.[12]

Cardiac Metastases

Incidence

The autopsy frequency of cardiac metastasis in patients with metastatic malignancies ranges from 8%[13] to ~30%.[14,15] In series of surgically resected cardiac tumors, metastatic lesions constitute 3% to 27% of all tumor resections and 22% to 61% of malignant tumors.[16]

Primary tumors in decreasing order of incidence include carcinomas of the lung, lymphomas, carcinomas of the breast, leukemia, carcinomas of the stomach, malignant melanoma, hepatocellular carcinoma, and carcinomas of the colon. The following tumors have

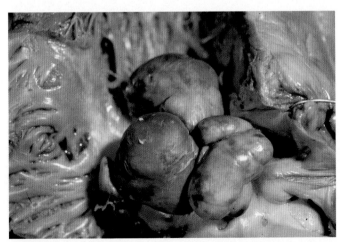

FIGURE 185.5 ▲ Metastatic carcinoid tumor, right atrium. The patient had multiple liver metastases; the primary tumor was in the ileum. Note the pectinate muscles of the right atrium (left).

an especially high rate of cardiac metastasis if the incidence of the primary tumor is considered: melanoma, thyroid carcinoma, extracardiac sarcomas, renal cell carcinomas, carcinoid tumors, and carcinomas of the lung and breast.[17]

Clinical

Clinical manifestations attributed to metastatic cardiac tumors are highly varied and include dyspnea, usually related to pericardial or pleural effusions; symptoms related to mass effect, such as outflow tract obstruction or obstruction of atrioventricular valves; syncope and conduction disturbances; heart failure; and embolic phenomena.

The time interval between diagnosis of the primary tumor and cardiac metastasis may be months or years. Cardiac metastasis of soft tissue sarcomas may occur as late as eight years after initial diagnosis[18] and even as late as 28 years for metastatic melanoma.[19]

In patients with carcinoid syndrome caused by metastatic carcinoid tumors of the bowel, the clinical distinction between carcinoid valve disease and metastatic carcinoid tumor to the heart may be difficult. Patients with metastatic carcinoid tumor to the heart usually have small bowel primaries, hepatic metastases, and concomitant carcinoid valve disease (see Chapter 38).[20]

Routes of Cardiac Spread of Metastases

Malignancies may spread to the heart by direct extension, usually from mediastinal tumors; hematogenously; via lymphatics, generally by retrograde extension; and by intracavitary extension from the inferior vena cava or pulmonary veins (Table 185.2).

The lymphatic spread of metastasis is associated with a high incidence of malignant pericardial effusions, in contrast to the hematogenous spread, which is associated with myocardial involvement. Lymphatic spread is generally accompanied by involvement and enlargement of pulmonary hilar or mediastinal lymph nodes and histologic evidence of pericardial lymphatic infiltration.

Melanoma, sarcomas, leukemia, as well as renal, adrenal, liver, and uterine tumors metastasize to the heart by a hematogenous route and therefore typically show myocardial involvement. Metastases via hematogenous spread represent the most frequent intracavitary tumors.

A subset of metastases is constituted by those tumors that grow as direct extensions into the cardiac chambers via the venae cavae or pulmonary veins. The most common route is the right atrium via the inferior vena cava, most commonly by renal cell carcinoma. The left atrium may be invaded by primary lung tumors or metastatic tumors to the lung.

TABLE 185.2   Metastatic Cardiac Tumors, Sites and Nodes of Spread

Right atrium	Direct extension	Renal cell carcinoma
		Hepatocellular carcinoma
		Uterine tumors (leiomyoma, stromal tumors, carcinomas)
		Renal tumors other than carcinoma
	Hematogenous metastasis	Melanomas
		Sarcomas
		Lymphoma
		Carcinoid tumors
		Carcinomas (rare)
Right ventricle	Direct extension	Via right atrial tumors
	Hematogenous metastases	Melanomas
		Sarcomas
		Lymphoma
		Carcinoid tumors
		Carcinomas (rare, usually as extension of pericardial metastases)
Left atrium	Direct extension	Lung carcinomas
		Lymphoma
		Lung metastases (osteosarcoma, other sarcomas)
	Hematogenous metastases	Melanoma
		Lymphoma
		Carcinomas (rare)
		Sarcomas (rare)[a]
Left ventricle	Hematogenous metastases	Melanoma
		Sarcoma (rare)
		Carcinomas (rare)
Pericardium	Direct extension	Thymoma
		Esophageal carcinoma
		Lung carcinoma
	Lymphatic spread	Lung carcinomas
		Breast carcinomas
		Lymphomas
		Other carcinomas (uncommon)

[a]Primary sarcomas are far more frequent in the left atrium than metastatic tumors.

Pathologic Findings

Metastatic deposits may be diffuse and multinodular or consist of a single dominant mass (Fig. 185.5). Histologically, the tumors resemble those of the primary (Figs. 185.6 to 185.9).

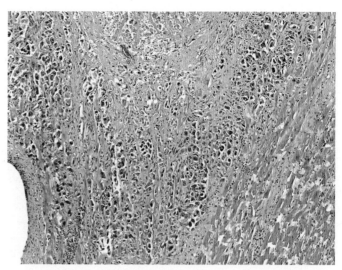

FIGURE 185.8 ▲ Metastatic non–small cell carcinoma of the lung. Note pleomorphic tumor cells infiltrating the ventricular myocardium.

Metastatic melanoma is the malignancy most likely to spread to the heart, particularly the right side; up to 64% of patients dying with melanoma will demonstrate cardiac involvement at autopsy.[21] In a surgical series at Mayo Clinic, there were seven patients with excisions of symptomatic metastatic cardiac melanoma, four female and three male (age 31 to 79 years). Remarkably, no patient had a history of metastatic melanoma elsewhere, and in 2, no primary lesion was ever identified. In four cases, the history of primary melanoma was remote, occurring 7, 9, 13, and 28 years prior to the discovery of their cardiac mass.[19]

Histologic types of sarcomas metastatic to the heart include osteosarcoma, uterine leiomyosarcoma, liposarcoma, pleomorphic sarcomas (previously termed "malignant fibrous histiocytoma"), synovial sarcoma, rhabdomyosarcoma, endometrial stromal sarcoma, and Ewing sarcoma.[16]

The cardiac site involved in most cases is the right ventricle, followed by the right atrium and left ventricle. One-third of patients have left atrial involvement as an extension of pulmonary metastasis.[23]

The diagnosis in surgical excisions is generally straightforward, as there is typically a history of previously excised sarcoma. Occasionally,

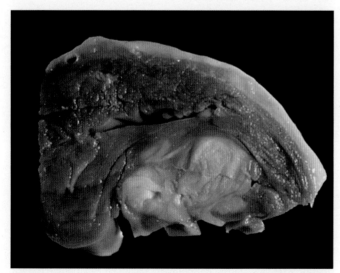

FIGURE 185.7 ▲ Metastatic rhabdomyosarcoma. The right ventricle shows fleshy tumor masses. The patient, a 22-year-old woman, had a history of metastatic rhabdomyosarcoma.

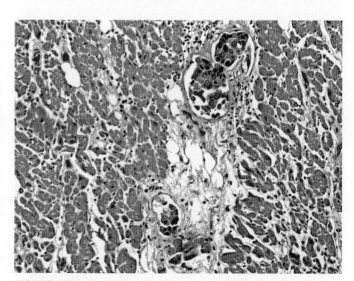

FIGURE 185.9 ▲ Metastatic non–small cell carcinoma, lung, the intramyocardial lymphatic invasion. There is lymphatic tumor spread within the right ventricular myocardium.

the heart can be the first manifestation, or a history of a remote tumor resection may not be known. Unlike the right atrium and ventricle, the left atrium is an extremely rare site of distant metastasis, however. If an unusual mesenchymal tumor is excised from the right side of the heart, a metastasis from a remote primary soft tissue lesion should always be considered.

REFERENCES

1. Gowda RM, Khan IA. Clinical perspectives of primary cardiac lymphoma. *Angiology.* 2003;54:599–604.

2. Jeudy J, Kirsch J, Tavora F, et al. From the radiologic pathology archives: cardiac lymphoma: radiologic-pathologic correlation. *Radiographics.* 2012;32:1369–1380.

3. Castelli MJ, Mihalov ML, Posniak HV, et al. Primary cardiac lymphoma initially diagnosed by routine cytology. Case report and literature review. *Acta Cytol.* 1989;33:355–358.

4. Tanaka PY, Atala MM, Pereira J, et al. Primary effusion lymphoma with cardiac involvement in HIV positive patient-complete response and long survival with chemotherapy and HAART. *J Clin Virol.* 2009;44:84–85.

5. Burke A, Virmani R. Hematologic tumors of heart and pericardium. In: *Atlas of Tumor Pathology. Tumors of the Heart and Great Vessels.* Washington, DC: Armed Forces Institute of Pathology; 1996:171–180.

6. Hsueh SC, Chung MT, Fang R, et al. Primary cardiac lymphoma. *J Chin Med Assoc.* 2006;69:169–174.

7. Haroche J, Amoura Z, Dion E, et al. Cardiovascular involvement, an overlooked feature of Erdheim-Chester disease: report of 6 new cases and a literature review. *Medicine (Baltimore).* 2004;83:371–392.

8. Cives M, Simone V, Rizzo FM, et al. Erdheim-Chester disease: a systematic review. *Crit Rev Oncol Hematol.* 2015;95:1–11.

9. Haroche J, Cluzel P, Toledano D, et al. Images in cardiovascular medicine. Cardiac involvement in Erdheim-Chester disease: magnetic resonance and computed tomographic scan imaging in a monocentric series of 37 patients. *Circulation.* 2009;119:e597–e978.

10. Maleszewski JJ, Hristov AC, Halushka MK, et al. Extranodal Rosai-Dorfman disease involving the heart: report of two cases. *Cardiovasc Pathol.* 2010;19:380–384.

11. Chen J, Tang H, Li B, et al. Rosai-Dorfman disease of multiple organs, including the epicardium: an unusual case with poor prognosis. *Heart Lung.* 2011;40:168–171.

12. Chen CY, Wu MH, Huang SF, et al. Langerhans' cell histiocytosis presenting with a para-aortic lesion and heart failure. *J Formos Med Assoc.* 2001;100:127–130.

13. MacGee W. Metastatic and invasive tumours involving the heart in a geriatric population: a necropsy study. *Virchows Arch A Pathol Anat Histopathol.* 1991;419:183–189.

14. Abraham DP, Reddy V, Gattusa P. Neoplasms metastatic to the heart: review of 3314 consecutive autopsies. *Am J Cardiovasc Pathol.* 1990;3:1958–1966.

15. Manojlovic S. Metastatic carcinomas involving the heart. Review of postmortem examination. *Zentralbl Allg Pathol.* 1990;136:657–661.

16. Burke AP, Tavora F, Maleszewski JJ, et al. Metastatic cardiac tumors. In: *Atlas of Tumor Pathology. Tumors of the Heart and Great Vessels.* Washington, DC: American Registry of Pathology; 2015.

17. Mukai K, Shinkai T, Tominaga K, et al. The incidence of secondary tumors of the heart and pericardium: a 10-year study. *Jpn J Clin Oncol.* 1988;18:195–201.

18. Shibata T, Suehiro S, Hattori K, et al. Metastatic synovial sarcoma of the left ventricle. *Jpn Heart J.* 2001;42:387–391.

19. Wood A, Markovic SN, Best PJ, et al. Metastatic malignant melanoma manifesting as an intracardiac mass. *Cardiovasc Pathol.* 2010;19:153–157.

20. Pandya UH, Pellikka PA, Enriquez-Sarano M, et al. Metastatic carcinoid tumor to the heart: echocardiographic-pathologic study of 11 patients. *J Am Coll Cardiol.* 2002;40:1328–1332.

21. Glancy DL, Roberts WC. The heart in malignant melanoma. A study of 70 autopsy cases. *Am J Cardiol.* 1968;21:555–571.

22. Hallahan DE, Vogelzang NJ, Borow KM, et al. Cardiac metastases from soft-tissue sarcomas. *J Clin Oncol.* 1986;4:1662–1669.

23. Platonov MA, Turner AR, Mullen JC, et al. Tumour on the tricuspid valve: metastatic osteosarcoma and the heart. *Can J Cardiol.* 2005;21:63–67.

186 Pericardial Cysts and Cystic Lesions

Allen P. Burke, M.D.

Mesothelial (Pericardial) Cysts

Mesothelial cysts account for ~20% to 30% of mediastinal cysts. Bronchogenic cysts are more common, but are usually paratracheal and outside the pericardial sac (see below).[1]

Pericardial cysts are mesothelial-lined structures that are either congenital or acquired and pose no diagnostic difficultly by imaging, unless there are superimposed degenerative or infectious changes. The mean age at presentation is about 50 years. Pericardial cysts may be incidentally discovered on chest x-ray or other imaging or cause symptoms of dyspnea, chest pain, or cough. The typical location is on the right side near the cardiophrenic angle and occasionally the left cardiophrenic angle.[1]

Grossly, the specimen will either be in pieces, and demonstrate nondescript fragments of fibrovascular tissue, or be removed intact, in which case there is a simple cyst with serous fluid (Fig. 186.1).

Histologically, the cysts are lined by mesothelial cells (Fig. 186.2), which can be confirmed by staining with anticalretinin, which is usually unnecessary. There may be fibrosis and chronic inflammation, with cholesterol clefts, if there was prior infection or inflammation, which occurs in a minority of cases.

Pericardial Lymphangioma

Also referred to as hygromas, lymphangiomas are composed of dilated lymphatic channels arising from sequestered lymphatic tissue, which fails to communicate normally with the lymphatic tree. Lymphangiomas are uncommon in the mediastinum, representing only 2% of mediastinal cysts.[2] Intrapericardial lymphangiomas are extremely rare and occur in infants, children, and young adults. Grossly, the surface is smooth with a bosselated surface. The histologic appearance of intrapericardial lymphangioma is identical to lymphangiomas of other soft tissue sites.

In contrast to mesothelial pericardial cysts, lymphangiomas are multilocular, are lined by flattened endothelial cells, contain proteinaceous fluid and lymphocytes, and often have smooth muscle cells and lymphoid aggregates within the cyst wall (Fig. 186.3).

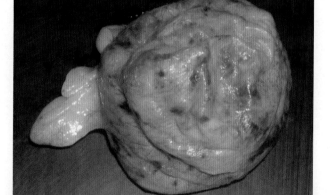

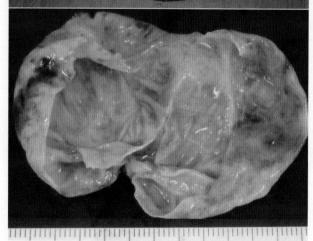

FIGURE 186.1 ▲ Pericardial (mesothelial) cyst. There is a multiloculated thin-walled cyst, which contains serous fluid. The patient was a middle-aged woman with atypical chest pain; CT scan showed a large cystic lesion in the right pericardium.

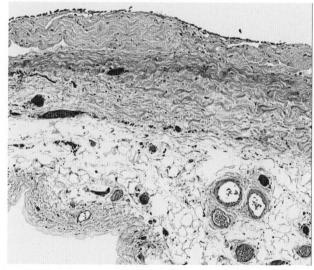

FIGURE 186.2 ▲ Pericardial (mesothelial) cyst. Histologically, the cyst wall resembles normal pericardium.

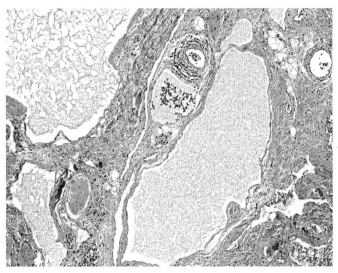

FIGURE 186.3 ▲ Lymphangioma. There are variable sized cysts lined by endothelial cells containing lymph fluid. There is prominent smooth muscle between them.

Immunohistochemical staining for factor VIII–related antigen and cytokeratin are helpful in distinguishing these tumors from mesothelial cysts. The cellular lining of lymphangiomas expresses endothelial markers, whereas the mesothelial lining cells of mesothelial cysts strongly express cytokeratins.

Bronchogenic Cysts

Bronchogenic cysts are the most common cystic lesions of the mediastinum and typically occur adjacent to the trachea, subcarinally, in the pulmonary hila, or adjacent to the esophagus.[3] They only rarely occur in the pericardium, where they often are attached to the ascending aorta.[4] They are typically discovered in children and young adults and may occasionally cause symptoms by pushing against the right atrium or superior vena cava or rupture.[5–7]

Pathologically, they resemble other mediastinal bronchogenic cysts (see Chapter 115).

Pericardial Germ Cell Tumors

Teratomas represent <5% of mediastinal cystic lesions and are usually outside the pericardium.[8] (see Chapter 24, Section 2). The rare reported intrapericardial germ cell tumors have all been teratomas (90%) or yolk sac tumors[9] (Fig. 186.4).

Most patients are infants or children. In adults, intrapericardial teratomas occur more frequently in men than in women. Intrapericardial yolk sac tumors are seen in the pediatric group, usually girls. Tumors are more likely symptomatic in children than adults.

Similar to bronchogenic cysts, teratomas are usually attached by a pedicle to one of the great vessels with arterial supply directly from the aorta.

Pure teratomas are benign in the pediatric population. Surgical excision is the treatment of choice. Yolk sac tumors may behave aggressively with metastatic potential.[9]

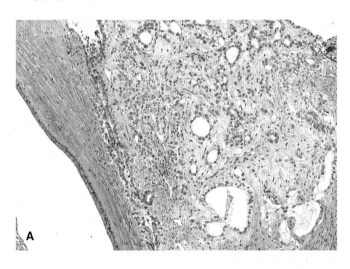

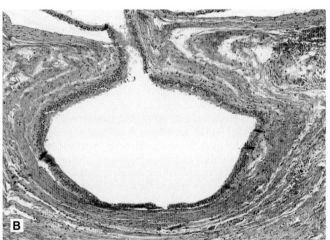

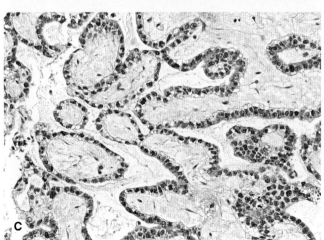

FIGURE 186.4 ▲ Intrapericardial teratoma and yolk sac tumor. The patient was a girl with an entirely intrapericardial multicystic mass with solid components. **A.** There are both components (yolk sac and teratoma). **B.** A higher magnification shows the teratoma. **C.** This figure demonstrates a papillary configuration of yolk sac tumor.

REFERENCES

1. Zambudio AR, Lanzas JT, Calvo MJ, et al. Non-neoplastic mediastinal cysts. *Eur J Cardiothorac Surg.* 2002;22:712–716.
2. Tajima S, Takanashi Y, Koda K. Enlarging cystic lymphangioma of the mediastinum in an adult: is this a neoplastic lesion related to the recently discovered PIK3CA mutation? *Int J Clin Exp Pathol.* 2015;8:5924–5928.
3. Muramatsu T, Shimamura M, Furuichi M, et al. Thoracoscopic resection of mediastinal bronchogenic cysts in adults. *Asian J Surg.* 2011;34:11–14.
4. Durieux R, Lavigne JP, Scagnol I, et al. Intrapericardial bronchogenic cyst adherent to the ascending aorta. *Thorac Cardiovasc Surg.* 2014;62:189–191.
5. Goksel OS, Sayin OA, Cinar T, et al. Bronchogenic cyst invading right atrium in a 5-year-old. *Thorac Cardiovasc Surg.* 2008;56:435–436.
6. Lu Q, Yang E, Wang W, et al. Spontaneous rupture of a giant intrapericardial bronchogenic cyst. *Ann Thorac Surg.* 2013;96:e109–e110.
7. Nair L, Ranawaka Y, Naidoo R. Intrapericardial bronchogenic duplication cyst. *Interact Cardiovasc Thorac Surg.* 2014;19:311–312.
8. Esme H, Eren S, Sezer M, et al. Primary mediastinal cysts: clinical evaluation and surgical results of 32 cases. *Tex Heart Inst J.* 2011;38:371–374.
9. Burke AP, Tavora F. Germ cell tumours. In: Travis WD, et al., eds. *WHO Classification of Tumours of the Lung, Pleura, Mediastinum and Heart.* Lyon, France: IARC Press; 2015:346–347.

187 Pericardial Mesothelioma

Allen P. Burke, M.D.

Terminology

Malignant mesotheliomas of the pericardium are malignant tumors derived from pericardial mesothelial cells and partly or completely encase the heart, with an absent or minor pleural component. The modifier "diffuse" is often applied to distinguish them from benign or low-grade more localized variants.

Of these unusual low-grade variants of mesothelioma, a case of multicystic mesothelioma of the pericardium has been reported,[1] as well as a single well-differentiated papillary mesothelioma.[2]

In general, the vast majority of reported pericardial mesotheliomas have been of the epithelioid type, with few sarcomatoid variants described, including one desmoplastic type.[3]

Clinical Findings

Pericardial mesotheliomas account for <2% of all mesotheliomas.[4] The mean patient age at presentation is in the fifth decade, with a male to female ratio of 2:1.[5] Because of the rarity of the disease, the extent of the link between pericardial mesothelioma and asbestos exposure is unclear.[6]

Pericardial effusion is often initially asymptomatic, and many patients are initially diagnosed with pericarditis. Pericardial constriction and tamponade may occur as the disease progresses. The tumors are locally aggressive tumors that may extend to the pleura, venae cavae, mediastinum, and great arteries. Distant metastasis, such as to the liver, is uncommon.[7,8]

Gross Findings

These tumors grow along the visceral and parietal surfaces of the pericardium, eventually encasing the heart. There is generally relatively minimal invasion of the heart itself (Figs. 187.1 to 187.3).

Microscopic Findings

Pericardial mesotheliomas are identical histologically to their pleural counterparts. Most are epithelioid, without sarcomatoid differentiation, which is rare, indicating biphasic growth.[9–11] Poorly differentiated epithelioid tumors are occasionally given designations such as "deciduoid" if there is abundant eosinophilic cytoplasm and a lack of tubulopapillary growth[12] (Figs. 187.4 and 187.5).

Differential Diagnosis

The initial diagnosis is often attempted on cytologic material from aspirated pericardial fluid and may be negative or inconclusive.[8,12] Mesothelioma should be considered with atypical epithelial proliferations in pericardial fluid or biopsies, despite its extreme rarity.

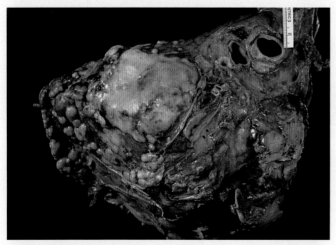

FIGURE 187.1 ▲ Pericardial mesothelioma. There is diffuse studding of the visceral pericardium.

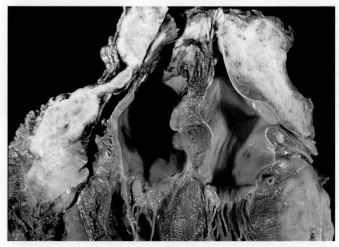

FIGURE 187.2 ▲ Pericardial mesothelioma. The tumor is invading the atrial walls.

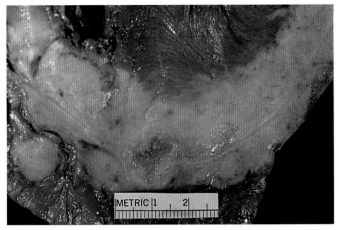

FIGURE 187.3 ▲ Pericardial mesothelioma. There is invasion into the subepicardial ventricular muscle.

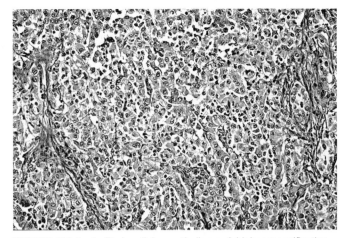

FIGURE 187.5 ▲ Pericardial mesothelioma. A higher magnification demonstrates sheets of epithelioid cells.

Most mesothelial proliferations in the pericardium are reactive. The distinction between mesothelioma and reactive mesothelial hyperplasia is based on similar criteria as in the pleura and requires demonstration of invasion into fat or stroma for an unequivocal diagnosis. Sheet-like or solid growth in the absence of significant inflammation or fibrinous reaction should raise the suspicion of mesothelioma. Reactive mesothelial nests tend to be oriented in a linear fashion.

Metastatic carcinoma is distinguished from mesothelioma based on immunohistochemical study (see Chapter 97).

Prognosis and Treatment

The prognosis of pericardial mesothelioma is poor, with a survival rate of <6 months after diagnosis.[8,13] Due to the rarity of the disease, reliable survival data are not available. A pericardial mesothelioma with metastasis has been reported to respond to pemetrexed.[7]

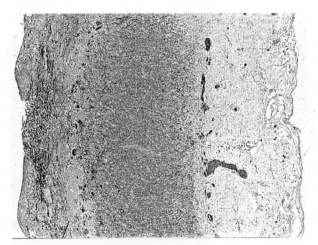

FIGURE 187.4 ▲ Pericardial mesothelioma. At low magnification, the tumor is growing along the pericardial surface, in sheets.

REFERENCES

1. Morita S, Goto A, Sakatani T, et al. Multicystic mesothelioma of the pericardium. *Pathol Int.* 2011;61:319–321.
2. Sane AC, Roggli VL. Curative resection of a well-differentiated papillary mesothelioma of the pericardium. *Arch Pathol Lab Med.* 1995;119:266–267.
3. Nicolini A, Perazzo A, Lanata S. Desmoplastic malignant mesothelioma of the pericardium: description of a case and review of the literature. *Lung India.* 2011;28:219–221.
4. Gemba K, Fujimoto N, Kato K, et al. National survey of malignant mesothelioma and asbestos exposure in Japan. *Cancer Sci.* 2012;103:483–490.
5. Thomason R, Schlegel W, Lucca M, et al. Primary malignant mesothelioma of the pericardium. Case report and literature review. *Tex Heart Inst J.* 1994;21:170–174.
6. Patel J, Sheppard MN. Primary malignant mesothelioma of the pericardium. *Cardiovasc Pathol.* 2011;20:107–109.
7. Doval DC, Pande SB, Sharma JB, et al. Report of a case of pericardial mesothelioma with liver metastases responding well to pemetrexed and platinum-based chemotherapy. *J Thorac Oncol.* 2007;2:780–781.
8. Nilsson A, Rasmuson T. Primary pericardial mesothelioma: report of a patient and literature review. *Case Rep Oncol.* 2009;2:125–132.
9. Jiang D, Kong M, Li J, et al. Primary sarcomatoid malignant pericardial mesothelioma. *Intern Med.* 2013;52:157–158.
10. Tateishi K, Ikeda M, Yokoyama T, et al. Primary malignant sarcomatoid mesothelioma in the pericardium. *Intern Med.* 2013;52:249–253.
11. Terada T. Primary sarcomatoid malignant mesothelioma of the pericardium. *Med Oncol.* 2012;29:1345–1346.
12. Reis-Filho JS, Pope LZ, Milanezi F, et al. Primary epithelial malignant mesothelioma of the pericardium with deciduoid features: cytohistologic and immunohistochemical study. *Diagn Cytopathol.* 2002;26:117–122.
13. Godar M, Liu J, Zhang P, et al. Primary pericardial mesothelioma: a rare entity. *Case Rep Oncol Med.* 2013;2013:283601.

188 Pericardial Metastases

Joseph J. Maleszewski, M.D., and Allen P. Burke, M.D.

Incidence and Histologic Types

About 10% of all patients with advanced-stage cancer develop cardiac metastasis, with the majority (about 75%) involving the epicardium and/or pericardium.[1,2] Metastases usually involve the pericardium by either direct extension or lymphatic spread. Lymphatic drainage of the heart usually flows from endocardium to epicardium. About two-thirds of metastases to the heart involve the pericardium, which can include the visceral pericardium (epicardium) or parietal pericardium.[3]

Metastatic tumors to the pericardium are most commonly carcinoma from the lung or breast. Other primary sites include the gastrointestinal tract, skin (melanoma) pancreas, kidney, thyroid, urinary bladder, ovary, endometrium, and thymus. Other nonepithelial metastases include lymphoma, angiosarcoma, and other metastatic sarcomas.[1–9]

The most common carcinoma to metastasize to the pericardium is non–small cell lung carcinomas, in both men and women. Adenocarcinomas form 75% of this group and small cell carcinoma, 12%.[10] In women, breast carcinoma is the second most common neoplasm to involve the pericardium, with breast and lung carcinomas collectively accounting for >90% of pericardial metastases.[5] In a series of pericardial metastases with postive fluid cytology, the most common tumor was lung cancer (52%), followed by breast cancer (13%), carcinoma of the esophagus (8%), non-Hodgkin lymphoma (8%), leukemia (5%) sarcoma (5%), and one each of thymoma, melanoma, carcinoma of the colon, testicular germ cell tumor, and squamous carcinoma of unknown origin.[11]

Clinical Findings

The clinical manifestations of pericardial metastasis are usually related to effusions, which are often hemorrhagic. Almost 90% of patients with malignant pericardial fluid specimens have a known prior history of malignancy.[10] However, rarely, the diagnosis is made first at biopsy, or even at autopsy, with pericardial tamponade.[12]

Pathologic Findings

Grossly, pericardial metastases result most frequently in hemorrhagic, fibrinous exudates covering various sized nodules on the surface of the pericardium. Diffuse pericardial thickening may also occur, in which case the differential diagnosis would include malignant mesothelioma (Fig. 188.1).

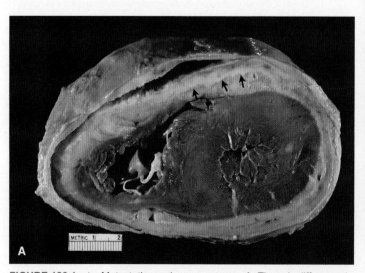
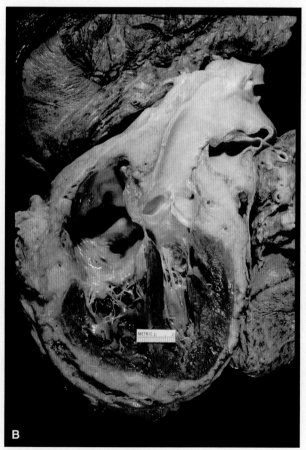

FIGURE 188.1 ▲ Metastatic carcinoma, autopsy. **A.** There is diffuse pericardial constriction with a layer of white tumor (*arrows*). **B.** The tumor is seen extending around the heart including the base and great arteries. The differential diagnosis would be malignant mesothelioma of the pericardium.

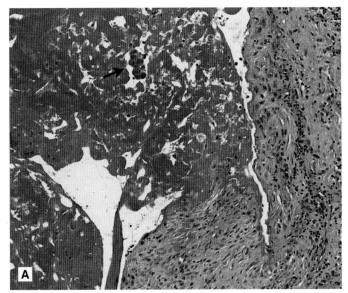
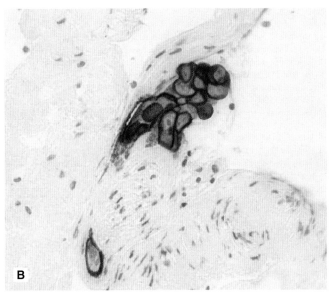

FIGURE 188.2 ▲ Metastatic carcinoma, lung primary, pericardial biopsy. **A.** There is a fibrinous exudate and a single malignant nest (*arrows*). **B.** The tumor stains for ber-EP4. TTF-1 was also positive (not shown).

The diagnosis of malignancy in hemorrhagic pericardial effusion is usually made by cytologic examination, with biopsies performed in about one-third of cases. The false-negative rate of cytology is low (<20%) and is more frequent in sarcomas and hematologic malignancies. The false-negative rate of biopsy is higher, about 40%.[5]

Microscopically, there is often a hemorrhagic exudate (Fig. 188.2). Epithelial tumors usually grow along the pericardial surface, with invasion and presence of tumor nests within the pericardial wall or epicardial angiolymphatic (Fig. 188.3). Immunohistochemistry can be very helpful in the distinction between metastatic disease and reactive mesothelial hyperplasia seen in organizing fibrinous pericarditis. The differential diagnosis is similar to that encountered in pleural biopsies (see Chapter 97).

Treatment and Prognosis

Pericardial metastasis, especially with tamponade imparts a very poor prognosis.[6] Treatment includes prolonged catheter drainage with or without pericardial sclerosis (often with tetracycline and steroids), local chemotherapy (often cis-platinum) systemic chemotherapy, combined chemotherapy, and, in some cases, local radiation therapy.[10] Although fewer than 25% of patients survive 1 year, treatment responses are achievable in the majority of patients who tolerate combined chemotherapy.[10]

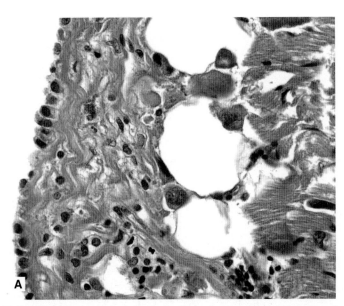
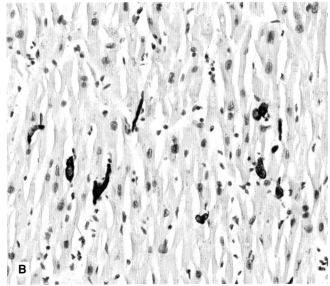

FIGURE 188.3 ▲ Metastatic cholangiocarcinoma, epicardial surface. **A.** There are enlarged atypical cells in the epicardial fat. The epicardial mesothelial surface is at the left. **B.** Cytokeratin 7 stain highlights tumor cells in the subepicardial lymphatics.

REFERENCES

1. Abraham KP, Reddy V, Gattuso P. Neoplasms metastatic to the heart: review of 3314 consecutive autopsies. *Am J Cardiovasc Pathol.* 1990;3:195–198.
2. Nakamura A, Suchi T, Mizuno Y. The effect of malignant neoplasms on the heart. A study on the electrocardiographic abnormalities and the anatomical findings in cases with and without cardiac involvement. *Jpn Circ J.* 1975;39:531–542.
3. Maleszewski JJ, Metastatic tumours. In: Travis WD, et al., eds. *WHO Classification of Tumours of the Lung, Pleura, Mediastinum and Heart.* Lyon, France: IARC Press; 2015:347–348.
4. Conway N, Hutchison S. Malignant pericardial effusion in a patient with prostate adenocarcinoma. *BMJ Case Rep.* 2012;2012. doi: 10.1136/bcr.01.2012.5570.
5. Dragoescu EA, Liu L. Pericardial fluid cytology: an analysis of 128 specimens over a 6-year period. *Cancer Cytopathol.* 2013;121:242–251.
6. Feferkorn I, Shai A, Gemer O, et al. The natural history of pericardial tamponade secondary to recurrent ovarian carcinoma—a case report and review of the literature. *Gynecol Oncol Rep.* 2014;10:53–55.
7. Lepska L, Pisiak S, Dudziak M. A case of carcinoid pericardial metastases and massive effusion. *Kardiol Pol.* 2013;71:881.
8. Nakazawa K, Kanemoto K, Suzuki H, et al. Purulent pericarditis with concurrent detection of *Streptococcus pneumoniae* and malignant squamous cells in pericardial fluid. *Intern Med.* 2013;52:1413–1416.
9. Nemeth H, Kuronya Z, Biro K, et al. Pericardial tamponade caused by tumor hemorrhage—a rare complication of metastatic testicular choriocarcinoma. *Pathol Oncol Res.* 2015;21:495–499.
10. Lestuzzi C, Bearz A, Lafaras C, et al. Neoplastic pericardial disease in lung cancer: impact on outcomes of different treatment strategies. A multicenter study. *Lung Cancer.* 2011;72:340–347.
11. Neragi-Miandoab S, Linden PA, Ducko CT, et al. VATS pericardiotomy for patients with known malignancy and pericardial effusion: survival and prognosis of positive cytology and metastatic involvement of the pericardium: a case control study. *Int J Surg.* 2008;6:110–114.
12. Cassady R, Prahlow JA. Sudden death due to cardiac tamponade from malignant pericardial involvement by metastatic lung cancer. *Forensic Sci Med Pathol.* 2015;11:127–129.

SECTION TEN
DISEASES OF THE THORACIC AORTA

189 Aortitis

Joseph J. Maleszewski, M.D., and Allen P. Burke, M.D.

Noninfectious Aortitis

Overview and Classification

Aortitis is broadly defined as inflammation of the aortic wall. Conditions that result in secondary inflammation are not typically considered aortitis. Aortic atherosclerosis, a disease that primarily affects the endothelium, is also typically not considered a form of aortitis, despite what is sometimes a considerable inflammatory component to the process.

Noninfectious aortitis is classified into several major disease classifications: giant cell/granulomatous aortitis (including Takayasu aortitis), lymphoplasmacytic aortitis (including IgG4-related sclerosing disease and that associated with rheumatologic disease), and more unusual aortic involvement by entities such as granulomatosis with polyangiitis (GPA; formerly known as Wegener granulomatosis), sarcoidosis, and Behçet disease[1-3] (Table 189.1). This chapter focuses on the more entities more commonly encountered by the surgical or autopsy pathologist.

In addition to the aforementioned traditional disease-specific classification of aortitis, a histologic pattern–based classification system has been recently proposed for use by pathologists.[4] Categories such as granulomatous/giant cell pattern–aortitis, lymphoplasmacytic pattern, mixed inflammatory pattern, suppurative pattern, and unclassified may be particularly helpful when limited clinical information is available.

Clinical Features

Most noninfectious forms of aortitis come to clinical attention because of ascending aortic dilatation/aneurysm formation and/or symptoms of secondary aortic valve regurgitation. Six to ten percent of surgical specimens for ascending aortic aneurysms demonstrate aortitis histologically. A small subset of individuals will experience aortic dissection or rupture, in which case sudden death may be the initial manifestation.

The etiology of noninfectious aortitis is unclear, but many instances are believed to be related to autoimmune phenomena and ~39% of cases are associated with frank autoimmune disorders (range from 13% to 84%).[2,5-10]

Gross Features

The gross features of noninfectious aortitis are similar across all of the histologic subtypes.[11] Aortitis can affect any site in the aorta, but has a predilection for the ascending aorta, which usually manifests the disease by increased diameter, dissection, and/or rupture.

Intimal wrinkling ("tree-barking") similar to infectious aortitis (Fig. 189.1). In many cases (particularly Takayasu aortitis), there is thickening of the aortic wall. Occasionally, there is minimal dilatation and even aortic narrowing (which may also be a curious feature of Takayasu aortitis) (Figs. 189.2 and 189.3).

TABLE 189.1 Aortitis: Clinical and Pathologic Findings

	Clinical	Site in Aorta and Other Sites of Involvement	Histologic Findings
Noninfectious			
Granulomatous (giant cell)	Association with polymyalgia rheumatica and temporal arteritis, always aneurysmal, often with aortic insufficiency, aortic dissection may occur female predilection; usually >60 y	Ascending aorta	Block-like zonal necrosis, media, with granulomatous giant cell reaction at the rim; intimal and adventitial fibrosis Diffuse, lymphoplasmacytic, nonnecrotizing (less common)
Takayasu	Hypertension, symptoms of vascular occlusion; young women, Asian descent aneurysms or stenoses	Ascending aneurysms, abdominal constriction; narrowing of coronary ostia, arch vessels, and mesenteric arteries	Similar to isolated with marked adventitial fibrosis and intimal fibrosis; zonal/laminar necrosis may not be as discrete
Lymphoplasmacytic	Rheumatoid arthritis, giant cell arteritis, others; slight female predilection, generally younger patients[a]; usually aneurysmal	Ascending aorta Descending thoracic (unusual)	Same as isolated; nonnecrotizing type may be more frequent; may have elevated IgG4-reactive plasma cell infiltrate
Infectious			
Syphilitic	Currently rare; occurs 10–15 y after untreated syphilis	Ascending, descending thoracic, massive aneurysms with erosion into surrounding structures	Necrotizing aortitis, prominent adventitial inflammation and scarring, similar features as isolated aortitis, possibly less discrete areas of necrosis
Purulent (mycotic)	History of bacteremia or osteomyelitis	Descending thoracic, mesenteric arteries, femoral arteries	Purulent inflammation with or without rupture and pseudoaneurysm

[a]Inflammatory aortic disease has been reported in patients with sarcoidosis, Behçet disease, rheumatoid arthritis, ankylosing spondylitis, lupus, and other autoimmune diseases. The link between the systemic rheumatologic disease and the aortic aneurysm is not always clear.

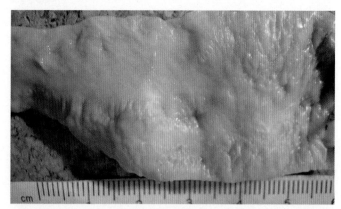

FIGURE 189.1 ▲ Ascending aortic aneurysm, aortitis. The specimen is a circumferential ring that is opened revealing marked dilatation of the aorta necessitating aortic repair with valve replacement. The characteristic feature is wrinkling or "tree-barking." This finding is secondary to intimal fibrosis, which is common in all types of aortitis, especially Takayasu or nonspecific isolated (necrotizing) aortitis. Tree-barking is classically associated with syphilis, currently a rare cause of aortitis in developed countries. The patient had no evidence of systemic vasculitis or Takayasu disease (isolated aortitis).

Granulomatous (Giant Cell) Aortitis

The most common type of encountered aortitis is granulomatous (giant cell) aortitis. The disease may be isolated to the aorta or occur in association with a systemic syndrome. Isolated aortitis refers to cases with no history or association with other rheumatic or vasculitic diseases and represents more than half of cases of ascending aortitis.[7,12] The majority of the subjects are elderly (mean age 69.1 years) although there is a large age range.[6,13] Most patients are asymptomatic and are referred for aortic aneurysm repair, with aortic valve replacement required in about half of cases.

The most common autoimmune disorder associated with ascending aortitis is giant cell *arteritis* of the temporal artery with or without polymyalgia rheumatica (PMR). The frequency of giant cell arteritis or PMR across 8 series is 19%.[2,5–10,13] Other rheumatologic disorders cause or are associated with aortitis. These include rheumatoid arthritis (~6%), systemic lupus erythematosus (3%), inflammatory bowel disease (2% to 3%), and ankylosing spondylitis/Reiter syndrome (1%).[2,5–10,13] There are also reports of associated Wegener granulomatosis, Behçet disease, polyarteritis nodosa, Cogan syndrome, Sjögren syndrome, and microscopic polyangiitis.[8]

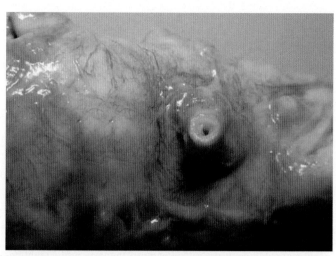

FIGURE 189.3 ▲ Takayasu disease. Takayasu disease is characterized by aortitis with extension into branch vessels resulting in the clinical syndrome, which for unknown reasons occurs almost exclusively in young women, in contrast to isolated necrotizing aortitis, which has no gender or age predominance and is usually aneurysmal. In this autopsy case of Takayasu disease and sudden death due to coronary ostial disease, there is also obstruction of aortic mesenteric ostia. (Photograph courtesy Dr. Erik Mont.)

Histologically, granulomatous aortitis is characterized by a granulomatous inflammatory infiltrate, involving the media, with a variable number of multinucleated giant cells (Figs. 189.4 to 189.7). A lymphoplasmacytic infiltrate may be present as well. The vessel frequently exhibits a "moth-eaten" appearance on elastic stain, due to the medial injury. The inflammation may involve the vasa vasorum and can even produce regional band-like infarction of the media. This is one mechanism of formation of so-called laminar medial necrosis (LMN). It is important to note, however, that LMN is neither specific for GCA nor an inflammatory process as it can be seen in noninflammatory aneurysms as well. The histologic appearance of the aortic valve only rarely shows valvulitis but rather changes secondary to insufficiency, such as mild fibrosis.[2,13]

Only a small proportion of patients diagnosed incidentally at surgery develop autoimmune syndromes or subsequent aneurysms in later years.[6,7,12]

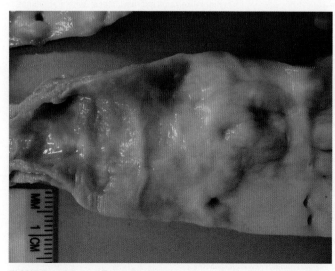

FIGURE 189.2 ▲ Takayasu disease. There is an area of constriction in the proximal abdominal aorta.

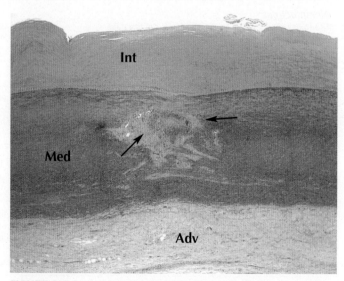

FIGURE 189.4 ▲ Necrotizing aortitis. The major findings are zonal necrosis (*arrows*) in the media (med), with intimal and adventitial fibrosis (adv). The intima is above (int). Movat pentachrome stain.

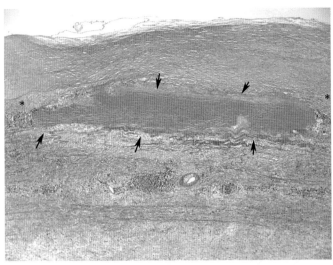

FIGURE 189.5 ▲ Necrotizing aortitis. A low magnification demonstrates a linear zone of hypereosinophilic coagulative necrosis in the media (*arrows*). There is pronounced intimal fibrosis **(above)** and adventitial scarring with pockets of chronic inflammation **(below)**, with areas of granulomatous inflammation at the lateral edges (*asterisks*).

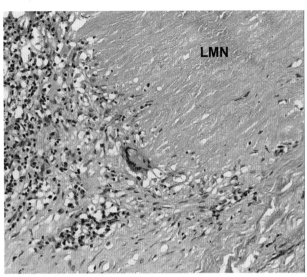

FIGURE 189.7 ▲ Necrotizing aortitis. A distinct area of necrosis of the elastic layers (laminar medial necrosis, LMN), rimmed by macrophage giant cell and lymphocytes.

Takayasu Aortitis

Takayasu aortitis was first described in 1908 by the Japanese ophthalmologist Takayasu. In 1951 Shimizu and Sano detailed the clinical features of this disorder, which they termed "pulseless disease."[14] The age at diagnosis, reported in the medical literature as Takayasu disease, ranges from 3.5 to 66 years, with a mean of 20 to 50 years. There is usually a nonspecific acute illness, but in many cases of pathologically documented aortitis, an acute phase of disease is not elicited by history. Symptoms of the late phase, which occurs from weeks to months after the initial phase, include diminished or absent pulses, bruits, and hypertension.

Histopathologic features are also dependent on the phase of the disease, though the late phase is more commonly encountered. Acutely, the disease can look identical to granulomatous aortitis and only the age of the patient can be used to reliably distinguish the two disease processes. A diagnosis of granulomatous aortitis is highly unlikely in an individual <50 years of age. In the chronic phase, there is fibrotic replacement of areas of the media with fibroplastic and fibrotic thickening of the intima and media, respectively.

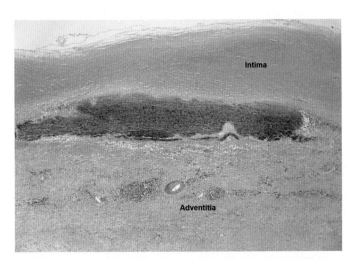

FIGURE 189.6 ▲ Necrotizing aortitis. The corresponding elastic stain (Movat pentachrome) to the area illustrated in Figure 189.5 shows that the necrotic area is still composed of stainable elastic tissue. Eventually, the elastic is destroyed and replaced by fibromuscular tissue with pools of proteoglycans that can mimic cystic medial necrosis.

Lymphoplasmacytic Aortitis (Including IgG4-Related Sclerosing Disease)

A less common pattern of aortitis is "nonnecrotizing" aortitis, which has been termed "diffuse" and "lymphoplasmacytic" aortitis (Figs. 189.8 and 189.9). Like granulomatous aortitis, there is an association with autoimmune states.

Approximately 5% to 20% of cases of thoracic aortitis may be related to IgG4-related sclerosing disease (IgG4-RSD). Although significant, it is much less than the 50% of cases of abdominal aortitis believed to be associated with IgG4-RSD. Complicating the issue, there is a lack of true consensus regarding diagnostic criteria for this entity. Many studies lack adequate serologic correlation and long-term follow-up, leading some authors to contend that elevated tissue IgG4 levels may not be specific for the diagnosis.

Histologically, lymphoplasmacytic aortitis lacks a granulomatous pattern of inflammation and, as the name would imply, is characterized by brisk lymphoplasmacytic infiltrate of the aortic media with associated damage. Tissue sections of aortic specimens with IgG4-RSD aortitis frequently exhibit a nongranulomatous lymphocytic aortitis with increased numbers of plasma cells. Eosinophils and obliterative phlebitis are also frequently observed. Storiform fibrosis, when present, is strongly suggestive of the diagnosis, though precise criteria defining such are lacking (Fig. 189.10).

Infectious Aortitis

Syphilitic Aortitis

Historical studies prior to the age of antibiotics have suggested that cardiac complications occur in ~10% of syphilitic patients. The latent period is usually 10 to 25 years. In the classic study by Heggtveit,[15] two-thirds of autopsy patients with cardiovascular syphilis had the classic triad of ascending aneurysm, aortic regurgitation, and coronary ostial stenosis. The clinical diagnosis of syphilis was made in only 20% of his cases, however.

Aneurysms are seen in over 90% of syphilitic aortitis (Fig. 189.11) and occur in the sinus of Valsalva (1%), ascending aorta (46%), transverse arch (24%), descending arch (5%), descending thoracic aorta (5%), abdominal aorta (7%), and multiple sites (4%).[15] The classic "tree-bark" appearance is shared with noninflammatory aortitis. Aortic rupture may occur, but dissections are unusual.[12]

Histologically, there are multifocal lymphoplasmacytic infiltrates in the adventitia and media (Fig. 189.12). Endarteritis obliterans can occur within the vasa vasorum. Microgummas may occur within the

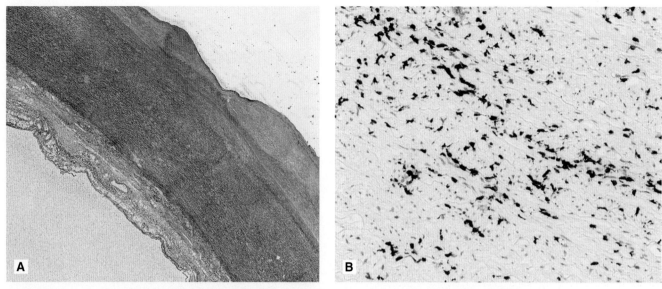

FIGURE 189.8 ▲ Nonnecrotizing aortitis. **A.** Elastic stain at lower power is unremarkable. **B.** CD3 immunohistochemical stain shows a diffuse infiltrate of T lymphocytes.

aortic media, but these are presumably identical to laminar necrosis of isolated necrotizing aortitis. Treponemes are usually impossible to demonstrate by silver impregnation stains. Uncommon complications of syphilitic aortitis include superior vena cava syndrome, bony erosion, aortopulmonary fistula, dissection, and stroke. Syphilitic aortitis is currently extremely rare in the United States and other developed countries. In general, syphilitic aortitis is more likely to cause massive aneurysm and erosion into adjacent structures, including bone, as compared with noninfectious aortitis of the proximal aorta.[12]

Pyogenic Aortitis (Infectious Aneurysm)

Nontreponemal infections of the aorta generally result in saccular, or less commonly fusiform aneurysms. The original designation "mycotic aneurysm" has been replaced by "infectious aneurysm." Bacteria most commonly invade the aorta implantation on the intimal surface,

occasionally in areas of atherosclerotic disruption, usually in patients with bacteremia caused by endocarditis. Other means include embolization into vasa vasorum, direct extension of infection from contiguous extravascular site, and iatrogenic inoculation of contaminated material into the vessel wall. Contiguous inoculation is often a complication of vertebral osteomyelitis. The formation of the aneurysm may evolve rapidly, over the course of days, after the initiation of the aortitis.

Infectious aneurysms often occur in the descending thoracic aorta. The most common organisms currently are *Staphylococcus aureus* (nearly half), *Salmonella* species, streptococci, Gram-negative rods, and fungi.[16-19] No organism is detected in up to 10% of cases. In addition to endocarditis, risk factors include prior surgery and transplantation.[16-19]

Grossly, infectious aneurysms are often saccular outpouchings measuring up to 5 cm in diameter. There is typically marked edema and inflammation of the adventitia, which results in characteristic soft

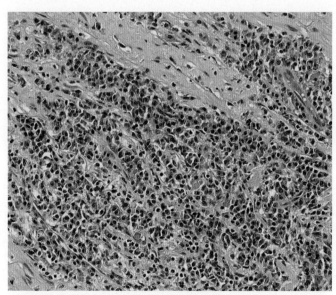

FIGURE 189.9 ▲ Nonnecrotizing aortitis. In some cases, there are abundant plasma cells (lymphoplasmacytic type).

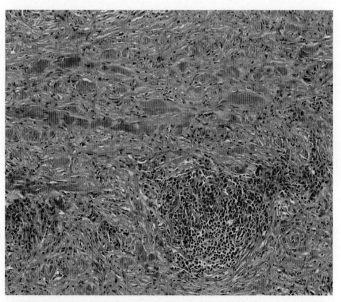

FIGURE 189.10 ▲ Sclerosing periaortitis. There is keloidal collagen and lymphoid aggregates. The fibrosis is vaguely storiform. There were areas of phlebosclerosis (not shown). These are features of IgG4-related disease.

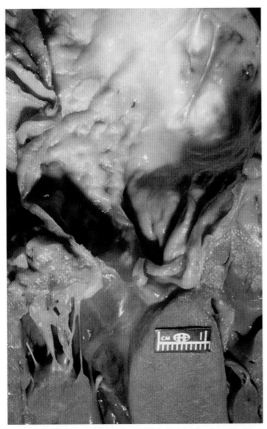

FIGURE 189.11 ▲ Syphilitic aneurysm. There is marked dilatation of the ascending aorta by an aneurysm, which is transilluminated. Syphilitic aneurysms are typically located in the ascending aorta, similar to those of isolated necrotizing aortitis, but are much rarer. They often show paper-thin walls and erode into surrounding structures.

tissue swelling on computed tomography or magnetic resonance imaging. Histologically, there are numerous neutrophils with extension into the adventitia. A rupture site may be seen in autopsies from patients dying with aortic rupture and pyogenic aneurysm.

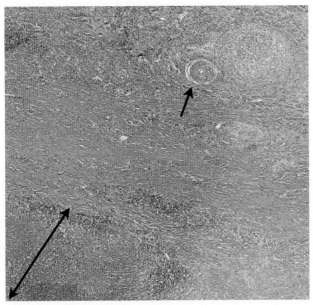

FIGURE 189.12 ▲ Syphilitic aortitis. There is marked fibrosis of the adventitia and destruction of the media (*two-sided arrow*). There is adventitial arterial thickening (*arrow*).

Practical Points

▶ There is no standardized classification of noninfectious aortitis, because the histologic findings are nonspecific, as well as clinical features of associated autoimmune syndromes, but there has been a recent shift to pattern-based classification.

▶ The surgical pathologist will see noninfectious aortitis primarily as an incidental finding in ascending aortic aneurysm repair; the histologic findings are those of necrosis of the media and variable inflammation and scarring of the adventitial and intima.

▶ The prognosis of isolated aortitis resulting in aortic aneurysm is excellent after repair, and most patients do not require anti-inflammatory treatment.

▶ Some cases of necrotizing aortitis are associated with autoimmune disease such as rheumatoid arthritis and inflammatory bowel disease; the histologic features are indistinguishable from isolated aortitis.

▶ Takayasu aortitis is a clinicopathologic term suggesting aortitis with stenosis of coronary ostia, arch vessels, or mesenteric arteries and is more likely to involve the descending and abdominal aorta with stenosis.

▶ Syphilitic aortitis is a rare cause of necrotizing aortitis and shares many histologic features with isolated aortitis; the diagnosis rests on serologic testing, as spirochetes are rarely seen in tissue sections.

REFERENCES

1. Stone JH, et al. IgG4-related systemic disease and lymphoplasmacytic aortitis. *Arthritis Rheum.* 2009;60(10):3139–3145.
2. Xu L, Heath J, Burke A. Ascending aortitis: a clinicopathological study of 21 cases in a series of 300 aortic repairs. *Pathology.* 2014;46(4):296–305.
3. Maleszewski JJ. Inflammatory ascending aortic disease: perspectives from pathology. *J Thorac Cardiovasc Surg.* 2015;149(2 suppl):S176–S183.
4. Stone JR, et al. Consensus statement on surgical pathology of the aorta from the Society for Cardiovascular Pathology and the Association for European Cardiovascular Pathology: I. Inflammatory diseases. *Cardiovasc Pathol.* 2015;24(5):267–278.
5. Fujimoto H, et al. Influence of aortitis on late outcomes after repair of ascending aortic aneurysms. *J Thorac Cardiovasc Surg.* 2015;150(3):589–594.
6. Liang KP, et al. Noninfectious ascending aortitis: a case series of 64 patients. *J Rheumatol.* 2009;36(10):2290–2297.
7. Miller DV, et al. Surgical pathology of noninfectious ascending aortitis: a study of 45 cases with emphasis on an isolated variant. *Am J Surg Pathol.* 2006;30(9):1150–1158.
8. Rojo-Leyva F, et al. Study of 52 patients with idiopathic aortitis from a cohort of 1,204 surgical cases. *Arthritis Rheum.* 2000;43(4):901–907.
9. Ryan C, et al. Non-infectious aortitis of the ascending aorta—a histological and clinical correlation of 71 cases including overlap with medial degeneration and atheroma—a challenge for the pathologist. *J Clin Pathol.* 2015;68(11):898–904.
10. Schmidt J, et al. Predictors for pathologically confirmed aortitis after resection of the ascending aorta: a 12-year Danish nationwide population-based cross-sectional study. *Arthritis Res Ther.* 2011;13(3):R87.
11. Miller DV, Maleszewski JJ. The pathology of large-vessel vasculitides. *Clin Exp Rheumatol.* 2011;29(1 suppl 64):S92–S98.
12. Tavora F, Burke A. Review of isolated ascending aortitis: differential diagnosis, including syphilitic, Takayasu's and giant cell aortitis. *Pathology.* 2006;38(4):302–308.
13. Burke AP, et al. Aortitis and ascending aortic aneurysm: description of 52 cases and proposal of a histologic classification. *Hum Pathol.* 2008;39(4):514–526.
14. Shimizu K, Sano K. Pulseless disease. *J Neuropathol.* 1951;1:37–47.
15. Heggtveit HA. Syphilitic aortitis. A clinicopathologic autopsy study of 100 cases, 1950–1960. *Circulation.* 1964;29:346–355.

16. Feltis BA, Lee DA, Beilman GJ. Mycotic aneurysm of the descending thoracic aorta caused by Pseudomonas aeruginosa in a solid organ transplant recipient: case report and review. *Surg Infect (Larchmt).* 2002;3(1):29–33.
17. Helleman JN, et al. Mycotic aneurysm of the descending thoracic aorta. Review and case report. *Acta Chir Belg.* 2007;107(5):544–547.
18. Pereira AA. Mycotic aneurysm as a result of severe salmonella infection in the adult intensive care unit: two case studies. *Dynamics.* 2006;17(4):16–18.
19. Silva ME, et al. Mycotic aneurysm of the thoracic aorta due to *Aspergillus terreus*: case report and review. *Clin Infect Dis.* 2000;31(5):1144–1148.

190 Noninflammatory Thoracic Aortic Aneurysms and Dissections

Allen P. Burke, M.D., and Joseph J. Maleszewski, M.D.

Terminology

The term aneurysm refers to a dilatation of a structure beyond its expected borders. Thus, the term is applied somewhat subjectively depending on the observer and modality used for observation. Aneurysms are broadly dichotomized into fusiform or saccular varieties by circumferential extent and shape. Saccular aortic aneurysms are a noncircumferential outpouching of the vessel wall and are typically seen outside the ascending aorta. Fusiform aortic aneurysms are circumferential and typically seen in the ascending aorta.

In addition to shape, aneurysms may also be classified based on the constituency of the aneurysm wall, as evidenced by histopathology. True aneurysms contain portions of all three layers of the vessel wall: intima, media, and adventitia. Dissections (so-called dissecting aneurysms) represent an intramedial channel of blood usually resulting from an intimal tear. False aneurysms (also called "contained ruptures") represent disruption of the vessel wall to the level of the adventitia, but not beyond. As such, the aneurysm wall of the latter will usually contain adventitia, intima (from reendothelialization), and occasionally mural thrombus (but *without* media).

Epidemiology

The incidence of thoracic aortic aneurysms is difficult to determine, as most patients are asymptomatic. The incidence is believed to be increasing and has been estimated at about 0.3% of the population, as defined by an aorta >5 cm in diameter.[1] There is an approximate 2:1 male predilection.[1]

The normal ascending aortic diameter as measured echocardiographically increases with age, from a mean of 3 cm at age 30 to 3.5 at age 80, and is related to body mass index.[2]

Location

Thoracic aortic aneurysms may involve the ascending aorta, aortic arch, descending aorta, or a combination of these locations. Proximal thoracic aortic aneurysms are usually fusiform dilatations of the ascending aorta that typically do not extend into the arch and are associated with systemic hypertension, inherited syndromes, and congenitally bicuspid aortic valves. Descending aneurysms may be fusiform or saccular and often extend into the abdominal aorta. Descending aneurysms are typically atherosclerotic. Other causes of descending thoracic aneurysms include postinfectious or mycotic aneurysms (see Chapter 189) and posttraumatic pseudoaneurysms. Posttraumatic pseudoaneurysms are typically located in the proximal descending thoracic aorta.

Etiology

Systemic hypertension is believed to be responsible for most ascending aortic aneurysms, but the exact mechanism is unknown.

Another major cause of noninflammatory thoracic aneurysms is the inherited connective tissue disease syndromes, specifically Marfan syndrome (MFS), Loeys-Dietz syndrome (LDS), and familial thoracic aortic aneurysm and dissection.[3] The major associations are bicuspid aortic valve and systemic hypertension. Approximately 25% of patients with thoracic aortic aneurysms have no known cause or association.

From a series of resected thoracic aneurysms at a referral center, 13% of noninflammatory aneurysms were associated with an inherited connective tissue disease, mostly MFS; 25% of patients had bicuspid aortic valves; and 51% had no association other than hypertension.[4]

Thoracic aortic aneurysms can be divided in four main categories regarding their association with genetic diseases (Table 190.1):
• Sporadic cases often associated with hypertension, with onset in mid or late adulthood. Approximately 20% of these patients have a family history, and the apparent inheritance is usually autosomal dominant and likely owing to multiple genetic and epigenetic factors.
• Cases associated with bicuspid aortic valve disease with familial aggregation; these constitute ~10% of patients and present in the 50s to 60s, with a strong male predominance.
• MFS; these constitute 3% to 15% of patients, depending on population.
• Other genetic conditions, including type IV Ehlers-Danlos syndrome and LDS (<1% of cases).

Many patients with aortic aneurysm and dissection do not fit any syndrome of collagen vascular disease, such as MFS, yet as many as 20% of those will have at least one first-degree family member with a known aneurysm in the arterial tree, usually with autosomal dominant inheritance.[5] In a series of patients with nonfamilial aortic aneurysms, only 3% carried mutations associated with aortic dissections, including *ACTA2* (α-actin2) or *FBN1* (fibrillin1). A higher rate (17%) of mutations, including *FBN1* and *TGFβR2*, was found in familial non-Marfan aneurysm patients.[3]

Bicuspid aortic valve disease is a common congenital cardiac defect that affects ~1% to 2% of the general population. There is a greater than fivefold risk for the development of proximal aortic aneurysms and

TABLE 190.1 Noninflammatory Thoracic Aneurysms: Characteristics by Associations

	Mean Age	Degree of Medial Degeneration	Aortic Root Involvement/ Sinotubular Junction Dilatation	Approximate Overall Frequency
Marfan syndrome	15–25	Severe	Usual	10%
Familial non-Marfan	20–40	Moderate to severe	Common	20%
Bicuspid aortic valve	30–40	Mild to moderate	Common	10%
Sporadic/hypertension	50–70	None to mild	Uncommon	60%

dissections.[6] Unicuspid aortic valve is associated with thoracic aortic aneurysm at an even higher rate.[6]

The cardiac manifestations of bicuspid aortic valve disease, which becomes manifest in most patients during the course of their lifetimes, are isolated aortic regurgitation (see Chapter 36), isolated ascending aortic aneurysm, aortic regurgitation associated with aortic aneurysm, isolated aortic stenosis (see Chapter 35), and aortic stenosis with aneurysm.[7] One-third of patients with bicuspid aortic valve and aortic aneurysms have aortic valve stenosis, and the other two-thirds valve insufficiency, with a small number having normal valve function.[8,9]

The genetic basis for bicuspid aortic valve syndrome, which is inherited as autosomal dominant disease in a minority of patients, is still unknown, although several cohorts with mutations in *GATA5, NKX2.5,* and *NOTCH1* have been reported.[10–12]

MFS is a disorder characterized by abnormalities of the eyes, skeleton, and cardiovascular system. MFS is an autosomal dominant disease, with 25% of patients having no family history (presumed *de novo* mutations). Cardiovascular manifestations of MFS include aortic root dilatation, ascending aortic dilatation, aortic dissections, other sites of aortic aneurysm, and mitral valve prolapse.[3] The histologic feature of aortic aneurysms in MFS is loss of elastic laminae with pooling of proteoglycans, so-called medial degeneration. The histologic findings are also seen to lesser degrees in familial non-Marfan aortic dissection and those associated with bicuspid aortic valve.

In the absence of surgical treatment, patients with MFS have a 50% risk of developing aortic dissection during their lifetime. The aortic dilatation observed in MFS is the result of defects in a specific component of the elastic fiber, fibrillin-1,[13] which is encoded by the *FBN1* gene on chromosome 15. An online database (http://omim.org/entry/134797) contains more than 250 mutations with variations of clinical expression. In a series of unrelated patients with suspected MFS and aortic aneurysms, a mutation could be found in 31%, mostly *FBN1*, and one mutation in *TGFβR1*, using sequencing and multiplex polymerase chain reaction techniques.[3]

LDS is an autosomal dominant Marfan-like connective tissue disorder that is an increasingly recognized cause of thoracic aortic aneurysm (http://omim.org/entry/6091912). It results from genetic mutations in the transforming growth factor beta receptors 1 and 2 (*TGFBR1* and *TGFBR2*). The syndrome is characterized by hypertelorism, bifid uvula, cleft palate, and arterial tortuosity with aneurysms and dissections. LDS has an earlier onset than does MFS, with recommendations for prophylactic aortic root replacement at younger ages and with smaller aortic dimensions. Histologically, there is diffuse medial degeneration, which may be subtle.[14] In a series of unrelated patients with suspected MFS and aortic aneurysms, a mutation could be found in 17%, mostly *TGFβR2*[3]

Type IV Ehlers-Danlos syndrome (EDS) (vascular type) is due to defects in the type III procollagen (*COL3A1*) (http://omim.org/entry/130050). It causes vascular fragility with aneurysm formation, rupture, and dissections. The aorta is involved in a small percentage, since this disease affects most often smaller arteries. Usually, there are multiple rupture sites in the aorta. Patients with type IV EDS may also have thoracic aortic aneurysms; however, the typical complication is rupture in normal-caliber artery. Coronary artery dissections, aortic rupture, iliac and femoral rupture, and coronary and other muscular arterial aneurysms are among the different complications seen in these patients. Generally, fewer than 1% of patients in series of thoracic aneurysms have EDS.

Osteogenesis imperfecta shares some clinical features with EDS. Type I osteogenesis imperfecta, the result of mutations in *COL1A1*, is weakly associated with aortic root dilatation, aortic insufficiency, and mitral valve prolapse (http://omim.org/entry/166200).

Ninety percent of descending thoracic aortic aneurysms are atherosclerotic. They are less frequently resected than ascending aortic aneurysms and are frequently treated medically or by endovascular repair.[15]

Clinical Features

A large percentage of patients with thoracic aortic aneurysms are asymptomatic. Thoracic aneurysms are usually found incidentally by imaging studies; the pathologist may encounter them at autopsy, some-

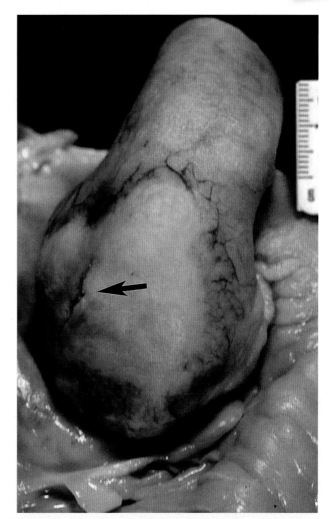

FIGURE 190.1 ▲ Proximal ascending aortic aneurysm, with rupture. The right side of the proximal ascending aorta is shown. There is a discrete area of saccular aneurysm, with a rupture site (*arrow*). There was no dissection. The histologic findings were those of marked cystic medial necrosis (not shown). Thoracic aneurysms with underlying cystic media necrosis have a variety of possible outcomes: dissection before significant dilatation, dilatation and then rupture without dissection, and dilatation with dissection. (Reproduced with permission from Virmani R, Burke AP, Farb A, et al. Cardiovascular pathology. In: Virmani R, Burke AP, Farb A, et al., eds. *Major Problems in Pathology Series.* Philadelphia, PA: WB Saunders; 2001;40:489.)

times after unexpected rupture (Figs. 190.1 and 190.2; Table 190.2). Symptoms develop in the setting of aortic insufficiency (aneurysms involving the aortic root or ascending aorta), dissection, or rupture.

The growth of aneurysm may be indolent, and there is debate as to the appropriate timing of surgical intervention, which typically occurs when the size reaches 5 cm. Serial imaging studies have shown a slow growth rate (about 1 mm yearly) until the diameter is about 5 cm, at which time it may be more rapid.[16,17]

Gross Findings

As noted above, uncomplicated thoracic aortic aneurysms can be divided grossly into saccular and fusiform. Fusiform aneurysms are most common and affect the entire circumference of the aorta and have tapered borders. Among the types of thoracic aneurysms, only infectious (mycotic) aneurysms, posttraumatic pseudoaneurysms, and penetrating atheromatous ulcers are typically saccular, all of which have a propensity for the distal thoracic aorta.

Aneurysms of the proximal portion of the aorta may stretch the aortic ring, resulting in aortic insufficiency (annuloaortic ectasia).

term has replaced legacy terminology such as cystic medial necrosis or cystic medial degeneration, which has largely fallen out of favor given that the observed lesions are neither cystic nor necrotic. Medial degeneration is characterized by an accumulation of basophilic ground substance in the media with areas of elastic fiber dropout[19] (Fig. 190.3). The pooling of proteoglycans is accompanied by extensive loss of elastic lamellae and smooth muscle cells. These changes result in the medial weakening that progresses to aneurysm, dissection, or both.

The greatest degrees of medial degeneration are often seen in the setting of inherited connective tissue disease, like MFS. Older patients with nonhereditary thoracic aortic aneurysms, and those associated with bicuspid aortic valve, have relatively small degrees of medial degeneration.[4]

Another histopathologic pattern is laminar medial necrosis or smooth muscle nuclear dropout. This nonspecific finding can be seen in all etiologies of aneurysm, even postinflammatory states. It is characterized by what is thought to be coagulative necrosis of medial smooth muscle cells, resulting in loss of nuclei and collapse of the elastic lamellae in a band-like pattern.[4]

Treatment and Prognosis

Ascending aortic aneurysms have several anatomic subsets, which affect surgical approach. Aortic root disease with or without ascending aortic involvement (annuloaortic ectasia) generally results in aortic insufficiency and often requires valve replacement with valved ascending aortic graft and reimplantation of coronary arteries (Bentall procedure) or valve-sparing aortic root repair with root reconstruction with or without valve reimplantation.[20]

Ascending aortic aneurysms not involving the root may cause aortic insufficiency due to dilatation of the sinotubular junction, but aortic valve insufficiency is generally corrected by aneurysm repair only and valve replacement is not necessary. In patients with valve disease (usually described as "floppy" or myxoid valve disease; Chapter 36), especially those with bicuspid aortic valves, valve repair or replacement may be necessary.[20] Among patients with ascending aneurysms and aortic insufficiency, two-thirds can be treated with ascending aortic aneurysm repair, and the remaining patients require valve replacement.[21]

The prognosis for patients with ascending aneurysm after aortic repair, with or without aortic valve surgery, is excellent, and is nearly that of an age-matched control population.[20]

The rate of rupture or dissection increases dramatically after 6-cm diameter is reached in a patient without a heritable connective tissue disease.[17] For those with a heritable connective tissue disease, 5 cm is considered the threshold for surgical repair to prevent complication.

Aortic Dissection
Background and Classification
Dissections are a potential complication of noninflammatory thoracic aortic aneurysms. An intimal tear results in splitting of the media, usually at or near the adventitial border, resulting in a *dissection plane*, or *false lumen*, that forms under pressure secondary to inherent medial weakness.

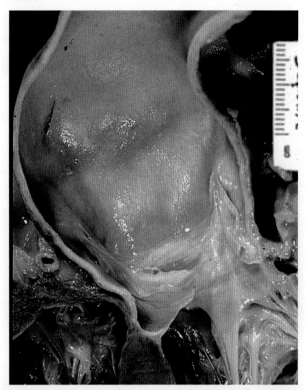

FIGURE 190.2 ▲ The aneurysm involves the ascending aorta with little involvement of the aortic root, explaining why there was no prior aortic valve insufficiency. (Reproduced with permission from Virmani R, Burke AP, Farb A, et al. Cardiovascular pathology. In: Virmani R, Burke AP, Farb A, et al., eds. *Major Problems in Pathology Series.* Philadelphia, PA: WB Saunders; 2001;40:489.)

Involvement of the aortic root is typical of MFS, syphilitic aneurysms, noninfectious aortitis, and bicuspid aortic valve disease. In noninflammatory aneurysms, the arch is generally spared, but aneurysms caused by aortitis[18] and atherosclerotic aneurysms frequently involve to the arch vessels.

The adventitial appearance of thoracic aneurysm is generally unremarkable, unless there is rupture without dissection, resulting in soft tissue hemorrhage. The intimal surface may exhibit atherosclerosis or occasionally mural thrombus in the region of the aneurysm.

Histologic Findings

Noninflammatory aortic aneurysms in adults are caused by myriad conditions, which may manifest as many histopathologic patterns, some subtle and others overt. No histopathologic patterns have been shown to exhibit disease specificity, and therefore, correlation with the presentation and clinical setting is paramount.

One of the more common histopathologic manifestations of noninflammatory aortic disease is so-called medial degeneration. This

TABLE 190.2 Percent Presence of Histologic Findings in Noninflammatory Aortic Aneurysm, Surgically Resected Specimens, Ascending Aorta[4]

	Connective Tissue Disorder[a]	Bicuspid Aortic Valve	Hypertension	Total
Cystic media necrosis[b]	63%	33%	42%	41%
Normal aorta	4%	40%	12%	18%
Acute dissection[c]	27%	18%	25%	21%

[a]Predominantly MFS, confirmed genetically in ½ of patients.
[b]Cystic medial necrosis has been graded as mild, moderate, or severe, when 5% to 25%, 26% to 75%, or >75%, respectively, of the medial thickness was involved.
[c]The uninvolved aorta shows medial degeneration in approximately the same frequencies as in nondissected aortas.
Data modified from Homme JL, Aubry MC, Edwards WD, et al. Surgical pathology of the ascending aorta: a clinicopathologic study of 513 cases. *Am J Surg Pathol.* 2006;30:1159–1168. Ref. [4].

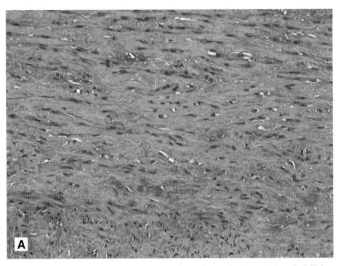

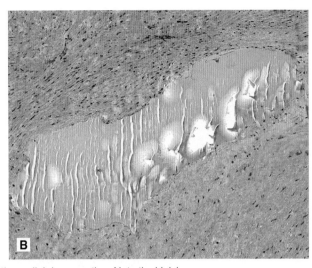

FIGURE 190.3 ▲ Medial degeneration, thoracic aneurysm. **A.** Mild cystic medial degeneration. Note the bluish accumulations of proteoglycans. **B.** There is a cyst-like area of proteoglycans in more severe medial degeneration.

The most commonly used classification is the one by DeBakey and colleagues[22]. Three major types are described (Fig. 190.4):

- Dissection involving both the ascending and descending aorta (type I), with the origin (intimal tear) in the ascending aorta
- Dissection only in the ascending aorta (type II) (intimal tear and dissection plane)

- Dissection involving only the descending aorta and rare examples of intimal tear in the descending aorta and dissection plane in both descending and ascending aorta (type III)

The Stanford classification simplifies this scheme into (A) dissections involving the ascending aorta and (B) dissections not involving the ascending aorta.[23] Sometimes considered in a separate category are those aortic dissections with the intimal tear in the aortic arch, which are clinically similar to type III dissections[24,25] (Figs. 190.5 and 190.6).

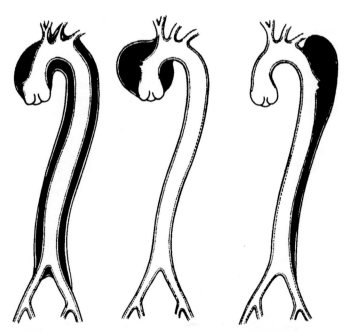

FIGURE 190.4 ▲ Patterns of aortic dissection. In DeBakey type I (**left**), dissection occurs both proximal and distal to the aortic arch, with the intimal tear proximal to the aortic arch. In type II (**center**), the dissection is contained proximal to the arch, and in type III (**right**), the intimal tear and dissection are distal to the arch. The approximate frequencies are 55%, 20%, and 25%, respectively. When the tear is distal with both proximal and distal dissection, the term IIIa is sometimes used. The Stanford classification is not based on intimal tear. Type A denotes dissection involving the ascending aorta, and type B not involving the ascending aorta. (Reproduced with permission from Isselbacher EM, Eagle KA, Desanctis RW. Diseases of the aorta. In: Braunwald E, ed. *Heart Disease. A Textbook of Cardiovascular Medicine.* Philadelphia, PA: WB Saunders; 1997:1555).

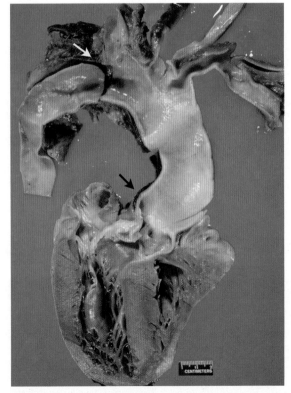

FIGURE 190.5 ▲ Acute dissection. The intimal tear is in the arch just distal to the arch vessels (*white arrow*). The dissection plane extended both distally and proximally to the level of the aortic valve (*black arrow*).

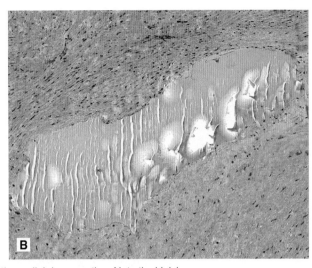

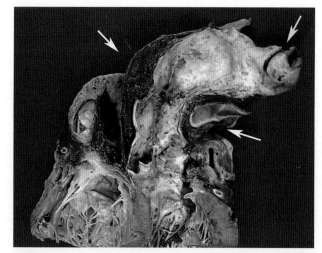

FIGURE 190.6 ▲ Ascending aortic aneurysm with acute dissection. The false lumen filled with partly clotted blood can be seen surrounding the aorta (*white arrows*). The intimal tear was distal to the arch (*yellow arrow*)

Clinical

Common associations with aortic dissection are presented in Table 190.3. Men are twice as likely as women to experience aortic dissections, which occur on average at age 60.[28] Patients with Marfan or other hereditary syndromes present at a far younger age, in the teens or early 20s. Only one-fifth of patients with acute aortic dissections who present for surgery have a prior history of aortic or valve disease.[29]

In autopsy series, type I and II dissections outnumber type III dissections, because they are more lethal.[6] The underlying causes and associations mirror those of noninflammatory aneurysms and vary similarly between ascending and descending aneurysms. There is a 9- and 18-fold increased risk for ascending aortic dissections in patients with bi- and unicuspid valves.[6]

For ascending aortic dissections, the most common symptom of the initial intimal tear is that of severe back pain, between the scapulae. Rupture of the false lumen, which occurs into the pericardial cavity in proximal dissections, results in cardiac tamponade and sudden death. The time interval between onset of symptoms and death, in patients who are not diagnosed, averages several days but can be only a few hours.[30] In two-thirds of patients undergoing operation, symptoms were present for 2 days or less.[29]

Ascending type A aortic dissections are missed clinically in over one-fourth of patients and can be initially discovered during coronary artery bypass surgery.[30] There is often a trigger for the initial intimal tear, such as sporting activity, lifting of heavy weights, or sexual intercourse in men.[28] In up to 15% of patients, no pain is reported.[31]

TABLE 190.3   Aortic Dissection, Associations, Autopsy Studies, % Frequency

	Marfan	Bicuspid AV	Hypertension	None
Type I/II (A)	5	16	52	27
Type III (B)	2	1-2[a]	78	20

[a]No difference from the general population.
Data from Larson EW, Edwards WD. Risk factors for aortic dissection: a necropsy study of 161 cases. *Am J Cardiol*. 1984;53:849–855. Ref. [6]; Roberts CS, Roberts WC. Aortic dissection with the entrance tear in transverse aorta: analysis of 12 autopsy patients. *Ann Thorac Surg*. 1990;50:762–766. Ref. [25]; Nakashima Y, Kurozumi T, Sueishi K, et al. Dissecting aneurysm: a clinicopathologic and histopathologic study of 111 autopsied cases. *Hum Pathol*. 1990;21:291–296. Ref. [26]; Wilson SK, Hutchins GM. Aortic dissecting aneurysms: causative factors in 204 subjects. *Arch Pathol Lab Med*. 1982;106:175–180. Ref. [27].

TABLE 190.4   Aortic Dissections, Causes of Death, and Sites of Rupture

	Type I and II (A)	Type III (B)
Pericardium	90	6
Mediastinum	2	6
Left pleural cavity	6	60
Right pleural cavity	2	24
Retroperitoneum	0	6

The causes of death related to aortic dissections are presented in Table 190.4.

Gross Pathologic Findings, Type I and II Aortic Dissections

Grossly, the intimal tear is usually within millimeters of the sinotubular junction and is most often transverse, perpendicular to blood flow, or may be somewhat angled (Fig. 190.7). Occasionally, it is circumferential, rarely resulting in intussusception of the artery. The aortic valve is bicuspid in about 10% of patients, an important feature to note, because of the heritable implications.

The degree of aneurysmal dilatation is variable, and often difficult to assess because of the tear, but should be estimated for clinical correlation in the case of imaging during life. Atherosclerosis is generally mild.

The false lumen rupture site is often overlooked but is generally near the intimal tear and results in hemopericardium.

The extent of the dissection plane, which is variably filled with blood, should be documented and forms the basis for classification. Extremely rare examples of "bloodless" dissections without intimal tears or significant blood in the false lumen have been reported causing sudden unexpected death, by unclear mechanisms.[32]

In chronic dissections, there is an intimal "flap" separating the normal intima from the dissected portion of the aorta, which typically has a mottled, coarse surface as opposed to the smooth normal intima (Fig. 190.8).

Most unoperated aortic dissections cause sudden unexpected death and are therefore medicolegal autopsies. Hospital autopsies of patients dying with aortic dissections have often been operated. The typical procedure is that of valve replacement with a Dacron tube graft that also replaces the ascending aorta. The distal portion of the false lumen

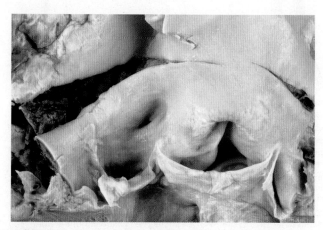

FIGURE 190.7 ▲ Intimal tear, proximal aorta. The tear is linear, near-circumferential, and just beyond the (tricuspid) aortic valve.

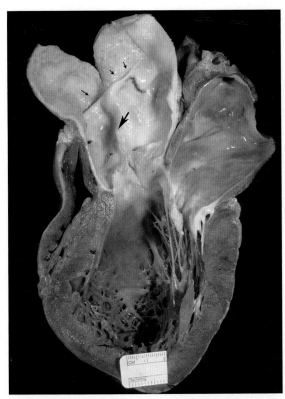

FIGURE 190.8 ▲ Ascending aortic aneurysm, Marfan syndrome. The *arrow* demonstrates the commissure between the right and noncoronary cusp, denoting the region of the sinotubular junction. The aortic root, proximal to this line, is dilated. The *small arrows* point to a shelf indicating the site of an old dissection.

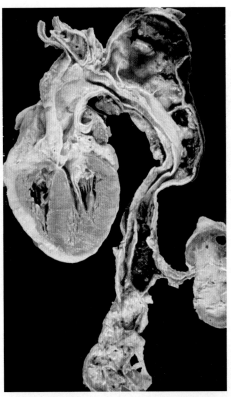

FIGURE 190.9 ▲ Aortic dissection, type III. The saccular dilated false lumen ruptured into the left pleural cavity. A healed dissection is present in the descending thoracic aorta, which extended just distal to the left renal artery. There is organizing thrombus in the false lumen near the subclavian as well as the left renal. Note fibrous tags in the false lumen at sites of intercostal artery origin. Type III dissections tend to have a more chronic course than types I and II and are more likely to show chronicity. (Reproduced with permission from Virmani R, Burke AP, Farb A, eds. *Atlas of Cardiovascular Pathology*. Philadelphia, PA: WB Saunders; 1996:130, Figure 15.11.)

is filled with a synthetic glue (BioGlue) in order to decrease the complication of redissection.[33]

The surgical pathology specimen is usually an intact ring of aorta, with adventitial hemorrhage and an evident false lumen. Occasionally, the inner and outer portions of the specimen are separate and the specimen is fragmented. It is optimal to attempt orientation of the aortic wall to allow for evaluation of reactive histologic changes secondary to the dissection and to document underlying medial disease.

Gross Pathologic Findings, Type III Aortic Dissections

Type III aortic dissections are far less common than type I or II dissections, as an unexpected cause of death at autopsy. More frequently, the diagnosis is known, and the patient has had medical therapy. Surgical intervention historically is performed in only 20% of patients with type III dissections, compared to 37% of type A dissections, because of a high risk of complications and success of antihypertensive treatment.[23]

Because of the chronicity of type III dissections, the false lumen is usually dilated and contains organized thrombus, with webs and fibrotic strands spanning the sides of the channel (Fig. 190.9). The parallel true and false lumens give the impression of a "double-barrel" aorta (Fig. 190.10).

Atherosclerosis is far more commonly seen at the entry tear of type III dissections than type A dissections and is present in four-fifths of cases.[6] Localized dissections with atherosclerosis at the intimal tear site have been termed aortic intramural hematomas that are diagnosed by imaging studies. They often regress with medical therapy but may extend to a full-blown type III dissection.[34] Histologic documentation has only rarely been reported as blood within the outer media.[35]

The distal portion of the false lumen will demonstrate a second communication with the true lumen, in the form of a reentry tear, similar to type I and II dissections (Fig. 190.11). The intimal tears associated with aortic dissections heal over time, in cases of prolonged survival, and have a white fibrous surface. The lining of the false lumen typically has a wrinkled, almost aortitis-like surface, in contrast to a true intima.

Type III dissections can be surgically corrected with placement of a Dacron conduit (Fig. 190.12). Percutaneous intervention, in the form of endografts, has become an alternate treatment of choice for chronic type III dissections, as well as nondissected noninflammatory and inflammatory thoracic aneurysms[36] (Fig. 190.13). The complications of paraparesis and paraplegia may be lower using thoracic endovascular aneurysm repairs (TEVARs) than for open thoracic aneurysm surgery.[37]

Histologic Findings

The histologic findings of acute ascending aortic dissections depend on the age of the dissection. Initially, within 12 hours, there is lining of fibrin and platelets along the tear, with sparse acute medial inflammation and no adventitial reaction (Fig. 190.14). From 12 hours to 2 days, there is a neutrophilic infiltrate in the media, with variable adventitial inflammation. Before 1 week, there is a phase of eosinophilic inflammation in the adventitia, after which macrophages and granulation tissue predominate (Fig. 190.15). Hemosiderin macrophages occur occasionally after 1 week.[29] The inflammatory changes in the media, in contrast to aortitis, occur primarily along the tear.[29]

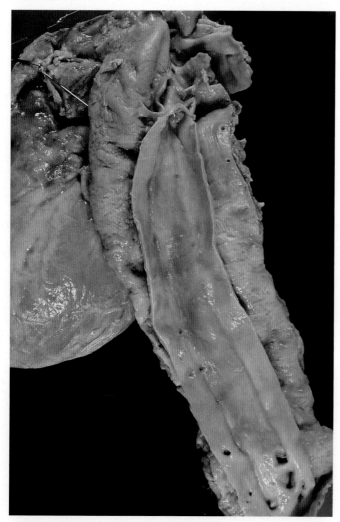

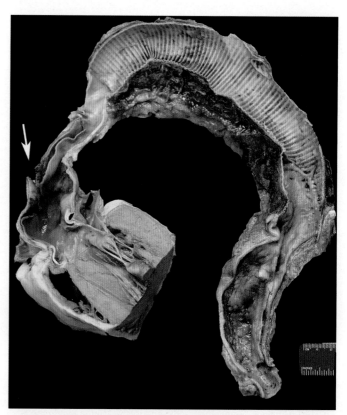

FIGURE 190.12 ▲ Marfan syndrome, ascending aortic aneurysm with dissection and rupture. The patient died suddenly with aortic dissection and rupture (*arrow*) with hemopericardium and sudden death. There was a prior history of abdominal aortic aneurysm repair with Dacron tube grafting. Any site of the aorta may be involved with aneurysms in Marfan syndrome, and multiple aneurysms are not rare, as in this case.

FIGURE 190.10 ▲ Recurrent chronic aortic dissection, distal to the anastomosis of a previous Bentall procedure. The true lumen of the descending thoracic and abdominal aorta is in the center, with the false lumen, with its characteristic wrinkled intimal surface, on both sides.

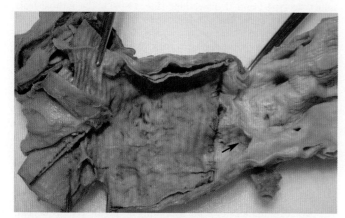

FIGURE 190.11 ▲ Aortic dissection, distal reentry tear, abdominal aorta. The patient had a type III dissection with proximal intimal tear distal to the subclavian artery (not shown). There was a prior history of Dacron bifurcating tube graft for abdominal aortic aneurysm (seen at left). The opened native aorta is the false lumen, with typical wrinkled appearance. Intimal wrinkling is characteristic of either aortitis or false lumen organization. The true lumen was compressed and is seen at the reentry site at the *arrow*, just proximal to the anastomosis. The right renal artery arose from the true lumen, and the left renal artery the false lumen.

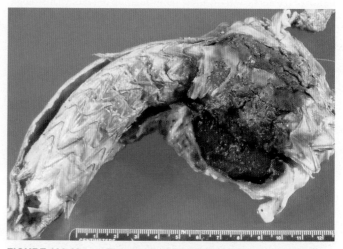

FIGURE 190.13 ▲ Thoracic aortic aneurysm, endograft repair. The stent is covered with synthetic material. The aneurysm, at the right, was leaking, prompting percutaneous intervention.

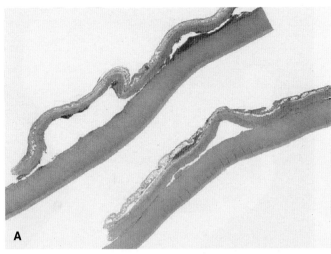
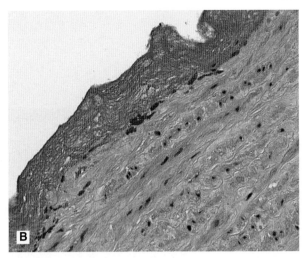

FIGURE 190.14 ▲ Acute aortic dissection. **A.** Low magnification demonstrates the separation at the outer media. **B.** A different example with slightly more organized fibrin along the lining of the false lumen.

Atherosclerosis is present in 14% of resected dissections and is typically focal. Healed dissections may also be occasionally present.[29] The uninvolved media typically shows some degree of cystic medial change.

In healed dissections, the organized thrombus lining the false lumen is rich in finely fibrillar elastic tissue (Fig. 190.16). Recanalized thrombi are frequently present in the chronic false lumen.

Treatment and Prognosis

Although patients with thoracic aneurysms of 6 cm or greater have a yearly rate of rupture or dissection of 7%, elective surgical repair restores survival to near normal.[17] Type A dissections are repaired with ascending aorta Dacron graft repair extending to the arch (hemiarch) and less commonly arch reconstructions with branched grafts. Aortic valve replacements are currently required in only a minority of patients, with a Bentall procedure (tube graft with reimplanted coronary arteries) or aortic valve replacement.[38]

Prior to endovascular repairs, the 30-day mortality of type B dissections that could be managed medically was <10%, compared to over 50% mortality for type A dissections that could not be operated.

There was an intermediate mortality (about 25%) for patients with all types of dissection treated surgically.[23] More recent studies showed a 56% 10-year survival for chronic type B dissections treated with either open surgery or TEVAR[39] and an 86% and 74% 1- and 10-year respective survival after operative repair for type A dissection, with only 7% hospital deaths.[38]

Aneurysm of the Sinus of Valsalva

The site in the aorta least likely to result in aneurysm is the most proximal portion, proximal to the annulus of the aortic valve or the aortic sinus. Aneurysm of the sinus of Valsalva was first described in 1839.[40] The aneurysm results from a weakness in the wall of the sinus leading to the dilatation or blind pouch (diverticulum) in one of the aortic sinuses, usually the right (Fig. 190.17). The pathologic diagnosis is generally made at autopsy, when the pathologist will identify a pouch-like structure bulging into the right atrium or ventricle, often in cases of sudden unexpected death due to rupture. In cases of surgical repair, the histologic findings are nonspecific and consist of bland connective tissue, sometimes with mucoid degeneration.[41]

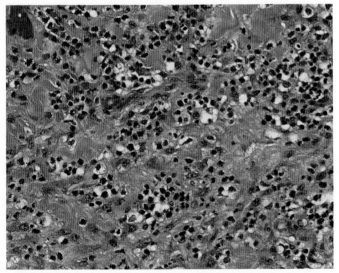

FIGURE 190.15 ▲ Acute aortic dissection, adventitial inflammation. There are prominent eosinophils, which occur between 2 and 7 days after the initial event.

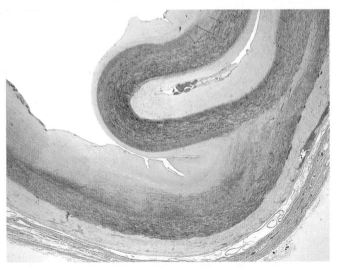

FIGURE 190.16 ▲ Chronic aortic dissection, Movat pentachrome stain. The false lumen is to the left and above and is lined by fibromuscular tissue rich in proteoglycans and elastic tissue. The intact aorta is to the right, and the adventitia below.

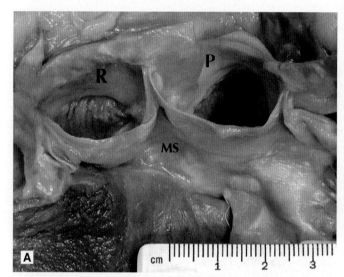

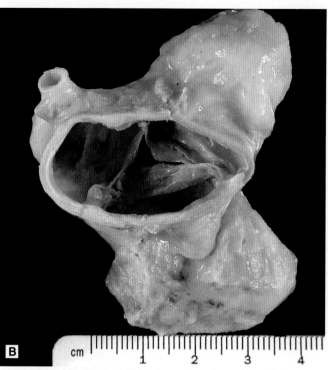

FIGURE 190.17 ▲ Sinus of Valsalva aneurysms, multiple. **A.** The right (R) and posterior (P) aortic sinuses had recesses barely visible. The membranous septum (MS) is located between the right and noncoronary cusps. **B.** The specimen is dissected out showing the right sinus aneurysm (top) and the noncoronary sinus aneurysm (below). The left coronary ostium is seen at the top left. The right sinus is the most common location for sinus of Valsalva aneurysms.

Calcification may occur.[42] Surgical repair of asymptomatic aneurysms of the sinus of Valsalva has been performed, and surface thrombus may be present.[41]

Most aneurysms of the sinus of Valsalva are congenital lesions with a strong association with ventricular septal defect. Other congenital anomalies that have been associated with sinus of Valsalva aneurysm are coarctation of aorta and bicuspid aortic valve. The congenital defect may result from a defect of fusion between the aortic media and the heart at the fibrous annulus of the aortic valve. Infective endocarditis and syphilis currently account for the majority of acquired aneurysms of sinus of Valsalva, representing fewer than 20% of total cases.

The age at presentation of congenital aneurysms ranges from 11 to 67 years, with a mean of 34 years. Asians and men appear more susceptible than Caucasians and women. Almost all are located in the right sinus and about half have an associated ventricular septal defect. Most of the remainder occurs in the noncoronary sinus, a site that is less frequently associated with ventricular septal defect.

The clinical course before rupture is that of a silent lesion. Cardiovascular collapse and sudden death may occur with rupture. The location within the right sinus of Valsalva is predictive of the site of rupture: those in the left portion of the right sinus of Valsalva protrude toward and rupture into the right ventricular outflow tract near the pulmonary valve. A ventricular septal defect is frequently associated with this particular anomaly. In those that arise in the middle of the right sinus of Valsalva and protrude and rupture into the inflow of the right ventricle, septal defects are uncommon. When the aneurysm originates from the posterior portion of the right sinus of Valsalva, it protrudes toward the plane of the tricuspid valve, rupture occurring mostly into the right atrium.

The diameter of the rupture site at the base of the sinus of Valsalva aneurysm ranges from 0.4 to 1.1 cm (mean 0.7 cm). The wall of the sinus of Valsalva is thin and consists of smooth muscle cells in a proteoglycan matrix; usually, no elastic fibers are identified.

REFERENCES

1. Kuzmik GA, Sang AX, Elefteriades JA. Natural history of thoracic aortic aneurysms. *J Vasc Surg.* 2012;56:565–571.
2. Goyal MS, Gottumukkala R, Bhalla S, et al. Bicuspid aortic valves and thoracic aortic aneurysms in patients with intracranial aneurysms. *Neurology.* 2015;84:46–49.
3. Lerner-Ellis JP, Aldubayan SH, Hernandez AL, et al. The spectrum of FBN1, TGFbetaR1, TGFbetaR2 and ACTA2 variants in 594 individuals with suspected Marfan Syndrome, Loeys-Dietz Syndrome or Thoracic Aortic Aneurysms and Dissections (TAAD). *Mol Genet Metab.* 2014;112:171–176.
4. Homme JL, Aubry MC, Edwards WD, et al. Surgical pathology of the ascending aorta: a clinicopathologic study of 513 cases. *Am J Surg Pathol.* 2006;30:1159–1168.
5. Milewicz DM, Chen H, Park ES, et al. Reduced penetrance and variable expressivity of familial thoracic aortic aneurysms/dissections. *Am J Cardiol.* 1998;82:474–479.
6. Larson EW, Edwards WD. Risk factors for aortic dissection: a necropsy study of 161 cases. *Am J Cardiol.* 1984;53:849–855.
7. Merlanti B, De Chiara B, Maggioni AP, et al. Rationale and design of GISSI OUTLIERS VAR Study in bicuspid aortic valve patients: prospective longitudinal, multicenter study to investigate correlation between surgical, echo distinctive features, histologic and genetic findings in phenotypically homogeneous outlier cases. *Int J Cardiol.* 2015;199:180–185.
8. Bauer M, Pasic M, Schaffarzyk R, et al. Reduction aortoplasty for dilatation of the ascending aorta in patients with bicuspid aortic valve. *Ann Thorac Surg.* 2002;73:720–723; discussion 724.
9. Auriemma S, Bortolotti U, Piccin C, et al. Suitability of stentless bioprostheses for combined replacement of the aortic valve and ascending aorta. *Ital Heart J.* 2004;5:673–677.
10. Martin LJ, Pilipenko V, Kaufman KM, et al. Whole exome sequencing for familial bicuspid aortic valve identifies putative variants. *Circ Cardiovasc Genet.* 2014;7:677–683.
11. Bonachea EM, Zender G, White P, et al. Use of a targeted, combinatorial next-generation sequencing approach for the study of bicuspid aortic valve. *BMC Med Genomics.* 2014;7:56.

12. Qu XK, Qiu XB, Yuan F, et al. A novel NKX2.5 loss-of-function mutation associated with congenital bicuspid aortic valve. *Am J Cardiol.* 2014;114:1891–1895.

13. Hasham SN, Willing MC, Guo DC, et al. Mapping a locus for familial thoracic aortic aneurysms and dissections (TAAD2) to 3p24-25. *Circulation.* 2003;107:3184–3190.

14. Maleszewski JJ, Miller DV, Lu J, et al. Histopathologic findings in ascending aortas from individuals with Loeys-Dietz syndrome (LDS). *Am J Surg Pathol.* 2009;33:194–201.

15. Czerny M, Funovics M, Sodeck G, et al. Long-term results of thoracic endovascular aortic repair in atherosclerotic aneurysms involving the descending aorta. *J Thorac Cardiovasc Surg.* 2010;140:S179–S184; discussion S185–S190.

16. McLarty AJ, Bishawi M, Yelika SB, et al. Surveillance of moderate-size aneurysms of the thoracic aorta. *J Cardiothorac Surg.* 2015;10:17.

17. Davies RR, Goldstein LJ, Coady MA, et al. Yearly rupture or dissection rates for thoracic aortic aneurysms: simple prediction based on size. *Ann Thorac Surg.* 2002;73:17–27; discussion 27–28.

18. Mennander AA, Miller DV, Liang KP, et al. Surgical management of ascending aortic aneurysm due to non-infectious aortitis. *Scand Cardiovasc J.* 2008;42:417–424.

19. Yuan SM, Jing H. Cystic medial necrosis: pathological findings and clinical implications. *Rev Bras Cir Cardiovasc.* 2011;26:107–115.

20. David TE. Surgical treatment of ascending aorta and aortic root aneurysms. *Prog Cardiovasc Dis.* 2010;52:438–444.

21. David TE, Feindel CM, Webb GD, et al. Long-term results of aortic valve-sparing operations for aortic root aneurysm. *J Thorac Cardiovasc Surg.* 2006;132:347–354.

22. Debakey ME, Henly WS, Cooley DA, et al. Surgical management of dissecting aneurysms of the aorta. *J Thorac Cardiovasc Surg.* 1965;49:130–149.

23. Nienaber CA, Eagle KA. Aortic dissection: new frontiers in diagnosis and management: Part I: from etiology to diagnostic strategies. *Circulation.* 2003;108:628–635.

24. Minatoya K, Ogino H, Matsuda H, et al. Surgical management of distal arch aneurysm: another approach with improved results. *Ann Thorac Surg.* 2006;81:1353–1356; discussion 1356–1357.

25. Roberts CS, Roberts WC. Aortic dissection with the entrance tear in transverse aorta: analysis of 12 autopsy patients. *Ann Thorac Surg.* 1990;50: 762–766.

26. Nakashima Y, Kurozumi T, Sueishi K, et al. Dissecting aneurysm: a clinico-pathologic and histopathologic study of 111 autopsied cases. *Hum Pathol.* 1990;21:291–296.

27. Wilson SK, Hutchins GM. Aortic dissecting aneurysms: causative factors in 204 subjects. *Arch Pathol Lab Med.* 1982;106:175–180.

28. Gansera L, Deutsch O, Szameitat L, et al. Aortic Dissections Type A during Sexual Intercourse in Male Patients: Accident or Systematic Coincidence? Examination of 365 Patients with Acute Aortic Dissection within 20 Years. *Thorac Cardiovasc Surg.* 2016;64:133–136.

29. Xu L and Burke A. Acute medial dissection of the ascending aorta: evolution of reactive histologic changes. *Am J Surg Pathol.* 2013;37:1275–1282.

30. Roberts WC, Vowels TJ, Ko JM, et al. Acute aortic dissection with tear in ascending aorta not diagnosed until necropsy or operation (for another condition) and comparison to similar cases receiving proper operative therapy. *Am J Cardiol.* 2012;110:728–735.

31. Spittell PC, Spittell JA Jr, Joyce JW, et al. Clinical features and differential diagnosis of aortic dissection: experience with 236 cases (1980 through 1990). *Mayo Clin Proc.* 1993;68:642–651.

32. Schyma C, Hagemeier L, Madea B. Bloodless aortic dissection. *Forensic Sci Med Pathol.* 2013;9:221–224.

33. Luk A, David TE, Butany J. Complications of Bioglue postsurgery for aortic dissections and aortic valve replacement. *J Clin Pathol.* 2012;65:1008–1012.

34. Song JK, Kim HS, Kang DH, et al. Different clinical features of aortic intramural hematoma versus dissection involving the ascending aorta. *J Am Coll Cardiol.* 2001;37:1604–1610.

35. Ibukuro K, Takeguchi T, Fukuda H, et al. An analysis of initial and follow-up CT findings in intramural hematoma, aortic double-lumen dissection, and mixed type lesions. *Acta Radiol.* 2015;56:1091–1099.

36. Thompson M, Ivaz S, Cheshire N, et al. Early results of endovascular treatment of the thoracic aorta using the Valiant endograft. *Cardiovasc Intervent Radiol.* 2007;30:1130–1138.

37. Bobadilla JL, Wynn M, Tefera G, et al. Low incidence of paraplegia after thoracic endovascular aneurysm repair with proactive spinal cord protective protocols. *J Vasc Surg.* 2013;57:1537–1542.

38. Tanaka M, Kimura N, Yamaguchi A, et al. In-hospital and long-term results of surgery for acute type A aortic dissection: 243 consecutive patients. *Ann Thorac Cardiovasc Surg.* 2012;18:18–23.

39. van Bogerijen GH, Patel HJ, Williams DM, et al. Propensity adjusted analysis of open and endovascular thoracic aortic repair for chronic type B dissection: a twenty-year evaluation. *Ann Thorac Surg.* 2015;99:1260–1266.

40. Isselbacher EM, Eagle KA, Desantis RW. Disease of the aorta. In: Braunwald E, ed. *A Textbook of Cardiovascular Medicine.* Philadelphia, PA: W.B. Saunders Co.; 1997: 1546–1581.

41. Yang Y, Zhou Y, Ma L, et al. Unruptured aneurysm of the sinus of Valsalva presenting with thrombosis and right ventricular outflow obstruction. *J Card Surg.* 2008;23:782–784.

42. Rhew JY, Jeong MH, Kang KT, et al. Huge calcified aneurysm of the sinus of Valsalva. *Jpn Circ J.* 2001;65:239–241.

191 Thoracic Aortic Atherosclerosis

Allen P. Burke, M.D.

Epidemiology and Risk Factors

In developed countries, atherosclerosis occurs in virtually every aorta, beginning in the second to third decades, with more rapid progression in the presence of genetic predisposition and acquired risk factors. Aortic atherosclerosis correlates with disease burden in other major arteries such as coronaries and carotids, with several histologic similarities. Autopsy studies have shown similar atherosclerotic plaque burden across arterial beds in a single patient.[1] In the aorta, there tends to be increasing atherosclerosis distally, with the formation of ulcerative plaques and aneurysms most common in the abdominal aorta and iliac arteries.

Epidemiologic studies have established the risk factors of age, male sex, obesity, smoking, and hypercholesterolemia for the development of aortic atherosclerosis. Those studies also highlighted the importance of reducing risk factors in decreasing the extent, severity, and complications of atherosclerosis. Results from the Pathological Determinants of Atherosclerosis in Youth (PDAY) study, a long-term cohort to identify lesions in patients 15 to 34 years old, found that fatty streaks begin earlier in the aorta compared to the coronaries and that the thoracic aorta are usually more involved by atherosclerosis than the abdominal aorta, but advanced lesions were more prevalent on the abdominal than in the thoracic aorta.[2]

Gross Findings

In contrast to the coronary arteries, aortic atherosclerosis has largely been classified and staged based on gross findings. The earliest lesion in the aorta is the fatty streak (presence in humans as early as in the first decade of life), which is seen as a yellowish, slightly elevated plaque on the surface of the intima. Fatty streaks in the aorta correspond roughly to intimal xanthomas, as described histologically in the coronary arteries. They usually start in the dorsal aorta, close to the ostia of the intercostal arteries, but in the abdominal aorta, close to the origin of the renal arteries, there is accumulation of fatty streaks in the ventral surface.

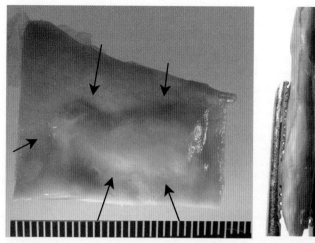

FIGURE 191.1 ▲ Raised lesion (fibrous plaque), aorta. Fibrous plaques occur at an early age and are precursors for ulcerated plaques. On cross section **(right)**, fibrous plaques usually demonstrate a lipid-rich core.

Occurring later than fatty streaks are raised lesions, or fibrous plaques. On cross section, they are often lipid rich (Fig. 191.1).

The characteristics of advanced aortic plaques are similar to those of the coronary arteries and include rupture, thrombosis, calcification, and aneurysm formation (Figs. 191.2 to 191.4). Because of the large caliber of the aorta, however, ruptured plaques are incidental findings and do not usually represent risk of embolization and death. Advanced lesions may, however, weaken the aortic media and result in aneurysm formation.

Microscopic Findings

Fatty streaks are histologically similar to intimal xanthomas of the coronaries. There is intracellular accumulation of lipids in macrophages and smooth muscle cells, forming foam cells. Fibrous plaques denote the formation of necrotic core with overlying fibrous cap (Fig. 191.5). Hemorrhage into plaque is common (Fig. 191.6). Ulcerated lesions result from rupture of a thin fibrous cap with luminal thrombus. Calcification of aortic atherosclerosis may be a prominent feature in the absence of atheroma, and progresses from a plate of intimal calcification to rupture of the calcified area and formation of calcified nodule.

Complications of Aortic Atherosclerosis

Although prevalent among all age groups in developed countries, aortic atherosclerosis remains asymptomatic until complications develop. Complications occur when there are advanced, ulcerative lesions. Symptoms result from aneurysmal change, especially in the abdominal aorta, with predisposition to rupture; embolic disease, from aortic arch vessels into the cerebral circulation, or abdominal aorta into visceral arteries; ulceration and intramural hematoma formation in the thoracic aorta; extension into mesenteric and renal arteries, with occlusion

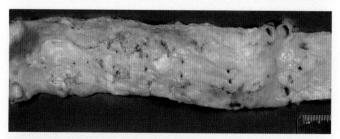

FIGURE 191.2 ▲ Moderate atherosclerosis, thoracic aorta. Raised lesions, with scattered ulcerated plaques, cover about 50% of the intima. The intercostal artery ostia are evident.

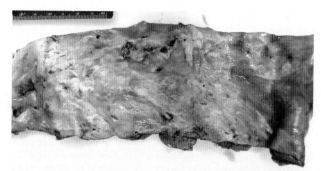

FIGURE 191.3 ▲ Severe atherosclerosis, thoracic aorta. Fibrous plaques, many of which are ulcerated, cover most of the intima.

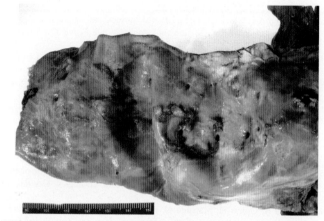

FIGURE 191.4 ▲ Severe atherosclerosis, thoracic aorta. In this example, there is early aneurysm formation. Note the ostia of the intercostal arteries indicating thoracic location.

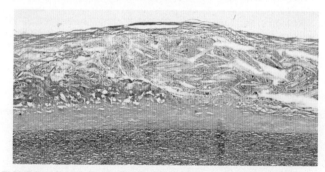

FIGURE 191.5 ▲ Thin-cap fibroatheroma, aorta. The media is below, and the fibroatheromatous core above. Movat pentachrome.

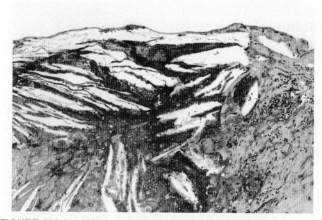

FIGURE 191.6 ▲ Thin-cap fibroatheroma, aorta. There is hemorrhage into plaque and large cholesterol crystal formation.

of these vessels and ischemic injury to the bowel or kidneys; and aortoiliac occlusive disease, without aneurysm formation. Occlusive aortoiliac disease may result in *Leriche syndrome*, characterized by impotence, claudication of the buttocks and thighs, leg weakness, and lack of palpable femoral pulses.

Thoracic Aortic Aneurysm

Atherosclerosis accounts for only 1% of ascending thoracic aortic aneurysms[3]; however, 90% of descending aortic aneurysms are atherosclerotic. Other causes of descending thoracic aneurysms include limited dissections (penetrating atherosclerotic ulcer/intramural hematoma), infectious (mycotic) aneurysms, and pseudoaneurysms, from either prior trauma or surgical interventions.

Grossly, atherosclerotic aneurysms may be saccular or fusiform (Fig. 191.7). The intima is covered with ulcerated plaques, and there is often laminated mural thrombus.

Atherosclerotic plaques are rare in proximal dissection intimal tears, but relatively common in type III dissection tears (see Chapter 190). When atherosclerotic plaques ulcerate and result in limited dissection, a so-called penetrating atherosclerotic ulcer ensues. These lesions typically are not aneurysmal, but show imaging characteristics of intramural hematoma and usually occur in the descending thoracic aorta.

Penetrating Atherosclerotic Ulcer

A complex atherosclerotic lesion sometimes ulcerates deep into the media and gives rise to a crater that is usually referred to as penetrating atherosclerotic ulcer. Most often, they occur in the descending thoracic aorta.[4] Patients are usually in the seventh and eighth decades of life and are virtually always hypertensive. Typical presenting symptoms include back pain and chest pain, and aortic dissection is usually the clinical diagnosis. There is an overlap between penetrating atherosclerotic ulcer and intramural hematoma in both pathologic and radiologic medical literature. Both entities probably represent a spectrum of the same disease that may sometimes terminate in acute aortic dissection. Patients with penetrating atherosclerotic ulcer are generally younger than those with aortic dissections and have a greater degree of atherosclerosis.[5-7]

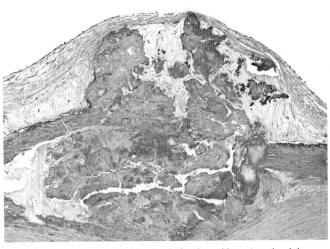

FIGURE 191.8 ▲ Aortic intimal calcification with rupture (nodular calcification). Ruptured calcium plates with fibrin and hemorrhage, which secondarily calcifies. Such lesions are common in the aorta and carotid arteries and uncommon in smaller caliber arteries such as the coronaries.

Histologically, they progress from nodular atherosclerotic plaques that begin in the intima and extend into the media (Figs. 191.8 and 191.9). The ulcerated plaque is similar to advanced atherosclerosis but deeper and more discrete (Fig. 191.10).

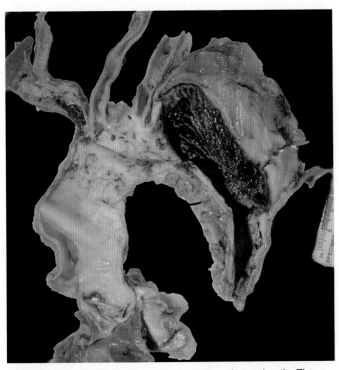

FIGURE 191.7 ▲ Thoracic aortic aneurysm, atherosclerotic. The aneurysm is just distal to the left subclavian artery and ruptured, resulting in hemothorax and sudden death.

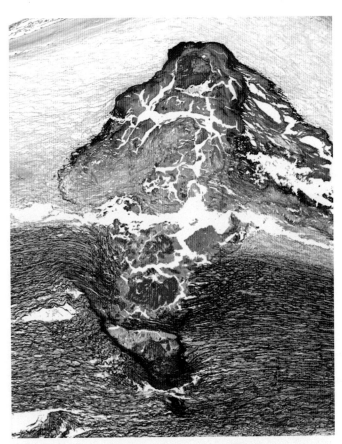

FIGURE 191.9 ▲ Nodular calcification, aorta, with medial involvement. Although atherosclerosis is primarily a disease of the intima, on occasion, there can be penetration into the media in cases of nodular calcification. Movat pentachrome stain. This lesion is the precursor for penetrating atherosclerotic ulcer and intramural hematoma.

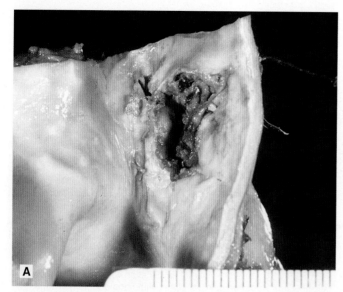
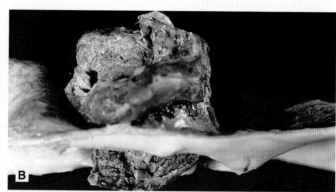

FIGURE 191.10 ▲ Penetrating atherosclerotic ulcer, aorta. **A.** In some cases, the plaque can penetrate the media and the full thickness of the wall. **B.** Penetrating atherosclerotic ulcer, aorta. A side view demonstrating rupture into the adventitia.

The treatment of penetrating atherosclerotic ulcer is not established, with some centers advocating an aggressive open or endovascular surgical intervention early, while others suggest medical treatment.[5-7]

The pathologist encounters penetrating ulcers generally at autopsy. Severe atherosclerosis with hemorrhage and some degree of dissection into the media can be seen grossly. Penetrating atherosclerotic ulcer can be the attributed cause of death in cases of ruptured wall with blood in the periaortic space. Hemothorax is usually present in these cases. Mycotic aneurysms are in the differential in cases of penetrating atherosclerotic ulcer, since both disease affect the same location and are associated with atherosclerosis. Histologic examination with identification of purulent inflammation will identify mycotic aneurysm, whereas hematoma and atheromatous material characterize penetrating ulcers.

Porcelain Aorta

One form of noninflammatory disease of the ascending aorta is the so-called "porcelain" aorta, a heterogeneous group of diseases defined by circumferential calcification that impedes surgical cross-clamping,

necessitating nonsurgical approaches to cardiac surgery, especially aortic valve replacements (Figs. 191.11 and 191.12).[8] It is encountered in about 1% of patients undergoing open heart surgery for coronary artery bypass grafting. It is likely most often caused by diffuse intimal calcification of preatheromas or early fibroatheromas and is associated with advanced age, kidney disease, risk factors for atherosclerosis, and radiation.[8]

Treatment

Aortic atherosclerosis is treated if there are complications of aneurysm or thrombotic occlusion. Occlusive atherosclerotic disease in the aorta occurs exclusively in the abdominal segment and is uncommon. Treatment for atherosclerotic thoracic aneurysms includes open repair and, increasingly, endovascular graft repair. Open repairs may require aortic arch reconstruction if there is involvement of the arch vessels, similar to ascending aortic aneurysm repair (see Chapter 53). Endovascular graft repair of descending thoracic aneurysms is generally done percutaneously. Similar to endograft repair of abdominal

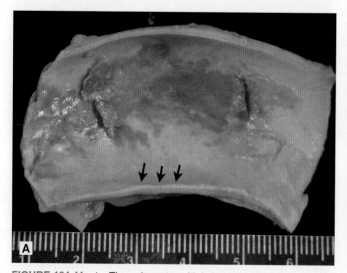
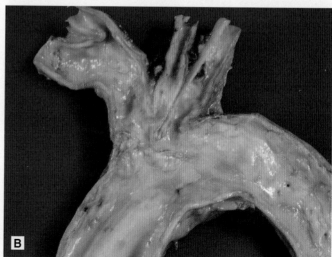

FIGURE 191.11 ▲ Thoracic aorta, with intimal calcification ("porcelain aorta"). **A.** A form of diffuse calcification (*arrows*) results in intimal calcium that results in a brittle aorta that is extremely difficult to cross-clamp during surgery without rupture. **B.** The calcification extends to the arch vessels.

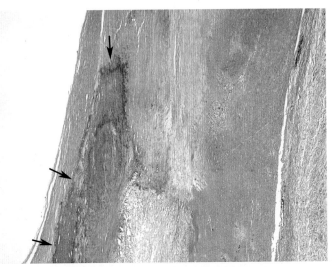

FIGURE 191.12 ▲ Thoracic aorta with intimal calcification. A histologic section of the aorta shows intimal calcification (*arrows*). The lumen is at the left.

aortic aneurysms, complications include endoleak or rupture of the contained aneurysm.

Endoleaks are generally classified by imaging as to source of blood accumulation within the space between the graft and aneurysm wall. Type I endoleak occurs when blood leaks at the proximal or distal edge of the endograft, if the seal is not adequate. Type II endoleaks result from an artery (usually lumbar in the case of the thoracic aorta) that is filling the original aneurysm sac around the graft. Type III and IV endoleaks result from leakage at a strut fracture or segment junction or flaw in the graft material, respectively.[9]

REFERENCES

1. Molnar S, Kerenyi L, Ritter MA, et al. Correlations between the atherosclerotic changes of femoral, carotid and coronary arteries: a post mortem study. *J Neurol Sci.* 2009;287:241–245.
2. McGill HC Jr, McMahan CA, Gidding SS. Preventing heart disease in the 21st century: implications of the pathobiological determinants of atherosclerosis in youth (PDAY) study. *Circulation.* 2008;117:1216–1227.
3. Homme JL, Aubry MC, Edwards WD, et al. Surgical pathology of the ascending aorta: a clinicopathologic study of 513 cases. *Am J Surg Pathol.* 2006;30:1159–1168.
4. Movsowitz HD, Lampert C, Jacobs LE, et al. Penetrating atherosclerotic aortic ulcers. *Am Heart J.* 1994;128:1210–1217.
5. Chuang CY, Chang TI, Lin YK, et al. Type A intramural hematoma and hemopericardium secondary to penetrating atherosclerotic ulcer. *Intern Emerg Med.* 2016;11:155–156.
6. Kovacevic P, Velicki L, Popovic D, et al. Surgical treatment of penetrating atherosclerotic ulcer of the descending aorta. *Vojnosanit Pregl.* 2013;70:874–877.
7. Siegel Y. Penetrating atherosclerotic aortic ulcer rupture causing a right hemothorax; a rare presentation of acute aortic syndrome. *Am J Emerg Med.* 2013;31:755 e5–e7.
8. Abramowitz Y, Jilaihawi H, Chakravarty T, et al. Porcelain aorta: a comprehensive review. *Circulation.* 2015;131:827–836.
9. Nakatamari H, Ueda T, Ishioka F, et al. Discriminant analysis of native thoracic aortic curvature: risk prediction for endoleak formation after thoracic endovascular aortic repair. *J Vasc Interv Radiol.* 2011;22:974–979 e2.

Index

Note: Page numbers in italics denote figures; those followed by t denote tables.